CONGRATULATIONS

You can now "Get Connected" to the MERLIN website for Comprehensive Neonatal Nursing!

Here's what's included to help you "Get Connected"

sign on at:

http://www.wbsaunders.com/MERLIN/Kenner

A website just for you as you learn neonatal nursing with the new 3rd edition of Comprehensive Neonatal Nursing

what you will receive:

Whether you're a student, an instructor, or a clinician, you'll find information just for you. Things like:
- Content Updates
- Links to Related Products
- Author Information... and more

plus:

Saunders WebLinks

An exciting new program that allows you to directly access hundreds of active websites keyed specifically to the content of this book. The WebLinks are continually updated, with new ones added as they develop.

Free CD-ROM Companion
with every copy of Comprehensive Neonatal Nursing, 3rd Edition

With Strong Emphasis on Clinical and Functional Relevance, this Valuable CD-ROM Features:

Competencies
Critical Thinking Case Studies
Study Questions
Supplemental Resources

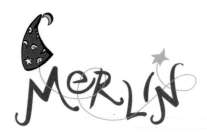

COMPREHENSIVE
NEONATAL
NURSING

A Physiologic Perspective

COMPREHENSIVE
NEONATAL
NURSING

A Physiologic Perspective

THIRD EDITION

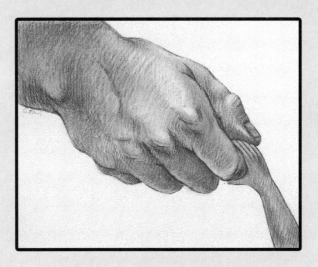

Carole Kenner, DNS, RNC, FAAN
Associate Dean for Academic Advancement
Professor, Clinical Nursing
University of Illinois at Chicago
Chicago, Illinois

Judy Wright Lott, DSN, RNC, NNP
Associate Professor and Acting Dean
Louise Herrington School of Nursing
Baylor University
Dallas, Texas

SAUNDERS
An Imprint of Elsevier Science
Philadelphia   London   New York   St. Louis   Syndey   Toronto

SAUNDERS
An Imprint of Elsevier Science

11830 Westline Industrial Drive
St. Louis, Missouri 63146

NOTICE

Nursing is an ever-changing field. Standard safety precautions must be followed, but as new research and clinical experience broaden our knowledge, changes in treatment and drug therapy may become necessary or appropriate. Readers are advised to check the most current product information provided by the manufacturer of each drug to be administered to verify the recommended dose, the method and duration of administration, and contraindications. It is the responsibility of the licensed prescriber, relying on experience and knowledge of the patient, to determine dosages and the best treatment for each individual patient. Neither the publisher nor the author assumes any liability for any injury and/or damage to persons or property arising from this publication.

Previous editions copyrighted 1998, 1993

International Standard Book Number 0-7216-9717-8

Vice President and Publishing Director, Nursing: Sally Schrefer
Executive Editor: Michael S. Ledbetter
Associate Developmental Editor: Amanda Sunderman Politte
Publishing Services Manager: Linda McKinley
Project Manager: Ellen Forest
Designer: Julia Dummitt
Cover Art: Clare Hirn

XX/YYY

Printed in the United States of America.

Last digit is the print number: 9 8 7 6 5 4 3 2 1

Contributors

Cynthia M. Acree, MSN, RNC, CNS, CRNP
Advanced Practice Nurse
Regional Perinatal Education Coordinator
Children's Hospital Medical Center of Cincinnati
Division of Neonatology and Pulmonary Biology
Cincinnati, OH

Leslie Altimier, MSN, RN
Manager, Neonatal Services
Good Samaritan Hospital
Cincinnati, OH

Gail A. Bagwell, MSN, RN
Clinical Nurse Specialist
Perinatal Outreach
Columbus, OH

Kathy Bergman, MSN, RNC, CNS
Nursing Faculty, Department of Nursing
Coordinator, Learning Resource Center
Xavier University
Cincinnati, OH

Susan Tucker Blackburn, PhD, RNC, FAAN
Professor
Department of Family and Child Nursing
University of Washington
Seattle, WA

Dorothy Brooten, PhD, RN, FAAN
School of Nursing
Florida International University
North Miami, FL

Joyce M. Butler, MSN, RNC, NNP
Neonatal Nurse Practitioner
Department of Pediatrics
University of Mississippi Medical Center
Jackson, MS

Waldemar A. Carlo, MD
Edwin M. Dixon Professor of Pediatrics
Director, Division of Neonatology
Director, Newborn Nurseries
University of Alabama at Birmingham
Birmingham, AL

Terri A. Cavaliere, MS, RNC, NNP
Neonatal Nurse Practitioner, North Shore University Hospital
Manhasset, NY;
Clinical Assistant Professor, School of Nursing
State University of New York at Stony Brook
Stony Brook, NY

Javier Cifuentes, MD
Neored Neonatal Group
Las Condes
Associate Professor, Department of Pediatrics
Catholic University of Chile
Santiago, Chile

Lana Conrad
IWK Health Centre for Children, Women and Families
Halifax, Nova Scotia
Canada

Marguerite Degenhardt, MS, ND, RN
Clinical Instructor
College of Nursing
University of Illinois at Chicago
Chicago, IL

Sergio DeMarini, MD
Director, Division of Neonatology
Ospedale S. Croce
Cuneo, Italy

Kathleen M. Driscoll, JD, MS, RN
Professor
Director, Accelerated Program
University of Cincinnati College of Nursing
Cincinnati, OH

Stephanie L. Durfor, RN, BSN, PHN
Public Health Nurse
Maternal Child Health
High Risk Infant Follow-Up
Goleta, CA

Jody A. Farrell, MSN, PNP
Nurse Coordinator/Specialist
University of California, San Francisco Medical Center
The Fetal Treatment Center
San Francisco, CA

Dianne M. Felblinger, EdD, MSN, CNS, RN
Associate Professor
Director, Women's Health Graduate Program
College of Nursing, University of Cincinnati
Cincinnati, OH

Deborah L. Fike, MSN, RNC, NNP
Neonatal Nurse Practitioner
Pediatrix Medical Group
Miami Valley Hospital
Dayton, OH

Linda Sturla Franck, PhD, RN, RGN, RSCN
Professor and Chair, Children's Nursing Research
King's College London School of Nursing and Midwifery
Great Ormond Street Hospital for Children
London, UK

Vivian C. Gamblian, MSN, RN
Owner, Gamblian Resources Company, Inc.
Director of Nurses, Healthy Homecomings of Texas
Allen, TX

Terry Griffin, MS, RNC, NNP
Rush Children's Hospital
Chicago, IL

Judith S. Harmon, MS, RN, CS, C-FNP
Perinatal Clinical Nurse Specialist
Phoenix Perinatal Associates, A Division of OBSTETRIX
Phoenix, AZ;
Consultant, Bereavement Services, RTS,
LaCrosse, WI

Rosanne C. Harrigan, EdD, APRN-Rx
Associate Dean for Integrative Health
School of Medicine
University of Hawaii
Honolulu, HI

Lynda Harrison, PhD, RN, FAAN
Professor and Associate Dean, Graduate Studies
School of Nursing
The University of Alabama at Birmingham
Birmingham, AL

Kathleen Haubrich, PhD, RN
Associate Professor, Department of Nursing
Miami University
Oxford, OH

J. Michael Hayes, PharmD
Drug Information Coordinator
Moffitt Cancer Center;
Clinical Assistant Professor
University of Florida College of Pharmacy
Tampa, FL

Diane Holditch-Davis, PhD, RN, FAAN
Professor and Director, Doctoral and Postdoctoral Program
School of Nursing
University of North Carolina at Chapel Hill
Chapel Hill, NC

Lori J. Howell, MS, RN
Program Coordinator
The Center for Fetal Diagnosis and Treatment at the
Children's Hospital of Philadelphia;
Director, Surgical Advance Practice Nurse Program,
Children's Surgical Associates;
Clinical Associate, School of Nursing
The University of Pennsylvania
Philadelphia, PA

Maribeth Inturrisi, MSN, RN, CNS
Obstetrical Clinical Nurse Specialist
Coordinator and Nurse Educator—California Diabetes
and Pregnancy Program
University of California
San Francisco, CA

Nia R. Johnson-Crowley, PhD, RN
Research Assistant Professor
Biobehavioral Nursing and Health Systems
University of Washington
Seattle, WA

Jamieson E. Jones, MD
Attending Neonatologist
University of California, San Diego Medical Center
San Diego, CA

Kristine A. Karlsen, MSN, RNC, NNP
Founder/Author of the S.T.A.B.L.E. Program
Neonatal Nurse Practitioner
Primary Children's Medical Center
Salt Lake City, UT

Nadine Annette Kassity, BSN, MSA, RN
Consultant for Integrative Medicine at Children's Hospital—
San Diego
Founder of Contemplative Care Consultants
San Diego, CA

Karen Kavanaugh, PhD, RN
Associate Professor
Department of Maternal and Child Nursing
University of Illinois at Chicago
Chicago, IL

Joanne McManus Kuller, MS, RN
Neonatal Research Assistant
Children's Hospital Oakland
Oakland, CA

Sharon Kwiecinski, RN
Children's Hospital Medical Center
Cincinnati, OH

Denise R. Lucas, MSN, RN, C
Staff Nurse, Labor and Delivery
Bethesda North Hospital
Cincinnati, OH

Carolyn Houska Lund, MSN, RN, FAAN
Neonatal Clinical Nurse Specialist
Children's Hospital Oakland
San Francisco, CA

Jill H. Malan, MS, RNC, NNP
Neonatal Nurse Practitioner—Special Care Nursery
Rush Presbyterian—St. Luke's Medical Center
Chicago, IL

Jacqueline M. McGrath, PhD, NNP, CCNS
Assistant Professor
Coordinator Neonatal Nurse Practitioner Program
College of Nursing, Arizona State University
Tempe, AZ

Scott D. Moniaci, PhD
Electrical Engineer
Huber Heights, OH

Valerie Kay Moniaci, MSN, RNC, NNP
Neonatal Nurse Practitioner
Pediatrix Medical Group of Ohio
Dayton, OH;
Director, NNP Program
University of Cincinnati
Cincinnati, OH

Sheryl Montrowl, ARNP, MSN
Neonatal Nurse Practitioner, Division of Neonatology
University of Florida
Gainesville, FL

Michele Murphy-Ratcliff, BSN, RN, PHN
Public Health Nurse, Maternal Child Health
High Risk Infant Follow-Up
Santa Barbara, CA

Nancy W. Park, MS, RNC, NNP
Consultant, Russell Klein Partners
Independent Contractor, Healthy Homecomings
Dallas, TX

Dennis J. Perez, PhD
Staff Psychologist
University of Illinois at Chicago
Chicago, IL

Judith Polak, MSN, RNC, NNP
Neonatal Nurse Practitioner
West Virginia University Department of Pediatrics
Morgantown, WV

Linda L. Rath, MSN, RN, CNNP
Assistant Professor
University of Texas School of Nursing
Galveston, TX

Karen L. Routzon, CRT
Clinical Therapist I
Neonatal/Pediatric Transport Team
Children's Hospital Medical Center
Cincinnati, OH

Debra A. Sansoucie, EdD, RNC, NNP
Director, Neonatal Nurse Practitioner Program
School of Nursing
State University of New York at Stony Brook
Stony Brook, NY

Kathleen Sandman, BSN, RN
Clinical Nurse II
Staff Nurse on Transport Team
Children's Hospital Medical Center
Cincinnati, OH

Jonathan E. Schwartz, MD
Neonatal Associates of Jacksonville
Staff Neonatologist
St. Luke's and St. Vincent's Hospital
Jacksonville, FL

Ashley Hodges Segars, MSN, CRNP, MA
Coordinator, Perinatal Outreach Education;
Administrator, Division of Neonatology
University of Alabama at Birmingham
Birmingham, AL

Julie Shaw, RN, MSN, MBA, CEN
Clinical Director II-Pediatric Intensive Care Unit
Children's Hospital Medical Center
Cincinnati, OH

Nancy M. Shaw, MSN, CNNP
Neonatal Nurse Practitioner
Primary Children's Medical Center
Salt Lake City, UT;
Voluntary Faculty
University of Utah School of Nursing
Salt Lake City, UT

Anna Sheets, BSN, RN
Clinical Nurse II
Children's Hospital Medical Center
Cincinnati, OH

Kie Shelley, RRT
Children's Hospital Medical Center
Cincinnati, OH

Beth Shields, PharmD
Clinical Pharmacist in Pediatrics
Department of Pharmacy
Rush-Presbyterian St. Luke's Medical Center
Chicago, IL

Kathleen R. Stevens, EdD, RN, FAAN
Professor and Director
Academic Center for Evidence-Based Nursing
University of Texas Health Science Center at San Antonio
San Antonio, TX

Frances Strodtbeck, DNS, RNC, NNP, FAAN
Associate Professor and Coordinator
Advanced Neonatal Nursing Program
Louise Herrington School of Nursing
Baylor University
Dallas, TX

Tanya M. Sudia-Robinson, PhD, RN
Faculty Associate in Healthcare Ethics
Center for Ethics
Emory University
Atlanta, GA

Karen Sweetwyne Thomas, MSN, RNC, NNP
Neonatal Outreach Education Coordinator
Carolinas Medical Center
Charlotte, NC

Catherine Theorell, MSN, RNC, NNP
Clinical Practice Specialist
University of Illinois
Neonatal Intensive Care Unit
Chicago, IL

Janet L. Thigpen, MN, RNC, CNNP
Neonatal Nurse Practitioner
Division of Neonatology
Department of Pediatrics
Emory University School of Medicine
Atlanta, GA

Lisa Spangler Torok, PhD, RN
Assistant Professor
Thomas More College
Crestview Hills, KY

Reginald Tsang, MD, MBBS
Professor of Pediatrics
University of Cincinnati
Cincinnati, OH

Armenda Turner, RN, CHTP
Certified Healing Touch Practitioner
Good Samaritan Hospital NICU
Cincinnati, OH

Kathleen VandenBerg, MA
Center Director, Stanford NIDCAP Training Center
Department of Pediatrics
Division Neonatal and Developmental Medicine
Cupertino, CA

Mary Duvall Vetter, MSN, CPNP
Children's Hospital Medical Center
Cincinnati, OH

Linda Waechter, RN
Clinical Nurse II
Children's Hospital Medical Center
Cincinnati, OH

Marlene Walden, PhD, RNC, NNP, CCNS
Assistant Professor, Department of Pediatrics/Division
of Neonatology
Baylor College of Medicine
Houston, TX;
The University of Texas Medical Branch School of Nursing
Galveston, TX;
Neonatal Nurse Practitioner
Texas Children's Hospital
Houston, TX

Jeanne Weiland, MSN, RN, CPNP
Cystic Fibrosis Clinical Nurse Specialist
Children's Hospital Medical Center
Cincinnati, OH

Elizabeth E. Weiner, PhD, RN, BC, FAAN
Associate Dean for Educational Informatics,
Professor in Nursing and Biomedical Informatics
Vanderbilt University
Nashville, TN

Tina Leigh Weitkamp, MSN, RNC
Associate Professor of Clinical Nursing
University of Cincinnati
Cincinnati, OH;
Staff Nurse, Mercy Hospital Anderson
Cincinnati, OH

Sara Rich Wheeler, DNS, RNCS, LCPC
Clinical Assistant Professor
College of Nursing
University of Illinois at Urbana-Champaign
Urbana, IL

Rosemary C. White-Traut, DNSc, RN
Associate Professor and Department Head
Department of Maternal/Child Nursing
University of Illinois at Chicago
Chicago, IL

Mary Mason Wyckoff, MSN, ARNP, C-FNP, NNP
Nurse Practitioner SICU
Jackson Health System
University of Miami
Miami, FL

Contributor to the Accompanying CD-ROM

Deborah Harris, RCpN, PG Dip (Nursing), FCNA (NZ)
Nurse Practitioner: Neonatology
Newborn Intensive Care
Health Waikato
Hamilton, New Zealand

Cover Image Illustrator

Clare Hirn, Illustrator
Louisville, KY

Reviewers

Kathleen Benjamin, MSN, RNC, NNP
Albany Medical Center Hospital
Albany, NY

Victoria Borges, NNP
Atlantic Regional Leader Pediatrix Program
Sunrise, FL

Susan Furdon, NNP
Neonatal Clinical Nurse Specialist/Nurse Practitioner
Albany Medical Center
Albany, NY

Rosanne C. Harrigan, EdD, APRN-Rx
Associate Dean for Integrative Health
School of Medicine
University of Hawaii
Honolulu, HI

Carol B. Jaeger, MS, PNP, CNNP, RNC
Vice President, Clinical Services—Neonatal
Children's Hospital
Columbus, OH

Marcia London, MSN, RNC, CNS, NNP
Senior Clinical Instructor and Director of NNP Program
Beth-El College of Nursing and Health Sciences
University of Colorado at Colorado Springs
Colorado Springs, CO

Ellen Mack, MSN, CNS, RNC
Cedars Sinai Hospital
Los Angeles, CA

Carol McNair, MN, RN
Sick Hospital in Toronto

Catherine McPherson, BSN, RN, NNP
Royal Alexandria Hospital
Edmonton, Alberta, Canada

Joy Hinson Penticuff, PhD, RN, FAAN
Assistant Dean
University of Texas at Austin
School of Nursing
Austin, TX

Debra A. Sansoucie, EdD, RNC, NNP
Director, Neonatal Nurse Practitioner Program
State University of New York at Stony Brook
Stony Brook, NY

Brenda Walker, BSN, RN
Neonatal Nurse
Blank Children's Hospital
Iowa City, Iowa

Foreword

Advances in management and treatment of newborns, in knowledge of their capabilities and development, in care of high-risk newborns and the need to extend support to families caring for smaller and sicker newborns have challenged health care providers in many ways. First, there is the need to keep abreast of advances in knowledge regarding care of newborns and support of their families. Equally important is the need to keep abreast of legal and health policy issues surrounding their care and the need for research to further improve care to this vulnerable group. We need evidence to support our practice. To accomplish this, textbooks for nurses caring for newborns and their families require both a comprehensive approach to care and a thorough discussion of problem areas of management and treatment. This book has both.

The authors address the breadth of issues in neonatal care, including high-risk pregnancy, fetal therapy, the need for changes in neonatal nursing education to include a competency base, evidence to support practice, care of the extremely-low-birth-weight infant, the impact of the Newborn Intensive Care Unit (NICU) on neonatal development, and use of complimentary therapies in newborn and infant care. Palliative care and end of life issues are included as the world increasingly recognizes the need for these discussions in neonatal nursing. While the breadth of content in the chapters is extensive, the text also covers major problems in depth, including respiratory, cardiovascular, metabolic, and gastrointestinal dysfunction, among many. Such breadth and depth will be an invaluable aid to health professionals providing care to neonates and their families and to educators preparing others to do so. The editors are to be applauded for contributing such an effort to the field of neonatal care.

Dorothy Brooten, PhD, RN, FAAN
Professor, Florida Atlantic University;
Principal, The Research A-Team, LLC, Miami, FL

Trends in neonatology encompass the survival of very-low-birth-weight premature infants and infants with multiple, severe congenital anomalies. Maternal risk factors have changed over the past decade. For example, more infants of mothers with chronic illnesses such as diabetes or sickle cell anemia or infants who are products of in vitro fertilization are found in today's neonatal units. More infants in neonatal intensive care units (NICUs) have been exposed to substances or are born to mothers with other risk factors such as delayed childbearing or childhood cancers. Often neonatal survival of these at-risk infants depends on the use of high-level technology. Surfactant administration, liquid ventilation, nitric oxide administration, high-frequency jet ventilators, dialysis, organ transplantation, and other extraordinary measures are rapidly becoming more commonplace. Yet in the midst of these high-tech interventions, developmentally supportive care interventions, such as dimming of the NICU lights, switching to visible alarms instead of audible ones, using nesting, encouraging kangaroo care, or even implementing co-bedding are emerging as important interventions, as there is increasing evidence to support the impact of the NICU environment on long-term infant/child outcomes.

A neonatal nurse is faced with a tremendous need for accurate, comprehensive information. This nurse must have a thorough understanding of normal physiology as well as the pathophysiology of disease processes. The neonatal nurse must be knowledgeable about associated risk factors, genetics, critical periods of development, principles of nutrition and pharmacology, and current neonatal research findings. The concepts of a family-centered approach to nursing care are important, too. No longer are parents considered visitors; they are an integral part of the care team. We have shifted to seeking evidence to support our practice instead of going by tradition. A multidisciplinary approach has been replaced by an integrated approach to care. All these elements form the solid foundation for assessment, planning, and implementation of comprehensive neonatal nursing care.

In the last decade, the nurse's role has broadened to include added responsibilities, which are recognized at both the staff and advanced practice levels. For the purposes of this book, two definitions of advanced practice are being used. They are the National Association of Neonatal Nurses' (NANN) definitions of clinical nurse specialist and neonatal nurse practitioner (NANN, Position Statement, 1990). The Association in 2000 reaffirmed these.

Clinical Nurse Specialist

The clinical nurse specialist (CNS) is a registered nurse with a master's degree who, through study and supervised practice at the graduate level, has become expert in the defined clinical area of nursing. The CNS provides for the diagnosis and treatment of human responses to actual or potential health problems of patients and their families within the specialized area

through direct patient care and clinical consultation. In addition, the CNS may act in an educational, research, liaison, or leadership role to promote optimal nursing care for the patients served.

Neonatal Nurse Practitioner

The neonatal nurse practitioner (NNP) is a registered nurse with clinical expertise in neonatal nursing who has received formal education with supervised clinical experience in the management of sick newborns and their families. The NNP manages a caseload of neonatal patients with consultation, collaboration, and general supervision from a physician. Utilizing the extensive knowledge of pathophysiology, pharmacology, and physiology, the NNP exercises independent or intradependent (in collaboration with other health professionals) judgment in the assessment, diagnosis, and initiation of certain delegated medical processes and procedures. As an advanced practice neonatal nurse, the NNP is additionally involved in education, consultation, and research at various levels.

Note: At the present time, the blurring of these two roles is being discussed. It has been proposed, but certainly not fully accepted, that a more appropriate term would be advanced practice nurse, or APN. This change is emotion laden, because although those involved in both practice and education have felt the difference was necessary in the past, it appears more critical for advanced practice nurses to work together rather than have a dichotomous title because of current health care reform. This statement appeared in the last edition of this book and as we go to press for the third edition, we have not made much progress towards resolving this issue.

The neonatal staff nurse role requires accurate and thorough assessment skills, excellent ability to communicate with other health professionals and patients' families, and a broad understanding of physiology and pathophysiology upon which to base management decisions. It requires highly developed technical skills as well as critical decision-making skills. With health care delivery changes, it also requires supervision of ancillary personnel and an informed delegation of certain patient-oriented tasks. These changes require the staff nurse to possess even better assessment skills and sound knowledge of physiology and pathophysiology than in the past because some decision-making will be done in concert with other, less highly trained personnel.

Purpose and Content

The third edition of this book again provides a comprehensive examination of neonatal nursing management from a physiologic and pathophysiologic approach appropriate for any health professional concerned with neonatal care. For the advanced practitioner and neonatal staff nurse, it provides a complete physiologic and embryologic foundation for each neonatal system. It includes medical, surgical, and psychosocial care, because the collaborative management approach is absolutely imperative to the well-being of the newborn and family. Appropriate diagnostic tests and their interpretation are included in each system chapter. There is extensive use of research findings in the chapters to provide evidence to support practice strategies and demonstrate rationale for clinical decision-making. Complete references for more in-depth reading are found at the end of each chapter so that the reader may pursue more specific information on a topical area. Inclusion of a CD and accompanying website with web linkages are new features. The CD contains competencies, critical thinking and study questions, case studies, and additional resources. Use of tables and illustrations to support material that is presented in the narrative portions is sure to be another help to the practicing neonatal nurse.

The thread of collaborative management is interwoven throughout the text. Foundational topics such as genetics, physiologically critical periods of development, nutrition, and parenting are included, as are topics of recent interest such as iatrogenic complications, neonatal pain, use of computers in nursing, and neonatal AIDS. Now more than ever, nursing must examine patient outcomes and nurse outcomes to meet the demands for providing cost-effective and high-quality care. Research is critical to support both the art and science of neonatal care. Whenever possible, the contributors remind the reader of areas in need of further study. New chapters have been added to address evidence-based practice and new trends in neonatal care. These include hospice and palliative care, management of the NICU environment, evidence-based nursing, care of the extremely-low-birth-weight infant, complementary therapies, and competency-based neonatal nursing education. Another feature is the Preemie Bill of Rights, which we felt was important as we put more emphasis on the consumer and his or her needs. Of course, for neonatal care, the consumer is the newborn/infant and family. This book is not a quick reference but provides comprehensive in-depth discussions along with detailed physiologic principles and collaborative management strategies. It provides a sound basis for safe and effective neonatal care.

The book begins with a discussion of general areas of neonatal nursing: the new health care delivery environment, regionalization today, evidence-based nursing, legal/ethical issues, collaborative research, competency-based neonatal nursing education, family-centered care, bereavement, and hospice and palliative care. Bereavement and chronic sorrow are discussed along with the newer field of neonatal hospice and palliative care because a happy ending is not always possible in perinatal and neonatal nursing. Human genetics is introduced, and the impact of environmental influences on the developing fetus, as well as the nursing implications of the Human Genome Project, are discussed. This provides the transition into the aspects of perinatal care, the high-risk pregnancy, and the effects of labor on the fetus. The text then deals with more specific neonatal topics, starting with stabilization, managing the NICU environment, newborn and infant neurobehavioral

development, monitoring neonatal biophysical parameters, computer technology, and assessment. This edition includes the most up-to-date information from the American Heart Association's Neonatal Resuscitation Program as well as elements of the S.T.A.B.L.E.® program used for infants undergoing transport. Each organ system is discussed in depth, including the respiratory system, its complications and new technologies, followed by assessment of and management strategies for the cardiovascular system; nutrition and the gastrointestinal system; and metabolic, endocrine, immunologic, hematopoietic, neurologic, musculoskeletal, genitourinary, integumentary, auditory, and ophthalmic systems. Diagnostic imaging and diagnostic text and laboratory values represent the section of the text that highlights the evaluative measures used by practitioners to identify the neonatal problem and its progress. This edition continues with the surgical neonate, neonatal pain, neonatal AIDS, the drug-exposed neonate, and care of the extremely-low-birth-weight infant. Because neonatal nurses are seeing more and more extremely-low-birth-weight infants, we wanted to address this population's unique care needs. The final group of chapters covers the discharge phase. Topics include principles of newborn and infant drug therapy, systematic assessment and home follow-up, neonatal behavior, assessment and management of neonatal behavior, the transition to home, and finally, home care. One topic that has been added in this edition is complementary therapies. Never has there been so much interest in or controversy over such interventions. We address what is known and where the gaps are in this area of neonatal care. This section recognizes that many neonatal nurses now care for infants through the first year of life. It also acknowledges the need for technology in the home and some guidelines for families who feel they have set up mini-NICUs in their homes.

In this edition, each of the chapters and sections has been updated to include the newest techniques, such as the latest trends in fetal therapy; progress with the mapping of human genes; use of computers, including Internet connections opening up global neonatal care issues for examination and discussion; inclusion of the latest issues in health care reform and its impact on nursing care; and the latest research findings appropriate to each of the sections.

To provide depth to these topical areas, physicians, nurses, infant developmental specialists, and other health professionals concerned with neonatal care from across the country and around the world were used as contributors in both editions. The attempt was made not only to tap the experts in the neonatal field but to have them represent as wide a geographic area as possible. We hope that the broad geographic distribution of contributors and reviewers will help minimize the effect of regional differences in clinical practice as reflected in the text.

Carole Kenner, DNS, RNC, FAAN
Judy Wright Lott, DSN, RNC, NNP

Acknowledgments

This book has been a major undertaking, one of which we are most proud. Even though this is the third edition, it still requires a lot of work to make sure the material is up-to-date and accurate. It would not have been possible without the support of many people who worked in many hidden ways. First we would like to thank our nursing developmental editor, Amanda Politte, who provided support and helpful suggestions, and whose organizational skills kept us all on target. Next, we thank Michael Ledbetter from Elsevier Science, who acquired this edition and encouraged us to try new avenues of learning for our readership.

We are truly grateful to our contributors, who in the midst of their very busy lives took on one more project. To those who stuck with us through a third edition, we are especially indebted. We also want to thank the new contributors who were willing to step in and share their expertise with us. We certainly recognize the time commitment that was made by each contributor. We believe that because of their efforts, we have been able to bring together the best and the brightest shining stars in neonatal care.

We would also like to thank our many reviewers for the constructive comments that helped structure the new content of the text. We recognize that your wisdom has guided us well in restructuring parts of the book to reflect changes in neonatal care worldwide.

We also want to thank Jan Zasada, The In Bin, for her hours of correcting our manuscripts, typing, and generally getting all our "ducks lined up" for this edition. She kept us moving along every step of the way.

Finally, but certainly not least, we would all like to acknowledge the support and encouragement of our families and friends: Les Kenner, George, Bill, and Tam Lott. Their strength and positive thoughts have kept us going throughout these many months. This edition is dedicated to our mothers who both died within days of each other and who were so proud of each of the previous editions, and to the memory of Blake Lott whose life ended much too soon.

We want to thank our readers who have validated the need for this text. We both appreciate when we hear from those of you who are using the text around the world. Without your support, there would be no need for a third edition.

Carole Kenner, DNS, RNC, FAAN
Judy Wright Lott, DSN, RNC, NNP

Contents

UNIT II
FAMILY DYNAMICS

UNIT IV

THE INTRAPARTAL ENVIRONMENT: MATERNAL-CHILD
INTERACTIONS

UNIT V

DEVELOPMENTALLY SUPPORTIVE CARE

UNIT VI
PHYSIOLOGIC ADAPTATION OF THE NEONATE

CHAPTER 1

NEONATAL NURSING IN THE NEW HEALTH CARE DELIVERY ENVIRONMENT

ROSANNE C. HARRIGAN, DENNIS J. PEREZ

The purpose of this chapter is to describe the role and career development pathway of the neonatal nurse in the health care delivery environment. The discussion focuses on the role and development of the neonatal nurse in comprehensive care; the contributions of neonatal nurse practitioners and specialists to the advancement of neonatal care; collaborative practice in the Neonatal Intensive Care Unit (NICU); the issues related to the practice, credentialing, and education of neonatal nurses; the influence of nursing management on neonatal outcomes; and the need for cultural sensitivity in neonatal nursing practice.

THE ROLE OF THE NEONATAL NURSE

NICU nurses provide expert and complex care to critically ill infants. In collaboration with the entire team of physicians, advanced practice nurses (APNs), respiratory therapists, pharmacists, and social workers, neonatal nurses nurture these infants to optimize their growth and development. Each day they use their commitment, passion, and expert skills to make a difference for patients and families (Maguire, 1999).

Neonatal nurses work in environments in which collegial relationships with physicians and nurse practitioners develop. Their professional practice model emphasizes and supports decision making at the bedside with those closest to the point of care. They share the values of family-centered care, professionalism, leadership, and participative management in everyday practice (Maguire, 1999).

Neonatal nursing practice consists of at least three elements: (1) implementing nursing therapy, (2) collaborating with other health care providers, and (3) assisting with medical care. The interrelationship of these three components centers on improving or maintaining neonatal and family health. Nursing therapy consists of assessment, planning, intervention, and evaluation of newborns and their families to provide developmentally appropriate environments, physical care, feeding, and parent care. Neonatal nursing care is protective, generative, and nurturing in nature and focuses on the needs of neonates as embodied persons rather than as biologic systems. The role of the neonatal nurse is described in Table 1-1. These roles evolve from beginning to advance practice levels. Progressive continuing and academic education is needed for role development.

CAREER DEVELOPMENTAL STAGES OF NEONATAL NURSES

Seven career developmental stages for neonatal nurses have been identified. Three occur at the RN practice level (providers of neonatal nursing care and communicators or managers of neonatal nursing practice), and four levels occur at the advanced practice level (expert practitioners, translators of research data into evidence-based practice, generators of knowledge for neonatal nursing practice, and shapers of policy related to neonatal health care). Each of these roles is explored in this chapter. Today neonatal nursing is promoting and adapting to changes in the management of the health of the fragile infants. Neonatal nursing skills are needed both within the NICU as well as in home-based delivery systems.

Although funds for education of neonatal nurses at all levels of career development have diminished because of cost containment, education for continued competency is also necessary. The impact of managed care on neonatal nursing roles has not been clearly delineated in the literature. However, neonates are being discharged earlier than ever, and the need for home care and advanced practice nurses with neonatal intensive care competencies that can provide transitional care is emerging. The provision by nurses of high-tech care in the home is also needed.

RN Practice Level

Beginning Practitioners of Neonatal Intensive Care: New Neonatal Nurses and Neonatal Nurses with Technical Competency.   A new neonatal nurse must be able to competently perform basic neonatal care delivery tasks. New neonatal nurse providers are both students and providers, as the nurse must perform while being observed for indications of competence and future potential. Support systems for new neonatal nurses are needed to reduce anxiety and job stress.

Because the new NICU nurse lacks experience and others on the staff do not know how much they can rely on the new nurse's judgment, direct supervision of the new nurse is essential. In other words, the new nurse must begin by sharing an assignment with an experienced neonatal nurse. Central activities of this role include helping, learning, and following directions. The entry-level neonatal nurse is a dependent practitioner. Home care nurses who manage neonates should spend a portion of their orientation in the NICU to experience this

TABLE 1-1	Role of the Neonatal Nurse Provider
Roles	**Activities**
Protect	Evaluate and identify risk factors
	Use screening tools to identify problems
	Initiate appropriate action and referral
	Provide anticipatory guidance
	Teach family about the neonate's health and developmental status
Generate	Promote development of new infant and family behaviors
	Modify environments or roles
	Help parents and neonates adjust to their developmental and health needs
Nurture	Provide surveillance of physiologic variables
	Provide infant comfort
	Provide family education about the infant's health and illness
	Conduct research
	Develop linkages with other hospitals' services
	Engage in interaction with community-based follow-up programs
	Provide education of other neonatal and home care providers

developmental stage and acquire associated competencies before accepting responsibility for the sick newborn in the home.

The primary outcome of the second developmental stage for neonatal nurses is technical competency and independence. Transition from the beginning practitioner stage is accomplished when the nurse can function as a technically competent professional who can work collaboratively and produce designated patient outcomes. At this developmental stage the nurse should have primary responsibility for a small number of patients. Close supervision is no longer needed, and technical skills have evolved to a high level. At this time the nurse often establishes an area of subspecialization in a defined area of practice—for example, transport (NANN, 1999d). This is the desired level of expertise for nurses who provide care for neonates at home.

Peer relationships take on increased importance during this stage of development. The nurse begins to rely less on experienced nurses for direction and becomes a peer rather than a subordinate. Transitions can be difficult because changes in attitudes and behavior are necessary on the part of the supervisor as well as the nurse.

To complete the developmental tasks associated with this stage, the nurse must go beyond dependence and develop personal ideas or views on what is required in a given situation. As individual standards of performance begin to develop, an awareness of a professional judgment and value system also begins.

Developing confidence in personal judgment is a difficult but necessary transition. Often the neonatal nurse takes a supervisory position during this stage. Although management opportunities are economically attractive, nurses who have not developed independence and technical competency will never be effective if they cannot understand the technical aspects of the work they supervise. Thus they face a high degree of risk. Lack of technologic expertise undermines the man-

ager's self-confidence and compromises the trust and confidence of his or her staff. Many nurses remain in this stage throughout their careers, making a substantial contribution to the well-being of infants and experiencing a high degree of professional satisfaction.

Communicators and Translators of Neonatal Nursing Care Practices. During this stage, nurses begin to take responsibility for influencing, guiding, directing, and developing the skills of other people and are ready to become full members of the collaborative practice team. Nurses also broaden their interest and begin to involve themselves in professional activities at the regional and national levels. Many return to school for additional education or graduate degrees. Nurses interact with others outside the unit for the benefit of those on the unit.

At this developmental stage the nurse becomes an informal mentor, an outgrowth of her or his personal esteem as a competent clinician. Increased productivity is expected because of the nurse's evolving capabilities; thus the nurse needs assistance from parents and other health professionals for both the detail work and the exploration of personal beliefs about neonatal care. The nurse becomes a mentor for less experienced nurses, and, in turn, he or she is mentored by more experienced nurses. The nurse also explores innovative solutions to problems at this stage as staffs begin to contact this mentor nurse for suggestions. At this developmental stage, the nurse influences other nurses. The most common role initiated during this stage is that of manager or supervisor. The nature of relationships must change significantly in this new role. The nurse becomes sensitive to the needs of other nurses and assumes responsibility for collaboration with a variety of disciplines. In addition, interpersonal skills in setting objectives, delegating, supervising, and coordinating must be developed.

At this point, the neonatal nurse has responsibilities to people at both higher and lower levels within the organization. The nurse must learn to cope with being in the middle of divided loyalties. This situation requires developing confidence in producing results and helping others do the same. This neonatal nurse can assist others in developing confidence by providing guidance and freedom and can experience success through the accomplishments of others. A delicate balance must be achieved by providing direction for others while allowing them the freedom to explore and develop their skills. Technical skill must be maintained in this stage.

Advanced Practice: Neonatal Nurses
Expert Practitioners, Translators, and Knowledge Developers. Following the completion of an advanced practice program, neonatal nurses provide expert neonatal nursing care as well as some aspects of neonatal medical care. These nurses assist with knowledge dissemination and development. The advanced practice neonatal nurse is essential today to ensure that practices are evidenced-based and are revised as new information is generated. Neonatal nurses who have completed doctoral programs are nurse scientists and independently or collaboratively conduct research to generate theory and test care-giving practices. These nurses also become teachers of neonatal nurses in academic educational programs.

Shapers of Neonatal Care Delivery Systems. Some nurses move onto another developmental stage. These nurses become shapers of health policy. They interface and negotiate with key segments of the health care system, developing new ideas, procedures, or services that lead to new areas of activity for the staff or directing the resources of the organization toward specific goals. The nurse at this developmental stage is politically astute and formulates policy for new initiatives and programs. Intense relationships outside the organization are developed. Skills needed to influence outcomes—such as personnel selection, resource allocation, and organizational design—are learned. Alliances are formed, and strong positions taken without feeling personal enmity toward people who have differing positions.

Implications for Career Development.   An understanding of the developmental stages for neonatal nurses has implications for career counseling. Neonatal nurses should be provided with an understanding of their career development path. Managers need the framework to establish unit structures and continuing educational programs that promote the neonatal nurses' development. The developmental stages also provide a structure for a career ladder.

THE CONTRIBUTIONS OF ADVANCED PRACTICE NEONATAL NURSES (APN)

History of Advanced Practice Nursing

In the 1970s, a national effort toward improving the outcome of care for high-risk neonates began. The development of effective NICUs has increased the demand for experienced personnel available on a 24-hour basis to manage emergency neonatal problems. To help meet this demand, the American Academy of Pediatrics (AAP) first recommended the use of neonatal nurse practitioners (NNPs) in the NICU (Harper et al, 1982). This endorsement of the practitioner's role was based partly on concerns about a potentially excessive exposure of the pediatric house officer to NICUs during residency training. To maintain a well-balanced residency and training program as well as an appropriate time commitment to newborn intensive care, the AAP proposed that extended-role nurses could adequately meet the demands for a portion of the personnel requirements. In 1999, the AAP revised their position on the use of NNPs to include support for the participation of NNPs in the care of hospitalized patients (AAP, 1999). The AAP recommends that NNPs caring for hospitalized patients should have appropriate credentials and clearly defined clinical privileges. Recommended credentials include specific education and experience—or both—for the position. This training may include experiences precepted by a qualified physician. They suggest that NNPs may take part in posthospitalization follow-up of patients by using written protocols for medical care and necessary patient education.

The employment of neonatal nurse practitioners, who would be responsible for the medical management of patients, required a redefinition of the traditional bounds of nursing practice. The scope of nursing practice in this role extends into the realm of medical practice and increases the need for collaborative planning of neonatal care.

No data that suggest the practice of neonatal nurse practitioners is any less efficacious than that of physician providers are available. However, in general, few data are available, and the data that are available are from studies with very small samples. In addition, in these investigations, the practice of nurses was compared with that of student physicians (Johnson et al, 1979; Mitchell-DiCenso et al, 1996). One fact is clear from a review of the literature; investigations to date have

evaluated the dependent component of these nursing roles—that is, their extended role into neonatal medicine—and not their expanded role in nursing nor their overall impact on the cost of achieving defined care outcomes.

Today, NNPs are used in 233 (55.3%) of neonatology practices. Of these, 77% of university practices use NNPs—along 52.9% of private practices, 46.3% of hospital practices, 33.3% of HMO practices, and 14.3% of military practices (Pollack et al, 1998). The percentage of NNPs increased with increasing size of practice and represented only 35% of practices with one neonatologist, whereas practices with more than 12 neonatologists represent 85.7% (Pollack et al, 1998). The concept of expanded and extended roles in nursing is not new. NNPs have been introduced into tertiary-level neonatal intensive care units in the United States, Canada, the United Kingdom, and New Zealand in response to increased survival rates of extremely low-birth-weight infants, shortage of physicians, and the nursing profession's emphasis on the development of advanced practice roles (DiCenso, 1998; Jones, 1999).

Nursing specialization is currently in its sixth decade. The term extended role was first used when nurse practitioners and physicians' assistants were referred to as physician extenders. Extended-role practices refer to the performance of practices previously considered medical; expanded practice refers to refinement and innovation within nursing. The difference between these two terms is more than semantic. In the past, much of the practitioner's practice has been in the extended role, whereas that of the specialist has been primarily in the expanded nursing role. However, practice is changing, and recognition of the importance of both these roles as well as the blurring of the distinction between medical and nursing practices has contributed to the merging of these roles and incorporation of both components into the interdependent advanced practice of neonatal nursing (Bates, 1970). Trotter & Danaher (1994) completed a descriptive evaluation of the advanced practice role and reported that both professionals and families were very satisfied with the clinical skills, knowledge base, and contributions to patient care that neonatal nurse practitioners provided.

The practitioner in the extended role has a legacy—nursing as a practicing profession. The practitioner and specialist roles have provided alternative developmental paths that lead not to administration but to advanced neonatal nursing practice. This exceedingly important aspect tends to be underplayed. Expanded and extended practice roles have provided an incredibly significant clinical renaissance, a quiet revolution within nursing that has helped the profession not only to survive and keep pace with technology and practice demands but also to progress and strengthen itself despite dramatic and far-reaching changes in health care. Nurse practitioners and clinical specialists have turned advanced neonatal nursing into a complex, highly technologic enterprise. The umbrella title, APN, should be used in public forums in reference to either the NNP or neonatal clinical nurse specialist (NANN, 1999a).

Based on changes in nursing practice and education, the following definitions have been adopted by NANN (1999a):

Advanced Practice Neonatal Nurse (APNN): A registered nurse (RN) with a graduate degree in nursing and a concentration in advanced practice neonatal nursing to include both didactic and clinical components. Included in didactic and clinical is advanced knowledge in nursing theory, research, physical and psychosocial assessment, appropriate interventions, case management, and care coordination.

The APNN is a clinically competent, expert practitioner who applies an expanded range of practice, theory, and research-based therapeutics in caring for infants and their families. APNN practice is further defined by the following core competencies:

1. Consulting and collaborating (intradisciplinary and interdisciplinary)
2. Clinical and professional leadership
3. Change agent skills
4. Ethical decision-making
5. Expert coaching and mentoring to families and colleagues
6. Evaluating, utilizing, and conducting research

Neonatal Nurse Practitioner (NNP): An RN who is an experienced, expert neonatal nurse and has obtained a graduate degree in the nursing specialty (or whose title/role has been grandfathered before January 1, 2000) with an emphasis in managing the health care needs of newborns and their families. The NNP diagnoses and treats in collaboration with neonatologists and other pediatric physicians. The NNP makes independent and interdependent decisions in the assessment, diagnosis, management, and evaluation of the health care needs of neonates and infants. In addition, the NNP selects and performs clinically indicated advanced diagnostic and therapeutic invasive procedures.

Neonatal Clinical Nurse Specialist (NCNS): A RN who is an experienced, expert neonatal nurse and has obtained a graduate degree in the nursing specialty with emphasis on the health care needs of newborns and their families. The NCNS promotes the delivery of quality neonatal nursing care by consulting, educating, researching, role modeling, developing staff, developing and supporting system structures for accreditation, fostering continuous quality improvement, and promoting cost containment. The NCNS makes independent and interdependent decisions to improve the quality of neonatal health care through the processes of change, consultation, education, modeling of expert care, leadership, case management, care coordination, and research utilization.

Contributions

The three activities of advanced practitioners that have contributed to the improvement of neonatal care are the following:

innovation and refinement of practice
acceptance of control of neonatal nursing practice
development of a research basis for practice

A review of literature reveals that the publication of research has significantly increased since the 1970s (Perez-Woods, 1991). The same is true of books on neonatal nursing. Of interest is that the majority of authors are clinically prepared neonatal nurses and that many have been educated as practitioners and specialists.

Nurse specialists and practitioners have extended the boundaries of neonatal nursing practice in relation to both independent and dependent functions and have developed innovative forms of service. Nurse practitioners and specialists have established consultation and practice services, thus demonstrating independence and autonomy in a visible way to the public. The nursing profession has always been ambivalent about specialized practice. On the face of it, specialization suggests that what the ordinary nurse does can be done better by a more educated nurse. The idea that "a nurse is a nurse is a nurse" has for almost a century been a blinding myth in a profession having the widest possible heterogeneity in demographic, educational, and other characteristics of its members. The profession has finally taken a position on level of educa-

tion and experience needed to deliver quality neonatal nursing care (NANN, 1999a; NANN, 1999c). NANN supports the position that the BSN should be the single entry point into RN practice (NANN, 2000). They have taken the position that advanced practice nurses (CNS and NNP) should be educated at the master's level. The previous ambivalence, uncertainty, and lack of clarity about specialization and the advanced practice of neonatal nursing are giving way to a valuing and commitment to the contributions of advanced practice nurses.

Responsibilities

Advanced practitioners of nursing have a responsibility to the profession and to society to know the field of neonatal nursing extremely well. In addition, advanced practice neonatal nurses have a responsibility to know a great deal about neonatal medicine. Nurse practitioners and specialists work together with neonatal nurse researchers toward mastering knowledge of practice at the boundaries of nursing's domains. Mastery over this domain yields public confidence in neonatal nurses.

COLLABORATIVE PRACTICE IN THE NEONATAL INTENSIVE CARE UNIT

The neonatal intensive care unit (NICU) has improved the prognosis for the critically ill newborn, particularly the low-birth-weight infant. This unique environment has brought together sophisticated technology and highly trained personnel, including physicians, nurses, laboratory technicians, respiratory therapists, and social workers. Today, the environment of the NICU has moved into the home, necessitating distance collaborative management strategies to ensure optimal outcome achievement from home care providers. The disciplined, professional group working in the high-technology environment of the home or NICU must develop a harmonious, collaborative spirit to achieve its aim—that is, improving the welfare of the very fragile newborn and the newborn's family. The development of a collaborative spirit is a significant challenge in this paradoxical environment, in which the source of greatest stress and greatest satisfaction—caring for desperately ill infants—is the same. Development of collaborative relationships can be both a satisfying and a productive experience.

The purpose of this section is to explore the concept of collaborative practice in achieving desirable neonatal management outcomes. Collaborative practice is the delivery of care to patients and their families by using the resources of a variety of health care providers. In collaborative practice environments, joint communication and decision making with the expressed goal of satisfying wellness and illness needs of infants and families while respecting the unique qualities and abilities of each professional is the norm. The basis for collaboration is the belief that quality patient care is achieved by the contribution of all health care providers. A true collaborative practice has no hierarchy. It is assumed that the unique contribution of each participant is based on expertise rather than the traditional employer/employee relationship. Collaborative practice involves a group of individuals with different educational backgrounds and skills who work together to provide care. Lamb & Napodano (1984) added that each person contributes to the decision-making process. The family is also an integral part of the team. The concept of collaboration does not assume that the contribution of each member of the group of providers is equal, but it acknowledges that each profession has something unique and important to contribute to the well-being of the infant and family. In addition, collaborative practice requires that professionals have mature role competence and highly developed technologic expertise. Leadership is decentralized, flexible, and problem-oriented (Ames & Perrin, 1980; Leininger, 1971; Shumaker & Goss, 1980).

Collaborative care requires that outcome goals and evidence-based practice guidelines be established for the major health problems and developmental needs experienced by the neonate and family. Today, management outcomes focus both on care in the NICU and on management at home. Strategies to achieve these goals are then identified in the form of practice guidelines. (For more information on the development and use of practice guidelines, see Chapter 4.)

The implementation and modification of the plan should be coordinated by a designated case manager. A case manager is an expert practitioner who serves to coordinate formal and informal health services for an individual child and family (Hickey, 1996). Identification of a case manager is essential because families experience significant anxiety during this period, and a consistent relationship with a consistent health care provider such as a case manager assists with communication and reduces anxiety. Case managers are also responsible for the consistency, efficiency, and timeliness of neonatal management (Harrigan, 1995).

In this section, the factors associated with the development of collaborative practice environments are described, and the strategies known to promote collaborative practice are explored.

The Context of Practice

In today's health care facilities, neonatal staff nurses are in short supply. Job satisfaction plummets when needed staff is unavailable and when moral and ethical conflict continue to create stress. On the other hand, opportunities for neonatal nurses have never been more diverse. APNs are managing low-risk and intermediate nurseries and taking on significant collaborative independence in the NICU (Ashworth et al, 1998). Opportunities for collaborative practice also are available in the community. Research data have affirmed the contribution of the advanced practice nurse in the provision of transitional care to both improved quality and cost containment for infants (Brooten et al, 1991; Genarro et al, 1991). Today, numerous health plans include provision for home follow-up following early discharge based on these data.

Systems of care also provide reimbursement for the services of APN at either an 85% of physician fee level if a physician is not on site or at 100% level if the service is incident to MD care. Many APNs also have prescriptive authority and can legally prescribe medications. More is also known about the practices of the APN in the NICU setting (Mitchell-DiCenso et al, 1996; Herman & Zeil, 1999; Griffith et al, 1999). These investigations affirm that the practices of the APN are at least as cost-effective as those of interns and residents and that the availability of reimbursement system demands additional investigations to determine the actual cost of APN providers.

The formulation of privileging systems and collaborative practice agreements is essential to ensure that legal issues are resolved before the implementation of advanced practice collaborative practice programs (Heith & Van Dinter, 2000; Kamajian et al, 1999). Numerous legal issues currently remain unresolved. The basic criteria seem to affirm that the APN

learned the practice or skill in the educational program and that continued competence has been maintained (Harrigan & Kooker, 2000).

Creating the Context.   Collaborative practice environments are based on the belief that the results of the collaborative efforts of a group of dedicated professionals are greater than the results achieved by each of the professionals acting independently. Collaborative practice environments result from the communication and cooperation among health care professionals (Herman & Zeil, 1999). Such professionals recognize that the collective effort of a number of talented professionals is needed to achieve neonatal outcomes efficiently and consistently. Because of the variety of backgrounds and experiences that each professional brings to the care of the neonate, there are more ideas, skills, and information with which to seek solutions. Collaboration requires dedicated, cooperative professionals (Herman & Zeil, 1999).

Viewing the developmental context in which collaboration occurs is essential. The context includes what the professionals bring to the care of the neonate and what they have to contribute. Professional development is influenced by interactions with others in the care-giving environment. Growth is influenced by the environmental and personal context within the unit. The developmental context is evolutionary and consists of a combination of factors specific to the situation and point in time. Philosophical, structural, and dynamic correlates of contexts support collaboration.

Philosophical Correlates.   Collaborative care environments require dedication on the part of professional providers to the process of identifying their values concerning patient care. The process used to define shared values requires professionals to recognize their own value systems, gain better understanding of themselves, and compare their beliefs with those of other providers. Ethical conflicts that exist are identified and discussed (Erlen, 1994). There is opportunity for compromise, resolution, or refinement; making the decision to leave the system is also an option.

The development of collaborative practice goals requires constancy. Constancy is the consistent implementation of principles as the basis for clinical decision making related to goal achievement. Consistency is needed for the development of trust, which is a basic element of collaboration. For example, for a collaborative health care team to function effectively, each of the team participants must generally agree on the basic concepts of professional practice. This understanding is important because areas that are unique to each profession as well as areas that overlap with other professions exist. For example, both a nurse and a psychologist may provide emotional support to a neonate's family, but their responsibilities concerning the administration of medication would not overlap (although nurses and physicians may have overlapping responsibilities in this area). Shared values are represented in the individualization of a practice guideline to a specific unit (Chapter 4).

Development of constancy is compromised in units affected by frequent nursing staff turnover; many rotating house staff, students, and faculty; and weak leadership. A significant investment of time is needed to reveal personal attitudes, clarify value systems, and develop trusting relationships. In a collaborative practice environment, additional time is also necessary to develop an understanding of the attitudes and values of others. Value conflicts often arise during the development or refinement of care maps or critical pathways. The consensus that evolves provides the foundation for the selection of principles that reflect unit values and goals that do not conflict with the beliefs of any individual staff member. The use of collaborative partnerships between service and academia for mediation may assist in resolving conflicts (Organek & Hegedus, 1993).

The principles also serve as a basis for the evaluation of patient care outcomes to be achieved by the unit staff. In mature collaborative systems, the principles and goals are written and formalized. Oral communication of outcome goals is no longer the norm (Harrigan, 1995); today, collaborative development of written care maps is the norm.

Philosophical belief systems are continuously evolving and are subject to change. Changes can result from the addition of new staff with values and beliefs different from those of the current staff, changes in the values and beliefs of the current staff, changes in the patient care environment, or changes in care models (i.e., managed care). Ongoing opportunity should be provided for input from new unit staff as well as for expression of the changing views of continuing staff members and administrators. Opportunity for participation should be available for all disciplines involved with outcome achievement, especially in managing long-term patient care outcome goals (Miller et al, 1993). Affirmation of identified belief systems at designated intervals is highly desirable.

Structural Correlates.   Both physical and organizational aspects of the neonatal care system structure affect the nature of the collaborative practice environment. Five aspects of the physical environment—the location of the equipment that provides care, the locations of offices of leadership personnel, the location of communication equipment, communication flow patterns, and traffic flow patterns—are primary concerns. Characteristics of the organization of medical, nursing, and allied health staff also can affect collaboration. The organization of the perinatal system or managed care network—as well as cultural characteristics of families—should be considered. Several investigations have related personnel stress and burnout with structural and organizational factors (Consolvo et al, 1989; Rosenthal et al, 1989). Nurses were often socialized into systems in which they lacked power to develop health care delivery patterns and were sheltered from the impact of health care decisions because of their place in the system structure. Passive acceptance of new care models such as managed care will only cause further problems associated with this role (Harrigan, 1995). Failure to provide data-based documentation of the value-added outcomes associated with professional nursing will result in diminished nursing resources within provider systems (Harrigan, 1995).

Physical factors such as the location of the offices of both nurse and physician leadership personnel can significantly affect availability and involvement with collaboration. The clinical specialist with an office on—rather than off—the unit is far more likely to be a collaborator. The use of space planners has significantly improved the flow of interactions on NICUs. In numerous NICUs across the country, however, the NICU staffs are separated both physically and organizationally. Although early discharge and referral to home care are now the norm, well-developed structures for collaborative planning and communication between the NICU staff and home care agencies are rare.

Anecdotal reports about the association between placement of equipment and supplies and a communication system at the bedside of individual infants as well as improved collaborative

decision making abound. However, little research to study the impact of physical environments in the NICU on the interactions of staff has been done. Well-designed studies that focus on the impact of physical space on caregiving would be of significant value to the profession (Brown & Taquino, 2001). Literature from other fields, such as business, certainly confirms the importance of space design on the development of human interactions. In some NICUs, overcrowding is a significant barrier to collaboration. Space planning should include consideration of the caregiving physical environment, work-flow patterns, location of offices for leadership personnel, and physical equipment for communication.

The organization of medical and nursing services can reveal a great deal about the probability of developing collaborative practice in the neonatal care system. Organizational structures that are centralized and hierarchical provide the greatest challenge for collaboration, whereas those that allow for decentralized decision making are the best. Collaboration requires that each individual's ability to contribute to clinical decision making be recognized. Collaborative practice is not a team for which the coach makes all the calls. Evaluation of the organizational structures and decision-making norms used by each group concerned with the patient outcomes in the neonatal care system is an important element of developing collaboration. The questions that are raised are 1) are the groups committed to collaboration? and 2) are the values, attitudes, and goals proposed by the members of the groups reflected in the organizational structure chosen to manage the group? Concern about the use of hierarchical models and residual concerns about territoriality have prohibited the development of organizational structures that integrate neonatal care services. In business literature this is called tearing down silos and leveling knowledge in an organization. Investigation of integrated organizational structures through the use of controlled research designs is warranted. Organizational models that are fully integrated and evaluated by use of quantitative measures of quality are needed. Successful collaborative systems require efficiency and recognized quality service at a low price. Systems must also be responsive to customers. High standards of care will be the hallmarks of successful competitors, and innovative structures to monitor, measure, and manage clinical performance will be the norm (Harrigan, 1995).

Organizational structures of groups of care providers are not static entities; they often reflect the developmental status of the group. Groups move from dependent centralized organizational structures to participative, self-directed, decentralized structures as they mature. However, stress caused by the demands of care provision, staff turnover, or availability can alter the organizational structure that a particular group prefers. As in other aspects of human development, organizational development occurs in stages, and stress may cause a return to an earlier stage of development. It is time for the discipline of nursing to experiment with new models of patient care management and to create cultures that embrace collaborative patient care management, continuous quality improvement, or the like. For the first time in the delivery of health care in the United States, a premium is associated with prevention and a profit associated with realigned incentives (Harrigan, 1995). Rewards will be provided to those who can eliminate operational efficiencies and inappropriate care giving practices. Collaborative structures are no longer just desirable; they are required. Regionalized perinatal system structures are disappearing and being replaced by systems that include primary care providers, home care services, and specialty services. Financing is needed to develop neonatal home care providers capable of managing technology, case finding, and providing social support.

Once an evaluation of the organizational structure of each professional group that provides service on the unit has occurred, identification of similarities, differences, and the potential for collaboration is possible. Collaboration does not work for all units; it requires a commitment to interdependence. Many professions function within primarily autonomous or primarily dependent types of organizational structures. Adherence to these types of organizational structures is not compatible with collaborative practice. Organizational characteristics that suggest successful collaboration include the following:

- Retention of qualified staff
- Low staff attrition rates
- Sharing decision making throughout the organization
- Delegation of tasks and authority as appropriate

Necessary systems include interdisciplinary community-based planning; integrated structure and accountability; integrated data collection, documentation, and evaluation; and innovative approaches to financing (AAP/ACOG Guidelines for Perinatal Care, 1997).

Dynamic Correlates.   Both professional and personal dynamics must be considered within the collaborative context. Professional dynamics that project mutual support, respect for persons, and recognition of each group's contribution to patient outcomes encourage collaboration. These professional characteristics usually reflect personal qualities that the individual brings to the caregiving setting. It is unusual for a person to display one set of values and attitudes as a professional and another set of values on a personal level. Evaluation of a potential staff member's values and beliefs can do a great deal to assist with the development of collaborative care environments. Concern with merely filling a vacancy with a qualified nurse or physician often prevents recognition of the potential impact of a values conflict on the dynamics of the group. Exploration of an applicant's value system should be an essential component of the interview process. No matter how brilliant the applicant, value conflicts can alter and potentially destroy a collaborative practice environment.

The evolution of collaborative practice is a developmental process. A new staff member focuses primarily on technical aspects of care and after 6 to 9 months begins to develop a notion of self as a professional provider in the NICU. At that point, the nurse often believes that he or she knows more than other professionals and parents about what is appropriate for an individual infant. During this developmental stage, the nurse has difficulty interacting with others and is not amenable to a collaborative mode of professional practice. However, transition to the communicator level of development soon occurs. The nurse in the first developmental stage (technician) practices in a dependent role, whereas during the second developmental stage, practice is characterized by independence and, at times, counter-independence. Territoriality is an additional characteristic of the second stage of professional development. This stage may persist for 1 to 2 years. During the first two developmental stages, professionals function best in associate care roles. Full participation in a collaborative care environment is difficult.

Collaborative practice requires participation from experienced neonatal staff—that is, those who are at the expert or contracted clinician level of development. At this level, professionals can identify their roles clearly, specify their limita-

tions, and accept responsibility for implementing their roles. Managers must have a vision of the ingredients needed to form a successful collaborative group and of the patient care goals to be achieved. The developmental process required before successful collaborative practice environments can be achieved needs to be anticipated. The expertise of experienced staff is needed to assist with the socialization of new members to the collaborative professional group.

Developing a Vision

Four major factors are associated with the development of a vision of a collaborative practice environment. These factors include the following:

- Realistic role expectations
- Acceptance of responsibility
- Recognition of limitations
- Resolution of territoriality (Maguire, 1999)

Mature clinicians with experience in the delivery of neonatal care develop an understanding of the contributions and limitations of all the different care providers. It is unfortunate that most nurses are not socialized into their roles in collaborative care environments in which mutual respect and role competence of the different types of care providers can be appreciated. Often the preceptor of the neonatal nurse is another staff nurse who is not ready to mentor. The development of collaborative care environments requires that managers appreciate the impact of socialization and mentorship on the development of professional values and attitudes. Internships or fellowships in collaborative practice settings assist with the development of realistic role expectations, as does the opportunity to be associated with mature, experienced practitioners. Collaborative practice is a role more appropriate for the experienced neonatal nurse (expert or contracted clinician). Nurses at the technical or surrogate parent level of development have significant difficulty with this role.

Once role expectations have been identified, responsibility for the role assumed must be accepted. This acceptance of responsibility is not as easy as it may seem. Collaborative practice roles are demanding and require a commitment that may extend beyond the traditional assigned scheduled shift. Traditional scheduling systems for patient management by nurses can be a barrier to collaboration because professionals must be present when they are needed by a particular newborn and family. In NICUs in which flexibility cannot be accommodated, a traditional case manager system may not be appropriate. Unit-based case managers have been tried with varying degrees of success. This model of care requires further exploration.

Collaborative practice requires that the expert practitioner recognize his or her limitations. Trust between members of the collaborative practice group depends on group members' ability to indicate when they are overwhelmed and need the expertise of another professional. Collaboration depends on the ability of members of the group to recognize their expertise and to acknowledge their limitations. Collaboration would be unnecessary if the skill of any single member of the group was sufficient to achieve the identified patient care goals.

Territoriality is a characteristic of most professional disciplines. Territoriality begins where the boundaries of a profession become clear. Collaboration requires that lines that box professions in separate containers be removed from time to time to serve the best interests of the patient. Territoriality also characterizes neonatal care systems environments in which truly expert or contracted clinicians are few and new group members are many. Most new members of a profession have been effectively socialized to believe that they have an independent practice mode and that dependency on others is a sign of weakness rather than a sign of strength. Learning to be interdependent takes time and trust. Mature, experienced clinicians can trust others in their group to provide care and recognize that they can seek assistance of other group members whenever it is needed. Nursing must reduce its focus on autonomy and develop a power structure within an integrated organizational system.

Communicating a Vision

In NICUs in which constant change in staff (e.g., academic medical centers) occurs, collaboration is possible only when empowering visionary health care professionals are present. Empowerment is the process of convincing staff that they can do their jobs and that what they do makes a difference. Visionary care providers must communicate their vision by using metaphors that are understandable to all members of the group. Each individual member of the group must be helped to value his or her contribution toward the achievement of patient care goals for the infants and their families. The neonatal care system is a challenging and often frustrating work environment, in which socialization of new staff members must include not only unit policies and procedures but also incorporation of a vision that reflects care goals for the unit. This socialization process takes at least a year, and expectations that a staff member will be a productive member of a collaborative practice group before this time are unreasonable. Socialization of new staff members is a responsibility for the most mature members of the collaborative practice group. The socialization experience should also include experience with all system components, including home care.

Visionary care providers are responsible for the empowerment of the infants and their families as well as members of the staff. Parents and community involvement in the care of high-risk neonates is essential for the achievement of both short-term and long-term developmental goals for these infants. The family establishes the primary value system for the infant; thus families must learn that they have significant contributions to make to the fragile humans for whom neonatal nurses care. In the neonatal care system, in which parents and staff are bombarded with information, the role of assertive health care professionals is to integrate information and facts into meaningful knowledge.

Collaboration reflects the communication of a vision—a vision so clear to the members of the staff that all are committed to the same goals as the infant and family. This commitment is made within an environment in which values and attitudes are shared. Approaches to the care of infants are consistent, and families believe that they play an important and valued role in management.

Factors that Impact Implementing a Vision

A number of factors significantly influence the implementation of a vision. These include federal and state statutes, guidelines generated by professional associations, educational requirements, and other regulations related to collaborative practice agreements, prescriptive authority, institutional regulations, and individual qualifications.

Federal Regulations. Before qualification for reimbursement of services, the APN must apply for a provider number both from Medicare as well as from third party insurance com-

panies and health maintenance organizations (HMOs) that commonly cover patients serviced in the unit. Before Congress passed the Balanced Budget Act (BBA) on August 5, 1997, the services provided by APNs were included in a complicated reimbursement system developed when Medicare was enacted in 1965. APNs were included in a category of "non-physician personnel," which included all RNs (not just APNs), Licensed Practice Nurses (LPNs), technicians, and other aides. A subset of these non-physician personnel is "non-physician practitioners" (NPP), which includes APNs (i.e., nurse practitioners, nurse-midwives, nurse anesthetists, clinical nurse specialists), clinical psychologists, clinical social workers, and physician assistants. Reimbursement (under Medicare Part B) was provided most often under an "incident to" rule, which requires meeting the following stipulations:

1. The APN has to be an employee of a physician or a physician practice; therefore Medicare is billed for the APN's services under the physician's name and at 100% of the physician rate.
2. The APN provides services furnished "incident to" the services of a physician—that is, they are considered physicians' services although they are provided by an APN.
3. The APN services must be provided under the physician's supervision.
4. The physician must be in the same suite of offices when the APN is providing "incident to" services. This does not mean the physician must witness the APNs providing care; however, it does not allow, for example, a physician to make rounds in the hospital while the APN is seeing Medicare patients in an adjacent office building.
5. For the services to be "incident to" that of a physician's, it is expected that a "direct, personal, professional service furnished by the physician to initiate the course of treatment of which the service being performed by the non-physician practitioner is an incidental part" has been provided (Medicare Part B Newsletter No. 012, August 30, 1996). Subsequent services by the physician of a frequency that reflects his or her continuing active participation and management of the course of treatment is also required.

Exceptions to "Incident to" in Rural Areas. The "incident to" rule was slightly modified as a result of the Omnibus Budget Reconciliation Act (OBRA) of 1990. At that time, the following modifications, applicable only to rural areas, were added:

- The services applied only to those provided by APNs, NPs, and CNSs.
- APN services were to be covered when performed in a team. A team consisted of an APN working in collaboration with a physician. "Collaboration" meant the APN was working with a physician to deliver health care services within the scope of the APN's professional expertise. These services were to be performed with medical direction and appropriate supervision, as provided for in jointly developed guidelines or other mechanisms defined by federal regulations and the laws of the state in which the services are performed.
- The physical presence of the physician on site while the APN delivered care was not required. Payment for services could be made directly to the APN rendering the care; however, the reimbursement rate was 85% of the physician rate.
- No restriction was placed on the APN's ability to assess and treat any new problems presented by the patient.

Balanced Budget Act of 1997. Beginning in 1990, it became eminently clear to APNs and legislators alike that it was illogical to allow certain clinical privileges and financial benefits to APNs solely based on the geographic location of their practices. As a result, the Balanced Budget Act (BBA) of 1997, which allowed all APNs and physician assistants (PAs) the same privileges and benefits previously limited to their rural colleagues, was passed. In other words, effective January 1, 1998, the following new provisions expanded part of the definition of "physicians' services" covered under Medicare Part B:

- Those that would be physicians' services if furnished by a physician.
- Those that are performed by an APN working in collaboration with a physician (as defined under the rural reimbursement system)
- Those that the APN is legally authorized to perform by the state in which the services are performed.
- Those that are reimbursable "only if no facility or other provider charges or is paid any amounts with respect to the furnishing of services" (Medicare Part B Newsletter No. 012, August 30, 1996). That is, Medicare would pay for APN services only once. As long as facilities do not include the cost of APN salaries in their formula for Medicare reimbursement, their services may be billed to Medicare on a fee-for-service basis. In outpatient settings, the salary costs of these clinicians can (and should) be broken out ("unbundled") from the hospital's overall costs.

This provision has been a *boon* to physician practices where such APNs are employed, even though reimbursement is 85%, rather than 100%, of the physician rate. Unlike in the "incident to" rule, under the new legislation the physician does not have to be in the same office suite when the APN is rendering care, and the restrictions regarding the physician's personal evaluation of every new patient and every new problem have been removed.

Nursing Home Services.   Coverage of APN services under the Medicare program was authorized by Omnibus Budget Reconcilliation Act (OBRA) 1989. This provision allowed the APN's employer to submit claims to the Medicare carrier for a service rendered by the APN to a resident in a nursing facility or a skilled nursing facility. The payment for this service was limited to 85% of the participating-physician fee schedule amount for the comparable service. All claims for these services had been made on an assignment basis, meaning that the APN's employer could not charge the nursing home resident beyond the Medicare-allowed fee. The provision called for the visits to be made by a member of a team—the APN, the collaborating physician, or a physician assistant. The team was allowed to make 1.5 visits per month on a routine basis. Additional visits could be made when the team member adequately substantiated the need for the more frequent visits.

However, as a result of BBA 1997, a provision specific to APN services in nursing homes no longer exists because these services are presumably covered as part of the overall reimbursement provision. Furthermore, APN services in nursing homes, which in the past were covered only in rural areas, are no longer restricted in that manner.

1998 Memorandum.   In a long-awaited memorandum dated April 1998, the Health Care Financing Administration (HCFA) explained that all APNs and PAs must have their own provider identification numbers (PIN) to bill Medicare, even if they are not self-employed and even if their employers have always billed for their services using the employer's PIN with a modifier.

State Regulations.   The APN's scope of practice is broadly defined and regulated by the Nurse Practice Act of each state under the authority of the state governments. Components of the practice act that define the scope of practice include definition of the role, title protection, reimbursement regulation, and prescriptive authority. The regulations vary by state; thus review of the Nurse Practice Act in the state related to advanced practice is essential. The reader is referred to the yearly publication "Annual Update on How Each State Stands on Legislative Issues Affecting Advanced Nursing Practice" in the Nurse Practitioner for specific state regulations (Pearson, 1999). This publication provides an overview of changes in state laws regarding advanced practice.

Guidelines Generated by Professional Organizations.
The National Association for Neonatal Nurses has provided guidelines for the education of advanced practice neonatal nurses (NANN, 1999a). This document can be used to broadly define the role and standards of clinical practice. The National Certification Corporation is the body that offers the certification examination for NNPs. Completion of a graduate program that contains the didactic content listed in the examination outline is required to sit for the examination. Specific continuing education requirements are required to maintain certification (NCC, 2000, www.nccnet.org).

Requirements Regarding Educational Preparation.   APNs are registered nurses (RNs) with graduate degrees in nursing and concentrations in advanced practice neonatal nursing to include both didactic and clinical components. Included in didactic and clinical is advanced knowledge in nursing theory, research, physical and psychosocial assessment, appropriate interventions, case management, and care coordination.

Other Regulations
Collaborative Practice Agreements.   Collaborative practice agreements are essential to implementing APN roles. A written agreement that describes physician collaboration is required by all states that employ NNPs. This agreement should describe the specific activities the NNP can perform. In addition, the agreement indicates those activities that can be performed autonomously and those that require supervision. Although some states require written protocols for operation, Hawaii is not one such state. Standards for developing skill competency may be useful adjuncts to the privileging process. The agreement must identify the physician and APN who are entering the arrangement. Figure 1-1 is an example of a collaborative practice agreement.

Prescriptive Authority.   The State Board of Nursing or The State Board of Medicine or a combination of the two governs the practice of APNs with prescriptive authority. These groups have promulgated regulations that permit qualified APNs to prescribe and dispense drugs. Most states require that applicants qualify for advanced practice recognition, complete not less than 45 hours of course work in advanced pharmacology, and have in place a written signed collaborative agreement between the prescribing APN and collaborating physician. Such agreements may require identification of the individuals, the area of practice in which the APN is certified, the categories of drugs the APN may (or may not) prescribe or dispense, affirmation by the physician that he or she has familiarity with the drug that the APN will prescribe, and documentation of professional liability insurance. Exclusionary formularies are recommended for prevention of continuous modifications to

I. General Information
  A. Nurse Practitioner Information
    1. Name _____
    2. Hawaii RN License Number _____
    3. Area of Certification _____
    4. Certifying Organization: _____
    5. Certification Expiration Date: _____
    6. Certification Number _____
    7. Practice Site Name and Address _____
    8. Hawaii Advanced Practice Recognition Number _____
    9. Expiration Date _____
    10. Hawaii Prescriptive Authority Number _____
    11. Expiration Date _____
  B. Physician(s) Information
    1. Name: _____
    2. Hawaii Registration Number _____
    3. Board Certification Area _____
    4. Certifying Organization _____
    5. Practice Site Name and Address _____
  C. Guidelines of Collaboration
    In this agreement, the term "collaboration" means that the nurse practitioner works with the collaborating physician(s) in an active practice to deliver health care services in accordance with the nurse practitioner's education and experience. These services are provided under medical direction in jointly formulated and approved guidelines as defined by the Hawaii Revised Statutes. The physician(s) shall file with the Board of Nursing notice of delegation of prescriptive authority and termination of such delegation
    The written collaborative agreement shall be reviewed and updated annually. A copy of this written collaborative agreement shall remain on file at all sites where the nurse practitioner renders service and shall be provided to the Hawaii State Board of Nursing upon request.

Signatures

_____   _____
Physician's Signature Date   Nurse Practitioner's Signature Date

II. References and Guidelines
  The nurse practitioner may use, but is not limited to, the following references, texts, or guidelines in providing care: credible texts and journals, AAP/ACOG Guidelines for Perinatal Care, and professional organizational statements.
III. Neonatal Nurse Practitioner Services
  Perform comprehensive physical assessments
  Provide services related to health maintenance and promotion
  Provide nutritional supplements
  Perform procedures (as privileged)
  Establish diagnoses for common short-term and chronic stable health conditions
  Order, interpret, and perform laboratory and radiology tests
  Prescribe medications, excluding controlled substances III-V (dependent on state)
  Provide stock and sample medications
  Perform other therapeutic or corrective measures as indicated
  Refer patients to licensed physicians or other health care providers as indicated
  Provide urgent care as indicated
IV. Nurse Practitioner & Physician Relationship
  The physician and nurse practitioner shall consult with each other either by telecommunication or in person as needed. The physician must be on site at least once a month to provide medical direction and consultation. In the absence of the designated collaborating physician(s), another physician shall be available for consultation.
  The nurse practitioner shall inform each collaborating physician of all written collaborative agreements that he or she has signed with other physicians and provide a copy of these to any collaborating physician upon request.

FIGURE 1-1
Sample nurse practitioner/physician written collaborative agreement from the state of Hawaii.

the agreement. To maintain prescriptive authority, an APN must demonstrate that he or she has maintained continued competency in advanced pharmacology. Specific requirements vary from state to state. An APN may not prescribe drugs without prior approval from the appropriate regulatory board.

Institutional Practice. Hospitals define the role of the APN through specific documents and institutional requirements that may include credentialing and privileging, written collaborative agreements, and job descriptions. Each institution may vary in their specific requirements. In general, tertiary care centers require APNs to complete the credentialing process. The process of delineating clinical privileges, however, is not standardized. The written collaborative agreement defines the APN's scope of practice. The job description further identifies the specific responsibilities of the APN within the institution and specifically within the NICU setting. The special needs of the NICU and the division shape the daily responsibilities of the APN.

Individual Qualifications. The knowledge, credentials, clinical experience, confidence, and ongoing competence of the individual APN also influence the scope of practice. Role development and expansion is common with increased experience and education.

Issues Related to Practice: Credentialing and Education of Neonatal Nurses

A relationship between the certification standards, licensing requirements and options, and titles and content of curricula used to prepare neonatal nurses should exist. Students and the public have the right to know whether and under what auspices the certification will be available and whether an acceptable level of congruence between program content and certification requirements exists. Legislation to control the development of advanced practice in neonatal nursing should not be sought. This control is a responsibility of the professional organization, and the National Association of Neonatal

Nurses (NANN) has accepted this responsibility (NANN, 1999a).

The public also has a right to reasonable expectations about the competencies of nurse providers of neonatal care. This right is based on the profession's social contract with society. The profession turns to the public for economic resources to carry out its socially delegated mandate. In return, the public needs to know the nature of specialized services provided by neonatal nurses to meet the needs of society. Authorized by society, the broadening field of practice of the neonatal nurse carries with it the profession's responsibility for maintaining high educational standards. The credibility and trustworthiness of all neonatal nurses is compromised when any nurse or specialist decides to call himself or herself an advanced practitioner without having credentials or skills and knowledge deemed appropriate by the profession. To represent oneself falsely to the public is indeed a gross violation of the public trust. The hallmark of an expert neonatal nurse is ability to recognize the limits of his or her professional knowledge and scope of practice. The profession has a responsibility to inform the public about advanced practitioners in neonatal nursing, and advanced practitioners have a responsibility to put before the public useful health information that they derive from their work. Employers have a right to know whether a nurse who claims to be a specialist is indeed so qualified, and they have a responsibility to verify credentials of neonatal nurse specialists.

The goals and norms of science are not identical to those of neonatal nurses. Scientists' work is primarily aimed at acquiring a body of knowledge that can help understand and explain the world around us. Neonatal nurses are primarily engaged in the delivery of care to newborns and the improvement of this care, and today these activities involve technology. The scientists' work is guided by the professional code of conduct. Although scientists and neonatal nurses may have similar perspectives, the relative importance of criteria that they use to assess data may be different, depending on whether the goal is to develop a body of knowledge or to solve a health-related problem. Both nurses and scientists develop knowledge as they attempt to explain phenomena. An understanding of science is necessary both for the nurse who is to contribute to the body of scientific knowledge and for the nurse who is going to use the information that is produced.

Expert neonatal nurses must possess specialized knowledge and expertise. They must consider how their role contributes to the advancement of neonatal nursing knowledge. The neonatal nurse must be competent in both a technical and a theoretical sense to achieve these goals. Education of neonatal nurses for advanced practice should occur in graduate schools. Graduate programs to prepare advanced practice neonatal nurses must be committed to integrating the practitioners' primary focus on the application of available knowledge with the scientists' interest in the expansion of knowledge. Neonatal nurses must be prepared to empirically investigate the adequacy of a statement's plausibility or the relevance of predictive factors associated with treatment approaches. Neonatal nurse research specialists are needed to conduct research and communicate the emerging evidenced-based foundation for neonatal nursing practice; this level of neonatal nurse education should occur in doctoral nursing programs.

Standardization of education at the master's level also serves the profession by gaining educational parity with other health care professions (e.g., social work, pharmacy). Policy makers are very aware of formal educational credentials. When the advanced practice nurse possesses a "universal degree," such as the master's of science, he or she gains credibility in negotiating issues surrounding scope of practice, such as prescriptive authority and third-party payment. Advanced practice graduate education must include biologic sciences, computer literacy, clinical reasoning, health policy, and financial management (NANN, 1999a). This educational process should parallel the career paths for nurses.

NURSING MANAGEMENT AND NEONATAL NURSING PRACTICE

The implementation of the neonatal positive pressure respirator in the 1970s and the development of the NICU forever changed the practice environment of the nursery. An environment that was once filled with the lusty cries of healthy newborns became a space-age life-support station for infants who previously would not have survived. The skills required of a neonatal nurse have continued to evolve since the mid-1970s to the point that the cost of orientation for a beginning role in neonatal intensive care usually exceeds $15,000 because nursing education programs do not prepare nurses specifically for this area of practice. In fact, a recent review of all levels of curricula from generic nursing programs (Harrigan, personal communication, 2001) suggests the content taught in these programs is related primarily to management of low-risk infants. Content related to the care of high-risk neonates is deemed the responsibility of continuing and graduate education. Thus the new neonatal staff nurse is often confronted with a role that demands the competence of an expert practitioner. Excellent orientation and quality management programs are essential to ensure that new nurses can provide quality care. Practice competence is one of a number of challenges that face the neonatal nurse administrator and that can significantly impact care outcomes. Other challenges include costs of nursing management, use of assistive personnel, characteristics of care-giving environments that promote job satisfaction, and ethical stressors in the NICU.

Costs of Nursing Services in the NICU

Nursing salaries account for 45% to 60% of NICU expenditures (Richardson et al, 2001). NICU care is labor-intensive because all newborns are totally dependent and require complex technological support for routine functions. A common rule that is used to calculate costs of nursing services is based on the belief that 5.2 nurses are needed to staff a 24-hour nursing position. This staff nurse position would be for bedside, direct care. These 5.2 nurses would provide continuous coverage for one year's worth of expenditures for a single position (Richardson et al, 2001). A simple calculation illustrates the magnitude of nursing cost. Assume 5.2 full-time equivalency (FTE) nurses, each costing $60,000 per annum ($50,000 salary and 20% benefits). This computes to $855/day in bedside nursing salary alone to cover a single patient in a 1:1 nurse to patient ratio. Thus the central issues for administrators are determining the number of patients for which a nurse can care concurrently and developing the ability to flex the number of nurse providers up and down with changes in patient volume. Non-contact nursing hours time dedicated to in-service training, orientation, quality improvement actions, intensive care unit wage differentials to attract the best nurses to this demanding practice area, and standby capacity (staff compensation for standby status) must also be considered in any cost calculations.

Nurse patient ratios range from 2:1 to (Extra Corporeal Membrane Oxygenation [ECMO] on dialysis, or immediately post-op) to 1:1 in certain cases. The average nurse:patient ratio is 1:2 or 1:3, depending on the infant's acuity level. Marshall et al (1989) describe the Australian estimates of nursing time (in hours/day) at 24.3, 15.8, 10.4, and 8.2 for intensive care, high dependency level 3, high dependency level 2, and low dependency level 2, respectively. Within a unit a continuum of patient need is managed by grouping of patients to constitute a manageable workload for each shift. A system should classify patients to rationalize allocation of nurses and assists in accounting or assigning charges. No empirical neonatal benchmarks for nursing ratios according to the complexity of the patient exist (NANN, 1999e).

Infants in the NICUs demand significant direct care. As resident physicians were withdrawn from training in intensive care settings, many hospitals are replacing them with NNPs. These highly skilled nurses earn salaries higher than those of the residents they replace. The economics of this situation may substantially increase costs. Evidence suggests that NNPs may be more cost-effective, as evidence exists to suggest that less experienced house officers order more tests and practice less efficiently and that these effects are aggravated by high census. Disruptions due to intern rotation also cause slippage in discharge time and increase costs (Rich et al, 1994).

Use of Assistive Personnel

As they view the impact of work redesigning and the use of assistive personnel on patient management, nurses are beginning to value each other. NANN has taken the position that appropriately educated nurses must be responsible for the assessment, planning, delivery, and evaluation of care provided to every newborn and family to ensure safe, high-quality care. Sick newborns require the care of specialized neonatal RNs who fully understand the disease process and treatment modalities involved. This professional nurse may assign or delegate tasks to assistive personnel based upon the assessed needs of the patient, the potential for harm, the complexity of the care to be provided, and the knowledge and skill of the personnel in question. Assistive personnel must have appropriate education in the care of the high-risk newborn and family, even when carrying out support services for the professional nurse. Systems for the delivery of care must be designed by RNs in collaboration with health care professionals, taking into consideration the needs of the patient population to be served, the resources available, and state and local regulations. With these requirements met, assistive personnel may be safely used to ensure delivery of high-quality care in the most cost-effective manner (NANN, 1999e).

Neonatal nurses are demanding that their tiny patients receive care from nurses.

Characteristics of Caregiving Environments that Promote Job Satisfaction

Increased job satisfaction is associated with improved recruitment and retention of nurses, whereas stressful practice environments reduce job satisfaction and retention. Creation of healthy practice environments should be a priority for neonatal nurse managers. Characteristics of a healthy work culture have been described by Walker (2001) and should be incorporated into the management goals for the NICU. The environment must contain opportunity for the following:

- Continuous learning
- Support for learning from mistakes
- Honoring the person-hood of each other
- Connecting people through shared purpose and meaning

- Forming partnerships
- Openness to understanding other points of view
- Respectful supportive relationships

The ability to listen without the need to analyze, prove, judge, rescue, fix, or blame is essential. Advocacy with the intention of revealing without defending is necessary. Nurses develop job satisfaction through involvement in decision making. Shared leadership at the unit level improves work environments, aids in retention, and defines accountability (Walker, 2001). A culture that supports reporting errors should be created. Mueller-Boyer (2001) suggests Root Cause Analysis (RCA) as a strategy to achieve this goal. This strategy can assist in doing the following:

- Identify near miss or what happened
- Identify the process or activity in which the event occurred
- Identify human factors, equipment factors, environmental factors, uncontrollable external factors, and other factors
- Indicate why the event happened
- Define the most proximate factors

Based on the analysis risk reduction, strategies are formulated. The strategy creates a trusting environment and allows for the formulation of risk reduction strategies.

To facilitate system integration, product line goals and objectives must support the service program, financial goals, and human resource objectives of the individual entities and the health system (Ropp, 2001). An awareness of system level commitment will assist with development, satisfaction, and commitment to vision for the neonatal nurse providers.

Brown & Taquino (2001) suggest that participation in the design of the neonatal care facility increases staff satisfaction and benefits infants and families as well. Planning based on a clear vision, building a dynamic design team, establishing realistic and achievable goals, identifying specific needs of individual groups, and implementing the realistic action plan are the suggested steps in the process.

Wolf et al (1994b) suggested the use of the transitional models (www.upmc.edu/beckwithinst) to position nursing in the center of patient care. She believes the model supports professional practice transformational leadership, improvement in the care delivery system, professional growth, and collaborative practice. The process components of the model include: critical thinking, negotiation, and decision making related to needs of patient, professional recommendations, and resource management (Arnold, 2001). Primary outcomes expected include: satisfaction, congruence, responsiveness, and patient participation. The outcomes related to the health care team include the following: a dynamic work environment, quality professional relationships, voice and power for caregivers, and a support system for personal and professional growth (Arnold, 2001).

Outcomes associated with using the Transitional Model include achieving the strategic direction of the health care organization (responsiveness, ability to financially compete, and enhanced reputation) and improving the professions ability to influence the growth of the members and profession as well as willingness of the organization to invest in the future of the profession. Nursing is the corner stone of high-quality, cost-efficient care (Wolf, 1994a).

Nurse providers of neonatal intensive care are primarily women. Women's health seems to be influenced by the type of leadership and existing organizational climate and culture (Bergman et al, 1996). Leadership and organizational climate influence how women are seen and valued. Incompetent leadership creates dissatisfaction and accentuates dependent relationships with other workers, whereas good leaders influence others for the benefit of the organization. Recipients of ridicule or demeaning comments display symptoms of frustration such as listlessness and sleeping problems and can become depressed (Bergman et al, 1996). Only a short period of time is necessary for the development of subjective symptoms of bad health or for recovery. An external channel for nurses to get assistance is needed (Bergman et al, 1996).

Kowalski (2001) has identified factors that influence current nursing workforce use. These factors are the competitive health marketplace, personnel shortages, financial limitations, and work environment (high turnover, flux, conflict, and intergenerational issues). Kowalski (2001) recommended recruitment and retention strategies based on understanding intergenerational differences, expenditure of resources to build teams, and increased attention to academic and continuing education. Unit-based educators, such as clinical specialists, are needed to provide for unit-based orientation as well as continued competency. Leadership and management styles that promote nurturing, growing, and coaching are also needed, as are work environments that honor, acknowledge, and respect workers and allow use of skills, tools, and critical thinking (Kowalski, 2001). MacPhee (1999) suggested that workplace networks are important to nurses with both flexible and traditional schedules. Nurses on flex schedules may form fewer social attachments to manage the increased demands of moving among multiple units. MacPhee (1999) reports no significant difference in social network composition.

A national shortage of neonatal nurses exists (Harrigan, personal communication, 2000); this situation is anticipated to become more problematic over the next 5 years. Nurses are discontent with their work environments, and the number of applicants to nursing programs is decreasing. Lack of job satisfaction and multiple opportunities in other employment markets are creating crisis situations in some areas where the supply of nurses is significantly smaller than the supply needed. This shortage is more severe in neonatal intensive care units than other nursing practice areas. Attention to factors critical to recruitment and retention of neonatal nurses is essential.

Ethical Stressors in the NICU

Moral stress is ever-present in the NICU. Neonatal nurses need support in developing personal qualities, integrated knowledge, and self-awareness. These qualities can be developed with clinical supervision; Severinsson & Kamaker (1999) found that moral sensitivity is increased in the presence of systematic clinical supervision.

Nurses are more likely to be involved in dilemma-resolution activities when they perceive higher levels of influence in their practice environments and higher levels of concern about the ethical aspects of individual patient situations. Nurses who emphasize consideration of morally relevant aspects of individual patient situations (that is, consequentialist value orientation) and underemphasize adherence to abstract standards, rules, and policies are more likely to be involved in dilemma resolution (Penticuff & Walden, 2000).

CULTURAL SENSITIVITY AND NEONATAL NURSING PRACTICE

Culturally sensitive care includes the ability to assess and incorporate into patient care those aspects of a culture significant to health and illness (NANN, 1999b). More education and re-

sources are needed to develop culturally sensitive nurses. To promote culturally sensitive care, NANN (1999b) has identified the following essential components:

- Education in how to provide culturally competent nursing care. This education is necessary in all levels of nursing education, in hospital/unit orientation, and in continuing education programs.
- The complete nursing assessment of a neonate must include a family cultural assessment. This assessment should identify cultural practices related to childbirth, infant care, health care preferences, family dynamics, sick child care, and perinatal loss.
- Neonatal nurses must have access to resources on cultural competence, readily available at all venues of practice.
- The performance review of the professional nurse should incorporate evaluation of cultural competence when providing care.
- Incorporation in nursing journals, publications, and media productions of information on culturally competent care.
- Development of programs for recruitment and retention of minority nurses. These should address the identified barriers of distance, discrimination, lack of financial assistance, and language.
- Increased federal and state funding for nursing education that includes emphasis on minority recruitment and employment in underserved areas.
- Collaboration between professional health care organizations is necessary to emphasize the importance of its scope of cultural competence.
- Further nursing research on cultural diversity and the impact on health care outcomes is needed. The word culture encompasses a multitude of concepts.

No single racial or ethnic group will constitute a majority in the United States by the end of the twenty-first century. Differences in language, socioeconomic status, and ethnicity may affect the outcomes of nursing management. "Ethical practice requires recognition of one's biases, a sensitivity to cultural differences, the avoidance of generalizations about cultures, and the provision of culturally relevant care" (NANN, 1999b). Nurses must recognize and understand the cultures of the families to whom they provide care. Respect for culture includes tolerance, understanding, support, acceptance, and validation of beliefs and practices of the patient's/family's culture (NANN, 1999b). Cultural sensitivity should be incorporated in nursing education, practice, and research.

SUMMARY

Several important issues have been discussed in this chapter, including the role and development of neonatal nurses, the contributions of advanced practice nurses to neonatal care, the merging of extended and expanded neonatal nursing roles into an advanced practice focus for neonatal nursing, the responsibility of students and practitioners to understand the basis for credentialing within the specialty, the education of neonatal nurses for advanced practice, the effect of nursing management on neonatal outcomes, and cultural sensitivity in neonatal nursing practice. Five groups of neonatal nurses have been identified—providers of neonatal nursing care, communicators or managers of neonatal nursing practice, translators of research data into useful practice information, generators of knowledge for neonatal nursing practice, and shapers of policy related to neonatal health care. Today, neonatal nursing is promoting and adapting to changes in the management of the health of the fragile infants. Neonatal nursing management skills are needed both within the NICU and in home care delivery systems. Neonatal nurses are in a unique position in this regard because of their significant impact on the family. Neonatal nursing roles will continue to evolve; we should therefore be flexible, systematic, and cogent in making practice decisions along the way.

Collaboration is the commitment of an entire group of care providers to shared values, approaches to care, and treatment goals. Collaborative care assumes that a group of disciplined professionals is present, each with a unique contribution to make to the well-being of the neonate and his or her family. Collaboration is the result of a developmental process through which the visions of talented health care professionals are communicated to the group and through which shared values and goals are developed. Collaborative practice demands responsibility and recognition of limitations from mature, expert clinicians. Collaborative practice is the practice model of choice for delivery of services to fragile, sick newborns in the highly technical intensive care unit and to their vulnerable families.

REFERENCES

American Academy of Pediatrics (AAP). (1999). *The role of the nurse practitioner and physicians assistant in the care of hospitalized children.* American Academy of Pediatrics Committee on Hospital Care Pediatrics, 103(5), 1050-1051.

American Academy of Pediatrics (AAD) and American College of Obstetrics and Gynecology (ACOG) (1997). *Guidelines for perinatal care,* ed 4, Elk Grove Village, IL: American Academy of Pediatrics.

Ames A, Perrin JM (1980). Collaborative practice: the joining of two professionals. *Journal of the Tennessee medical association,* 73(8), 557-560.

Arnold LS (2001). Transforming the health care system by transforming professional practice: A conversation with Gail Wolf, RN, DSN, FAAN. *Neonatal nursing,* 15(1), 8-15.

Ashworth C et al (1998). Providing opportunities for role development: ENB R23 'Enhancing Neonatal Nursing Practice'. *Journal of neonatal nursing,* (4)2, 8-11.

Bates B (1970). Doctor and nurse: changing roles and relations. *New England journal of medicine,* 283(3), 129-134.

Bergman B et al (1996). Women's work experiences and health in a male-dominated industry. *Journal of occupational and environmental medicine,* 38(7), 664-671.

Brooten D et al (1991). Functions of the CNS in early discharge and home follow up of very-low-birth-weight infants. *Clinical nurse specialist,* 5(4), 196-201.

Brown P, Taquino LT (2001). Designing and delivering neonatal care in single room. *Journal of perinatal neonatal nursing,* 15(1), 68-83.

Consolvo CA et al (1989). Profile of the hardy NICU nurse. *Journal of perinatology,* 9(3), 334-337.

DiCenso A (1998). The neonatal nurse practitioner. *Current opinion pediatrics,* 10(2), 151-155.

Erlen JA (1994). Ethical dilemmas in the high-risk nursery: wilderness experiences. *Journal of pediatric nursing,* 9(1), 21-26.

Gennaro S et al (1991). Postdischarge services for low-birth-weight infants. *Journal of obstetric, gynecological, and neonatal nursing,* 20(1), 29-36.

Griffith CH et al (1999). House staff workload and procedure frequency in the neonatal intensive care unit. *Critical care medicine,* 27(4), 815-820.

Harper RG et al (1982). The scope of nursing practice in level III neonatal intensive units. *Pediatrics,* 70(6), 875-878.

Harrigan RC, Kooker BM (2000). Health education needs in Hawaii: social work, dental hygiene and nursing. *Hawaii medical journal,* 59(2), 67-69.

Harrigan RC (1995). Health care reform: Impact of managed care on perinatal and neonatal care delivery and education. *Journal of perinatal neonatal nursing,* 8(4), 47-58.

Heith RM, Van Dinter M (2000). Developing collaborative practice agreements. *Journal of pediatric health care,* 14(4), 200-203.

Herman J, Zeil S (1999). Collaborative practice agreements for advanced practice nurses: what you should know. *AACN clinical issues,* 10(3), 337-342.

Hickey JV (1996). *Advanced practice nursing: moving into the 21st century in practice, education, and research.* In Hickey JV et al, editors: *Advanced practice nursing: changing roles and clinical application.* Philadelphia: JB Lippincott.

Johnson PJ et al (1979). Neonatal nurse practitioners: part 1. a new expanded nursing role. *Perinatology/Neonatology,* January-February, 34-36.

Jones B (1999). Neonatal nurse practitioners: a model for expanding the boundaries of nursing culture in New Zealand. *Nurse practice New Zealand,* 14(3), 28-35.

Kamajian MF et al (1999). Credentialing and privileging of advanced practice nurses. *AACN clinical issues,* 10(3), 316-336.

Kowalski K (2001). Nursing workforce of the future: the administrative perspective. *Journal of perinatal neonatal nursing,* 15(1), 8-15.

Lamb GS, Napodano RJ (1984). Physician-nurse practitioner interaction patterns in primary care practices. *American journal of public health,* 74(1), 26-29.

Leininger M (1971). This I believe: about interdisciplinary health education for the future. *Nursing outlook,* 19(12), 787-791.

MacPhee M (1999). Hospital networking: comparing the work of nurses with flexible and traditional schedules. *Journal of nursing administration,* 30(4), 190-198.

Maguire D (1999). Sharing the vision of NICU Nursing Practice. *Neonatal network,* 18(4), 71-72.

Marshall PB et al (1989). The cost of intensive and special care of the newborn. *Medical journal of Australia,* 150(1), 568-569, 572-574.

Medicare. Part B newsletter no. 012, August 30, 1996.

Miller M et al (1993). Collaborative experiences for NICU and early childhood education personnel. *Neonatal network,* 12(7), 37-42.

Mitchell-DiCenso A et al (1996). A controlled trial of nurse practitioners in neonatal intensive care. *Pediatrics,* 98(6), 1143-1156.

Mueller-Boyer M (2001). Root cause analysis in perinatal care: health care professionals creating safer health care systems. *Journal of perinatal neonatal nursing,* 15(1), 40-54.

NANN. (1999a). *Advanced practice neonatal nurse role* (No. 3000). Glenview, IL: National Association of Neonatal Nurses.

NANN. (1999b). *Position statement on cultural competence* (No. 3037). Glenview, IL: National Association of Neonatal Nurses.

NANN. (1999c). *Position statement on RN practice experience and neonatal advanced nursing practice* (No. 3011). Glenview, IL: National Association of Neonatal Nurses.

NANN. (1999d). *Position statement on transport of neonates across state lines* (No. 3020). Glenview, IL: National Association of Neonatal Nurses.

NANN. (1999e). *Position statement on the use of assistive personnel in providing care to the high-risk infant* (No. 3013). Glenview, IL: National Association of Neonatal Nurses.

NANN. (2000). *Position statement on BSN entry into practice* (No. 3014). Glenview, IL: National Association of Neonatal Nurses.

Omnibus Reconciliation Act of 1989. Washington, DC.

Organek N, Hegedus K (1993). Advanced practice: a model for neonatal/perinatal and woman/child nursing. *AACN clinical issues in critical care nursing,* 4(4), 631-636.

Pearson JH (1999). Regulation in the face of technological advance: Who makes these calls anyway? *Notre Dame journal of laws & ethics public policy,* 13(1), 1-8.

Penticuff JH, Walden M (2000). Influence of practice environment and nurse characteristics on perinatal nurses: responses to ethical dilemmas. *Nursing research,* 49(2), 64-72.

Perez-Woods R (1991). *Data based publications in maternal-child health.* Unpublished manuscript. (University of Hawaii, 2528 The Mall, Honolulu, HI).

Pollack LD et al (1998). United States neonatology practice survey: personnel, practice, hospital and NICU characteristics. *Pediatrics*, 101(3), 398-405.

Rich EC et al (1994). The effects of scheduled intern rotation on the cost and quality of teaching hospital care. *Evaluation of health professions*, 17(3), 259-272.

Richardson DK et al (2001). A critical review of cost reduction in neonatal intensive care: I: the structure of costs. *Journal of perinatology*, 21(2), 107-115.

Ropp A (2001). Managing women's and children's services: Contemporary models as a template for the future. *Journal of perinatal neonatal nursing*, 15(1), 55-67.

Rosenthal SL et al (1989). Stress and coping in a NICU. *Research in nursing and health*, 12(4), 257-265.

Severinsson EL, Kamaker D (1999). Clinical nursing supervision in the workplace: effects on moral stress and job satisfaction. *Journal of nursing management*, 7(2), 81-90.

Shumaker D, Goss V (1980). Toward collaboration: one small step. *Nursing and health care*, 1(4), 183-185.

Trotter C, Danaher R (1994). Neonatal nurse practitioners: a descriptive evaluation of an advanced practice role. *Neonatal network*, 13(1), 39-47.

Walker J (2001). Developing a shared leadership model at the unit level. *Journal of perinatal neonatal nursing*, 15(1), 26-39.

Wolf G et al (1994a). A transformational model for the practice of professional nursing: Part 1: the model. *Journal of nursing administration*, 24(4), 51-57.

Wolf G et al (1994b). A transformational model for the practice of professional nursing. Part 2. The model. *Journal of nursing administration*, 24(5), 38-46.

REGIONALIZATION IN TODAY'S HEALTH CARE DELIVERY SYSTEM

GAIL A. BAGWELL, CYNTHIA M. ACREE, KRISTINE A. KARLSEN, ANNA SHEETS, JULIE SHAW,

KATHLEEN SANDMAN, KAREN L. ROUTZON, LINDA WAECHTER, MARY DUVALL VETTER, KIE SHELLEY,

SHARON KWIECINSKI

In the late 1970s, guidelines describing a regionalized system of perinatal care were published and resulted in improved outcomes in pregnancy and survival of high-risk infants. Hospitals were divided into three levels, each with defined capabilities. Factors that influenced the level of designation were number of deliveries per year, location, training level of physicians and nurses, and availability of ancillary support systems. The goal was to promote access and quality care.

American health care delivery changed during the 1980s and 1990s. The growth of health maintenance organizations (HMOs), the implementation of diagnosis-related groups (DRGs) in certain states, changes in Medicaid and third-party reimbursement, the increasing number of medical specialists finishing fellowship programs, and a staffing crisis led to a deterioration in perinatal regional care in some areas. Within regions, hospitals began competing for patients rather than cooperating to provide optimal care (Finkelman, 2001). Regionalization depends on a strong transport system and very good stabilization methods in the field.

This chapter reviews the development of the regionalized system, the delineation of levels of care, the transport process, and various transport models. It outlines the responsibilities of the nursery staff at each level and the staff's role within the system, a detailed framework of the transport process including alternative types of transports, financial costs and legal issues. The S.T.A.B.L.E.® program's concepts towards promoting neonatal stability are described. The chapter concludes with a discussion of the challenges facing the regionalized system approach to care and the steps being taken to modify the system for the future and the effects on the transport process.

DEVELOPMENT OF THE REGIONALIZED SYSTEM

During the first half of the twentieth century, infant mortality rates decreased steadily worldwide. From 1950 to 1965, mortality rates continued to fall in western nations; in the United States, however, rates did not fall significantly. Barriers such as race, poverty, geographic location, and cultural and physical isolation kept high-risk pregnant women and infants from medical care. Research showed that persons at social and medical high risk were least likely to receive the necessary medical care. When these people received appropriate care, their outcomes improved. This relationship was demonstrated during

World War II, when more than 1,450,000 women and infants received medical care through the Emergency Maternity and Infant Care Program for the dependents of individuals in the Armed Forces. Perinatal and infant mortality rates improved. The program was discontinued in 1949, and a coincidental rise in mortality rates began in 1950.

As the medical community learned of the multiple causes affecting infant mortality, it began to change the delivery of perinatal care. High-risk maternal and neonatal care had a positive influence on mortality rates. Neonatal transport provided new access to intensive care nurseries. In the 1960's the American Medical Association (AMA) Committee on Maternal and Child Care was created to focus on identifying high-risk infants, the organization and delivery of high-risk care, problems of prematurity, need for perinatal research, education, and staffing requirements.

The AMA, the American Academy of Family Physicians (AAFP), the American Academy of Pediatrics (AAP), and the American College of Obstetricians and Gynecologists (ACOG) formed the Committee on Perinatal Health, which developed guidelines for a regional perinatal care system.

In 1976, the committee, supported by The National Foundation—March of Dimes, published *Toward Improving the Outcome of Pregnancy: Recommendations for the Regional Development of Maternal and Perinatal Health Service*. The committee determined that a "systems approach" would meet the objective of providing optimal care for the women and infants within a region. The committee defined regionalization as a geographic area's development of a coordinated, cooperative system of maternal and perinatal health care that identifies the complexity of maternal and perinatal health care each area hospital can provide. This identification comes about through mutual agreements between hospitals and physicians and on the basis of population needs and assists in achieving quality care for all pregnant women and newborns, maximal use of highly trained perinatal personnel and intensive care facilities, and reasonable cost effectiveness (The National Foundation—March of Dimes, 1976). According to the recommendations, a region would serve a population with 8,000 to 12,000 live births per year. Within each region, a medical center with over 2000 yearly deliveries would be designated a Level III, or tertiary center. These hospitals would care for pregnant women and infants at highest risk. Level II centers would serve as referral centers for hospitals that provided less specialized services. Level II hospitals would provide routine care and handle most obstetrical complications and short-term neonatal intensive care. Level I hospitals would serve a small population and provide care for uncomplicated deliveries and healthy newborns. Personnel would be trained to recognize obstetrical and neonatal emergencies and give competent care in these situations until the patient could be transported to another hospital.

Across the United States, the committee's recommendations were enacted, and regional systems were developed. The ACOG and AAP adopted the recommendations. The National Foundation—March of Dimes had already determined a relationship between perinatal events and crippling diseases of infants. The National Foundation committed administrative and financial support to the committee, financed projects to raise community awareness about the need for perinatal care, and designed educational programs for both pregnant women and health professionals.

The Robert Wood Johnson Foundation, a philanthropic organization, supported the committee's recommendations and financed eight regional programs (e.g., through the National Demonstration Program initiative) for a 5-year period. The foundation's goal was to evaluate the feasibility of the regional approach and its effect on improving health care. The results were positive on all fronts.

In 1989, the AAP and ACOG requested the March of Dimes to reconvene the Committee on Perinatal Health to make further recommendations for regional development. The document *Toward Improving the Outcome of Pregnancy: The 90s and Beyond (TIOP II)* (Committee on Perinatal Health, 1993) moves from a discussion of the past and current climate of care through indications of the problem to key recommendations considered essential for improving the outcome of pregnancy. The report continues to support the levels of care, stressed a new focus on prevention and ambulatory care, and emphasized the importance of data, documentation, and evaluation. They also recommended the designation of formalized perinatal regions and that each state have a perinatal board responsible for coordinating, planning, data collection, and education (Committee on Perinatal Health, 1993).

IMPACT OF REGIONALIZATION ON NEONATAL MORTALITY

A result of the development of the neonatal intensive care unit (NICU) and improved obstetrical care is the decline in neonatal mortality. The improvement in mortality rates must be examined by inspecting birth weight at delivery. The greatest impact is seen on the survival rates of extremely low-birth-weight (ELBW) neonates, or infants who weigh 750 to 1,000 grams at delivery. In 1960, the mortality rate of ELBW infants was 90%. In 1996, 86% of infants born weighing between 750 and 1000 grams and 54% infants weighing 500 to 750 grams at delivery survive (Lemons et al, 2001; Stevenson et al, 1998). ELBW infants born at Level I and Level II centers and then transferred to Level III centers have a lower rate of survival. The chance of survival improves when these infants are delivered at Level III centers (Phibbs et al, 1996, Kirby, 1996; Hernandez et al, 2000). Although the benefit of concentrating high-risk deliveries at Level III and designated Level II perinatal centers can be seen in improved survival rates, some physicians are reluctant to transfer their high-risk patients. The reasons given for this reluctance are financial issues, the competition among hospitals to attract patients by offering a full complement of services, and the obstetrician's or pediatrician's refusal based on his or her assessment of the ELBW infant's viability.

The voluntary cooperation of hospitals, physicians, and health officials to regionalize services had a positive impact on infant survival rates. Even today, the technology to determine at birth which handicaps, if any, ELBW infants will incur is not available. The opportunity for survival and normal development is influenced by the place of delivery. Kirby (1996) looked at neonatal mortality in a state with no regionalization system and found that infants with birth weights under 2000 grams have a lower mortality rate than those born in Level II facilities. Phibbs et al (1996) looked at neonatal mortality and morbidity and the effects of the level of the NICU and patient volume in non-federal hospitals with maternity units in California. They found that hospitals with Level III NICUs with an average daily census of 15 had the lowest risk-adjusted neonatal mortality rate. They also found no differences in costs for infants born at large Level III centers versus those born at other NICUs. Yeast et al (1998) examined the changing patterns of perinatal regionalization in the state of Missouri and the effect on neonatal mortality. They found that the deregionalization of care had not improved the outcomes for inborn infants less than 1500 grams, unless they were born at a Level III facility. Hernandez et al (2000) looked at the impact of infants on the threshold of viability on the neonatal mortality rate. They found that infants born at Level III tertiary perinatal centers had a better chance for survival to discharge than those born at a Level I or II facility. Studies have shown that the mortality rate among ELBW infants increases for those born at a Level I or II hospital. When possible, a high-risk pregnant woman should be transferred to a Level III hospital before delivery. For increased survival chances and influence on positive developmental outcome, ELBW infants should be transferred to a Level III NICU after stabilization following delivery. Changes are being implemented to continue the success of perinatal regionalization. The issues influencing the future of the program are explored later in this chapter.

THREE LEVELS OF PERINATAL CARE

In 1976, the Committee on Perinatal Health recommended division of the delivery of perinatal care into three levels. For the regionalized system to function effectively, a coordinated communication network was established within each region.

Level I hospitals were responsible for recognizing high-risk mothers and neonates and coordinating either their referrals or transports to a higher level of care. Level II hospitals had the Level I—hospital responsibility but also had intensive care facilities, usually used to care for sick neonates with a moderate degree of illness. The Level III hospital was responsible for the provision of comprehensive perinatal care services of all risk categories. A method of obtaining consultation and arranging maternal or neonatal transports was outlined. *TIOP II* calls for modifying the current system from being defined as levels to being identified as basic, specialty, and subspecialty perinatal centers. In the fourth edition of American Academy of Pediatrics (AAP) and American College of Obstetrics and Gynecology (ACOG) (1998) *Guidelines for Perinatal Care*, a change from using the traditional numerical designation to using the functional descriptive designations was made due to changes in the healthcare environment. However, most hospitals continue to use the designations of Level I, II, or III.

Through regionalization, outreach education programs became the responsibility of the regional centers for the basic and specialty hospitals in their region. *Guidelines for Perinatal Care* (fourth edition) continues to outline regional centers' responsibilities as organizers of educational programs to meet the needs of their region. The purpose of outreach was to educate perinatal personnel in recognizing high-risk conditions and to educate them in handling obstetrical and neonatal emergency complications when immediate transport was not possible.

The committee set guidelines for establishing a regionalized system and the responsibilities for hospitals at each level. The committee's framework was designed not as a standard of care but rather as an achievable goal of improving the outcome of pregnancy (The National Foundation—March of Dimes, 1976).

No defined national standard determines the difference between Level II and III care. In some states, individual hospitals classify their level of care; in others, the state sets the perinatal designation. The descriptions of care outlined below are those of the committee. Box 2-1 outlines the responsibilities for each level of care according to the AAP's/ACOG's (1998) *Guidelines for Perinatal Care*, using the new designations of basic, specialty, and subspecialty care.

Level I (Basic)

These facilities are located in communities with small populations, either suburban or rural. Because of their low number of births per year and their smaller economic base, these hospitals are responsible for managing uncomplicated maternal and newborn care. They must be able to give competent emergency care in unexpected situations. A strength of the Level I facility is its ability to recognize potential high-risk situations and provide both primary and preventive care or consultation and/or referral to an appropriate center.

The Level I hospital has a formal relationship with the regional Level III center. This relationship supports a method of consultation and communication and of patient transport between the two. The Level I hospital participates in an educational program to train its personnel in neonatal resuscitation and in stabilization of patients for transport. Infants can be transferred back to the community hospital from a Level II or III center after the acute illness has resolved. The community hospital promotes the infant's growth and development in a family-centered environment.

Level II (Specialty)

A wide variation in the abilities of Level II units exists, depending on the medical specialists and support services available in each institution. Level II facilities offer services for uncomplicated maternal and neonatal patients and are competent in handling certain obstetrical and neonatal complications (Figure 2-1). When needed specialists and services are not available, patients are transferred to the Level III center.

Either a neonatologist or a pediatrician with neonatal expertise directs the medical care in the special care nursery. The nursing staff is skilled in caring for sick infants and communicating effectively with the infant's parents. Infants either transported to or delivered at the Level III center can be transferred back to the Level II nursery when their conditions have stabilized. The Level II unit participates in collaborative educational programs with the Level III center. If the appropriate services are available, the Level II unit can serve as the referral site for Level I nurseries in the region.

BOX 2-1

Role Definitions in a Regional Perinatal Network*

Basic Care
Surveillance and care of all patients admitted to the obstetric service, with an established triage system for identifying high-risk patients who should be transferred to a facility that provides specialty or subspecialty care

Proper detection and supportive care of unanticipated maternal-fetal problems that occur during labor and delivery

Capability for emergency c-section within 30 minutes of decision to do one

Availability of blood and fresh-frozen plasma for transfusions

Availability of anesthesia, radiology, laboratory and ultrasound services 24 hour/day

Care of postpartum conditions

Evaluation of the condition of healthy neonates and continuing care of these neonates until discharge

Resuscitation and stabilization of all neonates born in hospital

Stabilization of small or ill neonates before transfer to a specialty or subspecialty care facility

Consultation and transfer agreements

Nursery care

Parent-sibling-neonate visitation

Collect and evaluate patient data

Specialty Care
Provide all services of basic care facility

Care of high-risk mothers and fetuses, both admitted and transferred from other facilities

Stabilization of ill newborns prior to transfer

Care of preterm infants with a birth weight of 1,500 grams or more

Subspeciality Care†

Provision of comprehensive perinatal care services for both admitted and transferred mothers and neonates of all risk categories, including basic and specialty care services as described above

Research and educational support

Analysis and evaluation of regional data, including those on complications

Initial evaluation of new high-risk technologies

Transport of neonates occurs to and from all facilities.
†*Level III NICUs located in children's hospitals may not offer services of basic and specialty care facilities.*
Adapted from American Academy of Pediatrics. (1997) Guidelines for perinatal care, ed 4, Elk Grove Village, Ill: American Academy of Pediatrics and American College of Obstetricians and Gynecologists. Used with permission.

Level III (Subspecialty)

Level III facilities serve as the region's referral sites for the most high-risk maternal and neonatal patients and provide routine obstetrical and newborn care. These institutions offer a full complement of consultants and ancillary services to care for their patients. Many children's hospitals have intensive care and specialized resources for neonates. The children's hospital is an appropriate referral site but should not be used as the sole Level III facility in the region. The Level III NICU has an equipped and trained team and is available around-the-clock

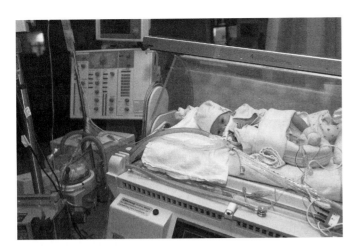

FIGURE **2-1**
Level II neonate who requires close supervision. Courtesy of Children's Hospital; Columbus, Ohio.

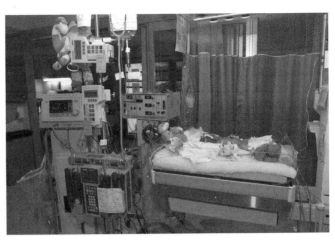

FIGURE **2-2**
Level III neonate who requires high-technology care. Courtesy of Children's Hospital; Columbus, Ohio.

for neonatal transport. A similar team may be available for transporting high-risk maternity patients. The team provides management and treatment during transport. It is also responsible for educating personnel at the referring hospital.

The Level III unit is responsible for instituting a continuing education program for the region. The regional center, often affiliated with an educational institution, serves as an educational training center for health care professionals. Perinatal personnel throughout the region may come to the Level III center to gain experience in caring for critically ill mothers and infants (Figure 2-2).

Nurses in the NICU have expertise in caring for the sickest neonates. They understand the physiology, the disease processes, and the necessary monitoring equipment. Communication with the infant's parents and offers of emotional support are essential skills for the NICU staff. This staff includes respiratory therapists, nutritionists, occupational and physical therapists, pharmacists, early intervention specialists, and perinatal social workers with expertise in working with neonates and their parents.

COORDINATION OF THE REGIONAL SYSTEM

Coordination of services and communication among institutions and personnel within the region is essential for the success of the system. All those involved must be aware of their responsibilities and roles within the system; they must have a working knowledge of how the system functions. Medical and nursing personnel, health departments, third-party payers, and consumer groups participate in the planning of care delivery within each region (The National Foundation—March of Dimes, 1976, Committee on Perinatal Health, 1993).

Interhospital conferences foster communication and continuity of care. These meetings provide the referring hospital with information on patients transferred to the regional center and information on learning opportunities (Hauth & Merenstein, 1997). The conferences give community physicians the chance to participate in case management, be updated on the latest research findings and care modalities, and learn the steps in obtaining consultations and patient transfers.

Evaluation of perinatal care plays an appropriate role in assessing whether the provision of care has been effective. Evaluation should include a perinatal data program to help monitor outcome, identify problem areas that require improvement, and assist in comparative studies.

FACTORS INFLUENCING PATIENT TRANSFER

The transport of sick neonates from their birth hospital to a perinatal center is a direct result of the regionalization system. The advantages and disadvantages of neonatal transport after delivery versus maternal transport before delivery continues to be debated. Studies that reported no significant differences between the mortality rates of premature infants transferred to Level III centers after delivery and those of infants born in Level III centers may have a built-in bias because the most critically ill and premature infants may not survive long enough to be transferred to a NICU and because premature infants with no morbidity are not always transferred. Other studies show a decrease in mortality when high-risk mothers are transferred to perinatal centers before delivery. Hernandez et al (2000) showed that the infant weighing less than 750 grams born in Level I centers had significantly greater mortality (84.4% versus 57.3% versus 60.6%) than those born at Level II and III centers, respectively. The neonatal mortality was higher at the Level III than at the Level II center because the sickest infants received care in the Level III center. A minimal difference exists between the survival rates of infants born after antenatal transport and those of deliveries scheduled at the referral center.

Both physical and financial barriers prevent the transfer of patients to perinatal centers. Competition between hospitals, especially in urban areas, may be a reason for Level II hospitals not to refer their patients to the Level III center. Hospitals use their ability to provide services for the entire family to attract clients; in addition, it provides continuity of care and promotes maternal-infant bonding. Childbirth may be a family's first experience with hospitalization. Hospitals want to develop a continuing relationship with the family, and a maternal or neonatal transport to a neighboring hospital for needed services can threaten this relationship. In addition to competition issues, the technology of neonatal intensive care is no longer the exclusive preserve of heavily funded academic centers (Pollack, 1996). The ease of technology transfer; the surplus of neonatologists and ancillary neonatal personnel, including neonatal nurse practitioners (NNPs)/advanced practice nurses (APNs); and reimbursement issues have enabled Level II NICUs to be established. Moreover, with the availability of skilled neonatal nursing staff to respond quickly to neonatal emergencies, the liability risks of hospitals and the medical staff have decreased (Sanders, 2000). A physician's decision to transfer a patient can also be influenced by the risk of nonpayment or loss of payment. Medicaid reimbursement for obstetrical care is more than 30% lower than reimbursement from a private paying patient. Obstetricians have been slower than other physicians to accept Medicaid patients. When the Level III hospital is university-affiliated and has a closed medical faculty, non-faculty obstetricians do not have admitting privileges. These physicians risk loss of payment by transferring patients to such a facility.

Other factors that can affect the transfer of patients to a Level III center include lack of bed space, unavailability of the needed resources, and unavailability of the needed equipment (e.g., extracorporeal membrane oxygenation [ECMO] and Inhaled Nitric Oxide [INO]). If one of these cases arises, the Level III center needs to assist the referring hospital to find another institution to accept the transfer of the infant and needs to assist with medical management of the infant by telephone until transfer. Finally, the Joint Commission on Accreditation of Healthcare Organizations (JCAHO)—although responsible for reviewing the operation guidelines of the NICU—does not have authority over access to treatment. Some NICUs were created under an individual state certificate-of-need legislation. The state does not have continuing authority over the operation of neonatal services once the certificate of need is granted. Institutions that received federal funding for construction and renovation under the 1946 Hill-Burton Act must provide charity care for patients who cannot pay. The Consolidated Omnibus Budget Reconciliation Act, enacted in March 1986, prohibits Medicare-participating hospitals from denying treatment to or transferring a woman in labor based on her socioeconomic status or inability to pay for health care.

With these regulations and concepts of regionalization came the need to develop a system of transport to ensure the safe transport of laboring women and critically ill infants to optimize outcomes. The details regarding the transport of the high-risk mother is beyond the scope of this chapter. Neonatal transport has developed as a dynamic and complex process trying to mimic the uterus because the uterus is the natural and best means of transport for the fetus. At birth, the infant leaves the uterus and the safety of the intricate physiologic environment that meets its every need. In the event of an unexpected outcome, health professionals are faced with the challenge of meeting the complex needs of the compromised infant. If the infant is born in a location without the resources to meet these special needs, transportation of the infant to a hospital with necessary resources becomes an additional challenge.

Transport services continue to evolve as a sophisticated process. This process is essential for providing optimal perinatal and neonatal care around the world.

HISTORICAL PERSPECTIVE

Written reports of the transport of ill individuals can be traced back to biblical times. In the Gospel Luke 5:18–19, a paralytic was brought on a mat to Jesus, who, according to the physician Luke, was the great healer (Salyer & Masi-Lynch, 1995).

Before the invention of the wheel, family members and friends used animals to carry individuals who required medical assistance. The wheel was then used in wagons created for patient transport. Wars and resulting casualties were the primary stimuli for the development of ambulance systems in the 1400s through modern times. The Vietnam War was the major impetus for the development of effective helicopter evacuation and transport.

During the Crimean War, Florence Nightingale brought to the public's attention the neglect of the sick and wounded by the British army. The Red Cross was formed in Europe in 1864, encouraging an organized method of rescuing the wounded from the various battlefields during the Crimean War.

The first electric ambulance was used in 1899 at the Michael Reese Hospital in Chicago; it was capable of traveling at a speed of up to 16 miles per hour. Neonatal ground transport started in the early 1900s with the use of horse-drawn carriages to transport premature infants to regional centers. French physician Martin Couney used such transports to display premature infants in London for public exhibits. British hospitals would not permit their infants to be used for exhibition, but they did not forbid others from being exhibited. Dr. Couney then decided to transport French infants across the English Channel by boat. The infants were transported in washbasins containing pillows and hot-water bottles to keep them warm and comfortable. By 1933, when Dr. Couney came to the United States with his exhibition, he had developed an ambulance for the transport of infants. One of his sources of neonates was the Chicago Premature Station. In 1948, an organized transport service was developed in New York City. The neonates were transported via a hand-carried aluminum incubator with hot-water bottles and a portable cylinder of oxygen (Chou & MacDonald, 1989). The average times were just over 2 hours for transport and 27 minutes for travel time, at a cost of $48.62. They experienced good outcomes, even with neonates who weighed less than 1,000 grams (Chou & MacDonald, 1989).

In the 1960s and 1970s, with regionalization of newborn intensive care becoming evident, the regional centers were developed to provide state-of-the-art care with well-trained staff and the highest technology and services available. The modern transport team evolved out of the need to take high-technology care to infants and transport infants to regional centers when the care they required was beyond the scope of the birth hospital. Such transports necessitated personnel who were skilled in caring for critically ill neonates.

NATIONAL STANDARDS AND GUIDELINES

Nationally recognized guidelines for Neonatal Transport have been established by both the American Academy of Pediatrics (AAP, 2000) and the National Association of Neonatal Nurses (NANN, 1998). Transport systems developed according to guidelines will be more responsive to the need for rapid access, will be better able to ensure delivery of high-quality care, and will function more safely and efficiently. The following topics are included in the guidelines:

- Administration
- Altitude physiology
- Communication and dispatch
- Equipment and medications
- Financial considerations
- Marketing

- Organization of neonatal interfacility transport service
- Outreach education
- Quality improvement
- Safety of the patient and team
- Team composition, selection, and training
- Transport database
- Vehicle selection

Professionals interested in forming a transport team, ensuring adherence to a basic national standard, developing team competencies, or establishing a sound quality improvement program will find these references a valuable resource.

TRANSPORT TEAM MODELS

Composition

Transport team composition varies from, depending on the number of transports per year, the acuity of the patient population, the medicolegal climate, and the availability of funding and personnel. Some hospitals with a low volume of transports commonly pull staff from the newborn unit when needed. Others may require a highly trained independent team to meet the transport needs. With the emphasis on cross-training and cost effectiveness, an increasing number of dedicated teams are also transporting pediatric, adult, or obstetric patients. The team must function as a unit regardless of team composition. Each team acknowledges the diversity of abilities, limitations, and scope of licensures for each individual who participates in the transport process.

Qualifications

Hospitals, infants, and families are best served by carefully selected of transport team members. Assessment of the applicants' suitability for the team might consider the following characteristics (NANN, 1998):

- Appreciation of public/community relations
- Critical thinking skills
- Educational and experiential background
- Leadership skills
- Proficient communication and interpersonal skills
- Technical and clinical competence

The best transport team members are skilled and creative at making critical decisions and being patient advocates. They are also diplomatic and effective communicators who realize their roles as ambassadors in the community and acknowledge the contribution of all participants in the transport process.

Team members must also be able to physically tolerate confined spaces, noise, motion, and vibration. Teams performing air transport often have weight requirements. The ideal team member is flexible enough to function professionally and effectively in any situation.

Orientation

The orientation of new transport team members varies according to the needs of each candidate. An individualized needs assessment tool helps determine the didactic and practical experiences helpful in preparing the potential team member for transporting intensely ill infants. The plan can be detailed enough to provide structure while flexible enough to enable revision as needed. Education and experience are combined most effectively in a one-on-one preceptor relationship. The preceptor uses fellow team members as resources in particular areas of skill, such as procedural or therapeutic communication skills. The program needs to be structured to encourage increasing independence, including building of rapport with current team members, and allowing for independent study time. After orientation, the new member should match his or her schedule with that of a veteran team member to aid in the completion of the role transition. Scheduled weekly evaluation with the preceptor and coordinator help ensure progress and address individual challenges or needs. Evaluations also give opportunities to commend and encourage unique skills that the new member may bring to the team. Content areas of orientation and competency need to include the following (NANN, 1998):

- Advanced airway management, including the skill of endotracheal intubation
- Artificial surfactant replacement therapy
- Assessment and stabilization of neonatal disorders and diseases
- Customer-oriented public relations
- Documentation of care and of process
- Equipment and monitoring
- Expectations of team member's participation in the work team
- Family-centered care
- Flight physiology
- Initiation of the transport process
- Interpretation of laboratory and diagnostic data
- Maternal health factors as they affect the neonate
- Medications/fluid management including: vasopressors, prostaglandins, and nitric oxide
- Medicolegal concerns
- Neonatal assessment
- Neonatal resuscitation program and or pediatric advanced life support course
- Patient and team safety
- Problem solving and triage
- Synchronized cardioversion
- Team performance improvement
- Therapeutic communication for handling crises
- Thermoregulation needle thoracotomy
- Transport policies and procedures
- Umbilical venous catheter placement

Continuing Education

Continuing education or a method of evaluating continued competence is a vital part of any transport program. Orientation and precepting should just be the beginning of a continuous education process for all transport team members. Continuing education helps to create a dynamic transport program that stimulates both personal and professional growth among team members and improves the quality of care that they deliver. Because transport team members often function in an environment of limited access to expert resources, they need to plan the time and funds to educate themselves to be as expert as possible for their work.

Team education days planned by the team members are essential for addressing learning needs, practicing skills, demonstrating competencies, and accomplishing required learning. Maintaining certification in neonatal resuscitation is nationally recognized and can be used as one check on competency for the team members. Specialty certifications can also be encouraged. By achieving certification, team members reinforce their knowledge base and attain recognition among their peers.

Competency checks of transport skill and knowledge can be creatively designed to provide bursts of fun and challenging learning. Checkpoints of learning should take place throughout the year. Accepted practice includes the demonstration of advanced skills such as endotracheal intubation, at least quarterly.

Team meetings where case reviews allow participants to gain an understanding of a variety of issues and to explore alternative methods of problem solving.

Attendance at national conferences benefits the team in many ways. In addition to supplying new knowledge, it provides a chance for the team to consider new ideas, view new equipment, establish resource contacts, and talk with transport experts.

Communication

To function effectively, transport team members must be expert communicators. Transport team members must speak clearly and concisely with the dispatch center, efficiently and respectfully with referral and receiving staff, and thoroughly with one another. Crisis communication skills with parents require yet another set of skills that are called upon quickly and adjust to each individual situation. Plans of care are based on the information that the transport team members bring and share with the receiving institution. Every aspect of the transport process depends completely on each individual's ability to communicate effectively.

Communication within the Team. Communication between team members is vital to the function and survival of a safe and effective transport program. Methods for sharing information on equipment readiness and repair, prescheduled transports, hospital memoranda, team meetings, and decisions are critical to daily operations. Voice mail, digital pagers, wireless communication systems, and email can all be used to keep the team apprised of transports in progress, changing needs, meeting reminders, and educational offerings.

Exercises and education in team building, personality profile identification, conflict resolution, and awareness of communication styles with coworkers are a valuable area of focus for continuing education. Interpersonal communication among members is complex. Respect for the diversity of one another's skills and appreciation of individual styles is necessary for teams to function well.

The Communication Center. A central dispatch center is required. The individual receiving the calls must be aware of team availability and obtain the initial information needed to mobilize the team using care to avoid "on-hold" waiting by referral staff who may need to continue to monitor and stabilize the infant. Experienced personnel—often a team member, the neonatologist, or neonatal fellow—complete the referral call to ensure stabilization of the infant until the team arrives. Some units choose to establish a designated hotline within the unit for direct access to neonatal experts by referral staff in the region. The opportunity for expert consultation and rapid team mobilization are the optimal goals for this portion of the transport process.

Communication of the Team with Others. Communication and rapport with the referral hospital can significantly affect patient outcome and the relationship between the referring and receiving hospitals. Each specializes in what they do most often; each wants a smooth transfer process; and each works for a good patient outcome. A climate of respect assures all parties that their input is valued and that the information they provide will be accepted. This respect must be genuine. Effective communication can be impaired when two people perceive the same information differently. In addition, time pressures caused by health care professionals' desire to resuscitate, stabilize, and transport sick infants as quickly as possible can limit their ability to send, receive, and validate information.

Transport team members are viewed as representatives of the care and quality of their institution. They must assume the responsibility of continually improving the quality of their communication skills and their interpersonal relationship skills.

Mobilization of the Team

The plan to mobilize the team must be devised in a manner that ensures the most efficient response time possible, usually 30 minutes or less. This time is measured from the time the referral hospital initiates the call to the time the team leaves the transport base. Information exchange, mobilization of team members, verification of vehicle availability, and ambulance loading of equipment and personnel all must take place within these 30 minutes. Each hospital must investigate its own challenges within this process. Documenting times and process problems are typically parts of a quality check performed by team members. Delays should be investigated. Extremely critical transports may require alterations in the usual mobilization process. Communication becomes critical as certain responsibilities are delegated and usual patterns are changed. Preplanning for challenging events is vital. The use of lights, sirens, and "hot" unloading (while helicopter blades are still in motion) require this type of preparation. The plan helps clarify what is acceptable to all parties and what is best for the patient.

MODES OF TRANSPORT

Transport teams throughout the country use various modes of transport. Most teams have access to both ground and/or air transport via helicopters and fixed wing planes (small propeller planes, small jet planes, and large commercial aircraft). The decision to use one mode of transport instead of another depends on the distance to be traveled, traffic and weather conditions, patient condition and diagnosis, crew and vehicle availability, and cost effectiveness. Each mode of transport is associated with unique advantages and disadvantages, making the best choice for each transport an important and at times complex decision. Each institution needs to have predetermined guidelines, policies, and lines of authority in order to prevent delays in response time related to the decision-making process.

Transport teams often use some means of ground transport if they are traveling within a 100-mile radius. Very little time is saved by flying within this range because of the arrangements that must be made for loading, unloading, and ground transport from the landing sites to and from the hospital.

Ambulance travel provides a more stable environment in which temperature is easily controlled, atmospheric pressure is not an issue, and space confinement is not drastic. This environment is more manageable, thus enabling the team to stop and perform any necessary procedures en route.

Helicopter transports have been most advantageous when used for transports for distances between 100 and 250 miles. Because helicopters can typically land close to the hospital, time is not lost on ground transport at each end of the flight.

The obvious advantage of helicopter transport is the speed of travel. Disadvantages of helicopter travel include the cost, noise level, inability to control temperature, changes in vibration and pressure, and severe space restrictions. Any transport over a distance of 250 miles usually requires some type of fixed-wing aircraft. The benefits of transport using fixed-wing aircraft are a long travel range. A major disadvantage is the additional time required to make arrangements, which include the need for ground transport to or from the institutions at the beginning and end of the trip.

Traffic and weather conditions must be taken into consideration when a transport is planned. Traffic conditions have an obvious influence on the amount of travel. Even though a referral hospital may be only 20 miles from the receiving hospital, a quick decision to transport by helicopter is justified to overcome obstacles to rapid ground transport. In other circumstances, ground transport is the best mode for a 200-mile trip if there are extreme weather conditions in the area. A decision to fly in inclement weather is the responsibility of the pilot. The safety of the team and well-being of the patient are serious considerations. Postponement of the transport is a viable option during these circumstances until it is considered safe for both the infant and the transport team to travel.

A patient's diagnosis or condition must be considered before a preferred mode of transport is chosen. When the referral call is initiated, vital information relating to the patient's condition is necessary. Phone consultation with a neonatal physician can facilitate appropriate stabilization and medical management while the transport team is en route. Considering the possible negative effects different modes of transport may have on the patient may alter an initial decision.

Crew and vehicle availability can affect the decision-making process. All transport vehicles have downtime for maintenance, repair, and inspection. In addition, the Federal Aviation Administration (FAA) has specific guidelines for flight hours for pilots in a given period of time. All aircraft have restrictions on the number of passengers permitted per flight. All such guidelines ensure safe transport practice and may limit the possible transport modes available at any given time.

At a time when cost containment is considered, expenditures generated by various modes of transport have an impact on the decision-making process. Ground transportation is typically less costly than air transport.

To prevent inconsistent decision-making and delayed response times, hospital policies and guidelines need to be established in advance. Then the complex decision of choosing the best mode of transport is less likely to cause negative outcomes.

EQUIPMENT

Standard

Standard neonatal transport equipment needs to include—but is not limited to—the transport incubator, monitoring equipment with the capability to monitor ECG, respirations, temperature, oxygen saturation, and invasive and non-invasive blood pressures, portable suction, compressed air and oxygen, air and oxygen blender box, neonatal ventilator, and medication infusion pumps (Figure 2-3). Some neonatal teams now use end-tidal CO_2 and handheld arterial blood gas analyzers to monitor the respiratory status of their intubated patients. Stethoscopes, cellular/digital phones, and a Polaroid® or digital camera round out the standard transport medical equipment.

Consideration toward conservation of both battery power and compressed gases takes on a new importance, as does AC/DC conversion capability. All equipment needs to be able to operate on battery power for twice the anticipated transport

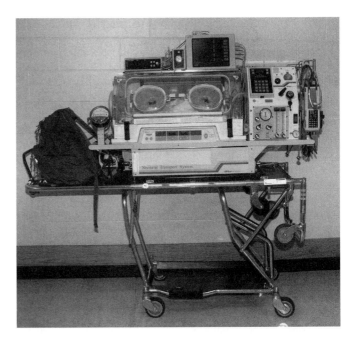

FIGURE **2-3**
Incubator. Equipment from Children's Hospital Medical Center; Cincinnati, OH. Photograph courtesy of T.L. Marcus.

time. Even then, teams needs to carry manual back-ups, in preparation for the unexpected.

Transport equipment should be chosen for portability, reliability, and expandability. This equipment must also be durable enough to function properly in adverse environmental conditions, such as motion, temperature, vibration, and atmospheric pressure changes. Air transports, narrow doorways, and small elevators necessitate consideration of weight and overall physical dimensions of transport equipment.

The clinical engineering department can help with decisions on equipment, especially on compatibility and the securing of equipment. Equipment with built-in attachments for securing, Velcro, tie-down straps, and individually designed securing measures help ensure the safety of both the patient and the team in the event of a sudden stop or accident. The clinical engineering department should test and regularly perform preventative maintenance on all equipment. They are also qualified to determine whether replacement parts are readily available and whether warranty and maintenance contracts are adequate.

Purchasing original and/or replacement durable medical equipment requires forethought. Advice from established teams or persons familiar with new equipment available on the market can prove invaluable. With budgetary constraints placed upon health care facilities, equipment priorities must be set and cost-benefit analysis determined. When selecting specific equipment, the ability to upgrade software and components can decrease the need to purchase new equipment at a later date.

Planning to replace the most expensive equipment every five to ten years can reduce unexpected emergency purchases. Once the proper equipment has been acquired, team members are responsible for maintaining the entire transport unit and associated equipment in a state of readiness. At the beginning of each shift and after the completion of each transport, all equipment should be checked for proper functioning, adequate battery power, and proper security to the incubator. Many teams have discovered that a checklist is the best way to ensure that each member takes responsibility for preparation and upkeep. In addition, appointing one member of the team to be responsible for handling equipment repair, concerns, and follow-up is an effective means of problem solving.

Transport Nitric Oxide

For many Level III nurseries, Inhaled Nitric Oxide (INO) has become a standard of care for treating persistent pulmonary hypertension of the newborn (PPHN). INO is a selective pulmonary vasodilator that, unlike many intravenous vasodilators, does not dilate the systemic vasculature system. If INO is abruptly discontinued, it can cause a severe rebound hypoxemia (AAP, 2000). Therefore the need to transfer neonatal patients with INO therapy has arisen. To answer this need, some neonatal transport teams have begun to offer portable INO therapy as an additional service.

Although INO equipment has become fairly standardized for in-hospital use, several variables must be considered when using INO therapy for interfacility transport. In the transport environment, the weight of transport equipment is of paramount importance. The addition of an INO system to an incubator can increase the total lifting weight by about 22 kilograms for loading into or out of a transport vehicle. This increase in weight may require additional personnel for safe lifting and loading procedure during the transport. The stretchers that support the incubator and other transport equipment need to be safety rated to carry this added weight. The INO unit must be mounted so as not to separate from the incubator in the event of an accident. For teams that transport by either plane or helicopter, the physical dimensions of the INO unit must be considered with regard to loading through aircraft doors and the interior dimensions of the flight cabin itself. Test fitting of the INO equipment into all modes of transport vehicles used by the team can identify the mounting modifications that must be made before a patient transport.

Another important consideration is the duration of the nitric oxide tanks. Care must be taken to determine that enough tanks are brought along to last at least twice the anticipated time of transport. These tanks should also be secured according to both the Department of Transportation (DOT) and the Federal Aviation Administration (FAA) standards. Material Safety and Data Sheets (MSDS) should be carried with the nitric oxide tanks. The providers of transport aircraft may also need to update their hazardous materials program to include inhaled nitric oxide.

Training for team members should include the physiologic effects of INO therapy, calibration and set-up of all nitric oxide equipment, and yearly competency testing to maintain proficiency in transporting INO therapy patients. One proposed method for maintaining familiarity with the equipment and set-up is to develop and annually review an INO training video. The medical director for the transport team should be consulted to establish standing order protocols for transporting patients on nitric oxide. In addition, having at least one transport team member as a resource person for INO therapy can enhance team training and equipment maintenance.

SUPPLIES

To be adequately prepared, the transport team must determine which supplies are needed to care for their particular patient

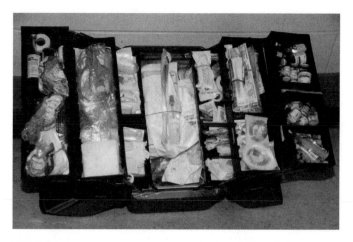

FIGURE **2-4**
Transport supply box. Equipment from Children's Hospital Medical Center; Cincinnati, OH. Photograph courtesy of T.L. Marcus.

population. At minimum, transport teams should be equipped with supplies for oxygen delivery, oxygen and air blenders, ventilation, airway maintenance, resuscitation, blood sampling, intravenous insertion, administration or narcotics or sedatives, chest tube and umbilical line placement, nutrition and fluid support, gastric decompression, wound dressing, and thermoregulation. Unusual diagnoses or circumstances may require items that must be readily available and added at the time of transport. These may include chest tube drainage supplies and Nitric Oxide with a Nitric Oxide delivery system. Additional completely stocked supply bags/boxes prevent delays in the event of closely spaced transport calls. Each supply bag/box needs to be stocked with the same supplies and organized in exactly the same manner so as to quickly retrieve supplies as needed. A checklist serves to organize and ensure complete supplies. A small disposable lock can be used to secure the container and complete set of contents. Figure 2-4 is an example of a supply box used by a transport team in the Midwest.

TRANSPORT AMBULANCES

An ambulance that is readily available and appropriately stocked for neonatal transports is needed to supplement the clinical expertise provided by the transport team. This can be accomplished in a variety of ways. Each team should examine their individual needs and determine the optimal arrangement for their service.

Often the simplest arrangement is to contact with an outside vendor of ambulance services in the area. In this case, the ambulance company provides the vehicle and a crew for driving and lifting, and the transport team provides the patient care and any needed specialized equipment. The ambulance company maintains any required licensing and bears the cost of operating the vehicle and the crew. The ambulance vendor may bill the patient for their costs directly, or they may bill the hospital. Advantages of the this type of an arrangement includes minimizing team operational expenses to personnel and equipment costs as well as leaving the administrative details of the ambulance operation to the outside vendor. The primary disadvantage is lack of control over ambulance operations and crew. Response times for the ambulance crew to meet the transport team and begin the transport vary widely and can impact service delivery. Ambulance drivers may vary from transport to transport and knowledge of referral hospital locations may be lacking especially if the team responds to locations outside the local hospital area.

Another alternative is ambulances owned and operated by the hospital. Because of maintenance requirements and unplanned vehicle down time, a minimum of two ambulances is typically necessary to maintain continuous service. Ambulances may be purchased specifically for the use of the transport team or may be part of a larger fleet used for pediatric and adult transports.

Many states require ambulance services obtain a license to operate. This process is primarily administrative and requires application and fee submission as well as an annual or semiannual renewal process. An inspection is usually required to ensure that mandated equipment is available and that the necessary paperwork is maintained. State requirements vary widely. Some states have specific licensure for neonatal transport units, and some license all ambulances with the same process and equipment requirements. Additionally, some states require a license to operate in their state even if the receiving hospital is not in that state. This should be a consideration for teams that transport neonates from referral hospitals in states other than their own. Advantages of ambulances owned and operated by the hospital include complete control over all aspects of the transport service, improved response times, customization of the vehicle, and commitment of personnel. Significant reduction in the mobilization time for the team, which yields a high degree of customer satisfaction from referral physicians and hospitals, is possible. The vehicle can be customized to include specialized cabinetry configurations, stretcher positions, oxygen and compressed air outlets, electrical outlets, and crew seating configurations that may be helpful for neonatal transports and that are not standard on most ambulances. Consistent personnel can be used for ambulance operations. Drivers can assist the patient care team with the equipment and basic aspects of care. Use of consistent personnel helps with efficiency and quality of care.

Disadvantages of hospital ambulances include cost and management of licensing and administrative responsibilities. Although the ambulance purchase price may seem expensive when first considering this option, ongoing personnel and operational expenses are the major disadvantage of this option. Systems must be put into place to ensure readiness of the vehicle and equipment and productivity of ambulance personnel during nontransport time. State licensing, if required, involves significant work in the beginning and ongoing attention annually. Initial licensing may take six months to a year to implement regulated processes and complete applications and inspections.

Other options that combine the aforementioned options may also be available. Each team should examine their service needs, transport volumes, and available resources to determine an appropriate ambulance option for their setting.

ROLE OF TRANSPORT PERSONNEL

The roles of the numerous types of transport personnel vary tremendously from state to state. The way in which a team member practices may depend on the individual's knowledge base, level of formal education, and level of experience and on state regulations, hospital policies, predetermined job descriptions, and team composition. Ideally, all transport personnel would be capable of providing holistic care for the neonate.

However, legal constraints prevent some transport personnel from independently providing all of the care that may be needed. Consequently, it is imperative that the transport members function as a team wherein each member provides quality care within the legal constraints designated by the position that he or she holds. All team members should be informed about the job descriptions for each type of health professional that could potentially serve on the transport team.

Medical Director

The medical director should be a specialist in the appropriate medical discipline. Teams that transport both neonatal and pediatric patients usually require codirectors or associate directors from neonatology and critical care or emergency medicine. These physicians are responsible for designing team training programs, developing or approving all transport team policies and procedures, reviewing all cases, and acting as liaison to other medical care providers.

Program Director

The program director is responsible for leadership in the day-to-day management, administration, budget development, and organization of the team. The director acts as a mentor to staff, oversees transport data collection, equipment selection and licensing and acts a team liaison to the medical director and hospital administration.

Medical Control Physician

A designated medical control physician (MCP) for an individual transport is responsible for immediate team composition and directing the clinical care provided by the team at the referral hospital and during transport. When a physician accompanies the team on a transport, that physician is the MCP. When a physician does not accompany the team, the MCP is available to the team via radio and/or cellular phone.

Transport Registered Nurse

The transport nurse is an experienced nurse with specific training in neonatal and pediatric critical care transport. In some cases, a neonatal nurse practitioner/advanced practice nurse may fill this role. The transport nurse is responsible for coordinating stabilization and management of the patient's care during transport. The transport nurse has the ultimate responsibility for the initial assessment and documentation of the patient's entire transport process. Ideally the nurse is cross-trained in respiratory therapy skills.

Transport Respiratory Therapist

The transport respiratory therapist is an experienced clinician with specific training in neonatal and pediatric critical care transport. The transport respiratory therapist provides ongoing assessment, airway stabilization, pulmonary care, and ventilator management. Ideally, the respiratory therapist is cross-trained in nursing skills.

Transport Technician

The transport technician is an experienced emergency medical technician or paramedic who has specific training in neonatal and pediatric critical care transport and interfacility transfer. The transport technician is responsible for maintaining and conserving the transport ambulances and assisting the team with the stabilization and preparation of the patient for transport. Transport technicians may augment staffing in the emergency department or other areas of the hospital when they are not actively engaged in transport duties.

SAFETY ISSUES

The following safety issues (AAP, 1999) should be of primary importance throughout the transport process. Safety policies, procedures, training, and monitoring must be ongoing and updated to ensure a high level of safety awareness among all team members. Teams may choose to appoint their own safety officers to provide accountability for this critical area. Securing or restraining of the patient, parent, team members, and equipment is a critical basic of personal safety. Considerations such as adequate lighting in the mobile environment cannot be taken for granted. Team familiarity with safety features of vehicles and training for "mock accidents" are also important in the mobile care environment. In dangerous weather, the safety of the team and infant must be a top priority. Development of disaster-planning guidelines will help the team to address what to do in the event of a transport vehicle crash, all types of inclement weather, and violence/social unrest in the city or region that the team services. Equipment and vehicles must meet safety standards and be kept safe and operational through regularly scheduled maintenance. Vehicles and aircraft must also meet guidelines set by the FAA and the United States Department of Transportation. Teams performing air transports should also follow guidelines established by the Association of Air Services and professional specialty organizations. Fitness and crew fatigue are issues that individual teams need to address through scheduling, policy, or other creative solutions.

Keeping current with the new safety guidelines and equipment and reviewing safety standards makes the team member perhaps the most valued resource for a smooth and safe patient transport. Training and use of body mechanics, hearing protection, and universal blood and body fluid precautions keep each team member safer. Attention to safety of the patient environment—including equipment, vehicle, and travel conditions—helps ensure patient safety.

THE TRANSPORT PROCESS

Assessment

The assessment of a neonate begins with the gathering of subjective data from referral hospital staff via telephone before transport. The amount of helpful information varies from basic to comprehensive, depending on the staff of the referral hospital. Objective assessment begins when the team arrives and does a system-by-system, head-to-toe examination. Cardiovascular assessment includes color; perfusion; capillary refill; quality of peripheral pulses; liver boundaries; precordial activity; and heart sounds, rate, and rhythm. Respiratory assessment includes color; rate; rhythm; use of accessory muscles; presence of grunting, retracting, flaring of nares, presence and quality of breath sounds; air exchange; and verification of airway patency. Neurologic assessment includes muscle tone, reactivity to stimuli, reflexes, fontanelles, quality of cry, and level of comfort at rest. Gastrointestinal and genitourinary assessment includes abdomen, genitalia, and history and specifics of meconium and urine output. Head-to-toe assessment includes gestational age, body and bone structure, nutritional status, skin, extremities, and pain assessment.

The treatment plan depends on the abnormalities found and the degree of neonatal compromise. Laboratory and radiographic data are helpful adjuncts to care in assessing the degree to which the neonate is compromised. Routine laboratory values include complete blood count (CBC) with differential blood count; blood cultures, if there is a setup for sepsis; blood glucose; and an arterial or capillary blood gas measurement. Routine radiographs include an anteroposterior (AP) view of the chest and abdomen. Data from lateral views may also be necessary. Physical assessment and laboratory and radiology results are valuable in establishing a database for determination of future treatment decisions.

Planning

Planning is vital to successful transport. Pretransport planning must consider desired optimal patient outcomes. Transport care can be at the beginning of any of the neonatal critical path or care maps that are developed to direct and monitor care. It includes not only patient and family needs but also logistics, communications, equipment, and vehicles.

The plan of care for the patient and family must be individualized and appropriate for the setting, distance from the regional center, and the mode of transport. Planning is a dynamic process that changes moment to moment on the basis of the patient's response. Protocols can serve as a resource from which to begin.

Implementation

If resuscitation is required, it is accomplished as quickly as possible. The main objectives of resuscitative efforts are to verify and maintain a patent airway, to provide effective oxygenation and ventilation, and to ensure that circulation is adequate to meet metabolic demands. Necessary neonatal resuscitation must begin immediately, even before Apgar scores are determined. Those scores and other evaluation measures were originally designed to assess the success of extrauterine adaptation with full-term babies. The American Heart Association (AHA) and AAP have an established Neonatal Resuscitation Program (NRP) and have made it available to health care workers for guidance in achieving these objectives (Kattwinkel, 2000). The program focuses on resuscitation in the delivery room; the same principles can be applied to resuscitation during the transport process. There is also an AAP program for Pediatric Advanced Life Support (PALS) that focuses on the more complex issues that a transport team may face, such as line placement, airway adjuncts, and synchronized cardioversion for the infant who is compromised as a result of supraventricular tachycardia. The course provides valuable, extensive resuscitation information (www.AAP.org). Many institutions use the NRP program in addition to training their personnel according to the S.T.A.B.L.E.® Program, developed by Kristine A. Karlsen. This program represents an acronym that stands for: Sugar, Temperature, Artificial/Assisted Breathing, Blood Pressure, Lab Work, and Emotional Support (Karlsen, 2001). This program is described in detail under the section "Outreach Education."

The process of stabilization is important and often determines the degree of success of the transition to extrauterine life and transport. Time spent seeking stabilization is vital to ensure optimal care for the neonate during the transport process. The team minimizes the time spent at the referral hospital in the stabilization process. Ideally, appropriate stabilization has occurred before the team arrives. The team completes procedures and provides care to prevent complications during the transport process to achieve the highest level of stability for each infant. The process of stabilization includes the following:

- Sugar/glucose levels—assessed, supported
- Temperature—assessed, supported
- Airway—assessed, secured, supported
- Respiratory effort—assessed, assisted/supported
- Ventilation—assessed, assisted/supported
- Oxygenation—assessed, facilitated
- Blood pressure/circulation—assessed, supported
- Acidosis—assessed, corrected
- Medications—need assessed, administered
- Nasogastric or orogastric tubes—need assessed, placed
- All other special interventions—need assessed, completed

Stabilization is accomplished according to the patient's need. Measures taken before transport—such as intubation, umbilical line or chest tube placement—are determined by how well the patient is adapting, the trend of the disease process, patient's age, time, distance, and mode of transport. Procedures are better performed in a hospital than in an ambulance at the side of the road or in a helicopter descended for an emergency landing in a cornfield. Care should be modified according to the patient's condition and the type of transport vehicle. Developing an optimally supportive environment during transport as may help decrease the stress of the transport process. Application of developmental care concepts to the transport process often helps to decrease the negative stimulation during this stressful transition. This care includes use of appropriate positioning, water mattresses, ear protection, pacifiers, Snuggle-Ups® (Children's Medical Ventures, Norwell, MA), minimal stimulation precautions, and, if necessary, sedation or analgesia. During the transport process, all aspects of care require constant monitoring, assessment and support, correction, intervention, and evaluation.

Patient Response to the Transport Process

The transport team generally arrives on the scene early in a neonate's hospital course and often during the most critical hours of his or her life. This time provides the transport team with the opportunity to reduce patient complications and improve the outcome of neonatal patients requiring transfer.

Conditions during transport are seldom ideal. Each patient needs to be constantly and carefully monitored for his or her unique response to stabilization and transport and treated accordingly. In addition to providing initial stabilization and performing complex procedures, the transport team must be proficient at the recognition and management of neonatal stress and pain. Minimizing sensory input for the neonate will decrease stress, reduce energy consumption, and result in improvement in oxygenation, respiration and heart rate (NANN, 2000). Use of developmental care techniques such as nesting or containment during procedures will help provide boundaries for the neonate to help him or her remain calm and comfortable. Positioning the neonate with his or her arms and legs centrally flexed or in a prone position with the hand to mouth during transport provides comfort and minimizes stress to the neonate (NANN, 2000).

The team needs to perform an appropriate pain assessment and provide safe pain management consistent with the total treatment plan. A neonatal pain assessment should be completed during the initial assessment. Intervention and reassessment should be performed throughout the transport and again on admission to the new nursery. The Neonatal Infant Pain Scale (NIPS) is a behavioral scale that can be used on both premature and term neonates (Lawrence et al, 1993).

Transition Into the Neonatal Intensive Care Unit

No transport can be considered complete until the infant is settled into a new bed at the receiving hospital and the admitting team of health care professionals has received a complete written and verbal report. To ensure a smooth transition, the admitting team must have a recent report of the infant's status and a reasonable estimated time of arrival. This type of communication can best be facilitated by the use of a mobile phone or two-way radio en route. However, if verbal contact cannot be established en route, the team needs to call the receiving hospital just before their departure from the referral hospital and provide the admitting team with the necessary information.

Upon arrival at the receiving hospital, the transport team should establish that the bed has been prewarmed and that all of the necessary equipment and supplies are available. Once it has been determined that the admitting team is adequately prepared for the arrival of the new infant, transport team members should prepare for the transfer of the infant from the incubator to the bed provided by the unit. Admitting nurses often prefer to weigh the infant before transferring him or her into the new bed. The transport team knows best whether the infant is stable enough to be weighed first. Consequently, the transport team members are responsible for making decisions about the most effective way to transfer the infant.

Once the decisions have been made and the infant and the equipment have been transferred to the new bed, the admitting team should take responsibility for getting the infant attached to all of the necessary equipment. Unless the infant needs immediate intervention, the transport team must begin a thorough, chronologic history of both the mother's pregnancy and the infant's hospital course. Any additional insights that the transport team has noted should be shared. In addition, a social history should be reported. It is important for the admitting team to know whether the mother is planning to breastfeed, whether the family has a social support network, or whether visitors can be expected. Once the infant has been settled and stabilized, the report has been given, and questions have been answered, the transport team members may leave the bedside to restock their equipment and complete their charting. Not until all written reports are completed and placed in the chart can the transition be considered complete. It is helpful to the mother and referral hospital staff for a call to be placed to the mother and nursery to inform them of how the infant tolerated the transport, his or her current status, and plans for care and to answer any last-minute questions.

Documentation

Thorough and accurate documentation is a critical form of communication in the transport process as well as a medicolegal necessity and essential quality improvement tool. The documentation process needs to begin as soon as contact has been made between the referral and the receiving institution. The infant's status, care, and response to that care must be thoroughly and accurately documented. The names of all the personnel involved in the care, stabilization, and transport of the infant must be noted. The mode of transport also must be noted.

The forms used to record the transport process vary from institution to institution. Each transport team needs to create its own checklists and flowsheets that specifically meet its needs. As hospital policies, patient population, and transport styles vary, the forms used to document the process also vary. Flowsheets are designed to include valuable information regarding prenatal care and condition, delivery and resuscitation efforts, team interventions and infant response, vital sign measurements, ventilator settings, comfort and developmental interventions, parent interactions with the infant, and consent for transport. Physician orders, history, and physical and transport summary allow the receiving institution to develop a clear picture of the events that transpired before the infant's arrival. All forms of documentation used for the transport process become a legal part of the infant's chart. Ideally, the team can collaborate so that only one document is used for the entire process. As computerized documentation becomes standard, teams will look to laptop programs that are able to interface with institutional systems.

The team should also maintain appropriate documentation when alternative types of transports are performed or when assistance within the hospital setting is rendered. Transport teams may find that a separate flowsheet for reverse transports or test runs is more efficient and practical. This form is best if made in triplicate so that the receiving hospital, the referral hospital, and the transport team each have copies. If no form is designated for documenting a specific transport function, team members must be aware of proper charting on the hospital's standard flowsheets. All transport functions must be documented thoroughly and accurately on an appropriate form that is a legal part of the chart.

Any information or action undocumented in the infant's chart is not considered in the legal arena. Regardless of the number of eyewitnesses available, if an uncharted action is considered not to have been done. Consequently, the legal ramifications of incomplete or inaccurate documentation are great. With the rise in the number of lawsuits being filed against health care professionals, meticulous documentation has become a medicolegal necessity. Documentation is also a vital part of any quality improvement program. Throughout the entire transport process, beginning with the initial phone contact made by the referral hospital until the infant has been smoothly transferred and admitted to the receiving institution, the transport team must meticulously consider time. Recording the time of initial referral, team mobilization and arrival at the referral institution and return to the receiving institution is very important. Reliable recordkeeping to maintain accurate transport statistics is an essential part of any quality improvement program.

To ensure documentation accuracy for both legal and quality assurance purposes, charting must be completed during and immediately after each transport. Without an appropriate documentation format established for every transport function, thorough and accurate recordkeeping may be compromised. Without a permanent, written account of the entire transport process and the quality of patient care, the legal security of the health care professionals and the maintenance of a quality transport program may be jeopardized.

IMPACT OF THE TRANSPORT PROCESS

Referral Hospital Staff

The referral hospital staff at times is forewarned of an impending delivery of a high-risk neonate who requires care beyond the scope provided by the referral hospital. When this is the case, a mother may be transported to a Level III care center, or arrangements may be made for a neonatal transport team to attend the delivery or to arrive shortly thereafter. Unexpected pregnancy outcomes, however, can be stressful events for the staff in the referral hospital nursery. The nursery nurses are called upon to meet the challenge of providing one-to-one nursing care for the intense stabilization period for a compromised neonate while maintaining care for the remaining patients in the nursery. This staffing pattern is usually not planned for in routine staffing numbers, and colleagues must pick up additional nursing assignments as well as help care for compromised neonates. The regional center's physician may request, by phone or in person, for a nurse to perform procedures that are infrequently experienced but are related to the care of the critically ill neonate, which add stress to an already stressful situation.

The neonate who initially does not meet transport criteria at birth but becomes progressively ill causes another stressful situation for the referral hospital because the amount of time for which the nurses at the referral hospital are responsible for the neonate is unpredictable. The attending physician may not be present or available for continual care demands. The nursing staff must carefully monitor the status of the compromised neonate and report changes as necessary. In an emergency, nursery nurses may have to call in physicians who do not specialize in neonatology to intubate a baby or aspirate a tension pneumothorax.

The referral staff needs to look upon these experiences as opportunities for growth and development in the area of intense neonatal care. From these experiences, protocols may be developed to guide staff through the next similar scenario. Different circumstances may prove to be opportunities to request outreach education from the regional center with regard to a certain problem or diagnosis that would help prepare staff for the care of the next critically ill neonate delivered in the referral hospital.

The referral hospital staff acts as a liaison to communicate with both the transport team and the family. It is ideal to assign one individual to work with and support the family during this dynamic time. Communication with the family, especially the mother, is especially important. The referral hospital staff and the transport team should collaborate closely regarding care and progress of the neonate before and after the time of admission to the regional center. The referral staff needs to assist the mother in the beginning of her grief work over the loss of the "perfect child" by letting her know that her feelings of sadness and depression are normal for her situation. Nursing care for the mother needs to also focus on elevating self-esteem, helping her to fully understand the situation to the best of her ability, providing strategies for dealing with other family members and friends, and understanding the myriad of information and new technology to which she has been and will be exposed during her child's stay in the neonatal intensive care unit.

Family

Because they will care for the neonate after discharge from the regional center, the involved family members must not be left out of the plan of care when an infant must be transported. In some cases the need for transport is planned, but in most cases it is unplanned and can be very stressful for the affected family.

Parents are often either in crisis or in a stage of grief over the loss of the perfect child at the time they are informed that their infant needs to be transported. Consequently, they may not remember what was said to them during the time of explanation about prognosis and impending transport. To assist in developing a therapeutic communication style with the parents, the team can introduce themselves and begin the questioning portion of interaction with the parents by congratulating them and asking whether they have chosen a name for their infant. This communication style lets the parents know that the infant is being considered as a special individual. The stress of the event can also prevent the parents from grasping the details of the medical diagnosis and plan of care for the infant at the birth hospital and the regional center. Emphasizing the diagnoses and plan of care more than one time is therefore necessary.

A preprinted parent information packet can help educate parents about diagnoses and the regional center's policies and procedures. The packet can also include simple maps, telephone numbers, lists of medical and nursing terminology, information on breastfeeding, and booklets on the care of the infant. Regional centers may also have videotapes for the parents to view the environment in which the infant will receive care. The informational needs of the parents at the time of transport are tremendous. If the infant will be transported by air, needs may center on the patient's condition, why the patient needs to be flown, where the patient will be admitted, and whether they can see the patient before the flight. Other informational needs include mode of travel, length of time of transport, care during transport, who can accompany the transport, regional center visiting and phoning policies, names of individuals caring for the patient, type of care to be rendered, costs involved, insurance coverage, directions to reach the center, and accommodations for parents.

Although all parents respond in unique ways, each of them considers transport a significant life event. Nurses must be nonjudgmental when a parent reacts dramatically to what the nurse may see as a minor problem. Parents do not have the experience that health care professionals have in the care of the compromised neonate.

Visiting the mother's room so that the parents can see and touch the infant must be a routine practice. This may be the first time—and perhaps the last time—that the parents and the family see the infant alive. When compromised infants are born, they are quickly whisked away from the parents at the delivery room table for resuscitation. The parents remember their child's quick removal from them and their inability to begin bonding. Seeing the infant—whom they could only imagine until birth—assists the parents with closure of the developmental tasks of pregnancy. Leaving an instant-developing photograph of the infant with the parents is an added courtesy; it can become a keepsake for the parents until they can actually see their infant at the regional center.

If the infant has any abnormalities, they need to be pointed out to the parents, because the defects are usually not as severe as the parents had imagined them to be during pregnancy or at the time of delivery. Positive features can also be pointed out at this time to encourage the parents to look at the whole infant, as opposed to only his or her defects.

The parents' response to this unexpected outcome of pregnancy depends on the context of the other events going on in their lives and the effectiveness of their coping strategies. Parents need to be encouraged to call and visit—with their other children if possible—as often as they can. They also need to be involved in care as is feasible. Breastfeeding can be encouraged if a mother has expressed an interest in providing milk for her infant. Mothers can be given specific information on pumping and storing breast milk. This information gives the mother something to do for her infant during this time, when she may feel the loss of her maternal caretaking role. The parents must be encouraged to seek as much support for their families as they need and should be informed of the support services at the regional center. Parents and family should be advised of the stress associated with these events and encouraged to ask questions and to ask for help as needed. No family should be expected to handle this crisis situation on their own. Working with families is in some cases the most difficult part of the transport. Concerns over the patient and the limited resources of battery, oxygen, and air prevail as the team works to support and inform the family of the current status and plans for care.

Post-transport Information Exchange

After the transport is completed and care is transferred to the receiving team of health care workers, it is good practice and professional courtesy to phone the birth hospital. This call is helpful to the referral hospital staff, who work with the mother and family left behind after the transport. These mothers and families are often in crisis or in a stage of grief or shock at the time of transport and are eager for information. The referral hospital staff, pediatrician, and obstetrician need as much information as possible to assist in facilitating communication between the referring and the receiving hospitals.

Staff at the birth hospital needs to encourage parents to call the regional center as often as needed. As information concerning condition and treatment is relayed to the birth hospital and the parents, the birth hospital staff can help the parents better understand the care and condition of the neonate and help establish community resources for the family. Compliance with recent federal restrictions through the Health Information Protection Act (HIPA) may limit information exchange with the referral hospital after the initial contact and transfer.

Multidisciplinary mortality and morbidity conferences can be scheduled on a regular basis between referral hospitals and the regional center to facilitate information exchange and learning. Outreach education can also be a means of development and growth in optimizing the care for the compromised infant.

ALTERNATIVE TYPES OF TRANSPORT

The main focus of this portion of the chapter is incoming neonatal transport. The emphasis on this particular type of transport is appropriate because stabilizing and transporting critically ill neonates remains a priority of transport teams across the country. However, the skills and expertise of the transport team members may be called upon for transporting patients of any age within medical care systems and to any destination, both regional and international.

International Transports

International transports provide one of the greatest challenges for a transport team. Planning must begin as soon as possible in order to ensure that all the logistic details are meticulously arranged. Finances must be arranged; airline or aircraft scheduled; visas or passports updated; an accepting institution and physician located; ground transport arrangements made both for departure and arrival.

Commercial airlines need to know the type, voltage, and amperage of all carry-on equipment. There may be limitations on when the equipment may be used. If supplemental oxygen is needed or is on standby, a physician's order is required, and the order must be placed with the airline as far in advance as possible. Airlines cannot provide heat or humidification for needed oxygen and may limit the amount delivered to the patient. If medications or special formula is required for the patient, the customs department may require specific documentation. The airline may require a written physician's statement regarding patient stability for the transport. A restraint system appropriate for the patient's age and size must meet the guidelines of the airline.

Supplies must be packed and arranged to be as accessible as possible. If a team is staying at the destination, lodging must be arranged. Currency must be exchanged. The need for translators must be considered, and culture-specific customs should be followed. Transports across time zones necessitate special attention to times and dates involved. Name and telephone numbers for contact personnel at the destination institution and the referral institution must be readily available.

A care conference should be arranged as soon as the transport is approved. At this time, the primary nurse, patient and family members can meet the transport members who will be involved in the transport, and together they can plan specifics for care, diversions, and developmentally appropriate activities. The well-being and safety of the patient, the team, and the family is of foremost importance as they travel. Careful planning is the key to success.

Back/Reverse Transports

When the demand for beds in the NICU in the local regional center exceeds availability, the results are overcrowding and the diversion of infants to Level III centers, farther from the delivery site. Therefore the return of convalescing infants to their community hospital—that is, back/reverse transport—has multiple benefits.

Back transports strengthen the referral system in the region by promoting communication and mutual trust among hospitals. Because the capabilities of Level I and II hospitals vary, it is important to learn each nursery's capabilities and limitations. The Level III transport team can ascertain this information during their transport calls. The Level III nursery can match the appropriate Level I or II nursery to the infant's continuing care needs when this information is available (Hauth & Merenstein, 1997). Care needs to be taken to determine follow-up availability of subspecialty services before the reverse transport is planned. These follow-up services include management of peripherally inserted central venous catheters, total parenteral nutrition administration, occupational therapy, opthalmology for eye exams for retinopathy of prematurity, head ultrasound follow-up, and hearing screening.

An efficient back transport program helps eliminate an acute shortage of NICU beds. Planning ahead for an infant's reverse transport to the community hospital optimizes the management of NICU beds during a shortage. The back transport of infants also promotes the sharing of fiscal responsibility within the region. *Per diem* costs are higher in the NICU than in the Level I or II nursery, and the occupancy of critical care beds by convalescing infants is not an effective use of NICU resources. Transferring convalescing infants improves the efficacy of use of Level I and II beds and provides the receiving hospital with a financial benefit of additional patient days.

The staff of the community hospital is able to maintain its expertise and skills by caring for convalescing infants. The result is an increase in pride and an investment in accountability in the care of these infants. In the less hectic environment of the nursery, the staff can focus on teaching the family how to care for the infant. Keeping the infant closer to the family allows for regular visits and greater involvement in the infant's care. The local physician can become involved with both infant and family sooner, which facilitates the transfer of trust from the Level III center to the local community hospital.

A successful back transport program depends on the involvement of personnel in both the transferring and receiving hospitals and the preparation of the family. A state's public health code and the receiving hospital's infection control policy must be understood before planning the back transfer. If the hospital has an isolation protocol that mandates the isolation of all patients coming in from the outside or other hospitals, the family should be informed of the policy, to alleviate last-minute surprises before the transport.

The financial issues surrounding back transport need to be clear before the transport is arranged. Parents may refuse a transfer if they are unable to pay or if the third-party payer is unwilling to reimburse them for the transport.

The physician and advanced practice nurses in the Level III center are responsible for defining the medical criteria for transfer and communicating the infant's care plan to the community physician. The community physician must agree to accept the infant and provide the medical supervision required. The physician at the Level III center provides the community physician with ongoing support and communication.

The NICU nursing staff has a major responsibility in the success of the program; they can identify infants who are ready for transfer. The Level III center staff is responsible for communicating the infant's nursing care needs, family needs, and any potential problems to a designated key contact person on staff at the receiving nursery staff. The communication between the nurses of both hospitals helps to strengthen collegiality throughout the region. The social workers in both hospitals must communicate to ensure the family of the available resources—physical, emotional, and financial—at the community hospital. This communication helps ease the family's transition to the new institution.

Family involvement and preparedness are essential to the success of the back transport. The idea of back transport needs to be presented when the infant or mother is initially transferred to the Level III center. Back transport needs to be presented as a positive step and a milestone for the infant. The family must be reassured that the infant is well enough for transfer and that the transfer is a safe procedure. It is important for the family to understand that policies and procedures may differ in the community hospital and that different methods are acceptable. The family needs to be encouraged to visit the community hospital and become acquainted with the staff before the infant's transfer.

The attitude of the Level III staff toward back transport is a major force in the success or failure of the program. Communicating confidence in and a commitment to back transport, along with support for the parents, helps to overcome the separation anxiety experienced by family and staff. However, the benefits of back transport are sabotaged when the Level III staff communicates uncertainty and lack of confidence in the community hospital to the parents.

Back transport of an infant to the home hospital has some disadvantages, such the potential for incomplete transfer of information with the change in care providers. However, this disadvantage lessens each year as technology such as FAX machines and computerization develops. This communication failure can disrupt the infant's continuing care. A family's problems with the changes in care providers, policies, and procedures are lessened with careful planning.

The Level III NICU faces two main disadvantages when all convalescing infants are back transported. The Level III center has fewer opportunities to learn to provide convalescent care, and the option to care for less critical infants provides both relief from intensive care nursing and enjoyment for the nursing staff.

For the regionalized system to function as designed, the transfer of patients must complete a circle. Level I and Level II nurseries rely on the Level III centers for sophisticated perinatal services. Level III centers, in turn, depend on Level I and Level II centers for needed resources to care for the convalescing infant and family.

Intra-hospital and Inter-hospital Procedure Runs and Inter-hospital Transfers

It is not uncommon for hospital personnel to request the expertise of transport team members when a critically ill patient needs to be moved either within or outside the institution for a specific test procedure. In most institutions, the transport team is a valuable resource for all staff members who need to monitor and move patients from one site to another. Transport team members familiar with the hospital policies and procedures pertaining to the transport process are knowledgeable about the equipment, supplies, and personnel needed to ensure a safe transport.

Postmortem Transports

On the occasion that an infant expires or death is imminent after transport to a tertiary care facility, arrangements can be made to reunite the infant and the mother. Transport of the infant to the mother is often requested not for medical reasons but to provide an important first step in the grieving process. Many parents want to see and hold their infant before life support is removed. Before the transport, the extent of further life support is decided; necessary paperwork completed, including consent to transport; and the parents are cautioned that the infant may possibly expire en route.

Several aspects of postmortem transports require special consideration. Changing the mindset from acute life-saving measures to the infant's comfort and the family's grief influences most aspects of the transport. The team composition often changes. Team members who originally transported the infant or those who have the best skills in the care of the dying may be requested to participate. The unit physician or nurse who cared for the infant often accompanies the team to answer parents' questions about the uniqueness or response of their infant. "What went wrong?," "Will it happen again?," "Did you try everything?," and "Was it something I did?" are a few questions that parents commonly ask. Clergy may also accompany and help to answer questions such as "Why me?" and "Why did God do this?" They are also a resource for funeral arrangements. Often, the parents appreciate a close family member or friend who can ride along so that someone they know is with the infant should the infant die en route.

The deposition of the body and the paperwork associated with a death require other considerations. Sometimes the infant's body is left at the birth hospital, which handles postmortem needs. This process can best be accomplished if no autopsy is planned, if the family physician is able to come to pronounce death and complete paperwork, and if the birth hospital is familiar with this situation. More often, the transport team returns the infant's body to the tertiary center, where paperwork, postmortem care, and an autopsy are performed.

When taking an infant to be with its family, the team must allow as much time as the parents need, including completely private time with their infant. The unit personnel need to be informed to arrange the care to support this sacred family gathering, which will never be forgotten. If a physician does not accompany the team, the nurse needs to note time and document assessment, especially the absence of the heart rate. On return, the physician can confirm and pronounce death.

Many nurseries provide a grief packet for parents. These packets are commercially available and can be individualized to institutional specifications. Contents may include footprints and handprints of the deceased infant, a lock of hair, photographs of the infant and sometimes items that may have been worn by the infant. Inclusion of information concerning support groups and the loss of an infant may also be helpful for parents and their families as they begin grieving.

Financial reimbursement for such a transport may also become an issue. Some insurance companies pay, considering it part of the care of the infant. Many that do not can be persuaded to pay, in view of the circumstances. When insurance companies refuse to pay, hospitals can choose to provide this compassionate service at no cost. Because postmortem transports are not common, investigating what works in a particular system and establishing a protocol are prudent. The transport team is often regarded as a resource for the many considerations necessary to a successful transport for all individuals involved.

THE BUSINESS OF TRANSPORT

The business of transport provides the support structure for a viable quality team. Administrative support, reimbursement, leadership, staffing, quality improvement, and program evaluation are key areas that, when functioning smoothly, allow the skilled team member to provide optimal care.

Administrative Support for a Transport Team

Transport is an expensive service that involves personnel, equipment, and vehicles. Hospitals are increasingly evaluating the cost versus benefit of transport services. Administration generally focuses on costs that are quantitative and more easily measured. Benefits of a transport service are qualitative and relate to patient outcomes. However, few objective quantitative studies on the effect of transport on patient outcome or length of stay exist (Brimhall, 1995).

Transport teams are low revenue producers, especially in comparison with the expense of 24-hour staffing, advanced training, and equipment purchases. The cost of staffing the team and providing necessary equipment and education for team members may be looked upon as the cost of doing business, inasmuch as the transport team services the hospital and community in the transport of patients that can potentially stay in the hospital for months. If expenses related specifically to team services can be determined, a billing structure can be established to attempt to bring in revenue to break even with needed expenditures.

Administrators understand the importance of a first-rate team for their image in the community. They also respond to the competitive need to maintain market position and the customer needs and requests for service. Level III nurseries not located in a delivery hospital often depend almost entirely on transport services to bring their patients to their institutions.

Reimbursement

Reimbursement for transport services varies tremendously. Contracts and alliances affect both patient costs and transport fees. Both managed care and governmental regulations impact reimbursement structure and dollar amounts. Actual collections for team services may be difficult to separate from collections for inpatient services. Payers may lump reimbursement dollars for transport into payment for inpatient services. This makes actual tracking of revenue specific to team functions difficult.

Precertification is increasingly requested. Some teams offer to help families with this necessity. Letters of medical necessity may be needed, as may a cost analysis justifying transfer of a patient to another institution. These issues can be anticipated for planned transports, especially for reverse transports or transports for planned surgeries if advance notice occurs during the insurance companies' business hours. Most often, however, precertification is impossible when stabilization and transfer of a critically ill neonate is needed. In those cases, understanding a region's general guidelines is important.

Land ambulance is the most inexpensive for local transports and generally the first choice. If environmental factors, extreme distances, or the patient's condition contraindicates land, air ambulance can be considered. Team members should be aware of travel time and costs of ground, fixed wing, and helicopter services in their area so that the mode most appropriate to patient need is used. Transports that require ground transport time of longer than two to three hours for the patient may be more cost-effective via fixed winged air. This may also be advantageous if it decreases out of the hospital time for the patient.

Those who review documentation for billing purposes should be able to ascertain necessity for transfer and choice of the receiving hospital. Choice of the receiving hospital is influenced by proximity, services offered, and possibly the insurance alliance of "preferred" hospitals. Reimbursement will occur more readily if transfer documentation regarding the reasons for the transport, choice of hospital, choice of transport service, and mode of transport are clear. Private insurance companies generally provide the best reimbursement. Coverage varies widely according to the plan. A physician describing the "medical necessity for a transport" can often make requests for increased reimbursement that are based on special need. Reimbursement from governmental providers is often much lower and varies from state to state. Governmental providers prefer the land ambulance. Reimbursement from governmental providers such as Medicaid may require the transporting hospital apply for a provider number and submit documentation of their services and any applicable licenses required for their state. This process is completed annually. Transport team leadership should work with the personnel in the department responsible for insurance contracts to determine the need for any special paperwork in their state to facilitate collections from governmental payers.

The billing system for the patient also varies. The hospital's patient accounts department, the ambulance company, and the transport team itself may also be involved. This process should be reviewed to meet both customer and provider needs. The team members' roles often involve gathering financial information for the patient from the referral hospital and determining charges for the transport so that appropriate billing can occur.

Staffing/Pay Issues

Providing a twenty-four hour service as well as coverage for simultaneous transports is a challenge for every team. Is the team unit-based and pulled from unit staffing or dedicated to transport services? How many teams are in-house or on call? Is the transport team large enough to provide flexible staffing but small enough to maintain each member's transport expertise? Decisions about team availability must incorporate volume and timing of transports, average length of transports, response time, needs for nontransport time, and maintenance of transport skills. Pay or compensation should match effort. Additional pay for hazardous duty or extended practice varies. Consideration should be given to keeping commitments during off-duty hours reasonable. Most teams use an on-call system to provide needed flexibility for high-volume times. If on-call requirements are common, morale and personal commitment may lessen, and increased turnover may result.

Justification for the needed full time equivalents for staffing may be challenging. Down time between transports leads to increased fixed costs that may seem impossible to spread over existing transport volume. Consideration of revenue generation from intensive care admissions that would not have occurred without the transport teams may help justify staffing needs when transport volumes do not generate adequate revenue.

Leadership

Transport team members are often considered mavericks that are confident, skilled, and stimulated by challenges. How does one lead such a group of individuals? Most programs have a manager whose specific responsibility is for transport.

Teams are, however, often well-suited for the self-directed work team approach. The work of the team is initiated, developed, and accomplished by team members. The program manager can then take the role of a coach, providing stability and guidance as a contact person as well as tracking the coordination of efforts.

Performance Improvement/Program Evaluation

The intent of any transport quality improvement program is to monitor and improve patient care in a cost-effective manner. Availability, accessibility, responsiveness, and effectiveness of the team are key issues. Because care is often provided for just a few hours, short-term outcome and patient response should be the focus of clinical indicators. Indicators should be established for high-volume, high-risk, and problem-prone transports.

The quality and effectiveness of patient care are tied closely to the quality and effectiveness of the transport team processes. Indicators tracking safety, competency, response times, unusual events, and communication help to highlight areas for improvement. Figure 2-5 provides a summary of quality indicators on neonatal transport. Staffing patterns may be changed to accommodate high-volume times for transports. New equipment may be purchased or training recommended.

Also important to quality is the customer's definition of quality. Major customers include the patient, the family, and referral personnel. Questionnaires directed to parents and referral hospitals provide valuable feedback regarding team pre-

Quality Indicators on Neonatal Transport

INDICATOR	APPLICATION
Intervention	Airway security
	ETT size and placement
	ETT placement confirmation
	Medication appropriateness and documentation
	IV access obtained and patent
	Vital sign assessment and documentation
	Neutral thermal environment
	Vital assessment upon arrival
Data collection and documentation	Compliance with policy and procedure
Timeliness of care	Response time
	Patient preparation time
Safety	Patient secured per procedure
Education	Training standards are met
Staffing	Staffing is comprehensively met
Professional competence	Prerequisite license and certification
	Continuing education met and documented
	Team effectiveness
Utilization review	Team composition per protocol
	Carrier selection per protocol
	Equipment use per protocol
	Procedure use per protocol
	Severity of illness versus appropriateness of orders
Unusual events reviewed	CPR during transport
	Mortality during transport
Customer's needs	Referring hospital staff competence
	Dispatch calls per protocol
	Follow-up calls per protocol
Program success/marketing	Referral demographics
	Revenue and billing projections

FIGURE **2-5**

Quality indicators for neonatal transport. From Dunn N (1995). Quality management strategies in interfacility transport. In *Current concepts in transport: neonatal obstetric, pediatric, and administrative, administrative subsection*, ed 7, Columbus, OH. Ross Laboratories.

sentation, explanations, and interactions. Focus group meetings with referral hospital personnel can give the team feedback on consumer service and learning needs that have become apparent. Customer input needs to be reflected in the team's plan to improve services.

A data collection system to track indicators needs to be built into the team documentation or into a team process that is easy for team members to complete. Problems that occur on a transport run should be documented immediately after transport, as should response times. Computers can be a valuable aid to recording and reporting data. Training all team members to master a user-friendly program increases involvement and accountability for quality of patient care.

Role of Outreach Education

To help ensure quality care for patients within the region, outreach education programs have been developed by the regional centers to assess educational needs, educate and train health care providers, implement and evaluate programs, collect and analyze perinatal data, provide patient follow-up to referral hospitals, and provide continuity of communication among hospitals. Education and training programs include physiologic

and technical information and a psychological component on the emotional issues of high-risk care and ways to promote parent-infant bonding during crises. These educational programs focus on meeting the goals of the regional approach (Hauth & Merenstein, 1997). The impact of the outreach programs is seen in the improvement of care and the decrease of mortality and morbidity in the region.

The development of outreach educational programs is an art and science in and of itself. There is a whole industry focused on the education, training, and development of the adult learner. Developers of such programs should consult with experts in their hospitals or regions and should obtain books or educational materials, some of which are available on the internet.

Outreach Education

With optimizing patient outcomes as a focus, the Guidelines for Perinatal Care (AAP & ACOG, 1997) and the Guidelines for Air and Ground Transport of Neonatal and Pediatric Patients (AAP, 1999) emphasized the importance of the regional centers providing outreach education for their referral hospitals. Objectives of this education including ensuring knowledge of basic stabilization for neonatal patients recognizing neonatal illnesses that require transfer to a higher level of care, and improving understanding of the physiologic basis for initiating care and stabilization before team arrival at the referring facility (AAP, 1999).

Several nationally recognized programs are available for neonatal resuscitation and transport-related education, particularly the neonatal resuscitation program (NRP) (AAP, 2000) and the S.T.A.B.L.E.® Program (Karlsen, 2001). Advance preparation of hospital staff in the postresuscitation care and stabilization of a sick newborn is critically important for optimizing patient outcome. A positive impact on the future pediatric life of a sick newborn may be achieved by providing anticipatory, prompt, and efficient care in the first "golden" hours after birth. This care is specific to the recognition and treatment of respiratory distress, infection, shock, and various congenital anomalies.

In the past, provision of education by the receiving hospital education department and/or transport team members has been an integral part of referral pattern marketing efforts. Today, however, referral patterns are often influenced by corporate affiliation and insurance plans. This trend may contribute to a decrease in educational offerings to referral facilities. Despite this challenge, the regional center is responsible for providing education through subspecialty experts, including neonatal outreach educators, transport team members, neonatologists, and perinatologists (AAP, 1997).

Due to decreased opportunities to care for sick neonates, hospital staff are often challenged to maintain knowledge, skills, and a high level of competency in this area. Two educational programs have been developed with these challenges in mind. The Neonatal Resuscitation Program (NRP) provides education in neonatal resuscitation. The S.T.A.B.L.E.® Program, first implemented in the United States in 1996, is a program that focuses on the postresuscitation and pretransport stabilization care of sick newborns including physical assessment, problem recognition and management. Mnemonics are memory tools that aid in retention and recall of information. When working under stressful conditions, as with an unstable neonate, a mnemonic may assist as a memory clue in the organization and provision of care. The S.T.A.B.L.E.® mnemonic stands for Sugar, Temperature, Artificial or Assisted breathing, Blood pressure, Lab work and Emotional support for the family. This mnemonic-based program serves as a concise guideline to organize the myriad of details and interventions for both stabilizing sick newborns and preparing them for transport when necessary. Any health care provider involved with the postresuscitation and/or pretransport care of potentially sick newborns would benefit from program participation. This includes RNs, physicians, respiratory therapists and pre-hospital providers.

S.T.A.B.L.E.® PROGRAM MODULES

The sugar section stresses the importance of withholding enteral feedings and providing intravenous fluids when an infant is sick. Initial IV fluid therapy, blood sugar monitoring and recognition, and treatment of hypoglycemia are discussed. Understanding the detrimental effects of hypothermia and prevention of cold stress are the focus of the temperature section. The concept of pulmonary vasoconstriction as a consequence of cold stress is covered in detail. The artificial/assisted breathing module is designed to help learners evaluate severity and treatment of respiratory distress, including blood gas interpretation, pneumothoraces, respiratory system warning signs, and

the management of intubated infants. Pulmonary vasoconstriction secondary to hypoxemia and hypoxia reinforces the temperature section module, in which this concept was first introduced. The instructional focus in the blood pressure section is on recognition and treatment of hypovolemic, cardiogenic, and septic shock, including appropriate volume boluses and Dopamine administration. The lab work module addresses neonatal sepsis, including infants at risk for infection; group B streptococcal infection; and maternal pretreatment with antibiotics, CBC interpretation, and initial antibiotic therapy. The emotional support section focuses on parental stress surrounding the birth of a sick and/or premature newborn and ways health care providers can support families that experience a newborn ICU admission. The final module in the program is quality improvement (QI). A case study relating to neonatal infection, respiratory distress, and communication issues follow a discussion on morbidity. The case study is designed to help the learner relate information learned in previous modules. The S.T.A.B.L.E.® Program recommends that pretransport stabilization care be evaluated through a QI process by the nursing and medical management team at the referral facility. Assistance in interpreting information should be available upon request from the receiving facility. The evaluation should occur in a timely fashion so that details are fresh in everyone's minds. The QI process should answer the following questions:

Was the patient well stabilized?

Were problems (e.g., communication, equipment, skills) that affected our ability to stabilize the infant encountered?

How did we perform as a team?

What could we do in the future to improve our performance in this situation?

What was the patient outcome?

Outreach education needs to also include information about common surgical, cardiac, neurologic, and genetic conditions that may be encountered and require pretransport stabilization. The S.T.A.B.L.E.® mnemonic has been adapted to address these issues and additional, new modules are intended to supplement the basic S.T.A.B.L.E.® Program. The following list is not all-inclusive but offers a brief overview of the module content.

S.T.A.B.L.E.®—Surgical

Identification and stabilization of newborns with intestinal obstruction, abdominal wall defects, tracheoesophageal fistula, and esophageal atresia.

S.T.A.B.L.E.®—Cardiac

Identification and stabilization of newborns with cyanotic congenital heart disease and left ventricular outflow obstruction.

S.T.A.B.L.E.®—Neurologic

Identification and stabilization of newborns with neural tube defects, birth asphyxia, and seizures.

S.T.A.B.L.E.®—Genetic and Other Conditions

Acute stabilization of newborns with hydrops fetalis; evaluation of newborns with various genetic disorders; trisomy 13, 18, 21; and anomalies.

Constant attention and work between regional centers and referral institutions focuses on the desire to improve care and outcomes and thus assists everyone involved with perinatal care in the region. As regional centers lead the initiative to strive for excellence in care, the patients, families and society benefit.

LEGAL ISSUES

The unique circumstances of critical care transport raise many questions of legal responsibility and liability. The dynamic acuity level of the patient, the dual responsibility of the transport team and the referral hospital, and the provision of care in unusual settings often with limited resources confuse the issues of duty and proximate cause.

Statutes and regulations historically have addressed first response teams and ambulance services. Regulations have not been issued for the critical care transport teams, whose composition and function differ significantly from those of the first-response teams. Most critical care transport teams are hospital-based, have mixed composition and skill sets, have a higher level of physician supervision, and transport more critically ill patients.

Transport team members are expected to adhere to the guidelines and protocols established by the base institution. They operate within the chain of command established by the medical director. Individual team members and the base institution may be liable if the team member does not perform within the defined guidelines of their department and their institution. All transport teams must follow standard resuscitation guidelines and have appropriate personnel, equipment, and supplies available for each transport (AAP, 1999).

Training, experience, and updated protocols are imperative in the maintenance of team expertise. Development of quality and safety indicators help track the effectiveness of training, quality of care, and adequacy of team processes. Team members are responsible for adhering to the requirements established by their professional licensure and practice acts.

The transport process usually begins when the referral call is received and the patient is accepted for admission. Because recommendations for care and intervention are often given during the referral call, some legal responsibility for the patient begins at this time. Lines of responsibility once the transport team is on the scene are less clear. Most institutions operate on the premise that once the team arrives at the referring institution, receives report, and begins to render care, they assume the greatest responsibility for the patient's care (AAP, 1999). Some institutions may want to consider a written agreement that defines levels of responsibility between the referring and the receiving institutions.

The dual responsibility of the transport team and referral hospitals also influences legal liability. The Consolidated Omnibus Reconciliation Act (COBRA) regulations generally affect referring hospitals more than transport teams. The act requires that the hospital evaluate all patients who present to the hospital with emergency conditions and that the hospital determine appropriate care, stabilize, and obtain informed consent to transfer.

Informed consent is a basic requirement for treatment, and treatment without consent constitutes battery. A signed and witnessed consent form generally includes agreement to treatments and admission to the hospital, excluding surgery, and should specify the mode of transport and name of the receiving institution. A common situation that raises questions of consent is that of a legal minor teenage mother's providing consent for her child. States vary in laws on the treatment of minors. Emancipated minors who are self-reliant, living apart from their parents, and are financially self-supporting can sign a consent form. Mature minors are deemed competent if they are of sufficient intellect and maturity to appreciate the benefits and risks of and alternatives to the proposed medical care (AAP, 1999). Cautious teams have both teenage mothers and one of their parents sign the consent form for transport. They also avoid signatures of fathers when the mothers are unwed or before responsibility is accepted on a signed birth certificate. Another situation is the unavailability of an ill or sedated

mother who is unable to sign the consent form. In emergency situations, both public policy and law support the assumption of implied consent for medical care. The responsible physician must document that an emergency situation exists, that treatment is for the patient's benefit, and that obtaining express consent is impossible. Choosing not to transport an infant because of presumed nonviability or futility of transfer and treatment raises both legal and ethical questions. In most cases, the duty is to transport until all involved parties can discuss these issues and the patient's condition becomes more clearly defined. If the patient is not transported, documentation of condition, parental wishes, and all considerations leading to this decision is essential.

The transport team is responsible for the integrity of the medical record throughout the transport. The medical record should contain an ongoing evaluation of the patient at the referring institution, during the transport, and on arrival at the receiving institution. Suggestions made at the time of referral, treatment efforts on the scene, and ongoing assessment of patient status should also be included in the documentation. Orders should be documented in real time and signed by the ordering physician as soon as possible. Transport teams without a physician in attendance must have the ability to contact the medical control physician at all times (AAP, 1999).

A focus on quality, training, and documentation of both care and process reduces legal risk. When high-quality care is provided and patients have positive outcomes, the liabilities associated with transport are negligible.

FUTURE TRENDS

The future of neonatal transport is most likely to be influenced by cost-benefit analysis as it relates to patient outcomes rather than by technologic advances, as it has been in the past. Current health reform is changing the paradigms of who provides care, where care is provided, and which care is considered appropriate.

Basic service parameters are undergoing very little change (Chester, 1995). Stabilization protocols are even more standardized as guidelines are published or information is rapidly shared on computer information highways.

The transported neonatal population is changing as the maternal transports increase. Fewer preterm infants are transported because more mothers are arriving at delivering hospitals that can also care for ventilated and ill preterm infants. Surfactant replacement therapy at referral hospitals has also influenced the need for transport to tertiary centers. In addition, capitation may influence where care can be provided with tertiary care for acute phases of illness and with intermediate nurseries for convalescent care. Maternal transports may not continue to increase if managed care contracts change the regionalization process. Mothers may be kept at outlying hospitals while their infants are transported only in the event of a postdelivery problem. Only time will tell.

Technologic advances continue to produce increasingly sophisticated yet very lightweight and transportable equipment to monitor the most delicate of vital signs. The future of most sophisticated treatments, including on-the-road extracorporeal membrane oxygenation, nitric oxide, and liquid ventilation will depend on improving patient outcomes, including cost-benefit concerns.

More certain is the increased use of complex information systems for documentation, dispatch, stabilization advice, data input, tracking of the transport process, patient outcomes, and communication between institutions. A national database is already being developed. Researchers and clinicians request information currently on the internet. Faxing patient information, which is becoming more common, may be replaced by relaying information from one computer to another by modem.

Team composition is also changing. Although teams are more often becoming dedicated strictly to transport, the number of members in each team is expected to decrease. With cross training, the job description may resemble less that of a registered nurse, respiratory therapist, or paramedic and more closely resemble a blended role with many common skill sets. Teams are increasingly physician-referred rather than physician-based. Tertiary care physicians will be less available as the emphasis on prevention and wellness increases. Use of certified nurse practitioners versus an expanded-role registered nurse varies depending on state practice acts and regional preferences and resources.

The high cost of air transport in comparison with ground transport is already causing a shift toward increased use of ground transport and is prompting a more critical look at the appropriateness of air transport for various conditions. Ground transport services are also experiencing the effect of mergers as private companies vie for contracts and as some hospitals decide whether it is cost-effective to have their own ambulance services.

To date, response time of 20 to 30 minutes to mobilize a team remains unchanged. Some teams may also be expected to find a way to break this paradigm.

Budget reductions are likely to affect all areas of neonatal care. Patient care hours are most likely to be supported, and training and daily operations will most likely be trimmed. However, teams around the country continue to place strong emphasis on education and training of team members. Some teams fear that administrators may not understand the unique challenges of transport and the critical importance of trained, skilled personnel in settings with limited resources. Evaluating team methods of training as well as all team processes to prove their value in the age of health care reform will continue to be a challenge.

CHALLENGES TO REGIONALIZATION IN TODAY'S HEALTH CARE ECONOMY

The primary goal of the Committee on Perinatal Health was improvement of patient outcomes. To accomplish this task, the committee recommended the regional structure for providing care. Inherent in the proposed regional system was a sense of altruism and the sharing of patients by physicians to benefit the patients at risk.

Toward Improving the Outcome of Pregnancy (The National Foundation—March of Dimes, 1976) outlined a regional concept but provided few details for implementation. The plan was to develop exemplary systems that would function as role models for others. Across the country, regional system organization was influenced by the geographic area, the personnel, and the political climate.

The health care environment has undergone dramatic changes since the implementation of regionalized care. Changes in the prospective reimbursement to hospitals in the 1980s affected the altruism and sharing inherent in regional systems and led to competition for patients. As a result, regional perinatal systems are breaking down.

The three levels of neonatal care established by the Committee on Perinatal Health have become blurred in the current environment. Level I nurseries are upgrading their services to Level II. The widest range of services is found in Level II nurseries, many of which provide services of a Level III NICU. With the advances in technology and services and the wide variation in levels of care, the traditional regional concept has become outdated. Meadow et al (2001) study showed no difference in outcome between infants born at Level II NICUs who were randomized in to obligatory transfer to a Level III center and infants randomized into the optional transfer group that stayed in the Level II NICU to be ventilated.

The prospective reimbursement to hospitals was altered with the introduction of Diagnosis Related Groups (DRGs). DRGs classify patients on the basis of principal diagnosis, age, surgical procedure, comorbidities, complications, and discharge status. Reimbursement to a hospital is relatively fixed according to a patient's classification. DRG reimbursement for Medicare patients began in 1983; a number of states followed, using DRGs for reimbursement of Medicaid patients. Blue Cross and some other national and regional commercial payers also implemented DRG reimbursement.

Neonatal care is contained in the Major Diagnostic Category 15: Newborns and Other Neonates with Conditions Originating in the Perinatal Period. This category is broken down into seven classifications.

Studies of infants transferred within the regional network showed that DRGs did not acknowledge differing levels of neonatal care or transport systems. As the federal DRG stood, regional systems would be disrupted.

Reimbursement policies favored Level I nurseries with shorter patient stays. Level II and III nurseries would be discouraged from returning stable neonates to Level I nurseries. This procedure creates potential for overcrowding of NICUs and lack of available Level III resources.

To maintain established regional networks, many states modified the federal DRGs to increase reimbursement for neonatal care. Although Medicaid reimbursement does not seriously affect perinatal regionalization, it affects ambulatory services by offering a lesser reimbursement for obstetricians, thus creating a barrier to accessible care.

Competition among hospitals for patients is the largest threat to existing regional networks. The increase in multihospital systems has made it difficult for one hospital to serve as the referral site within a defined region. This problem has led to the creation of new perinatal systems and the elimination of existing ones.

When insurance coverage is provided through HMOs and preferred provider organizations (PPOs), access is limited to contracted hospitals. Contracts—and hence transport patterns—are decided by the administrators of provider organizations, not by the physicians. In the past, physicians established professional relationships within the region, and patients were often transferred along the lines of those relationships.

The changing health care environment of the 1980s created a competitive atmosphere that has led to the breakdown of traditional regional alliances. The goal of decreasing perinatal mortality has been accomplished in infants with a birth weight greater than 1,000 grams but still needs improvement for infants weighing less than 1,000 grams. Although the future of regionalized care remains uncertain, subspecialty centers certainly remain crucial for infants weighing less than 1,000 grams because outcomes are better at these centers (Hernandez, 2000; Kirby, 1996; Phibbs, 1996; Yeast, 1998).

THE FUTURE OF REGIONALIZATION

The effects of a changing health care environment have resulted in a decreased commitment to regional networks and expansions in the hospital services developed to keep the hospitals competitive in the marketplace (Pollack, 1996).

The goals outlined by the Committee on Perinatal Health in *Toward Improving the Outcome of Pregnancy* (The National Foundation—March of Dimes, 1976) have been reached. A change in the health care environment, most notably competition among hospitals for patients, has weakened the regional systems developed in the 1970s. The future of perinatal regional care is in jeopardy. A broad-based Committee on Perinatal Health reconvened to analyze current definitions of care, identify problems with the existing system, and modify it to function through the 1990s and beyond. The focus of perinatal care has shifted from hospital-based care to overall health care awareness. Emphasis must be placed on preventative health care, education, and counseling. The goal of these emphases is quality health care that is accessible to all and economically efficient for the provider. Recommendations for improving the outcome of pregnancy were developed from these key areas. A recommendation from this committee is that the three levels of inpatient perinatal care be modified, enhanced, and promoted (Committee on Perinatal Health, 1993). Three types of perinatal centers have been defined—basic, specialty, and subspecialty. Basic perinatal centers provide basic inpatient care for pregnant women and newborns without complications; management of perinatal emergencies, including neonatal resuscitation; leadership in early risk identification before and at birth; consultation or referral for high-risk patients; and public and professional education (Committee on Perinatal Health, 1993; Maloni et al, 1996). Specialty perinatal centers provide management for certain high-risk pregnancies, including maternal referrals from basic care centers; services for newborns with selected complications, particularly those who are moderately ill; and appropriate continuing education (Committee on Perinatal Health, 1993). Subspecialty perinatal centers provide inpatient care for maternal and fetal complications; a NICU equipped to treat critically ill neonates; follow-up medical care of NICU graduates; consultation and referral arrangements with other hospitals (including transport arrangements); educational opportunities; a perinatal data base; and evaluation activities (Committee on Perinatal Health, 1993).

Recent studies on outcomes of the ELBW infant demonstrate a continuing need for a form of regionalization for this population. Because of increasing competition from hospitals to provide all services to their clientele, however, new and different ways to promote collaboration between basic, specialty, and subspecialty centers must be explored. One such way could be formation of a public and formal partnership between the hospitals to improve outcomes (Sanders, 2000). Pollack (1996) discussed the use of an integrated neonatology practice as a model for reorganization of perinatal services in Level II. In his model, the private practice neonatologists in the Level II unit function in coordination with the established Level III centers and neonatologists, and a strict set of guidelines are followed. Retrospective comparison of a Level II unit before and after establishment of this model showed a decrease in infants transported to the Level III unit, an increase in the number of infants transferred back, a reduction in the Level II neonatal mortalities associated with viability, and a decrease in the number of LBW and VLBW infants.

SUMMARY

The development of regional systems for providing perinatal care came in response to increasing perinatal mortality rates after World War II. Health care professionals recognized that achieving lower mortality rates requires that high-risk care for mothers and infants be accessible to all who need that level of care. The goals for regionalization, transport, and stabilization are still optimal health. Methods for achieving these goals in the future are still unclear. Neonatal nurses can affect the change in regionalization by collecting evidence to support models of care that include successful transport and stabilization algorithms.

In the twenty-first century, the regional approach and its three distinct levels of care face a challenge for survival that demands consideration of new ways to accomplish decreased neonatal mortality. Forming public and formalized partnerships with basic and specialty hospitals as well as with physicians may be one way of method. What will your role be? It is up to you; that is the challenge!

REFERENCES

American Academy of Pediatrics (1999). *Guidelines for air and ground transport of neonatal and pediatric patients.* ed 2, Elk Grove Village, IL, AAP.

American Academy of Pediatrics and American College of Obstetricians and Gynecologists (1998). *Guidelines for perinatal care.* ed 4, Elk Grove Village, IL, AAP.

American Academy of Pediatrics Committee on the Fetus and Newborn (2000). Use of Inhaled Nitric Oxide, *Pediatrics*, 106, 344-345.

Brimhall D (1995). Developing administrative support for transport. In Trautman MS (Ed.), Proceedings from *Current concepts in transport: neonatal, obstetric, pediatric, and administrative, administrative subsection,* ed 7, Columbus, OH: Ross Laboratories.

Chester G (1995). Neonatal ground transports—1994: a four-year evaluation of previous study. In MS Trautman (Ed.) *Current concepts in transport, administrative Subsection* (ed 7, pp. 150-151). Columbus, OH: Ross Laboratories.

Chou MM, MacDonald MG (1989). Landmarks in the development of patient transport systems. In MacDonald MM, Miller MK (Eds.), *Emergency transport of the perinatal patient* (pp. 2-31). Boston: Little, Brown.

Committee on Perinatal Health (1993). *Toward improving the outcome of pregnancy: the 90s and beyond.* White Plains, NY: March of Dimes Birth Defect Foundation.

Finkelman A (2001). *Managed care: a nursing perspective.* Upper Saddle River, NJ: Prentice Hall Health.

Hauth JC, Merenstein GB (Eds.) (1997). *Guidelines for perinatal care,* ed. 4, Elk Grove Village, IL: AAP.

Hernandez JA et al (2000). Impact of infants born at the threshold of viability on the neonatal mortality rate in Colorado. *Journal of perinatology,* 20(1), 21-6.

Karlsen KA (2001). *The S.T.A.B.L.E.® Program.* www.stableprogram.com. Salt Lake City, Utah.

Kattwinkel J (Ed.) (2000) *Textbook of neonatal resuscitation,* ed 4, Elk Grove Village, IL: American Academy of Pediatrics and American Heart Association.

Kirby RS (1996). Perinatal Mortality: the role of the hospital of birth. *Journal of perinatology,* 16(1), 43-49.

Lawrence J et al (1993). The development of a tool to assess neonatal pain. *Neonatal network,* 12(6), 59-66.

Lemons JA, Bauer CR (2001). Very low birth weight outcomes of the National Institute of Child Health and Human Development Neonatal Research Network, January 1995 to December 1996. *Pediatrics,* 107(1), E1-8.

Maloni JA et al (1996). Transforming prenatal care: Reflections on the past and present with implications for the future. *Journal of obstetric, gynecologic, and neonatal nursing*, 25(1), 17-23.

Meadow W et al (1996). Can and should level II nurseries care for newborns who require mechanical ventilation? *Clinical perinatology*, 23(3), 551-561.

National Association of Neonatal Nurses (2000). *Infant and family centered developmental guidelines*. Petaluma, CA: Author.

National Association of Neonatal Nurses. (1998). *Neonatal nursing transport standards and guidelines* ed 2, Petaluma, CA: Author.

The National Foundation—March of Dimes. (1976). *Toward improving the outcome of pregnancy: recommendations for the regional development of maternal and perinatal health services*. White Plains, NY: Committee on Perinatal Health.

Phibbs CS et al (1996). The effects of patient volume and level of care at the hospital of birth on neonatal mortality. *Journal of American Medical Association*, 276(13), 1054-1059.

Pollack LD (1996). An effective model for reorganization of perinatal services in a metropolitan area: a descriptive analysis and historical perspective. *Journal of perinatology*, 16(1), 3-8.

Salyer JW, Masi-Lynch J (1995). Respiratory care during the transport of infants and children. In Barnhart SL, Czervinske MP (Eds.), *Perinatal and pediatric respiratory care* (pp. 637-657). Philadelphia: WB Saunders.

Sanders MR (2000). Perinatal regionalization: Old lessons for the new millennium. *Connecticut medicine*, 64(2), 67-70.

Stevenson DK, Wright LL (1998). Very low birth weight outcomes of the National Institute of Child Health and Human Development Neonatal Research Network, January 1993 to December 1994. *American journal of obstetrics and gynecology*, 179(6), 1632-1639.

Yeast JD et al (1998). Changing patterns in regionalization of perinatal care and the impact on neonatal mortality. *American journal of obstetrics and gynecology*, 178(1), 131-135.

CHAPTER 3

EVIDENCE-BASED NEONATAL NURSING PRACTICE

Kathleen R. Stevens

Some type of knowledge guides every clinical action taken by a nurse. The underlying rationale for a nursing intervention may come from past experiences, trial and error, authority, a nursing procedure manual, a textbook, or science produced through systematic inquiry (research). Nursing care policies often represent a source of knowledge known as authority. Many sources of knowledge may underlie a policy—the policy-maker's own clinical experience, tradition ("we have always done it this way"), internal or external benchmarks, and textbooks. Whatever the knowledge base for the action, the nurse believes that the intervention will produce the desired health outcome for the patient or will accurately assess the patient's health status.

Each of these underlying rationales represents a "source of knowledge" used by the nurse to make clinical decisions to implement specific interventions. These sources of knowledge are the basis of clinical reasoning. However, not all sources of knowledge are highly reliable or consistently produce the desired patient outcome. Experience and trial and error are good teachers; however, the knowledge gained through these approaches contains bias. That is, the results may be due to something other than the intervention that is outside of the nurse's awareness, or the results from one situation may not be applicable to another situation or client. Conclusions drawn on experience and trial and error will not likely represent the full truth or validity of the broader reality

The quality of care improves when research results guide that care. The primary concept of Evidence-Based Practice (EBP) is that science is the most reliable source of knowledge upon which to base clinical decisions. Today, the measure of "best practice" is that interventions are based on "best evidence," that is, scientific findings. EBP is a new way of applying best evidence in clinical decision making to ensure the best outcome that science knows how to produce. Individual clinician decisions about care as well as agency policies about care standards should reflect the best evidence produced to date. The end result of applying state-of-the-science patient care is that health care status goals are effectively and efficiently met within the preferences of both the patient and health care provider (Sackett, 2000). This rapidly advancing trend of EBP embodies new methods and represents a new paradigm of research application in clinical care.

This chapter will define evidence-based practice. Examples of evidence to support neonatal and infant nursing care will be presented. Strategies for gaining support for the use of evidence in practice will be identified.

WHAT IS EVIDENCE-BASED PRACTICE?

Evidence-based practice is a process through which scientific evidence is identified, appraised, and applied in healthcare interventions (Ledbetter & Stevens, 2000). The definition of evidence-based practice is based on the definition of evidence-based medicine. Evidence-based medicine is defined as "the conscientious, explicit and judicious use of current best evidence in making decisions about the care of individual patients. The practice of evidence-based medicine means integrating individual clinical expertise with the best available external clinical evidence from systematic research" (Sackett, 2000). The objective of evidence-based practice is application of the best available evidence in clinical care.

Although evidence and knowledge can be drawn from a variety of sources, the best evidence is specifically identified as that evidence drawn from scientific investigation, or research (Guyatt & Rennie, 2002). Using research evidence as the basis for care increases certainty and predictability in the effect of the practice on the outcome. Implementation of evidence-based practices generates more accurate diagnosis, maximally effective and efficient intervention, and most favorable patient outcome. These ends can be accomplished through newly developed evidence-based practice methods, processes, and models.

A MODEL OF EVIDENCE-BASED NURSING

Evidence-based nursing can be described as a process of establishing research-based practice by transforming the evidence through a full cycle, into practice. The ACE Star Model depicts the Cycle of Knowledge Transformation (Stevens, 2001) as a five-step process (Figure 3-1). The steps are primary research, evidence summary, translation, implementation, and evaluation (Stevens, 2001).

Primary research is the research approach with which we are familiar—individual reports of research studies. Over the

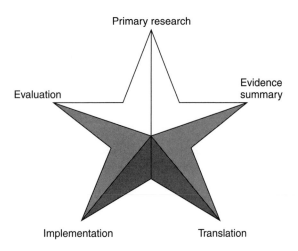

FIGURE **3-1**
ACE Star Model: Cycle of Knowledge Transformation. Copyright 2001, Kathleen R. Stevens. Used with expressed permission.

BOX **3-1**

Advantages of Systematic Reviews

A systematic review accomplishes the following:

Reduces large quantities of information into a manageable form

Integrates existing information for decisions about clinical care, economic decisions, future research design, and policy formation

Increases efficiency in time between research and clinical implementation

Establishes generalizability across participants, across settings, and treatment variations and different study designs

Assesses consistency and explains inconsistencies of relationships across studies

Increases power in suggesting the cause and effect relationship

Reduces bias from random and systematic error, improving true reflection of reality

Provides better continuous updates of new evidence

Adapted from Mulrow, 1994.

BOX **3-2**

Evidence Summaries on Neonatal Care from Credible Sources

Source: **Online Journal of Knowledge Synthesis for Nursing**

Hemingway M, Oliver S (2000). Bilateral head flattening in hospitalized premature infants. *Online journal of knowledge synthesis for nursing,* 7, 3, no pagination.

Stringer M, Hanes L (1999). Hydrotherapy use during labor: an integrative review. *Online journal of knowledge synthesis for nursing,* 6, 1, no pagination.

Andrade TM (1998). Sibling visitation: research implications for pediatric and neonatal patients. *Online journal of knowledge synthesis for nursing,* 5, 6, no pagination.

Rikli JM (1996). Parenting the premature infant: potential iatrogenesis from the neonatal intensive care experience. *Online journal of knowledge synthesis for nursing,* 3, 6, no pagination.

Source: Cochrane Library

Lemyre B, Davis PG, De Paoli AG (2000). Nasal intermittent positive pressure ventilation (NIPPV) versus nasal continuous positive airway pressure (NCPAP) for apnea of prematurity. The Cochrane Library (Oxford) issue 3.

Darlow BA, Graham PJ (2000). Vitamin A supplementation for preventing morbidity and mortality in very low birth weight infants. The Cochrane Library (Oxford) issue 3.

Shah V, Ohlsson A (2000). Venepuncture versus heel lance for blood sampling in term neonates. The Cochrane Library (Oxford) issue 3.

Craft AP, Finer NN, Barrington KJ (2000). Vancomycin for prophylaxis against sepsis in preterm neonates. The Cochrane Library (Oxford) issue 3.

Zupan J, Garner P (2000). Topical umbilical cord care at birth. The Cochrane Library (Oxford) issue 3.

Soll RF (2000). Synthetic surfactant for respiratory distress syndrome in preterm infants. The Cochrane Library (Oxford) issue 3.

Sinclair JC (2000). Servo-control for maintaining abdominal skin temperature at 36° C in low birth weight infants. The Cochrane Library (Oxford) issue 3.

---

past 30 decades, nurse researchers have produced literally thousands of research studies on a wide variety of nursing clinical topics. The cluster of primary research studies on any given topic may include both strong and weak study designs, small and large samples, and conflicting or converging results, leaving the clinician to wonder which study is the best reflection of truth.

To remedy this situation, evidence-based practice experts have developed the second step in evidence-based practice—evidence summary. In an evidence summary, all primary research on a given clinical topic is gathered together and summarized into a single statement about the state of the science. This summary step is the main feature that distinguishes evidence-based practice from simple research application and research utilization in clinical practice. The evidence summary offers distinct advantages, as are summarized in Box 3-1. Evidence summaries are also called evidence synthesis, systematic reviews, integrative reviews, and review of literature. The statistical procedure, meta-analysis, may also be used in an evidence summary. Evidence summaries communicate the latest scientific findings in a palatable and accessible form for the clinical nurse to readily apply the research in clinical decisions—that is, that evidence summaries establish the knowledge to guide our practices.

In the third step of EBP, experts are called on to consider the evidence summary, fill in gaps, and merge research knowledge with expertise to produce clinical practice guidelines. Clinical practice guidelines are commonly produced and sponsored by a clinical specialty organization. The International Lactation Consultant Association developed an excellent example of a clinical practice guideline. The association pulled together the evidence and expertise to produce evidence-based

TABLE 3-1	Alphabetical List of Sources of Systematic Reviews on the Internet
Systematic Review Source	**Address**
Agency for Healthcare Research and Quality (AHRQ)	http://www.ahrq.gov
Cochrane Collaboration	View introductory information at http://www.cochrane.org/cochrane/cc-broch.htm#CC Cochrane Reviewer's Handbook at http://www.update-software.com/ccweb/cochrane/hbook.htm

Cochrane Library	Subscription service, free browsing of abstract reviews, and alphabetical listing of all
	   titles in the Cochrane Library available at
	   http://www.update-software.com/cochrane/cochrane-frame.html

Online Journal of Knowledge Synthesis for Nursing (OJKSN)	For subscriptions, contact:
	   http://www.stti.iupui.edu/library/ajksn/subscrib_content.html
	Sample articles, editorials, and table of contents:
	   http://www.stti.iupui.edu/library/ojksn/

U.S. Preventive Services Task Force	http://www.ahrq.gov/clinic/uspsfact.htm

From Stevens KR, Pugh JA (1999). Evidence-based practice and perioperative nursing. Seminars in perioperative nursing, 8(3), 155-159.

multidisciplinary breastfeeding management strategies for the first 14 postpartum days to prevent premature weaning.

Once guidelines are produced, implementation plans are put into action to change both the individual clinician and organizational practices. Planned change approaches often are used to overcome resistance and move the individual and organization to a higher standard of practice based on evidence. In the cycle of knowledge transformation, practice changes are followed by evaluation of effectiveness, efficiency, health outcome, and satisfaction.

WHAT ARE THE MAJOR FEATURES OF EVIDENCE-BASED PRACTICE?

Major features of evidence-based practice include the following:
- It is heavily interdisciplinary.
- Development of clinical practice is based on evidence summary of the topic.
- Translation of evidence into clinical practice guidelines repackages the evidence for use by clinician.
- Individual provider and organizational factors guide implementation.
- Evaluation includes determining effectiveness and efficiency in terms of patient outcomes and economy. (Stevens, 2001).

Barriers to implementing research-based practice are removed by using evidence synthesis, when they exist. Systematic reviews "efficiently integrate valid information and provide a basis for rational decision making" in clinical care (Mulrow, 1994). Only in rare instances will a single research study offer highly reliable answers to a clinical question (Ledbetter & Stevens, 2000). It is most feasible for the nurse to use research evidence that has been summarized in the form of a systematic review. Because conducting evidence syntheses is a new, resource-intensive, and rigorous process, it is beyond the capacity of the typical clinician. For this reason, awareness of existing sources of synthesized evidence is critical for the clinician. Box 3-2 presents examples of evidence summaries from credible sources. In addition, Table 3-1 describes the most credible sources for evidence summaries to date.

In some cases, conclusions from the evidence summary support current practice and increase confidence that the nursing care will produce the desired outcome. In other cases, the evidence points to a needed change in practice. In either case, examining current practice in light of state of the science is becoming an expectation for health care.

SOURCES OF EVIDENCE FOR PRACTICE

Synthesis work is conducted by several organized agencies such as the Agency for Healthcare Research and Quality (AHRQ) and the Cochrane Collaboration. Because the conduct of a systematic review requires specialized scientific methods and significant resources, it is usually a sponsored activity conducted by groups of scientists. The prime sponsors are the Cochrane Collaboration (a global collaborative headquartered in the United Kingdom) and the Agency for Healthcare Research and Quality (a federally funded agency in the United States). In turn, these agencies disseminate the evidence summaries for use by clinicians, health policy makers, and consumers of health care.

APPLICATION TO NEONATAL NURSING CARE

Neonatal nursing is young in comparison to other nursing specialties. To date, much of the evidence to support care has been done by physicians. These studies have been represented in the systematic integrative reviews in the Vermont Oxford Database or Cochrane Collaborative. Nursing has just begun to systemically examine the nursing care. Some regarding developmental care are found in the Cochrane Collaborative Database. The National Association of Neonatal Nurses (NANN) submitted practice guidelines regarding many aspects of neonatal nursing care to the Agency for Healthcare Research and Quality. These guidelines represent evidence-based practice protocols. These activities are a start towards gaining a solid foundation in evidence to support our practice.

To date, little evidence from randomized control trials to support neonatal nursing care exist. What evidence there is normally falls in the realm of expert opinion or expert experiences. Although this foundation has some evidence beyond tradition, it does not possess the strength that findings from sound, scientifically grounded research studies have. This scarcity should not deter us from striving for evidence to support our practice nor should its lack serve as an excuse to accept tradition or the status quo. It means, rather, that as neonatal, newborn, and infant nurses we must conduct research studies to support our nursing interventions and care modalities. In the future all of our clinical standards and guidelines for practice should be grounded in scientific data. Support or the refutation of our nursing care interventions is necessary if we are to move neonatal and infant care to a higher level. When we can state that our practice base is grounded in scientific evidence, we will be in a stronger position to effectively collaborate with our physician colleagues who claim their practice base is more credible than ours. This statement is not meant to imply a competition with another discipline but rather that nurses support the need for "gold standards" in our care just as medicine does. We strive to base our clinical judgments on our expert knowledge and our scientific findings to provide the highest quality health care possible.

SUMMARY

Health care can be systematically improved through evidence-based practice. A number of groups provide credible evidence summaries on a variety of topics and offer conclusions about state of the science. The nurse can access these valuable summaries of clinical knowledge as a crucial part of moving research into practice.

REFERENCES

Guyatt G, Rennie D (2002). *Users' guides to the medical literature: essentials of evidence-based clinical practice*. Chicago: American Medical Association.

Ledbetter CA, Stevens KR (2000). Basics of evidence-based practice part 2: unscrambling the terms and processes. *Seminars in perioperative nursing*, 9, 3, 98-104.

Mulrow C (1994). Rationale for systematic reviews. *British medical journal*, 309, 597-599.

Sackett DL et al (2000). *Evidence-based medicine: how to practice and teach EBM*. Edinburgh: Churchill Livingstone.

Stevens KR, Pugh JA (1999). Evidence-based practice and perioperative nursing. *Seminars in perioperative nursing*, 8(3), 155-159.

Stevens KR (2001). An introduction to evidence-based practice. *Newborn and infant nursing reviews*, 1(1), 6-10.

Stevens KR (2001). ACE Star Model: Cycle of Knowledge Transformation. Available at www.acestar.uthscsa.edu.

CHAPTER 4

LEGAL AND ETHICAL ISSUES OF NEONATAL CARE

KATHLEEN M. DRISCOLL, TANYA SUDIA-ROBINSON

Ethical and legal situations are commonplace in the Neonatal Intensive Care Unit (NICU) today. Use of high technology to get pregnant, support a pregnancy, and finally to maintain a neonate make impossible situations of the past very possible today. The age of viability has decreased to almost midgestation. With genetic breakthroughs, "designer babies", clones, and the fixing of genetic defects in utero or in the NICU all are feasible. Use of stem cells from fetal or cord tissue represent a new horizon of care. This technology is causing more neonates to die after birth rather than in utero. These advances have lead to more ethical and legal dilemmas than ever before. Unfortunately, our ethical dilemmas precede our legal solutions. For the neonatal intensive care unit (NICU), these situations are complex and always increasing.

This chapter will highlight the most common situations that pose ethical or legal dilemmas for neonatal nurses. It will also provide an overview of ethical perspectives and highlight some of the salient ethical issues facing NICU health care providers and the families they serve. More questions than answers will be given; however, the reader will come away with a new sense of awareness of potential problems that may result in ethical or legal issues.

APPROACHES TO ETHICS

Approaches to and examinations of ethical issues vary. In the clinical arena, health care professionals look to applied ethics—a translation and direct application of ethical theories and rules—to provide guidance. This section discusses the more common of those approaches and thus is not all-inclusive. The reader is encouraged to explore ethical theories and models more deeply in ethics texts. All members of the NICU team must become more familiar with these and other perspectives that may further enlighten important ethical discussions and improve care delivery.

PRINCIPLES OF BIOMEDICAL ETHICS

Beauchamp and Childress (1979) introduced the application of four principles for biomedical ethics: beneficence, nonmaleficence, autonomy, and justice. Their selection of these four principles was designed to assist clinicians and others in their examination of the various biomedical issues they face.

Beneficence

The principle of beneficence is based upon performing beneficent acts, or doing good, and a balancing of benefits with risks and costs (Beauchamp & Childress, 2001). This obligates health care professionals to consider their actions in the context of potential risks or harms and the multifaceted costs that can be associated with their actions. Further, a particular treatment or therapy that was beneficial in one patient scenario does not necessarily mean that it will be equally beneficial in all circumstances. Weighing the potential benefits against the potential risks for each patient is necessary. Another important action is to frequently reevaluate the benefits and risks as the patient circumstances fluctuate.

Nonmaleficence

In concert with doing good, the principle of nonmaleficence carries the moral obligation to avoid causing harm to another person (Beauchamp & Childress, 2001). Guided by the Hippocratic oath, physicians and other health care professionals are obligated to help those in their care and not intentionally cause them harm.

The Rule of Double Effect. The rule of double effect (RDE), also referred to as the principle of double effect, holds that one may not do something that is intrinsically wrong to bring about a good end (Beauchamp & Childress, 2001). A classic example to illustrate this involves the administration of increasing amounts of morphine to provide a patient with adequate pain relief. If the patient's respiratory rate is slowed considerably and eventually to the point of cessation of breathing, the patient's death was not the intended outcome of the morphine administration. Rather, the intended or primary outcome was to relieve the patient's pain. In a case such as this, the relief of pain is of greater proportion or intended good than the unintended bad effect or patient's death. To further clarify this line of reasoning, an act that would constitute a wrong if directly administered (e.g., administering morphine with the explicit intent to end the patient's breathing) is an immoral evil if it is the unintended secondary or double effect of an otherwise good or permissible action (e.g., relief of pain).

To summarize, four requirements must be met for an act to be morally justifiable: (1) the act itself must be good or morally neutral; (2) the individual must only intend the good effect;

(3) the bad effect must not serve as the means to the good effect; and (4) the good effect must outweigh the bad effect (Beauchamp & Childress, 2001).

Current Clinical Relevance of the Rule of Double Effect.

Because the RDE focuses on an individual's intention with regard to a specific act, it has recently come under scrutiny regarding its applicability to current clinical ethical issues (Quill & Dresser, 1997). The RDE was intended to justify actions in situations that have clear bad and good effects (Beauchamp & Childress, 2001). The clear good effect in the above example is the relief of pain, whereas the clear bad effect is the cessation of respiration. Beauchamp and Childress (2001) have argued that by applying the RDE, one misses the more pressing question of whether death itself was good or bad for that patient. Thus ethicists such as Beauchamp and Childress (2001) note the limits of RDE in select clinical cases.

Autonomy

The principle of autonomy stresses an obligation to respect the decision-making capacity of persons. Further, it requires "respectful treatment in disclosing information and fostering autonomous decision making" (Beauchamp & Childress, 2001). Although the principle of autonomy obligates the health care provider to respect the patient's preferences, it is not an absolute right. This concept is particularly important in circumstances in which a patient's exercise of autonomy could potentially harm others. For example, if a patient with a highly contagious, deadly disease wants to refuse treatment and thus poses a public health hazard, his or her autonomy will be overridden by other competing moral obligations (e.g., protecting the health of the public).

Justice

The principle of justice is often equated with the concept of fairness (Rawls, 1971). In health care, the principle of justice provides a basis for the fair distribution of benefits, risks, and costs, as they exist in a particular scenario. Although many theoretical perspectives of justice exist, this section will address distributive justice.

Distributive justice examines how the needed goods or services should be distributed. The criteria for the distribution of these goods and services may determine each person's share through considerations of need, effort, contribution, merit, and free-market exchange (Beauchamp & Childress, 2001).

Examination of these criteria reveals that conflicts may occur with regard to priorities and the precise meaning of the terms of the criteria. For example, how will any given hospital define *need*? Should it be restricted to essential physiologic need, or could it also refer to need based on quality-of-life factors? These and many other questions require continued examination as they relate to further improving our health care system. It will continue to be important for health care professionals to explore the application of this principle in the NICU.

Use of Principles in the NICU

The following case discussion illustrates how the NICU team can use these four principles. An infant with hypoplastic left heart syndrome is admitted to the NICU. The parents want "everything" done for their infant. The health care team is concerned because in addition to the cardiac anomaly, the infant is only 24 weeks gestation, required vigorous resuscitation in the delivery room, and has coded since being brought to the NICU.

The principle of beneficence requires that the NICU team's actions benefit the infant. Among the questions to be explored are the following:

Will the treatment plan produce a favorable physiologic outcome for the infant?

For how long will the current treatment be beneficial?

What potential short- and long-term harm may occur from this treatment?

What is the cost of the proposed treatment?

Will the infant ever recover from the underlying disease condition that led to the need for this treatment?

What are the infant's chances of survival with this treatment?

What potential complications will arise from this treatment? (Sudia-Robinson, 1998a).

A careful examination of the answers to these and related questions is necessary as the NICU team weighs the potential benefits, harms, costs, and parental preferences for this infant. These questions are only a sample of those that need to be addressed. Other questions that focus on the parent's understanding of their infant's prognosis, the parents' meaning of doing "everything" for their infant, the availability of resources to continue the infant's care, and determinations of whether continued aggressive therapy is truly in this infant's best interest. The parents must be actively involved in the decisions at the level they desire.

ETHICAL THEORIES

Over the past two decades, the health care profession has focused much of its attention on applied ethics—in particular, on principlism. However, many other approaches to ethical inquiry exist, including theoretical models and clinical decision-making models. This section will briefly discuss the more widely known theories, and then the focus will turn to models that can be applied to ethical issues in health care.

Utilitarianism

Utilitarianism is a consequence-based theory, credited to the late seventeenth and early eighteenth century writings of Jeremy Bentham and John Stuart Mill. Utilitarianism focuses solely on the principle of utility (Beauchaump & Childress, 2001). From this theoretical perspective, one's course of action in any given circumstance focuses on maximization of utility or goodness. The challenge is to discover the greatest good by balancing the interests of all affected persons. As with other theoretical perspectives, utilitarianism has limitations. Depending on the precise circumstances, these limits can include overriding of an individual's rights for the sake of maximal social utility (Beauchamp & Childress, 2001). For example, the autonomy of parents could be overridden in a request for continuing care for their very ill neonate if the costs became too excessive. The social utility would take precedence over the individual's rights in this case. A related concern with this perspective is that the majority-consensus approach to defining utility can override the opinion of minority voices (Beauchamp & Childress, 2001). For example, parents of extremely premature infants could be considered a minority voice in the health care arena. Under the utilitarian approach to allocation, the distribution of health care dollars would go wherever it was felt to maximize utility—in this case to the sector of health care with the greatest number of patients with the most curable disease processes rather than to the infants in the NICU.

Kantianism

Kantianism is based on the mid-seventeenth century writings of Immanuel Kant. Also referred to as *deontology*, it is an obligation-based theory. Kant professed that individuals must act "not only in accordance with but for the sake of obligation" (Beauchamp & Childress, 2001). Kantianism stresses the moral imperative that individuals must always be viewed as an end and as such cannot be used as a means to an end. An example of the Kantian perspective could focus on a child who needs a bone marrow transplant. Testing indicates that this child's teenaged sibling is the best match; however, the sibling does not want to undergo bone marrow donation. Strict adherence to the Kantian perspective would prohibit the parents from forcing the adolescent to serve as the donor because that would make the adolescent merely a means (supplier of bone marrow) to the end (younger sibling's treatment and possibly cure).

One of the concerns with Kantianism is the inability to adequately address conflicting obligations (Beauchamp & Childress, 2001). For example, the parent of an infant in the NICU may have another child at home that requires specialized care. The parent has obligations to both and yet cannot possibly care for these children simultaneously. The theory does not provide guidance for how one could meet two competing obligations such as these.

Liberal Individualism

Liberal individualism is a rights-based theory that illuminates both the positive and negative rights of individuals. Positive rights focus on another's obligation to do something for the individual. For example, when a woman arrives at an Emergency Room in active labor, the health care team has an obligation to provide care for her. On the other hand, a negative right protects an individual from receiving unwanted treatment. For example, a patient who has been diagnosed with stage-4 carcinoma has a right to refuse further testing and treatment. Furthermore, a negative right prevents any care provider from performing surgery without explicit informed consent, except in a true emergency in which consent cannot be obtained). The rights discussed here are binding unless competing legal rights or moral obligations override these rights (Beauchamp & Childress, 2001).

A CASE ANALYSIS MODEL

Jonsen et al (1998) offer a case analysis approach to clinical ethics that focuses on four topics: medical indications, patient preferences, quality of life, and contextual features. This approach to case analysis provides an organizing framework for discussion and helps to illuminate pertinent ethical issues. A discussion of these four areas of focus follows.

Medical Indications

The medical indications section incorporates a discussion of the patient's history along with his or her diagnosis and prognosis. Also discussed are the treatment goals and probabilities for successful outcome. An important feature of this section is the discussion of how the patient will benefit from the medical and nursing care and how the health care team will avoid harming the patient (Jonsen et al, 1998).

Patient Preferences

Ascertaining patient preferences focuses on respect for the patient's autonomy. The gathering of data focuses on the patient's values and perspective of potential benefits and harms. In the NICU, the health care team assesses parental preferences for their infant's care and the parents' understanding of the risks and benefits.

Quality of Life

This section addresses the patient's quality of life by examining the potential physical, mental, and social deficits that might occur with the proposed treatment plan. The health care team is challenged to examine questions such as whether the patient would want to continue living in light of his or her condition or prognosis and whether any biases prejudice the provider's evaluation of the patient's quality of life (Jonsen et al, 1998). In the NICU, examining these and related questions provides additional insight into the parents' preferences and helps the NICU team consider their own perspectives and recognize potential biases.

Contextual Features

Examining the contextual features of a case provides an opportunity to consider the complexity of the patient's situation. Areas to be discussed include religious and cultural factors, financial and economic factors, legal implications of treatment decisions, provider or institutional conflicts of interest, and other family issues (Jonsen et al, 1998).

Proceeding to Resolution

After data for all four topical areas have been gathered, the next step is examination of the facts of the case. Additional questions may arise from this discussion, and additional data may be needed. Resultant discussion should focus on the convergence of facts and resolution of the issues that surface.

REST'S FOUR-COMPONENT MODEL

Rest (1979, 1986) developed a four-component model that outlines the processes necessary for ethical behavior. The components are moral sensitivity, moral reasoning, moral commitment, and moral character. This model has been used in studies of moral reasoning in nursing (Duckett et al, 1997; Olsen, 2001; Shuman et al, 1992; Wilson, 1995) and moral reasoning among medical students (Bishop & Wagner, 1997). Moral development in various professions also has been explored (Rest & Narvaez, 1994).

Moral Sensitivity

The first component of the model addresses the individual's sensitivity or recognition of a moral issue. Among the questions that could be asked in the NICU setting are whether the health care provider recognizes the ethical issue in the scenario and whether the health care provider perceives that he or she needs to further process and work through the situation to take action. For example, a nurse overhears two mothers talking at an infant's bedside. The first mother states, "We're in that study too . . . don't really know what they are doing . . . but, you know, you got to do it if you want the best for your baby."

Does the NICU nurse perceive any potential ethical issues inherent in this conversation?

Moral Reasoning

The next component or level is that of moral reasoning. Moral reasoning refers to the ability to develop an ethically appropriate course of action. The health care professional must also be able to articulate a justification for the ethical course of action they would recommend. To continue with the example of the two mothers discussing a study in the NICU, the nurse at this point would need to decide what to do and why. For example, the nurse may believe that the first mother does not have an adequate understanding of the research study. One course of action would be giving the mother a brochure about the study and telling her why the infant needs to be in the study. A more appropriate course of action would be to think about ethical principles and frameworks for analysis. The nurse should question whether informed consent actually occurred and whether the parents really want the proposed treatment plan for their infant. The nurse might then decide that a conference should be scheduled with the research team, or the nurse might recognize that both a significant knowledge gap and evidence of diminished autonomy or parental authority exist for both of these mothers. The nurse must then decide how to proceed.

Moral Motivation and Commitment

This component of the model emphasizes the commitment to an action plan. The nurse must decide to prioritize the moral values that exist alongside other competing values. In our example, the nurse would develop the plan of action for contacting the involved team members.

Moral Character

The moral character component of the model requires the actual implementation of the course of action. That action may require overcoming barriers or obstacles. For example, the nurse may contact a member of the research team who might tell the nurse that in his or her opinion the parents originally had and continue to have an adequate understanding of the proposed treatment plan. The nurse would then need to have the moral courage and perseverance to continue to try to act in the perceived best interests of these parents. Such action will not always be easy and may require a substantial amount of time and energy.

The necessary action in some cases may involve needed policy changes. It is important to note that, depending on the complexity of the issue, the nurse may not always be in a position to act alone. Many organizational and hierarchical aspects may bar direct action. An impasse may arise, at which point the nurse would need to determine alternate courses of action and gather additional support from other team members.

THE PRIMACY OF CARING

Benner (1996) contributes a unique nursing perspective to the ethics literature in her discussion of the primacy of caring. Benner (1996) examined everyday encounters of nurses and describes the ethical perspective as one of care, responsiveness, and responsibility. This "skilled know-how of relating to others in ways that are respectful, responsive, and supportive of their concerns" (Benner, 1996) is regarded as ethical comportment.

By attending to these aspects of relationships with patients and families, the nurse is able to view situations in ways that enhance understanding.

Benner (1996) identifies many types of narratives and what they teach the nurse about engagement with families. These narratives include how nurses learn the skill of involvement with patients and families (e.g., involvement and distance), narratives of disillusionment (e.g., limits of technology, ethical breaches), and narratives about death and suffering (Benner, 1996). Use of Benner's narratives (1984, 1996) in concert with the array of ethical perspectives can provide additional lenses from which to view the everyday ethical tensions that arise in the NICU.

ETHICS CONSULTATION

At times of impasse or perceived conflicts between members of the health care team and/or family members, an ethics consultation may be an appropriate course of action. Ethics consultations can be initiated by any member of the health care team or by the infant's parents. The specifics of case consultation will vary by institution. The essential features of an ethics case consultation include the request for consultation, identification of the problem or issues, review of the medical record, individual interviews with the parents and the involved NICU and other professional staff, facilitation of discussion of the case with the ethics committee, preparation of recommendations and follow-up as needed with involved persons (La Puma & Schiedermayer, 1994).

Ideally, an ethics consultation can improve the communication between everyone involved in the case, including the parents or other surrogate decision maker. Ethics consultations will be most beneficial when an ethicisit is on call, when all members of the health care team and of the family can initiate a consult, and when all individuals involved in the case are notified that a consult has been requested (Mitchell & Truog, 2000).

ETHICAL UNCERTAINTY AND THE MORAL IMPERATIVE FOR PARENTAL INVOLVEMENT

The NICU is an environment in which varying degrees of prognostic uncertainty exist. However, that uncertainty cannot become a barrier to discussion or disclosure of information, for "dealing with uncertainty is unquestionably the most difficult decisional task of medicine; yet it too is a task that is best shared with those for whom the decision matters most" (King, 1992).

Parents are legally and morally responsible for the health care of their infants. Health care professionals are also bound by professional codes of ethics to act in the best interests of those entrusted to their care. Furthermore, a developing body of literature focuses on the importance of parental involvement in decisions about the care of their infants in the NICU (Harrison, 1993; Jakobi et al, 1993; Pinch & Spielman, 1993, 1996; Raines, 1996; Stinson & Stinson, 1979; Sudia-Robinson, 1998b, 1999; Zaner & Bliton, 1991). Thus because both parents and NICU professionals have ethical obligations to do good for ill infants, it can be argued that an ethical imperative for them to collaborate in direct clinical decision making exists (Harrison, 1986, 1993; Jakobi et al, 1993; Penticuff, 1987, 1988).

Parents as Equal Partners

For parents to be adequately involved in the decision-making process, they must be recognized as equal partners or team members who bring a specialized expertise to the bedside. That unique expertise is the unconditional love for the child and their desire to ensure the child's well-being. It can be further argued that no one else on the team could better represent the child's best interest than the parents; thus the parents should be included in all discussions about their child's care. Additionally, the American Academy of Pediatrics (AAP) stresses that parents should be active participants in the decision-making process for their critically ill infants (AAP, 1996). This statement acknowledges that the parents may have a different perspective about what is right for their children.

To adequately engage parents in a collaborative manner, they must be respected for the expertise they possess. Traditionally, the NICU team members will discuss a proposed plan of care, weigh the risks and benefits, and determine a course of action. That course of action is arguably their responsibility. However, when the team then presents this plan to the parents, they usually engage in a one-way transfer of information rather than a dialogue.

A Collaborative Model

In an ideal collaborative model, the team members provide an opportunity for parents to weigh the potential risks and benefits of a given treatment plan prior to proceeding. The health care professionals would ensure that they render their thinking transparent to the parents (King, 1992). That is, they must explain their thought processes and how they reached the recommended plan of treatment. Parents should understand what compelled the team to choose path A over path B (King, 1992). This approach stresses the importance of not just sharing information with parents, but rather helping them to understand what their child's condition *means*.

Once parents can understand how to think about their children's conditions, they are better equipped to ask the necessary questions for their ongoing understanding and participation in the decision-making process. Parents would also be better prepared to interject their preferences so that alternate course of action can be considered as necessary. These suggestions and this advocacy for improved collaboration are not intended to diminish the roles or responsibilities of any member of the health care team. Rather, they are offered in an attempt to strengthen the relationship between the parents and the team. Although not all parents will be able to or will want to be as fully engaged as others, it seems prudent to advocate for mechanisms that will further empower parents to assume their rightful role.

ETHICAL ISSUES IN THE NICU

Countless ethical issues arise in the NICU. Among the more salient issues are pain management, futile treatments, home care of the technology-dependent infant, the allocation of resources, and infants as research participants. Ethical issues of pain management are discussed in chapters 9 and 42. The following section highlights these issues and offers additional challenges for NICU professionals.

Futility and Extreme Prematurity

Extremely premature infants (i.e., those born after fewer than 28 weeks gestation and with birth weights less than 750 grams)

account for 13,702 live annual births in the United States (CDC, 1995). These infants require neonatal intensive care for mechanical ventilation and other life-sustaining treatments. Infants born at the edge of viability and extremely premature raise ethical questions. These questions relate to quality of life and use of scare resources. The most immature and smallest of these infants have the highest likelihood of death within the first few days of life (Meadow & Reimshisel, 1996), and the survival rate for infants born at 23 weeks gestation is only 27% (Cooper et al, 1998). For infants who weigh 550 grams or less at birth, statistics indicate that fewer than 15% will survive (Lemons et al, 2001). The ethical questions consider whether the cost of survival is justifiable both the family and to society.

A mortality rate of nearly 85% is disconcerting and raises many ethical questions about the aggressiveness of care. Even infants with birth weights between 501 and 750 grams, a reported 40% to 50% mortality rate remains (Lemons et al, 2001). Additionally, continuing evidence suggests that most of the infants born at or before 25 weeks gestation will have neurologic and developmental disabilities (Lorenz et al, 1998; Wood et al, 2000).

Defining Futility.   Futility in the NICU has been defined in the recent literature (Penticuff, 1998; Pierce, 1998), yet continuing controversies (Avery, 1998) and complex moral issues have prevented the formation of a consensus regarding the precise point at which life-sustaining therapies become excessive (AAP, 1996). However, when a treatment cannot offer the patient direct benefit, health care providers are not ethically obligated to provide that treatment (Beauchamp & Childress, 2001).

Skilled Transitional Care.   Once it has been determined that continuing aggressive therapies is no longer in the infant's best interest, the NICU must be able to smoothly transition to palliative care. This is a skill that too few health care teams possess.

Brody et al (1997) identified the need for health care professionals to become skilled in the transition of care delivery from intensive life-support to end-of-life (EOL) care in those situations in which aggressive therapies have proven futile. When health care professionals lack training in the clinical aspects of withdrawing intensive life support, they could continue aggressive treatment beyond the point at which families would prefer to stop (Brody et al, 1997). Brody et al (1997) also identified concern about cessation of treatment in an unskilled manner, which may produce distressing patient symptoms that result in a negative experience for the patient, family and health care professionals. Although the focus of the Brody et al (1997) study was the adult ICU, compelling argument for the development of similar professional skill in neonatal EOL care exists.

Home Care of Technology-Dependent Infants

Only a decade ago, considering the home a suitable intensive care unit was a rare and fleeting thought that was used in few cases. Today, it is more the expectation than the exception. However, health care professionals and society in general may not have reached full acceptance and adequate accommodation of intensive home care. Many issues from caring for technology-dependent infants in the home (Kirk, 1998).

Parental Preparation. Despite our best efforts, can we ever *really* prepare parents for the change of their home into an intensive care unit? Should parents be told that although only one or two of their rooms may be designated the ICU, the entire house will be affected? Is it possible to explain the complete loss of privacy that will occur during the hours the home health nurses and therapists visit the home? Can they possibly be prepared for this type of parenthood?

Parental Challenges. Parents of infants who are technology-dependent face many challenges, including burden of care, lack of resources, and an uncertain future. Initially, parents are likely to receive support from friends and neighbors who are all interested in helping them through a difficult time. However, this necessary additional support will not last indefinitely. Friends and neighbors have experience in helping each other through difficult times and can pull together to provide dinner, babysitting, and assistance with running errands for a few weeks or months. Eventually, however, friends and neighbors will be seen less often as they refocus on their own families and responsibilities.

The impact of the responsibility of caring for a technology-dependent infant may not set in until weeks or months after the infant's discharge. The parents will struggle with competing demands for their resources and time (Sudia-Robinson, 1998b). The infant's siblings will strive for extra attention, yet their parents will struggle to be able to provide it. Often the amount of skilled nursing time is not sufficient for the mother to return to work if she needs to do so (Chapter 46).

Nursing Challenge. Issues about technological care in the home are ongoing. Neonatal nurses who provide in-home care can attest to the struggles that many families face. Exceptional models of homecare are needed to meet the comprehensive needs these families face. Attention is also needed in the policy arena to ensure that these families are not forgotten and that they are among those receive our special attention.

Allocation of Resources

The NICU continues to be one of the most expensive units in a hospital (Rogowski, 1998). The reimbursement standard, or DRG allotment, typically has been as low as one-sixth of the actual hospitalization costs (Tyson et al, 1996). Actual expenditures for a single infant in an NICU can exceed $600,000 (Stolz & McCormick, 1998). As health care costs continue to escalate and care intensifies, examining options for pairing resources with desirable outcomes becomes necessary (Sudia-Robinson, 1999b).

Few in the health care profession feel comfortable discussing the costs of care and resultant considerations for prioritizing care. A rising concern among some practitioners in the field is the potential for overuse of technology when the probability for successful outcome falls below 20% to 30% (Sudia-Robinson, 1999b). Concerns about needless suffering and engendering a false sense of hope may leave some with questions about the appropriateness of care in select situations in the NICU. Tyson et al (1996) express concern about extensive treatment for extremely premature neonates:

> Without mechanical ventilation, the most immature infants generally die shortly after birth. Mechanical ventilation can make the outcome worse—death after days to months of distress, or, for a small proportion of survivors, morbidity so severe that many parents consider it worse than death.

It seems inevitable that decisions regarding allocation of resources within the NICU will need to take precedence over other concerns. These discussions will best occur with many diverse voices representing various points of view all present at the table. Some of these discussions have begun to appear in the literature. Kliegman (1995) has advocated for a redirection of resources from extensive high-tech care for all to reducing the risks for prematurity and low birth weight. This line of thinking contends that medicine, nursing, and the best technology cannot eradicate the complex consequences of extreme prematurity. Researchers have noted that although the advent of surfactant therapy has increased chances of survival for those with extremely premature lungs, a simultaneously dramatic reduction in intraventricular hemorrhage or other significant sequelae has not occurred (Kliegman, 1995).

Among the voices for reforming health care are those who are concerned that too much money is spent in various intensive care settings on those who have the least likely chances of survival. For example, Daniels et al (1996) summarize description of fairness in health care:

> Fairness is at issue when health care dollars are spent in ways that do not produce health benefits. Those wasted resources will leave some people with unmet medical needs, or they may force us to spend money from elsewhere in our social budgets, leaving others with unmet educational or housing needs (Daniels et al, 1996)

An important closing comment on the examination of resource allocation is that nurses and other health care professionals must continue to strive for care that most directly meets the needs of those they serve. This may mean that some individuals need intensive palliative care rather than the current high-tech care for all models. No infant or family should ever receive less than our best care, but we must recognize that care is multi-faceted and that different emphases may be appropriate in different situations.

Infants as Research Participants

As health care moves toward evidence-based practice, research studies are becoming increasingly prevalent in NICUs. Many types of studies, ranging from interventional studies that test a drug or device to descriptive studies that use parent surveys to obtain information about their perspective of care, exist. Some studies will require more astute scrutiny from neonatal nurses than others. Some of the more pressing research issues include real or perceived pressure to participate and the balance of advances in knowledge that may not benefit the current participant but will likely benefit future infants.

Pressure to Participate. Parents of critically ill neonates may feel pressure to participate in research studies for their infants, regardless of whether this pressure is real or perceived. They may believe that these studies are the only way to ensure that their infants receive the best possible care. Nurses are often asked to witness the signing of research consent forms and are thus in a strategic position to observe behaviors or statements that may cause one to question the voluntary nature of their agreement. A parent may be afraid to decline participation, even if this is presented as a clear option. Thus if nurses sense at the time of consent—or, even more importantly, at a later time—that the parents felt pressured to participate, they can intervene on the parents' behalf. This may involve talking to the parents themselves or requesting that the study's principal investigator talk to the family about their decision.

Benefit to Future Infants.   Research in health care is designed to benefit future patients through the knowledge gained from the current participants. This is a critical point that is sometimes lost in the common perception that the research protocol represents a higher level of care. Indeed, sometimes individuals in a study will derive some direct benefits; however, they may also bear the burdens of the research without any significant benefit. This occurs because studies are designed with the concept of clinical equipoise, or the premise that the experts in the field do not know which treatment arm of the study is actually the best. The study's results will provide that answer.

The notion that one should volunteer for something that may cause some harm—and that furthermore that may not provide any benefit—seems at odds with the societal perception that whatever is new is usually better. Thus parents' understanding that no guarantee for success exists when they enroll their infants in studies—especially for Phase I clinical trials (which involve initial human dose testing)—is critical. The treatment being tested may be better, worse, or no different than the current standard of care. Nurses, physicians, and others involved in research in the NICU have a responsibility to ensure that the science of their disciplines is advanced but also must adequately explain to parents that no inherent pressure to participate exists.

SUMMARY OF ETHICAL ISSUES

This discussion of ethical issues has addressed some of the morally relevant issues for the care of neonates in the NICU and their families. Neonatal nursing has come of age with a display of superb clinical knowledge and skill in one of the most technologically advanced areas of health care. Neonatal nurses are recognized as collaborative team members who act in the best interests of infants and their families.

The current challenge for nurses is to become increasingly skilled in forming ethical arguments based on solid ethical foundations (ANA, 2001; Chinn, 2001) so that they can more effectively advocate for those in their care. Neonatal nurses have a rich history of dedicated care and advocacy. Thus it is crucial for neonatal nurses to continue to actively participate in discussions about the many pressing ethical issues that will shape future care delivered in their units.

LEGAL ISSUES IN NEONATAL CARE

Four decades ago, nurses in newborn care settings depended largely on vision and intuition as tools of assessment; technology in the newborn unit consisted of nasogastric tube feedings, an occasional intravenous infusion, and monitoring infant response to oxygen levels. Nursing policy and procedure manuals listed the "right way" to carry out nursing activities. Following the policy manual meant meeting the standard of care. In the 1960s, no risk management director existed because the risk of institutional financial loss through a malpractice suit was practically nonexistent. Two reasons for this lack exist—health care consumers viewed health care providers as doing their best for the consumer's benefit, and hospitals were generally insulated from law suits under the doctrine of charitable immunity. Nursing interventions were not identified, much less sub-

jected to scrutiny through measurement of the outcomes of care for the infant and the family.

Law was considered a societal institution that had little to do with nursing as a profession. One exception was periodic licensure renewal—a reminder to nurses that a law governed the scope of their practice. Prelicensure curricula, graduate programs, and continuing education programs did not address legal aspects of nursing practice.

Today, however, nurses must realize the potential for legal challenge to their practice through negligence or malpractice litigation. This discussion will focus first on the legal elements of negligence; sources for nursing standards of care; the process of litigation, including the role of the expert witness; risk management, emphasizing communication and documentation; and the counterparts of risk management, quality assurance, and improvement.

Litigation is not limited to negligence suits; wrongful birth and wrongful life litigation have arisen. The law also examines perinatal and neonatal intensive care nursing as a matter of social policy. The law as social policy addresses decision making about issues such as the use of life-sustaining measures, research, organ transplantation, drug abuse by expectant mothers, managed care, and the licensure and certification of nurse practitioners. Most recently the federal government has set guidelines for the privacy of patient records (HHS Fact Sheet: Protecting the Privacy of Patient Information). Expected in the future are specific regulations for addressing genetic privacy. Thus law acts as both a dispute resolution mechanism and as a social policy tool. Law consists of case, statutory, and regulatory laws. Each type of law balances competing perspectives to establish guidelines for relationships among individuals and groups in a society. The concept of law as a dispute resolution mechanism is the central theme of the first part of this section. The concept of law as a social policy tool will be addressed later in the chapter.

LAW AS A DISPUTE RESOLUTION MECHANISM

Elements of Negligence

In law, a negligence suit may be brought when careless—as opposed to intentional—acts or omissions of an individual bring about harm to a person to whom one has a duty of care. For example, a driver can be successfully sued under the legal theory of negligence if he or she carelessly proceeds through a stop sign, collides with another vehicle, and causes damage to the vehicle and injury to its occupants. The driver has violated his or her duty of care and caused injury. The four legal elements necessary to prove negligence are present in this situation. They are (1) duty, (2) breach of duty, (3) injury, and (4) causation. Litigation results when the presence of these elements is disputed. The process of litigation is an attempt by plaintiff and defendant to persuade a disinterested third party—a judge or a jury—to believe a particular version of the facts. The plaintiff seeks monetary damages; the defendant seeks exoneration.

In a negligence suit brought against a nurse in neonatal practice, the plaintiffs must show that the nurse owed the neonate a duty of care. Demonstration of employment by a health care facility, assignment to the NICU, and provision of direct or even supervisory care to the particular infant establishes the nurse's duty of care. The plaintiff must then show breach of that duty of care. Evidence of deviation from the expected standard of care through an action or omission of care establishes breach of duty. Violation of the standard of care must then be causally tied or connected to the actual injury. This connection is more difficult to demonstrate. For example, it may be difficult to prove that an already brain-damaged infant suffered additional damage as a result of deviation from the expected standard of care during a cardiac arrest. It is important to recognize that injury must always occur to prove negligence. Medication errors that result in no harm to an infant eliminate the possibility of legal liability in a negligence suit.

Malpractice Versus Negligence.   Malpractice is professional negligence. The law uses the term malpractice to describe negligence by individuals who violate a standard of care that can be known only by virtue of education in a field. Negligence that is not malpractice violates a standard of care that a lay person would know. Because neonatal nursing is a specialized area of practice, it would be rare for a nurse to deviate from the standard of care in such a way that a lay jury could understand the deviation without some explanation. Lay persons do not readily understand the implications of medication errors, equipment misuse, and fluid and oxygen administration misjudgments. However, a lay person would not need an expert witness to explain that leaving a side rail down on the crib of a normal 3-month-old child is a negligent act. Thus nurses can be simply negligent or be professionally negligent.

Statutes of Limitations.   Statutes of limitations set time frames during which certain legal actions must be brought. The purpose of the statutes is to prevent stale claims—that is, claims that have lost their credibility because information bases and persons knowledgeable about events are long removed from the event that precipitated the suit. The statutory time frames are intended to provide sufficient time for plaintiffs to discover injuries and bring suit while assuring potential defendants that they are not at risk forever. Statutes of limitations vary from state to state.

Statutes of limitations may be extended for cases that involve newborns because in many states the law has recognized that an injustice may occur if parents do not bring an action on behalf of their child during the usual statutory time frame. The remedy for this potential injustice is to permit the affected individuals themselves to bring actions on their own behalf within the ordinary statutory time frame after they reach the age of majority. For example, a child injured as a result of breach of the standard of care in a NICU might have until the age of 18 years plus the usual statutory time frame for bringing an action. Nurses in neonatal practice should be aware of the time frames for legal law suits for the states in which they practice.

Professional Liability Insurance.   Two types of professional liability coverage exist: claims-made coverage and occurrence coverage. Claims-made coverage pays damages only for claims brought during the period in which the policy is in force. Thus any claim in negligence brought during the policy period, even if the event occurred many years in the past, is covered. Occurrence coverage provides for claims brought many years after the precipitating event has occurred, even though the nurse no longer carries professional liability insurance.

Occurrence policies are advantageous to the nurse because continuing insurance coverage after ceasing to work or upon retirement is unnecessary. Nurses should examine their professional liability policies to determine whether coverage is the claims-made or occurrence type. If coverage is the claims-made type, nurses who leave the field should make arrangements to purchase a tail policy. The neonatal nurse should continue coverage through the duration of the statute of limitations.

The wise nurse maintains personal coverage even in the employ of a facility that would pay a claim (i.e., indemnify the nurse). Nursing actions outside of employment can give rise to litigation. The nurse that independently contracts with a facility—for example, a nurse who acts as a consultant—should carry personal professional liability insurance. The remote possibility that damages awarded might exceed facility policy limits, in which case the plaintiff could then tap the nurse's personal assets.

Personal professional liability insurance insulates the nurse from loss of personal possessions through negligence or malpractice suits. However, nurses should know that professional liability insurance does not insulate their assets from intentional acts. A nurse who defames a parent, threatens a parent, or deliberately harms an infant is not protected. This lack of protection is the case even if criminal charges have not been upheld before a civil suit is brought.

Standard of Care.   The nurse can positively channel the anxiety associated with fear of potential legal liability by increasing focus on professional accountability. Accountable professionals practice prudently and reasonably based on their education and experience. Knowing and practicing nursing according to current standards helps ensure that a legal challenge to one's practice can be successfully defended.

Box 4-1 defines professional accountability as "carrying out the nursing process." Legal accountability is then defined by giving a positive orientation to the legal elements of negligence. Nursing documentation provides evidence of both professional accountability and legal accountability.

The nurse can look to various sources to determine the relevant standard of care. The American Nurses' Association (ANA) uses the nursing process as a generic approach to guide nursing decision making for its clinical standards of practice. An attorney who represents a plaintiff wants to know whether the nurse assessed the infant's status, planned and carried out care, evaluated that care, and made appropriate revisions. Box 4-1 takes this approach to accountability. The current standards of practice also include professional performance stan-

---

BOX 4-1

Relationship of Professional and Legal Accountability

Professional Accountability		Legal Accountability
	D	
	O	
	C	
	U	
Assessment	M	Duty
Planning	E	Fulfilled
Implementation	N	Causes
Evaluation	T	Benefits
Revision	A	
	T	
	I	
	O	
	N	

dards that include accountability and ethical standards (American Nurses' Association, 1999).

Specialty professional associations may provide more specific guidelines to nurses in the neonatal area. These guidelines are updated by professional consensus mechanisms based on changing knowledge in the field. The National Association for Neonatal Nurses (NANN) has a series of standards in the form of guidelines. The association has chosen to write the guidelines in an instructional format with questions that address understandings critical to application of the knowledge in practice at the end. Examples of these guidelines include discharge guidelines for technology-dependent infants, early discharge guidelines for the term newborn, and guidelines for peripherally inserted central catheters (PICC). NANN position statements take a stand on nursing practice concerns. For NANN, these include pain management in infants, cultural diversity, and latex allergy. The practicing nurse is responsible for being aware of changing standards nationally, not just locally. The development and widespread distribution of guidelines in neonatal care set by professional associations are among the influences that have led states to recognize standards of care as being national rather than local in origin.

The internet provides ready accessibility to professional standards that affect perinatal care, such as those of the American Academy of Pediatrics (AAP) and the American College of Obstetricians and Gynecologists (ACOG) by simply typing in the name and searching for the organizations' web sites. Evidenced-based practice as standard of care derives from reports of research and outcome studies that are reported in professional journals. Standards also derive from the national facility accreditation standards set by the Joint Commission on Accreditation of Healthcare Organizations (JCAHO). Attending continuing education programs in the specialty area, referring to recognized texts when questions about care arise, and keeping abreast of state licensing standards are other methods of obtaining current information about standards of care.

Licensure and Certification.   Certification in one's specialty is a measure of specialty knowledge (Stanley & Bednash, 1998). Levels of certification are emerging. The baccalaureate degree is required for some recognition of specialty area expertise, and the master's degree is required for advanced practice roles. For individual practitioners, the National Certification Corporation (NCC) acts as the certification agency for neonatal nurses. The NCC also accredits neonatal nurse practitioner programs (Stanley & Bednash, 1998). Unlike in the medical profession, the advent of advanced practice nursing has led to the state board of nursing regulation of specialty practitioner, rather than strictly professional group (Anderson, 1999). In most states, advanced practice nursing licensure requires professional certification. Threats by the National Council of State Boards of Nursing (NCSBN) led certifying bodies to develop advanced practice examinations and to upgrade the quality or to demonstrate the soundness of their certification examinations (Stanley & Bednash, 1998).

Health care institutions have a corporate duty of care (Darling v. Charleston Community Memorial Hospital, 1966). One responsibility is ensuring conditions of employment that permit achievement of the expected standard of care in areas like NICUs. Plaintiffs will examine hospital policy and procedure to determine whether they reflect current standards of care. An example of a standard that must be met is ensuring that all staff understands the function and operation of new equipment.

Standards should be considered general guidelines to practice. Also important, however, is that any nurse be able to defend any action or inaction in relation to care of the neonate as reasonable and prudent. This defense means that the nurse must not only be able to identify what is regarded as the current general standard of care but also must have a rationale for decision making that adjusts care to the specific individual. For example, the general standard of practice may be to administer certain fluids at specific rates depending on the weight and maturity of the infant. This general standard does not excuse the nurse from failing to adjust the rate downward—even halting fluid administration—and seeking consultation in the event that the infant begins to show signs of fluid overload.

Changing Nursing Care Delivery Standards of Care.   The redesign of nursing care delivery systems to include the use of unlicensed assistive personnel (UAP) to perform nursing has led to concerns about patient safety. Boards of nursing may have specific rules regarding delegation of care. For example, Ohio created delegation rules under the statutory authority of Section 4723-13 of its nurse practice act. It is imperative for nurses to be aware that although tasks can be delegated, accountability cannot be delegated (Yoder-Wise, 1999).

Before delegating care to UAP, the nurse must be aware of the education and experience of the UAP. To ensure appropriate delegation, facilities are responsible for developing policies and procedures to ensure transmission of this vital information to staff nurses. Facilities should retain records of UAP education in respect to both content and competency, as in the Ohio Board of Nursing delegation rules. The nurse must keep in mind that he or she cannot delegate patient assessment. In other words, the nurse cannot delegate the judgment calls for changing nursing care plans and collaborating with other providers.

Consistency in patient care teams is one positive management approach. Consistent teams have knowledge of each member's strengths and weaknesses and can adjust for these differences to ensure patient safety. Cross-trained personnel from other units should be used with discretion because they disrupt team consistency and pose potential risks to patient safety.

At the national level, the ANA has called for nurses to advocate in alerting the public to unsafe staffing conditions (American Nurses' Association, 1995a). Concurrently, the ANA has called for an increasing focus on quality-of-care research (American Nurses' Association, 1995b).

Steps in the Litigation Process.   The steps of the litigation process are listed in Box 4-2. The first component of a malpractice suit is a dissatisfied person—either a parent, guardian or, as indicated previously, the neonate who has now achieved the age of majority. The dissatisfied person consults an attorney, who usually seeks the advice of an expert in the field to determine whether the plaintiff has sufficient cause to initiate a suit. The attorney will obtain the consent of the client to get copies of the patient's records for the expert's review.

Medical records are admissible in evidence as the business records of the health care facility. Records are presumed to be a true record of events. Evidence that records have been tampered with immediately raises questions about the credibility of the defendant facility and any nurse involved.

If the presence of the legal elements of negligence can be ascertained from a reading of the records, the attorney files a

---

BOX 4-2

Steps in the Litigation Process

Patient, guardian, parent believes the patient has been harmed by caregiver(s)
Consultation with attorney
Review of records by expert witness
Lawsuit initiated
Period of discovery
Settlement or trial
If trial, verdict
Possible appeal of verdict

---

complaint in the appropriate court of law. Simultaneously, the attorney serves the defendant—or sometimes multiple defendants—with copies of the complaint. The defendant provider or facility notifies its insurance carrier of the suit. The carrier notifies its defense law firm of the need for an answer to the complaint. Response must occur within a time period specified by the rules of civil procedure. An answer offers the opportunity to state a defense to the action or offer a motion to dismiss. If a motion to dismiss the complaint has accompanied the defendant's answer, the plaintiff will defend against the motion.

If the lawsuit moves forward, attorneys for both sides will seek to find out more about the circumstances surrounding the case in a process called discovery. Discovery consists of gathering information from both parties—for example, information about the injury or harm suffered by the plaintiff and about the standard of care in the defendant institution. Further scrutiny of the medical records will occur. This gathering of information may be accomplished through written questions—called interrogatories—to both parties and by obtaining depositions from persons involved in care and from expert witnesses.

The discovery period has several purposes. The process helps both lawyers and parties involved to prepare for trial. Discovery may lead to settlement. Facts may unfold that clearly favor either the plaintiff or the defendant. The favored party may move for a summary judgment. Settlement of a lawsuit can occur at any time before a trial or even during a trial. A trial is a formal process used to present a case to a judge or jury that includes testimony from fact and expert witnesses and actuaries in regard to damages. Motions for directed verdicts can end litigation if, following presentation of evidence, a party views the evidence as favorable to his or her case. In rare instances, the judge may even reverse a jury's judgment.

Verdicts may be appealed. Appellate courts generally defer to trial courts on matters of fact because appellate courts deal only with the written transcripts of a trial. Appellate court judges lack the benefit of observing the nonverbal communication of a trial witness. Thus a person who appeals on the weight of the evidence has a heavy burden to bear. Appellate courts generally rule on issues of law, such as whether the trial judge instructed the jury correctly as to the application of the law.

In trials, judges are responsible for the application of the law—hence the importance of their instruction to juries—and juries are responsible for applying the facts. Although parties in civil cases have a right to a jury trial, in some instances agreement may be reached to try a case before a judge alone. The judge then rules on both the law and the facts. In the legal

world, movements are afoot to use alternatives to this adversarial process as dispute resolution mechanisms. No-fault schemes for birth-related neurological injury are in place in Florida and Virginia (Studdert & Brennan, 2001). Other approaches include arbitration, mediation, and therapeutic jurisprudence.

Expert Witnesses. Expert witnesses supply opinions about the standard of practice in similar situations. They differ from witnesses of fact who supply "presence at the scene" knowledge—actual knowledge of the particular set of circumstances that led to litigation. The expert witness' knowledge of the particular facts is limited to a reading of the medical record. The more clearly the record reveals that the nurse practiced according to the standards of care current at the time of the situation in question, the more beneficial the expert witness can be to the nurse's defense. Nurses that act as expert witnesses must have practice experience and be knowledgeable about the practice area. Juries have discretion in the weight they accord the evidence provided by an expert witness.

Testifying as an expert witness for the defendant offers the opportunity to act as an advocate for the nurse who is arguably not negligent. Testifying as an expert witness for the plaintiff offers the opportunity to act as an advocate for the harmed person. Testifying as an expert witness also affords the opportunity to act as an advocate for society. This occurs when the expert, upon reviewing a record, determines that negligence has not occurred. In such an instance, the forthright report of the expert prevents the misuse of societal resources—namely, the court system.

A nurse who acts as an expert witness is entitled to charge for the service. The nurse should expect to be prepared by the attorney for deposition or trial. Preparation includes discussion about the line of questioning to be expected from attorneys for both sides and strategies for establishing credibility as a witness. Strategies include remaining calm despite the opposing attorney's attempt to shake the nurse's self-confidence, asking that ambiguous questions be repeated, answering only what is asked, and acknowledging the jury's presence both by looking at the jury and by using language that the jury can understand.

Management of Risk

The nurse in the NICU is at risk for lawsuit in a number of areas but can take measures to reduce exposure to this risk. Areas of particular concern are assessment, medication and fluid administration, equipment use, resuscitation, oxygen administration, and discharge planning with parents.

Individual Nursing Practice and Management of Risk. The 2000 Institute of Medicine Report on quality of care raised concerns of both providers and consumers of health care about safety in the delivery of health care. Leape (2001) noted that the figures of 44,000 to 98,000 annual deaths are disconcerting. More startling is the fact that nonfatal injuries may exceed one million. Health consumers experienced "affront and betrayal" from the health care providers in whom they had placed "a profound and personal trust" (Leape, 2001). Sound systems design can reduce the risk of many errors resulting in injury or death. Latham (2001) called for recognition that individual responsibility cannot be overlooked in the rush to blame systems. The content of the report, its context for consumers, and the need for individual professional accountability for care as well as accountability in systems of care is the message of the following paragraphs.

As the caregiver closest to the neonate, the nurse is best positioned to make and act on observations that reflect an abnormality in the neonate's system functions. The nurse reduces risk when he or she promptly records deviations and takes and records appropriate actions, such as the content of communication that occurs between caregivers and family of the neonate and consultation the nurse has with more experienced nurses, the nurse manager, a clinical specialist or neonatal nurse practitioner, and the responsible physician. Meticulous documentation maintains the professional accountability that deters litigation. Communication and documentation are the hallmarks of professional practice. Risk management literature indicates that the value of communication as a risk management tool cannot be overemphasized.

Nurses should take care that when following protocols they do not fail to take into consideration infant responses that are not covered by the protocol. "Cookbook" responses, to the extent that they are "by the book" rather than thoughtful reactions, are not good practice. For example, nurses are obligated to raise questions with the infant care team when they suspect that a new drug may be causing adverse reactions. This type of teamwork can lead to the timely withdrawal of a drug from the market. The withdrawal of the vitamin-E preparation E-Ferol is an example (Schorr, 1984).

The nurse must have sufficient working knowledge of equipment operation to recognize equipment malfunction. The nurse should leave the repair of malfunctions to trained persons. Faulty equipment altered by hospital personnel to make it work voids the manufacturer's strict liability for a defective product when an infant is harmed by equipment. Moreover, equipment must be used as directed by the manufacturer for its stated purpose. Equipment used for reasons other than its intended purpose makes the institution, rather than the manufacturer, liable for any infant harm attributed to the equipment's use.

Resuscitation events require careful documentation of both the sequence of events that precipitated resuscitation efforts and the sequence of interventions that occur during those resuscitation efforts. Assigning an individual to document the sequence of resuscitation efforts is critical to establishing the standard of care that was followed should questions later arise. Similarly, oxygen support for infants requires meticulous documentation to demonstrate that oxygen levels were commensurate with need and finely tuned to the infant's developmental stage.

As care patterns move infants home quickly, nurses become more vulnerable to law suits rooted in communication failure. Parents who have not adequately understood and practiced complicated technologic care—and even basic care, such as breastfeeding—may bring suit if their child suffers harm because of their lack of understanding or ability to provide care. Clear documentation of teaching that includes evidence of parent understanding, practice opportunities, written instructions to take home, and access to a nurse for questions decrease litigation risk. Interventions that reflect new professional thought or a more conservative standard of care than usual deserve a notation indicating their rationale. This is true for both nurse and physician progress notes.

The best documentation occurs concurrently or immediately following nursing actions. Practically speaking, however, notes may be written a few hours subsequent to nursing care events. Observations might, for example, be charted immediately on a checklist form, but narrative notes might be written later. Attorneys understand that this is the reality of nursing practice. Insertion of information some time subsequent to the shift on which an event has occurred also takes place. Such additions, known as late entries, although not ideal, may be acceptable. Late entries should be clearly identified as such in the medical record. If a long period of time lapses before the entry is made, it is appropriate to indicate briefly the reason for the delay (i.e., "first day back after 3 days off"). The reality is that late entries are often viewed with suspicion by the plaintiff's counsel. The underlying reason for acceptance of this practice is that it is better to have pertinent data that is admissible as evidence. If not present in the record, data may be inadmissible as evidence because the person who reports an event may not have actually witnessed the occurrence. Such information would be termed hearsay because of the witness's lack of firsthand knowledge. By precluding hearsay as evidence, legal procedure acknowledges that the truth is best known by a person who was at the scene of an event.

As the business record of the health care facility, the medical record is the enduring evidence of the activities of assessment, planning, implementation, and evaluation of the neonate's care. Documentation is the legal evidence of professional accountability. Assessments, interventions, evaluations and reevaluations, and communications not documented are presumed not to have occurred. Without documentation, the nurse who asserts at deposition or trial that an activity occurred can expect a deserved assault on his or her credibility.

Adverse Events. When adverse events occur, prompt corrective measures, followed by truthful explanations of the occurrence by the caregivers increase the parents' respect for the caregiver and ward off or provide a favorable climate for settlement should litigation occur. On discovery of an adverse event, the nurse should institute measures to remedy or minimize the harm. Institutions may absorb the cost of care for the extra procedures to treat the consequent condition. These two steps can minimize the actual monetary damages suffered by the neonate and the neonate's family. A forthright explanation to the family about the event and corrective actions that have been taken then serves to dispel the commonly held perception that caregivers cover up their errors. For example, failure to discover immediately the incorrect placement of a chest tube because of a delay in obtaining an x-ray film to check its location can result in severe compromise of the infant. Use of truth telling as a risk management tool would involve explanation of the error to the family. The health care facility would also absorb the costs of the second placement and any additional care required because of the error.

Incident or variance reports describe occurrences that pose a risk of harm or actual harm to patients and that risk monetary loss for a health care facility. Incident reports include both adverse events (in which actual harm occurs) and events in which potential for harm exists but actual harm (injury) does not occur. Malfunctioning equipment that has the potential for—but may not yet have caused—injury is a good example of the type of information included in the potential risk category, as is consistent failure to communicate or respond to communication in a timely manner about changes in patient status by nurses and other caregivers. Incident reports are not limited to the neonate; they include family, visitors, and staff. Even a highly effective risk management program cannot achieve zero risk, but incident reports afford facility staff and management the opportunity to identify areas of actual and potential risk so that steps can be taken to reduce such risk by changing practices or altering the environment.

Incident reporting is an aspect of the nurse's ethical obligation to provide safe care (American Nurses' Association, 1984, 1999, 2001). In the process of fulfilling this professional ethical obligation, the nurse also fulfills the obligation to the facility to assist it in meeting its corporate legal duty to provide a safe environment.

Incident reports that involve neonates should mirror descriptions found in the medical record by reporting the facts and the steps taken to assess and alleviate any actual injury. Conclusory or blaming statements should not be included in the report. Incident reporting systems should require professionals not only to disclose their own mistakes but also to report those of peers. The filing of an incident report should not be mentioned in the record because incident reports are not patient care documents and do not belong in the medical record.

A risk management maxim is that the incident reporting system should be separate from the system for nursing staff evaluation. Incident reports are administrative tools that provide the opportunity for adjustments to systems involved in delivering care to enhance the safety of patients, visitors, and staff. The incident reporting system itself should afford the opportunity for those involved to discuss the incident at the unit level as a health care delivery team. Occasion for discussion should provide opportunities to suggest strategies for avoiding similar incidents in the future. Staff evaluation, in contrast, focuses on the individual rather than on the system. The perception that incident reports are used for staff evaluation rather than system change may deter the completion of incident reports, thus reducing their effectiveness as a risk management tool. However, a series of incident reports involving one nurse and separate types of errors or multiple instances of the same type of error cannot be ignored in a performance review. Ignoring patterns of incidents is to potentially fail to deal with incompetent practice. Addressing incompetent practice is a professional obligation incurred according to the codes of nursing ethics of both 1984 and 2001 (American Nurses Association, 1984, 2001). Furthermore, failure to address incompetence puts health care facilities in the position of potentially being charged with failing to fulfill its corporate duty of care to staff with competent nurses. Thus although good reason exists for keeping the incident-reporting system and staff evaluation systems parallel, it would be poor corporate practice to make their separation a policy with no exceptions.

Incident reports allow management to take appropriate corrective actions to reduce risks and serve the useful purpose of prompting an immediate investigation following the occurrence of an incident, when memories are still fresh and the facts surrounding the incident are likely to be reported accurately. Should a lawsuit ensue, this timely follow-up can be valuable in preparing a case. The incident-reporting and claims-investigation process may be regarded as the workproduct of the defense and thus be immune from plaintiff scrutiny during the discovery period.

Accessibility of the incident report to the plaintiff's attorney does, however, vary from state to state and even from circumstance to circumstance. Sharing an incident report can be viewed as disadvantageous to the defendant because the plaintiff's attorney will attempt to show that the incident report was filed solely in anticipation of a lawsuit rather than for effective risk management. Conversely, when incident reports are subject to the discovery rule, they can also serve to enhance the credibility of the defendant when facts on incident report and medical record match.

Quality Programs. Quality assurance and improvement and total quality management programs can be considered the proactive counterpart of risk management efforts. Patient satisfaction surveys are a measure of quality. Rather than measure actual clinical care, however, they focus on environmental conditions such as waiting times and staff courtesy. Today the focus is on outcomes of care and measurable indicators in a process called continuous quality improvement. The Joint Commission on Accreditation of Health Care Organizations (JCAHO) looks for continuous quality improvement in its accreditation process.

A focus on outcomes of care generates new standards of care. Plaintiff's attorneys in the future will ask their expert witnesses in what percentage of cases a positive outcome could be expected in a given situation.

SOCIAL AND PUBLIC POLICY CONCERNS IN PERINATAL CARE

Decision-Making Infant Care

Treatment decisions are different for children than for adults. Infants in particular have no experience with life, so they cannot speak for themselves in relation to choice of treatment. Parents, as the natural guardians of children, are presumed to act in the child's best interests in making choices about treatment. Nurses and health care providers should assist parents in the decision-making process by providing appropriate and timely information. Unfortunately, providers sometimes may personally be at ethical or clinical odds with parental choices. This situation can and has generated legal action. Situations that give rise to legal action generally involve choice of treatment or the use of life-sustaining measures and the informed consent process. Informed consent is sought for invasive procedures and for other interventions that carry potential for serious risks to materialize as well as benefits to occur. Treatments that are within the usual course of care—such as measurement of weight, feeding, bathing, and observation of physiologic systems function—are part of the general consent to care signed by parents on the infant's admission to a health care facility. This section first reviews the formal consent procedure. It then discusses the use of life-sustaining measures for infants and focuses on the evolution of law in response to the Baby Doe cases.

Informed Consent. Neonates sometimes require surgical intervention (to correct defects), invasive diagnostic procedures, and invasive treatment procedures. Physicians or nurse practitioners may also suggest new interventions or interventions that are still part of a research protocol. The nurse has a legal role in the informed consent process; the legal role is generally limited to witnessing the consent form signed by the parents or legal guardian of the infant. By law, the responsibility for obtaining informed consent for treatments belongs to the physician or the researcher. In fact, the physician or researcher should witness the signing of the consent form if feasible. This practice has the advantage of placing the parents and physician together at a time when discussion regarding care could take place. Thus the nurse is not legally responsible for ascertaining whether the parents' consent is truly informed. However, the nurse is ethically responsible.

The physician must share information about the procedure to be undertaken, who will do the procedure, its benefits and risks, and alternatives to the procedure—including no treatment—must be shared with the consenting persons. Ethically, the physician should explain interventions so that the decision makers are rationally persuaded to agreement. Rational persuasion occurs when the decision maker arrives at the same conclusion as the advisor but bases the decision on the acceptance of reasoning presented by the advisor and when that reasoning concurs with the value system of the decision maker. With rational persuasion, the decision maker feels free to make a truly personal choice. This approach differs from manipulation, which occurs when the decision maker simply assumes the values of the physician and follows the physician's suggestion. Rational persuasion also differs from coercion, which occurs when the decision maker feels subjugated to the physician and powerless to choose. When coercion occurs, the decision maker keeps his or her own value system but goes along with the physician because he or she feels compelled to do so.

Although the nurse does not have a legal duty to obtain informed consent, the nurse can play an important risk management role by participating in the conference with the family in which the physician discusses treatment. Participation in the conference places the nurse in a position to clarify or amplify the family's understanding of the procedure when they have had time to reflect on—and possibly become confused about—the physician's explanations. Knowledge of the informed consent conversation also assists the nurse in supporting the family in their choices—that is, playing an advocate role, even when those choices may differ from the sincere and well-meaning recommendations of physicians. The nurse is never in a position to legally initiate medical recommendations or to comment on medical prognoses. When parents or other surrogate decision makers exhibit concern about prognoses, the nurse needs to reinvolve the physician in the consent process. Medical recommendations or discussion of prognoses by the nurse could easily become the basis of charges of practicing medicine without a license.

Obtaining informed consent is a process; lack of informed consent can cause a malpractice action. The occurrence of an undisclosed material risk—a risk that could cause reasonable decision makers to refuse the procedure—can result in lawsuit. Flores v. Flushing Hospital and Medical Center (1985) is a case in point. The family in that case was not told that the risks of providing oxygen to the premature neonate included blindness. They later sued both hospital and physicians. The outcome was a baby who was declared blind.

Legal Legacy of Baby Doe.   When withholding or withdrawing care from a disabled newborn becomes an issue, social policy introduces further constraint on the decision maker. A 1982 case precipitated public outcry against the parents' decision to forego treatment for their newborn who had Down's syndrome and esophageal fistula (Indiana *ex rel.* Infant Doe v. Monroe Circuit Court, 1982). Nutrition and treatment was withheld, and the child died. At the direction of then President Ronald Reagan, the Secretary of the Department of Health and Human Services (DHHS) notified hospitals that federal law prohibited discrimination on the basis of disability under the Rehabilitation Act of 1973. About a year later, the DHHS issued regulations titled "Interim Final Rules," or "Baby Doe Regulations." The regulations required the posting in delivery, maternity, pediatric, and nursing units of a notice stating that "Discriminatory failure to feed and care for handicapped infants in this facility is prohibited by federal law" (48 Federal Register 9630, 1983). The regulation contained instructions for any citizen to call a DHHS hotline if he or she knew of any severely defective newborn being denied food or customary medical care on the basis of a disability. This provision was particularly offensive to the health care provider community because the notice was required to be posted in places where the public would see it. The regulations were subsequently challenged and defeated because the procedure for promulgating regulations had not been followed (AAP v. Heckler, 1983). A later set of rules was also defeated with a court finding that Congress had never intended the Rehabilitation Act to apply to medical decisions affecting defective newborns (Bowen v. American Hospital Association, 1986).

In the midst of the legal controversy surrounding the federal regulations, Congress in 1984 chose to amend the Child Abuse Prevention and Treatment Act. Rules enacted under the amendment expanded the definition of child abuse to include "withholding medically indicated treatment" as "the . . . failure to respond to the infant's life-threatening conditions by providing treatment (including appropriate nutrition, hydration, and medication) which in the treating physician's or physicians' reasonable medical judgments will be most likely to be effective in ameliorating or correcting conditions" (45 Code of Federal Regulations S 1340.15 (b) (2), 1985). The rules reflected the balance in the Child Abuse Act Amendments "between the need for an effective program and the need to prevent unreasonable governmental intrusion" (49 Federal Register 14,879, 1984).

The Child Abuse Amendments tie federal funding to implementation of procedures designed to prevent instances of medical neglect, including withholding medically indicated treatment. The rules promulgated under the Child Abuse Amendments stress that infant care review committees are permissive rather than mandatory. Right-to-life constituencies are assured that decisions regarding treatment are not based on quality-of-life criteria.

The Child Abuse Amendments exempt three categories of infants from their provisions. These are reflected in the rules and include the following:

> when, in the treating physician's or physicians' reasonable medical judgment, (A) the infant is chronically and irreversibly comatose; (B) the provision of such treatment would (i) merely prolong dying, (ii) not be effective in ameliorating or correcting all of the infant's life-threatening conditions, or (iii) otherwise be futile in terms of survival of the infant; or (C) the provision of such treatment would be virtually futile in terms of survival of the infant and the treatment itself under the circumstances would be inhumane. (45 Code of Federal Regulations S 1340.15 (b) (2), 1985)

Under no circumstances is it permissible to withhold appropriate nutrition, hydration, and medication.

Brown and associates (1986) note these rules: (1) clarify when life-sustaining treatment may be withheld from a defective newborn; (2) affirm the parents or guardians as decision makers; (3) clarify the standard for decision makers; and (4) clarify the standard for decision making as the best interests of the infant. The gray area of decision making that remains for health care providers to determine is the term futility. Futility is defined as a situation in which the outcome seems without hope. It unfortunately is a very subjective determination. Judgments calls will differ as to when treatment is futile. The potential for differing judgment calls on futility are one reason to have a hospital ethics committee available as a source for consultation. In determining futility, collaborative decision making is more likely to lead to a judgment call that will not result in feelings of ethical comfort for all but more often than not will achieve consensus as to the most agreeable approach to resolving the dilemma.

Concerns about the use of life-sustaining measures with infants continue. Fairfax Hospital in Virginia requested a declaratory judgment that withholding a ventilator from an anencephalic infant when the infant suffered respiratory distress would not violate state or federal law. Both federal district and circuit courts found withholding the ventilator support would violate the Emergency Medical Treatment and Active Labor Treatment Act (1986) (*In the Matter of Baby K*, 1993; *In the Matter of Baby K*, 1994; Capron, 1994). The Supreme Court declined to hear the case. With ventilator support used when needed, the child lived to be 2½ years old.

In another case (Baby Ryan, cited in Capron [1995]), when parents sought a court order for life support for what physicians considered a futile situation, the hospital countered with a child abuse complaint against the parents. The child lived.

Treatment decisions are not made lightly; for every treatment issue reaching a court, many more issues are resolved through negotiation (Spielman, 1995). The occasional court decision simply adds to the framework within which those individual negotiations occur.

Research on Infants and Children

Nurses may find themselves conducting or participating in research conducted on neonates. Federal law establishes criteria for conduct of research on children according to varying degrees of risk (45 Code of Federal Regulations S 46.404-46.407, 1983). Familiarity with the provision of regulations guiding research is critical to the nurse who assumes an advocacy role for the child.

The four categories of risk are listed in Box 4-3.

The regulations in all four categories call for assent of children capable of participating in the decision-making process, with consent coming from parents or guardians. Clearly, assent does not apply to neonates. The second category, greater than minimal risk with possible benefit to subjects, requires that the risk be justified by the anticipated benefit and that the anticipated benefit be at least as favorable to the subjects as the available alternatives are. The third category, greater than minimal risk with no prospect of direct benefit, is approvable if (1) the

risk is only a minor increase over minimal risk; (2) the intervention presents experiences commensurate with what the subjects might experience in their actual or expected medical, dental, psychological, social, or educational situations; and (3) the intervention is likely to yield generalizable knowledge of vital importance for the understanding or amelioration of the subject's disorder or condition. Before approval of the fourth category of research, the Secretary of the DHHS must consult with a panel of experts and afford opportunity for public review. Following this review procedure, the research must satisfy either the conditions for the first three categories of risk or (1) be determined to present a reasonable opportunity of further understanding, prevention, or alleviation of a serious problem affecting the health or welfare of children (the category purpose); (2) be conducted in accordance with sound ethical principles; and (3) fulfill the necessary consent requirements.

Had the federal research regulations been in place in 1953, the infant plaintiff in a New York case might not have had cause to bring a lawsuit (Burton v. Brooklyn Doctors Hospital, 1982). Burton was born 2 days after the beginning of a national study known as the Cooperative Study of Retrolental Fibroplasia and the Use of Oxygen. The infant (Burton) was in good condition, and a resident physician later reduced initial higher oxygen levels. Later, however, another resident physician drastically increased the oxygen level as part of Burtons' random assignment in the study. The assignment of the infant to increased oxygen levels in his "good condition" was ethically questionable. Although retinopathy of prematurity might be regarded as a "serious problem affecting the health and welfare of children," one might argue that present requirements for review of the study by a panel of experts as well as public review might have resulted in a modification of the study design to exclude infants in "good condition." Of course, one might also argue from a justice or utilitarian perspective that the time involved in the current review process might have resulted in more infants suffering injury because dissemination of study results would have occurred later than 1954. In this case, however, the plaintiff recovered damages because the court found that the informed consent of the parents for oxygen administration should have been obtained because the treating physician's own study revealed that increased oxygen was dangerous for a healthy infant. Administration of the oxygen exposed the child to an unwarranted risk.

Only federally funded research falls under the law. However, most institutional review boards (IRBs) apply federal regulations to all research projects conducted within the institution. The IRBs review research proposals to ensure protection for human subjects under the regulations. Nurses working in institutions in which the review of human subjects does not apply to privately funded research may consider acting as advocates for children when research would violate the ethical tenets of the federal regulations. Nurse researchers who sit on IRBs bring the voice of the profession to board deliberations.

Organ Donation for Neonates

Infants often could benefit from whole-organ transplants. Unfortunately, the availability of suitable organs for infants is even more limited than it is for adults. One approach to resolving the scarcity has been using anencephalic infants as donors. Waiting until the natural death of the anencephalic infant precludes using organs for transplant because in the process of dying, vital oxygen delivery and blood flow to organs are increasingly compromised, which results in organ damage.

BOX 4-3

Categories of Risk for Research with Children

1. Research not involving greater than minimal risk
2. Research with greater than minimal risk but representing the prospect of direct benefit to individual subjects
3. Research involving greater than minimal risk and no prospect of direct benefit to individual subjects
4. Research not otherwise approvable that presents an opportunity to understand, prevent, or alleviate a serious problem that affects the health or welfare of children

What then are the legal vehicles that might be used for anencephalic donors, and what ethical problems do such donations raise? One legal approach is the use of a state's Anatomical Gift Act. All states have passed this type of legislation. These acts permit living adult donors to elect to donate one of a paired organ. The acts also provide for an individual to designate organ donation on his or her driver's license in the event of death. Amendments that permit parents to act as decision makers regarding donation of their anencephalic child's organs might be made to these acts. This approach avoids the larger societal concerns, raised by another approach—that is, amending acts that define death by adding a new category of anencephalic infant. Physiologically, anencephalic infants do not meet the criteria for brain death because brain stem function exists and therefore mechanical support for breathing via a respirator is generally unnecessary.

The development of brain death statutes actually originated with the need for transplantable organs as successful organ transplantation became a reality. Nonetheless, societal consensus does not exist to broaden brain death definitions; this lack of consensus is primarily because right-to-life groups would argue that the definition of anencephalic infants and persons who are in persistent vegetative states as "brain dead" may lead to societal condoning of euthanasia. The Baby K case mentioned earlier in relationship to the Baby Doe regulations illustrates the reluctance of two federal courts to begin forging such a trail.

Paliokas (1989) suggested that statutes should be specifically tailored to deal with anencephaly. Statutory safeguards against abuse would include (1) guidelines for establishing accurate diagnosis, (2) voluntary choice by the parents before birth, (3) review of each situation and the parental decision by a panel of legal and health professionals, and (4) court review when parents and panel body disagree. Policy statements in the statutes would emphasize their purpose as preservation of the child's dignity through minimization of any extraordinary medical interventions that simply prolong the dying process. In this respect, they would mirror current law, the Child Abuse amendments of 1986.

Capron (1987) discussed ethical problems associated with both approaches. First, amending anatomical gift or definition of death acts may set a poor precedent because similarly situated persons—the comatose, demented, or severely retarded—might also then be considered as sources for the harvest of organs. Second, if the rationale for the use of anencephalic infants is that they are non-persons because they will never be able to interact meaningfully with other persons, one might then destroy an anencephalic infant without being charged with homicide. In contrast, if anencephalic infants are recognized as persons, is it right to use one person as a means to save the life of another? This approach violates Kantian ethical principles, which do not permit the use of persons as a means to an end.

Capron suggested that the better alternative, in the ethical and legal sense, is to maintain both anatomical gift acts and definition of death statutes in their current form. He proposed that the medical profession work toward achieving approaches to maintaining anencephalic infant organs in a state viable for transplant when death eventually occurs.

Nurses working in NICUs should discuss these ethical and legal issues. Discussion and resultant understandings will put neonatal nurses in better positions to support not only the parents of a dying anencephalic infant but also those parents who wish to donate their anencephalic infant's organs and who are precluded from doing so by the current state of the law.

Litigation Surrounding Pregnancy

Nurses working in NICUs should be aware of wrongful pregnancy, wrongful birth, and wrongful life lawsuits. Nurses may need to support parents who feel wronged when negligently performed sterilization surgery results in a pregnancy or when parents are uninformed of infant defects that might have resulted in their electing abortion. In all instances, families face financial damage.

Courts have denied wrongful pregnancy claims on policy grounds, arguing that allowing the cause of action would generate fraudulent claims (Rieck v. Medical Protective Co. of Fort Wayne, Ind., 1974). Other courts have allowed damages for emotional distress of the mother, loss of consortium (loss of the companionship and services of husband and wife in marriage), and hospital and medical expenses associated with the pregnancy (Boone v. Mullendore, 1982). Most courts have denied costs of raising the healthy child on the basis that the child provides emotional benefit to the parents. This benefit rule, strictly followed, requires that the court ascribe a value to the benefit of having a child against the financial damage suffered by the family as the result of his or her birth (Restatement of Torts 2d, S 920, 1991). Massachusetts and Wisconsin high courts have permitted costs for raising a healthy child (Burke v. Rivo, 1990; Marciniak v. Lundborg, 1990).

Wrongful birth actions occur when the parents of a severely defective infant allege that the opportunity to choose to terminate or continue the pregnancy was lost because the physician failed to advise the parent of risk of defect or the means (genetic counseling or amniocentesis) available to determine potential or actual defects. In a 1979 case, Berman v. Allan, parents of a child with Down's syndrome alleged that the obstetrician had not met the standard of care because of a failure to alert the 38-year-old woman of the availability of amniocentesis. Parents recovered damages for mental and emotional anguish but did not recover the cost of child rearing. The court saw the disabled child as still being a benefit to the parents, and therefore the obstetrician was not found liable to the parents for child-rearing expenses.

In wrongful life lawsuits, the affected child seeks compensation for the burdens of a life that would not have been desired had a choice been available. Courts are reluctant to classify actions as "wrongful life" for two reasons: (1) no fundamental right to be born normal and whole exists; and (2) comparing life with the nonlife that the plaintiff claims would have been preferable is problematic (Becker v. Schwartz & Park v. Chessin, 1978; Elliott v. Brown, 1978). In California, Washington, and New Jersey, courts have resolved these difficulties by awarding the child only special damages—the cost of special care—rather than general damages that include pain and suffering. The courts have reasoned that special damages are congruent with what parents might recover in wrongful birth actions and that the actual injured party should not be in a lesser position than the parents for receiving damage awards. Courts have viewed denial of damages for pain and suffering as consistent with the difficulty of determining the value of nonlife over life with disabilities (Harbeson v. Parke-Davis, 1983; Procancik v. Cillo, 1984; Turpin v. Sortini, 1982).

Ohio courts do not award damages in wrongful life cases; consistent with previous case law, the Ohio Supreme Court recently refused to recognize the claim of a child born with spina bifida for damages. Instead, the court noted that a case in negligence on the part of the physicians who failed to inform the mother during her pregnancy of test results that indicated a possibility the child would be born with defects could be successfully pleaded only by the mother because the physicians' negligence was in no way causally connected to the child's spina bifida. In a dissent, one justice suggested the Ohio Supreme Court would have had more information on which to base a decision had it allowed the case to go to trial. He speculated that, for the child, a proper claim might be negligent infliction of emotional distress because of the difficulty of living with such a disability (Hester v. Dwivedi, 2000). As perinatal interventions improve—for example, intrauterine treatment of spina bifida—physicians must be increasingly alert to notifying patients of potential birth defects.

Nurses working in perinatal care may see potential plaintiffs in all these categories. The extension of compensation for wrongful pregnancy and wrongful birth to parents and sometimes to children affirms in law society's concern for the cost of raising disabled children and the mental and financial distress to parents and their other children caused by physician failure to adhere to the standard of care.

Perinatal Maternal Substance Abuse

Treatment. Concerns about infants suffering ill effects as a result of maternal drug abuse continue. Nurses should be aware of the legal issues raised by suggestions that the definition of child abuse be extended to include fetal abuse or that the substance-using mother be viewed as a criminal guilty of delivering drugs to a minor.

Until recently, however, the law has been satisfied to find women who abuse drugs during pregnancy in violation of child protective laws only. A common practice has been to wait until the child is born and then immediately move for child protective agencies to assume custody. Child protective laws generally do not involve criminal charges. Their policy goal is reunification of families. The law directs that this be achieved through development and implementation of reunification plans that call for the development of parental skills and, in the case of substance-abusing parents, successful completion of drug rehabilitation programs. A South Carolina court found legal authority lacking for a child abuse and neglect charge against a mother who used cocaine while pregnant. The court noted that in passing the law, the legislature did not intend to include "fetus" in the definition of "child" (Tolliver v. South Carolina, 1992).

Prosecutors have tried to bring criminal charges against drug-abusing pregnant women. The women have been charged under a number of criminal statutes: delivering cocaine to a newborn child through the umbilical cord, involuntary manslaughter, and criminal neglect. Jennifer Johnson, who was charged with delivering drugs to her child during the period after delivery and before the umbilical cord was cut, was found guilty by lower Florida courts (Key case on pregnant women and drug abuse going to trial, 1991). The Florida Supreme Court overturned the decision (Jos et al, 1995).

How does the law look at the fetus? An Ohio lower court case has chronicled the typical evolution of state law in response to this question (In re Ruiz, 1986). Common law, or case law, had for centuries recognized live birth as the prerequisite for legal protection. In the middle of the twentieth century, however, negligence law recognized separate recovery in damages for the child when a viable unborn child was injured

prenatally and was born alive (Williams v. Marion Rapid Transit, Inc., 1949). Ohio law and other states' laws later recognized not only negligence but also wrongful death actions for injuries suffered in utero if the child was born alive and later died (Jasinsky v. Potts, 1950). Stidam v. Ashmore (1959) extended this right to a wrongful death action even if a viable fetus was later stillborn. In the Ruiz case, the mother used drugs during pregnancy, and the issue was whether the unborn fetus might be considered a child under the child abuse statute. The court found that the state had a "compelling interest" in the welfare of children at the point of viability under Roe v. Wade (1973) and that therefore the child abuse and neglect statutes should apply. The potential deprivation of liberty for the defendant has led courts to defer to legislatures the task of defining the viable fetus as the victim under criminal law.

Jos and colleagues (1995) reported the development of an institutional policy at the Medical University of South Carolina that threatened criminal sanction if drug-abusing pregnant women failed to seek drug counseling and prenatal care. The policy applied only to women who attended university clinics—not to private obstetrical patients. In September 1994, the university discontinued the policy after encountering multiple legal difficulties. Dropping the policy was the condition of settlement in a suit brought by the Civil Rights Division of the DHHS. Several women who were jailed under the policy have brought a class action lawsuit. In addition, the Federal Office of Protection from Research Risks deemed the policy experimentation to have been conducted without IRB approval and therefore deferred renewal of the University's Multiple Project Assurance for at least 1 year. The results in this situation illustrated the wisdom of broad-based consultation before moving forward with controversial policy. In this case, the university surely never anticipated that such a policy would result in loss of research funding.

The Illinois legislature has criminalized drug abuse under its child protective legislation. The legislative response occurred when a prosecutor dropped involuntary manslaughter charges against a drug-abusing mother because case law that supported the charges was insufficient. The legislative response was to make the state's Child Abuse Act applicable to newborns. More specifically, the Illinois Infant Neglect and Controlled Substances Act of 1989 makes it a felony to "inflict or create a substantial risk of physical injury to a newborn infant by means of illegal drug use by the mother during pregnancy" (Curriden, 1990).

In general, those who support criminalization of prenatal substance abuse prefer to accomplish this under child protective statutes. They argue that this does not preclude the development of social policy supportive of substance abuse education and wider availability of drug abuse treatment centers to pregnant women. On the other side, however, are those who argue that, despite the symbiotic relationship of fetus and mother, the woman's right to choose her individual personal behaviors should be legally inviolate. According to this viewpoint, any attempt to criminalize a woman's behavior during pregnancy would be a violation of her fundamental rights. Beyond legalism and on a more practical level, opponents of criminalization argue that any threat of prosecution discourages substance abusers from seeking prenatal care and from providing accurate information to health care providers. Like their counterparts who support criminalization, advocates for women's rights suggest that the moral and proper approach is to increase the availability of health care services to pregnant women—including access to drug abuse treatment—in general. The American Civil Liberties Union (ACLU) and the American Public Health Association (APHA) take the women's rights approach. Jos and colleagues (1995) noted that the American Medical Association (AMA), the American Academy of Pediatrics (AAP), the American College of Obstetrics and Gynecology (ACOG), the American Society of Addiction Medicine (ASAM), and the American Nurses' Association (ANA) find criminal sanction inconsistent with the role of the health care provider as caregiver.

Research. In addition to questions of how the law should treat the substance-abusing mother, how the law should protect research subjects who participate in drug and alcohol abuse studies is another question. Generally, the nurse researcher must separate the research role from the clinician role. However, in studying maternal drug and alcohol abuse, a potential legal and ethical conflict arises when the researcher must decide whether the confidentiality of the research relationship overrides the nurse's obligation to report child abuse and neglect.

From a legal perspective, the answer is that "it depends." In 1988, Congress legislated confidentiality protection in section 301(d) of the Public Health Service Act (1988). Although researchers generally are ethically required to protect confidentiality, the act provides specific protection from being compelled to identify subjects in any federal, state, or local civil, criminal, administrative, legislative proceeding or in any other proceeding. Specifically the act provides that the Secretary of the DHHS (2001)

> may authorize persons engaged in biomedical, behavioral, clinical, or other research (including research on mental health as well as on the use and effect of alcohol and other psychoactive drugs) to protect the privacy of individuals who are the subject of such research by withholding from all persons not connected with the conduct of such research the names or other identifying characteristics of such individuals. (Section 301 [d])

Thus if a subject is prosecuted for child abuse, the nurse researcher need not testify that the subject was participating in a study on drug and alcohol abuse. If the researcher is unaware of the circumstances that led to the charges, he or she faces no dilemma. However, what if the nurse researcher's observations of the subject, the children, and the environment lead to a judgment that child neglect or abuse is occurring? Should the researcher regard the child neglect and abuse reporting laws with more weight than the confidentiality protection? The answer is *yes.* Researchers who seek confidentiality protection apply for confidentiality certificates for alcohol and drug abuse research through the National Institute on Alcohol Abuse and Alcoholism (NIAAA) or the National Institute on Drug Abuse (NIDA). For other biomedical research, confidentiality certificates must be sought through the Office of the Assistant Secretary for Health. The coverage and limitations of the certificate of confidentiality should be explained as part of the informed consent process of the research study. Although neither the Public Health Service Act (PHSA) nor regulations based on the act specifically state that reporting laws take precedence, the reporting laws do, in accordance with the DHHS Policy for Communicable Disease Reporting to the Centers for Disease Control and Prevention. The policy requires that in the research informed consent process potential subjects be advised of the child neglect and abuse law's reporting exception

to confidentiality. Furthermore, subjects must understand that confidentiality applies only to those data collected for research purposes. Observations that suggest child neglect or abuse may fall outside the scope of the research data. Overall, when child neglect or abuse becomes a concern, researchers should work cooperatively with local authorities.

When the researcher has both a treatment and research relationship with a subject, care must be taken to keep research and treatment data separate. Research data are reported in the aggregate, or the subject's identity is masked to assure confidentiality. Federal privacy protection applies to records of persons treated for drug and alcohol abuse problems (Comprehensive Alcohol Abuse and Alcoholism Prevention, Treatment and Rehabilitation Act, The Drug Abuse Office and Treatment Act, 1988). Under certain circumstances, information from these records must be revealed. Circumstances include court order, child abuse, medical emergency, or informed consent from the affected person. The researcher must be careful that in reporting research data he or she does not inadvertently disclose protected research data.

The Use of Health Information—The Federal Privacy Rules

In the Health Insurance Portability and Accountability Act (HIPAA) of 1996, Congress gave itself the deadline of August 21, 1999 to pass comprehensive health privacy legislation. Congress viewed the increasing reliance upon the electronic transmission of records as the stimulus for setting a national guideline for privacy standards in health care. When Congress failed to pass privacy legislation, the task fell by law to the rule-making process of the federal government through the DHHS. The final rule was issued December 28, 2000. Because a waiting period for the rules to take effect crossed over from the Clinton to the Bush administration, the rule was held up while the new Secretary of DHHS, Tommy Thompson, allowed 30 days for additional comments. On April 14, 2001 the rule went into effect with the proviso that it would be amended over the next year to clarify requirements and correct potential problems (HHS Fact Sheet: Protecting the Privacy of Patient's Health Information). The rule applies to health plans, health care clearinghouses, and certain health care providers (Federal Register: December 28, 2000). This last includes hospitals. The privacy rules cover health information in any form. The rules give patients more control over their health information, define boundaries for use and release of health care records, establish safeguards that health plans and providers must put into place to achieve privacy, establish accountability through civil and criminal penalties, and provide for exceptions to nondisclosure for purposes of public responsibility (Office of Civil Rights: General Overview). Law—rather than the discretion of the health plan or provider—now mandates that patients will be educated about privacy protections, ensured access to their records, and provided the opportunity to give consent before their information is released. Health information may not be used for purposes not related to health care such as by employers or financial institutions. Disclosure of health information will be limited to what is necessary. Those covered by the rules must develop procedures to safeguard protected information and must train employees and designate a privacy officer. The rules are administered by the DHHS Office of Civil Rights (HHS Fact Sheet: Protecting the Privacy of Patient's Health Information). Important for the perinatal nurse is that consent for release of information is not required for such situations as disclosure of abuse, neglect, or domestic violence, for public health activities, and for workers' compensation (Federal Register, December 28, 2000).

The Stem Cell Debate

Current law does not permit federal funding of stem cell research. Proponents of a change in the law argue that the potential for curing a number of debilitating chronic illnesses supports a change of position on the part of the federal government. In addition, they argue that only government-funded research has the financial capacity and ability to systematically support such a program of research. Because stem cells from fetal tissue have potential to be directed to develop into any cell, they appear to offer the most potential for success in treating illnesses. Other sources such as adult bone marrow and umbilical cord blood are more ethically acceptable to a number of political constituencies but are not susceptible to manipulating to the full range of cell types. The outcome of this debate will affect women treated for infertility who have in vitro fertilization of egg and sperm followed by implantation of only a few of the resulting embryos. Support for use of embryos would allow women to donate the unused embryos for research. This is a clear example of the intertwining of ethical and legal concerns because the center of ethical concern is destroying what many regard as the life of one as a means to enhance the life of another (The Cincinnati Enquirer, 2001).

Political and Legislative Activity

The neonatal nurse must become knowledgeable about the issues that concern the financing and delivery of neonatal care and become involved in proposed solutions. Involvement translates into citizen-nurse action that demands and then supports legislation that strikes a just balance between primary, secondary, and tertiary care needs. Activity in political campaigns, personal and written contacts with federal and state legislators, and testimony at legislative hearings are ways in which nurses can become involved. The nurse's role should not end at the legislative level. State and federal agencies develop rules not only for implementing payment mechanisms but also for guiding the standard of care in neonatal settings. Nurses are free to comment on rules proposed by federal agencies, which are published in the Federal Register, and on state agency rules, which appear in hearing notices published in newspapers and are sent to interested parties. Making sure that political candidates, members of state legislatures, and executive agency staff know that of the advocate's position as a nurse and a member of a professional association in nursing is key to ensuring that political involvement as a citizen is also viewed by those persons as involvement as a nurse.

SUMMARY

Although nurses are obligated to meet the current standard of perinatal nursing care in their own practice settings, they should view their practice in relation to the broader social policy concerns that encompass the delivery of perinatal care. Thus the range of the nurse's professional life should include engaging in the discourse—both in the employment setting and in society at large—about the impact of technologic change and social concerns on nursing education, practice, and research. As technology advances, so will the ethical and legal dilemmas. The best approach for health professionals to arm themselves against such situations is to increase their awareness of dilemmas and develop strategies to address them.

REFERENCES

American Academy of Pediatrics v. Heckler, 561 F. Supp. 395 (D.D.C. 1983).

American Academy of Pediatrics. (1996). Ethics and the care of critically ill infants and children (RE9624). Pediatrics, 98(1), 149-152.

American Nurses' Association (ANA). (1984). Code for nurses with interpretive statements. Washington, DC: ANA.

American Nurses' Association (ANA). (1995a). Nursing report card for acute care settings: A tool for protecting our patients, February 2, 1995. Washington, DC: Author.

American Nurses' Association (ANA). (1995b). Summary of the Lewin-VHI, Inc. Report: Nursing report card for acute care settings, February 2, 1995. Washington, DC: Author.

American Nurses' Association (ANA). (1999). Standards of clinical nursing practice (2nd ed.) Washington, DC: Author.

American Nurses' Association. (2001). The code of ethics for nurses. Retrieved from http://www.nursingworld.org.

Anderson C (1999). Advanced practice roles. In Sullivan EJ (Ed.), Creating nursing's future (pp. 76-81). St Louis: Mosby.

Avery GB (1998). Futility considerations in the neonatal intensive care unit. Seminars in perinatology, 22(3), 216-222.

Beauchamp TL, Childress JF (1979). Principles of biomedical ethics. New York: Oxford University Press.

Beauchamp TL, Childress JF (2001). Principles of biomedical ethics. ed. 5, New York: Oxford University Press.

Becker v. Schwartz and Park v. Chessin, 46 N.Y. 2d 401, 386 N.E. 2d 807 (1978).

Benner P (1984). From novice to expert: excellence and power in clinical nursing practice. Menlo Park, CA: Addison-Wesley.

Benner P et al. (1996). The primacy of caring and the role of experience, narrative and community in clinical and ethical expertise. In Benner P et al (Eds.). Expertise in nursing practice: caring, clinical judgment, and ethics. New York: Springer.

Berman v. Allan, 80 N.J. 421, 404 A.2d 8 (1979).

Bishop J, Wagner J (1997). Moral reasoning in medical students. Journal of general internal medicine, 12(S-1), 88.

Boone v. Mullendore, 416 So.2d 718 (Al. 1982).

Bowen v. American Hospital Association, 106 S. Ct. 2101 (1986).

Brody H et al. (1997). Withdrawing intensive, life-sustaining treatment—recommendations for compassionate clinical management. New England journal of medicine, 336(9), 652-657.

Brown H et al. (1986). Special project: Legal rights and issues surrounding conception, pregnancy, and birth (Baby Doe: The controversy surrounding withholding treatment from severely defective newborns). Vanderbilt law review, 39, 687-718.

Burke v. Rivo, No. SJC-5162 (Mass. S. Ct., March 1, 1990).

Burton v. Brooklyn Doctors Hospital, 88 A.D.2d 217, 452 N.Y.S.2d 875 (1982).

CDC (1995). Infant death and mortality rates by race of mother, birthweight, and gestational age: United States, 1991 birth cohort and 1995 period data. (LFWK46-1995).

Capron AM (1987). Anencephalic donors: Separate the dead from the dying. Hastings center report, 17(1), 5-9.

Capron AM (1994). At law—medical futility: Strike two. Hastings center report, 24(5), 42-43.

Capron AM (1995). Baby Ryan and virtual futility. Hastings center report, 25(2), 20-21.

Chinn PL (2001). Nursing and ethics: The maturing of a discipline. Advances in nursing science, 24(2), 5.

Cooper TR et al. (1998). Actuarial survival in the premature infant less than 30 weeks' gestation. Pediatrics, 101(6), 975-978.

Daniels N et al. (1996). *Benchmarks of fairness for health care reform.* New York: Oxford.

Darling v. Charleston Community Memorial Hospital, 33 Ill.2d 326, 211 N.E.2d 253 (1965), *cert. Denied,* 383 U.S. 946 (1966).

Department of Health and Human Services (DHHS). Protecting the privacy of patients' health information. Retrieved June 22, 2001 from Department of Health and Human Services website: http://www.hhs.gov/news/press/2001pres/01fsprivacy.html.

Duckett L et al. (1997). Progress in the moral reasoning of baccalaureate nursing students between program entry and exit. *Nursing research,* 46(4), 222-229.

Elliott v. Brown, 361 So.2d 546 (Al. 1978).

Emergency Medical Treatment and Active Labor Treatment Act of 1986, 42 U.S.C. S 1395 dd.

FitzGerald KT (1998). Proposals for Human Cloning: A Review and Ethical Evaluation. In Monagle JF, Thomasma DC (eds.). *Health care ethics: critical issues for the 21st century.* Gaithersburg, MD: Aspen Publications

Flores v. Flushing Hospital and Medical Center, 109 A.D.2d 198, 490 N.Y.S.2d 770 (1985). 45 CFR Parts 160 through 164: Retrieved July 7, 2001, from Department of Health and Human Services website: http://www.hhs.gov/ocr/part1.html.

45 C.F.R. S 46.404–46.407 (1983).

45 C.F.R. S 1340.15 (b) (2) (1985).

48 Fed. Reg. 9630 (1983).

49 Fed. Reg. 14,879 (1984).

Federal Register, Vol. 65, #250, December 28, 2000, (p 1–45).

Harbeson v. Parke-Davis, 98 Wash.2d 460, 656 P.2d 483 (1983).

Harrison H (1986). Neonatal intensive care: Parents' role in ethical decision making. *Birth,* 3, 165–175.

Harrison H (1993). The principles for family-centered neonatal care. *Pediatrics,* 92(5), 643–650.

Hester v. Dwivedi, 89 Ohio St.3d 575 (2000).

Indiana *ex rel.* Infant Doe v. Monroe Circuit Court, No. 482-5140 (Ind. Apr. 16, 1982), *cert. Denied,* 464 U.S. 961 (1982).

In the matter of Baby K, 832 F. Supp. 1022 (E.D. Va 1993); *In the matter of* Baby K, 16 F.3d 590 (4th Cir. 1994), *cert. Denied,* 115 U.S. 91 (1994).

In re Ruiz, 27 Ohio Misc.2d 31 (Ct. Comm. Pleas 1986).

Institute of Medicine, Committee on Quality of Health Care in America. (2000). *To err is human: building a safer health system.* Washington, DC: Author

Jakobi P et al. (1993). The extremely low birth weight infants: The twenty-first century dilemma. *American journal of perinatology,* 10(2), 155–159.

Jasinsky v. Potts, 153 Ohio St. 529 (1950).

Jonsen AR et al. (1998). *Clinical ethics,* ed. 4, New York: McGraw-Hill.

Jos PH et al. (1995). The Charleston policy on cocaine use during pregnancy: A cautionary tale. *The journal of law, medicine & ethics,* 23, 120–128.

King NMP (1992). Transparency in neonatal intensive care. *Hastings center report,* 22(2), 18–25.

Kirk S (1998). Families' experiences of caring at home for a technology-dependent child: A review of the literature. *Child care health development,* 24, 101–114.

Kliegman RM (1995). Neonatal technology, perinatal survival, social consequences, and the perinatal paradox. *American journal of public health,* 85(7), 909–913.

Key case on pregnant women and drug abuse going to trial. (1991, October). *The nation's health,* pp. 1, 20.

La Puma J, Schiedermayer D (1994). *Ethics consultation: a practical guide.* Boston: Jones & Bartlett.

Latham SR (2001). System and responsibility: Three readings of the IOM report on medical error. *American journal of law and medicine,* 27, 163–169.

Leape LL (2001). Foreword: Preventing medical accidents: Is systems analysis the answer? *American journal of law and medicine,* 27, 145–148.

Lemons JA et al. (2001). Very low birth weight outcomes of the National Institute of Child Health and Human Development Neonatal Research Network, January 1995 through December 1996. *Pediatrics,* 107(1), [Pediatrics Electronic Pages].

Lorenz JM et al. (1998). A quantitative review of mortality and developmental disability in extremely premature newborns. *Archives of pediatrics & adolescent medicine,* 152(5), 425–435. Magic seeds or innocent life? The stem cell debate. (2001, July 15). *The Cincinnati enquirer,* p. F1.

Marciniak v. Lundborg, No. 88-0088 (Wisc. S. Ct., January 16, 1990).

Meadow W et al. (1996). Birthweight-specific mortality for extremely low birth weight infants vanishes by four days of life: Epidemiology and ethics in the neonatal intensive care unit. *Pediatrics,* 97(5), 636–643.

Mitchell C, Truog RD (2000). From the files of a pediatric ethics committee. *The journal of clinical ethics,* 11(2), 112–120.

National Association of Neonatal Nurses: *Guidelines and Position Statements for neonatal nursing practice.* Glenview, IL: NANN.

Office of Civil Rights. General overview: 45 CFR Parts 160 and 164. Retrieved from Department of Health and Human Services website July 7, 2001: http://www.hhs.gov/ocr/hipaa/genoverview.html.

Office of Civil Rights (HHS Fact Sheet: protecting the privacy of patient's health information, p. 6) (Federal Register, December 28, 2000, p. 6).

Ohio Board of Nursing. Delegation rules 4723-13. Retrieved July 31, 2001, from http://www.state.oh.us/nur/4723-13 pdf.

Olsen DP (2001). Empathetic maturity: theory of moral point of view in clinical relations. *Advances in nursing science,* 24(1), 36–46.

Paliokas KL (1989). Anencephalic newborns as organ donors: an assessment of "death" and legislative policy. *William and Mary law review,* 31, 197–239.

Penticuff JH (1987). Neonatal nursing ethics: toward a consensus. *Neonatal network,* 5(6), 7–16.

Penticuff JH (1988). Neonatal intensive care: parental prerogatives. *Journal of perinatal and neonatal nursing,* 1(3), 77–86.

Penticuff JH (1998). Defining futility in neonatal intensive care. *Nursing clinics of North America,* 33(2), 339–352.

Pierce SF (1998). Neonatal intensive care: Decision making in the face of prognostic uncertainty. *Nursing clinics of North America,* 33(2), 287–297.

Pinch WJ, Spielman ML (1993). Parental perceptions of ethical issues post-NICU discharge. *Western journal of nursing research,* 15(4), 422–440.

Pinch WJ, Spielman ML (1996). Ethics in the neonatal intensive care unit: Parental perceptions at four years postdischarge. *Advances in nursing science,* 19(1), 72–85.

Procancik v. Cillo, 478 A.2d 755 (N.J. S. Ct. 1984). Restatement of Torts 2d, S 920 (1991 App.).

Public Health Service Act, S 301(d), 42 U.S.C. S 241(d), as added by Public Law No. 100-607, S 163 (November 4, 1988).

Quill TE et al. (1997). The rule of double-effect: a critique of its role in end-of-life decision making. *NEJM,* 337(24), 1768–1771.

Raines DA (1996). Parents' values: a missing link in the neonatal intensive care equation. *Neonatal Network,* 15(3), 1996.

Rawls J (1971). *A theory of justice.* Cambridge, MA: The Belknap Press of Harvard University Press.

Rest J (1979). *Development in judging moral issues.* Minneapolis: University of Minnesota Press.

Rest J (1986). *Moral development: advances in research and theory.* New York: Wiley.

Rest J, Narvaez D (Eds.). (1994). *Moral development in the professions: psychology and applied ethics.* Hillsdale, NJ: L Erlbaum Associates.

Restatement of Torts 2d, S920 (1991).

Rieck v. Medical Protective Co. of Fort Wayne, Ind., 64 Wis.2d 514, 219 N.W.2d 242 (1974).

Roe v. Wade, 410 U.S. 113 (1973).

Rogowski J (1998). Cost-effectiveness of care for very low birth weight infants. *Pediatrics,* 102(1), 35–43.

Schorr B (1984, May 7). Firm didn't disclose vitamin E item was linked to infant deaths, FDA says. *The Wall Street journal*, p. 6.

Shuman CR et al. (1992). Attitudes of registered nurses toward euthanasia. *Death studies*, 16, 1–15.

Spielman B (1995). Bargaining about futility. *The Journal of law, medicine & ethics*, 23, 136–142.

Stanley JM, Bednash G (1998). Formulation and approval of credentialing and clinical privileges. In Sheehy CM, McCarthy MC (Eds.), *Advanced practice nursing: emphasizing common roles*, pp. 138–167. Philadelphia, PA: FA Davis.

Stidam v. Ashmore, 109 Ohio App. 431, 11 O.O.2d 383 (1959).

Stinson R, Stinson P (1979). *The long dying of baby Andrew.* Boston: Little, Brown, & Co.

Stolz JW, McCormick MC (1998). Restricting access to neonatal intensive care: Effect on mortality and economic savings. *Pediatrics*, 101(3), 344–362.

Studdert DM, Brennan TA (2001). Toward a workable model of "No fault" compensation for medical injury in the United States. *American journal of law and medicine*, 27, 225–252.

Sudia-Robinson TM (1998a). An ethical examination of the case studies: dialysis in the newborn with chronic renal insufficiency (Currier, H.). *American nephrology nurses' association journal*, 25(1), 74–76.

Sudia-Robinson TM (1998b). Neonatal intensive care in the home. *Home care provider*, 3(6), 290–292.

Sudia-Robinson TM (1999). Survey of Level III NICUs regarding end-of-life care guidelines. (In review).

Sudia-Robinson TM (1999). Beyond standard care: An examination of care delivery for infants at the margins of viability. In Fowler JW (Ed.), Sawyer-Mellon Volume. (In review).

The Comprehensive Alcohol Abuse and Alcoholism Prevention, Treatment and Rehabilitation Act of 1970 (42 U.S.C. S 290dd-3) (1988).

The Drug Abuse Office and Treatment Act of 1972 (42 U.S.C. S 290ee-3) (1988).

Tolliver v. South Carolina, 90-CP-23-5178 (Cir. Ct. Mannin County, S.C. 1992).

Turpin v. Sortini, 643 P.2d 954 (Cal. S. Ct. 1982).

Tyson JE et al. (1996). Viability, morbidity, and resource use among newborns of 501-800-g birth weight. *Journal of the American Medical Association*, 276(20), 1645–1651.

Williams v. Marion Rapid Transit, Inc., 152 Ohio St. 114 (1949).

Wilson FL (1995). The effects of age, gender, and ethnic/cultural background on moral reasoning. *Journal of social behavior and personality*, 10, 67–78.

Wood NS et al. (2000). Neurologic and developmental disability after extremely preterm birth. *NEJM*, 343(6), 378–384.

Yoder-Wise PS (1999). Delegation: An art of professional practice. In Yoder-Wise PS (Ed.), *Leading and managing in nursing*, ed 2, St Louis: Mosby.

Zaner RM, Bliton MJ (1991). Decision in the NICU: The moral authority of parents. *Children's health care*, 20(1), 19–25.

CHAPTER 5

Collaborative Research in Neonatal Nursing

Lynda Harrison, Denise R. Lucas, Linda Sturla Franck

Practitioners, educators, and researchers can find a fertile ground for conducting research in the neonatal intensive care unit (NICU) or in neonatal follow-up settings. Neonatal nursing is an area that has evolved quickly, resulting in the use of techniques, equipment, and interventions that are not always research-based. Rather, many of the techniques are based on traditions, unsubstantiated methods, or trial-and-error approaches that have not been scientifically validated. With the many rapid advances in technology and treatments available to high-risk newborns and infants, it is increasingly important that neonatal nursing practice is evidence-based. Omery and Williams (1999) define evidence-based nursing practice as "the careful and practical use of current best evidence to guide health care decisions." To provide evidence-based nursing care, neonatal nurses must be knowledgeable consumers of research and must have a basic understanding of the process of research use.

Substantiation of neonatal nursing and neonatal care requires collaboration with other nurses and health professionals. The clinical nurse is often the first to recognize and identify newborn and infant care problems. With the guidance and assistance of other nurses, nurse specialists, and physicians, a collaborative investigation may be used to explore the problem. The combination of expertise from multiple disciplines can make a highly effective team.

Research is a formal, systematic inquiry or examination of a given problem. The outcome or goal of research is to discover new information or relationships or to verify existing knowledge. Other, less formal definitions of research focus on understanding an event by logically relating it to other events. Some types of research are designed to predict events by relating them empirically to antecedents in time. Still other types of research attempt to control or manipulate an event or procedure to determine its impact on other phenomena.

The focus of this chapter is on linking neonatal nursing practice and research. It discusses various research roles for neonatal nurses, including the use of consultation and collaboration for successful practice-based research and the process of research use. The chapter also discusses the identification of clinical problems amenable to research, different types of research designs, and the research process. Finally, the practical aspects of initiating a research project and using research findings in clinical practice are discussed.

WHY DO RESEARCH?

Using the research process to discover new information or to confirm empirical knowledge allows for the growth and evolution of nursing practice. Without research, nursing care would be based simply on tradition. The practice of nursing would change slowly and grow little because things would be done the way they have always been done. The failure to conduct research regarding neonatal care has taught us some sobering lessons. Judgments of efficacy based on observation of small numbers of infants or of treatments based on the principle "if a little is good, more is better" have resulted in significant morbidity and mortality for neonates. Misuses of oxygen therapy, chloramphenicol, and vitamin E are examples (Jain & Vidyasagar, 1989). From these experiences, the use of clinical research trials to evaluate new therapies scientifically before widespread application has become more common in neonatal care.

The research process also provides a vehicle for challenging accepted routines and theories. Nurses caring for neonates often identify issues for which inadequate scientific information on which to base clinical judgments does not exist.

RESEARCH ROLES FOR NEONATAL NURSES

The many different research roles for neonatal nurses include research consumer, participant, facilitator/coordinator, and investigator (Harrison, 2001b). All neonatal nurses should be knowledgeable consumers of research, should read reports of research, and ensure that their practice is research or evidence-based. To be a knowledgeable research consumer, the nurse must be a critical reader of research articles. A rigorous critique of research should also be carried out before one tries to use the findings in a practice situation. Box 5-1 lists questions identified by Beck (1990) that nurses should consider when critically reviewing research reports. These questions can also be applied to lay reports in local newspapers or magazines. The reader should consider who funded the project. If, for instance, a drug company supported the research and the findings were favorable, good questions to ask are whether the research may have been biased by the funding source or whether other investigators outside the company have replicated these findings. It is important to assess the validity of the conclusions and consider whether the researchers addressed intervening variables that

---

BOX 5-1

Some Current Neonatal Nursing Research Questions

Skin Care

How can epidermal damage from tape removal be reduced?

Can the permeable skin of preterm infants be used to deliver medication?

How can the barrier properties of the skin be improved to prevent infection and water loss?

Which cleansing agent and bathing techniques are best for preterm and full-term infants?

Do emollients prevent transepidermal water loss and dermatitis in premature infants?

Nutrition

How can breastfeeding practices be promoted among mothers of premature infants?

What are the most effective methods of delivering formula (e.g., continuous versus intermittent) to ill infants?

Does providing cheek and jaw support promote sucking patterns of preterm infants during feeding?

Is weight gain improved with demand versus scheduled feeding?

How can intravenous access be improved and complications minimized?

What is the effect of nonnutritive sucking on neonatal weight gain?

What is the effect of protein supplementation of breast milk on the weight gain of preterm infants?

Instruments and Procedures

What is the best method for collecting urine?

Which scale provides the most accurate weight?

What is the influence of equipment weights on neonatal daily weight measurements?

Which device provides the most accurate measure of temperature?

What is the effect of routine care tasks, such as suctioning, on cerebral blood flow velocity?

Which pulse oximeters are most effective in reducing the effects of motion artifact?

What is the efficacy of saline versus heparin locks for peripheral IV flushes in neonates?

Do temperature probe covers contribute to nosocomial infections by providing an environment for skin microbe colonization?

What is the effect of draw-up volume on the accuracy of electrolyte measurements from neonatal arterial lines?

Effect of the Environment

What is the impact of light, noise, and handling on infants in the NICU?

What is the appropriate level of stimulation for preterm infants?

What is the effect of supplemental massage and gentle touch on preterm infants?

What is the effect of cycled lighting on preterm infants?

What is the most appropriate method of positioning preterm infants to promote neuromuscular development?

What is the effect of swaddling preterm infants during painful procedures?

Extracorporeal Membrane Oxygenation ECMO

Is the initial training and ongoing education of ECMO specialists sufficient to maintain emergency management skills?

What are the long-term effects of ECMO's use?

What are the neurodevelopmental outcomes of infants who were treated with ECMO?

Endotracheal Tube Stabilization and Maintenance

How can slippage of the endotracheal tube within the trachea be measured?

How can movement of the endotracheal tube be minimized?

Is there a difference in the incidence of nosocomial infections, bronchopulmonary dysplasia, or frequency of suction when using closed versus open tracheal suctioning in neonates?

Management of Pain

How can neonatal pain be assessed?

When is pharmacologic treatment appropriate?

Are there long-term consequences of unrelieved pain experienced in the neonatal period?

What is the most effective method for weaning the infant from analgesics?

Does the use of premedication prior to intubation result in fewer signs of physiologic distress during intubation compared to intubation without premedication?

What are effective nonpharmacologic pain-management techniques for use with neonates?

---

might have affected the research outcomes. Ideally, studies should be replicated to make certain that the results would hold true in a different setting or with a new sample. Replication with similar findings lends credibility to the results. No single study's results should be accepted at face value without consideration of the potential biases.

The next decade will bring an increase in research with possible application to the nursing care of neonates. Each nurse caring for newborn or infant patients must first maintain an awareness of the research literature by keeping up to date with professional journals. Implementation of research innovations may be correlated with the reading of professional journals and attendance at research seminars (Luckenbill-Brett, 1987). Unfortunately, research findings are sometimes

used as a basis for practice without critical review (Perez-Woods & Tse, 1990). Omery & Williams (1999) and Walczak et al (1994) have identified a number of individual barriers to research utilization, including lack of time, lack of knowledge, and lack of appreciation for the value of research. Institutional barriers include inadequate staffing and failure to reward nurses who initiate change based on findings from research. Funk et al (1995) noted that additional barriers to using research include problems with the research and with the presentation of the research. Barriers related to the research itself include lack of replication of the research, uncertainty about the credibility of the research results, and methodological inadequacies of the research. Barriers related to the way the research was presented include problems with

---

BOX 5-1

Some Current Neonatal Nursing Research Questions—cont'd

Thermoregulation

Which techniques are most effective in minimizing insensible water loss and maintaining thermoregulation in the extremely premature infant?

What are the optimal procedures for maintaining thermoregulation when transferring infants from incubators or warmers to open cribs?

What are the effects of skin-to-skin holding (Kangaroo care) on thermoregulation of preterm infants?

Positioning

Which positions are most effective in promoting optimal oxygenation and in minimizing postural deformities?

Should all infants be turned every 2 hours?

Under what conditions is the prone position linked to sudden infant death syndrome?

What factors influence parents' decisions about sleep positions of their infants?

Effects of Cocaine

How is the behavior of a cocaine-exposed infant different from that of the nonexposed infant?

What is the appropriate level of environmental stimulation for these infants?

What types of intervention programs are effective for families of cocaine-exposed infants following hospital discharge?

Effective Parent Teaching Techniques

What are the most effective teaching methods for instructing parents in the care of their newborns?

Is computer-assisted instruction effective?

What type of posthospital follow-up is most helpful to parents of infants who are released from the NICU?

Are postdischarge telephone follow-up programs effective in promoting breastfeeding of preterm infants discharged from the NICU?

What are parents' perceptions of a parental care-by-parent program before NICU discharge of their infants?

Family Issues

What nursing interventions help to reduce stressors experienced by families who have infants in the NICU?

What interventions help to promote attachment and adaptive parenting between parents and preterm infants and between parents and infants with serious health problems?

What are the outcomes associated with participation in a parent support group for parents of preterm infants?

What are parents' perceptions of the NICU follow-up clinic?

Staff Education

What is the most effective method of orientation of new NICU nurses?

How should formal classroom teaching and clinical preceptorship be integrated?

Are self-paced learning modules an effective teaching methodology for neonatal nurses?

Can neonatal nurses use expert systems to support decision making?

Delivery of Nursing Care

What is the most effective model for delivery of nursing care in the NICU?

Can nonprofessional staff be used in the NICU to support the professional nurse?

Does the use of critical pathways facilitate "costing out" nursing services?

What is the effect of a structured neonatal resuscitation program on delivery room resuscitation practices?

Retention of Nurses in the Critical Care Setting

What are the factors that increase job satisfaction for nurses working in the NICU?

How do NICU nurses cope with stress?

What factors increase the likelihood that nursing jobs will be retained?

Do neonatal nurses perceive technology in the NICU as sources of stress?

---

understanding the statistical analysis, failure to identify the implications of the study, and failure to report the research clearly.

Neonatal nurses can participate in research in a variety of ways. One effective method to gain knowledge about the research process is to become involved in a colleague's project as a research participant.* Nurses can also participate in research as data collectors. Some neonatal nurses work as clinical research coordinators (CRCs) and assume primary responsibil-

ity for implementing clinical studies and protocols (McKinney & Vermuelen, 2000). The Association for Clinical Research Practitioners (ACRP) has a certification program for CRCs as well as for Clinical Research Associates. (For information see the ACRP web site at http://www.acrpnet.org.)

Another method of participating in the research process is to perform secondary analyses on data that were collected to answer another research question. Often answers to other research questions can be extracted from a single database without having to collect new data. Caution, however, must be used in the design of secondary analysis studies to minimize threats to validity and reliability inherent in the method.

Neonatal nurses prepared at the master's or doctoral level might also serve as research facilitators (McGee, 1996). Clini-

---

*In this chapter, the term "research participant"—instead of "research subject"—is used because many consider the term "subject" to connote that the researcher is in a position of power over the "subject."

cal Nurse Specialists (CNS) may promote research by coordinating research committees, promoting research utilization, coordinating research activities in the NICU, and providing educational programs to help nurses understand and use findings from research. According to the American Nurses' Association 1994 paper entitled *Education for Participation in Nursing Research*. Preparation of nurse scientists for principal investigator roles begins at the masters' level and is the focus of doctoral preparation. Nurses prepared at these levels assume primary responsibility as principal investigators in research (American Nurses' Association, 1994).

OBSTACLES TO INVOLVEMENT IN RESEARCH

The reluctance of nurses to become involved in research generally stems from two basic obstacles: lack of knowledge and lack of resources. Both of these obstacles can be overcome. To address these issues effectively, nurses must receive education regarding the research process, have the opportunity to participate in research projects (in data collection or as research participants), and participate with colleagues in sessions to stimulate the formulation of questions from their clinical experience. One can begin by asking the question "why?" of every NICU nursing practice.

Lack of resources—including time, money, and consultation—can be more difficult to address. In many institutions, the conduct of nursing research is still viewed as a frill and not central to the delivery of patient care. In such a setting, nurses who wish to conduct research may initially need to invest their own time and even money. However, once the research process has demonstrated clinical relevance, additional resources are often made available. Collaboration with colleagues within the institution, schools and universities, and industry can enhance resources. Writing grants with colleagues for the purposes of obtaining funds to support research is often the only way that clinical research can be conducted (Kenner & Walden, 2001).

USING RESEARCH TO CHANGE NEONATAL NURSING PRACTICE

Gennaro (1994) defined research utilization as "the process by which research knowledge is moved into the clinical arena." The first step in the research utilization process is the identification of a clinical problem to be addressed. Nurses might identify a problem of concern in their individual clinical setting, or specialty organizations might identify priorities for research utilization projects. For example, in 1990 the Association of Women's Health, Obstetric, and Neonatal Nurses (AWOHNN) convened a panel of nurse experts to identify areas with sufficient research to develop research-based protocols that could be tested in research utilization projects. Gennaro (1994) described the following neonatal research utilization topics that were identified by the AWOHNN panel:

1. Use of comfort measures such as non-nutritive sucking during or in anticipation of stressful procedures
2. Removal of barriers to successful breastfeeding and improving breastfeeding success in preterm infants
3. Improving skin integrity of low-birth-weight premature infants
4. Improving thermoregulation of infants
5. Reducing physiologic sequelae of infant suctioning
6. Using findings that indicate that infants do feel pain
7. Using telephone follow-up services for high-risk infants and families

Members of the AWOHNN Research Committee recommended that the organization fund a research utilization project to evaluate the best method for transition of preterm infants to open cribs and appointed a group of six neonatal nurse researchers to conduct the project (Meier, 1994). After reviewing the literature on the topic, the group held a series of meetings and ultimately developed a weaning protocol that was subsequently tested with 270 infants from 10 different hospitals (Medoff-Cooper, 1994). The results of this research utilization project demonstrated that preterm infants could be moved to an open crib at lower weights than had been suggested by results of previous studies.

A collaborative project developed by AWHONN and the National Association of Neonatal Nurses (NANN) used research findings to develop a protocol for neonatal skin care (Lund et al, 2001). As in the transition to open crib project, a group of researchers reviewed extant literature to develop a clinical practice guideline and data collection tools. Site recruitment resulted in participation of 65 coordinators from 60 clinical sites across 27 states. A total of 51 sites completed all phases of the project, which involved 2,820 infants in all levels of care. Results of the study indicated that the use of the clinical guideline resulted in improved skin condition of neonates in intensive, secondary and well-baby nurseries. Nurses also were better able to identify risk factors for impaired skin integrity in neonates.

Burns & Grove (2001) described a model of research utilization that is based on Rogers' (1995) model of diffusion of innovations (Table 5-1). This model includes five stages: knowledge, persuasion, decision, implementation, and confirmation. During the knowledge phase, existing research related to the clinical problem is reviewed and evaluated for scientific merit and relevance for the particular clinical setting. Haller and colleagues (1979) proposed the following criteria for determining whether research is ready for use in practice:

- Evaluation of the scientific merit of the study concerning validity, reliability, generalizability, and statistical significance
- Replication of findings to provide greater confidence in reliability and validity of results
- Determination of any potential risk to patients.

When reviewing research literature, one must keep in mind that negative findings can be as important to practice as positive results. However, negative findings tend not to be published.

During the persuasion stage of the research utilization process, Burns & Grove (2001) suggested that nurses encourage administrators as well as other health care providers to change their practice based on the findings of the research reviewed during the knowledge phase. Factors such as cost, potential benefits to the patient and to the institution, and the complexity of the change that is proposed will all influence the willingness of others to adopt the research-based change.

The decision to implement a research-based practice change often requires approval from others, including physicians, institutional committees, and administration (Burns & Grove, 2001). Using principles of change can help to promote success of this stage. Burns & Grove (2001) suggested involving all who would be affected by the change in the process of deciding whether to implement the change and also suggested enlisting the support of institutional leaders.

Implementation of the change might be done at the individual nurse, the unit, or the institutional level. A final and critical stage of the research utilization process is to confirm or evaluate the results of implementing the research-based change.

TABLE 5-1	A Model of Research Utilization
Phase	**Activities**
Knowledge	Review existing research on the problem. Evaluate existing research for scientific merit and for clinical relevance. Based on the review, determine whether to make a change in practice, considering factors such as feasibility, cost/benefit ration, innovativeness of the change, and norms of the social system which might influence openness/resistance to the change.
Persuasion	Identify key individuals who will be affected by the change, and include them in discussions about the change that is proposed; Educate key individuals about the problem and the need for change, as well as the advantages, compatibility, complexity, and expected results of the change.
Decision	Determine the scope of the change—e.g., will it be implemented on only one unit or system-wide? Obtain approval from necessary individuals and groups (e.g., physicians, nursing administrators, policy and procedure committees.
Implementation	Develop a protocol for implementing the change; Educate nurses and others who will implement the change; Plan for evaluating the outcomes of the change.
Confirmation	Evaluate the outcomes from the change (on patients, nurses, and others in the institution); Share results of outcomes with all interested parties (e.g., nurses, physicians, administrators) to increase the likelihood that the change will be continued.

Adapted from Burns N, Grove SK (2001). The practice of nursing research: conduct, critique, and utilization, ed 4, Philadelphia: WB Saunders.

This stage requires considerable planning before implementation and commitment to collect the data needed for evaluation. The case study at the end of this chapter illustrates the process of research utilization that might be followed to implement a research-based protocol related to handling preterm infants in the NICU.

IDENTIFYING THE RESEARCH PROBLEM OR QUESTION

Nurses in the clinical setting are often in the best position to identify and articulate research questions and to carry out research studies that improve the delivery of nursing care. The types of questions posed by clinical nurses range from basic physiologic mechanisms to comparisons of efficacy between different care giving techniques to identification and description of new phenomena. Box 5-2 lists topics of current research interest for neonatal nurses.

Many of these research questions are derived from the concern about the prevention of iatrogenic complications of treatments. Others emerge from systematic observation of clinical phenomena or from frustration with current practices. Ideas for research come from many different sources, including an individual nurse's experience, the nursing or health literature, discussions of social or health issues, or theory (Burns & Grove, 2001). Quality assurance and quality improvement activities often lead to the design and conduct of research. Nurses are often introduced to issues related to objective data collection through quality assurance audits. Issues of clinical consequence that are identified through quality assurance screening can lead to the articulation of research questions. Research principles can also be used in the evaluation of new procedures, protocols, and products. Evaluation is often an integral part of NICU nursing, but it is performed subjectively. Using research methodology to perform evaluation promotes scientific objectivity. Researchers and professional organizations sometimes conduct surveys or convene expert panels to identify research priorities. These priorities can also help researchers identify researchable problems. For example, the National Institute of Nursing Research (NINR) has identified the following priorities for funding during the period from 2000–2004: end-of-life and palliative care, chronic illness experiences, quality of life and quality of care, health promotion/disease prevention, symptom management, telehealth interventions, and cultural and ethnic considerations in health and illness (see the NINR website at http://www.nih.gov/ninr).

The nursing profession also demands research to address social issues and that research contributes to the overall societal health needs. The following questions, adapted from Fleming (1984), should be considered when selecting a research problem:

1. Is the problem important to the discipline of nursing?
2. Is the problem of interest to the investigator?
3. Does the problem reflect patterns of human behavior in interaction with the environment in critical life situations?
4. Does the problem reflect processes by which health status is affected?
5. Is the problem ethical?
6. Is the problem feasible to research?

The research process may appear intimidating at first, but it is not difficult to learn. Very simply, research is a method of problem solving that is similar to the nursing process itself. A major difference between research and problem solving is that the goal of research is to develop knowledge that can be generalized to other settings and populations.

When developing research problems, it is important to consider the significance, feasibility of research, and feasibility of the problem. Some problems may be highly significant but cannot be researched because they are of a moral or ethical nature. For example, the question "should preterm infants less than 22 weeks' gestational age be saved?" cannot be answered through research. It would be possible, however, to answer the question "What are attitudes of parents, physicians, and nurses towards treatment of preterm infants of less than 22 weeks' gestational age?" Factors that affect the feasibility of research include time, money, experience of the researcher and the research team, availability of study participants, and availability of appropriate facilities and equipment (Polit & Hungler, 1998).

BOX 5-2

General Criteria for Evaluating a Research Report

Step 1: Research Problem
1. Is the problem clearly and concisely stated?
2. Is the problem adequately narrowed down into a researchable problem?
3. Is the problem significant to nursing?
4. Is the relationship of the identified problem to previous research clear?

Step 2: Literature Review
1. Is the literature review logically organized?
2. Does the review provide a critique of the relevant studies?
3. Are the gaps in knowledge about the research problem identified?
4. Are important relevant references omitted?

Step 3: Theoretical or Conceptual Framework
1. Is the theoretical framework easily linked with the problem, or does it seem forced?
2. If a conceptual framework is used, are the concepts adequately defined and the relationships among these concepts clearly identified?

Step 4: Research Variables
1. Are the independent and dependent variables operationally defined?
2. Are any extraneous or intervening variables identified?

Step 5: Hypotheses
1. Is a predicted relationship between two or more variables included in each hypothesis?
2. Are the hypotheses clear, testable, and specific?
3. Do the hypotheses logically flow from the theoretical or conceptual framework?

Step 6: Sampling
1. Is the sample size adequate?
2. Is the sample representative of the defined population?
3. Is the method for selection of the sample appropriate?

4. Are the sample criteria for inclusion into the study identified?
5. Is there any sampling bias in the chosen method?

Step 7: Research Design
1. Is the design adequately described?
2. Does the research design control for threats in internal and external validity of the study?
3. Are the sample criteria for inclusion into the study identified?
4. Are the reliability and validity of the measurement tools adequate?

Step 8: Data Collection Methods
1. Are the data collection methods appropriate for study?
2. Are the data collection instruments described adequately?
3. Are the reliability and validity of the measurement tools adequate?

Step 9: Data Analysis
1. Is the results section clearly and logically organized?
2. Is the type of analysis appropriate for the level of measurement for each variable?
3. Are the tables and figures clear and understandable?
4. Is the statistical test correct for answering the research question?

Step 10: Interpretation and Discussion of the Findings
1. Are the interpretations based on the data?
2. Does the investigator clearly distinguish between actual findings and interpretations?
3. Are the findings discussed in relation to previous research and to the conceptual-theoretical framework?
4. Are unwarranted generalizations made beyond the study sample?
5. Are the limitations of the results identified?
6. Are implications of the results for clinical nursing practice discussed?
7. Are recommendations for future research identified?
8. Are the conclusions justified?

From Beck CT (1990). The research critique: general criteria for evaluating a research report. Journal of obstetric, gynecologic, and neonatal nursing, 19(1), 18-22. Reprinted with permission.

REVIEW OF THE LITERATURE

One of the first steps in the research process is to review the literature to bring together data and theories that pertain to the topic of interest. The relationships between the concepts and the major issues are uncovered, and the gaps or potential flaws in the current knowledge are identified. In essence, the review of the literature provides a logical step toward refining the research problem. The review also helps to formulate the research questions or hypotheses and direct the methodology or design of the study. Perhaps the question can be answered after the review. If not, the review of the literature will allow the practitioner to identify what has been studied, what suggestions on the same topic other researchers have made about

further research, and what instruments for measuring variables have been used or developed. Integrative research reviews and meta-analyses are two types of literature reviews that are particularly helpful in summarizing the available knowledge about a given problem or topic. A meta-analysis is a statistical summary of findings from a collection of studies of the same research problem. A meta-analysis is a type of research design in which individual studies are treated as study data. An example of a meta-analysis of relevance to neonatal nursing research was a review by Krywanio (1994) of physiological outcomes of hospital-based stimulation programs for preterm infants. An excellent source of meta-analyses on a variety of clinical problems is the Cochrane database. This database is developed and maintained by an international network of individuals who publish systematic meta-analyses of randomized clinical trials. Abstracts of all completed Cochrane reviews can be accessed at the following website: http://wwwcochrane.org. An example of a meta-analysis published in the Cochrane database that is of interest to neonatal nurses was a review published in 1998 by Vickers summarizing studies of preterm infants' responses to massage and touch interventions.

An integrative literature review is a narrative summary of related studies. The Online Journal of Knowledge Synthesis for Nursing is published by Sigma Theta Tau, International and includes integrative literature reviews on a variety of clinical nursing topics (see http://www.stti.iupui.edu/library/ojkns/). An example of an integrative review published in this journal is a summary of studies evaluating the effects of tactile stimulation on preterm infants published by Harrison and Bodin (1994). Table 5-2 lists a number of other websites that might provide information related to neonatal nursing research.

The next step is to explore appropriate methods for answering the question. The nature of the question dictates or determines the conceptual framework, methods, and design guiding the inquiry.

RESEARCH METHODS AND DESIGN

The research design is "a blueprint for conducting the study that maximizes control over factors that could interfere with the validity of the findings" (Burns & Grove, 2001). The researcher selects the type of design most appropriate for the study question and most feasible, based on available resources. The design guides the researcher in conducting the study and analyzing the findings. The paradigm, or worldview, that guides the research also influences designs. Polit and Hungler (1998) described the two predominant paradigms that have traditionally guided nursing research as the positivist and naturalistic paradigms. The positive paradigm underlies the traditional scientific approach and is based on an assumption that "nature is basically ordered and regular and that an objective reality exists independent of human observation" (Polit & Hungler, 1998). Research designs that are guided by the positivist paradigm are generally systematic and include mechanisms designed to control the research situation, to generate empirical (usually quantitative) data, and to generalize findings to a larger population. The naturalistic paradigm (also referred to as the phenomenological paradigm) is based on the assumption that "reality is not a fixed entity but rather is a construction of the individuals participating in the research; reality exists within a context, and many constructions are possible" (Polit & Hungler, 1998). Research designs that are guided by the naturalistic paradigm often use qualitative methods, collecting and analyzing data that are generally narrative (e.g., interviews, records of observations, textual analysis) to understand the holistic nature of human experience. Data collection methods in qualitative research designs are often more flexible and the sample sizes generally smaller than in designs guided by the positivist paradigm. The ultimate goal of research guided by the naturalistic paradigm is to gain a full understanding of a phenomenon—not necessarily to generalize to a larger population. The value of combining methods from both paradigms in nursing research (sometimes referred to as triangulation) is gaining increasingly recognition for obtaining more complete understanding of the phenomena under investigation.

PURPOSES OF RESEARCH

The level of inquiry is guided by the purpose of the research, which can be viewed as a continuum ranging from identification and description of phenomena, exploration of relationships, explanation of phenomena and relationships, and prediction and control of phenomena (Polit & Hungler, 1998). The purpose of the research guides the selection of the design and the methods for data collection. Some purposes are more amenable to designs based on the positivist paradigm (e.g., prediction and control), whereas others are more amenable to designs based on the naturalistic paradigm (e.g., identification of phenomena).

Research Focused on Identification of Phenomena
When the purpose of research is to identify or conceptualize a phenomenon, qualitative methods are often used. An example of a neonatal nursing study within this category was a study designed to identify challenges experienced by mothers in bottle-feeding their preterm infants (Thoyre, 2001). In this study, Thoyre videotaped 22 mothers as they were feeding their preterm infants. Following the feeding, the researcher interviewed the mothers as they observed the videotaped recording in order to identify the mothers' perceptions of the challenges they identified in bottlefeeding. Mothers identified three major challenges: ensuring safety, ensuring adequate caloric intake, and advancing the feeding once the infants were discharged home.

Research Focused on Description of Phenomena
If the purpose is to portray accurately the incidence, distribution, and characteristics of a group or situation, the research is descriptive. Descriptive research can be conducted within either a positivist or naturalistic paradigm and can use either quantitative or qualitative methods. Quantitative studies use numbers to categorize data. The data are reported via descriptive statistics such as frequencies, actual numbers, and percentages. Qualitative studies categorize and describe data according to patterns, themes, and categories of response at a nominal or naming level. Ethnographers, for example, attempt to describe characteristics of certain groups by qualitative methods. The data from these qualitative studies are analyzed through content analysis and report the categories or themes found. The sample may or may not be random. The subjects most likely are selected based on availability and for a specific purpose. The data are collected through either unstructured or semistructured methods. Examples of descriptive research include the following:
- Survey research
- Developmental studies
- Case studies

Quantitative descriptive research focuses on counting, describing, or classifying the measurable attributes of a phenomenon. For example, Altimier et al (1999) described temperature changes that occurred in preterm infants after transfer from a radiant warmer to the incubator. They found no significant differences in temperatures immediately after bed transfer; however, temperatures were lower 1 hour after the transfer. Qualitative descriptive research is focused on generating in-depth descriptions of various aspects of phenomena. For example, Miles et al (1999) conducted a retrospective descriptive study in which 19 African-American mothers shared their recollections about the hospitalization of their seriously ill preterm or

TABLE **5-2**	Internet Resources for Neonatal Nurse Researchers	
Source	**Web Address**	**Description**
Agency for Healthcare Research and Quality	www.ahcpr.gov	AHRQ (formerly known as the Agency for Healthcare Policy and Research) supports research to generate evidence-based information on health care outcomes, quality, cost, use, and access. Information from AHRQ's research helps people make more informed decisions and improve the quality of health care services.
Association for Clinical Research Practitioners (ACRP)	www.acrpnet.org	ACRP is a professional organization that has a certification program for Clinical Research Associates and for Clinical Research Practitioners.
Association of Women's Health, Obstetric, and Neonatal Nurses	www.AWHONN.org	The association provides nurses and the women and families for whom they care, with health promotion and prevention programs and resources that enhance health care practices and address the wide range of health care issues unique to women.
Journal of the Neonatal Nursing Association	www.neonatal-nursing.co.uk/	European journal for neonatal nurses. Includes jobs, resources, and a searchable database of articles.
Office of Human Subjects Research (OHSR)	http://ohsr.od.nih.gov/	OHSR operates within the NIH to help investigators understand and comply with ethical principles and regulatory requirements involved in human subjects research. An online training program on protection of human research participants is available at this web site.
The Academy of Neonatal Nursing	www.academyonline.org	The mission of The Academy of Neonatal Nursing is to provide quality neonatal nursing educational materials and programs at a reasonable cost to all neonatal nurses.
The Cochrane Collaboration	www.cochrane.org	Prepares, maintains, and promotes the accessibility of systematic reviews of the effects of health care interventions. Source for abstracts of all completed Cochrane reviews.
National Association of Neonatal Nurses	www.nann.org	NANN is a professional organization focused on promoting excellence in caring for newborns and infants. The association has a listserv to promote communication about neonatal nursing topics.
National Institute of Child Health and Human Development (NICHD)	www.nichd.nih.gov	The NICHD conducts and supports laboratory, clinical, and epidemiological research on the reproductive, neurobiologic, developmental, and behavioral processes that determine and maintain the health of children, adults, families, and populations.
National Institute of Health (NIH)	www.nih.gov	The NIH mission is to uncover new knowledge that will lead to better health for everyone.
National Institute of Nursing Research (NINR)	www.nih.gov/ninr	The NINR supports clinical and basic research to establish a scientific basis for the care of individuals across the lifespan—from management of patients during illness and recovery to the reduction of risks for disease and disability, the promotion of healthy lifestyles, promotion of quality of life in those with chronic illness, and care for individuals at the end of life.
Neonatal Intensive Care Unit	www.NICU.com	Publishes online discussions, published research, and events to promote better understanding of neonatal issues.
Neonatology on the Web	www.neonatology.com	Extensive directory of current literature, clinical resources, internet resource links, career information, nursing and other health professional job postings in NICUs nationwide.
NICU-WEB	http://neonatal.peds.washington.edu	Pediatric and neonatal common diagnoses, procedures, and interventions, as well as an extensive list of resources.

term infants. Mothers' greatest source of stress was being separated from their infants, and their highest source of satisfaction was support from health care providers.

Research Focused on Exploration

Exploratory studies can also be either qualitative or quantitative, and are focused on "investigating the full nature of the phenomenon, the manner in which it is manifested, and the other factors with which it is related" (Polit & Hungler, 1998). An example of a quantitative exploratory study is a study conducted by Vohr and colleagues (2000) to examine factors associated with neurodevelopmental and functional outcomes of extremely-low-birth-weight infants born between 1993 to 1994. Presence of chronic lung disease, grades 3 and 4 intraventricular hemorrhage, use of steroids for chronic lung disease, male gender, and presence of necrotizing enterocolitis were associated with more adverse outcomes. An example of a qualitative exploratory study is Costello & Chapman's (1998) exploration of the experiences of six mothers who participated in a care-by-parent program before hospital discharge of their preterm infants.

Research Focused on Explanation

Explanatory studies are often linked to theories and are focused on explaining relationships among phenomena. In quantitative explanatory studies, theories are generally used deductively, which means that predictions based on the theory form the basis for study questions or hypotheses that are tested in the research. In qualitative explanatory studies, theories are generally developed inductively, based on the specific data and observations collected during the research. An example of a quantitative explanatory study is a project conducted by Grunau et al (2000) to examine whether bodily movements identified as stress cues in the Neonatal Individualized Developmental Care and Assessment Program (NIDCAP) are cues of pain in low birth weight infants. The results suggested that finger splay and leg extension may be signals of distress, although the authors concluded that further study was needed. Holditch-Davis & Miles (2000) conducted a qualitative explanatory study in which they asked 31 mothers to tell stories about their NICU experiences. Data were analyzed to determine how well these stories fit with the Preterm Parental Distress Model.

Research Focused on Prediction and Control

In a practice profession such as nursing, an important goal of research is to predict and "control" patient outcomes and to identify effective nursing interventions that will promote optimal patient and family outcomes. Studies focused on prediction and control are generally based on the positivist paradigm and use quantitative research methods. Many of these studies use experimental designs that involve random assignment of study participants to either a treatment or "control" group, administration of an intervention, and control of extraneous variables that might affect study outcomes. The "gold standard" of experimental research is the randomized clinical trial. In this most rigorous of research designs, carefully controlled, prospective, blind trials can definitively establish risks and benefits of new treatments, minimizing bias and error. This method of clinical research is not without controversy, however. Ethical, financial, and social factors are often involved in decisions to introduce new treatments. The rigorous requirements for controlled evaluation of all new therapies may fail to acknowledge these clinical realities. The introduction of extra-

corporeal membrane oxygenation (ECMO) therapy in the NICU exemplifies the complex issues clinicians face in determining the need for and adequacy of clinical trials to determine benefits and risks of new therapies (Lantos & Frader, 1990). Westrup et al (2000) conducted a randomized clinical trial designed to evaluate the effects of a NIDCAP program in Sweden and reported a number of positive outcomes that favor the NIDCAP group including fewer days receiving continuous positive airway pressure (CPAP), and fewer cases of bronchopulmonary dysplasia (BPD). Harrison et al (2000) conducted an experimental study to evaluate the effects of a gentle human touch (GHT) intervention provided for 10 minutes, three times daily for 10 days to a group of preterm infants. A total of 84 preterm infants were randomly assigned to either the GHT or control group. Findings indicated significantly lower levels of active sleep, motor activity, and behavioral distress during the GHT periods compared to 10-minute baseline and post-touch periods, although no significant differences between the infants in the GHT and control groups on outcome variables that measured their developmental status, morbidity, or behavioral organization were found.

Researchers might also use quasi-experimental designs in studies designed to predict and/or control phenomena. Quasi-experimental designs have fewer controls than do true experimental designs and often do not involve random assignment of research participants to experimental and control groups. Kilbride et al (2000) reported findings from a quasi-experimental study designed to evaluate the effects of a case management intervention on infants who experienced prenatal cocaine exposure. Infants were alternately assigned to either a control group or the case management group, and a matched non-drug exposed group of infants was used for comparison purposes. Although infants in the case management group had higher mental development scores at age 6 months, there were no differences in developmental outcomes among the three groups of infants at age 36 months.

When experimental designs are used, the ethics of clinical research require that the investigator maintain a genuine state of uncertainty regarding the merits of one treatment over another (Freedman, 1989). This state of equipoise is often difficult to achieve, particularly if the clinicians strongly believe in the efficacy of one of the study treatments. Therefore study treatments must be randomized to minimize or eliminate bias. Education that concerns the statistical dangers of making decisions based on studies with insufficient sample size should assist who are all involved (other clinical staff and parents) in recognizing the merit of suspending judgment until all the data are collected. Criteria can be established to ensure that a study is not conducted longer than is necessary when clear benefit or harm becomes evident early on.

RESEARCH DESIGNS

Research designs can be classified along many different dimensions, including the purpose of the study (e.g., exploratory or descriptive research), the level of control over the independent variable (e.g., experimental, quasi-experimental, or nonexperimental), the number of data collection points (e.g., cross-sectional or longitudinal), and the timing of the independent variable in relation to the dependent variable (e.g., retrospective versus prospective) (Polit & Hungler, 1998). The use of a combination of research designs is common in today's research arena. Brink & Wood (1998) suggested that historical research, epidemiological research, instrument development, evaluative research, and philosophical research are examples of mixed designs.

Historical Research

Historical research is just coming into its own in nursing. Sarnecky defines this type of research as "a process of examining data from the past, integrating it into a coherent unity and putting it to some pragmatic use for the present and future" (Sarnecky, 1990). It uses previously recorded information to draw conclusions about past events and suggests present and past implications. Secondary analysis may also fall into this category because it represents the use of either secondary sources for information or a reexamination of previously collected data. An advantage to this method of data analysis is that it is cost-effective and allows the researcher to explore another research question that was not asked in the original study or studies. False inferences resulting from lack of random assignment, incomplete information, and inherent group differences are risks of this design.

Epidemiological Research

Epidemiological research has attracted much attention because the tracking of certain diseases, such as acquired immunodeficiency syndrome (AIDS), has significant public health implications. These studies are concerned with documenting the natural history, determining prevalence, and longitudinally following the evolution of phenomena. The objective of epidemiological studies is to follow the trend of diseases in specific populations. Although this type of research has historically been more medical in nature, many nurses are becoming interested in epidemiological methods to guide nursing interventions toward the promotion or restoration of health.

Instrument Development

Instrument development is a common nursing research design. It reflects the need for reliable and valid instruments to measure nursing phenomena. Qualitative as well as quantitative methods may be used to establish content validity of a preexisting or newly developed instrument. Instrument development takes considerable time and effort and may be a lifelong program of research itself if a valid and reliable instrument is truly developed. (Miles et al, 1993) conducted a study to develop an instrument to measure parental perceptions of stressors in the NICU. This instrument has been used widely in neonatal nursing research.

The focus group is a method used to identify items that should be included in questionnaires. Focus groups usually consist of 10 to 12 people from similar backgrounds with regard to the research area of interest. The group's homogeneity is desired so that the participants can generate ideas on a similar topic, such as the use of extracorporeal membrane oxygenation in the NICU and ethical dilemmas facing neonatal nurses.

Evaluative Research

Evaluative research has been conducted in education for many years. Nurse educators use evaluation methods in revising nursing curricula and provide documentation for National League for Nursing (NLN) or Commission on Collegiate Nursing Education (CCNE) accreditation visits. Nurse specialists provide in-service education and community workshops. Nurses have become more involved in these types of studies as quality assurance-quality improvement or total continuous quality improvement programs and the need for documentation of pa-

tient outcomes or nursing care costs have grown. These studies may be qualitative and concerned with why a program works, or quantitative, focusing on describing changes; or experimental, with an emphasis on establishing cause and effect relationships. Outcome-based research is a priority for the National Institutes of Health (NIH). It is also a priority of the Joint Commission for Accreditation of Healthcare Organizations (JCAHO). In part this is due to the mandate by third-party payers to receive validation that the treatment, procedure, and nursing care is cost-effective and appropriate to the outcome (Kachoyeanos, 1995, 1996). Research is a method of justifying neonatal nursing's role in care, "costing out" services, and validating patient outcomes. Patient outcome research teams are part of the initiative outlined by the Agency for Healthcare Research and Quality (AHRQ), which is concerned with studies evaluating outcomes of various health care practices (see the AHRQ website at www.ahrq.gov).

Philosophical Research

Philosophical research asks value questions. This type of research is more likely to be qualitative in nature, focusing on individual or cultural values and beliefs. Studies that address value questions can be most useful when nurses are concerned about how a group or individual may view a philosophical or ethical dilemma such as discontinuation of life support or the use of anencephalic infants for donor organs.

Replicating Studies

Nurses often feel that replicating or repeating a study is "cheating" and of no value. This feeling could not be further from the truth. Studies need to be repeated to support the findings from the original study. Replication lends credibility to previous results and allows the findings to be generalized. Researchers should provide accurate, detailed descriptions of how the research was performed so that others can replicate it.

Replication also provides an opportunity to learn from the experience of others—that is, to analyze what was done right as well as what was done wrong so that more accurate, precise studies can be designed. If a study that is replicated fails to produce the same results, it may mean that practice has changed, the study's original sample differs from the new sample, the methods in one or both studies were faulty, or the hypothesized relationships do not exist. In such cases, further exploration is needed. Replication of studies is an easy way to begin to learn the research process and is often less frustrating for the beginning researcher who does not feel capable of designing an original study.

RESEARCH TEAM COMPOSITION

The decision regarding the composition of the research team should be based on the type of research, the expertise needed to conduct a credible study, the type and amount of funds available to support the research, and the time expected to complete the study. The team may be a single investigator or a group of investigators.

Single Investigator Versus Co-Investigators

Single Investigator.   Advantages and disadvantages to conducting a research project as an individual exist. The single investigator has complete control of the project, conducts the project according to his or her own schedule, and does not depend on others for information about the progress of the project. One of the disadvantages is that no one else helps bear part of the research burden. Tasks such as writing the proposal, collecting data, and analyzing data can be facilitated through the use of a team. A single investigator may also be more vulnerable to bias.

Co-Investigators. Involving a team in planning and conducting research can be helpful and timesaving. Sharing knowledge and expertise has the potential for making a better project. The blend of an academician and clinician is often helpful in keeping theory in perspective while remaining based in reality in the clinical setting. However, working in a group is not always easy. It requires cooperation and often compromise on the project's purpose or plan. It is unrealistic to assume an equal distribution of work in such a collaborative effort; it does not often occur. Thus before entering into a collaborative venture, the group should outline precisely what tasks each member is to assume throughout the project as well as plans for publication of study findings and authorship credit. A contract may prevent misunderstandings during the project and prevent communication problems that may jeopardize the entire project's completion. During the proposal development stage, a time schedule for completion of each member's part of the project as well as a target for completion of the entire project should be established. If insurmountable problems arise among the members of the team, the principal investigator must decide how to proceed with the project, shift responsibilities, replace team members, or halt the project.

DEVELOPING THE RESEARCH PROJECT

Identifying Study Questions and/or Hypotheses
The purpose of the research project will dictate the form of the specific objectives, research questions, and/or hypotheses. Not all research investigations will have hypotheses. In descriptive studies, research questions direct the investigation (e.g., "What are parents' perceptions of stressors associated with having an infant in the NICU?"). In experimental studies, specific hypotheses are tested. The hypothesis is a statement of the predicted relationship between variables. Hypotheses may be stated in a null form (e.g., "There will be no difference in heart rate variability in an infant when suction is performed via an endotracheal tube adapter as compared with standard procedure") or in an alternative form (e.g., "Infants will have increased heart rate variability when suctioned via an endotracheal tube adapter as compared with standard procedure"). On the basis of the hypothesis, the investigator then sets out to test the stated relationship.

Defining Variables
Variables are those concepts that interest the researcher. They include the concepts that are to the researcher manipulates (the independent variables) and those that depend on the effect of the intervention (the dependent variables). Situational (or influencing or confounding) variables may influence or exert an effect on the variables of interest, and they may or may not be controlled for in the study's design. For instance, a study that evaluates an intervention designed to ease the transition of infants from the NICU to the home may have as an independent variable the intervention for parents following an infant's discharge from a level III nursery to the home. The dependent variables might be parental responses to the caring for the infant after discharge from the hospital to the home. The situational or influencing variables are those factors that may influence parental responses to having and caring for the in-

fant at home. These may include birth order of the infant, support systems available to the family, the family's socioeconomic status, previous experience with a NICU, and length of time the mother and infant were separated.

All variables must be defined conceptually as well as operationally. A conceptual definition is the general definition that is based on the theoretical framework that guides the study. An operational definition tells how the dependent variables are to be measured or how the independent variable is to be administered. For example, Short et al (1996) evaluated the effects of swaddling versus standard positioning on the neuromuscular development of infants less than 1,250 grams at birth. The operational definition of the swaddling intervention was "wrapping an infant in a blanket to maintain upper and lower extremities in flexion with hands positioned near the mouth." The operational definition of the dependent variable, neuromuscular development, was scores on the Morgan Neonatal Neurobehavioral Exam administered at 34 weeks' postconceptional age.

Selecting Research Instruments
Techniques or instruments used to measure the dependent variables or outcomes must be described according to the following:
1. Validity: Does the instrument measure what it purports to measure?
2. Reliability: Does the instrument provide consistent measures?
3. Suitability-utility: Is the instrument appropriate for the setting and subjects?
4. Sensitivity: Is the instrument sensitive enough to measure the phenomenon?
5. Specificity: Is the instrument specific enough to measure only the phenomenon?

If a well-established instrument is used, the instrument's validity and reliability in previous investigations must be addressed. If the investigator is developing an instrument, validity and reliability must be established. To establish validity and reliability, the instrument must be pilot-tested. A pilot test is a test run on a very small sample. This trial will provide the researcher with data to identify problems with the instrument, awkward wording of questions, or other methodological problems that need to be corrected before implementation of the full project. The investigator should document a detailed description of how the pilot test was conducted, the number of subjects, and their characteristics.

If interviews or observations are used to gather data, interrater and intrarater reliability must be established. Inter-rater reliability refers to consistent measurement across several observers, whereas intrarater reliability refers to consistent measurements on different occasions with the same observer. A number of ways exist to conduct interrater and intrarater reliability to ensure that there is consistency in the variable being measured. Generally, reliability coefficients should be at least 0.70.

Defining the Study Sample
The next step of the research project is to define the study sample. For example, if one wished to investigate respiratory procedures in preterm infants, the investigators would need to define the age, sex, and specific characteristics of the population of infants from which the sample will be selected for the study. In this case, the sample might be selected from the population of all premature infants less than 37 weeks' of gestation. Sample selection may be established in relation to exclusion criteria as well—for example, all infants except those on mechanical ventilation. The researcher must be able to explain why the

population is appropriate for the proposed investigation. However, it is seldom feasible to study the entire target population; therefore the researcher is left with the accessible population (e.g., all infants in a given nursery).

After the researcher determines the population and its characteristics, the specific methods for recruiting the research participants should be determined. The investigator needs to plan ahead to determine what will be done about participants who decline to participate, drop out, or do not participate in all parts of the study. For example, the investigator must consider what will be done about incomplete questionnaires or ones with obvious response sets, less than truthful responses, or unanswered items.

Because the birth of a high-risk infant represents a crisis for the family, special considerations for recruiting samples exist in neonatal research. For example, whenever possible, it is best to delay requesting consent for study participation until the infant's condition has stabilized and the parents have had a chance to adjust to the crisis of the unexpected pregnancy outcome. In some clinical trials, however, this may not be possible if the study focuses on an intervention that must be initiated soon after delivery. In these cases, it is sometimes necessary to approach parents during labor to request consent for study participation.

Power Calculations

The exact number of research participants necessary to achieve statistical significance in experimental investigations can be predicted by the use of power analysis. To calculate the number of participants needed for a given investigation, a brief review of the two types of statistical error, alpha and beta, is needed. Alpha, or a type I, error refers to the rejection of the null hypothesis when in fact it is true. Beta, or a type II, error refers to failure to accept the alternative hypothesis when in fact it is true. The "power" of a statistical test is an important concept. The more powerful the test, the less likely one is of committing a type II error. To apply the concept of power to an investigation, three aspects need to be considered: alpha level, sample size, and effect size. The effect size refers to the magnitude of the relationship between study variables, or magnitude of the difference between groups (when different groups are being compared). Knowledge of two of the three parameters will enable the investigator to calculate the missing value. Therefore, if one has determined the alpha level and if results from a previous investigation provide parameters for estimating the effect size, the overall estimate for sample size can be calculated mathematically. Samples should be large enough to result in a power of .80 to minimize the chances of a type II error. A good description of the procedure can be found in as well as statistical packages or websites for calculations can be found at http://www.im.nbs.gov/powcase/powlinks.html. Some of these web based programs will perform power calculations for the researcher who knows the alpha level, sample size, and effect size desired.

Setting

Investigations that focus on the neonate can occur in a variety of settings, including the nursery (level I, II, or III), the home, or the community. Research that is focused on the parents may take place in the delivery room, the nursery, the home, or the follow-up clinic. Most nursing studies are conducted in the field versus the laboratory setting. The term field refers to the world at large or to a more natural setting. The laboratory setting may be used for quasi-experimental or experimental designs, such as physiologic research or research using animal models. Regardless of the setting, the investigator needs to be very specific in describing the setting in which the study is conducted. Specificity in the description of the setting allows research consumers to determine the applicability of the study findings to their settings and allows others to replicate the study in the future.

Developing a Support Network

Whether one is conducting an investigation as the sole principal investigator or as part of a collaborative effort, clinical research is not an individual activity. High-quality research is most commonly the product of dialogue with experts and critique by colleagues. Of primary importance to the success of the project is the development of a support network. Some aspects of the research project will be tackled with enthusiasm, whereas other aspects will be put off or never completed. Whether one works alone or in a collaborative effort, a support network in which one receives assistance with refocusing on the goal, problem solving, or motivation eases the road to completion of the project.

Consultation

Although all members of a research team need a basic understanding of the entire research process, each member may contribute specific, unique expertise. The word statistics often freezes the potential researcher. Statistical consultation is an excellent example of using special expertise in the conduct of a research project to improve its scientific merit. Data cannot and should not be turned over to a statistician without consultation. The researcher must clarify with the statistician what is to be accomplished from the analysis; otherwise the study's results may be erroneous.

In a university setting, statistical consultants can be found in many departments, including biology, medicine, nursing, psychology, and sociology. Graduate students are often assigned the task of data entry and statistical analysis. The services of students can assist with the mechanics of data analysis but do not constitute and should not substitute for consultation with a statistician. Hospitals sometimes have statisticians within their own research departments, especially if they are involved in experimental or laboratory research.

Developing the Proposal

Clear identification of the elements that are expected in the proposal helps keep the development stage to a minimum. If a funding agency is to be involved, it may have a specific format for submission). Often this format is different from the proposal that will be submitted for institutional review.

Funding

Many sources of funds are available for research: local foundations, corporations, managed care or health maintenance organizations, university funding agencies, professional organizations such as the Association of Women's Health, Obstetrical and Neonatal Nurses, local chapters of Sigma Theta Tau, and the March of Dimes Birth Defects Foundation. The single most important item to determine prior to writing a proposal is the funding priorities of the agency. A critical element is the credentials needed by the principal investigator in order to qualify for funds. Some institutions require that a researcher be employed at that institution; other institutions require that a potential recipient of funds have a doctorate degree. Table 5-3 lists potential funding sources.

TABLE **5-3** Sources of Research Funding Information		
Source	**Address, Phone, Web Address**	**Type of Projects Funded**
American Association of Critical Care Nurses	AACN Department of Research 101 Columbia Aliso Viejo, CA 92656-1491 800-899-2256 www.aacn.org/	Grant is to encourage qualified nurses to contribute to the advancement of nursing through critical care nursing practice research.
American Nurses' Foundation	American Nurses' Foundation 600 Maryland Avenue, SW Suite 100 West Washington, DC 20024 202-651-7227 fax: 202-651-7354 www.nursingworld.org/anf	The purpose of the American Nurses Foundation (ANF) research Grants Program is to encourage the research career development of nurses, support scientific research for advancing the practice of nursing, promoting health, and preventing disease.
Association of Women's Health, Obstetric, and Neonatal Nurses (AWHONN)	Department of Education and Research 700 14th Street, NW Suite 600 Washington, DC 20005-2019 202-662-1600 fax: 202-737-0575 www.awhonn.org	Nursing research grants provide 'seed' monies for pilot research or total funding for small projects with potential to contribute to nursing knowledge and the clinical practice for the care of women and newborns.
National Institute of Child Health and Human Development (NICHD)	Bldg 31, Room 2A32, MSC 2425 31 Center Drive Bethesda, MD 20892-2425 www.nichd.nih.gov	The goal of NICHD's research programs is the improvement of maternal, infant, and child health through support of basic and clinical research to elucidate normal and abnormal growth, development, and maturation, from gametogenesis through maturity.
National Institute of Health Office of Extramural Research	Office of Extramural Research National Institute of Health Bethesda, MD 20892 301-435-0714 301-480-0525 http://grants1.mh.gov/grants/oer.htm Grantinfo@nih.gov	Extramural research grants are designed to fund projects that protect and improve human health, the NIH conducts and supports basic, applied, and clinical and health services research to understand the processes underlying human health and to acquire new knowledge to help prevent, diagnose, and treat human diseases and disabilities.
National Institute of Nursing Research	National Institute of Nursing Research Bethesda, MD 20892-2178 301-496-0207 www.nih.gov/ninr	The NINR extramural program (OEP) invites investigator-initiated applications that contain innovative ideas and sound methodology in all aspects of nursing research consistent with the NINR mission.
Sigma Theta Tau International	550 W. North Street Indianapolis, IN 46202 317-634-8171 fax: 317-634-8188 toll-free: 888-634-7575 toll-free: 800-634-7575 www.nursingsociety.org/research	Small grants to encourage nurses to contribute to the advancement of nursing through research.
The Academy of Neonatal Nursing	The Academy of Neonatal Nursing 2777 Yulupa Avenue #166 Santa Rosa, CA 95405-8584 707-568-2168 www.academyonline.org	Funds research projects related to neonatal nursing are provided through The Foundation of Neonatal Research and Education.
The Foundation Center	The Foundation Center 79 Fifth Avenue/16th Street New York, NY 10003-3076 212-620-4230 800-424-9836 fax: 212-807-3677 www.fdncenter.org	The Foundation Center provides print, CD-ROM, and online resources to help grantseekers identify appropriate funders and develop targeted proposals.

ETHICAL CONSIDERATIONS

Concerns related to ethical treatment of patients can be traced to the time of Hippocrates and the basic principle of "first do no harm." During World War II, prisoners in Nazi concentration camps were often subjects of experiments. They were exposed to altitude changes and extreme cold to determine their physiologic responses. They were injected with the malaria and typhus viruses without consideration about personal harm. These subjects had no ability to refuse and often died as a result of the experimentation (National Commission for the Protection of Human Subjects of Biomedical and Behavioral Research, 1979).

Once the war was over, the Nuremberg trials were held. The articles of the Nuremberg Tribunal of 1948 outlined what came to be known as the Nuremberg codes. This document was the First International Code of Research Ethics. It set the standards for research and described the need for informed consent. The responsibilities of the researcher were also highlighted. The code suggested that animal trials be performed before experimentation on human research participants. It further suggested that the researcher be scientifically expert and have some knowledge of the area of research. Furthermore, every research participant was to have the right to withdraw at any time during a study.

In the early 1960s in the United States that Congress mandated informed consent and the federal government for all research supported with federal funds. In 1964, the World Medical Association Declaration of Helsinki (revised in 1975) included ethical guidelines related to the use of humans in experiments. Following the first Helsinki Declaration, the United States Surgeon General in 1966 issued a policy statement on the protection of human subjects. During the same year, the American Medical Association published *Guidelines for Clinical Investigation*. The American Nurses' Association (1985) also published "Human Rights Guidelines for Nurses in Clinical and Other Research." These documents represent only broad guidelines about the conduct of general research and are not legally binding in and of them. They do not specify individual cases or situations.

The National Research Act of 1974 established the National Commission of Human Subjects of Biomedical and Behavioral Research (National Commission). Institutional review boards (IRBs) were then established. The commission was to look at the ethical underpinnings of research, specifically the boundaries between practice and research, risks and benefits, selection of subjects, and informed consent. They convened at the Belmont Center in Baltimore, Maryland. They encouraged debate among the membership to consider whether research could be performed without human subjects and to consider whether research is really necessary. These two questions are considered today by IRBs when research proposals are reviewed. In 1979, the commission issued the *Belmont Report* (National Commission, 1979). This report outlined three guiding principles for research: respect for persons, beneficence, and justice. Respect incorporates the idea that subjects are autonomous agents who can think clearly and make choices for themselves. If they cannot choose for themselves, they need special protection. This principle of special protection applies to children, the unborn, the poor or disadvantaged, the mentally retarded, or psychiatric and mental health clients who are considered mentally disabled. Respect also involves treating all subjects fairly and openly. All information, then, must be given through informed consent, which is implemented by the researcher by explaining the nature of the study, checking the understanding of the subject about his or her participation in the study, offering the right to withdraw at any time during the research, and ensuring freedom from coercion (i.e., no penalty will be attached if the potential subject refuses to participate or withdraws before the study ends). Respect includes privacy and confidentiality of information that the investigator obtains during the study's course.

The second principle outlined by the Belmont Report is beneficence, which involves the validation of trust and respect. Again, this relates to the principle of "first do no harm." Researchers as well as IRB members must realize that there may be unforeseen risks. Many of the medications and treatments currently used in practice may have long-range side effects that will not be recognized for years to come. The same holds true for research experimentation; however, the cost versus benefit must be considered. The currently known risks must be considered. The IRB and researcher share equal responsibility in protecting the human subject against untoward risks. The nature and scope of the risks must be weighed against the benefits of the study. Researchers must agree that the clinical trial will be stopped when the results are obvious.

The third ethical principle is justice, which is concerned with whether the risks are distributed equitably. This principle also guides the adjustment of protocols as problems are identified or more information becomes available, such as a recently discovered side effect of a treatment that makes an arm of the research protocol dangerous to continue. Any adjustment in the protocol for protection of the human subjects must go back to the IRB for approval.

The recommendations of the National Commission that was formed in 1974 served as the basis for a series of federal regulations governing involvement of human participants in research. These regulations were last revised in 1991 and serve as a basic guideline for researchers today (Harrison, 2001). An excellent resource for questions related to ethical aspects of research is the Office for Human Research Participants (OHRP) and the Office of Human Subjects Research (OHSR) within the United States Department of Health and Human Services (see http://ohsr.od.nih.gov/ for online computer-based training on the protection of human subjects).

Gaining access to research participants is often influenced by issues related to professional territoriality. Nurse researchers are often required to seek physician permission before inviting patients or families to participate in research. The American Nurses Association's Human Rights Guidelines for Nurses in Clinical and Other Research (1985) specify that "if subjects are patients of other practitioners, the investigator as an obligation to discuss the proposed study with that practitioner prior to its inception and to negotiate support for its successful completion" (American Nurses' Association, 1985). Although no consensus exists about whether nurses should be required to seek approval of physicians or other health team members before inviting families to participate in research, research projects are more likely to succeed if all members of the health care team are informed about the nature of the study.

INSTITUTIONAL REVIEW BOARDS

Review and approval of proposals must take place before the involvement of human or animal subjects can occur. This review may be by a committee within a department, or it may occur within an institution such as a hospital or a university. These reviews generally involve the departments of nursing, neonatology, and perinatology. The reviewers consider the merit of the design, feasibility, coherence with the institution's mission, and the protection of human research participants. In some institutions, review of the scientific merit of a study occurs separately from the review of the human research participants, whereas in others these two objectives are combined.

Institutional Review Boards (IRBs) were developed to ensure the rights and welfare of research participants. In general, these committees are multidisciplinary, including scientists, nonscientists, and lay public representatives. Each institution conducting research does not have to have its own board, but it must have access to one. Some institutions have human ethics committees to safeguard the rights of clients. If a research proposal for which no one on the committee has expertise is to be reviewed, an outside expert can be consulted to discuss the appropriateness of the protocol and whether any side effects of the treatment or research have been overlooked. Outside experts do not vote on the project, however.

The review process can benefit the researcher as well as the research participants because the committee can see problems that the researcher might not have considered before. A basic ethical concern in neonatal research is that the patient cannot speak and give informed consent. Parents sometimes feel vulnerable and unable to refuse a request for participation in research by the caregiver of their infants. It is then up to the collaborative health care team and the IRB to safeguard the neonates and their families. They must weigh the risks and benefits as well as the ethics of the proposed research. An informed consent process is the method of operationalizing the process of protection of human research participants (Harrison, 2001a). The basic elements are the following:

- An understandable explanation of the study and its procedures
- An explanation of any risk or discomfort to be encountered by a subject
- Identification of the cost versus the benefits of participation in the study
- Assurance that the researcher will be available to answer the subject's questions
- Assurance of confidentiality of information obtained
- Assurance of the right to withdraw from the study at any time during the project

The function of the IRB, then, is to review, approve, disapprove, or request revision of research protocols for the purposes of protecting human subjects and upholding the ethical principles of research. The actual review consists of examining the risks to the subjects in relation to the potential benefits. It also ensures that selection of subjects is equitable and nondiscriminatory. The informed consent is scrutinized for the previously mentioned basic elements and for readability. Today, the average United States citizen reads at less than a seventh-grade level. Many committees are suggesting that a fourth- to fifth-grade reading level be used for informed consent. This reading level is sometimes difficult to achieve because risk managers within institutions often dictate that legal language be incorporated into the informed consent. It is then up to the researcher or whoever obtains the informed consent to determine the level of comprehension of the potential subject. The researcher must also assure the IRB that the data collection

will be monitored to determine whether and when a research protocol should be terminated.

In some institutions, studies that involve minimal risk to subjects may be expedited or reviewed by a subcommittee rather than the full IRB. Survey research, retrospective chart reviews, and examination of data collected as part of clinical care, such as diagnostic specimens, may not require informed consent of the subjects.

The issues surrounding informed consent continue to change as questions about ethics and ethical decision-making arise. Genetic research, organ procurement, the use of anencephalic infants as organ donors, organ transplantation, as well as some behavioral research are all raising new concerns that IRBs must consider. Because of these changes and the concern over protection of human subjects, investigators who hold federal funding at certain institutions must undergo annual continuing education regarding IRB rules.

SUMMARY

Research must not be thought of as a discrete activity within neonatal nursing but rather as a way of thinking and an approach to each nursing encounter. Meier stated that "the evolving issue is not whether research in nursing is essential but rather how data that is crucially needed to guide clinical practice can be attained through systematic investigation" (Meier, 1983). Neonatal nurses, by virtue of their relatively new and rapidly evolving practice and their exposure to the research process, are in an excellent position to integrate research and practice to ensure that the care they provide to neonates and families is truly evidence-based.

REFERENCES

Altimier L et al (1999). Neonatal Thermoregulation: bed surface transfers. *Neonatal network*, 18(4), 35-38.

American Nurses' Association. (1985). *Human rights guidelines for nurses in clinical and other research.* Kansas City, MO: American Nurses' Association.

American Nurses' Association. (1994). *Education for participation in nursing research.* Kansas City, MO: American Nurses' Association.

Beck CT (1990). The research critique: general criteria for evaluating a research report. *Journal of obstetric, gynecologic, and neonatal nursing,* 19(1), 18-22.

Brink PJ, Wood MJ (Eds.). (1998). *Advanced design in nursing research,* ed 2, Newbury Park, CA: Sage Publications.

Burns N, Grove SK (2001). *The practice of nursing research: conduct, critique, & utilization,* ed 4, Philadelphia: WB Saunders.

Costello A, Chapman J (1998). Mothers' perceptions of the care-by-parent program prior to hospital discharge of their preterm infants. *Neonatal network,* 17(7), 37-42.

Fleming JW (1984). Selecting a clinical nursing problem for research. *Image: Journal of nursing scholarship,* 16(2), 62-64.

Funk SG et al (1995). Barriers and facilitators of research utilization: An integrative review. *Nursing clinics of North America,* 30(3), 395-407.

Gennaro S (1994). Research utilization: an overview. *JOGNN,* 23(4), 313-319.

Grunau RE et al (2000). Are twitches, startles, and body movements pain indicators in extremely low birth weight infants? *The clinical journal of pain,* 16, 37-45.

Haller KB et al (1979). Developing research based on innovative protocols. *Research in nursing & health,* 2, 45-57.

Harrison L (2001a) Informed Consent in Neonatal Nursing Practice and Research. *Central lines* 17(5).

Harrison L (2001b). Research roles for neonatal nurses. *Central lines*, 17(1), 18-20.

Harrison LL, Bodin MB (1994). Effects of tactile stimulation on preterm infants: An integrative review of the literature with practice implications. *The online journal of knowledge synthesis for nursing*, 1(6).

Harrison LL et al (2000). Physiologic and behavioral effects of gentle human touch on preterm infants. *Research in nursing & health*, 23, 435-446.

Holditch-Davis D, Miles MS (2000). Mothers' stories about their experiences in the neonatal intensive care unit. *Neonatal network*, 19, 13-21.

Jain L, Vidyasagar D (1989). Iatrogenic disorders in modern neonatology. *Clinics in perinatology*, 16(1), 255-273.

Kachoyeanos MK (1995). Opportunities in outcome evaluation research. *American journal of maternal child nursing*, 20(4), 223.

Kachoyeanos MK (1996). The current state of research in MCH nursing. *MCN; American journal of maternal child nursing*, 21(1), 13.

Kenner C, Walden M (2001). *Grantwriting tips*. Washington DC: American Nurses Publishing.

Kilbride H et al (2000). Thirty-six-month outcome of prenatal cocaine exposure for term or near-term infants: Impact of early case management. *Developmental and behavioral pediatrics*, 21, 19-26.

Krywanio ML: Meta-analysis of physiological outcomes of hospital-based infant intervention programs. *Nursing research*, 1994 May-Jun, 43(3), 133-137.

Lantos JD, Frader J (1990). Extracorporeal membrane oxygenation and the ethics of clinical research in pediatrics. *New England journal of medicine*, 323, 409-413.

Luckenbill-Brett JL (1987). Use of nursing practice research findings. *Nursing research*, 36(6), 344-349.

Lund CH et al (2001). Neonatal skin care: Clinical outcomes of the AWHONN/NANN evidence-based clinical practice guideline. *JOGNN*, 30, (1), 41-51.

McGee P (1996). The research role of the advanced nurse practitioner. *British journal of nursing*, 5, 290-292.

McKinney J, Vermuelen W (2000). Research nurses play a vital role in clinical trials. *Oncology nursing forum*, 27, 28.

Medoff-Cooper B (1994). Transition of the preterm infant to an open crib. *JOGNN*, 23(4), 329-335.

Meier P (1983). Research methodologies in neonatal nursing. *Neonatal network*, 2(2), 16-22.

Meier PF (1994). Transition of the preterm infant to an open crib: Process of the project group. *JOGNN*, 23(4), 321-326.

Miles MS et al (1993). Parental stressor scale: Neonatal intensive care unit. *Nursing research*, 42(3), 148-152.

Miles MS et al (1999). African American mothers' responses to hospitalization of an infant with serious health problems. *Neonatal network*, 18(8), 17-25.

National Commission for the Protection of Human Subjects of Biomedical and Behavioral Research. (1979). *The Belmont Report: Ethical principles and guidelines for the protection of human subjects of research* (DHEW Publication No. [OS] 78-0013 and No. [OS] 78-0014). Washington, DC: U.S. Government Printing Office.

Omery A, Williams RP (1999). An appraisal of research utilization across the U.S. *Journal of nursing administration*, 29, 50-56.

Perez-Woods R, Tse AM (1990). Research attitudes, activities, competencies, and interest of NANN members. *Neonatal network*, 8(5), 57-59.

Polit DE, Hungler BP (1998). *Nursing research: principles and methods*, ed 6, Philadelphia: Lippincott.

Rogers EM (1995). *Diffusion of innovations*, ed. 4, New York: Free Press.

Sarnecky MT (1990). Historiography: A legitimate research methodology for nursing. *Advances in nursing science*, 12(4), 1-10.

Short MA et al (1996). The effects of swaddling versus standard positioning on neuromuscular development in very low birth weight infants. *Neonatal network*, 15(4), 25-31.

Thoyre SM (2001). Challenges mothers identify in bottle feeding their preterm infants. *Neonatal network*, 20(1), 41-50.

Vickers A et al (1998). Massage therapy for preterm and/or low birth-weight infants. http://www.nichd.nih.gov/cochrane/vickers/vickers.html 10/6/98 (pages 1-30).

Vohr BR et al (2000). Neurodevelopmental and functional outcomes of extremely low birth weight infants in the National Institute of Child Health and Human Development Neonatal Research Network, 1993-1994. *Pediatrics*, 105, 1216-1226.

Walczak JR et al (1994). A survey of research-related activities and perceived barriers to research utilization among professional oncology nurses. *Oncology nursing forum*, 21, 710-715.

Westrup B et al (2000). A randomized, controlled trial to evaluate the effects of the newborn individualized developmental care and assessment program in a Swedish setting. *Pediatrics*, 105(1), 66-72.

CHAPTER 6

COMPETENCY-BASED EDUCATION IN NEONATAL NURSING

FRANCES STRODTBECK

As health care moves into the twenty-first century, the issue of developing, maintaining, and ensuring the competence of neonatal nurses remains at the forefront for many institutions and agencies concerned with the quality of neonatal health care. Although the emphasis on competence is not new, the topic gained prominence during the period of health care reform in the 1980s. As the American health care delivery system reorganized under the umbrella of health care reform, societal concerns about the quality of care received and the providers delivering that care increased (Whittaker et al, 2000). Responding to the escalating concern, credentialing agencies such as the Joint Commission on Accreditation of Healthcare Organizations (JCAHO) issued standards requiring documentation of the clinical competency of all nursing staff (JCAHO, 1999).

Hospitals now were faced with the need to develop systems for assessing both the initial competence of newly hired nurses and the ongoing competence of the existing nursing staff. Unfortunately, this regulatory push for documentation hit hospitals at a time when many were losing their unit-based educators or clinical nurse specialists (or both) as a result of downsizing. This loss was particularly hard for critical care units, such as the neonatal intensive care unit (NICU), that were short staffed and had high turnover rates for nurses at all educational levels. As this movement toward documentation of minimal competencies for hospital nurses was developing, educational institutions were looking at terminal program objectives and the ways in which these might translate into minimal competency statements for graduates. A strategy that gained acceptance during this period of upheaval was competency-based education (CBE). It offered a bridge between the academic center and the hospital or community health care center. The hope was that CBE offered a way to shorten orientation time while improving quality control for nurses' performance. The assumption was, if the academic centers could demonstrate that their graduates' competencies were closely tied to the minimal competencies expected by employers, the orientation could focus on the specialty content and needs in the area where the nurse eventually would work (Hodges & Hansen, 1999; Marrone, 1999).

This chapter traces the development of the competency movement in health care, discusses the advantages and disadvantages of competency-based education, and describes the impact of competency evaluation on neonatal nursing practice and education.

HISTORY OF THE COMPETENCY MOVEMENT

The first voice to link improvement in hospital care to the competence of its providers was Florence Nightingale's. In her books, *Notes on Nursing* (Nightingale, 1860) and *Notes on Hospitals* (Nightingale, 1859), she laid the foundation for changes that revolutionized nursing education and practice. The hospital-based education system that evolved from her teachings became the predominant model for nursing education in the United States. Hospital-based or diploma programs that used an apprentice model to integrate classroom learning and clinical performance dominated the American educational system for nurses until the late 1960s and early 1970s (Chapman, 1999). Subsequently, the growing importance of higher education shifted nursing education from the hospital-based school to the academic school or university and transferred responsibility for the competence of the new graduate nurse from the hospital or employer to the university and its educators (Bechtel et al, 1999). University-based nursing education gained in popularity, and the hospital-based programs began to disappear.

As the new paradigm of nursing education evolved, a gap appeared between the expectations in the practice arena (the hospitals and clinical agencies) and the expectations in the education arena; this gap persists as a major issue in nursing education today. According to Lenburg (1999a), "Employers are experiencing a widening gulf between the competencies required for practice and those new graduates learned in their education programs." This gap in competency adds to the cost of health care, because employers must spend more money on human resource time and expertise in orienting new nurses.

The landmark book, *On Competence: A Critical Analysis of Competence-Based Reforms in Higher Education*, paved the way for recommendations to reform the education of professionals in American universities and colleges (Grant, 1979). Although published more than 20 years ago, Grant's thoughts on competence are still relevant:

Today, in fact, belief in one's own competence is no longer enough, and a demand for demonstrated competence now motivates much of education. This demand underlies much of the insistence on continuing education and even relicensure in the major professions, and it aims both to uncover cases of self-delusion about one's competence and to prevent apathetic resignation about maintaining one's competence. There is more to know in general; there is more to know about the specialty on which one focuses; and there is more continuous production of new knowledge that requires sifting, even if much of it must be discarded as unproven or redundant.

Eventually government became concerned about the issue of education and competency. In 1986 the National Governors' Association tackled the tough issues of accreditation of institutions of higher learning and their accountability to the public for the competency of graduates (Lenburg, 1999b). As the pressure to become accountable for the competency of university graduates grew, academia responded. The journal of the American Association of Higher Education, *Change,* devoted the entire September/October issue in 1990 to addressing the problems of competence and higher education (Lenburg, 1999a, b, c). Over the next decade, academia imported total quality management concepts and strategies from the business world (Lenburg, 1999b, c). Academic accreditation agencies such as the National League for Nursing Accreditation Corporation (NLN) and the Commission for Collegiate Nursing Education (CCNE) incorporated competency language into their accreditation criteria (NLNAC, 1997; CCNE, 1998). State boards of nursing addressed the issue of ensuring competence and competency validation at the state regulatory level (National Council of State Boards of Nursing, 1998).

Multidisciplinary and consumer organizations concerned about the quality of health care also pushed for reforms to assure the public of the competency of those entering the health care professions and of those already in practice. In 1996 the Citizens Advocacy Center, an organization of public members of health care regulatory and governing boards, held a two-day conference titled, "Continuing Professional Competence: Can We Assure It?" The proceedings of the conference, published in 1997, called for stronger measures to assure the public of the continued competence of health care workers and to remove workers who may not be competent (CAC, 1997).

The Pew Health Professions Commission released several documents in the late 1990s calling for education reform and validation of the competency of existing practitioners (Pew Health Professions Commission, 1995 and 1998). The first report called for states to "require each board to develop, implement, and evaluate continuing competency requirements to assure the continuing competence of regulated health care professionals" (Pew Health Professions Commission, 1995). A subsequent report called for states to require that health care professionals "demonstrate their competence in the knowledge, judgment, technical skills, and interpersonal skills relevant to their jobs throughout their careers" (Pew Health Professions Commission, 1998). These reports proposed periodic reviews of professional competence at intervals not to exceed 7 years. In addition to mandatory continuing education, the commission advocated repeat testing of professionals using the initial licensing examination or a new examination in the specialty or practice area, chart or peer review (or both), and acceptance of professional credentialing such as certification and recertification.

Despite the differences in the issues of concern to employers, regulators, and politicians, academia, especially health care educators, clearly has been put on notice to shape up and provide society with a competent graduate. The key question for the nursing profession is, how should the nursing educational system be changed to meet this challenge, given the complexities of today's health care environment? The situation is well summarized by Lenburg (1999a): "Substantive reforms in academic and continuing education and in credentialing requirements are needed to accommodate consumer protection, technological innovations, sociodemographic and market forces, and the rising incidence of litigation related to health care."

A seemingly obvious solution would be to return to some variation of the apprentice model used in diploma nursing education; however, the logistics of implementing such a solution in a manner that would preserve the gains made by moving nursing education to institutions of higher learning would be insurmountable. Another obvious solution would be to narrow the gap between nursing education and nursing service. Bargagliotti and colleagues (1999) stressed the need to consider the stakeholders when considering competencies. They suggested that practice and education must work together to determine competencies. As Lenburg (1999b) observed:

> Nurse educators, whether responsible for classroom or clinical learning, are most effective when they engage in some form of clinical practice through which they adapt past skills to current circumstances and learn new ones now required in complex health care environments. Those who practice little, or not at all, are ill equipped to promote competence among students in the ever-changing contemporary work force.

Although a variety of models for integrating education and service have been tried across the country, most nursing academic programs remain separate from institutions that provide nursing services.

Other possible solutions offered have focused on changing the education model for entry into the nursing profession (i.e., requiring the professional doctorate) and on switching from the traditional pedagogy of lectures to alternative models, such as competency-based education and problem-based learning.

Proponents of the professional doctorate model cite the knowledge explosion, the proliferation of medical technology, the complexity of health care delivery systems, and the increasing need for nursing professionals to deal with sophisticated biomedical ethical situations as reasons for moving toward a longer basic nursing educational program (Carter, 1988; Fitzpatrick, 1988; Watson, 1988). The suggested curriculum would parallel the curriculum design for medicine and law; that is, the professional nursing education would be built on a foundation of study for the bachelor's degree in liberal arts or science and prescribed prenursing courses. Individuals interested in nursing careers then would apply for admission to a nursing school. Upon acceptance, the individual would complete a 3- to 4-year nursing curriculum, and graduates would be awarded a doctor of nursing (ND) degree. Although this model has many advantages, the reality is that the nursing profession is still arguing over the baccalaureate model for entry into practice.

As the competency movement gains strength, the need to prepare competent graduates becomes a de facto obligation for nursing schools. Changing from the traditional model of classroom teaching and learning to alternative models is both realistic and possible. Competency-based education and other similar models are growing in popularity in nursing academia and continuing education.

COMPETENCE AND COMPETENCY

What is competence? What is competency? What is the difference between the two? How is practice competence measured? These are some of the questions nursing educators and managers are asking.

Alspach (1992) defines competence as "the possession of knowledge, skills, and abilities necessary to perform the job" and competency as "the employee's ability to actually perform in the (work) environment in accordance with the role and standards of the institution." The National Institutes of Health (1995) defines competency as "a general statement that describes the knowledge, skills, and abilities necessary for safe nursing practice in a specific area." Competency, according to Benner (1984), is "the ability to perform the task with desirable outcomes under the varied circumstances of the real world." Jeffrey (2000) defines competency as a written statement established by expert opinion that identifies specific standards and direction for the professional's decision-making in health care.

In 1994 the American Nurses Association (ANA) defined competency as "the demonstration of knowledge and skills in meeting professional role expectations." More recently, an ANA Expert Panel (2000) published the following definitions of competence:

- Continuing competence: Ongoing professional nursing competence according to the level of expertise, responsibility, and domains of practice.
- Professional nursing competence: Behavior based on beliefs, attitudes, and knowledge matched to and in the context of a set of expected outcomes as defined by nursing scope of practice, policy, [the ANA] *Code for Nurses,* standards, guidelines, and benchmarks that assure safe performance of professional activities.
- Continuing professional nursing competence: Ongoing professional nursing competence according to level of expertise, responsibility, and domains of practice as evidenced by behavior based on beliefs, attitudes, and knowledge matched to and in the context of a set of expected outcomes as defined by nursing scope of practice, policy, *Code of Ethics,* standards, guidelines, and benchmarks that assure safe performance of professional activities.

Clearly, competence and competency are related but different. Competence refers to the skills and abilities of the individual; competency is the ability of the individual to demonstrate those skills and abilities in a work setting. Competence and competency are the two sides of one coin, and both are of concern to nursing educators and employers of new nurses.

Traditionally, individual competence is assessed during the interview and hiring process. This assessment usually consists of checking letters of recommendation; verifying educational and state recognition for practice as a registered nurse (RN); evaluating the applicant's self-reported information (e.g., résumé and job application); and conducting a personal interview. Advanced practice nurses (APN), especially nurse practitioners, often undergo an additional review of their skills and abilities during the credentialing process. The advanced practice skills and abilities are subjected to a peer-review process that often includes verification of previous employment, specialty certification, and state recognition of APN status, in addition to investigations for involvement in malpractice claims and disciplinary actions against the applicant's professional credentials.

Competency, on the other hand, is seen as an ongoing process, one that begins with employment and continues at periodic intervals for the duration of employment. Competency therefore is the issue of concern to employers, regulatory agencies, insurance companies, professional organizations, and society at large (Whittaker et al, 2000), whereas educators are concerned with preparing competent individuals.

Like many other practice disciplines, the profession of nursing has two dimensions, science and art. The science of nursing is imparted in formal educational programs and continuing education. The art of nursing is more elusive and is learned over time. The process of mastering both dimensions is essential. Benner (1984) details this process in her important book, *From Novice to Expert: Excellence and Power in Clinical Nursing Practice,* which is widely recognized within the profession. According to Benner, individuals go through five stages in the development of nursing expertise: novice, advanced beginner, competent, proficient, and expert.

It is noteworthy that competent is the third stage, not the final one. Two stages (proficient and expert) come after the development of competence. The new graduate nurse or the experienced nurse who is changing practice areas cannot reasonably be expected to be competent at the onset of employment in a new area such as the NICU; both will require some type of orientation before they can become contributing members of the NICU staff. It is reasonable to expect that both will acquire initial competency within a reasonable period of time as defined by the unit and the institution.

COMPETENCY-BASED EDUCATION

Understanding competency-based education (CBE) requires an understanding of what a competency is. A competency has three components: the knowledge that forms the basis of nursing practice; the performance skills (psychomotor and problem solving) to apply that knowledge to a clinical situation; and an affective response (Dunn et al, 2000).

Nursing competencies are often divided into levels. Fey & Miltner (2000) describe three levels: core, specialty, and patient care management competencies. Core competencies are the skills and knowledge required for the minimum safe level of nursing performance. Specialty competencies are the skills and knowledge required for the minimum safe level of nursing care for a specific patient population. Specialty competencies are often unit specific. Patient care management *competencies* demonstrate the integration of core and specialty competencies in the provision of safe patient care.

Competencies are often written in two parts: a statement that describes the performance standard and a list of performance criteria (Luttrell et al, 1999). The differences in the levels of competencies are illustrated in Table 6-1. Special attention should be paid to the progression from the broad (core) to the specific (patient care in a specific population).

Although some competencies are mandated by accreditation agencies such as JCAHO, most nursing competencies are derived from standards of practice developed by professional nursing organizations (Weinstein, 2000). Nursing standards of practice define the essential content competencies that form the foundation for CBE (Dozier, 1998). The National Organization of Nurse Practitioner Faculties (NONPF) has developed standardized general nursing competencies for advance practice nurses. These general competencies can be adapted to fit specialties within nursing. Specialty nursing organizations, such as the National Association of Neonatal Nurses (NANN), have a multifaceted role in the development of neonatal nursing competencies. Specialty organizations are responsible for developing the specific standards and clinical guidelines on which professional nursing practice is based (Whittaker et al, 2000). They also are responsible for monitoring issues that affect the practice of nursing, such as the development of an appropriate health care policy, and for supporting research to link nursing interventions to patient outcomes. Finally, nursing organizations support individual competence by

TABLE 6-1	Competency Levels Applied to Neonatal Nursing		
	Core Competency	**Specialty Competency**	**Patient Care Management Competency**
Performance standard	The nurse assesses the patient's level of pain.	The nurse recognizes the signs and symptoms of pain in neonates.	The nurse provides care for neonates in the immediate postoperative period.
Performance criteria	The nurse routinely assesses each patient's level of pain. The nurse implements a plan of care to provide pain relief.	The nurse assesses the neonates for signs and symptoms of pain every hour. The nurse initiates nonpharmacologic pain interventions per unit protocol.	The nurse cares for a neonate after gastrointestinal surgery for an abdominal wall defect. The nurse cares for the preterm neonate after surgery for a patent ductus ligation.

Modified from Fey MK, Miltner RS (2000). A competency-based orientation program for new graduate nurses. Journal of nursing administration 30(3), 126-132.

providing educational opportunities for nurses to maintain their skills and knowledge, by influencing changes in state nurse practice acts, and by participating in the credentialing process as appropriate (Weinstein, 2000; Whittaker et al, 2000).

Ensuring the competency of a nursing staff requires an organized approach to orientation to the unit and a system of verification and validation of the skills and knowledge applied. Because nurses have a variety of educational and experiential backgrounds, the traditional orientation involving lectures and procedural manuals is no longer an efficient and effective strategy (Dunn et al, 2000). Competency-based orientation (CBO) is one form of CBE and is the preferred model in many institutions because it allows for the variation in nurses' backgrounds. CBO is "the simultaneous integration of the knowledge, skills, and attitudes that are required for performance in a designated role and setting" (Alspach, 1984). Ideally, this type of orientation would be an extension of a generic, competency-based curriculum followed by the academic institutions, adapted to fit the clinical or practice setting.

Competency-based orientation has many advantages and few disadvantages. A major advantage is the shortened orientation for experienced nurses (Stewart & Vitello-Cicciu, 1989; O'Grady & O'Brien, 1992; Marrone, 1999). In the current economic environment, this can result in significant savings for the unit and the institution. Other advantages are (1) measurable performance standards; (2) increased quality control (because performance standards are consistent); (3) elimination of repetitive classroom lectures and presentations; (4) adaptability of the length of orientation to the needs of the new graduate or the experienced nurse; (5) personal accountability on the part of orientees for their own learning (or lack of it); and (6) treatment of orientees as adult learners.* The educator becomes the facilitator of the process rather than the master teacher and gatekeeper of learning (Mikos-Schild, 1999). As unit resources, preceptors serve as expert role models and facilitate the learning of the orientee.

Competency-based education has been criticized as emphasizing the science of nursing while paying little or no attention to the art of nursing. Communication skills, ethics, creative problem solving, and role development skills inherent in the art of nursing are difficult to quantify and to translate into objective, measurable competency statements (Mikos-Schild, 1999). Several authors have argued that the emphasis on skills and the technical aspects of nursing performance does not promote critical thinking and problem-solving skills (Mikos-Schild, 1999). Neary (2001) notes that measuring competency is difficult because of the subjective nature of evaluation and because of problems in measurability. Competencies often include a laundry list of skills and knowledge that must be attained. This application of competencies, more or less as tasks to be performed, may prolong orientation for the individual who is unable to set priorities or who is not motivated to complete the process (Mikos-Schild, 1999). Despite these disadvantages, CBE is widely used for orientation programs and some academic nursing programs. CBE is well suited to adult learners (Knowles, 1980).

One of the best-known approaches to CBE is the Competency Outcomes and Performance Assessment (COPA) model developed by Lenburg for the New York Regents College Nursing Program (Lenburg, 1999c). In the COPA model, traditional educational objectives are replaced with outcomes that are practice based, realistic, and measurable. The process of switching from the objective model to a competency-based model is governed by four key questions: What are the performance-based competency outcomes required for practice? What are the measurable indicators of competence for each outcome? What are the most effective learning strategies for achieving the outcomes? What are the most effective methods for assessing achievement of outcomes?

According to Lenburg, there are eight core practice competencies, each having subset skills (Table 6-2). The traditional learning objectives focused on the learning process (e.g., the student would be asked to discuss the role of the nurse in the NICU). Competency statements focus on the outcomes the institution desires in its graduates or employees. These statements are measurable performance outcomes that lend themselves to criterion-referenced performance evaluations. Objective evaluations based on psychometric concepts are developed to document learner competence for the core practice competencies. The psychometric concepts include critical elements, objectivity, sampling, acceptability, comparability, consistency, flexibility, and systematized conditions (Table 6-3).

---

*(Alspach, 1984; O'Grady & O'Brien, 1992; Chaisson, 1995; Marrone, 1999; Mikos-Schild, 1999; Smith, et al, 1996).

TABLE 6-2	Lenburg's Core Practice Competencies and Examples of Subset Skills
Core Competency	**Subset Skill Examples**
Assessment and intervention skills	Assessment
	Monitoring
	Therapeutic treatments
Communication skills	Oral
	Written
	Computer (information systems)
Critical thinking skills	Problem solving
	Evaluation
	Prioritizing
	Diagnostic reasoning
Human caring and relationship skills	Respect for cultural diversity
	Ethics
	Interpersonal relationships with patients, colleagues, and family
	Patient advocacy
Management skills	Delegation and supervision
	Materials resource management
	Accountability
	Quality improvement
Leadership skills	Professional accountability
	Role behaviors
	Risk taking
	Collaboration
Teaching skills	Health promotion
	Health restoration
	Group teaching
	Individual teaching
Knowledge integration skills	Nursing and related disciplines
	Liberal arts
	Natural and social sciences

Modified from Lenburg CB (1999c). COPA model. Online journal of issues in nursing. Available online at http://www.nursingworld.org/mods/mod110/copafull.htm.

TABLE 6-3	Psychometric Concepts Used with Competency Performance Assessments
Concept	**Definition**
Critical elements	Statements that collectively define competence for a particular skill; these are single, discrete, observable behaviors that are mandatory to demonstrate competence for the skill.
Objectivity	A procedure that minimizes subjectivity on the part of the assessor (evaluator); two components are used: (1) a written statement of what is expected (e.g., the content of a particular skill or critical element) and (2) the consensual agreement of all directly involved in any aspects of the testing process.
Sampling	The process of selecting the most frequently encountered or most essential skills for the test.
Acceptability	The determination of what percentage of skills will be considered passing (i.e., 85% must be achieved for acceptable performance).
Comparability	The development of procedures to ensure that each test episode is essentially the same with regard to extent and difficulty.
Consistency	The development of procedures to ensure that the testing process is the same regardless of who administers the examination.
Flexibility	The ability to adapt when the performance examination is given in an actual clinical environment rather than as a simulation.
Systematized conditions	The development of procedures for determining the actions to be taken in the event of unanticipated situations in the clinical environment so that evaluators (faculty) respond in a manner that is objective, comparable, and consistent.

Modified from Lenburg CB (1999b). COPA model. Online journal of issues in nursing. Available online at http://www.nursingworld.org/mods/mod110/copafull.htm.

Objective evaluations are developed for didactic and clinical learning. Didactic evaluations are called competency performance assessments (CPAs); clinical evaluations are called competency performance examinations (CPEs) (Luttrell et al, 1999). CPAs are used to evaluate didactic learning and classroom projects, such as poster presentations and written papers. CPEs are used in the clinical setting. They often are more exacting because the professional, legal, and ethical aspects of care all must be taken into account. An example of a CPE for newborn assessment is provided in Figure 6-1.

An element critical to the success of the COPA model of education is periodic program evaluation to determine the effectiveness of the learning plan in achieving the desired learning outcomes. This periodic review also allows for routine updates as practice or unit procedures change.

A major concern of academics is the measurability and standardization of their clinical evaluation tools. According to the COPA model, the criterion-referenced outcomes used as performance indicators would give faculty and clinic-based educa-

tors more confidence in their evaluations. Another advantage of the COPA model is that students could be moved through curricula as they demonstrate competencies, rather than on the basis of "seat time" amassed in a particular course. This means that it would not matter if it took 2 weeks or 20 weeks to master content and perform in a competent manner; passing the course would depend on mastery of the selected competencies (Kenner & Fernandes, 2001). Ideally, this arrangement would allow faculty members to spend more time with students having difficulty and would not hold back those with a solid grasp of the course content. Faculty members could hold back struggling students without feeling obligated to pass them on because the semester is ending. However, some problems arise with application of this model to that extent. Most of these problems center on faculty resources and on satisfying regulatory requirements for a certain number of hours spent in class

---

Competency Performance Assessment for Newborn Physical Examination

Name: _____ Date: _____ Examiner: _____

Start time: _____ Stop time: _____ Length of examination: _____

General Criteria

1. The student will maintain appropriate asepsis at all times during the examination.
2. The student will maintain patient safety at all times, including temperature control.
3. Skills marked with an asterisk (*) are required and must be performed to pass the performance examination.
4. The student will complete the examination within 30 minutes.

Competency	Met	Unmet
I. Vital Signs and Measurements		
A. Temperature	_____	_____
B. Heart rate	_____	_____
C. Respiratory rate	_____	_____
D. Weight	_____	_____
E. Length	_____	_____
F. Head circumference	_____	_____
II. General Appearance *(Inspection)*		
*A. Level of alertness/infant state	_____	_____
*B. Posture	_____	_____
*C. General proportions	_____	_____
*D. Symmetry	_____	_____
*E. Hydration/nutritional status	_____	_____
III. Integument *(Inspection, palpation)*		
*A. Skin (temperature, color, lesions)	_____	_____
*B. Hair (distribution, texture, patterns)	_____	_____
*C. Nails (presence, length)	_____	_____
IV. Head, Ears, Eyes, Nose, and Throat (HEENT) *(Inspection, palpation, auscultation)*		
*A. Head (size, shape)	_____	_____
1. Skull and scalp		
*2. Sutures (movement)		
*3. Fontanelles (number, size, position, bruits)		
*B. Face (features, symmetry)	_____	_____
*C. Eyes (shape, position, measurements, movements, red reflex, discharge, pupil response)	_____	_____
*D. Ears (shape, position, auditory canal, hearing)	_____	_____
*E. Throat (general appearance, color, lesions)	_____	_____

FIGURE **6-1**
Example of a competency performance examination (CPE) for newborn assessment.

or a clinical setting. These are hurdles that can be worked out with a little nursing creativity. Only time will tell if more academic settings will use these strategies to address the nursing shortage and the need to ensure the quality of their graduates.

Some programs are using competency statements to guide their neonatal nurse practitioner (NNP) protocols. This is done not to the extent of moving students through more quickly, but rather to address the need to demonstrate competencies in graduates. One such program is Arizona State University's NNP program. The terminal competencies identified for NNP graduates in the master of science program are listed in Box 6-1.

IMPLICATIONS FOR NEONATAL NURSING

Orientation to the NICU

Because neonatal nursing is a specialty area of practice, most graduate nurses complete their basic nursing education with very little clinical experience in the NICU. This places the burden of developing practice competence on the unit and the hospital. As a result of the projected nursing shortage, many NICUs will be employing new graduate nurses at a time when the supply of seasoned neonatal nurses may be diminished. The traditional orientation approach of classroom learning followed by a period of joint clinical practice with an assigned preceptor may not be possible. As the competition for new graduate nurses intensifies, many hospitals are developing internship or externship programs.

Internships and externships for the new graduate nurse are a viable option for NICUs. Most newly graduated nurses recognize the paucity of their knowledge and skills for intensive care units and want some type of formalized educational program to become staff nurses in these areas. Depending on the availability of staff development instructors and seasoned nurses willing to assume preceptor responsibilities, many internship and externship programs offer a mix of traditional classroom teaching and competency-based education. To maximize resources, hos-

BOX 6-1

Terminal Competencies for Neonatal Nurse Practitioner Graduates, Master of Science Program, Arizona State University College of Nursing

- Gathers pertinent information systematically and skillfully from all sources: perinatal history, diagnostic tests, and comprehensive physical examination with behavioral and developmental assessments and provides comprehensive health history and physical assessment.
- Differentiates normal and abnormal variations for all body systems.
- Accurately interprets diagnostic tests.
- Analyzes data from multiple sources in making clinical judgments and in determining the effectiveness of a plan of care.
- Develops problem lists with associated differential diagnoses.
- Provides holistic neonatal nursing care to high-risk infants in high-technology tertiary settings.
- Assesses family adaptation, coping skills, and the need for crisis and other interventions.
- Identifies educational needs of the family and assists with teaching.
- Ensures routine opportunities for neonate and parent relationships to emerge with development of bonding and attachment.
- Assists family to restructure daily living activities in ways that meet the needs of the infant and those of other family members.
- Evaluates infant physiologic and behavioral responses to interventions for revision of management plan.
- Communicates with family members regarding the changing health care needs of the infant.
- Initiates and performs measures necessary to resuscitate and stabilize a compromised infant.
- Accurately and appropriately performs routine diagnostic and therapeutic techniques according to established protocol and current standards for practice by neonatal nurse practitioners.
- Plans and implements appropriate pharmacologic therapies.
- Identifies ethical dilemmas in the evaluation and management of the high-risk infant.
- Develops therapeutic nurse-patient relationship.
- Demonstrates management of acute and chronic health alterations across the neonatal care continuum.
- Demonstrates health promotion and health maintenance strategies.

- Prioritizes and initiates pertinent diagnostic tests.
- Determines nursing and medical diagnoses and develops a prioritized comprehensive problem list.
- Establishes appropriate priorities of care.
- Collects patient data on an ongoing basis, prioritized according to immediate conditions or needs.
- In collaboration with the family, physician, staff nurse, and other members of the multidisciplinary health care team, formulates a plan of care that incorporates health care maintenance, discharge, and follow-up care.
- Demonstrates management of complex, rapidly changing clinical situations.
- Evaluates the patient's progress toward attainment of expected outcomes.
- Systemically evaluates and ensures quality and effectiveness of care.
- Demonstrates multidisciplinary consultation and collaboration.
- Initiates referrals based on the infant's and family's needs.
- Seeks appropriate consultation based on the infant's health care needs.
- Facilitates use of organizational resources in caring for the patient.
- Evaluates his or her clinical practice in relation to professional and ethical standards, relevant laws, statues, and regulations.
- Identifies the legal components of advanced neonatal nursing practice.
- Critiques theories and research and participates in research activities for the evaluation, modification, and enhancement of existing practice.
- Helps provide in-service education programs and functions as a neonatal clinical resource person within the institution.
- Assists in developing unit policies and procedures for nursing care of the high-risk infant and participates in quality assurance measures in the NICU.
- Develops and implements strategies that have a positive effect on the political and regulatory processes related to health care systems and the role of the neonatal nurse practitioner.
- Demonstrates commitment to the role of neonatal nurse practitioner and identifies mechanisms to determine the future direction of the profession.
- Demonstrates cultural sensitivity and cultural competence.

Modified from McGrath J, director, Neonatal Nurse Practitioner Program, Arizona State University, Tempe, Arizona. Personal communication, 2001.

pitals often combine nurse interns and externs for the classroom work. For example, a large tertiary hospital may offer a maternal-child nursing option, whereas a children's hospital may offer a critical care option. In the former case, the interns and extern may take classes together on maternity and pediatric nursing. In the latter case, the interns may be in class for the critical care core content.

CBE is also well suited to orientation for new graduate nurses and for experienced nurses who are changing their focus area. For the seasoned staff nurse who switches from adult intensive care, the orientation can focus on the neonatal-specific aspects of critical care. The orientation program for this nurse

can be individualized to allow credit for knowledge and skills previously learned. An experienced staff nurse who switches from the well baby nursery to the NICU needs to focus on the critical care aspects of newborns, because this individual already has a knowledge base about well infants and about concerns common to well babies and those in the NICU, such as thermoregulation and hypoglycemia.

Ongoing Staff Development

Although unit managers are responsible for documenting competency (i.e. validating skills and knowledge), the individual employee must pursue the necessary ongoing education. This can be done through continuing education programs offered by professional organizations and by staff development programs offered by the institution. Maintaining individual competence is a professional obligation of every neonatal nurse. This obligation is spelled out clearly in the ANA's *Code for Nurses* (ANA, 1985):

> The profession of nursing is obligated to provide adequate and competent nursing care. Therefore, it is the responsibility of each nurse to maintain competency in practice. The nurse must be aware of the need for continued professional learning and must assume personal responsibility for currency of knowledge and skills.

Voluntary certification is an excellent mechanism for staff nurses to document their ongoing competence in neonatal nursing. In addition to measuring specialty knowledge, national certification examinations require documentation of ongoing education to maintain the certified nurse's expertise. The National Certification Corporation for the Obstetric, Gynecologic, and Neonatal Nursing Specialties (NCC) offers several examinations for neonatal nurses. These include an examination for neonatal intensive care and low-risk newborn care. Subspecialty areas, such as lactation nursing, are also available to certified nurses (NCC, 2001). An examination in neonatal critical care is available from the American Association of Critical-Care Nurses (AACN) Certification Corporation (AACN, 2001). The findings of a recent study of 19,000 certified nurses indicated that certified nurses make fewer errors in patient care, have fewer adverse events, are more effective in interpersonal skills, and have more confidence in their ability to identify patient complications (Trossman, 2000).

Graduate Programs to Prepare Neonatal Nurse Practitioners

Ensuring the competence of neonatal nurse practitioners is a joint responsibility of the specialty organization that establishes the criteria for NNP programs, the academic institutions that provide this education, and the credentialing agencies that measure entry into practice knowledge. Currently, no specific education standards exist for NNP education programs. Nurse practitioner programs are evaluated against accreditation criteria developed for graduate nursing education. Under the leadership of the National Organization of Nurse Practitioner Faculties, a variety of nursing organizations concerned with nurse practitioner education standards and credentialing worked together to produce a document titled, *Criteria for Evaluation of Nurse Practitioner Programs* (NONPF, 1997). Although this document sets forth criteria for nurse practitioner programs, it does not address specialty-specific content, such as that required by a neonatal nurse practitioner. Although the National Association of Neonatal Nurses published guidelines for curriculum development for NNP programs, they are out of date (NANN, 1995). A NANN task force is developing educational standards for NNP programs, and these are due to be published in 2002. A critical step in this process is the identification of NNP core competencies. The core competencies will define the practice of the NNP and serve as the foundation for a quality educational program (Williams & Kelley, 1998).

Currently, the competence of new graduate neonatal nurse practitioners is a function of the individual's background in neonatal nursing and the quality of the NNP program attended. The quality of NNP programs varies and depends on a number of factors, including the experience and expertise of the program's faculty, the entrance requirements for students, and the amount of didactic and clinical experience obtained through the program.

Although the trend in academia is to reduce the amount of staff nursing experience required before graduate school, a recent survey of NNP program directors revealed that practice experience is considered essential for NNP education (NANN NNP Education Standards Task Force, 2000). Much work must be done before NNP competency can be ensured.

COMPETENCY VALIDATION

Hospitals are required to document initial competency and the ongoing competence of their nursing staff. Validation is essential to ensure both that the nurse continues to maintain the level of expertise necessary to provide safe care and that the nurse has the knowledge needed to provide the best possible care for the particular problems of patients (Gunn, 1999). Responsibility for validation often falls on the shoulders of the intensive care nursery's unit manager.

The frequency of validation may vary according to the specific skill. The interval for validation of such skills as neonatal resuscitation is determined by the national standard, as set by the Neonatal Resuscitation Program.* Other skills usually are validated annually or as required by accreditation criteria set forth by JCAHO.

Competency validation can be achieved through a variety of mechanisms, including self-assessment, direct observation of performance, objective examination, and documentation of the number of technical skills or procedures performed in a given time (Miller et al, 1998). For many skills, a combination of methods is used; for example, validation of neonatal resuscitation skills includes objective examinations and performance evaluations.

SUMMARY

Maintaining and ensuring the competence of neonatal nurses are major concerns of hospitals, regulators, insurance companies, and society at large. Changes in the health care industry as a result of managed care, mergers of provider institutions such as hospitals, and significant reorganization within the delivery system have placed new demands on the nursing profession to ensure the ongoing competence of its members. Individually and collectively, nurses are challenged by the need to keep current in the midst of a knowledge and technology explosion, by the demand from payers for greater productivity and efficiency in health care, and by consumers' growing sophistication about the consequences brought about by incompetent providers. Standards of nursing practice and accreditation criteria from agencies such as JCAHO are used to develop the nursing competencies.

Competency-based education provides a mechanism for contemporary nursing to provide a cost-effective, quality approach to nursing orientation. It also allows units and institutions to individualize the orientation program to meet the dif-

---

*Bloom, Cropley, American Heart Association and American Academy of Pediatrics (AHA/AAP) Neonatal Resuscitation Steering Committee, 2000.

fering needs of nurses who have significantly different backgrounds and levels of experience. Competency-based education shifts the focus of learning from the traditional model of objectives and classroom teaching to a new model based on competencies and outcomes.

The final aspect of ensuring competency of the nursing staff is the development of a mechanism for validating competencies. A variety of methods currently are used to validate nursing knowledge and skills, including skills checklists, performance appraisals, and formal testing (e.g., post-tests).

Ultimately, the individual nurse is responsible for maintaining professional knowledge and skills through continuing education and other educational activities. Educational institutions provide the nurse with the basic nursing education. Passing the registered nurse licensing examination is only the beginning of documentation of competence as a professional nurse. Ongoing competence requires each nurse to become accountable for his or her own practice.

REFERENCES

Alspach JG (1984). Designing a competency-based orientation for critical care nurses. *Heart lung* 13(6), 655-662.

Alspach JG (1992). Concern and confusion over competence. *Critical care nurse* 12(4), 9-11.

American Association of Critical Care Nurses (AACN) Certification Corporation (2001). *CCRN: certification for adult, pediatric, and neonatal critical care nurses.* Accessed online at www.certcorp. org/certcorp/certcorp.nsf/certcorp/ccrn?opendocument

American Nurses Association (ANA) (1985). *Code for nurses with interpretive statements.* ANA: Washington, DC.

American Nurses Association (1994). *Standards of nursing professional development: continuing education, and staff development.* ANA: Washington, DC.

American Nurses Association Expert Panel (2000). *Continuing competence: nursing's agenda for the twenty-first century.* ANA: Washington, DC.

Bargagliotti T et al (1999). Reducing the threats to the implementation of a competency-performance assessment system. *Online journal of issues in nursing.* Available online at http://www.nursingworld. org/ojin/topic10/tpc10_5.htm.

Bechtel GA, et al (1999). Problem-based learning in a competency-based world. *Nurse education today* 19(3), 182-187.

Benner P (1984). *From novice to expert: excellence and power in clinical nursing practice.* Addison-Wesley: Menlo Park, CA.

Bloom RS, Cropley C, AHA/AAP Neonatal Resuscitation Steering Committee (2000). *Textbook of neonatal resuscitation.* American Academy of Pediatrics/American Heart Association: Elk Grove Village, IL.

Carter MA (1988). The professional doctorate as an entry into clinical practice (pp 49-52). *Perspectives in nursing 1987-89: based on the presentations at the Eighteenth NLN Biennial Convention.* National League for Nursing (NLN) Publication #41-2199.

Chaisson SF (1995). Role of the CNS in developing a competency-based orientation program. *Clinical nurse specialist* 9(1), 32-37.

Chapman H (1999). Some important limitations of competency-based education with respect to nurse education: an Australian perspective. *Nurse education today* 19(2), 129-135.

Citizens Advocacy Center (CAC) (1997). *Continuing professional competence: can we assure it? Proceedings of a citizens advocacy center conference, December 16-17, 1996.* CAC: Washington, DC.

Commission for Collegiate Nursing Education (CCNE) (1998). *Standards for accreditation of baccalaureate and graduate nursing education programs.* CCNE: Washington, DC.

Dozier AM (1998). Professional standards: linking care, competence, and quality. *Journal of nursing care quality* 12(4), 22-29.

Dunn SV, et al (2000). The development of competency standards for specialist critical care nurses. *Journal of advanced nursing* 31(2), 339-346.

Fey MK, Miltner RS (2000). A competency-based orientation program for new graduate nurses. *Journal of nursing administration* 30(3), 126-132.

Fitzpatrick JJ (1988). The professional doctorate as an entry into clinical practice (pp 53-56). *Perspectives in nursing 1987-89: based on the presentations at the Eighteenth NLN Biennial Convention.* National League for Nursing (NLN) Publication #41-2199.

Grant G (1979). *On competence: a critical analysis of competence-based reforms in higher education.* Jossey-Bass: San Francisco.

Gunn IP (1999). Regulation of health care professionals. Part 2. Validation of continued competence. *CRNA: the clinical forum for nurse anesthetists* 10(3), 135-141.

Hodges J, Hansen L (1999). Restructuring a competency-based orientation for registered nurses. *Journal for nurses in staff development* 15(4), 152-158.

Jeffrey Y (2000). Using competencies to promote a learning environment in intensive care. *Nursing in critical care* 5(4), 194-198.

Joint Commission on Accreditation of Healthcare Organizations (JCAHO) (1999). *Comprehensive accreditation manual for hospitals: the official handbook.* JCAHO: Oakbrook Terrace, IL.

Kenner C, Fernandes JH (2001). Knowledge management and advanced nursing education. *Newborn and infant nursing reviews* 1(3), 192-198.

Knowles MS (1980). *The modern practice of adult education: from pedagogy to andragogy.* Follet: Chicago.

Lenburg CB (1999a). Redesigning expectations for initial and continuing competence for contemporary nursing practice. *Online journal of issues in nursing.* Available online at http://www.nursingworld. org/ojin/topic10/tpc10_1.htm

Lenburg CB (1999b). The framework, concepts, and methods of the competency outcomes and performance assessment (COPA) model. *Online journal of issues in nursing.* Available online at http:// www.nursingworld.org/ojin/topic10/tpc10_3.htm

Lenburg CB (1999c). COPA model. *Online journal of issues in nursing.* Available online at http://www.nursingworld.org/mods/mod110/ copafull.htm

Luttrell MF et al (1999). Competency outcomes for learning and performance assessment. *Nursing and health care perspectives* 20(3), 134-141.

Marrone SR (1999). Designing a competency-based nursing practice model in a multicultural setting. *Journal for nurses in staff development* 15(2), 56-62.

Mikos-Schild S (1999). Competency-based orientation. *Today's surgery nurse* 21(3), 3-17.

Miller E, Flynn et al (1998). Assessing, developing, and maintaining staff's competency in times of restructuring. *Journal of nursing care quality* 12(6), 9-17

National Association of Neonatal Nurses (NANN) (1995). *Program guidelines for NNP educational preparation.* NANN: Petaluma, CA.

National Association of Neonatal Nurses (NANN) NNP Education Standards Task Force. (2000). *Survey of NNP programs.* Unpublished data. NANN: Glenview, IL.

National Certification Corporation for the Obstetric, Gynecologic, and Neonatal Nursing Specialties (NCC) (2001). *NCC examinations.* Accessed online November 15, 2001, at www.necnet.org/ certification.examdesc.htm

National Council of State Boards of Nursing (NCSBN) (1998). *Assuring competence: a regulatory responsibility.* NCSBN: Chicago.

National Institutes of Health (NIH) Clinical Center Nursing Department (1995). *Nursing standards.* NIH: Rockville, MD.

National League for Nursing Accreditation Commission (NLNAC) (1997). *Accreditation manual and interpretive guidelines.* NLNAC: New York.

National Organization of Nurse Practitioner Faculties (NONPF) (1997). *Criteria for evaluation of nurse practitioner programs.* NONPF: Washington, DC.

Neary M (2001). Responsive assessment: assessing student nurses' clinical competence. *Nurse education today* 21(1), 3-17.

O'Grady TP, O'Brien A (1992). A guide to competency-based orientation: develop your own program. *Journal of nursing staff development* 8(3), 128-133.

Pew Health Professions Commission (1995). *Reforming health care work force regulation: policy considerations for the twenty-first century.* Pew Health Professions Commission: San Francisco.

Pew Health Professions Commission (1998). *Strengthening consumer protection: priorities for health care work force regulation: report of the Pew Health Professions Commission.* Pew Health Professions Commission: San Francisco.

Smith S et al (1996). Examining competency-based orientation implementation. *Journal of nursing staff development* 12(3), 139-143.

Stewart SL, Vitello-Cicciu KM (1989). Designing a competency-based orientation program for the care of cardiac surgery patients. *Journal of cardiovascular nursing* 3(3), 34-41.

Trossman S (2000). Certified nurses report fewer adverse events: Survey links certification with improved health care. *The american nurse* January-February 1, 9.

Watson J (1988). The professional doctorate as an entry into clinical practice (pp 41-47). *Perspectives in nursing 1987-89: based on the presentations at the Eighteenth NLN biennial convention.* National League for Nursing (NLN) Publication #41-2199.

Weinstein SM (2000). Certification and credentialing to define competency-based practice. *Journal of intravenous nursing* 23(1), 21-28.

Whittaker S et al (2000). Assuring continued competence. *Online journal of issues in nursing.* Available online at http://www.nursingworld.org/ojin/topic10_4.htm.

Williams DR, Kelley MA (1998). Core competency-based education, certification, and practice: the nurse-midwifery model. *Advanced practice nursing quarterly* 4(3), 63-71.

CHAPTER 7

FAMILY-CENTERED CARE

JACQUELINE M. McGRATH

Change is the most certain event in life. A moment of reflection on our own lives would validate the point that elements of change affect daily existence in varying degrees. A family experiencing the birth of an infant faces many changes. Some variations in lifestyle occur in the areas of employment, financial security, daily activities, relationships with others, and role. These changes in life roles have a major impact on each of the parents and on the family as a whole. When medical needs require admission of the new baby to the neonatal intensive care unit (NICU), the changes become even more significant because, for the most part, the needs of this child have not been planned for or expected. For the family, the changes can be devastating and challenging to manage without support from the NICU team.

In the NICU, it is wholly impossible to provide excellent health care to the infant without including the parents or family, or preferably both. Families provide the foundation for health concepts and are the child's portal to the health care system. Family beliefs and individual health values are highly correlated. Families are the constant for the child (Harrison, 1993) (Box 7-1). For these reasons, understanding the many influences of family on each of its members is an important concept for those caring for infants and children. Most professionals who work with children and families believe that family-centered care is the best approach, because this type of care likely will produce benefits for the child beyond those derived from high-quality technical care (Dunst & Trivette, 1996).

Defining family concepts and presenting the philosophy of family-centered care are the foundations of this chapter. Role theory also is explored as it relates specifically to parenting. Factors that influence parenting behaviors include personal experiences, medical and nursing staff expectations, environmental conditions, and peer relationships; these factors can either promote or interfere with the development of an intact family unit. A critically ill newborn complicates the learning of parenting skills, and a framework is provided for understanding what families need in the neonatal setting. The chapter concludes with family-centered care strategies that help the family unit function at its best during the NICU experience and that promote the discharge of intact families after the crisis has resolved. These strategies also cover issues related to sibling adaptation and involvement of extended family members in the care and decision making related to the infant.

FAMILY-CENTERED CARE

Family-centered care (FCC) is a philosophy of care in which the pivotal role of the family in the lives of children is recognized and respected. According to this philosophy, families are supported in their natural caregiving and decision-making roles by building on their unique strengths as people and as a family unit. FCC Family-centered care recognizes and promotes the normal patterns of a family's life at home and in the community. Rather than expecting the family to take on the medical culture of the institution, health care professionals recognize and reinforce the family's culture. Parents and professionals are seen as equals in a partnership committed to the child and to the development of optimum quality in the delivery of all levels of health care. Family-centered care strengthens the family unit through empowerment and by enabling the family to nurture and support their child's development (Dunst & Trivette, 1996; Levine, 1999) (Box 7-2). From the child's perspective, family-centered care is safe and familiar; even a newborn knows his or her family to some degree and needs their support. When the framework of family-centered care is the foundation of caregiving, the family is visible, available, and supportive of their infant's needs. The family also is empowered and intact as it functions in the health care system.

DEFINITION OF FAMILY

The concept of who and what family is to those who live in North America has changed significantly over the past several years. Families are expanding, contracting, and realigning at a rapid pace to keep up with the rapidly changing demands of our world. In modern times, dual career families, permanent single parent households, unmarried couples, homosexual couples, remarried couples, and sole parent adoptions have emerged as other models of family, in addition to the family units seen as "traditional" a century ago.

"Family" is a broad term that is best defined by the individual; however, in general, a family is made up of those people, both related and unrelated, who provide support, structure beliefs, and define values. Family has also been defined as a social system composed of two or more people who coexist in the context of some expectations of reciprocal affection, mutual responsibility, and temporal duration (Hanson & Boyd, 1996). Families provide the framework through which individuals en-

BOX 7-1

Key Elements of Family-Centered Care

The practice of family-centered care involves the following:
1. Recognizing the family as the constant in a child's life, whereas the service systems and those who work in them change.
2. Facilitating family-professional collaboration at all levels of health care.
3. Providing care for the individual child.
4. Participating in program development, implementation, and evaluation.
5. Contributing to policy formation.
6. Honoring the racial, ethnic, cultural, religious, and socioeconomic diversity of families.
7. Recognizing family strengths and individuality and respecting different methods of coping.
8. Sharing with families, on a continuing basis and in a supportive manner, complete and unbiased information.
9. Encouraging and facilitating family-to-family support and networking.
10. Understanding and incorporating the developmental needs of infants and their families into health care systems.
11. Implementing comprehensive policies and programs that provide emotional and financial support to meet the needs of families.
12. Designing accessible health care systems that are flexible, culturally competent, and responsive to family-identified needs.

Adapted from Johnson BH et al (1992). Caring for children and families: guidelines for hospitals. Association for the Care of Children's Health: Washington, DC.

BOX 7-2

Two Principles that Form the Foundation of Family-Centered Care

- Enabling: Creating opportunities and ways for families to use the abilities and competencies they already have to learn new ones as necessary to meet child and family needs.
- Empowering: Acknowledging and respecting the fact that the family has existing strengths and capabilities, and the professional builds on those strengths by supporting the family in meaningful decision making about issues that affect their welfare. Professionals who empower families interact and form partnerships with families in ways such that the family keeps or develops a sense of control over their own lives and attributes positive changes to their own strengths, abilities, and actions.

Modified from Dunst CJ, Trivette CM (1996). Empowerment, effective help-giving practices and family-centered care. Pediatric nursing 22(4), 334-337.

ter and interact with society at large. For infants and children, families are the means to resources, education, and society. Families bring their children to the health care system for care.

A family is defined by its members; "family" is an internal concept of how that particular group defines itself. It may be composed of family or friends; it may not depend on a blood bond but on the emotional tie or closeness felt among its members. It also may be an extended family that includes parents, grandparents, other relatives, and friends. Families nowadays are not necessarily defined as they have been in the past and not according to gender-specific roles. Families also can be defined by considering the degree to which the following five attributes are present (keeping in mind that these attributes also depend on the family's societal and cultural orientation) (Hanson & Boyd, 1996):
1. A family is a social system or unit.
2. Family members may or may not be related by birth, adoption, or marriage.
3. A family may or may not include dependent children.
4. Families involve commitment and attachment.
5. Family members usually have roles and caregiving functions (e.g., protection, nourishment, and socialization).

ROLE THEORY

Role theory, which appeared in the literature about 1930, offers a framework for understanding families and identifying the roles that individuals play within the family. As a broad term, role theory represents a collection of concepts, subtheories, and research that addresses certain aspects of social behavior. Over the years role theory has come to include two major theoretical perspectives: symbolic interaction and social structural role (Hardy & Conway, 1988). With both perspectives, role is a basic concept in the attempt to explain social order and interpersonal relationships.

The symbolic interaction theory relates to individuals who create and construct their personal environment as they interact with, shape, and adapt to their own social environment. These individual behaviors aid in constructing the meaning of roles. In contrast, social structural role theory has a broader base. It focuses on the ways in which society, social structure, and other social systems shape and determine an individual's behavior. Roles are social facts with patterned behaviors that develop over time, and they are predetermined by social forces (Hardy & Conway, 1988).

The term role has diverse uses. One definition of a role is overt and covert goal-directed patterns of behavior that result from individuals interacting with, shaping, and adapting to their social environment. Roles are dynamic, interactional, and reciprocal relationships among individuals, therefore values, attitudes, and behaviors influence these relationships (Linton, 1945). Examples of roles include sick, student, and maternal roles. Reciprocal relationships include the physician-nurse and parent-child roles. Each of these roles has specific behaviors and expectations placed on them by society, and these expectations guide individuals as to when, where, and in what manner they are to perform the role.

Each role also has specific demands. An individual learns these demands by maturing and advancing through the middle to later stages of the life cycle: (1) adolescence, (2) adulthood, (3) marriage and parenthood, and (4) middle and old age (Hardy & Conway, 1988). Individuals respond to the demands of a role differently based on their maturity and current stage in the life cycle. For example, a single, adolescent girl would be

TABLE **7-1**	Potential Role Problems
Role	**Potential Problems**
Role ambiguity	Role expectations are vague or lack clarity.
Role conflict	Role expectations are incompatible (conflicts exist between reality and expectations).
Role incongruity	Self-identity and subjective values are grossly incompatible with role expectations.
Role overload	Too much is expected in the time available.
Role underload	Role expectations are minimal and underuse the role occupant's abilities.
Role overqualification	Role occupant's motivation, skills, and knowledge far exceed those required.
Role underqualification	Role incompetence; the role occupant lacks one or more necessary resources (commitment, skill, knowledge).

From Hardy M, Conway ME (1988). Role theory: perspectives for health professionals, *ed 2. Appleton & Lange: Norwalk, CT.*

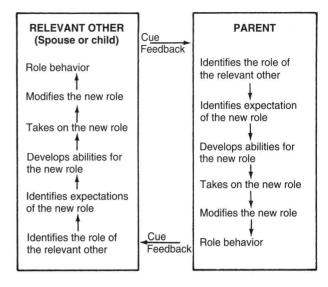

FIGURE **7-1**
Model of the role change process. (Hall-Johnson S (1986). *Nursing assessment and strategies for the family at risk,* ed 2. JB Lippincott: Philadelphia.)

expected to perform the maternal role differently from a married, adult woman.

Role theory identifies seven areas of distress associated with roles: (1) role ambiguity, (2) role conflict, (3) role incongruity, (4) role overload, (5) role underload, (6) role overqualification, and (7) role underqualification. These terms are defined in Table 7-1. These areas of distress are responsible for producing role stress and strain. Role stress is defined as either internal or external pressure that generates role strain. As a consequence, feelings of frustration, tension, or anxiety are produced in either the individual or the reciprocal partners (Hardy & Conway, 1988).

ROLE CHANGE

When problems occur with a role, a person or group may need to modify or completely change roles. As an individual changes roles and learns a new role, the required behavioral changes can be stressful. However, not changing roles results in intrapersonal and interpersonal role conflict and leads to further stress and anxiety.

The working mother is an example of role conflict and role overload problems. She struggles with her dual professional and maternal roles. A decision to quit work and devote all her time to mothering may contribute to a lack of self-worth or identity. A decision to continue both roles may generate feelings of guilt because she feels she is neglecting her family's needs. Reducing her work hours is a behavioral change she may make to allow more time for her family. She thus receives the positive reinforcement of employment, yet has more time for family and her maternal role. If she does not modify her roles, she experiences further stress and anxiety.

To be effective, role change requires several steps. Such change develops through gradual, continuous, and dynamic processes based on the individual's needs and those of relevant others. The steps to successful role change include identifying the role of the relevant other (or others), identifying the expectations of the new role, developing the abilities for it, taking on the new role, and modifying it. Figure 7-1 is a model for the role change process.

PARENTAL ROLE

Certain behaviors that are specific for both mother and father define the role of the parent. Several factors influence these behaviors: cultural background, personality, previous parenting and life experiences, the degree of attachment to the infant, and the expectations the parents have of themselves and the infant. The addition of a child changes everything in the close-knit relationship of the couple. Both must take on a new role; they are not just wife and husband, they are now mother and father as well. Feelings of inadequacy, conflict, and fatigue are often apparent during the transition and may adversely affect both existing relationships and those just developing between the parent and child. Parenting remains the only major role for which there is little preparation; difficulties encountered in the early stages of parenting may adversely affect all relationships but most especially the marital relationship. These difficulties can arise even if the new child is not the first child; each additional member of the family brings with it unique joys and challenges.

The situation in which a person must parent also influences behaviors. Parents faced with a crisis state must modify their roles and adapt to the necessary changes. Role and behavior changes can cause considerable stress, especially if these changes occur abruptly. Parents suffering from mental or physical illness or those who are chemically dependent can have limited coping abilities and social supports. Single, adolescent, or first-time parents also are at a disadvantage. They may lack maturity and coping skills because of limited life experiences and unavailable or inappropriate social support systems. These situations may inhibit the development of the parent-infant relationship and thus impair parenting behaviors.

Infant-related factors can also interfere with parental attachment and subsequent parenting behaviors. An example is an infant born with a congenital anomaly. Many of these infants may be mentally or physically disabled for a lifetime, which interferes with the parents' expectations of their infant. A visible anomaly is particularly difficult for parents because society places such emphasis on appearance. An infant with an easily correctable anomaly is tentatively unacceptable to society, until the anomaly has been corrected. A visible, noncorrectable anomaly has a greater impact on the parents and other family members. This stigma may include preterm infants who have deficits related to their untimely birth, such as blindness, deafness, or severe respiratory compromise. These parents may suffer from "chronic sorrow," and the child may grow up hindered by "vulnerable child syndrome."

A life-threatening or terminal illness in a child is another situation that may interfere with parenting attachment and behaviors. Parents may "hold back" their feelings for the child to try to protect themselves from loss and pain if the child dies. This inability to attach to their infant interferes with the parenting experience and may affect the child's development if the child lives past the expected life span.

At any birth the nurse must identify adaptive and maladaptive parenting behaviors. Adaptive behaviors indicate that both the infant's and parent's needs are met, and thus the parent-child relationship can be established. Mothers and fathers have different ways of expressing their parental roles based on gender differences alone. Tables 7-2 and 7-3 identify mothering and fathering behaviors the nurse can use in assessing adaptive or maladaptive behavior. These are guidelines and must be adapted to each parent based on the specific situation.

Parenting during Crisis

Taking on the parenting role is a major life task for a couple. The crisis of having a critically ill newborn in the NICU compounds the stress of that task. Whether the family unit attains growth from a positive resolution of this crisis or splinters because of a maladaptive adjustment largely depends on the quality of support provided by the nursing staff (Scharer & Brooks, 1994). The memory of what happens in the first days after a traumatic birth often stays with a family forever; just ask a mother to describe her birth experience, and she will talk for hours, explaining every detail (Wereszczak et al, 1997). Consequently, the interventions provided during the initial trauma can be critical to the adjustment and continued growth of the family unit.

Parents' Reactions

Crisis can be defined as an upset of a steady state. It is a period of disequilibrium precipitated by an inescapable demand to which the person is temporarily unable to respond adequately. The birth of a critically ill infant represents two types of crises for parents. The birth of any infant is a developmental crisis, a natural transitional phase in the lives of a couple. When the infant is premature or ill, parents also experience an accidental and unexpected crisis. The meaning of the event for the family and the resources available to deal with the event are variables that determine the scope of the crisis. With the technologic advances that have been made in medicine, some families now are able to better prepare for and make decisions about their child's prognosis and medical needs before birth. For example, many infants with gastrochisis are diagnosed during a prenatal ultrasound examination. In such cases, families have the opportunity to better plan for the birth and to make decisions with the health care team in a more conducive and supportive environment. The ability to anticipate the needs of the child reduces the sense of crisis for these families.

Families of a premature or sick newborn react in different and individual ways. Some common reactions are anxiety, guilt, fear, resentment, and anger. During the illness of a newborn, the parents must face many charged issues; two important ones are the loss of the perfect child they have anticipated and a fear that their infant may die.

In general, excitement and a flurry of preparation surround the birth of a child. Parties help families celebrate the anticipation of a new infant. Parents spend much time imagining what this child will look like and dreaming about the joys of parenting. The couple experience disappointment when the infant or pregnancy is not as anticipated. They may feel a sense of isolation from other couples who have had a normal pregnancy or infant. They may even have feelings of isolation from each other or from close family members. The inability to produce a healthy infant or to protect the infant from the invasive and painful environment necessary to sustain the child's life may cause feelings of inadequacy. The role the couple had thought they would assume as parents seems impossible to attain in the environment of the NICU, where everyone else seems to be making decisions about the fate of their infant. Parents seldom have had experience with the NICU before the intensity of the situation is heightened even more by the fact that they are center stage.

Parents must reconcile their idealized image of the child with the actual infant. They mourn the loss of the perfect child that was expected and feel anticipatory grief for the infant whose life is now in jeopardy (Olshansky, 1962) (Chapter 8). The birth of an ill or a premature infant places parents in a state of disequilibrium. Mothers of premature infants have had the emotional work of pregnancy cut short and are psychologically unprepared for the birth. If the mother had felt ambivalent about the pregnancy, she may believe that the infant's illness is a punishment for those emotions. A mother may also feel guilty that she could not carry the infant to term, even if no reason can be found for the baby's premature birth.

Many parents of sick newborns go through identifiable stages of emotional reaction. The initial response usually is one of overwhelming shock, characterized by irrational behavior, crying, and feelings of helplessness and despair. These families have difficulty with organization because their lives have been disrupted by the unexpected birth. They may feel as if everything is in chaos and the situation is out of their control. Substance abuse, teenage pregnancy, clinical depression, and domestic violence can increase the chaos and vulnerability of these families (Gale & Franck, 1998). Parents also may feel guilt over the premature delivery or the infant's illness. Self-blame often characterizes these feelings ("If only I had stayed home that day I noticed the spotting."). Parents may try to escape the situation by denial ("It will all be fine in just a few days."). At the bedside, parents may focus on facts they can understand and avoid issues they do not understand. To health care providers, this may seem as if the parents aren't listening or that they are unwilling to hear the information provided.

Intense feelings of resentment and anger follow denial. Parents may direct these feelings at themselves, the infant, members of the health care team, God, or even each other as parents. They may also experience feelings of ambiguity and may fear the infant's physical and mental outcome. For these reasons, they may avoid emotional involvement with the infant to protect themselves from the pain of possible loss. A lessening of the intense emotional reactions and an increased ability

TABLE 7-2	Guidelines for Assessing Adaptive and Maladaptive Mothering Behaviors
Adaptive Behavior	**Maladaptive Behavior**

DELIVERY

Adaptive Behavior	Maladaptive Behavior
Attempts to position head to see infant as soon as delivered and while infant is on warming table	Does not position head to see baby
When shown infant:	When shown infant:
Smiles	Frowns
Keeps eyes on infant, looking at all parts exposed	Stares at ceiling
Attempts en face position	Stares at baby without expression
Uses fingertip touch on face and extremities	Does not assume en face position
Asks to hold baby	Does not touch baby
Partly opens blanket to see more of infant	Does not ask to hold baby
Talks to baby	Declines offer to hold baby
Asks questions about baby	If infant is placed in her arms, lies still and does not touch or stroke baby's face or extremities
	May not look at infant
	Does not talk to baby
	Asks few or no questions
Makes positive statements about baby: "She's so cute!" "He's so soft!"	Makes no comments or makes only negative statements: "She looks awful." "He's ugly."
May cry out of joy or relief that infant is normal or of desired sex.	May cry, appearing unhappy or depressed.
May smile and cry at the same time. (To differentiate from crying out of disappointment, note facial expressions and verbal statements.)	When asked why she is crying, states she is disappointed in baby.
Expresses satisfaction with or acceptance of infant's gender: "We really wanted a girl, but it's more important that he's healthy." "I can't believe it; a boy, at last!"	Expresses dissatisfaction with baby's gender: "Not another girl. I should have known better than to try again for a boy." "I don't even want to see him." May use profanity when told gender.
Predominant affect: appears pleased and happy.	Predominant affect: appears sad, angry, or expressionless.
Suddenly decides she wants to breastfeed.	Suddenly decides against breastfeeding.

FIRST WEEK

Adaptive Behavior	Maladaptive Behavior
Initially uses fingertips on head and extremities. Progresses to using fingers and palm on infant's trunk. Eventually draws infant toward her, holding infant against her body.	Uses fingertip touch without progressing to palm on trunk or drawing infant toward her body.
Snuggles infant to neck and face.	Does not hold infant to neck or face.
Makes spontaneous movements, kissing, stroking, and rocking.	Makes few or no spontaneous movements with infant.
Attempts to establish eye contact by moving infant, assuming en face position, or shielding infant's eyes from light.	Does not use en face position or attempt to establish eye-to-eye contact.
Handles and holds baby at times other than when giving direct care.	Handles baby only as necessary to feed or change diapers.
Talks to infant.	Does not talk to infant.
Smiles at baby frequently; changes affect appropriately, such as when infant cries.	Rarely smiles at baby, or smiles all the time without change in affect.
Makes many specific observations of infant: "Her eyes look like they might turn brown." "One foot turns in just a bit."	Makes no observations.
	Makes few observations that are either general or negative.
Discusses infant's characteristics, attempting to relate them to others in the family: "He has my ears but his daddy's chin." "She really doesn't look like either of us, she just looks like herself."	Does not discuss infant's characteristics in relation to characteristics of family members.
With a positive manner, uses animal characteristics to describe baby: "She's just like a cuddly little kitten." "His hair feels like down."	In a negative or hostile manner, uses animal characteristics to describe baby: "She looks awful, just like a drowned rat." "He looks like an ape to me."
Asks questions about caring for infant discharge.	Asks no questions about care.

FIRST FEW WEEKS
(if infant remains hospitalized after mother has been discharged)

Adaptive Behavior	Maladaptive Behavior
Calls every day or every other day.	Calls less frequently than every other day or not at all.
Visits a minimum of twice a week.	Visits less frequently than twice a week or not at all.
Visits for a minimum of 30 minutes.	Visits for less than 30 minutes.

Modified from Hall-Johnson S (1986). Nursing assessment and strategies for the family at risk, ed 2. JB Lippincott: Philadelphia.   *Continued*

TABLE **7-2** Guidelines for Assessing Adaptive and Maladaptive Mothering Behaviors—cont'd	
Adaptive Behavior	**Maladaptive Behavior**
FIRST FEW WEEKS **(if infant remains hospitalized after mother has been discharged)—cont'd**	
Asks specific questions about infant's condition.	Asks no specific questions.
Asks appropriate questions frequently.	Asks inappropriate questions.
Spends most of visit looking at and handling infant.	Spends most of visit observing unit activities and other infants (this may be normal behavior for the first one or two visits); has little or no interaction with infant during visits.
Becomes involved with care when encouraged and supported by staff.	When encouraged by staff to participate in care, refuses, terminates visit, or performs only minimal care.
Although visits are frequent and last longer than 30 minutes, makes statements about missing infant (e.g., says that she misses infant at home or that she wishes she could visit more often and stay longer).	Makes no statements about missing infant, or states that she misses infant at home and wishes she could visit more often, but comments are not validated by frequent or lengthy visits.
Expresses reluctance to terminate visit.	Leaves nursery with little hesitation.
Waits until infant is asleep before leaving; touches or talks to baby just before leaving; may stand outside window and look at baby before leaving unit.	Frequently asks nurse to complete feeding or to change and settle infant.
FIRST MONTHS	
Holds infant close to her body.	Does not hold infant securely against her body.
Supports infant's trunk and head in position of comfort.	Head and body of infant are not well supported.
Muscles in her arms and hands are relaxed and conform to curvature of infant's body.	Shoulder, arm, and hand muscles appear tense; hands and fingers do not conform to infant's body.
During feedings, holds infant in well-supported position against her body.	Holds infant away from her body during feedings or props infant or bottle.
Positions during feeding so eye-to-eye contact can occur.	Position during feeding prevents eye-to-eye contact.
Minimizes talking to infant while baby is sucking.	Continues talking to infant during feeding even though infant is distracted and stops sucking.
Refers to infant using given or affectionate name.	Refers to infant in impersonal way (e.g., "the baby," "she," or "it").
Plays with infant at times unrelated to direct care.	Handles infant mainly during caretaking activities.
When infant is in infant seat, playpen, or crib, frequently interacts with baby.	Leaves infant for long periods in infant seat, playpen, or crib, interacting only after infant becomes fussy.
Places infant, when awake, in an area where baby can observe and interact with others.	Leaves infant, when awake, alone for long periods in bedroom or isolated area.
Occasionally leaves infant with someone else.	Frequently leaves baby with someone else or refuses to leave baby with someone else.
Uses discretion in selecting baby-sitter and provides instructions on baby's routines, likes, and dislikes.	Does not use good judgment in selecting baby-sitter; provides inadequate or no instructions for care.
Provides infant with routine well baby care. Carries out medical plan for management of specific problems or conditions (e.g., thrush, anemia, or ear infection).	Fails to provide infant with well baby care, seeking medical assistance only after problems, or keeps all appointments and makes additional phone calls or additional visits to physician or emergency room for imagined or insignificant problems.
Remains close to infant during physical examinations and attempts to soothe baby if infant becomes distressed.	Remains seated at a distance from the examination table; does not soothe infant during examination; frequently arranges for someone else to take infant for medical appointments.
Makes positive statements about mothering role.	Makes negative statements about mothering role.

Modified from Hall-Johnson S (1986). Nursing assessment and strategies for the family at risk, ed 2. JB Lippincott: Philadelphia.

to begin caring for their infant's emotional and physical needs are characteristic of adaptation and of taking on the parenting role. Reorganization is the final stage; at this point, parents come to terms with their infant's problems. This process can take a few days to several months. Unfortunately, in some cases it may never be successfully resolved.

Factors that Affect Parenting Skills

Certain factors affect a couple's ability to acquire parenting skills during the NICU experience (Box 7-3). Parents are un-

able to attach and detach at the same time; these two tasks are incongruent. Parents need time to detach or grieve for the lost perfect child before they can begin to attach to the ill infant. This adjustment may take days or even weeks, and for some families attachment may never occur.

Parents in the NICU environment face physical, mechanical, and psychologic or emotional obstacles. Miles and associates (1993) have developed a parental stressor scale for the parent with an infant in the NICU. Its purpose is to measure parental perceptions of stressors inherent to the NICU envi-

TABLE 7-3	Guidelines for Assessing Adaptive and Maladaptive Fathering Behaviors	
Situation	**Adaptive Behavior**	**Maladaptive Behavior**
Touches child	Freely, uses whole hand	Infrequent, uses fingertips, rough
Holds child	Holds child close to his body, relaxed posture	Holds child distant from his body, unrelaxed
Talks to child	Shows positive manner and tone; uses appropriate language, speech, content	Uses curt, loud, inappropriate language or content
Facial expression	Makes eye contact, expresses spectrum of emotions	Makes limited eye contact, little change in expression
Listens to child	Active listener, gives feedback	Inattentive or ignores child
Demonstrates concern for child's needs	Active, involves others, seeks information	Indifferent, asks few questions
Aware of own needs	Expresses feelings about self in relation to child	Gives no expression about self
Responds to child's cues	Responds promptly to verbal, nonverbal cues	Has limited awareness and response
Relaxed with child	Shows relaxed posture, muscle tone	Shows rigid posture, tension, fidgeting
Disciplines child	Initiates reasonable, appropriate discipline	Does not initiate discipline or uses measures too severe or too lax
Spends time with, visits child	Routinely, uses time so that child is involved	Has no routine, no emphasis on child during time spent
Plays with child	Uses appropriate level of play, active, both enjoy interaction	Uses inappropriate play, no obvious enjoyment
Gratification after interaction with child	Father states he is, appears gratified	Gives no statement or display of gratification
Initiates activity with child	Frequently	Infrequently
Seeks information and ask questions about child	Concerned, asks frequent, appropriate questions	Asks few questions, needs prompting
Responds to teaching	Positive, reinforces instructor, seeks more information	Has little interest
Knowledge of child's habits	Knowledgeable	Has little knowledge
Participates in physical care	Feeds, bathes, dresses child	Allow others to perform tasks
Protects child	Aware of environmental hazards, actively protects	Protective behaviors not exhibited
Reinforces child	Gives verbal-nonverbal responses to child's positive behaviors	Does not notice or acknowledge child's behavior
Teaches child	Initiates teaching	Shows no teaching behavior
Verbally communicates with mother about child	Uses positive, frequent verbal encounters	Gives negative, infrequent communication
Verbally and nonverbally supports mother	Demonstrates support; reassures, touches, guides	Support not obvious
Mother supports father, father responds	Gives positive response	Responds negatively or gives no response
Speaks of other children	Responds when asked, initiates	Shows no interest, no initiation

Modified from Hall-Johnson S (1986). Nursing assessment and strategies for the family at risk, ed 2. JB Lippincott: Philadelphia.

ronment. It has been found that an infant's appearance and experience of painful procedures, as well as the perceived severity of the child's illness, all contribute to the degree of stress experienced by parents (Miles & Carlson, 1996; Shields-Poe & Pinelli, 1997). A nurse who can properly identify the specific stressors for each family has the opportunity to assist the family in reducing those stressors and promoting adaptation for the family unit.

However, the nurse is still potentially the principal barrier to parenting in the NICU, because the nurse is the gatekeeper of the infant (Gale & Franck, 1998). The baby must in every aspect belong to the family and not to the medical team. For parents to attach to their infant, a welcoming, calming environment in which they feel comfortable is essential in the NICU (Box 7-4). This kind of environment encourages parents to become the primary caregivers and advocates for their

---

BOX 7-3

Factors that Influence Family Reactions to a Child's Hospitalization or Illness

- Severity of the illness and the threat to the child
- Previous experience with illness or hospitalization (or both)
- Familiarity with the medical procedures involved in diagnosis and treatment
- Available support systems
- Coping strategies of family members
- Other family stresses
- Cultural or religious beliefs
- Communication patterns of family members

BOX 7-4

Creating a Welcoming Environment in the Hospital for Families

1. When the opportunity presents before the birth, prepare the family for the infant's admission to the neonatal intensive care unit and hospital course.
2. Give a special orientation for families who have undergone an emergency admission.
3. Provide for the needs of families who travel long distances.
4. Make fathers as welcome as mothers.
5. Meet the needs of siblings and other family members.
6. Enable families to be together as much as possible; have open visiting hours 24 hours a day.
7. Encourage families to bring things from home that make their child feel more at home.
8. Provide privacy for family visiting.
9. Encourage family participation in the child's care.
10. Help the family stay in touch with extend family members and support givers in the community; isolation at the hospital is not helpful for the continued growth of the family.

Adapted from Johnson BH et al (1992). Caring for children and families: guidelines for hospitals. Association for the Care of Children's Health: Washington, DC.

---

child, and this advocacy is essential for the infant's continuing development, especially if the child has special needs (Gale & Franck, 1998).

Mothers and fathers react to stress and grief in different ways. A father may become engrossed in his work and may not share his feelings with the mother. A father often tries to be strong for the mother and may become protective, shielding her from painful information. The mother may view the husband's stoic behavior as cold and unfeeling. Both may have difficulty discussing the child because of guilt feelings. Normal postpartum blues can increase the mother's sensitivity and depression. She may cry for no real reason and feel embarrassed about irrational behavior. Existing weaknesses in a relationship may be magnified. Parents are separated at this time, and the fear may arise that their relationship will fall apart. Lack of communication can lead to isolation and feelings of resentment. Each may make assumptions about the other's feelings, resulting in misconceptions; these misconceptions, along with gender differences in coping, may continue for a lifetime if they are not recognized in this neonatal period, especially if the child has special needs or a developmental disability (Heaman, 1995).

Other stressors in the family, such as the needs of other children, financial concerns, illness of family members, or marital stress, can complicate the situation. For example, factors that can influence the degree of stress perceived by the family include the availability of appropriate emotional and psychologic support among family members and from friends and the availability and use of community resources. Maintaining a support system and using community resources and professional assistance are ways of dealing with the crisis. Coping abilities shown during previous crises often can predict how parents will cope with current crisis. In an acute crisis,

the family may be unable to use the resources available adequately because of lowered self-esteem, reduced family cohesiveness, and impaired family communication. Communication patterns could be impaired because of anger or emotion derived from the crisis situation. Therefore, at times when the family may require outside assistance, they may be unable to use or maintain the community resources required (Patterson, 1995).

A stressful situation has a specific meaning for each family and for each member of the family because of previous experiences and the family's perceptions of their demands and capabilities. Certain personality types thrive on stress and deal effectively with any crisis. Others are unable to deal with even the smallest crisis. For example, if a family acknowledges a stressor as a "challenge" or can bestow meaning on the situation, such as believing that "it is the Lord's will," adaptation will be successful. However, if the family interprets the stressor as threatening or undesirable, maladaptation results.

A stressful event has three levels of meaning within a family: the meaning of the stressful situation itself, the values inherent in the family identity, and the family's overall worldview (Patterson, 1995). The family's expectations for themselves and this new child affect parenting skills. The couple draws on childhood experience for parenting role models. The meaning the stressor has to the family also depends on the family's identity, cultural beliefs, and worldview. The family's identity comprises the values of the family, which are seen in the routines and rituals that develop in individual families. Stressors may disrupt these routines and rituals, threatening the development, maturation, and stability of the family system (Patterson, 1995). The family's worldview is based on how the family interprets reality, its core belief system (religious and cultural beliefs), and its purpose in life. The way a family handles its problems or deals with change often is based on the family identity and worldview. The family's worldview is the most stable of the three levels of meaning, but even it can be shattered by a severe crisis (Patterson, 1995).

The coping strategies are the cognitive and behavioral components of the effort to handle the stressful event; that is, what the family "does" to handle the stress. These strategies can be emotion focused (i.e., strategies for controlling the emotions the crisis has engendered, such as denial or anger) or problem focused (i.e., action-oriented strategies to manage the crisis) (Stevens, 1994). Coping behaviors are learned, and families can use any or all of the major coping functions. Emotion-focused strategies are used mostly in the adjustment phase of a crisis, and problem-focused strategies are used more in the adaptation phase.

CULTURAL PERSPECTIVES

Definitions

Some key definitions are important to an understanding of cultural perspectives.

- *Ethnicity:* A common ancestry through which individuals have evolved shared values and customs (McGoldrick & Giordano, 1996).
- *Culture:* Socially inherited characteristics, such as rituals; the thoughts, beliefs, behavior patterns, and traits inherent within a certain racial, religious, or social group.
- *Acculturation:* Changing one's cultural patterns and assimilating behaviors consistent with those of the society in which one

lives. This task can be done by learning the language, inter-mingling socially, or developing friendships, or through marriage or relationships formed in school or work places.

- *Religion:* A belief in divine powers; a system of beliefs, practices, and rituals.

The family has always been seen as the critical social unit for passing on beliefs and values in our society. Health care professionals must recognize and be sensitive to the influence of culture and ethnicity on a child's development and the family's response to illness or a chronic condition. The family's cultural ties provide support and a sense of stability during times of upheaval and stress.

The meaning of family varies with the ethnic or cultural background of the family. The concept of immediate family in Anglo-Americans means the nuclear family of mother, father, and children. For African-American families, this usually means extended family within the community. For Italians, family means a very strongly knit group of family and friends extending over three or four generations. The Chinese family consists of all their ancestors and all their descendents (McGoldrick & Giordano, 1996). Understanding and appreciating the differences in cultures and ethnic groups can assist the health care professional in promoting the family's health and supporting the family in times of illness or debilitating conditions.

Ethnic or cultural groups differ in the meaning of illness and disability and in when they seek health care. In general, Italians rely on the family for help when ill and seek medical help only as a last resort. They use words and emotion to convey the meaning of an experience to others (McGoldrick & Giordano, 1996). The close-knit family is of vital importance, and the nurse must respect the family as a cohesive unit. African Americans have an underlying distrust of the health care system. To effectively work with African American families, the nurse must help the family or empower the family to solve their own problems. Racism and oppression have left their marks on these families, and health care providers must enable the family to be the advocate for the ill child, to cope constructively with problems, and to deal with an unknown future if disabilities persist (Kaslow et al, 1995).

Some ethnic groups (e.g., Irish, African Americans, Norwegians) consider illness to be the result of an individual's own sins, actions, or inadequacies. Native American Indians consider illness or disability the result of misconduct, for which the family is being punished. The illness is part of the whole person. Native American Hawaiians view illness as an imbalance in the energy or harmony within the family. The illness is part of wellness, and this disharmony is a normal part of life. Anglo-Americans view illness as stemming from a scientific cause that is outside the family. The illness is foreign and intrusive to the individual and the family (McGoldrick & Giordano, 1996).

When a child is hospitalized, several important issues must be discussed with the family:

- What support the family wants
- Their preferences regarding language, food, holidays, religion, and kinship
- Their beliefs with regard to health, illness, and technologic advances
- Their health practices (e.g., immunizations, annual physical examinations)
- Their habits, customs, and rituals, which could affect their health

An understanding of family cultural differences can help the nurse provide care, determine the meaning of the illness or disability to the family, and assist the family in interventions appropriate to their culture. This understanding also shapes parent and staff expectations of each other and of the ways in which care is provided.

PARENT AND STAFF EXPECTATIONS

When parents have a sick infant in the NICU, they have certain expectations. They expect excellent medical and nursing care. They expect accurate and timely information throughout their child's illness, and they expect to be involved in decision making about the infant's care. The medical and nursing staff members, working as a team and supporting each other, instill confidence in the parents. The parents also benefit from communication that includes information about their infant and involvement in the decisions related to the child's care.

Members of the medical and nursing staffs also have expectations of the infants and families under their care. Sometimes these expectations are unrealistic. For example, the staff may expect parents to visit more often, even though the parents live far from the hospital, have other children, and must return to work, responsibilities that may prevent more frequent visits. The staff may expect the infant to nipple-feed more often or be weaned from oxygen faster. It can be distressing to parents to think that the medical staff is not pleased with their infant's progress, even though this attitude may not be verbalized. For this reason, incongruities should be avoided both in actions and in information.

Promoting Parenting in the Neonatal Intensive Care Unit

A major nursing goal in the NICU is to optimize parenting skills and discharge an intact family unit. There are different ways to ease parental anxiety during the NICU experience. Open visiting policies, especially 24-hour visiting, provides the parents more opportunities to be with their infant while allowing them to deal with other responsibilities. Restricted visiting may imply that the staff is hiding details of the infant's condition. Unrestricted access to the infant allows the bonding and parenting processes to begin.

One of the fundamentals of family-centered care is the belief that the family is an active member of the caregiving team right from admission (McGrath & Conliffe-Torres, 1996). Members of the caregiving team are not visitors. They are not asked to leave for rounds or procedures. In many NICUs the practice of inviting family members to participate in medical rounds is being explored. Families are part of the decision-making process and as such are given information so that they can decide when they would like to be present and when they feel they would rather not be involved (Raines, 1996). They are involved in the assessment of and planning for their child. Issues related to scheduling, teaching of medical staff, and confidentiality for families are still unresolved and remain a concern for care providers. However, for the most part, units where these practices are now common have found that the partnership between the family and the medical team is worth the effort required to implement such relationships. Providing for and facilitating the family's role as the constant in the child's life is the best approach for the child's long-term development.

Interventions with families must acknowledge the individuality of each of the members and of the family as a unit. Understanding that the needs of the whole are not equal to, greater than, or less than those of the parts is often a difficult concept for the neonatal nurse, who is involved more specifically with the care of the high-risk infant (Bruce & Ritchie, 1997). Researchers repeatedly have found that hospital-based neonatal nurses view caring for families as not within their realm of practice (and certainly not the priority in their practice) but as something extra they do "when there is time" (Bruce & Ritchie, 1997). These views are not congruent with family-centered care practices and need to be discarded. However, this can not happen without the support of the institution. Staffing plans that allow health care providers, especially nurses, time in their schedules to spend with families must be a priority if family-centered practices are to become the foundation for care (Johnson & Hanson, 1997).

Parents repeatedly have reported that they felt that health professionals did not recognize them as the expert caregivers of their child and the constant in their child's life (Scharer & Brooks, 1994). This perception may lead to mistrust in the relationships developing between the caregivers and the professionals and may intensify the stress for the child and parent during the hospitalization (McGrath, 2001). Acknowledging that parents are the experts and nurses are the consultants to whom parents may come for information or support is a shift that is still difficult for some professionals (Raines, 1998). Parents are empowered by nurses when they are respected, involved in the plan of care, provided with complete, unbiased information, and given a sense of control in the health care setting (Coyne, 1995; Raines, 1998; McGrath, 2001). Additional interventions that empower and support families include the following:

- Introducing the family to support systems in the form of families with children who are undergoing or have undergone similar experiences
- Providing the family with resources from the community (e.g., spiritual, economic, and social help, as well as information)
- Assisting the family in recognizing and using their strengths and coping skills or facilitating development of new coping strategies
- Encouraging the family to explore positive ways of coping with the situation
- Allowing and helping the family to resolve guilt feelings

Critical pathways have been developed to aid in the organization and evaluation of nursing assessments and interventions with children and families. These pathways help promote continuity of care and aid the nurse in prioritizing the needs of the child and family. They are outcome oriented and provide an excellent means of documenting nurses' actions. Critical pathways also are an excellent means of providing education and anticipatory guidance to parents and families, especially when teaching must be done over a long hospitalization or by several staff members.

Krebs (1998) has presented a clinical pathway nurses can use to enhance interaction between parents and their preterm infant. This pathway was designed for use in the NICU; however, it can be implemented with families wherever these infants are provided care. The pathway serves as a means to educate parents about the changing needs of their developing preterm infant. Implementation of the pathway increases parents' knowledge and responsiveness to their infant's behavior and helps parents develop independent, cue-based caregiving skills with their infant.

Gretebeck et al (1998) see the critical pathway as a way to implement developmentally sensitive caregiving into routine practices for all infants and families in the NICU. This critical pathway was developed with five areas of emphasis: environmental organization, the structure of caring, and feeding (all of which relate more to the infant), and family involvement and education (which relate more to the needs of the family). Outcomes for infants include physiologic stability, behavioral organization, and establishing predictable behavioral patterns; outcomes for the family include enhancing social support, increasing knowledge, and increasing involvement in the infant's care while preparing for discharge.

Family conferences can be used to evaluate the intervention strategies and how well they were able to meet the family's goals. Collaboration during conferences allows all present the opportunity to examine individual perspectives and goals while negotiating and reevaluating strategies to increase satisfaction with the treatment plan.

The attachment process begins at birth. With a sick or premature infant, this process is delayed until the parents can establish eye contact and begin touching their infant. Bonding is enhanced by allowing the parents to touch and hold the infant as soon as the child's condition allows. The preterm neonate's physical appearance, disorganized behavioral responses, and variable physiologic response to touch can cause much anxiety in the parents as they attempt to interact with their infant. Oehler and colleagues (1993) used a semistructured interview technique in their study of mothers of premature infants. They found that mothers interacted most often by talking and touching their infants and that mothers felt that their infants responded through body activity, eye opening, and orientation. However, it is important that the bedside nurse, who is well versed in what the sick or premature infant will tolerate, explain those limitations to the parents. It is vital that parents understand an infant's inability to respond or to tolerate eye contact or parental voice cues; otherwise parents may misinterpret cues or detach from their infant. It also is important for the nurse to teach the parents to recognize an infant's distress signals (e.g., hiccups, apnea, cyanosis, bradycardia, or mottling) so that parents can gauge their interactions by their infant's behavior.

A quiet, comforting atmosphere with low lighting helps calm both the infants and their families (Chapter 17). External stimuli in the NICU must be controlled; unnecessary stimuli aggravate these infants' already overwhelmed immature nervous systems, and loud monitor alarms and excessive staff noise can be upsetting and unnerving to parents (Brunssen, 1996; Gibbons et al, 1997; Gordin & Johnson, 1999; McGrath, 2000). Jamsa & Jamsa (1998) found that parents in the NICU felt that the technologic environment was frightening and that it delayed their ability to parent their children. In general, the equipment made the families feel like outsiders. Their discomfort inhibited interaction with their child and delayed their participation in caregiving. These researchers suggested changes in the technology of the NICU, such as use of different kinds of alarm signals with diminished volume; wireless, handheld information terminals; and remote monitoring. Some of this technology already is appearing in the NICU.

False alarms need to eliminated whenever possible in technologic design. Moreover, textual messages on equipment and monitors need to be examined. For example, Jamsa & Jamsa (1998) cited the fact that with some monitors, the textual message "Cardiac Arrest" appears on the monitor at times when the infant is just fine. The technology used in the NICU must be continually reevaluated and designed with a parent- and consumer-based perspective (Gordin & Johnson, 1999; McGrath, 2000). Achieving a balance between the high-technology environment and the need of parents to touch their infant frequently helps foster parental self-confidence. This balance must be a priority for the neonatal nurse (Kowalski et al, 1996).

Skin-to-skin holding, or "kangaroo care," is a "high-touch" avenue for promoting parenting, and it aids in the recovery of ill newborns. Skin-to-skin holding of even the sickest infants has been documented to provide many benefits, including decreased oxygen requirements, longer quiet sleep periods, and a shorter hospital stay (Drosten-Brooks, 1993). With skin-to-skin holding, the infant is held on the parent's chest. A cover gown may be put on backward with the opening in the front; this allows the infant to be snuggled next to the chest and the gown to be used as a cover over the infant. (For more information on environmental factors and how they affect neonatal development, see Chapter 17.) When parents are providing skin-to-skin holding for their infant, they are providing a warm bed with a familiar heartbeat. Besides the benefits to neonates, there are benefits to parents, including early bonding, increased confidence in parenting skills, and a sense of control; parents begin to have a sense of confidence that their infant is well cared for and may survive (Gale et al, 1993; Ludington-Hoe & Golant, 1993).

Staff members may resist skin-to-skin holding with extremely ill infants, fearing that intravenous lines or endotracheal tubes could become dislodged or that problems could occur while the infant was underneath the parent's clothes and the nurses would be blamed. Nurses must always consider the short-term losses of an intervention in addition to the long-term gains for the family and make a decision with the family that is in the best interest of the infant. Gale and associates (1993) found that nurses were reassured about skin-to-skin holding when the neonatal development nurse stayed at the bedside with the parent and the infant was returned to the bed immediately if any signs of compromise were noted. Nurses who were able to observe this technique first were less resistant as well, and after seeing the benefits to the infants and the limited problems, many nurses became supporters of kangaroo care. Established protocols and education of both staff members and parents help with the transition to skin-to-skin holding in the nursery (Paulsen-Bell & McGrath, 1996).

If an infant is being transferred to another hospital, parents need time to view their infant. This brief viewing reduces inaccurate fantasies about the neonate and promotes bonding and attachment behaviors. Occasionally, the mother's condition is unstable and she cannot visit the NICU soon after delivery. Instant pictures can be taken and given to the mother as soon as possible.

Many hospitals use volunteer "cuddlers" for the infants in stable condition in the NICU. Cuddling, singing, patting, and rocking are some of the soothing activities these volunteers provide for infants at times when nurses have other duties or when the infants' parents are not available. Many parents find it comforting to know that these "cuddlers" assist in consoling their infants while they are separated.

Throughout the infant's illness, parents need accurate, timely information about their child's condition (Box 7-5). Shellabarger & Thompson (1993) have identified specific information about the infant that parents feel they need. That information should be direct and honest and should not be contradictory. Parents also appreciate the use of drawings and diagrams when their infant's condition is explained to them, and they appreciate being encouraged by staff members to ask

---

BOX 7-5

Guidelines for Providing Information to Families of Ill Infants

Focus the teaching session so as to build confidence and foster independence in the family.

1. Begin by assessing what the family members already know.
2. Establish a working rapport with the family; work to ease their anxiety and fear and to convey confidence and assurance to family members.
3. Ask family members what they expect to learn from the session and provide information directed toward their concerns.
4. Initially, focus teaching on the diagnosis or current crisis.
5. Use language the family understands; avoid jargon.
6. Include the key characteristics of the plan of care and treatment.
7. Explain the ways in which the illness or medication regimen will affect daily life.
8. Use a variety of teaching materials and styles. All information should be provided orally and reinforced with handouts to be taken home.
9. Keep the information simple and concrete; reinforce oral communication with handouts. Expect to repeat the information and do so readily.
10. Avoid fear tactics but provide information on both benefits and detrimental effects.
11. Use praise to instill confidence.
12. Include anticipatory guidance.

---

questions. Presenting this information with some optimism allows the family some hope. Ideally, the information should be presented to both parents at the same time. It should be expressed in simple terms with short explanations. The parents are under much stress, and this information may be unfamiliar. Facts may have to be repeated several times before they are absorbed. Parents need a clear understanding of the information provided to make informed decisions about their infant's care. Family-friendly language in understandable terms should be used when delivering care and information. Medical information from a primary caregiver, such as a neonatal nurse practitioner or primary physician, provides consistency, especially when the news is difficult or "bad" (Box 7-6). Families also need information about visiting hours, unit policies, equipment, procedures, and treatments their infant is receiving. Direct telephone access allows an update from their nurse or physician at all times. After oral communication, written information helps parents remember important facts.

Many times the neonatal intensive care hospitalization is the beginning of chronicity for the infant and the family. Chronic illness challenges all members of the family (Diamond, 1994). Parenting a chronically ill child is qualitatively different from parenting a normal child. Nurses must promote the parents' and family's role as the caregiver for the child by determining the family's mode of coping and supporting those strategies while promoting family adaptation to the chronic illness. A major goal of care for these families is to integrate the child back into the family unit rather than making the child

---

BOX 7-6

Providing Difficult Information

Although difficult information most often is provided by physicians, nurses often are part of the team, especially if the information will be painful to the family. Nurses must know how to support families in these difficult situations.

1. Give unbiased information that is clear, direct, detailed, and understandable; during the discussion, get to the point quickly.
2. Provide the information with compassion and caring in a gentle but confident style; a private, quiet place free of distractions should be used for the discussion.
3. Personalize the information to this baby or child and this family.
4. Allow the family time to express feelings and ask questions, and provide support for those feelings and questions.
5. Provide information about resources and anticipatory guidance.
6. Arrange an opportunity for the family to meet another family who has experienced a similar situation or crisis.

Krahn GL et al (1993). Are there good ways to give "bad news"? Pediatrics 91(3), 578-582; Strauss RP et al (1995). Physicians and the communication of "bad news": parent experiences of being informed of their child's cleft lip and/or palate. Pediatrics 96(1), 82-88.

BOX 7-7

Principles of Family-Professional Collaboration

Family-professional collaboration accomplishes the following:
- Promotes a relationship in which family members and professionals work together to ensure the best services for the child and family.
- Recognizes and respects the knowledge, skills, and experience that families and professionals bring to the relationship.
- Acknowledges that the development of trust is an integral part of a collaborative relationship.
- Facilitates open communication so that families and professionals feel free to express themselves.
- Creates an atmosphere in which the cultural traditions, values, and diversity of families are acknowledged and honored.
- Recognizes that negotiation is essential in a collaborative relationship.
- Brings to the relationship the mutual commitment of families, professionals, and communities to meet the requirements of children with special health needs and their families.

Modified from Bishop KK et al (1993). Family-professional collaboration for children with special health care needs and their families. Department of Social Work, University of Vermont: Burlington, VT.

---

with a chronic illness a "special nucleus" that becomes the only priority or focus of family needs.

Family-centered care of an infant or child with any chronic illness is based on the premise that the family is the main source of support and caregiving for the child (Butcher, 1994). Thus family-centered care can be achieved through specific nursing strategies aimed at creating opportunities for families to use their own strengths and abilities to meet their child's and family's needs. Ultimately, family-centered interventions empower families to develop and maintain healthy lifestyles, leading to overall improvement of the family's quality of life.

The number of nursing or medical personnel in surgical outfits who interact with the parents can be overwhelming. Therefore introductions by name and position are important, and personnel should wear name tags to help families identify the staff members. Many institutions have adopted the primary nursing concept. Families often feel more secure knowing that one nurse directs their baby's nursing care throughout the hospitalization, and this allows a trusting, collaborative relationship to be established (Box 7-7). A friendly approach opens communication and demonstrates openness and approachability.

Using language that invites participation also is important (Box 7-8). The primary nurse can act as liaison between the family and the health care team (Scharer & Brooks, 1994). The liaison ensures that information about the infant's current condition, any changes in condition, and long-term outcomes for the infant are communicated to the family. The liaison role becomes essential if the infant is transported back to a community hospital. Parents need to know what to expect at that hospital and to understand that that agency now can handle the infant who was once too sick for them. Otherwise, parental mistrust of the community hospital may develop (Page & Lunyk-Child, 1995; McGrath, 2001).

Staff members' attitudes are an important part of the development of positive parenting (Box 7-9). Staff behaviors and attitudes can inhibit or encourage parenting skills. Conflict about parenting roles can exist between parents and staff members (Scharer & Brooks, 1994; Coyne, 1995), and this conflict may escalate into a struggle for control. Parents may view the staff members as acting as the infant's parents or the infant as belonging to the staff because staff members provide most of the care. The staff members' pet names for the neonate further reinforce parents' fears. Nursing staff can help the family by encouraging them to personalize the infant's care. Bringing in clothes, toys, and pictures of other family members and making cassette tapes of family voices are ways parents contribute to caretaking.

Nurses who care for families need to provide support and promote the family as a unit; however, overinvolvement of nurses can be detrimental to the family unit. Establishing appropriate relationships with families in our care can sometimes be difficult. It is necessary to identify inappropriate nursing behaviors and correct them. Educating the nursing staff about the parenting process facilitates identification of inappropriate nursing behaviors (Box 7-10). The education can be initiated during orientation of new staff members and reinforced at intervals with continuing education workshops on the subject (McGrath & Valenzuela, 1994; Walburn et al, 1997). Nurses must provide support while always acknowledging the boundaries of the family. Some families build walls and are so private about family matters it is difficult to obtain enough information to meet family needs, whereas other families become overly dependent on the nursing staff, needing their support at every moment. Interventions that promote independent family decision making include the following:

- Respecting the family as a unique unit
- Providing unbiased care to all families

BOX 7-8

Language that Facilitates Collaboration

"Do you prefer us to call you by your first name or your last name?"

"Here's what I'm thinking, but I'm wondering how this will work for you."

"Tell me how can I help you."

"Our institution usually does _____ this way. Would that work for you?"

"These are the things I plan to do for your child today. Would you like to do some of these activities?"

"What goals do you have for your child's care?"

"How does your child look to you today?"

"Do you have any questions or suggestions about your child's care?"

"This sounds important; help me understand your concern."

"Who would you like to have included in discussions about your child's care?"

"Let's talk about how much you want to be consulted."

Modified from Fialka J (1994). You can make a difference in our lives. Early on Michigan 3(4), 6-7, 11; Curley MA (1988). Effects of the nursing mutual participation model of care on parental stress in the pediatric intensive care unit. Heart lung 17(6), 682-688.

BOX 7-9

Key Content of Family-Centered Training Programs

- Principles of family-centered care
- Cultural competence
- Child development
- Family systems
- Communication with children and families
- Building of collaborative relationships with families
- Support for and strengthening of families in their caregiving roles
- Impact of hospitalization, illness, and injury on children and families, including the impact of health care costs on family resources
- Support for the developmental and psychosocial needs of children and families through hospital policies and programs
- Function and expertise of each discipline in the medical setting
- Multidisciplinary collaboration and team building
- Ethical issues and decision making
- Community resources for children and families

From the Association for the Care of Children's Health (ACCH), 19 Mantua Road, Mount Royal, NJ 08061; Johnson BH, Jeppson ES, Rudburn L (1992). Caring for children and families: guidelines for hospitals. ACCH: Bethesda, MD.

- Providing as much continuity in care provider as possible to promote family strengths
- Allowing the family to determine the implementation of the plan of care

With adequate staffing, nurses can promote parenting in the NICU. Overworked nurses can become frustrated and stressed, overwhelmed by their own anxieties. These feelings may impede their ability to interact calmly and therapeutically with a fragile family unit. Nursing management considerations should include provision for adequate staffing to allow nurses the time and emotional energy to meet the needs of parents in crisis (Scharer & Brooks, 1994). Patient assignments should be evaluated not only for the technical care an infant requires but also for the psychosocial demands of the family. Institutional policies should be carefully evaluated as to how they meet the needs of families (Figure 7-2).

Caretaking is a normal part of parenting. However, parents of sick or premature infants have been deprived of the time to prepare psychologically and to develop their caretaking skills. If nurses never allow the family to become involved in caretaking tasks, parents may feel inadequate or may resent the nurses. Positive reinforcement builds self-confidence in parenting abilities (Figure 7-3).

As the nurse prepares the parents for their infant's discharge from the NICU, it is important that the parents feel prepared to care for their infant. Nurses can use several key techniques to prepare parents for working with their infant and the technology in the NICU:

- Give constructive criticism.
- Encourage parents to discuss their concerns and emotions.
- Provide parents with information specific to their infant's care or condition.
- Clarify information that parents have received through other channels.

BOX 7-10

Nurse Behaviors that May Become Barriers to Positive Parenting

- Infant "belongs" to the nurse and the NICU rather than to the family; nurse refers to assignments or primaries as "my babies."
- Family is not considered a member of the caregiving team; for example, they are asked to leave for rounds and shift report.
- Family is not asked about the characteristics of their infant or included in discussions related the infant. Families are not seen as the expert about their infant. They are talked about rather than talked with.
- Care is task oriented, and staffing is acuity based rather than based on meeting the needs of families. Families are not invited to participate in the child's care.
- Infant's schedule belongs to the nurse and the NICU rather than to the family, so that feeding and caregiving might occur when the family is unavailable to participate. Scheduling is inflexible.
- Family is seen as an adjunct to the infant and his or her care. They are not the client or patient. Spending time with families is not considered a priority but rather a luxury. Spending time with families is not seen as essential to providing care for the infant.

Checklist for Family-Centered Care in Neonatal and Pediatric Critical Care Units

This checklist can be used by hospital administrators, care providers, and families to plan or evaluate policies, programs, and practices in critical care settings.

Environment and Design
- Are families' first impressions of the unit positive?
- Do the environment and design say that this is a caring place, a place for children and families?
- Are inappropriate, overwhelming stimuli minimized?
- Are maximum efforts made to control noise?
- Is the lighting comfortable for babies, children, and care providers?
- Does the lighting encourage normal diurnal rhythms?
- Is adequate, accessible work space available around the baby or child to allow staff members to provide care efficiently?
- Is a comfortable space available around the baby or child for families to provide care and nurturing?
- Is private space available for families (for day-to-day interactions, special situations, and meetings with health professionals)?
- Are families encouraged to make their baby's or child's immediate environment as homelike as possible?
- Are telephones, restrooms with diaper changing areas, breast-feeding rooms, water fountains, and food services nearby and easy to find?
- Are secure places available for families to hang coats and store other personal belongings such as purses, boots, and umbrellas?
- Is a comfortable space available near the unit in which the parents can sleep?
- Are space and support available for families to learn and practice new caregiving skills?
- Are there separate corridors for transporting critically ill children?

Patterns of Care
- Is care consistent and predictable?
- Do staffing patterns promote consistency and predictability of care?
- Does each child and family have a single, identified care coordinator?
- Are contributions from different disciplines coordinated and integrated into the care plan?
- Are care procedures and treatments planned to cluster and minimize unpleasant disturbances?
- Are measures taken to reduce the frequency and duration of painful treatments and procedures?
- Are pleasurable experiences routinely integrated into care?
- Are promoting and supporting family-child relationships seen as essential care practices?
- Are procedures in place to ensure smooth transitions from the unit to other settings, including home or home care or community services?

Family-Professional Partnerships
- Do staff members interact respectfully with *all* families?
- Do staff members view all families as having strengths and competencies?
- Are families who have experienced the unit involved in developing and evaluating the unit's policies, programs, and practices?
- Do unit practices promote parent-professional collaboration, beginning at the time of admission?
- Are families supported as full members of the health care team?
- Are all members of the team fully aware and respectful of the role the family has chosen on the team?
- Are the roles of the other team members clear to the family?
- Are families satisfied with the ways in which they are involved in decision making about their infant's or child's care?
- Are disputes between staff members and parents resolved in a positive and supportive manner?
- Is an ethics committee available to families and staff members?

Child and Family Support
- Does the unit define family in an inclusive way that incorporates all those who are most important in the child's life?
- Is the family encouraged to define itself?
- Is affordable temporary housing for families available near the hospital?
- Is financial support available (e.g., for parking, transportation, and lodging) to help families visit the hospital or stay nearby?
- Is the unit welcoming to parents 24 hours a day? To those in the parents' support network?
- Are visiting policies and practices supportive of children and families?
- Is staff or volunteer support available to ensure that visits by brothers and sisters and extended family members are positive experiences?
- Are translators and interpreters available for families who do not speak English or that use sign language?
- Are parents of newborns supported in their nurturing and caregiving roles?
- Are mothers who are hospitalized on another unit or in another hospital fully supported and kept informed about their baby?
- Are fathers and other men in fathering roles specifically supported and encouraged as partners in care?
- Is teaching parents about their baby's uniqueness and development an integral part of care?
- Are families encouraged to see positive physical and developmental progress in their baby or child and to celebrate milestones?
- Are opportunities facilitated for parent groups and for family-to-family support?
- Are a parent group and a family-to-family support group associated with the unit?
- Are referrals to such groups made on a regular basis?
- Is the NICU or PICU linked to a family-to-family support group in the community?
- Are children and families provided information and educational resources on topics of interest to them?
- Are written materials available in a language the family understands?
- Are materials for families written at a reading level no higher than a newspaper (about fifth grade)?
- Are audiovisual and other media available for families who cannot read?
- Are physical, emotional, and spiritual supports available to families to aid them in dealing with the intense feelings associated with having an infant or child in critical care?
- Are developmental specialists and staff members trained in family support regularly included on each child's health care team?

FIGURE **7-2**
Checklist for assessing family-centered care provided in neonatal and pediatric critical care units.

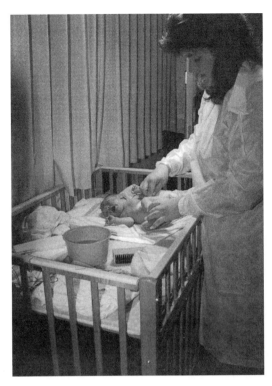

FIGURE **7-3**
Participation in infant care promotes self-confidence and supports the development of parenting skills.

- Draw the parents' attention to positive points about their infant, including how the child responds to the parents.
- Keep the channels of communication open by remaining nonjudgmental.

Parents can be given one last boost in confidence by allowing them to room-in with sick newborns before discharge. Parents feel secure knowing that nurses are close by if they are needed. This process also allows parents the assurance that they can care for their babies adequately.

Parent networking can be a vital tool for promoting parenting. Knowing that other families have survived this crisis can be reassuring. Support groups generally are helpful; however, they are not appropriate for every situation. Some couples need counseling. The primary nurse plays a key role in assessing signs that the family is not coping and needs therapeutic counseling. Support groups or counseling helps families look at problems objectively and learn alternative behavior for adaptive coping.

The nurse also can assist parents in identifying additional means of support. Ideally, parents should be permitted to define their "family" as needed to provide support during this crisis, allowing family members to visit as unit policy dictates. Grandparents, extended family, neighbors, and friends may constitute this group.

Grandparents may be a source of support in some instances. They may be forced into an uncomfortable role by seeing their own child in pain without a way to relieve that pain. Grandparents may also relive their own birthing experiences, which may result in associated anxieties and prevent them from providing support for the parents. Extended family members may be more helpful if discord exists between grandparents and the nuclear family.

Friends of the family can be an asset if they are effective listeners. They can offer to provide transportation for the mother and child care for brothers and sisters, or they can take over meal preparation and housekeeping chores to help alleviate family responsibilities. Just having someone to make telephone calls to other friends and family to update them on the infant's condition can be a great relief for the family.

Social workers involved early in the hospital stay provide parents with an objective person and contact with community resources. Families are reluctant to express dissatisfaction with their child's care to nurses. Social workers can help parents express concerns without fear of retaliation against their child. Clergy provide spiritual support for a family. Families often turn to religion for comfort and support at a time of crisis. It is important to offer parents privacy with the clergy to exercise their religious freedom.

SIBLINGS

Siblings have needs, because they are an important part of the new infant's life. Sibling visits may help relieve anxieties and make the birth a reality. Siblings have a variety of responses to a newborn's arrival in the home, especially after a lengthy hospitalization. Family routines are disrupted by a "normal" birth and are further disturbed by an admission to the NICU and then again at the time of discharge. Siblings may feel displaced while parents are visiting the ill infant. Siblings often are left with baby-sitters when they have rarely had experience with caretakers outside the immediate family. Fathers who may be uncertain about their family role may embrace their familiar work role and spend more time on the job. In these ways routines are disrupted, and parents are less available for their other children. These feelings may result in a variety of acting-out experiences. An example of a family's response to the homecoming of a new brother who had been in the NICU is presented in Box 7-11.

The birth of a new baby precipitates a family upheaval and the need for realignment of relationships and positions within the family constellation. Becoming a sibling is known to be a stressful or "crisis" experience for young children and can have an effect on their mental, emotional, and social development.

The birth of a preterm or critically ill neonate who requires intensive care constitutes a further crisis for parents and consequently disrupts the equilibrium of the family system (Bartlett & McGrath, 1999). Parents are reported to experience feelings of anxiety, grief, fear, anger, and guilt in response to the unanticipated events. Siblings are also affected and may experience helplessness, powerlessness, guilt, and anger in addition to the disruption of their daily routines and separation from their parents. The siblings may feel very alone because their worried parents are preoccupied with the newborn baby. Siblings feel like the forgotten family member at the very time they need attention most (Bartlett & McGrath, 1999).

Addressing the needs of families of hospitalized patients has gained acceptance and support among nurses since the advent of the concept of family-centered care (Ahmann, 1997; Hegedus & Madden, 1994; Plaas, 1994). Researchers have recognized the need for families of NICU patients to have increased psychosocial support and understanding during the crisis of hospitalization (McKim et al, 1995; Vasquez, 1995; Kowalski et al, 1996). All members of the family, parents and siblings, may exhaust their coping strategies and feel unsupported by those who are usually available emotionally and physically.

BOX **7-11**

Example of a Sibling Response to an Infant's Homecoming

John Jones was born at 33 weeks' gestation. The nurses described him as a typical preemie with respiratory distress syndrome (RDS) and intermittent apnea and bradycardia. He required Continuous positive airway pressure (CPAP) for several days and then hood oxygen for a week. After being weaned to room air, he was moved to the transitional nursery, where he stayed for another week until he mastered sucking, swallowing, and breathing. John's mother visited often. Mrs. Jones kept John supplied with breast milk and the latest drawings from his two sisters, Suzie, age 6, and Becky, age 4. John's father visited once in a while on his way home from work but did not take an active role in caretaking. He said that he was afraid to hold John but that he would once John got bigger and stronger. John was a cuddly little guy who had an uneventful recovery and was discharged after 3 weeks in the NICU.

Several days before discharge, John's mother confided in his primary nurse that she was about at the end of her rope because her husband was working longer hours and her daughters were acting up in ways they never had before. Becky had demonstrated regression behaviors of bed-wetting and thumb-sucking. She had also started carrying around her "blankie" again, something she had stopped doing long ago. Becky was particularly close to her mother, and after her mother's daily visit to the NICU, Becky would hit her mother, crying, "I hate you! I wish the baby would go away!" Mrs. Jones said that when she tried to console Becky, the child ran and hid under her bed, crying, "Leave me alone! You only love that baby!" If that weren't bad enough, Suzie had begun waking up with stomachaches and refusing to go to school. Suzie had always loved her teacher and classmates and now was frequently in trouble for misbehaving in class. When Mrs. Jones would make Suzie go to school, the little girl would cry and say, "I hate that baby! I'd like to run over him with Daddy's car!" Mr. Jones had withdrawn from family life and was spending long hours at work. Mrs. Jones was beside herself.

The nurse was able to reassure Mrs. Jones that the behaviors of her husband and daughters were typical. Although this reassurance didn't immediately alter the situation, at least Mrs. Jones knew that many families respond to NICU hospitalization in this way and that, given time, the family would reestablish equilibrium. Mrs. Jones was encouraged to take the weekend off from her NICU visiting routine. She was able to spend a couple of special days with her daughters and engage her husband in life outside the worries of the NICU.

However, this did not provide Mrs. Jones with emotional support or help with her feelings of being overwhelmed and depressed. The nurse was able to listen to her concerns and then put her in touch with a parent organization that had been formed to help support families through the transition home. The parent organization offered peer support from parents who had been through the experience. They were also able to help Mrs. Jones place the experience in its proper perspective.

The girls had enjoyed their weekend with their mother and were in a better frame of mind for the homecoming. Peer support helped Mrs. Jones so that she could in turn be available to her family. John was about ready for discharge and had progressed normally. Once John was home, Mrs. Jones included the girls in the baby's routine as much as possible by asking them to get his diapers and having them feed their dollies while she fed John. Suzie brought pictures of John to school for show and tell, and after Mrs. Jones called to speak to the teacher to explain the disruptions at home, Suzie gradually quit misbehaving. Becky continued to have problems with thumb-sucking and bed-wetting for several months while John was incorporated into the family and while a new family routine was established.

The philosophy of family-centered care in the NICU is reported to encourage not only parent participation but also involvement of the well sibling or siblings in the family process. This involvement allows children to see their new sibling and to feel as if they are a part of the family process. Feelings of isolation may engender fantasies about what is taking place in the NICU. At any age, it is easier to cope with reality than with what can be imagined.

Increasing numbers of hospitals are allowing the participation of children at a sibling's birth, sibling contact with the infant at birth, sibling contact with the infant on the postpartum unit, and sibling visiting in intensive care nurseries. For nurses facing these challenges, the philosophy of family-centered care can provide a firm foundation in striving toward excellence in the practice of caring for children and families (Ahmann, 1997). The development of a sibling-infant bond is vital to establishing and enhancing the relationship within the family unit. Holistic care surrounding childbirth may set up patterns or pathways that dramatically affect subsequent family interactions (Sherr, 1995).

Sibling Adaptation: A Review

Sibling relationships have often been viewed from a Freudian perspective, which emphasizes the concepts of sibling rivalry and displacement of the older child.

Increased engagement in fantasy play has been reported as children negotiate the stressful transition to becoming a sibling. Kramer & Schaefer-Hernan (1994) reported that children who exhibited fewer problems and accepted their siblings experienced a suppression in fantasy immediately after their siblings' birth; thus a temporary disruption in fantasy play may indicate adaptive coping.

The sequence in which siblings' touched the new infant varied between the school age and preschool groups; younger children tended to touch the newborn's head most commonly, whereas the older children touched the extremities first.

Gullicks & Crase (1993), examining parents' expectations and observations of their firstborn children's behavior before and after the birth of their second child, indicated that parents generally expected more negative behavior than they actually observed. The findings of Faller & Ratcliffe (1993), who described the development of early interaction between siblings, indicated that positive sibling relationships may be the norm rather than the exception. The literature indicates that reactions to the new arrival vary according to the family constellation, the emotional development of the older siblings and the age gap between them, and the gender of each sibling.

Sibling Visitation to the NICU

Sibling visitation in the hospital after the delivery of a newborn has become common practice. However, limited research has examined the consequences of permitting and prohibiting sibling visits in the NICU despite the argument that sibling involvement is consistent with the concept of family-centered perinatal care. Earlier studies of NICU sibling visitation programs provided valuable descriptive data on siblings' responses to the sick neonate. NICU visits provided an opportunity for the older brother or sister to see, touch, and talk to the newborn. This exposure was reported to help the children integrate the reality of the experience, to prepare for the possible loss of the newborn, and in some cases to reverse regressive behavior that had begun during the newborn's hospitalization.

Newman & McSweeney (1990) conducted a two-phase descriptive study designed to identify practices that fostered sibling involvement in the NICU. From interviews with national experts in neonatology, three factors were identified: (1) recognition of sibling's needs; (2) organization of sibling involvement programs; and (3) positive staff attitudes. The NICU head nurses further identified common themes in their unique programs that centered on families, the NICU atmosphere, and the promotion of sibling activities. A liberal visiting policy was recognized in all the units, promoting the concept of family-centered care and providing parents, siblings, and grandparents with the opportunity to be supportive together (Newman & McSweeney, 1990). However, the findings of this study focused on two areas of limitation: the results reflected the perceptions of providers and not necessarily those of the parents or siblings, and the exemplary NICUs, all level III units in teaching hospitals, may have been more technologically advanced and consequently may have had different practices or policies on family visiting.

Wolterman (1990) developed a Sibling Behavior Scale to study behavior in siblings after a visit to the NICU. The data suggested that siblings who were involved in the program demonstrated fewer overall negative behavior patterns than did siblings who were not involved. Preschool age siblings who visited the NICU appeared to be more interested in the environment, whereas school age siblings wanted to touch and hold the new baby. Wolterman also found that NICU visits gave siblings the opportunity to develop a "sense of history" from this early exposure to the infant, that they would remember when they first saw the baby and would be able to reflect on this experience for the rest of their lives. Although not intended to focus on the parent-child relationship, this study highlighted the importance of the NICU visit becoming a whole family experience.

The need for sibling education classes in the NICU is currently recognized. Speck and colleagues (1993) evaluated an NICU sibling education and visitation program implemented by nurses practicing in a 60-bed unit. Parents commented that the program encouraged family cohesiveness by allowing all family members to visit the infant together more frequently than the sibling visitation policy allowed. Parents also believed that it was important that siblings learned about the baby and the equipment in the NICU. To provide new learning experiences for children attending sibling classes, a variety of additional books and craft activities have been incorporated into the program. The results of a hospital-based sibling preparation class, reported by Spero (1993), indicated that the classes helped ease siblings' transition and increased parents' awareness of the crisis potential for the older children.

Implications for Practice.   Nurses have a unique opportunity to support the development of positive sibling relationships in the NICU environment. Evolving models of comprehensive care no longer overlook or delegate the care and needs of the whole family. Research on the families of NICU neonates has demonstrated parents' desire for a family-centered approach to care. Siblings are an integral part of any family, and their adjustment or lack of adjustment to the birth of a newborn greatly affects the well-being of the whole family. Siblings' adjustment to the once-sick infant needs further exploration.

When the birth of a sibling is further complicated by the baby's being ill or at risk, professionals caring for the baby are in a position to reassure parents that siblings will respond to the neonate in various ways based on each child's personality, age, and interests. Professional reassurance can help parents realize that siblings cannot help feeling angry and displaced by the baby. The parents' ability to accept their older children's competitive feelings and yet continue to love them helps those children to integrate ambivalence. Support through this ambivalence facilitates acceptance of the baby and the baby's incorporation into the family.

Increasing parents' knowledge about promoting positive sibling relationships through parent education programs may influence the parents' attitudes, thereby enhancing the future sibling relationship. In response to consumer demand, many hospitals have implemented sibling visitation and educational programs. This preparation can help siblings deal with the realities of the experience. Special attention from the NICU staff also can help siblings feel recognized, supported, and appreciated during this time of stress. Encouraging the sibling to gently touch and talk to the infant and allowing gifts of toys or even a drawing of themselves to be kept with the baby are activities that may foster attachment and growing connection with the newborn.

The death of a sibling usually has profound and lasting effects on surviving children. Surviving siblings, however young, may need some evidence that the baby existed; a visit to see the ill newborn in the incubator, a photograph, or a chance to participate in the funeral. Regardless of the child's age, it seems that the level of care offered to these siblings is crucial to determining the psychological and life adjustment of the bereaved child. Nurses need to be alert to the range and depth of childhood reactions.

Many of the research findings discussed here can serve as invaluable guides to help NICU nurses promote and facilitate effective sibling interactions and positive involvement between the sick neonate and the siblings. An appropriate environment in which nurses can assist children in coping with the profound changes that affect the sibling bond should also be provided, because such efforts help siblings fully integrate this major event into their young lives.

SUMMARY

The birth of any infant produces tremendous change in the lives of the parents. Normal adaptation can be complicated by the birth of a premature, critically ill infant or one with con-

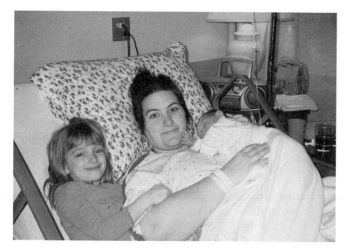

FIGURE **7-4**
The ultimate goal of the nurse is to ensure the integration of the infant into the changing family unit.

genital anomalies. If the family does not have adequate coping strategies or resources, this crisis could produce much role stress and strain, which ultimately can weaken or destroy the family unit. The nurse plays an integral role in guiding the family to appropriate resources and support services. By promoting adaptive rather than maladaptive roles, the nurse can ensure an intact family unit after the crisis (Figure 7-4).

REFERENCES

Ahmann E (1997). Kinship care: an emerging issue. *Pediatric nursing* 23(6), 598-600.

Bartlett L, McGrath JM (1999). Child's response to the birth of a sibling: myth versus reality. *Mother baby journal* 4(4), 1-5.

Bruce B, Ritchie J (1997). Nurses' practices and perceptions of family-centered care. *Journal of pediatric nursing* 12(4), 214-221.

Brunssen SH (1996). Sources of environmental stress experienced by mothers of hospitalized medically fragile infants. *Neonatal network* 15(3), 88-89.

Butcher LA (1994). A family-focused perspective on chronic illness. *Rehabilitation nursing* 19(2), 70-74.

Coyne IT (1995). Parental participation in care: a critical review of the literature. *Journal of advanced nursing* 21(4), 716-722.

Diamond J (1994). Family-centered care for children with chronic illness. *Journal of pediatric health care* 8(4), 196-197.

Drosten-Brooks F (1993). Kangaroo care: skin-to-skin contact in the NICU. *MCN: American journal of maternal child nursing* 18(5), 250-253.

Dunst CJ, Trivette CM (1996). Empowerment: effective help-giving practices and family-centered care. *Pediatric nursing* 22(4), 334-337.

Faller H, Ratcliffe L (1993). Sibling visitation: how far should the pendulum swing? *Journal of pediatric nursing* 8(2), 92-99.

Gale G, Franck LS (1998). Toward a standard of care for parents of infants in the neonatal intensive care unit. *Critical care nurse* 18(5), 62-73.

Gale G et al (1993). Skin-to-skin (kangaroo) holding of the intubated premature infant. *Neonatal network* 12(6), 49-57.

Gibbons C et al (1997). Biomedical equipment in the neonatal intensive care unit: Is it a stressor? *Journal of perinatal and neonatal nursing* 12(3), 67-73.

Gordin P, Johnson BH (1999). Technology and family-centered perinatal care: conflict or synergy? *Journal of obstetric, gynecologic, and neonatal nursing* 28, 401-408.

Gullicks J, Crase S (1993). Sibling behavior with a newborn: parent expectations and observations. *Journal of obstetric, gynecologic, and neonatal nursing* 22(5), 438-444.

Hanson SMH, Boyd ST (1996). Family nursing: an overview. In Cox L et al: *Family health care nursing: theory, practice, and research.* FA Davis: Philadelphia.

Hardy M, Conway ME (1988). *Role theory: perspectives for health professionals,* ed 2. Appleton & Lange: Norwalk, CT.

Heaman DJ (1995). Perceived stressors and coping strategies of parents who have children with developmental disabilities: a comparison of mothers with fathers. *Journal of pediatric nursing: nursing care of children and families* 10(5), 311-320.

Hegedus K, Madden J (1994). Caring in a neonatal intensive care unit: perspectives of providers and consumers. *Journal of perinatal and neonatal nursing* 8(2), 67-75.

Jamsa K, Jamsa T (1998). Technology in the neonatal intensive care: a study of parents' experiences. *Technology and healthcare* 6(4), 225-230.

Johnson BH et al (1997). *Newborn intensive care: changing practice, changing attitudes* (discussion guide). The Institute for Family Centered Care: Bethesda, MD.

Kaslow NJ et al (1995). A cultural perspective on family theory and therapy. *Psychiatric clinics of North America* 18(3), 621-633.

Kowalski K et al (1996). The high-touch paradigm: a twenty-first century model for maternal-child nursing. *MCN: American journal of maternal child nursing* 21(1), 43-51.

Kramer L, Schaefer-Hernan P (1994). Patterns of fantasy play engagement across the transition to becoming a sibling. *Journal of child psychology and psychiatry and allied disciplines* 35(4), 749-767.

Krebs TL (1998). Clinical pathway for enhanced parent and preterm interaction through parent education. *Journal of perinatal and neonatal nursing* 12(2), 38-49.

Levine A (1999). Humane neonatal intensive care initiative. *Acta paediatrica* 88, 353-355.

Linton R (1945). *The cultural background of personality.* Appleton-Century: New York.

Ludington-Hoe SM, Golant SK (1993). *Kangaroo care.* Bantam Books: New York.

McGoldrick M, Giordano J (1996). Overview: ethnicity and family therapy. In McGrath JM, editor (2001): Building relationships with families in the NICU: exploring the guarded alliance. *Journal of perinatal and neonatal nursing* 15(4), 1-10.

McGrath JM (2000). Developmentally supportive caregiving and technology: isolation or merger of intervention strategies? *Journal of perinatal and neonatal nursing* 14(3), 78-91.

McGrath JM, editor (2001). Building relationships with families in the NICU: exploring the guarded alliance. *Journal of perinatal and neonatal nursing* 15(4), 1-10.

McGrath JM, Conliff-Torres (1996). Integrating family-centered developmental assessment and intervention into routine care in the NICU. *Nursing clinics of North America* 31(2), 367-386.

McGrath JM, Valenzuela G (1994). Integrating developmentally supportive caregiving into practice through education. *Journal of perinatal and neonatal nursing* 8(3), 46-57.

McKim EM et al (1995). The transition to home for mothers of healthy and initially healthy newborns. *Midwifery* 11(4), 184-194.

Miles MS et al (1993). Parental stressor scale: neonatal intensive care unit. *Nursing research* 42(3), 148-152.

Miles MS et al (1996). Sources of support reported by mothers and fathers of infants hospitalized in a neonatal intensive care unit. *Neonatal network* 15(3), 45-52.

Newman CB, McSweeney ME (1990). A descriptive study of sibling visitation in the NICU. *Neonatal network* 9(4), 27-31.

Oehler JM et al (1993). Maternal views of preterm infants' responsiveness to social interaction. *Neonatal network* 12(6), 67-74.

Olshansky S (1962). Chronic sorrow: a response to having a mentally defective child. *Social case work* 43, 190-193.

Page J, Lunyk-Child O (1995). Parental perceptions of infant transfer from an NICU to a community nursery: implications for research and practice. *Neonatal network* 14(8), 69-71.

Patterson JM (1995). Promoting resilience in families experiencing stress. *Pediatric clinics of North America* 42(1), 47-63.

Paulsen-Bell R, McGrath JM (1996). Implementation of a research-based kangaroo care program in the NICU, *Nursing clinics of North America* 31(2), 387-403.

Plaas K (1994). The evolution of parental roles in the NICU. *Neonatal network* 13(6), 31-33.

Raines DA (1996). Parents values: a missing link in the neonatal care equation. *Neonatal network* 15(3), 7-12.

Raines DA (1998). Values of mothers of low birth weight infants in the NICU, *Neonatal network* 17(4), 41-46.

Scharer K, Brooks G (1994). Mothers of chronically ill neonates and primary nurses in the NICU: transfer of care. *Neonatal network* 13(5), 37-47.

Shellabarger S, Thompson T (1993). The critical times in meeting parental communication need throughout the NICU experience. *Neonatal network* 12(2), 39-45.

Sherr L (1995). *The psychology of pregnancy and childbirth*. Blackwell Science: Oxford, England.

Shields-Poe D, Pinelli J (1997). Variables associated with parental stress in neonatal intensive care units. *Neonatal network* 16(1), 29-37.

Speck L et al (1993). Sibling education: implementing a program for the NICU. *Neonatal network* 12(4), 49-52.

Spero D (1993). Sibling preparation classes. *AWHONNS: clinical issues in perinatal and women's health nursing* 4(1), 122-131.

Stevens MS (1994). Parents coping with infants requiring home cardiorespiratory monitoring. *Journal of pediatric nursing* 9(1), 2-11.

Trivette CM et al (1996). Key elements of empowerment and their implications for early intervention. *Infant toddler intervention* 6(1), 59-73.

Vasquez E (1995). Creating paths: living with a very-low-birth-weight infant. *Journal of obstetric, gynecologic, and neonatal nursing* 24(7), 619-624.

Walburn KS et al (1997). Training in family-focused developmental care: bridging the gap between traditional and family-centered care in the neonatal intensive care unit. *Infants and young children* 10(2), 46-56.

Wereszczak J et al (1997). Maternal recall of the neonatal intensive care unit. *Neonatal network* 16(4), 33-40.

Wolterman MC (1990). Validation of an instrument to study behaviors in siblings following sibling visitation on a neonatal intensive care unit. Doctoral dissertation. College of Education, University of Cincinnati: Cincinnati.

CHAPTER 8

WHEN A BABY DIES: CARING FOR BEREAVED FAMILIES

KAREN KAVANAUGH, SARA RICH WHEELER

The death of a newborn is a tragic and unexpected outcome of a pregnancy. Improvements in perinatal care and the focus on the use of technology during pregnancy (Layne, 1992) have led to the mistaken notion that newborn death has been eliminated. Little attention is given to newborn death in popular literature, and the news media focus on births of higher order multiples reinforces the public's impression that smaller, sicker infants survive. This media focus further reinforces the attitude that death is avoidable. Yet, despite drastic reductions in newborn and infant mortality in even the past 20 years (Guyer & Freedman, 2000), infant death is still a reality in the neonatal intensive care unit (NICU).

In 1998 there were approximately 28,486 infant deaths in the United States (Guyer & Hoyert, 1999). About half of these deaths were attributed to one of the following conditions: congenital anomalies, disorders related to short gestation and unspecified low birth weight, sudden infant death syndrome, and newborns affected by maternal complications of pregnancy (Guyer & Hoyert, 1999). In 1998 the infant mortality rate (IMR), which is the number of deaths in the first year of life, was 7.2 (per 1000 live births). The neonatal mortality rate (NMR), which is the number of deaths among infants under 28 days of age, was 4.8. These mortality rates remain much higher for African-American infants, among whom the IMR is 14.1 and the NMR is 9.3 (Guyer & Hoyert, 1999).

When death occurs in the NICU, the health care professionals should provide expert, compassionate care to the family of the newborn. To do so, they must understand the grief responses of family members and the issues unique to newborn death. This chapter discusses the grief process within the context of theoretic models and a framework for providing care to families.

THEORETIC MODELS

Theoretic models provide a framework for describing responses to loss and developing guidelines for caring for families. A knowledge of grief theory (classic and current), complicated grief, types of loss (sudden or anticipated), and a middle range theory of caring is important both for understanding the responses of families whose newborn has been diagnosed with a life-threatening or terminal illness and for providing care for these families. Selected classic theories of grief are included to highlight the theorist's contributions to the understanding of grief. However, these theories have been inappropriately applied to the grief of parents after a newborn death; these models have not been adequately tested with parents. Current models of grief are also reviewed, and these provide a fuller understanding of the complex, individual, and continuing nature of grief. These more recent models are based on research with bereaved individuals who have suffered various types of loss, including parental grief.

Classic Theories of Grief

Psychodynamic models of grief were heavily influenced by Freud (1961) and focused on grief as a dilemma resulting from the process of relinquishing a beloved object. Freud differentiated grief from depression and observed somatic distress in grievers, as well as a lack of interest in the outside world, an apparent loss of capacity to love, and painful dejection. Lindemann (1944), who conducted the first empirically based study of grief on adult survivors of a fire, found that the daily activities of the bereaved changed significantly and that the duration of grief seemed to depend on the person's willingness to mourn. Lindemann coined the term grief work to describe the mourning process. He characterized grief work as emancipation from the bondage of the deceased, readjustment to the environment in which the deceased is missing, and the formation of new relationships. Lindemann also described behaviors characterized as "pathologic grief"; however, use of such behaviors as criteria for pathologic grief in parents who have lost an infant recently has come under criticism (Janssen & Cuisinier, 1996).

Kubler-Ross (1969) studied the emotional responses of terminally ill adult patients as they anticipated their own deaths. In her pioneering work, *Death and Dying*, Kubler-Ross set forth a stage-based model for understanding the task of coping with dying and brought about significant changes in the way people thought about dying. Kubler-Ross reestablished death as a natural part of life and recognized that dying patients and their families want to discuss the impending death. The five-stage model of grief Kubler-Ross developed is her most frequently cited contribution to the literature. The stages she identified are denial, anger, bargaining, depression, and acceptance.

Over the years, many have mistakenly come to view the five-stage model as a predictive, developmental model in which the second stage cannot occur unless the first stage had been completed, and so on. The erroneous belief that the five stages are prescriptive in nature has fostered unrealistic expectations about grief on the part of those dying, the family members, and caregivers. Corr (1993) has identified other limitations with this model. Corr explained that the five stages are really defense mechanisms or ways of coping. Furthermore, these stages do not fully represent all ways of coping and especially do not fully account for the complex experience of dying. Nevertheless, an important lesson from Kubler-Ross's work is that knowledge about dying and grief must come firsthand from those who experience these life events; attentive listening, therefore, is critical to understanding people's responses and needs.

Current Models of Grief

More recently researchers have presented new views of grief, which stand in contrast to the classic view of a process of detaching from the deceased (Sanders, 1989; Solari-Twadell & Bunkers, 1995; Klass & Silverman, 1996). Current models of bereavement are founded primarily on attachment theory. Attachment models are rooted in the belief that attachment behavior is instinctive and that attachments are essential to human behavior. The goal of attachment behavior is to maintain effectual bonds; if the bonds are threatened, the individual seeks to preserve them (Bowlby, 1980).

Sanders.   Sanders (1989) offers a comprehensive framework for understanding grief as an integrative theory. Her work is based on previous studies by Bowlby (1980), Engel (1961), Fenichel (1945), Freud (1961), and Parks & Brown (1972). Integrative theory focuses on the interrelationship between the bereaved person and environmental factors (internal and external) that will affect the person's grief process. Internal factors include age, gender, personality, physical health, relationship with the deceased, and dependency behaviors. External factors include social support and the type of death (e.g., sudden, anticipated, or the result of long-term illness).

Sanders identified the following phases of bereavement. It is important to remember that the phases coexist, with one or more predominating.

Shock.   This phase is the expression of the impossibility of death. Sudden and unexpected loss may generate a greater degree of shock, but even when the death is anticipated, there is still some degree of shock and disbelief. The characteristics of shock are disbelief, confusion, restlessness, and feelings of unreality, regression, helplessness, and a state of alarm. Physical responses to shock may include dry mouth and throat, sighing, loss of strength, crying, uncontrollable trembling, easy startlement, upset stomach, loss of appetite, and sleep disturbances. Psychologic responses may be narrowing of the perceptual field, concern for self-needs, preoccupation with thoughts about the baby's death, and psychologic withdrawal. Sanders noted, "Shock can last from a few minutes to many days, but it usually passes into the next phase when the rituals of death are over and the emotions that have been constricted so tightly begin to release and overflow."

Awareness of Loss.   Separation anxiety predominates in this phase of bereavement. On a cognitive level, the bereaved knows the death has occurred, but on another level, the death is not perceived as real. Many environmental cues remind the bereaved of their loss (e.g., the baby's room, a car without a car seat, other parents with babies). The bereaved may feel physical pain and deep emotions when faced with these cues. There are many emotional struggles during this time. These conflicts are hard to resolve because they usually involve change. Grief takes time and energy that depletes the body's physical and emotional reserves. The immune system becomes impaired because of its response to the stress of grief. The bereaved are more susceptible to infectious diseases. Physical symptoms of this phase include aching arms, a gnawing in the stomach, heart palpitations, and sleep disturbances (e.g., nightmares, waking in the middle of the night thinking that they heard their deceased loved one, and difficulty falling asleep). The psychologic and emotional symptoms are yearning to see the loved one, sensing the presence of the baby, crying, anger, guilt, frustration, shame, oversensitivity, denial, and fear of another loved one's death. Physical and emotional exhaustion are paramount in this phase. This exhaustion motivates the bereaved to withdraw from others in an effort to conserve their strength and energy.

Conservation-Withdrawal.   This phase closely resembles clinical depression. The bereaved may feel as if they are "losing their minds." The withdrawal behavior may be reflected in a fatigued feeling and a need for rest. They feel as if they have little strength for everyday activities and need to conserve what energy they do have. Despair prevails because on both a conscious and an unconscious level, the bereaved are aware that the loved one has died and that their life together is over. Life as the bereaved knew it would never be the same. There is very little support for the bereaved at this time. Extended family members and friends have gone on with their lives and do not realize that the bereaved are still grieving their loss; they think that the bereaved have picked up the pieces and moved on with life. Immediate family members are mustering all their resources to keep themselves going and are unable to help each other. The bereaved may feel very helpless during this phase, especially if the deceased defined the bereaved's role.

Healing.   Healing occurs when the person's internal perceptions about himself or herself change from one who is bereaved to one who has experienced and survived the loss of a loved one. In the healing phase, the turning point becomes more defined in the person's thoughts. The bereaved begin to assume control of their lives and to make decisions about the future. This occurs slowly, over time. Men may feel a need to gain better control over their emotions; women may feel a greater need for control over their environment. Decisions about the future include developing a new identity, relinquishing old roles, assuming new roles in life and, for bereaved parents, whether to become pregnant again.

Throughout the grief process, the bereaved have searched for the meaning of their loss. What did the death mean? How will the deceased be remembered? Who will remember the loved one? What did the loved one's death mean to others? This search continues until some conclusion has been reached; this is known as loss integration. As time goes by, the bereaved develop different perspectives on their loss and the events surrounding the death. Kowalski (1991) called this change in how the bereaved remember their loved one and the circumstances of the death as "bittersweet grief." Bittersweet grief is the remembering of this experience and their loved one that stimulates a regrief for families. Anniversary dates, life milestones, special holidays may bring back the grief. Their loved one is not there to take part in the event or is unable to achieve a specific developmental task.

Renewal. This phase of bereavement occurs when the bereaved has dealt with the social consequences of bereavement, experienced an increase in self-esteem, taken charge and responsibility for their lives, and learned to live again. Renewal means new levels of functioning, a new awareness of self. Not all bereaved experience this phase of bereavement. The physical aspects are revitalization, stability in functioning, and the ability to care for one's physical needs. The psychologic aspects include feeling good about oneself again and living life with new vitality.

Klass, Silverman, & Nickman. In their respective research with families experiencing different types of loss (that of a child, spouse, or parent), Klass and colleagues (1996) found that bereaved children and bereaved adults struggle to maintain a connection to the one who has died; they form an inner sense of continuing bond with the deceased. This inner representation provides a connection with the physically absent but emotionally present loved one. Survivors remember the deceased lovingly for a long time, often forever. Remaining connected seems to facilitate the bereaved's ability to cope with the loss and accompanying changes in their lives. The connections provide comfort and support and ease the transition from past to future. This phenomenon cannot be accounted for in the early, classic models of grief.

In explaining parental grief, Klass said that grief involves changing the inner representations of the deceased children in the parent's inner and social worlds. The inner representation of the child is changed in the parent's life when the reality of a child's death and the reality of a parent's continuing bond with the child are made part of the socially shared reality. The end of grief is not breaking the bond with the deceased child; rather, it is integrating the child into the parent's life and into social networks in a different way from when the child was alive. Thus grief is the process by which the bereaved move from the equilibria in their inner and social worlds before a death to new equilibria after a death. Klass reported that it takes 3 to 4 years before the new equilibria seem steady enough to trust. In his work with bereaved parents, he found that, "You do not get over your grief," but it does not stay the same. Also, Klass did not find any prescribed stages of grief.

Cordell & Thomas. Cordell & Thomas (1997) have also expanded our understanding of parental grief. These authors presented their extended concept of parental grief because of the inadequacy of existing theories, particularly the stage models, in accounting for the grief of parents after the death of an infant. According to Cordell & Thomas, parental mourning is an enduring process that, rather than letting go, involves affirming the infant's life and the parent's role. Furthermore, the grief of parents is complex and individual; grief can be severe, complicated, and enduring and show many variations in emotional state over an extended period. As such, grief is an ongoing process. Parents work through their emotions from day to day and go through a continuous process of reexperiencing emotional reactions. Cordell & Thomas explained that parents are surprised at the intensity of their emotions, that mothers and fathers differ in their response, that this affects communication between them, and that parents perceive that others do not understand what they are going through and expect them to "get over" the death.

Pinwheel Model of Bereavement. Another current model of grief is the pinwheel model described by Solari-Twadell & Bunkers (1995). According to this model, loss and bereavement are unique, individually lived experiences that are based on the personal history of the bereaved (such as who the loved one was and what the person meant to the bereaved). Understanding the bereaved's history is critical for understanding the individual's loss. Personal history is the context in which other core themes are embedded. These core themes, which characterize the response to loss, include being stopped, pain and hurting, missing, holding, seeking, and valuing. Being stopped describes the interruption in one's life. A cluster of very intense painful emotions characterizes pain and hurting. Missing incorporates the awareness of all that has been lost. Holding is the desire to preserve all from the loved one's existence. Seeking is a search for help, and valuing implies the loss is cherished by the bereaved.

The individual moves out from these inner experiences through the process of surrender. Surrender occurs when a person begins to reach out to others and rejoin life. Rejoining life can be difficult, because life is different. Acceptance of the fact that life is different allows individuals to include new relationships and events in their lives. According to the pinwheel model, grief is a lifelong experience. It does not last for a specific amount of time, but rather continues indefinitely. Years after the loss, "waves" of feelings occur, even though they may not be as intense or as frequent as the initial period. Bereavement interphases with continuing life experiences, and when this occurs, the loss can be revisited, and the core themes are experienced intensely. Revisiting the loss is a normal part of grief and continues throughout a person's life.

"Pathologic" and Complicated Grief

No firm conclusions can be drawn about "pathologic" or "abnormal" responses to loss. Pathologic grief has not been defined universally. In their review of studies on pathologic grief after a perinatal loss, Janssen & Cuisinier (1996) concluded that psychologic and somatic complaints and behavioral changes are common in the first 6 months after a loss, therefore depressive reactions, somatic complaints, and impaired functioning are common for at least the first 6 months. Only about 10% to 15% of mothers of these infants have an extreme response and meet the criteria for a psychiatric mood disorder, and many of these mothers have a history of mental health problems.

Complicated bereavement occurs when the bereaved does not experience a decrease in the intensity and frequency of symptoms over time. Risk factors for complicated grief include a history of mental illness (Lasker & Toedter, 1991; Beutel & Deckardt, 1995; Hunfeld & Wladimiroff, 1995; Janssen & Cuisinier, 1997) and a lack of social support (Lasker & Toedter, 1991; Beutel & Deckardt, 1995). It is hard to differentiate between depression and grief because they look similar in the first weeks after a loss. Symptoms common to grief and depression include fatigue, sadness, tearfulness, lack of motivation, inability to enjoy oneself, and changes in sleep and appetite. Symptoms specific to depression are acute suicidality (preoccupation with dying, verbalization of purposelessness and a lack of hope, or a plan to hurt or kill oneself), hallucinations or guilt unrelated to the infant, and any one symptom that completely immobilizes a person. Although it is the responsibility of a qualified mental health professional to distinguish between uncomplicated bereavement, adjustment disorder, and clinical depression, nurses must be able to determine when a person needs to be referred to a mental health professional. Some symptoms that may serve as "red flags" to alert the nurse to the need for referral are presented in Box 8-1.

Types of Loss

Sudden Loss.   Sudden and unexpected death is very difficult for the family and for the professionals caring for them. There is no time to anticipate the loss, to prepare oneself emotionally, and to mobilize past coping skills. For these reasons, upon hearing the bad news many parents and their families find that they cannot comprehend what is being said and are immediately overwhelmed with raw coping and defense mechanisms (avoidance, denial, anger, withdrawal). It may appear as if they have not heard what they were just told. Health care professionals need to be quiet alongside families at this time, not judging what is said or done, but rather creating a safe environment for the expression of emotions of grief and feelings of loss.

Anticipated Loss.   Anticipatory grief may develop when a loss is anticipated in the near future. The family who has a critically ill member has the opportunity to entertain the idea that their loved one may die. While the loved one is in intensive

care, the pattern of the family's life begins to change from the expected homecoming; instead, they are going home from the hospital without their baby, staying at the hospital instead of being home, and experiencing severe emotional ups and downs with their baby's health. Families begin to learn how to cope with their critically ill baby; they learn the language and special nuances of the unit, where to find information to help them understand what is happening to their baby and, eventually, how to take care of themselves.

Rando (1986) identified family coping tasks for individuals who anticipate the death of a loved one as accepting versus denying the illness, establishing relationships with caregivers, regulating affect, renegotiating family relationships, meeting the needs of the dying, and coping with the postdeath phase. According to Rando, because the loss is anticipated, parents may begin to work through these phases before the death. Some families may even detach from their loved one too soon to protect themselves from the reality of the loved one's death. This may leave the dying baby alone and isolated, which can be frustrating to the health care staff members. During this time, families may be focused on relieving their infant's suffering. A program of hospice care can be an appropriate intervention at this time for all families whose infant is dying (Chapter 9).

Middle Range Theory of Caring

A middle range theory of caring (Swanson, 1991, 1993) can be used as a theoretic framework for providing care to bereaved families. The elements of this theory have been supported in studies of perinatal loss (Lemmer, 1991; Kavanaugh, 1997b; Kavanaugh & Robertson, 1999), have been tested in a caring-based counseling intervention study with women who miscarried (Swanson, 1999), and have been recommended as practice guidelines for perinatal bereavement support (Wheeler & Pike, 1991; Leon, 1992; Hersch & Gensch, 1993). According to Swanson (1993), caring is a "nurturing way of relating to a valued other toward whom one feels a personal sense of commitment and responsibility." For health care professionals, the ultimate goal of caring is to enable patients and their families to achieve well-being.

Caring consists of five therapeutic processes: maintaining belief, knowing, being with, doing for, and enabling. Maintaining belief is sustaining faith in the capacity of families to get through the experience of losing an infant and finding meaning in the experience. Behaviors for this caring process include believing in, offering a hope filled attitude, going the distance, offering realistic optimism, and helping find meaning. Knowing is striving to understand the experience through the parents' perspective. These behaviors include avoiding assumptions, assessing thoroughly, seeking cues, centering on the other, and engaging the self of both parents. Being with conveys the message of availability and ability to be emotionally and physically present. This includes being there, conveying availability, enduring with, sharing feelings, and not burdening. Doing for is doing for the parents what they would do for themselves and their infant if at all possible by anticipating their needs and preserving both the family's and the infant's dignity. Doing for includes performing skillfully, comforting, anticipating, protecting, and preserving dignity. Finally, enabling is facilitating the parents' passage through the experience by informing, explaining, and helping families to think through important decisions. Enabling includes generating alternatives, informing, validating, supporting, and focusing.

BOX 8-1

Signs that May Indicate a Need for Psychologic Referral

Physical Symptoms
Loss or gain of 15% of the person's body weight
Inability to maintain or initiate basic activities of daily living, including care of surviving children
Abuse of alcohol or mood altering chemicals
Symptoms of anxiety or depression that interfere with physical health
Worsening of symptoms over time

Emotional Symptoms
Symptoms of anxiety or depression that interfere with functioning at home or work or in social relationships (e.g., social withdrawl, inability to communicate)
Thoughts of suicide that become almost constant, expression of serious suicide intent, or development of a plan for suicide
Emotional responses (e.g., anger, guilt, self-blame) or obsessive thinking that worsens or does not change over time

Social Responses
Feeling of isolation because of inadequate support systems or lack of such systems
Difficulties in relationships with partner, children, family, or friends
Reclusiveness

GRIEF RESPONSES OF FAMILIES WHEN AN INFANT DIES

Women's Responses

"My arms still ache to hold our tiny baby."

"I have never been on such an emotional roller coaster; one day you think you're up and are going to make it through all this, and the next moment you're overwhelmed with all of your emotions."

The physical symptoms women report after a stillbirth or newborn death are emptiness, headaches, irritability, nausea, dizziness, backache, chest pains, nervousness, palpitations, muscle tension, aching arms, numbness and tingling, tachypnea, difficulty sleeping, and fatigue (Peppers & Knapp, 1980a, b; Lovell & Bakoula, 1987; Willis, 1991). The emotional feelings described by these women are disappointment, guilt, failure, embarrassment, emotional cocooning, inadequacy, and anger, especially at other women who have living children (Peppers & Knapp, 1980 a, b; Lovell & Bakoula, 1987; Hunfeld & Wladimiroff, 1997). Women may want to blame someone or something for the death of their baby, such as God, a member of the medical profession, or themselves, or all of these. Women report feeling cheated and that the death was unfair. Social responses include feeling lonely and ostracized (Cecil, 1994; Rajan, 1994; DeMontigny & Beaudet, 1999; Malacrida, 1999). Isolation and lack of social support occur, especially when family and friends had had the chance to know the infant and therefore minimize the loss. Other commonly described behaviors include loss of the future, shattered dreams, fears, inability to concentrate, and difficulty being with pregnant women and infants (Kavanaugh, 1997a).

Men's Responses

"Everyone kept telling me I needed to be strong for Jayne; no one ever asked about me."

"I'll tell you what my grief is like. It's like someone rammed their fist down my throat and ripped out my heart."

The physical responses reported by fathers are restlessness, emptiness, sleeping disturbances, nightmares, fatigue, weight gain, high blood pressure, diminished appetite, feelings of exhaustion, and arm pain (Kimble, 1991). The emotional responses of fathers include anger, avoidance of feelings, jealousy, guilt, sadness, unhappiness, crying, disappointment, helplessness, vulnerability, despair, and self-pity (Kimble, 1991; Puddifoot & Johnson, 1997). Some fathers express a feeling of powerlessness over their own lives and emotions (Kavanaugh, 1997a). The father's anger may be directed at God, himself, peers, or unrelated events that make him feel overwhelmed by the things he needs to do (e.g., arranging for the burial, or even carry out daily tasks) (Kimble, 1991). Social responses include feeling alone and a desire to withdraw from others. Some fathers report that they also feel the need to express concern for their spouse's well-being (Kavanaugh, 1997a). Some fathers have felt that their experiences were misunderstood by family, friends, and coworkers, which left them feeling unsupported by their family and community (Puddifoot & Johnson, 1997; Wagner & Higgins, 1997). Fathers' cognitive responses include difficulty concentrating, disorganized thoughts, and preoccupation with fears for their partner's well-being (Kimble, 1991; Puddifoot & Johnson, 1997).

Couples' Responses

"I really didn't want to go out after Jonathon died, but I would go because Jay would want me to . . . so we worked out a signal that I could let him know when I was ready to go home."

"I didn't know what to do . . . all she could do was cry, and someone needed to hold it all together or nothing would have gotten done."

Perinatal grief has been associated with marital discord (Wallerstedt & Higgins, 1996). Gilbert (1989) described the effects of perinatal loss on marital relationships. In that study, women appeared to have the additional experience of physically healing after a loss. Many men, however, had the burden not only of dealing with their own responses to the perinatal loss but also of coping with the threat to the wife's health. Couples looked to one another for confirmation of their feelings of loss and for support. Factors that influenced the marital relationship were the couple's ability to share their grief, to accept the differences in each other's grief responses, to be sensitive to each other's needs, to be flexible in role responsibilities, and to spend time together. In a study by Black (1991), women reported feeling that they shared a lot of commonalties with their partners; they felt understood and supported by them. However, the women also recognized that their grief responses to the loss were different from those of the men.

Feeley & Gottlieb (2000) found that after a stillbirth, a newborn death, or the death of an infant from sudden infant death syndrome (SIDS), mothers had a more difficult time communicating their grief, whereas fathers had difficulty expressing their emotions. These fathers also had difficulty coping with the mothers' emotional responses. Peppers & Knapp (1980b) had identified this response as incongruent grief, a term they used to describe the differences in a couple's responses after the death of an infant.

In summary, investigators have found that, compared with fathers, mothers grieve for a longer time and show more intense or a greater number of responses, such as guilt, depression, and crying (Theut & Zaslow, 1990; Black, 1991). Only a few investigators have reported that some fathers grieved for as long or longer than the mother or with greater intensity than the mother.

In addition to more intense, more prolonged grieving, mothers reported a longing to hold or to be with the infant and also difficulty being with other infants (Tudehope & Iredell, 1986; Kavanaugh, 1997a). In contrast, fathers described being concerned about their wives and reported feelings of helplessness and a need to be strong (Kavanaugh, 1997a). Several investigators have described different coping mechanisms for mothers and fathers. Mothers coped by talking about the loss (Black, 1991; Rajan, 1994), but fathers coped by returning to work or normalcy (Rajan, 1994) or by engaging in other physical activity (Black, 1991; Kavanaugh, 1997a).

Adolescents as Bereaved Parents

The few studies available on adolescent pregnancy loss (miscarriage, stillbirth, or newborn death) suggest that adolescent girls may show a wide range of responses, and many of these girls become pregnant again soon after their loss (Barglow & Istphan, 1973; Stevens-Simon & Kelly, 1996; Wheeler, 1997). Barglow & Istphan (1973) found that adolescent girls moved through stages resembling a mourning process. A yearning that was characterized by daydreaming about their infant and a desire to become pregnant again followed initial feelings of shock.

Adolescent parents, both females and males, also experienced guilt, anger, and many somatic complaints. Apathy typically was expressed by a neglect of self-care or by an inability to visualize the future, responses researchers perceived as a way for these young people to cover their pain and despair. Recovery occurred when adolescents became more purposeful in their behavior and began to think about their future.

Adolescent girls who experienced miscarriage, stillbirth, or newborn death had physical disturbances such as exhaustion, change in appetite, aches and pains, dry mouth, and feeling a lump in the throat (Wheeler, 1997). Emotional responses included guilt, anger, irritability, fear of failure, crying easily, frequent mood changes, an increase in emotional sensitivity, a desire to scream, and feelings of emptiness or of being barren. Not all adolescents cried at the time of the loss, and some believed that they could have "done something" to prevent the loss. The social responses of the adolescents included isolating themselves from others and feeling "different." Cognitive responses reflected a disbelief that the loss had occurred, confusion, difficulty concentrating, and preoccupation with thoughts about the baby, the experience itself, and how life would have been different if the pregnancy had continued. Some adolescents viewed the experience as having a positive outcome; they believed that the loss was for the best, that they had a better understanding of the fragility of life, or that they felt more mature. Only a few indicated a desire to die or to be dead.

These studies suggest that miscarriage, stillbirth, or newborn death is a significant life event for most adolescents, and for some it might be followed by grief responses, a bereavement process, and perhaps a rapid repeat pregnancy.

Children's Responses

Little research has been done in the area of children's responses to the death of a newborn sibling. Children's grief responses are influenced by their ability to conceptualize death, their age and vocabulary at the time of the death, their parents' responses to the death, and previous social and cultural experiences with death. Even very young children (i.e., those under the age of 2) can perceive the changes in their family's routines and their parents' feelings and can observe the emotions that accompany the death of an infant. Young children may not understand the concept of death and its irreversibility, but they do understand separation. When children see their parents sad, tense, irritable, and upset, they want to know what made them feel this way. It is very easy for children at any age to interpret their parents' responses to the death of an infant, or even the death itself, as being their fault.

Children cannot cope with the death of a sibling unless their parents can. Parents naturally model behavior for their children. In addition, if parents are withdrawn and remote, the children may suffer a significant secondary loss, the functional loss of their parents (Dowden, 1995). Initially, all children react to the death of their sibling. There are common responses among children that can build on each other based on the child's age. Younger children might become more demanding, cling more to their parents, cry or fuss more, express fears of abandonment, have nightmares, or feel guilty. School age children may become more aggressive at school, withdraw from others, make poorer grades, feel rejected, be angry, or worry more. Adolescents may react similarly to school age children and may also act confused or stay away from home or become overly involved in taking care of their parents to the exclusion of other friendships. Typically, when children feel that they are not receiving the time and attention they need

from their parents, they "act out" in ways that attract the parents' attention.

Both caregivers and parents need to be mindful of the individuality of each child when planning interventions. It is important for parents to explain to their children in language and concrete examples that the children will understand. Age-appropriate books can be used to assist with the explanation. It is critical to be honest and not to tell stories that must be changed as the child grows. It is important to answer all questions, even if the answer is "I don't know." Children who have never experienced a death need to be told about death in terms of the body being unable to work any more. Young children understand that toys break, do not work in the same way, and cannot be fixed. Children then will want to know what happens after death. Parents should explain about the rituals they are following in saying goodbye and should include their children if the children want to be included.

One of the most difficult concepts for children to understand is how people get to heaven when they are buried in the ground (if that is the family's spiritual belief) (Schaefer & Lyons, 1993). To explain how souls get to heaven, parents can put a glove, which represents the body, on their hand, and then take the glove off and lay it down, demonstrating staying on earth; they then move the hand that was in the glove in a fluttering motion to show how the soul gets to heaven.

Over time children's grief responses slowly abate. Professional help might be needed if a child is consistently having problems, if the responses worsen instead of improve over time, if the child's responses change suddenly or dramatically, or if the parents feel that they cannot cope.

Grandparents' Responses

A 10-year study by DeFrain (1991) of parents who experienced a stillbirth, newborn death, or SIDS included extended family members, primarily grandparents. Grandparents have a double burden of grief. They see their child suffering from the loss of the baby and are unable to make the situation better for their child. They cannot carry the burden of their own child's grief. They also are grieving for the grandchild who died. They, too, had hopes and dreams of being a grandparent and of whom the baby would resemble and would grow to be like. Grandparents have their own grief process and in their search to determine what happened may inadvertently blame themselves for "bad genes" or their children for not doing all they could during the pregnancy or after birth. DeFrain found that grandparents need information on how they can help their children recover from their loss, how long grief lasts, and the differences between men's and women's grief responses.

NURSING CARE OF BEREAVED FAMILIES

Standardized checklists for caring for families who experience a loss are available (Ryan & Cote-Arsenault, 1991). These checklists focus on tasks, such as providing infant mementos and encouraging parents to see and hold their infant. However, using only checklists does not always allow for adequate assessment and individualized care (Leon, 1992), nor do the checklists provide guidelines for the way these tasks should be carried out. Caring behaviors should be used in conjunction with checklists to guide care for bereaved families.

In her study of parents' perceptions of caring after a stillbirth or newborn death, Lemmer (1991) identified two categories of caring: taking care of, which involved providing expert care and information, and caring for or about, which involved providing direct emotional support and individualized, family-centered care; acting as a surrogate parent; facilitating the creation of memories; and respecting the rights of parents. These caring behaviors are similar to those described in Swanson's middle range theory of caring. Together with the rights of the parents when a baby dies (Box 8-2) and the rights of the deceased infant (Box 8-3), these behaviors can serve as the basis for supportive care of families.

Caring Behaviors

Providing Expert Care.   Families expect nurses to be knowledgeable, competent, efficient, and able to anticipate and manage problems in the care of their sick newborn. The nurse must recognize significant signs and symptoms that reflect a change in the baby and report appropriately to the neonatologist and must be able to identify comfort needs and pain relief for both mother and newborn. Nurses in the NICU should remember that many mothers who have an infant in their unit have recently given birth, and their needs are the same as those of any woman who has given birth (e.g., peri-pads, milk expression or suppression, pain relief, rest, nutrition). Food and fluids for families must be available on the unit or in the parents' lounge to help the mother replenish her physical strength after birth. Beverages should be noncaffeinated, to reduce physical stress

and promote rest. Comfortable chairs and couches that make up into beds must be available to further ensure adequate rest. Mothers who have experienced a cesarean birth or difficult delivery may have additional physical needs (e.g., pain medication in the NICU, wheelchair access, and outlets for plugging in intravenous pumps).

Families need to be reassured that the nurses and doctors are knowledgeable and technically competent. Parents expect the staff members to talk with each other about the care of their baby so that their child receives consistent care between caregivers, between shifts, and from shift to shift. When the nurses give special attention to their baby, families appreciate this gesture. Some examples of special attention are notes written on behalf of the baby to the parent or parents, special pictures, remembering holidays celebrated by the family, and unrestricted visitation for siblings, extended family, and friends.

Providing Information.   The importance of communicating with parents who experience a perinatal loss has been documented repeatedly in the research literature.* Nurses need to remember that when families have an infant in the NICU, they are in crisis. When families perceive themselves as being in crisis, their behavior and understanding of what is being discussed may be different from what the nurses or physicians think it should be or from how they might be under normal circumstances. It is important for nurses to look for cues that tell them the parents or family members have heard what has been said; such cues include eye contact, questions that reflect the information just given, and responses to that information. In most cases the infant's birth has been the only hospital experience the parents have had before the baby's admission to the NICU, and they may not be knowledgeable about the culture of health care (e.g., when their physician will make rounds, how the health care system works, medical terminology, or the purposes of technical equipment and medications). Most parents are either unaware of the questions or are afraid to ask them. Nurses can help parents determine what questions they need to ask, how to ask them, and when.

Several researchers have offered guidelines for communicating painful medical news.† These guidelines include the following:

- Prepare the parents by giving them a warning before actually giving the painful information.

---

*Dunn & Goldbach, 1991; Lemmer, 1991; Covington & Theut, 1993; Calhoun, 1994; Lasker & Toedter, 1994; Crowther, 1995; Kavanaugh, 1997b; Malacrida, 1997; Radestad & Nordin, 1998.
†Sharp & Strauss, 1992; Krahn & Hallum, 1993; Shellabarger & Thompson, 1993; Girgis & Sanson-Fisher, 1995; Ptacek & Eberhardt, 1996; Serwint & Rutherford, 2000.

BOX 8-2

Rights of Parents when a Baby Dies

To be given the opportunity to see, hold, and touch their baby at any time before and after death, within reason

To have photographs of their baby taken and made available to the parents or held in security until the parents wish to see them

To be given as many mementos as possible (e.g., crib card, baby beads, ultrasound and other photographs, lock of hair, footprints and handprints, record of weight and length)

To name their child and bond with him or her

To observe cultural and religious practices

To be cared for by empathetic staff members who will respect their feelings, thoughts, beliefs, and individual requests

To be with each other throughout the hospitalization as much as possible

To be given time alone with their baby, allowing for individual needs

To request an autopsy; in the case of miscarriage, to request to have or not have an autopsy or pathology examination as determined by law

To have information presented in terminology understandable to the parents regarding their baby's status and cause of death, including autopsy and pathology reports and medical records

To plan a farewell ritual, burial, or cremation in compliance with local state regulations and according to their personal beliefs or religious or cultural tradition

To be provided with information on support resources that assist in the healing process (e.g., support groups, counseling, reading material, perinatal loss newsletters)

BOX 8-3

Rights of the Deceased Baby

To be recognized as a person who was born and died
To be named
To be seen, touched, and held by the family
To have life-ending acknowledgment
To be put to rest with dignity

From SHARE, Pregnancy and Infant Loss Support, Inc., St. Joseph's Health Center, 300 First Capital Drive, St. Charles, MO 63301.

From SHARE, Pregnancy and Infant Loss Support, Inc., St. Joseph's Health Center, 300 First Capital Drive, St. Charles, MO 63301.

- Have a person who is known to the parents and who knows their baby deliver the news.
- Give the news in person in a private, quiet, comfortable location free of distraction.
- Give the news as soon as possible when problems are suspected.
- Give the news when the parents are with the baby and are together or when other supportive individuals are present.
- Give the news with compassion and caring, paying attention to body position and language.
- Give clear, accurate, information and present it with certainty (or the appropriate degree of certainty); use diagrams and illustrations to include positive characteristics of the baby.
- Give the news at a pace the parents can follow and with an approach that elicits the parents' understanding of the situation.
- Give specific information on referrals, services, and support and a summary of what will be done for the baby.

Nurses and physicians need to communicate with parents at regular intervals; bad news should not come as a surprise at the last minute (Kavanaugh & Paton, 2001). The words used to describe how their baby is doing should be individualized and should convey respect. Nontechnical language should be used, and the infant should be referred to by name, not as "the fetus" or "it" or by any other abbreviation that leaves the impression the child is less than human (Box 8-4). Expert nurses anticipate the information needs of the parents, offer explanations more than once, and are patient with the process of parents "learning the system." Parents need to be informed of their baby's treatment plan, how it will change with the condition of their infant, possible problems that have a reasonable chance of occurring, and their responsibilities as parents in treatment decisions. They need to be informed about the purposes of the equipment and medication used for their infant. Finally, parents need to know how they can be involved in caring for their infant while in the NICU and after the death.

Providing Direct Emotional Support.   Nonverbal communication of support is shared through eye contact, attentive listening, concerned facial expressions and, most important,

---

BOX **8-4**
What to Say and What Not to Say to Bereaved Parents

What to Say
"I'm sad for you."
"How are you doing with all of this?"
"This must be hard for you."
"What can I do for you?"
"I'm sorry."
"I'm here, and I want to listen."

What Not to Say
"You're young, you can have others."
"You have an angel in heaven."
"This happened for the best."
"Better for this to happen now, before you knew the baby."
"There was something wrong with the baby anyway."
"Fetus" or "it" in referring to the baby

Gundersen Lutheran Medical Foundation; provided by RTS Bereavement Services, 1910 South Avenue, La Crosse, WI 54601.

---

through the nurse's physical presence and willingness to be alongside grieving families. Nurses who wipe their tears, shed a tear for them, check on them often, and used empathetic touch are perceived as caring.

Actualizing the Loss.   Some bereaved parents and family members may need help in expressing the experience of their loss. The nurse should always use the name of their baby or refer to the child as their son or daughter. Open-ended questions or comments that encourage the family to talk about their experience can be helpful, such as the following:
"What has the doctor told you?"
"What have you noticed that's different about Mariah?"
"Whom in your family does Juan look like?"
"I know you were with Laura when she died; what was that like for you?"
"Tell me about your daughter's funeral."
Any statements that minimize the loss, judge the parents, or increase the parent's guilt should be avoided, such as the following:
"Your baby would have been severely damaged. It is better that she only lived an hour."
"Why didn't you go to a specialist during your pregnancy?"
"Didn't you know you were in preterm labor?"

Helping the Survivor Identify and Express Feelings.   A grieving family's emotions and expressions of grief can seem overwhelming to nurses. Feelings of anger, guilt, and sadness are heightened in the early moments, days, and months after a death. When a bereaved person expresses feelings of anger, the nurse should identify those feelings by saying, "You look angry" or "What happened to make you feel so angry?" Typically, anger is a surface response for feeling powerless or helpless in their current situation. Once the nurse accepts the feelings of anger and conveys willingness to listen, the anger dissipates, and some problems can be solved.

When an infant dies, families typically have many questions about the loss. "What did I do?" "I did this; did that cause it to happen?" "Do you think I should (could) have done _____?" These questions represent the phase of bereavement known as awareness of the loss. Parents, family members, and friends all need to find a reason and sometimes a purpose for what happened. This is a major concept of the grief process called loss integration. Part of the grief process is to determine what happened, what the parents' or family's role was, why it happened to them, why it happened to their baby and, ultimately, for some parents, why God let it happen. The nurse should recognize that the bereaved need to find their own answers to these questions, because that process is a part of their healing. For this reason, instead of just answering the questions, the nurse should encourage the bereaved to talk about their experience more. For example, a mother says, "I hung the wash on the line the day before I went into labor; did that cause the cord to be wrapped around the baby's neck so tight?" The nurse's response should be, "You sound like you are feeling guilty for what happened; I'd be trying to find a reason, too. What else have you thought about?" Only giving the bereaved advice or answering their questions does not help them process their grief. Many times the nurse could pinpoint what physically happened to cause the baby's death and answer the parent's questions; however, the ultimate questions of "why, why me, why my child, why God" remain.

The research of Davidson (1984) reveals that the overpowering emotions that occur with the loss of a child, such as sobbing, crying, and anger, come in waves that typically last only 15 minutes at a time. However, being with someone who is sobbing, crying, choking on their tears, or angry can be extremely difficult. The initial response is to touch the person who is crying or to hand them a tissue. Although such a response may seem supportive at the time, the expression of emotion may be halted or stifled.

Careful assessment must be made when touch is used as a therapeutic technique to convey empathy. When touch is used appropriately, the bereaved continues to cry, although perhaps not as strongly. Inappropriate touch distracts the bereaved from the expression of emotion and causes the person to stiffen, pull way, startle, freeze, look at the spot that was touched or, more important, stop the expression of emotion. Nurses should quietly support the bereaved by being present, sitting quietly alongside and accepting any expressed emotion, with their hands folded, mouth shut, and body positioned in a mirroring, empathetic manner. This presence leaves the mourners with the feeling of being cared for. Safe means of touching when caring for the bereaved might be placing an arm around the shoulder; clasping an elbow, knee, or hand; or wiping the person's tears when they have stopped crying. In handing a tissue, the nurse needs to watch for signals that the bereaved is ready to wipe away the tears (e.g., the person wipes the eyes or nose, raises the head, looks around, or reaches for a tissue). Telling someone it is all right to cry, handing them a tissue, and patting them on the back does not create an open atmosphere for expressing feelings.

Providing Time to Grieve. On a busy unit it may be hard for the nurse to slow the system down for families to say good-bye to their baby. When an infant dies, parents are no longer aware of shift changes or any needs the hospital system might have. Having a special room or area available to the family is ideal. In less than ideal circumstances, curtains could be drawn, or the family and baby could be moved off the unit. When families are pushed or rushed into making decisions, they typically respond to the health care system's needs, not their own. Nurses must be sensitive to the family's needs at this time. Providing time for them to see and hold their baby in private, for taking pictures, and for making arrangements for their baby to be returned to them helps the family create special memories. Delaying the processing of consent forms for autopsy or removal from the hospital can help the family have more time with their baby, as well as help mobilize support systems. These strategies help further the family's acceptance of the loss and offer the opportunity for a last good-bye before returning to the real world; they also leave the family feeling well cared for.

Interpreting Normal Feelings. Many of the parents whose baby dies in the NICU have never experienced a loss of this magnitude. The physical, emotional, and cognitive grief responses they experience at the time of their loss are so overwhelming they may be afraid of losing control, or they may feel that they are going crazy or losing their mind. Because most parents have never felt this way before, they have little understanding of normal grief responses. It is important for the nurse to remember that the grief responses bereaved parents have after a loss for the most part are new coping mechanisms and that initially any response should be considered normal unless the person has had a previous mental health diagnosis. Some parents may respond to their baby's death with comments or behavior that seem inappropriate to the nurse.

The importance of giving anticipatory guidance about grief has been documented consistently in the literature.* Therefore, when the time is right and definitely before the parents leave the hospital, nurses need to reassure and educate them about the grief process, their feelings, the differences between men's and women's grief responses, and how other family members and friends may respond. Reading material on the grief process and on the differences between men's and women's grief, talking with children, accepting the responses of family and friends, and planning a special good-bye can satisfy some of the educational needs of bereaved families. Other strategies for providing parents with information and education can be pursued through follow-up phone calls, by having the parents talk with other parents who have suffered a similar loss, by referring the parents to a perinatal bereavement support group (Box 8-5), and by providing a suggested reading list for the parents or their children.

Allowing for Individual Differences. Grief is very personal, and many families want to keep it private. How a person responds to loss and grief depends on the individual's age, gender, culture, religion, socioeconomic status, and perception of loss, as well as on the expectations of others, previous experiences with loss, and many other factors. Nurses may observe many different types of response in a single family. Men typically want to protect their partners; grandparents want to protect their children from further hurt; and bereaved parents are not sure they can share their grief with their children. Family members' feelings of powerlessness and helplessness may be hidden behind behaviors such as expressing anger, resisting ideas, overcontrolling the situation, or blaming others. Using an individual family member as an example, the nurse can respond to these underlying feelings in the following ways:

1. Position yourself as being on the same side as the resistant person.
   - Recognize how painful this time is for the parent, grandparent, or child.
   - Acknowledge how difficult it must be to feel so responsible for making sure that everything and everyone is taken care of.
   - Ask about the individual's personal hopes, dreams, and feeling of loss.
2. Use self-disclosure carefully in terms of your own experience or your experiences in caring for other families in similar situations.
3. Gently confront when necessary. (e.g., "I can see how you are struggling to help your ____.")

These techniques can help the nurse guide the resistant person to a position where the individual's needs can be meet. Some families need to be asked more than once (but should not be asked more than three times during the initial phase of grief) when important decisions need to be made. This gives them the opportunity to change their minds, to express their needs to each other, and to make decisions based on their individual needs, as well as the family's needs.

Respecting the Rights of the Parents. Parents must make many decisions after their infant's death. They need to be guided through this process (Figure 8-1), and their rights must

---

*Lemmer, 1991; Sexton & Stephen, 1991; Calhoun, 1994; Harper & Wisian, 1994; Lasker & Toedter, 1994; Malacrida, 1997.

BOX 8-5

Resources and Web Addresses for Perinatal Loss

Center for Loss in Multiple Birth, Inc.
(CLIMB; www.climb-support.org)
Jean Kollantai
PO Box 1064
Palmer, AK 99645
(907) 746-6123
CLIMB provides support by and for the parents of twins, triplets, or higher order multiple birth children who have experienced the death of one or more child during pregnancy, at birth, in infancy, or in childhood.

Centering Corporation (www.centering.org)
Box 3367
Omaha, NE 68103-0367
(402) 553-1200
The Centering Corporation provides more than 100 books for children and adults, videos, and sympathy cards, including cards for bereaved parents. They will develop needed books and provide caring workshops.

Center for Loss & Life Transition (www.centerforloss.com)
3735 Broken Bow Road
Fort Collins, CO 80526
(970) 226-6050
The Center for Loss & Life Transition is a private organization dedicated to helping both the bereaved, by walking with them in their unique life journeys, and bereavement caregivers, by serving as their educational liaison and professional forum.

The Compassionate Friends (www.compassionatefriends.org)
PO Box 3696
Oak Brook, IL 60652-3690
(630) 990-0010
(877) 969-0010
The mission of the Compassionate Friends is to assist families in the positive resolution of grief after the death of a child and to provide information to help others support the bereaved family.

Hygeia (http://hygeia.org)
Hygeia is the largest international online website to offer comprehensive resources and references for bereaved families. It also offers a large database and in-person consultation.

Memory Boxes
Memories Unlimited
Martha and Bill Wittgow
9511 Johnson Point Loop NE
Olympia, WA 98516-9529
(360) 491-9819
(360) 491-9827 (fax)
info@memoriesunlimited.com
www.memoriesunlimited.com
This organization provides memory boxes and pamphlets that support grieving families.

Parents of Stillborn
5570 South Langston Road
Seattle, WA 98178
(206) 772-5338
Information line: (206) 782-0054
Parents of Stillborn is a support group for parents who have lost a child due to miscarriage or newborn death.

RTS Perinatal Bereavement Program (formerly known as Resolve through Sharing) (www.gundluth.org/bereave)
RTS Bereavement Services
1910 South Avenue
La Crosse, WI 54601
(608) 791-4747
RTS is part of Bereavement Services, a professional, interdisciplinary approach to bereavement care across the life span. RTS provides training and support materials to health care professionals working with parents who have lost an infant during pregnancy or shortly after birth.

SHARE, Pregnancy and Infant Loss Support, Inc.
(www.nationalshareoffice.com)
St. Joseph's Health Center
300 First Capital Drive
St. Charles, MO 63301
(636) 947-6164
The primary purpose of this organization is to provide support to help parents achieve a positive resolution of their grief at the time of or after the death of an infant. The secondary purpose is to provide information, education, and resources on the needs and rights of bereaved parents and siblings.

The UK-Based Child Bereavement Trust
(http://www.childbereavement.org.uk)
Aston House, West Wycombe
High Wycombe, Bucks HP14 3AG
(0) (149) 444-6648
This organization is a charity that provides specialized training and support for professionals to enable them to improve their response to the needs of bereaved families.

Checklist for Assisting Parents Experiencing Stillbirth or Newborn Death

_____

Mother's discharge date: _____   Religion: _____

Mother's name: _____   Age _____ Gr _____ Para _____ L.C. _____ Due Date _____

Address: _____   Previous loss: _____

Phone number: (___) _____   Date/time of birth: _____

Father's name: _____   Date/time of death: _____

Address: _____   Baby's name: _____ Sex: _____

Phone number: (___) _____   Children's name(s): _____ Age: _____

Optimal call time _____   _____ Age: _____

RTS Counselor: _____   _____ Age: _____

Unit: _____ Ext. _____   Support people: _____

Regular OB MD/Midwife _____   Attending MD &/or pediatrician _____

Date	Time	Follow Protocol in RTS manual Sec. II, p 3-8			Comments	Initials
		Notify/assign RTS counselor:	□Yes	□No		
		Pastoral Care notified:	□Yes	□No		
		Communications notified:	□Yes	□No		
		Saw baby when born and/or after birth:	□Mother	□Father		
		Touched and/or held baby □Mother □Father □Siblings □Grandparents □Friends Offered private time with their baby:	□Yes	□No		
		Baptism offered: (use seashell as vessel, give to parents)				
		Remembrance of Blessing offered:	□Yes	□No		
		Given option to transfer off Maternity Unit:	□Yes	□No		
		Patient's room flagged with door card:	□Yes	□No		
		Autopsy: □Yes □No Genetic studies:	□Yes	□No		
		Genetic associate notified (see note):	□Yes	□No		
		Regular physician/midwife notified of death:	□Yes	□No		
		Memo sent to physician/midwife:	□Yes	□No		
		Section of fetal monitor strip:	□Given to parents	□On file		
		ID bands/crib cards/tape measure:	□Given to parents	□On file		
		Footprints/handprints/weight/length recorded on "In Memory Of" sheet:	□Given to parents	□On file		
		Lock of hair offered:	□Yes	□No		
			□Given to parents	□On file		

FIGURE **8-1**
Sample checklist for helping parents whose infant was stillborn or whose newborn has died. (RTS Bereavement Services, 1910 South Avenue, La Crosse, WI 54601.)

Date	Time	Follow Protocol in RTS manual Sec. II, p 3-8			Comments	Initials
		Mementos (clothing, hat, blanket, pacifier, crib cards, basin, thermometer, silk flower)	☐Given to parents	☐On file		
		Complimentary birth certificate:	☐Given to parents	☐On file		
		Resolve through sharing photographs taken (clothed, unclothed, with props, family photo):				
		Polaroid (3 or more)	☐Given to parents	☐On file		
		35 mm (6-12 pictures)	☐Given to parents	☐On file		
		Medical photographs:	☐Yes	☐No		
		Informed about postponing funeral until mother is able to attend:	☐Yes	☐No		
		Services/funeral arrangements, options discussed: ☐Self-transport ☐Gravesite services ☐Visitation ☐Hospital chapel ☐Cremation ☐Funeral home ☐Burial at foot or head of relative's grave ☐Specific area for babies in cemetery				
		Funeral arrangements made by:	☐Mother	☐Father		
		Discussed: ☐Seeing baby at funeral home ☐Taking pictures there ☐Providing outfit or toy for baby ☐Dressing baby at funeral home				
		Follow protocol in RTS manual (Sec. II, p. 3-8)	☐Mother	☐Father		
		Grief information packet given to:	☐Mother	☐Father		
		Discussed grief process and incongruent grief with:	☐Mother	☐Father		
		Discussed grief conference:	☐Yes	☐No		
		RTS Parents Support Group brochure given to:	☐Mother	☐Father		
		RTS business card given to:	☐Mother	☐Father		
		Pregnancy & Infant Loss Card sent to RTS secretary:	☐Yes	☐No		
		Follow-up calls: 1 week _____ 3 weeks _____ Due date _____ 6-10 months _____ Anniversary date: _____				
		Grief conference planned with parents: Date: ____ Time: ____ Place: ____ Letter of confirmation sent:	☐Yes	☐No		
		Parent Support Group, first meeting attended: Date _____ Follow-up meetings attended: Dates: _____				
		Would like another parent to call: ☐Ask later	☐Yes	☐No		
		Parent contact: _____				

(From RTS Perinatal Bereavement Program [formerly known as Resolve through Sharing], La Crosse, WI.)

FIGURE **8-1, cont'd**
For legend see opposite page.

be respected.* Families need to be involved in the decision-making process because the decisions made at the time of the loss and over the next few days will provide them with memories for a lifetime. Parents must be given adequate time to make the necessary decisions and must be given an opportunity to change their minds within a time period appropriate to the decision. Many bereaved parents are clueless as to their needs for memories or their rights as parents. It sometimes is difficult for the nurse to create an environment in which information and options are offered to parents without making them feel guilty if they do not choose to exercise those rights or if the parents' choices are not the ones the nurse would make. Finally, whenever a bereaved parent expresses a need, regardless of how unusual the request may sound to the nurse, the nurse must try to meet the request. Unmet needs can lay the groundwork for the development of complicated bereavement, and they leave the parents feeling unimportant and not valued.

Seeing, Holding, and Caring for the Infant. Parents need the opportunity to "parent" their baby after death. For some parents this may be their first opportunity to bathe, diaper, or dress the child. Bereaved parents need to have time alone with their baby to say and do the things they would have done had their baby been able to go home (Figure 8-2). Asking parents about what they had dreamed of doing for or with their baby after birth can offer insight into arranging for special memories. The following are a few examples of special memories that some families have requested:

- Taking their son to the park with their dogs for the afternoon because they wanted him to feel the sun on his face before he died.
- Allowing them to spend the night sleeping with their daughter skin to skin.
- Rocking both babies at the same time when a death occurred with a multiple birth.
- Bathing their son, rubbing lotion on him, dressing him, wrapping him in his blanket, and then placing him in his bassinet.
- Reading a "Golden Books" story while rocking her daughter.
- Listening to her son's heartbeat for one last time.
- Having the infant brought back to the unit from the morgue so that her brother could spend special time with his sister.

Visitation with Other Family Members and Friends. Bereaved parents need to be offered the opportunity to include their children (regardless of age), grandparents, extended family members, and friends, allowing them to see and hold their baby. Such visits afford others the opportunity to become acquainted with their son or daughter, to understand the parents' loss, to offer their support, and to say good-bye. This experience can help parents explain to their surviving children who their brother or sister was and what death means, and it offers the opportunity for siblings to ask questions. Involving extended family and friends enables parents to mobilize their social support system of people who will be with them at the time of the loss and in the future, and it gives the nurse an opportunity to recommend concrete ways that family and friends can help the parents. Nurses should provide specific information on ways family and friends can provide the various types of so-

*Lemmer, 1991; Sexton & Stephen, 1991; Calhoun, 1994; Kavanaugh, 1997b; Malacrida, 1997.

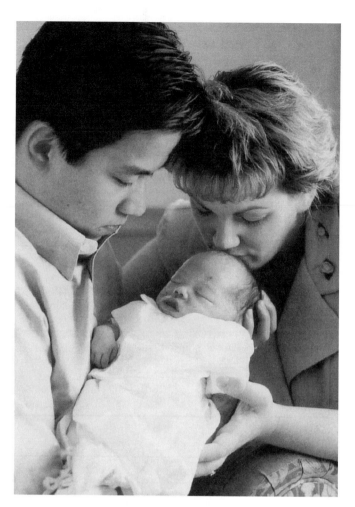

FIGURE **8-2**
Parents with deceased infant.

cial support, including emotional support, practical help, guidance, and possibly financial assistance.

Special Memories. Parents need tangible memories of their baby to allow them to actualize the loss. Parents may want to bring in a previously purchased baby book to be completed during their baby's hospitalization. Memory books, cards, and information on grief and mourning are available for purchase by families, hospitals, or clinics through national perinatal bereavement organizations (Box 8-5).

Pictures are often the most important memento a parent can have. Photographs should be taken whenever possible while the infant is alive and after the infant has died. However, cultural practices should be respected. For example, it may be inappropriate to take pictures for some Native American families (Table 8-1). The most important principle regarding cultural and religious practices is that the nurse should determine the cultural and religious practices the family wishes to carry out. The nurse should not assume that all members of a certain religious or cultural group maintain and practice similar beliefs.

Pictures should include close-ups of the infant's face, hands, and feet. The infant should be clothed in a gown and hat and wrapped in a blanket, and pictures should be taken with the parents, siblings, extended family members, and friends (Figure 8-3). Other photographs of the infant unclothed can be taken at the parents' request. Flowers, blocks, stuffed animals, or toys

TABLE 8-1	Selected Cultural and Religious Aspects of Perinatal Death Practices
Perinatal Death Practice	**Cultural/Religious Practice**
Burial options	Cremation is forbidden, discouraged, or allowed only under unusual circumstances for Baha'is, Jews, and members of the Christian and Missionary Alliance, Church of Jesus Christ of Latter-Day Saints, and Greek Orthodox Church. Cremation is customary for Hindus and Unitarian Universalists.
Embalming	The body is not to be embalmed for Jews and Baha'is unless required by state law.
Pictures	Picture taking may conflict with the beliefs of some cultures, such as those of Native Americans, Eskimos, Amish, Hindus, and Muslims. It is important to offer these families a choice; within the culture as a whole, a photograph may not be acceptable.
Sacraments	Most Protestant denominations and some Roman Catholics perform baptism usually only if the infant is living. Judaism, Hinduism, and Islam have rituals for preparing the body for burial.

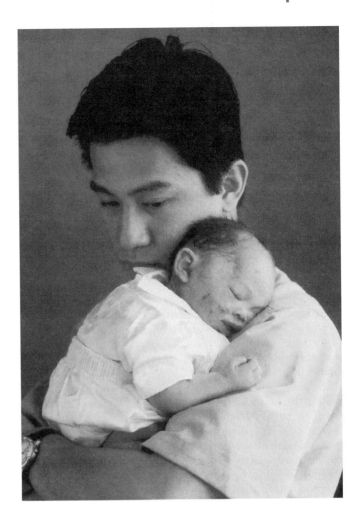

FIGURE 8-3
Father with deceased infant.

can be placed in the background to make the picture seem less stark. Black and white film can be used when it would be sensitive to minimize the harshness of colored photographs (e.g., with severe bruising). Keeping a camera nearby and taking pictures when parents are spending special time with their baby can provide families with important memories. Disposable cameras can be purchased so that parents can take numerous photographs of the infant and family. Some families may have their own camera or video equipment and may prefer that the nurse record them parenting their baby as they bathe, dress, or diaper. Asking families what their dreams were for parenting their baby can give the nurse insight into creating a memorable pictorial history of the infant's short life.

The nurse should provide the family with the infant's weight, length, and head circumference. Footprints and handprints can be taken and placed with the other information on a memorial card or in a memory book or baby book. If the footprint or handprint does not turn out, the nurse can trace around the desired body part, or an impression can be made by using a product similar to plaster of paris called Orthostone (Dentsply International, York, PA). Any article that comes in contact with the infant during care (e.g., tape measure, blanket, hat, hospital undershirt, lotion, shampoo, comb, pacifier, identification bands, crib cards) should be saved, placed in a resealable bag, and given to the parents. Articles should not be washed or cleaned beforehand, so that the parents can keep the smell of their baby. A lock of hair may be an important keepsake for the parents' memories. The nurse must ask one or both parents' permission before cutting a lock of hair, which can be removed from the nape of the neck, where it is not noticeable.

Rituals of Remembrance.   Many families may have spiritual needs at the time of a loss, and these needs can be an important part of their care, support, and memories. Support from the clergy is an option that should be offered to all families. Families may wish to have their own pastor, priest, rabbi, or spiritual leader contacted, or they may wish to see the hospital's chaplain. Nurses can offer the opportunity for the presence of clergy by saying, "It's customary in our hospital when a family is experiencing (a crisis or loss of a loved one) that we notify pastoral care. Can I do this for you?" Members of the clergy may offer families the opportunity for baptism, sacrament of the sick, anointing, a naming ceremony, a blessing, special prayers, a memorial service, or other rituals relevant to their spiritual belief. For many families, having the clergy involved in their care can bring a sense of peace in a crisis situation. It is important that the nurse not impose personal religious practices, such as baptism, on the infant without a parent's request or consent.

Autopsy and Organ Donation.   Parents have described the importance of autopsy and burial counseling.* Health care professionals must acknowledge to parents that although these decisions are difficult, the consequences become more important

*Dunn & Goldbach, 1991; Sexton & Stephen, 1991; Calhoun, 1994; Harper & Wisian, 1994; Lasker & Toedter, 1994; Crowther, 1995; Primeau & Lamb, 1995; Kavanaugh, 1997b; Khong, 1997; Malacrida, 1997; Limbo & Wheeler, 1998; Radestad & Nordin, 1998.

as time passes. A good understanding of the differences between a partial and a complete autopsy and of which organs typically are used in infant organ donation is necessary. Health care professionals also should examine their feelings and attitudes concerning autopsies, because these might influence the way in which the consent is obtained (Chiswick, 1995; Khong, 1997). An autopsy can be instrumental in determining the cause of death. For some families this information is helpful for understanding why their loss occurred, for processing their grief, and perhaps for preventing another loss. Other families may feel that their baby has been through enough, and they may prefer not to have further information about the cause of death. Some religions prohibit autopsy. These decisions are difficult for families to make, and they will need time to discuss this option.

Organ or tissue donation can be an aid to grieving, an opportunity for the family to see something positive associated with this experience. Before this option is offered to the family, however, the nurse should contact the regional organ bank so that it can be determined whether the infant is a candidate for organ donation. This determination actually should be made before the infant has died. Donation of selected organs may be possible if the infant was born at 36 weeks' gestation or later.

Taking the Infant to the Morgue. Before taking the infant to the morgue, nurses should prepare the child's skin by gently putting cold cream on the eyelids, hands, and face to keep the skin from dehydrating during refrigeration. The infant should be undressed, placed on a large, smooth blanket with the arms at the side (as infants are seen in the nursery), and carefully wrapped with a smooth blanket to prevent impressions from being made on the face.

The nurse should transport the child to the morgue according to hospital protocol, usually by placing the infant in a crib or by carrying the infant in the arms. The infant should be placed face up, with the blanket loose over the face, in the refrigeration unit of the morgue. If the infant is to be placed in a casket, the child should be positioned comfortably. If the infant is too large for the casket, the arms can be positioned on the chest, or the infant can be placed on the abdomen with the head turned and the knees tucked under the chest in the fetal position.

Funeral Arrangements. In making final arrangements for their baby, families may want a special service. They may choose to have a service in the hospital chapel, visitation at a funeral home or their own home, a funeral service, or a graveside service. Families can make any of these services as special, personal, and memorable as they like through music, poems, or readings. Some families may want to buy an outfit for their baby to be buried in, or they may want to use something already purchased. They also may want to bathe and dress their baby again at the funeral home, hold their baby one last time, and place their son or daughter comfortably in the casket. This can be done even if an autopsy has been performed on the infant. However, families need to know what to expect (e.g., the incisions, coolness, and rigidity of the body after embalming). Meaningful mementos chosen by the parents or the baby's siblings can be placed in the casket with the infant. Some parents may want to carry the casket to the vehicle used for transport or to the gravesite. Caskets used for babies typically are made of Styrofoam, therefore the outside can be decorated with magic markers or spray-painted by family members or siblings.

Some parents or grandparents may want to build a casket from wood or dig the grave, which would depend on the rules and requirements of the cemetery.

Parents should be given information about choices for the final disposition of their baby, and cultural practices should be respected (Table 8-1). Final disposition can include burial or cremation. Depending on the cemetery's policies, babies who are placed in a casket or the ashes from babies who are cremated can be buried in a special place designated for babies, at the foot of an already deceased relative, in a separate plot, or in a mausoleum. The remains may also be scattered in a designated area (many states have regulations regarding where ashes can be scattered). A local funeral director or a state's Bureau of Vital Statistics should have information about the state's rules, codes, and regulations regarding live births, death certificates, burial requirements, transportation of the deceased by parents, and cremation. Parents who will bury their baby a distance from where they live or where the infant died may want to transport their baby to the funeral home in the area where the infant is to be buried. Nurses should be knowledgeable about the process of self-transport and the required forms.

Follow-Up Care

Some investigators have recommended follow-up care for parents who experience a perinatal loss (Harper & Wisian, 1994; Malacrida, 1997). Follow-up care is a necessary component of a program of support because of the documented social isolation of the parents after discharge (Rajan, 1994; Kavanaugh & Robertson, 1999; Malacrida, 1999) and the frequent accounts of parents' lack of understanding of the events surrounding the loss (Covington & Theut, 1993; Crowther, 1995; Radestad & Nordin, 1998; Kavanaugh & Robertson, 1999). Some investigators have documented the importance parents ascribe to follow-up contact with a health care professional (Harper & Wisian, 1994; Malacrida, 1997) and the importance of providing information on support groups (Sexton & Stephen, 1991; Calhoun, 1994).

Follow-up phone calls or visits (or both) should be made to the family after a newborn death. Phone calls made within 1 week after a loss and again in 1 to 2 weeks, or in conjunction with the mother's postpartum appointment, are critical components of follow-up. Sample questions for the initial telephone call are presented in Box 8-6. During this follow-up contact, the health care professional should clarify information, validate the parents' feelings, and help the parents identify effective ways of coping and sources of support (Friedrichs & Daly, 2000).

If the parents have consented to an autopsy, the health care professional that has maintained contact with the family should be a part of the autopsy conference. It is helpful for institutions to develop specialized perinatal loss clinics where families meet with an interdisciplinary team of health care professionals (e.g., perinatologist, neonatologist, nurse, mental health professional, and genetic counselor) to have their questions answered and their emotional needs assessed and met. Parents may want to review the previous pregnancy and loss to understand what happened, how it happened, and what they might do differently during a subsequent pregnancy. Also, it is important to remember that even though parents might not bring up the previous loss during a routine follow-up postpartum appointment, the health care professional should not be afraid to discuss the loss with them and ask them if they have any concerns. The health care team must be honest and must not hedge when questions are asked. It is important to instill

---

BOX 8-6

Questions for an Initial Follow-up Telephone Call after the Death of a Baby

"You might recall that you were told that someone from the hospital would call you in (number) weeks."

"Is this a good time to talk?"

"Are there any issues that you have been thinking about that perhaps I could follow-up on for you?"

"Have you been back yet for a postpartum check-up?"

"Some parents have noticed a change in their sleeping or eating habits. Has this been a problem for you?"

"How has (name of other parent) responded to your loss? Sometimes it is hard for both parents to talk about it. How has it been for you?"

"Do you have other family members or friends that you have been able to talk to? What types of things have they been able to do for you?"

"Do you have plans to work outside your home? The first few days at work can be especially difficult. Have you thought about how it might be for you?"

"Did you receive any information on support groups for parents?"

"Are there any other materials you received in the hospital that you have questions about?"

"Are there any other questions that I can answer for you?"

"During the call you stated that. . . ."

"I will call you again on (date)."

Friedrichs J, Daly MI et al (2000). Follow-up of parents who experience a perinatal loss: facilitating grief and assessing for grief complicated by depression. Illness, crisis & loss 8(3), 302.

---

confidence in the woman and in her body's ability to have a successful pregnancy. This helps create an atmosphere of trust and helps the woman and her partner to be more open.

SPECIAL CONSIDERATIONS

Multiples

"When I have the girls out in the stroller and everyone is remarking how cute our twins are, I just want to scream, 'They're triplets . . . their brother died!'"

Technologic advances in perinatal care and reproductive technology have led to a subsequent increase in twin and higher order multiple births (Guyer & Hoyert, 1999). Since 1980 the number of twin births has increased 52%, and the number of triplet and other higher order multiple births has increased 404% (Guyer & Hoyert, 1999). Experiencing the death of an infant who is a multiple is often referred to as "bittersweet" because of the dual emotions of joy and grief that parents experience. Having multiples is a special parenting experience, and with the death of an infant who was a multiple, parents lose the unique opportunity to parent the multiples (Swanson-Kauffman, 1988). Yet, the results of research with parents of twins have shown that it is critical for parents to be recognized as parents of multiples even after one infant has died (Sychowski, 1998) (Figure 8-4).

When parents experience the death of a twin or higher order multiple, they also are parenting the surviving infant (or

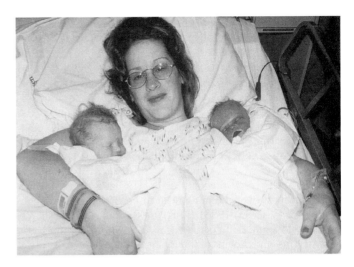

FIGURE **8-4**
Mother with surviving twin and deceased twin.

infants), who often is being cared for in the NICU. Thus parents are undergoing the stress of the NICU experience in addition to their grief, and they may fear that something will happen to their surviving infant. Parents have reported that family and friends expect them to move on with their grief and focus on their surviving infant (Sychowski, 1998). Anecdotal reports also show that health care professionals fail to acknowledge the deceased infant and instead focus on the survivor, especially if the survivor is in the NICU. Therefore it is critical to recognize the special needs of parents of multiples:

- Some parents may find it difficult to be around other multiples in the NICU; consideration should be given to moving the surviving multiple away from other multiples in the nursery if this approach would be supportive to the parents.
- Nurses must remember that a surviving multiple is still a multiple and should be referred to appropriately. For example, a surviving triplet should be referred to as a triplet, not a twin, no matter when the loss occurred. The only exception is when parents use different language to refer to their surviving infant, which sometimes occurs when the loss has occurred during the first trimester of the pregnancy.
- Sensitivity should be shown by leaving the letters marking the difference between multiples on the crib (e.g., "A," "B," or "C").
- Parents should be allowed time to see and hold all multiples together.
- Similar kinds of infant mementos should be created for all infants as desired by the parents. A variety of pictures should be taken of the infants, including pictures of all multiples together even if one infant has already died. Parents have often superimposed their infants' pictures at a later date when these pictures were not taken in the hospital.
- The parents should be given a copy of a newsletter from the Center for Loss in Multiple Birth (Box 8-5).
- Nurses should not be reluctant to talk about the infant who died when the parents visit their surviving multiple in the NICU.

Parents worry about the grief of the surviving multiple as the child grows up (Sychowski, 1998). Also, the surviving multiple serves as a constant reminder of the other child (Swanson-Kauffman, 1988; Sychowski, 1998). These concerns are an important part of anticipatory counseling for the parents, especially in regard to the milestone events in the survivor's life.

Subsequent Pregnancy After a Loss

"We wanted to get pregnant right away . . . so we had sex every day and sometimes several times a day. I began to feel like a robot . . . what used to be special became routine."

"God made a terrible mistake, and he wouldn't do it again."

"I knew when the baby was inside of me, it was safe; it was when he would come out everything could change."

"My body doesn't do pregnancy well. I hated to have to be pregnant again to get what I wanted most."

One of the questions most asked by bereaved parents who have suffered a miscarriage, stillbirth, or SIDS death is when or if they should become pregnant again (DeFrain, 1991). Many parents feel an overwhelming need to become pregnant again (Limbo & Wheeler, 1998). This obsession may occur shortly after the loss and is perpetuated by the feelings of emptiness, aching arms, and dreams of the infant that are part of the physical and emotional grief responses. Some fathers may think that another pregnancy may be something they can do to help their partners feel better. The reasons for getting pregnant again may vary from not wanting to hurt anymore to wanting to have a family.

Physicians may recommend that the couple wait 3 to 6 months before trying to conceive (Kowalski, 1991). Davis & Stewart (1989) studied physicians' recommendations for attempting to conceive after a perinatal loss and found that most physicians recommended a specific waiting period before trying to conceive. However, most parents did not want to be told when to get pregnant again and followed their own ideas about when to conceive. If couples who have experienced a stillbirth or newborn death conceive soon after their loss, they may experience an anniversary of the infant's death and the birthday of their subsequent baby within a relatively short period. Some mothers and fathers experience emotional flashbacks of the previous pregnancy, labor and delivery, and time spent in the NICU. These flashbacks can be frightening and confusing and may cause them to be concerned about their mental health. Investigators have also consistently documented increased anxiety in mothers during a pregnancy subsequent to a perinatal loss (Theut & Pedersen, 1988; Davis & Stewart, 1989; Armstrong & Hutti, 1998; Cote-Arsenault & Marshall, 2000). Parents in these studies also were more reserved with social customs during the pregnancy (e.g., announcing the pregnancy, having a baby shower). For these parents, pregnancy was seen as a task with a goal, to produce a healthy baby, rather than as a time of enjoyment. Despite these findings, investigators have also demonstrated that a subsequent pregnancy after a loss diminishes the intensity of the parents' grief response (Zeanah, 1989). Nurses should provide anticipatory counseling to parents who are contemplating a subsequent pregnancy and to their families, so that they are aware of the feelings they may experience (Robertson & Kavanaugh, 1998).

CARE FOR THE CAREGIVER

Nurses experience varying degrees of stress in their work. The major source of stress for those who work on a continuing basis with the dying can be organizational, work related, interpersonal, or intrapersonal (Marino, 1998). Working with the dying and the bereaved can touch health care professionals in profound ways (Worden, 1982, 1991). Nurses who have children at home, who are pregnant, or who want to have children can strongly identify with parents when their baby dies. It increases anxiety in terms of their personal relationships and

death awareness. Working with the dying can affect nurses' sense of power, mastery, and control (Rando, 1986). Nurses who have not worked through their grief for their professional losses are more vulnerable to unresolved grief. The reasons for not beginning or not completing the grief process often are not addressed in the work place or at home and are difficult for some nurses to articulate. Furthermore, nurses who express their grief might be perceived by their peers or the hospital administration as not being in control of their feelings and emotions, therefore those behaviors would not be supported.

Newborn deaths in an NICU can occur at the same time or serially within a short period. This can lead to bereavement overload, or cumulative grief. Cumulative grief can lead to emotional exhaustion, depression, anxiety, displacement, feelings of decreased professional competency, or a generalized lowering of self-esteem. One of the more serious effects of cumulative grief is denial. As Marino (1998) found, "Distorted or masked grief, which is the grief exhibited in terms of physical illness, substance abuse, or risk-taking behaviors, also can occur."

Learning how to cope with feelings and emotions that occur as a result of infant death is difficult. The loss needs to be dealt with personally, psychologically, socially, and institutionally. Fortinash & Holoday-Worret (2000) have identified personal coping measures and techniques for adapting to stress. Exercise, recreational activities, music therapy, humor, relaxation exercises (e.g., progressive, guided imagery and biofeedback), and yoga all can provide a sense of well-being and of being in control of life events. Psychologic and social supports need to be a blend of both personal and institutional resources.

Nurses generally do not receive adequate preparation for coping with the stress of the work place and of caring for the dying (Feldstein & Gemma, 1995). Adequate education about death and dying, grief theory, feelings associated with loss, and coping strategies help nurses to understand their feelings and the need to develop adaptive coping mechanisms. Health care professionals who care for families who experience a perinatal loss should be well informed about the behaviors and needs of families members. Educational programs on perinatal loss and support of families should be included in employee orientation programs. Health care professionals skilled at caring for families who experience a loss should serve as mentors for their colleagues to ensure the availability of competent health care professionals. Continuing education programs centered on death and grief, including staff feelings about loss, should be offered routinely. Case reviews could be used to provide both novices and experts with the opportunity to learn. This approach would also underscore the importance of meeting the educational and support needs of the professional staff, so that they can provide bereaved families with the best possible care.

Institutions should develop guidelines, policies, and procedures to help the nurse cope when a life can no longer be saved. These processes are aimed at helping the nurse to feel confident and competent in caring for an infant who is dying and at the time of death. Institutions should also formally offer grief support to nurses whose patients have died. This can be done through team debriefing after the death and continuing opportunities to share, offer, and receive support; these measures further enhance nurses' feelings of competency and their sense of mastery and control over their work.

Flexibility in scheduling should allow nurses to attend the funeral, memorial service, or gravesite service for a patient. Nurses should be given time to participate in any institution-sponsored memorial service for infants or other individuals who have died and to take time off to recover or regroup after a stressful period at work. Also, the need for referral for counseling should be assessed if a nurse appears to be experiencing cumulative grief and is unable to cope.

SUMMARY

Because of their continuous presence in the NICU, nurses bear witness to deeply personal experiences with families of infants. When an infant dies, the nurse is in a critical position to provide supportive care to the families. Adequate knowledge of the responses and needs of family members who experience a newborn death can help the nurse provide optimum care and can make a profound difference in how the family experiences this tragic event.

REFERENCES

Armstrong D, Hutti M (1998). Pregnancy after perinatal loss: the relationship between anxiety and prenatal attachment. *Journal of obstetric, gynecologic, and neonatal nursing* 27(2), 183-189.

Barglow P et al (1973). Responses of unmarried adolescent mothers to infant or fetal death. *Adolescent psychiatry* 2, 285-300.

Beutel MR, Deckardt R (1995). Grief and depression after miscarriage: their separation, antecedents, and course. *Psychosomatic medicine* 57(6), 517-526.

Black RB (1991). Women's voices after pregnancy loss: couples' patterns of communication and support. *Social work in health care* 16(2), 19-36.

Bowlby J (1980). Loss, sadness, and depression. In Bowlby J, editor. *Attachment and loss*, vol 3. Basic Books: New York.

Calhoun LK (1994). Parents' perceptions of nursing support following neonatal loss. *Journal of perinatal and neonatal nursing* 8(2), 57-66.

Cecil R (1994). "I wouldn't have minded a wee one running about:" miscarriage and the family. *Social science and medicine* 38(10), 1415-1422.

Chiswick M (1995). Perinatal and infant postmortem examination: difficult to ask for but potentially valuable. *British medical journal* 310(6973), 141-142.

Cordell AS, Thomas N (1997). Perinatal loss: intensity and duration of emotional recovery. *Omega: journal of death and dying* 35(3), 297-308.

Corr CA (1993). Coping with dying: lessons that we should and should not learn from the work of Elisabeth Kubler-Ross. *Death studies* 17, 69-83.

Cote-Arsenault D, Marshall P (2000). One foot in, one foot out. Weathering the storm of pregnancy after perinatal loss. *Research in nursing and health* 23(4), 473-485.

Covington SN, Theut SK (1993). Reactions to perinatal loss: a qualitative analysis of the National Maternal and Infant Health Survey. *American journal of orthopsychiatry* 63(2), 215-222.

Crowther ME (1995). Communication following a stillbirth or neonatal death: room for improvement. *British journal of obstetrics and gynecology* 102(12), 952-956.

Davidson GW (1984). *Understanding mourning*. Ausburg: Minneapolis.

Davis DL, Stewart M (1989). Postponing pregnancy after perinatal death: perspectives on doctors' advice. *Journal of the American academy of child and adolescent psychiatry* 28(4), 481-487.

DeFrain J (1991). Learning about grief from normal families: SIDS, stillbirth, and miscarriage. *Journal of marital and family therapy* 7(3), 215-234.

DeMontigny F, Beaudet L (1999). A baby has died: the impact of perinatal loss on family social networks. *Journal of obstetric, gynecologic, and neonatal nursing* 28(2), 151-156.

Dowden S (1995). Young children's experience of sibling death. *Journal of pediatric nursing* 10(1), 72-79.

Dunn DS, Goldbach DRC (1991). Explaining pregnancy loss: parents' and physicians' attributions. *Omega: journal of death and dying* 23(1), 13-23.

Engel GL (1961). Is grief a disease? A challenge for medical research. *Psychosomatic medicine* 23, 18-22.

Feeley N, Gottlieb LN (2000). Nursing approaches for working with family strengths. *Journal of family nursing* 6(1), 9-24.

Feldstein MA, Gemma PB (1995). Oncology nurses and chronic compounded grief. *Cancer nursing* 18(3), 228-236.

Fenichel O (1945). *The psychoanalytic theory of neurosis*. Norton: New York.

Fortinash KM, Holoday-Worret PA (2000). *Psychiatric mental health nursing*, ed 2. Mosby: St Louis.

Freud S (1961). Mourning and melancholia. In Strachey J, editor. *The standard edition of the complete psychological works of Sigmund Freud*, vol 14. Hogarth Press: London.

Friedrichs J, Daly M (2000). Follow-up of parents who experience a perinatal loss: facilitating grief and assessing for grief complicated by depression. *Illness, crisis, and loss* 8, 296-309.

Gilbert KR (1989). Interactive grief and coping in the marital dyad. *Death studies* 13(6), 605-626.

Girgis A, Sanson-Fisher RW (1995). Breaking bad news: consensus guidelines for medical practitioners. *Journal of clinical oncology* 13(9), 2449-2456.

Guyer B, Freedman MA (2000). Annual summary of vital statistics: trends in the health of Americans during the twentieth century. *Pediatrics* 106(6), 1307-1317.

Guyer B, Hoyert DL (1999). Annual summary of vital statistics: 1998. *Pediatrics* 104(6), 1229-1246.

Harper MB, Wisian NB (1994). Care for bereaved parents: a study of patient satisfaction. *Journal of reproductive medicine* 39(2), 80-86.

Hersch L, Gensch B (1993). *RTS counselor manual*, ed 3. Lutheran Hospital: La Crosse, WI.

Hunfeld JAJ, Wladimiroff JW (1997). The grief of late pregnancy loss. *Patient education and counseling* 31(1), 57-64.

Hunfeld JAJ, Wladimiroff JW (1995). Previous stress and acute psychological defense as predictors of perinatal grief: an exploratory study. *Social science and medicine* 40(6), 829-835.

Janssen HJEM, Cuisinier MCJ (1996). A critical review of the concept of pathological grief following pregnancy loss. *Omega: journal of death and dying* 33(1), 21-42.

Janssen HJEM, Cuisinier MCJ (1997). A prospective study of risk factors predicting grief intensity following pregnancy loss. *Archives of general psychiatry* 54(1), 56-61.

Kavanaugh K (1997a). Gender differences among parents who experience the death of an infant weighing less than 500 grams at birth. *Omega: journal of death and dying* 35(3), 281-296.

Kavanaugh K (1997b). Parents' experience surrounding the death of a newborn infant whose birth is at the margin of viability. *Journal of obstetric, gynecologic, and neonatal nursing* 26(1), 43-51.

Kavanaugh K, Paton J (2001). Communicating with parents who experience a perinatal loss. *Illness, crisis, and loss* 9, 369-380.

Kavanaugh K, Robertson PA (1999). Recurrent perinatal loss: a case study. *Omega: journal of death and dying* 39(2), 133-147.

Khong TY (1997). Improving perinatal autopsy rates: who is counseling bereaved parents for autopsy consent? *Birth* 24, 55-57.

Kimble DL (1991). Neonatal death: a descriptive study of fathers' experiences. *Neonatal network* 9(81), 45-50.

Klass D, Silverman PR, editors (1996). *Continuing bonds: new understandings of grief*. Taylor & Francis: Washington, DC.

Kowalski K (1991). No happy ending: pregnancy loss and bereavement. *NAACOG critical issues* 2(3), 368-380.

Krahn GL, Hallum A (1993). Are there good ways to give "bad news"? *Pediatrics* 91(3), 578-582.

Kubler-Ross E (1969). *On death and dying*. Macmillan: New York.

Lasker JN, Toedter LJ (1991). Acute versus chronic grief: the case of pregnancy loss. *American journal of orthopsychiatry* 61(4), 510-522.

Lasker JN, Toedter L (1994). Satisfaction with hospital care and interventions after pregnancy loss. *Death studies* 18(1), 41-64.

Layne LL (1992). Of fetuses and angels: fragmentation and integration in narratives of pregnancy loss. *Knowledge and society: the anthropology of science and technology* 9, 29-58.

Lemmer SCM (1991). Parental perceptions of caring following perinatal bereavement. *Western journal of nursing research* 13(4), 475-493.

Leon IG (1992). A critique of current hospital practices. *Clinical pediatrics* 31(6), 366-374.

Limbo RK, Wheeler SR (1998). *When a baby dies: a handbook for healing and helping.* Lutheran Hospital: La Crosse, WI.

Lindemann E (1944). Symptomatology and management of acute grief. *American journal of psychiatry* 101, 141-149.

Lovell H, Bakoula C (1987). Mothers' reactions to a perinatal death. *Nursing times*, 40-42.

Malacrida CA (1997). Perinatal death: helping parents find their way. *Journal of family nursing* 3, 130-148.

Malacrida C (1999). Complicating mourning: the social economy of perinatal death. *Qualitative health research* 9, 504-519.

Marino PA (1998). The effects of cumulative grief in the nurse. *Journal of intravenous nursing* 21(2), 101-104.

Parks CM, Brown RJ (1972). Health after bereavement: a controlled study of young Boston widows and widowers. *Psychosomatic medicine* 34(5), 449-461.

Peppers L, Knapp RJ (1980a). *Motherhood and mourning a perinatal death.* Praeger: New York.

Peppers LG, Knapp RJ (1980b). Maternal reactions to involuntary fetal/infant death. *Psychiatry* 43(2), 155-159.

Primeau MR, Lamb JM (1995). When a baby dies: rights of the baby and parents. *Journal of obstetric, gynecologic, and neonatal nursing* 24(3), 206-208.

Ptacek JT, Eberhardt TL (1996). Breaking bad news: a review of the literature. *Journal of the American medical association* 276(6), 496-502.

Puddifoot JE, Johnson MP (1997). The legitimacy of grieving: the partner's experience at miscarriage. *Social science and medicine* 45(6), 837.

Radestad I, Nordin C (1998). A comparison of women's memories of care during pregnancy, labour, and delivery after stillbirth or live birth. *Midwifery* 14(2), 111-117.

Rajan L (1994). Social isolation and support in pregnancy loss. *Health visitor* 6(33), 97-101.

Rando TA, editor (1986). *Parental loss of a child.* Research Press: Champaign, IL.

Robertson P, Kavanaugh K (1998). Supporting parents during and after a pregnancy subsequent to perinatal loss. *Journal of perinatal and neonatal nursing* 12(2), 63-71.

Ryan PF et al (1991). Facilitating care after perinatal loss: a comprehensive checklist. *Journal of obstetric, gynecologic, and neonatal nursing* 20(5), 385-389.

Sanders CM (1989). *Grief: the mourning after—dealing with adult bereavement.* Wiley Interscience: New York.

Schaefer D, Lyons C (1993). *How do we tell the children?* Newmarket Press: New York.

Serwint JR, Rutherford L (2000). Sharing bad news with parents. *Contemporary pediatrics* 17, 45-46, 49-50, 53-54, 56, 59-60, 62, 64, 66.

Sexton PR, Stephen SB (1991). Postpartum mothers' perceptions of nursing interventions for perinatal grief. *Neonatal network* 9, 47-51.

Sharp MC, Strauss RP (1992). Communicating medical bad news: parents' experiences and preferences. *Journal of pediatrics* 121(4), 529-546.

Shellabarger SG, Thompson TL (1993). The critical times: meeting parental communication needs throughout the NICU experience. *Neonatal network* 12(2), 39-44.

Solari-Twadell PA, Bunkers SS (1995). The pinwheel model of bereavement. *Image: journal of nursing scholarship* 27(4), 323-326.

Stevens-Simon C et al (1996). Absence of negative attitudes toward childbearing among pregnant teenagers. A risk factor for a rapid repeat pregnancy? *Arch pediatr adolesc med* 150 (10), 1037-1043.

Swanson KM (1991). Empirical development of middle range theory of caring. *Nursing research* 40(3), 161-166.

Swanson KM (1993). Nursing as informed caring for the well-being of others. *Image: journal of nursing scholarship* 25(4), 352-357.

Swanson KM (1999). Effects of caring, measurement, and time on miscarriage: impact on women's well-being. *Nursing research* 48(6), 288-298.

Swanson-Kauffman K (1988). There should have been two: nursing care of parents experiencing the perinatal death of a twin. *Journal of perinatal and neonatal nursing* 2(2), 78-86.

Sychowski SMP (1998). Life and death: in the all at once. *Mother baby journal* 3(1), 33-39.

Theut SK, Pedersen FA (1988). Pregnancy subsequent to perinatal loss: parental anxiety and depression. *Journal of the American academy of child and adolescent psychiatry* 27(3), 289-292.

Theut SK, Zaslow MJ (1990). Resolution of parental bereavement after a perinatal loss. *Journal of the American academy of child and adolescent psychiatry* 29(4), 521-525.

Tudehope DI, Iredell J (1986). Neonatal death: grieving families. *Medical journal of Australia* 144(6), 290-292.

Wagner T, Higgins PG (1997). Perinatal death: how fathers grieve. *Journal of perinatal education* 6(4), 9-16.

Wallerstedt C, Higgins PG (1996). Facilitating perinatal grieving between the mother and the father. *Journal of obstetric, gynecologic, and neonatal nursing* 25(5), 389-394.

Wheeler SM, Pike M (1991). *Grief resources manual.* Grief, Ltd: Danville, IL.

Wheeler SR (1997). Adolescent pregnancy loss. In Woods JR, Woods JL, editors. *Loss during or in the newborn period: principles of care with clinical cases and analyses.* Janetti: Pitman, NJ.

Willis L (1991). A comparison of grief responses and physical health changes in Caucasian and African-American women following a third trimester stillbirth. Unpublished doctoral dissertation. Ohio State University: Columbus.

Worden JW (1982). *Grief counseling and grief therapy.* Springer: New York.

Worden JW (1991). *Grief counseling and therapy.* Springer: New York.

Zeanah CH (1989). Adaptation following perinatal loss: a critical review. *Journal of the American academy of child and adolescent psychiatry* 28(3), 467-480.

HOSPICE AND PALLIATIVE CARE

TANYA SUDIA-ROBINSON

In the neonatal intensive care unit (NICU), the assurance that "everything possible is being done" often is interpreted as meaning that the patient is receiving state-of-the-art technologic care. Yet the health care system fails both infants and their families when death occurs. The failure lies not in the infant's death itself, but rather in the neglect to emphasize state-of-the-art palliative care. Until it is evident that all dying infants receive highly skilled palliative care, as well as advanced technologic care, modern medicine cannot say that the best possible care has been provided to these infants and their families. This chapter focuses on the care of infants who are dying and the urgent need for exemplary neonatal and pediatric hospice and palliative care programs.

ETHICAL OBLIGATION TO PROVIDE OPTIMUM END-OF-LIFE CARE

It can be argued that all members of the health care team have an ethical obligation to plan and implement end-of-life (EOL) care; to provide highly skilled care at all times except at the end of life is to ignore the essence of comprehensive health care. The ethical dimensions of neonatal EOL care include an obligation to provide compassionate care; beneficent and nonmaleficent care, especially in regard to infant pain; and recognition of the moral authority of caring, informed parents as surrogate decision makers for their infants.

Compassionate Care at the End of Life

Almost a decade ago, Pellegrino & Thomasma (1993) argued that health care professionals have a special responsibility to provide compassionate care at the end of life. They identified compassion and temperance as among the essential virtues of medical practice and cautioned against overuse of high-technology equipment in place of human engagement with patients. They noted that particularly at the end of life, health care professionals can become so focused on technologic processes that they use them as "substitutes for human and compassionate care."

Even today, infants in the NICU frequently die while still intubated and still connected to various pieces of equipment. A recent study of childhood deaths in Canadian hospitals found that the acuity of care was high before death and that most of the decisions about EOL issues were made very close to

the actual time of death (McCallum et al, 2000). In that study, most of the children were intubated at death (73%), and most died in the intensive care unit (83%). In the United States most pediatric deaths also occur in hospital intensive care units (Kerr, 2001), and there is evidence that children often suffer needlessly before death (Stephenson, 2000; Wolfe et al, 2000). A random survey of 30 NICUs across the United States indicated that although most of these units had policies regarding postmortem and bereavement care services, none had procedural guidelines for EOL care (Sudia-Robinson, 1999).

New approaches must be taken to establish compassionate EOL care for all infants in the NICU. This challenge is intensified in a system in which health care professionals are oriented toward active intervention with technologic devices rather than toward an acceptance of death (Jecker & Pagon, 1995). As Jecker & Pagon said, health care professionals are "applauded for acting, intervening, and forestalling death. Once set in motion, these active, goal-directed virtues can easily acquire a momentum of their own." These researchers urge an increased understanding and application of virtues such as patience, cautiousness, and humility in the perinatal setting.

Wolfe (2000) also serves as an advocate for compassionate care for children at the end of life. She identified the "principle of family" in pediatric EOL care; that is, an obligation to treat the whole family. Wolfe saw the health care staff as having an ethical obligation to "pursue comfort aggressively" and to fully engage the parents in the decision-making process for their child.

Obligation to Provide Beneficent Care

The widely accepted principle of beneficence requires that health care professionals actively provide care that directly benefits their patients. As defined by Beauchamp & Childress (2001), the principle of beneficence encompasses both positive beneficence and actively providing benefit and utility, which requires a balancing of benefits and adverse effects. Professional codes of ethics require that nurses and physicians act in a manner that benefits those entrusted to their care. Health care professionals therefore are obligated to examine their actions with regard to intended beneficial outcomes while simultaneously considering the drawbacks or adverse consequences of their actions.

Obligation of Nonmaleficence

Health care professionals also have a legal and moral obligation to avoid inflicting harm on their patients (Beauchamp & Childress, 2001). Adherence to this principle, known as nonmaleficence, may encompass the provision of life-sustaining treatment, as well as the cessation of such treatment. For example, when a treatment ceases to provide the intended benefit for a patient, it may be considered futile, and the health care professional therefore is no longer obligated to continue that treatment (Beauchamp & Childress, 2001).

Health care professionals who continue to provide futile and burdensome treatments may be viewed as doing more harm than good. The distinction is made by meticulously balancing the benefits and burdens to the patient. For critically ill infants in the NICU, procedures or treatments can be considered inhumane if they inflict pain or discomfort on the infant without actual benefit (Jecker & Pagon, 1995). Jecker & Pagon noted, "Medical interventions provided without benefit rob patients of their very humanity. Inhumanity implies that medical care aimlessly prolongs a patient's pain or suffering, making the use of medical technologies a torture or punishment. Inhumanity suggests a failure to empathize with the sufferings of patients."

Despite these arguments for humane care, burdensome, futile treatments sometimes still are given in the NICU. Weir (1984, 1995) has argued that death should not be considered the worst outcome for some infants, particularly when the chances for survival are remote or when physiologic survival is accompanied by unrelieved pain and suffering. In such cases, health care providers may be merely prolonging dying.

Recognition of Parents' Moral Authority

Parents have both legal and moral authority to serve as surrogate decision makers for their infants. A growing body of literature supports parental decision-making authority, particularly for extremely premature or near-viable infants (Jecker & Pagon, 1995; Raines, 1996; Pinkerton et al, 1997); however, few studies have examined ways to empower parents to exercise this authority fully. Furthermore, a body of literature written by both parents and health care professionals suggests that parents may not be involved adequately in decisions about prolonged, aggressive treatments for their infants (Stinson & Stinson, 1979; Harrison, 1993; Pinch & Spielman, 1993, 1996; Raines, 1996). It can be argued that parents may not be as fully involved in decisions about their infant's care as they would like and have the authority to be, especially in cases in which aggressive therapies are of uncertain benefit to the infant.

A consensus is growing among ethicists, clinicians, and families that when the benefits of life-sustaining therapies are questionable, parental involvement in treatment decision making is an ethical imperative.* When life-sustaining therapies have proved futile, parents and professionals often are uncertain how to provide end-of-life care. The following quote is from Robert Stinson, father of Andrew, who was born in 1976 at 24 weeks' gestation. At that time Andrew's survival was unprecedented. He underwent intensive care for 6 months, was critically ill throughout this time, and was resuscitated numerous times before his death.

What they never understood was that one can care deeply enough about a child like Andrew to want his misery ended. Allowing Andrew to die naturally was what we wanted for him, not just to him. I thought often, when I did go in to see him, about his massive pain. He was sometimes crying then; a nearly soundless, aimless cry of pain, undirected and unlistened to except, I sometimes thought, by me. As often as I wanted to gather him into my arms, I wanted him to be allowed to die. What is the name for that? (Stinson & Stinson, 1979).

Although the Stinsons' experience occurred more than 25 years ago, there still is evidence that professionals do not always incorporate the parental perspective into care decisions,* particularly with regard to burdensome, futile treatments (Yellin et al, 1998).

Burden of Treatment

The burden of treatment experienced by extremely premature infants in the NICU, especially those with minimal chance for survival, requires further ethical examination. In a national survey of physicians certified in neonatal-perinatal medicine, Yellin and colleagues (1998) found that many neonatologists believe that "there is an ethical or legal obligation to perform treatments that are not in the infant's best interests, regardless of parental preference." Yellin and coworkers concluded that because some neonatologists are unwilling to withdraw treatments, they may be overtreating some infants in the NICU.

The inordinate medical intervention that occurs for some infants stems from the lack of consensus surrounding the issue of futility (Avery, 1998; Penticuff, 1998). Penticuff (1998) identified harm that ensues for infants, families, the health care team, and society when there is no accepted definition of futility. Such harm includes "needless infant suffering through prolongation of the process of dying" and "psychologic entrapment of the medical team and the family," in which initial aggressive therapies lead inexorably to more aggressive therapies, with only death as the stopping point.

Brody and colleagues (1997) call for compassionate clinical management during the withdrawal of intensive life-sustaining treatment for adult patients using a strategic approach with well-defined goals that dictate the plan of care. Once the goals have been identified, the team examines both the benefits and burdens of the proposed treatment plan with the family. With this approach, any treatment that is more burdensome than beneficial is limited or eliminated. Brody and coworkers identified pain and discomfort as components of treatment burden and said that there is "no sound rationale for withholding adequate analgesia or sedation" during EOL care. This is an area that requires further examination as it relates to critically ill neonates at the end of life.

NEONATAL PAIN MANAGEMENT AT THE END OF LIFE

Research is limited on the provision of analgesia and sedation for infants at the end of life. One study focused on medications administered during life-support (e.g., ventilator) withdrawal. Partridge & Wall (1997) conducted a retrospective chart review to examine the practice of opioid analgesia administration in one NICU at the time of life-support withdrawal. They found that, of infants who had a known painful condi-

---

*President's Commission for the Study of Ethical Problems in Medicine and Biomedical and Behavioral Research, 1983; Harrison, 1993; Jakobi et al, 1993; Penticuff, 1987, 1988, 1995, 1998).

---

*Mehren, 1991; King, 1992; Harrison, 1993; Pinch & Spielman, 1996; Raines, 1996.

tion (e.g., acute abdominal or surgical pain) and were receiving analgesia before the decision was made to withhold further life-sustaining treatment, 84% received opioid analgesia during life-support withdrawal. An interesting finding of this study was that the infants who did not receive any analgesia at the time of life-support withdrawal had also not received any pain medication before the decision was made to discontinue life support. These findings suggest that analgesia is not being given to ease the possible suffering associated with withdrawal of life support, but rather to manage specific disease processes. (Additional aspects of neonatal pain management are discussed in Chapter 42.)

HOSPICE CARE

The use of hospice and palliative care has made a significant difference in EOL care for adults. However, the movement toward hospice care for neonates and young children has been slow to take hold.

Hospice is both a philosophy and a system of compassionate, team-oriented care for individuals at the end of life. According to the National Hospice and Palliative Care Organization (2000), the guiding philosophy of hospice is that "each of us has the right to die pain free and with dignity, and that our families will receive the necessary support to allow us to do so." Hospice care can be provided in select hospitals, in individual hospice facilities, or in a person's home. Although there has been a national movement toward making hospice care available to most adults, there are few examples of hospice centers specifically designed for children and their families.

Pediatric Hospice Care

Although there are few pediatric hospices in the United States, those that exist provide exemplary care for children and their families. One example of a model program is the newly opened Kids Path Hospice and Palliative Care of Greensboro, North Carolina. At Kids Path, care is provided for children with acquired immune deficiency syndrome (AIDS), congenital anomalies, chromosomal disorders, and cancer (Kerr, 2001). It is the only children's hospice facility in North Carolina and among the fewer than 25 such facilities in the United States. Kids Path uses an interdisciplinary care team that includes a pediatric nurse practitioner, registered nurses, medical director, social worker, counselors, and a chaplain.

Barriers to Pediatric Hospice Service

Unfortunately, many barriers obstruct the availability and provision of hospice care to all children and families who could benefit from it. The National Hospice and Palliative Care Organization (2000) has described psychologic, financial, educational, and regulatory barriers to pediatric palliative care (NHPCO, 2000). One of the psychologic barriers is the association of palliative care with the concept of giving up. Families often avoid palliative care, rather than identifying with the life-enhancing benefits it offers. Financial barriers arise because the home-based, multidisciplinary care is often not reimbursed. The educational barriers for care providers are evident in the lack of palliative care training for most physicians and the avoidance of discussing hospice care with parents. Regulatory barriers also exist because the reimbursement system is based on the needs of adults. Ignoring the differences in care needs between children and adults creates barriers to hospice as an option for many families.

PEDIATRIC PALLIATIVE CARE

The American Academy of Pediatrics (AAP) (2000) has issued guidelines for the care of children with life-threatening and terminal conditions. The AAP recommends palliative care for infants when "no treatment has been shown to alter substantially the expected progression toward death." According to the AAP guidelines, palliative care incorporates control of pain, symptom management, and care of the psychologic, social, and spiritual needs of children and their families. The AAP also has established five principles of palliative care: (1) respect for the dignity of patients and families, (2) access to competent and compassionate palliative care, (3) support for the caregivers, (4) improved professional and social support for pediatric palliative care, and (5) continued improvement of pediatric palliative care through research and education.

Respect for the Dignity of Patients and Families

Respect for patients' and families' dignity means that information about palliative care should be provided, and the parents' ability to make their own choice of a program should be respected. Also, the plan of care must incorporate and respect the parents' expressed wishes for their child's care, specifically with regard to testing, monitoring, and treatment (AAP, 2000).

Access to Competent and Compassionate Palliative Care

Compassionate palliative care includes alleviation of pain and other symptoms and access to supportive therapies, such as grief counseling and spiritual support. This principle includes provision of adequate respite care for parents (AAP, 2000).

Support for the Caregivers

The AAP recognizes the importance of support for health care professionals involved in the child's care. This support may include paid funeral leave, peer counseling, or remembrance ceremonies (AAP, 2000).

Improved Professional and Social Support for Pediatric Palliative Care

A number of barriers can prevent families from obtaining pediatric palliative care, including the obstacles discussed previously. Health care professionals must help families overcome these obstacles (AAP, 2000).

Continued Improvement of Pediatric Palliative Care through Research and Education

Health care professionals need continuing education on ways to provide comprehensive palliative care. Also, research is needed that focuses on the effectiveness of palliative care interventions and on models of pediatric palliative care delivery (AAP, 2000). A list of hospice and palliative care resources is provided in Box 9-1.

INCORPORATING PEDIATRIC PALLIATIVE CARE INTO THE NICU

The AAP recommends that palliative care begin at the time of diagnosis of a life-threatening or terminal condition (AAP, 2000). In the NICU, particularly for extremely premature neonates and for neonates with life-threatening anomalies, palliative care should begin at the time of admission. For many health care professionals, this requires a rather dramatic shift

Pediatric Hospice and Palliative Care Resources

American Academy of Pediatrics (www.aap.org)
141 Northwest Point Boulevard
Elk Grove Village, IL 60007
(847) 434-4000
The American Academy of Pediatrics guidelines for palliative care and care guidelines for terminally ill children can be viewed at this site.

Children's Hospice International (www.chionline.org)
901 North Pitt Street, Suite 230
Alexandria, VA 22314
(800) 242-4453
This site provides information about hospice care for children and has links to related sites for families and care providers.

Children's International Project on Palliative and Hospice Services (www.nhpco.org)
National Hospice and Palliative Care Organization
1700 Diagonal Road, Suite 625
Alexandria, VA 22314
(877) 557-2847
This site discusses the hospice philosophy and provides links to related sites.

Footprints Program (www.footprintsatglennon.org)
Cardinal Glennon Children's Hospital
1465 South Grand Boulevard
St. Louis, MO 63104
(877) 557-2847
This is an interdisciplinary program that coordinates community services, bereavement support, and consultation regarding pain and symptom management.

Innovations in End-of-Life Care (www.edc.org/lastacts)
This is an online international journal and forum for leaders in end-of-life care.
Volume 2, issue No. 2, 2000, focuses on pediatric palliative care.

Pediatric Palliative Care Project (www.seattlechildrens.org)
Seattle Children's Hospital
4800 Sand Point Way NE
Seattle, WA 98105
(206) 527-5732
This site provides an example of a statewide pediatric palliative care project.

evitable point at which intensive efforts to prolong life merely serve to prolong the infant's dying. In such cases, both infants and their families would benefit from a smooth transition to intensive palliative care. This requires a level of skilled care that is not always present in the NICU. The care providers must be able quickly to recognize the futility of sustained therapies and must be expert at providing palliative care to both infant and family. Unfortunately, as research has indicated, all too often infants and children die while still intubated (McCallum et al, 2000); suffer from pain that is inadequately controlled (Stevens & Johnston, 1995; Partridge & Wall, 1997); and have not received the benefits of palliative care measures (Byock, 1997; Goldman, 1998; Rushton, 2000; Stephenson, 2000).

The National Association of Neonatal Nurses (NANN), the Association of Pediatric Oncology Nurses (APON), and the Society of Pediatric Nurses (SPN) have stated that this area of neonatal care is very important. Under the auspices of the National Leadership Academy on EOL Issues, which is sponsored by Johns Hopkins University (www.son.jhmi.edu/newsandmedia/endoflife.html), these three organizations are adapting the *Last Acts Precepts* (www.lastacts.org) for neonatal and pediatric patients. The Last Acts organization provides support for health professionals and families through publications and taking action on EOL issues. It believes that appropriate language must be included to reflect cases such as an infant who is literally born dying, as well as the family's unique needs in such cases. This collaboration is a milestone in efforts to recognize that neonatal and pediatric patients and their families deserve the same level of care that adults have received.

Worldwide, recognition of the need for neonatal and pediatric palliative care is growing, thanks to funding from the Soros Foundation, the Robert Wood Johnson Foundation, City of Hope, Johns Hopkins University, the Association of American Colleges of Nursing, and other organizations that support educational efforts about EOL and palliative care. Nursing curricula are being revised to include content and competencies on EOL care. Training programs, such as the End of Life Nursing Education Consortium (ELNEC) (www.aacn.nche.edu/elnec), are broadening nurses' knowledge in this specialty. Organizations such as the International Association of Hospice and Palliative Care, the NHPCO, and the Hospice and Palliative Care Nurses Association, which traditionally have focused primarily on adult issues, have begun incorporating pediatric palliative care concerns into their initiatives. All these actions bode well for the integration of EOL care into customary pediatric and neonatal care as a standard that is expected and demanded.

BEREAVEMENT

The grief process is unique to each individual and varies in expression, duration, and meaning. Parents often move through the grief process differently. The infant's mother may express her grief by crying, whereas the father may express his grief by isolating himself.

For many parents, the grief process is lifelong. Significant life events can trigger their grieving, as can such routine childhood milestones as seeing a neighbor's child get on the school bus for her first day of kindergarten or, many years later, receiving a high school graduation announcement for what would have been their child's class.

from providing intensive high-technology care to providing intensive palliative care. At times, particularly during the early diagnostic phase, palliative care can be provided along with technologic care; this arrangement allows the staff to focus on symptom management and pain control while weighing the benefits and harm of treatment. It also provides for interdisciplinary team members who can provide the support the family needs.

Often, when a neonate is born at the edge of viability, the clinical course shows a downward trend. The neonate's physiologic parameters cause concern as evidence mounts that the organ systems are failing. This scenario represents the in-

As parents progress through the first year after their loss, it is important to prepare them for the grief they are likely to experience in the future and to help them develop a plan for themselves. Every family is unique and determines their own milestone days, those days that bring special remembrance of their child. Milestone days may include the child's birthday, the anniversary of the child's death, or holidays. It sometimes is helpful for parents to schedule time off on these milestone days so that they can plan a special activity. Some parents may want to be alone and take a quiet walk together. Others may prefer to be surrounded by relatives or a few close friends. Still others may want to spend the day with another parent who has experienced similar grief.

The nurse should stress three important points to bereaved families: (1) grief is individualized; (2) grief is a process; and (3) family members should not hesitate to seek assistance with their grief, even years after the child's death. (A comprehensive discussion of bereavement is provided in Chapter 8.)

SUMMARY

Even when death approaches quickly in the NICU, measures can be taken to ease the infant's transition and adequately assist the family. It is no longer enough to provide quality bereavement and postmortem care to infants and their families. Research into and evaluation of care guidelines are needed so that infants can receive the same quality of EOL care afforded other members of society. Neonatal nurses have been at the forefront of this movement and now have the opportunity to serve as leaders in the design and implementation of exemplary neonatal palliative care programs.

REFERENCES

American Academy of Pediatrics (2000). Palliative care for children. *Pediatrics* 106(2), 351-357.

Avery GB (1998). Futility considerations in the neonatal intensive care unit. *Seminars in perinatology* 22(3), 216-222.

Beauchamp TL, Childress JF (2001). *Principles of biomedical ethics*, ed 5. Oxford University Press: New York.

Brody H et al (1997). Withdrawing intensive life-sustaining treatment: recommendations for compassionate clinical management. *New England journal of medicine* 336(9), 652-657.

Byock I (1997). *Dying well: peace and possibilities at the end of life*. New York: Riverhead Books: New York.

Goldman A (1998). ABC of palliative care: special problems of children. *British medical journal* 316(7124), 49-52.

Harrison H (1993). The principles for family-centered neonatal care. *Pediatrics* 92(5), 643-650.

Jakobi P et al (1993). The extremely low birth weight infants: the twenty-first century dilemma. *American journal of perinatology* 10(2), 155-159.

Jecker NS, Pagon RA (1995). Medical futility: decision making in the context of probability and uncertainty. In Goldworth A et al, editors. *Ethics and perinatology*. Oxford University Press: New York.

Kerr E (2001). Kids Path cares for children coping with illness or loss. *MD news Piedmont triad* (5), 24-26.

King NMP (1992). Transparency in neonatal intensive care. *Hastings Center report* 22(2), 18-25.

McCallum DE et al (2000). How children die in hospital. *Journal of pain and symptom management* 20(6), 417-423.

Mehren E (1991). *Born too soon*. Doubleday: New York.

National Hospice and Palliative Care Organization (NHPCO) (2000). *Compendium of pediatric palliative care*. NHPCO: New Orleans.

Partridge JC, Wall SN (1997). Analgesia for dying infants whose life support is withdrawn or withheld. *Pediatrics* 99(1), 76-79.

Pellegrino ED, Thomasma DC (1993). *The virtues in medical practice*. Oxford University Press: New York.

Penticuff JH (1987). Neonatal nursing ethics: toward a consensus. *Neonatal network* 5(6), 7-16.

Penticuff JH (1988). Neonatal intensive care: parental prerogatives. *Journal of perinatal and neonatal nursing* 1(3), 77-86.

Penticuff JH (1995). Nursing ethics in perinatal care. In Goldworth A et al, editors. *Ethics and perinatology*. Oxford University Press: New York.

Penticuff JH (1998). Defining futility in neonatal intensive care. *Nursing clinics of North America* 33(2), 339-352.

Pinch WJ, Spielman ML (1993). Parental perceptions of ethical issues post-NICU discharge. *Western journal of nursing research* 15(4), 422-440.

Pinch WJ, Spielman ML (1996). Ethics in the neonatal intensive care unit: parental perceptions at 4 years postdischarge. *Advances in nursing science* 19(1), 72-85.

Pinkerton JV et al (1997). Parental rights at the birth of a near-viable infant: conflicting perspectives. *American journal of obstetrics and gynecology* 177(2), 283-288.

President's Commission for the Study of Ethical Problems in Medicine and Biomedical and Behavioral Research (1983). *Deciding to forego life-sustaining treatment*. US Government Printing Office: Washington, DC.

Raines DA (1996). Parents' values: a missing link in the neonatal intensive care equation. *Neonatal network* 15(3), 1996.

Rushton CH (2000). Pediatric palliative care: coming of age. *Innovations in end-of-life care*, 2(2) (online journal).

Stephenson J (2000). Palliative and hospice care needed for children with life-threatening conditions. *Journal of the American medical association* 284(19), 2437-2438.

Stevens BJ et al (1995). Issues of assessment of pain and discomfort in neonates. *Journal of obstetric, gynecologic, and neonatal nursing* 24(9), 849-855.

Stinson R, Stinson P (1979). *The long dying of baby Andrew*. Little, Brown: Boston.

Sudia-Robinson TM (in press). Survey of level III NICUs regarding end-of-life care guidelines. (In review).

Weir RF (1984). *Selective nontreatment of handicapped newborns*. Oxford University Press: New York.

Weir RF (1995). Withholding and withdrawing therapy and actively hastening death. II. In Goldworth A et al, editors. *Ethics and perinatology*. Oxford University Press: New York.

Wolfe J (2000). Suffering in children at the end of life: recognizing an ethical duty to palliate. *Journal of clinical ethics* 11(2), 157-161.

Wolfe J et al (2000). Symptoms and suffering at the end of life in children with cancer. *New England journal of medicine*, 342(5), 326-333.

Yellin PB et al (1998). Neonatologists' decisions about withholding and withdrawing treatments from critically ill newborns. *Pediatrics* 102(3), 757.

CHAPTER 10

HUMAN GENETICS AND IMPLICATIONS FOR NEONATAL CARE

CAROLE KENNER

No one can pick up a newspaper, listen to a radio, or watch the news without hearing the word "genetics." Since 1986, when the National Academy of Sciences first explored the possibility of unraveling the human genetic code, the belief has grown that all diseases probably stem from the chromosome and the gene. Today, with the human genome demystified, we know that specific genes are responsible for specific diseases. Although not all diseases or anomalies are directly linked to a specific gene or set of genes, evidence is growing that genetics plays a significant role in every clinical facet of health care.

Approximately 2% to 3% of newborns in the United States have a congenital anomaly (Scheuerle, 2001), such as trisomies 13, 18, or 21, or Treacher Collins syndrome. Some newborns have birth defects that have a genetic basis, whereas other newborns suffer from a genetic disease. The distinction is that a genetic disease results from an aberration in the infant's deoxyribonucleic acid (DNA), such as occurs with cystic fibrosis and sickle cell anemia (Scheuerle, 2001). All these newborn problems are familiar to the neonatal nurse. For many neonatal nurses, the genetic mechanisms and the role of genes in disease were not part of basic nursing education. Typically, little information about genetics was included in the curricula beyond the mendelian laws of inheritance. With the exponential increase in genetics information, that is no longer sufficient. Families can easily obtain a lot of highly technical (and sometimes wrong) information about their infant's condition and the possible genetic basis for that condition. Health professionals must be knowledgeable about genetics and must be certain that families clearly understand their infant's condition. This chapter briefly reviews the historical perspective and then discusses the new frontier of genetics as it relates to neonatal and infant care.

HISTORICAL PERSPECTIVE

Long before DNA was discovered or any of the intracellular contents of cells were known, scientists noted that the basic traits of certain organisms were passed down to succeeding generations with varying degrees of constancy. This observation was noted not only among human beings and other "higher order" species of animals but also among plants and simple forms of animal life. In general, the physical characteristics of offspring usually resembled the physical characteristics of the parent organism. This fact was explained as a basic "mix-

ing" of maternal and paternal characteristics in the formation of a new individual or new generation. More difficult to explain was how a child could resemble or have a specific characteristic found only in a more remote family member, such as a great grandmother or an uncle, rather than in one of the parents. In observing variations in inheritable characteristics over many generations among plants, Gregor Mendel, a nineteenth century botanist, proposed a mechanism that essentially involved the "strength" of some characteristics to explain variations in patterns of inheritance. Even at this point, no one cell structure was identified as responsible for the transmission of these patterns of inheritance.

In the late nineteenth century, biologists discovered small "chromatic elements" in the nucleus of a cell that stained differently from other cell components. In addition, these elements, called chromosomes, were present only at specific times in the cell cycle. It was determined that chromosomes were composed of homologous pairs that split longitudinally during cell division. Chromosomes were thought to be responsible for mendelian heredity. One half of each pair of chromosomes was derived from the maternal gamete and the other half from the paternal gamete.

In 1914 researchers discovered that chromosomes disappeared during the interphase of the cell cycle, only to reappear at mitosis in the same number and with the same morphologic features as at the previous mitosis. As a result of these observations, chromosome formation was speculated to be an organized process from one cell generation to another and not merely a result of random meshing of nuclear material. It was observed that when the chromosomes were abnormal in shape or number, subsequent development was abnormal. This led to the hypothesis that chromosomes were the carriers of heredity and that aberrations in chromosomes (both numeric aberrations and structural aberrations) would result in aberrant development. Normal functioning of cells and whole organisms depended on the equilibrium of this genetic material.

Even though these concepts were proposed more than 70 years ago, testing was limited by the dearth of technologic advances in cytogenetics (the analysis of chromosomes and their genes) and molecular genetics until relatively recently. Cytogenetic advancements occurred first and led to a means of diagnosing some specific genetic abnormalities. The early cytogenetic work increased the precision and clinical application of molecular genetic advancements.

HUMAN GENOME PROJECT

In the near future the Human Genome Project (HGP), a project conducted under the auspices of the National Institutes Health, will revolutionize thinking about health care. The goal of the project is to determine the location of the genes that make up the human genetic code, and this goal has almost been reached.

About 100,000 genes are believed to encode approximately 3 billion bits of information (National Human Genome Research Institute [NHGRI], 2001). The genetic code directs the body's cells in how to perform, what to produce, and even when to die. It carries the "recipe" for the body's proteins, the building blocks of all tissues. When this recipe fails or is altered, so is the structure of the body. In some cases this alteration is so subtle that only the cellular level or genetic level is affected. In other cases, however, the mistake results in a disease or structural defect, such as occurs with neurofibromatosis or some forms of cancer.

Errors in the genes are linked to about 3000 to 4000 conditions (NHGRI, 2001). A genetic map now exists that shows which genes are located on what chromosome, and a region on the chromosome where defective genes lie can even be pinpointed. Although a condition may be known to be dependent on these defective genes for expression, the genes surrounding the defective ones may or may not be affected. However, the location gives the health professional a starting point to do some detective work about possible health risks.

Through the efforts of the HGP, medical science has gained a knowledge of the specific locations of genes on specific chromosomes; this creates the opportunity to design therapies directly targeted to the defective gene or its results. Therapy in the future may involve drugs genetically designed to treat a person's unique genetic makeup. Therapies could be targeted at the specific cause rather than at easing symptoms (NHGRI, 2001). Such specific knowledge also gives health professionals the opportunity to predict the likelihood that specific family members will develop certain conditions. Prenatal teaching or preconception education becomes more important in light of this new information. True health promotion, and in some cases disease prevention, can be a reality. Unfortunately, the exact genetic linkage of some diseases will be difficult to determine for some time to come, because often a sequence of genes is required to produce a condition, and the genes involved in the sequence may or may not be located on one chromosome. The HGP will reveal these genetic complexities at some time, but not all will be easily uncovered.

Not all of this newfound knowledge is positive; health professionals have raised many concerns about the ethical dilemmas arising from the HGP. The Ethical, Legal, and Social Implications (ELSI) Branch of the HGP has launched studies to determine some of the situations that pose problems for health professionals and for the children and families they serve. As the NHGRI has pointed out:

> For some diseases . . . our ability to detect the nonfunctional gene has outpaced our ability to do anything about the disease it causes. Huntington disease is a case in point. Although a predictive test for high-risk families has been available for years, only a minority of these individuals has decided to be tested. The reason? There is no way to cure or prevent Huntington disease, and some individuals would rather live with the uncertainty than with the knowledge they will be struck, sometime in midlife, with a fatal disease. And what might happen if a health insurance company or a potential employer learns that

an individual is destined to develop Huntington disease; might that person be denied coverage or a job? (NHGRI, 2001)

The same issues are being raised by newborn screening and testing. The Secretary's Advisory Committee on Genetic Testing (SACGT) has examined the issue of genetic testing, including the possible implications of such tests, how the tests should be regulated, and what issues must be considered in counseling patients and families (SACGT, 2001). The committee received position statements from many specialty health professional organizations, including neonatal and maternal child nursing groups. Among the concerns to emerge were whether the tests should be mandatory or remain voluntary, and who would have access to the information. Discrimination in insurance coverage, as mentioned above, also was a major ethical issue. Only time will tell the outcome of these ethical issues. However, when headlines in the popular press and the health professional literature proclaim, "Genetic Deficiency May Explain Sudden Infant Death Syndrome," it is difficult to view the negatives; if this linkage between a missing enzyme and SIDS is true, much good could be derived from this testing. (Conn & Wright, 2001).

Nurses must continue to advocate for their infants and families; to do this, they must have a solid grounding in genetic knowledge, including foundational genetics starting at the molecular level. Knowledge of the molecular level starts with the structure of the DNA molecule and includes the coding pattern for a protein.

Deoxyribonucleic Acid

DNA is composed of two very long chains (strands) of interlocking nucleotides (Figure 10-1). Each nucleotide is composed of a molecule of any one of the following four bases: ade-

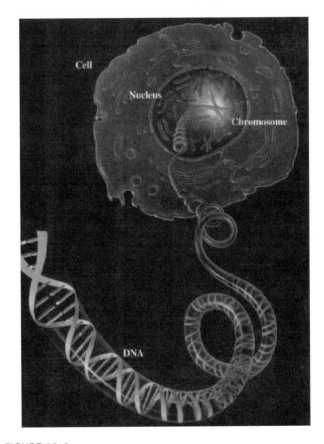

FIGURE **10-1**
DNA structure. Courtesy National Human Genome Research Institute, Bethesda, MD.

nine (A), guanine (G), thymine (T), and cytosine (C). Adenine and guanine are purine bases; thymine and cytosine are pyrimidine bases. These bases are attached to a five-carbon sugar (a pentose arrangement called a ribose), which is connected to a phosphate group. The phosphate groups actually provide the linkage between the individual bases, forming the long strands. The phosphate connections therefore are the actual "backbone" of the DNA strand.

In human beings, DNA does not exist as a single strand; rather, the DNA is double stranded in an antiparallel arrangement. The two strands are not directly physically connected; instead, a number of relatively weak ionic forces hold the two strands in proximity. These ionic forces are different for the two groups of bases, and these differences are responsible for adenine always pairing with thymine (and vice versa) and guanine always pairing with cytosine (and vice versa). Thus the two strands of DNA are lined up together and are composed of interacting bases that form base pairs. Because the bases are specific in their attractions, the two strands of DNA are complementary in terms of their nucleotide sequence. If the sequence of one DNA strand is known, the sequence of the complementary DNA strand can be accurately predicted.

In its native state during the reproductive resting state of the cell (G$_0$), the double-stranded DNA has a loosely coiled helical (double strand) arrangement. At various times in the cell cycle, the DNA becomes more tightly packed together by further coiling at well-regulated intervals around protein substances called histones; this gives the DNA the appearance of beads on a string. The complex of DNA wound around each histone is called a nucleosome. In addition to the histone proteins that come into contact with the DNA at specific points in the strand and at certain times in the cell cycle, nonhistone proteins are associated with the DNA. During cell division, the DNA must become even more tightly packed together to form dense structures called chromosomes. Each chromosome is composed of a relatively large section of DNA containing many genes.

The basic structure of chromosomes is presented in Figure 10-2. Most of the nomenclature currently used to describe specific areas or features of chromosomes is derived from the 1971 Paris Conference of the International Human Genetics Congress.

Chromatids are the two long structures that make up the two longitudinal halves of the chromosome, present during metaphase of cell division. Chromatids on the same chromosome are called sister chromatids. The point at which the two sister chromatids are joined is called the centromere. Many chromosome features are described in relation to the centromere. The portions of the chromatids above the centromere are shorter than those below the centromere and are called the p arms (or "short" arms). The portions of the chromatids below the centromere are called the q arms (or "long" arms). The distal ends of the chromosome are called the *telomeres* or the terminals.

Normally, human beings have 46 chromosomes (23 different pairs) in all cells except mature red blood cells and the mature sex cells (sperm and ova). This number, called the diploid number (2N) of chromosomes for human beings, constitutes the genome, or the complete set of human genes. Of the 23 pairs, 22 pairs are autosomal chromosomes (autosomes), which code for and regulate somatic cell development and function. One pair of chromosomes constitutes the sex chromosomes, which code for and regulate sexual development and function. Mature red blood cells have no nucleus and therefore have no chromosomes. Mature sex cells (gametes) have only 23 chromosomes (half of each pair). This number is known as the haploid number (1N) of chromosomes for human beings.

Genetic Testing

The constitutional chromosomes of an individual can be studied through a process called chromosome analysis (karyotyping), which can be performed only on dividing cells. This process involves obtaining a sample of sterile, living tissue that is capable of relatively rapid cell division. Blood lymphocytes or skin fibroblasts are most often used for this purpose. The tissue is incubated with nutrient fluids at 37° C for several hours to several days to encourage more cells to enter the reproductive cycle and proceed to the mitotic phase. The dividing cells are artificially trapped in the metaphase stage of mitosis, fixed with preservative, placed on microscope slides, stained, and evaluated under the microscope.

Chromosome analysis then is carried out through examination of karyotypes. Microscopic photographs of metaphase chromosomes are made, and from these photographs the chromosomes are karyotyped; that is, grouped in sequences of pairs according to the size of the chromosome pairs and the positions of the centromeres. Each group begins with the largest pair of chromosomes that has the centromeres most centrally located. Subsequent chromosome pairs are ordered according to descending size and more distally located centromeres. Analysis of such a karyotype can determine numeric chromosome aberrations. However, this method of chromosome analysis is haphazard because specific individual chromosomes cannot be identified precisely. There are approximately 1000 genes on each chromosome but only about 100 genes in each band (i.e., the light and dark areas of the chromosome that appear when DNA is examined in a laboratory setting) (Scheuerle, 2001).

A more accurate chromosome analysis is obtained when standard cytogenetic techniques are combined with the process of banding. Giemsa banding (G-banding) is the banding technique most often used for chromosome analysis. In G-banding, the fixed slides are exposed to a proteolytic enzyme

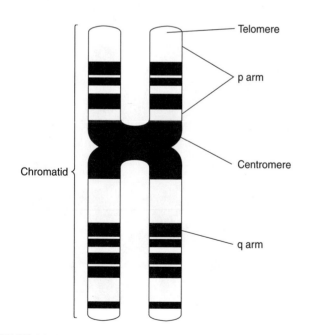

FIGURE **10-2**
Basic structure of chromosomes (Giemsa-banded chromosome 11).

(usually trypsin), which selectively digests areas of the chromosome, and the slide is then stained with Giemsa stain. The areas in which protein has been digested do not take up the stain, which leaves a white space (negative band) on the chromosome. The areas in which protein was not digested do take up the stain, leaving a dark area (positive band) on the chromosome. As a result of this process, each chromosome pair has a unique banded or striped appearance, which permits absolute identification of specific chromosomes (Figure 10-3).

Chromosome analysis that uses banding techniques can identify structural chromosomal abnormalities within individual chromosomes, as well as numeric chromosome abnormalities. However, even this technique has severe limitations, because the smallest chromosome area that can be observed under standard light microscopy has at least 10,000 base pairs. Many genetic disorders are known to involve deletions or rearrangements of genes much smaller than 10,000 base pairs.

Molecular testing is also used to determine if an aberration is present; this technique involves examining the DNA directly. Another form of testing involves examining the gene directly; this test requires a knowledge of which gene alteration results in a specific disease process. A mutation that results in sickle cell anemia, for example, can be detected by this method of analysis, which uses allele-specific oligonucleotide (ASO) techniques (Scheuerle, 2001). The direct mutation technique depends on a knowledge of the sequence of base pairs that is altered in a suspected disease. This technique can detect fragile

X or a breakable area (Scheurerle, 2001). Linkage testing is used when a family member has a known genetic problem and the health professional wants to determine if the condition exists in the infant. The results of linkage testing are not considered diagnostic in the first person affected, but rather only after a second possibly affected family member has been identified. This testing is useful for diseases such as cystic fibrosis and Duchenne muscular dystrophy.

Blood tests for DNA analysis are also used. These have been popularized for paternity issues and for use in criminal cases. The test is considered diagnostic. Protein tests performed on blood examine the structure of the protein. The test helps when a suspected protein structural defect is believed to be involved in the defect or disease. This test would assist in the diagnosis of diseases such as Ehlers-Danlos syndrome, osteogenesis imperfecta, and Marfan syndrome. Each of these conditions is a connective tissue or protein abnormality (Scheurele, 2001).

Biochemical testing is used when a defect in the metabolic enzymes is suspected. Measurement of amino or organic acids results in identification of an abnormality. The technique is considered a screening test, not a diagnostic test, and is followed by direct measurement of the enzymes.

Cellular Division

For human beings, development begins when one haploid egg is fertilized by a single haploid sperm. The result of this union is a single cell containing the entire human genome, 23 pairs of

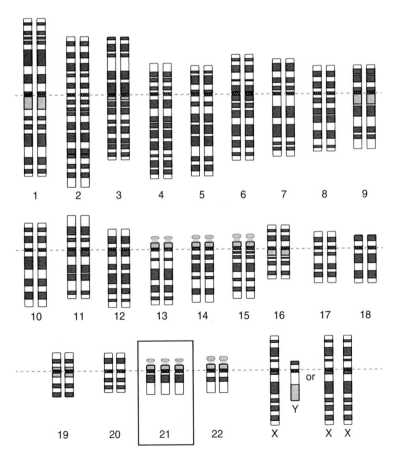

FIGURE **10-3**

Trisomy. One chromosome set (*boxed area*) contains three copies of a chromosome instead of the normal two copies. Courtesy National Human Genome Research Institute, Bethesda, MD.

chromosomes, half of each pair from the maternal gamete (egg or ovum) and half from the paternal gamete (sperm). For the one-celled organism to develop successfully into a complete human being, cell division by duplication is necessary. Duplication divisions occur through the process of mitosis.

Mitosis. Mitosis permits duplication division of one cell to form two daughter cells, which are identical to each other and to the original cell. The complete process of cellular reproduction, including actual mitosis, involves four phases, which collectively are called the cell cycle (Figure 10-4). The primary purpose of the processes involved in mitosis is to ensure that each daughter cell precisely inherits the exact human genome. Although the process of mitosis usually results in an equal division of all cellular structures and contents for the two daughter cells, it is absolutely essential for function that the genetic material inherited by each daughter cell be identical to that of the original cell. The DNA synthesis phase, therefore, is a critical stage of cell division.

The cell cycle is actually a model depicting various activities that cells must accomplish for successful cell division that results in high-fidelity duplication. It is important to remember that the cell cycle refers only to the reproductive cycle of a cell; it does not take into consideration the cell's total life cycle. After development is complete, most cell types do not spend much time in the actual reproductive cycle. Rather, they

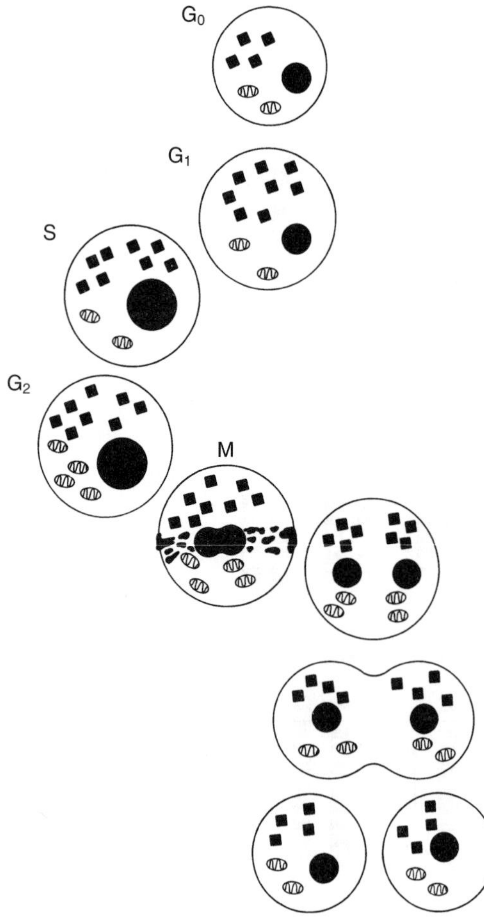

exist as functional cell citizens that are performing all their specific and appropriate duties except reproduction. This non-reproductive state is called G_0. Normal cells leave this state and enter the reproductive cycle only if (1) they are a specific cell type that is capable of cell division (some cells, such as neurons, skeletal muscle cells, and cardiac muscle cells, do not divide after development is complete); and (2) the particular cell type is needed for normal growth or replacement of dead or damaged cells.

G_1 Phase. On entering the G_1 phase of the cell cycle, the cell is committed to divide; this is an irreversible step for normal cells. At this time the cell takes on added nutrients to form energy substances needed for the strenuous processes involved in actual cell division. In addition, the cell increases the fluid and membrane content to accommodate the needs of two cells.

S Phase. For each daughter cell to inherit the proper human genome, the DNA content of the original cell must first duplicate itself. The process of making more DNA to form a new cell is called DNA synthesis (S phase of the cell cycle), and it occurs entirely within the nucleus. The original strands of DNA temporarily loosen from the tight helical arrangement. The loosened strands separate into two single strands so that each single strand can be used as a template for the new DNA (Figure 10-5). A series of enzymes is required for this process.

To achieve duplication the DNA strands relax; the strands unwind from the histones; and the helix straightens out slightly. An additional enzyme enters the straightened area and separates the two strands over a limited area. Another enzyme enters and prevents the two strands from rejoining. A different enzyme attaches itself to one strand, travels down it, "reads" the base sequence of this strand, and forms a new strand of DNA that is complementary to the one being read. This process is called the semiconservative mode of DNA synthesis because it results in two identical double helices, each containing one original strand of DNA and one newly created strand of DNA.

After the strands of DNA have been duplicated (replicated), they pack back down into supercoiled chromosomes and line up so that they are ready to be pulled apart (split) during the M phase of the cell cycle. This splitting permits the two sets of DNA to become part of two new cells instead of just one cell.

G_2 Phase. The G_2 phase of the cell cycle is characterized by intense protein synthesis. The cell synthesizes all the enzymes and other complexes necessary to carry out the actual division of the cell, as well as the proteins needed for the regular "housekeeping" duties of the cell. Increased amounts of various organelles also are synthesized to meet the needs of two future cells.

M Phase. The actual part of the cell cycle in which two new cells are formed from the original cell is called mitosis, and it is the only time when the DNA is organized into chromosomes. This phase is further divided into subphases.

From the time the cell's DNA is duplicated in the S phase through the G_2 phase, the cell's nucleus is said to be in interphase. During interphase the DNA is loosely coiled into nucleosomes and is widely dispersed throughout the nucleus. Only the nucleolus and two centrioles are distinguishable under standard light microscopy. At this time the two centrioles each begin to form a daughter centriole. As the cell leaves the

FIGURE **10-4**
Four phases of cellular reproduction: the cell cycle. The four phases of this cycle include G1, S, G2, and M.

G_2 phase and begins the M phase, the DNA begins to condense. In early prophase, long spaghetti-like strands of newly formed chromosomes are discernible. Throughout prophase, the DNA continues to condense until recognizable chromosomes are present. Later in prophase, the centrioles move to opposite poles of the cell and begin to synthesize spindle fibers. During prometaphase, these spindle fibers attach to the kinetochores of chromosomes on or near the centromeres, and the nuclear membrane begins to disintegrate. During metaphase of mitosis, the chromosomes are at their most compact and most readily visible structural forms. The chromosomes line up in the middle of the cell along the equatorial plane. At this point the cell enters anaphase of mitosis, during which the two sister chromatids of each chromosome are pulled apart toward the pole to which each is attached. This process is called nucleokinesis, indicating that the nucleus has moved and separated into two nuclei within the one cell. Under normal conditions, the chromosomes separate in such a way that the two daughter cells receive genetic components identical to each other and identical to the originating cell. The spindle fibers continue their pulling motion, and the cell begins *cytokinesis*, or the separation of the single cell body into two separate cell bodies, each with one nucleus. Cytokinesis is completed during telophase of mitosis, and at this time the DNA begins to loosen from the compacted chromatids. When the nuclear material is completely dispersed throughout the nucleus with only the centrioles and nucleolus discernible, the two new daughter cells are in interphase.

During early embryonic development, the initial fertilized egg with 46 chromosomes undergoes many duplication divisions, resulting in a large, hollow ball of cells (blastocyte), each with the same amount and organization of genetic material in its nucleus and exactly the same appearance and function. Although individual genes can undergo mutations after conception that result in altered gene expression, the actual genetic fate of this future human being, determined at the time of conception, is irreversible and cannot be changed.

At this point, these early embryonic cells are called undifferentiated because none of these cells has yet taken on the specific appearance (morphologic characteristics) and function or functions of the mature cell type it eventually will become. Obviously, something has to change during the course of development, because normal human infants are not born as large balls of undifferentiated cells.

Between 8 and 10 days after conception, the human embryonic cells initiate the steps that lead to differentiation. In response to an unknown signal or signals, each cell commits itself to a specific maturational outcome. At the time of commitment, the cell has not taken on any differentiated features or functions, but it now positions itself within a group that eventually will take on specific morphologic characteristics and functional behavior. The process of commitment involves turning off specific genes that regulated and directed the early rapid growth and turning on other specific genes that control the expression of particular differentiated functions. The uncommitted, pluripotent cell is referred to as the stem cell. Stem cell transplants are used to treat leukemia and other forms of autoimmune suppression. Stem cell research has sparked considerable controversy over the use of fetal tissue in such experimental situations. Only time will resolve these issues.

It is critical to remember that all differentiated somatic cells (body cells, not including sex cells) retain all the genes in the human genome. At one time the differences in appearance and function between cell types were explained by the theory that different cells actually "lost" the genes it did not need and retained only those it required to reproduce itself and to perform its special functions. We now know that this is not the way differentiation occurs and is maintained. Instead, all cells (excluding the sex cells) retain all genes. However, genes are selectively expressed or repressed in different cell types. For example, the gene for insulin is present in all cells; however, only in the beta cells of the pancreas is the insulin gene expressed, or "turned on," to meet the body's need for insulin production. There is nothing wrong with the insulin genes in other cell types (e.g., in skin cells or skeletal muscle cells); simply put, because the special functions of these other cells do not include the production of insulin, the insulin gene in these cells is maintained in a repressed, or "turned off," state. This turning off of early embryonic genes appears to be accomplished through the activity of special repressor genes that function solely to repress the activity of the early embryonic genes so that they can no longer be freely expressed. This knowledge offers potential for future genetic treatment for many diseases.

Meiosis. The process by which early embryonic cells destined to become mature sex cells achieve maturation is somewhat different from that for somatic cells. Early in development, the committed sex cells continue to undergo mitotic cell

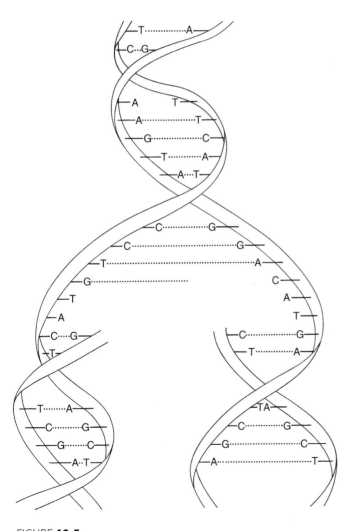

FIGURE **10-5**
DNA synthesis.

division to increase their overall numbers. The cells resulting from these mitotic divisions continue to be diploid. Before the sex cells can completely mature, however, they must reduce their chromosome complement to the haploid rather than the diploid number through meiotic cell division.

Meiosis is the form of cell division that reduces the genetic complement of the cells by half, an actual reduction division that is different from the duplication division of mitosis. The result of meiosis is the production of new daughter cells that are identical to each other (in terms of their autosomes) but different from the originating cell. This process is necessary for gametogenesis, the final formation of sex cells. To accomplish this, the entire process of meiosis involves two completely separate series of cell divisions, one stage of which closely resembles a mitotic cell division. As a result of meiosis, four haploid cells are formed from a single diploid precursor sex cell.

As the precursor gametes (sex cells) prepare to become haploid gametes, each diploid precursor undergoes one round of DNA replication (synthesis), just as mitotic cells do in the S phase of mitosis. At this point in the process, the diploid precursor cell is now tetraploid (4N), with twice the normal number of chromosomes (92).

The cell now enters prophase of the first meiotic division. Each chromosome has two sister chromatids joined only at the centromere. Early in prophase, or meiosis I, the chromosomes condense and coil up, and the homologous pairs of chromosomes form a synapse. During synapse the homologous pairs of chromosomes associate with each other, lying side by side to form a tetrad with four chromatids. Because they are so close and because they are not yet compacted completely, some "crossing over" of genetic material occurs, both from the chromatids on the same chromosome (sister chromatids) and from the chromatids on the homologous pair (nonsister chromatids). Many genes are located on each chromatid. This crossing over of genetic material from nonsister chromatids has the effect of randomly "reshuffling" the maternally and paternally derived genes within the chromatids of homologous pairs, producing a wide variety of new combinations.

All the autosomes undergo this reshuffling process during synapse. The sex chromosomes have only a few limited exchanges at the telomeres. This limitation of exchanges is necessary because the chromatids of the X and Y chromosomes are different, each with unique areas. By not exchanging unique areas, the integrity of the sex chromosomes is maintained. In this way, the species continues with only two genders.

After synapse the two centrioles in the cell move to opposite poles on the nucleus and begin to form spindles. The synaptic pairs of chromosomes further condense and move to the equatorial plane of the nucleus, where metaphase of meiosis I begins; this stage is similar to metaphase in mitosis. The newly created spindles attach to the centromeres of the chromosomes. Contraction of the spindles causes whole chromosomes to be separated from chromosome pairs, but the newly reorganized chromatids of each chromosome remain together (anaphase I). At this point, dysfunction occurs as the chromosomes form dyads or pairs of sister chromosomes, and the cell completes cytokinesis so that two new cells with 46 chromosomes each are formed. However, because of the crossing over that occurred during synapse and because the new chromosomes randomly assort into pairs, the two newly created cells do not contain the identical gene complement of the precursor sex cell that began the process of meiosis. The new combina-

tion of chromosomes cannot be equally separated by maternal and paternal origin. Although the two new cells each contain 22 pairs of autosomes and one pair of sex chromosomes, some of the pairs may be composed wholly of maternally derived chromosomes; others may be composed wholly of paternal chromosomes; and still others may be composed of varying combinations of maternal and paternal genetic material.

These two cells, which contain 46 chromosomes each (two copies of each chromatid), now spend some time in interphase before completing meiosis. The amount of time spent in interphase varies, with secondary oocytes remaining considerably longer in interphase (years) than secondary spermatocytes. No further duplication or synthesis of DNA occurs in these cells.

Meiosis is completed after the second meiotic division. In meiosis II, the two new interphase diploid cells created in meiosis I enter prophase and begin condensing their DNA so that chromatids are formed. The centrioles in each of the two nuclei separate to opposite poles and form spindles that attach to the centromere of each chromosome. The cells now enter metaphase as the nuclear membrane begins to disintegrate.

The chromosomes in each of the two cells move to the equatorial plane and line up. The spindles separate the chromatids. Each pair of chromosomes has four chromatids. When these chromatids separate, one chromatid from each chromosome is segregated to each new daughter cell; each daughter cell therefore receives two chromatids from each pair of chromosomes. However, because the four chromatids segregate independently to the two daughter cells, there is no guarantee that each daughter cell will receive a chromatid from each chromosome of the chromosome pair. It is highly likely that for some chromosome pairs, the daughter cell will inherit two chromatids from one chromosome of a pair and none from the other chromosome.

The result of the entire process of meiosis is the formation of four haploid gamete cells from one diploid precursor sex cell. The crossing over of genetic material from homologous pairs of chromosomes during synapse with random assortment of chromatids in meiosis I, followed by independent segregation of chromatids in meiosis II, has some intriguing consequences. Even though all gametes are descended from the same clone of precursor sex cells and have identical genetic constitutions, the reshuffling of paternal and maternal whole genes and alleles (recessive as well as dominant) can result in hundreds or even thousands of possible minor variations in the genetic makeup of the gametes. Given this range of possibilities, the astounding fact is not that brothers and sisters sometimes do not resemble each other, but rather that they ever do.

PROTEIN SYNTHESIS

All cells that make some protein have in their DNA the code for that protein, the actual gene for that protein. The unique DNA pattern (gene) for that specific protein is first converted into a piece of ribonucleic acid (RNA). RNA is similar to DNA, but instead of containing thymine (T), RNA contains uracil (U).

Proteins are formed by the linkage of individual nitrogen units, called *amino acids*, into a linear strand. There are 22 different amino acids; each has a unique three-base code sequence, called a *codon*, that identifies the DNA and RNA pieces specific for that amino acid. Some amino acids have only one codon, whereas others have as many as four different but closely related codons:

Amino Acid	RNA Codon
Methionine	AUG
Alanine	GCU, GCC
Valine	GUU, GUC, GUA, GUG
Phenylalanine	UUU, UUC

The total number of amino acids in a specific protein and the exact order in which they are connected help determine the nature and activity of the protein. The making of protein, or protein synthesis, is similar to some of the steps in DNA synthesis, although carried out on a smaller scale.

When a cell begins to make a specific protein (e.g., insulin), the cell must loosen the area of DNA that contains the amino acid code (gene) for insulin. The DNA in the region of the gene to be read loosens and unwinds slightly from the histones, using enzymes that are similar to those involved in DNA synthesis. Once the appropriate area of DNA has unwound and the two strands are separated and held open, a special RNA enzyme binds to the gene area of the DNA and reads it. When the enzyme recognizes a "start" signal, it moves along the strand and synthesizes a new strand of RNA complementary to the gene area of the DNA. When the enzyme reaches the end of the gene sequence, a "stop" signal tells the enzyme to stop making new RNA. The newly created RNA strand moves away from the gene. The DNA closes back together and recoils into the normal helical formation. The new piece of RNA is called messenger RNA (mRNA or sometimes just the "message") because it contains the special coded pattern sequence (the message) for building the specific protein (in this case, insulin).

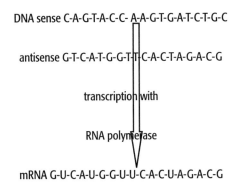

DNA sense C-A-G-T-A-C-C- A-A-G-T-G-A-T-C-T-G-C

antisense G-T-C-A-T-G-G-T-T-C-A-C-T-A-G-A-C-G

transcription with

RNA polymerase

mRNA G-U-C-A-U-G-G-U-U-C-A-C-U-A-G-A-C-G

After the mRNA has been transcribed from the gene areas of the DNA, it moves from the nucleus to the cytoplasm. In an active cell, the message becomes very busy here in conjunction with two other types of RNA. A lot of individual amino acids are present inside the cytoplasm, waiting to be properly lined up and hooked together to form a protein, in a process called translation. Substances called ribosomes, which are made up of special bunches of ribosomal RNA, also are present, along with yet another type of RNA called transfer RNA (tRNA).

Transfer RNAs are adapter molecules that assist in bringing the correct amino acid into the lineup at the proper time. Each tRNA can carry or hold only one amino acid at a time, and the tRNA has an anticodon that is complementary to that specific amino acid's codon. Therefore, because each tRNA can bind to only one of the 22 different amino acids, there must be at least 22 different types of tRNA.

In the cytoplasm, the ribosome attaches to the mRNA strand and begins to move along the strand, reading it as it moves along. When a three-base code is read and interpreted by the ribosome as a specific codon for a specific amino acid, the ribosome allows the tRNAs to come in and attempt to match their anticodons to the codon. When the correct tRNA matches up with the codon on the mRNA, that tRNA releases its amino acid and allows the amino acid to bind to the growing protein strand. This process is repeated all the way down the mRNA until all the correct amino acids are lined up and hooked together in the right order to make the specific protein.

PATTERNS OF INHERITANCE

Gregor Mendel and others established general rules or concepts concerning the inheritance of specific traits governed by single genes before gene composition was determined. Much of the preliminary information was obtained through observation and manipulation of many generations of plant reproduction; however, these concepts also appear generally accurate for the transmission of some human traits.

Mendelian Laws of Gene Expression

Mendel's work explained the concept of dominant and recessive traits. Through his observations of different types of garden peas, Mendel determined that specific varieties of peas had unique traits. For example, one variety of peas always produced wrinkled seeds when fertilized with pollen from the same pea type, whereas another variety of peas always produced smooth seeds when fertilized with pollen from its same pea type. Modeling out this information yielded the following table, in which P_1 indicates the original parent generation; F_1 indicates the first-generation offspring or progeny; F_2 indicates the second-generation offspring or progeny; F_3 indicates the third-generation offspring or progeny; and so forth for succeeding generations. Each generation of progeny was fertilized with pollen from the same generation.

Generation	Smooth Seeds	Wrinkled Seeds
P_1	Smooth × smooth	Wrinkled × wrinkled
	↓	↓
F_1	All smooth seeds	All wrinkled seeds
	↓Self-pollination	↓Self-pollination
F_2	All smooth seeds	All wrinkled seeds
	↓Self-pollination	↓Self-pollination
F_3	All smooth seeds	All wrinkled seeds
	↓Self-pollination	↓Self-pollination
F_4	All smooth seeds	All wrinkled seeds

When Mendel experimented with cross-pollination (cross-breeding) of pea varieties, the inheritance of the traits came out differently than expected. The following model depicts Mendel's results when he fertilized a smooth pea variety with the pollen of a wrinkled pea variety.

P_1	Smooth × wrinkled
F_1	All smooth seeds
	Self-pollination
F_2	Smooth and wrinkled seeds
	(3:1 ratio of smooth to wrinkled)

Mendel's explanation for this observation was that the trait for seed texture was determined by the inheritance of a pair of hereditary elements, now known as gene alleles (an allele is any possible alternative form of a gene), and that the relative "strength" of these two elements varied. This variation in strength resulted in variable expression of the trait when the pair of hereditary elements was mixed (heterogeneous). When both parent seeds had the same hereditary element or genotypes (homogeneous), all the offspring in succeeding generations had the same appearance, or phenotype, of the expression of that element. For homogeneous pairs, the phenotypes and the genotypes were identical. When the parent seeds were heterogeneous for a particular hereditary element, the first-generation offspring expressed only the stronger or dominant element, even though both elements were present in all offspring. In this situation, the phenotype was different from the genotype; that is, the appearance of the peas in the F_1 generation was smooth even though the hereditary elements for texture of these peas consisted of one gene allele for smooth texture and one gene allele for wrinkled texture.

The mixed appearance of the peas in the second self-fertilized generation led Mendel to determine that the hereditary element (gene allele) for smooth texture was dominant and the hereditary element for wrinkled texture was recessive. Dominant traits could be expressed in the phenotype when the genotype for that trait was either homogeneous or heterogeneous, but recessive traits could be expressed in the phenotype only when the genotype for that trait was homogeneous.

Further experimentation with cross-pollination of plants led to the determination of codominance or incomplete dominance. In cross-pollinating red roses with white roses in the parental generation, Mendel predicted that only the dominant color trait would be expressed in the F_1 generation, with both colors being expressed in the F_2 generation (in a 3:1 ratio). Because red was a stronger, bolder color, Mendel expected that the first-generation flowers from this cross-pollination would all be red. Instead, the roses in the first-generation progeny were all pink, indicating that the gene for red and the gene for white were equally dominant. Roses in the second generation of this cross-pollination were red, pink, and white in a 1:2:1 ratio. Therefore in codominance, the phenotype accurately expresses the genotype. Red roses must have two red gene alleles (homogeneous), pink roses must have one red gene allele and one white gene allele (heterogeneous), and white roses must have two white gene alleles (homogeneous).

The mendelian rules for patterns of inheritance apply only to traits or characteristics regulated by a single gene with multiple possible alleles. The relationship between genotypic and phenotypic expression, as well as predictability, can be explained with the use of the Punnett square, in which the known maternal genotype for one or more specific traits is plotted against the known paternal genotype for the same specific trait or traits. The examples in Figure 10-6 use blood type to demonstrate this relationship. The alleles for type O blood are recessive, and the alleles for both type A and type B blood are dominant.

In Figure 10-6, A, the mother is phenotypically and genotypically type O (OO); the father is phenotypically and genotypically type B (BB). The expected genotypes for all first-generation offspring is BO, with the expressed phenotype for all first-generation offspring being type B blood.

In Figure 10-6, B, the mother is phenotypically and genotypically type O (OO), and the father is phenotypically and

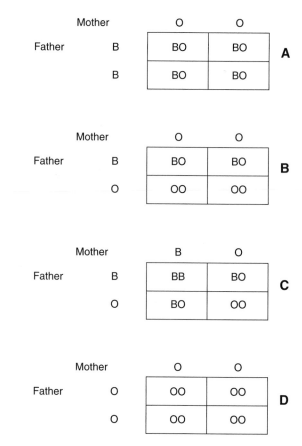

FIGURE **10-6**
Punnett squares of single-gene traits.

genotypically heterozygous (BO). The expected expression and genotypes for the first-generation offspring of this mating would be 50% heterozygous (BO) with a type B phenotype and 50% homozygous (OO) with a type O phenotype.

In Figure 10-6, C, the mother and father are both phenotypically type B and genotypically heterozygous (BO). The expected phenotypes and genotypes for the first-generation offspring of this mating would be type B (25% homozygous [BB] and 50% heterozygous [BO]) and 25% type O (homozygous OO). Therefore two parents expressing type B blood can produce a child with type O blood if they are both genotypically heterozygous for that blood type.

In Figure 10-6, D, the mother and father both express type O blood. Because the alleles for type O blood are recessive, the presumed genotype for this pair is OO, with the expected phenotypes and genotypes in all the first-generation offspring being type O homozygous (OO). According to mendelian patterns of inheritance, it is not possible for parents with a type O phenotype to produce a child with type B blood. However, in rare cases two type O parents have produced a child with blood type B (with absolute parentage established by tissue typing and the presence of identifying polymorphic chromosomes). One explanation for this phenomenon is incomplete penetrance of a dominant trait. In such a situation one of the parents with phenotypically type O blood could have a BO genotype, but the type B blood allele would not have completely penetrated and therefore would not be expressed. Because the B gene was present, it was transmitted to the offspring, in whom penetrance was complete and the gene was expressed.

Patterns of Traits Inherited by Single-Gene Transmission

A single gene, whether dominant or recessive, may control a trait. The locations of some genes have been specifically identified, or mapped, on human chromosomes; the exact locations of many genes have not yet been identified. Even without establishing a gene's chromosomal location, it is possible to determine the way the gene for a specific trait is transmitted. The way in which the trait is expressed through multiple generations of a family reveals specific patterns that indicate whether the gene is dominant, recessive, located on an autosomal chromosome, or located on one of the sex chromosomes. This information can be elucidated without identifying the specific gene through the use of pedigree analysis. Determination of inheritance patterns for a specific trait allows more accurate prediction of the risk that any one individual will transmit that trait or characteristic.

The pedigree is a schematic drawing of a family history, which allows a pictorial representation of patterns of inheritance over many generations. In analyzing a pedigree, the answers to the following specific questions are noted:

1. Is any pattern of inheritance present or does the trait appear sporadic?
2. Is the trait transmitted equally or unequally to males and females?
3. Is the trait present in every generation or does it skip a generation?
4. Do only affected individuals have children affected with the trait or can unaffected individuals also have children who express the trait?

Figure 10-7 shows a variety of typical pedigrees for a number of inherited traits. Construction of a pedigree as part of history taking has a number of advantages:

- It facilitates note taking, increasing the accuracy of the history and serving as a means to organize collected information.
- It serves as a means of communication, allowing information collected by one health team member to be shared with other professionals working with the individual or family so that information is not repeated.
- It provides a means for professionals working with an individual or family to visualize and validate the relationships of affected individuals within a family scope. Creating a visual image of relationships may assist family members in clarifying who is or is not a blood relative of an affected individual.
- It facilitates the emergence of patterns of inheritance for a specific trait in a specific family.
- It enhances analysis of gene expression and transmission of more than one trait through linkage studies.
- It helps to identify individuals at risk within a kinship more accurately (these individuals then can undergo examination or receive counseling).

Construction of a pedigree involves the use of a symbol key (some symbols vary with region, institution, and organization). A typical key for pedigree construction and analysis is presented in Figure 10-8. The pedigree usually is started with the proband (also known as the prepositus), the individual who draws medical (genetic) attention to the family. The proband usually is indicated with an arrow.

The four types of inheritance patterns associated with traits controlled by a single gene are autosomal dominant, autosomal recessive, sex-linked dominant, and sex-linked recessive. Each of these inheritance patterns is defined by specific criteria.

Traits with an Autosomal Dominant Pattern of Inheritance

Autosomal dominant single-gene traits require that the gene controlling the trait be located on an autosomal chromosome, and the trait usually is expressed even when the gene is present on only one chromosome of a chromosome pair. A typical autosomal dominant pattern of inheritance that meets all the defining criteria would be:

1. The trait appears in every generation with no skipping. When the trait is a result of a new mutation (de novo), this criterion is demonstrated only in the branch of the pedigree stemming from the person who first exhibited the new mutation.
2. The risk for affected individuals to have affected children is 50% with each pregnancy.
3. Unaffected individuals do not have affected children; therefore their risk is 0%.
4. The trait is found equally in males and females.

Autosomal dominant patterns of inheritance are associated with many normal variations in body structure, such as brown eye color, widow's peak hairline, and curly hair. In addition, this pattern of inheritance has been demonstrated in a variety of genetically transmitted problems, including achondroplasia, familial hypercholesterolemia, Huntington disease, dentinogenesis imperfecta, brachydactyly, allergic hypersensitivity, Marfan syndrome, and familial hypercalcemia.

Traits with an Autosomal Recessive Pattern of Inheritance

Autosomal recessive single-gene traits require that the gene controlling the trait be located on an autosomal chromosome, and the trait can be expressed only when the gene is present on both chromosomes of a chromosome pair. A typical autosomal recessive pattern of inheritance that meets all the defining criteria would be:

1. The trait appears in alternate generations of any one branch of a kinship.
2. The trait or characteristic usually first appears only in siblings (progeny of unaffected parents) rather than in the parents themselves.
3. Approximately 25% of a kinship is affected and expresses the trait.
4. The children of an affected father and an affected mother are always affected (risk is 100% for each pregnancy). Two affected individuals cannot have an unaffected child.
5. Unaffected individuals who are carriers (have the gene on only one chromosome of a chromosome pair) and do not express the trait themselves can transmit the trait to their offspring if their mate either is also a carrier or is affected. The risk of a carrier having a child who expresses the trait is 25% with each pregnancy when the carrier is married to another carrier, 50% with each pregnancy when the carrier is married to an affected individual, and 0% with each pregnancy when the carrier is married to a noncarrier. The risk of the unaffected carrier having a child who is a carrier for the trait is 50% with each pregnancy.
6. The trait is found equally in males and females.

Autosomal recessive patterns of inheritance are associated with many normal characteristics and variations in body structure and function, such as blue eye color, straight hair, and the Rh-negative blood type. In addition, this pattern of inheritance has been demonstrated in a variety of genetically transmitted conditions, including albinism, sickle cell anemia, cystic fibrosis, phenylketonuria, Tay-Sachs disease, Hurler

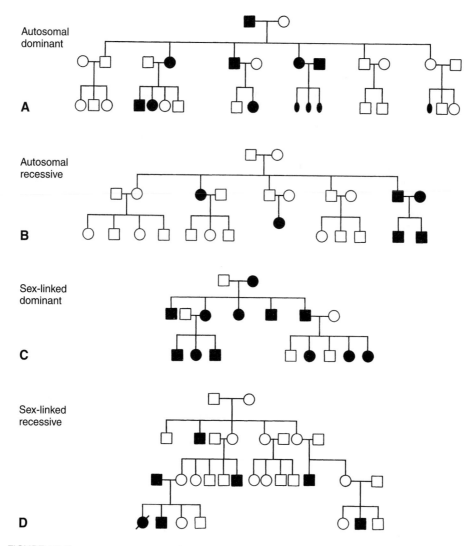

FIGURE **10-7**

A variety of typical pedigrees for a number of inherited traits.

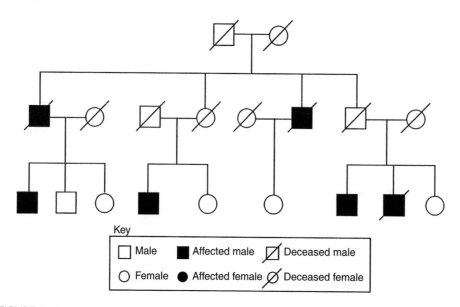

FIGURE **10-8**

Typical key for pedigree construction and analysis. Courtesy National Human Genome Research Institute.

syndrome, Bloom syndrome, Fanconi anemia, galactosemia, and hyperextensible thumb.

For some of these diseases, the carrier has no symptom of the trait, and in other conditions the carrier does not express the full-blown condition but may express a milder form when predisposing environmental or personal events are present. For example, carriers of sickle cell anemia may have some sickling of their red blood cells under conditions of extreme hypoxia, although the sickling is never as severe or widespread as it is in the person who is homozygous for sickle cell anemia.

Sex-Linked Patterns of Inheritance

Some genes are present only on the sex chromosomes. The Y chromosome appears to have few genes that are not also present on the X chromosome. However, the X chromosome has many single genes that do not appear to be present elsewhere in the human genome. For all intents and purposes, then, the discussion of sex-linked patterns of inheritance is really a discussion of X-linked patterns of inheritance.

Because X chromosomes are distributed unequally between males and females (1:2 ratio, respectively), the X-linked chromosome genes likewise are distributed unequally between the two genders. Males have only one X chromosome and are said to be hemizygous for any gene on the X chromosome. As a result, X-linked recessive genes have a dominant expressive pattern of inheritance in males and a recessive expressive pattern in females. This difference in expression occurs because males do not have a second X chromosome to balance the expression of any recessive gene on the first X chromosome.

Dominant Patterns.   For a sex-linked (X-linked) dominant single-gene trait to be expressed, the gene controlling the trait must be located on only one of the X chromosomes. A typical sex-linked dominant pattern of inheritance meets certain criteria that are obvious in the pedigree. The defining criteria are:

1. There is no carrier status; all individuals with the gene are affected.
2. Female children of affected males are all affected (risk is 100%), whereas male children of affected males are unaffected (risk is 0%). Therefore the overall risk of an affected male having affected children is 50% for each pregnancy, since the probability of having a female is also 50%. It is the inheritance of the trait by female offspring of affected males that defines the problem as X-linked dominant, because the inheritance pattern among the offspring of affected females is identical to an autosomal dominant pattern.
3. The trait appears in every generation.
4. For homozygous females, the risk of having an affected child is 100% with each pregnancy, and offspring of both genders are affected equally. For heterozygous females, the risk of having an affected child is 50% with each pregnancy, and children of both genders are equally at risk.
5. In the general population, X-linked dominant problems affect twice as many females as males, but heterozygous females usually express a milder form of the problem than do hemizygous males.

The most common X-linked dominant problem is hypophosphatemia.

Recessive Patterns.   X-linked recessive single-gene traits are among the best-defined inherited health problems. This pattern of inheritance requires that the gene controlling the trait be present on both X chromosomes for the trait to be fully expressed in females (females must be homozygous for the trait) and on only one of the X chromosomes for the trait to be expressed in males (males must be hemizygous). A typical sex-linked recessive pattern of inheritance meets all the following defining criteria:

1. Expression, or incidence, of the trait is much higher among males in a kinship (and in the general population) than among females.
2. The trait cannot be transmitted from father to son because the father contributes only the Y chromosome to his son's sex chromosome pair.
3. Transmission of the trait occurs from father to all daughters (who are all carriers but either do not express any of the trait or express it in a very mild form).
4. Female carriers have a 50% risk (with each pregnancy) of transmitting the gene to their offspring. Female offspring who inherit the trait are carriers, and male offspring who inherit the trait are affected.

Sex-linked recessive inheritance patterns may be responsible for normal variation of some secondary female sex characteristics. This pattern of inheritance also has been associated with a variety of disorders, including hemophilia (A and B), Duchenne muscular dystrophy, ichthyosis, Lesch-Nyhan syndrome, color blindness and, probably, fragile X syndrome. For some of these disorders, females who are heterozygous for the gene express no overt symptoms (such as color blindness). For other disorders, female heterozygotes express some mild aberrations (increased bleeding tendency in carriers of hemophilia, mild retardation in fragile X syndrome). Few females who express homozygosity for these disorders have been found; it may be that homozygosity leads to such a severe disorder that it is lethal in embryonic or early fetal life.

Multifactorial Inheritance

Some single-gene traits have a consistently predictable pattern of gene expression that follows strict mendelian law for patterns of inheritance and degree of expression in affected individuals. Other single-gene traits, especially autosomal dominant traits, have a relatively high degree of variability, with no established reason for the variation of expression. One of the theories proposed to explain this is the concept of evolution. This concept suggests that developmental interactions over time (generations) may modify the response of the individual to an abnormal gene. Another theory is that although a particular trait may be the result of the expression of one gene, other genes may act in concert to regulate the activity and expression of that gene. This theory suggests that for expression of an aberrant gene to cause severe problems, a regulating gene or genes must also have abnormal expression.

In addition to variation in the expression of single genes, a single gene may be responsible for the expression of many effects that appear unrelated. This concept, known as pleiotropy, probably involves changes or aberrations in regulatory genes rather than in structural genes. One example of pleiotropy is Marfan syndrome. This syndrome is transmitted as an autosomal dominant trait, but the expression involves a variety of aberrations in unrelated tissue types. These aberrations include excessive growth of long bones, the presence of or predisposition to development of an aortic aneurysm, and severe nearsightedness.

Some heritable problems are associated with more than one gene. For example, congenital deafness is an outcome associated with a variety of abnormal genes, although not all of the genes have to be abnormal for deafness to result. A possible explanation for this phenomenon is that ear development and hearing involve complex structures and functions that require the input of many genes working in concert for proper development during embryonic and fetal life. An aberration in any one of these genes may result in a failure of one specific aspect of development that leads to overt deafness, although the exact mechanism causing the deafness is different for each gene aberration. Therefore more than one factor can cause the aberrant development. When more than one gene is responsible for a specific characteristic or trait, the trait is controlled through polygenic expression. Cleft palate and neural tube defects are other examples of developing tissues that require polygenic expression for normal development and that can develop abnormally if any of the required genes is not normal.

CHROMOSOMAL ABERRATIONS

As discussed previously, chromosomes are formed during the metaphase of mitosis from tightly packed, supercoiled DNA. Each chromosome contains hundreds of genes; detectable aberrations of any chromosome can result in aberration in the structure or expression of one or more genes.

Numeric Aberrations

The normal diploid number of human chromosomes at metaphase of mitosis is 46; that is, 23 pairs. Some individuals have missing or extra whole chromosomes. This type of aberration usually is the result of abnormal or delayed disjunction (nondisjunction) in gamete formation during meiosis I or meiosis II. Instead of all gametes having 23 chromosomes each, some gametes have 24, some have 22, and some have the normal 23. When a 24-chromosome gamete is united with a 23-chromosome gamete of the opposite sex during fertilization, the resulting new individual has 47 chromosomes. One chromosome set contains three copies of a chromosome instead of the normal two copies; this situation is called a trisomy. When a 22-chromosome gamete from one parent is united with a 23-chromosome gamete of the other parent during fertilization, the resulting new individual has 45 chromosomes. One chromosome set contains only one copy of a chromosome instead of the normal two copies; this is called a monosomy. Whenever the individual has more or fewer chromosomes than normal, some malformations and abnormal developmental processes are expressed. Nondisjunction is most commonly associated with advanced maternal age at the time of conception, presumably as a result of primary oocytes spending years in prophase of meiosis I. Nondisjunction can occur at any age.

In theory, nondisjunction can occur within any chromosome pair. However, examination of the chromosomes of individuals who survive into the fetal period has shown that nondisjunction of some chromosome pairs must lead to embryolethal consequences. The most common chromosomal aberration found among all conceptuses is a missing X chromosome, or Turner syndrome (45,XO). Evidently most conceptuses with a chromosome constitution of 45,XO do not survive beyond the embryonic period. The most common chromosomal aberration observed among newborns is trisomy 21 (Down syndrome) (47,XX or XY, 21). Other syndromes of trisomy that can be observed among newborns are trisomy 13, trisomy 15, trisomy 18, and sex chromosome trisomies (47,XXX; 47,XXY; 47,XYY). Trisomy 16 has been identified in embryonic and

early fetal wastage, but this abnormality does not usually lead to a fully developed individual. Autosomal monosomes may be conceived but rarely survive to the stage of birth, although monosomy 21 has been reported among newborns.

All individuals with autosomal trisomies experience some degree of mental retardation. In addition, each trisomy is associated with a specific set of abnormalities, malformations, and unique developmental patterns. This is why individuals with trisomy may share heritable characteristics with their normal family members (e.g., hair color and texture, skin tone, eye color), but many of their structural features tend to resemble those of unrelated individuals who have the same trisomy.

Individuals with missing or extra whole sex chromosomes tend to be intellectually normal and have fewer recognizable physical malformations compared with individuals with autosomal numeric aberrations. Somewhat controversial is the concept that these individuals have behavioral patterns that are not completely normal, such as attention deficit problems and other learning disorders.

Structural Aberrations

Structural aberrations can occur in one of two ways: (1) parts of chromosomes can break off and either become lost or attach themselves to other chromosomes, an actual translocation of chromosomal material from one chromosome to another; or (2) one whole chromosome can become joined to another whole chromosome, a translocation of chromosomes called robertsonian translocation.

When chromosomes are broken and translocated to other chromosomes, the total amount of chromosomal material may be balanced (normal) or unbalanced (abnormal). If the total amount of chromosomal material present in the individual's cells is balanced, even though it is not located in the usual positions, the individual phenotypically is normal. Problems do not arise until this individual reproduces. Because some of this individual's gametes are not normal (i.e., not balanced) as a result of random assortment and independent segregation of chromatids during gametogenesis, the person is at risk for having chromosomally unbalanced and abnormal offspring. This individual should be referred for genetic counseling. The same situation is true for individuals with robertsonian translocations. As long as the normal amount of chromosomal material is present in all the individual's cells, the individual is phenotypically normal, even though the chromosomes' locations might be abnormal.

PRENATAL TESTING AND SCREENING

For some heritable conditions, prenatal screening is available for determining if a fetus is affected. The issue of prenatal diagnosis is complex. Many of the tests are expensive, carry some degree of risk to the pregnancy, and cannot always provide conclusive results. Tests may be performed directly on fetal cells or indirectly on products synthesized by the fetus, or by imaging. Some tests are even done before implantation.

Preimplantation Genetic Diagnosis

Preimplantation genetic diagnosis (PGD) is used with in vitro fertilization (IVF), oftentimes to determine if the zygote has any readily detectable genetic abnormalities. The cells from the zygote are biopsied and analyzed using a polymerase chain reaction (which consists of a series of events or reactions that occur as a substance moves down the strands of DNA) or fluorescence in situ hybridization (FISH) (see explanation below). The FISH test can detect conditions such as Duchenne muscular dystrophy, cystic fibrosis, and severe combined immunodeficiency (SCID) (Harris and Verp, 2001). More commonly, tests are performed on fetal cells or enzymes.

Fetal Ultrasonography

Fetal ultrasonography involves the use of high-frequency sound waves that are reflected differently in various media and in tissues of different densities. With computer enhancement, ultrasonography can provide a relatively detailed image of the embryo and fetus. Interpretation of the images produced has been refined to such a degree that even minor structural aberrations can be detected. Ultrasonography often is used to locate the placenta, cord, embryo or fetus, amniotic fluid pockets, and other associated structures before more invasive diagnostic procedures are performed. Fetal ultrasonography can provide information about fetal age, the amount of amniotic fluid present, and a variety of structural abnormalities (Hata et al, 1998). Many abnormalities can be identified with fetal ultrasonography, including the following:

- Neural tube defects (spina bifida, encephaloceles, microcephaly, anencephaly, hydrocephaly)
- Skeletal dysplasia (fractures, disproportions, bowing)
- Gastrointestinal anomalies (gastroschisis, atresias, tracheoesophageal fistulas)
- Congenital heart disease (coarctation of the aorta, transposition of the great vessels); echocardiograms can be performed in conjunction with ultrasonography to determine chamber and valvular abnormalities, hypoplastic ventricles, and septal defects
- Genitourinary problems (horseshoe kidneys, polycystic kidneys, exstrophy of the bladder, Potter syndrome or sequence)
- Cystic hygromas

Tests on Fetally Derived Cells

A wide variety of tests can be performed directly on fetal cells. The most common methods of obtaining fetal cells are through amniocentesis and chorionic villus sampling.

Chromosome Analysis by Amniocentesis. Amniocentesis is an invasive procedure in which the amniotic cavity is accessed under sterile conditions through the abdominal wall of the mother. This procedure usually is performed in conjunction with fetal ultrasonography to minimize the risk of puncturing vital fetal structures with the relatively large-bore amniocentesis needle. The ideal gestational age for safe amniocentesis is 16 weeks after conception has occurred. At this time considerable amniotic fluid is present, and the fetus is capable of shedding many viable cells. Once the needle is in place, approximately 20 ml of amniotic fluid is withdrawn. Some viable fetal cells will be present in the fluid. This test sometimes is referred to as midtrimester testing, because it is used from 15 to 20 weeks' gestation.

Early amniocentesis, which is performed before 14 weeks' gestation, also is used. Usually, not enough fetal cells are obtained to ensure an adequate sample size for most tests, therefore the cells are cultivated in tissue culture. The amniotic fluid is centrifuged under sterile conditions, and the dense cells separate from the fluid and migrate to the bottom of the tube. These cells are gently transferred from the tube to tissue culture plates or flasks, and a nutrient medium is added. The cells are incubated for 3 to 10 days. When sufficient mitoses have occurred to increase the original number of cells by at least a factor of 10, most tests for abnormal conditions can be performed. The tests most often performed include chromosome analysis, enzyme analysis, tests for the presence or absence of a specific product, and examination of genes using molecular probes. When sufficient fetal cells are present in the cultures, a substance is added to trap cells in metaphase of mitosis (the stage during which chromosomes are visible). The cells are then harvested and the chromosomes analyzed.

Chromosome Analysis by Chorionic Villus Sampling. Chromosome analysis can also be performed on fetal tissue obtained through chorionic villus sampling (CVS). This technique involves removing a piece of tissue from the growing placenta after its location has been identified through ultrasonography. The needle can be inserted either through the cervical os (more common method) or by transabdominal puncture. This procedure can be performed during the first trimester, as early as 9 to 10 weeks' gestation.

Enzyme Analysis. Some genetic metabolic diseases are caused by a deficiency of a specific enzyme in the fetus. Often these children are normal at birth because maternal enzymes crossed the placenta and performed the specific function in the fetus. However, after birth, maternal enzymes can no longer be used. The pathway affected by the missing or inactive enzyme malfunctions, and the body begins to demonstrate abnormal buildup of products or abnormal metabolism.

Fetal cells cultured for several weeks without the influence of maternal enzymes can express the same metabolic abnormalities that the child would show after birth. Enzyme analysis of the cells or culture fluid (or both) can determine whether a specific enzyme is present at all or whether it is present in normal concentrations. Some genetic metabolic problems that can be identified through enzyme analysis of fetal cells are Tay-Sachs disease, Hurler syndrome, metachromatic leukodystrophy, galactosemia, and homocystinuria.

Alpha-Fetoprotein. Alpha-fetoprotein (AFP) is normally synthesized in measurable quantities only during embryonic and fetal life. In the early embryo, the yolk sac synthesizes AFP; later the fetal liver and gastrointestinal cells assume this function. AFP is present in fetal blood and in some extracellular fluids, and it serves the same function that albumin does in human blood after birth. Because the fetal and maternal circulations are integrated, substances made by the fetus that are small enough move down their concentration gradients into maternal serum. AFP also is present in fetal urine and therefore in amniotic fluid. The synthesis of AFP is well regulated, and the pattern of normal amniotic fluid levels specific to gestational age is known. Variation from this normal pattern is associated with developmental problems.

AFP can be measured in the amniotic fluid (requires amniocentesis) or in maternal serum. The maternal serum alpha-fetoprotein (MSAFP) test is one of the more commonly used prenatal screening tests. The accuracy of both the amniotic fluid and MSAFP measurements requires exact identification of gestational age at the time the fluid or serum is obtained. An AFP value is considered elevated if it is at least twice the mean for that specific gestational age. The most common problem associated with elevated AFP is an open neural tube defect (the open tube provides a means for extra AFP to leak into the amniotic fluid). A lower than normal AFP value also has been associated with fetal developmental problems, although this phenomenon shows more variability. The most common condition consistently associated with low AFP is Down syndrome, although the phenomenon is not consistent enough to be used as the only screening test for Down syndrome. Other conditions associated with low AFP are gestational diabetes and spontaneous abortion.

Multiple Marker Screen.

The multiple marker screen, or triple screen, is more sensitive for aneuploidy than is AFP by itself. This screen can detect changes in the maternal AFP, human chorionic gonadotropin (hCG), and unconjugated estriol (uE_3) (Harris & Verp, 2001). These values are particularly useful in detecting conditions such as trisomies. The same factors that can affect AFP levels, of course, can cause inaccurate results in the multiple screen, including wrongly estimated dates of confinement and multiple gestations (twins). Low levels of AFP, uE_3, and hCG may indicate trisomy 18, whereas a high level of hCG with low levels of AFP and uE_3 are found in Down syndrome.

The multiple marker screen is performed between 15 and 20 weeks' gestation. If an abnormality is found, ultrasonography should be used to confirm the problem. The exact mechanism involved in the alteration of AFP and hCG levels when a chromosomal problem exists is unknown, although it probably relates to a problem with the fetal liver (Harris & Verp, 2001).

Percutaneous Umbilical Blood Sampling.

Percutaneous umbilical blood sampling (PUBS) is another test that can be useful from 18 weeks' gestation. PUBS requires use of ultrasonography to visualize the positioning of the catheter into the umbilical cord. Blood is withdrawn and tested for genetic abnormalities. PUBS is an invasive procedure through which fetal blood can be obtained for karyotyping, but FISH is replacing it in many perinatal centers.

Fluorescence in Situ Hybridization.

FISH uses DNA probes that resemble chromosomal sequences or regions. These probes are fluorescent, and when they bind with areas in or on the chromosome, they are visible when viewed 24 hours later. FISH probes are available for chromosomes 13, 18, 21, and X and Y (Harris & Verp, 2001). The conditions for which they are used include Prader-Willi syndrome and aneuploidy (Harris & Verp, 2001).

Other Molecular or DNA Probes.

In some cases the actual gene associated with a specific problem has been identified, and molecular probes complementary to the gene have been made. These probes can be used to determine whether the gene is present in the fetal cells. Use of molecular probes does not require dividing fetal cells, although a sufficient volume of cells is necessary. In some cases, enough fetal cells can be obtained through amniocentesis or CVS so that the test can be performed directly on the DNA of the tissue. At other times, a greater volume of fetal cells is required, and the fetal cells must be grown in culture before the DNA can be extracted and probed.

Some molecular probes are commercially available, which makes testing more accessible and less costly. Genetic metabolic diseases for which molecular probes are commercially available are cystic fibrosis, hemophilia B, Huntington disease, retinoblastoma, sickle cell anemia, and thalassemia. Molecular probes for other genetic metabolic diseases are not commer-

cially available, and the tests can be performed only in certain university research centers. These genetic metabolic diseases include Duchenne muscular dystrophy, hemophilia A, Lesch-Nyhan syndrome, neurofibromatosis, and phenylketonuria. Table 10-1 presents a list of testing methods currently available for prenatal diagnosis.

NURSE'S ROLE IN GENETICS

Genetics is a complex topic that touches on many aspects of perinatal and neonatal nursing. It involves prenatal screening and diagnosis, assistance with infertility testing and intervention, diagnosis of congenital syndromes and associations and metabolic disease, identification of reproductive hazards in the work place and the surrounding environment both for health professionals and the public, identification of congenital problems that occur secondary to substance abuse, and fetal therapy and surgery and the neonatal implications of such procedures (Jones, 1994; Wright, 1994).

Neonatal nurses must be knowledgeable about the critical periods of development, about prenatal testing procedures, and about long-term neonatal outcomes. Over the past 25 years, advances in genetic knowledge, resulting especially from the findings of the Human Genome Project, coupled with technologic advances, have made prenatal screening and diagnosis available as part of conventional prenatal care. In time it is believed that most of our modern diseases will be linked with a genetic problem.

A positive family history for a disorder, as well as identification of ethnic, racial, or age groups at risk for genetic conditions, may encourage couples to seek prenatal testing. Carrier status screening is available for many disorders, such as cystic fibrosis, hemophilia, and sickle cell and thalassemia trait or disease. There have been 370 disorders identified. A woman who is a carrier of an X-linked disorder has a 50% chance of passing the affected gene to her child; this could have devastating results, such as severe mental retardation in fragile X syndrome or muscular degeneration and death in Duchenne muscular dystrophy.

Through education, the public is becoming more aware of the possible reproductive risks that may be encountered in everyday life. For example, isotretinoin (Accutane), a drug released in 1982 for the treatment of severe acne, is known to cause miscarriages and birth defects if used during pregnancy or within 1 month of becoming pregnant. Anomalies reported to be associated with the use of isotretinoin are hydrocephaly, microcephaly, small and malformed ears, severe congenital heart defects, and cleft palate. The mutagenic effects of the drug occur during the early weeks of pregnancy, frequently before a woman knows she is pregnant.

Reproductive risks are of special concern in teenagers, who often are risk takers and are not knowledgeable about the harmful fetal and neonatal effects of street drugs, tobacco, or alcohol or of huffing (breathing in of substances) during a pregnancy. With the current high rate of teenage pregnancy, this may have a major impact on the future genetic well-being of children in the United States.

The number of alcohol and substance abusers is increasing, as is the number of birth defects. Fetal alcohol syndrome and fetal alcohol effects are growing problems. The incidence of fetal alcohol syndrome and fetal alcohol effects in the United States is estimated at 1 to 3 cases per 1000 births. Frequently

TABLE 10-1	Technologic Advances that Aid Prenatal Diagnosis			
Procedure	**When Performed**	**Method and Accuracy**	**Risk to Mother**	**Risks to Fetus or Embryo**
Ultrasonography	During first or second trimester	Ultrasound waves are emitted by a transducer in pulses; sound waves bounce off structures and return to the transducer. Accuracy depends on the examiner and the nature of the structures (e.g., defect, if one is present).	No physical risks	No known physical risks
Multiple marker screen	15-21 weeks' gestation	Maternal serum sample is screened for AFP, estriol, and hCG. Sensitivity for Down syndrome is 60%; false-positive rate is 6%.	Usual risks of venipuncture	None
Midtrimester amniocentesis	15-20 weeks' gestation	Needle is inserted into uterus to aspirate 20 ml of amniotic fluid. False-positive and false-negative rates are less than 0.5%.	Vaginal bleeding, amniotic fluid leak, infection	Fetal loss rate is 0.5%; other risks are needle puncture and Rh sensitization.
Chorionic villus sampling	10-13 weeks' gestation	Transcervical catheter or transabdominal needle is inserted into the placenta, and tissue is aspirated. Diagnostic success rate is 99.6%.	Vaginal bleeding, infection	Fetal loss rate is 0.5% to 1%.
Early amniocentesis	Before 14 weeks' gestation	Same method and accuracy as midtrimester amniocentesis, but less fluid is aspirated.	Same as midtrimester amniocentesis, with increased risk of amniotic fluid leak	Fetal loss rate is 1.7%; talipes equinovarus risk is 1.2%; culture failure rate is 1.3%.
Percutaneous umbilical blood sampling	18 weeks' gestation to term	Needle is guided by ultrasonography into the umbilical cord, and fetal blood is aspirated. Accuracy approaches 100%.	Fetal-maternal hemorrhage, infection; premature rupture of membranes; labor	Fetal loss rate is 1% to 2%; other risks are fetal bleeding, umbilical cord hematoma, fetal bradycardia, fetal trauma, and placental abruption.
Fetal skin or liver biopsy	17-20 weeks' gestation	Ultrasonography is used to guide biopsy of fetal tissues. Accuracy has not been established.	Bleeding in the uterus, infection, premature rupture of membranes, labor	Fetal loss rate is probably below 5%; scarring is another risk.
Preimplantation genetic testing	Before implantation	IVF is performed, and cells biopsied from the zygote are analyzed before transfer into the uterus. Polar bodies can be analyzed before oocyte insemination. Accuracy is high.	Risks related to IVF procedure	No increase in anomalies, but loss rate in vitro and after transfer is uncertain.
Fetal cells in maternal serum	First trimester; currently investigational	Maternal blood sample are drawn, and fetal cells are separated and analyzed using FISH with chromosome-specific DNA probes.	Usual risks of venipuncture	None

From Harris CM, Verp MS (2001). *Prenatal testing and interventions*. In Mahowald MB et al, editors. Genetics in the clinic: clinical, ethical, and social implications for primary care. *Mosby: St Louis.*
AFP, *Alpha-fetoprotein;* FISH, *fluorescence in situ hybridization;* hCG, *human chorionic gonadotropin;* IVF, *in vitro fertilization.*

the diagnosis is not made until later in life in relation to learning disabilities and developmental delays. Signs of fetal alcohol syndrome may include (1) prenatal or postnatal growth retardation; (2) central nervous system involvement, such as neurologic abnormalities, developmental delays, or intellectual deficits; and (3) dysmorphologic facial features, which may include microcephaly, microphthalmia or short palpebral fissures, poorly developed philtrum, thin upper lip, or flattened maxillary area (Lashley, 1998).

It is estimated that 4 million to 6 million individuals in the United States are regular cocaine users and that 1 in 10 pregnant women uses cocaine (the rate is significantly higher in some urban areas). It is difficult to show a cause and effect relationship between cocaine use in pregnancy and specific birth defects because so many of these women smoke heavily, drink coffee to excess, use a number of drugs, have poor nutritional status, and receive little prenatal care. Cocaine therefore is associated with, rather than marked as the direct cause of, poor maternal, fetal, and neonatal findings. Two cases of anomalies that have been reported in association with cocaine use in pregnancy include severe ocular malformation and Turner syndrome with bilateral foot defects.

The neonatal nurse may be the first health care professional to identify an infant who is a victim of substance abuse. Knowledge in this field may enable a nurse to obtain early interventional care for mother and child and thereby reduce the debilitating effects of substance abuse on the family (see Chapter 39).

The nurse may be involved preconceptually with families who have a history of risky behaviors or with other families who for some unknown reason have had little success at becoming pregnant. The use of assisted reproductive technology for in vitro fertilization is having an impact on the field of genetics as never before. This technology not only has had a significant impact on the achievement of successful pregnancies but also has helped develop techniques that allow health professionals to perform sophisticated prenatal genetic testing. Preconceptual and preimplantation genetic testing offer the opportunity for prenatal diagnosis earlier than can be done with CVS. Gamete analysis is possible through micromanipulation of the oocyte and aspiration of the first polar body after the first meiotic division. If the polar body containing the abnormal gene for a single-gene disorder (e.g., cystic fibrosis) is found in a heterozygous woman, the woman can be assured that the remaining oocyte will carry the normal gene. A preimplant biopsy is performed when the single cell has changed into an eight-cell embryo (approximately 72 hours after conception). This test can detect Y-specific DNA (as in the case of some X-linked disorders) or other genetic disorders. This technique would allow only unaffected embryos to be transferred.

No longer is a specialty in genetics for nurses considered necessary only as a major or option at the master's level; all health professionals at every level of education must have a knowledge of genetics. In 2001 the National Coalition of Health Professional Education in Genetics (NCHPEG) published a list of core competencies, which are considered necessary for all health professionals in all disciplines (Jenkins, 2001). The nursing profession led this movement, recognizing the importance of genetics to all areas of nursing practice.

Neonatal nurses, whether registered nurses or advanced practitioners with more extensive genetic knowledge, are on the cutting edge of the new technology. They also are in the midst of some of the most intense ethical and legal dilemmas facing the nursing profession. For example, fetal therapy and surgery now are possible for a variety of conditions, but these capabilities raise such questions as in which cases should the therapy or surgery be performed and who should decide.

Potentially disabling or lethal conditions now can be treated in utero. For example, fetal surgery is used to correct urinary obstructions that, if allowed to continue, could result in hypoplastic lungs. This treatment generally amounts to fixing an anomaly that occurs secondary to a genetic problem. Gene therapy has gained national recognition as a viable option for fixing defective somatic cells, and stem cells can be injected to treat immune problems such as SCIDS. Other, less successful therapies have been tried for cystic fibrosis. More research is needed in this area (see Chapter 13).

Conditions such as hydrocephaly, obstructive uropathy, congenital diaphragmatic hernia, gastroschisis, and omphalocele have been successfully treated surgically during fetal life.

Certain criteria have been established for fetal surgery, including the following:

1. The surgery must allow elimination of a genetic condition that might be lethal or might complicate in utero treatment.
2. Fetal patients must be carefully selected by a multidisciplinary team involved in the prenatal care and natural history of the fetal defect.
3. The family must make a commitment to involvement in long-term care.
4. The family must understand that the treatment is experimental (see Chapter 13).

Nurses in neonatal intensive care units will have more such patients as fetal therapy and surgery centers spread across the country.

Assessment of the neonatal skin may reveal a genetic problem. A whole area of genetics called genodermatology focuses on genetic skin disorders (Spitz, 1996). Genetic diseases such as Turner syndrome, Marfan syndrome, Sturge-Weber syndrome, epidermolysis bullosa, and phenylketonuria are just a few examples of dysfunctions that have skin or dermatologic manifestations. Although not conclusive, these manifestations give the nurse another "genetic" clue of a complex neonatal problem. Consumers want health professionals to be knowledgeable about the treatment of these conditions and the long-term prognoses for their infants. Families expect nurses to help them prepare for these treatments and to understand the emotions and trauma involved.

The field of genetics puts emphasis on prevention and on reducing the long-term complications associated with a disorder. Prevention includes the "family of the future"; this involves identifying the diagnosis of the proband (the affected individual) and determining the risks to other family members and offspring. The hope is to prevent illness and to avoid complications that might result in chronic illness or hospitalization.

Community-based screening programs can be cost-effective if disorders (e.g., sickle cell disease, Tay-Sachs disease) are detected preconceptually. Infants with neural tube defects may be delivered at a tertiary care center, where immediate care is available, thus reducing cost, preventing injury to the neonate, and allowing treatment to begin immediately after birth.

Where does nursing fit into all of this? A nurse with a subspecialty in genetics may act as a genetic counselor, informing families of their genetic risks, providing information, and giving support during the initial diagnosis and through follow-up. However, the holistic nature of nursing, which takes in the biopsychosocial needs, extends beyond just counseling measures as they often are defined; it includes a broader perspective of care. The six roles of the professional nurse—advocate, practitioner, collaborator, investigator, educator, and leader—are all essential in working with patients and families with genetic and congenital disorders.

Families identified through prenatal testing or at the birth of their child as having a genetic problem are shocked by the news. They experience a grief reaction. Loss of the "perfect child" triggers grief and begins the mourning over the unfulfilled expectations for their fantasy child. The nurse can support the family in assimilating the information given by other disciplines. The grief response can turn into chronic sorrow as grief is prolonged (see Chapter 8). Without psychologic support and intervention, the family's grief eventually may interfere with their ability to carry out their daily responsibilities.

The nurse can help the family recognize the normalcy of such a reaction and can anticipate its occurrence when planning care.

The nurse can also act as an advocate for the family and refer them to community resources such as genetics clinics, family support groups, or specialized home health care services. Access to care is an important aspect of advocacy for these families. They need to mobilize themselves psychologically in order to use these community supports, and such mobilization is difficult when grief has taken away hope and the ability to move forward. Without active intervention and professional support, many of these families will not progress beyond this stage of immobility. Health professionals must recognize this need early in care to be most effective with intervention.

As specialization and technology improve in health care, the professional often appears to the family as an expert who is too busy or too knowledgeable to answer seemingly less important questions or concerns. Can our efficiency and knowledge as practitioners actually become barriers to communication? Owing to our expertise, we are valued as important to care, but if we do not make ourselves accessible to the family or investigate their concerns, many of these concerns or misconceptions are not verbalized. Parents sometimes express the feeling that the physician or genetics counselor is too focused on the person with the disorder to be bothered with their other questions. These feelings are not usually shared with the health professional at the time. The nurse involved in follow-up, especially community-based follow-up, often senses these feelings. Collaboration and a sharing of information are needed if the family is to receive holistic care. The family may need referral to a support group, and referrals for assessment of developmental disabilities will be needed so that early intervention can be started. Use of the nursing process allows identification of the needs of the family that are not addressed by other disciplines.

Positive family histories for certain familial or genetic conditions often are identified through community-based health care. A familial problem can also be identified in an inpatient setting or in any type of care unit. Pedigree analysis can be a useful investigative tool in the prevention or detection of a familial problem. Subtle changes in expressivity of a genetic disorder may be detected if this tool is used to obtain and document a family history. Visual charts are more likely to be looked at than are several written pages. This timesaving technique is especially important in this era of shortened hospital stays and reduced staffing, because less time is spent in actually reading charts. A pedigree analysis might also be the key to more aggressive treatment or follow-up on information that might otherwise not be identified. It may also form the basis of health education and teaching, in which the nurse often is involved.

It should also be evident that the educator and collaborator roles do not stop with the immediate patient population but must extend to the community at large. There is a tremendous need for interpretation of the information the public receives. Not a day goes by without some television or newspaper item relating to genetics. This information must be clarified, and a nurse with a specialized knowledge in genetics can carry out this public education effectively. Other health professionals who lack this specialized knowledge will also need education about recent genetic developments. Outreach education is an important aspect of nursing practice. Nurses as educators and leaders provide role models for mentoring of their peers. They may lead others into formal education in the genetics field and can provide accurate and timely information to nursing and the public.

The neonatal nurse involved in community-based follow-up care has a special need for updated genetic information. Prenatal and newborn screening and early identification of genetic, congenital, or familial problems often occurs in this practice setting. This nurse is also involved in the treatment of the actual disease, such as phenylketonuria or cystic fibrosis, and must help educate the family about the need for complying with treatment and for continuing follow-up care. The nurse should also be aware of community resources, for both the public and the professional, that provide treatment, support, and education for such medical-genetic disorders.

The genetics clinical nurse specialist or the neonatal nurse involved with infants and families experiencing genetic problems must use this knowledge in the area of nursing research. Such research might include epidemiologic studies that follow the natural history of a disease or the environmental factors that may be involved, as well as qualitative studies that describe families' perceptions. Genetic problems are still a part of the Healthy People 2010 objectives (US Department of Health and Human Services, 2001). Educational studies may include a family's knowledge of their specific disease. Evaluative studies may also be conducted to determine the quality of genetics-based nursing services and their impact on families' needs. Evaluation of nursing care based on outcome criteria is essential for determining the need for revision or expansion of this form of care.

Nursing research could have an impact on patients' morbidity and mortality. The development of protocols and standards based on nursing research findings may be instrumental in significantly reducing long-term complications in very-low-birth-weight (VLBW) infants. Developmental supportive environmental studies, the impact of positive parent-infant interaction, and aspects of skin care for this population have all been linked with reduced morbidity in the VLBW group.

Along with the positive aspects of nursing practice and research findings, genetic advances produce ethical dilemmas. Technologic advances frequently precede ethical considerations and decision making. Issues of maternal versus fetal rights arise in cases involving fetal therapy and surgery. Tort liability of wrongful birth and death cases is becoming more common in the judicial system. Fetal abuse cases regarding cocaine ingestion during pregnancy are also occurring more frequently. These ethical and legal considerations only add to the concerns nurses face today, and they may cause burnout related to stress in the work place. The end result may be that fewer nurses will stay in neonatal nursing. Collaboration with other disciplines is essential to keeping abreast of the most current information. There is a critical need for the blending of neonatal nursing with sound genetic knowledge, and this blending may even increase the retention of nurses in the field.

REFERENCES

Conn R, Wright M (2001). Genetic deficiency may explain sudden infant death syndrome. www.eurekalert.org/pub_releases/2001-05/wfub-gdme-3005101.php.

Harris CM, Verp MS (2001). Prenatal testing and interventions. In Mahowald MB et al, editors. *Genetics in the clinics: clinical, ethical, and social implications for primary care.* Mosby: St Louis.

Hata T et al. (1998). Three-dimensional ultrasonographic assessments of fetal development. *Obstetrics and gynecology* 91(2), 218-223.

Jenkins J (2001). *Core competencies in genetics essential for all health care professionals.* National Coalition for Health Professional Education in Genetics (NCHPEG): Rockville, MD.

Jones SL (1994). Assisted reproductive technologies: genetic and nursing implications. *Journal of obstetric, gynecologic and neonatal nursing* 23(6), 492-497.

Lashley FRC (1998). *Clinical genetics in nursing practice*, ed 2. Springer: New York.

National Human Genome Research Institute (NHGRI) (2001). About the human genome project. (http://www.nhgri.nih.gov/policy_and_public_affairs). The Human Genome Research Project: From Maps to Medicine.

Scheuerle AE (2001). Diagnosis of genetic disease. In Mahowald MB et al, editor. *Genetics in the clinics: clinical, ethical, and social implications for primary care*. Mosby: St Louis.

Secretary's Advisory Committee on Genetic Testing (SACGT). (2001). What's new: TGAC [The Genome Action Coalition] Hotline, 2000. http://www.tgac.org/archive/November_15__2000. html.

Spitz JL (1996). *Genodermatoses: a full-color clinical guide to genetic skin disorders*. Williams & Wilkins: Baltimore.

US Department of Health and Human Services (DHHS) (2001). *Healthy people 2010*. DHHS: Washington, DC.

Wright L (1994). Prenatal diagnosis in the 1990s. *Journal of obstetric, gynecologic, and neonatal nursing* 23(6), 506-515.

CHAPTER 11

FETAL DEVELOPMENT: ENVIRONMENTAL INFLUENCES AND CRITICAL PERIODS

JUDY WRIGHT LOTT

In this chapter, the major events of prenatal development are described and critical development periods for the major organ systems are identified. A brief review of the events beginning with fertilization is included, but the reader is referred to an embryology text for a more thorough account. Human genetics is discussed in Chapter 10.

EARLY FETAL DEVELOPMENT

The process of human development begins with the fertilization of an ovum (female gamete) by a spermatocyte (male gamete). The fusion of the ovum and sperm initiates a sequence of events that causes the single-celled zygote to develop into a new human being. During the 38th to 42nd weeks of gestation, dramatic growth and development occur at a pace unequaled during any other period of life.

Fertilization

Approximately 200 million to 500 million sperm are deposited in the posterior fornix of the vagina during ejaculation; large numbers of spermatozoa are necessary to increase the chances for conception, because the spermatozoa must traverse the cervical canal, the uterus, and the uterine (fallopian) tubes to reach the ovum. The ovum usually is fertilized in the ampulla, the widest portion of the uterine tubes, which is located near the ovaries. The tails of the spermatozoa propel them, and this movement is aided by muscular contractions of the uterus.

Spermatozoa undergo two physiologic changes in order to penetrate the corona radiata and the zona pellucida, the barriers around the secondary oocyte. The first change is capacitation, an enzymatic reaction that removes the glycoprotein coating from the spermatozoa and plasma proteins from the seminal fluid. Capacitation generally occurs in the uterus or uterine tubes and takes about 7 hours. The second change, the acrosome reaction, occurs when a capacitated sperm passes through the corona radiata, causing structural changes that result in fusion of the plasma membranes of the sperm and the oocyte. Progesterone released from the follicle at ovulation stimulates the acrosome reaction. Three enzymes are released from the acrosome to facilitate entry of the sperm into the ovum: hyaluronidase allows the sperm to penetrate the corona radiata, and trypsin-like enzymes and zona lysin digest a pathway across the zona pellucida.*

Only about 300 to 500 spermatozoa actually reach the ovum. When a spermatozoon comes into contact with the ovum, the zona pellucida and the plasma membrane fuse, preventing entry by other sperm. After penetration by a single sperm, the oocyte completes the second meiotic cell division, resulting in the haploid number of chromosomes (22,X) and the second polar body. The chromosomes are arranged to form the female pronucleus.*

As the spermatozoon moves close to the female pronucleus, the tail detaches and the nucleus enlarges to form the male pronucleus. The male and female pronuclei fuse, forming a diploid cell called the zygote. The zygote contains 23 autosomes and one sex chromosome from each parent (46,XX or 46,XY). The genetic sex of the new individual is determined at fertilization by the contribution of the father. The male parent (XY) may contribute either an X or a Y chromosome. If the spermatozoon contains an X chromosome, the offspring is female (46,XX). If the spermatozoon receives one Y chromosome, the offspring is male (46,XY). Individual variation is the result of random or independent assortment of the autosomal chromosomes.*

Cleavage

Mitotic cell division occurs after fertilization as the zygote passes down the uterine tube, resulting in the formation of two blastomeres (Figure 11-1). The cells continue to divide, increasing in number but decreasing in size. The term cleavage is used to describe the mitotic cell division of the zygote (Figure 11-2). When the number of cells reaches approximately 16 (usually on the third day), the zygote is called a morula because of its resemblance to a mulberry. The zygote reaches the morula stage about the time it enters the uterus. The morula consists of groups of centrally located cells, called the inner cell mass, and an outer cell layer. At this stage the individual cells are called blastomeres. The outer cell layer forms the trophoblast, from which the placenta develops. The inner cell mass, called the embryoblast, gives rise to the embryo.*

---

*Larsen, 1997; Moore & Persaud, 1998 a and b; Sadler & Langman, 2000; Jirasek et al, 2001.

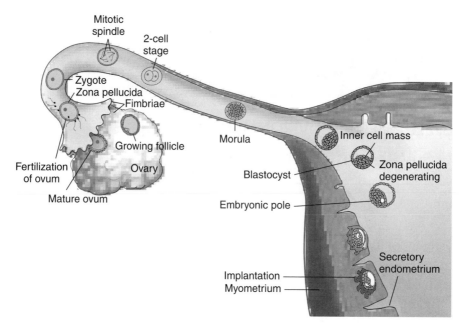

FIGURE **11-1**

Fantastic voyage: from fertilization to implantation. The journey through the fallopian tubes takes approximately 4 days. During this time, mitotic cell division occurs. Implantation occurs on about day 9 through day 12.

After the morula penetrates the uterine cavity, fluid enters through the zona pellucida into the intercellular spaces of the inner cell mass. About the fourth day after fertilization, the fluid-filled spaces fuse, forming a large cavity known as the blastocyst cavity. The morula is now called the blastocyst. The trophoblast forms the wall of the blastocyst, and the embryoblast projects from the wall of the blastocyst into the blastocyst cavity. The uterine secretions nourish the blastocyst until implantation occurs.*

Implantation

The zona pellucida degenerates on about the fifth day after fertilization, allowing the blastocyst to attach to the endothelium of the endometrium on about the sixth day. The trophoblasts then secrete proteolytic enzymes that destroy the endometrial endothelium and invade the endometrium. Two layers of trophoblasts develop; the inner layer is made up of cytotrophoblasts, and the outer layer is composed of syncytiotrophoblasts. The syncytiotrophoblast has fingerlike projections that produce enzymes capable of further eroding the endometrial tissues. By the end of the seventh day, the blastocyst is superficially implanted (Figure 11-3).*

Formation of the Bilaminar Disk

Implantation is completed during the second week. The syncytiotrophoblast continues to invade the endometrium and becomes embedded. Spaces in the syncytiotrophoblast, called lacunae, fill with blood from ruptured maternal capillaries and secretions from eroded endometrial glands. This fluid nourishes the embryoblast by diffusion. The lacunae give rise to the uteroplacental circulation. The lacunae fuse to form a network

that then becomes the intervillous spaces of the placenta. The endometrial capillaries near the implanted embryoblast become dilated and eroded by the syncytiotrophoblast. Maternal blood enters the lacunar network and provides circulation and nutrients to the embryo. The maternal-embryonic blood circulation provides the developing embryo with nutrition and oxygenation and removes waste products before the development of the placenta. Fingerlike projections of the chorion, the primary chorionic villi, develop into the chorionic villi of the placenta at about the same time.*

The inner cell mass differentiates into two layers: the hypoblast, or endoderm, a layer of small cuboidal cells, and the epiblast, or ectoderm, a layer of high columnar cells. The two layers form a flattened, circular bilaminar embryonic disk. The amniotic cavity is derived from spaces within the epiblast. As the amniotic cavity enlarges, it is covered by a thin layer of epithelial cells. During the development of the amniotic cavity, other trophoblastic cells form a thin extracoelomic membrane, which encloses the primitive yolk sac. The yolk sac produces fetal red blood cells. Other trophoblastic cells form a layer of mesenchymal tissue, called the extraembryonic mesoderm, around the amnion and primitive yolk sac. Isolated coelomic spaces in the extraembryonic mesoderm fuse to form a single, large, fluid-filled cavity surrounding the amnion and yolk sac, with the exception of the area where the amnion is attached to the chorion by the connecting stalk. The primitive yolk sac diminishes in size, creating a smaller secondary yolk sac.*

Two layers of extraembryonic mesoderm result from the formation of the extraembryonic cavity. The extraembryonic somatic mesoderm lines the trophoblast and covers the amnion, and the extraembryonic splanchnic mesoderm covers the yolk sac. The chorion is made up of the extraembryonic somatic mesoderm, the cytotrophoblast, and the syncytiotrophoblast. The chorion forms the chorionic sac, in which the embryo and the amniotic and yolk sacs are located. By the end of the

---

*Larsen, 1997; Moore & Persaud, 1998 a and b; Sadler & Langman, 2000; Jirasek et al, 2001.

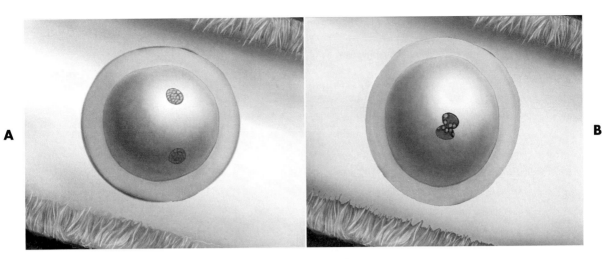

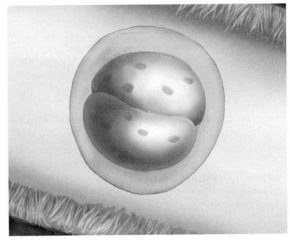

FIGURE **11-2**
Cleavage stage of cell division. **A,** Zygote. **B,** Zygote undergoing first cleavage. **C,** Two-cell blastomere state.

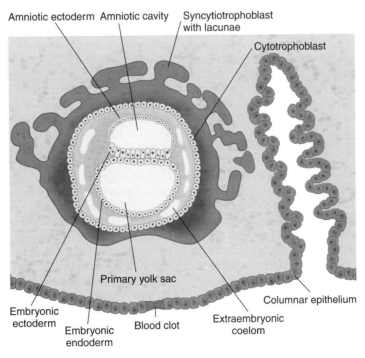

FIGURE **11-3**
Cross section of a blastocyst at 11 days. Two germ layers are present. The trophoblast has differentiated into the syncytiotrophoblast and the cytotrophoblast.

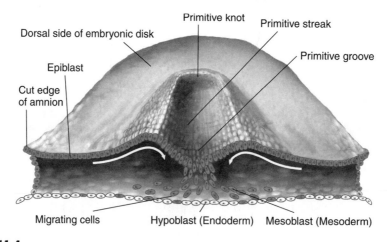

FIGURE **11-4**

Formation of the trilaminar embryonic disk: gastrulation. During gastrulation, the bilaminar embryonic disk becomes a trilaminar embryonic disk consisting of the epiblast (ectoderm), the hypoblast (endoderm), and the mesoblast (mesoderm). Redrawn from Moore KL, Persaud TVN (1998). *Before we are born: essentials of embryology and birth defects*, ed 5. Philadelphia: WB Saunders.

second week, a slightly thickened area has formed near the cephalic region of the hypoblastic disk; this area, known as the prochordal plate, marks the location of the mouth.

Formation of the Trilaminar Embryonic Disk: Week 3

The third week of development is marked by rapid growth, the formation of the primitive streak, and the differentiation of the three germ layers, from which all fetal tissue and organs are derived (Figure 11-4).*

Gastrulation.   Gastrulation is the process through which the bilaminar disk develops into a trilaminar embryonic disk. Gastrulation is the most important event of early fetal formation; it affects all the rest of embryologic development. During the third week, epiblast cells separate from their original location and migrate inward, forming the mesoblast, which spreads cranially and laterally to form a layer between the ectoderm and the endoderm called the intraembryonic mesoderm. Other mesoblastic cells invade the endoderm, displacing the endodermal cells laterally and forming a new layer, the embryonic ectoderm. The hypoblastic ectoderm therefore produces the embryonic ectoderm, the embryonic mesoderm, and most of the embryonic endoderm. These three germ layers are the source of the tissue and organs of the embryo.*

Primitive Streak.   Over days 14 to 15, a groove and thickening of the ectoderm (epiblast), called the primitive streak, appears caudally in the center of the dorsum of the embryonic disk. The primitive streak results from the migration of ectodermal cells toward the midline in the posterior portion of the embryonic disk. The primitive groove develops in the primitive streak. When the primitive streak begins to produce mesoblastic cells that become intraembryonic mesoderm, the epiblast is referred to as the embryonic ectoderm and the hypoblast is referred to as the embryonic mesoderm.*

Notochordal Process.   Cells from the primitive knot migrate cranially and form the midline cellular notochordal process. This process grows cranially between the ectoderm and the endoderm until it reaches the prochordal plate, which is attached to the overlying ectoderm, thus forming the oropharyngeal membrane. The cloacal membrane, caudal to the primitive streak, develops into the anus.

The primitive streak produces mesenchyme (mesoblasts) until the end of the fourth week. The primitive streak does not grow as rapidly as the other cells, making it relatively insignificant in size compared with the other structures that continue to grow. Persistence of the primitive streak or remnants of it are the cause of sacrococcygeal teratomas.*

The notochord is a cellular rod that develops from the notochordal process; it is the structure around which the vertebral column is formed. The notochord forms the nucleus pulposus of the intervertebral bodies of the spinal column (Figure 11-5).*

Neurulation.   Neurulation is the process through which the neural plate, neural folds, and neural tube are formed. The developing notochord stimulates the embryonic ectoderm to thicken, forming the neural plate. The neuroectoderm of the neural plate gives rise to the central nervous system. The neural plate develops cranial to the primitive knot. As the neural plate elongates, the neural plate gets wider and extends cranially to the oropharyngeal membrane. The neural plate invaginates along the central axis to form a neural groove with neural folds on each side. The neural folds move together and fuse, forming the neural tube (Figure 11-6). The neural tube detaches from the surface ectoderm, and the free edges of the ectoderm fuse, covering the posterior portion of the embryo. With formation of the neural tube, nearby ectodermal cells lying along the crest of each neural fold migrate inward, invading the mesoblast on each side of the neural tube. These irregular, flattened masses are called the neural crest. This structure's cells give rise to the spinal ganglia, the ganglia of the autonomic nervous system, and a portion of the cranial nerves. Neural crest cells also form the meningeal covering of the brain and spinal cord and the sheaves that protect nerves. Neural crest cells contribute to the

*Larsen, 1997; Moore & Persaud, 1998 a and b; Sadler & Langman, 2000; Jirasek et al, 2001.

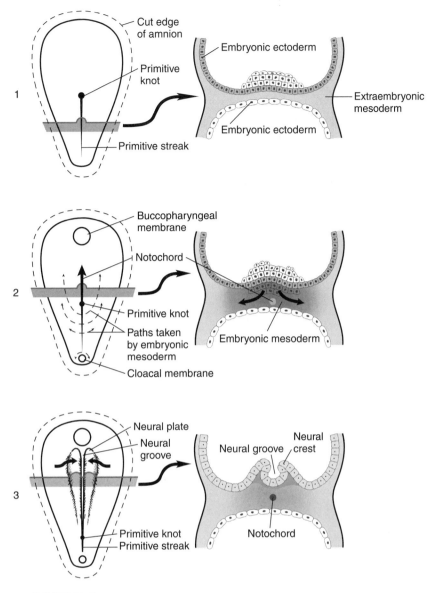

FIGURE **11-5**
Formation of the primitive streak, primitive knot, notochord, and neural groove.

formation of pigment-producing cells and the adrenal medulla, and to skeletal and muscular development in the head.*

Development of Somites.   Another important event of the third week is the development of somites, which give rise to most of the skeleton and associated musculature and much of the dermis of the skin. During formation of the neural tube, the intraembryonic mesoderm on each side thickens, forming longitudinal columns of paraxial mesoderm. At about 20 days, the paraxial mesoderm begins to divide into paired cuboidal bodies known as somites. In all, 42 to 44 somites develop, in a craniocaudal sequence, although only 38 develop during the "somite period." These somite pairs can be counted, and they can provide an estimate of fetal age before a crown-rump measurement is possible.*

Intraembryonic Cavity.   Another significant process is the formation of the intraembryonic cavity. This structure first appears as a number of small spaces within the lateral mesoderm and the cardiogenic mesoderm. These spaces combine to form the intraembryonic cavity; it is horseshoe shaped and lined with flattened epithelial cells that eventually line the peritoneal cavity. The intraembryonic cavity divides the lateral mesoderm into the parietal (somatic) and visceral (splanchnic) layers. It gives rise to the pericardial cavity, the pleural cavity, and the peritoneal cavity.*

PLACENTAL DEVELOPMENT AND FUNCTION

The rudimentary maternal-fetal circulation is intact by the fourth week of gestation. Growth of the trophoblast results in numerous primary and secondary chorionic villi, which cover the surface of the chorionic sac until about the eighth week of gestation. At about the eighth week, the villi overlying the conceptus (decidua capsularis) degenerate, leaving a smooth

*Larsen, 1997; Moore & Persaud, 1998 a and b; Sadler & Langman, 2000; Jirasek et al, 2001.

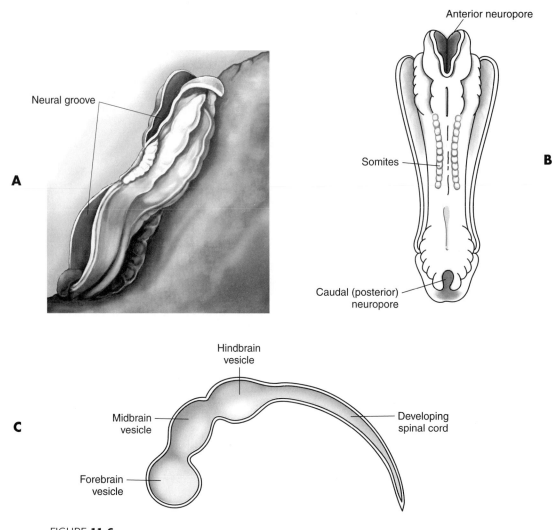

FIGURE **11-6**
Formation of the neural tube. **A,** Neural groove. **B,** Closure of the neural tube is almost complete.
C, Dilation of the neural tube forms the forebrain, midbrain, and hindbrain.

area (smooth chorion). The villi underlying the conceptus (decidua basalis) remain and increase in size, producing the chorion frondosum, or fetal side of the placenta. The maternal side of the placenta is made up of the chorion and the chorionic villi. Upon implantation of the conceptus, maternal capillaries of the decidua basalis rupture, causing maternal blood to circulate through the developing fetal placenta (chorion frondosum). As growth and differentiation progress, extensions from the cytotrophoblast invade the syncytial layer and form a cytotrophoblastic shell, surrounding the conceptus and chorionic villi. This shell is continuous but has communications between maternal blood vessels in the decidua basalis and the intervillous spaces of the chorion frondosum. The latter is attached to the maternal side of the placenta (decidua basalis) by the cytotrophoblastic shell and anchoring villi. The placenta is mature and completely functional by 16 weeks of development (Figure 11-7). If the corpus luteum begins to regress before the sixteenth week and fails to produce enough progesterone (the hormone responsible for readying the uterine cavity for the pregnancy), the pregnancy is aborted because the placenta is not capable of supporting the pregnancy on its own until about this time.*

Placental-Fetal Circulation

A simple ebb and flow circulation is present in the embryo, yolk sac, connecting stalk, and chorion by 21 days' gestation. By 28 days, unidirectional circulation has been established. Deoxygenated fetal blood leaves the fetus via the umbilical arteries and enters the capillaries in the chorionic villi, where gaseous and nutrient exchange takes place. Oxygenated blood returns to the fetus through the umbilical veins. At first there are two arteries and two veins, but one vein gradually degenerates, leaving two arteries and one vein. If only one artery is present, a congenital anomaly, especially a renal one, should be suspected.*

Placental Function

Normal growth and development of the embryo depend on adequate placental function. The placenta is responsible for oxygenation, nutrition, elimination of wastes, production of hormones essential for maintenance of the pregnancy, and transport of substances. In addition, the placenta synthesizes

*Larsen, 1997; Moore & Persaud, 1998 a and b; Sadler & Langman, 2000; Jirasek et al, 2001.

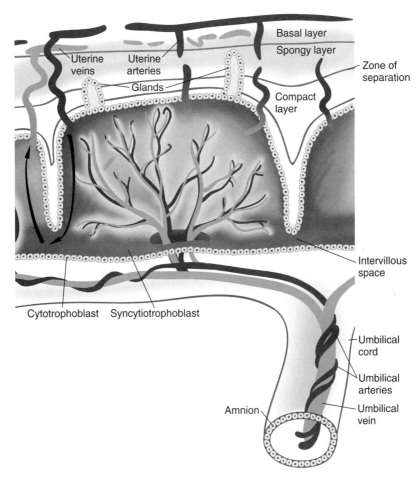

FIGURE **11-7**
Formation of the placenta, showing the fetal and maternal sides. The placenta separates from the uterus at the site indicated by the black line, which marks the zone of separation.

glycogen, cholesterol, and fatty acids, which provide nutrients and energy for early fetal development. Transport across the placental membrane occurs primarily through simple and facilitated diffusion, active transport, and pinocytosis. Oxygen, carbon dioxide, and carbon monoxide cross the placenta through simple diffusion. The fetus is dependent on a continuous supply of oxygenated blood flowing from the placenta.*

Water and electrolytes cross the placenta freely in both directions. Glucose is converted to glycogen in the placenta as a carbohydrate source for the fetus. Amino acids move readily across the placental membranes for protein synthesis in the fetus. Free fatty acids are transferred across the placenta by pinocytosis. There is limited or no transfer of maternal cholesterol, triglycerides, and phospholipids. Water- and fat-soluble vitamins cross the placenta and are essential for normal development (Moore & Persaud, 1998a, b).

The placenta produces and transports hormones that maintain the pregnancy and promote growth and development of the fetus. Chorionic gonadotropin, a protein hormone produced by the syncytiotrophoblast, is excreted in maternal serum and urine. The presence of human chorionic gonadotropin is used as a test for pregnancy. Human placental lactogen, also a protein hormone produced by the placenta, acts as a fetal growth-promoting hormone by giving the fetus priority for receiving maternal glucose.*

The placenta also produces steroid hormones. Progesterone, produced by the placenta throughout gestation, is responsible for maintaining the pregnancy. Estrogen production by the placenta depends on stimulation by the fetal adrenal cortex and liver. Placental transport of maternal antibodies provides the fetus with passive immunity to certain viruses. IgG antibodies are actively transported across the placental barrier, providing humoral immunity for the fetus. IgA and IgM antibodies do not cross the placental barrier, placing the neonate at risk for neonatal sepsis. However, failure of IgM antibodies to cross the placental membrane explains the lower incidence of a severe hemolytic process in ABO blood type incompatibilities compared with Rh incompatibilities. The latter result when an Rh-negative mother has an Rh-positive fetus. If the mother is sensitized to the Rh-positive fetal blood cells, the mother produces IgG antibodies. IgG is transferred from the maternal to the fetal circulation, and hemolysis of fetal red blood cells occurs.*

The placenta is selective in allowing the transfer of substances; however, this selectivity does not screen out all potentially harmful substances. Viral, bacterial, and protozoal

*Larsen, 1997; Moore & Persaud, 1998 a and b; Sadler & Langman, 2000; Jirasek et al, 2001.

BOX 11-1

Germ Cell Derivatives

Ectoderm
Central nervous system (brain, spinal cord)
Peripheral nervous system
Sensory epithelia of eye, ear, and nose
Epidermis and its appendages (hair and nails)
Mammary glands
Subcutaneous glands
Tooth enamel
Neural crest cells
Spinal, cranial, and autonomic ganglia cells
Nerve sheaths of peripheral nervous system
Pigment cells
Muscle, connective tissue, and bone of branchial arch origin
Adrenal medulla
Meninges

Mesoderm
Cartilage
Bone
Connective tissue
Striated and smooth muscle
Heart, blood, and lymph vessels and cells
Gonads
Genital ducts
Pericardial, pleural, and peritoneal lining
Spleen
Cortex of adrenal gland

Endoderm
Epithelial lining of respiratory and gastrointestinal tracts
Parenchyma of tonsils, thyroid, parathyroid, liver, thymus, and pancreas
Epithelial lining of bladder and urethra
Epithelial lining of tympanic cavity, tympanic antrum, and auditory tube

---

organisms can be transferred to the fetus through the placenta. Toxic substances such as drugs and alcohol can also be transferred to the fetus. The effects of these substances depend on the stage of gestation and the type and duration of exposure, as well as the interaction of these and other factors, such as nutrition.

EMBRYONIC PERIOD: WEEKS 4 THROUGH 8

The embryonic period lasts from the beginning of gestational week 4 through the end of week 8. All major organ systems are formed during this period. The embryo changes in shape as the organs develop, taking a more human shape by the end of the eighth week. The major events of the embryonic period are the folding of the embryo and organogenesis (Figure 11-8).

Folding of the Embryo

In the trilaminar embryonic disk, the growth rate of the central region exceeds that of the periphery such that the slower growing areas fold under the faster growing areas, forming body folds. The head fold appears first, as a result of craniocaudal

elongation of the notochord and growth of the brain, which projects into the amniotic cavity. The folding downward of the cranial end of the embryo forces the septum transversum (primitive heart), the pericardial cavity, and the oropharyngeal membrane to turn under onto the ventral surface. After the embryo has folded, the mass of mesoderm cranial to the pericardial cavity, the septum transversum, lies caudal to the heart. The septum transversum later develops into a portion of the diaphragm. Part of the yolk sac is incorporated as the foregut, lying between the heart and the brain. The foregut ends blindly at the oropharyngeal membrane, which separates the foregut from the primitive mouth cavity (stomodeum).*

The tail fold occurs after the head fold as a result of craniocaudal growth progression. Growth of the embryo causes the caudal area to project over the cloacal membrane. During the tail folding, part of the yolk sac is incorporated into the embryo as the hindgut. After completion of the head and tail folding, the connecting stalk is attached to the ventral surface of the embryo, forming the umbilical cord. Folding also occurs laterally, producing right and left lateral folds. The lateral body wall on each side folds toward the median plane, causing the embryo to assume a cylindric shape. During the lateral body folding, a portion of the yolk sac is incorporated as the midgut. The attachment of the midgut to the yolk sac is minimal after this fold develops. After folding, the amnion is attached to the embryo in a narrow area where the umbilical cord attaches to the ventral surface.*

Organogenesis: Germ Cell Derivatives

The three germ cell layers (ectoderm, mesoderm, and endoderm) give rise to all tissues and organs of the embryo (the main germ cell derivatives are listed in Box 11-1). The germ cells follow specific patterns during the process of organogenesis, and the development of each major organ system is discussed separately. The embryonic period is the most critical period of development because it encompasses the formation of internal and external structures. The critical periods of development for the organs are also discussed in the section on specific organ development.

FETAL PERIOD: WEEK 9 THROUGH BIRTH

The fetal period begins at the start of the ninth week of gestation and extends through the rest of the pregnancy. It is characterized by further growth and development of the fetus and of the organs formed during the embryonic period. Other changes that occur include the appearance of vernix caseosa, lanugo, and scalp hair. The eyelids open at about 24 to 26 weeks' gestation. The fetus has the potential for survival at approximately 24 weeks, but the preterm newborn experiences many difficult physiologic adjustments for intact survival. Closer to term, subcutaneous fat is deposited, giving the skin a smooth, firm, plump appearance and texture. The last part of the fetal period provides preparation for transition to the extrauterine environment.*

The fetus is at less risk for structural defects caused by teratogenic factors than the embryo; however, the risk still exists for functional impairment of existing structures.

Text continued on p. 163

---

*Larsen, 1997; Moore & Persaud, 1998 a and b; Sadler & Langman, 2000; Jirasek et al, 2001.

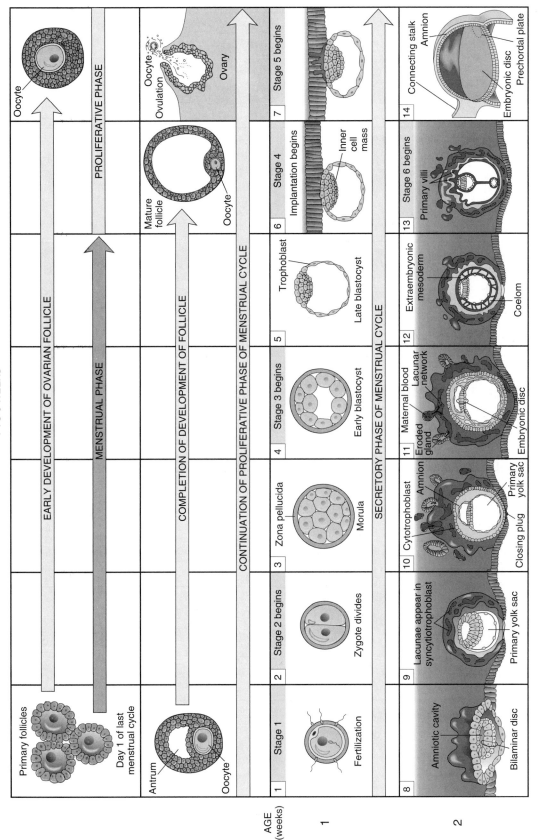

FIGURE **11-8**
Critical periods of development. From Moore KL, Persaud TVN (1998). *Before we are born: essentials of embryology and birth defects*, ed 5. WB Saunders: Philadelphia.

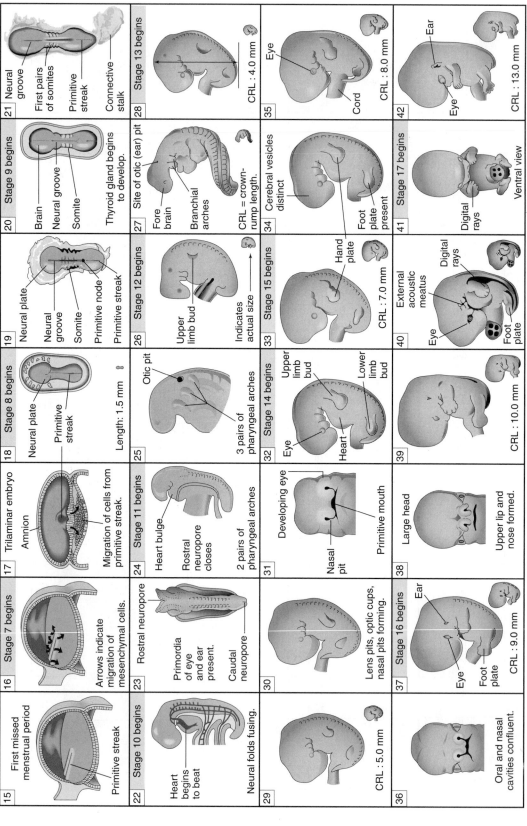

FIGURE **11-8, cont'd**
For legend see page 159.

TIMETABLE OF HUMAN PRENATAL DEVELOPMENT
7 to 38 weeks

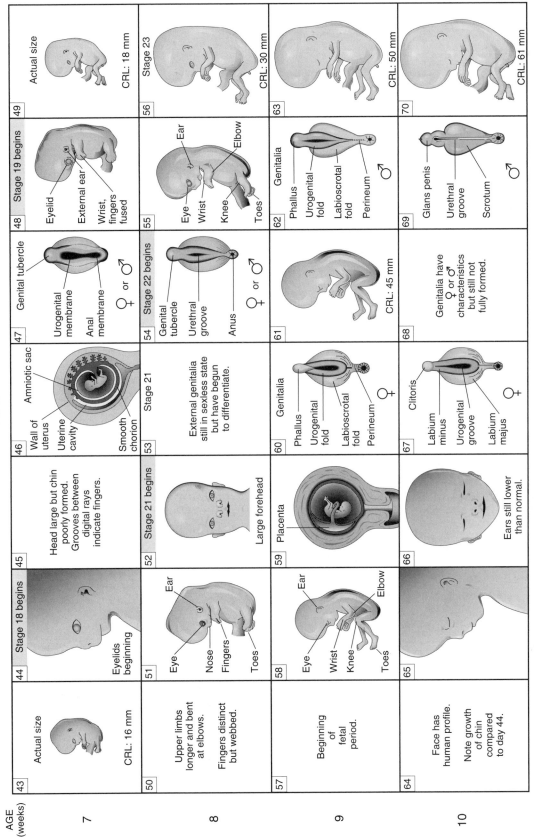

FIGURE **11-8, cont'd**
For legend see page 159.

Eleventh Week to Full Term

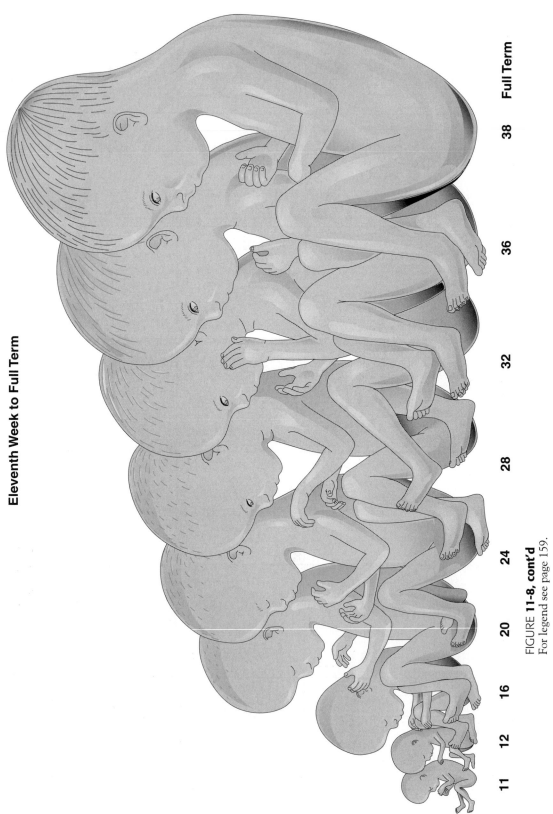

11   12   16   20   24   28   32   36   38   Full Term

FIGURE **11-8, cont'd**
For legend see page 159.

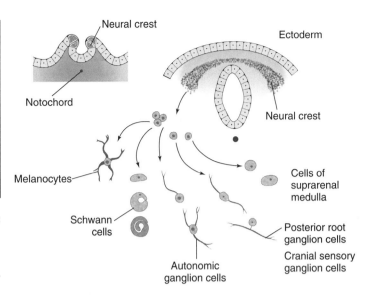

FIGURE **11-9**

Differentiation of the nervous system. The cells of the neural crest differentiate into cells of the ganglia, Schwann cells, cells of the suprarenal medulla, and melanocytes.

BOX **11-2**

Three Periods of Fetal Development

Preembryonic period (weeks 1 through 3): Extends from fertilization of the ovum to formation of the embryonic disk with three germ layers.
Embryonic period (weeks 4 through 8): Period of rapid growth and differentiation; formation of major organ systems.
Fetal period (weeks 9 to 40 [term]): Continued growth and development of organ systems.

Data from Moore KL, Persaud TVN (1998). The developing human: clinically oriented embryology, ed 6. WB Saunders: Philadelphia.

Box 11-2 presents a summary of the important stages of prenatal development.

DEVELOPMENT OF SPECIFIC ORGANS AND STRUCTURES

Nervous System

The nervous system originates in the neural plate, which arises as a thickening of the ectodermal tissue about the middle of the third week of gestation. The neural plate further differentiates into the neural tube and the neural crest. The neural tube gives rise to the central nervous system, and the neural crest cells give rise to the peripheral nervous system (Figure 11-9). The cranial end of the neural tube forms the three divisions of the brain: the forebrain, the midbrain, and the hindbrain. The cerebral hemispheres and the diencephalon arise from the forebrain; the pons, cerebellum, and medulla oblongata arise from the hindbrain. The midbrain makes up the adult midbrain.*

The cavity of the neural tube develops into the ventricles of the brain and the central canal of the spinal column. The neuroepithelial cells lining the neural tube give rise to nerves and glial cells of the central nervous system. The peripheral nervous system consists of the cranial, spinal, and visceral nerves and the ganglia. The somatic and visceral sensory cells of the peripheral nervous system arise from neural crest cells. Cells that form the myelin sheaths of the axons, called Schwann cells, also arise from the neural crest cells.*

Cardiovascular System

The fetal cardiac system appears at about 18 to 19 days' gestation, and circulation is present by about 21 days. The cardiovascular system is the first organ system to function in utero. The heart and blood develop from the middle layer (mesoderm) of the trilaminar embryonic disk. Tissue from the lateral mesoderm migrates up the sides of the embryonic disk, forming a horseshoe-shaped structure that arches and meets above the oropharyngeal membrane. With further development, paired heart tubes form, which then fuse into a single heart tube (Figure 11-10). The vessels that make up the vascular system throughout the body develop from mesodermal cells that connect to each other, with the developing heart tube and the placenta. Thus, by the end of the third week of gestation, a functional cardiovascular system exists.*

As the heart tube grows, the folding of the embryonic disk results in the movement of the heart tube into the chest cavity.

---

*Larsen, 1997; Moore & Persaud, 1998 a and b; Breier, 2000; Sadler & Langman, 2000; Jirasek et al, 2001.

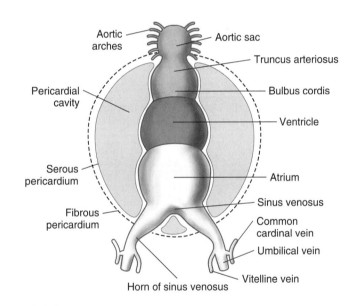

FIGURE **11-10**

Formation of the single heart tube (the tube is shown as it appears inside the pericardial cavity). Note that the atrium and sinus venosus are outside the pericardial cavity.

The heart tube differentiates into three layers: the endocardial layer, which becomes the endothelium; the cardiac jelly, which is a loose tissue layer; and the myoepicardial mantle, which becomes the myocardium and pericardium. The single heart tube is attached at its cephalic end by the aortic arches and at the caudal end by the septum transversum. The attachments limit the length of the heart tube. Continued growth results in dilated areas and bulges, which become specific components of the heart. The atrium, ventricle, and bulbus cordis can be identified first, followed by the sinus venosus and truncus arteriosus. To accommodate continued growth, two separate bends in the heart occur. It first bends to the right to form a U shape; the next bend results in an S-shaped heart. The bending of the heart is responsible for the typical location of cardiac structures (Figure 11-11).*

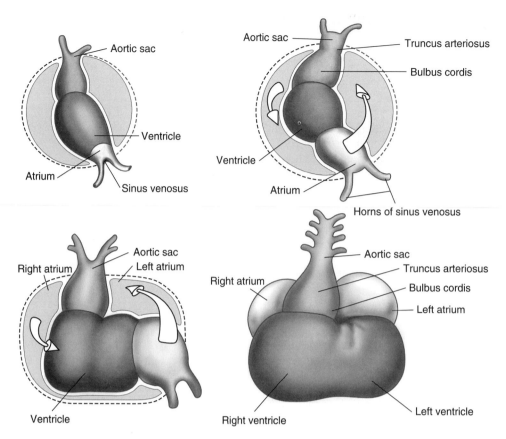

FIGURE **11-11**
Bending of the heart tube inside the pericardial cavity. The bending of the tube brings the atrium into the pericardial cavity. The sinus venosus is taken into the right atrium and the coronary sinus.

Initially, the heart is a single chamber; partitioning of the heart into four chambers occurs from the fourth to sixth weeks of gestation. The changes that cause the partitioning of the heart occur simultaneously. The atrium is separated from the ventricle by endocardial cushions, which are thickened areas of endothelium that develop on the dorsal and ventral walls of the open area between the atrium and the ventricle. The endocardial cushions fuse with each other to divide the atrioventricular canals into right and left atrioventricular canals. Partitioning of the atrium occurs through invagination of tissue toward the endocardial cushions, which forms the septum primum. As the septum primum grows toward the endocardial cushions, it becomes very thin and perforates, becoming the foramen ovale. The septum primum does not fuse completely with the endocardial cushions; it has a lower portion that lies beside the endocardial cushions. Overlapping of the septum primum and the septum secundum forms a wall if the pressure in both atria is equal. In utero, the pressure on the right side is increased, allowing blood to flow across the foramen ovale from the right side of the heart to the left side (Figure 11-12).*

The ventricle is also partitioned by a membranous and muscular septum. The muscular portion of the septum develops from the fold of the floor of the ventricle. With blood flowing through the atrioventricular canal, ventricular dilation occurs on either side of the fold or ridge, causing it to become a sep-tum. The membranous septum arises from ridges inside the bulbus cordis. These ridges, continuous into the bulbus cordis, form the wall that divides the bulbus cordis into the pulmonary artery and the aorta. The bulbar ridges fuse with the endocardial cushions to form the membranous septum. The membranous and muscular septa fuse to close the intraventricular foramen, resulting in two parallel circuits of blood flow. The pulmonary artery is continuous with the right ventricle, and the aorta is continuous with the left ventricle (Figure 11-13).*

The blood flowing through the bulbus cordis and truncus arteriosus in a spiral causes the formation of ridges. The ridges fuse to form two separate vessels that twist around each other once. Thus the pulmonary artery exits the right side of the heart and is in the left upper chest, and the aorta exits the left side of the heart and is located close to the sternum.*

The pulmonary veins grow from the lungs to a cardinal vein plexus. Concurrently, a vessel develops from the smooth wall of the left atrium. As the atrium grows, the pulmonary vein is incorporated into the atrial wall. The atrium and its branches give rise to four pulmonary veins that enter the left atrium. These pulmonary vessels, connected to the plexus of the cardinal vein, provide a continuous circulation from lung to heart. The pulmonary and aortic valves (semilunar valves) develop from dilations within the pulmonary artery and aorta. The ebb and flow circulation through these structures causes them to

*Larsen, 1997; Moore & Persaud, 1998 a and b; Breier, 2000; Sadler & Langman, 2000; Jirasek et al, 2001.

*Larsen, 1997; Moore & Persaud, 1998 a and b; Sadler & Langman, 2000; Jirasek et al, 2001.

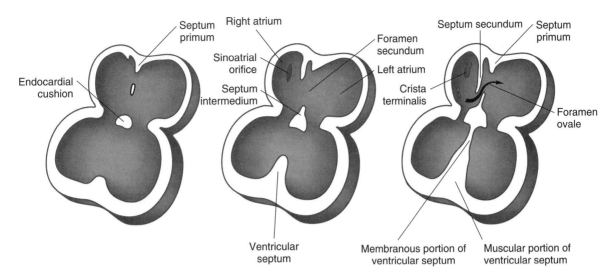

FIGURE 11-12
Partitioning of the atrium. Through the process of septation, the atrium is partitioned into the right and left atria.

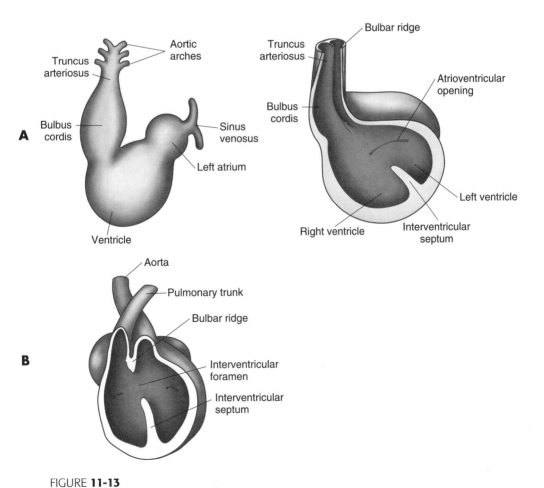

FIGURE 11-13
Partitioning of the ventricles. **A,** Five chambers are present in the heart at 5 weeks' gestation. **B,** At 6 weeks, the bulbus cordis has been taken into the ventricles, and the interventricular septum has partitioned the ventricles into right and left sides.

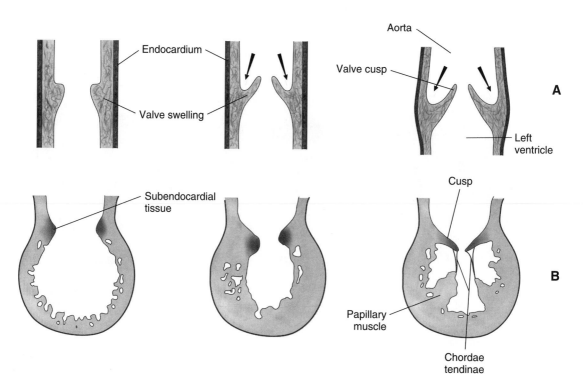

FIGURE **11-14**
Formation of the heart valve. **A,** Formation of the semilunar valves of the aorta and the pulmonary artery. **B,** Formation of the cusps of the atrioventricular valves.

hollow out, forming the cusps of the valves. The tricuspid and mitral valves develop from tissue around the atrioventricular canals that thickens and then thins out on the ventricular sides, forming the valves (Figure 11-14).*

Respiratory System

The development of the respiratory system is linked to the development of the face and the digestive system. The respiratory system is composed of the nasal cavities, nasopharynx, oropharynx, larynx, trachea, bronchi, and lungs (Figure 11-15). The lungs develop in four overlapping stages that extend from the fifth week of gestation until about 8 years of life (Table 11-1). At term birth, the normal respiratory system functions immediately. Adequate functioning of the respiratory system requires a sufficient number of alveoli, adequate capillary blood flow, and an adequate amount of surfactant produced by the secretory epithelial cells or the type II pneumocytes. Surfactant prevents alveolar collapse and aids in respiratory gas exchange. Research into the role of epidermal growth factor (EGF) in the development of the fetal respiratory system has determined that EGF indirectly promotes branching morphogenesis of the lung epithelium through a direct effect on the mesenchyme.†

Through recent advances in genetics, researchers have come to realize that airway pressure plays a role by altering effector cells (epithelial, mesenchymal, or both). Through signal conduction, pathways turn "on" or "off" the regulatory genes

that play key roles in the regulation of lung development through induction of transcription factors, growth factors, and other regulatory proteins (Ciley et al, 2000). Further research into genetics may result in ways to promote lung maturity in preterm infants.

Muscular System

The muscular system develops from mesodermal cells called myoblasts. Striated skeletal muscles are derived from myotomal mesoderm (myotomes) of the somites. Most striated skeletal muscle fibers develop in utero, and almost all striated skeletal muscles are formed by 1 year of age. Growth is achieved by an increase in the diameter of the muscle fibers rather than by growth of new muscle tissue. Smooth muscle fibers arise from the splanchnic mesenchyme surrounding the endoderm of the primitive gut. The smooth muscles lining the vessel walls of the blood and lymphatic systems arise from somatic mesoderm. As smooth muscle cells differentiate, contractile filaments develop in the cytoplasm, and the external surface is covered by an external lamina. As the smooth muscle fibers develop into sheets or bundles, the muscle cells synthesize and release collagenous, elastic, or reticular fibers (Figure 11-16).*

Cardiac muscle develops from splanchnic mesenchyme from the outside of the endocardial heart tube. Cells from the myoepicardial mantle differentiate into the myocardium. Cardiac muscle fibers develop from differentiation and growth of single cells rather than from fusion of cells. Cardiac muscle grows through the formation of new filaments. The Purkinje fibers, which are larger and have fewer myofibrils than other

---

*Larsen, 1997; Moore & Persaud, 1998 a and b; Sadler & Langman, 2000; Jirasek et al, 2001.
†Larsen, 1997; Gresik et al, 1998; Moore & Persaud, 1998 a and b; Sadler & Langman, 2000; Jirasek et al, 2001.

*Larsen, 1997; Moore & Persaud, 1998 a and b; Sadler & Langman, 2000; Jirasek et al, 2001.

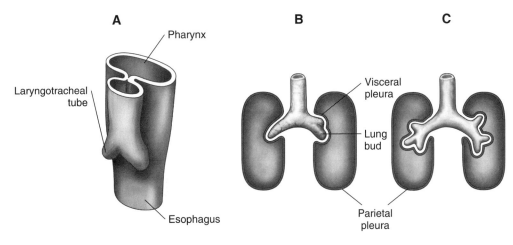

FIGURE **11-15**
Development of the pulmonary system. **A,** Formation of the laryngotracheal tube through fusion of the margins of the laryngotracheal groove. **B,** Invagination of the lung buds into the intraembryonic cavity. **C,** Division of the lung buds into the right and left mainstem bronchi.

TABLE **11-1**	Stages of Lung Development
Stage	**Critical Events**
Stage 1: Pseudoglandular period Weeks 5 to 7	Conducting airway develops.
Stage 2: Canalicular period Weeks 13 to 25	Bronchial lumina and terminal bronchioles enlarge. Lung tissue becomes vascularized. Respiratory bronchioles and alveolar ducts develop. Limited number of primitive alveoli develop.
Stage 3: Terminal sac period Week 24 to birth	Primitive pulmonary alveoli develop from alveolar ducts. Vascularity increases. Type II pneumocytes begin to produce surfactant by about week 24.
Stage 4: Alveolar period Late fetal period until about 8 years of age	Pulmonary alveoli are formed by thinning of the terminal air sac lining. One eighth to one sixth of the adult number of alveoli are present at term birth; number of alveoli increases until age 8 years.

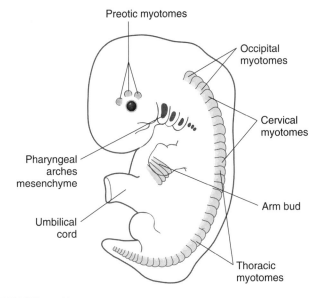

FIGURE **11-16**
Origin of the muscles of the head and neck.

cardiac muscle cells, develop late in the embryonic period. Purkinje fibers function in the electrical conduction system of the heart.*

Skeletal System

The skeletal system develops from mesenchymal cells. In the long bones, condensed mesenchyme forms hyaline cartilage

models of bones. By the end of the embryonic period, ossification centers appear, and these bones ossify by endochondral ossification. Other bones, such as the skull bones, are ossified by membranous ossification, in which the mesenchyme cells become osteoblasts (Figure 11-17).

The vertebral column and the ribs arise from the sclerotome compartments of the somites. The spinal column is formed by the fusion of a condensation of the cranial half of one pair of sclerotomes with the caudal half of the next pair of sclerotomes. The skull can be divided into the neurocranium and the viscerocranium. The neurocranium forms the protective covering around the brain. The viscerocranium forms the skeleton of the face. The neurocranium is made up of the flat bones that surround the brain and the cartilaginous structure, or chondrocranium, that forms the bones of the base of the skull. The neurocranium is made up of a number of separate cartilages, which fuse and ossify by endochondral ossification to form the base of the skull.*

*Larsen, 1997; Moore & Persaud, 1998 a and b; Sadler & Langman, 2000; Jirasek et al, 2001.

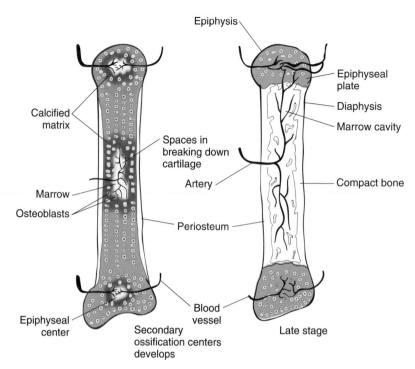

FIGURE **11-17**
Endochondral ossification of bones.

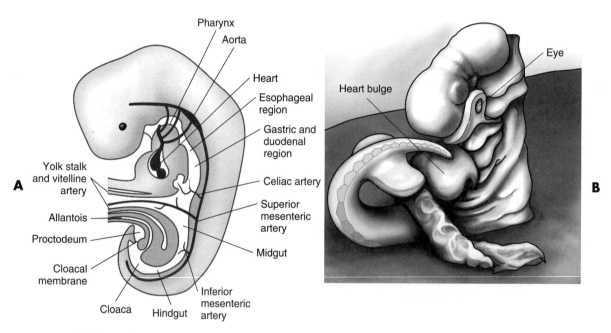

FIGURE **11-18**
Primitive gut. The early gastrointestinal system is present in an embryo at about 4 weeks' gestation.

Gastrointestinal System

The gastrointestinal system is primarily derived from the lining of the roof of the yolk sac. The primitive gut, consisting of the foregut, midgut, and hindgut, is formed during the fourth gestational week (Figure 11-18). The structures that arise from the foregut include the pharynx, esophagus, stomach, liver, pancreas, gallbladder, and part of the duodenum. The esophagus and trachea have a common origin, the laryngotracheal diverticulum. A septum, formed by the growing tracheoesophageal folds, divides the cranial part of the foregut into the laryngotracheal tube and the esophagus. Smooth muscle develops from the splanchnic mesenchyme that surrounds the esophagus. The epithelial lining of the esophagus, derived from the endoderm, proliferates, partly obliterating the esophageal lumen. The esophagus undergoes recanalization by the end of the embryonic period.*

*Larsen, 1997; Moore & Persaud, 1998 a and b; Sadler & Langman, 2000; Jirasek et al, 2001.

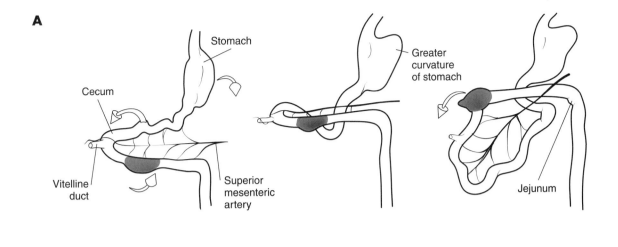

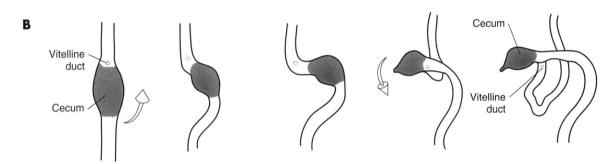

FIGURE **11-19**
Migration and rotation of the midgut. **A,** Counterclockwise 90-degree rotation of midgut loop and
"herniation" into extraembryonic cavity. **B,** Counterclockwise 180-degree rotation of midgut loop
on return to the abdominal cavity.

The stomach originates as a dilation of the caudal portion of the foregut. The characteristic greater curvature of the stomach develops because the dorsal border grows faster than the ventral border. As the stomach develops further, it rotates in a clockwise direction around the longitudinal axis. The duodenum is derived from the caudal and cranial portions of the foregut and the cranial portion of the midgut. The junction of the foregut and midgut portions of the duodenum is normally distal to the common bile duct.*

The liver, gallbladder, and biliary ducts originate as a bud from the caudal end of the foregut. The liver is formed by growth of the hepatic diverticulum, which grows between the layers of the ventral mesentery, forming two parts. The liver forms from the largest, cranial portion. Hepatic cells originate from the hepatic diverticulum. Hematopoietic tissue and Kupffer cells are derived from the splanchnic mesenchyme of the septum transversum. The liver develops rapidly and fills the abdominal cavity; it begins its hematopoietic function by the sixth gestational week. Primitive erythropoiesis is characterized by large, nucleated erythrocytes that contain embryonic hemoglobin and are not dependent on erythropoietin (Dame & Juul, 2000).

The smaller portion of the hepatic diverticulum forms the gallbladder. The common bile duct is formed from the stalk connecting the hepatic and cystic ducts to the duodenum. The

pancreas is derived from the pancreatic buds that arise from the caudal part of the foregut.*

The structures that are derived from the midgut include the remainder of the duodenum, the cecum, the appendix, the ascending colon, and most of the transverse colon. The intestines undergo extensive growth during the first weeks of development. The liver and kidneys occupy the abdominal cavity, restricting the space available for intestinal growth. The growth of the intestines is accommodated through a migration out of the abdominal cavity via the umbilical cord. A series of rotations occurs before the intestines return to the abdomen. The first rotation is counterclockwise, around the axis of the superior mesenteric artery. At about the tenth week, the intestines return to the abdomen, undergoing further rotation. When the colon returns to the abdomen, the cecal end rotates to the right side, entering the lower right quadrant of the abdomen. The cecum and appendix arise from the cecal diverticulum, a pouch that appears in the fifth week of gestation on the caudal limb of the midgut loop (Figure 11-19).*

The hindgut is that portion of the intestines from the midgut to the cloacal membrane. The latter structure consists of the endoderm of the cloaca and the ectoderm of the anal pit. The cloaca is divided by the urorectal septum. As the septum grows toward the cloacal membrane, folds from the lateral walls of the cloaca grow together, dividing the cloaca into the rectum and upper anal canal dorsally and the urogenital sinus ventrally. By the end of the sixth week, the urorectal septum fuses with the cloacal membrane, forming a dorsal anal membrane and a larger ventral urogenital membrane. At about the end of

*Larsen, 1997; Moore & Persaud, 1998 a and b; Sadler & Langman, 2000; Jirasek et al, 2001.

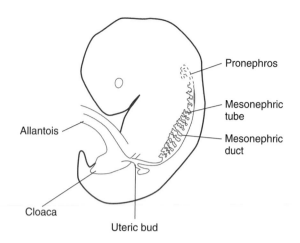

FIGURE **11-20**
Development of the kidney: location of the pronephros, and the mesonephric tube and duct (which make up the mesonephros).

the seventh gestational week, these two membranes rupture, forming the anal canal.*

Urogenital System

The development of the urinary and genital systems is closely related. The urogenital system develops from the intermediate mesoderm, which extends along the dorsal body wall of the embryo. During embryonic folding in the horizontal plane, the intermediate mesoderm is moved forward and is no longer connected to the somites. This mesoderm forms the urogenital ridge on each side of the primitive aorta. Both the urinary and genital systems arise from this urogenital ridge. The area from which the urinary system is derived is called the nephrogenic cord. The genital ridge is the area from which the reproductive system is derived.*

The kidney passes through three stages of development: the pronephros, the mesonephros, and the metanephros. The pronephros, a nonfunctional organ, appears in the first month of gestation and then degenerates, contributing only a duct system for the next developmental stage. The mesonephros uses the duct of the pronephros and develops caudal to the pronephros (Figure 11-20). The mesonephros begins to produce urine during development of the metanephros. The mesonephros degenerates by the end of the embryonic period, and remnants of it persist as genital ducts in males or as vestigial structures in females. The metanephros appears in the fifth week of gestation and becomes the permanent kidney; it begins to produce urine by about the eleventh week of gestation. The urinary bladder and the urethra arise from the urogenital sinus and the splanchnic mesenchyme. The caudal portion of the mesonephric duct is incorporated into the bladder, giving rise to the ureters.*

Although the genetic sex of the embryo is determined at conception, the early development of the genital system is indistinguishable until the seventh week of gestation. Beginning in the seventh week, the gonads begin to be differentiated. The ovaries and the testes are derived from the coelomic epithelium, the mesenchyme, and the primordial germ cells. Development of female sexual organs occurs in the absence of hormonal stimulation precipitated by the H-Y antigen gene

*Larsen, 1997; Moore & Persaud, 1998 a and b; Sadler & Langman, 2000; Jirasek et al, 2001.

carried on the Y chromosome. If the Y chromosome is present, testes develop; otherwise, ovaries develop.*

CONGENITAL DEFECTS

Congenital defects or anomalies are structural or anatomic abnormalities present at birth that are attributed to genetic or chromosomal abnormalities or to maternal or environmental factors. Congenital defects vary in severity and location, ranging from insignificant flaws to major organ system deformities. Most congenital defects result from an interaction between genetic and environmental factors or from multifactorial inheritance. The generally reported incidence of congenital defects is about 2% to 3%. The actual incidence is higher because some defects are not apparent at birth. Close to 12% of birth defects are not discovered until after the newborn period. (Felix, et al, 2000). The incidence of all defects (both minor and major) is approximately 14%. Almost 20% of all perinatal deaths are caused by congenital defects. Congenital defects caused by single-gene disorders and chromosomal abnormalities are discussed in Chapter 10.

Moore & Persaud (1998a) listed six mechanisms by which congenital defects occur: (1) too little growth, (2) too little resorption, (3) too much resorption, (4) resorption in the wrong location, (5) normal growth in an abnormal position, and (6) overgrowth of a tissue or structure. Embryonic organs are most sensitive to noxious agents during a period of rapid cell growth and differentiation. Damage to the primitive streak at about 15 days' gestation could cause severe congenital malformations of the embryo because of the primitive streak's role in the production of intraembryonic mesoderm, from which all connective tissue is formed. Because biochemical differentiation occurs before morphologic differentiation, organs or structures are sensitive to the action of teratogens before they can be identified.

Critical Periods of Human Development

Environmental influences during the first 2 weeks after conception may prevent successful implantation of the blastocyst and cause abortion of the embryo. The most sensitive period for the embryo is the period of organogenesis, especially from day 15 to day 60. Each organ has a critical period during which its development is most likely to be adversely affected by the presence of teratogenic agents (see Figure 11-8 for the critical periods for each major organ system).

Teratogens

Teratogens are agents that may adversely affect embryonic development, and about 7% of all congenital defects are caused by exposure to teratogenic agents. Known teratogens include drugs or other chemicals, radiation, and infectious organisms. Very few agents have been proved to be teratogenic, primarily because the risks to human beings make scientific study difficult. Some agents have been tested on animal models, but caution must be used when extrapolating these findings to human beings. Some agents were identified as teratogenic after exposure to the agent resulted in an increased incidence of defects. Limited knowledge about the safety of all substances makes it prudent for women to avoid all possible teratogens before conception and during pregnancy.

Drugs and Chemicals.   Drugs and chemicals account for about 2% to 3% of congenital defects. Few drugs are known to be teratogenic, but no drug can be considered completely safe;

therefore all drugs should be avoided unless the benefit of taking the drug outweighs the possible risks. Drugs of various classifications have been identified as being teratogenic.

Alcohol has been associated with congenital defects, including craniofacial abnormalities, limb deformities, and cardiovascular defects. Associated abnormalities include growth deficiency and mental retardation. The term fetal alcohol syndrome is used to describe the cluster of defects characteristic of maternal ingestion of alcohol. No level of alcohol consumption can be considered safe, therefore alcohol should be avoided throughout the perinatal period (Baraitser & Winter, 1996).

Certain antibiotics have been identified as teratogens. Tetracycline is deposited in the embryo's bones and teeth, leading to a brown discoloration of the teeth and diminished growth of the long bones. Antitubercular agents, such as streptomycin and dihydrostreptomycin, have been associated with hearing deficits and damage to cranial nerve VIII. Sulfonamides have been associated with an increased incidence of kernicterus in the newborn. Currently, the safest antibiotic for use in pregnant women appears to be penicillin. This drug has not been associated with an increased incidence of congenital defects (Sanders, 1996).

Several anticonvulsant drugs have been implicated in the presence of congenital defects (Sanders, 1996). The use of phenytoin may cause craniofacial defects, nail and digital hypoplasia, intrauterine growth retardation, microcephaly, and mental retardation. Other anticonvulsant drugs identified as teratogens are trimethadione (Tridione) and paramethadione (Paradione). The defects caused by these drugs include fetal facial dysmorphia, cardiac defects, cleft palate, and intrauterine growth restriction.

Warfarin, an anticoagulant, can cause craniofacial abnormalities, optic atrophy, microcephaly, and mental retardation. Other anticoagulants, although not specifically teratogenic, cross the placental barrier and may lead to hemorrhage in the fetus. Heparin does not cross the placental barrier and is used for anticoagulation in pregnant women.

Antineoplastic agents are particularly teratogenic. Aminopterin and methotrexate both have been associated with major congenital malformations, especially central nervous system defects. Antineoplastic drugs may be harmful to health care workers exposed to them during routine nursing interventions. Women who are pregnant or trying to conceive should not administer antineoplastic agents (Sanders, 1996).

Antipsychotic and antianxiety agents are also suspected of being teratogenic agents. Phenothiazine and lithium have been linked to congenital defects. Diazepam (Valium), meprobamate, and chlordiazepoxide may cause congenital defects. Diazepam is associated with an increased incidence of cleft lip with or without cleft palate.

Hormonal agents are also implicated in the incidence of congenital defects. Androgenic agents (progestins) may cause masculinization of female fetuses. Diethylstilbestrol (DES), a synthetic estrogen used to prevent abortion in the 1940s and 1950s, has been found to cause an increased incidence of vaginal and cervical cancer in female children exposed to the drug in utero, and associated abnormalities of the reproductive system often cause reproductive dysfunction (Sadler & Langman, 2000). Cortisone has been shown to cause cleft palate in animal models but has not been implicated as a factor in cleft palate in human newborns.

Social or recreational drugs are highly suspected of contributing to congenital defects. Drugs such as lysergic acid di-

ethylamide (LSD) have been associated with limb and central nervous system abnormalities. Other drugs that may be teratogenic are phencyclidine and marijuana. "Crack" cocaine, a relative newcomer to the social drug inventory, has been associated with congenital abnormalities. The recreational drug Ecstasy has been linked to heart and limb defects. However, because drug abusers tend to use several drugs, have poor nutritional habits, and lack prenatal care, it is difficult to establish the effects of the drugs individually.

Miscellaneous drugs from other categories that are suspected of leading to congenital defects include propylthiouracil and potassium iodide, which are associated with neonatal goiter and mental retardation. Amphetamines are associated with oral clefts and heart defects. Salicylates (aspirin), the medication most commonly used during pregnancy, may be harmful to the fetus if taken in large amounts. Retinoic acid (vitamin A) is teratogenic in high doses in human beings. Isotretinoin, a drug used to treat acne, causes craniofacial abnormalities, cleft palate, thymic aplasia defects, and neural tube defects (Sadler & Langman, 2000).

Environmental chemicals such as pollutants, fungicides, food additives, and defoliants have been suspected of causing congenital defects. The claim most strongly supported is that mercury causes neurologic manifestations similar to those seen in cerebral palsy, blindness, and mental retardation (Sadler & Langman, 2000). Although little evidence is available to prove that other environmental agents are teratogenic, no data prove that environmental chemicals are not dangerous. Therefore pregnant women should avoid exposure to possibly toxic chemicals. Unfortunately, recognizing exposure to potentially hazardous products is difficult because they are so widely used (Sadler & Langman, 2000).

Radiation.   Exposure to high levels of ionizing radiation can result in microcephaly, skull defects, spina bifida, blindness, and cleft palate. Studies of the outcomes of women who were pregnant during the atomic bombing of Hiroshima and Nagasaki showed that 28% had abortions, 25% had liveborn infants who died within 1 year, and 25% of the survivors gave birth to children with central nervous system disorders (Sadler & Langman, 2000). There is no established "safe" level for radiation. The severity of the radiation-induced defects depends on the duration and timing of exposure. There is no evidence that the small amount of radiation required for modern x-ray studies is harmful; however, caution is used to minimize exposure of the fetus because of the potential for cumulative effects of radiation exposure throughout the life span.

Infectious Agents.   Three viral agents have been identified as teratogenic to the developing fetus: rubella, cytomegalovirus (CMV), and herpes simplex. The incidence of congenital malformations in newborns of women who had rubella in the first trimester of pregnancy is 15% to 20%. Typical malformations include heart defects, deafness, and cataracts. CMV is thought to be the most commonly occurring viral infection of the human fetus. CMV in early embryonic development probably results in spontaneous abortion; infection during the second or third trimester may cause microcephaly and microphthalmia. Herpes simplex infection of the fetus primarily occurs late in the pregnancy, commonly during delivery. Congenital abnormalities in fetuses infected before delivery include microcephaly, microphthalmia, retinal dysplasia, and mental retardation.

Maternal infection with *Toxoplasma gondii*, a protozoal parasite, can cause hydrocephalus, cerebral calcification, microphthalmia, and ocular defects. *T. gondii* can be contracted from undercooked meat, by handling the feces of infected cats, or from the soil. Untreated primary maternal infection with *Treponema pallidum*, the microorganism that causes syphilis, results in serious fetal infection, but adequate treatment kills the organism, preventing serious defects. Untreated syphilis can lead to congenital deafness and mental retardation.

Other viral agents also have been implicated as causes of congenital malformations. Defects have been reported after maternal infection with mumps, varicella, echovirus, coxsackie virus, and influenza virus. The incidence of congenital malformations with these infections is unknown but is thought to be low (Sadler & Langman, 2000). Further information on viral agents is presented in Chapter 29.

Another teratogenic factor is hyperthermia. Hyperthermia may be the causative factor in congenital defects associated with viral agents because of the fever produced by the viruses. Hyperthermia can also be caused by maternal use of hot tubs or saunas.

Maternal Substances. The effects of substances present in pregnant women in inappropriate amounts (high or low) may contribute to congenital defects in the fetus. Evidence indicates that high maternal levels of certain physiologic compounds may have a deleterious effect on fetal development. High maternal levels of phenylalanine during pregnancy can result in neurologic damage resembling that from untreated phenylketonuria (PKU), even though the fetus does not have genotypic PKU. Thyroid deficiency during the last two trimesters of pregnancy and can result in mental retardation or other neurologic deficits. Thus untreated maternal hypothyroidism can also adversely affect the developing fetus (Utiger, 1999). Recently, researchers have postulated that high maternal levels of trans fatty acids may adversely affect fetal development, although more research is needed before specific recommendations can be made. (Carlson, et al, 1997).

Good nutrition has long been considered essential for proper growth and development of the fetus. However, with the exception of folic acid, for which studies indicate that deficiencies are causally related to defects of the neural tube, little evidence is available on the role of micronutrients in fetal development. Supplementation of vitamins and minerals must occur within the appropriate critical period of development to be effective, or it may be harmful (McArdle & Ashworth, 1999). Environmental factors that have yet to be identified may influence the development of the fetus. In assessing the influences on fetal development, it is essential to consider the fetus's environment, in terms both of the uterine environment and the mother's environment.

REFERENCES

Baraitser M, Winter RM (1996). *Color atlas of congenital malformation syndromes*. Mosby: St Louis.

Breier G (2000). Angiogenesis in embryonic development: a review. *Placenta*, 21(suppl A), S11-S15.

Carlson SE, et al (1997). Trans fatty acids: infant and fetal development: report of an Expert Panel on Trans Fatty Acids and Early Development. *American journal of clinical nutrition*, 66 (3), 715S-736S.

Ciley RE, et al (2000). Fetal lung development: airway pressure enhances expression of developmental genes. *Journal of pediatric surgery*, 35(1), 113-119.

Dame C, Juul SE (2000). The switch from fetal to adult erythropoiesis. *Clinics in perinatology*, 27(3), 507-526.

Felix JF, et al (2000). Birth defects in children with newborn encephalopathy. *Developmental medicine and child neurology*, 42(12), 803-808.

Gresik EW, et al (1998). The EGF system in fetal development. *European journal of morphology*, 36(suppl), 92-97.

Jirasek JE, et al (2001). *An atlas of the human embryo and fetus: a photographic review of human prenatal development*. Parthenon: New York.

Larsen WJ (1997). *Essentials of human embryology*. Churchill Livingstone: Philadelphia.

McArdle HJ, Ashworth CJ (1999). Micronutrients in fetal growth and development. *British medical journal*, 55(3), 499-510.

Moore KL, Persaud TVN (1998a). *Before we are born: essentials of embryology and birth defects*, ed 5. WB Saunders: Philadelphia.

Moore KL, Persaud TVN (1998b). *The developing human: clinically oriented embryology*, ed 6. WB Saunders: Philadelphia.

Sadler TW, Langman J (2000). *Langman's medical embryology*, ed 8. Lippincott Williams & Wilkins: Baltimore.

Sanders RC, editor (1996). *Structural fetal abnormalities: the total picture*. Mosby: St Louis.

Utiger RD (1999). Maternal hypothyroidism and fetal development. *New England journal of medicine*, 341(8), 601-602.

CHAPTER 12

HIGH-RISK PREGNANCY

JUDITH S. HARMON

Perinatal nursing is advancing rapidly. In light of some of those changes, greater emphasis is being placed on identification of maternal risk factors, early preventive and therapeutic treatment, patient education, stabilization of maternal conditions, and transport before delivery.

MATERNAL-FETAL UNIT

Placenta

From the beginning of cell division and the formation of the morula, certain cells are destined to form the placenta. As the morula passes through the fallopian tube, it becomes the blastocyst. The outer layer of the blastocyst is called the trophoblast. The trophoblast invades the lining of the uterus (the endometrium), forming three layers of cells; the outermost layer sends out fingerlike projections called villi. For the villi to embed successfully, the endometrium must be richly supplied with nutritive substances (Gilbert & Harmon, 2003).

Previous scarring from incisions into the uterus or from infection in the lining may adversely affect where implantation occurs. Typically, the blastocyte implants and develops into the placenta, which implants in the posterior portion of the fundus of the uterus. If it implants in the lower portion of the uterus or does not implant securely, bleeding and separation may occur in the third trimester.

The placenta serves four main organ or system functions: (1) it acts as a respiratory organ, exchanging oxygen and carbon dioxide through the simple diffusion process (this action depends on adequate uteroplacental blood flow); (2) it serves as a fetal kidney for the metabolic side of acid-base balance, regulating the excretion of wastes and electrolyte balance; (3) it acts as the gastrointestinal tract for storage and release of nutrients, based on fetal need; (4) it functions as a fetal skin for temperature control.

The circulation of essential components to and from the fetus depends on a number of factors, including the surface area of the placenta (specifically the integration of the villi dictates) and the amount and rate of diffusion of necessary nutrients and other biochemical components. Depending on the point of gestation, from the twentieth week on, approximately 400 to 700 ml of maternal blood flows through the uterus; approximately 80% of this blood flow goes into the intervillous space. There, in the "lake" surrounding the peninsula-like villi, the maternal blood, through villous tissue, exchanges nutrients and oxygen for wastes and carbon dioxide. Nutrients are stored in the placenta and released as needed by the fetus, independent of blood flow or concentration.

The umbilical cord consists of two arteries and one vein encased in Wharton jelly. The umbilical cord delivers biochemical components to the fetus and also removes them. Because the placenta functions as the fetal lung, the arteries carry the relatively unoxygenated blood from the fetus to the placenta, and the vein carries reoxygenated blood from the placenta to the fetus. The arteries have a thicker wall than the vein, therefore the vein (with the more oxygenated blood flow) constricts more easily. Under healthy circumstances, all blood flow to the uterus and through the placenta forms a low-pressure system through widely dilated vessels. Maternal disease and pregnancy complications that affect the mother's cardiac or vascular systems inevitably affect the mother's nutrition and ultimately affect oxygen and carbon dioxide exchange across the placental membrane.

Amniotic Fluid

The amnion is a membranous sac that surrounds the fetus. As the amnion enlarges, it gradually sheaths the umbilical cord. Initially, most of the fluid in the amnion is derived from maternal blood. Later, the fetus contributes to the amount by excreting urine into the amniotic fluid. Amniotic fluid is also normally swallowed by the fetus and absorbed into the gastrointestinal (GI) tract. Through fetal surgery and follow-up of infants that have had this procedure, we now know that the amniotic fluid contains growth factors that enhance the maturation of the respiratory and GI tracts (Creasy & Resnik, 1999).

Certain fetal or maternal conditions may affect the quantity of amniotic fluid. Fetal renal malfunctions may lead to less amniotic fluid as a result of decreased urine volume from the fetus; GI anomalies may result in increased amniotic fluid because of the fetus's inability to swallow amniotic fluid. Certain maternal conditions, especially nutritional deficiencies, often are associated with a smaller placenta and smaller amniotic fluid volume. These factors, in turn, can lead to nutritional growth restriction of the fetus. Decreased amniotic fluid most commonly is a concern with postterm pregnancy in which both the fetal and maternal contributions to the volume are reduced.

Amniotic fluid has a number of functions. It permits symmetric growth and development and prevents the amnion from adhering to the embryo. It also cushions the fetus against jolts by distributing any impact on the mother's body. It helps to control fetal body temperature by maintaining a relatively constant temperature and enables the fetus to move freely, thus aiding musculoskeletal development. It protects the umbilical cord against injury and the fetus against microbial agents. However, these functions may be impaired with oligohydramnios (inadequate amniotic fluid) or polyhydramnios (excess amniotic fluid) (Moore & Persaud, 1998; Creasy & Resnik, 1999; Gilbert & Harmon, 2003).

Maternal Nutrition

Maternal nutrition plays a significant role in fetal well-being and in the prevention and treatment of high-risk pregnancies. A 25% deficit in needed calories and protein can interfere with the synthesis of deoxyribonucleic acid (DNA). A nutritional deficiency during the first 2 to 3 months of pregnancy can have teratogenic effects or can lead to spontaneous loss of the pregnancy. After 2 to 3 months, a maternal nutritional deficiency can impede fetal growth, resulting in a fetus that is small for gestational age, or the fetus may have diminished brain growth. These infants may be unable to attain their optimum potential in stature, intellect, and future health.

Specific maternal nutritional deficiencies can have deleterious effects on the fetus. Protein (75 to 100 g daily) is important for supporting embryonic-fetal cell growth, for promoting necessary increased maternal blood volume, and possibly for helping prevent pregnancy-induced hypertension (PIH). To prevent maternal anemia, which adversely affects oxygenation and neonatal red blood cell mass, the mother must have an adequate intake of iron, folic acid, and vitamins B_6 and B_{12}. Supplemental iron of at least 300 mg in maternal stores is necessary, because the fetus draws upon these stores.

During pregnancy the mother's diet should contain 30 to 50 mg of zinc each day. Zinc is found in such foods as nuts, meats, whole grains, legumes, and dairy products. A deficiency of zinc during pregnancy increases the risk of premature rupture of membranes and preterm labor. A maternal zinc deficiency also may be the result of a related deficiency in the antimicrobial properties of the amniotic fluid (Davis & Sherer, 1993; Gilbert & Harmon, 2003).

Changes in sodium intake also can create problems in pregnancy. A restricted sodium intake (less than 2.5 g per 24 hours) can impede an adequate increase in maternal blood volume, which in turn can activate the renin-angiotensin-aldosterone cycle and lead to vasoconstriction. Excess sodium intake can cause vasoconstriction through increased sensitivity of the blood vessel wall to angiotensin.

To meet the growing needs of the fetus for maternal storage of fat and protein, an increase of 300 to 500 calories per day above normal caloric requirements is required. The fat and lean body tissue stored serve as reserves for the fetus during the last part of pregnancy and provide an energy source for labor, delivery, and lactation. Intake of harmful substances such as alcohol, tobacco, and illegal drugs interferes with adequate absorption of nutrients by the fetus and the mother (Gilbert & Harmon, 2003).

MATERNAL HEALTH AND EFFECTS ON THE FETUS

Postterm Pregnancy

Incidence.   Postterm pregnancy has long been reported in human beings. Postmaturity in the fetus is the second leading cause of intrapartum asphyxia. Approximately 10% of all pregnancies continue 14 or more days beyond term. Of these, 20%

to 40% result in postmature neonates, among whom the perinatal mortality rate is three times that of term newborns. Mortality rates show that 35% of the deaths occur antepartum, 47% intrapartum, and 18% in the neonatal period (Creasy & Resnik, 1999) (Box 12-1).

Etiology.   It is widely accepted that the postmature neonate is affected by some degree of placental insufficiency; however, this does not explain the prolongation of pregnancy past term. The actual onset of labor appears to be the result of changes in the estrogen-progesterone ratio; these substances ultimately release prostaglandins from the uterine muscle through contractions. Prostaglandins, in turn, pave the way for release of oxytocin to increase the intensity of the contractions. An increase in mature fetal adrenocortical activity stimulates the release of maternal oxytocin (Gilbert & Harmon, 2003).

Pathophysiology.   After 36 weeks the placenta begins to age, laying down fibrinoid material on the surface of the villi. By about 42 weeks, the surface area of the placenta available for oxygen and carbon dioxide exchange is diminished. In addition, the amount of amniotic fluid declines because of diminished maternal blood flow; thus the fetus is at risk both for uteroplacental insufficiency and for cord entrapment (Gilbert & Harmon, 2003).

Signs and Symptoms.   A number of warning signs may indicate postterm problems, including maternal weight loss of more than 2 pounds a week, oligohydramnios of less than 300 ml, meconium-stained amniotic fluid, advanced bony maturation of the fetal head, and prolonged labor (Gilbert & Harmon, 2003).

Effects on the Fetus and Neonate.   The effects of postterm pregnancy on the fetus and neonate include failure of growth; dehydration; dry, cracked, wrinkled, parchment-like skin as a result of reduction of subcutaneous fat; long, thin arms and legs; advanced hardness of the skull; absence of vernix and lanugo; skin maceration, especially in folds; brownish-green discoloration of the skin caused by meconium staining; and increased appearance of alertness (Gilbert & Harmon, 2003). Postmaturity syndrome is considered an imbalance between continued placental capacity to function and fetal nutritive and respiratory demands.

Treatment.   Between 40 and 42 completed weeks of gestation, decisions should be made about intervening in the pregnancy. If the physician and the pregnant woman elect to continue the pregnancy and await the onset of labor, antepartum fetal heart rate (FHR) and ultrasonographic monitoring tests are ordered; these may involve biweekly nonstress tests, contraction stress tests, amniotic fluid volume indices, biophysical profiles, or some combination of these tests.

Medical management includes decisions about the type and time of delivery. With careful antepartum FHR monitoring and a fetus who demonstrates well-being in utero, the pregnancy can continue uninterrupted until 42 weeks. At 42 weeks, a trial induction is recommended so that rapid placental aging is less likely to adversely affect the outcome. Induction usually is preceded by prostaglandin gel ripening of the cervix or immediately by oxytocin drip. Careful FHR and maternal monitoring during the intrapartum period improves the outcome, but a cesarean birth is more likely if the fetus does not tolerate labor

BOX **12-1**

Antepartum and Intrapartum Complications of Postterm Pregnancy

Antepartum Complications
- Failure of growth
- Cord accident
- Hypoxia manifested by decreased fetal movement, late deceleration with contraction stress testing, or absent long- and short-term variability on fetal heart rate (FHR) monitoring strips

Intrapartum Complications
- Increase in cesarean birth rate as a result of lack of cephalic molding and high arrest of fetal head or as a result of fetal response to labor stressors
- Intrauterine fetal hypoxia caused by placental insufficiency or cord compression
- Traumatic vaginal birth

or if the mother does not progress in labor (Creasy & Resnik, 1999).

Nursing Management.   Prenatal care requires careful collection of data to ensure accurate dating. This information should include the first day of the last menstrual period; whether conception was preceded by normal menses; the results of ultrasonographic dating before 20 weeks; the date of the first felt fetal movement between 18 and 20 weeks; the findings of doptone FHR monitoring at 12 to 13 weeks; the findings of fetoscope FHR monitoring at 18 to 19 weeks; and the fundal height growth rate at 22 weeks (which should not vary by 3 cm or more from the number of weeks of gestation) (Gilbert & Harmon, 2003).

The pregnant woman should be taught how to count fetal movements; usually a count of four kicks per hour is adequate. Nurses should also explain the FHR monitoring tests. The woman should understand the purpose of challenging fetal well-being, as well as the interpretation of good, bad, and equivocal results. She also should be prepared for the possibility of a cesarean birth.

As the woman approaches 40 weeks, her history of previous pregnancies should be reassessed for increased risk. Factors that increase risk are previous postterm delivery, cesarean birth for failure to progress, and unexplained stillbirth before the estimated date of confinement. This reassessment should be done before 40 weeks' gestation if the mother notices a decline in fetal movements by daily count; if maternal weight loss is more than 2 to 3 pounds in 1 week without an identifiable cause; and if the hard, bony fetal head can be palpated at the symphysis with no early cervical changes.

Intrapartum care should include (1) a careful review of all dating information and the mother's general health history, including a genetic or family history, as well as any FHR monitoring results; (2) evaluation of fundal height, fetal position, and engagement, with use of the Leopold maneuver to estimate the fetus's size, presentation, and position; and (3) careful electronic FHR monitoring or intermittent auscultation to rule out FHR patterns of cord compression or insufficient uteroplacental transfer of oxygen.

Troublesome patterns require prompt nursing treatment, including turning the patient to her left side or from side to side; improving the maternal circulating volume with intravenous fluid challenge (usually with lactated Ringer's solution); discontinuing labor stimulation, if used; administering oxygen at 8 to 10 L by face mask; notifying the physician or midwife; preparing for expeditious delivery if the condition does not improve within 30 minutes; and using suction equipment if meconium is present in the amniotic fluid.

Preterm Delivery

Incidence.   Preterm delivery occurs in 10% to 12% of all live births in the United States. Despite current therapies for halting preterm labor, this incidence has risen for the past 30 years. Preterm delivery accounts for 75% to 80% of all neonatal morbidity and mortality (Gabbe et al, 1996; James et al, 2000; Gilbert & Harmon, 2003).

Etiology.   The exact etiology of preterm labor has continued to elude health professionals. However, screening for risk factors can now be done. Risk factors fall into four main categories: medical and past pregnancy history, current pregnancy history, socioeconomic factors, and daily habits and lifestyle (Gilbert & Harmon, 2003).

Medical and past pregnancy history factors that contribute to a risk for preterm labor or preterm delivery or both include conditions such as diabetes, hypertension, renal disease, heart disease, or systemic lupus erythematosus; more than two spontaneous or elective abortions; previous preterm labor or preterm delivery or both (increasing the likelihood of repetitive preterm labor or preterm delivery or both by 40%); diethylstilbestrol (DES) exposure; and uterine anomalies.

The current pregnancy may reveal problems that may lead to preterm labor or preterm delivery or both, such as abruptio placentae, placenta previa, preeclampsia, multiple gestation, urinary tract infection, febrile illness, abdominal or cervical surgery, and small stature or low weight (under 5 feet tall or less than 100 pounds).

Maternal socioeconomic factors that contribute to the risk of preterm labor or delivery include employment outside the home, less than a twelfth-grade education, single mother, younger than 17 or older than 39 years of age, late prenatal care, poor nutritional resources, and two or more toddlers in the home.

Daily habits or lifestyles that may contribute to preterm labor include smoking more than half a pack of cigarettes per day; use or abuse of hazardous substances (e.g., nicotine, alcohol, cocaine, heroin); long commute to work or to obtain health care; inadequate rest during the day, and poor nutritional habits (Creasy & Resnik, 1999; James et al, 2000).

Pathophysiology.   Preterm events may trigger preterm labor, such as an increase in estrogen in relation to progesterone; increased stretching of uterine muscle, leading to release of arachidonic acid; fetal stress, leading to an increase in fetal cortisol; an increase in prostaglandins; and increased release of maternal oxytocin (Svigos et al, 2000; Gilbert & Harmon, 2003).

Signs and Symptoms.   Preterm labor is the occurrence of the following conditions between 20 and 37 weeks of gestation: painless or mildly uncomfortable contractions; more than four contractions per hour; contractions lasting longer than 30 seconds; and contractions that lead to cervical changes.

The signs and symptoms of preterm labor may vary from specific to vague complaints; the pregnant woman may report low abdominal cramping or pressure, rhythmic tightening and relaxation of the abdomen, aching of the lower back, tingling down the thighs, an increase in or watery vaginal discharge, brownish or pink vaginal discharge, diarrhea with or without abdominal cramping, and generally "feeling bad" (Gilbert & Harmon, 2003).

Effects on the Fetus and Neonate.

In general, preterm labor itself is not harmful to the fetus. Exceptions occur when preterm labor leads to increased stress on the fetus, such as cord compression with contractions or diminished blood supply that exceeds the fetal-placental ability to compensate. Preterm delivery, especially before 32 completed gestational weeks, may result in increased neonatal morbidity and fatality. The primary problem is lung immaturity, which is marked by insufficient production of surfactant and a diminished number of functional alveoli. Because of these deficiencies, the neonate is unable to perform vital respiratory functions. Technologic improvements, such as advances in ventilatory management, have improved outcomes, yet these interventions can lead to consequent morbidity.

Hypoxia can lead to intracranial hemorrhage, necrotizing enterocolitis, renal damage, and other serious system failures. Neonates can experience serious birth injuries, lifetime disabilities, intellectual compromise, and death (Gilbert & Harmon, 2003).

Treatment.

A number of drugs are available that suppress labor (tocolytics), and these can be used to halt preterm labor. However, effective use of these drugs requires that the mother be able to identify the early signs and symptoms of preterm labor and that health care providers respond promptly to the patient's reports of these signs and symptoms.

Some of the tocolytic agents are magnesium sulfate, beta-sympathomimetics (terbutaline), prostaglandin inhibitors (indomethacin, ibuprofen, sulindac), and calcium channel blockers. Magnesium sulfate and terbutaline are the most commonly accepted drugs for halting labor; prostaglandin inhibitors and calcium channel blockers most often are used after the first two drugs have failed. With the exception of intravenous magnesium sulfate, these drugs can halt preterm labor only for brief periods of time.

An exception to the effectiveness of tocolytics is multiple gestation, because the abdomen and uterus grow taut faster and more intensely. When the symptoms are treated in the early stages of preterm labor, better outcomes have been reported with home use of tocolytic drugs, given orally or subcutaneously through an infusion pump. Otherwise, as in a singleton pregnancy, oral agents have been reported to have only anecdotal success at best.

Other adjunct treatments also can help, such as cervical cerclage and early bed rest or a restriction on activities. However, these measures depend on early access to health care, adequate screening, and the patient's willingness to follow health care recommendations (Creasy & Resnik, 1999; Gilbert & Harmon, 2003).

Cortisol has been administered as an adjunct when success in halting labor has been in doubt. It is theorized that between 28 and 32 weeks' gestation, cortisol stimulates a cascade of events that stabilizes lecithin, stimulating production of fetal surfactant and thereby promoting lung function. The use of cortisol has been widely researched, with diverse opinions about its efficacy (Gabbe et al, 1996; Creasy & Resnik, 1999; James et al, 2000).

Medical management may also involve use of home uterine contraction monitors or terbutaline pumps for subcutaneous infusion therapy. Neither of these has proved effective without professional nursing care and education of the patient (Creasy & Resnik, 1999; James et al, 2000; Gilbert & Harmon, 2003).

Nursing Management.

Although the exact cause of premature delivery is not known and most likely involves several factors, nurses play a major role in the attempt to reduce the number of these deliveries. Early prenatal care should be accessible and acceptable to all pregnant women. Nurses working in maternity clinics and offices should implement creative programs that meet the needs of the population served both for accessibility and acceptability. Once into the health care system, all pregnant women should be systematically screened for the risk factors discussed previously. All pregnant women should be taught the physical signs of preterm contractions and how to use their hands to detect rhythmic abdominal tightening. Finally, they should be taught and supported in self-advocacy when reporting signs and symptoms of preterm labor (Gabbe et al, 1996; Creasy & Resnik, 1999; James et al, 2000; Gilbert & Harmon, 2003).

Third-Trimester Bleeding

The two major causes of third-trimester bleeding are placental adherence and implantation problems. These may result in placental abruption or placenta previa.

Incidence.

The risk of placental abruption is 0.5% to 2.5%, and the risk of recurrence in subsequent pregnancies is 5.6%. The risk of placenta previa is 0.5%. Women who have been pregnant several times (multigravidas) have a slightly higher risk of placenta previa, and their risk of recurrence increases fivefold (Gabbe et al, 1996; Creasy & Resnik, 1999; James et al, 2000; Gilbert & Harmon, 2003).

Etiology.

The cause of placental abruption is unknown. Conditions associated with abruption are PIH or chronic hypertension, present in 4% of patients; maternal age over 35 years; multiparity of more than five pregnancies; previous abruption (the risk is increased 10% after one abruption and 25% after two abruptions); trauma from a direct blow to the abdomen or needle puncture during amniocentesis; short umbilical cord; folic acid deficiency; and cigarette smoking, cocaine use, or polysubstance abuse, which cause vasoconstriction of spiral arterioles and lead to decidual necrosis (Gilbert & Harmon, 2003). The cause of placenta previa also is unknown. It frequently is associated with conditions that cause uterine scarring or that interfere with blood supply to the endometrium. Predisposing factors include abortion, cesarean birth, increased parity, prior previa, uterine infection, closely spaced pregnancies, uterine tumors, multiple pregnancy, and maternal age over 35 years (Creasy & Resnik, 1999; James et al, 2000; Gilbert & Harmon, 2003).

Pathophysiology.

Abruption of the placenta is thought to occur when the spiral arterioles, which nourish the decidua (endometrium) and the placenta, begin the process of degeneration. As necrosis takes place, the blood vessels rupture and bleed into the site, leading to separation of the placenta as pressure from the bleeding increases. Abruption may occur at the marginal edges of the placenta, outward to the edges. An abruption is classified, according to the amount of surface involved, as mild (less than 15%), moderate (15% to 60%), or severe (more than 60%) (Creasy & Resnik, 1999; Gilbert & Harmon, 2003).

Signs and Symptoms. Signs and symptoms of placental abruption include uterine tenderness or rigidity and low back pain; dark red vaginal bleeding; fetal symptoms of stress; and maternal signs of shock and disseminated intravascular coagulation (DIC). Signs and symptoms of placenta previa rarely occur before the early third trimester. The onset of symptoms usually is mild, and their recurrence is unpredictable. Signs and symptoms include painless bleeding, usually bright red and initially slight in amount; high presenting fetal part; and subsequent recurrences of bleeding in increasingly significant amounts and associated signs of fetal stress (Gilbert & Harmon, 2003).

Effects on the Fetus and Neonate. The major effects of third-trimester bleeding on the fetus are related to inadequate oxygen-carbon dioxide exchange via the placenta, the potential maternal imperative for premature delivery, or a combination of factors (Gilbert & Harmon, 2003).

Treatment. Treatment of placental abruptions or placenta previa depends on three major factors: the severity of the blood loss, fetal maturity, and fetal well-being (Box 12-2). If the bleeding is mild and stops readily and the fetus is immature and shows no sign of distress, expectant management is chosen. This plan includes hospitalization; bed rest for at least 72 hours; close observation for bleeding; continuous FHR monitoring; maternal red blood cell replacement as necessary; no maternal vaginal examinations; preparation for cesarean birth (vaginal birth is not safe for mother or infant with continual abruption or partial or complete placenta previa); discharge to home, undelivered, only if bleeding subsides and stops (or if placenta previa, if present, is incomplete); and instructions given to the mother for bed rest, restricted activity, and measures to prevent preterm labor (Creasy & Resnik, 1999). Fetal maturity is assessed to determine the risks and benefits of prolonging the

pregnancy with a compromised uteroplacental unit. If fetal well-being is compromised by maternal bleeding, emergency cesarean section is indicated.

Hypertensive Disorders of Pregnancy

The Committee on Terminology of the American College of Obstetricians and Gynecologists has developed the following classification system for hypertensive and prehypertensive states in pregnancy:

- **PIH, or gestational hypertension:** Development of hypertension after 20 weeks' gestation without proteinuria; normotensive blood pressure within 10 postpartum days
- **Preeclampsia:** Development of hypertension with or without edema after 20 weeks' gestation or early postpartum
- **Eclampsia:** Development of convulsions or coma in a patient with preeclampsia, or superimposed preeclampsia or eclampsia in a patient with chronic hypertension
- **Concurrent hypertension and pregnancy (CHP):** Chronic hypertension that develops before pregnancy or before 20 weeks' gestation and is not associated with pregnancy
- **Hemolysis, elevated liver enzymes, and low platelets (HELLP) syndrome:** A complex of symptoms described as a severe forerunner of PIH that has a sudden onset and is diagnosed from the signs and symptoms of hemolysis, elevated liver enzymes, and low platelets

Incidence. Approximately 6% to 30% of all pregnant women have hypertensive disorder. A woman pregnant for the first time (primigravida) is six times more likely than a multigravida to develop PIH, and PIH is five times more prevalent in lower socioeconomic groups. Other factors associated with a higher incidence of PIH include a family history, diabetes mellitus, multiple gestation, polyhydramnios, persistent hypertension, hydatidiform mole, and RH incompatibility (Gilbert & Harmon, 2003).

Etiology. The etiology of PIH is largely unknown. However, four factors are widely accepted as being associated with PIH: nutritional deficiency, immunologic deficiency, genetics, and uterine ischemia. For example, a woman may be at risk for PIH if she has a diet low in protein and sodium, a suppressed immune system, a family history of a genetic dysfunction that might lead to vascular changes or hypertension, or signs of uterine ischemia.

Pathophysiology. In PIH disorders, vascular sensitivity to angiotensin II increases. This increase in sensitivity occurs before the onset of hypertension; when the normal pregnancy-related resistance to angiotensin II is lost, blood vessel spasms occur, causing vasoconstriction and a rise in blood pressure. Blood flow to most organs is diminished, especially to the uterus, placenta, kidneys, liver, and brain, impairing their function by 40% to 60%. Impaired blood flow results in pathophysiologic changes, including decreased uterine and placental blood flow, resulting in premature, exaggerated degeneration of the placenta; increased uterine activity; decreased blood supply to the kidneys and a reduced glomerular filtration rate, causing degenerative changes in the glomerulus and sodium and water retention; decreased serum albumin and decreased plasma colloid osmotic pressure; fluid shifts and generalized edema; decreased blood supply to the liver, impairing liver function, and to the eyes, resulting in retinal arteriolar spasms and blurred vision; loss of fluid from blood vessels in the brain, leading to cerebral edema and hemorrhages; and damage to blood vessel

---

BOX 12-2

Nursing Management for Third-Trimester Bleeding

Assessments
- Risk screening in early prenatal care
- Fetal heart rate monitoring for presence, absence, or compromise of fetal well-being in the presence of maternal bleeding
- Visual inspection
- Quantification of maternal blood loss
- Rapid change in fundal height or maternal vital signs or both in association with abdominal or back pain

Interventions
- If bleeding threatens mother's life or stresses fetus, prepare for emergency delivery, usually by cesarean birth.
- If expectant management is chosen, teach pregnant woman ways to prevent preterm labor.
- Prepare parents for possible preterm delivery.

Modified from Gilbert E, Harmon J (2003). Manual of high risk pregnancy and delivery, ed 3. Mosby: St Louis.

walls, which occurs with progression of the disease (Creasy & Resnik, 1999). Platelets, fibrinogen, immunoglobulin, and components of complement are deposited at the damaged sites, and DIC occurs.

Signs and Symptoms. The two cardinal signs of PIH are proteinuria and a blood pressure of 140/90 or higher on two occasions within 6 hours, or an increase of 50 mm systolic or 15 mm diastolic or both over the baseline blood pressure (Gilbert & Harmon, 2003).

Effects on the Fetus and Neonate. Perinatal mortality related to PIH usually ranges from 1% to 8%; if the condition is allowed to progress to eclampsia or HELLP syndrome, the incidence is as high as 35%. Most perinatal losses are directly related to placental insufficiency, resulting in intrauterine fetal demise or early neonatal death in an already compromised premature infant.

Placental insufficiency in PIH usually leads to some degree of nutritional intrauterine growth restriction. The fetus is asymmetrically affected in that head size is close to normal for gestation, but general body size and fat deposition are decreased. This nutritional deprivation causes the fetus to be more vulnerable to the effects of labor contractions and other stressors. During antepartum or intrapartum monitoring, the fetus is more likely to show signs of fetal stress when oxygen and carbon dioxide exchange is mildly compromised over a shorter period.

Growth restriction of the fetus is more often associated with a decrease in the amount of amniotic fluid as well. Any repetitive occlusion of the umbilical cord during contractions or with fetal movement may cause stress. Signs of fetal stress with FHR monitoring may include tachycardia (a rate over 160 beats per minute, or an increase of more than 20 beats per minute over the previous baseline); absence of long- or short-term variability; or late decelerations with or without cord compression (variable decelerations) (Gilbert & Harmon, 2003).

Treatment. The only cure for PIH is delivery. Treatment is aimed at stabilizing the mother's condition and at reducing the immediate risks to the fetus, which include prematurity and fetal compromise caused by maternal hypertension (Box 12-3).

BOX 12-3

Nursing Management of Hypertensive Disorders of Pregnancy

Assessments
- Fetus: Monitor for signs of fetal stress intermittently during antepartum period (i.e., with contraction stress tests or nonstress tests); monitor continuously during intrapartum period.
- Mother: Monitor blood pressure and laboratory studies.

Interventions
- Treat signs of fetal stress with maternal bed rest in left lateral position. Provide oxygen therapy and prevent volume depletion.
- Administer antihypertensive drugs intravenously only in conjunction with continuous fetal heart rate monitoring.
- Teach pregnant women at risk for pregnancy-induced hypertension to recognize and report early signs and symptoms.

Because the maternal intravascular volume is depleted through loss of intravascular fluid into interstitial tissue, absolute bed rest facilitates optimum use of the existing intravascular volume. Other treatment methods vary in relation to antepartum, intrapartum, or postpartum complications.

Antepartum. Treatment is directed at improving maternal status to gain gestational time for the fetus. Treatment consists of the following (Creasy & Resnik, 1999):
- Pharmacologic treatment of maternal hypertension with drugs such as hydralazine, alpha-methyldopa, clonidine, or sodium nitroprusside. There has been long-term experience with the use of hydralazine for rapid response to hypertension and with alpha-methyldopa for long-term effects.
- Intermittent evaluation of fetal well-being through contraction stress or nonstress tests or biophysical profiles.
- Ultrasound evaluation for growth of fetus every 2 to 3 weeks.
- High-protein diet for the mother (more than 100 g per day).
- Monitoring of maternal laboratory studies (i.e., uric acid, platelets, liver enzymes) and clinical signs for worsening of the disease.

Diuretics and severe sodium restriction have no place in the treatment of PIH and in fact may worsen the disease. Likewise, long-term expectant management is not likely to result in improved maternal or fetal status and therefore is not practiced in most centers (Creasy & Resnik, 1999).

Intrapartum. Treatment is aimed at obtaining and maintaining immediate stabilization of the mother's condition and then delivering the premature or mature fetus. Stabilization consists of the following (Creasy & Resnik, 1999):
- Pharmacologic therapy with intravenous magnesium sulfate to prevent central nervous system irritability and treatment of maternal hypertension above 160/100 with hydralazine or other fast-acting antihypertensives.
- Plasma volume expanders, which may be used as a temporary therapy.
- Determination of a delivery route based on whether labor can be induced (cervical ripening), the gestation of the fetus, and fetal tolerance to the stress of labor. A surgical delivery may not be safe for a woman with signs of DIC or HELLP syndrome because of the potential for hemorrhage. On the other hand, continuing the pregnancy through labor may not be tolerated by the fetus or may progress to eclampsia in a mother with HELLP syndrome because of diminished clotting factors; an epidural may be contraindicated because of the increased potential for epidural space bleeding. Given these circumstances, a surgical delivery with general anesthesia would be the best choice.

Diabetes in Pregnancy

In pregnancy, diabetes is classified according to White's classification system (Table 12-1) (Gilbert & Harmon, 2003). This system originally was intended to prognosticate neonatal outcome. It subsequently was modified and is now used primarily to make decisions on timing fetal surveillance and to evaluate for maternal complications.

Incidence. Diabetes is a factor in 1% to 2% of all pregnancies. Women can readily be screened for gestational onset with a 50-g glucola load and a 1-hour post-blood glucose study. Levels above 120 to 140 mg are evaluated for insulin requirement with a 3-hour glucose tolerance test that yields two or more abnormal results or when the fasting blood glucose level rises above 110 mg/% while the patient is treated with diet.

Etiology.   Diabetes exists when insufficient effective insulin is produced by the beta cells in the islets of Langerhans' in the pancreas. Pregnancy has been likened to a diabetogenic state because of increases in the metabolism of protein, fat, and carbohydrate that require additional insulin. The increased production of estrogen, progesterone, human placental lactogen (HPL), and cortisol has an antagonistic effect on insulin made by the body or taken exogenously. Women at risk for developing gestational-onset diabetes are those who are over age 35 years; chronically hypertensive; obese; a multigravida with a previous unexplained stillbirth, more than two or three spontaneous miscarriages, or a previous macrosomic infant at term (especially if larger than 9 pounds); and women who have a strong family history of diabetes or a history of frequent vaginal monilial infections, or a current history of glucosuria (Gilbert & Harmon, 2003).

Pathophysiology.   During the first trimester, changes in maternal metabolism foster rapid cell division and organ differentiation in the embryo. Thyroid function enhances the metabolic rate, increasing the need for protein and fat stores and rapid glucose use. The need for insulin commonly declines, and this may be further complicated by a decrease in food intake because of early pregnancy nausea and vomiting.

TABLE **12-1**	White's Classification System for Diabetes in Pregnancy
Category	**Description**
Class A	Gestational onset, normal fasting blood glucose level: diet control required
	Gestational onset, abnormal fasting blood glucose level: insulin therapy required
Class B	Onset after age 20: insulin therapy required (This is type II diabetes mellitus, even if it is not discovered until the pregnancy is confirmed; the diagnosis is revealed by a glycolysated hemoglobin test in the first trimester.)
Class C	Strong family or patient history points to early screening for diabetes: in these cases, a glycolysated hemoglobin test aids in more timely control of blood sugar early in the pregnancy and in postpartum follow-up of the mother (Gilbert & Harmon, 2003)
Class D	Onset after age 10, duration less than 10 years, no vascular complications: insulin therapy required
Class F	Onset before age 10, or duration longer than 10 years, or early vascular complications: insulin therapy required
Class H	Renal and retinal changes: insulin therapy required
Class R	Renal changes: insulin therapy required
Class T	Heart complications, mother often over age 35 with early age onset of diabetes, 50% risk of obstetrical maternal mortality: insulin therapy required
	Postrenal transplantation: insulin therapy required

The placenta begins to function as its own endocrine organ in the second trimester, producing increasing amounts of estrogen, progesterone, human placental lactogen (HPL) and cortisol. These hormones work antagonistically against the effectiveness of insulin for carrying glucose into cells. The pancreas must produce more insulin to overcome the antagonistic effects of the four hormones. If it is unable to do so, glucose builds up in the maternal bloodstream, and metabolism is diverted to an anaerobic route. Amino acids and fats are burned in excess during anaerobic metabolism, leading eventually to ketoacidemia in the mother. Because the normal fetal pH is lower and derived solely from the maternal blood in the intervillous space, fetal acidemia is likely.

Excess glucose from the maternal circulation is used and stored in the placenta. As the fetus draws on the glucose, the fetal pancreas is stimulated to produce increased amounts of insulin. The increased fetal insulin acts as a growth promoter, causing the fetus to grow large and to increase the deposition of body adipose tissue.

As a vascular organ, the placenta is vulnerable to the vascular complications of maternal diabetes. It may age earlier or faster, or it may not develop sufficiently to provide the fetus with an adequate blood supply. The placenta may also swell with added fluid, resulting in poor diffusion of necessary substrates, carbon dioxide, and oxygen (Gilbert & Harmon, 2003).

Effects on the Fetus and Neonate.   One of the possible fetal effects is interference with DNA-RNA transfer as a result of maternal high blood glucose before and at the time of conception. This effect probably explains the high incidence of neonatal congenital heart defects, lethal and nonlethal neurologic malformations, GI defects, and renal polycystic disease. If the blood glucose level remained high for longer than 3 months before conception, DNA-RNA transfer is interrupted, and the problems just mentioned, as well as other more minor defects, may result. The mechanisms of these defects are still poorly understood and only theoretic (James, et al, 2000; Gilbert & Harmon, 2003). Increased, rapid fetal body growth and decreased fetal brain and body growth also are possible.

Neonatal effects include hypoglycemia in the transitional period because of high insulin production but loss of maternal glucose supply; hyperbilirubinemia from increased "glucose saturated" fetal hemoglobin and breakdown of this in the early neonatal period; hypercalcemia, hypokalemia, and other abnormalities in electrolytes; increased incidence of cesarean birth or traumatic vaginal birth, usually from shoulder dystocias; neonatal respiratory distress syndrome even after 36 weeks; and high maternal blood glucose, high placental glucose storage, high placental production of cortisol, low fetal production of cortisol, and low surfactant production, all leading to decreased lung maturity at expected gestation (Creasy & Resnik, 1999; Gilbert & Harmon, 2003).

Treatment.   Medical treatment of a pregnancy complicated by diabetes is aimed at maintenance of euglycemia before conception and throughout the pregnancy (Box 12-4). Euglycemia requires a careful balance of diet, insulin, and activity (Creasy & Resnik, 1999). The diet should consist of 1800 to 2400 calories, divided into four to six meals made up of 50% complex carbohydrate, 30% fat, and 20% protein. Insulin, when required, is given in a split-dose regimen, usually consisting of some combination of regular and intermediate insulin based on a prospective regulation of blood glucose levels between 60 mg/% and

---

BOX 12-4

Antepartum Nursing Management of Diabetes in Pregnancy

Assessment
- Maternal educational needs
- Fetal assessment with evaluation of fetal movement counts, nonstress tests, or contraction stress tests
- Maternal complications of polyhydramnios, pregnancy-induced hypertension, urinary tract infection, preterm labor, or persistent abnormal blood glucose levels

Intervention
- Education of the pregnant woman and those in her support system for the following:
  - □ Dietary management
  - □ Blood glucose determination four to six times daily
  - □ Insulin injections and changes in dosage
  - □ Activity schedule and necessary modification
  - □ Effects of diabetes and pregnancy on herself and the fetus
  - □ Reason for testing for maternal and fetal complications
- Support and assistance with time management problems and financial stressors arising from increase in testing.

TABLE 12-2 Cardiac Disease Classification

Category	Description
Class I	Asymptomatic
Class II	Symptomatic with increased exercise
Class III	Symptomatic with normal exercise
Class IV	Symptomatic at rest

for about 50% of cases, and congenital heart disease is responsible for the other half.

Etiology. Cardiac disease in pregnancy may take one of several forms: rheumatic fever, valve deformities, congenital heart disease, congestive cardiomyopathies, or cardiac dysrhythmias. Several conditions may predispose pregnant women to a mortality rate above 50%, including Marfan syndrome with aortic arch dissection; primary pulmonary hypertension, manifested by Eisenmenger syndrome (pulmonary hypertension); and diabetes complicated by heart disease.

Pathophysiology. When the heart fails as an efficient pump, blood volume is shunted to essential organ systems in the body. During pregnancy, a diseased heart may be unable to respond efficiently to the increased circulating volume. As blood is shunted to essential organs for the mother, it may bypass the growing uterus, placenta, and intervillous space, and thus the fetus to some extent.

Effects on the Fetus and Neonate. The fetus or neonate may suffer adverse effects as a result of decreased maternal placental blood flow, including diminished fetal body growth, diminished brain growth, and a higher incidence of fetal wastage and pregnancy loss. During the intrapartum period, the fetus may be stressed beyond capacity to demonstrate the ability to withstand labor. Signs of fetal stress may include deceleration patterns, such as late decelerations because of insufficient uteroplacental blood flow or variable decelerations because of insufficient amniotic fluid to protect the umbilical cord from compression.

If delivered prematurely for maternal reasons, the neonate has the additional difficulties of premature birth. If congenital heart disease is present in the mother, the risk is greater of congenital heart abnormalities in the neonate as well (Gilbert & Harmon, 2003).

Fetal Assessment

Antepartum. Fetal assessment during the antepartum period consists of ultrasonography for growth rate and nonstress or contraction stress tests, biophysical profiles, or some combination of these on a weekly or biweekly basis after 26 weeks' gestation. It is important to try to prevent associated maternal complications such as anemia or severe preeclampsia, which might further compromise fetal well-being.

Intrapartum. Fetal assessment during the intrapartal period includes carefully monitored labor for problems with maternal cardiac preload or afterload, often with central line hemodynamic invasive monitoring; continuous FHR monitoring, often with the pregnant woman on her left side with oxygen therapy; and a shortened and assisted second stage of labor, usually with epidural anesthesia or analgesia to reduce pain and cardiac workload as well as preload. Because pain is a com-

---

150 mg/% and an activity schedule that does not vary much from day to day or week to week.

Careful evaluation of the maternal estimated date of delivery is required before fetal surveillance parameters can be ordered. In general, this estimate is made with an early prenatal examination, history, and ultrasound confirmation. Further early maternal evaluation for diabetic vascular complications in insulin-dependent diabetes may include glycosylated hemoglobin, 24-hour urine tests for protein and creatinine, recent eye examination, and an electrocardiogram.

Antepartum fetal surveillance includes maternal serum alpha-fetoprotein measurement to screen for neural tube defects; ultrasound evaluation between 15 and 20 weeks' gestation for congenital developmental problems and also for growth rate, usually between 26 and 30 weeks and near expected delivery (37 to 38 weeks); amniocentesis for fetal lung maturity at the time of the last ultrasound evaluation; and fetal movement counts ("kick counts") daily, biweekly nonstress tests, weekly contraction stress tests, weekly ultrasound biophysical profile evaluation, or some combination of testing weekly. These tests may begin anytime after 25 weeks and before 38 weeks, depending on the risk to the fetus and maternal complications.

Intrapartum management usually consists of an insulin drip for an insulin-dependent labor patient. If laboring for an anticipated vaginal birth, continuous FHR monitoring should be evaluated for the onset of signs of fetal stress.

Cardiac Disease and Pregnancy

Although a patient's classification for cardiac disease (Table 12-2) does not change for the worse with pregnancy, the increased workload on the heart may increase symptoms by one or two classification levels (Gilbert & Harmon, 2003).

Incidence. The incidence of cardiac disease in pregnant women varies from 0.5% to 2%. Rheumatic fever is responsible

plex interaction of physiologic and psychologic factors, pain management requires pharmacologic agents and good communication. Good communication may include cognitive management through thorough explanation of the next anticipated step (Lowe, 1996).

Urinary Tract Disease in Pregnancy

Urinary tract infection (UTI) occurs in 4% to 7.5% of childbearing women. Approximately 30% of pregnant women with untreated asymptomatic bacteriuria develop pyelonephritis during pregnancy. The organisms usually responsible for UTI are *Escherichia coli*, staphylococci, or streptococci. An inflammation in bladder or renal tissue may result in fever and increased production of prostaglandins. An increase in prostaglandin production predisposes a pregnant woman to preterm labor and thus the fetus to preterm delivery. If maternal sepsis develops, fetal fever and infection from amnionitis often result.

Renal disease in pregnancy is infrequently the result of diabetic glomerulonephritis or maternal connective tissue disease, especially if end-stage renal disease has occurred. In general, women with end-stage renal disease do not ovulate. When they do become pregnant, fetal wastage is high because of the increase in urea byproducts in the maternal bloodstream and amniotic fluid. As a result, the fetus grows poorly and often succumbs to the hostile maternal environment.

UTIs and fever must be treated with appropriate antibiotics therapeutically or prophylactically or both. Treatment of renal disease, which may temporarily worsen in pregnancy in response to increased renal blood flow and work, usually is aimed at clearing the maternal blood of urea wastes. Most recently, some success has been reported with continuous ambulatory peritoneal dialysis for end-stage renal disease in pregnancy (Gilbert & Harmon, 2003).

Nursing Management.   Nursing management for UTI is primarily aimed at preventing infection, reinfection, and preterm labor. This management is best accomplished through prenatal education regarding an increased oral fluid intake of 6 to 8 ounces per waking hour; perineal hygiene, with cleaning front to back and urination after intercourse; recognition of early signs of preterm labor; and reporting of early signs of infection and preterm labor.

MATERNAL TRANSPORT

Many states have regionalized care centers for newborns and pregnant women. Hospitals or care centers may be designated as level I, II, or III, depending on the extent and complexity of prenatal care available (Table 12-3).

Identification of Need

A level III perinatal service provides services for all mothers and neonates, has research support, and is able to compile, analyze, and evaluate regional data. It is desirable to have a level III regionalized center available and centrally located in relation to several level I and level II facilities. Transport equipment and educated team members should be accessible within a reasonable time. Ideally, maternal transport should occur, because the mother is the best incubator. The availability of research and resources makes this a more likely reality in a level III facility than in a level I or level II facility.

TABLE 12-3	Level of Care According to Pregnancy Risk
Care Level	**Pregnancy Risk**
Level I	Low-risk pregnant women and their healthy newborns
Level II	Moderate-risk pregnant women likely to deliver newborns without need for ventilatory assistance; also low-risk pregnant women and their newborns
Level III	High-risk pregnant women likely to deliver high-risk newborns requiring specialized technologic care; also moderate- and low-risk pregnant women and their newborns

Modified from Gilbert E, Harmon J (2003). Manual of high risk pregnancy and delivery, ed 3. Mosby: St Louis.

Population

Assignment of maternity patients into high-risk and low-risk categories is useful for defining patient acuity and determining staffing patterns. Determinations of staffing requirements should be related to patient acuity, numbers, staff education and experience, and facility resources.

Equipment

A level III center should have state of the art equipment available for monitoring fetal well-being. This monitoring includes antepartum and intrapartum FHR monitoring and ultrasonography. Immediate cesarean delivery should be available in the delivery suites and ideally in the labor, delivery, and recovery areas. Antepartum maternal care requiring invasive hemodynamic monitoring should be a technical resource.

Evaluation or Maternal-Fetal Stabilization

Ideally, the fetus is incubated maternally until fetal lung maturity is determined. However, certain maternal conditions (e.g., HELLP syndrome, connective tissue disease, cardiac compromise) may unbalance the risk-benefit ratio in such a way that delivery of a premature infant would result in the best neonatal outcome. These decisions are best made when sophisticated maternal and fetal surveillance techniques are available and level III nursery facilities can be used. Stabilization is used when that ratio is weighted toward either "better off delivered" or "better off undelivered." Depending on the maternal or fetal condition and the treatment methods available, the decision may take hours or days (Beauchamp & Childress, 2001; Gilbert and Harmon, 2003).

Care during Transport

Fixed-wing airplane, helicopter, and ground transport should all be options for maternal transport from level I or level II facilities to level III centers. Teams composed of qualified staff members, a nurse, and a physician should respond to the request for transport. Fetal monitoring equipment should be used when appropriate during transport. Transport staff must have education and experience in labor and delivery care of high-risk mothers and neonates (Gilbert & Harmon, 2003).

> ### BOX 12-5
>
> #### Possible Legal Pitfalls in a High-Risk Obstetric Practice
>
> - Staff fails to keep current in knowledge and skills.
> - Risks for mother or neonate are not adequately identified.
> - New or unexpected complications are not anticipated, and no preparations are made for such complications.
> - Families are not included in decision making and are not informed about risks or consequences.
> - Consultation is not sought although clearly available—and consultation is *always* available as a result of technologic advances in means of communication.

Modified from Gilbert E, Harmon J (2003). Manual of high risk pregnancy and delivery, ed 3. Mosby: St Louis.

LEGAL ISSUES

Obstetric litigation leads in major medical malpractice cases (Box 12-5). The four elements necessary for successful litigation are duty, breach of duty, causation, and proven damage. Duty is the particular relationship that arises when a hospital, nursing staff, and physician agree to assume the care of a particular patient. Breach of duty occurs when one or more members of that group do not meet the minimum agreed-upon standard of care. Causation is shown when the breach of duty has a direct link to the proven cause of the actual damages. Proven damage generally is physical and often lasting (Chapter 4).

The best defense is always to consider the risk-benefit ratio to the mother and unborn infant. Professional behavior demands that caregivers act as advocates for patients unable to do so themselves and that they safeguard patients from harm that may result from the unsafe, illegal, or unethical conduct of others.

SUMMARY

This chapter has presented a brief overview of the most common maternal high-risk conditions and the effects on the fetus and neonate. It has presented information in a manner to help neonatal nurses understand how the neonate comes to need special care.

REFERENCES

Beauchamp T, Childress J (2001). *Principles of biomedical ethics.* Oxford Press: New York.

Brent N (2000). *Nurses and the law,* ed 2. WB Saunders: Philadelphia.

Creasy R, Resnik M (1999). *Maternal fetal medicine: principles and practice,* ed 3. WB Saunders: Philadelphia.

Davis J, Sherer K (1993). *Applied nutrition and diet therapy for nurses.* WB Saunders: Philadelphia.

Gabbe S et al (1996): *Obstetrics: normal and problem pregnancies.* Churchill Livingstone: New York.

Gilbert E, Harmon J (2003). *Manual of high risk pregnancy and delivery,* ed 3. Mosby: St Louis.

James D et al, editors (2000). *High risk pregnancy: management options,* ed 2. WB Saunders: Philadelphia.

Lowe NK (1996). The pain and discomfort of labor and birth. *Journal of obstetric, gynecologic, and neonatal nursing* 25(1), 82-92.

Moore KL, Persaud TVN (1998). *Before we are born: essentials of embryology and birth defects,* ed 5. WB Saunders: Philadelphia.

Svigos J et al (2000): Threatened and actual preterm labor, including mode of delivery. In James D et al, editors. *High risk pregnancy: management options,* ed 2. WB Saunders: Philadelphia.

FETAL THERAPY

JODY A. FARRELL, MARIBETH INTURRISI, KATHY BERGMAN, CAROLE KENNER, LORI J. HOWELL

Throughout history, human fetal development has been viewed as a mysterious and secretive process, held in such awe that some ancient cultural rituals focused on protecting the pregnant woman from evil spirits in order to shield the fetus from harm. To a large extent, ultrasonography has unveiled that mystery, altered attitudes about the developing fetus, and become the medium by which the fetal growth and development unfolding in the womb are accurately documented. In addition, and perhaps more importantly, in the past two decades major advances in fetal imaging and diagnostic techniques have dramatically improved our ability to identify, comprehend, and manage many prenatally diagnosed malformations, ironically by providing a means of following the natural history of the untreated disease. Early diagnosis and close follow-up of fetuses with congenital malformations have been the keys to determining which clinical features affect the outcome, as well as the management approaches that improve the prognosis and outcome. Increasingly sophisticated ultrasonographic equipment and techniques aid in identifying a growing number of fetal disorders and structural defects at a stage early enough to allow prenatal intervention. For a number of these fetal defects, selection criteria for in utero intervention have been defined, and anesthesia, tocolysis, and surgical techniques for hysterotomy and fetal surgery have been developed and refined (Harrison, 1996). As a result of these advances, the fetus has claimed a role as a patient in its own right.

For the nursing profession specifically, fetal therapy presents a wide variety of interesting and complex challenges. The nurse is called on to provide counseling, educational, organizational, and technical skills to the treatment team and to patients and their families. Nurses also provide significant insight on the ethical and moral considerations that arise in this evolving field of medicine. This chapter provides an historical perspective of fetal treatment, including fetal surgery, and describes in some detail the key events of this multifaceted, complex area of fetal treatment, recognizing that the number of congenital anomalies amenable to in utero intervention is increasing and that approaches to treatment are improving. It also describes collaborative health team management of patients undergoing fetal therapy and outlines future trends in the field.

HISTORICAL OVERVIEW

A possible strategy for treating erythroblastosis fetalis, a life-threatening fetal and neonatal complication, prompted the first attempt at amelioration of a fetal condition. In 1963, New Zealand clinician-scientist A.W. Liley performed an in utero, fluoroscopy-guided exchange transfusion of red blood cells into the abdomen of a 32-week fetus. He believed that the red blood cells would be carried into the fetal bloodstream via the lymphatics, and he proved to be correct (Liley, 1963). The attempt of this procedure, let alone its success, was heralded as opening a new direction and a new era in obstetric and pediatric care; it effectively marked the birth of fetal treatment, the in utero medical intervention or correction of a fetal condition. As a result of Liley's work, not only have treatments for erythroblastosis fetalis and other fetal anemias been refined and improved (Laifer & Kuller, 1996), but other researchers have been encouraged to pursue and develop therapies helpful to their fetal patients.

Advances and improvements in imaging technology have been the hallmarks of the evolving field of fetal treatment. In the 1950s and 1960s, the use of ultrasonography as a diagnostic and imaging tool gave rise to farther-reaching implications in health care, and Ian Donald specifically is credited with developing its application in obstetrics. Ultrasonography now can be reliably used to determine gestational age, fetal growth patterns, fetal well-being, amniotic fluid levels, and the position of the placenta. It also can detect certain congenital anomalies (especially structural malformations when imaging is performed before 24 weeks' gestation), and it is this capability that particularly links ultrasonography to fetal diagnosis and treatment.

Ultrasonography has also proved to be an essential adjunct to other prenatal diagnostic procedures such as amniocentesis, chorionic villus sampling, and percutaneous umbilical blood sampling (Chapter 41). These techniques, coupled with ultrasonography, laid the groundwork for the new frontier of fetal treatment. Once abnormal fetal conditions could be detected early, many then became amenable to prenatal treatment. No longer were management options limited to termination of the pregnancy or postnatal treatment. Table 13-1 lists the fetal conditions that often prove amenable to medical or surgical treatment in utero.

TABLE 13-1	Fetal Conditions Amenable to In Utero Treatment
Condition	**Intervention**
FETAL THERAPY: MEDICAL TREATMENT	
Rh sensitization	Red cell transfusion (into umbilical vessel or intraperitoneal)
Pulmonary immaturity	Betamethasone (transplacental)
Vitamin B_{12} deficiency	Vitamin B_{12} (transplacental)
Carboxylase deficiency	Biotin (transplacental)
Supraventricular tachycardia (SVT)	Digoxin, flecainide, or similar drug (transplacental)
Heart block	Betamimetics (transplacental)
Hypothyroidism	Thyroxine (transplacental)
Adrenal hyperplasia	Steroids
Intrauterine growth restriction (IUGR)	Protein calories (transamniotic)
Severe combined immunodeficiency syndrome (SCID)	Stem cell transplantation into umbilical vessel
FETAL THERAPY: SURGICAL TREATMENT	
Urinary tract obstructions	Closed procedure (i.e., percutaneous catheter placement) or open procedure (i.e., vesicostomy)
Hydronephrosis	
Lung hypoplasia	
Renal and respiratory failure	
Diaphragmatic hernia	Open procedure (i.e., decompression of chest contents); placement of Gore-Tex patch; repair of diaphragm
Lung hypoplasia	
Respiratory failure	
Cystic adenoma formation	Closed procedure (i.e., placement of catheter for decompression) or open procedure (i.e., correction of malformation)
Lung hypoplasia	
Respiratory failure	

In 1981 Michael Harrison and a multidisciplinary team of perinatologists, geneticists, anesthesiologists, neonatologists, and nurses at the University of California at San Francisco became the first group to clinically attempt correction of urinary tract obstruction in utero. As clinicians, these researchers often were faced with the reality that infants diagnosed with bilateral congenital hydronephrosis were delivered stillborn or died during the neonatal period as a result of severe pulmonary hypoplasia (i.e., failure of the lungs to develop) or renal failure (Chapter 33). Having thoroughly documented the natural history of the untreated disease in animals, Harrison and his co-investigators hypothesized that if the outlet obstruction could be corrected before birth, the fatal pulmonary hypoplasia or renal failure could be averted. The hypothesis was extensively and successfully tested in fetal sheep, and the surgical and anesthesia techniques were worked out. This paved the way for the first attempt at a closed surgical procedure in a human fetus with urinary tract obstruction.

In the 1981 case, a catheter needle was passed through the maternal abdominal wall into the fetal bladder (Figure 13-1). An indwelling bladder catheter then was secured to drain fluid from the bladder into the amniotic sac; this catheter remained in place until birth. The procedure was successful at decompressing the bladder and restoring amniotic fluid volume. Then (as now), although the cause of the obstruction was not corrected until the neonatal period, the deleterious effects of the obstruction were averted while the fetus continued to grow and develop.

The success of the intervention expanded the possibilities of fetal and neonatal medicine. Other physicians began to consider using this type of rationale for treatment and this type of surgery for other anomalies. By the early 1980s, it became evident that this therapeutic approach was not just a passing trend.

About the same time, an international group of physicians and scientists met in Santa Ynez, California, to discuss new directions in the medical sciences. This meeting resulted in the formation of the International Fetal Surgery Society, later renamed the International Fetal Medicine and Surgery Society (Manning, 1986). The organization created an International Fetal Surgery Registry to track the number, type, and outcome of fetal surgical attempts. Because reporting is voluntary, the registry by no means represents all cases of fetal surgery; however, it is a means of much-needed data collection that yields insight into the many variables of fetal disease.

Three registries now exist, collecting data from around the world on many types of fetal disorders. In the United States, the only centers that currently perform open procedures involving hysterotomy and direct fetal surgery are the fetal treatment centers of the University of California at San Francisco, Children's Hospital of Philadelphia, and Vanderbilt University Medical Center. However, the number of institutions that offer fetal therapy as a treatment option has grown considerably and includes Boston Children's Hospital, Georgetown University, Wayne State University, the University of Manitoba, the University of Toronto, the University of Montreal, and many more. Fetal therapy also is offered at centers in Italy, Germany, France, Denmark, England, New Zealand, Australia, Israel, Chile, Argentina, and Yugoslavia.

Fetus as Patient: Maternal-Fetal Risks and Benefits

Fetal surgery is predicated first and foremost on a responsibility to the mother to ensure her safety, because she, along with her unborn child, is a patient in this endeavor. The risk-benefit ratio favors the fetus with a lethal malformation, because without intervention, the mortality rate is 100%, and with intervention, survival is possible. The risks, however, are not that easily justified for the mother, who essentially is an innocent bystander whose physical health usually is not jeopardized by her unborn baby's condition. For this reason, before clinical application of fetal surgery could be considered, it had to be proved that any intervention through the mother would not imperil her safety. As a result, fetal surgical procedures were tested first in the most rigorous animal model, the nonhuman primate (monkey), whose anatomy and physiology most closely resembles that of the human pregnancy.

The first technical issue addressed was how to safely open and close the gravid uterus such that bleeding and chorioamnion membrane separation were prevented and a watertight closure could be attained. The University of California at San Francisco (UCSF) group solved this problem by developing an absorbable stapling device and special back-biting retractors for the uterine edges. The uterus then could be closed in two layers with absorbable sutures supplemented with fibrin glue.

Next, a way had to be found to monitor the fetus and uterine activity after the procedure. Consequently, a relatively large radiotelemeter was developed that could be placed inside the fetus in a submuscular pocket. This device monitored fetal heart rate and temperature and uterine pressure (contrac-

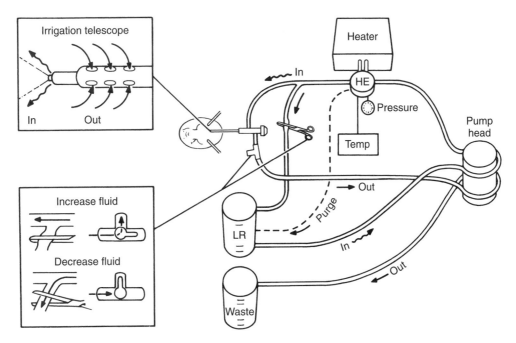

FIGURE **13-1**
Warmed lactated Ringer's solution is circulated through the inner sheath of the hysteroscope and exits at the lighted tip. Amniotic fluid can be suctioned via the outer sheath. The irrigation and aspiration volumes can be carefully regulated with the pump.

tions). The radiotelemeter now has been miniaturized to the point that it can be passed down a trocar during fetoscopic procedures; it floats in the amniotic fluid, emitting signals that are translated onto a real-time bedside computer.

Although there have been no reports of maternal death during or after fetal intervention, maternal morbidity associated with preterm labor and its treatment remains an issue. The most common side effect of the tocolytic therapy, pulmonary edema, occurs while women are receiving high doses of these medications to stop preterm labor. Although reversible, this complication emphasizes the need for close monitoring in an intensive care setting (DiFederico et al, 1998; Farrell et al, 1999). The move toward fetoscopic procedures (discussed later in this chapter) has been a tremendous advance in fetal intervention. Pulmonary edema has rarely been reported after fetoscopic procedures, because these minimally invasive techniques incite less uterine irritability than does open fetal surgery (which requires an open hysterotomy), and they therefore usually require lower doses and combinations of tocolytics (Kiatano et al, 1999).

Another important consideration was preservation of the mother's reproductive capability. During open fetal surgery, the hysterotomy often is not performed in the lower uterine segment because of fetal or placental positioning (or both) and because the lower uterine segment is not fully developed in the second trimester. To avoid the risk of uterine scar dehiscence during labor, delivery by means of cesarean section is advised after fetal surgery and for all future pregnancies. However, this is not necessary after fetoscopic procedures.

The ability to carry and deliver subsequent pregnancies does not appear to be jeopardized by fetal surgery; a recent survey of fetal surgery patients revealed that of the 27 mothers who attempted pregnancy after fetal surgery, 25 conceived and delivered normal children. The two women who failed to conceive both had a strong preoperative history of infertility (Farrell et al, 1999).

Ethical Considerations
Fetal therapy presents new and often complex ethical dilemmas to the health care system and to society. Some fetal procedures are still considered experimental, and for these, ethical considerations can be addressed through the process of obtaining approval from the center's institutional review board and developing an informed consent procedure. Many fetal treatment centers find discussion and review by an ethics committee or fetal surgery oversight committee useful in developing protocols for complex or controversial treatments and for evaluating challenging clinical cases. A clear requirement, however, is that the proposed course of action must respect the patient's authority, elicit the patient's preferences, and acknowledge the patient's life values. Every institution has an established protocol for offering and providing an experimental treatment, and these guidelines should always be followed to guarantee ethical conduct with regard to the procedure and, more important, to safeguard the patient's rights.

FETAL SURGICAL TECHNIQUES

Open Fetal Surgery
The timing of open fetal surgery depends on the malformation and its pathophysiologic course. Difficulty determining an accurate diagnosis and the fragility of fetal tissue are limiting factors for performing procedures at less than 18 weeks' gestation. After 30 weeks' gestation, manipulation of the uterus is associated with a high risk of premature rupture of the membranes (PROM) and preterm labor; if these occur, delivery of the fetus and treatment of the malformation with standard postnatal care becomes a more reasonable approach.

In open fetal surgery, a general anesthetic is administered to the mother (and transferred to the fetus through the placenta), and a low abdominal transverse (Pfannenstiel) incision is made to open the maternal abdomen and visualize the uterus.

Intraoperative ultrasound is then used to identify the position of the fetus and the location of the placenta. Depending on the placenta's location, an anterior or posterior hysterotomy is performed with a specially developed, absorbable uterine stapling device that provides hemostasis and seals the membranes to the myometrium. The fetus is given a narcotic and paralytic agent intramuscularly, and the appropriate fetal part or parts are exposed.

Throughout the procedure, warm lactated Ringer's solution is continuously infused around the fetus and open uterus to maintain fetal body temperature. Fetal monitoring during the surgery is done with a sterile pulse oximeter and a radiotelemetric device (usually implanted under the pectoral muscle), which records the fetal electrocardiogram and temperature and the intrauterine amniotic pressure. After the defect has been repaired, the fetus is returned to the womb, and amniotic fluid is restored with warm saline containing an antibiotic, such as nafcillin. The uterine incision is closed with two layers of absorbable suture, and fibrin glue is used to help seal the incision and prevent leakage of amniotic fluid.

Minimally Invasive Fetal Surgery

Although fetoscopic techniques for direct visualization of the fetus are not new, recent modifications of postnatal endoscopic techniques and the development of new fetoscopic instruments have resulted in minimal access fetal surgery (FETENDO). The FETENDO technique has proved successful at preserving fetal homeostasis by protecting the intrauterine physiologic milieu, and the maternal morbidity associated uterine incision (e.g., preterm labor, postoperative bleeding) has been avoided (Albanese & Harrison, 1998a).

For a FETENDO procedure, the mother is placed in a modified lithotomy position. Anesthetic techniques, tocolytic therapy, and maternal monitoring are the same as for open fetal surgery. Preoperative and intraoperative sonography map the position of the placenta and the fetus and guide placement of the trocar. An anterior placenta usually requires a low transverse abdominal incision to expose the uterus, and the trocars are placed superiorly and posteriorly. Continuous irrigation using a pump irrigation system via the sheath of the hysteroscope is crucial to optimizing visibility (Figure 13-1). This system maintains a constant intrauterine fluid volume, avoids the risk of air embolus with gas distention of the uterus, ensures a continuously washed operative field, improves visibility by exchanging the cloudy amniotic fluid with lactated Ringer's solution, and keeps the fetus warm.

One of the obstacles with the FETENDO technique is manipulating the fetus into the correct position and keeping it there for the duration of the procedure. This very often frustrating problem is best illustrated by the development of FETENDO tracheal occlusion to treat congenital diaphragmatic hernia, in which a chin stitch (Figure 13-2) is used to keep the fetal neck exposed by extending the head (Albanese et al, 1998a; Harrison et al, 1998). At the end of the procedure, the amniotic fluid volume is assessed by sonography and optimized. Antibiotics are subsequently infused, the trocars are withdrawn, and the puncture site is closed with absorbable suture and fibrin glue.

Anesthesia

Anesthesia is necessary regardless of the approach to fetal intervention (i.e., percutaneous or as an open surgical procedure). The situation is complex because the anesthesiologist must consider the two patients who are being anesthetized simultaneously. The particular hazards of anesthesia during pregnancy are related to physiologic changes in the mother and possible adverse effects on the fetus. Therefore anesthetizing a pregnant woman during major surgery requires specially trained anesthesiologists who can provide low-level anesthesia and pain management for the maternal-fetal unit while ensur-

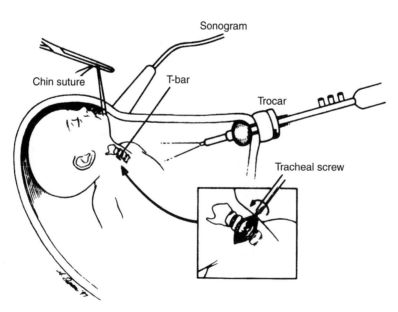

FIGURE **13-2**
Under sonographic guidance, (1) the fetus's neck is exposed, and the head is stabilized by placing a transuterine chin suture; (2) a T-bar is placed in the fetal trachea to help localize the midline of the neck. After anterior tracheal dissection has been performed, a tracheal "screw" (inset) is placed in the tracheal wall and anterior traction is applied, allowing safe posterolateral tracheal dissection. The trachea subsequently is occluded with a titanium clip. Courtesy The Fetal Treatment Center, University of California, San Francisco.

ing the mother's safety and minimal side effects for both patients (Collins, 1994).

In developing anesthetic techniques for fetal surgery, researchers had to consider the physiologic differences between healthy pregnant women and healthy nonpregnant women. A pregnant woman shows a decrease in peripheral vascular resistance (cardiac output increases with no increase in blood pressure, resulting in a decrease in peripheral vascular resistance); a decrease in functional residual capacity and an increase in alveolar ventilation (which speeds up induction with inhalation anesthetics); an increase in oxygen consumption (decreased functional residual capacity combined with increased oxygen consumption makes pregnant women more likely to become hypoxic); and hypotension as a result of aortocaval compression (lying supine, a pregnant woman in the second and third trimesters experiences reduced blood flow back to the heart because of aortocaval compression by the gravid uterus). Direct compression of the great vessels by the gravid uterus reduces uterine blood flow, therefore the operating table is tilted laterally for all procedures to prevent uterine hypoperfusion. Finally, the anesthesiologist and the surgeons must maintain a continuous exchange of information throughout the procedure about the status of mother and fetus to ensure both patients' well-being.

As the pregnant uterus grows, the stomach is displaced cephalad and horizontally, which changes the angle of the gastroesophageal junction and predisposes the mother to passive regurgitation. This, along with an increase in gastric acid production, makes her more susceptible to regurgitation and aspiration when anesthetized. To reduce the acidity of the gastric juice, oral antacids are administered before general anesthesia is induced.

Pregnant women are also more sensitive to inhalation anesthetics because the endorphin level is elevated, and they therefore are more susceptible to overdosing. Regional anesthetics also require special attention. The increase in femoral venous and intraabdominal pressure enlarges the epidural veins, which decreases the epidural space, thus less anesthetic is needed.

Fetal oxygenation depends on the maternal arterial oxygen content. If the mother's partial pressure of arterial oxygen, partial pressure of arterial carbon dioxide, and uterine blood flow are maintained within normal limits, fetal asphyxia does not occur. Although elevated maternal oxygen tension (which commonly occurs during anesthesia) is safe for the fetus, maternal hyperventilation can also cause fetal hypoxia and acidosis. Other causes of fetal asphyxia are maternal hypotension, which causes a decrease in uterine blood flow, as well as uterine vasoconstriction caused by anxiety, insufficient anesthesia, or vasoactive drugs.

When the mother is anesthetized for fetal surgery, the fetus also receives the anesthetic by means of placental transfer. Operating on an unanesthetized fetus results in stimulation of the autonomic nervous system and increases in hormonal activity and motor activity; for these reasons, general anesthesia is used for all open procedures to provide both maternal and fetal anesthesia.

Anesthesia of the mother and her baby is established with halogenated agents that also provide profound uterine relaxation. Insertion of an epidural catheter enhances postoperative pain control. In the operating room, the mother is placed in left lateral decubitus position to prevent compression of the inferior vena cava by the gravid uterus. Maternal monitoring is accomplished with standard techniques, including pulse oximetry, a radial arterial catheter, a blood pressure cuff, large-bore intravenous catheters, measurement of urine output, and an electrocardiogram.

FETAL MALFORMATIONS AMENABLE TO SURGICAL CORRECTION

Prenatal diagnosis has defined a "hidden" mortality rate for some lesions, such as congenital diaphragmatic hernia, bilateral hydronephrosis, sacrococcygeal teratoma, and congenital cystic adenomatoid malformation of the lung. These lesions, when first evaluated and treated postnatally, demonstrated a favorable selection bias (and thus generated skewed, inaccurate, usually lower mortality rates) because the most severely affected fetuses often died in utero or immediately after birth. These deaths, often unaccounted for, represent the hidden, often increased mortality for some anomalies. Although most prenatally diagnosed malformations are best managed by appropriate medical and surgical therapy after maternal transport and planned delivery at a tertiary care center, an expanding number of simple anatomic abnormalities with predictable, lethal consequences have been corrected before birth. The development of minimum access fetal surgery techniques, along with improvements in the treatment and prevention of preterm labor, may enable the transition from treating only life-threatening defects to treating those that are not life-threatening but substantially morbid, such as myelomeningocele and cleft lip/palate.

Obstructive Uropathy

Obstructive uropathy occurs in 1 in 1000 live births. Unilateral urinary obstruction (e.g., ureteropelvic junction obstruction) has a good prognosis and usually does not require fetal intervention. Fetuses with bilateral obstruction, principally male fetuses with posterior urethral valves, are potential candidates for prenatal intervention based on the degree and duration of the obstruction. Newborns with partial bilateral obstruction may have only mild and reversible hydronephrosis. However, children born at term with a high-grade obstruction may already have advanced hydronephrosis and renal dysplasia, which are incompatible with life.

The outcome for patients with urinary tract obstruction depends primarily on whether oligohydramnios develops; this condition is the result of decreased fetal urine production and can lead to possibly fatal pulmonary hypoplasia (Potter sequence). Fetuses in the early second trimester that are identified with oligohydramnios have a mortality rate that is higher than 90%.

Prenatal ultrasound examination is reliable for detecting fetal hydronephrosis and for determining the level of the urinary obstruction. When sonography demonstrates bilateral hydronephrosis, the initial assessment for fetal renal function is determining the amount of amniotic fluid. Because most of the amniotic fluid in middle and late pregnancy is the product of fetal urination, a normal amniotic fluid volume implies production and excretion of urine by at least one functioning kidney. A diminished amniotic fluid volume on serial ultrasound examinations with bilateral hydronephrosis usually indicates deteriorating renal function.

Renal function then can be assessed in two ways, by the appearance of the renal tissue on ultrasound examination and by laboratory analysis of urine obtained by bladder aspiration. The presence of cortical cysts or increased echogenicity is highly predictive of renal dysplasia; however, the absence of these findings does not preclude it. Direct sampling of the fetal urine provides critical information about fetal renal function. Normal fetal urinary chemistry levels are: sodium below 100 mEq/dl, chloride below 90 mEq/dl, osmolarity below 200 mOsm/L, and beta$_2$-microglobulin below 4 mg/dl. Higher levels, which indicate that the fetal kidney is unable to reabsorb these molecules, are predictors of poor postnatal renal function. Three bladder aspirations must be performed, separated from each other by at least 24 hours. The first one empties stagnant bladder urine, and the second empties stagnant urine in the collecting system; the third specimen is most reflective of current kidney function.

The important dilemma in the treatment of fetuses with hydronephrosis is how to select those with dilated urinary tracts that have a problem so severe that renal and pulmonary function may be compromised at birth, yet that still have sufficient renal function to profit from prenatal intervention. Only fetuses that have or develop oligohydramnios with normal renal function (as shown by urine electrolyte and protein values), are less than 30 weeks' gestation, and have no associated anomalies are considered for prenatal intervention.

The aim of prenatal intervention is to bypass or directly treat the obstruction. If the urinary tract is adequately drained, restoration of amniotic fluid enhances fetal lung growth and prevents further deterioration of renal function. Methods of urinary tract decompression include percutaneous placement of a vesicoamniotic shunt, fetoscopic vesicostomy, open vesicostomy, and fetoscopic fulguration of posterior urethral valves (Quintero et al, 1995).

Currently the most widely used method of treating bladder outlet obstruction is percutaneous insertion of a double-J vesicoamniotic shunt. The surgical procedure varies, depending on the fetal renal disorder or the surgical team's preference. Posterior urethral valve obstruction may be treated by percutaneous placement of a shunt (catheter) from the fetal bladder to the amniotic sac (closed procedure). This shunt uses a Harrison French double-reversed pigtail catheter (Figure 13-1). The catheter or stent is shaped like a pigtail and has openings at either end. The diameters of the two ends are dissimilar, a safety feature in case the catheter becomes dislodged. The larger end is located in the amniotic cavity, so that the catheter would be more likely to move back into this cavity rather than into the fetal bladder.

A polyethylene catheter sometimes is used because it is more rigid and therefore less likely to bend or kink. The catheter is introduced through the maternal abdomen and uterus into the fetal abdomen and bladder by means of a needle and trocar guidance system, much as angiocatheters are used for intravenous therapy. When the catheter is in place, one end is in the renal pelvis and the other end is in the amniotic sac, providing a means to increase the amount of amniotic fluid. The guidance system is withdrawn, leaving the tubing in place. More than one insertion attempt may be necessary for successful placement. During the neonatal period, the fetus must undergo corrective surgery to repair the bladder and abdominal wall and relieve the urethral obstruction.

An open technique can be used to correct hydronephrosis in the fetus. For an open procedure, a maternal hysterotomy is performed after induction of general anesthesia. The uterine cavity is opened under ultrasonographic guidance to avoid the placenta and to guide the incision over the fetal abdomen. The fetal abdomen and thorax are exposed, but the fetus is

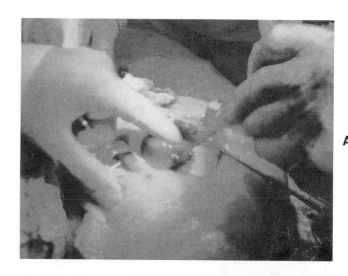

A

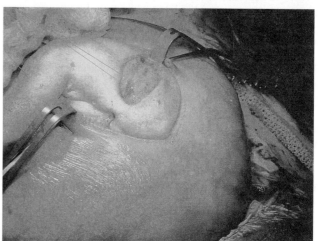

B

FIGURE **13-3**

A, Fetus with a congenital cystic adenomatoid malformation (CCAM) at 22 weeks' gestation. B, Resection of the CCAM. Courtesy The Fetal Treatment Center, University of California, San Francisco.

not removed (Figure 13-3). A pulse oximeter is taped to the fetus's hand to monitor the fetal heart rate and oxygenation and uterine activity during the procedure (at the end of the procedure, a telemetric device is sewn under the skin of the fetal thorax to provide continuous fetal heart rate and intrauterine pressure measurements; this device is left in place until delivery). A vesicostomy is performed, and a large volume of urine is drained from the fetal bladder. This vesicostomy is used in postnatal life to drain urine from the bladder (Figure 13-4). The bladder is marsupialized to the fetal abdominal wall, leaving an avenue for urine to flow from the fetal bladder into the amniotic sac. On closure of the uterus, lactated Ringer's solution is infused into the amniotic space via a red Robinson catheter, returning the amniotic fluid volume to normal and correcting the oligohydramnios. The membranes and uterus are closed by suture and sealed with fibrin glue to prevent intraabdominal leakage of amnio-tic fluid.

To prevent long-term renal and pulmonary problems, treatment must be undertaken early. Fetal surgery for posterior urethral valve obstruction has been performed early as 18 weeks' and as late as 26 weeks' gestation. The ultimate goal

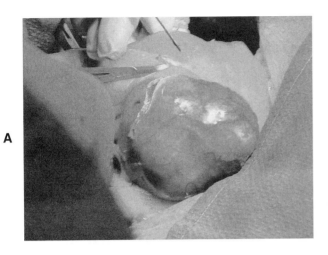

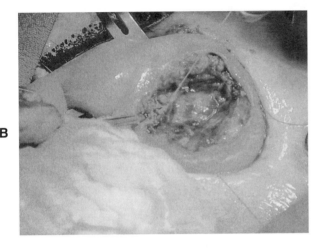

FIGURE **13-4**
A, Fetus with a sacrococcygeal teratoma undergoing in utero resection at 23 weeks' gestation. **B,** Fetus after excision of the tumor. Courtesy The Fetal Treatment Center, University of California, San Francisco.

is to prevent irreversible renal damage and pulmonary hypoplasia.

Congenital Diaphragmatic Hernia

Congenital diaphragmatic hernia (CDH) is a simple anatomic defect in which abdominal viscera herniate into the hemithorax, most often through a posterolateral defect in the diaphragm. Despite advances in prenatal care, maternal transport, neonatal resuscitation, and the availability of extracorporeal membrane oxygenation (ECMO), the devastating physiologic consequences of pulmonary hypoplasia and hypertension are associated with a high neonatal mortality rate and long-term morbidity (Harrison et al, 2001). In fetal sheep, compression of the lungs during the last trimester, either with an intrathoracic balloon or by creation of a diaphragmatic hernia, resulted in fatal pulmonary hypoplasia. Removal of the compression allowed pulmonary growth and development to progress and increased the chances of survival.

The prenatal diagnosis of CDH is established by ultrasonography, which shows herniation of abdominal contents (e.g., loops of bowel, the stomach, or the left lobe of the liver) into

the fetal thorax. The function of certain fetal organs, such as the heart and kidneys, can be assessed in utero, but the fetal lungs do not exchange gas and therefore cannot be assessed directly. Several sonographically detectable predictors of the severity of CDH have been proposed; the two most important parameters are the lung to head ratio (LHR) (Lipshutz et al, 1997) and the position of the left lobe of the liver (Albanese et al, 1998b). The LHR is the calculated volume of the contralateral lung (the ipsilateral lung cannot be identified with CDH) indexed to head circumference to adjust for gestational age. Fetuses with an LHR of more than 1.4 have a favorable prognosis with tertiary postnatal care and therefore are not candidates for fetal intervention. For fetuses in which a major portion of the left lobe of the liver has herniated into the hemithorax, the survival rate is approximately 50%; for those in which the liver is in the normal abdominal position, the survival rate is over 90% (Albanese et al, 1998b). This determination is technically challenging and requires color Doppler ultrasonography to visualize the position of the branches of the left portal vein. These prognostic indicators allow careful selection of severely affected fetuses that may benefit from fetal intervention.

Prenatal treatment of CDH has continued to evolve since the first attempted CDH repair in 1986 at the University of California at San Francisco (Figure 13-5). Open fetal surgery, in which a hysterotomy was performed and the diaphragm was repaired directly, presented many technical problems. Reduction of a herniated lobe of the liver during repair resulted in kinking of the intraabdominal umbilical vein; this cut off blood flow from the placenta and led to fetal demise. Data from a 1994 study at the University of California at San Francisco showed that repair of the diaphragm for fetuses without liver herniation worked but was no better than standard postnatal care (Harrison et al, 1997). For those with the more severe form of CDH (i.e., liver herniation), complete repair was not technically feasible. This forced a redirection in thinking about how to treat fetuses with the most severe CDH.

An accident of nature supplied a new paradigm for treating these fetuses. It has long been noted that fetuses with congenital high airway obstruction syndrome (CHAOS) caused by laryngeal or tracheal atresia have large, hyperplastic lungs as a result of overdistention from lung fluid (Hedrick et al, 1994). Laboratory studies not only confirmed that this model is reproducible but also showed that lungs that are physically larger are also functionally larger. This concept was tested using fetoscopic techniques for temporary occlusion of the fetal trachea using a balloon to accelerate fetal lung growth (Bealer et al, 1995; Harrison et al, 1996, 1998; Skarsgard et al, 1996). The preliminary data showed this technique to have great promise and formed the basis for a 1999 clinical trial sponsored by the National Institutes of Health (NIH) in which tracheal occlusion at 26 weeks' gestation was compared with standard postnatal care for fetuses with an LHR below 1.4 and liver herniation.

The technique for removing the tracheal balloon is called the ex utero intrapartum treatment (EXIT) procedure (Figure 13-6) (Mychaliska et al, 1997). A hysterotomy is performed and the fetal head and shoulders are delivered, but the cord is not clamped. During this period of placental support, the pediatric surgeon inserts a bronchoscope and then pops and removes the balloon with suction. The neonate is intubated, surfactant is administered, and mechanical ventilation (by hand) is begun. Once the oxygen saturation increases, the cord is cut and the infant is delivered.

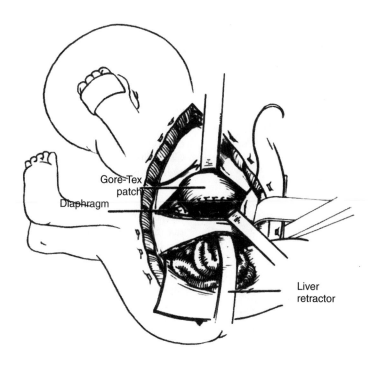

FIGURE **13-5**

The arm and left side of the fetus's chest are brought out of the uterus so that the surgeon can operate. The intestines and stomach are pushed out of the lung cavity to give the lung room to grow. Finally, the hole in the diaphragm is repaired with a patch. Courtesy The Fetal Treatment Center, University of California, San Francisco.

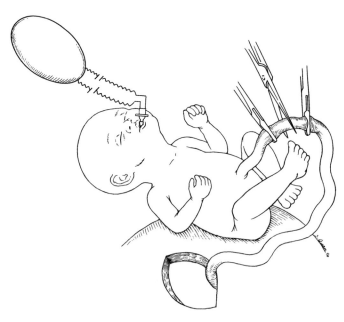

FIGURE **13-6**

Essential elements of ex utero intrapartum treatment (EXIT) procedure. Courtesy The Fetal Treatment Center, University of California, San Francisco.

Congenital Cystic Adenomatoid Malformation

Congenital cystic adenomatoid malformation (CCAM) of the lung is the most common type of fetal thoracic mass that can be detected by prenatal ultrasound examination as early as 16 weeks' gestation. Most cases are diagnosed before 22 weeks'

gestation. CCAM is a hamartoma of the lung that usually is unilateral and lobar. The differential diagnoses include pulmonary sequestration, CDH, other congenital cystic malformations (e.g., bronchogenic, enteric, or neurogenic cysts), and CHAOS. CCAMs have a broad spectrum of clinical severity and usually follow one of three courses: they may enlarge significantly, leading to fetal hydrops; they may remain unchanged; or they may shrink and disappear prenatally. These malformations lead to fetal demise in 100% of pregnancies when sufficient cardiac and great vessel compression lead to hydrops. However, the size and degree of mediastinal shift alone is not predictive of hydrops, which occurs in only the minority of prenatally diagnosed CCAMs.

Experimentally, the pathophysiologic consequences and the rationale for in utero treatment of CCAM have been clarified (Rice et al, 1994). The only indication for fetal intervention is the presence of hydrops, manifested by fetal ascites, pericardial or pleural effusions, and scalp and integumentary edema. If this condition occurs before 32 weeks' gestation, the fetus may be a candidate for intervention.

Macrocystic lesions can be treated using minimally invasive introduction of a percutaneous thoracoamniotic catheter, which drains and decompresses the mass to allow fetal lung growth (Morin et al, 1994). Microcystic lesions have been removed by the open (hysterotomy) technique, with subsequent resolution of hydrops. Solid masses require surgical resection between 21 and 27 weeks' gestation, when lung growth continues and can resume a normal growth pattern for optimal lung development (Morin et al, 1994). At this gestational age, as well, type II cells are producing surfactant, therefore the fetus may tolerate the surgical procedure better than at an earlier stage. This fetus-neonate should be delivered at a tertiary care center where ECMO is available, because the possibility of pulmonary hypoplasia still exists (Morin et al, 1994). Postnatal radiographic studies are needed to detect any residual or return of the CCAM.

Sacrococcygeal Teratoma

Sacrococcygeal teratoma (SCT) is the most common tumor in newborns, occurring in 1 in 35,000 to 40,000 live births. SCT, a neural tube defect that can be detected by ultrasonography, is the growth of a tumor in the sacral and coccygeal areas of the spinal cord or at the base of the tailbone (coccyx). The natural history of prenatally diagnosed SCT is very different from that of neonatal SCT, and the well-established prognostic indicators for the latter do not apply for fetal SCT. Malignancy is the primary cause of death in neonatal SCT but is rare in these tumors in utero (Graf et al, 1998). The life-threatening consequences of fetal SCT are associated with the development of high output cardiac failure, which results from a "vascular steal" phenomenon through the solid, highly vascular tumors.

Only 10% of fetal SCTs cause hydrops; if left untreated, the mortality rate is 100%. SCT also may lead to a potentially devastating maternal complication called maternal mirror (Ballantine) syndrome, in which the mother experiences progressive symptoms suggestive of preeclampsia, including hypertension, peripheral edema, proteinuria, and pulmonary edema, because of the release of endothelial cell toxins from the edematous placenta. This syndrome is reversed not by removing the SCT prenatally, but only by delivering the fetus and the placenta.

Prenatal sonographic diagnosis of SCT is based on detection of a characteristic sacral and/or intraabdominal mass, which can be seen as early as 14 weeks' gestation. With widespread use of sophisticated obstetric sonography during midgestation, most SCTs can be diagnosed in utero. Fetal SCTs can be cystic, solid, or mixed in appearance (Westerburg et al, 2000); differential diagnoses include myelomeningocele and obstructive uropathy. Color flow Doppler ultrasonographic examination of large vascular tumors may show markedly increased distal aortic blood flow and shunting of blood away from the placenta to the tumor, a condition that almost uniformly leads to hydrops and makes the fetus a possible candidate for surgical intervention. Of the reported cases undergoing open fetal surgical resection of an SCT, there are few long-term survivors to date (Adzick et al, 1997; Graf et al, 2000).

Fetal surgery for SCT involves tumor resection. Briefly, a maternal hysterotomy is performed, and the fetal buttocks and lower spinal cord are exposed. If the lesion is small, a stapling device is used to apply pressure to the highly vascular tissue, gradually cutting off the blood supply to the tumor; this technique minimizes fetal blood loss. If the tumor is too large to be safely handled by stapling, umbilical tape can be pulled tightly over the tumor mass, binding it and cutting off the blood supply. The surgeon then can remove or resect the tumor with little risk of bleeding. Because these tumors sometimes recur or are not removed completely, further surgery may be required during the neonatal period.

Currently, research efforts are directed toward developing a minimally invasive approach to treatment; rather than debulking the mass, the tumor's blood supply would be interrupted by coagulating the major feeding blood vessels (Westerburg et al, 1998). This approach can be accomplished percutaneously using a radio frequency ablation device. The UCSF fetal treatment team has used an ultrasonographically guided,

percutaneous, minimally invasive technique to coagulate the blood vessels in three fetuses, two of whom survived the procedure. The third fetus died due to complications (Paek et al, 2001a).

Twin to Twin Transfusion Syndrome

Twin to twin transfusion syndrome (TTTS) is the most common complication in monochorionic-diamniotic twin pregnancies, occurring in 5% to 35% of these pregnancies. Although associated anomalies are rare, TTTS is associated with a high risk of miscarriage, brain damage, perinatal death, and morbidity in survivors.

In TTTS, unequal sharing of the monochorionic placenta usually can be seen sonographically, because the insertion of the smaller (or donor) twin's placental cord often is marginal or velamentous, whereas the larger (or recipient) twin's cord inserts into the placenta centrally. Vascular connections on the placental surface exist between the twins, and if these are unbalanced, a net shunting of blood occurs as a result of arteriovenous anastomoses, which sometimes can be detected by Doppler ultrasonography.

Ultrasonography commonly demonstrates severe oligohydramnios or anhydramnios in the sac of the donor twin (also known as the "pump" or "stuck" twin). The differential diagnoses for a "stuck twin" include uteroplacental dysfunction, discordant aneuploidy, structural urinary tract malformations, or congenital infection. The recipient twin, on the other hand, develops polyhydramnios, pulmonary hypertension, and cardiomyopathy caused by chronic blood volume overload. The vessels in question are unpaired vessels with flow from the donor fetus to the recipient fetus. Doppler studies demonstrate the characteristic pulsatile arterial blood flow on the donor's side, whereas the vessel shows a continuous venous flow on the recipient's side.

The initial treatment for TTTS is one or more large-volume amniocenteses of the recipient's polyhydramniotic sac. In nonresponders and in recipients who have or develop hydrops as a result of blood volume overload, additional fetoscopic ablation of communicating vessel anastomoses is performed with a yttrium aluminum garnet (YAG) laser. The surgical procedure varies, because some surgeons coagulate all vessels seen crossing the intertwin septum on the placental surface (Hecher et al, 1999), whereas others coagulate only the unpaired intertwin communicating vessels (De Lia et al, 1995; Feldstein et al, 2000).

Neural Tube Defects

Myelomeningocele (MMC), or spina bifida, is a midline defect that results in exposure of the contents of the spinal column. The defect usually is located in the lumbosacral portion of the vertebrae. In the United States alone, 1500 to 2000 babies are born with MMC every year. Routine maternal serum alphafetoprotein (MSAFP) screening identifies more than 80% of children with MMC. When MSAFP values are outside the normal range, direct sonographic visualization of the fetal spine can be performed by 16 weeks' gestation to confirm the presence of an MMC and other possible associated findings, including frontal bone scalloping (lemon sign), abnormality of the cerebellum (banana sign), Chiari II malformation (hindbrain herniation), hydrocephaly, microcephaly, and encephalocele.

The clinical observation that, in fetuses with MMC, lower extremity function present early in the pregnancy was progressively lost in later gestation provided the rationale for considering prenatal intervention. Creation and repair of the defect in animals showed that intrauterine repair of myelomeningocele may preserve peripheral neurologic function (Meuli et al, 1995 a, b; Hutchins et al, 1996). Experimental studies also indicated that the Chiari II malformation, which is nearly always associated with MMC, may be prevented by prenatal repair (Paek et al, 2000).

Recent clinical experience has shown that open fetal surgery may improve neurologic function and more dramatically resolve the hindbrain herniation associated with myelomeningocele (Adzick et al, 1998; Tulipan et al, 1998; Bruner et al, 1999 a, b; Sutton et al, 1999). This early experience appears promising, but the variable natural history of myelomeningocele, the lack of accurate prenatal indicators of neurologic function, and the absence of matched controls and long-term follow-up data hamper assessment of the benefits of prenatal intervention. The NIH has encouraged a controlled, randomized, multicenter trial of fetal myelomeningocele repair to assess the safety and efficacy of the procedure and to address the deficiencies in data.

Congenital High Airway Obstructive Syndrome

Congenital high airway obstruction syndrome usually is caused by laryngeal or tracheal atresia and in rare cases by isolated tracheal stenosis, mucosal web, or extrinsic compression by a large cervical mass (e.g., teratoma or lymphangioma). Regardless of the etiology, fetal upper airway obstruction prevents egress of the fluid produced in the lungs, which normally travels from the airways into the amniotic space. This fluid usually is produced under a pressure that favors movement out through the fetal mouth, partly aided by fetal breathing movements. Sonographic findings of CHAOS include a bilaterally flattened or everted diaphragm; large, overdistended (i.e., fluid filled), echogenic lungs that compress the mediastinum; dilated large airways distal to the obstruction; and fetal ascites or hydrops (or both) resulting from compression of the heart and great vessel or vessels (Hedrick et al, 1994). If hydrops does not develop in utero, a fetus with CHAOS may be treated with the EXIT procedure, which maintains the baby on placental support until an airway is established via orotracheal intubation or tracheostomy (Mychaliska et al, 1997). However, if fetal hydrops develops, early delivery or prenatal tracheostomy is an option for treatment, depending on the gestational age. Three known survivors of prenatally diagnosed CHAOS have been reported in the literature (DeCou et al, 1998; Crombleholme et al, 2000; Paek et al, 2001b).

Amniotic Band Syndrome

The incidence of amniotic band syndrome is 1 in 1200 to 15,000 live births. Early rupture of the amnion results in mesodermic bands that emanate from the chorionic side of the amnion and insert onto the fetal body. These bands may lead to amputations, constrictions, and postural deformities that occur secondary to immobilization. Crombleholme and colleagues produced amniotic band syndrome in fetal sheep so as to study the effects of fetoscopic release on morphometric outcome (Crombleholme et al, 1995).

It has been shown that the earlier the band occurs, the more severe is the resulting lesion (Strauss et al, 2000). For example, amniotic rupture in the first weeks of pregnancy may result in craniofacial and visceral defects; with rupture during the second trimester, fetal morbidity ranges from formation of syndactyly to limb amputation. Umbilical cord constriction at any time in gestation may result in fetal death. Given the risks for fetal and maternal morbidity, fetoscopic intervention for mild

forms of amniotic band syndrome is not warranted at this time. However, for more severe forms, fetoscopic lysis of the bands may be useful (Quintero et al, 1997).

MULTIDISCIPLINARY COLLABORATIVE APPROACH TO FETAL THERAPY

The complexity of fetal surgery obviously requires a multidisciplinary team approach to care of the mother and fetus undergoing prenatal intervention; both patients also require continuous monitoring in an intensive care setting. A fetal treatment team should include a perinatologist, neonatologist, pediatric surgeon, sonographer, anesthesiologist, operating room and perinatal nurse specialists, and social worker, as well as a nurse coordinator who can serve as a liaison with the family (Sullivan & Adzick, 1994).

Time generally is of the essence with fetal surgery cases; the legal window that allows the option of pregnancy termination may be closing, and delays can lead to substantial fetal morbidity and even mortality. For maximum possible benefit, candidates for fetal surgery should be identified and referred before 23 weeks' gestation. Early referral allows the fetal surgery team adequate time to consider the clinical situation carefully and to perform appropriately timed interventions. Box 13-1 outlines the multidisciplinary approach to specific interventions developed by the fetal surgery team at the University of California at San Francisco.

Considerations for Collaborative Care Planning

When fetal surgery is the chosen treatment, the clinical case may be broken down into six phases: diagnosis, information and decision making, perioperative and postoperative care, home care and follow-up, delivery, and neonatal period. Each stage involves distinct and important nursing input and responsibilities.

Diagnosis. The diagnostic phase generally covers the period from referral to the fetal treatment center through the evaluation process. For the families, who often are given limited information about the reason for referral, this typically is a waiting period, first for an appointment and then for the results of the evaluation. For many families this is the most difficult time, and the nurse should provide appropriate and sufficient information about the process and suggest resources (e.g., social services, support groups, counseling services) to help the family cushion themselves against the fears and anxiety inherent in this stressful situation. The nurse must recognize that the family is enduring the loss of a normal pregnancy and experiencing the anxiety of an uncertain future. Also, in this initial phase the family's major concerns often center on the diagnosis and the cause of the fetal problem and their possible role in that cause. Families need explicit reassurance that the cause is unknown.

Information and Decision Making. Once the perinatologist and pediatric surgeon have established the differential diagnoses, the family is presented with the treatment options. These may include termination of the pregnancy (if still early enough in gestation), surgical intervention, or simply waiting to term for standard postnatal care. The question of whether invasive therapy should be offered and recommended or offered but not recommended is posed at this point. Such therapy should be offered and recommended only if two criteria are met: (1) the therapy is judged to have a high likelihood of

BOX 13-1

Sample Care Plan for Women Undergoing Fetal Surgery (Clinical Pathway)

The following care plan is used at the Fetal Treatment Center at the University of California, San Francisco.

1. *Informed consent and counseling:* All members of the team are included (perinatologist, fetal treatment center nurse coordinator, pediatric surgeon, operating room nurse specialist, sonographer, obstetric anesthesiologist, perinatal nurse specialist, perinatal social worker)
2. *Admission:* Evening before procedure.
3. *Preoperative assessment:* Assessment includes baseline cervical examination (digital and by sonogram), baseline maternal vitals and oxygen saturation levels, electronic fetal heart rate, and maternal uterine activity strip
4. *Tocolysis:* All patients receive tocolysis as follows:
   - **Indomethacin:** 50 mg by rectum (pr) given at 10 PM before surgery and on call to operating room, then every 4 to 6 hours for at least 24 to 48 hours after procedure.
   - **Magnesium sulfate:** 2 g/hour given intravenously, initiated intraoperatively and continued until uterine activity has been controlled for 24 to 48 hours.
   - **Terbutaline:** If the subcutaneous pump is used, it is initiated before the magnesium sulfate is stopped and is continued until delivery.
   - **Nifedipine (oral):** If used, it is begun when the magnesium sulfate is discontinued and given every 4 to 6 hours until delivery.
5. *Coping and supportive care:* The nurse specialists and the perinatal social worker provide continuity for issues of coping.
6. *Pain management:* All patients undergo general anesthesia for the procedure and have an epidural catheter placed postoperatively for pain management via epidurally administered narcotics and *-caine* anesthetics.
7. *Medications:* Postoperatively patients receive intravenous antibiotics until they are afebrile for 48 hours.
8. *Monitoring:* Patients receive one to one care for 24 hours; electronic uterine-fetal monitoring is continuous.
9. *Fluid management:* Strict measurement of intake and output (I&O) measurement and total fluid restriction to 2400 ml in 24 hours are necessary to prevent or limit pulmonary edema. Weighing the patient daily and continuous pulse oximetry help detect pulmonary edema early. Adventitious lung sounds are a late sign.
10. *Oxygen therapy:* Oxygen is provided via nonrebreather mask for the first 2 hours after surgery and then by naso-pharyngeal prongs to keep the arterial oxygen saturation above 95%. Incentive spirometer is performed every 3 to 4 hours while awake. Lungs are assessed every 6 hours.
11. *Activity:* Complete bed rest is required until uterine activity is controlled. Thigh-high TEDs and Venodyne boots with a sequential compression device are used while the patient is on complete bed rest to reduce the risk of emboli.
12. *Follow-up:* The patient should return weekly for sonographic evaluation and examination by a perinatologist. Biweekly nonstress test and amniotic fluid index (NST/AFI) should begin a 26 weeks.

From information provided by The Fetal Treatment Center, University of California, San Francisco.

being life-saving or of preventing serious, irreversible disease, injury, or disability for the fetus and the child to come; and (2) the therapy has a low risk of mortality and a low or manageable risk of disease, injury, or disability to the fetus. Although the risk to the mother is expected to be low or at least manageable, any surgical procedure carries some risk of morbidity and mortality, and this should be stated explicitly in the counseling and informed consent processes.

The decision-making phase often is the time the family's worst fears are confirmed. As the grief reaction begins, the family's emotions and feelings may become more intense; they may react rather than respond in various situations. They also must face the religious, moral, and ethical implications of the decision, as well as the financial and practical considerations. TTTS best illustrates this situation. As described earlier, these cases involve a recipient twin and a "pump" twin, and the latter usually is structurally normal but faces a high probability of death without intervention. Although several fetal therapeutic techniques have been used successfully to correct this problem, the family must still wrestle with the issue of possible risk to both twins (i.e., subjecting to possible risk the one twin who would most likely do well during extrauterine life) in choosing a treatment.

In practice, before deciding what is best for them, the family meets with all members of the fetal treatment team. Team members provide detailed information about preoperative, intraoperative, and perioperative hospital and home care and answer questions and address concerns. The family also meets privately with the perinatal social worker, who makes a psychosocial assessment and evaluates the family's ability to cope with each of the treatment choices. This evaluation includes assessment of the marital relationship, available support systems, coping strategies used in previous crises, previous experience of loss, current stress factors (e.g., concern for care of children at home), recent unemployment or financial constraints, and other health problems. Collectively, this information assists in the team's assessment of how well the family will cope with the current crisis and what resources may be helpful in working with them.

Perioperative and Postoperative Care. If fetal intervention is chosen, nurses help prepare the family for the procedure and provide them with extensive preoperative teaching. It may also be an appropriate time for to suggest and discuss with the family seeing, holding, and naming their infant, in case fetal loss occurs at any time during the perioperative period. Box 13-1 details patient management during the preoperative and postoperative periods.

Postoperative Management. In lieu of direct physical examination in the postoperative stage, daily fetal sonography and echocardiography provide necessary insight and information about fetal status. During this 5- to 7-day period, too, continuous epidural analgesics are given to the mother to ease maternal stress and aid tocolysis. Nurses provide key support, encouragement, education, and confidence at this critical time, when the mother and family face uncertainty about their fetus's survival and the possibility and consequences of uncontrollable preterm labor. Additional attention to the mother is important, because she must endure the effects of medications that may disrupt her mental status, postoperative comfort, and ability to sleep. She also may feel intimidated by the array of technologic equipment used in postoperative care. To minimize the mother's sense of depersonalization, the nurse should help promote flexible visiting hours, personalization of the room or bedside, and physical contact with significant others (Howell & Dunphy, 1999).

Preterm Labor. Preterm labor is the Achilles heel of fetal intervention and the primary cause of maternal morbidity and fetal death. Its pathophysiology after hysterotomy is not yet clearly understood, and effective postoperative tocolysis (with minimum side effects) remains a frustrating clinical problem (Albanese & Harrison, 1998). Currently the tocolytic regimen begins with administration of indomethacin to the mother before surgery and over the next several days. Of the available tocolytics, indomethacin was chosen because of its ability to inhibit the synthesis of prostaglandins released during uterine manipulation. In contrast to their value in spontaneous labor, terbutaline, magnesium sulfate, and nifedipine have been relatively ineffective and offer little advantage in the treatment of preterm labor induced by hysterotomy. Outpatient tocolysis consists of oral or subcutaneous terbutaline (administered via a pump) or oral nifedipine. If membranes rupture or labor cannot be controlled, cesarean delivery is performed, usually before 36 weeks' gestation (Harrison et al, 2001).

The mother, for her part, may be constantly concerned that something she does or fails to do will lead to preterm labor, premature rupture of membranes, or some other harm to the fetus. If possible, home care nursing generally is provided once a week to ensure continuing instruction in self-care, management, and support, if these are not accomplished through outpatient visits.

Home Care and Follow-Up. The discharge to home can be a particularly anxious time for the family for several reasons. For example, the mother often is restricted to complete bed rest and tocolytic therapy and, as mentioned previously, she may be fearful that something she does or fails to do will harm the fetus. For this reason, the patient and a family member or friend are encouraged and sometimes required to stay near the medical center so that they can return once or twice a week for fetal evaluation (i.e., nonstress test [NST] and amniotic fluid index [AFI]) and sonographic evaluation and assessment for signs of preterm labor. In some instances plans may be made for patients to stay at a nearby facility, such as a Ronald McDonald House (Harrison et al, 2001). If membranes rupture or shred (i.e., chorioamniotic separation) or if preterm labor cannot be controlled, the mother can be rehospitalized, kept on bed rest, and continuously monitored.

Extended separation from children, family, and friends during this follow-up phase may be a significant emotional strain on the patient, and time away from work and lost wages may be a tremendous financial hardship. The nurse coordinator should remain in daily contact with the family to maintain a good sense of their emotional well-being and should suggest or provide whatever resources are appropriate to help ease the burden of their particular situation.

Delivery. Delivery of the infant may take place any time after fetal surgery but most often occurs 4 to 10 weeks after the procedure, depending on a number of factors. The lesion for which the surgery was performed also determines the conditions that must be satisfied in anticipation of delivery. For example, for fetuses that have undergone fetoscopic tracheal occlusion, delivery must take place under highly controlled circumstances with the entire fetal treatment team available or present when the EXIT procedure is performed.

During this phase, the parents' major concerns focus on the infant's chances of survival, both short term and long term, and interestingly but not surprisingly on the infant's physical appearance at birth as a result of having undergone a surgical procedure. The parents should have the opportunity to see and touch the infant as soon as possible after birth, regardless of the outcome. If the infant does not survive, one of the nurse specialists should encourage the parents to hold, look at, and take pictures with their infant, because these actions help them accept the outcome and experience closure. If the infant survives, it is equally important for parents to see and touch the baby as soon as possible after delivery, to provide reassurance. If the physical conditions of both mother and infant make this contact difficult or impossible, a member of the treatment team should take pictures that can be given to the family immediately.

Neonatal Period. The final phase, the neonatal period, requires the team to work closely with the family's long-term health care providers to ensure appropriate management of the case once the family leaves the fetal treatment center. Even if the infant does not survive, the nurse coordinator should maintain contact with the family so that autopsy results and genetic counseling can be provided. One of the nurse specialists may want to initiate discussion of the various stages of the grief process with the parents to alleviate feelings and fears of never "getting back to normal." This is also an appropriate time to discuss the reactions of friends and family.

For the family whose infant has survived, the realization that the baby may require further surgery surfaces during this period, or the family may learn that the infant may not live long despite the fetal surgery. Even when the infant is doing well and has minimal risk of further illness, the family may not readily accept the information given. For example, they may anticipate the infant's death, even though any number of health care professionals may explain that it is not a concern. The family may require significant psychosocial support after the discharge of the mother and infant to ensure a successful transition to home. This support can be provided through telephone contact, home visits, and clinic visits soon after discharge to assess the family's adjustment. Referrals to support groups, psychologists, or professionals of other disciplines should be made immediately if the family appears to be have trouble coping with having the infant home.

As can clearly be seen, the fetus with an anomaly requires the attention of a team of specialists (Harrison et al, 2001). Not only are there ethical issues that require the balancing of risks and benefits, but there are two patients, the mother and the fetus (Spitzer, 1996). Fetal surgery requires a collective approach to caregiving. The multidisciplinary team at a fetal treatment center requires meaningful collaboration involving the pediatric surgeon, perinatal obstetrician, sonographer, anesthesiologist, operating room and obstetrical nurses, geneticist, social worker, ethicist, and nurse coordinator (Taeusch & Ballard, 1998). Various defects require more subspecialties (e.g., when the defect involves the central nervous system, a pediatric neurosurgeon is involved). Despite the multiple talents in the group, the role of the nurse in the team must not be discounted. Nursing represents a source of continuity in maternal-child care sessions; nurses provide care through all stages of fetal surgery and can be critical advocates for maternal and fetal surgery patients (Collins, 1994).

The multidisciplinary approach continues through the waiting period for delivery and through follow-up care. The infant may require future surgery and specialized follow-up care, depending on the severity of the fetal/neonatal problem. The family also requires intensive follow-up care. A team approach helps alleviate additional stress caused by inconsistencies in care plans and physical and financial demands. As technology and scientific knowledge expand, the need for team care will only increase.

FETAL THERAPY: NEW HORIZONS

As mentioned previously, treatments for genetic problems are being attempted through fetal therapy. For example, with errors of metabolism, the mother is given medication, vitamins, or the substance the infant lacks, and that substance passes through the placenta to the fetus (Chapter 27). Other therapies have been aimed at blood incompatibility problems.

One of the newer fetal therapies with exciting potential is the treatment for SCID, a disorder that carries a high mortality rate and that forces infants and children to live in protective bubbles to avoid exposure to infectious agents because their own immune systems are essentially nonfunctional. Stem cell transplantation has been successful in treating this condition in utero, although its application in medicine is in jeopardy as controversy surrounding its use mounts. However, these stem cells can be obtained from a parent and transfused through the umbilical cord of the fetus, from which the cells migrate to the spaces in the fetal bone marrow. Abundant space exists there because the liver is the primary hematopoietic organ during gestational development. These transplanted cells (which do not trigger rejection in the fetus because it is in a preimmune state at this stage in gestation) proliferate and replace the fetal stem cells and become differentiated into the various cell types of the immune system (Wiley, 1996).

In the neonatal period, tests can be performed to identify, in particular, T lymphocytes, which in turn can be tested to determine cell origin. In a successful treatment case at Wayne State Medical Center in Detroit, the cells were paternal in origin and were sufficient in number to suggest a cure for SCID (Flake, 1995). If this therapy continues to be successful, the treatment method may be attempted for all forms of hemoglobinopathies, particularly sickle cell anemia and thalassemia. Already a national network of cord blood banks gives families the opportunity to save cord blood for use later in life in the event that an immune problem arises. The movement to embrace this new therapy brings with it ethical considerations of which the nurse must remain aware (McMillan, 1996).

Future of Fetal Surgery

Increasingly sophisticated techniques for prenatal diagnosis have revolutionized the field of fetal medicine. The fetus has come a long way from the biblical "seed" and mystical "homunculus" to an individual with medical problems that can be diagnosed and treated. The short but eventful history of fetal surgical intervention offers new hope for the fetus with an isolated congenital malformation. The great promise of fetal therapy is that for some diseases, the earliest possible intervention (i.e., before birth) produces the best possible outcome (i.e., the best quality of life for the resources expended). However, the promise of cost-effective preventive fetal therapy can be subverted by misguided clinical applications, such as performing a complex in utero procedure that "half saves" an otherwise doomed fetus for a life of intensive (and expensive) care. Enthusiasm for fetal intervention must be tempered by reverence for the interests of the mother and her family, by careful study of the disease in experimental fetal animals and untreated human fetuses, and by a willingness to abandon therapy that does not prove effective and cost-effective in properly controlled trials.

Some hospitals, such as Children's Hospital of Philadelphia, have hired nurses with expertise in fetal surgery to work with the staff of the neonatal intensive care unit (NICU) to provide care once the baby is born. Follow-up for this population is individualized according to the type of fetal surgery or therapy. Follow-up for the families focuses on general care needs but acknowledges the trauma of the fetal treatment and the effect it has on their lives after the birth and discharge. This type of specialized care currently is found in only a few NICUs, but it is likely to become more widespread as technology and knowledge of genetics expand. Nursing will have a significant role in shaping the future care of these patients.

SUMMARY

The overall goal of this chapter has been to provide a comprehensive description of fetal treatment and, in particular, fetal surgery and a delineation of milestones achieved to date in this specialized area of perinatal and neonatal health care. As this field of clinical practice and laboratory research rapidly evolves and expands, it is reasonable to assume that more neonatal health care professionals will be approached with questions and asked to comment on fetal treatment and surgery. It therefore is important that neonatal nurses, including community hospital-based nurses, have a basic understanding of this relatively recent and burgeoning area of medicine and its associated technology. The overview of fetal therapy offered in this chapter may provide a basis for that understanding and may spark enough interest in the reader to seek additional information. Finally, this chapter recognizes the critical, complex, and often-difficult role nurse specialists fulfill in fetal treatment. The nurse is both patient advocate and fetal treatment team representative. It is not that other health care professionals on the team do not have this same responsibility, nor is it that these are dual roles with mutually exclusive agendas. It is, however, an entirely singular role in which the responsibilities are complex and multifaceted; the nurse specialist who fulfills them must be able to weigh, balance, interpret, and act on a variety of issues from an equally multifaceted perspective. This chapter, then, is an acknowledgement of the tremendous talent, intellect, skill, and compassion that nursing professionals bring to the field of fetal treatment, key elements in the success of this new therapy.

REFERENCES

Adzick NS et al (1997). A rapidly growing fetal teratoma. *Lancet* 349:538.

Adzick NS et al (1998). Successful fetal surgery for spina bifida. *Lancet* 352:1675-1676.

Albanese CT, Harrison MR (1998a). Surgical treatment for fetal disease: the state of the art. *Annals of the New York academy of science* 847:74-85.

Albanese CT et al (1998a). Endoscopic fetal tracheal occlusion procedure: evolution of techniques. *Pediatric endosurgery and innovative techniques* 2:47-53.

Albanese CT et al (1998b). Fetal liver position and perinatal outcome for congenital diaphragmatic hernia. *Prenatal diagnosis* 18:1138-1142.

Bealer JF et al (1995). The "PLUG" odyssey: adventures in experimental fetal tracheal occlusion. *Journal of pediatric surgery* 30:361-364.

Bruner JP et al (1999a). Endoscopic coverage of fetal myelomeningocele in utero. *American journal of obstetrics and gynecology* 180:153-158.

Bruner JP et al (1999b). Fetal surgery for myelomeningocele and the incidence of shunt-dependent hydrocephalus. *Journal of the American Medical Association* 282:1819-1825.

Collins JE (1994). Fetal surgery: changing the outcome before birth. *Journal of obstetric, gynecologic, and neonatal nursing* 23:166-169.

Crombleholme TM et al (1995). Amniotic band syndrome in fetal lambs. I. Fetoscopic release and morphometric outcome. *Journal of pediatric surgery* 30:974-978.

Crombleholme TM et al (2000). Salvage of a fetus with congenital high airway obstruction syndrome by ex utero intrapartum treatment (EXIT) procedure. *Fetal diagnosis and therapy* 15:280-282.

DeCou JM et al (1998). Successful ex utero intrapartum treatment (EXIT) procedure for congenital high airway obstruction syndrome (CHAOS) owing to laryngeal atresia. *Journal of pediatric surgery* 33:1563-1565.

De Lia JE et al (1995). Fetoscopic laser ablation of placental vessels in severe previable twin-twin transfusion syndrome. *American journal of obstetrics and gynecology* 172:1202-1208.

DiFederico EM et al (1998). Pulmonary edema in obstetric patients is rapidly resolved except in the presence of infection or of nitroglycerin tocolysis after open fetal surgery. *American journal of obstetrics and gynecology* 179:925-933.

Farrell JA et al (1999). Maternal fertility is not affected by fetal surgery. *Fetal diagnosis and therapy* 14:190-192.

Feldstein VA et al (2000). Twin-twin transfusion syndrome: the "SELECT" procedure. *Fetal diagnosis and therapy* 15(5):257-261.

Flake A (1995). Fetal surgery. Presentation given at the National Association of Neonatal Nurses Regional Conference: From Conception to Kindergarten, October 1995, Chicago.

Graf JL et al (1998). A surprising histological evolution of preterm sacrococcygeal teratoma. *Journal of pediatric surgery* 33:177-179.

Graf JL et al (2000). Successful fetal sacrococcygeal teratoma resection in a hydropic fetus. *Journal of pediatric surgery* 35:1489-1491.

Harrison MR (1996). Fetal surgery. *American journal of obstetrics and gynecology* 174:1255-1264.

Harrison MR et al (1996). Correction of congenital diaphragmatic hernia in utero. VIII. Response of the hyperplastic lung to tracheal occlusion. *Journal of pediatric surgery* 31:1339-1348.

Harrison MR et al (1997). Correction of congenital diaphragmatic hernia in utero. VII. A prospective trial. *Journal of pediatric surgery* 32:1637-1642.

Harrison MR et al (1998). Correction of congenital diaphragmatic hernia in utero. IX. Fetuses with poor prognosis (liver herniation and low lung to head ratio) can be saved by fetoscopic temporary tracheal occlusion. *Journal of pediatric surgery* 33:1017-1022.

Harrison MR et al (2001). *The unborn patient: the art and science of fetal therapy*, ed 3. WB Saunders: Philadelphia.

Hecher K (1999). Endoscopic laser surgery versus serial amniocentesis in the treatment of severe twin-twin transfusion syndrome. *American journal of obstetrics and gynecology* 180:717-724.

Hedrick MH et al (1994). Congenital high airway obstruction syndrome (CHAOS): a potential for perinatal intervention. *Journal of pediatric surgery* 29:271-274.

Howell LJ, Dunphy PM (1999). Fetal surgery: exploring the challenges in nursing care. *Journal of obstetric, gynecologic, and neonatal nursing* 28:427-432.

Hutchins GM (1996). Acquired spinal cord injury in human fetuses with myelomeningocele. *Pediatric pathology and laboratory medicine* 16:701-702.

Kiatano Y (1999). Open fetal surgery for life-threatening fetal malformations. *Seminars in perinatology* 23:448-461.

Laifer SA, Kuller JA (1996). Percutaneous umbilical blood sampling. In Kuller JA et al, editors. *Prenatal diagnosis and reproductive genetics*. Mosby: St Louis.

Liley AW (1963). Intrauterine transfusion of foetus in haemolytic disease. *British medical journal* 5365:1107-1109.

Lipshutz GS et al (1997). Prospective analysis of lung to head ratio predicts survival for patients with prenatally diagnosed congenital diaphragmatic hernia. *Journal of pediatric surgery* 32:1634-1636.

Manning FA (1986). International Fetal Surgery Registry: 1985 update. *Clinical obstetrics and gynecology* 29:551-557.

McMillan MP (1996). Banking on cord blood. *Journal of obstetric, gynecologic, and neonatal nursing* 25:115.

Meuli M et al (1995a). In utero surgery rescues neurologic function at birth in sheep with spina bifida. *Journal of pediatric surgery* 30:342-347.

Meuli M et al (1995b). Creation of myelomeningocele in utero: a model of functional damage from spinal cord exposure in fetal sheep. *Journal of pediatric surgery* 30:1028-1032.

Morin L et al (1994). Prenatal diagnosis and management of fetal thoracic lesions. *Seminars in perinatology* 18:228-253.

Mychaliska GB et al (1997). Operating on placental support: the ex utero intrapartum treatment (EXIT) procedure. *Journal of pediatric surgery* 32:227-231.

Paek BW et al (2000). Hindbrain herniation develops in surgically created myelomeningocele but is absent after repair in fetal lambs. *American journal of obstetrics and gynecology* 183:1119-1123.

Paek B et al (2001a). Radiofrequency ablation of human fetal sacrococcygeal teratoma. *American journal of obstetrics and gynecology*.

Paek B et al (2001b). CHAOS controlled: successful fetal intervention for complete high airway obstruction syndrome. *Fetal diagnosis and therapy*.

Quintero RA et al (1995). In utero percutaneous cystoscopy in the management of fetal lower obstructive uropathy. *Lancet* 346:537-540.

Quintero RA et al (1997). In utero lysis of amniotic bands. *Ultrasound in obstetrics and gynecology* 10:316-320.

Rice HE et al (1994). Congenital cystic adenomatoid malformation: a sheep model of fetal hydrops. *Journal of pediatric surgery* 29:692-696.

Skarsgard ED et al (1996). Fetal endoscopic tracheal occlusion (FETENDO-PLUG) for congenital diaphragmatic hernia. *Journal of pediatric surgery* 31:1335-1338.

Spitzer AR (1996). *Intensive care of the fetus and neonate*. Mosby: St Louis.

Strauss A et al (2000). Intrauterine fetal demise caused by amniotic band syndrome after standard amniocentesis. *Fetal diagnosis and therapy* 15:4-7.

Sullivan KM, Adzick NS (1994). Fetal surgery. *Clinical obstetrics and gynecology* 37:355-371.

Sutton LN et al (1999). Improvement in hindbrain herniation demonstrated by serial fetal magnetic resonance imaging following fetal surgery for myelomeningocele. *Journal of the American Medical Association* 282:1826-1831.

Taeusch HW, Ballard RA (1998). *Avery's diseases of the newborn*, ed 7. WB Saunders: Philadelphia.

Tulipan N et al (1998). Reduced hindbrain herniation after intrauterine myelomeningocele repair: a report of four cases. *Pediatric neurosurgery* 29:274-278.

Westerburg BW et al (1998). Radio frequency ablation of the liver in the fetal sheep: a model for treatment of sacrococcygeal teratoma in the fetus. *Surgery forum* 49:461-463.

Westerburg B et al (2000). Sonographic prognostic factors in fetuses with sacrococcygeal teratoma. *Journal of pediatric surgery* 35:322-326.

Wiley JM (1996). Stem cell transplantation for the treatment of genetic disease. In Kuller JA et al, editors. *Prenatal diagnosis and reproductive genetics*. Mosby: St Louis.

CHAPTER 14

EFFECTS OF LABOR ON THE FETUS AND NEONATE

TINA LEIGH WEITKAMP, DIANNE M. FELBLINGER

While caring for the pregnant mother, nurses also must be concerned for the welfare of the fetus. Whether the pregnancy has progressed normally or has been complicated, labor and delivery place the greatest stress on the fetus.

Even though the human body has a tremendous resilience to the stress of labor, research to determine the factors related to fetal stress during labor has expanded. The advent of electronic fetal monitoring (EFM) has provided nurses both with a wealth of knowledge about the fetus's status and ways to support fetal well-being. When this general state of normalcy gives way to a more critical or complicated labor scenario, the nurse can provide the appropriate care immediately. This chapter gives an overview of the effects of labor on the fetus and ways to monitor fetal well-being during the intrapartal period.

FETAL DEVELOPMENT AND FETAL MONITORING

With implantation of the blastocyst in the decidua, the placenta begins to develop. As the trophoblast grows, it develops into two layers, the cytotrophoblast and the syncytiotrophoblast. The syncytiotrophoblast forms the primitive uteroplacental circulation through erosion of the maternal blood vessels of the decidua, resulting in formation of the intervillous space. The intervillous space allows for transfer of oxygen (O_2) and nutrients from the maternal circulation to the fetal circulation and the return of carbon dioxide (CO_2) and waste products to the maternal circulation. By the end of the second week of development, chorionic villi begin to form. During the third week, rapid growth occurs, resulting in an increase in the surface area for maternal and fetal circulation. Chorionic villi cover the entire surface of the chorionic sac until the eighth week, at which time those on the decidua capsularis stretch and gradually disappear, giving the chorion a smooth appearance. The chorionic villi attached to the decidua basalis increase rapidly in size and complexity and are known as the villous chorion. The placenta is formed from both fetal (villous chorion) and maternal (decidua basalis) portions, which are held together by stem villi or anchoring villi.

Blood leaving the fetus through the umbilical arteries enters and moves through the placental arteriocapillary-venous network to the chorionic villi, where it comes in contact with the placental membrane, and gas and nutrient exchange occurs. Oxygen and nutrients reach the fetus through the umbilical vein.

During pregnancy, the maternal and fetal circulations are separated by the placental membrane. Until midpregnancy this membrane consists of four layers: syncytiotrophoblast, cytotrophoblast, connective tissue, and endothelium from the fetal capillary. As the pregnancy progresses, the cytotrophoblast disappears and the syncytiotrophoblast thins (Moore & Persaud, 1998). Oxygenated blood enters the intervillous space through the ends of the eroded maternal spiral arteries of the decidua basalis. The maternal blood pressure forces the maternal blood toward the placental membrane, allowing for exchange of gases and metabolic products. These products cross the placental membrane by means of several different types of transport: simple diffusion, facilitated transport, active transport, pinocytosis, and bulk flow (Table 14-1). Factors that affect the rate of transfer include molecular size, electrical charge, lipid solubility, placental size, placental blood flow, level of saturation, and metabolism of the substance by the mother, fetus, and placenta. Waste products from the placenta quickly cross the placental barrier into the maternal circulation (Moore & Persaud, 1998).

The fetal cardiovascular system begins to develop in the wall of the yolk sac during the third week of gestation. Formation of primitive fetal blood also begins in the wall of the yolk sac during the third week. Blood vessels from the yolk sac connect with those in the connecting stalk and chorion to form the primitive cardiovascular system. As development progresses, the blood travels throughout the entire fetus in a unique pattern.

The umbilical vein divides as it enters the fetus, and a small amount of the blood circulates through the liver and then empties into the inferior vena cava. Most of the blood entering the fetus bypasses the liver through the ductus venosus and enters the inferior vena cava. From the inferior vena cava, the blood enters the right atrium and passes through the foramen ovale into the left atrium, left ventricle, and aorta. From the aorta, the blood travels to the head and upper extremities or to the trunk and lower extremities. Blood returning from the head enters the superior vena cava and then the right atrium and right ventricle. From the right ventricle, a small amount of blood enters the pulmonary circulation; most of the blood enters the pulmonary artery through the ductus arteriosus and flows to the descending aorta and the placenta through the two umbilical arteries.

TABLE **14-1**	Types of Placental Transport and Affected Substances
Type of Transport	**Substances**
Simple diffusion	Water, electrolytes, carbon dioxide, anesthetic gases, free fatty acids
Facilitated transport	Glucose, galactose, oxygen
Active transport	Amino acids, calcium, iron, iodine, water-soluble vitamins, glucose
Pinocytosis	Albumin, gamma globulins, fat-soluble vitamins
Bulk flow	Water

The heart forms at 18 or 19 days' gestation, when the cardiogenic cords appear and lay the foundation of the endocardial heart tube. Heart pulsations begin as peristaltic waves forcing blood through the tube at day 22. As the fetal heart develops, the beating of the heart comes under the control of the sinoatrial node, which sets the heart rate. The normal fetal heart rate (FHR) is 120 to 160 beats per minute (bpm). As in adults, both the sinoatrial and atrioventricular nodes are under the influence of the vagus nerve.

The FHR is regulated by the parasympathetic and sympathetic branches of the autonomic nervous system, along with baroreceptors and chemoreceptors. Parasympathetic nervous stimulation of the heart (stimulation of the vagus nerve) results in a decrease in the heart rate. This system is responsible for producing long-term and short-term variability in the heart rate. Sympathetic nervous stimulation of the heart occurs when norepinephrine is released by the fetus and results in an increase in the FHR, myocardial contraction, and blood pressure. Chemoreceptors respond to changes in oxygen and carbon dioxide levels, and baroreceptors increase the FHR in response to an increase in blood pressure. This increase is often counteracted through stimulation of the baroreceptors found in the internal and external carotid arteries, which in turn stimulates the vagus and glossopharyngeal nerves, resulting in a decrease in FHR and blood pressure.

Fetal Heart Rate

The fetal heart rate can be auscultated with a fetoscope between 16 and 20 weeks' gestation. With a Doptone unit, the FHR can be auscultated when the uterus is above the pelvis. The fetal heart is heard loudest through the fetus's back. As the fetus matures and reaches term, the back can be easily identified through the Leopold maneuvers.

Electronic Fetal Heart Monitoring

Electronic fetal monitoring gained widespread use during the 1970s and has become the standard of care in many communities. The original goal of fetal monitoring was to identify changes in the fetal heart that indicated hypoxia. However, after almost three decades of research, the purpose of fetal monitoring has changed; the focus has shifted to health, with the goal of identifying whether the fetus is healthy or unhealthy.

Baseline Fetal Heart Rate.   The baseline FHR is defined as the fetal heart rate between contractions as measured over a period of at least 10 minutes. This baseline does not include periodic or episodic changes. A fetus usually has a baseline FHR of 110 to 160 bpm at term, although a term or postterm fetus may have a baseline FHR as low as 100 bpm. The lower heart rate is a result of maturation of the neurologic system (see Chapter 31 for more information on the neurologic system).

Fetal Bradycardia.   Fetal bradycardia is an FHR below 110 bpm for 10 minutes or longer (National Institute of Child Health and Human Development, Research Planning Workshop, 1997). Maternal causes of fetal bradycardia can include anesthesia, hypotension, position, hypothermia, and systemic lupus erythematosus. Fetal causes include prolonged cord compression, prolapse of the umbilical cord, congenital cardiac conduction and structural defects, hypothermia, fetal hypoxia, and continuous pressure on the fetal head during descent (terminal or end-stage bradycardia). A continuous FHR of 100 to 120 bpm in a term or postterm infant may be due to a mature parasympathetic system.

Fetal Tachycardia.   Fetal tachycardia is an FHR above 160 bpm for 10 minutes or longer (National Institute of Child Health and Human Development, Research Planning Workshop, 1997). An FHR above 180 bpm has been associated with fetal hypoxia. Other causes of tachycardia often are unknown; known causes include extreme prematurity, maternal hyperthermia, fetal or maternal infection, fetal or maternal anemia, ingestion of beta-sympathomimetic drugs, use of inotropic drugs or drugs that inhibit vagal response (atropine, hydroxyzine, and phenothiazine), cocaine use, maternal anxiety, hyperthyroidism, chronic hypoxia, fetal cardiac anomalies, fetal heart failure, supraventricular tachycardia, and excessive fetal activity.

Variability.   Variability is caused by the interaction between the sympathetic and parasympathetic nervous systems (Figure 14-1). For variability to occur, an unimpaired autonomic nervous system, a medulla oblongata, and a heart must be present. The interplay of the sympathetic and parasympathetic systems is then communicated to the medulla and the heart and is recorded as variability on the fetal heart tracing. This interplay is more evident as the fetus matures. The changes between each beat or between the R-waves are known as short-term variability. Short-term variability is mostly influenced by the parasympathetic system, which innervates both the sinoatrial and atrioventricular nodes. Short-term variability is evaluated only through internal electronic fetal monitoring and is noted as being present or absent. Long-term variability is seen as larger or cyclic changes that occur over a 1-minute period (Association of Women's Health, Obstetrics, and Neonatal Nurses [AWHONN], 1997). As with short-term variability, long-term variability can be evaluated only through internal electronic fetal monitoring.

Long-term variability is an indicator of fetal wellness and is evaluated in the following manner (National Institute of Child Health and Human Development, Research Planning Workshop, 1997):

- Undetectable: No variability
- Minimal: Below 5 bpm but greater than undetectable
- Moderate: 6 to 25 bpm
- Marked: Above 25 bpm

Many factors affect the variability of the fetal heart rate, including prematurity, severe fetal tachycardia, maternal drug ingestion (e.g., analgesics, hypnotics, and parasympathetic

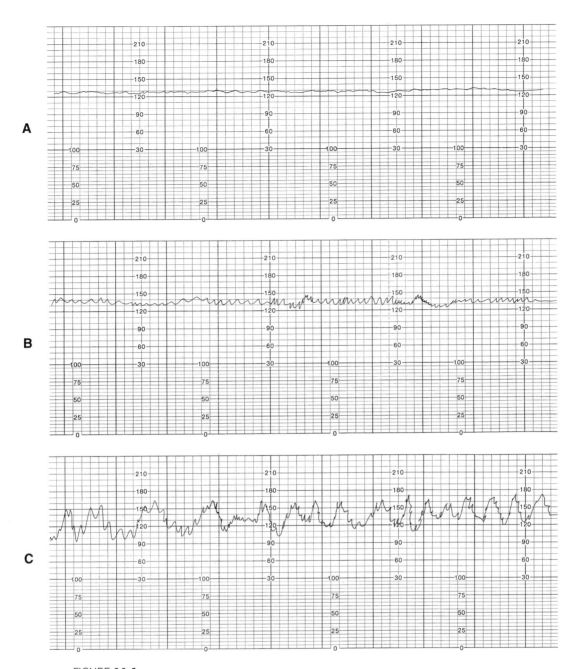

FIGURE **14-1**
Variability in fetal heart rate. **A,** Decreased or minimal variability. **B,** Average variability.
C, Marked, or saltatory, variability.

blocking agents), quiet fetal sleep, fetal hypoxia, congenital anomalies, anencephaly, and fetal acidosis.

A decrease in variability or minimal variability requires evaluation of possible causes. Fetal anomalies, maternal medications, and fetal behavioral states all can reduce variability. Interventions to correct decreased variability include position changes, hydration, changes in breathing techniques, stress reduction methods, and discontinuation of oxytocin. Marked variability may result from a sympathetic response to an acute hypoxic episode; possible interventions to correct this include position change, hydration, oxygen, stress-reduction methods, and discontinuation of oxytocin. Research indicates that long-term variability is decreased before significant fetal acidemia develops (Fox & Kilpatrick, 2000). In most cases, variability changes related to hypoxia develop gradually and are usually related to periodic or episodic changes. Prolonged continuous bradycardia of 60 bpms or less and life-threatening events (prolapsed cord and placental abruption) can quickly produce severe fetal acidosis, with rapid changes in variability (Fox & Kilpatrick, 2000).

Periodic Heart Rate Changes.   Periodic changes are changes that occur in the baseline FHR during a contraction or as the result of a contraction. The two types of periodic changes are accelerations and decelerations. Accelerations are visually apparent, abrupt increases in the FHR that reach their peak less than 30 seconds after onset; they often are associated with fetal movement (National Institute of Child Health and Human Development, Research Planning Workshop, 1997). In a fetus over 30 weeks' gestation, the peak is more than 15 bpm above the baseline, lasts longer than 15 seconds, and returns to baseline in less than 2 minutes. In a fetus under 30 weeks' gestation, the peak is 10 bpm or more over baseline and lasts longer than 10 seconds (National Institute of Child Health and Human Development, Research Planning Workshop, 1997). Prolonged accelerations last longer than 2 minutes but less than 10; an acceleration that lasts longer than 10 minutes is a change in baseline (National Institute of Child Health and Human Development, Research Planning Workshop, 1997). Accelerations are a product of the beta-adrenergic sympathetic nervous system and indicate an intact nervous system. Most accelerations are reassuring signs. However, repetitive, uniformly shaped accelerations may be an early response to mild hypoxia caused by cord compression.

Decelerations are transitory decreases from the baseline FHR that last less than 10 minutes (AWHONN, 1997). The three types of deceleration, early, variable, and late, are defined by their timing in relation to a uterine contraction and their general shape. Studies evaluating the relationship between FHR patterns, acidemia, and neonatal morbidity have shown that decelerations are a poor predictor of significant fetal acidemia except when the FHR remains below 60 bpm for 10 minutes or longer (Fox & Kilpatrick, 2000). The evidence indicates that the degree of variability that accompanies the deceleration is the most sensitive predictor of neonatal outcome (Fox & Kilpatrick, 2000).

FHR dysrhythmias are irregularities in the FHR, usually as a result of electrical firing in the heart that causes ectopic or premature beats. Dysrhythmias are best detected with a fetoscope, because irregularities often appear as artifacts with external monitoring.

Accelerations. Accelerations of the FHR occur with stimulation of the sympathetic nervous system. They appear as an increase in the FHR above the baseline, and their shape may resemble that of the uterine contraction pattern (when contractions are present), or they may occur after fetal movement. The onset of an acceleration depends on the stimuli, which may include spontaneous movement, stimulation of the fetal scalp, abdominal palpation, fundal pressure, uterine contractions, or mild umbilical cord compression. Figure 14-2 presents a fetal heart tracing showing accelerations.

Decelerations

Early Decelerations. Early decelerations occur as a result of pressure, usually on the fetal head, which stimulates the vagus nerve, resulting in a decrease in the FHR; recovery occurs once the pressure is removed from the head. When visualized, early decelerations appear as mirror images of the contraction pattern. The gradual deceleration starts early in the contraction, peaks at about the acme of the contraction, and returns to baseline by the time the contraction is complete. The shape is uniform in early decelerations, and variability is present. The FHR typically does not drop more than 25 bpm from the baseline. The depth of the deceleration increases as the length of the contraction increases. Early decelerations are seen during active labor as the fetus descends into and through the pelvis and frequently are seen with cephalopelvic disproportion. If the head is high, no caput or molding is present, and cervical dilation is less than 4 cm, it is not an early deceleration (Murray, 1997). Treatment of early decelerations begins with identification of the pattern and assessment of the fetus's status. Figure 14-3 presents a fetal heart tracing showing early decelerations.

Late Decelerations. Late decelerations are a result of uteroplacental insufficiency, a condition that occurs when gas exchange is restricted anywhere between the uterus, placenta, and fetus, resulting in fetal hypoxia. When late decelerations are a result of decreased maternal circulation, the underlying causes may include preeclampsia, diabetes, anemia, cardiac disease, respiratory disease, or regional anesthesia. When impaired uterine circulation results in late deceleration, the cause often is related to hyperstimulation of the uterine musculature from oxytocin or prostaglandin stimulation. Placental gas exchange often is jeopardized by a decrease in the placental area or by increased distance between the fetal capillaries and the maternal blood supply. Placental problems usually arise from a small placenta (as seen with intrauterine growth restriction) or from separation of part of the placenta (as seen with premature separation of the placenta or placenta previa). Postmaturity, malformations, and placental fibrin deposits and calcification also reduce the surface area. Small placentas also are found in women with a history of diabetes, collagen diseases, herpes, poor nutrition, smoking, multiple gestations, and preeclampsia

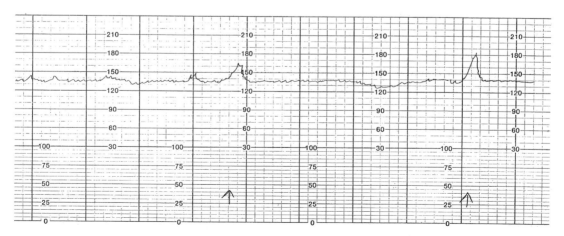

FIGURE **14-2**
Acceleration in fetal heart rate.

experience late decelerations. Late decelerations are preceded by altered blood flow to the placenta, a reduction in the maternal oxygen saturation, or placental changes that alter the maternal-fetal gas exchange. These conditions cause a decrease in uterine blood flow with contractions and a reduction in the partial pressure of oxygen (pO_2) after the acme of a contraction, which slow the fetal heart rate.

Late decelerations have a smooth, uniform appearance and occur after the contraction has begun, usually around the acme of the contraction. The lowest point of the deceleration generally comes well after the acme, and the return to baseline is gradual (requiring longer than 30 seconds) after uterine resting tone has returned to normal. Late decelerations often are seen with a loss of variability and a rising baseline FHR (Figure 14-4).

Treatment of late decelerations involves increasing the uterine blood flow and gas exchange. The methods used depend on the possible causes and current maternal status; they include correcting maternal hypotension (increasing intravenous fluids), reducing uterine stimulation (stopping or reducing oxytocic medication or administering tocolytic agents), position changes, or administration of oxygen by tight face mask. Other interventions may include checking for a prolapsed cord and insertion of an internal spiral electrode and an intrauterine pressure gauge to obtain an accurate picture of the FHR pattern, uterine activity, and the relationship of the de-celeration to uterine activity and an amnioinfusion (administration of a warmed normal saline solution into the uterus via a hollow intrauterine pressure catheter, a procedure discussed later in the chapter). The physician or nurse-midwife should be notified, and the actions should be documented.

Variable Decelerations.   Variable decelerations usually are caused by umbilical cord compression. They usually appear in patterns of FHR decrease that differ in size, duration, and shape from contraction to contraction. Variable decelerations occur in approximately half of all women in labor and are most common during the second stage. The duration and depth of the deceleration are directly related to the fetal hypotension, hypoxia, and hypertension that result (Murray, 1997). The onset of the deceleration usually is rapid, with the onset differing in relation to the contraction. First the umbilical vein is compressed, which slows the oxygenated blood flow to the fetus, causing a decrease in cardiac output and a fall in blood pressure. As the umbilical artery is compressed, the blood flow from the fetus is occluded and the blood pressure rises, stimulating the baroreceptor response. These changes are thought to trigger the vagal response, which causes the sudden drop in the fetal heart rate. Recovery of the baseline FHR usually is rapid as the pressure of the contraction diminishes. These decelerations may be U-, V-, or W-shaped with a rapid drop in the FHR (Figure 14-5).

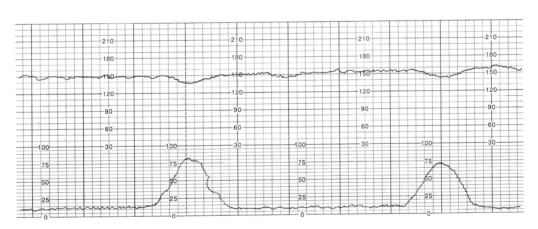

FIGURE **14-3**
Early deceleration in fetal heart rate.

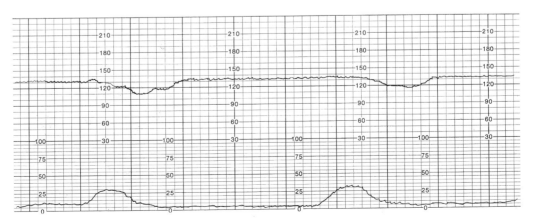

FIGURE **14-4**
Late deceleration in fetal heart rate.

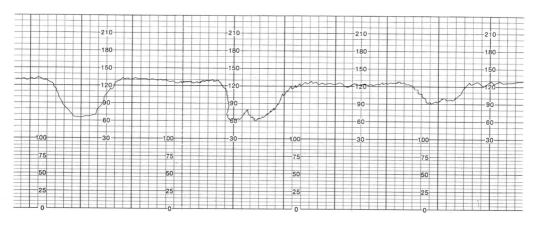

FIGURE **14-5**
Variable deceleration in fetal heart rate.

A shoulder is a compensatory acceleration (less than 20 bpm above baseline for less than 20 seconds) that precedes or follows a deceleration, and when short-term variability is present, the pattern is reassuring. (AWHONN, 1997). However, repeated hypoxic episodes that stress the fetus can result in an overshoot. Overshoots are smooth compensatory accelerations that follow a variable deceleration; they generally are more than 20 bpm above baseline and last longer than 20 seconds. When the overshoot is repetitive and short-term variability is absent, the pattern is not reassuring.

Treatment of variable decelerations involves changing the mother's position in hopes of relieving the pressure on the umbilical cord. A fluid bolus is given to increase the maternal vascular bed. If previous actions do not improve the fetus's status, uterine activity is reduced by discontinuing or reducing oxytocic agents. A spiral electrode may be applied to enhance the quality of the monitor strip, and an amnioinfusion may be done. The physician or nurse-midwife should be notified and appropriate documentation recorded.

During the antepartal and intrapartal periods, the fetus is susceptible to hypoxia, which may occur in an acute or a chronic form. When hypoxia is acute, decelerations appear on the fetal monitor. If the hypoxia is chronic, fetal growth is diminished. Evaluation for chronic hypoxia requires a biophysical profile, which has five parameters: reaction to a nonstress test, fetal breathing motions, gross fetal body movements, fetal body tone, and volume of amniotic fluid.

FETAL PULSE OXIMETRY

Pulse oximetry, which has been used successfully in other areas of medicine, has become available for use in labor. Pulse oximetry is based on two main principles: (1) oxygen hemoglobin (O_2Hb) and hemoglobin (Hb), which differ in their ability to absorb light, and (2) the amount of arterial blood in tissues changes during each pulse beat in the cardiac cycle. Fetal pulse oximetry notes changes in fetal oxygenation, and the accuracy of results depends on the placement of the sensor. If hair prevents the sensor from coming into direct contact with the skin, the light signals are impaired. Caput, vernix, and skin thickness all may affect readings. The normal range for the fetal scalp partial pressure of oxygen ($FspO_2$) is 30% to 70% and depends on the placement of the sensor. Most studies have been done with the fetus in the cephalic presentation, and the reliability of readings in other presentations is unknown. Fetal

pulse oximetry is becoming more widely available and may be a major factor in intrapartal care in years to come.

PLACENTAL FACTORS CONTRIBUTING TO FETAL COMPROMISE DURING LABOR

The placenta plays a vital role throughout the pregnancy. Numerous placental factors can directly or indirectly cause fetal compromise during labor. Maternal perfusion of the placenta may be diminished, or fetal uptake from the placenta may be reduced; both these factors affect the fetal outcome of the labor process.

Diminished Maternal Perfusion of the Placenta

Diminished maternal perfusion of the placenta can be caused by such factors as hypotension, hypertension, abruptio placentae, and hypertonic contractions. Because any of these factors can adversely affect the maternal-fetal dyad, indicating a decrease in maternal-placental perfusion during the labor process, the nurse must be vigilant in assessing for them.

Hypotension. Hypotension can develop in conjunction with numerous conditions, including maternal blood loss, drug ingestion or exposure, or position changes, such as placement of the mother in the supine position for administration of anesthetic agents. Any of these complications can affect fetal well-being adversely.

Maternal Blood Loss. Maternal blood loss, or obstetric hemorrhage, has been documented as one of the leading causes of maternal mortality. Except for pregnancies linked to abortive outcomes, postpartum hemorrhage has been implicated in 50% of hemorrhagic deaths (Berg et al, 1996). Bleeding after 20 weeks complicates approximately 6% of all pregnancies and may be a life-threatening condition (Creasy & Resnik, 1999). Obstetric hemorrhage may require cesarean section; conditions that may be involved include obstetric lacerations, uterine atony, retained placenta, uterine inversion and, in rare cases, placenta accreta. The nurse must be able to manage any of these potentially dangerous situations.

The goals for management of conditions that can result in hypotension and consequent hemorrhagic shock generally are twofold. The primary goal is to restore the blood volume and the oxygen-carrying capacity immediately. The second goal is to provide the specific nursing interventions required for the condition causing the hemorrhage. Stabilization of the patient's condition is of paramount importance (Creasy & Resnik, 1999). The mother's condition must be stabilized, or the effects of blood loss on the fetus may be ominous. Uteroplacental insufficiency can leave the fetus incapable of a life-sustaining physiologic response. The fetal response to acute blood loss is similar to the maternal reaction: hypoxemia and acidosis result in bradycardia, vasospasm, and the initial shunting of blood to vital organs. As the mother's condition worsens, these compensatory mechanisms become inadequate, and brain damage and fetal demise may result (May & Mahlmeister, 1994).

Drug Ingestion and Exposure.   Exposure to certain drugs may have hypotensive effects on the mother and thus may adversely affect the fetus in utero. The nurse caring for the patient must be aware of the pharmacologic action of any drugs the patient receives during hospitalization, as well as the action of any drugs the patient has taken before admission. Medications known to have hypotensive effects include ritodrine, magnesium sulfate, and narcotic substances.

Ritodrine (Yutopar) and terbutaline often are given as tocolytic agents in an effort to arrest labor. Because these drugs cross the placenta, the nurse must be aware of their effects on both the mother and the fetus. The drugs may result not only in a drop in maternal blood pressure but also in an increase in the maternal and fetal heart rates. Magnesium sulfate ($MgSO_4$) is another drug used for its tocolytic effect that depresses myometrial contractility, and it also may be given to treat preeclampsia. The nurse must be aware that $MgSO_4$ can cause a drop in blood pressure as a result of splanchnic dilation and that severe maternal hypotension may occur. A decrease in the FHR may occur when $MgSO_4$ is given to the mother. The neonatal toxic effects of maternal $MgSO_4$ administration generally are minimal; however, decreased muscle tone and drowsiness may be noted in newborns whose mothers received $MgSO_4$ for tocolysis.

Narcotic drugs, particularly those used in conjunction with administration of an anesthetic, may cause respiratory depression and hypotensive episodes in the laboring patient. Whether these substances are administered in therapeutic doses in a controlled labor setting or ingested by a drug-addicted mother before admission, the nurse must be aware that placental transfer of these drugs usually occurs quickly. Narcotic addiction during pregnancy may lead to premature delivery, stillbirth, or addiction in infants, who may experience neonatal abstinence reactions. The nurse caring for the drug-addicted mother must understand that the narcotic-exposed infant may demonstrate severe withdrawal symptoms in utero, at birth, or during the 10- to 15-day period immediately after birth. Some drug-exposed infants experience subacute withdrawal for 4 to 6 months after birth. Because of the potential for depressant and hypotensive effects of therapeutic narcotic administration and the magnitude of the complications associated with illicit maternal use of these drugs, the nurse must be alert to the impact these drugs may have on the mother, the fetus, and the infant.

Maternal Position Changes During Labor.   The relative position of the mother during the labor and delivery process may affect her hypotensive state and thereby the response of the fetus. It has been well documented that the supine position is not ideal for the mother in labor. Supine positioning of the mother affects cardiac output through compression of the aorta and the vena cava, thus adversely affecting the circulatory response of the fetus. The laboring mother generally is placed in the left lateral recumbent position to avoid a hypotensive state, known as supine hypotensive syndrome. When supine hypotensive syndrome occurs, the decrease in maternal cardiac output may be harmful to the fetus; uterine arterial pressure also may decline, which could be especially detrimental to the fetus if it occurs concomitantly with extensive blood loss or administration of an anesthetic during delivery.

Hypertension.   The nurse must be alert to an existing or impending hypertensive state during labor. Hypertension may be a factor in numerous situations, such as in patients with chronic hypertension, in those with preeclampsia (onset usually after 20 weeks' gestation), and in patients who have taken certain drugs. Hypertension can compromise placental function and thus adversely affect fetal health. Infants of all hypertensive women should be treated and monitored as possible high-risk infants. Intrauterine growth retardation and perinatal mortality are more prevalent among pregnancies of hypertensive women.

Ideally, hypertension is documented early in the pregnancy of women who have a history of chronic hypertension. Early recognition of this chronic state allows time for adequate blood pressure monitoring and provides baseline data that later help the nurse differentiate the chronic hypertensive state from a superimposed state of preeclampsia. The nurse must understand that the fetal effects of these two hypertensive states are different. The perinatal mortality rate for infants of women with superimposed preeclampsia is higher than that for infants of women in whom the hypertension exists alone. The decidual vessels of women with mild to severe hypertension may show changes similar to those noted in the renal arterioles of women with an extensive history of hypertension. The diminished uteroplacental perfusion that occurs secondary to this change is at least additive and perhaps synergistic with the decidual vascular changes of preeclampsia. These additional decidual vascular changes also may be associated with the higher rate of abruptio placentae in women with superimposed preeclampsia. Creasy and Resnik (1999) noted that, "Preeclampsia also has been seen earlier in the pregnancies of hypertensive women than in the pregnancies of normotensive women." In view of the difficulties that arise in recognizing and treating superimposed preeclampsia, all infants of hypertensive women should be considered at risk, and their nursing care should be planned accordingly.

To treat the patient with pregnancy-induced hypertension (PIH), the nurse first must be aware of the classic symptoms associated with this condition, which include the following:

- Hypertension: A sustained blood pressure increase to 140 mm Hg systolic or 90 mm Hg diastolic (American College of Obstetricians and Gynecologists, [ACOG], 1996).
- Proteinuria: 0.5 g/L in a 24-hour period (normal is less than 300 mg/24 hours) or a dipstick reading of +1 or +2. Proteinuria usually is the last symptom to appear.
- Edema: Clinically evident swelling or a sudden, rapid weight gain in the second or third trimester; nondependent edema of the hands and face is significant. Edema may or may not be present and should not be the pivotal factor for diagnosis of PIH. Clinical manifestations of severe PIH may include an elevated serum creatinine, grand mal seizures (eclampsia), pulmonary edema, oliguria (less than 500 ml in 24 hours), microangiopathic hemolysis, thrombocytopenia, hepatocellular dysfunction, intrauterine growth retardation or oligohydramnios, and symptoms indicative of significant end-organ involvement such as headache, visual disturbances, and epigastric or right upper quadrant pain (ACOG, 1996).

PIH often is seen in conjunction with intrauterine growth restriction and an increase in the rate of preterm delivery among the surviving infants (May & Mahlmeister, 1994). The nurse must assess for uterine growth in relation to gestational age by using McDonald's measurements (fundal heights). The nurse must also be familiar with the results of the mother's ultrasound examination, nonstress test, and amniocentesis. Understanding the effects of hypertension on the fetus can help the nurse develop an individualized plan of care for the mother and the fetus during the prenatal and labor periods.

Certain drugs also may produce an untoward hypertensive effect on the mother and thus adversely affect fetal health. Stimulants such as cocaine, amphetamines, and methamphetamines may induce an increase in the maternal heart and respiratory rates and may elevate her blood pressure. Cocaine may diffuse across the placenta and reduce placental blood flow, hampering fetal gas and nutrient exchange. Cocaine-exposed infants have a higher incidence of impaired fetal growth, premature birth, and neonatal seizures (Chapter 39). Because many mothers who use illicit substances may be polydrug users, the nurse must be able to assess the infant for multiple indications of maternal substance use or abuse. The infant may show signs of central nervous system (CNS) hyperirritability, gastrointestinal disturbance, and respiratory distress, as well as vague autonomic symptoms (Lowdermilk et al, 2000).

Abruptio Placentae. Diminished maternal perfusion of the placenta may also occur with abruptio placentae, or separation of the normally implanted placenta before the birth of the fetus (Creasy & Resnik, 1999). The diminished perfusion of the placenta may result in untoward fetal effects, and abruption of the placenta during labor may contribute to fetal compromise. Although not every case of abruptio placentae results in fetal death, three major causes of fetal demise are related to abruptio placentae: fetal anoxia, neonatal prematurity, and fetal exsanguination. The neonatal intensive care unit (NICU) nurse must be aware that an abruption that occurs before 28 weeks lessens the fetus's chance for survival. More than 20% of births resulting from abruption occur between 28 and 32 weeks' gestation, and these neonates present a challenge in nursing care.

The method and timing of delivery and consequently the labor period of the patient with abruptio placentae are of paramount concern to the nurse. The factors that affect the progression of the labor period are related to fetal gestational age, maternal condition, and the status of the cervix. If the gestational age is early and the abruption is only mild, an observational approach is acceptable. In the absence of maternal complications or fetal compromise, the nurse may cautiously administer tocolytic agents while continually assessing the maternal and fetal status. Early pregnancy may be prolonged with careful continuing assessment for signs of abruptio placentae, which may manifest with concealed or apparent hemorrhage. When hemorrhage is concealed, no vaginal bleeding is seen, but the nurse must be alert for sudden, pronounced uterine or abdominal pain, a rapid increase in the rigidity or size of the uterus, absence of fetal heart tones, and signs of acute fetal compromise. When hemorrhage is apparent, the nurse also assesses for bright red or dark clotted vaginal bleeding. Uterine tonicity may increase, and the uterus may fail to relax between contractions. Abruptio placentae can progress to hypovolemia and shock secondary to the hemorrhagic state, and disseminated intravascular coagulation also may occur.

When the placental separation is moderate or severe, the nurse must be ready to prepare the patient for delivery. In the event of fetal demise, vaginal delivery is indicated as a means of reducing the chance of maternal morbidity. If the fetal heart tracing is within normal parameters and the uterus relaxes between contractions, the mother may be prepared for a vaginal delivery. If intravenous oxytocin is used to augment uterine activity, extreme caution must be exercised, because the uterine response may be unpredictable and the threat of uterine rupture is greater.

If the fetus is alive but shows signs of acute fetal compromise, immediate cesarean section is indicated. Signs of fetal compromise may include changes in the FHR (tachycardia, bradycardia), late decelerations, and decreasing or absent variability. The rate of fetal death secondary to abruption has been estimated as 1 in 420 deliveries (Creasy & Resnik, 1999), and this condition remains a leading cause of maternal death (Lowdermilk et al, 2000).

Hypertonic Contractions. Hypertonic contractions may also be a factor in diminished maternal perfusion of the placenta. Hypertonic contractions may occur in conjunction with excessive administration of oxytocin and precipitous labor.

Oxytocin usually is released from the posterior lobe of the pituitary gland, but intravenous oxytocin may be given to augment the labor process. Synthetic oxytocin preparations (e.g., Pitocin) act on the uterine muscle to stimulate uterine contractions. Pitocin is a powerful drug and must be used judiciously. Administration of oxytocin carries the risk of producing abnormally strong or tetanic uterine contractions secondary to uterine overstimulation, therefore an intravenous infusion pump must be used to ensure safe administration of Pitocin. The nurse must be alert for signs of fetal compromise and must be aware of the possibility of uterine rupture. The fetus must be monitored constantly, and the internal uterine pressure monitor is used as indicated. If signs of hypertonicity are evident, the nurse should immediately discontinue the oxytocin infusion and notify the physician.

Hyperstimulation of the uterus may cause fetal compromise as a result of impaired uteroplacental perfusion, abruption of the placenta, amniotic fluid embolism, cervical laceration or uterine rupture, and neonatal trauma (May & Mahlmeister, 1994). The nurse must be aware of these complications and must assess the patient for risks and benefits to the mother and her fetus.

Precipitous labor also may result from a pattern of unusually strong and frequent uterine contractions. Precipitous labor generally lasts less than 3 hours before the spontaneous delivery of the fetus. The fetus may pass quickly through the pelvis because of relatively low resistance of the maternal tissues. Factors that may signal the possibility of precipitous labor include multiparity; a large, bony pelvis; soft, pliable genital tissue; a small fetus in vertex position; previous precipitous labor; or cocaine abuse (May & Mahlmeister, 1994).

The fetus may survive a precipitous labor if there is little resistance to fetal descent and if placental perfusion is adequate. If the fetus experiences chronic distress, however, the fetal status may deteriorate during a precipitous delivery because perfusion is diminished by uterine hypermobility. With bony or soft tissue resistance to the delivery, trauma to the fetal head may occur on descent. In any unassisted birth situation, the possibility also exists of neonatal aspiration and hypothermia. The nurse must be alert to these risk factors and carefully monitor the labor progress of the mother at risk for precipitous labor. The mother's contractions, cervical dilation, and effacement, as well as the fetal station and presentation, must be assessed continually. The consistent attention of the nurse during the labor period is vitally important to the safe delivery of the fetus in this situation.

Diminished Fetal Uptake from the Placenta

Diminished fetal uptake from the placenta may also cause or contribute to fetal compromise during labor. A decrease in fetal uptake may occur in situations such as umbilical cord compression and fetal anemia.

Umbilical Cord Compression. Partial, brief compression of the umbilical cord may occur during the first stage of labor and may be indicated by variable decelerations on the electronic fetal monitor. A change in maternal position, such as turning the mother from side to side, may eliminate or lessen the compression pattern. Maternal vital signs must be closely monitored.

During the second stage of labor, compression may occur during fetal descent. Variable decelerations are associated with fetal complications only when these heart rate changes are severe or prolonged. Repeated stress diminishes the fetal oxygen reserve. Fetal depression occurs when the nuchal cord is tight. Severe variable decelerations may result in fetal acidosis. The fetal blood pH is sampled, and oxygen is administered to the mother at 8 to 10 L/minute by face mask. Severe, persistent fetal bradycardia with recurrent or diminished variability after a uterine contraction may indicate cord compression and the need for immediate delivery. The nurse must be able to react quickly while displaying a supportive demeanor for the patient and her family. Intrauterine amnioinfusion may be attempted to relieve cord compression, particularly in certain cases of oligohydramnios or premature rupture of membranes. Amnioinfusion involves the administration of a warmed normal saline solution into the uterus via a hollow intrauterine pressure catheter. The complications of this procedure include uterine overdistention and an increase in the uterine resting tonus. Continuous fetal and maternal monitoring is essential during this procedure (Murray, 1997).

Fetal Anemia. Another factor that can cause or contribute to fetal compromise during labor is hemolytic disease of the newborn, or fetal anemia (also called erythroblastosis fetalis or nonimmune hydrops). Fetal anemia may occur in conjunction with Rh incompatibility. Rh is a genetically determined factor. Rh disease is present when the mother is Rh negative, the father is Rh positive, and the fetus is Rh positive. When fetal Rh positive red blood cells come in contact with the mother's circulating blood, an antigen-antibody response may be stimulated. In general, the mother becomes sensitized during her first pregnancy, and the Rh-positive fetus of a subsequent pregnancy is affected. Rh-positive antibodies are produced and transferred across the placenta, and they subsequently attach to the fetal red blood cells, which are destroyed. In response to the red blood cell destruction, the fetus produces many immature red blood cells, a condition known as erythroblastosis fetalis. In the most severe form of the disease, known as hydrops fetalis, the fetus may become severely anemic.

Although this condition is not as common as it was in years past, the complications can be devastating. Ascites and generalized edema may develop. Half of these fetuses become hydropic between 20 and 34 weeks' gestation; the other half, between 34 and 40 weeks. Hydrops fetalis is not due to fetal heart failure, nor is the fetus hypervolemic or in heart failure at birth. Heart failure may develop after birth. Hepatic enlargement and hepatocellular damage are the more likely etiologic factors (Creasy & Resnik, 1999). Although most hydropic fetuses show evidence of severe anemia, the nurse must be aware that some may have hemoglobin levels well above 7 g/dl (see Chapter 30 for a complete discussion).

During labor, the mother who is Rh negative should be crossmatched for Rh immunoglobulin to be given after the delivery. If a sensitized mother has some degree of erythroblastosis, the labor nurse and the neonatal team must work together during the delivery. The infant is transfused with Rh-negative blood soon after the fetal hemoglobin, hematocrit, and blood type are determined. The hydropic infant probably will be transferred to the NICU for follow-up care. The nurse must be aware of the needs of both the infant and the family and make every effort to explain the rationale for the infant's care in a supportive manner. The explanation should be given in terms the family can understand and should be repeated often, soon after delivery and again before discharge. Because of the stress of labor and delivery and the effects of medication that may have been used during delivery and the postpartum period, the mother may not remember the explanation, regardless of her educational level. Providing written information to the mother and another family member helps the family process the information.

ADMINISTRATION OF ANESTHETIC AGENTS DURING LABOR

The pain caused by the contractions that occur during labor is difficult for many women to tolerate. Beginning with Queen Victoria in the mid-1800s, pain control during childbirth became accepted, and since that time many drugs and methods of pain control have been used. Almost all medications are administered to the mother, and they then cross the placenta and enter the fetal circulation. The type of drug, the maternal dose, the route, and the fetus's age all play a role in the effect the drug has on the fetus. Pain-controlling drugs are rarely given orally during labor because absorption from the maternal gastrointestinal tract is diminished. To reduce the chance of acid aspiration in labor, it is common practice to use antacids to neutralize stomach contents. The current standard of care uses sodium citrate and a gastric histamine receptor antagonist (Sleutel & Golden, 1999). These drugs have minimal if any effect on the fetus during labor.

Either anesthetic or analgesic agents may be administered during labor. An analgesic diminishes pain sensation and thereby raises the pain threshold; an anesthetic not only provides analgesia but also inhibits pain perception and increases muscle relaxation. The analgesic agents used during labor usually belong to one of the following classifications: sedatives, H_1 receptor antagonists, opioids, narcotic antagonists, or a mixed compound.

Sedatives do not reduce pain. They are used during early labor to reduce maternal anxiety by sedation. However, sedatives may increase apprehension if they are given without analgesic agents. Use of sedatives should be limited to the early phase of the first stage of labor. These drugs may cause maternal CNS depression, including respiratory and vasomotor depression and drowsiness. Hypotension, nausea, vomiting, vertigo, and lethargy also are often seen. Because of the risk of maternal hypotension, close monitoring of maternal and fetal status is essential. If sedatives are administered shortly before delivery, neonatal depression may result.

Benzodiazepines (Diazepam, Valium) are similar to ataractics (tranquilizers) in that they do not relieve pain during labor but they do increase relaxation and may produce sleep in some women. These medications pass through the placenta and may result in fetal respiratory depression. FHR variability declines with these medications (Faucher & Brucker, 2000).

H_1 receptor antagonists block the action of histamine at the receptor site. Promethazine (Phenergan) causes marked sedation and may decrease FHR variability. Hydroxyine (Vistaril) does not potentiate opioid-induced analgesia, and it has not been shown to increase neonatal respiratory depression. (Faucher & Brucker, 2000) The major side effect of H_1 antagonists is hypotension, which can impede the uteroplacental circulation. After administration of these drugs, the fetal status must be closely monitored, and methods to increase uteroplacental circulation should be used as necessary. Infants born shortly after administration of the drug may be hypotonic, drowsy, and prone to hypothermia. A decrease in bilirubin binding sites has been associated with promethazine use, placing the neonate at risk for hyperbilirubinemia.

Opioids produce a high level of pain relief without amnesic effects. The drugs rapidly cross into fetal circulation, where they are metabolized by the fetal liver and kidneys. Some maternal breakdown of the drugs also occurs. Because the fetal and neonatal liver and kidneys are less effective than the adult organ systems, the metabolism is much slower if the fetus is delivered before complete drug metabolism. Fetal side effects include decreased FHR variability and respiratory depression. Neonatal neurobehavioral changes can occur for several days. The most commonly give opioids are butorphanol, fentanyl (Sublimaze), morphine, meperidine, (Demerol), and nalbuphine (Nubain). Butorphanol and nalbuphine are combination agonist-antagonists. The combination drugs cause drug withdrawal symptoms in narcotic-dependent mothers and fetuses.

Narcotic antagonists, such as naloxone (Narcan), reverse the effects of narcotic-induced respiratory depression by displacing the narcotic at the receptor sites of the central nervous system. After delivery, naloxone may be given directly to the neonate through the umbilical vein or through an endotracheal tube. Intramuscular or subcutaneous administration has a delayed onset of action. Because the action of the antagonist is quick and the duration short, repeat doses often are needed if respiratory depression recurs. Naloxone should not be given if the mother is addicted to narcotics or is taking methadone, because neonatal seizures may result (Kattwinkel, 2000).

During the 1950s regional anesthesia was introduced into obstetrics. Regional anesthetics provide pain relief by blocking the nerve impulses. In obstetrics, regional anesthetics are administered by epidural block, spinal block, combined spinal-epidural saddle block, subarachnoid block, caudal block, paracervical block, pudendal block, and local perineal infiltration.

With an epidural block, analgesia is achieved within 10 to 30 minutes of administration. The medication is administered into the epidural space, where pain nervous innervations are blocked. The advantage is that the mother can remain awake and participate actively in the birth process. The disadvantages are due to the sympathectomy, which results in peripheral vasodilation. Maternal hypotension and decreased uterine blood flow may result in changes in the fetal heart pattern. Hypotension can be prevented or minimized by hydrating the

woman before inducing anesthesia and by placing her on her side with a wedge under her to relieve the pressure on the vena cava. It is important to remember than a normotensive reading may be obtained with a decrease in uteroplacental resistance, therefore monitoring of the fetal response is essential. If the hypotension is moderate, the laboring woman may also be treated with O_2 by face mask. If this does not solve the problem, the woman's legs may be elevated to promote blood return, and ephedrine may be administered.

Other side effects of an epidural block include nausea, vomiting, urinary retention, shivering, headache, and fever. Research has shown that women who have had an epidural for longer than 5 hours gradually show a temperature increase of 0.8° to 1° C. The cause of this increase is unclear, but it is thought that the epidural anesthesia might alter the thermoregulatory threshold for vasodilation and sweating.

The medications used for an epidural block may be administered intermittently or continuously. The advantages of continuous infusion are consistency of the anesthesia level, lower blood concentrations, and a reduced incidence of hypotension. The drugs can be administered intermittently in boluses or with patient-controlled bolus injections. The catheter may remain in place after delivery for pain control during the immediate postpartum period.

A walking epidural or intrathecal block places a narcotic at the opioid receptor sites on the spinal cord, which results in analgesic effect without interfering with motor function. This is a one-time administration of medication for pain relief.

A combination spinal-epidural block offers the advantages of both epidural and spinal anesthesia. This method allows opioids to be placed intrathecally where they work best and also allows administration of epidural analgesia as labor progresses. The fetal-neonatal effects are related to hypotension. No significant change is seen in the American Pediatric Gross Assessment Record (APGAR) scores or neurobehavioral examinations (Camann, 2000).

Spinal, saddle, and subarachnoid blocks are administered by injecting a local anesthetic into the spinal canal to provide anesthesia for delivery. These methods are used primarily for repeat cesarean birth and in many cases have been replaced by the epidural block. If the delivery is to be vaginal, the anesthetic is administered at the level of the T10 vertebra; for a cesarean birth, it is given at the level of T8. For a saddle block, the anesthetic is injected into the spinal area such that nerve impulses through the perineal area and upper inner thighs (areas that touch a saddle) are blocked. The major advantage of this type of anesthesia is the immediate onset and small dose of medication needed. The major disadvantage is the hypotension that results from blocking the sympathetic nerves.

For a caudal block, the anesthetic is administered through the caudal area of the spine, providing anesthesia to the cervix, vagina, and perineum by blocking the sacral nerve. This method has been largely replaced by the epidural block.

A paracervical block results in interruption of the nerve impulses of the inferior hypogastric plexus and ganglia. This provides pain relief from cervical dilation but not from uterine contractions, and it does not anesthetize the lower vagina or perineum. The major advantage is the speedy onset of the anesthesia. The disadvantages, related to the high vascularity of the area, include possible hematoma formation, either as a result of labor or delivery trauma or of the injection itself; rapid absorption of the medication; and fetal bradycardia as a result of absorption of the medication. Fetal injury from direct injection of the local anesthetic into the fetal scalp also may occur, especially if cervical dilation is advanced (Chestnut, 1999).

The pudendal block provides anesthesia for the second and third stages of delivery and during repair of the episiotomy. The anesthetic agent is injected below the pudendal plexus, blocking the nerve impulse of the perineal muscles, lower vagina, vulva, urethral sphincter, perineum, and perianal muscles. It does not provide pain relief from uterine contractions. The major advantage is the lack of maternal hypotension, and effects on the fetus are rare except when the anesthetic is injected into the vascular system.

Perineal infiltration provides anesthesia for the episiotomy only and provides no muscle relaxation.

All regional anesthesia techniques involve the use of a local anesthetic. All local anesthetics are potent vasodilators, and absorption into the maternal circulation occurs within 10 to 15 minutes (Faucher & Brucker, 2000). The three types of local anesthetics are the ester-linked anesthetics, the amide-linked anesthetics, and the opiate anesthetics. The ester-linked agents are short acting and quickly metabolized by plasma cholinesterase. They do not cross the placenta to the fetus. The ester-linked anesthetic tetracaine (Pontocaine) is more slowly metabolized and has a long duration. Procaine (Novocain) is good for local infiltration but not for large areas because it lasts approximately 1 hour. Chloroprocaine (Nesacaine) is used when fetal respiratory depression must be avoided. It lasts approximately 1 hour and has a rapid onset; however, injection into the spinal fluid should be avoided.

Liver enzymes metabolize the amide-linked agents, which cross the placenta. Because the fetal liver does not produce the same amounts of liver enzymes as those found in maternal circulation, the fetus and neonate slowly metabolize the amide-linked agents. Lidocaine (Xylocaine), mepivacaine (Carbocaine), bupivacaine (Marcaine), and ropivacaine (Naropin) all last at least 1 hour, and bupivacaine may last as long as 3 hours. Epinephrine in low doses sometimes is added to accelerate the onset of analgesia. Amide-linked agents are good for prolonged pain relief. However, they affect the fetus, and the effects include neurobehavioral changes, jaundice, and late decelerations.

Because the pain of labor is a complex response with both physiologic and psychologic aspects, many nurses encourage women to use a combination of pharmacologic agents as described earlier and cognitive management to reduce anxiety and tension (Lowe, 1996). Keeping the woman focused and participating in the process of pain control helps reduce the need for medication, thus reducing the fetal-neonatal side effects of such therapies. Cultural aspects of childbearing pain should also be considered in the management plan. A Chinese woman may experience a great deal of pain but may remain stoic according to her tradition (Weber, 1996). The nurse, in this case, must rely on knowledge of the laboring process and subtle cues to assess the degree of pain.

INDICATIONS FOR TESTING FETAL WELL-BEING

The effects of labor on the fetus are numerous and frequently unpredictable. The nurse must remain constantly alert for any subtle changes in maternal or fetal condition that signify fetal compromise or distress. These changes may occur suddenly and with very little warning, and often only a short time is available for nursing intervention. For these reasons, tests for fetal well-being are performed routinely on the mother with a high-risk pregnancy during the antenatal period. Ideally the mother is observed closely during this period, and the information gathered can be useful for planning care during the crucial labor and delivery period.

The nurse must be aware of situations in which antenatal testing is indicated. Antenatal testing for fetal well-being is indicated with certain maternal conditions that could result in diminished uteroplacental perfusion (e.g., chronic hypertension and PIH, renal disease, collagen vascular disease, cardiac disease, diabetes mellitus). Testing is also indicated if maternal conditions may cause intrinsic placental disease that leads to placental insufficiency, as in diabetes mellitus or postdates pregnancy. Other high-risk pregnancies that require close monitoring include multiple pregnancy and those involving intrauterine growth retardation or hemolytic disease. Situations that would entail higher than usual risk for fetal death include decreased perception of fetal movement and a history of previous unexplained stillbirth. The tests for fetal well-being have been divided into two categories, biochemical tests and the biophysical profile.

Biochemical Tests

Biochemical tests are appealing because they can be performed simply and quickly at intervals during the antenatal and labor periods. The search continues for serum and urine indicators of fetal compromise. Human placental lactogen (HPL) and estriol levels have been investigated for their usefulness in managing high-risk pregnancies, but neither measurement has been found to ensure fetal well-being or to predict fetal compromise. The trend in maternal-child testing has been away from reliance on biochemical parameters and toward the antenatal biophysical profile system.

Biophysical Profile

The biophysical profile is a noninvasive assessment system that evaluates the fetus's status on the basis of five or six parameters, with each area receiving a score. This system is based on the premise that varying degrees of hypoxia affect different brain centers, and the longer the hypoxia is present, the more systems are affected. The later in gestation a fetal system develops, the more sensitive that system is to decreasing amounts of oxygen. Because the central nervous system develops late in gestation, it is most sensitive to oxygen deprivation. Development of the medulla is completed during the end of the second trimester or the beginning of the third trimester, therefore it is capable of responding to decreased oxygen concentration by losing heart rate variability. The ventral surface of the fourth ventricle completes development at 20 to 21 weeks and is responsible for fetal breathing movements, which cease after loss of heart rate variability. Fetal motor movement begins after development of the cortex nuclei at about 9 weeks' gestation, and fetal muscle begins to develop tone at about 7½ to 8½ weeks.

Except for the nonstress test (NST), all the components of the biophysical profile are done with ultrasonographic visualization. One of the first evaluations was the NST, which gauges the response of the FHR to fetal activity or stimulation. With activity, the fetal heart rate normally increases by at least 15 beats for 15 seconds. This test normally is performed several times over a 10- to 20-minute period.

Other components of the biophysical profile are fetal breath movements (FBMs), fetal movement (FM), fetal tone (FT), and the amniotic fluid volume (AFV). FBMs are evaluated by using ultrasonographic visualization to assess the fetal chest and abdomen for breathing movements; movement of the fetal trunk (FM) also is assessed. FT is assessed by evaluating the extension and flexion of the fetal body or extremities. AFV is a measurement of the amount of amniotic fluid present. The amniotic sac is scanned for pockets of fluid measuring at least 2 mm in two different planes.

Placental grading was added later to the biophysical profile. It entails examination of the basal and chorionic plates of the placenta. A grade 0 placenta is immature; a grade III placenta is significantly aged and may not be functioning optimally.

Each area is evaluated using specific criteria, and a score of 0, 1, or 2 is assigned. The scores are totaled and evaluated. A total score of 8 to 10 indicates a normal infant with low risk of chronic asphyxia. With a total score of 4 to 7, chronic asphyxia is suspected, and a score below 4 strongly suggests chronic asphyxia. A score of 6 represents an abnormal biophysical profile.

Ultrasonography

Ultrasonography has been used as a diagnostic tool in obstetrics since the 1960s. Current uses include diagnosis and evaluation of early pregnancy; determination of gestational age and size; and identification of multiple pregnancies, placental location, amniotic fluid volume, fetal presentation and position, and fetal malformations. A variety of methods are available, including transvaginal scanning, Doppler ultrasonography, color imaging, and three-dimensional ultrasonography.

PREPARATION FOR BIRTH

Each of the numerous delivery options has implications for fetal well-being. Spontaneous vaginal delivery, when feasible, is the option of choice. However, circumstances may require a cesarean section or the use of forceps or vacuum extraction.

Although cesarean section has become a relatively safe procedure, it is associated with a higher risk of morbidity and mortality than vaginal delivery. Cesarean delivery has been associated with increases in neonatal respiratory morbidity at all gestational ages; with fetal asphyxia related to uteroplacental hypoperfusion secondary to anesthesia induction or maternal position; and with inadvertent scalpel lacerations (Creasy & Resnik, 1999). The neonatal nurse must be aware of the possible complications of cesarean section and must immediately and thoroughly assess the neonate for such complications.

Low forceps or midforceps delivery may be used to facilitate the birth of the infant's head. The use of forceps may help avoid maternal exhaustion from prolonged pushing and may allow a vaginal birth in a mother who otherwise might have to undergo a cesarean section. Possible complications for which the nurse must be alert include vaginal, cervical, and perineal laceration; uterine rupture; uterine atony and bleeding; bladder trauma; infection; and trauma to the fetal head. The nurse must emotionally support the mother during the procedure, monitor the fetus during the delivery, and assess carefully for any postpartum complications.

The indications for vacuum extraction are similar to those for use of forceps: arrest of labor during the second stage and maternal need for shortening of the second stage because of maternal exhaustion, cerebral or cardiovascular disease, or fetal compromise. Contraindications to the use of the vacuum extractor may include an unengaged fetal head; face, brow, or breech presentation; cephalopelvic disproportion; incomplete dilation of the cervix; and prematurity. Fetal complications may include cephalohematoma, retinal hemorrhage and, in rare cases, intracranial hemorrhage (Creasy & Resnik, 1999). In 1998 the U.S. Food and Drug Administration released a public health advisory alert regarding the risks of vacuum extraction. Vacuum extraction has been associated with serious or fatal complications, including subgaleal (subaponeurotic) hematoma and intracranial hemorrhage (ACOG, 2000). The nurse must closely monitor the mother, fetus, and neonate for any possible complications and for any device-related injuries. The nurse also must explain to the patient and family that the presence of a caput succedaneum at the suction site is normal and should resolve within about 24 hours.

Regardless of the mode of delivery, the nurse should explain to the family the rationale for the delivery option and should be present to provide support for the family during the actual birth process. The nurse also has a responsibility to be well aware of the advantages and possible complications of each type of delivery and to assess the mother and fetus accordingly.

CRITICAL CARE OBSTETRICS

The increase in acuity of many patients, coupled with rapid growth in knowledge and technology, has laid the foundation for critical care obstetrics. Preterm and consequently high-risk infants are surviving for longer periods after birth at earlier gestations than ever before. Both these infants and their mothers are at high risk and in need of more complex care that is based on an expanded level of knowledge and skill. In addition to electronic fetal monitoring, nurses now are asked to monitor the mother with cardiac monitors, invasive hemodynamic monitoring catheters (e.g., Swan-Ganz catheters), central venous pressure catheters, and arterial lines. In complicated cases, mechanical ventilatory assistance also is introduced into the labor and delivery or recovery suite.

Nurses in all types of settings now are responsible for developing a plan of care to be used in critical care situations. In some settings the roles of the traditional labor and delivery nurse and the traditional critical care nurse are merging. Some nurses welcome the challenge of developing their expertise in both specialties. Nurses respond to the challenge by combining experience in high-risk labor and delivery settings with experience in critical care units. Obstetric intensive or special care units are an emerging trend, one that provides an opportunity for expansion of clinical nursing collaboration and for expansion of nursing knowledge through collaborative nursing research.

SUMMARY

Many neonatal nurses do not have the opportunity to work in an antenatal or intrapartal area; however, what happens during these periods directly affects the type of neonatal problems encountered. With a brief review of some of the effects of labor on the fetus, anticipatory care can be given either by the practitioner trying to stabilize the neonate's condition in the delivery room or by the neonatal nurse trying to prevent complications in the NICU. This chapter, along with Chapter 12, gives a good overview of the perinatal conditions that may compromise neonatal well-being.

REFERENCES

American College of Obstetricians and Gynecologists (ACOG) (1996). Women's Health Care Physicians: Compendium 2001: hypertension in pregnancy. ACOG Technical Bulletin No 219, 533-540.

American College of Obstetricians and Gynecologists (ACOG) (2000). Women's Health Care Physicians: Compendium 2001: clinical management guidelines for obstetrician-gynecologists. ACOG Practice Bulletin No 17, 998-1005.

Association of Women's Health, Obstetrics, and Neonatal Nurses (AWHONN) (1997). *Fetal heart monitoring: principles and practice*. AWHONN: Washington, DC.

Berg CJ et al (1996). Pregnancy-related mortality in the United States, 1987-1990. *Obstetrics and gynecology* 88:166.

Camann W (2000). Combined spinal-epidural anesthesia in obstetrics. *Current Reviews for Nurse Anesthetists* 23:129-140.

Chestnut D (1999). Alternative regional anesthetic techniques: paracervical block, lumbar sympathetic block, pudendal block, and perineal infiltration. In Chestnut DH, editor: *Obstetric anesthesia: principles and practice*, ed 2, Mosby: St Louis.

Creasy RK, Resnik R (1999). *Maternal-fetal medicine*, ed 4. WB Saunders: Philadelphia.

Faucher MA, Brucker MC (2000). Intrapartum pain: pharmacologic management. *Journal of obstetric, gynecologic, and neonatal nursing* 29:169-180.

Fox M et al (2000). Fetal heart rate monitoring: interpretation and collaborative management. *Journal of midwifery and women's health* 45:498-506.

Kattwinkel J (ed) (2000). *Textbook of neonatal resuscitation*, ed 4. American Academy of Pediatrics and American Heart Association: Elk Grove Village, IL, and Dallas, TX.

Lowdermilk DL et al (2000). *Maternity and women's health care*, ed 7. Mosby: St Louis.

Lowe NK (1996). The pain and discomfort of labor and birth. *Journal of obstetric, gynecologic, and neonatal nursing* 25:82-92.

May KA, Mahlmeister LR (1994). *Maternal and neonatal nursing: family-centered care*, ed 3. JB Lippincott: Philadelphia.

Moore KL, Persaud TVN (1998). *Before we are born: basic embryology and birth defects*, ed 5. WB Saunders: Philadelphia.

Murray M (1997). *Antepartal and intrapartal fetal monitoring*, ed 2. Learning Resources International: Albuquerque.

National Institute of Child Health and Human Development, Research Planning Workshop (1997). Electronic fetal heart rate monitoring: research guidelines for interpretation. *American journal of obstetrics and gynecology* 177:1385-1390.

Sleutel M, Golden S (1999). Fasting in labor: relic or requirement? *Journal of obstetric, gynecologic, and neonatal nursing* 28:507-512.

Weber SE (1996). Cultural aspects of pain in childbearing women. *Journal of obstetric, gynecologic, and neonatal nursing* 25:67-72.

CHAPTER 15

RESUSCITATION AND STABILIZATION OF THE NEWBORN

CAROLE KENNER

The transition from intrauterine to extrauterine life is perhaps the greatest challenge any human being can face in the course of a lifetime. This transition is made with little difficulty if the fetus is healthy and is born at or near term. However, if the fetus is premature or compromised, some assistance may be needed. Approximately 3% to 7% of all newborns require some form of support (Niermeyer & Keenan, 2001). This support may be as simple as ensuring thermoregulation or clearing the airway. However, if an infant is born prematurely, the level of support usually is more complex.

CARDIOPULMONARY EXTRAUTERINE ADAPTATION

Successful transition to extrauterine life requires spontaneous breathing, independent system functioning, and successive cardiopulmonary changes. Before delivery the fetus relies solely on the placenta for all gas exchange and for excretion of metabolic wastes. Oxygenated blood flows from the placenta to the fetus through the umbilical vein. Once the vein has penetrated the fetal abdominal wall, it divides into two branches. One branch, the ductus venosus, carries about half of the blood directly to the inferior vena cava just below the diaphragm. The other branch carries the remaining incoming blood to the hepatic microcirculation; after perfusing the liver, this blood is drained by the hepatic vein into the inferior vena cava, where it joins blood returning from the lower body.

Interestingly, flow studies have shown relatively little mixing of blood coming from different sites. The ductal blood that bypassed the liver tends to flow along the dorsal and left wall of the inferior vena cava, whereas the blood from the liver and lower body flows along the ventral and right wall. When the blood reaches the right atrium, a flap of tissue known as the eustachian valve directs the better oxygenated ductal blood across the foramen ovale into the left atrium (right-to-left shunting). The desaturated blood from the liver and lower body, as well as the desaturated blood in the superior vena cava (from the head and upper body) and the coronary sinus (from the heart), is directed across the tricuspid valve into the right ventricle.

In the left atrium, the blood that flowed across the foramen ovale is mixed with the small amount of blood returning from the collapsed, dormant fetal lungs. This mixture flows across the mitral valve into the left ventricle and then across the aor-

tic valve, to be carried away from the heart by the ascending aorta. Because of the transport mechanism comprising the ductus venosus, eustachian valve, and foramen ovale, most blood in the aorta comes directly from the umbilical vein and is relatively well oxygenated. As this blood moves to and through the aortic arch, the arterial branches carry the oxygenated blood to the heart, brain, head, and upper torso. The small amount of remaining blood continues into the descending aorta.

The desaturated blood in the right ventricle crosses the pulmonary valve to enter the pulmonary arteries. However, because the pulmonary vasculature is constricted and highly resistant to flow, only about 12% of this blood actually enters the pulmonary circulation. The remaining 88% follows the path of least resistance through the ductus arteriosus into the descending aorta.

Blood to the descending aorta has two sources: the small amount of blood that was carried through the aortic arch from the left ventricle, and the large amount of blood that was carried through the ductus arteriosus from the right ventricle. About one third of this mixture is carried through the trunk, abdomen, and lower extremities; the remaining two thirds enters the umbilical artery and is returned to the placenta to be reoxygenated.

Circulatory flow in the fetus, then, is determined by anatomic ducts, which allow the most highly oxygenated blood to be directed toward the myocardium and brain and which channel desaturated blood to bypass the highly resistant lung beds in favor of the low-resistance pathway back to the placenta. With the clamping of the cord and the infant's first breath, this flow pattern changes drastically. As the chest is squeezed during delivery, the bulk of pulmonary lung fluid is evacuated up and out through the mouth. When the chest recoils, air is drawn into the lungs. With this first breath, the partial pressure of oxygen (pO_2) and the hydrogen ion concentration (pH) begin to rise, and the pulmonary vessels begin to dilate. This progressive vasodilation causes a steady drop in pulmonary resistance, and the pressure in the pulmonary artery and right side of the heart falls. At this same time, systemic resistance abruptly rises when the placenta is lost. This increase in systemic resistance causes the blood pressure in the aorta and the left side of the heart to rise. The peripheral vasoconstriction that occurs in response to skin cooling, combined with the increased amount of blood flowing through the lungs and returning to the left atrium, further accentuates the increase in left-sided heart pressures.

As the right atrial pressure falls and the left atrial pressure rises, the flap of the foramen ovale is pushed against the atrial septum and is effectively closed. Simple mechanical forces also close the ductus venosus, and vessel walls collapse on themselves as umbilical venous return is terminated. Constriction and closure of the ductus arteriosus, however, depend primarily on the net effects of rising oxygen levels and falling prostaglandin E_2 (PGE_2) levels. The rise in oxygen tension, of course, is associated with the onset of spontaneous, regular respirations. The fall in PGE_2 (which held the ductus arteriosus open in utero) is thought to be due to the removal of the placenta, a site of PGE_2 production, and to the increased blood flow to the lungs, where PGE_2 is metabolized.

ASPHYXIA

Asphyxia occurs when the organ of gas exchange fails or in some way is prevented from performing its function. For the fetus, the organ of gas exchange is the placenta; for the neonate, it is the lungs. When infants become asphyxiated, either in utero or after delivery, the immediate consequence is progressive hypoxia and hypercarbia with mixed (metabolic and respiratory) acidosis. Under conditions of profound hypoxemia, the body shifts from aerobic to anaerobic metabolism. The final product of this alternative energy-producing pathway is lactic acid. As this strong acid accumulates, metabolic acidosis develops. At the same time, the carbon dioxide levels in the blood build steadily. Excess carbon dioxide combines with water to form carbonic acid, which leads to the development of respiratory acidosis. As the mixed acidosis worsens, the myocardium fails. The heart rate falls, followed shortly thereafter by a drop in blood pressure. Blood flow to the tissues is reduced, and the hypoxia, hypercarbia, and acidosis worsen.

The closest model of the human response to asphyxia was provided by Dawes' 1968 study of the rhesus monkey fetus and asphyxia. Figure 15-1 presents the well-defined sequence of events observed. Shortly after the onset of asphyxia, rapid gasping begins and often is associated with thrashing movements of the arms and legs and brief elevation of the heart rate. If the gasping does not relieve the asphyxia within about

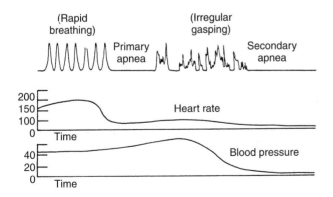

FIGURE **15-1**
Effect of asphyxia on fetal breathing, heart rate, and blood pressure. From Kattwinkel J, ed. (2000). *Textbook of neonatal resuscitation, ed. 4.* American Academy of Pediatrics and American Heart Association: Elk Grove Village, IL.

1 minute, all respiratory activity ceases (primary apnea) and the heart rate begins to fall. Primary apnea lasts about 60 seconds and is followed by a series of spontaneous deep gasps. If the asphyxia persists, the gasping respirations become progressively weaker, stopping altogether after about 4 to 5 minutes. Secondary apnea (terminal apnea) follows the last gasp, beginning approximately 8 minutes after the onset of the anoxic event. The heart rate continues to fall, and hypotension develops; if the asphyxia is not reversed within several minutes, extensive organ damage and, ultimately, death occur.

In the early stages of asphyxia in adults and children, the body at least initially attempts to maintain perfusion (and hence oxygen delivery) by increasing cardiac output through the mechanism of increasing both the heart rate and the stroke volume. The fetus and newborn, however, have relatively fewer myofibrils, and the heart is unable to stretch sufficiently to hold a greater volume. The inability to effectively increase the stroke volume means that cardiac output can be increased only by increasing the heart rate. Unfortunately, because the heart rate of the normal fetus and newborn already is relatively high, 100 to 160 beats per minute (bpm), there is little room for improvement. Instead, the fetal system compensates by massive peripheral vasoconstriction, preferentially shunting and maintaining blood flow to the heart, brain, and adrenal glands at the expense of organs such as the gastrointestinal tract, kidneys, skin, and skeletal muscle. This compensatory mechanism is somewhat akin to the diving reflex of submerging mammals. The fetal brain and heart normally receive approximately 7% of the cardiac output, but during fetal hypoxemia, almost 25% may be shunted to those organs to ensure adequate tissue oxygenation. The placenta also receives a greater proportion of the cardiac output in cases of hypoxemia accompanied by acidosis. However, with worsening fetal hypoxemia and hypercarbia, even this compensatory mechanism fails, and the familiar cascade of events (acidosis, bradycardia, and hypotension) is set into motion.

The passage of meconium in utero is estimated to occur in 10% to 15% of all fetuses and is considered a marker of antepartum or intrapartum asphyxia. Gasping by the fetus in utero can result in aspiration. The pathophysiologic stimuli that trigger meconium passage are not clearly understood, although some combination of vagal stimulation and hyperperistalsis after an episode of intestinal ischemia generally is thought to be the cause. Meconium-stained amniotic fluid, as well as its possible sequela, meconium aspiration syndrome, therefore may be an unfortunate side effect of the diving reflex.

Continuous (uninterrupted) monitoring of fetal status (by heart rate monitoring, scalp pH, or observation of meconium) allows early identification of the major clinical manifestations of fetal asphyxia. Once the condition is identified, every effort must be made to expedite delivery so that the gas exchange functions can be transferred from the placenta to the lungs. Depending on how quickly this can be done, the fetus already may have gone through primary apnea and may be in secondary apnea at the time of birth. Practically speaking, it is difficult to differentiate primary from secondary apnea until after the event. Consequently, all newborns who are apneic or who show evidence of cardiorespiratory depression should be treated as if they were in secondary apnea and should be given urgent resuscitative care. Most infants in primary apnea resume breathing when they are stimulated and given supplemental oxygen. However, infants in secondary apnea have been subjected to the asphyxiating event for a much longer time, long enough to show signs of central nervous system involvement. They are hyporeflexive, hypotonic, and unresponsive to stimulation alone because the reflexes have been lost. These infants require ventilation and perhaps more aggressive therapy to maintain and improve cardiorespiratory function.

The urgency of intervention cannot be overstressed. The closure of the foramen ovale and ductus arteriosus is at best tenuous until fibrinous bands of tissue anatomically close the sites. Consequently, any event that delays the onset of respiration could lead to hypoxia, hypercarbia, and acidosis. Under these circumstances the pulmonary vasculature remains constricted and the pulmonary vascular resistance remains high, which may cause a return to right-to-left shunting across the foramen ovale and ductus arteriosus, as in perinatal circulation. In such cases blood again largely bypasses the lungs, but the placenta is no longer available for gas exchange. If this condition persists, the infant becomes progressively more hypoxic, hypercarbic, and acidotic, giving rise to a vicious circle of asphyxia from which the infant may not be able to escape.

THERMOREGULATION

All newly born infants require temperature stabilization. Therefore one of the first steps in stabilization and resuscitation or support in the delivery room is maintenance of the newborn's temperature. Before birth, the infant's core temperature is slightly higher than the maternal core temperature. If the mother experiences hypothermia, depending on the severity, the fetus also may be cold. The physiologic mechanism that dictates a fetal temperature higher than the maternal temperature has not been established. After birth, the neonate is exposed to the relatively cold environment of the delivery room. The infant experiences a sudden increase in demand to produce heat to maintain a stable body temperature. Although delivery rooms use various methods to prevent heat loss after birth, the infant's temperature can fall as much as 2.6° C. In the course of a normal delivery, the wet infant can lose as much as 200 calories of heat for every 1 kg of body weight for each minute that heat loss is allowed to continue. One of the vital points of neonatal stabilization in the delivery room, then, is drying the neonate quickly so as to reduce the chance of iatrogenic hypothermia.

Neonatal peripheral cooling stimulates heat production even before a drop in core temperature is detected. Facial cooling alone is sufficient to initiate this response. The response results from stimulation of the skin receptors, especially in the area of the facial trigeminal nerve. These receptors transmit the stimuli to the pituitary gland to begin heat production. The same stimuli are transmitted to the respiratory center at the time of birth. Contraction of the diaphragm, in turn, is initiated to trigger respiration. (This mechanism has implications for neonatal resuscitation, because blowing cold air across the newborn's face can produce respirations; however, it also can result in significant heat loss.)

Heat Loss
Heat can be lost through four processes: conduction, convection, evaporation, and radiation. Heat loss resulting from conduction losses at the time of birth occurs in two stages. In the first stage, interior body heat is lost to the skin's surface via the tissues and body organs. In the second stage, heat is released from the skin's surface to environmental surfaces, such as a

cold infant scale. Minimal heat losses may also occur through the urine and feces.

Convective losses are due to air flowing across body surfaces, and evaporative losses occur with heat rising from the skin to the air. These types of heat loss usually are related to differences in water concentrations between the skin and the air. Convective and evaporative losses occur in three ways. First, heat is lost from the interior body to the skin through the blood's circulation. Second, further heat loss occurs as air moves over the neonate's wet skin. Third, inspired air is heated and moistened in the pulmonary capillary bed and then exhaled.

Radiant losses result when the neonate is placed near objects that are cooler than the skin's surface.

Most heat loss in the neonate occurs through radiation and convective losses. Preventing heat loss is the first goal in neonatal thermoregulation. The secondary goal is to minimize the energy required for the infant to produce heat.

Heat Production
The neonate produces heat by three methods: voluntary muscle activity, shivering, and nonshivering (chemical) thermogenesis. Of these, shivering is the most inefficient method. Although shivering is the primary method of heat production in adults, a full-term infant has limited ability to produce heat in this manner, and a preterm infant has virtually no ability to generate heat through shivering.

In a full-term neonate, voluntary muscle activity is used to some extent to generate heat. This activity generally is related to positioning to reduce heat losses. Full-term infants can assume a flexed position to retard heat loss from exposed surfaces. Preterm infants, however, have a limited ability to assume a flexed position; they more commonly assume a relaxed posture, leaving the skin's surface exposed. Heat loss is inevitable unless steps are taken to protect these vulnerable infants. Critically ill or sick neonates, another group of vulnerable infants, assume a flaccid, outstretched position.

The main method of heat production for the infant, therefore, is chemical thermogenesis. Norepinephrine stimulates brown fat metabolism, resulting in heat energy. The availability of glucose initiates glycolysis, and digestion also may play a limited role in heat production. Without adequate sources of brown fat and glucose or in the absence of enteral feeding, the neonate is at risk for thermal instability secondary to inability to carry out effective thermogenesis.

Once the heat generation response has been initiated, oxygen consumption rises as the infant's body metabolizes brown fat. Infants who require resuscitation or who are unable to meet the demands of increased oxygen intake are at greatest risk of a diminished ability to achieve early thermoregulation.

Thermoneutrality
The goals of maintaining a stable body temperature are to ensure normal growth and to meet energy needs. In this thermoneutral state, body temperature is maintained within a normal range, and caloric expenditure and oxygen consumption are minimal. What constitutes the normal range has not yet been defined precisely, and further research is needed. The thermoneutral body temperature of a full-term infant may range from 36.6° to 37° C, but it may be as low as 35° C for a preterm infant. The broad range of what constitutes normal body temperature relates more to gestational age than to birth weight, because infants who are small for gestational age (SGA) may have a better ability to self-regulate than their size indicates.

In very premature infants, determining a thermoneutral temperature may be complicated. In such neonates, oxygen uptake may not increase sufficiently to meet heat production needs, especially in the first few weeks of life.

Thermoneutrality may be difficult to achieve in very-low-birth-weight (VLBW) and extremely-low-birth-weight (ELBW) infants in the first few days after delivery. Despite an inability to sweat, premature infants (less than 37 weeks' gestational age) have high evaporative heat losses because of the increased permeability of their skin. The very thin, gelatinous epidermis, typical of gestationally immature neonates, affords very little protection against heat loss. The thermoneutral ambient temperature range that best meets the infant's metabolic needs may be narrow and may fluctuate less than 0.5° C. In some cases the environmental temperatures tolerated by a premature infant may have a range of less than 3° C, depending on the heat source and the degree of humidity. Humidification in the range of 40% to 60% may lower the environmental temperature needs of a premature infant by 1° C or more. Research in this area is underway.

The determination of appropriate environmental temperatures is based on the infant's ability to maintain a satisfactory body temperature using the least amount of energy. A thermoneutral environment can be maintained for a full-term infant in an incubator with an air temperature between 32° and 35° C. A premature infant often needs an air temperature between 35° and 37° C. If the infant is clothed, the air temperature often can be reduced by 2 to 4° C. As the infant matures, the air temperature needed to maintain thermoneutrality declines.

Mechanisms of Neonatal Heat Regulation

Infants have a much greater potential for heat loss than adults because their body surface is greater in relation to their weight. A decline in neonatal fat stores impairs insulation from heat loss caused by external environmental changes. Heat production by the neonate and environmental control by the health care team together meet the infant's thermoregulatory needs.

When clothed and fed, healthy full-term babies (appropriate for gestational age [AGA]) can produce heat to self-thermoregulate. In a cold environment, these infants can increase basal heat production by two to three times the normal rate within a day or two of birth.

It would seem that neonates who are large in comparison with the normal weight and size for their gestational age (large for gestational age [LGA]) would be able to generate sufficient heat to maintain self-thermoregulation. In reality, these infants may lack sufficient brown fat stores. They also may be poor feeders whose oral intake is insufficient for generating heat.

Several other factors may limit an infant's ability to thermally self-regulate. Hypoxia or hypoglycemia may prevent the infant from generating sufficient heat through metabolism. Infants also are at risk after episodes of stress or prolonged periods of increased metabolic demand; these infants may have depleted stores of brown fat and glucose and therefore may be unable to generate heat.

Central nervous system (CNS) defects or infection may alter the temperature-regulating ability of the brain. In an infant with CNS alterations, hypothalamic control may be absent. Anencephalic infants and infants with intracranial defects or hemorrhage (or both) may be unable to produce heat. Use of maternal analgesia may inhibit the infant's ability to generate

heat in the first few days of life because metabolism is slowed by these drugs. The use of anesthetics or muscle relaxants in infants also may alter thermal response through neural inhibition of temperature response.

Heat production in the newborn gradually improves during the first few days of life with the institution of feedings. Oral feedings have been shown to cause an increase in neonatal heat production that is not present when protein hydrolysate is administered parenterally.

Providing thermoregulatory care for SGA infants can be especially difficult. Many nurseries use an infant's weight to determine whether care should be provided in an incubator or under a radiant warmer. In other units, weight is considered less important than the infant's condition.

Preterm infants are at risk for difficulty generating heat and energy because of a large body surface area in relation to weight, limited brown fat stores, and delayed or absent mediating responses to initiate heat production. Brown fats stores begin to develop around 26 to 30 weeks' gestation and continue to develop after birth. Another problem in preterm infants, in addition to limited stores of fat, glucose, liver enzymes, and hormones, is that norepinephrine may not be released in sufficient amounts to initiate metabolic thermogenesis.

Although sweat glands are almost nonexistent in preterm infants, enormous amounts of water are lost through the skin's surface. These losses rise dramatically when radiant heating sources are used or when the infant is placed under phototherapy lights. Under these circumstances, premature infants can lose as much as 120 ml of water per kilogram per day. Humidification of the environment in the range of 40% to 60% may protect premature infants from heat loss caused by evaporative losses.

Heat conservation is limited in most infants 24 to 25 weeks' gestational age because of their flaccid posture. Limited heat sources and the inability to conserve heat place these infants at risk for cold stress, and they are very sensitive to even the slightest change in environmental temperature.

Gluconeogenesis

Although glycogenolysis is the main source of energy for the infant after birth, gluconeogenesis plays a role in energy stabilization. The process of gluconeogenesis converts proteins and lipids into glucose for the body's use. In this process, the anterior pituitary gland releases corticotropin, which stimulates the release of the glucocorticoid hormone cortisol from the adrenal cortex. Cortisol mobilizes proteins in the cells for metabolism into glucose. Glycogen stores in the SGA infant are limited. Because of hepatic immaturity, the preterm infant's ability to initiate gluconeogenesis is delayed. Hormonal levels also may be inadequate to initiate gluconeogenesis. Premature infants thus have difficulty meeting metabolic needs and maintaining body temperature.

Glycolysis

As explained previously, infants derive most of their heat production from the metabolism of brown fat. However, because this tissue does not begin to develop around the neck, along the spinal column, around the scapulae, across the clavicle line, and down the sternal line until the twenty-sixth week of gestation, premature infants have difficulty with glycolysis. Full-term infants have sufficient brown fat to meet minimum heat needs for 2 to 4 days after birth. Heat production is activated when a cold stimulus is transmitted to the hypothalamus (the anterior hypothalamus regulates the body's set point temperature). Heat loss triggers this reaction.

Heat Transfer

Hypothermia is the most common concern for neonatal nurses. Hyperthermia, although a serious concern, occurs less frequently. Heat is transferred through four basic mechanisms: radiation, convection, conduction, and evaporation. Heat can be gained through radiation, conduction, and convection.

Radiation. Radiant energy is transferred between two objects in the environment that are not in direct contact. The infant can readily gain heat from a warm object in the immediate environment, such as a radiant heater. An unprotected infant can also lose heat to objects in the immediate surroundings. Incubator walls, crib walls, and unwarmed objects placed near the infant all may be avenues of heat loss.

The ambient air temperature of the incubator is only one factor in the assessment of the infant's environmental status, because large radiant heat losses may occur even with seemingly normal ambient air temperatures. Radiant heat loss is the most common type of heat loss in infants less than 25 weeks' gestation after the first postnatal week; it also is the main type of heat loss for all infants throughout the neonatal period. Radiant heat commonly is used to warm infants because it is fast and efficient. It is especially useful in the period immediately after birth, when easy access to the infant is vital. Furthermore, radiant heat sources can be used in tandem with other heat sources.

Convection. Convection occurs when heat is exchanged between the environment and an object in that environment. For example, in an open crib the infant loses heat into the atmosphere. The amount of exposed skin determines the amount of heat lost through convection. To maintain a normal body temperature, a clothed infant who is exposed to air currents or cool air temperatures may be required to use a great deal of energy that is needed for growth.

In radiant warming beds, a cool room or high air currents may counterbalance the effect of high heat output from radiant warmers, thus cooling the infant. Inside the incubator, the infant gains heat from the warm internal environment. Clothed or unclothed, the infant is prevented from losing heat in this warmed setting.

Conduction. Conduction is the transfer of heat from one object to another when the two are in contact. Conduction losses occur when the infant is placed on a cool surface. In the delivery room, the infant should be placed on a prewarmed surface, and linens also should be prewarmed. Once stabilization has occurred, strict care must be taken to avoid conductive heat losses. Radiographic plates and weight scales, although used only briefly, may cause a drop in temperature in a premature or clinically unstable infant.

Evaporation. Evaporation is the loss of heat through water lost from the skin into the environment. Evaporative heat loss is the chief form of heat loss in premature infants during the first week of life. High evaporative loss is counterbalanced by a decrease in radiant and convective losses. The evaporation mechanism cannot be used to provide heat for the infant.

Evaporative heat loss occurs most commonly after delivery and after bathing; during these times the cool room air is most likely to cause heat loss through moist, uncovered skin. How-

ever, heat loss through excessive evaporation can be prevented or minimized by protecting the infant's body surfaces from the cooling effects of the environment with protective clothing and skin barrier creams and by maintaining a high humidity level in the infant's environment.

Environmental Effects

The infant's immediate environment can play a major role in thermoregulation. The room temperature often is kept slightly warmer than would be expected in the home, and air currents must be monitored. Thermoregulation considerations are being incorporated into the design of neonatal intensive care units (NICUs) (Chapter 16). For example, external windows, especially during cool weather, may serve as sources of radiant heat loss for an infant in a warm room.

The thermal environment also plays a role in insensible water loss. As the ambient temperature rises to the maximum level for thermoneutrality or even surpasses it, the infant's insensible water loss also rises. Premature infants have greater insensible water loss than do full-term infants.

THERMAL MANAGEMENT

There is no single normal temperature for an infant. A normal range for an individual infant must be broad enough to allow for temperature variations that can occur during sleep or feedings. Premature infants often are stabilized at temperatures slightly lower than those considered acceptable for full-term infants.

A healthy term infant can initiate heat production within a few hours after birth, although the infant usually requires assistance in maintaining body temperature during this time. After delivery, infants often are cared for in a warming bed until the body temperature has stabilized. Once stabilization has occurred, the infant may be dressed in a shirt and diaper and wrapped in one or two cotton blankets. If the ambient temperature is cool or if drafts are felt in the immediate area, the infant's head may be covered with a cotton stocking-knit cap.

The thermal management of a low-birth-weight (LBW) or premature infant requires special attention. There is no set temperature at which an infant is considered to be in a neutral thermal environment. For some LBW infants, a skin temperature of 36° to 36.5° C may be acceptable. For others, a lower temperature range may be more appropriate as long as adequate calorie needs are met, especially in the form of gastric feedings.

Interventions

Radiant Warmer Beds. Radiant warmer beds have the advantage of being a powerful, efficient means of providing heat for the newborn. However, they allow a great deal of convective heat loss in the infant. In the delivery room, use of the radiant warmer bed allows thorough assessment of the infant, because clothing would obstruct careful head to toe analysis. Once the infant has been dried and wrapped, the heat from a radiant warmer may serve as adjunct warmth for the infant attempting to achieve self-regulation.

Stabilized infants in radiant heaters have shown a significantly higher insensible water loss and a higher oxygen intake than infants cared for in incubators. Evaporative heat losses can be reduced by using plastic blankets, which also help prevent convective losses. Many NICUs use radiant warmers regardless of the infant's size. Such units prefer to compensate for the insensible water losses seen in even the smallest infants. Liberalization of fluids, however, requires meticulous monitoring of intake and output to avoid fluid overload. Some units also use a technique known as "swamping" (described later in the chapter) to reduce insensible water losses.

Incubators. The incubator is the ideal environment for an infant who is unable to self-thermoregulate. Radiant and convective heat losses are kept to a minimum because the ambient temperature is high, warming the incubator walls. Appropriate nursing care and assessment can be performed whether the infant is naked or dressed and wrapped. The air temperature of the incubator is adjusted according to the infant's needs.

Portholes and doors must be kept closed except for specific interventions. The incubator temperature may drop several degrees if the portholes are left open for several minutes, and the temperature drops dramatically if the door is left open for any period of time. It can take 10 to 20 minutes for the incubator temperature to reach the previous level and stabilize.

Computer-assisted temperature control in incubators has proven effective at reducing the mortality rate for infants whose temperatures are closely monitored. Computer regulation of servocontrolled incubators reduces the amount of ambient temperature variations, thus reducing physiologic responses to cold stress. However, these systems are quite costly and have not been widely adopted.

Premature infants having difficulty establishing thermoregulation in an incubator may have better results in a double-walled incubator. The double wall prevents radiant heat loss to the cool walls, because the inside wall is warmed by the ambient air temperature of the incubator. Double-walled incubators may lead to high convective heat losses in some infants, even though radiant heat loss may be diminished. The temperature stabilization of the infant must be monitored to determine the effectiveness of the incubator. A double-walled transport incubator may be more effective at maintaining infant temperature than a single-walled incubator. Incubators can be heated with either conduction or radiation sources. Oxygen consumption is not significantly different between infants in radiant-heat incubators and those in conductive-heat models.

The nurse often is the one who reminds other health professionals to cluster the times when the incubator is opened. Collaboration is necessary if heat is to be preserved and the neonate is to be protected from temperature fluctuations. Some bed manufacturers combine radiant warmers and incubators in a single unit. This configuration is meant to alleviate heat loss when access to the baby requires long-term opening of the portholes. When the sides of the combination bed are lifted for the procedure, the unit converts to a radiant warmer, keeping the temperature steady. Research is needed to determine if the claims about temperature stability for this device are accurate.

Heat Shields. Heat shields have proved effective in some cases when thermoregulation could not be achieved with radiant or convective heat sources alone. Plexiglas tents have been used to shield the infant in the incubator. Infants in radiant warmers have been shielded with plastic sheeting placed over the area of the infant. It must be remembered, however, that effective heat shields may block the warming equipment, preventing it from providing heat to the infant. In a cold-stressed infant, heat shields may be inappropriate.

Warming Pads. Heated water pads have proved effective for reducing the heater output when used on infants cared for under radiant warmers. A decline in heater output may reduce

the ill effects of radiant heat on infants. Heated mattress pads also are effective at maintaining heat in transport incubators before and during transport.

Head Coverings. The infant's head is the largest heat-losing body surface. Traditionally, the head was left uncovered, resulting in heat loss. In current thermoregulatory care, head coverings are used for most newborns. In the delivery room, the infant is dried and wrapped in a prewarmed blanket, and the head is covered, most often with a cotton stocking-knit cap. If the cap becomes moist, it should be removed and replaced with a clean, dry one, otherwise the wet material of the cap will increase heat loss.

Once the infant has been stabilized, the hat may be used to prevent heat loss in drafty rooms or during exposure for nursing care or examination. A premature infant may benefit from the addition of a plastic lining in the cap, which further insulates the head against evaporative and conductive heat loss. If the infant has become cool, however, a lined cap may prevent the child from gaining heat through radiation or conduction. In such cases the insulated cap should be removed, and a plain cotton cap may be used. Some institutions prefer to use woolen caps, but these sometimes cause skin irritation and should be discontinued if this occurs.

Plastic Wraps and Coverings. Plastic wraps have been used on infants to reduce evaporative heat loss in the early postdelivery stage of life. Bubble plastic has proved to be an effective insulator that still allows visualization of the infant. For infants under radiant warmers, loosely fitting plastic wraps have been effective at reducing insensible water loss and oxygen consumption and at allowing the heater temperature setting to be lowered. In some cases high humidity (up to 80%) is piped into this plastic bubble, a practice called swamping, which reduces evaporative and insensible water losses, especially in VLBW and ELBW infants.

Skin Protectors. Paraffin has been used with some success as a skin barrier to prevent evaporative heat loss. Although helpful in some infants, its use must be balanced with other methods of thermoregulation. Skin irritation is possible and requires termination of treatment with this method.

Barrier creams have also been used to reduce evaporative heat loss. However, in preterm infants, the body's thin layer of skin may allow considerable absorption of the chemicals in the cream.

Skin protector treatments may require repeated applications that disturb the infant. Also, the infant's skin must be assessed regularly for irritation. The contents of the products used must be double-checked to prevent complications.

Skin-to-Skin Care. Skin-to-skin (kangaroo) care involves placing the infant skin to skin with the parent; this allows the transfer of heat from the parent's body to the infant's body. In the delivery room, skin-to-skin care can be part of the stabilization process to maintain thermoregulation (see Chapter 44 for more information on skin-to-skin care).

THERMAL STRESS

Despite attempts to maintain thermoneutrality, the infant may experience temperature changes that may cause physiologic stress. Changes that lead to an increase or decrease in temperature produce changes in the infant that may be difficult to regulate. Brief episodes of cold stress in the first few days of life, however, may help the infant self-thermoregulate when cold stress occurs after the third day of life. Even full-term infants experience cold stress and must be assessed for it by simultaneous temperature site comparisons. Preterm infants may not show a similar response. A decrease in stress and conservation of calories places the infant at less risk for temperature instability, or at least for instability resulting from depleted energy stores.

Cold Stress

Infants are at risk for cold stress when in transport from one warmed environment to another. Cold stress can occur in a premature infant who is being transferred from one incubator to another. Cold stress also is a common problem in infants who must be transported from one hospital to another, because environmental temperature changes cannot be easily controlled. Infants who require surgery are at risk for cold stress from the time they are transported to the operating room until they are returned to the unit, and anesthetic agents may inhibit an infant's ability to generate heat or maintain thermoneutrality. For these reasons, in some institutions surgery is performed in the confines of the NICU or immediately adjacent to the main NICU room.

Three mechanisms are at work in cold stress. The first mechanism involves the sympathetic nervous system; specifically, peripheral vasoconstriction occurs to limit the loss of heat. Also, the heart rate increases to compensate for the increased demand for metabolism to maintain heat. The second mechanism involves shivering and posturing. Although infants have limited ability to shiver, some heat may be generated in this manner. Posture changes, chiefly toward a more flexed position, also help the infant retain body heat. Preterm infants have no ability to shiver and extremely limited ability to change position. The third mechanism involves stimulation of the pituitary gland and the release of chemicals that initiate other chemical responses to produce heat energy.

The effects of cold stress can be detected in all aspects of body functioning. Each system affected by the cold stress has a feedback mechanism that affects another body system. Even before temperature changes are recorded, oxygen consumption has already increased. Preventing cold stress is essential to protecting the infant from multisystem stress.

The cardiorespiratory system manifests the most obvious symptoms when an infant is suffering from cold stress. As the temperature drops, peripheral vasoconstriction ensues to conserve heat. As the central blood volume increases, the pulse and blood pressure rise. Once central cooling has occurred diuresis may result, with a decline in pulse and blood pressure, leading to diminished cardiac output. Arrhythmias may occur secondary to acidosis as fatty acids break down in an attempt to generate heat.

The central nervous system can be affected by cold stress as a result of cardiovascular changes. Peripheral vasoconstriction diminishes cerebral blood flow, and electroencephalographic activity may decline (for an accurate electroencephalogram, the body temperature must be in the normal range). Peripheral nerve conduction may also be delayed. The pupils may become dilated and fixed.

The metabolic response to cold stress encompasses fluid, electrolyte, and glucose aberrations. In the early stages, diuresis occurs. If cold stress continues, additional changes take place.

With diminished perfusion of the kidneys, glomerular filtration declines, along with reabsorption of sodium, water, and glucose. Hypoglycemia results as the consumption of glucose increases with the rise in the metabolic rate. Unstable glucose levels can lead to further acidosis and neurologic damage. As the release of nonesterified fatty acids (NEFAs) increases, the liver slows metabolism of glucose, inhibiting thermogenesis. As liver function declines, drugs are metabolized and excreted more slowly.

Acidosis occurs because of a variety of factors. As tissue perfusion declines, lactic, pyruvic, and organic acids build. The kidneys and liver are unable to metabolize and secrete these products. The enzymatic action in the kidneys is blocked, and diminished excretion of hydrogen ions disrupts acid-base regulation. Fluid balance is further complicated by poor gastrointestinal absorption and decreased peristalsis.

As acidosis continues, dissociation of indirect bilirubin from albumin-binding sites increases. The increase in NEFAs is caused by their high affinity for the albumin-binding sites. If NEFA levels are high, kernicterus can occur in a cold-stressed infant with relatively low bilirubin levels.

A cold-stressed infant may be at risk for bleeding, because clotting factors may be altered. Besides the development of thrombocytopenia, hematocrit increases, and the blood becomes more viscous. This may be secondary to fluid shifts that occur with cold stress.

Clinically, a cold-stressed infant becomes lethargic and refuses to eat. Respirations become slow and shallow, and if stimulated, the infant has a weak cry. The response to painful stimuli is diminished. A ruddy coloring that occurs secondary to the failure of dissociation of oxyhemoglobin belies the seriousness of the infant's condition. If the condition continues, the infant becomes edematous or scleremic.

Methods of Rewarming

To keep oxygen consumption to a minimum during rewarming, the incubator temperature should be adjusted to 1° to 1.5° higher than the infant's temperature. The incubator temperature may be increased by 1° degree every hour until the infant's temperature has been stabilized. If the infant has been severely cold stressed, the child's temperature may continue to decline during the early stages of rewarming. Caps, plastic wrap, and heat shields should be removed so that they do not prevent heat gain.

Ingested fluids can be warmed before administration to the infant. Feedings should always be warmed before being given to a premature or cold-stressed infant. In most cases, feedings should be withheld from a cold-stressed infant to prevent problems caused by a decrease in gastrointestinal motility. Intravenous fluids also may be warmed using blood-warming devices or by placing an extra length of tubing inside the incubator to allow the warmed environment to warm the fluids.

High serum sodium levels are associated with an increase in body temperature, whereas high calcium levels indicate a decrease in body temperature. The exact mechanism for this is unknown, but the phenomenon may be related to the ratio of sodium to calcium and not to isolated elevation of either electrolyte. Normal saline may be given intravenously during the rewarming process to help raise the infant's body temperature.

Heat Stress

Excluding the febrile state, heat stress should never be allowed in neonates. When it does occur, it generally is caused by improper use or monitoring of equipment to warm infants. Occasionally the neutral thermal temperature for the infant may be overestimated, resulting in heat stress when the body temperature climbs too high for that infant.

Overheating often can be differentiated from febrile episodes by determining the difference between the core or rectal temperature and the skin temperature of the central body and distal extremities. When the core temperature is elevated in febrile conditions, the skin temperature of the distal extremities remains cool compared with the skin temperature of the trunk. This difference may also be evident in VLBW infants if thermoregulation has not been satisfactorily achieved.

Overheating can lead to a variety of responses. All infants tend to be less active as the environmental temperature increases. Heat stress may be evident in a preterm infant at a temperature below 36° C. Mature infants may become more restless or irritable. Both preterm and full-term infants generally attempt to assume an extended posture and become more flaccid. Cardiovascular changes may be subtle; elevations in the heart rate and respiratory rate may be negligible.

Color changes may be more evident in infants than in adults and more indicative of heat stress. Color changes in an overheated infant often occur first on the soles of the feet, which become more pink to red. An overall increase in redness may not occur until the infant is heat stressed. A febrile infant often becomes paler and has cool extremities.

A heat-stressed infant should be assisted in keeping metabolic heat production to a minimum. The infant who assumes an extended position should be left in this position to encourage heat loss. Skin surfaces can be left exposed to enhance evaporative loss. Active temperature reduction methods should be kept to a minimum to prevent a dramatic loss of heat, which could lead to cold stress and shock.

Apnea. Apnea is a problem associated with temperature changes, especially in premature infants. Sudden or dramatic infant temperature changes can lead to apnea. Overheating can increase the number of apneic spells in premature infants.

Special attention must be paid to infants during rewarming to prevent complications from rapid body and environmental temperature changes. A sudden increase in ambient temperature may lead to an increase in apneic spells and to overly rapid rewarming of cold-stressed infants.

Thermoregulation is the cornerstone of neonatal care; it is essential to the infant's stability. Scrupulous temperature control can make resuscitative efforts more effective and successful and in some cases can avoid the progression to aggressive resuscitation, which otherwise may become necessary if temperature instability leads to cardiorespiratory depression.

CAUSES OF CARDIORESPIRATORY DEPRESSION IN THE NEWBORN

The combined effects of numerous maternal, fetal, and intrauterine factors determine the condition of an infant at birth (some of these factors are listed in Table 15-1). Although some of these factors emerge only during labor and delivery (e.g., cord prolapse), most arise during gestation (e.g., placenta previa) or even before conception (e.g., maternal diabetes). Regardless of the site or time of origin, the influence of each of these problems can become manifest as cardiorespiratory depression in the newborn.

To provide effective care, the nurse must be able not only to recognize potential risk factors but also to understand the ways

TABLE 15-1	Conditions Associated with Asphyxiation of Newborns
Source of Problem	**Conditions**
Maternal	Amnionitis, anemia, diabetes mellitus, pregnancy-induced hypertension, heart disease, hypotension, respiratory disease, maternal genetic cause, drugs, infection, maternal deformities
Uterine	Preterm labor, prolonged labor, multiple pregnancies, abnormal fetal presentation
Placental	Placenta previa, abruptio placentae, placental insufficiency, postterm pregnancy
Umbilical	Cord prolapse, entanglement, or compression

Fetal	Cephalopelvic disproportion, congenital abnormalities, erythroblastosis fetalis, intrauterine infection
	Iatrogenic causes:
	  Mechanical (difficult forceps delivery)
	  Drugs

in which they disrupt cardiorespiratory function. Ideally, the nurse determines that cardiorespiratory depression may occur and is thoroughly prepared to intervene. Although many risk factors come into play, the underlying pathogenic processes can be divided into six major categories. The mnemonic TAMMSS can be used as a simple but effective means of remembering these etiologic groups:

- *T* Trauma
- *A* Asphyxia (intrauterine)
- *M* Medication
- *M* Malformation
- *S* Sepsis
- *S* Shock (hypovolemia)

Trauma

Traumatic injury to the central or peripheral nervous system is an uncommon occurrence that can result in immediate or delayed respiratory depression. Because the skull is incompletely mineralized and has open sutures, it can undergo considerable distortion without fracture. However, the underlying membranes and vessels are much less resilient and are easily stretched or torn if overly compressed, particularly if the pressure is abruptly applied. Similarly, forced traction or torsion of the neck during delivery may damage the spinal cord or the phrenic nerve, with consequent paralysis of the diaphragm. An unusually long and difficult labor, a precipitous delivery, multiple gestation, abnormal presentation (especially breech), cephalopelvic disproportion (secondary to macrosomatia or a small or contracted pelvis), shoulder dystocia, or rapid extraction by forceps (as may be required for fetal distress) frequently is involved. Despite their generally low birth weight, premature infants also may be at risk because of the unusual compliance of their skulls.

Asphyxia (Intrauterine)

The most common cause of cardiorespiratory depression at birth is fetal hypoxia and asphyxia. Any condition that reduces oxygen delivery to the fetus may be the cause. Such conditions include maternal hypoxia (from hypoventilation or hyperventilation, respiratory or heart disease, anemia, postural hypotension); maternal vascular disease that results in placental insufficiency (from preexisting or pregnancy-induced diabetes, primary or pregnancy-induced hypertension); and accidents involving the umbilical cord (compression, entanglement, or prolapse). Postterm pregnancies also are at risk, perhaps because of placental aging and progressive placental insufficiency. An asphyxial episode occasionally may trigger the passage and aspiration of meconium in utero.

Medication

Pharmacologic agents given to the mother during labor and delivery may affect the fetus both directly and indirectly. Indirectly, these agents may cause maternal hypoventilation and hypotension or adversely affect placental perfusion. Hypnotic, analgesic, or anesthetic drugs may depress maternal respirations, resulting in reduced oxygen intake and delivery to the tissues and organs, including the uterus and placenta. Anesthetic agents, because of their effect on the sympathetic nervous system, may also cause peripheral vasodilation, diminished cardiac output, and hypotension with decreased placental perfusion. Oxytocin (Pitocin), on the other hand, may cause uterine hyperstimulation and shorten placental perfusion time. Each of these conditions places the fetus at greater risk of fetal hypoxia and asphyxia. In addition, narcotic analgesics, which rapidly cross the placenta, may directly depress neonatal respiratory drive.

Malformation

Infants may have any of a vast array of congenital anomalies, but the ones that cause the most concern during the first few minutes of life are those with associated facial or upper airway deformities and conditions that lead to pulmonary hypoplasia. Many of these conditions can be diagnosed through antenatal ultrasonographic examinations and other screening techniques, but suspicion also should be raised if oligohydramnios or polyhydramnios is reported.

Oligohydramnios is seen with prolonged rupture or leakage of membranes and in infants with renal agenesis or dysplasia or urethral obstruction. If fluid is lost or diminished, the developing fetal structures may be compressed, leading to characteristic Potter facies (including micrognathia) or pulmonary hypoplasia. Polyhydramnios is seen in infants with impaired swallowing ability (as in anencephaly and neuromuscular disorders); in those with real or functional obstruction high in the gastrointestinal tract (as with esophageal atresia); and in those with profuse leakage of cerebrospinal fluid (as in neural tube defects), which contributes to the volume of amniotic fluid. Polyhydramnios is also noted with diaphragmatic hernia and hydrops fetalis.

Sepsis

The fetus may acquire bacterial or viral agents from infected amniotic fluid, from maternal blood crossing the placenta, or by direct contact on passage through the birth canal. An infant is especially susceptible to infection if born prematurely (because these infants are relatively immunocompromised) or if born to a mother who had premature rupture of membranes or a history of infection or chorioamnionitis. If infection is acquired in utero, the lungs tend to be heavily involved, and the alveoli may be filled with exudate. The infant may be apneic at birth, may be slow to establish a spontaneous and regular breathing pattern, or may show frank signs of respiratory distress.

Shock (Hypovolemia)

Most of the blood lost during delivery is from the maternal side of the placenta and therefore is of no consequence to the newborn. However, blood loss from the fetal side of the placenta as a result of abruptio placentae or placenta previa can lead to acute hypovolemia and cardiovascular collapse. Normally the umbilical cord is unusually strong, but ruptures are possible if cord tension increases suddenly, as in a precipitous delivery, or if the vessels are superficially implanted in the placenta (velamentous insertions). In rare cases acute hypovolemia may occur without frank hemorrhage. With severe cord compression, for example, blood flow to the fetus is impeded. The umbilical arteries, however, are much more resistant to compression and continue to pump blood back to the placenta. In this case, the effects of hypovolemia and asphyxia may be superimposed. Infants with chronic blood loss (as in fetal to maternal hemorrhage or twin to twin transfusions) generally are asymptomatic immediately after delivery.

PREPARATION FOR DELIVERY

The success of resuscitative efforts depends on three factors: (1) anticipation of the need, (2) the presence of trained personnel, and (3) ready availability of necessary equipment and supplies. The most competent personnel and the finest equipment are useless if they are not present in the delivery room. Frantic calls for assistance or a scavenger hunt for equipment should never occur; they needlessly delay intervention and can compromise the patient's outcome.

Anticipation

The antepartum and intrapartum history of each pregnant woman must be carefully reviewed to identify those at risk of delivering a depressed infant. Especially worrisome is a fetus that clinically demonstrates the effects of asphyxia (i.e., a nonreassuring fetal heart rate pattern, particularly bradycardia and loss of beat to beat variability; acidosis, as determined by fetal scalp blood sampling; or meconium-stained amniotic fluid).

Personnel

Although most risk factors can be identified at some time during the pregnancy, many may not become apparent until birth. Delivery through meconium-stained amniotic fluid and unexpected diaphragmatic hernia are just two cases in point. Consequently, at least one person competent in neonatal resuscitation should be present at every delivery. Obviously, additional personnel should be made available if a depressed newborn is expected (Bloom & Cropley, 1994; Kattwinkel, 2000).

When a team is required, the role each member is to play in the resuscitative effort should be predetermined. The head of the team generally is the person who will establish and maintain the airway, the one responsible for ventilation and intubation. A second person is responsible for monitoring the heart rate and for initiating chest compressions if needed. If intravenous (IV) medications are required, two additional individuals are needed, one to catheterize the umbilical cord and administer the drugs and the other to pass equipment and prepare the medications. The person who passes equipment and prepares the medications may also be responsible for documenting the resuscitation process, but a fifth person is preferable for this because minute to minute notations must be made. The individual delivering the baby is not considered part of this resuscitative team.

Equipment and Supplies

A newly born infant is predisposed to heat loss (particularly evaporative and radiant losses) and, if unprotected, can quickly become cold stressed. The consequences of such stress include hypoxemia, metabolic acidosis, and rapid depletion of glycogen stores with hypoglycemia. All are conditions that may exacerbate asphyxia and thus complicate resuscitation. Clearly, measures to prevent hypothermia must be part of any resuscitative effort. The delivery room should be kept warm, and the radiant bed should be preheated if possible. Prewarming of linens, towels, and caps or other head coverings also is helpful.

Possible exposure to blood and body fluids is of particular concern in the delivery room. Gloves, gowns, masks, and protective eyewear should be worn during procedures that are likely to generate droplets or splashes of blood or other body fluids (Kattwinkel, 2000).

The additional equipment and supplies needed to carry out a full resuscitation (Box 15-1) should be checked as a part of the daily routine. Small supplies should be organized according to frequency of use and may be displayed on a wall board kept in the radiant warmer (if there is sufficient drawer space) or stored in a cart or specially designed tackle box. Breakaway security clips may be used to safeguard materials when they are not in use, but foolproof or locking closures that require a key are not appropriate in delivery rooms, birthing rooms, or nurseries. A bedside table or flat surface (other than the bed) should be within reach to provide space for catheter trays and medication preparation.

As the delivery nears, the team should double-check all supplies and make sure the equipment is in working order. Hospital infection control policies dictate how far in advance packaged supplies can be opened, connected to tubing, and otherwise prepared. A back-up or duplicate set of materials should be maintained in case of equipment failure, contamination, or multiple births. All items used should be restocked as soon as possible after a resuscitation.

BOX 15-1

Equipment and Supplies Needed for Full Resuscitation

Suction Equipment
Bulb syringe
Mechanical suction and tubing
Suction catheters (5 or 6 French, 8 French, 10 French or 12 French)
8 French feeding tube and 20-ml syringe
Meconium aspirator

Bag and Mask Equipment
Neonatal resuscitation bag with pressure-release valve or pressure manometer (the bag must be capable of delivering 90% to 100% oxygen)
Face masks, newborn and premature sizes (cushioned rim masks preferred)
Oxygen with flowmeter (flow rate up to 10 L/min.) and tubing

Intubation Equipment
Laryngoscope with straight blades, No. 0 (preterm) and No. 1 (term)
Extra bulbs and batteries for laryngoscope
Endotracheal tubes (2.5, 3, 3.5, and 4 mm internal diameter)
Stylet
Scissors
Tape or securing device for endotracheal tube
Alcohol sponges
CO_2 detector (optional)
Laryngeal mask airway (optional)

Medications
Epinephrine 1:10,000 (3-ml or 10-ml ampules)
Isotonic crystalloid (normal saline or Ringer's lactate) for volume expansion

Sodium bicarbonate 4.2% (5 mEq/10 mL) 10-ml ampules
Naloxone hydrochloride (0.4 mg/ml, 1-ml ampules; or 1 mg/ml, 2-ml ampules)
Dextrose 10% (250 ml)
Normal saline (for flushes)
Feeding tube, 5 French (optional)
Umbilical vessel catheterization supplies
　Sterile gloves
　Scalpel or scissors
　Povidone-iodine solution
　Umbilical tape
　Umbilical catheters, 3.5 French, 5 French
　Three-way stopcock
Syringes, 1, 3, 5, 10, 20, 50 ml
Needles, 25, 21, 18 gauge, or puncture device for needleless system

Miscellaneous
Gloves and appropriate personal protection
Radiant warmer or other heat source
Firm, padded resuscitation surface
Clock (timer optional)
Warmed linens
Stethoscope (neonatal head preferred)
Tape, 1/2 or 3/4 inch
Cardiac monitor and electrodes or pulse oximeter and probe (optional for delivery room)
Oropharyngeal airways (0, 00, 000 sizes or 30, 40, and 50 mm lengths)

From Kattwinkel J, ed (2000). Textbook of neonatal resuscitation ed. 4. *American Academy of Pediatrics and American Heart Association: Elk Grove Village, IL.*

GENERAL CONSIDERATIONS

The two goals of resuscitation are (1) to remove or ameliorate the underlying cause of asphyxia and (2) to reverse or correct the associated chain of events (hypoxia, hypercarbia, acidosis, bradycardia, and hypotension). To achieve these ends, resuscitation management should be centered on attempts to expand, ventilate, and oxygenate the lungs, with cardiac assistance provided as necessary. However, intervention must be specific to each infant in extent and form and must be determined by appropriate assessment.

The APGAR score provides a shorthand description of the infant's condition at specific intervals after birth and may be useful as a rough prognostic indicator of long-term outcome; however, it does have limitations. Although it is a quantitative tool, the scoring often is subjectively or retrospectively applied. It often is poorly correlated with other indicators of well-being, such as cord pH. Its usefulness is suspect with extremely preterm infants who may have poor respiratory drive and who may be relatively hyporeflexive and hypotonic because of immaturity rather than distress. Finally, waiting until the first APGAR score is assigned at 1 minute of age causes unnecessary delay in care. For these reasons, the APGAR score should not be used to determine the need for or course of resuscitation (Bloom & Cropley, 1994; Kattwinkel, 2000).

The initiation and progression of resuscitation are based on three signs: respiratory effort, heart rate, and color. As soon as the infant has been positioned under a radiant warmer, thoroughly dried, and suctioned, these signs are assessed at 30-second intervals and interventions are carried out as needed.

The basics of neonatal resuscitation are as easy as ABC: *airway*, *breathing*, and *circulation*. These are the critical elements of any resuscitative effort.

Airway Control
Positioning. Airway control is a fundamental prerequisite for effective oxygenation and ventilation. To achieve this, the infant should be placed in a flat supine position. The practice of placing the infant in a slight head-down tilt (Trendelenburg position) has been abandoned. This maneuver historically was used under the presumption that fluids from the lower extremities would be redistributed to the intrathoracic compartment. Studies with healthy adults in the Trendelenburg position have demonstrated improvement, albeit transient (lasting less than 10 minutes), in the stroke volume of the heart, but they have also indicated that a tilt as slight as 10 degrees may cause blood to pool in the dependent cerebrovascular bed (Terai et al, 1995). Infants have only a limited ability to increase stroke volume but are at greater risk than older children or adults for intraventricular hemorrhage secondary to rupture of the vulnerable microvessels of the germinal matrix; consequently, the potential benefit, if any, of the head-down tilt position is not believed to be worth the risk.

Once the infant is in the supine position, the neck is placed in a neutral or slightly extended "sniff" position (Bloom & Cropley, 1994; Kattwinkel, 2000). Compared with the adult tongue, an infant's tongue is relatively large in proportion to the mouth, and this slight extension moves the tongue and epiglottis away from the posterior pharyngeal wall and opens the airway. Care must be taken to avoid full extension, however, which reduces the circumference of the airway and increases airway resistance. The reasonably safe extension pos-

ture appears to be no more than 15 to 30 degrees from neutral (Reiterer et al, 1994). An oral airway should be placed if the tongue is unusually large (as in Beckwith-Wiedemann syndrome) or if the chin is unusually small, causing posterior displacement of the tongue (as in Pierre Robin sequence or Potter association). Because newborns also have a relatively large head in comparison with the chest and tend naturally to fall into a flexed position, a shoulder roll, $\frac{3}{4}$ to 1 inch thick may be used to raise the chest and align the cervical vertebrae. This roll may be particularly helpful if the occiput is exaggerated in size by molding or edema. If these procedures fail to provide an unobstructed airway, intubation is indicated (Bloom & Cropley, 1994).

Suctioning. If time permits, the mouth, nose, and posterior pharynx should be suctioned while the head is on the perineum before the thorax has been delivered. After delivery the infant is placed on the warming bed and quickly dried and positioned, and the airway is more thoroughly cleared with a bulb syringe. Because suctioning may cause inadvertent stimulation and gasping, the mouth should always be suctioned before the nose. Mechanical suction often is mentioned as an alternative to the bulb syringe, but it generally should not be used immediately after delivery. If infants are suctioned vigorously within the first 5 minutes of life, apnea or arrhythmias may follow. These symptoms probably are due to vagal stimulation, with reflex bradycardia. If a bulb syringe can be used instead of a suction catheter, this situation usually can be avoided. If mechanical suction is required (i.e., for meconium removal), it should be applied for no longer than 5 seconds at a time with an 8 or 10 French suction catheter and with the equipment set to produce no more than 100 mm Hg (136 cm H_2O) negative pressure (Bloom & Cropley, 1994).

If meconium is present in the amniotic fluid, the first step is to suction the nasohypopharynx with a bulb syringe or a 10 or 12 French suction catheter as soon as the head is delivered and before the shoulders appear. Endotracheal (ET) suctioning may be needed for the most thorough clearing of the airway if the infant is depressed or not rigorous (Niermeyer & Keenan, 2001). This suctioning is performed *before* the infant is dried or otherwise stimulated and is conducted under laryngoscopy with suction directly applied to the trachea, with the ET tube used as a suction catheter. There is some controversy over the benefit of ET suctioning if the infant is vigorous and the meconium is thin; however, suctioning generally is recommended if the infant is depressed (heart rate below 100 bpm and the infant is not rigorous) or the meconium is thick or particulate. The suction is applied as the ET tube is slowly withdrawn, and the procedure is repeated as needed until the meconium has been cleared. Techniques involving mouth suction should not be used because of the risk of exposure of personnel to blood and other body fluids. Also, passing a suction catheter through the ET tube or directly intubating the trachea with a suction catheter is an inadequate substitute for the ET tube, because the small bore of these catheters is easily clogged with the thick, tenacious meconium (Bloom & Cropley, 1994).

Tactile Stimulation
In a mildly depressed infant, drying and suctioning generally produce enough stimulation to induce effective respirations. If the respiratory rate and depth are nevertheless diminished, rubbing the spine or flicking or slapping the soles of the feet can briefly stimulate the infant. If the infant's reflexes are in-

tact, 10 to 15 seconds of stimulation should be sufficient to elicit a response. Longer and more vigorous methods of stimulation should be avoided (Bloom & Cropley, 1994).

OXYGENATION AND VENTILATION

Oxygenation and ventilation are the sine qua non of neonatal resuscitation. In fact, most infants who require resuscitation can be revived with oxygen and ventilation alone. Even when more aggressive therapies are required, they ultimately are undertaken to support oxygen delivery to the tissues, either by optimizing the airway (i.e., intubation) or by supporting the "pump" that "pushes" oxygen to the periphery (i.e., chest compressions, medications). Early administration of 100% oxygen is critical and may be accomplished by several techniques. The risks associated with oxygen excess should not be a concern during the brief period required for resuscitation.

Free-Flow Administration of Oxygen

An infant who is breathing spontaneously but fails to become pink in room air needs supplemental oxygen. The oxygen can be provided directly from the end of the oxygen tube held in a cupped hand, by a funnel or face mask attached to the tubing, or by an anesthesia-type ventilation bag. The flow should be set to deliver at least 5 L/minute, and the tubing, funnel, or mask should be held close to the infant's face to maximize the inhaled concentration (Bloom & Cropley, 1994).

Ventilation

If the infant fails to become pink with free-flow oxygen or shows other signs of cardiorespiratory decompensation (apnea or gasping respirations or a heart rate below 100 bpm), positive-pressure ventilation should be instituted. The initial breaths generally require pressures of 30 to 40 cm H_2O to inflate the lungs. Pressures for succeeding breaths vary with the infant's condition. A ventilation rate of 40 to 60 breaths per minute should be used.

Ventilation Bags

Two types of ventilation bags are available for neonatal use, the self-inflating bag and the anesthesia bag. Self-inflating bags do not require gas flow but do require a reservoir to deliver high concentrations of oxygen. Traditionally these bags have been fitted with a pressure release "pop off" valve preset at 30 to 40 cm H_2O to prevent overinflation of the lungs and the risk of pneumothorax. Most self-inflating bags must be squeezed to move gas through the circuit and may not be capable of passive, free-flow oxygen delivery.

Anesthesia bags that are flow inflating, on the other hand, are closed systems and therefore must be connected to a compressed gas source. Although self-inflating bags have the advantages of being both easy to operate and gas flow independent, anesthesia bags provide more reliable oxygen concentrations (particularly at low flow rates), better control of inspiratory times, and a greater range of peak inspiratory pressures, and they can be used to provide free-flow oxygen.

Both types of bags can be used to provide ventilation by mask or ET tube. Both can also be equipped with a manometer to monitor airway pressure, but visualization of the chest is equally if not more important. The degree of chest rise should simulate that seen when a normal newborn takes an easy breath. Excessive chest rise reflects overzealous delivery of tidal volume; if there is no movement, delivery is inadequate. A self-inflating or flow-inflating bag that has a regulatory valve with a maximum volume of 750 ml should be more than sufficient to deliver the normal tidal volume of 20 to 30 ml for the average newborn (Bloom & Cropley, 1994; Niermeyer & Keenan, 2001).

Methods of Ventilation

For mask ventilation, a face mask is used to provide an oxygen-enriched "microenvironment." An anatomically shaped mask with a cushioned rim is preferred for this purpose. Because masks are available in a variety of sizes, care must be taken to select one that covers the tip of the chin, the mouth, and the nose but not the eyes. Mask ventilation is a simple, noninvasive method of oxygen delivery that can be initiated without delay, but use of a mask has disadvantages. First, it may be difficult to obtain and maintain a good seal between the mask and the infant's face, particularly around the nose. Any leakage of air results in underventilation, which is aggravated if low lung compliance or high airway resistance is a factor. The seal should be "airtight" without excessive pressure applied. Second, the mask itself has a considerable amount of dead space. Consequently, a sufficient tidal volume must be delivered to prevent accumulation and rebreathing of carbon dioxide. Masks used for neonatal resuscitation ideally should have a dead space of less than 5 ml. Finally, prolonged bag and mask ventilation may produce gastric distention from swallowed gas, which in turn impedes diaphragmatic excursions and places the infant at risk of regurgitation and aspiration. However, this problem can be easily avoided by inserting an 8 French orogastric tube if mask ventilation continues beyond 2 minutes. The gastric contents should be suctioned and the tube left in place as a vent as long as mask ventilation is provided (Bloom & Cropley, 1994).

Mask ventilation suffices for most infants, but if it proves ineffective (as evidenced by poor chest rise or continuing bradycardia) or if prolonged ventilation is expected, an ET tube should be inserted. Premature infants (certainly those weighing less than 1000 g) who have diminished lung compliance, immature respiratory musculature, and decreased respiratory drive may also benefit from early intubation (Bloom & Cropley, 1994). In research comparing outcomes for VLBW infants (those weighing less than 1500 g) who were selectively intubated at delivery or given a trial of spontaneous ventilation, the results showed that the infants who were immediately intubated had higher 5-minute APGAR scores, less acidosis, less hypoglycemia, and fewer pneumothoraces and required slower ventilatory rates.

Infants suspected of having a diaphragmatic hernia, hydrops fetalis, or certain airway or gastrointestinal abnormalities also benefit from immediate intubation. Uncuffed tubes with a uniform internal diameter should be used. The proper tube size and depth of insertion are determined by the infant's size by weight (Table 15-2). Most neonatal ET tubes have a black line (vocal cord guide) near the tip of the tube that serves as a guide for insertion. When this guide is placed at the level of the vocal cords, the tube should be properly positioned with its tip in the midtrachea. As an alternative, the distance from the midtrachea (tube tip) to the infant's upper lip may be estimated using the simple tip-to-lip formula:

$$\text{Weight (kg)} + 6 = \text{Tip-to-lip distance}$$

When the tube is properly situated, the centimeter marking on the side of the tube at the level of the upper lip should be at or

TABLE **15-2**	Endotracheal Tube Size and Placement	
Infant's Weight (kg)	**Tube Size (mm)**	**Insertion Depth (cm)**
<1	2.5	<7
1-2	3	7-8
2-3	3.5	8-9
>3	3.5-4	>9

Data from the American Heart Association Emergency Cardiac Care Committee and Subcommittees (1992). Guidelines for cardiopulmonary resuscitation and emergency cardiac care. VII. Neonatal resuscitation. Journal of the American Medical Association 268:2276-2281; and from Bloom RS, Cropley C (1994). Textbook of neonatal resuscitation. American Academy of Pediatrics and American Heart Association: Elk Grove Village, IL.

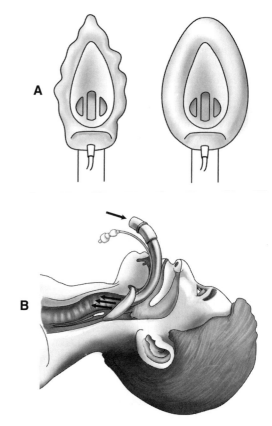

FIGURE **15-2**

A, Laryngeal mask airway deflated for insertion *(left)* and with cuff inflated *(right)*. **B,** Laryngeal mask airway in position with cuff inflated around laryngeal inlet. From Efrat R et al (1994). The laryngeal mask airway in pediatric anesthesia: experience with 120 patients undergoing elective groin surgery. *Journal of pediatric surgery* 29(1):23-41; 29(2):206-208.

near the tip-to-lip distance. For example, infants weighing 1 kg are intubated to a depth of 7 cm ($1 + 6 = 7$); those weighing 2 kg to a depth of 8 cm ($2 + 6 = 8$), and so on. Tubes with metallic markers or fiberoptic illumination at the tip may make it possible to determine the depth of the tube transdermally (i.e., by observing a circle of light on the skin or by hearing an audible signal from a transcutaneous locator instrument), but these modifications do not allow differentiation between ET intubation and esophageal intubation and therefore offer no advantage in an emergency situation (Heller & Heller, 1994). Similarly, capnometers used during resuscitation to measure end-tidal carbon dioxide and thus confirm tube placement in the trachea may be inaccurate when pulmonary blood flow is poor or absent (Bhende & Thompson, 1995).

Correct placement is best demonstrated by the tried and true methods: improved clinical signs (heart rate, color, and activity), symmetric chest rise, bilateral and equal breath sounds (as auscultated in the axillae), and fogging of the tube on exhalation. Air should not be heard entering the stomach, and the abdomen should not be distended. If any doubts exist, tube placement can be checked by repeated laryngoscopy; the tube should be clearly seen passing through the glottic opening (Bloom & Cropley, 1994).

ET intubation is the definitive technique for airway management and ventilation. However, agility and accuracy in placement require continual practice. Also, many hospital personnel are restricted by policy or statute from learning or using this skill. The laryngeal mask airway (LMA), which was approved by the U.S. Food and Drug Administration in 1991, has been enthusiastically accepted in some settings as an alternative that offers most of the advantages of intubation but does not require laryngoscopy for placement.

The LMA (Figure 15-2) is a relatively long tube with a bag connector and an inflation port at one end and an inflatable soft cuff at the other. The tube is blindly passed into the hypopharynx so that the tip of the cuff lodges in the esophageal opening. Inflated, the cuff creates a seal around the larynx. The tube then is connected to a bag that delivers oxygen by ventilation through the central aperture of the laryngeal mask.

Little research has been done comparing the LMA with ET intubation, particularly in neonates. However, it appears that for ventilation purposes, the LMA, under controlled circumstances, can be as effective as but never more effective than in-

tubation. Also, placement of the LMA is not necessarily easier than intubation. Studies have indicated wide variability in successful placement of the LMA on the first attempt (68% to 100% for those with expertise in airway management), whereas reported success rates for intubation generally are always about 90% to 95%. Even with successful placement, nearly a quarter of infants with a laryngeal mask airway subsequently develop airway obstruction, probably because of displacement during patient movement. The cuff provides only a low-pressure seal around the larynx, which limits the airway pressures that can be achieved during ventilation. The risks of gastric insufflation and regurgitation of gastric contents are reduced but not eliminated. Because of its size, the LMA currently is restricted to term infants, although there have been anecdotal reports of successful use in very small infants (1 to 1.5 kg). The LMA does not provide access to the lower airway and therefore is not suitable for meconium removal or drug administration, nor does it preserve the airway during laryngospasm. Its usefulness in neonates who require chest compressions and in those with oropharyngeal disease or diaphragmatic hernia has yet to be assessed.*

---

*Brimacombe, 1994 and 1995; Efrat et al, 1994; Paterson et al, 1994; Brimacombe & Berry, 1995; Brimacombe & Gandini, 1995; Williams, 1995.

CHEST COMPRESSIONS

Chest compressions rarely are required for resuscitation in the delivery room. They are performed in only 1 of every 1000 deliveries but probably are avoidable even in most of these cases. According to some authorities, approximately one third of the infants who received chest compressions have showed biochemical evidence of asphyxia (acidemia), but the remaining two thirds were found to have a malpositioned ET tube or inadequate ventilatory support (i.e., insufficient rate or pressure). Clearly, the airway should be reassessed and respiratory support should be optimized before chest compressions are initiated (Perlman & Risser, 1995). Assuming that these components are satisfactory, chest compressions are begun if the heart rate drops below 60 bpm or if it is between 60 and 80 bpm but is not improving (Bloom & Cropley, 1994).

Chest compressions provide temporary support for circulation and oxygen delivery. Pressing on the sternum has two effects: it compresses the heart against the vertebral column, and it increases intrathoracic pressure. Both effects cause blood to be pushed out of the heart into the arterial circulation. When the sternal pressure is released, the ventricles return to their original shape; intrathoracic pressure falls toward zero; and venous blood is pulled into the heart by a suction effect (Bloom & Cropley, 1994; Elliott, 1994).

Either of two techniques may be used to perform chest compressions. For the thumb method, both hands encircle the chest; the fingers support the back, and the thumbs (pointing cephalad either side by side or one on top of the other, depending on the infant's size) are used to press the sternum downward. For the two-finger method, one hand supports the back from below while two fingers of the free hand are held perpendicular to the chest and the fingertips are used to apply downward pressure on the sternum. Comparative studies have shown that higher systolic blood pressure, higher diastolic blood pressure, higher mean arterial pressure, and higher coronary perfusion pressure are generated with less external compression force when the thumb method is used. This method also has had fewer reports of trauma to the liver and other abdominal organs. Moreover, the thumb method is perhaps easier and certainly less tiring to perform. The thumb method therefore is preferred, but the two-finger method may be necessary if the nurse's hands are too small to encircle the chest properly or if access to the umbilicus is needed to facilitate placement of an umbilical venous catheter (UVC) for administration of emergency drugs (Bloom & Cropley, 1994; Elliott, 1994).

For both methods, the pressure is applied to the lower third of the sternum (just below the nipple line but above the xiphoid process) where the right ventricle lies closest to the sternum. Just enough force is used to depress the sternum 1/2 to 3/4 of an inch (Bloom & Cropley, 1994). Research indicates that myocardial and cerebral blood flow are optimal when the downward stroke and release phases of the compression are equal in time (Niermeyer and Keenan, 2001). This equalization is best accomplished with a smooth stroke and release rhythm.

Positive-pressure ventilation with 100% oxygen must be continued while chest compressions are performed. The most recent guidelines recommend interposing chest compressions with ventilations at a 3:1 ratio. Every fourth compression is dropped to allow delivery of a single, effective breath. During the course of a full minute, 90 compressions and 30 ventila-tions are given (Bloom & Cropley, 1994). Faster rates were recommended in the past, but they only increase the chance of administering simultaneous compressions and ventilations (Bloom & Cropley, 1994; Trautman, 1995). Most research indicates that simultaneous delivery increases the intrathoracic pressure to a level at which ventilation is impeded and coronary perfusion is reduced. Whether there is any effect on cerebral blood flow is equivocal, but there have been other reports of lower survival rates when simultaneous compression and ventilation was used.

Experimental techniques, such as external circulatory assist devices (e.g., mechanical "thumpers," pneumatic vests, and abdominal binders), counterpoint abdominal compressions (e.g., cough cardiopulmonary resuscitation), and active decompression (e.g., plumber's plunger), have shown promise in animal studies. However, few large-scale clinical trials have been done, and most of those used adults. Consequently, these methods cannot be advocated for neonatal resuscitation at this time.

MEDICATIONS

Epinephrine

Epinephrine is a direct-acting catecholamine with both alpha-adrenergic and beta-adrenergic effects. These effects lead to peripheral vasoconstriction, acceleration of the heart rate, and an increase in the forcefulness of cardiac contractions. The net effect is a sharp rise in blood pressure (pressor effect) and an increase in cardiac output. The marked pressor effect combined with the increased aortic diastolic pressure increases the cerebral and myocardial perfusion pressures, maintaining blood flow to these critical organs during resuscitation. Epinephrine therefore is considered the drug of choice with asystole or persistent bradycardia (heart rate below 80 bpm) despite adequate ventilation with 100% oxygen and chest compressions. For newborns the recommended dosage is 0.1 to 0.3 ml/kg of 1:10,000 solution (0.01 to 0.03 mg/kg) (Bloom & Cropley, 1994; Niermeyer & Keenan, 2001). The drug is rapidly inactivated by an enzymatically driven process known as sulfoconjugation, in which the active compound is bound to (conjugated with) sulfate (Schwab & von Stockhausen, 1994). The half-life of infused epinephrine is approximately 3 minutes. Consequently, the dose may be repeated every 3 to 5 minutes as clinically indicated.

Epinephrine is administered by ET tube or by the IV/UVC route. Because IV/UVC placement may be difficult and time-consuming during resuscitation, initial doses tend to be given by ET tube. Unfortunately, absorption into the circulation from the pulmonary capillary bed may be highly variable because of the low blood flow state associated with resuscitation. In addition, much of the ET-instilled drug remains along the walls of the ET tube and in the conducting airways, with a relatively small amount finding its way into the deep absorptive surfaces of the alveoli.

A number of steps can be taken to aid delivery when the ET route is necessary. First, to optimize blood flow to the lungs, every effort must be made to ensure that chest compressions are performed effectively. Second, epinephrine may be dispersed more quickly to deeper pulmonary tissues by diluting the drug and following the instillation with a few forceful ventilations or a small amount of flush. When diluted, the medication should be mixed with a sufficient amount of normal saline to produce a final volume of 1 to 2 ml (Bloom & Cropley, 1994). As an alternative, some individuals prefer to administer the drug through a 5 French feeding tube positioned through the ET tube. Theoretically, the smaller lumen feeding tube would have less surface area to which the drug could cling, but the actual clinical significance, if any, is unknown. In view of this erratic absorption, subsequent doses should be given by the IV/UVC route as soon as access is achieved. In the rare cases in which line placement is unattainable and the infant has failed to respond to standard doses given by the ET route, higher dosages of 1 to 2 ml/kg (0.1 to 0.2 mg/kg) may be considered (Bloom & Cropley, 1994).

Although higher doses of epinephrine administered by the ET route may have a role in exceptional situations, routine IV/UVC administration of high-dose epinephrine is not recommended in newborns. Studies with adults and older children have shown a dose-response relationship, with higher doses bringing about greater improvements in coronary and cerebral blood flow; in neonates, however, the efficacy and safety of high-dose IV/UVC epinephrine have not been adequately evaluated. Most of these studies have been done with patients with a history of coronary artery disease who demonstrate ventricular fibrillation. Neonates, however, more commonly have bradycardia caused by hypoxia. These pathophysiologic differences prevent extrapolation of findings. Furthermore, administration of high doses generally has been followed by a prolonged period of hypertension. Because the newborn, particularly the prematurely born, has a vascular germinal matrix, the risk may be greater for intraventricular hemorrhage. In fact, this area of the brain is most susceptible to hemorrhage when hypertension is preceded by hypotension, which is the case with resuscitation. For this reason, only the standard dose of epinephrine (0.1 to 0.3 ml/kg) should be given by the IV/UVC route.

Volume Expanders

Volume expanders are indicated with evidence or suspicion of acute blood loss with signs of hypovolemia. These signs include pallor despite oxygen therapy, hypotension with weak pulses despite a normal heart rate, and failure to respond to resuscitation (Bloom & Cropley, 1994). Low hematocrit and hemoglobin concentrations are diagnostic of blood loss, but the levels may be misleadingly normal immediately after acute loss. In general, it takes about 3 hours for a sufficient amount of fluid to shift from the interstitial to the intravascular space to produce the degree of compensatory hemodilution reflected by a fall in laboratory values.

The basic requirement for any replacement solution is that the electrolyte and protein composition be roughly equivalent to that which was lost. Otherwise, an osmotic pressure gradient is created, and fluids are driven out of the capillaries into the interstitial tissue. The expansion of circulatory volume is only transient, and the infant is put at risk for secondary problems, particularly pulmonary edema. Clearly, whole blood is the fluid of choice for volume replacement, and it offers the added benefit of oxygen-carrying capacity. Fresh O-negative blood crossmatched against the mother should be used. When blood is not readily available, 5% albumin-saline (or other plasma substitute) or isotonic fluids (normal saline or Ringer's lactate) may also be used (Bloom & Cropley, 1994). Glucose-containing fluids (e.g., D_5W or $D_{10}W$) should not be given by bolus because of the risk of profound hyperglycemia. Hyperglycemia with untreated asphyxia may aggravate metabolic acidosis.

For emergency treatment of hypovolemia, 10 ml/kg of volume expander is given slowly over 5 to 10 minutes by the IV/UVC route (Bloom & Cropley, 1994). Rapid infusion must be avoided, because abrupt changes in vascular pressure in the

vulnerable matrix capillaries place the infant (especially a preterm infant) at greater risk of intraventricular hemorrhage. The response usually is dramatic, with a prompt improvement in blood pressure, pulses, and color. If the signs of hypovolemia continue, however, a second volume replacement may be given. Persistent failure beyond this point probably indicates some degree of "pump failure," and further improvement is not likely until cardiac function is improved. In fact, excessive volume administration may so engorge the heart and overstretch the cardiac muscle fibers that the strength of contractions is actually diminished. In such cases, administration of sodium bicarbo-nate (to correct metabolic acidosis) or an inotropic agent (such as dopamine) should be considered (Bloom & Cropley, 1994).

Dopamine

When vascular volume has been restored but hypotension still exists because of myocardial decompensation (pump failure), dopamine may be used to increase cardiac output, blood pressure, and peripheral and organ perfusion. A precursor of norepinephrine, dopamine is a naturally occurring catecholamine with alpha-adrenergic, beta-adrenergic, and dopaminergic effects. The beta effects are elicited both directly (by direct interaction with the receptors) and indirectly (by releasing norepinephrine, which interacts with receptors). The effects of dopamine are complex and dose related. In general, low doses (less than 2 μg/kg/minute) primarily stimulate dopaminergic receptors. Moderate doses (2 to 10 μg/kg/minute) activate dopaminergic receptors. High doses (over 15 to 20 μg/kg/minute) activate all three adrenergic receptors, but alpha stimulation negates the effect of beta stimulation (Young & Mangum, 2001).

Dopamine is metabolized rapidly, having a serum half-life of 2 to 5 minutes. The duration of action is less than 10 minutes. Consequently, the drug must be given by continuous IV infusion. When used after a prolonged resuscitation, dopamine is infused at an initial dosage of 5 μg/kg/minute and titrated in increments of 3 to 5 μg/kg/minute to a maximum of 20 μg/kg/minute until blood pressure and perfusion improve. Heart rate and rhythm and blood pressure must be monitored continuously. Like all catecholamines, dopamine is inactivated by an alkaline solution and therefore should not be mixed with sodium bicarbonate (Bloom & Cropley, 1994; Young & Mangum, 2001).

Sodium Bicarbonate

Of the biochemical events that arise from asphyxia, the most significant is the conversion from aerobic to anaerobic metabolism with the production of lactic acid. As this strong acid accumulates, metabolic acidosis develops, myocardial contractility declines, hypotension worsens, and the cardiac response to catecholamines weakens (Leuthner et al, 1994). In such cases, the best treatment for acidosis is directed at its cause, hypoxemia. Immediate therapy includes ventilation with 100% oxygen and cardiac compressions to restore blood flow and tissue oxygenation. However, if the resuscitation is prolonged and the infant remains unresponsive, alkali therapy may be helpful (Bloom & Cropley, 1994). Sodium bicarbonate is the most frequently used alkalinizing agent, but its use remains controversial, therefore it should be used only when no improvement is seen (Niermeyer & Keenan, 2001).

Sodium bicarbonate ($NaHCO_3$) is a physiologic buffer. When it is added to a solution of strong acid, such as hydrochloric acid (HCl), the bicarbonate anion (HCO_3^-) combines with the hydrogen ion (H^+) from the acid to form the weaker carbonic acid (H_2CO_3) and a neutral salt, such as sodium chloride (NaCl):

$$HCl + NaHCO_3 \rightarrow H_2CO_3 + NaCl$$

The carbonic acid rapidly dissociates into water (H_2O) and carbon dioxide (CO_2), and the blood transports the dissolved carbon dioxide to the lungs, where it is eliminated:

$$H_2CO_3 \rightarrow H_2O + CO_2$$

Although sodium bicarbonate historically was considered a pharmacologic mainstay of neonatal resuscitation, a growing body of research suggests that sodium bicarbonate administration may actually be counterproductive and possibly injurious. First and foremost, effective removal of carbon dioxide by the lungs depends on both ventilation and pulmonary blood flow. If either is inadequate (which frequently is the case during resuscitation), CO_2 accumulates, with a shift from metabolic to respiratory acidosis without any real resolution of acid-base imbalance (Leuthner et al, 1994). Second, CO_2 diffuses across cell membranes much more rapidly and easily than does bicarbonate. That is, CO_2 quickly moves out of the capillaries into cells, whereas bicarbonate lags behind in the intravascular space. The blood pH rises, but intracellular pH transiently falls. Therefore, when the cells of the heart are involved, intramyocardial acidosis worsens and cardiac performance declines further (Leuthner et al, 1994). Other possible consequences of sodium bicarbonate administration are intraventricular hemorrhage (as a result of rapid infusion of hypertonic solution) and hypernatremia.

Administration of sodium bicarbonate should not be undertaken lightly and is in fact discouraged for brief resuscitation or episodes of bradycardia. It should be reserved for prolonged arrest unresponsive to other therapy and then used only after effective ventilation and compressions have been established. The dosage currently recommended is 4 ml/kg of 4.2% solution (2 mEq/kg) by the IV/UVC route. This hypertonic solution contains 0.5 mEq/ml and therefore should be given slowly over at least 2 minutes (1 mEq/kg/minute) (Bloom & Cropley, 1994). At the first opportunity, samples for blood gas analysis should be drawn from whatever site is available to confirm metabolic acidosis.

Naloxone

For the mother, narcotic analgesics are an effective means of pain control during labor. Unfortunately, these lipid-soluble drugs rapidly cross the placenta and can cause neonatal respiratory depression. Peak fetal narcotic levels occur 30 minutes to 2 hours after administration to the mother. The degree and duration of depression shown by the newborn depend on the dose, the route, and how soon before delivery the drug is given. Affected infants show decreased respiratory effort and muscle tone but typically have a good heart rate and perfusion. If these signs are noted and the mother was given a narcotic within 4 hours of delivery, the infant should be given a narcotic antagonist (Bloom & Cropley, 1994; Wimmer, 1994).

Naloxone hydrochloride is a synthetic narcotic antagonist designed to reverse narcotic-induced respiratory depression. It acts by competing with narcotics for receptor sites in the central nervous system. As a pure competitive antagonist, it binds with but does not activate receptors. Consequently, in the absence of narcotics, naloxone exhibits essentially no pharmacologic activity. As always, ventilatory support is still the first defense against respiratory depression (Niermeyer & Keenan, 2001).

Naloxone is available in a variety of concentrations; however, the American Academy of Pediatrics Committee on Drugs (1990) currently recommends use of either the 0.4 mg/ml preparation or the 1 mg/ml preparation. Neonatal naloxone (0.02 mg/ml) should not be used because of the fluid volume that would be given. The dosage is 0.1 mg/kg, which may be repeated every 2 to 3 minutes as needed. Administration by the IV/UVC or ET route is preferred, but the drug also can be given intramuscularly (IM) or subcutaneously (SQ), because affected newborns generally have good perfusion. The IV/UVC route provides the quickest onset of action (generally apparent within 2 minutes), but IM injection produces a more prolonged effect. Adequate ventilatory assistance must be provided until reversal is complete. Close monitoring should continue for 4 to 6 hours after administration. Because the liver rapidly metabolizes naloxone, its duration of effect may be shorter than that of some narcotics, and respiratory depression may recur. If signs reappear, additional doses of naloxone should be given (Bloom & Cropley, 1994; Wimmer, 1994). Although naloxone has no known short-term toxic effects, it is contraindicated in infants born to narcotic-dependent mothers. Because abrupt and complete reversal of narcotic effect may precipitate seizures (withdrawal reaction), assisted ventilation is provided in this circumstance until the respiratory drive is adequate (Bloom & Cropley, 1994).

Because several studies have suggested that hypoxia and acidosis stimulate the release of endogenous opiates (endorphins), it has been theorized that these endorphins might accentuate the depressing effect of hypoxemia on the cardiorespiratory system. However, clinical trials of naloxone administration to infants with 1-minute APGAR scores of 6 or lower have shown no effect on spontaneous respiratory frequency or heart rate.

Other Drugs

Calcium ions play a critical role in the depolarization of cardiac pacemaker cells in the sinoatrial and atrioventricular nodes, and the movement of calcium into and within the cells of the cardiac and vascular smooth muscle accelerates and maintains the chemical reactions necessary for muscle contraction. As a result, administration of calcium salt (e.g., calcium gluconate, calcium chloride) has been widely recommended in the past to increase heart rate, improve myocardial contractility, and raise blood pressure during resuscitation (Proano et al, 1995). Although these effects are theoretically plausible, several studies have failed to show the anticipated improvement in cardiovascular function. However, adverse side effects have been reported even at standard doses. Although preterm and sick newborns may develop hypocalcemia in the first week of life from a variety of causes, low calcium levels are rarely if ever a factor at birth because calcium is actively transported across the placenta from mother to fetus. Administration of calcium in the first few minutes of life therefore may produce dangerously high serum calcium levels. Pacemaker blockade, bradycardia, and even arrest may result from fatigue after excessive and sustained stimulation. Moreover, high intracellular free calcium levels have been implicated in the activation of aberrant enzyme systems, intracellular release of free fatty acids, generation of oxidative free radicals, and cerebral arterial spasm, which may trigger many of the undesirable consequences of asphyxia. In summary, no data currently are available to support the use of calcium, but a considerable amount of evidence indicates that it may actually be deleterious. Although calcium administration may be appropriate under other circumstances as therapy for documented hypocalcemia or to antagonize the adverse effects of hyperkalemia or hypermagnesemia, calcium should not be used for neonatal resuscitation in the delivery room (Bloom & Cropley, 1994; Keenan, 1994).

Another drug that has fallen out of use in neonatal resuscitation is atropine. Atropine is an anticholinergic drug that blocks the action of acetylcholine at cholinergic receptor sites. Parasympathetic (vagal) stimulation of the heart normally inhibits and decelerates cardiac function (Table 15-3). If this stimulation is blocked, cardiac tone and activity returns to normal. Although atropine may be useful for reversing bradycardia of vagal origin (as from airway manipulation during intubation), infants who require resuscitation in the delivery room are typically bradycardic because of hypoxia. Administration of atropine in this situation has a transient effect at best, and bradycardia will return if the hypoxia persists (Burchfield, 1994).

SPECIAL CIRCUMSTANCES

For some infants, changes in or variations of the usual resuscitative measures are needed. Most of these infants have congenital anomalies, structural defects, or conditions that compromise the cardiovascular system, such as neural tube defects, abdominal wall defects, diaphragmatic hernias, hydrops fetalis, esophageal atresia, pneumothorax, choanal atresia, and laryngeal anomalies. Resuscitative measures with these disorders are discussed in greater detail elsewhere in this text.

Termination of Resuscitation

The law and its underlying ethical principles require that treatment be provided and continued as long as it is judged to be effective in ameliorating or correcting an underlying pathophysiologic process. Unfortunately, the data are insufficient to allow a general recommendation for how long resuscitation should be performed before continuation can be deemed futile and efforts are terminated. Evidence indicates that neonates with a birth weight below 750 g who require cardiac compressions in the delivery room do not survive to discharge. Survival also is unlikely at any birth weight if the APGAR score remains zero after 10 minutes of aggressive resuscitation.

Although many hospitals have guidelines for withholding full resuscitation for ELBW infants and those with lethal anomalies, early and well-documented discussion with parents is recommended when such events are anticipated prenatally. If the event was not anticipated, great attention should be given to postmortem evaluation. Blood for chromosome examination and other pertinent laboratory work, radiographs, and an autopsy are important both for family counseling and for evaluation of the resuscitation process.

Postresuscitation Stabilization

A successfully resuscitated neonate requires special consideration during stabilization. The goal of care after resuscitation is to reverse the causes of cell death and tissue injury (hypoxia, ischemia, acidosis) and avoid any exacerbating conditions (hypothermia, hypoglycemia). The mnemonic STABLE can aid the nurse in remembering the basic components of the stabilization process (Karlsen, 2001):

S Sugar
T Temperature
A Artificial breathing
B Blood pressure
L Laboratory work
E Emotional support for the family

A full description of the STABLE program can be found in Chapter 2.

Documentation

No resuscitative event can go unrecorded. Unfortunately, the circumstances surrounding resuscitation are fraught with medicolegal hazards. Assessment of the infant generally is limited to the most basic measurements (respiratory rate, heart rate, and color). Immediate response may be affected by many factors unrelated to professional competence. Furthermore, the

TABLE 15-3	Effects of Stimulation of the Autonomic Nervous System			
	ADRENERGIC (SYMPATHETIC) EFFECTS			Predominant Parasympathetic (Cholinergic) Effects
Site	Alpha Receptors	Beta Receptors	Dopaminergic Receptors	
Heart				
SA node	—	↑Heart rate	—	↓Heart rate
AV node	—	↑Conduction velocity	—	↓Conduction velocity
Cardiac muscle	—	↑Contractility	—	↓Contractility
Lungs				
Bronchial muscle	Constrict	Relax		Constrict
Arteries				
Coronary	Constrict	Dilate	Dilate	Constrict
Pulmonary	Constrict	Dilate	?	—
Cerebral	Constrict	—	Dilate	Dilate
Renal	Constrict	Dilate	Dilate	—
Veins				
	Constrict	Dilate	Constrict	—

Data from Zaritsky A, Chernow B (1984). Use of catecholamines in pediatrics. Journal of pediatrics 105:341-350.
SA, Sinoatrial; AV, atrioventricular.

ultimate outcome may not become apparent for years. Even the best, most appropriate care can look "bad" in retrospect if documentation is incomplete or inaccurate. Yet no area of the hospital is perhaps less conducive to quality documentation than the delivery room, where a variety of professionals (nurses, physicians, and respiratory therapists) from different clinical areas (obstetrics, neonatology, anesthesiology), each with a unique perspective on the situation, are brought together in an emergency. Notes are jotted on bed linen, scrub clothes, paper towels, or anything at hand. More often than not, these brief notes are so hastily written that they are little more than a list of the medications given. When transcribed, the events may be documented in two totally separate charts, one for the mother, another for the infant. Great care must be taken with record keeping so that events and actions can be accurately reconstructed many years in the future (Thigpen, 1995).

Descriptive charting is most appropriate in this situation. The record should include the pertinent perinatal factors, the physical findings, the activities performed, and the infant's response, but definitive diagnoses should not be offered. It is particularly important that information concerning the pregnancy, labor, and delivery be based on fact and not hearsay. Terms such as "fetal distress" and "asphyxia" tend to take on a life of their own once they have been committed to paper, even if they are not supported by clinical evidence. It is best to record factual data, such as vital signs and blood gas determinations, without adding an interpretation. Ventilation, chest compressions, and administration of medications are essential items for documentation, but the basics should not be dismissed. It is just as important to note that attempts were made to keep the infant dry and warm.

Accurate timing of notes can be critical, because actions are judged by the minute to minute changes noted in the chart. A preprinted recording form not only helps in this regard but also can provide a structure for evaluation and decision making. Any form used should be printed in triplicate: one copy (the original) is retained for the medical record; the second copy is sent to the pharmacy so that medications can be quickly restocked; and the third copy is used for quality assessment (Thigpen, 1995).

SUMMARY

Although most depressed infants respond to drying, warming, positioning, suctioning, and tactile stimulation, every obstetric and neonatal unit should be adequately equipped and well prepared to handle neonatal emergencies. To provide neonatal care effectively, nurses must understand the cardiorespiratory transition and must be able to identify factors that may interfere with successful transition, comprehend the principles of resuscitation, and intervene based on assessment of respirations, heart rate, and color.

REFERENCES

American Academy of Pediatrics Committee on Drugs (1990). Naloxone dosage and route of administration for infants and children: addendum to emergency drug doses for infants and children. *Pediatrics* 86:484-485.

American Heart Association Emergency Cardiac Care Committee and Subcommittees (1992). Guidelines for cardiopulmonary resuscitation and emergency cardiac care. VII. Neonatal resuscitation. *Journal of the American Medical Association* 268:2276-2281.

Bhende MS, Thompson AE (1995). Evaluation of an end-tidal CO_2 detector during pediatric cardiopulmonary resuscitation. *Pediatrics* 95:395-399.

Bloom RS, Cropley C (1994). *Textbook of neonatal resuscitation.* American Academy of Pediatrics and American Heart Association: Elk Grove Village, IL.

Brimacombe J (1994). The laryngeal mask airway for neonatal resuscitation [letter]. *Pediatrics* 93:874.

Brimacombe J (1995). Laryngeal mask airway for emergency medicine. *American journal of emergency medicine* 13:111-112.

Brimacombe J, Berry A (1995). The laryngeal mask airway: a consideration for the Neonatal Resuscitation Programme guidelines? *Canadian journal of anaesthesia* 42:88-89.

Brimacombe J, Gandini D (1995). Resuscitation of neonates with the laryngeal mask airway: a caution. *Pediatrics* 95:453-454.

Burchfield DJ (1994). Why *not* use atropine in neonatal resuscitation? *NRP news intermountain west* 1:1.

Dawes GS (1968). *Fetal and neonatal physiology.* Chicago: Year Book Medical Publishers.

Efrat R et al (1994). The laryngeal mask airway in pediatric anesthesia: experience with 120 patients undergoing elective groin surgery. *Journal of pediatric surgery* 29:206-208.

Elliott RD (1994). Neonatal resuscitation: the NRP guidelines. *Canadian journal of anaesthesia* 41:742-753.

Heller RM, Heller TW (1994). Experience with the illuminated endotracheal tube in the prevention of unsafe intubations in the premature and full-term newborn. *Pediatrics* 93:389-391.

Karlsen KA (2001). *A mnemonic approach to neonatal stabilization: transporting newborns the S.T.A.B.L.E. way. Development of an outreach educational program* (abstract). Available online at http://www.stableprogram.com/courses.html

Kattwinkel J, editor (2000). *Textbook of neonatal resuscitation,* ed 4. American Academy of Pediatrics and American Heart Association: Elk Grove Village, IL; Dallas.

Keenan B (1994). Calcium use for neonatal resuscitation. *NRP news intermountain west* 1:1-2.

Leuthner SR et al (1994). Cardiopulmonary resuscitation of the newborn: an update. *Pediatric clinics of North America* 41:893-907.

Niermeyer S, Keenan W (2001). Resuscitation of the newborn infant. In Klaus MG, Fanaroff AA, editors. *Care of the high-risk neonate,* ed 5. WB Saunders: Philadelphia.

Paterson SJ et al (1994). Neonatal resuscitation using the laryngeal mask airway. *Anesthesiology* 80:1248-1253.

Perlman JM, Risser R (1995). Cardiopulmonary resuscitation in the delivery room: associated clinical events. *Archives of pediatric and adolescent medicine* 149:20-25.

Proano L et al (1995). Calcium channel blocker overdose. *American journal of emergency medicine* 13:444-450.

Reiterer F et al (1994). Influence of head-neck posture on airflow and pulmonary mechanics in preterm neonates. *Pediatric pulmonology* 17:149-154.

Schwab KO, von Stockhausen HB (1994). Plasma catecholamines after endotracheal administration of adrenaline during postnatal resuscitation. *Archives of disease in childhood* 70:F213-F217.

Terai C et al (1995). Effects of mild Trendelenburg on central hemodynamics and internal jugular vein velocity, cross-sectional area, and flow. *American journal of emergency medicine* 13:255-258.

Thigpen J (1995). Neonatal resuscitation record. *Neonatal network* 14:57-58.

Trautman MS (1995). Neonatal resuscitation: be prepared. *Contemporary pediatrics* 12:101-110, 113.

Williams RK (1995). Resuscitation of neonates with the laryngeal mask airway: a caution. *Pediatrics* 95:454.

Wimmer JE (1994). Neonatal resuscitation. *Pediatrics in review* 15:255-265.

Young TE, Mangum OB (2001). *Neofax '901: a manual of drugs used in neonatal care,* ed 12. Ross Products Division, Abbott Laboratories: Columbus, OH.

CHAPTER 16

MANAGEMENT OF THE NICU ENVIRONMENT

LESLIE BRINLEY ALTIMIER

One of the earliest systems to develop in the embryo is the neurological system. Neurological development begins in the third week of gestation with the formation of the neural plate, neural folds, and neural tube during dorsal introduction. Once the tube is formed and becomes a closed system, different regions of the brain begin to develop (McGrath, 2000). As these different regions of the brain begin to develop, the following distinct overlapping processes characterize the Central Nervous System (CNS) development: neuronal proliferation, migration, synapses formation, organization, and myelination (Blackburn, 2003). The forebrain, thalamus, hypothalamus, cerebral hemispheres, and basal ganglia are the first areas to develop in the fetal brain (Volpe, 2001). Although this development begins before birth, it does not fully mature until adulthood. (For more detailed information on neurobehavioral development and the neurologic system, see Chapters 17 and 31.)

The infant's neurological system needs to perform at birth. Understanding of support for the fragile neurological system can be a first step toward helping the infant better manage within the extrauterine environment. A part of this support is the adoption of the conceptual framework and philosophy of developmental care. The ideal Neonatal Intensive Care Unit (NICU) environment will support and promote the premature infant's adaptability to extrauterine life—known as neurobehavioral organization. This chapter will briefly review the neurologic developmental of the infant. It will highlight aspects of developmental care and the impact of the NICU environment on neurologic development.

NEUROLOGIC DEVELOPMENT

The five dimensions of neurobehavioral organization are autonomic, motor, state, attention/interaction, and self-regulatory (Als, 1986). The goal for each dimension is an "organized" infant who responds to environmental demands without disruption in physiologic and behavioral responses (Ludington-Hoe, 1996).

Autonomic Dimension

The first dimension the infant faces is the autonomic dimension. The premature infant's physiologic parameters vacillate greatly. With age, infants gain physiologic stability. An auto-

nomically organized infant maintains autonomic stability despite disturbances from the environment.

Motor Dimension

The motor system includes behaviors associated with muscle tone, posture, and generalized body movements (Als, 1986). Premature infants have less control over purposeless movements. Random, disorganized body movements indicate motor disorganization. Preterm infants tend to overreact to environmental stimuli by exhibiting gross motor movements. The goal of developmental care is to minimize purposeless movements to conserve energy.

State Dimension

The state organization system incorporated the different ranges of state from sleep to the aroused state. A state-organized infant can transition between states appropriately and has the physiologic and behavioral conditions to reach or withdraw from any state. For the premature infant who is overstimulated in the NICU environment, 60% to 70% of sleep time is active sleep (Holditch-Davis, 1990). Interventions that increase sleep and maximize quiet sleep are needed to protect the infant from environmental stimulants and consequently foster motor control (Yecco, 1993).

Attention/Interaction Dimension

The attentive/interactive dimension incorporates attentiveness. Alertness is an exciting milestone. An organized infant has the ability to attain, maintain, and withdraw from attentiveness.

Self-Regulatory Dimension

The self-regulatory dimension is associated with the infant's ability to achieve and maintain a balance of all neurobehavioral dimensions through the use of self-consoling behaviors, such as sucking or hand-to-mouth maneuvers (Als, 1986).

The birth process brings new experiences to infants. The ability to adapt to the extrauterine environment is poorly developed in the premature infant; thus the goal of the NICU environment is to support the infant in this new extrauterine life. Sick infants are very vulnerable to external stimuli. They can become sensory overloaded very quickly. Premature infants need support to achieve state organization to respond appropriately to the new environment. As the infant transitions from the warm, dark, quiet, and cushioned intrauterine environment to the cold, bright, noisy extrauterine environment, the emphasis becomes how to best support the infant's developing brain in the NICU environment. The NICU environment is dominated by ever-increasing technology. In the midst of such technology, more attention is needed to strike a balance between the developing human brain and the NICU environment.

Advances in medical management of premature infants have resulted in decreased infant mortality, especially among extremely low-birth-weight infants. NICUs and Special Care Nurseries are uniquely positioned to support the infant's continued neurobehavioral development by modifying the high-risk neonatal environment.

Additionally, NICU staffs use new caregiving strategies that promote developmentally supportive care principles into traditional models of care. Premature infants have markedly improved outcomes when the stress of overstimulation is reduced in their environment. Reducing light, sound, and activity levels in the NICU as well as enhancing the proper positioning and handling of infants can achieve this goal.

ENVIRONMENTAL FACTORS/MACRO ENVIRONMENT

Light

Lighting needs to be balanced between dimmed ambient lighting, natural lighting, and brighter task lighting. Premature infants are photophobic but will open their eyes in dim lights. Lighting in most NICUs is continuous, high-level, and fluorescent. Because of the concern about potential retinal damage in premature infants, NICUs should provide ambient lighting at levels recommended by the Illuminating Engineering Society (i.e., 10 to 20 foot candles) (Illuminating Engineering Society of North America, 1995). Ambient light levels need to be adjustable at each bedside. The level should range from 1- to 60-foot candles (White, 1998). Bright lights in the NICU can disrupt sleep/wake states. Studies have demonstrated benefits to NICU infants who are exposed to diurnal variations in ambient lighting that reduces nighttime levels as low as 0.5-foot candles. NICUs should try to reduce ambient lighting to 0.5-foot candles. Lighting at this level encourages diurnal variation. Both natural and electrical light sources should have controls that allow immediate, sufficient darkening of any bed space for transillumination when necessary. Use of multiple switches on individual dimmers to allow different levels of illumination is helpful.

Procedural lighting should be available at each bedside to evaluate an infant or to perform a procedure. This increased illumination should not increase light levels of adjacent babies. Placing all lights on individually controlled dimmer switches is helpful. Illumination of support areas—such as charting areas, medication preparation areas, and reception areas—should be adequate to perform important or critical tasks. This light level should conform to Illuminating Engineering Society specifications (Illuminating Engineering Society of North America, 1995). When possible, independent controls should be used to accommodate sleeping infants and working nurses.

Windows provide a psychological benefit to NICU staff as well as families. Daylighting is desirable for charting as well as for the evaluation of infant skin tone. Serious problems with radiant heat loss or gain and glare can occur by placing infants too close to external windows even though window treatments are commercially available to alleviate some of these problems.

Exterior windows provide the recommended natural light and assist with diurnal cycling. It is recommended that exterior lighting be available throughout the NICU. These windows can be placed away from direct patient areas—for example, high up on the walls, as skylights, or in other locations that provide indirect light to the patient area. The latter might be a window in a hallway that secondarily allows light to pass into the NICU. All windows, including skylights, should have retractable covers when light is not desired.

At least one source of daylight should be visible from the patient care area. External windows should be at least two feet away from the infant's bed. These windows should be insulated and have shading devices in a neutral color to minimize color distortion from transmitted light (White, 1998).

Sound

High noise levels in NICUs affect infants, staff, and families (Table 16-1) (Graven et al, 1992; Glass, 1999). Excessive noise can damage delicate auditory structures and can have adverse physiological effects such as hypoxia, increased intracranial pressure, increased blood pressure, apnea, bradycardia, and color changes (Graven et al, 1992). These high noise levels are often a result of equipment, alarms, ceiling and flooring material, communication devices, talking or the underlying heating and air conditioning ventilation systems. Personnel and equipment also generate transient sounds.

Sound levels in NICUs have been documented to range from 50 to 90 decibels (dB) with peaks to 120 decibels (Lotas, 1992). Safety standards for sound exposure in adults have long been established, yet this area is relatively new for infants (Thomas, 1989).

Both intensity and duration of sound exposure should be considered when evaluating the noise level in a NICU. Some units are placing microphones in the ceiling above infant care areas to determine the sound levels that are filtering to the infant. These microphones are wired to an alarm device that feeds a signal to a ceiling light or light panel at a central nurses' station if the sound level exceeds a predetermined level. This system helps alert staff and parents to sounds that exceed a reasonable level, such as 65 dB. This alarm helps modify behavior and ensures better monitoring of all noise sources. If a sound detection system such as this cannot be installed, handheld devices can be used periodically or at the time of certain procedures to monitor sound levels—including the human voice.

TABLE **16-1**	Records of Various Examples of NICU Equipment	
Equipment	dB levels
IV pump alarm	60-78
Tapping incubator with fingers	70-95
Closing incubator drawer	70-95
Bubbling water in ventilator/hood tubing	62-87
Closing a solid plastic porthole	80-111
Pulse oximeter alarm	86

From Thomas K (1989). How the NICU Environment Sounds to a Preterm Infant. Maternal child nursing, 14, 249-251.

Equipment should be selected with a noise criterion rating of ≤40 dB. Infant bed areas should be situated to produce minimal background noise and to contain and absorb as much transient noise as possible. Many sound control features should be considered in the design of a NICU. The current air duct and ventilation system should be evaluated for noise and dust. Air ventilation systems are a challenge in a unit that attempts to provide private, separate areas that require a full ceiling-to-floor separation. From a budgetary perspective, it may substantially increase the cost of the unit renovation/construction. Those units that have met the fiscal and physical challenges of providing adequate ventilation have done so in an attempt to provide a more homelike atmosphere. Acoustic ceiling tiles in direct patient care areas with a noise reduction coefficient (NRC) rating of at least 0.90 should be considered (American Society for Testing and Materials, 1992). Raised ceilings were used to create an open atmosphere. Porcelain sinks rather than stainless steel sinks can also minimize noise. Carpet decreases the noise level and promotes a homelike environment, yet vinyl-flooring material directly at the bedside can ease the routine cleaning. Despite concerns over carpet use in NICUs, no documented studies or evidence to support increased infection rates exist. One important issue is the noise created by the equipment used to clean the carpet. When industrial-sized vacuum cleaners are used, the noise level exceeds the recommended sound level in the immediate area of the infant's and decreases the dust level. Acoustical partitions may be additionally used to minimize noise (American Society of Heating, Refrigerating, and Air-Conditioning Engineers, 1995).

A wireless phone system carried by each health care provider in place of bedside phones can also limit noise. The ringer can be set on vibrate to minimize the noise level. Decibel monitoring systems can help regulate the levels of conversation and incidental noise throughout the NICU by activating a light alarm. A decibel-monitoring limit should be set at 65 dB and can then be dialed strategically down as staff changes their behavior.

Music therapy is used in some units to calm and soothe the environment. This therapy works for infants, families, and staff alike. However, the sound must be monitored for safe and reasonable levels.

The following Acoustical Design Guidelines should be considered:

Background noise, 50 dB (Environmental Protection Agency)

Transient noise <70 dB (American Academy of Pediatrics)

Equipment with NC (Noise Control) Rating <40 dB

Incubator motor noise <50 dB (AAP)

Voice levels 60 to 70 dB

Noise levels (work-related) 90 dB (Occupational Safety and Health Administration)

These guidelines include environmental factors that should also be considered throughout renovation:

Temperature 75° to 79° F (23.8° to 26.1° C)

Humidity 30% to 60%

Air exchange 6 per hour / 2 with outside air exchange

All air filtered at 90% efficiency

Activity

The unborn infant lives in a warm, cushioned, amniotic fluid environment. Once born, the infant is exposed to a multitude of intrusive and stress-producing activity. Infants may exhibit adverse physiologic symptoms to this stimulation such as tachycardia, bradycardia, color changes, and oxygen desatura-

tions. More profound infant distress signals such as retractions, vomiting, or seizure activity may occur with over stimulation (Graven et al, 1992).

Infants should be handled gently without sudden changes in movement. Pharmacologic as well as nonpharmacologic comfort measures should be provided with painful procedures. Infants may be placed on sheepskins or waterbed to stimulate the intrauterine environment (Lawhon & Melzar, 1998). Infants should be placed in a position of comfort to promote flexion with well-defined boundaries.

Opportunities should be provided for non-nutritive sucking when the infant shows an interest in sucking and is medically stable. Health professionals have asked whether activities such as non-nutritive sucking may create stability that, when withheld until the infant is stable, causes stress. More studies are needed to examine the effects of developmental care on creating or contributing to physiologic stability.

Parents should be encouraged to provide gentle touch and containment by cupping the infant's head and buttocks rather than lightly stroking his skin. Offering parents the opportunity to "kangaroo" their infant skin-to-skin may help facilitate the family's psychological healing, enhance parent-infant bonding, and improve lactation (Alfonso et al, 1993). The increase in recommended space for each infant care area allows for the placement of a comfortable chair for the parent just to sit and to provide kangaroo care.

Infants' senses of smell are stimulated primarily by unpleasant odors. Betadine®, skin preps, and alcohol smells are often present. Additionally, the infant is exposed to fragrances worn by staff members. Infants may respond to olfactory stimuli with altered respirations, increased heart rate, and physical movements to push away from the unpleasant stimulus (Gardner & Lubchenco, 1998). Behaviorally, staff should be educated on this topic to prevent olfactory overstimulation.

CAREGIVING FACTORS/MICRO ENVIRONMENT

In utero, the infant is confined to an enclosed space with relatively well-defined boundaries. As the infant grows, his or her available space for free movement decreases, and his or her body becomes more flexed (i.e., physiologic flexion). The developing infant can extend his arms and legs, meet resistance, and pull his extremities back into a gentle flexion. Physiologic flexion is believed to be vital for the development of normal body movement and control (Gardner & Lubchenco, 1998). Additionally, prone flexion may promote physiologic subsystem stability as evidenced by improved oxygenation and stable heart rate and respirations (Als, 1986).

After delivery, the infant is generally placed on a flat surface with limited physical boundaries to enhance or support flexion. Providing opportunities for both flexion and extension is essential in helping the infant achieve motor stabilization and may decrease the incidence of musculoskeletal abnormalities.

The premature infant often makes repeated yet unsuccessful attempts to seek boundaries by extending his or her arms and legs. In addition, he or she may try to return to a tucked and flexed position. These repeated motoric efforts may exhaust the infant, thus using much of an already limited energy supply. Developmentally supportive care giving is aimed at minimizing energy expenditure while promoting a balance between flexion and extension for any infant. Proper positioning and handling have been shown to affect many physiological and neurobehavioral parameters in the preterm infant. Appropriate positioning—such as midline orientation, hand-to-mouth activity, flexion, self-soothing, and self-regulatory abilities—contributes to neurobehavioral development. Correct body positioning can prevent postural deformities such as hip abduction and external rotation, ankle eversion, retracted and abducted shoulders, increased neck hyperextension and shoulder elevation, and cranial molding. Prone positioning increases oxygenation, tidal volume, and the compliance of the lungs. Positioning can also affect visual coordination (Lutes, 1996).

Body containment is also an important factor because it increases the infant's feelings of security and self-control and decreases stress. Infants who are contained tend to be calmer, require less medication, and gain weight more rapidly.

The long-term effects of improper positioning can be very expensive for parents and the tax-payer. In proper positioning and alignment (regardless of prone, supine, or side-lying position), the knees and nipples should be in the same plane. If the hips are unsupported, gravity will pull the knees apart, and the infant will exhibit "frog like" positioning, which enables the gluteous muscles (i.e., muscles in the buttock) and latissimus dorsi (i.e., muscles in the lower back) to shorten, thus decreasing the ability of those muscles to elongate in a sitting position. Diapers that do not fit appropriately can also cause this damage. Scapular retraction can occur if the shoulder girdle is not supported in a flexed position.

Handling

Frequent handling and touching disturbs sleep, which leads to decreased weight gain and decreased state regulation. In one study, premature infants were found to be disturbed an average of more than 23 times in 24 hours (Altimier et al, 1999). The premature infant in the NICU achieves an average of five to fifteen minutes of deep, undisturbed sleep within a 24-hour day Altimier et al, 1999). Routine procedures often result in significant hypoxia. Most episodes of hypoxemia happen during handling by care-givers. The extent of hypoxemia was greatly reduced when care-giving was modified. The developmentally supportive care-giver identifies the importance of minimizing the frequency of interruptions to help promote uninterrupted sleep as well as providing the appropriate quality and intensity of stimulation during wakefulness (Als & Duffy, 1982).

Deep sleep is characterized by regular breathing, no evidence of rapid eye movements, relaxed facial expression, no spontaneous motor activity, and occasional startles (Als & Duffy, 1996). Light sleep is characterized by rapid eye movements under closed eyelids, periods of irregular and regular breathing, and low-level activity. In addition, occasional startles, whimpers, smiles, mouthing, and sucking behaviors may be observed (Als & Duffy, 1996).

If the infant is receiving too much or too little stimulation, he or she may demonstrate behaviors of state disorganization, including fussing, yawning, frowning, and involuntary eye movements. If the infant's behavioral cues are not addressed and stimulation modified, further signs of physiologic and motoric disorganization may result (Als, 1996).

Self-regulation is the ability to move smoothly between states and to achieve a balance of all neurobehavioral dimensions through use of self-consoling behaviors (Als, 1986). Infants can achieve self-regulation when a developmentally appropriate setting is provided for the infants and families. By assessing the infant's behavioral responses to caregivers and other aspects of the physical environment, one can support the infant's neurodevelopment and can decrease stress.

PHYSICAL ENVIRONMENT

Quiet, less obtrusive havens promote better sleep, less crying, faster weight gain, and earlier discharge than traditional NICUs do (Volpe, 2001; Als, 1986). When designing a NICU, one should consider providing a developmentally appropriate setting for high-risk infants and families. This design must provide a functional environment for families and staff.

With advances in new technology and the promotion of family-centered care in the NICU, many hospitals throughout the world are planning and building new units. When new design or redesign occurs, a shared vision and common goals must exist among all disciplines. The goal with any renovation or construction is to optimize design and to consider infant physiology as well as physical and financial opportunities and constraints. NICU design shall be driven by systematic program goals and objectives that define the purpose of the unit, service provision, space use, projected bed space needs, staffing requirements, and other information related to the mission of the unit (White, 2002).

Mandatory Regulations

Mandatory federal, state, and/or provincial regulations should be considered as well as the Recommended Standards for Newborn ICU Design. The following mandatory regulations are guidelines to consider as well as Newborn ICU Design:
Certificate of Need (CON)
State licensure
Building codes
Fire and Safety Standards
American Disabilities Act (ADA)
Food and Drug Administration (FDA)
Occupational Safety and Health Administration (OSHA)
Joint Commission on Accreditation of Health Organizations (JCAHO)

Planning a Design Project

When initiating a renovation process, one can be overwhelmed with the amount of information to learn. The goal of this section is to guide an optimal physical design of one renovation while considering physiological, developmental, and financial constraints. NICU planners should start a minimum of one year before a renovation or construction and create a detailed time line. A multidisciplinary health care team—Registered Nurses (RNs), Medical Doctors (MDs), nutritionists, Respiratory Therapists (RTs), radiograph personnel, pharmacists, Occupational Therapists (OTS), Physical Therapists (PTs), administration, educators, patient care assistants, unit coordinators, lab personnel, audiology, architects, construction team, sound consultants, project managers, environmental consultants, and developmental consultants—should be selected to meet weekly. Environmental consultants are helpful to monitor air quality and conduct real-time dust-level monitoring if renovation or construction is phased and a NICU is going to remain operational throughout the renovation process.

The literature should be reviewed for the most current information about scientifically supportable practices regarding the high-risk infant's environment. Funding needs to be addressed through the hospital and/or philanthropic campaigns. Signage can demonstrate recognition for different dollar amounts.

Focus groups should be included to solicit staff, family, and physician input. The team should tour various facilities to share insight on what does and does not work and to benchmark various units. Predetermined site questions can help focus the renovation team. Top reasons to renovate should be ranked to keep all committee members focused on the renovation priorities.

The NICU environment should appeal not only to its tiny residents but also adults. The bed layout, lighting sound control, and traffic patterns that support the developmental needs of sick infants and soothing spaces for families and staff to interact should be considered (Figure 16-1). During demolition and construction, frequent walkthroughs provide feedback for ongoing changes and improvements.

Patient Care Areas

The NICU should be a distinct, controlled area immediately adjacent to perinatal services, except in freestanding children's hospitals. When perinatal and neonatal services are on separate floors, direct dedicated elevator access should be provided (White, 2000).

Each infant care space should be 120 to 150 square feet. This space must accommodate the equipment for monitoring and delivering care. There should also be enough space to allow parents to sit together at the bedside and to hold their infants. The infant care space should allow privacy for the infant and family. The developing family unit needs privacy to encourage relationship building, care-giving activities, and initiation of customs and ethnic traditions. Separation and privacy of the infant space can be accomplished by use of half- or whole-walls, movable curtains or screens, or adjustable walls. Some units are now designed as single rooms with unit control stations or a centralized nurses' station. The single room concept designs have been built as NICUs or Special, Transitional, or Developmental Care Units. The NICU should have an identified entrance and reception area for families.

A corridor design entrance should be family-friendly, which can offer hope. A "Wall of Fame" can be created to offer a sense of soothing comfort and hope to parents and visitors. A family lounge can provide a vending area, refrigerator, microwave, and eating area. A computer with Internet capabilities for families can offer additional resources and/or e-mail capabilities. Some units actually set up kiosks with computer desk and terminals so that families can access information in a somewhat private area. A children's library is a valuable area for parents to read books to infants or for their siblings to explore and read. An isolette with a baby doll can help siblings adapt to their new baby's little world. Dolls that represent the cultural diversity of the patient population should be chosen.

The scrub room, where all families enter, can be designated as the communication area. An educational board (rotated weekly) may provide developmental or educational tips. A communication board, which provides family support, group information, and/or parent classes, is also helpful.

A rooming inn area (just like an inn) that can provide hotel-type rooms or care-by-parent rooms is essential. Each room should be supplied with a refrigerator, television, telephone, and bathroom (Figure 16-2). Overnight stays by parents in rooms that are in close proximity to the NICU should provide parents a sense of encouragement so that they support their infants in the NICU.

A combined lounge for all disciplines with windows and bright lights are helpful for staff. The lounge needs to be in close proximity to the unit. The staff restroom should be separate from the lounge (Figure 16-3). Mailboxes and purse lockers should also be provided in the lounge.

Families can use window seats placed wherever possible to step away from the bedside if desired or for staff to conduct private conversations. Alcoves or areas of privacy can be supportive to families coping with stress and for staff needing areas to conduct confidential conversations.

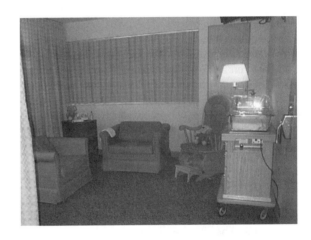

FIGURE **16-2**
Rooming inn.

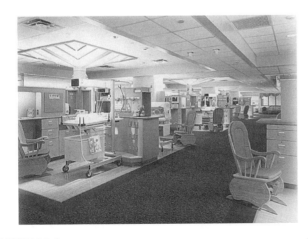

FIGURE **16-1**
Nursery.

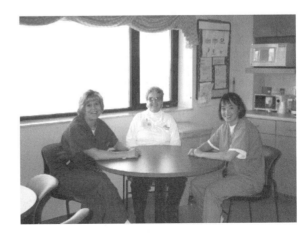

FIGURE **16-3**
Staff lounge.

A main supply area central to the patient care area can be designed with moveable shelves to augment space. It is space- and time-efficient to locate a "dirty" equipment room adjacent to the "clean" equipment room. Storage areas and cabinets should be placed throughout the unit to provide ample storage space. Storage should be calculated to include supplies and all beds in and out of use. This storage space is essential to the efficient and effective operation of a NICU.

Office space for interdisciplinary team members needs to be integrated in the design. Flexible meeting and conference areas are essential to staff, parent, and support group activities. Another aspect of space includes a combined practitioner and resident office designed with a separate desk area for each person. Additionally, binder bins can provide each an area to store personal belongings. The attending physicians like their "own" space to consult with subspecialties.

A treatment/procedure room should be included in the unit design with operating room (OR) capabilities. Flip-down headwalls provide the capability of surgery on either side. This room can double as an overflow room for high census periods or additional isolation room space. This room can also decrease the need for use of the main OR or Caesarian section rooms.

A library/conference area should be ranked high as a priority. Staff meetings, in-services, parent meetings, and conferences can take place in this area. This library can have built-in shelves, television, VCR, a big expo board, and teleconference capabilities.

The headwall design process should include the creation of a full-scale headwall mock-up for all staff to evaluate. It should be ergonomic with individual workstations. Computer outlets should be placed at each workstation. The layouts of outlets, medical gasses, drawers, trash, and linen can be changed frequently by the use of post-it notes. This process allows staff the opportunity to test the functionality of the bed space. Parents should have space at the bedside for personal belongings and should have a bulletin board to personalize their infant's room.

Breast-feeding rooms should be available and close to the NICU for mothers to pump while they are in the NICU. These should be larger than a small closet because the size and lack of windows in some breastfeeding rooms have inhibited their use. Ideally the room should provide comfortable seating within a private setting. The lighting level should be moderate to decrease stress but high enough to facilitate clear visualization of the breast pump, equipment, and infant. A sink is necessary for hand washing. Educational material is valuable to a parent who feels the need to learn all that he or she can to adequately care for her infant.

With the increase in multiple births, NICUs should consider areas specifically designed for multiples. The hindrances of current NICU design—such as limited electrical, gas, and vacuum outlets as well as space limitations—can be identified and addressed in the design of the "multiple pod." The "multiple pod" is the first unit in the world designed specifically for multiples. With a rise in multiples, being proactive in meeting the unique needs of infants and families of multiples was important. Current technology and space allows for care of singletons. The multiple pod can efficiently and comfortably care for twins, triplets, and quadruplets. The current NICU standards and guidelines indicate that space can be allocated for multiples to be together in separate beds or to co-bed in one bed. The design of the space can accommodate families to be with all infants at the same time rather than going from room to room.

The "multiple pod" is a unique design to accommodate the needs of multiple birth infants and their families. Other designs also are used to accomplish the same goal—meeting physical and psychosocial care needs. These designs may be single rooms with toilet facilities to specialized units.

An example is Rainbow Babies and Children in Cleveland, Ohio, which has a designated developmental care unit with rooms to accommodate family care. This example is but one of many others that are now becoming a popular NICU design feature. Whatever the design, the room should be ample to accommodate large cribs for two, three, four, or more infants at the same time.

Every multiple bedside is wired so that up to four monitors can be networked and used simultaneously and so that the number of electrical, medical gas, and suction outlets can be supplied to comply with state regulations for the volume of equipment needed for multiples who are co-bedding.

Family restrooms that provide medicine cabinets stocked with feminine pads and breast pads are a nice amenity. A grieving/bereavement area is a private area with hidden gasses to ventilate babies before ending support. This area can accommodate families without their feeling out in the open. Two doors—one to enter and one to exit the unit without having to walk by babies—is of great value to families (Figure 16-4).

Some hospitals are buying the BabyCare Links® program (www.babycarelink.com; Framingham, Mass.). This computerized/web-based program allows parents who cannot visit the unit to log on to the computer and see a photo gallery of their infants' progress. One section offers a personal journal that is kept by the nurses for the parents. Some hospitals have real-time video capabilities so the parents can actually see their infants in real time. This example is just one of the many growing resources to keep parents connected, even at a distance, to their infants.

Radiograph personnel should be consulted early in the renovation process. An example of an radiograph area designed by radiograph personnel includes a digital machine work area and room for the portable radiograph machine.

SUMMARY

To provide developmentally supportive care and to optimize the experience of infants in intensive care, an understanding of their behavioral capabilities as well as their surrounding physi-

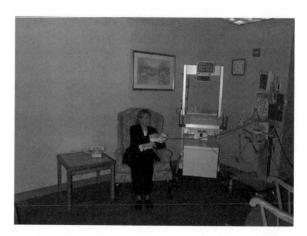

FIGURE **16-4**
Grief room.

cal environment is essential. Participation by all disciplines is vital for the success of any NICU design project. High-tech and high-touch care can be provided with low lighting and acoustic levels. The production of an efficient, peaceful, and satisfying environment for both administering and receiving care is an optimal goal for each high-risk infant.

REFERENCES

Alfonso D, et al. (1993). Reconciliation and healing for mothers through skin-to-skin contact provided in an American tertiary level Intensive Care Nursery. *Neonatal network*, 12(3), 25-32.

Als H (1982). Toward a synactive theory of development: Promise for the assessment and support of infant individuality. *Infant mental health journal*, 3(4), 229-243.

Als H (1986). A synactive model of neonatal behavioral organization: Framework for the assessment of neurobehavioral development in the premature infant and for support of infants and parents in the neonatal intensive care environment. *Physical and occupational therapy in pediatrics*, 6 (3/4), 3-53.

Als H, Duffy F (1996). Effectiveness of individualized neurodevelopmental care in the newborn intensive care unit, (NICU). *Acta, paediatric supplemental* 416, 21-30.

Altimier L, et al. (1999). Value Study. *Neonatal network*, 18(4), 35-38.

American Society of Heating, Refrigerating, and Air-Conditioning Engineers. (1995). *Sound and vibration control. In ASHRAE Handbook*. Atlanta: American Society of Heating, Refrigerating, and Air-Conditioning Engineers.

American Society for Testing and Materials. (1992). *Standard Definitions of Terms Relating to Environmental Acoustics*. Philadelphia: American Society for Testing and Materials; Publication ASTM C-634.

Blackburn ST (2003). *Maternal, fetal, and neonatal physiology: a clinical perspective*, St Louis: Mosby.

Gardner SL, Lubchenco LO (1998). *The neonate and the environment: impact on development.* (pp. 197-242). In Merenstein GB, Gardner SL, *Handbook of neonatal intensive care*, ed 4, St Louis: Mosby.

Glass P (1999). The vulnerable neonate and the neonatal intensive care environment. In Avery GB, et al, editors. *Neonatology: pathophysiology and management of the newborn*, ed 5, Philadelphia: JB Lippincott.

Graven S, et al. (1992). The high-risk infant environment, Part 1. *Journal of perinatology*, 12(2), 164-172.

Holditch-Davis D (1990). The development of sleeping and waking states in high-risk preterm infants. *Infant behavior & development*, 13, 513-531.

Illuminating Engineering Society of North America (1995). Lighting for health care facilities, RP29. New York: Illuminating Engineering Society of North America.

Lawhon G, Melzar A (1988). Developmental care of the very low birth weight infant. *Journal of perinatal/neonatal nursing*, 2(1), 56-65.

Lotas MJ (1992). Effects of light and sound in the neonatal intensive care unit environment on the low birth weight infant. *NAACOG's (Nurses Association of the American College of Obstetrics and Gynecology) clinical issues in perinatal & women's health nursing*, 3(1). 34-44.

Ludington-Hoe SM, Swinth JY (1996). Developmental aspects of kangaroo care. *Journal of obstetrical-gynecological neonatal nursing*, 25(8), 691-703.

Lutes L (1996). Developmental care: bedding twins/multiples together. *Neonatal network*, 15(7), 61-62.

McGrath J (October/November, 2000). Developmental Physiology of the Neurological System, *Central lines*, 16, 4, 1-16.

Thomas K (1989). How the NICU Environment Sounds to a Preterm Infant. *Maternal child nursing*, 14, 249-251.

Volpe JJ (2001). *Neurology of the newborn*, ed 4, Philadelphia: WB Saunders.

White R (2000). Recommended Standards for Newborn ICU Design. Report of the Fifth Consensus Conference by the Committee to Establish Recommended Standards for Newborn ICU Design. http://www.nd.edu/nkkblberg/designstandards.htm; http://www.nann.org/resource/publctns/ctrlline/ju198/design.htm.

Yecco GJ (1993). Neurobehavioral development and developmental support of premature infants. *Journal of perinatal and neonatal nursing*, 7(1), 56-65.

NEWBORN AND INFANT NEUROBEHAVIORAL DEVELOPMENT

DIANE HOLDITCH-DAVIS, SUSAN TUCKER BLACKBURN, AND KATHLEEN VANDENBERG

The care of high-risk infants, both those born prematurely and those with medical, surgical, or developmental problems, has long been a major focus of health care concern. Efforts to increase the understanding of the pathophysiologic problems encountered by these infants, along with new management strategies and technologies, have markedly improved the outcome of these infants. Much of the focus of the neonatal intensive care unit (NICU) has been on meeting the physiologic needs of these infants, with less attention, until recently, on the social interactive consequences of this environment. Thus the advances in neonatal care have been accompanied by increasing concerns and documentation regarding the impact of the NICU environment on the infant's physiologic and neurobehavioral functioning, the lack of sensory input geared to meet the individual infant's needs and current level of developmental function, and the effects of stress and overstimulation.

Although tremendous progress has been made in reducing mortality and morbidity in high-risk infants, these infants, especially those born prematurely, are still vulnerable to a wide variety of neurodevelopmental problems. These problems have been referred to as the "new morbidities of low birth weight infants" and include behavioral disorganization, attention deficit disorders, hyperexcitability, language problems, sensory/perceptual and higher-order cognitive problems, regulatory disorders, and school dysfunction (Blackburn, 1995; McGrath et al, 2000). Adverse outcomes of high-risk infants may be related to a variety of factors, including immaturity, perinatal trauma, the early NICU environment, the home environment in which the child is raised, and parent-child interactional considerations. The development of many of these infants is characterized by an unevenness that can lead to later difficulties. This unevenness may be as much the result of the impact of the early environment and its incongruencies as the effects of perinatal stress.

The immature infant differs in two important ways from the healthy full-term infant. First, these infants are born early and therefore must deal with and adapt to the extrauterine environment with bodily systems, including a central nervous system (CNS), that are not yet mature. Second, this interruption of intrauterine life significantly modifies the environment of the infant (Blackburn, 1998). Thus the preterm infant spends the last weeks or months of gestation in an environment—the

NICU—that is much different from that of the uterus or that of a healthy full-term infant. The NICU environment has similar implications for the more mature, although still vulnerable, ill full-term infant. For these infants, this environment is also abnormal and quite different from that experienced by healthy infants who go home with their parents soon after birth.

Neonatal nurses are very familiar with interpreting the physiologic status of infants and basing their interventions on physiologic changes. Nurses have placed increased emphasis on the importance of understanding the behaviors of infants under their care because behavior is the only way infants can communicate their needs and their responses to nursing interventions (Als, 1986; Catlett & Holditch-Davis, 1990). However, two factors make this understanding difficult. First, newborn infants have very limited behavioral repertoires. The same behavior may have different meanings in different situations, but busy neonatal nurses may not have the time necessary to correctly interpret infants' behaviors by comprehensively assessing both the infants' actions and the environmental stimulation. Second, the behavior of critically ill infants is even more difficult to interpret because they lack the energy to display characteristic behavioral responses. Thus neonatal nurses can never rely totally on infants' behaviors to determine infants' needs, but in combination with physiologic parameters, understanding infant behavior enriches both nursing assessment and the evaluation of nursing interventions.

In considering the vulnerabilities of ill and immature infants, it is useful to examine the implications of each of these areas: the state of CNS development, neonatal neurobehavioral development, and the NICU environment. This chapter will discuss each of these topics and examine the sleeping and waking states—and its relevance for neonatal nursing.

FETAL AND NEONATAL CENTRAL NERVOUS SYSTEM DEVELOPMENT

As noted in Chapter 31, the development of the CNS can be divided into six overlapping stages (see Table 31-1). These stages are important to consider in examining the effects of the NICU environment because the stage of development influences the effect of any insult. In addition, several areas of the CNS continue to undergo significant changes during the period when preterm infants are in the NICU, increasing their vulnerability to insult. The stage of development is also reflected by the behaviors characteristic of immature infants (Box 17-1). The first three stages of CNS development (dorsal induction, ventral induction, and neuronogenesis) are completed before the fourth month of gestation. The last three stages (neuron migration, synaptogenesis and arborization, and myelinization) of CNS development continue during the time many infants are in the NICU (Volpe, 2001). Myelinization, although vulnerable to perinatal insults, is a process that continues for many years. Therefore unless insults are severe or prolonged, their effects may be mitigated.

Areas of development during the last part of gestation that are particularly critical in considering neurobehavioral vulnerabilities of ill or immature infants include: (1) autonomic homeostatic control; (2) alterations in the germinal matrix and migration of neurons and glial cells; (3) CNS organizational processes; and (4) growth of the cortex and cerebellum. From about 28 to 32 weeks' gestational age, preterm infants begin to achieve some degree of physiologic homeostasis, with increasing control of the sympathetic system over their autonomic functioning. With increasing autonomic control, the infant develops greater autonomic stability. This autonomic stability can be seen, for example, in the decreasing incidence of apnea and bradycardia. As these infants move to greater cortical control over the next months, their development is characterized by periods of temporary organization followed by periods of disorganization as new levels of maturation and control are achieved These periods of disorganization are reflected in the infant's sleep-wake patterns, proportion of transitional or indeterminate sleep, and fragmented behavioral responses and reflexes.

The germinal matrix in the periventricular subependymal area is a site of origin for neuronal and glial cells. The maximal rate of neuronal proliferation occurs between 12 and 18 weeks of gestational age, although neurons continue to proliferate, particularly in the cerebellum, until after term (Volpe, 2001). Neurons and glial cells migrate from the germinal matrix to their eventual loci within the CNS, where they further differentiate and take on unique and individual functions (Moore & Persaud, 1998). Initially the neurons migrate to areas deep within the cortex; later neurons migrate further toward the surface of the cortex. Thus neurons formed early come to lie in deeper layers of cortex and subcortex; those formed later are found in more superficial layers. The cortex generally has a complete component of neurons by 33 weeks' gestation. Until 32 to 34 weeks' gestational age, the fragile, poorly supported blood vessels in this area receive a significant proportion of cerebral blood flow (Volpe, 2001). Insults to this area before this period may lead to periventricular and intraventricular hemorrhage (Chapter 31).

Organization, or "the processes by which the nervous system takes on the capacity to operate as an integrated whole" (Blackburn, 2003), begins during the sixth month of gestation and extends many years after birth. Neuron growth and connections lead to development of brain sulci and gyri. A brain growth spurt occurs from 26 to 30 weeks, leading to more complex behaviors (Als, 1999; Volpe, 2001). Organization of the CNS is critical for cortical and cognitive development. These processes may be particularly vulnerable to insults from the effects of the NICU environment.

Subplate neurons differentiate early and migrate to cortex from the germinal matrix to serve as guides for ascending and descending projections to target neurons. The subplate neurons provide critical connection sites for axons ascending from thalamus and other sites, until the neurons that these axons will eventually connect with have migrated from the germinal matrix (Blackburn, 2003). The subplate reaches its peak from 22 to 34 weeks (Volpe, 2001). Once cortical neurons have reached their eventual loci, they become arranged in layers and develop dendrites and axons that undergo extensive branching. The pattern of dendritic connections between neurons is a critical growth process that constitute the "wiring" of the brain (also called arborization). These interconnections are critical for processing of impulses, cell-to-cell communication, and communication throughout the nervous system. Lack of connections can result in hypersensitivity, poorly modulated behaviors, and all-or-nothing responses, which can often be observed in preterm infants in the NICU (Box 17-1). Similar behavior patterns can also be seen in some children in later infancy and childhood.

Another component of organization is the formation of connections or synapses between neurons and development of intracellular structures and enzymes for neurotransmitter production. Synaptogenesis is critical for integration across all areas of the nervous system. Synapses continue to restructure throughout development, and this process is thought to be the basis for memory and learning. Synaptogenesis is mediated by excitatory neurotransmitters such as glutamate (Fox et al, 1996). Glutamate acts on N-methyl-D-asparate (NMDA) receptors to enhance neuronal proliferation, migration and synaptic plasticity (Fox et al, 1996; Ikonomidou et al, 2001; Sanchez & Jensen, 2001). Another component of organization is reduction in the

---

BOX 17-1

Neurodevelopmental Limitations of the Very-Low-Birth-Weight Infant and Related Behavioral Manifestations

Limitations in Neurologic Function

Sparse myelin
Lung refractory period
Weak transmission
Decreased inhibitory potential
Decreased functional validation (ability to utilize various systems)
Slow nerve conduction
Slow synaptic potential
Unable to sustain high firing rates
Incomplete cell differentiation
Decreased synaptogenesis and dendritic arborization

Behaviors of Immature Infants

Irregular state regulation
Increased and decreased tone
Alterations in primitive reflexes
Easily exhausted
Irritable, difficult to soothe
Inability to inhibit
Jerky movements
Low arousal, inability to sustain an alert state
Poor coordination
Altered autonomic regulation
Asymmetrical, uncoordinated posture and movement

number of neurons and their connections through the death of many neurons and regression of dendrites and synapses. Neuronal death assists in elimination of errors within the nervous system, such as neurons that are improperly located, that fail to achieve adequate connections, or that are underused.

Organizational processes and modification of neurons continue into adulthood but are particularly vulnerable during infancy. The ability of a neuron to change structure and function has been called plasticity.

> The more immature the infant at birth the greater the impact of neural plasticity. There is considerable evidence in animal studies that sensory input influences later neuronal structure and function; for instance, an enriched environment during infancy improves developmental outcome by maximizing brain potential. This plasticity is both an advantage and a liability. Although sensory input may increase cellular processes and interconnections, the sensory environment may also produce undesired changes in structure and function (Black, 1998; DiPietro, 2000). The preterm infant in the NICU may be particularly vulnerable to these alterations (Blackburn, 2003).

Neuronal differentiation and organization are controlled by the interaction of genes with the environment. Each neuron has many synaptic connections that allow the brain to integrate and organize information. There is initially an overproduction of neurons and nerve connections. Many of these neurons and connections are later eliminated Whether or not a connection is retained or eliminated is influenced by the infant's early environment and experiences (Black, 1998; DiPietro, 2000). For example, the brain is more likely to strengthen and retain connections that are used repeatedly and to eliminate underused connections. Improper sensory input (too much or too little) or input that is inappropriate in terms of timing may alter brain development (Black, 1998). Thus the environment of the immature infants in the NICU and in the early months following discharge is critical for brain development and later cognitive function.

Greenough and Black have postulated that there are two types of neural plasticity: experience-expectant and experience-dependent (Black, 1998; Greenough, 1987). Experience-expectant plasticity is linked to brain developmental timetable. Thus specific sensory experiences and input are needed at specific times for neural development and maturation. Altered sequences or types of sensory input can alter or disrupt development. Experience-dependent plasticity involves interaction with the environment to develop specific skills for later use. This form of plasticity involves memory and learning and allows development of flexibility, adaptation, and individual differences in social and intellectual development (Black, 1998; Greenough, 1987).

The cerebellum is also vulnerable to insults from the early environment. The cerebellum is primarily concerned with control of muscles and coordination of movements; it undergoes a critical growth spurt at 30 to 32 weeks' gestation. This spurt includes an increase in dendritic arborization, which is complete earlier than many other areas of the brain. Insults may lead to the altered sequences of motor development seen in some preterm infants (Volpe, 2001).

NEONATAL NEUROBEHAVIORAL DEVELOPMENT

To provide developmentally supportive, family-focused care for high-risk infants in the NICU, the nurse must understand behavioral and developmental issues as they impact the infant and the family. In the last 20 years, our knowledge of early childhood development has been dramatically altered by an avalanche of new research in neurobiological, behavioral, and social sciences that has led to major advances in understanding the conditions that influence the well being and early development of infants and young children. A deeper understanding of the importance of early life experience and the highly interactive influences of genetics and the environment on the developing brain has deepened our understanding of the early years. Attention to the powerful influence of the role of early relationships and the capabilities of the development of emotions in young children has finally taken center stage. Add to this the changes in our social structures and changes in our families—culturally and economically—including the shifting of parenting roles, along with changes in the workplace and in child care services for the very youngest, the continuing high levels of economic hardship in many families, and it becomes clear that a professional review and rethinking of policy and practice required dedicated attention and a thoughtful response (Shonkoff & Phillips, 2000).

One of the first requirements of early development is the process of acquiring the capacity to self-regulate. This capacity refers to the mastery of tasks that were in the beginning carried out and accomplished by the mother's body while the infant was in the womb; after birth and the transition out of the womb, the task becomes the infant's job. This ability to transition from external regulation to the ability to accomplish regulation on one's own is a lengthy process in infant development. The tasks involved initially include physiological regulation such as maintaining normal body temperature, regulating day night cycles, and learning to calm oneself and relax after basic needs are met. Later, self-regulation means controlling one's own emotions and managing to keep one's attention focused (Shonkoff & Phillips, 2000).

Shonkoff and Phillips (2000) refer to this process as reacting and regulating one's range of developmental function. The process is deeply related to one's relationships with others. Parents become the "co-regulators" or extensions of the infant's internal regulatory systems working to regulate function in the young child just as he or she is working towards the same. This requires of caregivers the ability to read and understand the infant's needs and the sensitivity, knowledge, and energy to respond in helpful satisfying ways. Parents must establish "regulatory connections" with young children and then gradually shift the independent task of regulation gradually over to them, one domain and one day at a time, being forever watchful that the balance in the child is not seriously disrupted The ways that infants and young children learn about self-management involves behavioral, emotional, and cognitive self-control; which must evolve for competent functioning.

During early child development (birth to six years) children become consistently independent and develop the ability to manage their own behavior. Two concerns related to these developmental processes that have been thoroughly covered in developmental literature are concerns over sleep behavior and crying behavior. Infants with serious medical conditions that require intensive care nursery stays, including preterm or medical fragile infants, have more difficult transitions to regulatory competence. Immature sick newborns are much less able to organize and stabilize sleep, waking, and feeding. They tend to be unpredictable, to cry more, and be fussier. They tend to make less eye contact, smile less, vocalize less, show less positive affect, and are generally more difficult and harder for parents to read (Barnard, 1999; Beckwith & Rodning, 1992). During the first three months after birth for a full-term newborn, the infant depends on the relationship with the primary caregiver. The infant takes on an extensive undertaking that requires that he or she learn to get to sleep on his own, stop crying when consoled, respond to the caregiver, and establish day-night, wake-sleep rhythms. Once the rapid developmental changes of the first three months of life after full-term birth accomplish its developmental changes, the infant faces another level of regulation in controlling his or her emotions and behavior. Followed by the regulation of attention and the regulation of mental processes, a process known as executive function emerges and involves the ability to think, retrieve, and remember information, solve problems and engage in complex activities, which involve oral language, reading and writing, math, and social behavior.

A key concept that is emerging from this synthesis of the most recent research reveals that early experiences clearly affect the development of the brain. Development is beginning during early fetal life and will lay a foundation for all that is to follow. Als and colleagues (1982, 1986) have developed a model for understanding the organization of neurobehavioral capabilities in the development of the fetus and newborn infant. This model describes emerging behavioral organizational abilities of the neonate. This model is based on the assumption that infants actively communicate via their behavior, which becomes an important route for understanding thresholds of stress or stability. Behavior of the infant not only is the main route of communication but also provides the basis for the structure of developmental assessment and provision of developmentally appropriate care (Als, 1986).

This synactive theory of development (Als, 1982) provides a model through which one can specify the degree of differentiation of behavior and the ability of infants to organize and control their behavior. The focus is not on assessment of skills but on the unique way each individual infant deals with the world around her or him. The synactive theory of development specifies the range of neonatal behavior as the infant matures as well as the ability of the infant to regulate behavior. This model is based on the assumption that the infant's primary route of communicating both functional stability and the limits for stress is through behavior (Als, 1986). For example, infants who extend their limbs after being turned to supine to have their diaper changed may be communicating that they cannot control their limbs and movement in that position. Containing the limbs of these infants helps them to develop control and reduces stress over the loss of control.

Infants are seen as being in continual interaction with their environment via five subsystems: autonomic/physiologic; motor; state/organizational; attentional/interactive, and self-regulatory. These subsystems mature simultaneously, and within each subsystem a developmental sequence can be observed. Thus at each stage of development, new tasks and organizations are learned against the backdrop of previous development. The subsystems are interdependent and interrelated. For example, physiologic stability provides the foundation for motor and state control; the infant cannot respond socially to caregivers until motor and state control is achieved. The loss of integrity in one subsystem can influence the organization of other subsystems in response to environmental demands. In the preterm, less organized infant, the systems interplay, con-

tinuously influencing each other. In the healthy full-term infant, these systems are synchronized and function smoothly. Thus full-term infants can regulate their autonomic, motor, state, and attentional systems with ease and without apparent stress. However, less mature infants tend to be able to tolerate only one or minimal activity at a time and may easily lose control if their individual thresholds are exceeded.

Instability in the autonomic system can be seen in the pattern of respiration (pauses, tachypnea), color changes (red, pale, dusky, mottled), and various visceral signs (regurgitation, twitching, stooling). Organization of the motor system is assessed by observing the infant's tone and posture (flexed, extended, hyperflexed, flaccid); specific movement patterns of the extremities, head, trunk and face; and level of activity. The development of motor responses is closely linked to state organization (Als, 1986, 1996).

The state system is understood by noting the available range of states of consciousness (sleep to arousal, awake to alert, crying), how well each state is defined (in terms of behavioral and physiologic parameters), transitions between states, and the quality of organization of these states. States may be poorly defined at first, especially in the immature infant. For example, jerky body twitches and fussing may accompany sleep and wake states. In addition, the immature infant may not be able to achieve clearly defined states as seen in the mature infant (Als, 1982).

Initially, preterm infants tend to be unstable and fragile, with sudden changes in their autonomic, motor, and state systems. These infants often have minimal response to handling or other sensory input until a threshold is reached, then quickly develop a cascade of responses, ending in several color changes, flaccidity, bradycardia, and apnea. As the infant matures, the responses are more variable, and the infant is less likely to totally decompensate (Als, 1986, 1999). Changes within the autonomic, motor, and state systems at all stages of development are not just reactions to stress and overstimulation but can signal that the infant's tolerance threshold has been exceeded by recognizing these signs early, the nurse can intervene to prevent mild to severe decompensation.

The attentional/interactive system involves the infant's ability to orient and focus on sensory stimuli, such as faces, sounds, or objects—that is, the external environment. This system also includes the range of abilities in states of consciousness: how well periods of alertness are defined and how transitions into and out of alertness are handled At first, this alertness may be very brief with a dull look or glassy-eyed stare. As this system matures, the infant is able to interact with greater ease and for longer periods. Social responsiveness requires that the infant have enough state control to sustain some awake and alert states (Als, 1982).

The self-regulatory system includes behaviors the infant uses to maintain the integrity and balance of the other subsystems, to integrate the other systems, and to move smoothly between states. For example, some infants can tuck their limbs close to their body in an effort to gain control when stressed, whereas others seem to relax if they can brace a foot against the side of the crib.

In summary,

the process of development appears to be that of stabilization and integration of some subsystems, which allows the differentiation and emergence of others which in turn feed back on the integrated system. In this process the whole system is reopened and transformed to a new level of more differentiated integration from which the next newly emerging subsystem can further differentiate and press to actualization and realization. (Als, 1982, 1996).

By observing and assessing the newborn infant's responses to the caregiver and other aspects of the environment across these five subsystems of behavioral functioning, one can develop and implement a plan of care to support the infant's emerging neurodevelopmental organization and reduce stress.

Assessment of Neonatal Neurobehavioral Development

Developmental assessment of newborn functioning emerged with the awareness of the amazing capabilities of neonates. The newborn infant, who for years was thought to be nonreactive and incapable of social participation, is now seen as an active participant in social interaction and capable of self-regulation (Als, 1984, 1996; Brazelton & Nugent, 1995). Even with a greater understanding of newborn capabilities, researchers and clinicians have been unable to accurately predict the future course of an infant's development from early neurologic or behavioral assessments.

Historically, two types of neonatal assessments have evolved—the neurologic examination and the behavioral examination. The neurologic examination assesses the function of the CNS and typically includes assessment of motor tone and reflex behaviors within the context of infant state. The behavioral examination complements and elaborates on the neurologic assessment. An assumption underlying the behavioral examination is that the observable behavior of an infant is a reflection of his or her underlying neurologic status. The behavioral examination seeks to describe the quality of behavioral performance. More recently, these two forms of assessment have been combined into the neurodevelopmental or neurobehavioral assessment.

The neurodevelopmental examination is important because it yields a large pool of early observable behavior, including information about the infant's neurologic status and abilities to cope and interact with the environment. In addition, data from this examination can assist the clinician in estimating maturity and in identifying and evaluating problems that could be precursors to later developmental problems. Because the neurodevelopmental examination provides an immediate basis for determining the status of the infant's development, the results can be used for planning intervention strategies as well as for screening for infants in need of further diagnostic assessments.

Who Needs To Be Assessed?

All neonates and their caregivers can benefit from ongoing neurobehavioral assessment. These assessments provide information on the infant's behavioral capabilities, interactive qualities, and adaptations to the extrauterine environment. This information can be used in planning care, developing individualized intervention strategies, modifying care as the infant matures, and in parent teaching and other activities to promote parent-infant interaction. However, for some infants, neurodevelopmental assessment is critical for documentation of neurodevelopmental status, screening, and early case finding.

Certain groups of infants are at increased risk for developmental disabilities and later cognitive impairment (Leonard et al, 1990). Infants that fall into the highest risk category include very-low-birth-weight (VLBW) infants and those with significant intracranial hemorrhages. Preterm infants with known sensory impairment and chronic illness are also at risk for later cognitive dysfunction. Infants with respiratory distress syndrome (RDS) are at greater risk if they also develop chronic lung disease. Severe bronchopulmonary dysplasia (BPD) is generally associated with a prolonged and complicated hospital course, increasing the risk for later neurodevelopmental problems (Ariagno et al, 1996a; Bull & Dodge, 1996).

Neurobehavioral Assessment in the NICU. Neurobehavioral assessment can be performed at several different levels and is an essential part of comprehensive care of the high-risk infant in the NICU. Individuals such as Brazelton, Als, and their colleagues have sought to assess preterm and full-term newborn behavior and adaptations. Their work is based on an understanding of newborns as competent individuals with emerging developmental processes who are engaged in dynamic interactions and negotiations with their environment. As a result, several tools have been developed to describe and quantify neurobehavioral organization of both preterm and full-term newborns. The tools that are described here are the Brazelton Neonatal Behavioral Assessment Scale (NBAS) (Brazelton & Nugent, 1995) and the Assessment of Preterm Infant Behavior (APIB) (Als et al, 1982), which is a component of the neonatal individualized development care and assessment program (NIDCAP®) (Als, 2001), and Family and Infant Relationship Support Training (FIRST) (Browne et al, 1996).

Brazelton Neonatal Behavioral Assessment Scale (NBAS). The NBAS is a comprehensive behavioral assessment of the healthy full-term neonate. The NBAS combines evaluation of basic reflex responses with the integration of motor capacity, state regulation, and interactive abilities (Brazelton & Nugent, 1995). Infants are followed through the various states of sleep, arousal, and wakefulness and assessed on their ability to self-regulate in the face of increasingly vigorous activity. A primary focus is observation of the infant's individual and unique ability to respond to outside stimulation while regulating responses to and coping with pleasurable or stressful situations. The infant's best performance is scored. The results are an assessment of the infant's ability to (1) organize states; (2) habituate to external stimulation; (3) regulate motoric activity in the face of increasing sensory input; (4) respond to reflex testing; (5) alert and orient to visual and auditory stimuli; (6) interact with a caregiver; and (7) self-console. Individuals planning to use the NBAS for clinical or research purposes must establish reliability with a recognized trainer. Training in the use of the NBAS is provided in various locations throughout the United States (Table 17-1).

The NBAS has been used in numerous studies of neonatal behavior, including investigations of cross-cultural differences, characteristics of drug-addicted infants, effects of obstetric medication, and aspects of maternal-infant interaction (Brazelton & Nugent, 1995). An especially valuable use of the NBAS for nurses and other clinicians is as an intervention. For example, by performing an NBAS in front of the infant's parents, the parents become increasingly aware of and amazed at the remarkable abilities of their infant. An understanding of their newborn's capacity to interact visually, turn to their voices, regulate state and motor activity, and self-console expands the parent's perception of the infant as a unique, competent individual and enhances parent-infant interaction (Als, 1999; Blackburn & Kang, 1991; Brazelton & Nugent, 1995).

Included *add 19 Centers email*

TABLE 17-1	Training Centers for Training in Newborn or Infant Behavior		
Assessment	**Training Center**	**Location**	**Contact** *email*
Brazelton Neonatal Behavioral Assessment Scale (NBAS)	The Brazelton Institute	Boston, MA	617-355-5794
Newborn Individualized Developmental Care and Assessment Program® (NIDCAP®)	National NIDCAP® Center	Boston, MA	617-355-8249
	Sooner NIDCAP® Center	Oklahoma City, OK	405-271-6625
	Carolina NIDCAP® Center	Raleigh, NC	919-350-8276
	Colorado NIDCAP® Center	Denver, CO	303-861-6546
	Stanford NIDCAP® Center	Palo Alto, CA	650-498-7473
	SAPTA NIDCAP® Center	Toledo, OH	800-464-3227
	Center at Boston Medical Center	Boston, MA	617-414-5461
	St. Luke NIDCAP® Center	Boise, ID	208-381-4374
	Mid-Atlantic NIDCAP® Center	Camden, NJ	856-963-6708
	NIDCAP® Center of Milwaukee	Milwaukee, WI	414-219-5523
	Scandinavian NIDCAP® Center	Lund and Stockholm, Sweden	Nidcap.Scandinavia@telia.com +46-08-5177-2370
Assessment of Preterm Infant Behavior (APIB)	National Center Stanford APIB Center	Boston, MA Palo Alto, CA	617-355-8249
Family Infant Relationship Support Training (FIRST)	Center for Family and Infant Interaction	Denver, CO	www.uchsc.edu/sm/peds/cf

All NIDCAP® information can be found at www.nidcap.com/pub/program_guide.doc.

In response to a need to identify the preterm infant's neurobehavioral repertoire, the NBAS was expanded and modified for use with low-birth-weight infants. Items were added to the original scale, including difficulty of elicitation of alerting, degree of facilitation necessary to support the infant, control over stimulation, robustness, endurance, degree of exhaustion, quality of alertness, and balance of tone (Brazelton & Nugent, 1995). These subscales are also useful in describing at-risk full-term infants, such as drug-exposed infants.

Assessment of Preterm Infant Behavior (APIB).   The APIB was developed to respond to the need for a more discrete assessment of preterm infant functioning. Als (1984) felt that the additional items on the NBAS encompassed only the range of behavior close to that of the full-term infant and did not provide a comprehensive description of the subtler differences seen in less mature neonates. The APIB is based on the synactive theory of development, which describes the early behavioral organization and development of the neonate. The APIB is particularly useful for the preterm and full-term high-risk infant from birth to 44 weeks' post-conceptional age. The purpose of this assessment is to determine organization of the CNS and how infants cope with the intense environment of the NICU. The focus of the APIB is not only assessment of skill performance or specific responses to various stimuli but also the unique way each individual infant deals and interacts with the world around him or her. As described previously, infants are seen as being in continual interaction with their environment and as communicating their responsiveness via five subsystems (autonomic, motor, state, attentional, and self-regulatory) (Als, 1986).

The APIB consists of six packages or sets of maneuvers adapted from the NBAS. The packages are organized to provide increasing input with which the infant must react starting with stimulation while the infant is asleep to assess habituation. Subsequent packages move through maneuvers ranging

from low and medium tactile manipulations to high tactile and vestibular handling. Throughout the assessment, the infant is continually observed for responses related to each of the five subsystems. Thus the infant is observed and scored on each of the five subsystems and for examiner facilitation (ability to use support) before, during, and after administration of the items in each package. These responses are called the system scores and range on a 9-point scale from organized (1) to disorganized (9).

The APIB has been used for research and clinical purposes. As a research tool, it has been used to describe and identify neonatal behavioral organization in preterm and other high-risk infants (Als, 1986). Clinically, psychologists, neonatologists, neurologists, nurses, developmental specialists, and therapists have used the APIB in providing consultation in the NICU regarding developmental interventions for specific infants. The APIB is useful in determining an infant's degree of fragility and ability to tolerate different caregiving parameters. By measuring maturity of the five subsystems, one can determine maturity of each system and tolerance for handling as well as generate developmental care plans specific to each infant at that stage of development. The APIB is also useful in assessing infant readiness for changes in caregiving routines and in the physical and social environment. Assessing the degree of fragility and tolerance for activities can provide an invaluable piece of information about the infant's functional level and assist staff in making decisions about whether to protect the infant or to advance to the next level of care, as is illustrated in the following case.

A 28-week preterm infant had just been extubated and graduated to oxygen by nasal cannula and moved from the open bed to the incubator. An APIB revealed a responsive infant but one who was working extremely hard to regulate his system amidst two major changes: extubation and change of physical environment. Although successful regulation was noted, it was also apparent that the infant was at maximal capacity in organizing himself. He showed efforts to tuck and maintain hand to mouth; however, he could not maintain these postures for long without help. It was apparent that the infant's threshold had been reached and that any more change or stress would have caused a loss of control in his system's integrity. Immediately after the assessment, the neonatologists ordered nipple-feedings once a day. With this new demand, the examiner felt that this infant would exceed his threshold and be unable to regulate himself. The developmental specialist recommended waiting 1 week for the infant to stabilize and to integrate his new experiences before taking on any new demands. This recommendation was not followed, and feeding continued two days later, the developmental specialist returned and noted that the infant had a trial of nippling. He had desaturated, become bradycardic, required bag-and-mouth ventilation, and was considered to have "flunked" nippling. The order was terminated, with the plan to try again in a week. When feeding was reordered a week later, the infant tolerated it well.

Training in the APIB (see Table 17-1) is extensive and requires knowledge of the NICU, including care practices and routines, staffing patterns, and typical infant experiences in that setting as well as physiologic limitations and medical problems.

Neonatal Individualized Development Care and Assessment Program (NIDCAP®).

The NIDCAP® incorporates several levels of developmental training in assessment techniques and intervention planning for high-risk preterm and full-term infants. Included in this program is an observation tool (level 1 NIDCAP®—naturalistic behavioral observation), which is extremely useful for the NICU nurse. This assessment involves an observation of the infant before, during, and after a routine caregiving episode. It provides the NICU nurse with information on the infant's individual cues for both stress and stable, organized function. The nurse can then structure the infant's experiences, including caregiving interventions and the physical and social environment, to support the infant at the current level of tolerance. This support includes an awareness of the timing of caregiving events, sequencing events and interventions to prevent or reduce stress as well as to enhance stable behavior. Support for parents in understanding their infant's unique behavior and needs is also provided.

NIDCAP® training (see Table 17-1) involves a one-day didactic session and clinical demonstration of the observational tool, after which the trainee completes a specified number of observations on infants of different gestational age, post-birth age, and health status. This observation period is followed by an assessment of reliability for certification by the trainer.

Family Infant Relationship Support Training (FIRST).

The FIRST, adapted from the NIDCAP®, is an observation of the high-risk newborn infant and caregiver behavior in the context of their relationship immediately after discharge from the intensive care nursery (Browne et al, 1996). The FIRST is used with infants and caregivers in the home and community up to eight months of age. Once the observation can be completed, provision of appropriate developmentally supportive care is outlined by observing typical routine caregiving events such as diaper changing or feeding. Developmentally supporting the newborn and caregiver during the transition from hospital to home and through these early crucial stages of recovery from intensive care not only smooths the transition but also supports the emerging relationship between infants and parents.

Training (Table 17-1) involves a one day didactic workshop followed by a practicum in which observations are practiced with extensive videotapes and clinical practice utilizing supportive developmental strategies are presented. After practice with 10 infants, trainees return for a skills check evaluation to determine independent use of the tool.

Assessment Beyond Neonatal Development in the NICU.

As the infant matures, moves out of the neonatal period, and becomes a "long termer" in the NICU with chronic respiratory or other problems, neurodevelopmental assessments continue to provide important information. For the infant who requires prolonged hospitalization, a developmental assessment at the bedside can provide information on how the infant interacts with objects and people, organizes behavior, and copes with the environment as well as on the infant's neurologic status. No formal developmental assessments have been standardized for these NICU populations. Most developmental psychologists or specialists adapt items from other examinations such as the Bayley Scales of Infant Development (Bayley, 1969).

Because of the nature and severity of their illnesses, these infants may not be able to tolerate a complete examination at one session. To learn about the infant's behavioral capabilities and coping abilities adequately, the examiner must consider events that occurred for several hours before the assessment and be aware of the environment in which the infant normally lives and of his or her usual types of sensory experiences. Important areas of assessment include (1) availability of alerting; (2) ability to use interventions for consoling or developmental activities; (3) self-soothing capacity; (4) motor activities and strengths; (5) tolerance for handling (how long? with whom?); (6) degree of fragility; (7) degree of distractibility; (8) hand use; (9) parts of body available for use; and (10) respiratory capacity and tolerance.

NEONATAL INTENSIVE CARE ENVIRONMENT

The high-risk infant in a NICU lives in a highly unusual environment that provides markedly different experiences than the home environment of the healthy full-term neonate. The full-term healthy infant generally has access to a consistent nurturing caregiver and an appropriate variety of stimulation. The full-term infant with 40 weeks of intrauterine development is ready for a variety of sensory experiences, including the visual, tactile, auditory, kinesthetic, proprioceptive, olfactory, and gustatory. When these competencies to process sensory information interplay with experience, appropriate patterns of adaptation, cognitive learning, and motor control are formed. The impact of illness on an immature CNS—with accompanying restriction of movement, exposure to high levels of inappropriately patterned sensory input, and loss of a consistent primary caregiver—can alter adaptation patterns and lead to distortions in functioning (Bull & Dodge, 1996).

The NICU is often a stressful environment for infants, parents, and staff. Source of stress for infants in the NICU include the physical environment, caregiver interventions, medical and surgical procedures, pain, distress, pathologic processes, temperature changes, handling, and multiple simultaneous modes of stimulation (Blackburn, 1998). Consequences of neonatal stress include energy expenditure, altered healing and recovery, risk of iatrogenic complications, altered growth, and altered organization. Stress can also effect interactions and parenting. Chronic stress can produce long term changes in stress response systems, leading to decreases in adaptive capacity and increased risk for physical and psychological disorders. In the NICU the infant may experience significant stress during a period of critical brain development. An infant's stress tolerance may be reached or exceeded repeatedly, contributing to short- and long-term morbidity. Baseline responses to stress are set early in life and can influence later responses and adaptation. Recent reports suggest that early stress in the fetus and neonate may produce permanent changes in neural pathways increasing the risk of later disorders such as adult psychopathology and hypertension (Anand, 2000; Anand & Scalzo, 2000; Nelson & Carver, 1998; Porte et al, 1999).

To better understand the possible contributions of early environmental factors to the developmental problems associated with prematurity and other high-risk events and to the development of attachment between high-risk infants and their parents, it is essential to examine the environment in which these infants spend the critical period of their development. White-Traut and colleagues (1994) noted that although the last two sensory systems to become functional are the visual and auditory systems, these two systems commonly receive the most, and often random, stimulation in the NICU environment (Figure 17-1). Thus the NICU environment is inconsistent with the preterm infant's level of development and quite different from the intrauterine one.

Intrauterine Environment

The intrauterine environment, with few exceptions, is recognized as the optimal environment to foster the growth and development of the fetus. This environment provides a variety of stimuli to the fetus while modifying the intensity and nature of the sensory input. Characteristics of the intrauterine milieu include (1) auditory input such as the blood flow through the umbilical cord, maternal bowel sounds, and muffled sounds from the extrauterine environment; (2) vestibular, tactile, and kinesthetic stimuli from maternal and fetal movements; and (3) rhythmic and cyclic recurrent stimuli such as the maternal heartbeat, maternal sleep and activity patterns, and neurohormonal cycles (Blackburn, 1998; Graven, 1996).

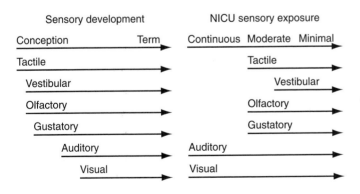

FIGURE **17-1**

Comparison of sensory development to sensory experience in the NICU. From White-Traut R et al (1994). Environmental influences on the developing premature infant: theoretical issues and applications to practice. *Journal of obstetric, gynecologic and neonatal nursing,* 23, 393-401.

Touch in utero entails contact with warm amniotic fluid and contact with body parts or the wall of the uterus. Maternal movement and buoyant amniotic fluid provide rich vestibular stimulation for the fetus in utero. Fragrant molecules in amniotic fluid stimulate oral and nasal chemoreceptors (Hepper, 1995; Lecanuet & Schaal, 1996). Sound in utero is fluid and bone-conducted rather than air-conducted, which attenuates the sound and modulates its intensity. The uterus provides rhythmic, structured, patterned sound—primarily from the mother—at frequencies that parallel and support cochlea development (Glass, 1999). Intrauterine sounds tend to be of low frequency and intensity compared to extrauterine sounds (Lecanuet & Schaal, 1996). Less than 2% of external light is transmitted into the uterus. The light that is transmitted is primarily red, long wave-length light, whereas in the extrauterine environment, the infant is exposed to light across the spectrum and particularly shorter blue wave-length light (Glass, 1999).

NICU Environment: Overview

Birth represents an obligatory change of environments. For high-risk infants, this new environment is the NICU. The infant is thrust into a world of bright lights, sudden and loud noises, and rapid temperature changes, an environment without the containment and movement of the uterus. The infant is exposed to painful and aversive experiences. There is often an irregular pattern of handling and an absence of handling in response to the infant's emerging behavioral organization. Immaturity and health status make the high-risk infant both dependent on and vulnerable to this environment to maintain vital functions, promote growth and development, and provide opportunities for the development and organization of the infant's state and behavior (Blackburn, 1998).

Characteristics of the NICU Environment

In examining the environment of the high-risk neonate, one must consider both the physical and social interactive (animate) environment. Interactions between the infant and environment are influenced by infant physiologic, maturational, and behavioral differences and by caregiver factors such as timing, sensitivity to infant cues, and contingency of caregiver actions. Korner (1973) suggested that, ideally, the early environment of preterm infants should create a situation in which infant maturation can take place with a minimum of interference. The more intact the infant at discharge, the more capable he or she will be of coping with the home environment and responding appropriately to parents.

Potential adverse effects of the physical aspects, social experiences, and hazards associated with neonatal intensive care and the NICU environment are numerous. Every treatment and every characteristic present in the NICU has the potential to be detrimental as well as beneficial to the infant (Peabody & Lewis, 1985). Environmental stimuli in the NICU may be an important factor that contributes to the developmental problems associated with prematurity. Recent interest in the NICU environment has yielded documentation of the stresses and hazards existing in today's NICUs and their impact on the high-risk infant. Additional research is needed to further define effects of this environment and to identify the most effective interventions.

Unfortunately, the medical and nursing management of sick neonates often becomes a source of excessive and disjunctive stimulation at a time when the neonate needs an organizing influence to promote neurobehavioral organization. Environmental conditions also affect the infant's physiologic status. Studies have shown that infants respond to events in the NICU with both behavioral and physiologic responses. The earliest may be a sudden or abrupt fluctuation in heart rate, respiratory rate, or oxygenation in response to specific environmental or caregiving events such as door slamming, suctioning, bathing, or even too close presentation of a caregiver's face (Evans, 1991; Peters, 1992, 1998). Commonly no efforts are made to include modifications in patterns of physical and social stimuli in caregiving routines. NICU patients, staff, and parents are often exposed to an ongoing intense and bizarre onslaught of unpatterned sensory stimuli that have important implications for the physiologic and developmental outcome of infants who require NICU care.

Physical Environment

Sound. Sound and noise levels in the NICU are of concern due to potential damage to the developing cochlea with hearing loss and arousal. Arousal is a particular concern with immature infants who are unable to inhibit responses. In addition, arousal may deplete the infant's physiologic resources and energy reserves and waste calories over time. Noise interferes with sleep and causes fatigue in adults and older infants. It increases heart rate, blood pressure, leads to vasoconstriction, and alters respiratory patterns and endocrine function (Ariagno, 1996b; Blackburn 1998; Glass, 1999; Philbin & Klass, 2000a, 2000b). Concerns have also been raised about the possible additive effects of drugs and environmental noise. In addition, background sound levels in the NICU may interfere with the ability of the infant to discriminate speech of parents and other caregivers.

Several studies have documented the newborn's physiologic and behavioral responses to frequent and low and high intensive noises in the NICU (Morris et al, 2000; Philbin, 2000). The infant's behavioral and physiologic responses to loud noises can lead to several physiological issues, including hypoxemia, blood pressure instability, cardiorespiratory liability, and altered cerebral blood flow. This then increases the risk of intraventricular hemorrhage or periventricular leukomalacia.

In addition to the immature neuronal organization in the preterm, the size, length, shape, and diameter of the infant's ear canal significantly influences the standing wave frequencies and resonant peaks in the ear canal. As a result, the cochlea of preterm infants may be affected more easily from exposure to loud noises of both low and high intensity. Long et al (1980) reported physiologic effects of sudden noise on premature infants. The noise resulted in agitation and crying, which led to increases in intracranial pressure, heart rate, and respiratory rate changes and decrease in the transcutaneous oxygen tension. In addition, desaturation episodes have been correlated with peak noise bursts (Satish & Doll-Speck, 1993). Long et al (1980) postulated that these physiological changes might be the effects on the fragile vasculature and neurons of the developing neonatal brain. Changes such as these may have indirect effects on the neonatal brain because of altered perfusion or oxygenation of the brain tissue exacerbated by immature autoregulation of the infant. But, as these researchers emphasize, direct pathologic effects of sound on the neonatal brain have not been documented. Well-designed research is needed to determine the qualities of the ideal auditory environment in the NICU.

Sound is measured across two parameters: intensity (how much sound) and frequency (what kind of sound). Loudness of sound is measured in decibels (dB). Ambient sound levels in the NICU have been documented at 50 to 90 dB, which is higher than in the average office or home. Due to concern over these levels, many units have worked hard to decrease ambient background sound levels to closer to 50 to 60 dB. Normal adult speech in conversation is usually recorded at a loudness of 45 to 50 dB (Table 17-2). Sound levels inside infant incubators have been reported to range from 50 to 80 dB (Philbin, 2000; Philbin et al, 1999). In adults, levels above 80 to 85 dB have been associated with hearing loss in some individuals. Decibel levels are even higher inside incubators of infants with ventilatory support equipment. However, the incubator does muffle external sounds, an advantage that is not experienced by infants in open radiant warmers.

Transported infants are exposed to both high noise levels and vibration. Rotary wing aircraft have the most vibration and noise, often exceeding 90 dB, followed by fixed wing air and ground transport (Campbell et al, 1984). Infants on high-

TABLE 17-2	Sound Levels and Potential Effects	
Source	**Sound Level (dB)**	**Potential Effects (in Adults)**
Airplane engine	130	Pain
Rock music	120	
Heavy traffic	90 to 80	
	80	Potential for hearing damage in adults
Placing bottle on incubator	84	
Closing incubator portholes	80	
Factory	80	
NICU (general)	70 to 60	
Closing incubator cabinet	70	Annoying
Adult ICU or recovery room	68 to 50	
Incubator alarm or opening a plastic sleeve	67	
NICU radio	62 to 60	
Bubbling water in ventilator tubing	62	
Normal conversation	50 to 45	
Light traffic	50	
	40	Ambient background noise
Whisper	30	

dB, *decibels*; NICU, *neonatal intensive care unit*; ICU, *intensive care unit. Compiled from Baker CF (1984). Sensory overload and noise in the ICU: Sources of environmental stress.* Critical care quarterly, 66-80; *Gottfried A, Gaiter J (1985). Infant stress under intensive care. Baltimore, MD: University Park Press; Hilton BA (1985). Noise in acute patient areas.* Research nursing & health, 8:283-292; *and Thomas K (1989). How the NICU environment sounds to a preterm infant.* American journal of maternal child nursing, 14:249-251.

frequency ventilation are also exposed to vibration and noise. Specific effects of these conditions on infants are not known; however, noise and vibration may have a synergistic effect on hearing loss (Hamernik et al, 1989).

Sound levels in NICUs have two characteristic patterns. There is the continuous pattern of background noise previously described, which has little diurnal rhythm. Interposed with this constant background noise are peak noises, which can significantly increase the decibel level. These noises are generated by activities such as monitor alarms, telephones, radios, hitting or setting items on the Plexiglas top of the incubator, intercoms, staff calling across the room, equipment dropping, or banging the doors of the incubator cabinet. Reports of peak noise levels as heard by infants inside standard hospital incubators noted that some of the highest levels were associated with events such as dropping the head of the mattress, closing portholes with a snap, tapping fingers or placing a bottle on the Plexiglas top of the incubator or bedside table, banging trash can lids, and closing cabinet doors (DePaul & Chambers, 1995). What is striking is that the noise from all of these activities is easily preventable. Table 17-2 gives additional examples of NICU sound levels.

Light.   Exposure of infants in NICUs to high-intensity, continuous light has also been of considerable concern. If the light intensity is seldom changed, as is the case in many NICUs in the past, infants never experience diurnal rhythmic patterns necessary for development. Another concern is that intense stimuli, whether light or noise, have a potentially arousing effect on the CNS. This effect may be especially problematic for neonates, who cannot regulate incoming stimuli, leading to wasted energy and sensory overload.

The effects of intense, ambient, cool white fluorescent lights on neonates are unknown, although exposure of animals, older children, and adults has been reported to lead to biochemical and physiologic effects. Concerns about light in the NICU include the effects on eye development and vision, development of the visual cortex, neurosensory development, and on circadian rhythms and sleep-wake cycle development. Light may also degrade nutrients such as riboflavin and vitamin A in exposed parenteral nutrition solutions.

Environmental lighting has been suggested as a factor increasing risks of ophthalmologic problems in premature infants, particularly retinopathy of prematurity. Studies have reported varying outcomes and had many methodological differences and limitations (Blackburn, 1996b; Fielder & Moseley, 2000). A recent prospective, multi-center randomized clinical trial reported no difference in the frequency of ROP in experimental versus control infants born at <1251 grams and <31 weeks gestation (Reynolds et al, 1998). Experimental infants wore goggles that decreased visible light by 97% and ultraviolet light by 100% starting no later than 24 hours after birth until they reached 31 weeks post-conceptional age or four weeks after birth, whichever came first. Ambient lighting adjacent to the infant's faces was 399 lux for experimental infants and 447 lux for control infants. Concern about the effects of light is not limited to ROP, however. As a group preterm infants are at risk for multiple structural and growth alterations of the eye (such as ROP, amblyopia, myopia, strabismus, astigmatism) as well as alterations in visual function that may reflect alterations in the visual cortex (Blackburn, 1995; Fielder & Moseley, 2000; Glass, 1999). These alterations include alterations in visual acuity, color vision, and problems with visual processing such as visual attention and pattern discrimination, visual recognition memory, and visual-motor regulation. Thus the visual environment of the NICU—which is markedly different from what the infant's neurosensory system is expecting at that stage of eye and CNS visual cortex development—may alter organization of the visual cortex and modify responses of cortical neurons.

Preterm infants are also more vulnerable to retinal light damage. Factors influencing the amount of light reaching the retina include lens translucency (increased in preterm infants), amount of time the eye is open (increased in very-low-birthweight infants), pupil reactivity (decreased <30 weeks' gestational age), density of optic media (less dense in preterms), macular pigment (immature retinal structures and vascularity) as well as infant position (e.g., facing artificial light sources or windows) and bed position in relation to windows (Blackburn, 1996a; Fielder & Moseley, 2000; Glotzbach et al, 1993; Robinson & Fielder, 1992).

Common measurements used in describing light environments are irradiance ("what kind of light") or the amount of radiant energy (w/cm^2) emitted over specific wavelength bands and illuminance ("how much light") in lux (lumens/m^2) or footcandles (ftc). Lux divided by 10 is roughly equivalent to footcandles. Light intensity in the NICU ranges from 192 to 1488 lux (approximately 19 to 148 ftc), with greater intensity during day than night hours (Fielder & Moseley, 2000). Treatment lights and warming lamps used in the NICU average 200 to 350 ftc (or higher), and bilirubin lights may be as high as 10,000 ftc (Glass, 1999).

For many years, NICU lighting was bright and continuous throughout the 24-hour day. This lack of diurnal rhythmicity may interfere with the development of natural rhythms. More recently, many nurseries have instituted some dimming of lights at night. The studies done to date have reported that infants experiencing reduced light levels for a portion of the 24-hour period had reduced heart rate, decreased activity, enhanced biologic rhythms, increased sleep, and improved feeding and weight gain (Blackburn & Patteson, 1991; Brandon, 2000; Miller et al, 1995). Thus reducing light levels may facilitate rest and subsequent energy conservation and promote organization and growth. However these studies are characterized by small sample sizes, lack of consistency regarding light intensity and length of cycling, and other methodological problems.

Safe levels of light and sound in NICUs have not been established and warrant additional study. Until such data are available, baseline levels should be monitored in units, and staff should be informed as to current knowledge about patterns of intense stimuli exposure and the effects on newborn animals and on adults. Working to decrease light and sound in NICUs is an important part of providing developmental supportive and safe care.

Animate Environment.   For the high-risk infant, the major early caregiver is usually the nurse in the NICU. For any infant, the caregivers, whether parent, nurse, or other individual, have major influences on the amount and variety of sensory input the infant receives. The caregiver selects the specific sensory input to which the infant is exposed, thus helping to shape the sensory environment. In addition to carrying out specific infant care techniques, the caregiver functions by increasing and decreasing sensory thresholds, modulating arousal, and fostering attentional and alerting behaviors. Initial adaptation of the infant to the extrauterine environment is enhanced by synchrony between infant behaviors and caregiver action.

The majority of caregiving experienced by infants in NICUs involves medical or other caregiving interventions associated with high levels of sensory input. In comparison with healthy full-term infants, these infants experience less adult speech directed toward them, spend more time alone, and are more often asleep during "social" interactions. Most studies have reported that, on average, infants in intensive or intermediate care nurseries are handled for anywhere from 11 to 23 of the 24-hour day, although there are wide variations for individual infants (Blackburn & Barnard, 1985). In most cases, this is probably less than that received by the full-term infant at home. What characterizes NICU caregiving is that infants in these settings are handled more frequently with fewer periods for uninterrupted rest and sleep (Ariagno, 1996b).

Caregiver-infant interactions often have an all-or-nothing form, ranging from no contact to repeated, frequent, stressful, and often painful interventions. Social interaction with the caregiver may be stressful for the immature or ill infant. For these infants, the critical factor is whether the infant can tolerate the level of sensory input, regardless of whether that input is supposed to be positive or is painful. Many "sudden" physiologic crises are preventable if the caregiver recognizes and responds to infant cues and provides interventions to allow infant recovery and reorganization. For example, during sponge bathing of very-low-birth-weight infants, Peters (1998) noted that behavioral cues indicating stress often preceded physiologic changes.

Patterns of caregiving in the NICU can profoundly affect the development of infant state organization and biologic rhythms. Infants entrain their physical and physiologic activities to regularly recurring endogenous (hunger, secretion of hormones, respiration, elimination) and exogenous (sound, care-taking activities, patterns of light) events. The patterns of care can either enhance or interfere with the infant's neurobehavioral organization. These organizations will be enhanced by caregiving that is based on infant cues.

An important component of the infant's animate environment is the opportunity for contingent caregiving—that is, caring in which the experiences and caregiver responses depend on the infant's behavior. In this way, infants begin to learn that their behavior influences their environment and vice versa (Blackburn & Barnard, 1985). Contingent interaction between the infant and caregiver depends on three characteristics: (1) readability or clarity of behaviors and cues; (2) predictability of the other in anticipating behavior from immediately preceding behaviors; and (3) responsiveness or reactions of the other with appropriate behaviors within a short latency period (Sammons & Lewis, 1985). These characteristics are inherent in both the infant and the environment, including caregivers. The more readable, predictable, and responsive the infant and the physical environment, the smoother and more rewarding the infant and parent interactions will be. However, the traditional NICU environment is far from being easily readable, is often unresponsive, and is highly unpredictable. At the same time, the NICU infant, due to immaturity or illness, is also not easily readable, is unpredictable, and appears unresponsive. The first step in rectifying this situation is for caregivers to learn to recognize infant cues and to respond appropriately to provide a more readable, predictable, and responsive environment for the infant.

DEVELOPMENTAL INTERVENTION APPROACH

The developmental intervention approach is based on the synactive theory (Als, 1982) and focuses on fostering neurobehavioral and physiologic organization. Intervention strategies are individualized for each infant and based on ongoing assessment of that infant. An assumption underlying this approach is that the high-risk infant is vulnerable to sensory overload and overstimulation and that he or she demonstrates this via a variety of physiologic, state, motoric, and attentional cues. Therefore the goal is not to focus on achievement of developmental milestones or to offer stimulation to foster specific skills but rather to help the infant stabilize at each stage of maturation and to support the infant's emerging behaviors and organization while reducing stress.

The developmental intervention approach does not mean that sensory input is never provided. Sensory input is an important and critical parameter in fostering CNS development. However, sensory input is provided only when appropriate to the infant's physiologic a behavioral status and is individualized to the needs and abilities of the infant at that time. There is also recognition that for the ill, unstable, or fragile infant, the best form of sensory input may be no input but protection. In addition, infants are assessed for early signs of sensory overload so appropriate interventions can be initiated to avoid overstimulation.

Cue-Based Care

Caregiving based on infant cues is an important parameter of providing developmentally appropriate care. These cues provide communication about an infant's needs and status at any given time. Both full-term and preterm infants provide us with specific cues that can be used in planning care. These cues include infant state, sensory capabilities (Tables 17-3 and 17-4), and signs of stability, instability and stress (Tables 17-5 and 17-6). Caregiving based on infant cues involves attention to messages from the infant that may indicate timing for interventions, such as when to provide care, or opportunities for sensory input and interaction. These cues also indicate how the infant handles stimuli, signals sensory overload, and tolerates stimulation. Thus information is available as to when the infants cannot tolerate additional handling or stimuli and needs time out to regroup and reorganize.

Neonatal Sensory Abilities. The sensory systems develop in a specific sequence: somatosensory (tactile and proprioceptive), vestibular, chemoreceptive, auditory, and visual (Figure 17-1). During fetal life there is a lack of competing stimuli during rapid maturation of each system. For example the infant develops chemoreception before the structures for hearing and vision are in place and after somatosensory and vestibular function has matured. Similarly the hearing maturation in the fetus is most rapid during a time when vision is still immature and in an environment where vision is not being stimulated by light. Animal studies have demonstrated that out of sequence stimulation of one system interferes with development of not only that system but also other systems that are still immature (Graven, 2000). For example, in animal models inappropriate visual stimulation while hearing and vision are still developing may alter not only vision but also hearing development (Glass, 1999).

Somatosensory and vestibular sensations mature early. The fetus responds to touch around the mouth by 2 months of gestational age; hands become touch sensitive by 10 to 11 weeks.

TABLE 17-3	Development of Hearing in Preterm and Term Infants
Age	**Anatomic and Functional Development**
Preterm infants <28 weeks	Fetal hearing begins at by 23 to 24 weeks Threshold about 65 db, 500 to 1000 Hz Auditory brain stem responses by 26 to 28 weeks
Preterm infants 28 to 30 weeks	Rapid maturation of cochlea and auditory nerve Responses rapidly fatigue Initial auditory processing by 30 weeks Threshold 40 db with an increased frequency range
Preterm infants 32 to 34 weeks	Outer hair cells mature by 32 weeks Rapid maturation of cochlea and auditory nerve
Preterm infants >34 weeks	Increased speed of conduction Ossicles and electrophysiology complete by 36 weeks Hearing threshold 30 db, increasing range Increasing ability to localize and discriminate
Term infants	Ability to localize and discriminate sounds Hearing threshold 25 db Range 500 to 4000 Hz

Compiled from Glass P (1999). The vulnerable neonate and the neonatal intensive care environment. In Avery GB et al (Eds.). Neonatology: pathophysiology and management of the newborn, ed. 5, Philadelphia, Lippincott, Williams & Wilkins; Hall JW (2000). Development of the ear and hearing. Journal of perionatology 20:S12; Lecanuet J-P & Schaal B (1996). Fetal sensory competencies. European journal of obstetrics and gynecology, 68:1; Philbin MK & Klaas P (2000). Hearing and behavioral responses to sound in full-term newborns. Journal of perinatology, 20:S68.

Receptors are present throughout the fetal body by 20 weeks (Glass, 1999). Vestibular stimulation is mediated by receptors in the ear that detect changes in directions and rate of head movement and rotation. The vestibular system maturation begins by 14 to 15 weeks gestation with responses to vestibular stimulation seen as early as 25 weeks gestation (Glass, 1999). Oral (taste) and nasal (smell) chemoreception, develop during the second trimester. The taste buds are present by 12 to 13 weeks and receptors by 16 weeks. By term the infant has adult numbers of receptors. Nasal chemoreceptors develop from 7 to 20 weeks' gestation and respond to the fragrant molecules in amniotic fluid. The composition of amniotic fluid varies with maternal diet and baths both oral and nasal chemoreceptors. Fetal swallowing rates have been reported to change with exposure to different taste in amniotic fluid. Preterm infants respond to different tastes and smells by at least 28 weeks gestation (Lecanuet & Schaal, 1996). Term infants are able to detect, localize, and discriminate a variety of distinct odors and tastes. They respond preferentially to breast odors, their mothers' scents, and other odors associated with positive reinforcements (Varendi et al, 1997; Winberg & Porter, 1998).

The structures of the auditory system, including the inner ear and cochlea, are mature enough to support hearing by approximately 20 weeks' gestation. Fetal hearing is thought to begin at 24 to 25 weeks. In preterm infants, auditory evoked potentials can be recorded and responses to sound observed as early as 25 to 26 weeks (Hall, 2000). Between 28 and 34 weeks, the preterm infant develops the ability to begin to orient to sound, turning the head in the direction of auditory stimulus and showing evidence of arousal and attention (Glass, 1999). During the third trimester the cochlea continues to mature and develop its ability to hear sounds across frequencies. The hearing threshold decreases with gestational age. Anatomic and functional development of hearing in preterm and term infants is summarized in Table 17-3.

The eyes begin to develop early in the embryonic period but continue anatomic and functional maturation into the third trimester and early infants. Vision is the least mature sense at birth, and even full-term infants undergo significant continued maturation during infancy. By 22 weeks' gestation, the layers of the retina have formed rod differentiation and retinal vascularization begin by 25 weeks' gestational age; myelinization of the optic nerve begins at 24 weeks. By 26 weeks, visual cortex neurons are in place with rapid development of visual neuronal connections and processes between 28 and 34 weeks' gestation (Glass, 1999). Anatomic and functional development of hearing in preterm and term infants is summarized in Table 17-3.

Behavioral Cues: Stress and Stability. The NICU staff—especially nurses—play a significant role in shaping the environment and making caregiving more responsive to infants. This requires as careful observation and documentation of infant behavior as is given to physiologic status and development of an individualized plan of care (Box 17-2). Infant responses to the environment will be influenced by factors such as state; basic needs (e.g., hunger); sensory threshold; parameters of the animate and inanimate environment, including readability, predictability and responsivity; infant health status; and level of neurobehavioral maturity (Blackburn, 1998). Infant behavioral responses include specific autonomic, motoric, and state cues, which indicate stress and the need for immediate intervention, and stability cues, which indicate that the infant is coping positively. Tables 17-6 and 17-7 summarize infant stability and instability/stress cues. Examples of selected cues are illustrated in Figures 17-2 and 17-3.

Guidelines for Providing Developmental Support

An understanding of behavioral cues and attentions to signs of stress are only the first steps in providing developmentally appropriate interventions. Strategies to ameliorate stress and behavioral disorganization must be individualized and appropriate to the infant's level of development and health status. Applying developmental interventions in this manner may increase the infant's tolerance for stimulation and reduce stressful events that are costly in terms of energy expenditure, caloric utilization, and physiologic homeostasis (Figure 17-4). This approach may also reduce the need for pharmacologic interventions, including sedatives and promote adaptation and organization (Heller et al, 1997; VandenBerg & Franck, 1990).

As infants become better able to self-regulate through appropriately planned handling and reduction or modulation of stressful events, their behavior will reflect a pattern of emerg-

TABLE 17-4	Development of Vision in Preterm and Term Infants

Age	Anatomic and Functional Development
Preterm infants 24 to 28 weeks	Eyelids: unfuse at 24 to 26 weeks
	Lens: cloudy, second of four layers forming
	Cornea: hazy until 27 weeks
	Retina: rod differentiation by 25 weeks, vascularization begins
	Visual cortex: rapid dendritic growth
	No pupillary response
	Eyelid tightening to bright light but quickly fatigues
	VER to bright light but quickly fatigues
	Very myopic
Preterm infants 30 to 34 weeks	Lens: clearing, second layer complete, third forming
	Retina: rod complete except for fovea by 32 weeks, cone differentiation begins
	Visual cortex: rapid dendritic and synapse development
	VER more complex, latency decreases
	Bright light causes sustained pupil closure
	Abrupt reduction may cause eye opening
	Pupillary response sluggish but more mature
	Spontaneous eye opening, brief fixation in low light
Preterm infants 34 to 36 weeks	Pupils: complete pupillary reflex by 36 weeks
	Retina: cone numbers in fovea increase
	Blood vessels reach nasal retina
	Visual cortex: morphologically similar to term
	Increased alertness, less sustained than term
	VER resembles that of term infant with longer latency
	Spontaneous orientation toward soft light
	Beginning to track, show visual preferences
	Less myopic
Term infants	Still immature with much development from 0-6 months
	Retinal vessels reach periphery of temporal retina
	Lens transmits more short-wave light than adult
	Acuity approximately 20/200 to 20/1600
	Attend to form, object, face, track horizontally and some vertically
	See objects to at least 2½ feet, attend best at 8 to 12 inches

Adapted from Glass P (1999). The vulnerable neonate and the neonatal intensive care environment. In Avery GB et al (Eds.). Neonatology: pathophysiology and management of the newborn, ed 5, pp. 91-108. Philadelphia: Lippincott, Williams & Wilkins.

ing competency in responding to and interacting with their environment, of which their parents are a critical part. Goals of developmental interventions are to (1) promote an understanding with the parents of their infant's behaviors, including manifestations of stress and stability; (2) facilitate neurobehavioral organization based on individualized assessment of the infant's capacity; (3) enhance infant recovery; (4) promote CNS organization; (5) facilitate self-regulatory capabilities; (6) preserve energy and promote growth; (7) reduce stress and prevent agitation; and (8) normalize the environment to the extent that medical care permits (VandenBerg, 1985, 1995).

Because infants in NICUs face challenges to their survival and do not have fully functional biological systems, the goal is to support these infants and stabilize each of their subsystems, described by Als (1982), as they mature. This requires that a behavioral assessment that describes the infant's current level of organization, the infant's individual coping mechanisms, and the impact of the infant's illness on neurodevelopmental functioning be completed before interventions are offered.

Once the infant's current level of organization has been documented, a plan of care that delineates the degree and kind of environmental support necessary to promote organization

and development can be developed. This plan should be based on the following guidelines:

1. Interventions must seek to normalize or modify the NICU environment to the extent that medical care permits.
2. Interventions must be consistent with the infant's level of maturity and gestational age.
3. Interventions must be appropriately times in terms of the infant's state, physiologic status, and behavioral responses.
4. Interventions must be individualized to a given infant and be altered with changes in the infant's health status and neurobehavioral maturation.
5. Interventions must be sensitive to the infant's cues.
6. Interventions must take into account how much stimuli each infant can tolerate.

Box 17-2 illustrates questions the nurse can ask and areas to assess in preparing for care during care and in the recovery period after care is completed.

Effectiveness of Individualized Developmental Care
The individualized developmental care approach as been tested in several studies (Tables 17-7 and 17-8). In these studies, specially trained developmental care professionals served

oh

TABLE 17-5	Signs of Stress in Intensive Care Nursery Infants			
Autonomic System	**Motor System**	**State System**	**Attentional-Interaction System**	**Self-Regulatory System**
Respiration: • Pauses • Tachypnea • Gasping Color Changes: • Paling around nostrils • Perioral duskiness • Mottled • Cyanosis • Gray • Flushed • Ruddy Visceral: • Hiccups • Gasping • Grunting • Spitting up • Straining as if actually producing a bowel movement Motor: • Seizures • Tremoring/startling • Twitching • Coughing • Sneezing • Yawning • Sighing	Fluctuating tone: Flaccidity of: • Trunk • Extremities • Face Hypertonicity: • Leg extensions • Salutes • Airplaning • Sitting on air • Arching • Finger splays • Tongue extensions • Fisting Hyperflexions: • Trunk • Extremities • Fetal tuck Frantic, diffuse activity	Diffuse states: Sleep: • Twitches • Sounds • Jerky moves • Irregular respirations • Whimpers • Grimacing • Fussy in sleep Awake: • Eye floating • Glassy eyed • Strained/fussy • Staring • Gaze aversion • Panicked, worried, or dull look • Weak cry • Irritability • Abrupt state changes	May demonstrate stress signals of other systems: • Irregular respirations • Color changes • Visceral responses • Coughing, twitches • Sneezing • Yawning • Sighing • Eye floating • Glassy eyed • Staring • Straining • Gaze aversion • Panicked, worried or dull look • Weak cry • Irritability • Abrupt state changes • Fluctuating tone • Frantic diffuse activity • Becomes more stressed with more than one mode of stimuli	May use the following to attempt to gain balance: • Lowers state • Postural changes • Motoric strategies: leg/foot bracing, hand clasping, foot clasping, finger folding, hand to mouth, sucking, grasping, hand holding, tucking • Good self-quieting and consolability • Rhythmic, robust crying • Clear sleep states • Focused alertness with shiny-eyed and focused expression, frowning, cheek softening, "ooh" face, cooing, smiling
INTERVENTION STRATEGIES TO REDUCE STRESS				
Modify environment (light, noise, traffic) Positioning Minimal handling Swaddling, covering	Positioning Handling to contain limbs Handling slow/gentle Blanket rolls Containment, nesting	Clustering care Primary nursing to accurately read infant cues Appropriate timing of activities and daily routines Autonomic and motoric subsystems must have reached stability	Modulate interactions to infant's tolerance level Provide supports necessary to bring out best alertness Offer 1 mode of stimulation at a time Use modulated voice, face, rattle, face and voice together (Baby responds best to animate stimuli)	

Adapted from VandenBerg KA, Franck L (1990). Behavioral issues for infants with BPD. In Lund C (Ed). BPD: strategies for total patient care. Petaluma, CA: Neonatal Network, p. 124. Reprinted by permission of NICU Ink®, Santa Rosa, CA. Derived from Assessment of Preterm Infant Behavior, Als, 1982.

as the educators, catalysts, and supporters of the bedside teams caring for infants in the NICU. Each infant and family in these studies was assured a process-oriented, individualized perspective that emphasizes the continuous neurobiological emotional regulation of infant and parent. Care teams include parents, key nurses, primary physicians, developmental spe-cialists, respiratory therapists, social workers, and other med-ical staff. Emphasis is on shifting from a protocol-based care focus to a relationship-based care focus in which the care-givers (parents and nurses) are encouraged to view the infant with respect and as able to communicate his or her needs via behavior.

TABLE 17-6	Signs of Stability in Intensive Care Nursery Infants			
Autonomic System	**Motor System**	**State System**	**Attentional-Interaction System**	**Self-Regulatory System**
Smooth, regular respirations Pink, stable color Stable visceral with **no** evidence of: • seizures • gagging • emesis • grunting • tremors • startles • twitches • coughing • sneezing • yawning • sighing	Smooth, controlled posture Smooth movements of extremities and head seen in: • hand clasp • leg/foot brace • foot clasp • finger folding • hand to mouth • grasping • sucking • tucking • hand holding Good, consistent tone throughout body	Clear, well-defined sleep states Good self-quieting and consolability Robust crying Focused, clear alertness with animated expressions such as: • frowning • cheek softening • "ooh" face • cooing • smiling	Responsivity to auditory and visual stimuli bright and of long duration Actively seeks out auditory and shifts attention smoothly on his or her own from one stimulus to another Face demonstrates bright-eyed, purposeful interest varying between arousal and relaxation	Infants has sophisticated, well-differentiated repertoire of successful strategies to maintain each system, autonomic, motor, state, and attention, such as: • autonomic: sucking, grasping • motor: tucking, foot bracing • state: visual tracking, sucking • attention: hand to mouth, hand holding
INTERVENTIONS				
Interventions not necessary to reduce stress, but to enhance and facilitate normal development				

From VandenBerg KA, Franck L (1990). Behavioral issues for infants with BPD. In Lund C. (Ed). BPD: strategies for total patient care. Petaluma, CA: Neonatal Network, p. 125. Reprinted by permission of NICU Ink®, Santa Rosa, CA. Derived from Assessment of Preterm Infant Behavior, Als, 1982.

Studies that focus on understanding behavioral cues and documenting the infant's current level of functioning have been conducted at the Brigham and Woman's Hospital in Boston, (Als et al, 1986; Als et al, 1994). These studies demonstrated the usefulness of ongoing behavioral management of the high-risk neonate in the NICU. Parents carried out planned, consistent interventions, and primary care nurses focused on environmental modifications, such as handling and positioning. In general, both the parents and nurse focused on reducing stress and enhancing stable functioning. Results from the first randomized controlled trial (Als et al, 1994) involved infants weighing <1251 grams at birth before 30 weeks' gestation who were intubated within three hours after delivery and required mechanical ventilation for at least 24 of the first 48 hours. The 20 experimental infants demonstrated significant reduction in hospitalization length, age at discharge, improved weight gain to 2 weeks after due date, lower hospital costs, and reduced incidence of IVH and severity of chronic lung disease. These infants also were reported to have faster weaning from the respirator, from supplemental oxygen, and from gavage feedings. Improved developmental outcomes at ages 2 weeks and 9 months after the due date were also noted. Systematic electrophysiological group differences by quantified EEG (qEEG) with topographic mapping or Brain Electrical Activity Mapping (BEAM) were also found between control and experimental group infants at 2 weeks post term. Outcomes at age 8 years are preliminarily available and encouraging.

A second randomized controlled trial, done after the availability of surfactant, found similarly encouraging results (Fleisher et al, 1995; Heller et al, 1997). Experimental infants once again demonstrated fewer days on positive pressure, fewer days in the hospital, and significantly reduced hospital costs ($128,000 per experimental infant × 17 = $2.18 million saved in hospital charges). One third of the control infants went home several months after the experimental infants, thus indicating a reduction in chronicity in the experimental group. This study also demonstrated that these results could be obtained even when a developmental care program was new to the staff.

Other studies have focused on providing a quiet, calm, and darkened environment as well as individualized gentle nursing care at the bedside. These studies also reported positive results (Becker et al, 1991a; Becker et al, 1993). Improvement in medical and growth outcomes and motor and behavioral state organization in experimental infants were also reported.

A recent, as yet unpublished, multisite project that involved four NICUs and one intermediate nursery (n = 94) again showed effectiveness in the developmental care model in the NICUs in terms of significant reduction in morbidity and hospital stay. Developmental outcome as measured with the APIB showed significant improvement, as did family functioning. Buehler et al (1995) studied the intermediate population of premature infants and implemented individualized developmental care. Once again the APIB and Prechtl examinations and qEEG results showed significant neurobehavioral and electrophysiological improvement of the preterm experimental group when compared with the preterm control group. The preterm experimental group reached developmental function comparable to full-term newborns at 2 weeks.

From these studies, it is becoming evident that several components are needed in order to effectively implement a comprehensive model of developmental care within a nursery

OK revised 2014

BOX 17-2

NIDCAP® Outline of Components for Direct Caregiving

Preparation for Care
   Assess your readiness to begin:
- Are my materials appropriate? (Gather all items needed.)
- Is the room appropriate? (Check light, noise, temperature, and traffic.)
- Am I ready?
- Is the baby in a good state to begin?
- Are self-regulatory supports in place? (Does the baby have something to suck? Something against which to brace its feet? Something to grasp and hold onto? [or whatever else the baby needs])

During Care
   As you begin:
- Gently introduce yourself.
- Observe the baby's state as you begin.
- Plan to be vigilant of the baby's reactions—watch for the following:
      State changes
      RR, HR, O_2, color changes
      Changes in position, or remains in flexed position
      Baby's use of self-regulatory supports (e.g., sucks pacifier, holds finger, braces feet, etc.)
- If these happen as stress reactions, stop, break, and provide support until the baby returns to stable levels.
- If the infant loses control, stop and resupport (if possible)

Important: Note the following:
- How does the baby manifest stress?
- How can you prevent onset of stress reactions?

- What strategies work best?
- How far can you go with care and pace?
- Where does the baby become disorganized? How is this manifested?
- What can be done to help avoid these stress behaviors? To minimize them?
- How much stress is exhibited? What behaviors are seen? What stability is seen?

Recovery
   Energy:
- Assess level of fatigue, tolerance, and energy.
- Can I get the baby's energy to return? How?
- Is the baby exhausted or tired? Or fatigued, with some energy left?
- How could we avoid loss of energy or work at a successful level for the baby?
   Environment:
- Adjust noise or light to support resting or waking position.
- Reposition and add supports.
- What supports go in place to support transition to sleep or wakefulness?
   Transition to stability:
Transitions are events in themselves. Do not underestimate the energy they make take from the baby!
- Make the transition to sleep (reposition first, adjust environment and room).
- Stay with the baby until transition is complete (organized state).

Note: *Transitioning to an organized state means to organized calm sleep or an awake state, which is deep sleep or quiet alert.*
Developed by Kathleen VandenBerg, 2001.

---

system. These include development of staff positions for trained developmental specialists as well as for developmental nurse educators. Additional requisites include training of interdisciplinary leadership professionals who can ensure the survival and funding of the developmental program. Training in developmental concepts is essential for all staff, and the development of a parent council is recommended. A process for reflection and provision of continuing education opportunities must be available. Consultation and training is currently available from eleven NIDCAP® training centers, ten in the USA and one in Europe (several are under development) (Table 17-1). Based on the extensive experience of these centers, moving towards successful delivery of newborn intensive care in a developmental framework is typically a 5-year process.

Individualized developmentally supportive family-focused care has been shown to stabilize the infant and reduce stress during NICU hospitalization. Study results indicate that neurodevelopmental and medical outcome following premature birth are improved. Additional randomized trials are currently underway in Europe and Canada to further validate this approach and provide long term outcome results. Bowden (2000) and associates conducted a systematic review of developmental care

and provided a nice summary of the state of the science of these interventions.

INTERVENTION STRATEGIES

Environmental Modifications

Auditory Environment: Reducing Noise Levels.   Several recommendations have resulted from a recent review by an expert panel on sound of available research that describes newborn hearing ability and newborn behavioral responses to sound in the intensive care nursery (Graven, 2000; Morris et al, 2000; Philbin, 2000; Philbin et al, 1999). These researchers warn that although findings from the available studies—which are of poor quality and poor design and lack validity and reliability—are tempting to apply, they yield very little reliable clinical evidence or guidance as to the effects of sound on premature behavior in the intensive care nursery. They point out that even the full-term newborn who is acknowledged to be an active listener and learner may demonstrate some immaturity in the developing auditory system. The full-term healthy newborn would even have difficulty sleeping, self-quieting, and paying attention with high noise levels such as exist in the NICU (Morris et al, 2000).

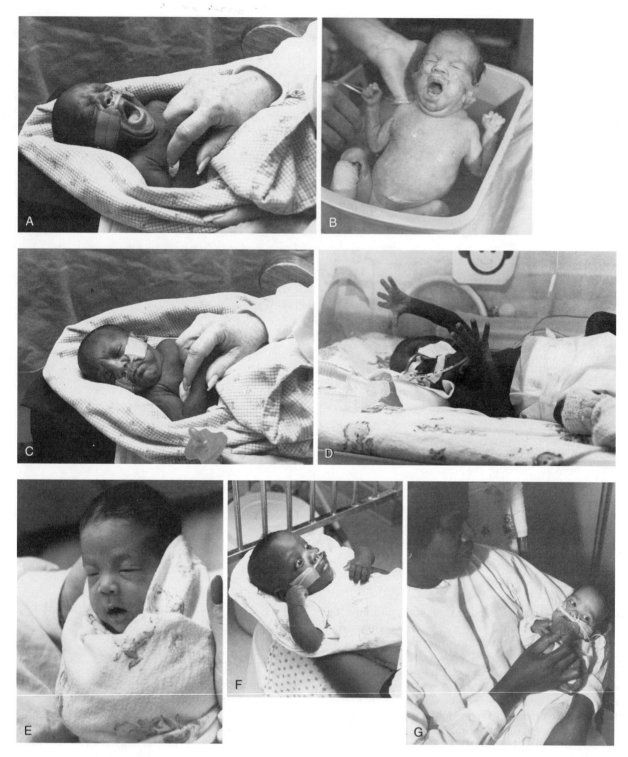

FIGURE **17-2**
Examples of selected instability cues. From the autonomic system: **A,** yawning; **B,** mottling. From the motor system: **B,** fussing; **C,** straining; **D,** finger splay; **E,** facial hypotonia. From the state system: **F,** glassy-eyed hyperalertness; **G,** gaze aversion. (Courtesy of Children's Hospital, Oakland, CA.)

Several efforts in the nursery have attempted to change staff behavior, but most have met with only limited success. Evans and Philbin (2000) suggest achieving quiet in the nursery by first changing the crowded, reverberant nature of the physical space. Efforts to reduce noise in the nursery have included special teaching sessions on measuring infant sleep, repairing and replacing of noisy equipment, efforts to introduce quiet hour,

and day-night cycling. None of these interventions has met with consistent success in controlling noise. Some studies have sought to directly block sound from the infant's ears (Zahr & de Traversay, 1995) with minimal success. Ear coverings pose potential problems for the infant because they alter only some of the sounds, require a tight seal around the ear, and can cause skin breakdown. In a review of these studies, Philbin et al

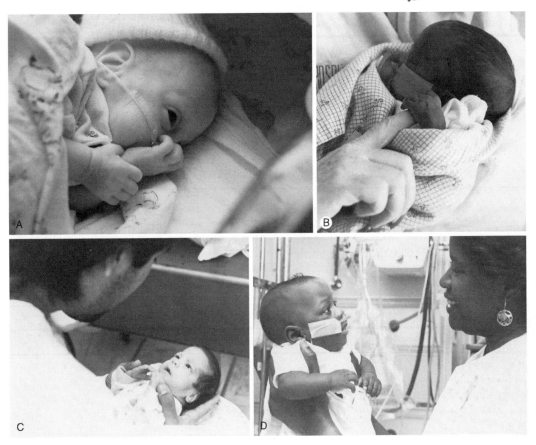

FIGURE **17-3**
Examples of selected stability cues. From the motor system: **A,** hand clasp and hand-to-mouth activity; **B,** grasping; **C,** hands together at midline. From the state system: **A,** active self-quieting; **C** and **D,** focused, shiny-eyed alertness. (Courtesy of Children's Hospital, Oakland, CA.)

ENERGY IN +	PHYSIOLOGIC ENERGY OUT +	BEHAVIORAL ENERGY OUT=	GROWTH ENERGY RETAINED
Food calories	Thermocontrol	Recycling	Weight gain
	Respiration	Stress	Growth
	Cardiovascular system	Overland	Formation of new tissues: muscle, fat dendrites
	Digestion		Development and organization of subsystems
	Other processes		

FIGURE **17-4**
Energy conservation model. Adapted with permission from Sammons WAH, Lewis JM (1985). *Premature babies: a different beginning.* St Louis: Mosby.

(1999) note that evidence from the literature and clinical experience reveals that a behavior change in altering noise in the nursery is not enough to fully control the noise levels and concludes that the traditional design for NICUs has not addressed noise levels because they were not designed to be quiet.

Sound levels vary in different NICUs and over time within a unit. These levels should be monitored regularly so that problem areas can be identified and modified (Gray & Philbin, 2000). Sound-level meters can be purchased at most electronic stores and are easy to use, or a professional acoustical engineer in the hospital may take sound levels and measurements. The reason for doing this would be to work toward reducing nursery sounds and their effects on newborns, as well as on staff in the unit. Adult work-related errors have been noted to be higher in the noisy nursery environment (Thomas & Martin, 2000).

Acoustical conditions cause constant high levels of reverberation of sound in NICUs. In other words, sounds bounce off surfaces and walls and keep bouncing repeating the effects of one stimulus over and over. Attention to sources of sound in the unit and to one's own contribution to the sound level at the bedside may facilitate a quieter environment for the infant. Closing incubator portholes, cabinets, or nursery doors gently and removing water bubbling in oxygen and ventilator tubing may decrease background noise. Eliminating radios is also helpful. Putting telephones and as many alarms as possible on low levels is another effective strategy for reducing background noise. Some nurseries use light cues that signal to staff that the sound alarm is sounding at the bedside without any noise. Peak noises can be reduced by avoiding tapping or banging on tops of incubators. Paying attention to location of cribs in relation to equipment, doorways, and traffic paths is also important. Providing staff with pagers that vibrate can reduce the effect of the loud overhead speaker system.

Recent studies reviewing the literature for "music therapy" raises concerns about the methodology of presenting sound stimuli without evaluating the appropriate the levels of music stimuli or the developmental level of the infant receiving the exposure (Cassidy & Ditty, 1998). The paucity of evidence

TABLE 17-7. Summary of Data Supporting Developmental Supportive Care: Medical and Cost Outcomes

	Becker, 1991	Als, 1986	Als, 1994	Fleisher, 1995	Westrup, 2000	Buehler, 1995
Type of study	Phase lag	Phase lag	RCT	RCT	RCT	RCT
Weight at birth	<1500 gm	<1250 gm	1250 gm	<1250 gm	<32 wks	<2500 gm
Days on ventilator or CPAP	⇓	⇔	⇓	⇓	⇓	n/a
Days on oxygen	⇓	⇓	⇓	⇓	⇓	n/a
Days to nipple	⇓	⇓	⇓	⇓	n/a	n/a
Weight gain	⇔	⇔	⇑	⇑	⇔	⇔
Hospital stay	⇓	⇔	⇓	⇔	⇔	⇔
Savings per child	$12,250	$114,000	$93,000	$128,000	n/a	⇔

Research investigating the effectiveness of developmentally supportive care on medical and cost outcomes demonstrates significant differences in favor of the experimental group. Only the first author is referenced in the table; full references are in the chapter reference list. ⇑ = *significant increase;* ⇓ = *significant decrease;* ⇔ = *no significant difference; n/a = not investigated. RCT = randomized controlled trial. From Browne JV et al (1996). Family Infant Relationship Support Training.* Denver: The Center for Family and Infant Interaction.

TABLE 17-8 Summary of Data Supporting Developmental Supportive Care: Developmental Outcomes

	Becker, 1991	Als, 1986	Als, 1994	Fleisher, 1995	Buehler, 1995
Development at 42 weeks	⇑	⇑	⇑	⇑	⇑
Brain activity at 42 weeks	n/a	n/a	⇑	n/a	⇑
Development within 12 months	n/a	⇑	⇑	n/a	n/a
Development at 3 years	n/a	⇑	⇑		n/a
Development at 8 years	n/a	⇑			

Research investigating the effectiveness of developmentally supportive care on developmental outcomes demonstrates significant differences in favor of the experimental group. Only the first author is referenced in the table, full references are in the chapter reference list. ⇑ = *significant increase; n/a = not investigated. From Browne JV et al (1996). Family infant relationship support training.* Denver: The Center for Family and Infant Interaction.

regarding use of music to sick newborns makes questionable the safeguards for validity and reliability of this mode of exposure for newborns in the NICU (Philbin, 2000; Philbin & Klass, 2000a, b). Regardless of their content, tape recordings have little basis for being used with newborns in the NICU. Negative consequences have not been evaluated, and possible benefits have not been demonstrated (Philbin, 2000). The concern from a behavioral perspective relates to exposing a hospitalized infant to recordings and musical toys while the infant has little control over his or her environment. The infant faces a nonresponsive music box or recording device playing freely, which places him or her in a situation in which he or she cannot regulate the input or his or her response.

The current national trend is moving towards remodeling of hospital environments, with intensive care nurseries becoming redesigned with acoustical surfaces and quieter walls, floors, and ceilings. Thus an environment that absorbs rather than reverberates sound can be built (Philbin et al, 1999). The development of single-room-design NICUs increases options for modification of sound and noise reduction (Brown & Taquino, 2001).

Recommendations of an expert panel on sound (Graven, 2000) include the following:

1. Avoid prolonged exposure to low-frequency sound levels (<250 Hz) above 65 db (a) during pregnancy.
2. Earphones or other devices for sound production should not be directly attached to the pregnant woman's abdomen.

3. The voice of the mother during normal daily activities and the sounds produced by her body and her usual surroundings is sufficient for normal fetal auditory development.
4. The fetus does not require supplemental stimulation; therefore programs to supplement the fetal auditory experience are not recommended.
5. NICUs should incorporate a system of regular noise assessment.
6. NICU sound limit recommendations are to maintain an hourly Leq of 50 db (a), an hourly L10 of 55 db (a), and a 1-second Lmax of 70 db (a), all a-weighted, slow-response scale.
7. NICUs should develop and maintain a program of noise control and abatement to operate within the above recommended sound limit recommendations.
8. Infants must have ample opportunities to hear their parents' voices (live, not recorded) during interaction between parent and infant at the bedside.
9. Earphones and similar devices attached to the infant's ears for sound transmission should never be used.
10. There is little evidence to support the use of recorded music or speech in the environment of the high-risk infant. Audio recordings should not be used routinely and, if used, should never be left unattended in the infant's environment.

Visual Environment: Reducing Light Levels. Individual lights at each bedside allow the nurse to individualize lighting for each infant. Diffuse lighting is preferable to high brightness lighting fixtures. Covering incubators, radiant warmers, and cribs reduces infant exposure to bright overhead lights or daylight. Complete covering can be used for sleep periods, with partial covering, during wakeful times. Advantages of covers include reduction in ambient light and environmental noise and opportunities for diurnal variation, protection, and insulation of the incubator. Concerns include safety (e.g., infant may not be visible if incubator is completely covered), sensory isolation, lack of diurnal variability, overprotection, and overheating. As with other interventions, it is critical to individualize to each infant based on assessment of that individual infant's status.

Dimmer switches, window shades, and curtains increase staff control over the light environment. Dimming lights at night may promote development of diurnal cycles. Adjusting lighting levels during other periods fosters state transition and periods of alertness or sleep. Infants who are having brief, predictable alert periods need semidim light until they are ready to maintain longer periods of alertness. Infants should be placed in dim light while the pupils are dilated before and after ophthalmologic examinations. Light can damage certain nutrients in human milk, formula, and parenteral nutrition solutions; therefore prolonged exposure of milk and nutrition solutions to bright light should be avoided (van Zoeren-Grobben et al, 1993). Abrupt changes from dark to light have been associated with physiologic changes and thus should be avoided when possible (Brandon, 2000). The entire visual environment of the infant needs to be evaluated regularly and simplified. Infants in the NICU can accumulate an amazing clutter of toys, pictures, and other equipment that may be overstimulating for an individual infant.

Specific recommendations regarding the NICU light environment have not been published, and there is paucity of well-designed research that examines specific interventions. The light environment intervention that has been studied most often is cycled lighting. However, a paucity of studies in this area remains, and the available studies have significant methodological limitations and inconsistent findings (Blackburn, 1996a, b; Blackburn & Patteson, 1991; Lotus, 1992; Miller et al, 1995). Continuing issues in management of the light environment of the high-risk infant include at what gestational ages to include use of cycled vs. non-cycled lighting, the amount of light and dark, cycle length, use of dim vs. dark vs. light, light spectrum and intensity, and light environments at different ages (Brandon, 2000; Blackburn, 1996b).

Brandon (2000) recently studied three groups of infants born at <31 weeks' gestation who received (1) near dark until 32 weeks, then cycled light to discharge (n = 19); (2) cycled light from birth to discharge (n = 21); or (3) near dark to 36 weeks then cycled light to discharge (n = 22). Her data suggest advantages of cycled lighting over continuous dark. Her "light" period used an intensity of 200 to 225 lux (approximately 20 to 25 ftc), and "near dark" was 5 to 10 lux (approximately 0.5 to 1 ftc). These values are of much lower intensity and with greater differences between light and dark intensities than were used in previous studies. Brandon found no significant advantages of long-term (i.e., to 36 weeks' gestation) near darkness in the hospitalized preterm infant over cycled lighting. Exposure to cycled light from birth versus from 32 weeks gestation produced similar findings for this sample in terms of length of hospitalization and growth. Thus the available cycled light studies yield little reliable clinical evidence or guidance as to what the staff should do with regard to light in the intensive care nursery.

Preliminary suggestions from the expert panel on light (Blackburn, 1996; Glass, 1999) and the NICU Design Standards (White, 2002) suggest the following recommendations may be appropriate:

1. Light levels should be regularly monitored and documented, both for the unit as a whole and for individual infants. Because accurate light measurement can be difficult, this is probably best done by a professional engineer from hospital environmental services.
2. The amount of light to which infant is exposed must be able to be individually controlled for each infant. This includes sources of light, covers, eye shields, and other devices that control retinal light exposure and includes delivery room, transport, and other locations where the infant receives care.
3. Ambient lighting levels in newborn intensive care rooms and at infant bedsides should be adjustable (range from 10 to 60 ftc) (White, 2002). Although optimal levels of light are unknown, White (2002) suggests that recommendations for newly constructed or renovated units meet Illuminating Engineering Society (1995) guidelines for ambient lighting of 10 to 20 ftc with the ability to go as low as 0.5 ftc.
4. Infants should be placed (or screened) so they do not look directly at focused procedure lamps or at natural sunlight that provides significantly higher illuminations that ambient lighting. Procedure and heat lamps should be placed so that they are not directed toward the infant's eyes (or the eyes of infants in adjacent beds), and caregivers should consider use of eye shields when a procedure spotlight is being directed at any part of an infant.
5. The clinical use of visual stimulation programs with preterm infants should await further investigation, including proof of efficacy and absence of harm both short and long-term effects.

Congestion and Traffic Patterns. The remodeling of many intensive care nurseries with new configuration of space along with additional space for families has reduced the congestion and traffic issues in many NICUs. Increased activity and disorganized movements of staff and families—with resulting congestion and increased noise levels—can increase stress and arousal for infant and even adults. Much of the data regarding the responses of newborns to congestion and rounds in the NICU is anecdotal. However, these observations suggest that for some infants, these events my lead to physiologic and motoric disorganization, apnea, and bradycardia. Infants need to be assessed, observed, and monitored to identify that environmental events, such as change of shift report and nursing or medical rounds, are not disruptive. Infants for whom these events are problematic can be moved out of the unit traffic pattern, and reporting and rounds can be moved away from the bedside.

Altering Patterns of Care

As the infant's primary caregiver in the NICU, the nurse has a predominant role in controlling patterns of care. Caregiving patterns can be altered to respond more appropriately to an infant by evaluating the need for routine orders and caregiving interventions. The need for specific non-emergency interventions must be evaluated for their urgency and the potential impact on the infant. Most NICU infants are being monitored for a variety of physiologic parameters with sophisticated equipment. The data from this equipment can be used to decrease disruption of the infants by routine activities such as monitoring of vital signs. Non-emergency interventions—including monitoring of vital signs, feeding, bathing, diapering, and administration of routine medications—can be performed in states other than quiet sleep (infants do not stay in quiet sleep periods for long—often for less than 5 to 10 minutes). In as much as infants spend very little time in the quiet alert state, aversive procedures should be avoided during this state. Duxbury et al (1984) found that infants who received care (except for emergency procedures) only after beginning to awaken spontaneously had improved growth and physiologic function and a significantly decreased length of hospital stay.

Caregiving interventions can also be grouped or clustered to provide longer uninterrupted rest periods. Caregiving involves a significant amount of sensory input and energy. Although some infants do well with clustering of care, others become exhausted and overloaded. Some infants tolerate the clustering of aversive interventions (e.g., blood drawing, injections, suctioning); others do not. Some infants tolerate clustering of these procedures with infant care interventions (e.g., feedings, diapering, and so on); others do not. The amount of time between clusters must be monitored to provide adequate time for recovery and rest (Evans, 1994). Time of interventions within a cluster is also an important consideration, not only in terms of potential side effects but also in terms of avoiding exhausting an infant before feeding her or him (VandenBerg, 1990). Therefore clustering of care must be accompanied by ongoing individualized assessment of the infant's responses and may not be appropriate for the very-low-birth-weight or very fragile infant. In addition, all infants must be observed carefully for signs of stress during caregiving and provided with recovery time as needed. Interventions such as containment can assist the infant in tolerating necessary caregiving interventions.

Interventions with Overstimulated or Stressed Infants

All infants in a NICU will have periods when they cannot cope with environmental stressors and caregiving interventions and will demonstrate signs of sensory overload (Table 17-5). For the immature or fragile infant, any handling may be stressful—even handling that staff or parents perceive as positive, such as holding, stroking, or talking to the infant. When an infant becomes overloaded, a behavioral observation is essential to evaluate the levels of stress and the behavioral repertoire available to the infant for self-regulation. From this information interventions can be proposed and implemented to facilitate the infant's reorganizing and recovery before, during, and after handing events. Interventions with overstimulated infants include time out with minimal or no handling or sensory input, containment or swaddling the infant with one's hands or a blanket, holding the infant quietly and providing no other sensory input (e.g., do not talk to, stroke, or jiggle the infant), placing blanket rolls at the infant's back and feet, or placing one's hands on the soles of the infant's feet.

Positioning

Positioning has been studied in relation to physiologic variables such as arterial oxygen tension, respiratory rate, lung compliance, oxygenation, physical activity, and energy expenditure. To improve the mechanics of breathing, these studies recommend the prone position as the preferred position for low-birth-weight infants in the NICU. Prone positioning has also been associated with more organized state control, enhancing quiet sleep, and reducing wake states and crying.

Positioning of the sick or immature infant includes consideration of the effects of gravity along with neuromuscular char-

acteristics such as variable weak muscle tone and decreased flexion in the limbs, trunk, and pelvis. These infants are at risk for positioning disorders such as widely abducted hips (frog-leg position); retracted and abducted shoulders; ankle and foot eversion; increased neck extension with a right-sided head preference; and increased trunk extension with arching of the neck and back. These positioning disorders affect later development because of their impact on the ability of the child to bear weight, bring the shoulders forward and hands to midline, and rotate the head. Therefore, in addition to improved physiologic status, developmental goals of positioning include enhancement of flexion in the limbs and trunk, extensor balance, and facilitation of midline skills.

These goals are superseded, however, by the importance of stress reduction and enhancement of organized motor system function. This means prevention of ongoing frantic activity (flailing) and frequent recurrent extensions of the extremities and neck. These responses are very costly to the infant in terms of energy expenditure, respiratory function, and oxygenation. Thus the immature or sick neonate requires support from caregivers to facilitate and maintain postures that enhance motor control and physiologic functioning and reduce stress. Most infants can be routinely placed in side-lying and prone positions and rotated every 2 to 3 hours. Supine positions are generally avoided. Infants who must be placed supine should be positioned to promote flexion and proper alignment.

Covering, swaddling, and placing blanket rolls around the infant help him or her maintain the desired posture and prevent loss of control of the flexed position. The use of these rolls provides containment and boundaries for the infant and promotes feelings of security, quiescence, and energy conservation. Many infants will seek out boundaries by moving around in their incubator until they rest against its sides, foot, or head. Infants who do so and are resting or sleeping should be left undisturbed in these positions—unless they are unsafe—until the next caregiving period. At that time, the infant can be repositioned and provided with boundaries or nested with blanket rolls along his or her side and at the feet and head. Nesting is often an effective way of reducing agitation. Placing rolls at the infant's feet also provides him or her with something against which to brace during stressful interventions. Care must be taken to not nest infants so tightly that their movements are severely restricted.

When infants need to be moved and or repositioned, either to provide an alternate position or for caregiving procedures or holding, the infant should be unwrapped and repositioned slowly with containment of the limbs and support of the head and neck. Stress responses are avoided by maintenance of the posture. When repositioning the infant, the nurse should ensure that the infant is covered or swaddled if possible. If covering is not possible for medical reasons, partial wrapping is encouraged. Swaddling with blankets or containment with the caregiver's hands also reduces stress during procedures. Several investigations have suggested that the use of containment with preterm infants during procedures such as endotracheal suctioning may modify the procedure's physiologic and behavioral consequences by reducing the decrease in arterial blood pressure, heart rate, and oxygenation, thus promoting more stable intracranial pressure and decreasing behavioral stress cues (Taquino & Blackburn, 1994; Corff et al, 1995). Swaddling is also appropriate before and after procedures to minimize motor and physiologic changes. Infants can also be placed on soft foam or in slings to promote flexion, provides tactile input, and reduce skin abrasion. Positioning interventions are illustrated in Figure 17-5.

Handling

Intervention strategies related to handling must be based on two critical components: individualization and timing. The individualization of caregiving for each infant includes flexibility and willingness on the part of the caregiver to adapt handling to specific infant needs to reduce stress and prevent agitation. The caregiver must also recognize that infants' needs change, so that what may be a well-chosen, appropriate intervention during one shift may not work at all during the next one.

Appropriate timing of handling is also essential to avoid overtiring, overstimulating infants, or increasing stress. Infants can improve their abilities to regulate their own movements, states, and autonomic function when caregiving activities are offered in sequence and with sensitivity to the infant's degree of tolerance. Examples of timing include stopping and letting the infant gain control of his or her physiologic or motoric status before completing an assessment or procedure or pacing the infant by removing the nipple during oral feeding when respiratory rate exceeds usual limits.

Infants in a NICU—no matter how sick or how small—experience and react to every aspect of care and the surrounding environment. A goal of neonatal care is to avoid costly stress in these infants. Slow, sensitive handling for medical procedures and routine caregiving is required to accomplish this goal. Sensitive handling is based on an understanding of infant state and cues (Table 17-5). Before gently touching an infant, the caregiver should talk softly. This reduces startling. Tremors or "hands out of nowhere" are suddenly moving other stress responses from the infant. Minimal handling protocols are necessary for immature, fragile infants (VandenBerg & Franck, 1990). Minimal handling protocols allow infants to have extended sleep periods, which facilitate autonomic and state control.

State Modulation

One of the primary functions of the caregiver during the infant's early life is modulation of levels of arousal in the infant. Lack of interactions organized around soothing or attempts to decrease arousal may contribute to impairment of the high-risk infant's ability to modulate his or her state organization, thus resulting in an infant who presents fewer or less clear cues to his or her parents.

Initially, state modulation efforts are directed toward protecting the infant from environmental stressors and aversive sensory input by reducing arousal through implementing time-out maneuvers. These early interventions are directed toward protecting the infant from disorganization and decompensation. Infants cannot truly maintain mature states until they achieve control over their autonomic and motoric systems (Als, 1986).

Interventions to organize state include evaluating caregiving activity schedules with regard to their necessity and appropriateness for a particular infant with the goal of working to-

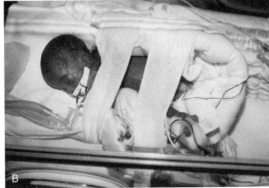
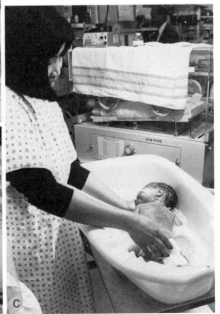
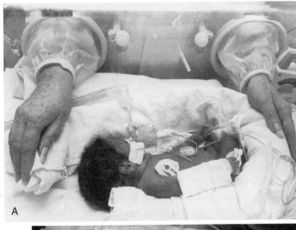

FIGURE **17-5**
Handling and positioning of infants in the NICU. **A,** Creating a nest using blankets; **B,** nesting using Snuggle-up. Courtesy of Children's Medical Ventures, Boston, MA; **C,** positioning during a bath. Courtesy of Children's Hospital, Oakland, CA.

ward restfulness and supporting growth (Als, 1999). Infants' caregiving schedules are coordinated with the family schedules to support the integration of the infant into the family and foster family involvement. During delivery of care, caregivers can approach the infant with calm attention, including the family by explaining the sequence of care components to be addressed. Observation of the infant's level of sleep or wakefulness is necessary to facilitate organization of sleep, alerting, and crying. Introducing themselves to the infant using a soft voice and gentle touch, providing periods of rest and recovery between handling events, and containing the infant in a gentle embrace with their hands support the infant's regulation of state. To promote sleep, the caregiver can modify the environment to reduce light, noise, and traffic around the infant's bed. Use of boundaries, prone positioning, minimal handling, predictable routines, and support of flexion will also facilitate sleep organization. Interventions to prevent irritability and crying include predictable routines, reducing environmental stress, timing procedures or other caregiving according to infant cues, and soothing infants when they become stressed. Periods of irritability can be minimized if signs of stress and sensory overload are recognized early and appropriate interventions are initiated. Soothing interventions for the immature or ill infant include containment and swaddling, providing time out for recovery, reducing stimulation, holding the infant's hands or feet, prone positioning, and providing sucking opportunities (Als, 1986; Lawhon, 1986; VandenBerg, 1990, 1995).

Immature infants will initially spend very little time in alert states. When they do achieve an alert state, these states are transient and easily disrupted. Caregivers need to approach infants who have reached a quiet alert state carefully. It is often an exciting event when an infant finally opens his or her eyes and reaches a quiet alert state. Unfortunately, caregivers often try to capitalize on this time by providing input and reinforcement that is "too much, too soon." A more appropriate response to interacting with these infants is to allow the infant to initiate and control the interaction. This can be done by slowly approaching the infant with low-keyed input, using one mode of stimuli at a time, then gradually increasing the input based on the infant's cues. If the infant begins to show signs of stress, the caregivers should provide time out and begin the interaction again after the infant recovers. Shielding the infant's eyes from overhead lights can facilitate alert states.

As infants mature and their health status improves, they will be able to handle more mature interactions with their parents, nurses, and other caregivers. State modulation activities can then be introduced around caregiving events such as feeding. Fuhrman (1984) studied the effects of a parent-initiated state modulation intervention in which parents were taught to arouse their preterm infants before feeding and to soothe the infants after feeding. These infants were all stable and ready for discharge home. Fuhrman found that at follow-up 4 weeks after discharge, infants who received this intervention were significantly more alert before feeding, had shorter feeding times, and had higher scores on the Nurse Child Assessment Feeding Scale (NCAFS) for both infant and parent subscales.

Alerting activities with healthy full-term or more mature, stable preterm infants include talking to the infant; varying the pitch and intensity of one's voice; unwrapping the infant, even if only the upper extremities; providing a drowsy infant with visual or auditory stimuli; putting the infant in an upright position such as up on one's shoulder; and eliciting the rooting or sucking reflexes. Activities to soothe include talking in a slow, steady monotone; swaddling the infant with hands or blanket; providing a pacifier or helping the infant get his or her fingers or hand into the mouth; and placing one's hands against the soles of the infant's feet (Blackburn & Kang, 1991). As with the more fragile infants, these infants should also be observed for their stress and stability cues in response to each intervention.

Provision of Sensory Input

As the preterm infant matures and the ill preterm or full-term infant recovers and stabilizes, provision of sensory input becomes an important parameter to foster neurologic development. Provision of sensory input is not just providing additional stimulation; careful thought needs to be given to the appropriate types of sensory input based on the infant's state, health status, maturity, developmental level, and cues.

Caregivers must be cautious when providing sensory input and must be sensitive to infant responses and abilities to tolerate stimuli. Inasmuch as optimal levels, amount, complexity, and type of sensory input have not yet been established, efforts to stimulate the high-risk infant can quickly result in overstimulation with physiologic, motoric, and behavioral decompensation. The old adage "if a little is good, more must be better" must be avoided to protect the infant from stimulus bombardment. As noted earlier, for the immature or fragile infant, the best form of additional stimulation is none.

Specific considerations for providing sensory input to high-risk infants include (1) protect the infant from aversive sensory experiences; (2) sensory input should be biologically meaningful; (3) sensory input should be provided only if the infants is medically stale and has had no recent care changes; (4) sensory input should be introduced in the order of development of the senses (i.e., tactile first and visual only after the infant is stable; see Figure 17-2); (5) monitor infant responses and tolerance to all sensory input and modify based on infant cues; (6) support— but do not accelerate—normal maturational processes; (7) remember these infants are vulnerable to sensory overload; (8) most infants can deal only with a small amount of stimuli at a time and at a slower rate; and (9) the infant may be able to handle only unimodal rather than multimodal stimuli. If the infant demonstrates signs of stress when presented with sensory input, it should be eliminated and tried again at a later date. Philbin (1996) notes that responsiveness to a stimulus does not imply that it was received, perceived, needed, or beneficial. The optimal sensory input for any infant is that provided by a knowledgeable, sensitive parent. Thus care should be directed at helping parents learn about their infants' cues and needs.

Feeding

The NICU patient encounters many factors that are likely to jeopardize the development of normal healthy feeding patterns. Treatment factors include prolonged use of endotracheal tubes and gavage feeding and tape placed on the face to hold tubing. These procedures contribute to noxious oral sensations and may lead to oral defensive behaviors such as hypersensitivity to touch. Other factors related to the environment and caregiving routines affect the development of feeding skills. These include inconsistent caregivers, intense stimuli, and varied patterns of handling, which disorganize sensory experience. Intense environmental stimuli may over-stimulate the infant and interfere with the infant's ability to organize motor activity for efficient sucking.

In addition, because of the severity of their illness or immaturity, many neonates will not have the energy for feeding.

Feeding is a very demanding task, often exceeding what has been asked of an infant up to that point in his or her care. If the infant is preterm, he or she has an immature CNS with weak movement patterns, disorganized states, and oral structures that do not function as those of a full-term neonate. Tongue and jaw movements are affected by immature development, thus leading to poorer control of suck, swallow, and breathing patterns. Behavioral patterns include weak, poorly sustained sucking and inadequate state control during feeding. This interferes with coordination of suck and swallow with breathing. Nippling even small amounts can lead to exhaustion and flaccidity with disruption of respiratory control. Compounding the problem is staff and parental anxiety over weight gain and growth.

Usually, these infants can suck and swallow a small amount adequately. They then lose control, developing poor coordination of sucking and swallowing with breathing, an inability to sustain sucking, poor suck and swallow rhythm, respiratory irregularities, or exhaustion. This pattern of behavior has been termed the disorganized feeder, as opposed to the dysfunctional feeder (VandenBerg, 1990).

Recently, an assessment tool that analyzes jaw and tongue movements during neonatal sucking has been used by a high percentage of feeding specialists in the intensive care nursery. The Neonatal Oral Motor Assessment of Sucking (NOMAS) separates 13 characteristics of jaw movement and 13 characteristics of tongue movement into categories of normal, disorganized, and dysfunctional sucking (Palmer, 1993; Palmer et al, 1993). A disorganized suck refers to a lack of rhythm of the total sucking activity, whereas dysfunction refers to the interruption of the feeding process by abnormal movements off the tongue and jaw. The NOMAS has been used clinically in the nursery and in research. The NOMAS—along with the training offered by its author, Marjorie M. Palmer—has enlightened NICU staff to the developmental needs of newborns as they undertake a most demanding task in their developmental journey thus far—sucking and oral feeding. The NOMAS has already demonstrated its usefulness and has been used as a measure of the effectiveness of intervention with poor feeders in the nursery and as an indicator of oral motor disorganization versus dysfunction during early feeding (Palmer & Heyman, 1999; VandenBerg, 1990). Training courses in the use of the NOMAS are available through Therapeutic Media, San Juan Bautista, California (510-651-2285).

The dysfunctional feeder is the neurologically abnormal feeder with abnormal jaw and tongue movements during nutritive sucking (Braun & Palmer, 1982). This pattern does not spontaneously improve over time and requires intense therapeutic intervention. A specialist trained in feeding neonates should assess dysfunctional feeders. This specialist is usually an occupational, physical, or speech therapist or an infant educator. Abnormal oral muscle tone and reflexes commonly are present in this group of infants; professional intervention is required for improvement.

The disorganized feeder pattern usually improves as the infant recovers from neonatal illness and does not require specific therapeutic intervention (Braun & Palmer, 1982; VandenBerg, 1990). However, these infants do require sensitive pacing and accurate reading of their behavioral cues for signs of stress or stability to facilitate adequate nippling (Cagan, 1996).

The goal for the disorganized feeder is to learn self-regulation of autonomic, motoric, and state systems to eventually nipple adequately. To do this, the infant must be able to simultaneously (1) coordinate suck and swallow with respira-

tions while maintaining heart rate and color; (2) coordinate movement patterns, posture, and tone; and (3) remain in a calm, organized state. To help the infant achieve this level of functioning, the caregiver needs to respect the infant's neurobehavioral functional level and not push feeding beyond the infant's capabilities. Fostering state control, timing the feeding, pacing the feeding, positioning the infant, modifying the environment, sxneurodevelopmental approach to feeding infants in the NICU (Cagan, 1996; VandenBerg, 1990). Environmental modifications include creating a quiet setting with indirect lighting and minimal congestion and traffic. Position to facilitate feeding includes promoting generalized body flexion to reduce hypertonia and to assist with swallowing, maintaining the head in midline with hands close to face, providing hip flexion, and swaddling. Feeding disorganization is a temporary problem that caregivers can easily facilitate with adequate awareness of the appropriate interventions.

Nonnutritive Sucking

Sucking is one of the earliest coordinated behaviors of the fetus. Sucking is necessary for biologic survival and is an important parameter of caregiver-infant interaction, self-gratification, and soothing. Human infants demonstrate two modes of sucking—nutritive and nonnutritive—each with a specific pattern of organization (Medoff-Cooper, 1991). Nonnutritive sucking has a pattern of short, alternating bursts of sucking and rest in contrast to the longer, continuous, rhythmic patterns characteristic of nutritive sucking (Medoff-Cooper et al, 1989). Nonnutritive sucking is present in the fetus as early as 4.5 months of gestation and is seen in very-low-birth-weight infants. The presence of nonnutritive sucking in these infants does not mean that they have the ability to coordinate and maintain nutritive sucking. The ability to maintain, regulate, and organize the pattern and rhythm of nutritive and nonnutritive sucking is affected by the infant's maturity, illness, and experience.

Nonnutritive sucking is induced by placing a nipple in the infant's mouth without presentation of food. Nonnutritive sucking and rhythmic mouthing (seen in quiet sleep) have similar temporal organization, with regularity of the sucking-pause pattern. Nonnutritive sucking is a state modulation and organizing activity that is used during gavage feeding and interfeeding intervals. It has been associated with improved oxygenation; decreased, more stable intracranial pressure; increased quiet sleep; decreased activity and crying; increased alertness; increased readiness for nipple feeding; better weight gain; and shorter hospital stays (DiPietro et al, 1994; Pickler et al, 1996, Shiao et al, 1997).

As noted earlier, infants who spend their first months after birth in a NICU or special care nursery experience many factors that may interfere with the acquisition of normal oral functioning and thus condition the infant to respond defensively to any oral stimuli. Nonnutritive sucking can be used to provide the infant with a source of self-consolation and self-regulation and to provide pleasant oral sensation that will serve as a basis for a positive introduction to nutritive sucking and feeding.

Strategies to facilitate development of nonnutritive sucking in intubated infants include (1) using nasal rather than oral intubation; (2) minimizing touch and stress to the oral musculature (and, when necessary, using gentle, slow touch); (3) placing in side-lying position with hands together; (4) positioning with hands tucked under chin or so that hands touch parts of face; and (5) providing pacifiers. After extubation, infants can be positioned with their hands together at the mouth or hands touching their face. In addition, pacifiers can be provided during nasogastric feedings and between feedings.

Kangaroo Care

Kangaroo care is a form of parental caregiving that grew out of a crisis in the newborn intensive care nursery in Bogota, Colombia. Two pediatricians working in a large, understaffed, poorly equipped hospital where mortality of low-birth-weight infants was high, pioneered this type of care. Along with the economic problems, cross-infection was rampant. Their mothers often abandoned infants in the hospital. Kangaroo care was developed for mothers with stable preterm neonates. This type of care has become, in a modified form, a standard of care in many countries.

The kangaroo method of care involves placing a stable full-term or preterm newborn skin-to-skin in a vertical position between the mother's breasts or on the father's chest. The warmth of the skin-to-skin contact and other sensations fosters close contact between parent and infant. The infant usually wears only a diaper. The parent wears a loose blouse/shirt, dress, or gown that opens in the front and that can be easily wrapped around the infant once placed on his or her chest (Figure 17-6). The infant is kept warm by the heat generated by the parent's body and is covered by their clothing, so heat loss is avoided. In fact, most nurses report that close monitoring of the infant's temperature is important during kangaroo care so as to avoid overheating rather than under-heating.

Kangaroo care has been studied in many countries. Positive effects of kangaroo care include decreased variation in heart rate, improved oxygenation, reduction in apneic and bradycardic episodes, improved lung mechanics, decreased activity and perhaps energy expenditure, decreased arousal, increased quiet sleep, reduced maternal stress, and an increased number of mothers still breastfeeding at the time of infant discharge from the hospital (Anderson, 1999; Bell & McGrath, 1996; Gale et al, 1993; Gale & VandenBerg, 1998; Ludington, 1990; Ludington-Hoe et al, 1991; Ludington-Hoe et al, 1994; Ludington-Hoe & Swinth, 1996; Moran et al, 1999). The vertical positioning with kangaroo care may also provide vestibular stimulation, relieve horizontal pressure on the head and body, and help and reduce cranial flattening (Gale & VandenBerg, 1998). The close contact between infant and parent provides a source of contingent stimulation and exposure to the sensory environment (i.e., tactile, smell) of the breast. Several variations of kangaroo care allow the procedure to be adapted to the infant, parent, and unit (Table 17-9). Infants can receive kangaroo care for extended periods of the 24-hour day or periodically, depending on parental visiting patterns. Box 17-3 describes preparation of infant and parent for kangaroo care.

Family-Centered Care

Family-centered care addresses the delivery of health care. This emphasis has risen out of the concern that the family and its influence on the patient in hospital settings, whether that patient be a newborn infant, an adolescent or adult, was diminishing or not being considered Parents of infants and young children in hospitals were complaining that they were not being consulted or included in discussions or in the decision-making process for their loved ones. Families and parents in both pediatrics and obstetric facilities were expressing a loss of control and helplessness. Thus consumer voices and professional organizations concerned about health issues for women and infants and children have taken a stand in support of family-centered approaches.

To date many changes have taken place, and the actual national focus of implementing family-centered care has become very well known in many hospitals, including intensive care nurseries, as well as in maternity care and clinics and in practices affiliated with them. Medical care systems are being shaped and revitalized by a collaborative model of planning, implementation, and evaluation of maternity and newborn services.

There is a growing research base that demonstrates that family-centered care works by improving outcomes in health and psychosocial areas for infants and their parents. Data to support the efficacy of family-centered care for newborns is reported by Buehler et al (1995) and Fleisher et al (1995), who have investigated the effects of family-focused developmental care with premature infants in the intensive care nursery. "Family-centered care is a neurobiologic imperative for fragile infants. Family-centered care and developmental care are inextricably linked" (Als & Gilkerson, 1997).

Family-centered care in the newborn intensive care nursery offers a philosophy of care that acknowledges that the family has the greatest influence over an infant's health and well-being. All families, even those that are struggling with difficulties, are seen as bringing important strengths to their infants' experiences in the health care system. Key concepts in the de-

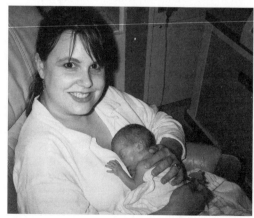

A

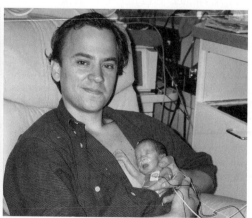

B

FIGURE **17-6**

Skin-to-skin "kangaroo" method of holding preterm infants by **A,** mother and **B,** father. Courtesy of Kristin Geen, St. Louis, MO.

livery of family-centered care include respect for the infant and parents, provision of opportunities for regular sharing of information, and parent planning. Supports that acknowledge the importance of parental decisions, which are valued and addressed with flexibility, are in place. Implementing a meaningful family-centered care focus involves educating administrators, clinicians, researchers, and all staff in collaborative efforts that build relationships and facilitate involvement in the emotional, social, and developmental support of children.

Implementation of family-centered care can be practiced in numerous ways—from offering a weekly one-hour dinner on site at the hospital for parents to ask for their input in hospital committees and to contribute the family perspective to the decision-making process. Several medical schools, training programs and hospitals have involved families as faculty in inservice education. The family perspective gives unique insight into the effects of medical care, practices, and services. The most well known source of information and training for hospitals has emerged from the Institute for Family-Centered Care in Washington, D.C. This organization provides technical assistance, training seminars, and direct consultation in developing this focus in specific hospital settings. Several hospitals and units have rewritten their mission statements to reflect the new awareness that the child is part of the family and the family is the constant in the child's life (Box 17-4). Not only have both professionals and families found these collaborations effective but they have also led to permanent changes in attitudes and knowledge in the health care delivery system.

BOX 17-3

Example of a Protocol for Kangaroo Holding

1. Explain the procedure to the parent so that she or he understands kangaroo holding before starting. Confirm that this is an activity that the parent wants to participate in. Prepare a chair and area where the parent can relax in privacy.
2. To prepare the infant:
   a. Remove the infant's clothing except for a diaper.
   b. Place the infant vertically on the mother or father's chest between the breasts.
   c. Close the parent's gown around the baby and place a blanket over the infant.
3. To prepare the parent:
   a. Have the parent wear a scrub gown open in front with no other clothing over the chest.
   b. Assist the infant to position the head comfortably once placed on the parent's chest.
4. Monitor auxillary temperatures of the infant every 15 minutes. Remove the blanket if the infant's temperature is >37.3° C (99.2° F). Do not use heat lamps. Most infants will stay very warm next to their parents' skin.

TABLE 17-9	Levels of Kangaroo Care
Level	**Description**
Late K	Begins after the infant has survived the intensive care phase, has stable respirations, and is breathing room air. This can be days or weeks postbirth. This method is being studied experimentally in the United States and Europe.
Intermediate K	Begins after the infant has survived early intensive care, usually about 1 week postbirth. These infants often still require oxygen and may have periods of apnea and bradycardia. This method is being studied anecdotally and experimentally in Europe and the United States.
Early K	Begins as soon as the infant is stable postbirth, usually during the first day and often the first hours after birth. This is the method used in Bogotá, Colombia.
Very early K	Used with stable infants with Apgars above 6 who are returned to their mothers during the first minutes following birth. If the mothers are lying down, the infants are placed prone on their abdomens. These infants then stay with their mothers thereafter. This is being used by a few obstetricians.

From Anderson GC (1987). Personal communication. Used with permission. For updated information, please refer to Kenner C, Lott JW (2003): Neonatal nursing handbook. St Louis: Mosby.

BOX 17-4

Sample Mission Statements for Intensive Care Nurseries that Practice Family-Centered Care

Vision for the Special Care Nursery

The needs of a family, whose tiniest member has been admitted to our Special Care Nursery, are unique and may often seem indefinable. The moments of fear, helplessness, pain, and joy are common along this journey. It is our mission to assist you, the family, along each step of this journey and to prepare you for your return home. With this goal in mind, we offer the following beliefs as the foundation of our care:

- We recognize that the family is the constant in a child's life.
- We believe that the most essential component in the long-term outcome of an infant is the parent-child relationship.
- We believe that the parents do not "visit" their babies in the Special Care Nursery; rather, they provide care and parenting.
- We will create an environment that supports and protects the baby's individual abilities and the family's emerging parenting behavior.
- We believe that a partnership exists between families and health care professionals—a partnership that recognizes the expertise of each.
- We recognize that the family is a culture unto itself with different values and unique ways of realizing its dreams.
- We are committed to providing health care services that are flexible, culturally competent, and responsive to the family's identified needs.
- We believe that the goal of Special Care Nursery is to bring the baby back within the family's embrace by developing and nurturing the family's rightful role as primary care giver.

Interventions with Parents

The ability of the high-risk infant to organize physiologic responses and neurobehavioral activity after birth is crucial (1) in allowing the infant to respond more appropriately to his or her environment, of which the parents are an important part; (2) in providing the parents with a better understanding of their infant's unique rhythms; and (3) in supporting the infant's emerging organization and integration, making her or him more capable of coping with the home environment. Thus interventions with parents can help not only to enhance the infant's neurobehavioral organization and development but also to promote parent-infant interaction. To intervene with an infant without involving the parents ignores a major component of the infant's environment and self-regulatory capacities. In the long run, infants spend more time with their parents than with NICU staff. In many studies, the best predictors of later infant outcomes are not the NICU environment *per se* nor in the infant's health status but rather in parental variables and the home environment. Interventions with parents include the following recommendations: (1) personify the infant as a unique individual with strengths as well as limitations; (2) never discourage parent from touching the infant but help them know how to touch and to speak to infant before touching; (3) help parents identify, interpret, and respond to infant cues; (4) verify and confirm parent's observations about infant cues; (5) assist in identifying effective techniques for interacting with the infant; (6) model approaches appropriate to infant's status and maturity; (7) avoid remarks unfavorably comparing infant responses to parents versus staff; (8) encourage parents to personalize infant's environment; (9) involve parents in planning infant's care; (10) involve parents as early as possible in infant's care; (11) encourage and support touching and holding the infant as well as other caregiving; (12) encourage and support decision making and advocacy; (13) provide privacy; (14) provide anticipatory guidance as infant recovers and matures (Blackburn & Kang, 1991; Gale & Franck, 1998; McGrath & Conliffe-Torres, 1996).

APPLICATIONS OF INTERVENTION STRATEGIES TO SPECIFIC SITUATIONS

This section describes a variety of intervention strategies that can be used with individual infants according to their level of neurobehavioral development and health status. This section examines developmental interventions that the nurse might consider in planning care for infants that fall within specific groups: extremely preterm (very-low-birth-weight), growing preterm, and ill full-term infants; infants with BPD or requiring prolonged or repeated hospitalization; and infants born to mothers with a history of perinatal substance abuse. These areas are only for consideration, because, as emphasized earlier in the chapter, each infant needs to be assessed on an ongoing basis so that the plan of developmental care is individualized to that infant's unique needs, level of developmental function, and ability to tolerate environmental stimuli and other sensory input. Developmental interventions are also an important component in the management of infants experiencing pain (Chapter 42).

Extremely Preterm Infants

The traumatic and abrupt early transition from intrauterine to extrauterine life places the underdeveloped fetus in an incongruent and stressful situation (Als, 1982). In utero, this infant experienced a warm, comfortable, dimly lit, fluid-filled, and gently oscillating environment where basic physiologic, sensory, and motor needs were met. The extrauterine experience, in sharp contrast, provides a noisy, non-adaptive environment for which the fetus is unprepared but on which he or she must depend for survival. In utero, when he or she functions in an environment for which he or she is well adapted, the fetus is quite competent. However, a preterm infant in a NICU must cope with a continuous bombardment of inappropriate stimuli. Thus neonates who are born early must struggle to develop and maintain their autonomic, motor, and sensory systems in organized patterns of functioning in the midst of inappropriate, overwhelming stimuli. If the autonomic system is extremely immature, the infant is often overwhelmed just by the tasks of stabilizing this system, much less by achieving organization or recovering from illness.

The CNS of the preterm infant is well adapted for the intrauterine world at a time when the infant is forced to deal with the extrauterine environment. This leads to an environmental mismatch that influences brain development. The infant brain is undergoing major development and organization during this period. Als (1986, 1999) describes the brain of the immature infant as overly sensitive and at the mercy of sensory information, unable to buffer input because of the lack of inhibitory controls. Therefore the extrauterine environment strongly influences the development of the immature infant. Experiences such as repeated hypoxic events secondary to handling or environmental stimuli may negatively affect the infant's vulnerable brain, leading to permanent insults (Als, 1999; Als et al, 1986).

Inasmuch as the possibility of CNS dysfunction increases when the environment of the nursery provides overwhelming or inappropriate stimuli to an immature organism, caregivers must be aware of and seek to modify these experiences in relation to stressors from the physical environment (e.g., light, sound), caregiving activities and routines, and medical procedures. Very-low-birth-weight infants must first stabilize physiologically, and their behaviors are directed toward this end. Conservation of energy is critical in accomplishing this task and achieving homeostasis. If the tiny amounts of energy available are consumed in coping with overwhelming stimuli and handling, the infant will operate at a deficiency with no reserve. It becomes essential that caregivers interpret the infant's cues for stress and instability and work to protect the infant from the environment and the effects of caregiving interventions. Thus the primary goal in intervening to promote developmental competence in the very-low-birth-weight infant is to alter the environment and caregiving events that cause stress and interfere with physiologic homeostasis (VandenBerg & Franck, 1990).

This alteration can be accomplished by identifying the behaviors in the infant that indicate stress and disorganization and the events in the physical environment or associated with caregiving that trigger these behaviors. Interventions can then be provided that reduce the incidence of these stressful behaviors. This approach seeks to support the emergence of developmental maturation, energy conservation, and eventual recovery from acute illness. A primary area of intervention is to work with the parents to promote understanding of the infant's behavior and needs. Parents also need a participatory role in caregiving and in planning and carrying out the developmental protections. Specific intervention strategies for the very-low-birth-weight neonate are summarized in Table 17-10.

TABLE 17-10	Guide for Prevention and Management of Stress in Very-Low-Birth-Weight Infants	
Problem	**Goal**	**Method**

Environmental
Immature, vulnerable CNS
	Infant will be protected from environmental stimulation.	Reduce light:
		   Cover all bedsides, table beds, cribs, etc. with dark cloths or covers.
		Reduce noise:
		   Implement quiet hour and post signs at bedside to remind staff; pad trash cans, doors, drawers; pad loudspeakers at bedside.

Handling
Easily stressed by all or any procedures
	Infant will be prepared to tolerate and recover from procedures with minimal stress as expressed in autonomic/motoric reactions.	Before procedure:
		   Carry out procedure in stages if possible, allowing recovery and return to appropriate heart and respiratory rates or TcPO$_2$ after each step. Cluster care only as appropriate for individual infants. Some may need slow, continuous, gently efficient carrying out of all procedures, followed by rest. Pace according to individual cues.
		After procedure:
		   Continue positioning and containment up to 10 minutes or until infant is stable again, with heart and respiratory rates or TcPO$_2$ back to baseline, and has recovered tone.

Positioning Extended flaccid unsupported limbs Abducted hips Retracted shoulder Poor and variable muscle tone (from flaccid to hypertonicity)	Infant's limbs will be flexed; infant will be positioned in postures that permit flexion and minimize flailing, arching, and squirming.	Minimal handling protocol. Position prone/side lying. Support with blanket rolls. Swaddle, wrap to maintain flexion.
State Regulation Frequent agitation Erratic sleep Exhaustion/excessive fatigue *alertness*	Infant's sleep will be organized, agitation prevented, and energy and calories preserved for growth, not stress.	Modify environment to reduce stimulation. Position. Provide boundaries. Swaddle, contain. Handle slowly and gently. Cluster care and leave protected/undisturbed for 2- to 3-hour intervals (see minimal handling protocol). Avoid unnecessary stimulation.

From VandenBerg KA (1995). Behaviorally supportive care for the extremely premature infant. In Gunderson LP, Kenner C (Eds.). Care of the 24-25 week gestational age infant (small baby protocol), ed 2. Petaluma, CA: Neonatal Network. Reprinted by permission of NICU Ink®, Santa Rosa, CA.

Growing Preterm Infants

As preterm infants recover from their initial health problems and develop increasing neurobehavioral organization, their developmental needs change. Although these infants still need protection from aversive aspects of the environment, they also need increasing opportunities for positive interaction with that environment. Environmental interventions for these infants are directed at modifications to approximate the home environment, including diurnal cycling of light and sound.

By approximately 32 weeks' postconceptional age, infants have achieved enough autonomic regulation and homeostasis to begin to interact more actively with specific aspects of the environment, including caregivers. A primary focus during this period is promotion of state organization. Specific techniques are described in the previous section on state modulation. These infants will also benefit from opportunities for nonnutritive sucking and kangaroo care, both of which also influence state organization.

Interaction with caregivers and the physical environment can be facilitated by opportunities for increasing sensory input. Initially, this input must be unimodal, low-keyed, brief, and matched to the infant's behavioral capabilities and ability to tolerate. Social interaction and provision of sensory input should be matched with the appropriate state and should proceed in a graded fashion. Infants should be continuously observed for signs of sensory overload, and, if these occur, the stimuli should be reduced or removed (Als, 1999).

Parents and other caregivers must recognize that even when these infants are ready for discharge in terms of their physiologic status, they are still immature neurobehaviorally. Therefore it is critical that before discharge, parents learn to recognize how their infant indicates that he or she is stressed or sensorially overloaded, what circumstances and events tend to stress the infant, and what interventions are most effective to help the infant deal with stressful situations and reorganize. Table 17-11 provides suggestions for parents in providing routine care for their infant.

Full-Term Ill Infants

Full-term infants have an advantage over preterm infants in that they are better organized because of a more mature CNS. As a result, the full-term infant is better able to deal with the extrauterine environment and is ready for active social interaction. If this infant is critically ill, he or she may not be able to tolerate and interact with the environment in ways similar to a healthy infant's interactions. The major focus of developmental care for the ill full-term infant is on conservation of energy and reduction of stress so as not to further compromise physiologic stability and recovery processes while meeting the infant's developmental needs in a manner that is appropriate to his or her health status.

Environmental stressors from light, noise, traffic, and congestion must be reduced. Prone or side-lying positioning of the infant to maintain flexion, use of boundaries, and swaddling can facilitate energy conservation and stress reduction. Full-term infants are often irritable and commonly cry. Soothing interventions include containing and swaddling, reducing stimulation, holding the infant's hands and/or feet, positioning prone, and providing sucking opportunities. These infants may need minimal handling and sensory input during the period in which they are critically ill. The above recommendations are also appropriate for infants with cardiac problems.

As the infant recovers, he or she will be ready for more active interaction with caregivers and able to tolerate increased sensory input. Considerations in providing sensory input and in facilitating social responsiveness during the recovery period

TABLE **17-11**	Guidelines for Incorporating Developmental Principles into Daily Care for the Stable Growing Infant	
Caregiving	**Easily Stressed Infant**	**Well-Organized Infant**
Waking	Enter room slowly, turn on light, and open curtains or pull up shades slowly. Avoid arousing if in sleep. Vocalize softly. Uncover or unwrap gently. Avoid overstimulating, even if infant is difficult to arouse.	No special adjustment is required. Proceed slowly, noting stress and stability cues and helping infant maintain equilibrium.
Changing	Adjust room temperature. Avoid sudden changes in position. Contain limbs while shifting position. Keep tactile stimulation mild. Frequent consoling may be necessary, but allow infant to use own self-quieting mechanisms. Stop changing if infant demonstrates signs of instability.	As above.
Feeding	Attend to unique demands for feeding. Time feeding to coincide with spontaneous alert periods. Avoid unessential noise. Inhibit disorganized motor activity by wrapping or holding infant close to body. Adjust distance from caregiver to suit infant.	As above.
Bathing	As above, proceed slowly, watching for signs of exhaustion and disorganization (stress cues). Ventral openness may be disruptive. Ventral body surface inhibition may be needed, bracing hands or feet against hand or bedside. Cover body parts not being bathed. Offer support as needed in the form of a finger or pacifier. Allow frequent rests. Allow infant to organize self when possible.	As above.

Adapted from Rauh VA et al (1990). The mother-infant transactional program: The content and implications of an intervention for the mothers of low-birth weight infants. Clinics in perinatology, 17, 31-45.

are similar to those for the growing preterm infant. Intervention strategies for the full-term neonate are summarized in Table 17-12.

Infants with Bronchopulmonary Dysplasia (BPD)

The diagnosis of bronchopulmonary dysplasia (BPD) has significant serious consequences for the parents and staff as well as the infant. BPD is a disorder associated with a prolonged and complicated hospital course. Although BPD can develop in full-term infants, it is seen most frequently in preterm and low-birth-weight infants. Prolonged hospitalization jeopardizes developmental progress, as infants experience daily exposure to high levels of inappropriate patterns of sensory input from the hospital environment. This is compounded by restriction of movement from prolonged ventilation or need for supplemental oxygen and the loss of a consistent primary caregiver. These factors contribute to the higher incidence of developmental problems seen in these infants.

Infants with BPD demonstrate many complex behavioral difficulties, often in relation to signs of physiologic compromise. These infants' caregivers frequently identify agitation and stressful episodes as areas of major concern. Other problems include excessive energy expenditure, overreactivity to stimuli, poor self-regulation, repetitive motor behaviors, motor abnormalities, defensive behaviors, frantic activity, and poor feeding (VandenBerg & Franck, 1990).

Because of these behavioral difficulties, the infant with BPD presents several challenges to the NICU nurse. These infants are often unable to provide easily readable cues to signal the onset of severe stress, which often leads to physiologic compromise. The infant with BPD often has an all-or-nothing response to care. These infants may become quickly overstimulated, even from the most benign, routine handling. Instead of a grad-

ual arousal to crying, the infant will abruptly become hypoxic and dusky and will require immediate physiologic support. These infants do not typically demonstrate a gradual build-up of irritability or other signs of stress. It is extremely difficult to plan or organize care for such an unpredictable patient. State transitions are often unpredictable as well, which is frustrating for the caregiver, who must try to provide care while dealing with an infant who is calm one minute and severely stressed the next. Moreover, the usual soothing techniques of rocking, holding, and talking are not only ineffective; they often exacerbate the infant's stress (VandenBerg & Franck, 1990).

The preterm infant with BPD must also cope with an immature, vulnerable CNS. These infants may be behaviorally disorganized and thus overreact to their environment, unable to shut out stimuli effectively. This may occur at great physiologic cost to their systems and manifest in poor respiratory control, frequent desaturation, and/or a period of duskiness and cyanosis. The infant with BPD also has other physiologic stressors. The contribution of hypoxia, pain, bronchospasm, gastroesophageal reflux, and pharmacologic therapies such as diuretics and xanthine to the agitated state and behavioral disorganization must also be considered.

TABLE 17-12	Developmental Care for Full-Term Ill Neonates
Type of Strategy	**Examples of Interventions**
Minimize environment stress	Reduce noise levels
	Reduce light levels
	Reduce congestion
Energy conservation	Minimize environmental stress (see above)
	Individualize handling and use with appropriate timing
	Position infant to foster physiologic stability and state control and prevent agitation
	Provide opportunities for nonnutritive sucking
	Reduce pain (Chapter 42)
Promote neuro-behavioral organization	Incorporate developmental care principles into routine care activities (see Table 17-11)
	Promote state organization and state modulation
	Provide sensory experiences appropriate to infant's health status
	Involve parents in planning and implementing care

TABLE 17-13	Developmental Care for Infants with Bronchopulmonary Dysplasia
Type of Strategy	**Examples of Interventions**
Strategies for behavioral management	Modify environment (light, noise, etc.)
	Time handling to avoid overtiring and overstimulating
	Time daily events with appropriate infant states
	Adapt caregiving routines to individual infant's needs
	Read infant's subtle cues and provide prompt responses to prevent escalation of stress
	Minimize handling
Soothing strategies	Reduce activity around bedside
	Allow 2 to 3 hours of undisturbed rest between caregiving routines
	Plan nursing care activities around infant states
	Minimize stressful routines (i.e., suction PRN rather than per a schedule)
	Reduce activity at first subtle sign of stress (if holding, put back in bed prone; if playing with toys, hold quietly)
	Swaddle prone or side-lying with pacifier
	Make a ring of blanket rolls around baby and tuck in
	Provide sucking opportunities
	Provide opportunities for grasping

Adapted from Lund C (Ed), BPD: strategies for total patient care. Petaluma, CA: Neonatal Network. Reprinted by permission of NICU Ink®, Santa Rosa, CA.

The complex associations between the infant's behavior and physiologic compromise are not yet fully understood. Sedation is often used to manage the agitation of infants with chronic lung disease. The long-term implications of this type of management are unknown. Developmental care for the infant with BPD is essential for preventing and managing agitation in these infants. Applying behavioral and environmental interventions before pharmacologic interventions can, in many cases, prevent stress and eliminate or reduce the need for medication (VandenBerg & Franck, 1990).

The goals of developmental care for the infant with BPD include fostering self-regulation, which will help reduce agitation; preserving energy to promote growth; and supporting CNS organization and recovery. Specific strategies for working with these infants are listed in Table 17-13. An essential component of care of these infants is promoting understanding by parents of their infants' behavioral needs and providing opportunities for positive parent-infant interaction.

Infants who Require Prolonged or Repeated Hospitalization

The infant with BPD or the extremely-low-birth-weight ill infant (<800 g) will frequently have a lengthy hospital course that is often complicated by developmental delays. These infants must recover and achieve physiologic intactness before adequate developmental progress can be expected. Even after discharge, repeated hospitalizations accompanied by disruptions in feeding and recurring infections and other illness will certainly have an impact on a child's overall development and level of functioning. These delays are often transient, but they need careful and ongoing evaluation. As these infants recover, developmental progress usually escalates. Developmental care focuses on continued amelioration and resolution of the stresses of the family as well as on promotion of CNS organization in the infant.

Developmental interventions for these infants and their parents do not require the aggressive high-level approach necessary with the developmentally disabled infant who needs therapeutic enrichment. This population needs an approach that seeks to facilitate the normal acquisition of developmental skills while taking into account the individual coping behaviors and capacities of the recovering infant.

Developmental care of infants requiring prolonged or repeated hospitalization during infancy presents special challenges to caregivers in dealing with both physiologic and growth and developmental needs. Goldberger (1990) suggests that the goals of stimulation programs for these infants should be to modify the environment to provide adequate and appropriate developmental opportunities and maximized comfort and to enhance the parent's sense of competence and control. Interventions include: (1) limiting the number of caregivers; (2) encouraging internal and external rhythmicity and development of diurnal cycles; (3) responding appropriately, rapidly, and consistently to infant crying and other cues; (4) reducing fragmented sensory events, such as stomach filling by tube feeding, without opportunity for sucking and being held; (5) providing opportunities for coordinated multi-sensory events such as establishing eye contact with the infant while talking to him or her or reducing the use of radios to provide stimulation, when in actuality this becomes just white background noise; (6) providing predictability in routines and people and providing opportunities for learning cause and effect; (7) providing opportunity for variety, change, and novel situations;

(8) respecting the infant's personal space; and (9) providing age-appropriate play materials and opportunities for exploration (Goldberger, 1990).

COLLABORATIVE CARE

Both the assessment and management of neurobehavioral development involve a multidisciplinary, collaborative approach. Although the nurse is the primary early caregiver who will transfer care to the parents as the baby' recovers, most of the hands-on care is delivered by the nurse in the hospital. The nurse and parents practice in consultation and partnership, with members of other disciplines who can provide assessments, recommend family-focused developmental interventions and/ or specific therapies. Other professionals involved may include physical therapists, occupational therapists, infant educators, developmental specialists, neonatologists, and developmental psychologists. In addition, provision of consistent and individualized family-focused developmental care and modifications of the NICU environment require the support, understanding, and cooperation of all individuals in the nursery, including those who have direct (e.g., physicians, nurses, therapists, laboratory and x-ray technicians) and indirect (e.g., unit secretaries, cleaners) patient contact—all in collaboration with the parents and family.

To provide developmentally appropriate care, the NICU environment, caregiving practices, and caregiving routines must be evaluated on a regular basis. Barriers to providing this type of care can be identified, and strategies can be developed for changes. In most settings, it is unrealistic to expect to institute major changes all at once. Priorities for changes in the environment and care practices along with their advantages to the institution, staff, patients, and family need to be identified. The typical length of time to institute a fully implemented family-focused developmental program takes approximately five years (Als, 1999). It is often best to start with those practices that are likely to be the easiest to change, will generate the least resistance, and will lead to success immediately. The initial proposal for changes in family-focused developmental care can begin with a small group of committed nurse and other professionals.

The NIDCAP® Program

The NIDCAP® model is based upon implementing family-focused developmental care by using a specially trained developmental leadership staff. Family-focused developmental care becomes an established priority that is reflected in the NICU mission statement, allocation of staff and resources, and caregiving practices. Staff positions—including a developmental specialist and a developmental care nurse educator—are recommended. Training for staff is provided, and a developmental multidisciplinary team meets regularly to coordinate the programs. Time for reflective processing is recommended for evaluation of the process of implementation for individuals as well as the team.

The Wee Care® Program

The Wee Care® Program is a commercial program, which, as part of Children's Medical Ventures (CMV), offers a broad-based overview of developmental care theory and application of basic principles. Didactic classroom teaching activities are offered along with workshops to provide opportunities for participants to practice delivery of developmental care principles.

Small group discussions, role-playing, and hands-on practice are part of the methodology. Wee Care® consultants monitor and support the progress of implementation of developmental principles in the unit and provide additional mentoring for up to one year. Participants purchase developmental care products from CMV as part of their agreement.

SLEEP-WAKE STATES

Another aspect of neurobehavioral development that is considered as part of any developmental program is the sleep-wake states and how they impact on the response to stimuli. Sleeping and waking states are clusters of behaviors that tend to occur together and represent the level of arousal of the individual, the individual's responsivity to external stimulation, and the underlying activation of the central nervous system. Three states have been identified in adults: wakefulness, non-REM (rapid eye movement) sleep, and REM sleep. In infants, it is also possible to identify states within waking and states that are transitional between waking and sleeping because infants are less able to make rapid changes between states than are adults. Infants also have more difficulty sustaining alertness when awake. Because the electrophysiologic patterns associated with sleeping and waking states in infants are somewhat different from those in adults, the sleep states are usually designated active and quiet sleep, rather than REM and non-REM sleep.

Neonatal nurses need to be aware of the infant's present sleep-wake state and typical sleep-wake patterns when making assessments because infant behavior and physiology is affected by state. The functioning of cardiovascular, respiratory, neurologic, endocrine, and gastrointestinal systems differ in different states. Moreover, sleeping and waking states affect the infant's ability to respond to stimulation (Ariagno, 1996a, b). Thus infant responses to nursing interventions and to parental interactions depend to a great deal on the infant's when the stimulation begins. Timing routine interventions to occur when the infant is most responsive is an important aspect of some current systems of individualized nursing care (Als et al, 1986; Becker et al, 1991a) Finally, studies have indicated that sleeping and waking patterns are closely related to neurologic status. Thus aberrant sleep-wake patterns could potentially be used to identify infants at risk for neurologic complications or poor developmental outcome.

STATE SCORING SYSTEMS

In adults, sleeping and waking are usually scored by electroencephalography (EEG). However, because of the neurologic immaturity of infants, EEG is less reliable and needs to be combined with observation. When EEG and behavioral scoring of states in preterm infants are compared, there is a high degree of agreement (Sahni et al, 1995). Thus directly observing the infant and identifying global categories that are made up of a number of specific behaviors that tend to occur together and reflect a similar level of arousal and responsiveness to the environment, whether full-term or preterm, can validly score sleeping and waking states in newborn infants. Nurse researchers currently use four standardized systems for scoring behavioral observations of sleep-wake states. The systems were developed by Brazelton (1984), Thoman (1990), Als et al (1982), Anderson (1999), and Gill et al (1988). These systems define states in very similar ways and are probably equally useful for clinical purposes. Figure 17-7 presents a comparison of the state definitions used in these systems.

Clinicians and researchers differ in the ways they use these scoring systems. Neonatal nurses spend a lot of time observing infants and altering their care by assessing infant behavioral changes. Experienced clinicians are undoubtedly already familiar with the characteristics of sleeping and waking states in these infants even though they may be unable to name specific states. Thus all they need to do to include judgments of sleeping and waking states clinically is to use the state definitions of any standardized scoring system to systematize their clinical impressions.

For research, however, it is essential that the investigator receive training in the use of a particular scale so that the investigator is using it reliably. It is also important that clinicians reading research understand the differences among the scoring systems so that they can better interpret the findings and understand reports using different names for the same sleep-wake state.

Early State Scoring Systems

Sleeping and waking scoring systems for infants originate in the work of neurologists, pediatricians, and behaviorists in the 1960s. The neurologists needed a way to systematize the observations they made along with EEG studies, and behaviorists and pediatricians were particularly interested in the waking states and the effect of state on responsiveness to stimulation. Wolff (1959, 1966), a pediatrician, conducted extensive observations of newborn infants in the hospital and at home. As the result of his observations, he proposed a seven-state system. Prechtl and Beintema (1968), pediatric neurologists, proposed a simple five-state system that could be used either to score observations made along with EEG or to ensure that motor reflexes were elicited under optimal conditions. Finally, a team of pediatricians and neurologists at the University of California at Los Angeles (UCLA) developed a manual to define the behavioral and EEG criteria for sleeping and waking (Anders et al, 1971). Each of the state scoring systems currently in use is a refinement of these earlier systems.

Brazelton's State Scoring System

T. Berry Brazelton is a pediatrician from Harvard University in Cambridge, Massachusetts. He and his colleagues developed a state scoring system to be used as part of a behavioral evaluation of newborn infants, the Neonatal Behavioral Assessment Scale or NBAS (Brazelton, 1984). The purpose of this tool was to assess the individuality of the infant within the interactional process. This state scale was derived both from Dr. Brazelton's clinical experiences and from the existing state systems of Prechtl and Beintema (1968) and Thoman (1975). Brazelton's state scoring system consists of six states: deep sleep, light sleep, drowsy, alert, considerable motor activity, and crying. During the administration of the NBAS, this scoring system is used to identify predominant states, state transitions, and the quality of the alertness. However, it can also be used for scoring sleep-wake states during other situations. As of 1983, more than 100 papers had been published using the NBAS and Brazelton's state scale (Brazelton, 1984), and many more have been published since then.

Brazelton's state scoring system has a number of advantages that make it the scoring system of choice for clinicians and also useful for researchers. This state system is easy to learn because the differences between the states are fairly obvious and there are only six states. Because of the widespread use of Brazelton's state scoring system, individuals experienced with this scale are

Brazelton	Thoman	Als	Anderson
6. Crying	Cry	6B. Lusty crying	12. Hard crying
		6A. Crying	11. Crying
5. Considerable motor activity	Fuss	5B. Considerable activity	10. Fussing
	Non-alert waking	5A. Active	9. Very restless awake
			8. Restless awake
4. Alert	Alert	4B. Bright alert	7. Alert inactivity
		4AH. Hyper-alert	
		4AL. Awake and quiet	
3. Drowsy	Daze	3B. Drowsy	6. Quiet awake
	Drowse		5. Drowsy
	Sleep-wake transition	3A. Drowsy with more activity	4. Very restless sleep
2. Light sleep	Active sleep	2B. "Noisy" light sleep	3. Restless sleep
	Active-quiet transitional sleep	2A. Light sleep	2. Quiet sleep: irregular respiration
1. Deep sleep	Quiet sleep	1B. Deep sleep	1. Very quiet sleep
		1A. Very still deep sleep	

FIGURE **17-7**

Approximate equivalence of the four major sleep-wake state scoring systems. *Note:* Because the criteria used by these systems differ and because they are based on different conceptual frameworks, exact equivalence among them is not possible. Isolated instances of infant behavior may be scored quite differently than suggested by this table.

located in virtually every part of the United States. In addition, there are six reliability-training centers located throughout the country for those who want to use the entire NBAS or plan to use the state scoring system in research. Thus obtaining training in this scoring system is relatively easy. Finally, most researchers and experienced clinicians are familiar with the state definitions from this scale so that findings of sleeping and waking observations made with this scoring system are readily understood.

On the other hand, this state scoring system does have some limitations for use in research. First, because of the small number of states, it is not always sensitive enough to identify differences between normal full-term infants and infants with perinatal complications. Moreover, the NBAS state scoring system is appropriate for use only with infants between 36 and 44 weeks' gestational age (GA). The sleeping and waking states of infants born before 36 weeks' gestation and those born after 44 weeks' gestation will not be completely captured with this system. For example, older infants frequently are motorically active and alert during play, but in Brazelton's system, alertness is scored only when the infant is motorically quiet. Young preterm infants are frequently unable to make much sound when crying; thus their cry periods would be scored as considerable motor activity.

Thoman's State Scoring System

Evelyn B. Thoman is a psychobiologist who worked at the University of Connecticut. Although trained as an experimental psychologist to work with animals, she became interested in the interactions between human infants and their mothers when she went to work with Dr. Anneliese Korner at Stanford University in 1969 and has been studying them ever since. She developed her first state scoring system in 1975 (Thoman, 1975) based on the work of Wolff (1966) and Korner (1972). Although some researchers continue to use this system today, it has undergone considerable revision (Thoman, 1990). The Thoman state scoring system consists of 10 sleeping and waking states: alert, non-alert waking activity, fuss, cry, daze, drowse, sleep-wake transition, active sleep, active-quiet transitional sleep, and quiet sleep. Dr. Thoman and others have shown that both acceptable interrater reliability and test-retest reliability can be obtained with her system (Acebo, 1987; Holditch-Davis, 1990a; Holditch-Davis & Edwards, 1998a; Holditch-Davis & Thoman, 1987; Thoman et al, 1987). Predictive validity is demonstrated by evidence that early sleeping and waking behaviors scored on Thoman's scale are related to later developmental outcome (Becker & Thoman, 1981; Thoman et al, 1981).

Thoman's state scoring system has a number of advantages. The documented reliability and validity of this system is of value to researchers. The sleeping and waking states are differentiated enough that they can be used with infants with perinatal complications (Holditch-Davis and Thoman, 1987; Thoman et al, 1985, 1988). This system has been used with preterm infants (Holditch-Davis, 1990a) and with infants older than one month after term (Acebo, 1987; Holditch-Davis et al, 2000). The states in this system can also be combined when an investigator does not need such fine discriminations.

This scoring system has two disadvantages. First, a 10-state system is somewhat more difficult to learn than a 6-state system because it requires more subtle discriminations. However, individuals experienced in using a 6-state system, such as Brazelton's, can readily learn this system. Also, because this state scoring system is not used as widely used as Brazelton's, it is more difficult to obtain training in its use.

Als' State Scoring System

Heidelise Als is a psychologist working at Harvard Medical School with Dr. Brazelton and his colleagues. For a number of years, she has worked with these colleagues to modify the NBAS (Brazelton, 1984) to make it more appropriate for use with premature infants. The Assessment of Preterm Infants' Behavior (APIB) is administered in much the same way as the NBAS, but the infant's behavior is scored in much greater detail so as to quantify not only the infant's skills but also the infant's reactivity and stress in response to environmental stimulation (Als et al, 1982). Like the NBAS, the APIB is best administered to infants between 36 and 44 weeks' GA, but the observational portion of the tool can be used with younger preterm infants (Als, 1986). The state scale from the NBAS has been expanded into a 13-state system by subdividing each of the six states so that the immature and unclear sleeping and waking states of premature infants can be more adequately described. These 13 states are very still deep sleep, deep sleep, light sleep, "noisy" light sleep, drowsy with more activity, drowsy, awake and quiet, hyper-alert, bright alert, active, considerable activity, crying, and lusty crying. The state subscale of the APIB has been shown to differentiate between premature and full-term infants after term (Als et al, 1988; Mouradian et al, 2000) and to correlate with electrophysiologic measures of brain activity (Duffy et al, 1990). In addition, the APIB and the state subscale are used to provide assessments that are the basis for planning individualized interventions as part of the Neonatal Individualized Developmental Care and Assessment Program (NIDCAP) (Als, 1986; Als et al, 1986).

The Als' state scoring system has a number of advantages and disadvantages for clinicians and researchers. First, a 13-state system is more difficult to learn than a 6-state system such as Brazelton's (1984). However, since the Als system was developed from the Brazelton states, individuals familiar with the Brazelton system should have no difficulty learning it, and when the complexity of the 13 states is not needed they can be collapsed to the 6 states from the NBAS. Second, inasmuch as the APIB, like the NBAS, was never intended for use with infants older than 1 month after term, the state scale may not adequately capture the states of older infants. Finally, because the APIB is a relatively new scale, only a few research reports have been published using this state scoring system separately from the APIB (e.g., Van Cleve et al, 1995). The amounts of individual states exhibited by different groups of infants and developmental changes in each state have not been reported. Thus it is not yet clear how useful the Als scoring system is in describing the sleeping and waking patterns of infants.

Anderson's State Scoring System

Gene Cranston Anderson is a doctorally prepared nurse researcher working at Case Western Reserve University in Cleveland, Ohio. She has long been interested in interventions that keep mother and infant together after birth, reduce infant crying, and promote feeding. She developed a 12-state scoring system, the Anderson Behavioral State Scale (ABSS), to be used with preterm infants based on her own observations of these infants and on the work of Parmelee and Stern (1972). Parmelee was one of the contributors to the UCLA state manual (Anders et al, 1971). The ABSS consists of very quiet sleep, quiet sleep with irregular respirations, restless sleep, very restless sleep, drowsy, quiet awake, alert inactivity, restless awake, very restless awake, fussing, crying, and hard crying. The states are arranged so that there is a linear relationship between the states and heart rate and energy consumption, with the states with the lowest numbers having the lowest mean heart rates. The ABSS has been used to show the effects of prefeeding nonnutritive sucking (Gill et al, 1988) and kangaroo care (Ludington, 1990) on preterm infant state patterns.

As with the other scoring systems, the ABSS has a number of advantages and disadvantages for clinicians and researchers. As the newest state scoring scale, it has had only limited use outside of nursing. Thus the reliability and validity of this scale are not well established Because the ABSS was designed for use with preterm infants, the utility of this scale for full-term infants and older infants is unknown, although its similarity to other state scoring systems suggests that it should be applicable for healthy full-term newborn infants. The ABSS may also be difficult to learn because of the complexity of 12 states. As Figure 17-7 illustrates, the sleep states in this system differ markedly from the sleep states defined in other state scoring systems, so this is not a good scoring system to use if one is primarily interested in studying sleep states and wants to compare findings with other studies. Finally, the linear relationship between the states in this system and heart rate may make it the ideal choice for researchers who are primarily interested in studying the energy consumption of infants. However, this feature means the ABSS has a very different theoretical basis than the other state scales. The other state scoring systems differentiate among states based on qualitatively different aspects of the infant's behavior, but the ABSS emphasizes quantitative differences among the states, although Anderson has recently emphasized qualitative differences between states.

Description of Individual States

Because the definitions of sleep-wake states are so similar among these scoring systems (see Figure 17-7), it is possible to describe in general the sleeping and waking states displayed by infants. For clarity's sake, generic state names will be used in all further descriptions. When they are not available, the state names from the Thoman system will be used. Each sleeping and waking state is made up a different constellation of behaviors and serves a different function for the infant. Physiologic functioning is also different in each of these states.

Infants are most responsive to the environment when in the waking states, and, in particular, when alert. When the infant is alert, the eyes are open and scanning. Motor activity is typically low, particularly in full-term newborns, but premature infants and infants older than 1 month after term may be motorically active. Alertness is the state in which the infant exhibits focused attention on sources of stimulation (Brazelton, 1984). Thus this is the best state in which to test reflexes (Prechtl & Beintema, 1968) and take measures of attention. Alertness has been suggested to be the optimal state for feeding. This state is also the one in which infants are most receptive to interactions with their parents and other adults. Yet alertness rarely occurs in the preterm period (Holditch-Davis, 1990a; Holditch-Davis & Edwards, 1998a) and occurs relatively infrequently during the first month after term, only about 10 to 15% of the total day.

Crying, another waking state, serves a communication function. However, the meaning of cries differs in different situations and may depend on their intensity. Although crying that occurs when the infant is alone may elicit parental attention, crying that occurs during social exchanges may actually disrupt the parent-infant relationship. In full-term infants, crying during social interactions is related to the overall amount of maternal stimulation and to consistency in the patterning of maternal activities over weeks. In both studies, infants exhibiting the highest amounts of social crying received less appropriate maternal stimulation. Crying in ill infants can have adverse effects.

The final waking state, non-alert waking activity, is characterized by periods when the infant is motorically active but not alert or crying. Usually the infant's eyes are open. One study of non-alert activity found that excess amounts of this state in full-term infants is associated with inconsistency in the patterning of states over weeks and, in turn, inconsistency in state patterning is related to poor developmental outcome. Premature infants, after term, exhibit elevated levels of this state (Holditch-Davis & Thoman, 1987) and are known to be at increased risk of poor developmental outcome (Hack et al, 2000; Rickards et al, 2001). However, whether there is a relationship between these findings is unknown.

The states transitional between sleeping and waking have rarely been studied. In fact, the Prechtl scoring system omits them altogether on the grounds that they are not true states but just transitions between states. However, newborn infants, both term and preterm, actually spend significant amounts of time in them, ranging from about 6% of the day at 29 weeks' GA to 14% in the first month after term (Holditch-Davis, 1990a; Holditch-Davis & Thoman, 1987). Thoman (1985) describes three states transitional between waking and sleeping: drowse, when the infant is quiet and appears sleepy with eyes opening and closing slowly; daze, when the infant is quiet with eyes that are open but dazed in appearance; and sleep-wake transition, when the infant exhibits mixed signals of waking and sleeping, is motorically active, and may appear to be waking up. Drowse and daze typically occur in the midst of periods of waking or as the infant is falling asleep. Sleep-wake transition typically occurs at the end of sleeping as the infant is awakening but may also occur in the middle of sleep particularly in premature infants. Drowse, daze, and sleep-wake transition are often combined in research reports. However, studies have indicated that these states have different patterns of correlations with other states (Thoman et al, 1987). During the first month after term, premature infants have been found to spend significantly more time in sleep-wake transition and less time in drowse or daze than full-term infants (Holditch-Davis & Thoman, 1987). If these three states had been combined, these differences would have been missed. In addition, hospitalized preterm infants spend more time in sleep-wake transition when they are with nurses rather than parents but do not differ in the amount of drowsiness that occurs with these different caregivers (Miller & Holditch-Davis, 1992). They also exhibit more sleep wake-transition and less drowsiness during procedural care than during feeding and changing (Brandon et al, 1999).

There are two major sleep states—active sleep and quiet sleep—although some state systems define a transitional state between them. In active sleep, the infant's respiration is uneven and primarily costal in nature. Sporadic motor movements occur, but muscle tone is low between these movements. The most distinct characteristic of this state is rapid eye movements that occur intermittently.

Active sleep is the most common state from birth throughout infancy, but it occurs only during about 20% of sleep in adults. Because of this dramatic developmental decrease and the frequent movements seen in infants during active sleep, many clinicians think of active sleep as a disorganized and primitive state. Surprisingly, this state has relatively recent phylogenetic origins, occurring only in birds and mammals. Thus it has been hypothesized to be necessary for brain development. This hypothesis has received support in full-term infants (Denenberg & Thoman, 1981). In animal studies, prolonged deprivation of active sleep in infancy permanently altered brain functioning and resulted in hyperactivity, distractibility, and altered sexual performance (Mirmiran, 1986). Inasmuch as respiratory patterns are relatively unstable in active sleep (Haddad et al, 1987) and oxygenation is lower and more variable (Gabriel et al, 1980; Martin et al, 1979), the large amount of active sleep seen in young preterm infants (Holditch-Davis, 1990a; Holditch-Davis & Edwards, 1998a) may contribute to their respiratory difficulties.

The other sleep state, quiet sleep, is characterized by a lack of body movements and the presence of regular respiration. A tonic level of motor tone is maintained in this state. The major purpose of quiet sleep seems to be rest and restoration. This state has been hypothesized to be necessary for healing. Quiet sleep may also be needed for growth because it is in this state that growth hormone is secreted in adults. However, a study of full-term infants did not find any relationship between growth hormone secretion and quiet sleep. Oxygenation is higher during this sleep state; thus quiet sleep may be beneficial for infants with respiratory problems.

The amount of quiet sleep is also very sensitive to the environment. Infant stimulation studies, for example, have found that quiet sleep is the state most likely to be increased by vestibular and kinesthetic interventions (Ingersoll & Thoman, 1994). The stimulation provided by routine nursing care, on the other hand, results in significantly less quiet sleep as compared with times when the preterm infant is undisturbed (Brandon et al, 1999; Holditch-Davis, 1990b), and the amount of this state is further reduced when the infant experiences painful or uncomfortable procedures (Holditch-Davis & Calhoun, 1989). Thus this is the state most likely to be affected by the NICU environment.

EFFECT OF PHYSIOLOGIC PARAMETERS ON STATE

Physiologic functioning varies in different states. In turn, abnormalities in physiologic functioning can alter the sleeping and waking states of infants. This discussion focuses on the interrelationship of sleeping and waking and four areas of physiologic functioning of interest to neonatal nurses—perinatal illness, the central nervous system, circulatory system, and respiration.

Perinatal Illness

The state patterns of infants who experienced perinatal complications may differ markedly from the state patterns of healthy full-term infants. Small-for-gestational-age full-term infants, for example, have more disorganized sleep as evidenced by more active sleep without rapid eye movements than healthy full-term infants and more quiet sleep with ocular movements. They also exhibited poorer responsiveness during alertness as measured by the NBAS.

The sleep of premature infants after term is known to differ from that of full-term infants of the same corrected ages, in that there is a decreased total amount of sleep, longer episodes of quiet sleep, more body movements, more frequent REM episodes, and somewhat lower correlation among the various behavioral criteria of the sleep states. Premature infants show day-night differentiation in their sleeping and waking patterns

at the same or an earlier post-conceptional age than full-term infants (Shimada et al, 1993; Whitney & Thoman, 1994). In addition, their EEG patterns differ from those of full-term infants. Premature infants display longer bursts during trace alternans, earlier sleep spindle appearance, more immature EEG patterns, and poorer phase stability for EEG frequencies. Premature and full-term infants also differ on architectural, phasic, continuity, spectral, and autonomic measures (Scher et al, 1992b, 1994b, 1994c).

The ways that the waking states differ between full-term and premature infants of similar post-conceptional ages are less well established. The results of studies using relatively brief assessments have been contradictory. Premature infants have been found to be less, more, or equally alert and less, more, or equally irritable than full-term infants. However, over prolonged observation periods, premature infants exhibited more alertness and non-alert waking activity and less drowsiness than full-term infants (Holditch-Davis & Thoman, 1987).

The severity of illness that the infant experiences during the perinatal period has relatively small additional effects on sleeping and waking. In general, critical illness has immediate effects on sleeping and waking patterns, but these effects disappear after the infant recovers as long as there are no neurologic complications and as long as infants are observed at same ages corrected for GA at birth. Karch and colleagues (1982) studied healthy and ill preterm infants at comparable ages and found that ill infants exhibited more quiet sleep, more indeterminate sleep, and less wakefulness. The ill infants in this study were examined while on mechanical ventilation. Thus the state differences reflect the immediate influence of critical illness and mechanical ventilation. Preterm infants ill with respiratory distress syndrome have been found to exhibit delayed state development but show state patterns comparable to healthy preterm infants' once they recover. Doussard-Roosevelt et al (1996) found that preterm infants with more medical complications showed more active sleep during brief sleep observations at 33 to 35 weeks than healthier preterm infants. Curzi-Dascalova et al (1993) found that the longest sleep cycle of mechanically ventilated preterm infants was shorter than that of non-ventilated infants. Holditch-Davis and Hudson (1995) used changes in sleep-wake to identify a wide variety of acute medical complications in preterm infants, including hydrocephalus, sepsis, and cold stress. Infant medical complications also affected the scores of infants on standardized neurobehavioral assessments but only on items requiring vigorous responses (e.g., vigor of crying, irritability, and motor development) but not on other state items, including alertness and percent sleeping (Korner et al, 1994).

Studies of infants who have recovered from their illnesses have found fewer differences. High and Gorski (1985) did not find any differences in the sleeping and waking patterns of convalescent premature infants differing in the severity of their previous illness. Likewise, Holditch-Davis (1990a) found that the only difference in the development of sleeping and waking states in convalescent preterm infants was that more severely ill infants showed less fussing and somewhat poorer organization of quiet sleep. Als et al (1988) found no difference in the state organization of premature infants born at less than 33 weeks' GA and premature infants born between 33 and 37 weeks' GA when state organization was measured two weeks after term. In addition, scores on the NBAS state scale did not differ significantly between sick and healthy full-term infants at the time of hospital discharge.

Infants with chronic lung disease are more likely than other premature infants to have oxygen desaturations when sleeping. Yet it is unclear whether this illness has any effect on sleeping and waking patterns. Holditch-Davis and Lee (1993) compared high-risk preterm infants with and without chronic lung disease from 32 to 36 weeks' post-conceptional age on sleep-wake states and sleep organization exhibited over 4-hour observations in the intermediate care unit. The only difference between the infants with and without chronic lung disease was that infants with chronic lung disease had more irregular respiration in quiet sleep. Despite the fact that many clinicians believe that infants with chronic lung disease are more sensitive to stimulation, there were also no differences in sleeping and waking when the infants with and without chronic lung disease were with caregivers (Holditch-Davis, 1995). However, at term age, premature infants with chronic lung disease had less active sleep, more frequent arousals, and more frequent body movements in sleep than premature infants who never experienced any respiratory illnesses and performed more poorly on the interactive and motor clusters of the NBAS (Myers et al, 1992).

Neurologic System

Because sleeping and waking states are assumed to reflect the underlying activation of the central nervous system (CNS), it is not surprising that close relationship exists between sleep-wake states and CNS functioning. Four factors illustrate this interrelationship. First, sleeping and waking exhibit a large amount of development in the first year of life, the time of the most rapid CNS development. Sleeping and waking state affect neurologic responses. Infants with neurologic abnormalities exhibit abnormal sleeping and waking patterns. Finally, sleeping and waking states can be used to predict developmental outcome.

Development of Sleeping and Waking States. Infants exhibit definite developmental changes in their sleeping and waking state patterns throughout the first year of life. The age at which sleep-wake states first appear is unknown. The earliest study of sleeping and waking in preterm infants younger than 30 weeks' GA found that these infants had only a single active sleep-like state, but these findings are questionable because all of the infants in this study were dying at the time of the state recordings. More recent studies of preterm infants have found that by 24 weeks' GA, cycling between waking and sleeping can be identified by EEG in some preterm infants. By 27 weeks' GA (the earliest age studied), infants exhibit distinct waking and sleeping states (Holditch-Davis, 1990a; Holditch-Davis & Edwards, 1998a). However, before 30 weeks' GA, the various behaviors associated with sleep and waking—eye movements, body movements, respiration, and muscle tone—are not well coordinated; not until at least 36 weeks' GA do preterm infants exhibit the same degree of correlation between these parameters as do full-term infants. Studies of sleeping and waking states in fetuses conducted using observations made during ultrasound examinations have had similar findings (DiPietro et al, 1996).

Infants exhibit greater amounts of active sleep and indeterminate states during the preterm period and lower amounts of waking states than after term (Holditch-Davis, 1990a; Holditch-Davis & Edwards, 1998a). Active sleep occupies as much as 60% to 70% of the day for young preterm infants (Holditch-Davis, 1990a; Holditch-Davis and Edwards, 1998a) and is further increased during acute illness. The major devel-

opmental change during the preterm period is a decrease in the amount of sleep due a decrease in active sleep (Holditch-Davis, 1990a; Holditch-Davis & Edwards, 1998a; Ingersoll & Thoman, 1999). In addition, quiet sleep and waking states, especially crying, increase (Holditch-Davis, 1990a; Holditch-Davis & Edwards, 1998a; Vles et al, 1992). The organization of the sleep states, as measured by the percentages of the state with typical state criteria or by the correlation between criteria, also increases throughout the preterm period (Holditch-Davis, 1990a; Holditch-Davis & Edwards, 1998a). The mean duration and frequency of episodes of each state also change over the preterm period: quiet waking, active waking, and sleep-wake transition episodes occurred more frequently than active waking and quiet sleep but length of these periods increased over age (Ariagno, 1996a, b; Holditch-Davis & Edwards, 1998b; Ingersoll & Thoman, 1999).

The sleeping and waking states of infants in the first month after term differ dramatically from those of preterm infants. Healthy full-term neonates spend approximately 40% of the daytime in active sleep and 20% in quiet sleep. Slightly higher amounts of sleep states occur at night (Thoman & Whitney, 1989; Whitney & Thoman, 1994). Waking states make up the rest of the day, with alertness (14%) and drowsiness (13%) being the most common (Holditch-Davis & Thoman, 1987).

The major developmental trends exhibited by full-term infants in the first month are a decrease in active sleep and an increase in the amount of alertness. Moreover, the mean lengths of episodes of the sleep states change, with active sleep decreasing and quiet sleep increasing. Similar trends occur for premature infants during this period (Holditch-Davis & Thoman, 1987; Whitney & Thoman, 1994). In addition, both full-term and premature infants begin to show entrainment to a day-night schedule of sleeping and waking by about a month after term (Shimada et al, 1999).

Sleeping and waking states continue to develop throughout the first year. Waking periods become longer and more consolidated. The infant spends an increasing proportion of wakefulness in the alert state and gains the ability to remain alert while crying (Acebo, 1987). The amount of time spent crying decreases (Michelsson et al, 1990; St. James-Roberts & Plewis, 1996). In addition, total sleep time decreases, with almost all of this decrease due to a decrease in active sleep time (Holditch-Davis et al, 1999; St. James-Roberts & Plewis, 1996). The amount of quiet sleep remains the same or increases from term age on; thus by about 6 months of age, the amount of quiet sleep exceeds the amount of active sleep. The nature of these changes depends somewhat on feeding type, as breastfed infants exhibit longer sleep latency, more non-REM sleep, and shorter duration of REM sleep than formula-fed infants do (Butte et al, 1992). In addition, the number of sleep episodes decreases and becomes consolidated primarily into nighttime, although most infants continue to exhibit some amount of night waking (Ottaviano et al, 1996; Scher, 1991). By 1 year, the infant is taking about two daytime naps (Weissbluth, 1995) and sleeping about 10 to 12 hours through the night. Prematurely born infants may display shorter night sleep and more night wakenings than full-term infants.

Other developmental changes during the first year affect the organization of sleep. The cycling between active and quiet becomes more consistent over the first few months, and by 4 months of age, the complete sleep cycle first exhibits a standard length of about 1 hour. Many preterm infants display hour-long sleep cycles by 36-week post-conceptional age

(Borghese et al, 1995). The sleep states also develop the EEG patterns typical of adults. By 3 months of age, the EEG stages within quiet sleep can be identified, and this sleep state can now be called non-REM sleep.

Neurologic Responses.   Infants exhibit different neurologic responses in different sleeping and waking states. The magnitude of neurologic reflexes is known to differ greatly in different states. Therefore standardized infant assessments and neurologic examinations specify which states are optimal for testing each reflex (Brazelton, 1984; Prechtl & Beintema, 1968). The amplitude, wave form, and latency of visual evoked potentials are different in different sleeping and waking states with the greatest differences being between sleep and waking (Apkarian et al, 1991).

Neurologic Problems.   The state patterns of infants with neurologic insults differ markedly from those of healthy infants. Infants with Down syndrome have been found to spend more time awake and to have abnormally long periods of quiet sleep. At term, premature infants with intraventricular hemorrhage have been found to have lower arousal using the NBAS than healthy full-term infants. Full-term infants with hyperbilirubinemia show decreased amounts of wakefulness. As compared to full-term infants with only mild bilirubin elevations, infants with moderately elevated bilirubin values exhibit significantly lower scores in state regulation and range on the NBAS and exhibit minor neurologic abnormalities as shown by increased latency of brain stem auditory evoked potentials. Infants who eventually died from sudden infant death syndrome (SIDS) moved less during sleep, had more REM in the newborn period, and showed less waking in the early morning hours than control infants (Kahn et al, 1992; Schechtman et al, 1992), and male infants at high risk for SIDS fail to show an increase in wakefulness with age (Cornwell, 1993). Abnormal cry patterns have been found in infants who have neurologic injuries or hyperbilirubinemia or are at risk for SIDS (Corwin et al, 1995). Milder insults, such as slight hyperbilirubinemia not requiring phototherapy, have not been found to affect infant sleeping and waking.

In addition, infants exposed prenatally to drugs or alcohol exhibit abnormalities in their state patterns possibly as the result of neurologic insults caused by the drugs. For example, alcohol-exposed infants exhibit sleep disruptions and abnormal cries (Nugent et al, 1996). Infants exposed to marijuana have shorter, higher cries with more variation in frequency (Lester & Dreher, 1989) and exhibit a decrease in quiet sleep time. Methadone-exposed infants exhibit abnormal cries with short first expirations. They are more irritable and less able to sustain a high quality alert state. Newborn infants of mothers who smoked during pregnancy spend less time in active and quiet sleep and less time awake and have higher cries than did infants whose mothers did not smoke (Kotzer, 1994; Nugent et al, 1996). Infants who were prenatally exposed to cocaine showed less active sleep and more indeterminate sleep. They also scored less positively on NBAS in the areas of orientation, state regulation, and autonomic regulation clusters than drug-free infants (Black et al, 1993; Regalado et al, 1995). On the other hand, Woods and colleagues (1993) did not find any differences on the NBAS between cocaine-exposed and drug-free infants (Chapter 39).

Prediction of Developmental Outcome.   Finally, the organization of sleeping and waking, as indicated by individual state criteria or the overall patterning of states, can be used to predict the developmental outcome of infants. In healthy preterm infants, lower spectral EEG energies predicted lower neurodevelopmental performance at 12 and 24 months (Scher et al, 1994a). Low levels of trace alternans, an EEG pattern seen during quiet sleep in neonates, is predictive of lower intelligence quotients (IQs) in premature infants (Beckwith & Parmelee, 1986), and delayed maturity of EEG patterns of preterm infants was found to be associated with poor neurologic outcome. More sleep-wake transition, shorter sleep periods, and fewer arousals from quiet sleep during the first day of life in full-term infants are associated with lower developmental scores at 6 months. Elevated amounts of intense bursts of rapid eye movements and long sleep-cycle lengths at 6 months are associated with developmental problems in full-term infants (Borghese et al, 1995). Acoustic characteristics of infant cries have been used to predict developmental outcome in preterm infants and infants who were prenatally exposed to drugs. Measures of sleep-wake states during the preterm period—including the amount of crying during gavage feedings, the overall quality of state organization as compared with other infants, sleep cycle length—have been found to predict Bayley scores during the first year and measures at term have been shown to relate to developmental outcome at age 8. However, the amount of indeterminate sleep—any period not meeting the criteria for one of the five states defined by Prechtl and Beintema (1968)—in premature infants at term was not related to developmental status at 2 years (Maas et al, 2000). The development of particular sleep behaviors during the first year after term was related to the outcome of premature infants. In apparently normal full-term infants, the stability of state patterns in the first month has been found to predict developmental outcome. This finding has been replicated using EEG measures of state in groups of hospitalized preterm infants, in premature infants after term (Whitney & Thoman, 1993), and in siblings of infants who died from SIDS (Thoman et al, 1988).

Circulatory System

Sleeping and waking states affect the infant's circulatory system. Overall, heart rate is higher in waking than sleeping states, and particularly during crying (Ludington, 1990). Mean heart rates in the two sleep states are very similar, but heart rate is more variable in active sleep (Galland et al, 2000). This difference in variability is large enough that it is possible to differentiate between the two sleep states on the basis of heart rate variability. Thus neonatal nurses need to be aware of the infant's state when determining heart rate, and routine vital signs probably should not be obtained while the infant is crying.

Sleeping and waking states also affect the infant's circulation. Cerebral blood flow is highest in waking. It is significantly higher in active sleep than in quiet sleep in full-term infants but not in infants less than term age. Variability in cerebral blood flow velocity is lowest in quiet sleep, whereas marked fluctuations occur in active waking (fussing and non-alert waking activity). Minor variations in cerebral blood flow velocity occur in active sleep. Blood pressure is slightly higher when the infant is awake than when asleep.

Respiration

The effect of sleeping and waking states on the respiratory system is even greater than on the circulatory system. The nervous system controls of breathing are different in different states (Phillipson, 1978). During wakefulness, breathing is regulated by metabolic controls, general stimulation from the reticular activating system, and voluntary activities. In quiet sleep, metabolic controls predominate, and maintaining acid-base and oxygen homeostasis is the primary stimulus for breathing. Medullary respiratory center activity varies during active asleep depending on whether the infant is experiencing rapid eye movements and motor activity (phasic active sleep) or not (tonic active sleep), indicating that these two types of active sleep include different controls on breathing. During phasic active sleep, behavioral controls, similar to the voluntary controls in waking, predominate. In tonic, active sleep, the major respiratory control results from direct stimulation of the state in a manner similar to the reticular stimulation of respiration during wakefulness. As a result of these different controls, infants exhibit higher respiratory rates and lower tidal volumes in phasic active sleep than in tonic active sleep.

Respiratory activity responds differently to chemical stimulation in different states. Baseline arterial oxygen and carbon dioxide levels are lower in active sleep than in either waking or quiet sleep, possibly because of hypoventilation or ventilation-perfusion inequalities in this state. Ventilation is increased in response to hypoxia in all states, but this hyperventilation is not maintained in active sleep. In addition, arousal in response to hypoxia is slower in active sleep. Response to hypercapnia is also different in different states. There is a shift to the right in the carbon dioxide response curve in quiet sleep as compared to waking. This response is further reduced in tonic active sleep and is absent in phasic active sleep.

As a result of these differing neurologic controls on breathing, a number of respiratory variables in both full-term and preterm infants are influenced by sleep and waking states. Respiration rates are higher and more variable in active sleep. Active sleep has also been shown to result in hypoventilation in preterm infants because of central inhibition of spinal motoneurons and poor coordination between chest and abdominal muscles. Thus paradoxic movements of the chest wall and abdominal muscles during breathing are common during active sleep in preterm infants. However, it is not clear whether lung volume is decreased in active sleep in full-term infants. Expiratory volumes and flow rates are larger in waking than in sleeping infants.

The frequency of central apnea is also different in different sleep states. Central apnea rarely occurs during waking. Most studies indicate that brief apneic pauses of less than 20 seconds in length occur more frequently in active sleep than quiet sleep in both full-term and preterm infants (Holditch-Davis et al, 1994; Vecchierini et al, 2001). The effects of sleep state on the frequency of periodic respiration (cyclic breathing alternating with brief apneic pauses) are less clear. Some studies found that periodic respiration occurs more frequently in active sleep, whereas others found no difference in periodic respiration frequency in the two sleep states (Holditch-Davis et al, 1994). The mean length of apneic pauses is longer in quiet sleep (Holditch-Davis et al, 1994), apparently because of a lower incidence of apneas less than 6 seconds in length in quiet sleep rather than because of an increased incidence of longer apneas. In addition, a variety of stresses, including an increase in body temperature and sleep deprivation, have been shown to increase apnea frequency, primarily in active sleep (Gaultier, 1994).

However, it cannot be concluded from these studies that pathologic apneas (apneic episodes longer than 20 seconds and usually associated with bradycardia and hypoxemia) are more common in active sleep because these studies rarely included episodes of pathologic apnea. Infants in these studies were usually older than 36 weeks' GA, even though the peak age for pathologic apnea is less than 32 weeks' GA. Even when infants of the correct ages are studied, pathologic apnea is often too rare to permit statistical analyses comparing states (Holditch-Davis et al, 1994). One study of older infants being treated for prolonged apnea did not find any difference in the rate of brief respiratory pauses in the two sleep states, nor did the frequency of brief pauses differ from that found in healthy infants. Yet some association may exist between active sleep and pathologic apnea inasmuch as the methylxanthines, caffeine and theophylline, used to treat this condition are known to increase the amount of wakefulness and decrease the amount of active sleep in addition to their direct effects on respiration.

EFFECT OF NURSING INTERVENTIONS ON STATE

Sleeping and waking states are also affected by the types and timing of stimulation that the infant receives from the environment. Thus nursing interventions have the potential to either promote state organization or to disrupt it. The effects of four common nursing interventions—routine NICU care, painful procedures, social interaction, and infant stimulation—on infant sleeping and waking are examined in this section.

Effect of Environmental Stimulation

Investigators have suggested that the hospital provides stimulation that is inappropriate for the development of premature infants and is likely to result in disorganized sleeping and waking patterns. The NICU provides infants with an extremely bright and noisy environment with little diurnal variation and frequent interventions for technical procedures but little positive handling (Zahr & Balian, 1995). The sickest infants actually receive the most handling (Zahr & Balian, 1995) even though they lack the physiologic reserves to cope with it. These infants become hypoxic in response to virtually any form of stimulation: noise, technical procedures, and social touches. The severity of the negative physiological responses to one procedure, endotracheal suctioning, has been related to the infant's state during the procedure (Bernert et al, 1997). Preterm infants who cried during suctioning had greater changes in oxygenation and heart rate than infants who slept through suctioning. Moreover, some researchers have suggested that these reductions in oxygenation in response to handling may actually be the result of changes in sleeping and waking states. Convalescent infants receive less handling than ill infants but do experience social interactions as a greater proportion of their care.

Several of the aspects of routine NICU care are known to contribute to disruption of infant sleeping and waking patterns. Nursing and medical interventions frequently result in state changes. The frequency of these interventions in the NICU has been found to be as high as five times per hour. Preterm infants change their sleep-wake states about six times per hour, and 78% of these changes are associated with either nursing interventions or NICU noise (Zahr & Balian, 1995). Preterm infants are rarely able to sustain quiet sleep during nursing interventions (Brandon et al, 1999; Holditch-Davis, 1990b) and usually awaken with each intervention. Inasmuch as infants fall asleep in active sleep, frequent nursing interventions are particularly likely to reduce the amount of quiet sleep that the infant experiences. These sleep disruptions result in increased waking and, in particular, crying time. Preterm infants normally spend only a small percentage of their time in waking states (Holditch-Davis, 1990a), but this percentage increases significantly when they are with nurses (Brandon et al, 1999; Holditch-Davis, 1990b). Also, developmental changes in the amount of waking occur only over the time infants are with nurses, and the distribution of states differs depending on the nursing activity with active waking more common and drowsiness less common during more intrusive care (Brandon et al, 1999).

In addition, neonatal nurses and physicians seldom consider infant sleep-wake states and other infant cues when choosing the time for routine interventions. Although two studies found relationships between nursing care and sleeping and waking for groups of preterm infants (Barnard & Blackburn, 1985; Lawson et al, 1985), these results probably represent infant reactions to nursing care or infants conditioned to anticipate regular nursing procedures rather than nurses responding to infant states. Infant activity has been found to decrease after nursing interventions (Blackburn & Barnard, 1985). Gottfried (1985) found that nurses responded to fewer than half the cries of convalescent premature infants. Then too, meeting infant social needs is not a nursing priority. Linn et al (1985) found no relation between staff-patient ratio and the amount of positive handling infants received. Yet a lack of responsiveness to infant cues may serve to slow the development of stable diurnal patterns of sleeping and waking that several investigators have suggested is the first task of infancy (Barnard & Blackburn, 1985). Full-term infants receiving responsive care develop day-night differentiation in their sleeping and waking in 5 to 7 days, whereas this differentiation is delayed when the care is not responsive.

In light of the American Academy of Pediatrics (1992) recommendation that infants be placed on their backs to sleep, the effects of positioning on infant sleep-wake states also need to be considered. Full-term infants in the supine position show greater wakefulness, less quiet sleep, lower heart rates, higher rates of brief respiratory pauses, and better airway protection during sleep than when prone (Jeffrey et al, 1999; Skadberg & Markestad, 1997). Similar effects on sleeping and waking, heart rate, and oxygenation have been found in growing preterm infants and in preterm infants with chronic lung disease (Goto et al, 1999; Martin et al, 1995; McEvoy et al, 1997; Myers et al, 1998). Thus supine positioning may not be appropriate for preterm infants with respiratory compromise; moreover, in preterm infants who are no longer acutely ill, positioning decisions will require balancing infant needs for rest and oxygenation with the need to provide an example for parents.

Finally, the lighting of the NICU, as discussed earlier in this chapter, contributes to sleeping and waking problems in infants. Lighting in most NICUs is continuous, high-level, and fluorescent. However, researchers have hypothesized that continuous light can result in endocrine changes, changes in biologic rhythms, and sleep deprivation during the NICU stay (Blackburn, 1996). The frequency of eye opening and waking states is related to the level of illumination in the NICU; less eye opening occurs when the lights are brightest. Sudden decreases in lighting result in increased eye opening (Moseley et al, 1988). This finding supports the common nursing and parental intervention of shading infant eyes with one's hand to elicit alertness. In addition, infants exposed to NICUs that vary the intensity of lighting on a diurnal pattern open their eyes significantly more than those exposed to continuous illumination.

In view of the problems with routine NICU care, it is not surprising that several researchers have attempted to alter this environment to promote better sleeping and waking patterns in infants. When Gabriel and associates (1981) consolidated nursing care so that convalescent premature infants were disturbed less often, the infants were awake less often and had longer sleep episodes. Als and colleagues (1986) developed a system of individualized interventions for preterm infants that included sensitivity to infant cues and careful avoidance of sleep disruptions. Their experimental infants did not exhibit different state patterns than the control infants, but the experimental infants did have fewer medical complications and improved performance on the APIB. A replication found improved state regulation and state stability as measured on the APIB (Buehler et al, 1995). Using a modification of Als' intervention system, Becker and associates (1991a, 1991b) also found improvements in infant morbidity but did not find differences in state behaviors on the NBAS at the time of hospital discharge; however, the experimental infants showed higher oxygen saturations, fewer disorganized movements, and more alertness during nursing care than did controls (Becker et al, 1993). Fajardo et al (1990) cared for premature infants in a quiet, private room with a day-night cycle, demand feedings, and social interactions by the nurses. These babies showed an increase in the mean length of active sleep and an increase in the organization of sleep states as evidenced by a decreased number of state changes and increased number of enduring state episodes.

A number of researchers altered NICU lighting patterns. Mann et al (1986) cared for preterm infants in a nursery in which light and noise intensities were reduced between 7:00 AM and 7:00 PM. As compared with infants from a control nursery, the experimental infants were found to sleep more but not until after hospital discharge. Blackburn and Patteson (1991) compared preterm infants in a nursery with continuous lighting with infants in a nursery with lighting that was dimmed at night. Infants in cycled light exhibited less motor activity during the night and lower heart rates over the entire day than the control infants. When preterm infants in the intermediate care unit were given four half-hour nap periods a day during which their incubators were covered and they received no nursing or medical procedures, they exhibited less quiet waking and longer uninterrupted sleep bouts than preterm infants without naps (Holditch-Davis et al, 1995), and they experienced a more rapid decline in apnea and more rapid weight gain (Torres et al, 1997). Brandon (2000) compared preterm infants who received care in near darkness with infants who received cycled light. Although there were no differences in state patterns (Brandon, 2000), the infants receiving cycled light showed more rapid weight gain (Brandon et al, 2001). Altogether, these findings suggest that neonatal nurses need to examine their routine practices to see if changes could be made to better promote stable sleeping and waking patterns in infants.

Painful Procedures

Infants in intensive care inevitably experience painful procedures. Neonatal nurses need to be alert to the effects of these procedures on infant sleeping and waking states. During painful procedures, infants are more likely to be awake and less likely to be in quiet sleep than during routine nursing care (Fearon et al, 1997; Van Cleve et al, 1995). All but the youngest and sickest preterm infants are likely to cry (Van Cleve et al,

1995), although the length of time until the cry begins depends on the infant's sleeping and waking state at the beginning of the procedure. Healthy full-term infants have the longest latency to cry when in quiet sleep, and young, preterm infants who are asleep at the beginning of the procedure and have recently undergone another painful procedure are the most likely to show only a minimal behavioral response to a painful procedure (Johnston et al, 1999a; Stevens et al, 1994). Immediately after the painful procedure, the full-term infant is likely to remain awake. However, in preterm infants, this tendency is not any greater than the tendency to stay awake after routine handling. At times longer than an hour after the procedure, full-term infants who experienced the severe pain of circumcision have been found to exhibit more quiet sleep, possibly in an effort to shut out the pain.

Nursing comfort measures have the potential to minimize some of these state effects. Yet it is not clear how frequently practicing nurses actually use them. In one study, nurses were not found to use positive touches or talking any more frequently during painful procedures than during routine care. Franck (1987) identified nine different comfort measures that nurses reported using to soothe infants who were receiving painful procedures (Chapter 42). To date, only a few of them have studied. Tactile stimulation, music, and intrauterine sounds were found ineffective for both preterm and full-term infants when given during the painful procedure. However, pacifiers were found to reduce crying and arousal in full-term and preterm infants when given during and after the procedure (Fearon et al, 1997). A sucrose-flavored pacifier was found to be even more effective than a plain pacifier in reducing the amount of crying by full-term and preterm infants during blood drawing and circumcision (Abad et al, 1996; Blass & Hoffmeyer, 1991; Johnston et al, 1997; Johnston et al, 1999). Swaddling has also been shown to be effective with full-term infants but less so than pacifiers, and the infants were more likely to be alert if given pacifiers. Facilitated tucking—a modified form of swaddling in which the infant's arms and legs are contained in a flexed position next to the trunk—was effective in reducing responses to heelsticks (Corff et al, 1995). Preterm infants who received facilitated tucking during and after heelsticks exhibited less crying, less sleep disruption, and fewer state changes after the heelstick than without tucking. Rocking was not effective in reducing cry facial expressions in preterm infants in response to a heelstick although the infants were in quiet sleep more (Johnston et al, 1997). Thus there is evidence that use of swaddling and pacifiers with sucrose can help reduce the sleeping and waking changes caused by painful procedures. However, additional research is needed to determine the effects of other comfort measures and how comfort measures affect more severe pain, such as postoperative pain.

Social Interaction

Sleeping and waking states are known to influence the interactions between full-term and premature infants and their mothers after term age, and in turn maternal interactions alter infant sleep-wake patterns. For example, infant crying may lead the mother to pick up the infant. At another time, a mother may awaken a sleeping infant for a feeding, thereby altering the infant's sleeping and waking patterns. Mothers have been found to exhibit different patterns of interactions when infants are in different states. Aspects of the infant's state organization, including the degree to which he or she shows different patterns of crying and alertness in different situations, are related to the overall quality of the mother-infant interaction. A responsive style of mothering results in infants developing day-night differentiation in their sleeping and waking patterns sooner. In addition, maternal emotional stress has been found to relate to the amount of night sleeping that full-term infants exhibit at 4 and 12 months (Becker et al, 1991a, 1991b).

Social interaction is known to affect sleep-wake patterns of premature infants after hospital discharge. At 4 to 6 weeks corrected age, breast-fed premature infants exhibited more crying, especially during daytime, than formula-fed infants did (Thomas, 2000). At 6 months corrected age, premature infants were more likely to be drowsy or asleep during feeding and alert during nonfeeding periods, and the behaviors of mothers differed during feeding and nonfeeding (Holditch-Davis et al, 2000). Mothers were more likely to engage in behaviors that involved close contact during feeding—such as holding, having body contact, and rocking their infants, whereas during nonfeeding periods, they were more likely to engage in more distal behaviors—such as gesturing and playing with the infant.

Less is known about the effect of social interaction in the hospital on infant sleeping and waking states. Minde et al (1983) found that ill preterm infants exhibited less eye opening—and thus probably less waking—when they were interacting with their mothers than did healthier preterm infants. Mothers report being aware of the sleeping and waking behaviors of their preterm infants—especially eye movements, orientation, and body movements—when they attempt to interact; they also report having used specific infant responses as guides to increase or decrease their interactive activity (Oehler et al, 1993). Waking, eye opening, increased body movements, positive facial expressions, and calming encouraged increased interaction; body movements, negative facial expressions, and withdrawing discouraged maternal interaction. However, preterm infants exhibit the positive interactive behaviors rather small portions of the time with their mothers (Oehler, 1995).

Moreover, social stimulation affects the physiologic status of preterm infants. The variation in infant oxygen saturation during parent touching was related to behavioral state and gestational age, such that infants who were more aroused and awake at the beginning of touch and had younger gestational ages at birth showed greater variation in their oxygen saturations (Harrison et al, 1991). Using a standardized protocol of social stimulation, Eckerman and colleagues (1994) found that preterm infants of at least 33 weeks' post-conceptional age responded to talking by eye opening and arousal, but when touching was added to the talking, the infants showed increased periods of closed eyes and negative facial expressions. Infants with more neurologic insults showed even greater negative responses to touching. This finding suggests that preterm infants are responsive to social stimulation of low intensity but that if the intensity of social stimulation is increased, they are no longer able to cope with it. Furthermore, medical complications further decrease infants' ability to cope with moderate-intensity social stimulation.

Preterm infants have also been found to respond differently to nurses and parents. In one study, preterm infants opened their eyes more when interacting with parents than when interacting with nurses. In another study with sicker infants, preterm infants spent more time in active sleep and less time in sleep-wake transition when with their parents than when with nurses (Miller & Holditch-Davis, 1992). In both of these studies, parents and nurses behaved differently toward infants, with nurses more likely to engage in routine nursing and medical procedures and parents more likely to hold infants and provide positive social stimulation. These findings suggest that preterm infants respond to the less active, more social stimulation provided by parents at first by sleeping and then, as they mature, by awakening to engage in interaction. The early sleeping may serve to conserve energy consumption and promote growth.

Kangaroo care, a recent nursing intervention to promote mothers' holding their preterm infants in skin-to-skin contact, has been found, in many studies, to increase amount of sleeping—and especially quiet sleep—as compared with periods when the infant is alone in the incubator (Ludington, 1990; Ludington et al, 1992; Luddington-Hoe et al, 1994, 1999; Messmer et al, 1997). Other researchers, however, have not found any changes in state patterns during kangaroo care (de Leeuw et al, 1991) or have found a decrease in active sleep and an increase in transitional sleep but no change in quiet sleep (Bosque et al, 1995).

Infant Stimulation

A number of the stimulation interventions used with infants are known to affect sleeping and waking states. In some cases, the goal of the intervention is to alter sleeping and waking states either to lower the infant's arousal so as to provide more energy for growth or to promote more mature state patterns. In other cases, the state effects are side effects of interventions that were designed to alter other aspects of the infant's functioning. This section examines the effects of several different types of infant stimulation interventions currently in use in NICUs.

Nonnutritive sucking is an intervention that has been variously used to soothe irritable infants and to promote feedings and growth. It is known to decrease restlessness and increase sleep time in full-term and preterm infants. However, these effects only last while it is being used. The BNAS state scores were not altered in preterm infants offered regular nonnutritive sucking during tube feedings as compared to control infants (Field et al, 1982). Nonnutritive sucking is effective in reducing crying after painful procedures and promoting either alertness or sleeping (Fearon et al, 1997). When given to preterm infants just before feedings, nonnutritive sucking helps them to arouse into a quiet, waking state and then maintain this state, in which they are most likely to feed effectively (McCain, 1992, 1995; Pickler et al, 1996). Nonnutritive sucking is more effective in this arousal than stroking (McCain, 1992). Other researchers did not find a change of state with nonnutritive sucking but did find that preterm infants who received nonnutritive sucking before feedings had higher feeding performance scores and more sleep after feedings (Pickler et al, 1993).

Waterbeds are another common infant stimulation intervention known to affect the sleeping and waking states of preterm infants. The purpose of this intervention is to provide compensatory vestibular-proprioceptive stimulation for preterm infants who are largely deprived of this form of stimulation in the NICU. Infants on waterbeds exhibit increased amounts of active and quiet sleep, less irritability, fewer state changes, and decreased crying (Deiriggi, 1990; Korner et al, 1990). These effects are enhanced if the waterbed oscillates (Korner et al, 1990), but even infants on plain waterbeds exhibit more sleep than they do on regular incubator mattresses (Deiriggi, 1990). When infants have been on waterbeds for prolonged periods of time, state effects continue even during periods when the infant is off the waterbed, as evidenced by decreased irritability

and increased alertness during a standardized assessment of preterm infant behavior. It has also been suggested that waterbeds reduce apnea. However, it is unlikely that this effect has clinical significance. When infants treated with theophylline for apnea of prematurity were placed on waterbeds, they showed the same state effects as found in infants without this complication, but they did not exhibit decreased apnea.

Gentle touching is another form of infant stimulation. Harrison et al (1996) provided 15 minutes of daily gentle human touch to preterm infants in the first 2 weeks of life. Infants had significantly less active sleep and motor activity during the periods of gentle touching. When the frequency of this intervention was increased to three times a day, preterm infants exhibited less active sleep, motor activity, and distress during gentle touching periods but did not differ from control infants on any outcome variable (Harrison et al, 2000).

Infant massage is another common infant stimulation technique. It provides both tactile and kinesthetic stimulation because it is necessary to move the infant to provide tactile stimulation to different parts of the body. The purpose of this type of stimulation is primarily to promote growth and augment development, but it also affects infant sleeping and waking states. White-Traut and Pate (1987) used the Rice Infant Sensomotor Stimulation, a 10-minute structured massage of the infant's entire body from head to toe, to provide extra stimulation for growing preterm infants. They found that during massage infants were more alert, but it is not clear that this effect was due to the massage. In this study, infants were taken out of the incubator for the massage, so the state changes might be the result of changes in the thermal environment. In another study, the intervention protocol was altered to be more contingent to infant cues (White-Traut et al, 1993). Again, the experimental infants showed increased alertness during the intervention and continued to be alert for 30 minutes afterwards. In another study, the massage intervention was compared with auditory stimulation alone; auditory stimulation along with massage; and auditory, massage, and rocking combined (White-Traut et al, 1997). Infants showed increasing alertness during the intervention in the massage and massage plus auditory groups, whereas the auditory group showed more quiet sleep. The massage, auditory, and rocking group showed minimal changes during the intervention but sustained alertness for 30 minutes afterwards. The combined auditory, massage, and rocking intervention was then tested on preterm infants with periventricular leukomalacia (White-Traut et al, 1999). Infants who received this combined intervention showed an increase in alertness over the intervention period and were hospitalized for 9 fewer days.

In other studies, stroking of the infant's body followed by passive flexion and extension of the extremities for 15 minutes 3 times a day for 10 days was shown to result in increased weight gain in preterm infants (Scafidi et al, 1990). During the massage treatments, infants exhibited more active sleep (Scafidi et al, 1990), but it is questionable whether any state effects persisted after the treatment period. In one study, massage-treated infants exhibited better scores on the NBAS and spent more time awake and active, whereas in the replication, no differences in the state organization of treated and control infants were found (Scafidi et al, 1990).

Rocking is a form of infant stimulation usually performed in order to soothe the infant. It has been administered either directly while holding the infant or by placing the infant in special cribs or incubators modified to rock at specific speeds. The immediate effects of rocking are reduced crying. However, the rhythm and direction of rocking are important in determining which of the other states the infant was most likely to exhibit. Exposing preterm infants to rocking over a 2-week period had longer-lasting results. They exhibited increased quiet sleep and decreased active sleep.

In yet another study, preterm infants were placed in a non-rigid reclining chair twice a day for 3 hours from about 30 weeks' post-conceptional age until hospital discharge (Provasi & Lequien, 1993). Sleeping and waking states were observed for a 2-hour period for control infants and two 2-hour periods for the experimental infants (once in their beds and once in the infant seat) shortly before discharge. Experimental infants spent more time in quiet sleep and active sleep and less time in quiet and agitated waking than the control infants, but no differences in the state patterns of the experimental infants when in their beds and in the infant seat were found.

In a final type of infant stimulation, Thoman and Graham (1986) placed a "breathing" stuffed bear in the incubator with a preterm infant. The goal of this intervention was to provide a form of rhythmic stimulation that would help the infant organize his or her sleeping and waking patterns. In addition, this form of stimulation was voluntary. Because the bear took up only a small part of the incubator and babies were usually put to sleep in positions in which they were not in physical contact with the bear, infants could choose whether or not to remain in contact with the bear whenever their random movements brought them into contact with it. As compared with controls, experimental infants spent a much greater percentage of time in contact with the area of the incubator with the bear. By the end of the intervention period, experimental infants exhibited significantly increased quiet sleep time. This study has been replicated with two additional samples, and both have shown increased contact with the breathing bear as well as more quiet sleep and less active sleep than infants given a nonbreathing bear (Ingersoll & Thoman, 1994; Thoman et al, 1991).

USEFULNESS OF NEONATAL SLEEP-WAKE STATES FOR ASSESSMENT

Sleeping and waking states are ubiquitous characteristics of neonates. The infant's behavioral and physiologic responses are filtered through neural controls mediated by the sleeping and waking states. Although it is certainly possible to give competent nursing care to high-risk infants without considering their sleep-wake states, recognizing specific states will enable the nurse to better interpret both physiologic and behavioral changes. By observing sleeping and waking, the nurse will be able to determine whether physiologic parameters are consistent with those expected in a particular state. Changes in sleeping and waking patterns can be used to help the nurse identify the need for interventions and to aid the evaluation of these interventions. Most importantly, by observing sleeping and waking behaviors, the nurse will come to know each infant better and thus be better able to provide individualized care. This knowledge of individual infants can then be shared with parents to help them develop positive interactions with their children.

SUMMARY

High-risk infants are both dependent on and vulnerable to their early environment—the NICU and intermediate nursery—to maintain their physiologic function, to promote growth and development, and to provide opportunities for the organization of state, behavioral, and social responsiveness. The immaturity and physiologic and neurobehavioral instability of these infants make them particularly vulnerable to environments that do not support their emerging organization and patterns or that do not attend to their cues and respond appropriately. Nurses can and do play a big role in controlling sleep in the NICU environment. It is important that parents are included in these efforts to promote positive sleep-wake patterns in the NICU and once the infant is home.

In summary, the goals in addressing the neurobehavioral needs of high-risk infants are the following:

1. Provide an environment that enhances and supports the infant's developing capabilities.
2. Protect the infant from sensory overload and minimize stressors.
3. Assist parents in understanding their infant's unique abilities.
4. Help parents interact with their infant in ways appropriate to the infant's health status, state, and level of maturity.

Use the infant's needs and capabilities to foster more positive parent-infant interaction will need to be assessed. These needs will have to be considered within the formal and informal power structures within the unit. Changes in developmental care can often begin with a few nurses altering the way they care for the infants assigned to them. Role modeling, mentoring, and positive reinforcement, along with regular educational opportunities and case discussions, are useful strategies (McGrath & Valenzuela, 1994). Various models for implementing developmental supportive care programs have been described (Als, 1986; Browne et al, 1996; Cole et al, 1990; Grunwald & Becker, 1990; McGrath & Valenzuela, 1994; Tribotti & Stein, 1992).

REFERENCES

Abad F et al (1996). Oral sweet solution reduces pain-related behaviour in preterm infants. *Acta paediatricia*, 85, 854-858.

Acebo C (1987). Naturalistic observations of mothers and infants: descriptions of mother and infant responsiveness and sleep-wake development. *Dissertation Abstracts International*, 48, 2134B (University Microfilms No. DA8722598).

Als H (1982). Toward a synactive theory of development: promise for the assessment and support of infant individuality. *Infant mental health journal*, 3(4), 229-243.

Als H (1984). Newborn behavioral assessment. In Burns WJ, Lavigne JV (Eds.). *Progress in pediatric psychology*. New York: Grune & Stratton.

Als H (1986). A synactive model of neonatal behavioral organization: framework for assessment of neurobehavioral development in the premature infant and for support of infants and parents in the neonatal intensive care environment. part 1: theoretical framework. *Physical and occupational therapy in pediatrics*, 6(3-4), 3-53.

Als H (1996). *The very immature infant—environmental and care issues*. Paper presented at The Physical and Developmental Environment of the High Risk Neonate. Clearwater Beach, FL: University of South Florida College of Medicine.

Als H (1999). Reading the premature infant. In Goldson E (Ed). *Nurturing the premature infant: developmental interventions in the neonatal intensive care nursery* (pp. 18-85). New York: Oxford University Press.

Als H (2001, Revision). Program Guide: Newborn Individualized Developmental Care and Assessment Program (NIDCAP®), an education and training program for health care professionals. Boston Children's Medical Center Corporation.

Als H et al (1982). Assessment of preterm infant behavior (APIB). In Fitzgerald HE, Yogman M (Eds.). *Theory and research in behavioral pediatrics* (Vol. 1, pp. 64-133). New York: Plenum Press.

Als H et al (1986). Individualized behavioral and environmental care for the very-low-birth-weight preterm infant at high risk for bronchopulmonary dysplasia: neonatal intensive care unit and developmental outcome. *Pediatrics*, 78(6), 1123-1132.

Als H et al (1988). Behavioral differences between preterm and full-term newborns as measured on the APIB System scores. *Infant behavior and development*, 11(3), 305-318.

Als H et al (1994). Individualized developmental care for the very-low-birth-weight preterm infants: medical and neurofunctional effects. *Journal of the American medical association*, 272(11), 853-858.

Als H, Gilkerson L (1997). The role of relationship-based developmentally supportive newborn intensive care in strengthening outcome of preterm infants. *Seminars in perinatology*, 21, 178-189.

American Academy of Pediatrics. Task Force on Infant Positioning and SIDS. (1992). Positioning and SIDS. *Pediatrics*, 89, 1120-1126.

Anand KJS (2000). Effects of perinatal pain and stress. *Progress in brain research*, 122, 117.

Anand KJ, Scalzo FM (2000). Can adverse neonatal experiences alter brain development and subsequent behavior? *Biology of the neonate*, 77, 69.

Anders T et al (Eds.). (1971). *A manual of standardized terminology, techniques and criteria for scoring of states of sleep and wakefulness in newborn infants*. Los Angeles: UCLA Brain Information Service/BRI Publications Office.

Anderson GC (1999). Kangaroo care of the premature infant. In Goldson E (Ed). *Nurturing the premature infant: developmental interventions in the neonatal intensive care nursery* (pp. 131-160). NY: Oxford University Press.

Apkarian P et al (1991). Effects of behavioural state on visual processing in neonates. *Neuropediatrics*, 22(2), 85-91.

Ariagno R (1996a). *Sleep, sleep cycles, and sleep deprivation*. Paper presented at The Physical and Developmental Environment of the High Risk Neonate. Clearwater Beach, FL: University of South Florida College of Medicine.

Ariagno R (1996b). *Sleep, sleep cycles, and sleep deprivation*. Paper presented at The Physical and Developmental Environment of the High Risk Neonate. Clearwater Beach, FL: University of South Florida College of Medicine.

Ariagno R et al (1996). *A comparison of polysomnographic vs. motility monitoring system sleep state determination during naps in infants*. Paper presented at The Physical and Developmental Environment of the High Risk Neonate. Clearwater Beach, FL: University of South Florida College of Medicine.

Barnard KE (1999). *Beginning rhythms: the emerging process of sleep-wake behaviors and self-regulation*. Seattle: NCAST, University of Washington.

Barnard KE, Blackburn S (1985). Making a case for studying the ecological niche of the newborn. In Raff BS, Paul NW (Eds). *NAACOG Invitational Research Conference. Birth Defects: Original Article Series*, 21(3), 71-88.

Bayley N (1969). *Bayley scales of infant development*. New York: The Psychological Corporation.

Becker PT et al (1991a). Correlates of diurnal sleep patterns in infants of adolescent and adult single mothers. *Research in nursing and health*, 14(2), 97-108.

Becker PT et al (1993). Effects of developmental care on behavioral organization in very-low-birth-weight infants. *Nursing research*, 42(4), 214-220.

Becker PT, Thoman EB (1981). Rapid eye movement storms in infants: Rate of occurrence at 6 months predicts mental development at one year. *Science*, 212(4501), 1415-1416.

Becker PT, Thoman EB (1982). Waking activity: The neglected state of infancy. *Brain research*, 256(4), 395-400.

Beckwith L, Parmelee AH, Jr. (1986). EEG patterns of preterm infants, home environment, and later IQ. *Child development*, 57(3), 777-789.

Beckwith L, Rodning C (1992). Evaluating effects of intervention with parents of preterm infants. In Friedman SI, Sigman MD (Eds.). *The psychological development of low-birth-weight children*. Norwood, NJ: Ablex Publishing Corporation.

Bell RP, McGrath JM (1996). Implementing a research-based kangaroo care program in the NICU. *Nursing clinics of North America*, 31, 387-403.

Bernert G et al (1997). The effect of behavioural states on cerebral oxygenation during endotracheal suctioning of preterm babies. *Neuropediatrics*, 28, 111-115.

Black JE (1998). How a child builds its brain: some lessons from animal studies of neural plasticity. *Preventative medicine*, 27, 168-171.

Black M et al (1993). Prenatal drug exposure: neurodevelopmental outcome and parenting environment. *Journal of pediatric psychology*, 18(5), 605-620.

Blackburn S (1995). Problems of preterm infants after discharge. *Journal of obstetric, gynecologic, and neonatal nursing*, 24(1), 43-49.

Blackburn S (1996a, January). *Studies of light and its application to clinical practice*. Paper presented at The Physical and Developmental Environment of the High Risk Neonate. Clearwater Beach, FL: University of South Florida College of Medicine.

Blackburn ST (1996b). Research utilization: modifying the NICU light environment. *Neonatal network*, 15(4), 63-66.

Blackburn ST (1998). Environmental impact of the NICU on developmental outcomes. *Journal of pediatric nursing*, 13, 279-289.

Blackburn S, Barnard KE (1985). Analysis of caregiving events in preterm infants in the special care unit. In Gottfried A, Gaiter J (Eds.). *Infants under stress: Environmental neonatology* (pp. 113-129). Baltimore: University Park Press.

Blackburn S, Kang RE (1991). *Early parent-infant relationships*, ed 2. White Plains, NY: March of Dimes Birth Defects Foundation.

Blackburn ST (2003). *Maternal, fetal and neonatal physiology: a clinical perspective*, ed 2, Philadelphia: WB Saunders.

Blackburn S, Patteson D (1991). Effects of cycled lighting on activity state and cardiorespiratory function in preterm infants. *Journal of perinatal and neonatal nursing*, 4(4), 47-54.

Blass EM, Hoffmeyer LB (1991). Sucrose as an analgesic for newborn infants. *Pediatrics*, 87(2), 215-218.

Borghese IF et al (1995). Sleep rhythmicity in premature infants: implications for developmental status. *Sleep*, 18, 523-530.

Bosque EM et al (1995). Physiologic measures of kangaroo versus incubator care in a tertiary-level nursery. *Journal of obstetric, gynecologic, and neonatal nursing*, 24(3), 219-226.

Bowden VR et al (2000). Developmental care of the newborn: *Online journal of clinical innovations*, 3, 1-77.

Brandon DH (2000). The effect of cycled light versus near darkness on growth and development of preterm infants born at less than 31 weeks' gestation. (Doctoral Dissertation, University of North Carolina). *Dissertation abstracts international*, 61(05B 2000), 2468.

Brandon DH et al (1999). Nursing care and the development of sleeping and waking behaviors in preterm infants. *Research in nursing and health*, 22, 217-229.

Brandon DH et al (2001). The effects of cycled light vs. continuous near darkness on health outcomes in preterm infants born at <31 weeks gestation. Manuscript under review.

Braun M, Palmer M (1982). *Early detection and treatment of infants and young children with neuromuscular disorders*. New York: Therapeutic Media.

Brazelton TB (1984). *Neonatal behavioral assessment scale*, ed 2, Spastics International Medical Publications, in association with William Heinemann Medical Books Ltd., London, and JB Lippincott Co., Philadelphia.

Brazelton TB, Nugent JK (1995). *Neonatal behavioral assessment scale*, ed 3, London: MacKeith Press.

Brown P, Taquino LT (2001). Designing and delivering neonatal care in single rooms. *Journal of perinatal and neonatal nursing*, 15(1), 68-83.

Browne J et al (1996). *Family infant relationship support training*. Denver: The Center for Family and Infant Interaction.

Buehler DM et al (1995). Effectiveness of individualized developmental care for low-risk preterm infants: Behavioral and electrophysiological evidence. *Pediatrics*, 96, 923-932.

Bull MJ, Dodge NN (1996). *Physical and developmental environment of high-risk infants requiring prolonged hospitalization.* Paper presented at The Physical and Developmental Environment of the High Risk Neonate. Clearwater Beach, FL: University of South Florida College of Medicine.

Butte NF et al (1992). Sleep organization and energy expenditure of breast-fed and formula-fed infants. *Pediatric research,* 32(5), 514-519.

Cagan JB (1996). *Feeding readiness behavior in preterm infants.* Paper presented at The Physical and Developmental Environment of the High Risk Neonate. Clearwater Beach, FL: University of South Florida College of Medicine.

Campbell AN et al (1984). Mechanical vibration and sound levels experienced in neonatal transport. *American journal of diseases of children,* 138(10), 967-970.

Cassidy JW, Ditty KM (1998). Presentation of aural stimuli to newborns and premature infants: an audiological perspective. *Journal of music therapy,* 35, 70-87.

Catlett AT, Holditch-Davis D (1990). Environmental stimulation of the acutely ill preterm infant: Physiological effects and nursing implications. *Neonatal network,* 8(6), 19-26.

Cole JG et al (1990). Changing the NICU environment: The Boston City Hospital model. *Neonatal network,* 9(2), 15-23.

Corff KE et al (1995). Facilitated tucking: A non-pharmacologic comfort measure for pain in preterm neonates. *Journal of obstetric, gynecologic and neonatal nursing,* 24, 143-147.

Cornwell AC (1993). Sex differences in the maturation of sleep/wake patterns in high risk for SIDS infants. *Neuropediatrics,* 24(1), 8-14.

Corwin MJ et al (1995). Newborn acoustic cry characterisitics of infants subsequently dying of sudden infant death syndrome. *Pediatrics,* 96, 73-77.

Curzi-Dascalova L et al (1993). Sleep state organization in premature infants of less than 35 weeks' gestational age. *Pediatric research,* 34, 624-628.

Deiriggi PM (1990). Effects of waterbed flotation on indicators of energy expenditure in preterm infants. *Nursing research,* 39(3), 140-146.

Denenberg VH, Thoman EB (1981). Evidence for a functional role for active (REM) sleep in infancy. *Sleep,* 4(2), 185-191.

DePaul D, Chambers SE (1995). Environmental noise in the neonatal intensive care unit: Implications for nursing practice. *Journal of perinatal and neonatal nursing,* 8(4), 71-78.

DiPietro JA (2000). Baby and the brain: advances in child development. *Annual review of public health,* 21, 455-471.

DiPietro JA et al (1994). Behavioral and physiologic effects of nonnutritive sucking during gavage feeding in preterm infants. *Pediatric research,* 36, 207-214.

DiPietro JA et al (1996). Fetal neurobehavioral development. *Child development,* 67, 2553-2567.

Doussard-Roosevelt J et al (1996). Behavioral sleep states in very low birth-weight preterm neonates: Relation to neonatal health and vagal maturation. *Journal of pediatric psychology,* 21, 785-802.

Duffy FH et al (1990). Behavioral and electrophysiological evidence for gestational age effects in healthy preterm and fullterm infants studied two weeks after expected due date. *Child development,* 61(4), 271-286.

Duxbury ML et al (1984). Caregiver disruptions and sleep of high-risk infants. *Heart and lung,* 13(2), 141-147.

Eckerman CO et al (1994). Premature newborns as social partners before term age. *Infant behavior and development,* 17(1), 55-70.

Evans JC (1991). Incidence of hypoxemia associated with caregiving in premature infants. *Neonatal network,* 10(2), 17-24.

Evans JC (1994). Comparison of two NICU patterns of caregiving over 24-hours for preterm infants. *Neonatal network,* 13(5), 87.

Evans JB, Philbin MK (2000). Facility and operations planning for quiet hospital nurseries. *Journal of perinatology,* 20, S105-S112.

Fajardo B et al (1990). Effect of nursery environment on state regulation in very-low-birth-weight premature infants. *Infant behavior and development,* 13(3), 287-303.

Fearon I et al (1997). Swaddling after heel lance, age-specific effects on behavioral recovery in preterm infants. *Journal of developmental and behavioral pediatrics,* 18, 222-232.

Field T et al (1982). Nonnutritive sucking during tube feedings: Effects on preterm neonates in an intensive care unit. *Pediatrics,* 70(3), 381-384.

Fielder AR, Moseley MJ (2000). Environmental light and the preterm infant. *Seminars in perinatology,* 24, 291-298.

Fleisher RF et al (1995). Individualized developmental care for very-low-birth-weight premature infants. *Clinical pediatrics,* 34(10), 523-529.

Fox K et al (1996). Glutamate receptor blockage at cortical synapses disrupts development of thalamocortical and columnar organization in somatosensory cortex. *Proceedings of the National Academy of Science USA,* 93, 5584-5589.

Franck LS (1987). A national survey of the assessment and treatment of pain and agitation in the neonatal intensive care unit. *Journal of obstetric, gynecologic, and neonatal nursing,* 16(6), 387-393.

Fuhrman P (1984). *The effect of preterm infant state regulation on parent-child interaction.* Unpublished master's thesis, University of Washington, Seattle.

Gabriel M et al (1981). Sleep-wake pattern in preterm infants under two different care schedules during four-day polygraphic recording. *Neuropediatrics,* 12(4), 366-373.

Gabriel M et al (1980). Sleep induced pO_2 changes in preterm infants. *European journal of pediatrics,* 134(2), 153-154.

Gale G et al (1993). Skin-to-skin (kangaroo care) holding of the intubated premature infant. *Neonatal network,* 12(6), 49-57.

Gale G, Franck LS (1998). Toward a standard of care for parents of infants in the neonatal intensive care unit. *Critical care nurse,* 18(5), 62-64, 66-74.

Gale G, VandenBerg KA (1998). Kangaroo care. *Neonatal network,* 17(5), 69-71.

Galland BC et al (2000). Factors affecting heart rate variability and heart rate responses to tilting in infants aged 1 and 3 months. *Pediatric research,* 48, 360-368.

Gaultier CL (1994). Apnea and sleep state in newborns and infants [Review]. *Biology of the neonate,* 65(3-4), 231-234.

Gill NE et al (1988). Effect of nonnutritive sucking on behavioral state in preterm infants before feeding. *Nursing research,* 37(6), 347-350.

Glass P (1999). The vulnerable neonate and the neonatal intensive care environment. In Avery GB et al (eds.). *Neonatology: pathophysiology and management of the newborn,* ed 5, pp. 91-108. Philadelphia: Lippincott, Williams & Wilkins.

Glotzbach SF et al (1993). Light variability in the modern neonatal nursery: Chronobiological issues. *Medical hypotheses* 41(3), 217-224.

Goldberger J (1990). Lengthy or repeated hospitalization in infancy: Issues in stimulation and intervention [Review]. *Clinics in perinatology,* 17(1), 197-206.

Goto K et al (1999). More awakenings and heart rate variability during supine sleep in preterm infants. *Pediatrics,* 103, 603-609.

Gottfried AW (1985). Environment of newborn infants in special care units. In Gottfried AW, Gaiter JL (Eds.). *Infant stress under intensive care: Environmental neonatology* (pp. 23-54). Baltimore: University Park Press.

Graven SN (1996, January). *Concepts of fetal sensory development.* Paper presented at The Physical and Developmental Environment of the High Risk Neonate. Clearwater Beach, FL: University of South Florida College of Medicine.

Graven SN (2000). Sound and the developing infant in the NICU: conclusions and recommendations for care. *Journal of perinatology,* 20(8 Pt 2), S88-S93.

Gray L, Philbin MK (2000). Measuring sound in hospital nurseries. *Journal of perinatology,* 20, S100-S104.

Greenough WT et al (1987). Experience and brain development. *Child development,* 58, 539-559.

Grunwald PC, Becker PT (1990). Developmental enhancement: Implementing a program for the NICU. *Neonatal network,* 9(6), 29-30, 39-45.

Hack MM et al (2000). Neurodevelopment and predictors of outcomes of children with birthweights of less than 1000g: 1992-1995. *Archives of pediatric and adolescent medicine,* 134, 725-731.

Haddad GG et al (1987). Determination of sleep state in infants using respiratory variability. *Pediatric research,* 21(6), 556-562.

Hall JW (2000). Development of the ear and hearing. *Journal of perinatology,* 20, S12-S20.

Hamernik RP et al (1989). Noise and vibration interactions: Effects on hearing. *Journal of acoustic society of America,* 86(6), 2129-2137.

Harrison LL et al (1991). Preterm infants' physiologic responses to early parent touch. *Western journal of nursing research,* 13(6), 698-713.

Harrison L et al (1996). Effects of gentle human touch on preterm infants: pilot study results. *Neonatal network,* 15(2), 35-42.

Harrison LL et al (2000). Physiologic and behavioral effects of gentle human touch on preterm infants. *Research in nursing and health,* 23, 435-446.

Heller C et al (1997). Sedation administered to very-low-birth-weight premature infants. *Journal of perinatology,* 17, 107-112.

Hepper PG (1995). Human fetal "olfactory" learning. *International journal of prenatal and perinatal psychology and medicine,* 7, 147.

High PC, Gorski PA (1985). Recording environmental influences on infant development in the intensive care nursery: womb for improvement. In Gottfried AW, Gaiter JL (Eds.). *Infant stress under intensive care: environmental neonatology* (pp. 131-155). Baltimore: University Park Press.

Holditch-Davis D (1990a). The development of sleeping and waking states in high-risk preterm infants. *Infant behavior and development,* 13(4), 513-531.

Holditch-Davis D (1990b). The effect of hospital caregiving on preterm infants' sleeping and waking states. In Funk SG et al (Eds.). *Key aspects of recovery: improving nutrition, rest, and mobility* (pp. 110-122). New York: Springer.

Holditch-Davis D (1995). Behaviors of preterm infants with and without chronic lung disease when alone and when with nurses. *Neonatal network,* 14(7), 51-57.

Holditch-Davis D et al (1994). Pathologic apnea and brief respiratory pauses in preterm infants: relation to sleep state. *Nursing research,* 43(5), 293-300.

Holditch-Davis D et al (1995). The effect of standardized rest periods on convalescent preterm infants. *Journal of obstetric, gynecologic and neonatal nursing,* 24(5), 424-432.

Holditch-Davis D et al (1999). Early interactions between mothers and their medically fragile infants. *Applied developmental science,* 3, 155-167.

Holditch-Davis D et al (2000). Feeding and non-feeding interactions of mothers and prematures. *Western journal of nursing research,* 22(3), 320-334.

Holditch-Davis D, Calhoun M (1989). Do preterm infants show behavioral responses to painful procedures? In Funk SG et al (Eds.). *Key aspects of comfort: management of pain, fatigue, and nausea* (pp. 35-43). New York: Springer.

Holditch-Davis D, Edwards L (1998a). Modeling development of sleep-wake behaviors: II. results of 2 cohorts of preterms. *Physiology and behavior,* 63(3), 319-328.

Holditch-Davis D, Edwards L (1998b). Temporal organization of sleep-wake states in preterm infants. *Developmental psychobiology,* 33, 257-269.

Holditch-Davis D, Hudson DC (1995). Using preterm infant behaviors to identify acute medical complications. In Funk SG et al (Eds.). *Key aspects of caring for the acutely ill: technological aspects, patient education, and quality of life* (pp. 95-120). New York: Springer.

Holditch-Davis D, Lee DA (1993). The behaviors and nursing care of preterm infants with chronic lung disease. In Funk SG et al (Eds.). *Key aspects of caring for the chronically ill: Hospital and home* (pp. 250-270). New York: Springer.

Holditch-Davis D, Thoman EB (1987). Behavioral states of premature infants: Implications for neural and behavioral development. *Developmental psychobiology,* 20(1), 25-38.

Ikonomidou C et al (2001). Neurotransmitters and apoptosis in the developing brain. *Biochemical pharmacology,* 62, 401-405.

Illuminating Engineering Society of North America. (1995). *Lighting for healthcare facilities,* RP29. New York: Illuminating Engineering Society of North America.

Ingersoll EW, Thoman EB (1994). The breathing bear: effects on respiration in premature infants. *Physiology and behavior,* 56(5), 855-859.

Ingersoll EW, Thoman EB (1999). Sleep/wake states of preterm infants: Stability, developmental change, diurnal variation, and relation with caregiving activity. *Child development,* 70, 1-10.

Jeffery HE et al (1999). Why the prone position is a risk factor of sudden infant death syndrome. *Pediatrics,* 104, 263-269.

Johnston CC et al (1997). Effectiveness of oral sucrose and simulated rocking on pain response in preterm neonates. *Pain,* 72, 193-199.

Johnston CC et al (1999a). Do cry features reflect pain intensity in preterm neonates? *Biology of the neonate,* 76, 120-124.

Johnston CC et al (1999b). Factors explaining lack of response to heelstick in preterm newborns. *Journal of obstetric, gynecologic and neonatal nursing,* 28, 587-594.

Kahn A et al (1992). Sleep and cardiorespiratory characteristics of infant victims of sudden death: A prospective case-control study. *Sleep,* 15(4), 287-292.

Karch D et al (1982). Behavioural changes and bioelectric brain maturation of preterm and fullterm newborn infants: a polygraphic study. *Developmental medicine and child neurology,* 24(1), 30-47.

Korner AF (1972). State as variable, obstacle, and as mediator of stimulation in infant research. *Merrill-Palmer quarterly,* 18(2), 77-94.

Korner AF (1973). Early stimulation and maternal care as related to infant capabilities and individual differences. *Early child development and care,* 2(3), 307-327.

Korner AF et al (1990). Sleep enhanced and irritability reduced in preterm infants: differential efficacy of three types of waterbeds. *Journal of behavioral and developmental pediatrics,* 11(5), 240-246.

Korner AF et al (1994). Preterm medical complications differentially affect neurobehavioral functions: Results from a new neonatal medical index. *Infant behavior and development,* 17(1), 37-43.

Kotzer AM (1994). Maternal smoking and infant sleep behavior. *Neonatal network,* 13(1), 65.

Lawhon G (1986). Management of stress in premature infants. In Angelini DJ et al (Eds.). *Perinatal/neonatal nursing: a clinical handbook* (pp. 319-328). Boston: Blackwell Scientific Publications.

Lawson KR et al (1985). Infant state in relation to its environmental context. *Infant behavior and development,* 8(3), 269-281.

Lecanuet J-P, Schaal B (1996). Fetal sensory competencies. *European journal of obstetrics, gynecology and reproductive biology,* 68, 1-23.

de Leeuw R et al (1991). Physiological effects of kangaroo care in very small preterm infants. *Biology of the neonate,* 59(3), 149-155.

Leonard CH et al (1990). Effect of medical and social risk factors on the outcome of premature and very-low-birth-weight infants. *Pediatrics,* 116(4), 620-626.

Lester BM, Dreher M (1989). Effects of marijuana use during pregnancy on newborn cry. *Child development,* 60(4), 765-771.

Linn PL et al (1985). An ecological description of a neonatal intensive care unit. In Gottfried AW, Gaiter JL (Eds.). *Infant stress under intensive care: environmental neonatology* (pp. 83-111). Baltimore: University Park Press.

Long JG et al (1980). Noise and hypoxemia in the intensive care nursery. *Pediatrics,* 65(1), 143-145.

Lotus MJ (1992). Effects of light and sound in the neonatal intensive care unit environment on the low-birth-weight infants. *NAACOG's clinical issues in perinatal and women's health nursing,* 3(1), 34-44.

Ludington SM (1990). Energy conservation during skin-to-skin contact between premature infants and their mothers. *Heart and lung,* 19(5, Part 1), 445-451.

Ludington SM et al (1992). Efficacy of kangaroo care with preterm infants in open-air cribs. *Neonatal network,* 11(6), 101.

Ludington-Hoe SM et al (1991). Physiologic responses to skin-to-skin contact in hospitalized premature infants. *Journal of perinatology,* 11(1), 19-24.

Ludington-Hoe SM et al (1994). Kangaroo care: research results, and practice implications and guidelines; findings of two research projects. *Neonatal network,* 13(1), 19-27, 29-34.

Ludington-Hoe SM et al (1999). Birth-related fatigue in 34-36-week preterm neonates: Rapid recovery with very early kangaroo (skin-to-skin) care. *Journal of obstetric, gynecologic and neonatal nursing,* 28, 94-103.

Ludington-Hoe SM, Swinth JY (1996). Developmental aspects of kangaroo care. *Journal of obstetric, gynecologic and neonatal nursing,* 25, 691-703.

Maas YGH et al (2000). Predictive value of neonatal neurological tests for developmental outcome of preterm infants. *Journal of pediatrics,* 137, 100-106.

Mann NP et al (1986). Effect of night and day on preterm infants in a newborn nursery: Randomised trial. *British medical journal: clinical research edition,* 293(6557), 1265-1267.

Martin R et al (1979). Changes in arterial oxygen tension during quiet and active sleep in the neonate. *Birth defects: original article series,* 15(4), 493-494.

Martin RJ et al (1995). Vulnerability of respiratory control in healthy preterm infants placed supine. *Journal of pediatrics,* 127, 609-614.

McCain GC (1992). Facilitating inactive awake states in preterm infants: A study of three interventions. *Nursing research,* 41(3), 157-160.

McCain GC (1995). Promotion of preterm infant nipple feeding with nonnutritive sucking. *Journal of pediatric nursing,* 10, 3-8.

McEvoy C et al (1997). Prone positioning decreases episodes of hypoxemia in extremely low birth weight infants (1000 grams or less) with chronic lung disease. *Journal of pediatrics,* 130, 305-309.

McGrath JM, Conliffe-Torres S (1996). Integrating family-centered developmental assessment and intervention into routine care in the neonatal intensive care unit. *Journal of perinatal and neonatal nursing,* 8(3), 46-57.

McGrath JM, Valenzuela G (1994). Integrating developmentally supportive caregiving into practice through education. *Journal of perinatal and neonatal nursing,* 8(3), 46-57.

McGrath MM et al (2000). Longitudinal neurologic follow-up in neonatal intensive care unit survivors with various neonatal morbidities. *Pediatrics,* 106, 1397-1405.

Medoff-Cooper B (1991). Changes in nutritive sucking patterns with increasing gestational age. *Nursing research,* 40(4), 245-247.

Medoff-Cooper B et al (1989). Neonatal sucking as a clinical assessment tool: Preliminary findings. *Nursing research,* 38(3), 162-165.

Messmer PR et al (1997). Effect of kangaroo care on sleep time for neonates. *Pediatric nursing,* 23, 408-414.

Michelsson K et al (1990). Crying, feeding and sleeping patterns in 1 to 12-month-old infants. *Child: care, health and development,* 16(2), 99-111.

Miller CL et al (1995). The effects of cycled and noncycled lighting on growth and development in preterm infants. *Infant behavior and development,* 18(1), 87-95.

Miller DB, Holditch-Davis D (1992). Interactions of parents and nurses with high-risk preterm infants. *Research in nursing and health,* 15(3), 187-197.

Minde K et al (1983). Effect of neonatal complications in premature infants on early parent-infant interactions. *Developmental medicine and child neurology,* 25(6), 763-777.

Mirmiran M (1986). The importance of fetal/neonatal REM sleep. *European journal of obstetrics, gynecology, and reproductive biology,* 21(5-6), 283-291.

Moore KL, Persaud TVN (1998). *The developing human: clinically oriented embryology,* ed 6, Philadelphia: WB Saunders.

Moran M et al (1999). Maternal kangaroo (skin-to-skin) care in the NICU beginning 4 hours postbirth. *American journal of maternal child nursing,* 24, 74-79.

Morris BH et al (2000). Physiological effects of sound on the newborn. *Journal of perinatology* 20, S55-S60.

Moseley MJ et al (1988). Effects of nursery illumination on frequency of eyelid opening and state in preterm infants. *Early human development,* 18(1), 13-26.

Mouradian LE et al (2000). Neurobehavioral functioning of healthy preterm infants of varying gestational ages. *Journal of developmental and behavioral pediatrics,* 21, 408-416.

Myers BJ et al (1992). Prematurity and respiratory illness: Brazelton Scale (NBAS) performance of preterm infants with bronchopulmonary displasia (BPD), respiratory distress syndrome (RDS), or no respiratory illness. *Infant behavior and development,* 15(1), 27-42.

Myers MM et al (1998). Effects of sleeping position and time after feeding on the organization of sleep/wake states in prematurely born infants. *Sleep,* 21, 343-349.

Nelson CA, Carver LJ (1998). The effects of stress and trauma on brain and memory: a view from developmental cognitive neuroscience. *Developmental psychopathology,* 10, 793-809.

Nugent JK et al (1996). The effects of maternal alcohol consumption and cigarette smoking during pregnancy on acoustic cry analysis. *Child development,* 67, 1806-1815.

Oehler JM (1995). Development of mother-child interaction in very low birth weight infants. In Funk SG et al (Eds.). *Key aspects of caring for the acutely ill: technological aspects, patient education, and quality of life* (pp. 120-133). New York: Springer.

Oehler JM et al (1993). Maternal views of preterm infants' responsiveness to social interaction. *Neonatal network,* 12(6), 67-74.

Ottaviano S et al (1996). Sleep characteristics in healthy children from birth to 6 years of age in the urban area of Rome. *Sleep,* 19, 1-3.

Palmer MM (1993). Identification and management of the transitional suck pattern in premature infants, *Journal of perinatal and neonatal nursing,* 7(1), 66-75.

Palmer MM et al (1993). The Neonatal Oral-Motor Assessment Scale: a reliability study, *Journal of perinatology,* 13, 28-35.

Palmer MM, Heyman MB (1999). Developmental outcome for neonates with dysfunctional and disorganized sucking patterns: preliminary findings. *Infant and toddler intervention: the transdisciplinary journal,* 9(3), 299-308.

Parmelee AH, Jr., Stern E (1972). Development of states in infants. In Clemente CD et al (Eds.). *Sleep and the maturing nervous system* (pp. 200-215). New York: Academic Press.

Peabody JL, Lewis K (1985). Consequences of neonatal intensive care. In Gottfried A, Gaiter J (Eds.). *Infants under stress: environmental neonatology* (pp. 199-226). Baltimore: University Park Press.

Peters K (1998). Bathing the premature infant: The physiologic and behavioral consequences. *American journal of critical care,* 7, 90-100.

Peters KL (1992). Does routine nursing care complicate the physiologic stability of the premature neonate with respiratory distress syndrome? *Journal of perinatal and neonatal nursing,* 6(2), 67-84.

Philbin MK (1996). Some implications of early auditory development for the environment of hospitalized preterm infants. *Neonatal network,* 15(8), 71-73.

Philbin MK (2000). The influence of auditory experience on the behavior of preterm newborns. *Journal of perinatology,* 20, S77-S87.

Philbin MK et al (1999). Recommended permissible noise criteria for occupied, newly constructed or renovated hospital nurseries. *Journal of perinatology,* 19 (Part 1), 559-563.

Philbin MK, Klass P (2000a). Hearing and behavioral responses to sound in full term newborns. *Journal of perinatology,* 20, S68-S76.

Philbin MK, Klass P (2000b). Evaluating studies of behavioral effects of sound on newborns. *Journal of perinatology,* 20, S68-S76.

Phillipson EA (1978). Control of breathing during sleep. *American review of respiratory disease,* 118(5), 909-939.

Pickler RH et al (1993). The effect of nonnutritive sucking on bottle-feeding stress in preterm infants. *Journal of obstetric, gynecologic and neonatal nursing,* 22(3), 230-234.

Pickler RH et al (1996). Effects of nonnutritive sucking on behavioral organization and feeding performance in preterm infants. *Nursing research*, 45, 132-138.

Porte FL et al (1999). Long-term effects of pain in infants. *Journal of developmental and behavioral pediatrics*, 20, 253.

Prechtl HFR, Beintema J (1968). *The neurological examination of the full-term newborn infant*. Spastics International Medical Publications, in association with William Heinemann Medical Books, Ltd., London, and JB Lippincott Co., Philadelphia.

Provasi J, Lequien P (1993). Effects of nonrigid reclining infant seat on preterm behavioral states and motor activity. *Early human development*, 35(2), 129-140.

Regalado MG et al (1995). Sleep disorganization in cocaine-exposed neonates. *Infant behavior and development*, 18, 319-327.

Reynolds JD et al (1998). Lack of efficacy of light reduction in preventing retinopathy of prematurely. Light Reduction in Retinopathy of Prematurely (LIGHT-ROP) Cooperative Group. *New England journal of medicine*, 338, 1572-1576.

Rickards AL et al (2001). Cognition, academic progress, behavior and self-concept at 14 years of very low birth weight children. *Journal of developmental and behavioral pediatrics*, 22, 11-18.

Robinson J, Fielder AR (1992). Light and the immature visual system. *Eye*, 6, 166-172.

Sahni R et al (1995). Methodological issues in coding sleep states in immature infants. *Developmental psychobiology*, 28(2), 85-101.

St. James-Roberts I, Plewis I (1996). Individual differences, daily fluctuations, and developmental changes in amounts of infant waking, fussing, crying, and sleeping. *Child development*, 67, 2527-2540.

Sammons WAH, Lewis JM (1985). *Premature babies: a different beginning*. St Louis: Mosby.

Sanchez RM, Jensen FE (2001). Maturational aspects of epilepsy mechanisms and consequences for the immature brain. *Epilepsia*, 42, 577.

Sander LW et al (1970). Early mother-infant interaction and 24-hour patterns of activity and sleep. *Journal of American academy of child psychiatry*, 9(1), 103-123.

Sander LW et al (1979). Changes in infant and caregiver variables over the first two months of life: regulation and adaptation in the organization of the infant-caregiver system. In Thoman EB (Ed). *Origins of the infant's social responsiveness* (pp. 349-407). Hillsdale, NJ: Lawrence Erlbaum.

Satish M, Doll-Speck L (1993). *Elevated sound levels increase desaturation episodes in sick preterm infants*. Paper presented at the Annual Meeting, American Academy of Pediatrics, Washington, DC.

Scafidi FA et al (1990). Massage stimulates growth in preterm infants: A replication. *Infant behavior and development*, 13, 167-168.

Schechtman VL et al (1992). Sleep state organization in normal infants and victims of the sudden infant death syndrome. *Pediatrics*, 89(5), 865-870.

Scher A (1991). A longitudinal study of night waking in the first year. *Child: care, health and development*, 17(5), 295-302.

Scher MS et al (1994a). Lower neurodevelopmental performance at 2 years in healthy preterm neonates. *Pediatric neurology*, 11, 121.

Scher MS et al (1992a) Comparisons of EEG sleep measures in healthy full-term and preterm infants of matched conceptional ages. *Sleep*, 15(5), 442-448.

Scher MS et al (1994b). Comparison of EEG sleep state specific spectral values between healthy full-term and preterm infants at comparable postconceptional ages. *Sleep*, 17(1), 47-51.

Scher MS et al (1994c). Comparisons of EEG spectral and correlation measures between healthy term and preterm infants. *Pediatric neurology*, 10(2), 104-108.

Shiao SY et al (1997). Meta-analysis of the effects of nonnutritive sucking on heart rate and peripheral oxygenation: research from the past 30 years. *Issues in comprehensive pediatric nursing*, 20, 11-24.

Shimada M et al (1993). Development of the sleep and wakefulness rhythm in preterm infants discharged from a neonatal intensive care unit. *Pediatric research*, 33(2), 159-163.

Shimada M et al (1999). Emerging and entraining patterns of sleep-wake rhythm in preterm and term infants. *Brain & development*, 21, 468-473.

Shonkoff JP, Phillips DA (2000). *From neurons to neighborhoods: the science of early childhood development*. Washington, DC: National Academy Press.

Skadberg BT, Markestad T (1997). Behavior and physiological responses during prone and supine sleep in early infancy. *Archives of disease in childhood*, 76, 320-324.

Stevens BJ et al (1994). Factors that influence the behavioral pain responses of premature infants. *Pain*, 59, 101-109.

Taquino L, Blackburn S (1994). The effects of containment during heelstick and suctioning on the physiologic and behavioral responses of preterm infants. *Neonatal network*, 13(7), 55.

Thoman EB (1975). Early development of sleeping behaviors in infants. In Ellis NR (Ed). *Aberrant development in infancy: human and animal studies* (pp. 122-138). New York: John Wiley & Sons.

Thoman EB (1985). Sleep and waking states of the neonate (rev. ed). (Unpublished manuscript, available from Thoman EB, Box U-154, Graduate Program in Biobehavioral Sciences, 3107 Horsebarn Hill Road, University of Connecticut, Storrs, CT 06268.)

Thoman EB (1990). Sleeping and waking states in infancy: A functional perspective. *Neuroscience and biobehavioral reviews*, 14(1), 93-107.

Thoman EB et al (1981). State organization in neonates: Developmental inconsistency indicates risk for developmental dysfunction. *Neuropediatrics*, 12(1), 45-54.

Thoman EB et al (1985). Theophylline affects sleep-wake state development in premature infants. *Neuropediatrics*, 16(1), 13-18.

Thoman EB et al (1987). The sleeping and waking states of infants: Correlations across time and person. *Physiology and behavior*, 41(6), 531-537.

Thoman EB et al (1988). Infants at risk for sudden infant death syndrome (SIDS): Differential prediction for three siblings of SIDS infants. *Journal of behavioral medicine*, 11(6), 565-583.

Thoman EB et al (1991). Premature infants seek rhythmic stimulation, and the experience facilitates neurobehavioral development. *Journal of behavioral and developmental pediatrics*, 12(1), 11-18.

Thoman EB, Becker PT (1979). Issues in assessment and prediction for the infant born at risk. In Field T et al (Eds.). *Infants born at risk: behavior and development* (pp. 461-483). New York: SP Medical and Scientific Books.

Thoman EB, Graham SE (1986). Self-regulation of stimulation by premature infants. *Pediatrics*, 78(5), 855-860.

Thoman EB, Whitney MP (1989). Sleep states of infants monitored in the home: Individual differences, developmental trends, and origins of diurnal cyclicity. *Infant behavior and development*, 12(1), 59-75.

Thomas KA (2000). Differential effects of breast- and formula-feeding on preterms' sleep-wake patterns. *Journal of obstetric, gynecologic and neonatal nursing*, 29, 145-152.

Thomas KA, Martin PA (2000). NICU sound environment and the potential problems for caregivers. *Journal of perinatology*, 20, S94-S99.

Torres C et al (1997). Effect of standardized rest periods on apnea and weight gain of convalescent preterm infants. *Neonatal network*, 16(8), 35-43.

Tribotti SJ, Stein M (1992). From research to clinical practice: Implementing the NIDCAP. *Neonatal network*, 11(2), 35-40.

Van Cleve L et al (1995). Pain responses of hospitalized neonates to venipuncture. *Neonatal network*, 14(6), 31-36.

van Zoeren-Grobben D et al (1993). Lipid peroxidation in human milk and infant formula: effect of storage, tube feedings, and exposure to phototherapy. *Acta paediatrica*, 82, 645-649.

VandenBerg K (1990). The management of oral nippling in the sick neonate: The disorganized feeder. *Neonatal network*, 9(1), 9-16.

VandenBerg KA (1985). Revising the traditional model: An individualized approach to developmental interventions in the intensive care nursery. *Neonatal network*, 3(5), 32-38.

VandenBerg KA (1995). Behaviorally supportive care for the extremely premature infant. In Gunderson LP, Kenner C (Eds.). *Care of the 24-25 week gestational age infant (small baby protocol)* (ed 2, pp. 145-170). Petaluma, CA: NICU Ink.

VandenBerg KA, Franck L (1990). Behavioral issues for infants with BPD. In Lund C (Ed). *BPD: strategies for total patient care*. Petaluma, CA: Neonatal Network.

Varendi H et al (1997). Natural odour preferences of newborn infants change over time. *Acta paediatrica*, 86, 985-990.

Vecchierini M-F et al (2001). Patterns of EEG frequency, movement, heart rate, and oxygenation after isolated short apneas in infants. *Pediatric research*, 49, 220-226.

Vles JS et al (1992). State profile in low-risk pre-term infants: a longitudinal study of 7 infants from 32-36 weeks of postmenstrual age. *Brain and development*, 14(1), 12-17.

Volpe JJ (2001). *Neurology of the newborn*, ed 4, Philadelphia: WB Saunders.

Weissbluth M (1995). Naps in children: 6 months-7 years. *Sleep*, 18(2), 82-87.

White R (1999). Recommended standards for newborn ICU design. *Journal of perinatology*, 19 (pt 2), S2-S12.

White-Traut RC et al (1993). Patterns of physiologic and behavioral response of intermediate care preterm infants to intervention. *Pediatric nursing*, 1(6), 625-629.

White-Traut R et al (1994). Environmental influences on the developing premature infant: theoretical issues and applications to practice. *Journal of obstetric, gynecologic and neonatal nursing*, 23, 393-401.

White-Traut RC et al (1997). Response of preterm infants to unimodal and multimodal sensory intervention. *Pediatric nursing*, 23, 169-175, 193.

White-Traut RC et al (1999). Developmental intervention for preterm infants diagnosed with periventricular leukomalcia. *Research in nursing and health*, 22, 131-143.

White-Traut RC, Pate CM (1987). Modulating infant state in premature infants. *Journal of pediatric nursing*, 2(2), 96-101.

Whitney MP, Thoman EB (1993). Early sleep patterns of premature infants are differentially related to later developmental disabilities. *Journal of developmental and behavioral pediatrics*, 14(2), 71-80.

Whitney MP, Thoman EB (1994). Sleep in premature and full term infants from 24-hour home recordings. *Infant behavior and development*, 17, 223-234.

Winberg J, Porter RH (1998). Olfaction and human neonatal behaviour: clinical implications. *Acta paediatrica*, 87, 6-10.

Wolff PH (1959). Observations on newborn infants. *Psychosomatic medicine*, 21, 110-118.

Wolff PH (1966). The causes, controls, and organization of behavior in the neonate. *Psychological issues*, 5(1), 1-105.

Woods NS et al (1993). Cocaine use during pregnancy: maternal depressive symptoms and infant neurobehavior over the first month. *Infant behavior and development*, 16(1), 83-98.

Zahr LK, de Traversay J (1995). Premature infant responses to noise reduction by earmuffs: Effects on behavioral and physiologic measures. *Journal of perinatology*, 15, 514.

Zahr LK, Balian S (1995). Responses of premature infants to routine nursing interventions and noise in the NICU. *Nursing research*, 44(3), 179-185.

CHAPTER 18

Monitoring Neonatal Biophysical Parameters in a Developmentally Supportive Environment

Valerie Kay Moniaci, Scott D. Moniaci

BIRTH ENVIRONMENT

Knowledge and technology in the neonatal field have advanced rapidly over the past 10 years. We have learned that the environment into which infants are born has a significant impact on their overall outcome. Neonatal intensive care units (NICUs) are being built so that they are more baby and family friendly. Neonatal nurses must constantly update their skills in the newest treatment methods and technologic advances, and all health care professionals in the NICU must have a basic understanding of the way each piece of equipment works.

For all infants, successful adaptation to extrauterine life depends on timely assessment of their physiologic and biochemical status in the immediate postnatal period. Warmers, resuscitation bags, and cardiorespiratory and saturation monitors are aids in the successful transition to extrauterine life. Also, continuous monitoring of all physiologic and biochemical parameters immediately provides caregivers with important data on which to base their response.

The infant considered nonviable 10 years ago now has a greater than 80% chance of life. However, monitoring these infants is difficult because of their small size and physical limitations. The extremely-low-birth-weight (ELBW) infant is even more of a challenge; these neonates have a greater risk of skin breakdown, and placing monitoring leads and saturation probes can damage their fragile skin.

Bedside monitoring of physiologic parameters has become standard in the NICU. Different types of equipment may be used, but all provide continuous monitoring of vital signs (temperature, heart rate, blood pressure, respiratory rate, and carbon dioxide and oxygen levels). Advances in computer technology have provided not only bedside charting, which allows the nurse more time with the baby, but also systems that coordinate and maintain patient data in one program that can easily be retrieved when needed. Remote access monitoring allows continuous monitoring in different areas of the unit based on a central computerized system. This system also allows physicians to access the information from their home computers.

Transcutaneous oxygen and carbon dioxide monitors are slowly being replaced by inline sensors that provide continuous readouts of oxygen and carbon dioxide levels via the umbilical arterial catheter. These sensors have reduced the cost of neonatal care by reducing the number of times blood must be drawn for blood gas determinations in sick and premature babies. The sensors also may affect the total number of blood transfusions because they greatly reduce the amount of blood removed and tested. Continuous data readouts for oxygen and carbon dioxide, variables that are important for every organ system, allow the nurse to make nearly instantaneous changes in oxygen and ventilator settings.

The neonate presents numerous obstacles to transduction that make it difficult to obtain data instantaneously. Clinical medicine often adapts technologic devices that have proved accurate and reliable in other research fields. The measurement of biophysical parameters in a living organism does pose some problems that may not be encountered elsewhere. However, regardless of the signal to be measured and monitored, a number of fundamental principles must be applied to ensure the results are accurate and reproducible. This chapter discusses those principles, and the physics and engineering bases for their implementation.

BIOLOGIC SIGNALS

Continuous monitoring of all biophysical parameters has become the hallmark of intensive care units, and the NICU is no exception. Continuous monitoring provides instantaneous information on the patient's biologic status so that interventions can be carried out without delay, improving the outcome of care. Monitoring of the heart rate (by means of an electrocardiogram [ECG]), blood pressure (via central and peripheral routes), respiratory rate, temperature (continuous and intermittent), and oxygen levels is commonplace in most NICUs. Many different types of equipment are available with a variety of biophysical monitoring capabilities. Understanding when to use specific equipment and the reason for using it helps nurses achieve positive outcomes for patients.

Signals from the body must be "transduced" to the monitoring equipment in order for it to "read out" the information. In some cases a stimulus to the body system may be needed to generate a transducible signal that can be processed for interpretation. A common example of this is blood pressure measurement with a sphygmomanometer.

Accurate measurement of a biologic signal depends on the sensing system's ability to detect a specific transducible property of the signal and convert it to electrical energy, which can then

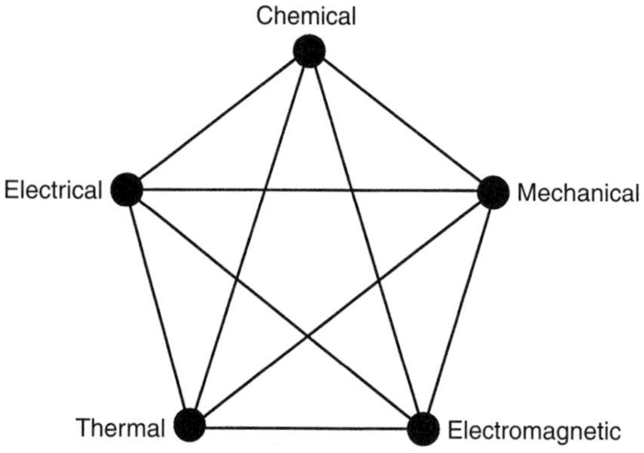

FIGURE **18-1**

Biologic signal types. Interconnecting lines represent biologic events that could have a cascade of physical properties.

TABLE **18-1**	Types of Sensors Used for Monitoring Various Biophysical Parameters
Sensor Type	**Biophysical Parameter**
Chemical	PO_2, PCO_2
Electrical	Heart rate, respiration rate
Mechanical	Blood pressure, intracranial pressure
Electromagnetic	Skin temperature, oxygen saturation
Thermal	Temperature, metabolic rate

PO_2, *Partial pressure of oxygen*; PCO_2, *partial pressure of carbon dioxide.*

be processed to provide some type of visual presentation. This is what is "seen," for example, on the ECG monitor. The transducer must have a high degree of specificity so that it can distinguish the targeted signal from other biologic signals, and it must also filter out extraneous or biologic noise, such as muscle movement artifact. Biologic signals can be categorized according to physical properties described by chemical, electrical, mechanical, electromagnetic, or thermal behavior (Figure 18-1).

Many biologic processes involve chemical reactions. The actual reaction or the end product of the reaction may provide some detectable difference in chemical state that forms a basis for detection and signal generation. In most cases, biochemical reactions and associated signals are inaccessible to in vivo transduction with current methods and require the removal of the tissue or fluid for processing and analysis.

Because of its ionic origin, the bioelectrical signal can be considered a special type of biochemical signal. Bioelectrical signals range from the low-voltage transmembrane potentials in cells to the medium-voltage electrocardiographic signals of the heart. Bioelectrical signals are the type most widely used in clinical medicine, because they can be transduced and manipulated with relative ease to provide information using conventional signal processing tools such as the amplifier and the computer.

The pressure, flow, and velocity of the blood are important biomechanical signals that are easily transduced.

Electromagnetic signals have energies in the wavelength region of nonionizing radiation. In some cases electromagnetic signals can be detected by a change in energy at some wavelength or by a shift in the wavelength of peak energy emission.

Because most biochemical reactions result in the release or consumption of energy, biologic status can be assessed by the transduction of specific thermal properties, such as by measuring temperature changes or the amount of heat released. Temperature is the most widely used biophysical indicator of health status (Table 18-1).

Although not accessible noninvasively, each cell has its own state of electrical activity, which can characterize its biologic status. Single-cell membrane potentials form the basis for all biopotentials; that is, together, the cell membrane potentials for a particular type of tissue produce that tissue's biopotential. Biopotentials are the most frequently transduced physiologic parameters. The ECG, for example, measures the biopotential generated by cardiac tissue, which is detectable

even on the surface of the skin. In biologic systems, the movement of ions in an electrolyte solution produces electrical activity. (This same principle explains the generation of current in the typical lead-acid car battery.) Biopotentials are used to communicate or stimulate specific responses. They also can be converted into electrical voltages (e.g., using ECG electrodes to transduce an electrical response).

The body is composed of a wide range of physical systems that communicate with each other, and it adjusts and controls these systems to obtain a specific response or state. Electrical, mechanical, chemical, and thermal systems are used for communication and stimulation in living biologic systems. The cardiovascular, respiratory, and nervous systems have been studied in depth using biophysical transduction techniques. The transducers and monitoring systems for these body systems form the basis for most inline continuous monitoring tools.

The biochemical system that controls energy output for body activity and the messenger system for cellular communication are the most inaccessible to noninvasive transduction. Biophysical transducers have been developed to obtain indirect measurements from these biochemical systems. For example, the oxygen saturation level of hemoglobin can be determined using optical techniques. Light pulses are timed to the cardiac pulse wave, and the differences in absorption between oxygenated and unoxygenated hemoglobin are detected as changes in the intensity of transmitted optical levels. These light level differences can be correlated with the level of oxygen saturation.

In particular, at the biochemical level, much is unknown about the interaction and interrelationship both of individual cell types and of overall systems. This interaction among cell types and higher order physiologic systems makes the detection of parameters in nonisolated intact biologic systems extremely difficult. Consequently, clinical assessment of biochemical status still relies heavily on analysis of isolated tissue or body fluids. However, as our understanding of the body's interactions improves, noninvasive optical techniques could be developed, expanding the use of noninvasive biophysical transduction at the bedside.

BIOPHYSICAL MONITORING SYSTEM

Biophysical monitoring systems can be described as open-loop or closed-loop architecture (Figure 18-2, A). Open-loop systems (Figure 18-2, B) are the simplest and are used to transduce spontaneous events, as in ECG monitoring. In closed-loop systems (Figure 18-2, C), the patient receives a stimulus, and a feedback signal adjusts the stimulus in response to the level of the transduced signal from the patient. The closed-loop system

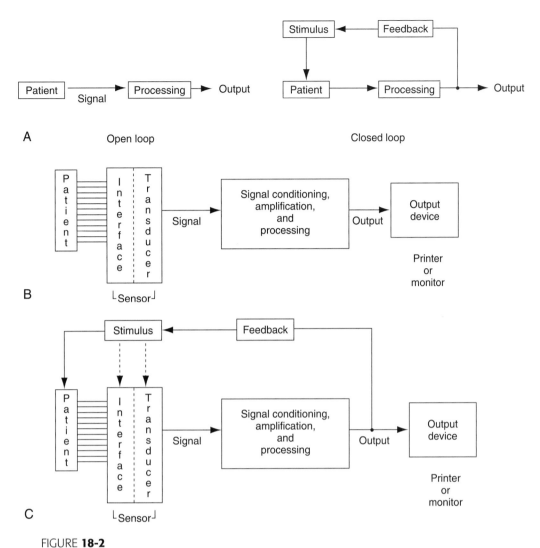

FIGURE **18-2**
A, Types of monitoring system architecture. **B,** Open-loop biophysical monitoring system.
C, Closed-loop biophysical monitoring system.

is used when a transducible response is not normally present; a good example of this type of system is the automated, noninvasive blood pressure monitor, which uses controlled deflation of cuff pressure to transduce blood pressure.

With open-loop biophysical monitoring systems, the basic components are the same for most types of in vivo monitoring setups. The system consists of three main components: a sensor that is connected to the patient, signal conditioning equipment that conditions and processes the signal, and an output device, such as a computer terminal or printer, to present the transduced information to the caregiver.

The sensor typically has two main components: the interface and the transducing element. The interface is in contact with the patient (e.g., electrically conductive paste on an ECG electrode). The transducing element is designed to be responsive to and to recognize the specific parameter of interest and to generate some type of electrical signal (e.g., the oxygen electrode used in transcutaneous oxygen measurement). The electrical signal is sent to the signal conditioning and processing equipment. For some transduction applications, a membrane must be incorporated between the patient and the sensor to filter out noise or to allow only a specific analyte to reach the sensing element; in such cases the membrane becomes the in-

terface to the patient. Using a membrane increases the specificity of the sensor. For example, a transcutaneous oxygen transducer's sensitivity to oxygen is controlled by placing an oxygen-permeable membrane between the patient and the sensing element.

Some biophysical parameters are best measured when electronic filters are used in the transducer to remove noise and to make the sensor more sensitive to signals with a particular frequency response. The disadvantage of this approach is that it can be used only to remove noise in frequency ranges above and below the actual physiologic response measured. Electronic filters are also used when the amplitude of the sensor signal is low and could be subject to interference from ambient radio waves. In addition, in applications involving low biologic signal power, local amplification at the transducer is used to boost the strength of the signal, making it less sensitive to external interferences.

The output from the transducer is always some form of analog signal, which usually is carried through wires to the signal conditioning equipment. Although not widely used in neonatal monitoring, telemetry in the radio frequency or optical ranges can be used to send the transduced signal to the conditioning equipment. Telemetry eliminates the need for wires between the transducer and the conditioning or display equipment.

The signal conditioning system processes the signal and converts it into a form that can be displayed on a cathode-ray tube or sent to some other type of output device, such as a printer or strip chart recorder. The signal conditioning section of the system is where the transduced signal is converted from some type of voltage signal to clinically relevant units; for example, the output from a blood pressure transducer is an analog voltage that is processed to provide a readout in millimeters of mercury.

When a biophysical parameter of interest cannot be transduced from spontaneous occurrence, it may be possible to elicit a transducible response by using some type of external stimulus (e.g., using light to produce a visual evoked response, which is an electrical signal that can be transduced and recorded). In other types of evoked response transduction, it may be desirable or necessary to control the degree of stimulation. This can be accomplished by modifying the level of stimulation according to the strength of the transduced signal. This type of feedback control is used in noninvasive blood pressure monitoring, in which the cuff pressure is progressively increased to occlude blood flow. The occlusion force is patient dependent, and the use of closed-loop control of the cuff pressure makes this type of transduction feasible for automated continuous or intermittent blood pressure monitoring. In Figure 18-2, C, the dotted lines from the stimulus to the sensor indicate a feedback system in which the sensor itself is actuated or adjusted in response to the transduced signal.

Factors that Influence Monitoring Reliability

Computers have greatly influenced biophysical monitoring systems, but computer processing and manipulation capabilities are limited and ultimately depend on the quality of the transduced signal. The computer cannot add physiologic information to the transduced biophysical signal or compensate for unforeseen errors in the transduction processes. Even though electrical monitoring devices are readily available and widely used, they still can provide false or inaccurate data. Even the best electrical equipment cannot replace an accurate, complete assessment of the patient's status. Effective use of measurement systems in biophysical monitoring depends on how error-free the process can be. Errors can occur in the transducer at the site of signal detection, in the conditioning and processing equipment, or in both. The conventional approach to eliminating errors is to calibrate the system using a known standard. The performance of the monitoring system is based on the types and magnitude of the errors that may be encountered in the application. Calibration is an effective means of detecting and correcting for amplitude errors. Errors usually are defined in the manufacturer's specifications for the specific monitoring system.

Because the biologic system primarily generates AC or time-varying complex periodic signals, the monitoring system architecture must accurately reproduce the transduced signals in both amplitude and frequency. The ECG waveform is a complex periodic biologic signal. The primary frequency of this wave is the heart rate. However, the basic wave is complex in that the amplitude of the wave changes at different rates over one cycle. If the biophysical transduction or signal conditioning system does not have adequate frequency response, the signal may be distorted. The frequency response of the system is defined as the range of frequencies over which the amplitude and phase of the biologic signal can be detected accurately (Figure 18-3). As the preferred response, the amplitude ratio of the signal should be constant over the range of frequencies

encountered in the signal. The signal is attenuated when the system absorbs more energy at one set of frequencies than at other frequencies. At some frequencies the system also can exhibit resonance, an undesirable type of signal amplification. All of this means that it is important to know the frequency content of the biologic signal to be measured and to select a monitoring system with an adequate frequency response or bandwidth.

The important aspect with respect to the bandwidth of a signal is to determine the fastest changing portion of the signal. Analysis of this fast-changing part yields the highest frequency component of the signal. For complex biologic signals, spectral analysis tools are used to dissect the signal. This process is based on the Fourier theorem, which states that it is always possible to decompose a complex periodic waveform into a series of simple sine waves of varying frequencies. Each of the sinusoids contributes to the original signal. These sinusoids are called harmonics, and the contribution of each harmonic to the original signal is weighted as a function of its amplitude. The bandwidth of the signal is defined by the frequency range of the simple sinusoids required to recreate the signal. This type of analysis is widely used and is referred to as spectral or Fourier analysis. Fourier analysis also yields information on the phase angle characteristics of the signal. The phase angle of the signal is a function of the capacitive and inductive components of the signal source. Distortion of the phase angle by the monitoring system can cause shifts in the timing of the signal. In most cases, however, phase angle distortion only delays the signal, it does not alter its actual shape. Table 18-2 presents some routine physiologic determinations and their associated biophysical systems, as well as the amplitude and frequency ranges of the signals encountered in these systems.

Most monitoring systems can have expected errors that incorrectly represent the amplitude of the signal (Figure 18-4). Some such errors occur over time and are referred to as drift errors. Drift can be caused by changes in the transducer properties with time and usually occurs slowly. A drift error usually starts out small and increases gradually with time. These types of errors can increase or decrease the amplitude of the signal, but they are different from offset errors because the magnitude of the error changes with time (with offset error, the magnitude remains constant).

Another type of error can occur when there is a change in the degree of error based on the amplitude of the signal; this is called a proportional error. Proportional errors can also be nonlinear, which makes them extremely difficult to correct. Hysteresis errors are caused when the current measurement

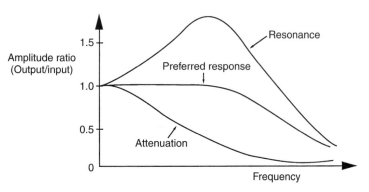

FIGURE **18-3**
Influence of frequency response on a signal.

depends on the previous measurement level. The error may be different when the signal goes from a low to a higher level or from a high to a lower level. Most electronic devices are susceptible to hysteresis errors.

Computer processing of the transduced signal can compensate and correct for some of these errors when they are nonrandom. However, in some monitoring systems these errors are small and cannot be corrected or compensated for in the conditioning and processing components. In such cases, the error is used to quantify the accuracy of the system in the form of a tolerance for the output. Tolerances are expressed as a percentage of the range or are assigned limits to the range. For example, the output for a transcutaneous monitor could be specified as accurate within 5 mm Hg.

In the transduction of information from the biologic system, the positioning of the transducer may alter the response and introduce errors. This is the major practical limitation of using transducers that must make physical contact with the living tissue. Another important factor in the performance of measurement systems is the signal to noise ratio, which expresses the level of noise in a system in reference to the level of signal. This ratio should be as high as possible to minimize the effect of noise on the monitoring system. Sometimes wires used to connect a transducer to the patient act as an antenna and pick up electrical noise from the environment, which could cause interference, for example, in an ECG. Biologic noise may affect the actual transducer if the sensing element cannot be protected from biologic matter that generates characteristics similar to those of the anolyte of interest.

Stability is another important criterion when assessing the performance of a monitoring system. Stability can be affected by temperature changes in the operating environment. In addition, the monitoring system may depend on its own operating temperature, which may change as a function of the length of time power is supplied. This operating temperature change is characterized as warm-up time.

In neonatal monitoring, the effect of temperature must be considered for all types of transduction, because nursing care for nearly all neonates is carried out in warming beds. In most cases these environments are convectively warmed enclosed incubators or open bassinet infrared radiant heaters. It is also important to consider how high-intensity optical radiation from phototherapy or examination lights may affect the transducers or conditioning and processing devices.

Specific Applications

Temperature Measurement.   Contact thermometry is the prevalent technique for the routine measurement of body temperature. The neonatal body temperature can be measured using a rectal or skin surface technique. The rectal temperature is the best indictor of the "core" body temperature; however, in neonates this technique is not used every time vital signs are

TABLE 18-2	Amplitude and Frequency Ranges of Frequently Monitored Biophysical Parameters		
		Amplitude Range	Frequency Range
Cardiovascular System **Electrocardiogram (ECG)**			
Skin surface		0-5 mV	0.05-80 Hz
Direct cardiac		0-20 mV	0.05-80 Hz
Pressure			
Arterial		20-300 mm Hg	0-15 Hz
Ventricular		5-300 mm Hg	0-15 Hz
Blood Flow			
Cardiac output		0-1 L/second	0-15 Hz
Velocity		0-5 m/second	0-15 Hz
Respiratory System			
Flow rate		0-1 L/second	0-5 Hz
Blood gases			
PO_2		10-650 mm Hg	0-2 Hz
PCO_2		10-90 mm Hg	0-2 Hz
pH		6.9-7.7	0-2 Hz
Neuromuscular System **Electroencephalogram (EEG)**			
Body surface		5-300 mV	0.2-50 Hz
Brain surface		10-5000 µV	0.2-50 Hz
Evoked potentials		0-50 mV	10-500 Hz
Core temperature		30°-40° C	DC
Skin temperature		20°-42° C	DC
Water evaporation rate		0-70 g/m²/hour	0-5 Hz

pH, *hydrogen ion concentration*; PO_2, *partial pressure of oxygen*; PCO_2, *partial pressure of carbon dioxide*.

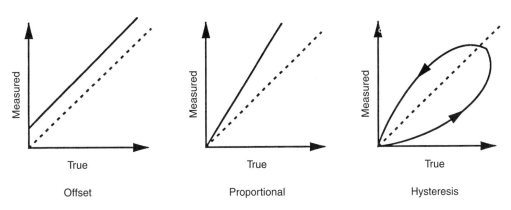

FIGURE **18-4**
Amplitude errors. The dotted lines represent a linear response.

measured because of the risk of gastrointestinal perforation and vagal response. Skin temperature monitoring is the most commonly used technique for temperature measurement in the NICU. Auxiliary temperature measurement often is used in conjunction with continuous monitoring by means of a skin temperature probe attached to an open bed warmer or incubator. A continuous readout of the infant's temperature provides current and accurate information for the caregiver *providing* the probe is attached securely and placed appropriately. If the infant is found lying on the probe or if the probe becomes loose, the temperature displayed may not reflect the infant's true temperature. Probes placed on bony prominences do not contact enough of the skin surface to display an accurate temperature. In most clinical situations, however, skin temperature alone provides no real quantitative assessment of the patient's status. The skin temperature, the core temperature, and the ambient air or environmental temperature, considered together, provide a more effective indicator of the infant's thermal balance.

An important consideration in the temperature regulation of neonates is the relationship between body temperature and oxygen consumption or metabolic demand. Unfortunately, metabolic effects (as measured by oxygen consumption) cannot be continuously monitored in babies. Intermittent temperature measurement in newborns merely tells us how efficient the neonate's body is at maintaining its temperature; it does not provide information about the amount of energy the body expends to maintain that "normal" temperature. For example, infants who are dressed or swaddled in an incubator on either air or skin temperature mode may have a normal temperature, but it may be at the expense of growth because of an increased metabolic demand to provide heat. If the air and skin temperature set points are significantly lower than might be expected for gestational age, the infant's body must maintain its own temperature instead of relying on the incubator to do its job (Lyon et al, 1997, Narendran & Hoath, 1999).

ELBW infants pose special problems with temperature regulation because they have very little subcutaneous fat, an immature epidermis, an increased surface area to body weight ratio, and poor vasomotor control (Vohra et al, 1999). It is becoming common practice in this age group to add humidity to incubators in an attempt to maintain normal body temperatures by reducing insensible water losses and limiting the metabolic demand for oxygen (Narendran & Hoath, 1999).

Temperature is one of the crucial indicators of the health status of newborns. Glass thermometers gradually have been replaced by electronic thermometers. Using an individual thermometer for each baby is inexpensive, ensures sterility, and prevents cross-contamination. Parents can easily be taught how to take their infant's temperature as early as the first day of life. Protective plastic sleeves can be used on the sensing element; in some cases, the sensing element itself is a single-use disposable item.

Heat loss in the neonate occurs by four methods: radiation, conduction, convection, and evaporation. Radiant heat loss occurs when heat from the infant is transferred to a nearby object, such as a cool window. Double-walled incubators help prevent radiant heat loss. Conductive heat loss occurs when the infant is placed directly on a cooler object and the baby's body heat is transferred to the object. This occurs when infants are placed in open bed warmers that have not been preheated or when they are laid on cool blankets or cold radiographic plates. Convective heat loss occurs when the infant is placed

in a cool room or corridor or is exposed to outside air (e.g., when nursing care is provided with the incubator door open). Maintaining room temperature in the nursery in a neutral thermal environment (22.2° to 24.4° C) (Blackburn & Loper, 1992) helps eliminate convective heat loss. Evaporative heat loss occurs with evaporation of moisture from a wet object into surrounding cooler air. This type of heat loss is most evident during the immediate postnatal period, when the infant is wet from the delivery, but it also can happen during bathing. After delivery, drying the infant immediately with a warm blanket helps prevent evaporative heat loss. During bathing, shielding the baby with a warm blanket and drying the infant rapidly helps limit evaporative heat loss.

A common problem with all types of contact thermometry is that the indicated temperature is a reflection of the entire surface in contact with the sensing element. A large sensing element indicates an average temperature for its entire surface contact area. The temperature-sensing device must have adequate time to equilibrate with its environment before a reliable temperature can be measured. This time to an acceptable response is a function of the time constant of the sensor. The time constant is the standard notation for classifying how fast a temperature is sensed and is defined as the time to reach 63% of the final value in response to an abrupt change in temperature. The length of time required to reach the final temperature usually is multiple time constants. The time constant is primarily a function of the physical size and density of the temperature-sensing element. Devices with large time constants cannot be used to monitor temperature when rapid changes are expected.

Electronic thermometers are based on the principle that most materials show some type of physical change in response to temperature. The thermistor, the platinum resistance temperature device (RTD), and the thermocouple are the most common temperature-sensing elements used in electronic thermometers. The temperature-dependent physical changes in each of these devices are reversible and can be transduced with repeatability and acceptable accuracy for biologic applications.

The thermistor is a thermally sensitive resistor in which the resistance changes as a function of temperature. Thermistors are made from semiconductor materials. Semiconductor materials usually are some form of metal oxide and are similar to the basic materials used to produce the semiconductor components of electronic instruments (e.g., transistors, integrated circuits). The electrical conduction and resistance properties of these materials change exponentially with temperature. This exponential change makes these devices very sensitive to temperature, but the exponential nature of the change makes the resistance curve for the thermistor nonlinear. To obtain useful temperature data, the nonlinear change in resistance with temperature must be corrected in the signal conditioning and processing component of the monitoring system. When a constant current is passed through a thermistor, changes in resistance caused by temperature change produce a change in the voltage measured across the thermistor. Thermistors can be made very small and, with laser cutting techniques, can be produced in large quantities with low variability in the resistance temperature response.

Platinum RTDs are based on the resistance change of metal wire with temperature changes. The wire is wound on an insulating core for physical support. The mechanical winding process requires much larger dimensions than for thermistors. The resistance change of an RTD is always linear, and this linear response to temperature is the significant advantage of RTDs over thermistors. Because they are much larger than thermistors, RTDs have larger time constants. Also, RTDs cannot be used for invasive applications as easily as the much smaller thermistors.

Unlike the thermistor or RTD, a thermocouple does not require an applied voltage or current at the transducing element to measure temperature. The thermocouple is based on the principle that when two dissimilar metals are placed in contact, a voltage difference is created across this metal contact. Because the thermocouple is made from metals, the voltage difference is a function of temperature. This difference in voltage results in current flow through the circuit, which can then be transduced and processed. Thermocouples can be made as small as the available wire diameters. Its small size gives the thermocouple a faster response time than either the thermistor or the RTD. However, for biologic in vivo tissue exposure, the metals must be protected from oxidation, and the protective coating can adversely affect the time constant of the thermocouple because of the increased thermal mass.

Advances in manufacturing have greatly reduced the cost of thermistors, RTDs, and thermocouples, to the extent that these sensing elements can be designed as single-use or disposable items. For example, because the actual resistance of a thermistor is a function of its physical size, automated cutting equipment can adjust the size to meet a very specific resistance range. This type of manufacturing process can ensure that each thermistor produced is virtually the same.

The use of these types of temperature-sensing elements in disposable thermometers can also overcome an inherent problem in that each of these devices deteriorates with age. In particular, the resistance of a thermistor changes over time. This type of failure is gradual and can go undetected if calibration is not checked regularly. Calibration of equipment using thermistors should be closely monitored if the thermistors are not replaced routinely.

The most common failure for thermistors, RTDs, and thermocouples is an open circuit or short circuit. For a thermistor, a short circuit occurs as a very high temperature reading (zero resistance). Most clinical thermometers provide some type of alarm that indicates when a catastrophic failure such as this has occurred.

The most common problem with temperature measurement is ensuring that the sensor has good contact with the surface being measured. Measuring the skin temperature of a newborn in the delivery room is difficult because it is virtually impossible to attach a skin probe to the wet infant. When the sensor is not in intimate contact with the skin surface, the temperature measured is greatly influenced by the environmental temperature. The skin probe used on an infant under a radiant warmer does not accurately indicate the infant's skin temperature if the temperature sensor is not shielded from the direct radiation of the heating system by a reflective pad. The pad reflects the incident radiation and prevents the absorption of energy, which would heat the sensor and elevate the detected temperature.

As their name implies, noncontact infrared thermometers and infrared thermographic cameras can measure temperatures without being in contact with the surface to be measured; this ensures a high level of sterility and of protection for the infant's skin. Noncontact thermometers work on the principle that all materials emit radiation. The intensity and wavelength of the emitted radiation are a function of the object's temperature; as the temperature increases, so does the intensity or power at a given wavelength. The peak of the energy curve moves toward the shorter wavelengths as the temperature increases (Figure 18-5).

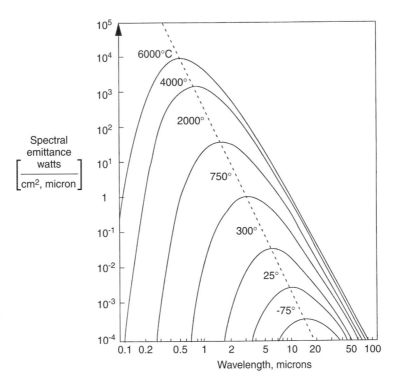

FIGURE **18-5**
Blackbody radiation curves. Intensity increases with temperature, and the peak of the energy curve moves toward shorter wavelengths.

The temperature of the surface emitting the radiation can be determined by measuring the power of the radiation over a range of wavelengths. For temperatures in the physiologic range, energy is emitted in the infrared region. The infrared detectors used to measure human body temperatures are designed for wavelengths in the 5- to 25-mm range. These devices can be used for single-point temperature measurement, or they can provide thermal images for an entire surface. Infrared detectors (e.g., all optical measurement systems) can have interference either from reflections from other objects or from infrared energy transmitted through the surface being observed. The total energy received at the detector is a combination of the emitted, reflected, and transmitted energies (Figure 18-6).

When using infrared thermometers, the nurse must make sure that no other sources of heat can interfere with the surface being measured. Infrared energies are reflected, just like visible light. Infrared thermometers are used to measure the tympanic membrane temperature, because the tympanic membrane has proved to be a good indicator of core temperature. However, the size of the optic head on these temperature monitors makes it difficult to position the thermometer in the ear canal to ensure good alignment with the tympanic membrane, particularly in premature infants. If not aligned properly, the thermometer may read the temperature of the ear canal rather than the tympanic membrane. Also, this type of temperature measuring device can be affected by the depth the probe is inserted into the ear canal and possibly by the presence of vernix or other debris. Some NICUs are using tympanic temperature measurements, reportedly with good results, but clinical trials have yet to be conducted with premature and term infants of various gestational ages and under various conditions.

Electrocardiographic Monitoring. Biophysical signals are derived from the electrical activity of the body at a cellular level. The human body is composed of approximately 75 trillion cells, which vary in size, shape, construction, and physical properties. The internal structures of the cell are separated from the surrounding body fluid by a cell wall membrane. Bioelectricity is generated because the cell wall membrane is semipermeable, meaning that electrolytes (sodium and potassium) can move freely into and out of the cell, each cell generating an electrical charge or transduced signal that is observed on monitoring equipment. The difference in ionic concentration between the inside and the outside of the cell produces an electrical membrane potential across the cell wall. When a cell is at rest (polarized), the concentration of ions is such that the interior of the cell is more negative than the exterior. (Sodium and potassium are both present inside and outside the cell. Inside the cell the concentration of potassium is approximately 30 times that of sodium, whereas outside the cell, the concentration of sodium is approximately 10 times that of potassium. This creates an electrical potential difference across the cell wall of −90 mV, with the inside being the negative reference point.) Stimulated cells become "depolarized," which changes the makeup of the cell membrane. At this time, potassium is moved out of the cell, and sodium moves inside. Depolarization lasts several milliseconds and changes the membrane potential of the cell from −70/91 mV to +20/40 mV. This change in potential is called the action potential. During the action potential, the cell cannot be retriggered by stimulation; this period is called the refractory period. Different cells in the body elicit different action potentials (Carr, 1992).

Bioelectrical potentials are transduced from the skin surface for ECG, electroencephalogram (EEG), and evoked potentials. The potentials on the body range from 1 V to 1 mV. Body surface electrodes attached to the skin (Figure 18-7) are used to convert the ionic potentials produced by the ionic current flow in tissue into electronic potentials. The surface electrode uses a metal-electrolyte interface. The electrolyte for biologic transduction can be the fluid around the tissue. Artificial electrolytes in a gel substance usually are incorporated into commercial electrodes. An electrical potential is generated at the

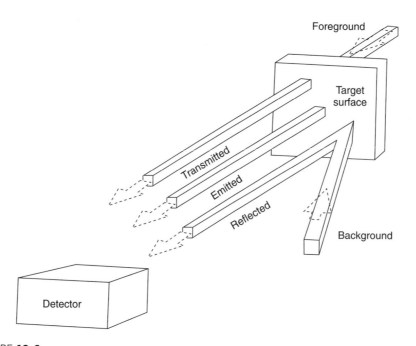

FIGURE **18-6**
The total amount of energy received at the detector is a combination of the emitted, reflected, and transmitted energies.

metal-electrolyte interface when there is a difference in the diffusion rates of ions into and out of the metal. Metallic ions in solution with their associated metals always develop an electrode potential, known as a half-cell potential. The most common electrode is the silver–silver chloride electrode. Pairs of these electrodes can be coupled to produce a voltage source, just as in a battery.

Two electrodes are necessary to measure bioelectrical potentials, and the voltage measured is actually the instantaneous potentials of the two electrodes. If the two electrodes are exactly the same, the voltage difference depends on the biologic ionic difference between the two electrodes. If the two electrodes are different, there is a potential, or DC, voltage between them. This DC voltage, referred to as electrode offset, affects the transduction of ionic potentials. Offsets such as this sometimes are caused by drying of the electrolyte gel in one of the electrodes. Microelectrodes and needle electrodes used to penetrate the skin function on the same basic principle as ECG electrodes. The premature infant has a poorly developed stratum corneum. Because this immature skin has a low resistance to current flow, a good electrical signal is easy to obtain during the early postnatal period. As the stratum corneum develops and the skin becomes less moist, it is important to check and replace the electrodes to ensure that there is sufficient electrolyte for good electrical conduction. Difficulties with the ECG baseline usually can be attributed to drying of the electrolyte. Also, during the neonate's first week of life, the electrodes are very sensitive to motion artifact and baseline drift.

Respiratory Rate Monitoring. Impedance electrodes generate an electrical field around tissue. The electrodes are the same as those used for biopotential transduction, such as with the ECG. Measured distortions or changes in the electrical field can be attributed to specific tissue effects. Impedance electrodes are applied in the form of an impedance bridge, and the electrodes are excited with low-voltage, high-frequency AC. The high frequencies used pose no risk of ventricular fibrillation.

Impedance is the transduction principle used to measure respiratory rate and cardiac output. Two electrodes placed at the extremes of the thoracic cavity can be used to detect volume changes caused by respiration (Figure 18-8). The expansion and contraction of the intervening tissue mass during each respiratory cycle cause detectable changes in the electrical conducting path. This change is referred to as impedance and is transducible if the changes are large enough. In the three-lead ECG configuration, impedance transduction usually is applied to two of the electrodes to determine the respiratory

rate. Because the electrodes detect resistance to current flow, it is extremely important that they be in intimate contact with the skin surface. In these cases, also, drying of the electrolyte gel results in impedance changes that can cause baseline drift. This method of monitoring the respiratory rate is widely used because it does not require any electrodes or connections to the infant other than those needed for ECG monitoring.

Pulse Oximetry (Transcutaneous Oxygen Saturation) Monitoring. Transcutaneous measurement of the oxygen saturation of the blood ($TcSaO_2$), known as pulse oximetry, is widely used in the NICU. Pulse oximetry provides a continuous readout of the oxygen saturation but is not without limitations. Poor perfusion, as seen with cool extremities or diminished cardiac output, results in a significant underestimation of the saturation value. The accuracy of measurements also is affected by the proportions of hemoglobin A and hemoglobin F, the partial pressure of arterial carbon dioxide ($PaCO_2$), the hydrogen ion concentration (pH), and the infant's temperature (Grieve et al, 1997).

The concentration of hemoglobin also can affect the readout of the pulse oximeter. For example, an infant born with a low hemoglobin (less than 5 g) will display falsely elevated saturation levels because the small amount of hemoglobin present is easily saturated with oxygen. Despite this full saturation of the hemoglobin with oxygen, the infant may still be hypoxemic because the amount of available oxygen (and ultimately hemoglobin) is inadequate for metabolic purposes.

Pulse oximetry is easy to use, but the probe site must be moved frequently between the extremities to maintain the integrity of the skin. This may be problematic with ELBW infants, whose skin is fragile and friable. Artifact movement can produce falsely high or low values, and infant movement and poor attachment of the probe are frequently the cause of false readings from the monitor. The accuracy of readings generally is accepted if the pulse rate readings are within 10% of each other on both the saturation monitor and the cardiorespiratory monitor (Grieve et al, 1997). The monitors from different manufacturers display differences in artifact presence and slight differences in saturation readings. (In one clinical trial, the Nellcor pulse oximeter showed a mean saturation level approximately 2% higher than the Ohmeda oximeter [Grieve et al, 1997].) It is a constant struggle to maintain saturation levels within set ordered limits to provide adequate oxygenation, yet not impose the risks of hyperoxia on the newborn infant.

Oximetry uses spectrophotometric analysis of light transmitted through or reflected back from light-absorbing substances. Light-absorbing substances have an absorption coefficient for

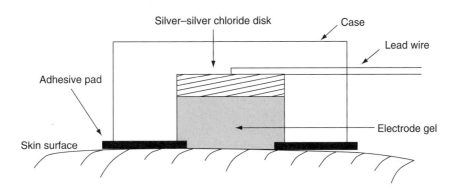

FIGURE **18-7**
Diagram of a skin surface electrode.

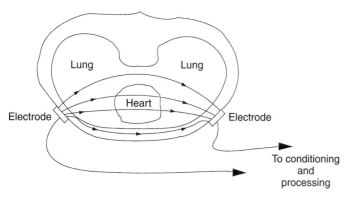

FIGURE **18-8**
Electrodes placed on the extremities of the thoracic cavity are sensitive to volume changes caused by respiration. The arrows show the current path between the electrodes.

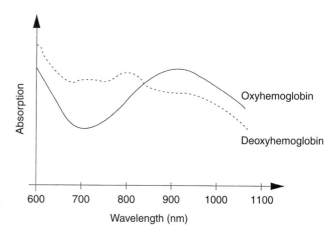

FIGURE **18-9**
Absorption characteristics for oxyhemoglobin and deoxyhemoglobin as a function of wavelength.

each wavelength. Therefore, the amount of light absorbed at any wavelength is a function of the concentration of the substances that have high absorption coefficients at that wavelength. When the distance that the light travels is kept constant, only the concentration of light-absorbing substances affects the levels of transmitted or reflected light. Using this basic optical technique, the concentration of substances can be determined if some unique absorption characteristics are present at a specific wavelength. Other substances with similar absorption characteristics must be removed or must always be at a constant or known concentration.

Because oxyhemoglobin and deoxyhemoglobin have distinctively different absorption characteristics (Figure 18-9), the concentration of each in a sample of blood can be determined in vitro. This is done by irradiating the blood sample with light at a wavelength that has different absorption characteristics for oxyhemoglobin and deoxyhemoglobin (approximately 650 nm) and at a wavelength for which the absorption characteristics are the same for oxyhemoglobin and deoxyhemoglobin (805 nm). The percentage of hemoglobin saturated with oxygen can be calculated from these intensities.

This same principle is used in pulse oximetry to determine the percent saturation of arterial blood in vivo. Changes in the intensity of light transmitted through or reflected from tissue during the inflow phase of the cardiac cycle (systole) are assumed to be attributable to arterial blood alone, as shown in Figure 18-10. If light intensity is measured during systole and also during the period between heart beats (diastole), the difference between the light intensities can be attributed to arterial blood flow alone. Measurements of light intensities at 650 nm and 805 nm are taken for systole and diastole. The light intensities are corrected for tissue variations, and the pulsatile variation can then be attributed to arterial flow only. The sensor does not require calibration; the ratio of the corrected light intensities gives the beat to beat percent saturation.

The first generation of oxygen saturation devices used fiberoptic cables to deliver the light to the sensor tip and another fiberoptic cable to return the transmitted light to the detector. Currently, monochromatic light-emitting diodes and photodetectors are small enough to encapsulate in self-contained sensors.

With the optical technique, the percent saturation can be influenced by venous pulsatile flow and motion artifact, which can change the effective thickness of the tissue between the light source and the detector. Ambient lights with high intensities in the levels used for saturation can be detected by the saturation detector if they are not adequately shielded. Also, the absorption characteristics of fetal hemoglobin are slightly different from those of adult hemoglobin, therefore saturation monitors used in the early postnatal period must be corrected to compensate for these differences. The timing of the activation of the light pulses is critical to the accuracy of the derived percent saturation; addition of an independent source for timing of the pulse wave can improve accuracy if triggering of the light pulses is linked to this independent source. To compensate for poor or variable arterial perfusion, the light intensities on the transmitters of most oximeters can be adjusted so that the level of light received at the detector provides an acceptable pulse wave.

Pulse oximetry is widely used in both the adult and neonatal fields of medicine, but it can be unreliable in certain circumstances. Patient motion, low peripheral perfusion, shock states, intense ambient light, and electrical interference can result in inaccurate readings and false alarms, which are bothersome for caregivers and pose a safety hazard for patients. Manufacturers Mallinckrodt and Masimo both have updated their machines to provide highly accurate oxygen saturation monitoring while minimizing false alarms. Masimo's Signal Extraction Technology alarms have proved to be true 100% of the time, compared with a rate of 70% to 90% for conventional pulse oximeters. In 1993 Mallinckrodt introduced the Oxisensor II, a high-performance, low-noise sensor that provides enhanced signal acquisition and detection of in-band motion artifact to reduce false alarms.

Partial Pressure of Oxygen. Transcutaneous measurement of the partial pressure of oxygen in arterial blood ($TcPaO_2$) can be achieved using oxygen polarographic techniques. Figure 18-11 presents a general schematic of this technique that is based on the Clark oxygen electrode.

The polarographic cell has a cathode (usually platinum) and an anode (usually silver–silver chloride, or Ag-AgCl), the surfaces of which are in contact with an electrolyte, such as potassium chloride (KCl). The anode and cathode are polarized with 600 mV DC. Oxygen molecules, which can reach and dissolve in the electrolyte, are electrochemically reduced

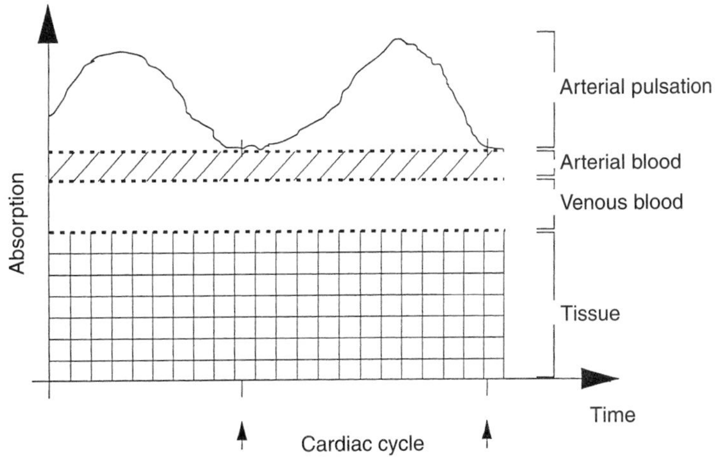

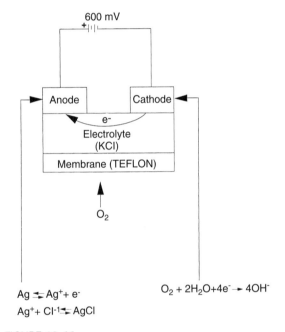

FIGURE 18-10
Changes in the intensity of transmitted or reflected light area function of (1) the absorption characteristics of the tissue at the measurement site, (2) absorption changes caused by venous blood flow, and (3) absorption changes caused by arterial pulsation.

FIGURE 18-11
Schematic of a partial pressure of oxygen (PO_2) transducer.

at the cathode. Each O_2 molecule takes four electrons (e^-) from the cathode and combines with two water molecules (H_2O) to form four hydroxyl ions (OH^-). At the anode, silver is oxidized, and electrons are liberated. The silver ions combine with chloride ions to form silver chloride. These reactions provide a continuous flow of electrons between the cathode and the anode. Because the supply of electrons to the cathode depends on the supply of oxygen molecules, the partial pressure of oxygen (PO_2) can be determined. The flow of electrons generates a detectable current, which can be processed to provide its output in millimeters of mercury. A membrane permeable only to oxygen must be used to protect the electrode from all other molecules. A thin membrane of Teflon is used in most commercial devices. Because they affect the flow of oxygen to the electrodes, the thickness and composition of the membrane ultimately determine the response time of the sensor.

These oxygen electrodes must be calibrated at two reference levels before use because the buildup of charge on the electrodes over time causes drift.

$TcPaO_2$ is based on the concept that the rate of oxygen diffusion through the skin can be changed by elevating the skin temperature above 40° C. (Normally, very little or no oxygen is transported through the skin.) The skin usually is heated to 43° to 44° C, at which temperature diffusion increases even through the outer barrier of the skin, the stratum corneum. Because heating also causes vasodilation, blood flow to the dermal capillaries increases, raising the oxygen tension in these vessels close to the levels of the deeper arterial vessels. To protect the sensor from the effects of oxygen in the air, the probe assembly is attached to the skin with an adhesive that provides a good mechanical airtight seal. The heating of the skin to promote oxygen diffusion causes mild erythema. Extreme care must be taken because of the high temperatures used at the surface of the sensor, which is in contact with the very immature skin of the premature infant. For this reason, many units use this form of monitoring only on term or near-term infants whose skin is not so much at risk of breakdown. $TcPaO_2$ is still not an absolute measurement system and is used primarily as a trending tool in conjunction with absolute gas tensions measured in arterial blood with a laboratory analyzer.

Partial Pressure of Carbon Dioxide.   Transcutaneous measurement of the partial pressure of carbon dioxide in arterial blood ($TcPaCO_2$) can be performed using transduction techniques based on the Severinghaus principle; in short, the effect of CO_2 on the pH of a solution is transduced. The resultant pH is measured using standard glass pH electrodes. Figure 18-12 presents a general schematic of this type of transduction.

The CO_2 molecules are absorbed in an electrolyte (HCO_3), forming hydrogen and bicarbonate ions. A potential is generated between the pH electrode and the reference electrode. The potential is proportional to the concentration of CO_2. The CO_2 sensor must be calibrated at two points using reference gases (usually 5% and 10% CO_2). Heat is also used in the PO_2 sensor to increase the diffusion of CO_2 across the stratum corneum. Because the transduction mechanism is based on the

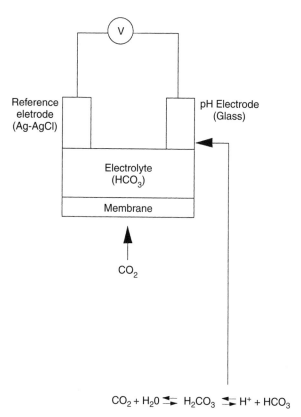

$$CO_2 + H_2O \rightleftharpoons H_2CO_3 \rightleftharpoons H^+ + HCO_3$$

FIGURE 18-12
Schematic of a partial pressure of carbon dioxide (PCO_2) transducer.

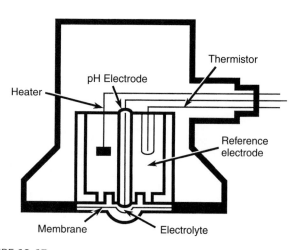

FIGURE 18-13
Cross sectional diagram of a transcutaneous partial pressure of carbon dioxide (PCO_2) sensor. Courtesy Hoffmann-La Roche, Basel, Switzerland.

pH glass electrode, the sensor is extremely sensitive to temperature (Figure 18-13). Both the $TcPaO_2$ and $TcPaCO_2$ are highly influenced by skin perfusion. Also, unlike with $TcSaO_2$ measurement systems, the sensors' response time is slow, making it difficult to use data for anything other than gross trending of gas tensions.

Another type of CO_2 monitoring is the open circuit, flow-through indirect calorimetry technique used to measure oxygen consumption and carbon dioxide production in neonates. Bauer and coworkers (1997) compared the use of a face mask, head hood, and canopy for breath sampling to determine oxygen consumption and carbon dioxide production in nonventilated infants. Breath sampling in premature infants is difficult because of the need for low flows to prevent excessive dilution of expired air and because the low sampling flow increases the risk of inadequate gas sampling, which can underestimate the results. Results can be overestimated with increased activity or body temperature (Bauer et al, 1997).

A portable infrared end-tidal CO_2 monitor has been used most widely for induction of anesthesia in children and for transport of critically ill adults. The problem with this type of monitoring in infants is that a 38-ml dead space may result in very small infants rebreathing the air. Biochem International in Waukesha, Wisconsin, has devised the Biochem 520 CO_2 breath indicator, a sidestream infrared capnometer with only a 2-ml dead space. One reason this form of monitoring is used during transport is to determine if the endotracheal tube is in proper position for ventilation.

Blood Pressure Monitoring. The most common blood pressure measurement is the arterial blood pressure, which routinely is measured by a central/direct method (through placement of an umbilical or a peripheral arterial catheter) or by a peripheral method (i.e., a blood pressure cuff attached to a blood pressure machine). The gold standard is direct blood pressure measurement by means of a central line. Continuous readouts of blood pressure can be obtained by either direct or peripheral means. The central venous pressure (CVP) can be measured in newborns, but this is not a routine form of measurement in most NICUs. Because of neonates' small size and low blood pressure values (in comparison with adults), these infants' blood pressure cannot be taken with a regular stethoscope and blood pressure cuff. A variety of electrical blood pressure machines are available for use in these small patients.

The true definition of pressure is force per unit area. When the force in a system is constant, the pressure is said to be hydrostatic. When the force varies, the pressure is said to be dynamic or hydrodynamic. Human blood pressure is an example of hydrodynamic pressure. In physiologic systems, a multitude of factors can influence blood pressure results. Blood contains cells and other materials that can adhere to cell vessel walls. Blood vessel walls are distensible and can constrict and dilate at will. Especially in older adults, the walls are not smooth but often are clogged with plaque or tiny clots that impede normal blood flow. The viscosity of the blood changes under different circumstances, and this can affect the heart's ability to move the blood through the system.

Other factors also complicate blood pressure monitoring. For example, the diameter of the blood vessels changes constantly in an attempt to regulate systemic blood pressure, and cardiac pumping creates pulsatile waves that are not static.

Based on the human arterial waveform, several components of blood pressure can be measured: the systolic (peak) pressure, the diastolic (minimum) pressure, the dynamic average pressure (one-half peak minus minimum), and the mean (average) blood pressure.

In the medical field, the mean arterial pressure is equal to the diastolic pressure (P1) plus one third the difference between the systolic and diastolic pressures (P2 − P1). The average adult spends one third of the cardiac cycle in systole and two thirds in diastole. The average heart rate of an adult is much slower than that of a neonate, and spending two thirds of

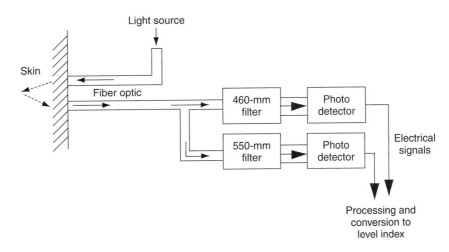

FIGURE **18-14**
Block diagram of an optical device used to measure bilirubin. The arrows indicate the direction of light flow.

the cardiac cycle in diastole increases the filling time of the chambers, which ultimately affects cardiac output. In the neonate, whose heart rate is well over 100 bpm, this equation may not prove true. It may be more acceptable to consider the neonate as spending approximately one half the cardiac cycle in systole and one half in diastole. This reduces the filling time of the chambers and may affect overall cardiac output, especially if the heart rate is well over 200 bpm. Significant tachycardia may affect the blood pressure monitor's ability to appropriately determine blood pressure values because of inadequate filling time and, ultimately, decreased cardiac output.

Direct measurement of blood pressure is based mostly on strain gauge transduction principles. Strain is the change in length of an object per unit length. Strain gauges usually are constructed of materials that can detect changes in electrical resistance for small changes in length. The sensitivity of the strain gauge is a function of the force necessary to cause a detectable deflection in the gauge membrane. Attaching an object to the gauge can facilitate the transduction of force. If a fluid exerts force on the active surface of the gauge, movement of the gauge can be expressed as a pressure. Blood pressure measurement with a catheter is based on this principle. With a sterile saline solution in the catheter, the pressure of the blood for each cardiac cycle is transmitted through the fluid column to the active face of the pressure transducer. The length and the type of material used in the catheter can affect the frequency response in this type of pressure measurement system. The transducer must be located at the level of the heart to avoid pressure offsets.

In all direct pressure measurement systems in which a fluid-filled catheter is used to transmit the pressure wave to the strain gauge, the catheter must be free of air bubbles. If a significant amount of air is present in the system, the pressure waveform is distorted, because air, unlike saline, can be compressed. The loss of energy from compression in the catheter can dampen the actual pressure wave, resulting in an inaccurate blood pressure reading. Bubbles usually can be dislodged by gently tapping the pressure transducer manifold.

Semiconductor strain gauges, which can be made in very small sizes, are extremely sensitive and produce measurable outputs with little distortion in the gauge membrane. Displace-

ments as small as a few microns can be detected. Semiconductor-based strain gauges are used in catheters with the pressure transducer at the tip. In these catheter-tip pressure transducers, the pressure variations are transduced at the measurement site itself and not through a fluid column.

Sphygmomanometry is an indirect method of measuring blood pressure. A blood pressure cuff is placed around the extremity and inflated to the point where it totally occludes the blood flow through the artery. Pressure in the cuff is released slowly until sharp, snapping Korotkoff sounds are heard. These sounds occur when turbulent blood flow, under pressure, breaks through the occlusion into the downstream artery; this represents systolic pressure. When the turbulence resolves, diastolic pressure is recorded. These systems have automated inflation and deflation mechanisms and are designed to measure cuff pressures at the systolic and diastolic end points of the cardiac cycle. With the availability of small, sensitive pressure transducers and suitable plastics for the cuff, this technique has gained acceptance as a screening tool for infants. When a timer is incorporated to activate the inflation and deflation pumps at discrete intervals (e.g., every 30 minutes), the technique can be used in an almost continuous, noninvasive way to track pressure. The widespread availability of low-cost, sophisticated electronics allows incorporation of fail-safe alarms to prevent overinflation or continuous inflation of the cuffs.

All types of pressure monitoring, direct and indirect, are extremely sensitive to motion artifact and positioning of the pressure transducer. Pressure transducers usually are extremely temperature sensitive because they rely on the detection of small mechanical changes in metals as the transduction mechanism.

Serum Bilirubin.   Total bilirubin can be measured with a device that uses a simple optical system (Figure 18-14). The device is designed to quantify the degree of yellowing of the tissue underlying the skin. Because bilirubin has unique absorption spectra, the concentration of bilirubin can be determined in vivo by analyzing the reflected light from a source directed at the skin. The reflected light is split into two beams with a dichroic mirror. The light is then passed through 460- and 550-mm filters and is converted to electrical energy by photodetectors. The relative energies of the reflected light can be correlated to the concentration of total bilirubin at the measurement site.

Cerebral Blood Flow Velocity.   Cerebral blood flow (CBF) velocity monitoring is becoming more widely used in the NICU for both clinical and research purposes. The critical minimum level of CBF has not yet been defined by research, but in neonates it affects the overall patient outcome. Newborns, especially premature infants, are most vulnerable during the first 3 days of life. Because the brain is sensitive to ischemia, its circulation depends on adequate autoregulation of CBF to prevent intracranial insults, which means that the infant's body must vary the amount of blood flow to the brain to maintain a constant level.

In newborns, the body's ability to regulate blood flow to the brain varies according to gestational age and is affected by fluctuations in the systemic blood pressure, oxygenation, CO_2 levels, and the degree of metabolic activity. The ideal situation is a constant CBF level that changes only minimally with alterations in systemic blood pressure. Unfortunately, because the premature infant's body lacks the ability to regulate CBF, these babies are at risk of dramatic increases and decreases in CBF and perfusion, which places them at risk of intraventricular hemorrhage (IVH) and periventricular leukomalacia (PVL). Routine aspects of neonatal care (e.g., suctioning, mechanical ventilation, fluid administration, repositioning, bathing) alter CBF in the newborn, which can have dramatic results in ELBW infants (Borch & Greisen, 1998).

Cerebral blood flow can be monitored noninvasively with Doppler flow velocity monitors. Measurements usually are taken with the neonate in a supine position. A pulsed Doppler flow velocity meter with a 7.5 MHz frequency and continuous multifrequency scanner with a 7.5 MHz shore focus probe are used. Noise from the movement of the blood in the vessel is filtered with a 100 Hz high-pass filter. The probe is positioned transcranially over the temporal bone to "catch" the vessel as it leaves the circle of Willis. Sagittal and coronal measurements are taken "through" the open fontanelle. Audio and visual signals are detectable and projected. Direct measurement can be obtained with an analog output system. These measurements include the systolic velocity, diastolic velocity, and integration of the area under the curve, which is considered a close approximation of the blood flow volume.

Meek and colleagues (1998) used cerebral blood velocity values to measure changes in hemodynamics over the first 3 days of life in preterm infants with normal head scans. They suggest that the increases in CBF in the first 3 days of life are a normal adaptive response of the cerebral circulation to extrauterine life rather than a direct result of changes in blood pressure, $PaCO_2$, or hematocrit. The sample size of this study was small, but the study does suggest that questions have yet to be answered in this area, and continued research is imperative to improve our understanding of both the process and the outcomes of changes in CBF in neonates.

New Techniques for Monitoring the Neonate

Ventilator technology has evolved dramatically over the years. For example, some new ventilators now include components for testing pulmonary function, allowing continuous measurement of tidal volume, pressure, and flow wave forms. These technologic advances have led to changes in the way infants are ventilated. Thirty years ago, ventilators were adapted from the adult model and used with some success for infants. Current ventilators have a variety of modes of ventilation, which can be adapted to the baby and the disease being treated. Many of these new modes of ventilation, with continuous display of tidal volumes and the pressures required to generate a set tidal volume, allow the baby to self-wean. This should reduce overall morbidity and mortality in these tiny patients.

SUMMARY

New monitoring equipment is becoming available almost daily, and its integration into the NICU creates a need for educational programs to ensure that the equipment is used safely and efficiently. It is imperative that all health care workers in the unit have a basic understanding of the equipment's capabilities and limitations. Because treatment often is modified according to the values obtained from monitoring devices, the health professional must know both the factors that may influence monitoring values and also how to distinguish between artifact and actual physical changes in the neonate's status. The ability to make this distinction is critical.

REFERENCES

Bauer K et al (1997). Comparison of face mask, head hood, and canopy for breath sampling in flow-through indirect calorimetry to measure oxygen consumption and carbon dioxide production of preterm infants <1500 grams. *Pediatric research* 41:139-144.

Blackburn S, Loper D (2003). Thermoregulation. In Blackburn S, Loper D, editors. *Maternal, fetal, and neonatal physiology: a clinical perspective*. WB Saunders: Philadelphia.

Borch K, Greisen G (1998). Blood flow distribution in the normal human preterm brain. *Pediatric research* 43:28-34.

Carr J (1992a). Sensors for biomedical devices, medical and laboratory oscilloscopes, ECG and EEG signals: where do they come from? In Carr J: *Biomedical equipment use, maintenance, and management*. Prentice Hall: Upper Saddle River, NJ.

Carr J (1992b). Bioelectric amplifiers, electrocardiograph machines, medical pressure measurements, patient monitoring systems, temperature sensors, respiration monitors, and apnea alarms. In Carr J: *Biomedical equipment use, maintenance, and management*. Prentice Hall: Upper Saddle River, NJ.

Carr J (1992c). Computers in medical instruments. In Carr J: *Biomedical equipment use, maintenance, and management*. Prentice Hall: Upper Saddle River, NJ.

Carr J (1992d); Electromagnetic interference to medical electronic equipment; Electrical safety: your job! In Carr J: *Biomedical equipment use, maintenance, and management*. Prentice Hall: Upper Saddle River, NJ.

Grieve S et al (1997). Comparison of two different pulse oximeters in monitoring preterm infants. *Critical care medicine* 25:2051-2054.

Lyon AJ et al (1997). Temperature control in very-low-birth-weight infants during first five days of life. *Archives of disease in childhood* 76:F47-F50.

Meek J et al (1998). Cerebral blood flow increases over the first three days of life in extremely preterm neonates. *Archives of disease in childhood (fetal/neonatal edition)* 78:F33-F37.

Narendran V, Hoath S (1999). Thermal management of the low birth weight infant: a cornerstone of neonatology. *Journal of pediatrics* 134:529-531.

Vohra S et al (1999). Effect of polyethylene occlusive skin wrapping on heat loss in very-low-birth-weight infants at delivery: a randomized trial. *Journal of pediatrics* 134:547-550.

CHAPTER 19

COMPUTER TECHNOLOGY USE IN NEWBORN AND INFANT NURSING

ELIZABETH E. WEINER, LINDA STURLA FRANCK

Gathering data and managing information have always been key nursing functions. Nearly 150 years ago, Florence Nightingale set forth the rationale for this: "In dwelling upon the vital importance of sound observation, it must never be lost sight of what observation is for. The collection of data is not for the sake of piling up miscellaneous or curious facts, but for the sake of saving life and increasing health and comfort."

If nurses are to give data collection a high priority, the data must be meaningful to patient care. Computer technology has become essential to the processes of recording data and transforming it into usable nursing information. Nurses in neonatal units rely heavily on monitoring devices, information systems, web resources, and communications systems to provide up-to-date care efficiently. However, the technology must make care more efficient and effective and not simply create more machines to "nurse." The ultimate goal is to provide nurses with the time and the information that quality nursing care demands.

The complexity of patient care in the neonatal intensive care unit (NICU) presents some of the greatest challenges, as well as the greatest potential benefits, for the use of technology. This chapter describes the impact of computer technology on data gathering and management in nursing; provides a resource for developing or using computer technology in the NICU; and explains the process and strategies for finding current information related to care of the neonate and infant.

NURSING INFORMATICS

The term "nursing informatics" often is interpreted to mean the use of technology in providing nursing care in clinical, administrative, practice, and educational settings. However, "nursing informatics" is not synonymous with "use of technology"; rather, technology is simply a tool used in the practice of nursing informatics.

In their classic article, "The Combination of Nursing Science, Information Science, and Computer Science," Graves & Corcoran (1989) first defined nursing informatics as the transformation of data into information and then into knowledge, a necessary transformation for all professional domains. As advances in technology have increased the possible applications, the roles of the informatics nurse also have expanded, requiring an updated definition of nursing informatics.

The most recent Scope and Standards of Nursing Informatics Practice (2001) defines nursing informatics as a specialty that integrates nursing science, computer science, and information science to manage and communicate data, information, and knowledge in nursing practice. Nursing informatics facilitates the integration of data, information, and knowledge to support patients, nurses, and other providers in decision making in all roles and settings. This support is accomplished through the use of information structures, processes, and technology.

The Scope and Standards guidelines also describe the role of the advanced practice informatics nurse, or informatics nurse specialist. Among this nurse's responsibilities are using the information systems life cycle and other tools and processes to analyze data, information, and the requirements of the information system; designing, selecting, and evaluating information technology, data structures, and decision-support mechanisms and then integrating them into a smoothly functioning information system; and aiding in the discovery of new aspects of nursing knowledge.

In the United States the American Medical Informatics Association (AMIA) provides an organizational structure for those interested in informatics applications across the various health care professions. This organization, which holds fall and spring meetings, belongs to the International Medical Informatics Association (IMIA). A working group in nursing meets during the national conferences; the group's goals and objectives can be found on their web page (http://www.amia-niwg.org/). A helpful resource found on the group's page is a list of informatics programs. These programs include academic degrees, certificate programs, or continuing education. The University of Maryland and the University of Utah were the first to offer informatics degrees. Duke University offers a popular online certificate program, with a brief visit to the campus for face-to-face conferences. Loyola University in Chicago just received a grant to build a Nursing Informatics program, and the University of Illinois at Chicago offers a certificate program between the College of Nursing and the School of Public Health. Most informatics programs have focused on the clinical area; however, Vanderbilt University plans to open a nursing informatics program in the fall of 2002 with subspecialties in clinical and educational informatics.

Nurses practicing in any setting who consistently contribute to informatics solutions should consider becoming certified in nursing informatics. The American Nurses Credentialing Center (ANCC) is responsible for the certification process, and the examination is taken at local computerized testing centers. (For further information on eligibility, see the ANCC web site at http://www.ana.org/ancc/.)

PRACTICE USES OF TECHNOLOGY

Nurses who care for neonates and infants depend heavily on data collection and interpretation devices. Because of the volatile clinical situations that can arise with such tiny patients, this equipment must be able to collect and display data quickly.

A stable health care environment through the 1960s and 1970s and the increasing availability and lower cost of computer technology prompted health care leaders to begin investigating the use of technology to address health care needs (Staggers & Thompson, 2001). Early efforts were directed at developing hospital information systems (often proprietary in nature). These systems usually had different functions in different institutions, but their primary purpose was to support acute care. During the 1970s and 1980s, the focus became fee-for-service reimbursement with advanced billing features rather than the provision of clinical care.

In the 1990s computerization efforts centered on longitudinal patient care data across the life span, although development fell short of this goal. Staggers & Thompson (2001) have described the trend toward development of computer-based patient record (CPR) systems. This trend can be attributed in part to the Health Insurance Portability and Accountability Act of 1996 (HIPAA), which strictly limits the disclosure and use of health care information, with criminal penalties possible for violations (Christiansen, 1999). Committees are present at all health care facilities to determine the institutional response to the HIPAA legislation.

Not surprisingly, as health care needs expanded, so did the ability of the technology to meet those needs. Weiner & Trangenstein (1999) have described the crosscurrents of clinical nursing practice and technology. The needs of nursing have grown from an emphasis on collecting data and information (which could be task automated) to establishing relationships by creating databases. As technology advances, a virtual practice arena is emerging, with advanced communication and decision-making capabilities.

Ozbolt & Bakken (2001) described patient care systems in great detail, pointing out that the systems enhance or detract from patient care according to their "goodness of fit." They also described the societal forces that have influenced the design and implementation of patient care systems. The key to performing a necessary clinical function is data standards, based on a standard vocabulary for nursing. Unfortunately, in the past, nurses' data about patients often were recorded as narrative notes, with content and phrasing as varied and individual as the nurses. The researchers concluded that patient care systems are changing in two ways. First, legacy systems, designed primarily for administrative functions, are being replaced by systems designed to support and improve clinical practice. Second, integrated, multidisciplinary systems are replacing those designed to support one discipline.

Patient monitoring systems have also undergone a revolution in design. The latest bedside monitors have multiple microcomputers and much more computing power and memory than the early systems (Gardner & Shabot, 2001). In addition, there has been widespread commercial development of computer-based monitoring and information systems for intensive care units (ICUs), to the extent that well over 2000 such systems are in use in ICUs worldwide. Nurses in the neonatal intensive care unit (NICU) must be well versed in the operation of the unit's information management system. Care in the NICU requires prompt, accurate treatment decisions that are based on compact, well-organized information patterns.

EDUCATIONAL USES OF TECHNOLOGY

The impact of technology on the teaching and learning processes has dramatically changed the roles of both students and faculty. Although most nursing schools in the 1980s and 1990s incorporated the use of technology into their programs, the growth of the world wide web over the past 5 years has far extended the reach of earlier programs.

Much of the early use of technology in nursing education can be directly attributed to the generous donations of the Helene Fuld Foundation. Many schools have instructional media laboratories that were begun with funds from the foundation, and the name appears in a number of different institutions. In addition, the Fuld Institute for Technology in Nursing Education (FITNE) has been a leader in providing hardware and software resources for nursing education programs. The FITNE group was perhaps best known for creating the Nightingale tracker, a handheld device designed for use in community health that could upload data to a server in a central location. The device is still used in a limited number of settings.

Another major thrust in the development of simulation software was the introduction of a series of software titles that used the video disk to deliver short video sequences driven by user input via the computer. These programs were launched by a grant from IBM, which provided for a consortium of developers from 14 universities in the United States and Canada who actively produced cases during the early 1990s. Some of these titles are being converted to the more popular CD-ROM format that uses digitized video files, again driven by user input.

It was not until the development of web-based authoring templates that most nursing faculties became willing to change their teaching strategies. Programs such as Blackboard and WebCT, developed in 1995, currently have the market share of classes, hosted locally on a central campus server or on the server hosted by those organizations. These "virtual electronic classrooms" generally are password protected so that only those registered for the class can use the collected electronic resources. Faculty members design the classes so that the students can interact with the program, just as in the more typical classroom. Minimal use of these templates results when faculty members choose only to place their syllabuses online. A better use involves threaded discussions, active web links, small group exercises, interactive modules, and other creative exercises.

Englebardt (2002) distinguished between "distributed education" and "distance education." Distance education refers to educational events that occur with the instructor and the students in different geographic locations. Distributed education denotes a learner-center environment that uses technology to supplement traditional courses or deliver distance education. These strategies can be used in real-time (synchronous) or different times (asynchronous). Electronic mail has become a popular form of asynchronous communication for all age groups, thus extending the need for better access from home. Electronic discussion forums, listservs, and virtual office hours are just a few examples of communication strategies available to nursing faculty members and students today. Instead of serving as a preparer and presenter of lectures, the faculty member has become a moderator and guide.

Another way to extend the walls of the classroom is through the use of streaming video. Recording and encoding video into the course is possible. The classes presented in the typical classroom can view the session viewed synchronously (with the software Real Video) or asynchronously if archived or distributed for later use via CD-ROM. This is a popular technique, because it requires less effort to change the typical class to one that is more interactive in nature. As students begin to realize that distance options are increasing, there will be even more pressure to convert passive content to interactive learning exercises.

No evidence indicates how much of either the face to face or the distance method provides the best learning experience. Most faculty members use a hybrid approach that combines the two. This hybrid approach, sometimes referred to as a web-enhanced course, takes advantage of the web for a portion of the course, but students are not totally dependent on electronic media for their coursework.

RESEARCH USES OF TECHNOLOGY

The information age has created a unique challenge for today's researchers: how are they to make sense of all the information that has become available? The first difficulty is that the researcher must collect as many data sources as possible. This data gathering process is complicated by the fact that the Internet and the world wide web have introduced a number of sites that must be carefully assessed for credibility.

At the same time, use of the world wide web has extended publication possibilities. Data and information can be posted immediately upon receipt. Unlike in the publishing process for print formats, publication lags are rare.

The computer's capability for storing large data sets for purposes of analysis and query makes it an ideal tool to help capture nursing knowledge. Through the use of other software tools, data and information can be organized and presented in a way that leads to the discovery of further knowledge framed within a domain.

Sigma Theta Tau International (STTI) is a 79-year-old honor society for nursing with a membership numbering more than a quarter million (the web homepage is www.nursingsociety.org). Its mission is to improve the health of people worldwide by improving nursing scholarship. Central to accomplishing this mission is the Virginia Henderson International Nursing Library, an electronic library that provides a variety of services to scholars around the world. These services began in 1990 with the Registry of Nursing Research, which consisted of a database that would allow queries by a researcher's name, the subject of the project, and the findings of the research.

A secondary aspect of online services was the unveiling of the first online journal in nursing, the *Online Journal of Knowledge Synthesis for Nursing* (OJKSN). This peer-reviewed, full-text electronic journal gave nurses access to integrative reviews of research pertinent to clinical practice. Recognizing that most practicing nurses have limited time to gather and synthesize studies about certain topics, the journal's leadership has encouraged the pairing of nurse researchers with practicing nurses, and the two together present their interpretation of knowledge synthesized from the literature. Recent examples of topics pertinent to neonates and infants include, "Sibling Visitation: Research Implications for Pediatric and Neonatal Pa-

tients" (Andrade, 1998); "Bilateral Head Flattening in Hospitalized Premature Infants" (Hemingway & Oliver, 2000); and "Mother-Infant Interaction and Maternal Substance Use/Abuse: an Integrative Review of Research Literature in the 1990s" (Johnson, 2001). All these articles have tables that briefly describe the reviewed studies, as well as bibliographic references linked to those references that can be found online with the click of a mouse.

A new indexing paradigm is being used in the Virginia Henderson International Nursing Library. STTI contracts for processing services from 24th Century Press for the development and maintenance of indices called "literature indexes." The indexing strategy uses *pairs* of research-salient terms in the sentences of selected abstracts. After finding a term of interest, the user sees all terms related to the focal term. Selecting a related term of interest takes the user to all the abstract sentences in which that exact pair of terms is found. From there, the user can go directly to the citation in PubMed, a free National Library of Medicine reference database. This type of search provides a context that makes it much easier for the user to determine relevancy. The nursing research literature (indexing from 1996 to the present) and the acquired immunodeficiency syndrome/human immunodeficiency virus (AIDS/HIV) literature (indexing from 1998 to the present) were the first of these indices introduced in 1999. Both are updated monthly. This indexing system covers all nursing journals in which 50% or more of the articles are research articles. Other journals that publish nursing research (interdisciplinary, national, and international) are being invited to submit nursing research abstracts for free indexing by STTI.

This new search paradigm has given rise to the beginning of a research vocabulary of nursing, which may provide a means of linking nursing research to the patient record (Harris et al, 2000).

In the area of neonatal nursing, use of the literature index revealed 1624 studies using the term "infant" and 174 using "neonate" (as accessed via the web on November 19, 2001). Cross-linking the term "neonate" with "hospital" resulted in the studies found in Box 19-1.

A more advanced method of data management based on empiric knowledge allows the researcher to craft a unique knowledge base in a selected area of study. The software *arcs* (developed by Judith Graves) provides the knowledgebase management and knowledge modeling system. After selecting and recording aspects of various studies, the researcher can begin to develop models illustrating clear variable relationships and others less clear requiring further study.

The researcher thus becomes the knowledge base builder. As such, the builder determines what details are important in the subject domain and makes certain that those details are entered into the software program. The knowledge is then graphically represented in causal/associational models. These models may be better known to various users as relational maps or models, concept maps, domain maps, theoretic models, or knowledge models. Graphically representing the knowledge of a domain in the form of traditional scientific models facilitates scientific discovery. Gaps and conflicts in knowledge and levels of research control become visible through the maps, which collect and illustrate variables studied together and the category of statistical relationship studied, and the direction of findings. Summaries of salient features of a domain, such as types of research design, variables and how they were operationalized, treatment outcome methods, and even

BOX 19-1

Search Results Linking "Neonate" and "Hospital" in Nursing Research Literature

Aylott M (1997). Expanding the role of the neonatal transport nurse: nurse-led teams. *British journal of nursing* 13:800-804.

Nottingham Neonatal Service provides a unit-based inter**hospital** transport program for the stabilization and transportation of critically ill **neonates** in the Trent region.

Do a PubMed search of abstract number 97428953.

Huffines B, Logsdon MC (1997). The neonatal skin risk assessment scale for predicting skin breakdown in neonates. *Issues in comprehensive pediatric nursing* 20:103-114.

Using this scale to predict and prevent skin breakdown could reduce costs associated with a prolonged **hospital** stay for **neonates.**

Do a PubMed search of abstract number 98085435.

Pleasure L et al (1997). An expanded neonatal morbidity scale for premature infants. *Journal of nursing measures* (2)5: 119-138.

Revision of a neonatal morbidity scale (NMS) that has served as a means for comparison of neonatal illness in studies of high-risk **neonates** after initial **hospital** discharge.

Do a PubMed search of abstract number 98199411.

Fowler S et al (1998). Evidence of person-to-person transmission of *Candida lusitaniae* in a neonatal intensive care unit. *Infection control and hospital epidemiology* 19(5):343-345.

Epidemiologic investigation and molecular typing techniques identified three **neonates** infected with identical strains of *Candida lusitaniae* that were distinguished readily from epidemiologically unrelated strains from other locations in the **hospital.**

Do a PubMed search of abstract number 98273752.

Franck LS et al (1998). Opioid withdrawal in neonataes after continuous infusions of morphine or bentamyl during extracorporeal membrane oxygenate. *American journal of critical care* 7:364-369.

Neonates receiving morphine were discharged from the **hospital** a mean of 9.6 days sooner than **neonates** who had received fentanyl.

Do a PubMed search of abstract number 98413320.

Al-Reubea AA et al: *Klebsiella pneumoniae* bloodstream infections in neonates in a hospital in the Kingdom of Saudi Arabia. *Infection control and hospital epidemiology* (1998). 19:674-679.

Objective: To identify risk factors for *Klebsiella pneumoniae* bloodstream infections in **neonates** in a **hospital** in the Kingdom of Saudi Arabia.

Design: Two case-control studies among **hospital**ized **neonates** from February 15 to May 14, 1991 and a procedural and microbiologic investigation.

Do a PubMed search of abstract number 98449616.

funding, become obvious using the text retrieval features of the software.

The exemplar is the HIV/AIDS knowledge base, which is now available at the STTI web site (www.nursingsociety.org/library). The knowledge stored in this knowledge base comes from nursing research studies and was built by Dr. Judith Baigis and Barbara Goldrich with the help of graduate students at Georgetown University. The Helene Fuld Foundation funded the project through STTI. The honor society will provide a publication venue for future electronic knowledge bases, and the HIV/AIDS knowledge base is a prototype for publishing research electronically via the web.

PERSONAL DIGITAL ASSISTANTS

Personal digital assistants (PDAs) allow clinicians to enter and manage critical information at the point of care. The ability to link data on a PDA to a central database on a server allows for near-unlimited potential in developing point of care applications and systems for patient data management. The PDA currently most popular with health care providers uses the Palm operating system, which originally was developed for the PALM Pilot line of PDAs.

The web site of RNpalm.com (http://www.rnpalm.com/) provides an excellent overview of recent trends in mobile computing for nurses. The web site includes software titles, recent hardware upgrades, a discussion group for PDAs (PDAs in Nursing Listserv), the RNPalm Newsletter, and reviews of both hardware and software. Most of the software available for medical PDAs is found on the web. Table 19-1 lists some of the software sites as of this writing. Drug formularies for newborns and infants are just one example of a PDA program that can be used in the NICU.

Carroll, Saluja, and Tarczy-Hornoch (2001) described the design, software and hardware selection, and preliminary testing of a PDA-based patient data and charting system for use in the University of Washington NICU. The study found that a PDA-based electronic charting and work flow management system allows physicians to record patient information at the point of care and later to synchronize it to a central database. These researchers plan further study of the impact of PDA use on patient outcomes and clinician efficiency.

ONLINE RESOURCES

The increased use of the Internet has transformed the clinician's role from health expert into information broker (Clark, 2000). As such, clinicians have the responsibility to be knowledgeable about sources of information and to be able to explain them for patients and families. Patients and family members already are challenging clinicians with information from the Internet, and nurses must be able to assist consumers by directing them to valid web sites and helping them identify reliable sources of information.

Other forms of electronic communication are becoming prevalent. E-mail often is sent between families and health care providers. Much online support can be gained from others who have had similar experiences and who share those experiences through chat rooms or listserv support groups. Wootton (1999) described this phenomenon as the creation of a new genre of online self-help. Online support groups offer patients and families shared information, time to listen, and warm acknowledgment of their physical and emotional challenges. Wootton describes the web as a combination of a global library, an enormous set of Yellow Pages, and a community network or town meeting.

With so many sources of information available, neonatal nurses be aware of resources that might aid in the provision of quality nursing care. Box 19-2 lists the web addresses of some of these resources.

TABLE 19-1	Personal Digital Assistant (PDA) Software Applications	
Applications	**Description**	**Source and Cost**
Anatomic Images		
Anatomy	Quick reference for human anatomy; 10 databases describe the different body systems.	http://www.medicalpiloteer.com/ $10
Clinical References		
5 Minute Pediatric Consult	Designed for quick consultation on problems seen in infants, children, and adolescents; more than 500 clinical topics are covered.	http://www.skyscape.com/products/products.cgi $64.95
PediatricDrugs (Handbook of Pediatric Drug Therapy)	A sophisticated but easy to use pediatric drug resource for handheld devices.	http://www.skyscape.com/products/products.cgi $49.95
Medical Management of Biological Causalities	A concise, pocket-size guide for prophylaxis and management of biologic casualties; intended as a quick reference and overview, not a definitive text.	http://www.usamriid.army.mil/education/ bluebook.html Free
Pocket Psychiatry	Comprehensive collection of 11 databases.	http://www.handango.com $29.99
Merck Manual	Widely used general medical textbook.	http://www.pdamd.com/ $79.95
Tabers Cyclopedic Medical Dictionary	Leading nursing and allied health dictionary.	http://www.skyscape.com/products/products.cgi $49.95
Harrison's Principles of Internal Medicine	The pocket-size book of choice for quick information on the pathophysiology, clinical presentation, diagnosis, and treatment of all disorders.	http://www.handheldmed.com $79.95
ABG Decoder	Aids quick analysis of laboratory values for arterial blood gases.	http://www.rnpalm.com/software_RNpalm.htm Free
ICD (Coder)	An ICD9 diagnosis code lookup program.	http://www.nnk.com/icd/index.htm Free for individual use
Surgical Knots, Sutures and Stitches	Comprehensive textbook on closing wounds; has more than 20 illustrations showing different types of sutures, needles, knots, and closure techniques.	http://www.handango.com $10
Diagnosis and Screening		
Glascow Coma Scale	A commonly used standardized test, the Glasgow Coma Scale evaluates brain injuries by rating three categories of patient responses: eye opening, best motor response, and best verbal response. Levels of responses indicate the degree of nervous system or brain impairment.	http://www.rnpalm.com/software_RNpalm.htm Free
PreOperative Evaluation	Chapters are arranged by organ systems.	http://hsc.unm.edu/medicine/gim/etext.htm Free
Clinical Tools		
MedMath	Medical calculator for the Palm Computing Platform; designed for rapid calculation of equations commonly used in adult internal medicine.	http://www.stanford.edu/~pmcheng/medmath/ index.html Free
STAT Growth Charts	Automates the June 2000 revision of the Centers for Disease Control Growth Charts; rapidly calculates exact growth percentiles, z-scores, and new BMI for age scores.	http://www.statcoder.com/growthcharts.htm Free
O_2 Tank	Calculates how long O_2 cylinders will last; can calculate for D, E, M, and H cylinders.	http://www.rnpalm.com/software_RNpalm.htm Free
BMI Calculator	Contains a chart that shows the categories of BMI values for adults.	http://www.rnpalm.com/software_NFP.htm Free
IV Rate Calc	Calculates intravenous (IV) drip rates in milliliters per hour (ml/hour); features a user-editable database of drugs to speed calculations.	http://www.spazthecat.com/palm.html $5
Outlines in Clinical Medicine	Extensive resource covering 850 clinical topics; indexed with more than 12,500 terms and medications.	http://www.collectivemed.com/p_outli.html $94.95

Continued

TABLE 19-1	Personal Digital Assistant (PDA) Software Applications—cont'd	
Applications	**Description**	**Source and Cost**
Neurologic Exam	A guide to the neurologic examination.	http://psych.colorado.edu/~brez/pilot/pilotpsy.htm Free
The Full Physical	Series of 13 comprehensive but succinct guides for performing medical examinations.	http://members.home.net/drpilot/software/ titles.html $14.99
The Complete History	A comprehensive guide to performing medical histories.	http://members.home.net/drpilot/software/ titles.html $7.99
Immunization Guide	TealInfo folio includes the 2000 American Academy of Pediatrics immunization schedule; also includes detailed information on each vaccine, including adverse effects, dosing intervals, contraindications, catch-up schedules, and travel requirements.	http://www.keepkidshealthy.com/ pediatricpilotpage/tealinfo.html Free
MedCalc	Allows rapid calculation of equations commonly used in internal medicine.	http://medcalc.med-ia.net/ Free
Pedisuite	Seven modules that provide both calculations and information for pediatric health care professionals.	http://www.medicalwizards.com/ $39.99
Educational Programs		
Code Blue!	A realistic patient case simulator and educational tool; starts with the history and electrocardiogram (ECG), then user must try to save the patient by ordering drugs and other treatments; cardiac module uses American Heart Association ACLS guidelines (program is not associated with the AHA or ACLS course).	http://www.rnpalm.com/software_free.htm Free
Med Rules	Award-winning application featuring useful clinical prediction rules taken from the medical literature; for educational use only.	http://pbrain.hypermart.net/ Free
Drug References		
ePocrates qid (Infectious Disease)	A quick guide to antimicrobial recommendations.	http://www.epocrates.com/products/ Free
EPocrates qRx	Lists more than 1500 drugs, along with interactions, adverse reactions, pregnancy and lactation cautions, and special dosing recommendations.	http://www.epocrates.com/products/ Free
Davis Drug Guide for Nurses	Includes more than 5000 trade name and generic drugs, nearly 140 drug classifications, more than 1000 drug monographs, and 700 commonly used combination drugs.	http://www.skyscape.com/products/products.cgi $49.95
Davis Drug Guide for Physicians	Includes more than 4000 trade name and generic drugs, nearly 50 drug classifications, more than 1500 drug monographs, and 475 commonly used combination drugs.	http://www.skyscape.com/products/products.cgi $49.95
Davis Guide to IV Medications	A pocket guide to IV medications that lists the drugs alphabetically by generic name. Entries provide information on administration, clinical precautions, laboratory test considerations, pharmacologic profile, and adverse reactions for all ages of patients. Numerous appendices offer schedules of controlled substances, tables and formulas, and various guidelines and test values. It also covers recent infusion control devices and precautions for geriatric patients.	http://www.handheldmed.com/ $49.95

TABLE 19-1	Personal Digital Assistant (PDA) Software Applications—cont'd	
Applications	**Description**	**Source and Cost**
Electronic Organizers		
On-Time Rx (medication management application)	A patient medication management tool; all patient information is conveniently stored and easily maintained in the system and can be updated frequently as conditions change.	http://www.ontimerx.com/ $29.95
Data Management		
PatientKeeper 2.20.4	Stores patient information.	http://www.patientkeeper.com/demos/pkp233/pk2.asp Personal version: $35
PocketMD	Designed to replace 3 × 5 pocket note cards; quickly displays patient information and facilitates flexible, efficient patient data layout.	http://www.pocketmd.com $5 ($30 with full formulary)
Databases		
PEPID (portable emergency physician information database)	A comprehensive reference tool for those in the field of emergency medicine.	http://www.pepid.com/ $39.95 for 6-month subscription

Special thanks to Patricia Trangenstein, PhD, RN, University of Cincinnati, for contributing the data for this table.

BOX 19-2

Web Resources for Neonatal Nursing

Academy of Neonatal Nursing
http://www.academyonline.org/page493797.htm

Advanced Practice of Neonatal Nursing
http://www.aap.org/policy/024.html

Association of Women's Health, Obstetric, and Neonatal Nurses
http://www.awhonn.org/

Birth: Issues in Perinatal Care
http://www.blackwell-science.com/

Hygeia:Online Journal for Pregnancy and Neonatal Loss
http://www.hygeia.org/index11.htm

Journal of Neonatal Nursing
http://www.neonatal-nursing.co.uk/

Journal of Obstetric, Gynecologic, and Neonatal Nursing
http://www.sagepub.co.uk/

National Association of Neonatal Nurses
http://www.nann.org/

Neonatal Network
http://neonatalnetwork.com/

Neonatal Nursing Positions
http://www.jobneonatal.net/

Neonatal Resuscitation Program
http://www.nrp.mb.ca/

Neonatology on the Web
http://www.neonatology.org/neo.links.nursing.html

Newborn Screening Practitioner's Manual
http://www.mostgene.org/pract/praclist.htm

NICU - Web
    Also has links to NICU-NET (neonatology list server) and Neonatal-talk (neonatal nursing list server); organized under sections of common diagnoses, procedures, reference, pediatric and neonatal resources, other web resources
http://neonatal.peds.washington.edu/

Premature Infant Resources
http://premature-infant.com/

Recommended Design Standards
For NICUs
http://www.nd.edu/~kkolberg/DesignStandards.htm

General Sites
CINAHL
http://www.cinahl.com/

Cochrane Collaboration
http://hiru.mcmaster.ca/cochrane/default.htm

National Human Genome Research Institute
http://www.nhgri.nih.gov/

National Library of Medicine
http://www.nlm.nih.gov/

PubMed
http://www.ncbi.nlm.nih.gov/entrez/query.fcgi

Sigma Theta Tau Virginia Henderson International Nursing Library
http://www.nursingsociety.org/

Note: All Web addresses were current as indicated in the entries. Should you receive an addressing error message, use one or more of the various search engines now available with web browsing software to locate the source.

TABLE 19-2	Discussion Lists in Perinatal and Neonatal Nursing*	
List	**Address for Commands**	**Subscribe Command**
Childbirth Education (BIRTHED)	listserv@puvm.psu.edu	subscribe birthed Firstname Lastname
Perinatal Nursing (PNATALRN)	listserv@listserv.acsu.buffalo.edu	subscribe pnatalrn Firstname Lastname
Neonatal Nursing	Neonatal-talk@liststar.bizjet.com	Subscribe (type this in subject line and leave message blank)
Nursing Informatics (NRSING-L)	listserv@library.umed.edu	Subscribe nrsing-l Firstname Lastname

Those interested in these lists must subscribe to receive the electronic mailings and also must unsubscribe to stop delivery of the messages.

The increased use of electronic communication has had social implications. McCartney (1999) described Netiquette, or good manners on the Internet, a basic guideline to promote courtesy and efficiency in local e-mail, Internet communication, and discussion lists. Table 19-2 describes the information needed to subscribe to nursing discussion lists of interest.

EVIDENCE-BASED OUTCOMES AND CLINICAL PATHWAYS

Clinical pathways provide a foundation for multidisciplinary documentation that focuses on the attainment of a specific outcome within a given period (Thede, 1999). The pathway identifies the desired outcomes for the patient according to the clinical diagnoses. Most of these pathways have been based on the principles of evidence-based practice.

Because nurses are advocates for their patients and are also committed to the research knowledge base to guide nursing practice, the movement of evidence-based practice has reached new heights. Ledbetter (2000) stated that for nursing practice to be "evidence-based best practice," nurses must apply the same rigor and vigilance seen in the conduct of research. The zeal to provide the tightest randomly controlled trials (RCTs) may have resulted in the loss of some information that would help guide nursing practice. Stevens (2001) points out:

Our challenge is to design rigorous systems that synthesize "other than RCT" knowledge into a pragmatic and unbiased representation of the state of the science on a topic—one with relevance for the clinician. Nursing must rise to the challenge of this significant opportunity to contribute our scientific know-how in developing methods that amalgamate qualitative research, theoretical knowledge, clinical expertise, and research results across disciplines.

Groups such as the Cochrane Collaboration and the Agency for Healthcare Research and Quality have invited nurses to design methods and evidence summaries that reflect rigorous, reliable, valid, and unbiased scientific conclusions. Nurses have the mandate to improve the quality of care based on this science.

The evidence-based practice movement will see new growth in the future. Readers are encouraged to contribute to the movement in their own institutions.

SUMMARY

Because nurses function in such an information-rich environment, they must learn to use technologic devices appropriately. These devices are particularly important in the care of infants and neonates, whose small size and rapid response to both positive and negative events create significant nursing challenges.

Furthermore, the massive influx of technology into all nursing settings has changed the role nurses must fulfill to be effective, contemporary practitioners. By shifting to the role of knowledge broker, nurses will be in the best position to serve as both advocates and clinicians in the practice, education, and research arenas. In addition, the rapid growth of the Internet provides nurses with the unique opportunity to partner with patients' families and support groups.

REFERENCES

American Nurses Association (ANA) (2001). *Scope and standards of nursing information practice*. Washington, DC: ANA.

Andrade TM (1998). Sibling visitation: research implications for pediatric and neonatal patients. *The online journal of knowledge synthesis for nursing* 5, Document No 6. Available online at http://www.stti.iupui.edu/library/ojksn/e.html

Carroll AE et al (2001). Development of a personal digital assistant (PDA)-based client/server NICU patient data and charting system. *Proceedings of the American medical informatics association symposium 2001*, pp 100-104.

Christiansen J (1999). Health IT and privacy: the legal perspective. *MD computing* 16:15-16.

Clark D (2000). Old wine in new bottles: delivering nursing in the twenty-first century. *Journal of nursing scholarship* 32:11-15.

Englebardt SP (2002). Technology and distributed education. In Englebardt SP, Nelson R, editors. *Healthcare informatics: an interdisciplinary approach*. Mosby: St Louis.

Gardner RM, Shabot MM (2001). Patient-monitoring systems. In Shortliffe EH et al, editors: *Medical informatics: computer applications in health care and biomedicine*, ed 2. Springer-Verlag: New York.

Graves JR, Corcoran S (1989). The study of nursing informatics. *Image: journal of nursing scholarship* 21:227-231.

Harris MR et al (2000). Embedded structures and representation of nursing knowledge. *Journal of the American medical informatics association* 7:539-549.

Hemingway M, Oliver S (2000). Bilateral head flattening in hospitalized premature infants. *The online journal of knowledge synthesis for nursing* 7, Document No 3. Available online at http://www.stti.iupui.edu/library/ojksn/e.html.

Johnson MO (2001). Mother-infant interaction and maternal substance use/abuse: an integrative review of research literature in the 1990s. *The online journal of knowledge synthesis for nursing* 8, Document No 2. Available online at http://www.stti.iupui.edu/library/ojksn/e.html.

Ledbetter C (2000). Evidence-based best practice. *The online journal of knowledge synthesis for nursing*. Available online at http://www.stti.iupui.edu/library/ojksn/e.html.

McCartney PR (1999). Internet communication and discussion lists for perinatal nurses. *Journal of perinatal and neonatal nursing* 12:26-40.

Nightingale F (1860). *Notes on nursing: what it is and what it is not*. Appleton & Co: New York.

Ozbolt JG, Bakken S (2001). Patient care systems. In Shortliffe EH et al, editors: *Medical informatics: computer applications in health care and biomedicine*, ed 2. Springer-Verlag: New York.

Staggers N et al (2001). History and trends in clinical information systems in the United States. *Journal of nursing scholarship* 33(1):75-81.

Stevens KR. (2001). The truth, the whole truth, about EBP and RCTs. *The online journal of knowledge synthesis for nursing.* Available online at http://www.stti.iupui.edu/library/ojksn/e.html.

Thede LQ (1999). *Computers in nursing: bridges to the future.* JB Lippincott: Philadelphia.

Weiner BE, Trangenstein PA (1999). The third wave of information technology. In Sullivan EJ, editor. *Creating nursing's future: issues, opportunities, and challenges.* St Louis: Mosby.

Wootton JC (1999). Worldwide web resources for perinatal nursing. *Journal of perinatal and neonatal nursing* 12:15-25.

CHAPTER

20

NEWBORN AND INFANT ASSESSMENT

DEBRA A. SANSOUCIE, TERRI A. CAVALIERE

Assessment is a continuous process of evaluation throughout the course of routine care of the neonate and infant. However, periodically a more formalized, comprehensive examination must be undertaken to determine wellness or to evaluate a specific problem. The results of the comprehensive physical assessment serve as the database upon which clinical judgments about diagnosis and treatment are based.

A comprehensive physical assessment is performed for various reasons. The assessment may be the initial examination at birth, assessment of extrauterine transition, determination of gestational age, comprehensive assessment after transition, discharge examination, well-baby outpatient examination, or evaluation of an illness or injury. Although these assessments have many commonalities, each has a somewhat different purpose.

FIRST NEONATAL ASSESSMENT AND THE APGAR SCORE

The initial neonatal assessment occurs immediately after delivery with the assignment of Apgar scores. These scores were devised in 1952 by Virginia Apgar as a means of assessing the clinical status of infants immediately after delivery (Apgar, 1953). The Apgar score consists of five components—heart rate, respiratory effort, muscle tone, reflex irritability, and color—and each component is given a score of zero, one, or two; the scores are then added to obtain a total score (Table 20-1). Although the total score originally was assigned at 1 minute after birth, the current recommendation is that it be assigned at 1 and 5 minutes. If the total score is below seven at 5 minutes, the assessment is repeated every 5 minutes for 20 minutes or until a score above seven has been achieved twice consecutively.

The value of the Apgar score has been challenged because of its misuse in the identification of birth asphyxia and prediction of neurologic outcome. It is important to recognize that elements of the Apgar score may be influenced by a variety of factors besides birth asphyxia, including, among others, preterm birth, administration of drugs to the mother, and congenital anomalies. A low 1 minute Apgar score does not correlate with the newborn's future outcome. The 5 minute Apgar score, especially the change in the score between 1 and 5 minutes, is a useful indicator of the effectiveness of resuscitation efforts. However, even a 5 minute score of zero to three, although possibly a result of hypoxia, is limited as an indicator of

the severity of the problem and correlates poorly with future neurologic outcome (Stanley, 1994). Apgar scores are still useful for assessing the condition of the newborn at birth; however, as recognized by the American Academy of Pediatrics (AAP) Committee on the Fetus and Newborn and the American College of Obstetricians and Gynecologists Committee on Obstetrics (1996), additional information is required to properly interpret the scores of infants who require immediate resuscitation.

OTHER CONSIDERATIONS FOR THE INITIAL NEONATAL ASSESSMENT

A brief physical examination should be performed before the infant leaves the delivery area. Considerations for this assessment include inspection for birth injuries and major congenital anomalies and evaluation of pulmonary and cardiovascular adjustment to extrauterine life. Evaluation of early transition to extrauterine life includes observation of color for adequacy of perfusion and oxygenation, appraisal of respiratory effort, auscultation of breath sounds and heart sounds, and inspection of the amount, color, and consistency of secretions. The infant's tone, activity, and appropriateness of state should also be noted at this time. A cursory inspection of all external areas should be performed before the infant leaves the delivery area, including a general inspection of the external genitalia and, in males, palpation for testes in the scrotum. The entire examination should be performed under a radiant heat source to prevent significant heat loss from the infant.

EVALUATION OF TRANSITION

The transition from a fetal to an extrauterine environment reflects adaptation to both intrapartum and neonatal events. These events result in sympathetic activity that affects the infant's color, respiration, heart rate, behavioral state, gastrointestinal function, and temperature (Aucott, 1997). It is important to remember that the physiologic and biochemical changes peculiar to the period of transition to extrauterine life affect the physical findings of early examinations. The examination performed during transition is described separately because characteristics that are normal during transition may be abnormal if they appear at other times.

TABLE 20-1	Apgar Scoring System		
	ASSIGNED POINTS		
Sign	**0**	**1**	**2**
Heart rate	Absent	Slow (under 100 bpm)	100 bpm
Respirations	Absent	Weak cry; hypoventilation	Good, strong cry
Muscle tone	Limp	Some flexion	Active motion
Reflex irritability (response to brisk slap on soles of feet)	No response	Grimace	Cough or sneeze
Color	Blue or pale	Body pink; extremities blue	Completely pink

Used with permission of American Academy of Pediatrics Committee on the Fetus and Newborn and the American College of Obstetricians and Gynecologists Committee on Obstetrics (1996). Use and abuse of the Apgar score. Pediatrics 98:141-142.

As the neonate's circulation converts from the fetal route, there may be a period in which pulmonary vascular resistance remains greater than systemic vascular resistance, resulting in a right to left shunt across the ductus arteriosus. Higher preductal oxygen saturation causes the neonate's face and upper body to appear pink while the lower body and legs appear pale or blue; this creates a visible demarcation across the chest. As the fetal circulation successfully converts to the neonatal pathway, this transitional differential cyanosis disappears (Aucott, 1997).

Acrocyanosis is common during this period. To evaluate babies with deeper skin pigmentation, the nurse should observe the color of the mucous membranes. When the neonate is stimulated, the skin may appear blushed or bright red; this change in color is called erythema neonatorum, or generalized hyperemia, which develops a few hours after birth. It generally resolves within several minutes to an hour and rarely appears with the same intensity. According to Fletcher (1998), "This event of total blushing is noteworthy in that it likely signals the successful completion of fetal to neonatal transition in the cardiopulmonary system and provides some reassurance of health in that infant." Erythema neonatorum is not synonymous with erythema toxicum neonatorum.

The neonatal heart rate may range from 160 to 180 beats per minute (bpm) in the first 15 minutes of life; it slowly falls to a baseline rate of 100 to 120 bpm by 30 minutes of life. The heart rate is labile, and brief periods of asymptomatic, irregular heart rates are not pathologic. Murmurs are common, because the ductus arteriosus may still be patent. Respirations are also irregular during the first 15 minutes, with rates ranging from 60 to 100 breaths per minute. Grunting, flaring, retractions, and brief periods of apnea may also be seen in the neonate. Crackles may be present on auscultation (Aucott, 1997).

Despite the changes in the heart and respiratory rates during the initial 15 to 30 minutes of life, healthy term infants are awake and alert. They may rest quietly, cry periodically, startle spontaneously, and breastfeed during this period. Full-term babies often show flexed posture with good muscle tone; preterm newborns, in comparison, have less flexion and tone (Katz & Nishioka, 1998). Temperature is decreased, and gastrointestinal activity includes the establishment of bowel sounds and the production of saliva. This first period of reactivity may be prolonged in infants who have experienced difficult labor and delivery, in sick term infants, and in well premature infants (Aucott, 1997).

After the first period of reactivity, the infant is relatively unresponsive or sleeping, and the heart rate drops to a baseline of

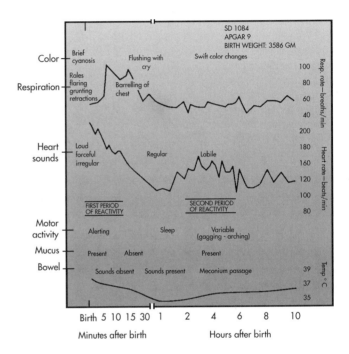

FIGURE **20-1**
Normal transition period. From Lowdermilk DL et al (2000): *Maternity and women's health care*, ed 7. Mosby: St Louis.

100 to 120 bpm. This interval, which lasts approximately 60 to 100 minutes, is followed by a second period of reactivity, which lasts anywhere from 10 minutes to several hours. During this time the infant may show rapid color changes, intermittent tachypnea and tachycardia, and changes in tone. Healthy infants may have periods during which the respiratory rate is considerably higher than 60 breaths per minute; however, the infant does not appear distressed and can slow this rate enough to nipple feed successfully. Meconium often is passed during this period (Aucott, 1997). The chart in Figure 20-1 summarizes some of the physical changes seen during the transition period.

NEWBORN EXAMINATION

The comprehensive newborn examination generally is performed within the first 12 to 18 hours of life, after transition has been completed successfully. The examination should be initiated when the infant is quiet and should progress from assessments that are least likely to bother the infant to those that

TABLE **20-2**	Examination Sequence Based on Infant's State		
Assessment Technique	**Required State**	**Arousing Maneuver**	**Equipment**
Observe general appearance			
Observe color			
Observe resting posture	Quiet		
Observe spontaneous activity	Active		
Count respirations	Quiet		
Count heart beats	Quiet		Clock
Inspect facies at rest	Quiet		Clock
Auscultate heart sounds	Quiet		Stethoscope
Auscultate breath sounds	Quiet		Stethoscope
Measure blood pressure	Quiet		Blood pressure cuff
Inspect head and neck region			
Stimulate response to sound	Quiet		Calibrated noise maker
Inspect trunk anteriorly			
Palpate abdomen, cardiac impulse	Quiet		
Feel pulses			
Examine genitalia			Lubricant for rectal examination
Inspect trunk posteriorly			
Inspect arms and hands			
Inspect legs and feet			
Assess passive tone			
Assess active tone	Active	X	
Elicit primitive reflexes	Active	X	
Assess muscle strength	Active	X	
Assess gestational age			
Test range in major joints		X	
Manipulate hips	Quiet	X	
Measure temperature			Thermometer
Examine ears			Otoscope
Determine pupil response			Bright light
Examine fundi	Quiet	X	
Elicit tendon reflexes		X	Percussion hammer
Stimulate response to pain		X	
Weigh infant	Quiet	X	Scales, growth chart
Measure head circumference			Tape measure, growth chart
Measure chest and abdomen circumferences		X	Tape measure
Measure length			Tape measure, growth chart
Transilluminate head		X	High-intensity light
Percuss abdomen	Quiet		
Percuss lungs	Quiet		

Data from Fletcher MA (1998). Physical diagnosis in neonatology. *Lippincott-Raven: Philadelphia.*

are most irritating. An examination sequence based on the infant's state is outlined in Table 20-2.

DISCHARGE EXAMINATION

The purpose of the discharge examination is to assess the infant's ability to be cared for outside the controlled environment of the hospital. The focus of the assessment depends primarily on how long the infant has been hospitalized and for what reasons. The needs of a healthy, full-term infant being discharged home with the mother are different from those of a growing, preterm infant who has been hospitalized for weeks or months and who has significant sequelae. Evaluating the caretaker's capability to care for and observe changes in the infant is an important aspect of the discharge assessment and follow-up plan. Anticipatory guidance regarding feedings, sleep-

ing position and environment, skin care, safety practices, and recognition of signs and symptoms of illness should be provided at this time.

OUTPATIENT EXAMINATION

The focus of the first outpatient examination is the infant's adaptation to the home environment. This examination includes assessment of any issues highlighted at discharge. Some factors to be considered in the infant are temperature stability, ability and success at feeding and elimination, sleep patterns, normal color, drying of the umbilical cord, reassessment of hip stability, and normal state and behavior. Any areas that may have been relatively inaccessible during earlier examinations should be included, such as the eyes, ear canals, and eardrums (Fletcher, 1998).

The birth history, including the birth weight, gestational age, and any problems should be reviewed. As part of the complete physical examination, height, weight, and head circumference should be plotted and developmental progress observed. The results of newborn metabolic screening and the infant's immunization status should be reviewed. For sick infants, general assessment assists in the establishment of priorities. For example, if a child is experiencing pronounced respiratory problems, assessment of this area is a priority. Anticipatory guidance issues include nutrition, elimination, sleep patterns, development and behavior, social and family relationships, and injury prevention (AAP, 1997a). A more detailed description of health maintenance for high-risk infants during the first year of life is presented later in this chapter.

ENVIRONMENT

The routine neonatal assessment should take place in a quiet, warm environment. The room should be lighted well enough for appropriate observation, but the light should not be so strong that the infant is deterred from opening the eyes. Prevention of heat loss is critical to the infant's comfort and to the maintenance of thermal neutrality and glucose homeostasis. Most healthy term infants can tolerate being undressed in a reasonably warm room for the 5 to 10 minutes required to perform the physical assessment. If the environment is cool or drafty or if the infant is sick or preterm, an external heat source should be provided, such as a radiant warmer or heat lamps. If heat lamps are used, the infant's eyes should be shielded to prevent adverse effects from prolonged exposure of the infant's eyes to the bright light of the lamps. Warming the hands and examination equipment before beginning not only prevents heat loss but also avoids upsetting an otherwise quiet and cooperative infant.

The examination should be conducted in a quiet environment with a calm infant. A placid infant provides the best opportunity for gathering meaningful data. Extraneous environmental noise hampers auscultation and assessment of bodily sounds and may overwhelm a sick or immature infant, causing changes in state and cardiovascular status (Fletcher, 1998). Handling the infant gently and speaking in a soothing voice may allow the examiner to complete most of the assessment without distressing the infant. Disturbing components of the examination, such as deep palpation of the abdomen and assessment of the hips, should be performed last.

Having one or both parents present during the routine neonatal assessment offers the opportunity to assess their competence in caregiving and to educate them about the unique physical traits, behavior, and coping skills of their infant. The examiner may also use this time to build rapport and trust with the parents, to listen to their concerns, and to offer pertinent information. Some issues may require privacy for discussion, therefore confidentiality should be considered when conversing with parents in the presence of others.

COMPONENTS OF A COMPREHENSIVE HISTORY

The neonatal history is very similar to that for an older child or adult, including information about the past medical history, the current condition, and the family. For a newly delivered infant, the initial neonatal assessment probably will be conducted before the nurse speaks to the parents. Basic information about the pregnancy and delivery should be available in the maternal records, but a complete history lays the founda-

tion for the comprehensive newborn examination and should be elicited directly from the parents. Without a complete history, the examiner may lack adequate information to formulate an accurate impression.

The components of a complete history are the identifying data; chief complaint; interim neonatal history or history of presenting problem or illness; antepartum history; obstetric history; intrapartum history; and the maternal medical, family medical, and social histories (Table 20-3). After data collected from the complete history and physical assessment are organized and all expected and unexpected findings have been reviewed, areas of concern are identified and prioritized for further evaluation and attention. This forms the framework for the clinical diagnosis and plan of care.

INTERVIEWING THE PARENTS

The interview with the parents is a vital component of the health assessment of a newborn or an infant. This interview offers the nurse an excellent opportunity to develop a therapeutic partnership with the parents in the care of their baby. Ideally, the interview is conducted in a quiet, comfortable setting; if it takes place at the bedside in a busy intensive care unit, the parents may be distracted and overwhelmed by the sounds and sights customary to this environment. If the ideal setting is not possible, the nurse can provide a focal point of warmth and attention by using a conversational tone of voice, maintaining eye contact, and concentrating fully on the parents. However, this can be done only with a discipline that dispels both personal and professional distractions.

It is important that nurses introduce themselves and clearly state their name and role in the baby's care. Nurses should make sure they understand the parents' names and should pronounce them correctly. They should ask the baby's name and use it often during the conversation. During this session, the purposes of the health interview and physical assessment should be clarified. Cooperation and sharing are more likely if the parents understand that the questions lead to better care for their infant.

The use of silence and listening, as well as allowing ample time for response to questions, is crucial to reassuring parents that what they say is worthwhile. Also, the parents can easily be shown that the interview is important and will not be rushed. Nurses should fix their attention on the parents and listen and should not interrupt unless necessary. They also should avoid asking the next questions before listening to the complete answer to the current question. They should indicate that they understand the responses and should request clarification if necessary. Nurses should take care to avoid overly technical language, medical jargon, and the tendency to inundate the parents with information. They should attempt to verify that the parents understand what has happened and what they have been told and that they seem to be coping. Nurses should always discuss and explain what the parents can expect to happen next, methods of keeping in touch, pertinent telephone numbers, and the visitation policy, if appropriate.

It often is difficult to approach parents about sensitive matters, such as drug or alcohol use or concerns about the death of their infant. The following suggestions may assist in the discussion of sensitive issues (Seidel & Ball, 1999). Nurses should:

- Respect the individual's privacy
- Avoid discussing sensitive topics where the conversation might be overheard

TABLE **20-3**	Components of a Comprehensive Neonatal History
Component	**Data Required**
Identifying data	Infant's name, parents' names, parents' telephone numbers (home and work), infant's date of birth, gender, and race; source of referral (obstetric or pediatric provider) if any.
Chief complaint	Statement of initial known status (age, gender, birth and current weights, gestational age by dates and examination) and problems infant might have; for a newborn or well-baby examination, the statement simply reflects the current health status (e.g., "Full-term male infant, now 1 week of age, for well-baby follow-up.").
Interim history/history of presenting problem	Chronologic record of newborn's history from time of delivery to present or, if older infant, chronologic narrative of chief complaint. Narrative should answer questions related to where (location), what (quality, factors that aggravate or relieve symptoms), when (onset, duration, frequency), and how much (intensity, severity).
Antepartum history	Historical data about the pregnancy, including maternal age, gravidity, parity, last menstrual period, and estimated date of delivery. Date and gestational age at which prenatal care began, provider of care, and number of visits should be recorded here. Mother's health during pregnancy, infections, medications taken, use of illicit drugs or alcohol, abnormal bleeding, and results of prenatal screening tests also should be included.
Obstetric history	Significant history regarding previous pregnancies; neonatal problems or subsequent major medical problems of previous children and current age and health status of living children should be noted.
Intrapartum history	Duration of labor, whether it was spontaneous or induced, duration of rupture of membranes, type of delivery, complications; infant's birth weight, presentation at delivery, and Apgar scores; resuscitative measures if required and response to those measures.
Past medical history	Significant maternal history of chronic health problems or diseases treated in the past or during the pregnancy, including surgical procedures and hospitalizations before or during the pregnancy. For older infants, also obtain information about infant's history, including feeding, development, illness, and immunizations.
Family medical history	Significant family medical history of chronic disorders, disabilities, known hereditary diseases, or consanguinity.
Social history	Parents' marital status, paternal involvement, parents' occupations and educational level; sources of financial support, housing accommodations, and insurance status must be noted, as well as any support agencies involved. Family unit should be defined and religious and cultural affiliations noted, along with number of individuals living in the home. Plans for child care should be elicited, as well as any current family stressors (e.g., moving, death in the family).

- Begin the discussion with open-ended questions and ask the least threatening questions first
- Take a direct and firm approach
- Avoid apologizing for asking a question (the nurse is doing nothing wrong)
- Avoid lecturing (the nurse is not there to pass judgment)
- Understand that defensive behavior might be the individual's way of coping
- Proceed slowly and take care not to demean the individual's behavior

It is vital that, in communicating with parents from diverse cultures, nurses appreciate and respect differences in communication patterns and in childbearing and health practices. A knowledge of cultural variations in family and health practices assists nurses in developing sensitivity to differences; however, the family must be observed carefully for cues to family practices and relationships with children and one another.

PHYSICAL ASSESSMENT TECHNIQUES

The techniques used for physical assessment are inspection, palpation, percussion, and auscultation. Learning these skills requires patience and practice, and the inability of the newborn to provide verbal cues presents an additional challenge.

With experience, the practitioner learns to process a multitude of observations while assessing individual systems and then to use this data to form a clinical impression and plan of care.

Inspection

Inspection is a crucial skill in the physical assessment of neonates, but it also is a difficult one to master. Inspection is the simple yet intricate use of the auditory and visual senses to evaluate an infant's state, color, respiratory effort, posture, and activity, as well as the shape and symmetry of various body regions. The sense of smell may be used to note unusual odors. The impression obtained from methodical observation establishes priorities for the remainder of the systematic assessment. In the physical examination, thoughtful observation, rather than simple looking, is the most efficient means of detecting changes. Inspection should be used throughout the physical assessment and should continue as long as the infant remains in the nurse's care.

Auscultation

Auscultation is the process of listening for sounds made by the body. The bell of the stethoscope is used for low-pitched sounds (e.g., cardiovascular sounds) and the diaphragm for higher pitched sounds (e.g., lung and bowel sounds). The

TABLE 20-4	Percussion Sounds				
Type of Sound	**Intensity**	**Pitch**	**Duration**	**Quality**	**Common Locations**
Tympany	Loud	High	Moderate	Drumlike	Gastric bubble; air-filled intestine (simulate by tapping puffed out cheeks)
Resonance	Moderate to loud	Low	Long	Hollow	Lungs
Hyperresonance	Very loud	Very low	Long	Booming	Lungs with trapped air; lungs of a young child
Dullness	Soft to moderate	High	Moderate	Thudlike	Liver, fluid-filled space (e.g., stomach)
Flatness	Soft	High	Short	Flat	Muscle

Data from Engel J (1997). Pocket guide to pediatric assessment, ed 3. Mosby: St Louis.

stethoscope should be placed lightly but firmly against the wall of the body part being assessed. A calm infant and quiet environment facilitate auscultation. Practice in recognizing normal body sounds is required before abnormal sounds can be identified accurately.

Palpation

With palpation, the examiner uses the sense of touch to determine hydration, texture, tension, pulsation, vibration, amplitude, and tenderness, as well as the depth, size, shape, and location of deep structures. The touch used for palpation must be gentle and is performed with the flats of the finger pads rather than the fingertips (Fletcher, 1998). To gather the most accurate information, the infant should be calm at the onset of the abdominal examination. Relaxing the abdominal musculature by flexing the infant's knees and hips with one hand facilitates palpation of the liver and spleen. Gentle pressure must be emphasized during palpation of sensitive organs (e.g., liver, spleen, and skin) that are at greater risk for injury and bleeding in neonates, particular preterm infants or those that have hepatomegaly. Warming of the examiner's hands, use of a pacifier, and progression from superficial to deep palpation help maintain the infant's comfort throughout most of the examination. Tender areas should always be palpated last.

Percussion

Percussion is the use of tapping to produce sound waves that may be assessed according to intensity, pitch, duration, and quality (Table 20-4). Percussion may be direct or indirect. For direct percussion, the examiner directly strikes the body part to be assessed with the tip of the middle right finger. For indirect percussion, the examiner places the middle finger of the nondominant hand against the skin of the body part to be assessed and strikes the distal joint with the tip of the middle finger of the dominant hand. The wrist must make a snapping motion, creating a brisk thump with the tip of the right middle finger against the left middle finger's distal joint. Vibrations are transmitted from the bones of the finger joint touching the infant's body to the underlying tissue (Figure 20-2). Although percussion is rarely used in neonatal assessment, it may be a useful technique for examining the older infant or child.

ASSESSMENT OF SIZE AND GROWTH

A normal growth pattern reflects well-being in the fetal and neonatal periods. Fetal and neonatal growth rates are predictable and can be measured by various methods. To determine if an individual infant's growth is adequate, an appropri-

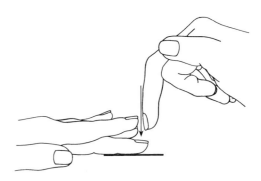

FIGURE 20-2
Percussion. Note the position of the fingers. From Engel J (1997). *Pocket guide to pediatric assessment*, ed 3. Mosby: St Louis.

ate standard must be used with which the child's measurements can be compared. The growth curves used must match the patient as closely as possible in gender, race, gestational age, genetic potential, and environmental factors, such as altitude. A discussion of the techniques used to estimate and assess fetal growth is beyond the scope of this chapter and can be found elsewhere in this text. Two methods of evaluating adequacy of growth in the newborn are the gestational age assessment and the clinical assessment of nutritional status (CANSCORE.).

ASSESSMENT OF GESTATIONAL AGE

A determination of gestational age (GA) is part of the physical examination of every newborn. Classification of newborns by gestational age enables the health care provider to determine the neonatal mortality risk (Figure 20-3) and to identify possible disorders (Figure 20-4) and initiate intervention or screening (Lepley & Gardner, 1998). Figure 20-5 shows the classification of newborns by intrauterine growth and gestational age. Table 20-5 presents terms used in GA assessment and in determining the adequacy of in utero growth.

As was previously mentioned, morbidity and mortality can be predicted from the GA assessment (Figures 20-3 and 20-4). Neonates with the lowest risk of problems associated with morbidity and mortality are term infants who developmentally are appropriate for gestational age (AGA). Risks associated with categories of gestational age and intrauterine growth retardation/restriction are shown in Table 20-6.

After birth, gestational age is determined by the evaluation of physical, neurologic, and neuromuscular characteristics. A number of methods have been developed to assess gestational

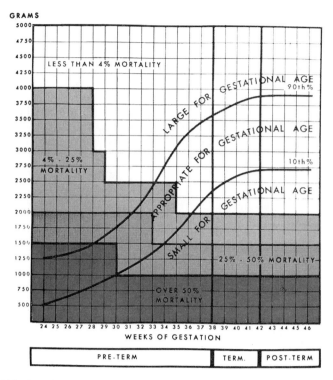

FIGURE **20-3**

University of Colorado Medical Center classification of newborns by birth weight and gestational age and by neonatal mortality risk. From Battaglia FC, Lubchenco LO (1967). A practical classification of newborn infants by weight and gestational age. *Journal of pediatrics* 71:159-163.

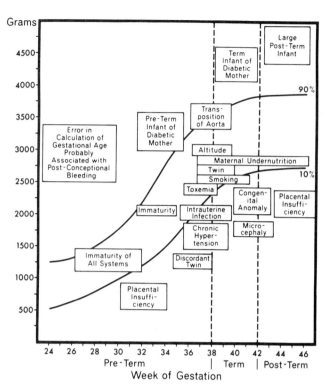

FIGURE **20-4**

Deviations of intrauterine growth: neonatal morbidity by birth weight and gestational age. From Lubchenco LO (1967). *The high risk infant.* WB Saunders: Philadelphia; as adapted from Lubchenco LO et al [1968]. In Jonxis JHP et al, editors: *Aspects of prematurity and dysmaturity.* Charles C Thomas: Springfield, IL.

TABLE **20-5**	Terms and Abbreviations Used in Assessment of Gestational Age and Adequacy of Intrauterine Growth
Term and Abbreviation	**Description**
Low birth weight (LBW)	Infant weighing less than 2500 g*
Very low birth weight (VLBW)	Infant weighing less than 1500 g*
Extremely low birth weight (ELBW)	Infant weighing less than 1000 g*
Appropriate for gestational age (AGA)	Parameter (weight) within the tenth to ninetieth percentile for gestational age
Large for gestational age (LGA)	Parameter above the ninetieth percentile for gestational age
Small for gestational age (SGA)	Parameter below the tenth percentile for gestational age
Intrauterine growth restriction (IUGR)	Slowing of intrauterine growth documented by ultrasound; a neonate may be IUGR without being SGA
Symmetric IUGR	Measurements for weight, length, and head circumference all within the same growth curve even if neonate is AGA, LGA, or SGA
Asymmetric IUGR	Measurements for weight, length, and head circumference in different growth curves
Term gestation	Neonate born between 37 and 42 weeks' gestation
Preterm gestation	Neonate delivered before completion of week 37 of gestation
Postterm gestation	Neonate delivered after completion of week 42 of gestation

*Regardless of length of gestation.

CLASSIFICATION OF NEWBORNS—
BASED ON MATURITY AND INTRAUTERINE GROWTH
Symbols: X - 1st Examination O - 2nd Examination

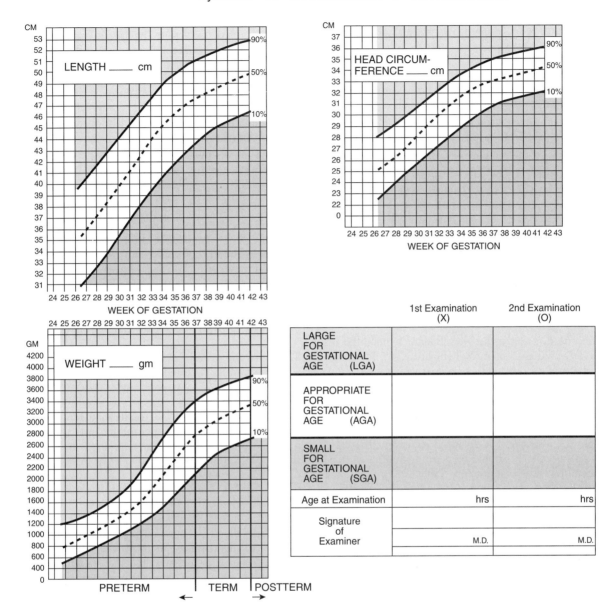

FIGURE **20-5**

Estimating gestational age: newborn classification based on maturity and intrauterine growth. In Lowdermilk DL et al (2000). *Maternity and women's health care*, ed 7. Mosby: St Louis. Modified from Lubchenco L et al (1966). Intrauterine growth in length and head circumference as estimated from live births at gestational ages from 26 to 42 weeks. *Journal of pediatrics* 37:403; Battaglia F, Lubchenco L (1967): A practical classification of newborn infants by weight and gestational age. *Journal of pediatrics* 71:159.

TABLE **20-6**	Risks Associated with Gestational Age and Intrauterine Growth Restriction
Category	**Risks**
Small for gestational age (SGA), large for gestational age (LGA), intrauterine growth retardation/restriction (IUGR)	Perinatal and long-term problems
Preterm SGA	Problems associated with immaturity of body systems and placental insufficiency
Preterm	Problems associated with immaturity of body systems
Postterm	Problems associated with placental insufficiency
Term LGA	Risks are greatest in perinatal period, but long-term problems can develop.

age in newborns. Currently, the New Ballard score (NBS) is the most widely used assessment tool (Figure 20-6). Its advantages over the other scoring systems are its wide range (20 to 44 weeks) and its accuracy (within 1 week) of GA measurement (Southgate & Pittard, 2001). Performing the examination as soon as possible in the first 12 hours of life enhances its accuracy.

Although GA assessment is discussed separately, the components of the assessment should be performed as part of the infant's general physical examination. Table 20-7 presents the essentials of the NBS; each component is scored as shown in Figure 20-6. The total score is calculated, and the resulting GA is plotted on a graph (see Figure 20-5).

CLINICAL ASSESSMENT OF NUTRITIONAL STATUS (CANSCORE)

GA assessment does not identify all infants with intrauterine malnutrition. Although the terms small for gestational age (SGA) and intrauterine growth retardation/restriction (IUGR) are related, they are not synonymous. IUGR represents a reduction in the expected fetal growth pattern, whereas SGA refers to an infant whose birth weight is less than population norms. All IUGR infants are not SGA, and all SGA infants are not IUGR (Kliegman & Das, 2002).

Many but not all infants who are either SGA or IUGR are malnourished in utero. However, malnutrition can occur in neonates of any birth weight. Because malnutrition alters body composition and can prevent adequate brain growth, it is important to identify infants who have been affected in utero. These infants may be at risk for problems associated with aberrant growth (Fletcher, 1998).

McLean and Usher (1970) described physical findings that are suggestive of weight loss or poor nutrition. These physical characteristics form the basis of the CANSCORE used in the clinical evaluation of nutritional status in newborns at term (Figure 20-7).

MEASUREMENT TECHNIQUES

For most infants the parameters of weight, length, and occipitofrontal circumference (OFC) are adequate for the basic physical assessment. These measurements are compared against standard growth curves. If the infant has any abnormalities in the size of a body component or shows disproportionate growth, the involved areas should be measured and compared with established norms (Fletcher, 1998).

Weight and Length

The infant should be weighed while unclothed and quiet. Weight can be falsely increased by a significant amount of infant motion (Fletcher, 1998). The weight of the average full-term newborn that is AGA is 3.5 kg, with a range of 2500 to 4000 g (Tappero, 1996; Grover, 2000a).

The crown to heel length can be obtained using a measurement board or a standard tape measure. With the infant supine and legs extended, the nurse draws a line on the bed at the baby's head and another at the heels and then measures the distance between these two points (Figure 20-8). The average full-term newborn is 50 cm long with a range of 45 to 55 cm (Tappero, 1996; Grover, 2000a). Other measurement techniques are described in the appropriate sections.

PHYSICAL EXAMINATION OF THE NEONATE

The following sections describe the newborn examination beyond the transition period.

Vital Signs

Once transition is complete, the neonate has a respiratory rate between 40 and 60 breaths per minute, and the rate may be irregular. Respirations are easy and unlabored; breath sounds should be clear on auscultation. The heart rate ranges from 80 to 160 bpm, depending on the infant's state and gestational age (Vargo, 1996). Premature neonates have a higher baseline heart rate. The resting heart rate is the most representative for any baby.

Normal blood pressure ranges depend on gestational and chronologic ages and the methods used. Blood pressure in premature babies is proportional to size; therefore normal values are lower than for term babies (Hegyi et al, 1994). Figures 20-9 and 20-10 and Tables 20-8, 20-9, and 20-10 show normal blood pressure values over various time frames and gestational ages.

Temperature is determined by axillary measurement; acceptable values range from 35.5° to 37.5° C (Blake & Murray, 1998; Southgate & Pittard, 2001).

Cardiovascular Values

The heart is assessed for rate, rhythm, character of heart sounds, and presence of murmurs. During infancy the position of the heart changes, and the point of maximum impulse (PMI) shifts (Fletcher, 1998). In the first few days of life the PMI is located at the fourth intercostal space at or to the left of the midclavicular line (Vargo, 1996). Auscultation should be performed at the second and fourth intercostal spaces, cardiac apex, and axilla (D'Harlingue & Durand, 2001). Murmurs are commonly heard before the ductus arteriosus closes completely. However, murmurs that are persistent may not be normal and require evaluation (Katz & Nishioka, 1998). Brief asymptomatic irregularities in rate and rhythm are not uncommon, especially in the preterm baby. The most common benign

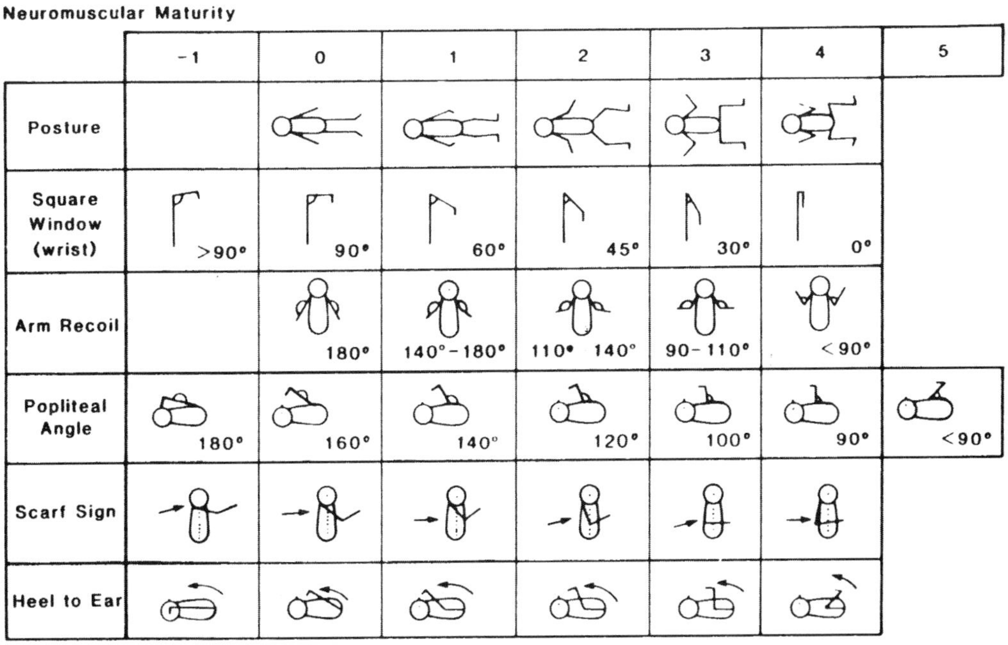

Neuromuscular Maturity

	-1	0	1	2	3	4	5
Posture							
Square Window (wrist)	>90°	90°	60°	45°	30°	0°	
Arm Recoil		180°	140°-180°	110° 140°	90-110°	<90°	
Popliteal Angle	180°	160°	140°	120°	100°	90°	<90°
Scarf Sign							
Heel to Ear							

Physical Maturity

Skin	sticky friable transparent	gelatinous red, translucent	smooth pink, visible veins	superficial peeling &/or rash. few veins	cracking pale areas rare veins	parchment deep cracking no vessels	leathery cracked wrinkled
Lanugo	none	sparse	abundant	thinning	bald areas	mostly bald	
Plantar Surface	heel-toe 40-50mm: -1 <40mm: -2	>50mm no crease	faint red marks	anterior transverse crease only	creases ant. 2/3	creases over entire sole	
Breast	imperceptible	barely perceptible	flat areola no bud	stippled areola 1-2mm bud	raised areola 3-4mm bud	full areola 5-10mm bud	
Eye/Ear	lids fused loosely: -1 tightly: -2	lids open pinna flat stays folded	sl. curved pinna; soft; slow recoil	well-curved pinna; soft but ready recoil	formed & firm instant recoil	thick cartilage ear stiff	
Genitals male	scrotum flat, smooth	scrotum empty faint rugae	testes in upper canal rare rugae	testes descending few rugae	testes down good rugae	testes pendulous deep rugae	
Genitals female	clitoris prominent labia flat	prominent clitoris small labia minora	prominent clitoris enlarging minora	majora & minora equally prominent	majora large minora small	majora cover clitoris & minora	

Maturity Rating

score	weeks
-10	20
-5	22
0	24
5	26
10	28
15	30
20	32
25	34
30	36
35	38
40	40
45	42
50	44

FIGURE **20-6**
Maturational assessment of gestational age: New Ballard scoring system. From Ballard JL et al (1991). New Ballard Score, expanded to include extremely premature infants. *Journal of pediatrics* 119:417-423.

dysrhythmias are sinus bradycardia or tachycardia and premature atrial or ventricular contractions (Vargo, 1996). An electrocardiogram (ECG) or heart monitor is needed to properly identify the abnormality. Exact identification of the abnormality cannot be made solely by auscultation.

A precordial impulse may be visible along the left sternal border during the first 6 hours (Fletcher, 1998; Southgate & Pittard, 2001). In premature neonates, because of their thin skin and absence of subcutaneous fat, the precordial impulse may be visible for a longer period.

Pulses are palpated for rate, strength, and synchrony. Figure 20-11 shows the location of pulses in the neonate (Vargo, 1996). Radial or brachial pulses are compared for timing and intensity, and the same is then done for bilateral femoral pulses. Finally, the preductal and postductal pulses are examined.

TABLE **20-7**	New Ballard Scoring System		
Component	**Assessment Technique**	**Effect of Maturity**	**Comments**
Neuromuscular Maturity			
Posture	Observe infant while baby is unrestrained and supine; note amount of flexion and extension of extremities.	Extensor tone is replaced by flexor tone in a cephalocaudal progression.	Knees may be hyperextended in a frank breech delivery.
Square window	Flex wrist; measure minimum angle formed by ventral surface of forearm and palm.	Angle decreases; at term no space exists between palm and forearm.	Response depends on muscle tone and intrauterine position.
Arm recoil	Place infant in supine position with head in midline. Flex elbow and hold forearm against arm for 5 seconds; fully extend elbow, then release; note time required for infant to resume flexed position.	Angle decreases and recoil becomes more rapid.	
Popliteal angle	Flex hips, placing thighs on abdomen; keeping hips on surface of bed, extend knee as far as possible until resistance is met; estimate popliteal angle.	Popliteal angle decreases.	Amount of extension can be overestimated if knee is extended beyond point where resistance is first met; this assessment also is affected by intrauterine position and hip dislocation.
Scarf sign	With head in midline, pull hand across chest to encircle neck; note position of elbow relative to midline.	Increased resistance to crossing the midline.	Reflects muscle tone; response is altered by obesity, hydrops, or fractured clavicle.
Heel to ear	Keep infant supine with pelvis on mattress; press feet as far as possible toward head, allowing knees to be positioned beside abdomen; estimate angle created by arc from back of heel to mattress.	Angle decreases; hip flexion decreases toward term.	Reflects muscle tone.
Physical Maturity			
Skin	Observe translucency of skin over abdominal wall.	Skin becomes thicker and ultimately dry and peeling; pigmentation increases.	Skin becomes drier hours after birth; phototherapy or sunlight enhances pigmentation.

Based on Fletcher MA (1998). *Physical diagnosis in neonatology. Lippincott-Raven: Philadelphia; and Southgate WM, Pittard WB (2001). Classification and physical examination of the newborn infant. In Klaus MH, Fanaroff AA, editors. Care of the high risk neonate, ed 5. WB Saunders: Philadelphia.*

Capillary refill reflects the adequacy of perfusion. This is assessed by depressing the skin over the abdomen or on an extremity until the area blanches. The capillary refill time is the number of seconds that elapse until the color returns to the area. This should be less than 3 seconds.

General Appearance

The infant's general appearance is indicative of nutritional status, maturity, and overall well-being. Term neonates normally are well formed and rounded and have stores of subcutaneous fat. They assume the fetal position at rest. Premature babies may display less flexion than those born at term. Movement should be spontaneous and tremulous. Neonates range in mood from quiet to alert; they are consolable when crying. The cry is strong and sustained (Katz & Nishioka, 1998).

Skin

The skin is assessed for maturity, consistency, and color. Discolored areas, variations, or abnormalities are noted for size and location. The skin of a full-term newborn contains subcutaneous fat that provides insulation against heat loss. It is smooth, pink, and wrinkle free. Premature infants lack subcutaneous fat; their skin is thinner than that of term babies and has visible blood vessels over the chest and abdomen. Extremely immature babies often have a gelatinous appearance with transparent skin. They commonly have a red, ruddy color caused by underdevelopment of the stratum corneum. Subcutaneous fat also is lacking in neonates who are IUGR. This group of babies may have loose skin folds, particularly around the knees.

Vernix is the greasy yellow or white substance found on fetal skin, particularly in the axillary, nuchal, and inguinal folds.

TABLE 20-7	New Ballard Scoring System—cont'd		
Component	**Assessment Technique**	**Effect of Maturity**	**Comments**
Lanugo	Assess for presence and length of hair over back.	Lanugo emerges at 19 to 20 weeks and is most prominent at 27 to 28 weeks; it then gradually disappears, first from the lower back and then from at least half of the back.	The degree of pigmentation and quantity of hair are related to race, gender, and nutritional status.
Plantar surface	Measure length of foot; determine presence or absence of true deep creases (not merely wrinkles).	Early in gestation, foot length correlates with fetal growth; creases develop from toes to heel, and absence of creases correlates with immaturity.	Plantar creases also reflect intrauterine fetal activity; accelerated creasing is seen with oligohydramnios; diminished creasing suggests lack of activity in a mature fetus.
Breast	Estimate diameter of breast bud; assess color and stippling of areola.	Definition and stippling of areola and pigmentation are evident near term; bud size increases because of maternal hormones and fat accumulation.	With intrauterine growth restriction, breast tissue may be diminished, but development of areola proceeds regardless of malnutrition.
Ear cartilage	Fold top of auricle; observe speed of recoil.	Cartilage becomes stiff, and auricle thickens.	Compression in utero and absence or dysfunction of auricular muscles diminishes firmness.
Eyelid opening	Without attempting to separate eyelids, evaluate degree of fusion.	Opening begins at 22 weeks; lids are completely unfused by 28 weeks.	Fused eyelids should not be considered a sign of nonviability; lids may be fused at term with anophthalmia.
External genitalia Male	Palpate scrotum to assess degree of descent of testes; observe rugae and suspension of scrotum.	At 27 to 28 weeks, testes begin to descend into scrotum; rugae formation begins at about 28 weeks; by term rugae are well defined, and scrotum is pendulous.	Rugae are decreased with scrotal edema; testes may be absent (cryptorchidism).
Female	Assess size of labia minora and labia majora.	Labia minora increase in size before labia majora; at term labia majora cover labia minora completely.	Size of labia majora depends on amount of body fat; with malnutrition, size may be diminished; edema may increase size of labia majora.

Composed of sebaceous gland secretions, lanugo, and desquamated epithelial cells, it protects against fluid loss and bacterial invasion (Fletcher, 1998). Vernix is most abundant during the third trimester and decreases in amount as the fetus approaches 40 weeks.

Lanugo is fine, downy hair that first appears on the fetus at 19 to 20 weeks' gestation and becomes most prominent at 27 to 28 weeks. It begins to disappear from the lower back and usually is not present at term.

Head
The head is inspected for shape, symmetry, bruises, and lesions. Neonates delivered by cesarean section generally have a rounded head. Infants born vaginally in vertex position can have overriding sutures; this results in an irregularly shaped head that persists only for a few days in full-term neonates but may be evident for several weeks in premature babies (Katz & Nishioka, 1998). The head circumference is measured in the occipitofrontal plane and is the largest diameter around the head. It is obtained with the tape measure placed snugly above the ears, the eyebrow ridges, and the occiput of the head. The average OFC in a full-term neonate is 35 cm, with a normal range of 31 to 38 cm (Katz & Nishioka, 1998). The major bones of the head, as well as sutures and fontanels, are shown in Figure 20-12.

The head should be palpated to assess the firmness of bone and the size and configuration of fontanels and sutures and also to detect swelling, masses, or bony defects. The amount of overlap of sutures may vary, depending on the extent of molding. Normally the sutures should move freely when gentle pres-

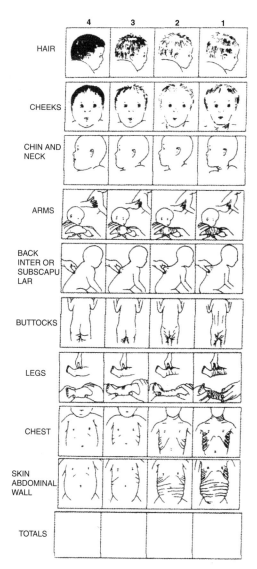

FIGURE **20-7**

Clinical assessment of nutritional status at birth (CANSCORE system). Nine signs are used to assess the nutritional status of newborn term infants. Each sign is rated from 4 (best) to 1 (worst). The CANSCORE is the sum of the nine signs. *Hair:* Large amount, smooth, silky, easily groomed (4 points); thinner, some straight "starring" hair (3 points); still thinner, more straight, with depigmented stripe (flag sign). *Cheeks:* Progression from full buccal pads and round face (4 points) to significantly reduced buccal fat with narrow, flat face (1 point). *Chin and neck:* Double or triple chin fat folds, neck not evident (4 points) to thin chin, no fat folds, neck with loose, wrinkled skin very evident (1 point). *Arms:* Full, round, cannot elicit accordion folds or lift folds of skin from elbow or triceps area (4 points) to striking accordion folding of lower arm (to elicit this sign, the examiner uses the thumb and fingers of the left hand to grasp the infant's arm just below the elbow, and the thumb and fingers of the right hand to encircle the infant's wrist, and then moves the two hands toward each other); skin loose, easy to grasp and pull away from the elbow (1 point). *Back:* Skin in interscapular area difficult to grasp and lift (4 points) to skin in interscapular area loose, easily lifted in a thin fold (1 point). *Buttocks:* Full, round gluteal fat pads (4 points) to virtually no evident gluteal fat, skin of buttocks and upper, posterior thigh loose and deeply wrinkled (1 point). *Legs:* Same as for arms. *Chest:* Full and round, ribs not seen (4 points) to progressive prominence of ribs with obvious loss of intercostal tissue (1 point). *Abdomen:* Full, round, no loose skin (4 points) to distended or scaploid but with very loose, easily lifted, wrinkled skin with accordion folds demonstrable (1 point). From Metcoff J (1994). Clinical assessment of nutritional status at birth, *Pediatric clinics of North America* 41:875-891.

sure is applied to the bones on opposite sides of the suture lines. Directly after birth it may be difficult to determine if the sutures are fused or merely overlapping. Reevaluation when molding and overlap have resolved may yield more reliable information about the presence of craniosynostosis (Fletcher, 1998).

The anterior fontanel is 2 to 3 cm wide, 3 to 4 cm long, and diamond shaped (Figure 20-12). The posterior fontanel is 1 to 2 cm wide and triangular. It may be difficult to palpate the fontanels directly after birth because of cranial molding (Katz & Nishioka, 1998). Tension in the fontanel should be assessed with the infant both recumbent and upright. Serial measurements of the width of the anterior fontanel are more helpful than a single measurement because of wide variations in size and differences in measurement techniques (Fletcher, 1998).

Hair is evaluated for color, length, continuity, texture, quantity, position and number of hair whorls, and hairlines. Term newborns have fine hair with identifiable individual strands. Hair may appear disheveled for the first several weeks to months (Fletcher, 1998). In premature neonates the hair is more widely dispersed and is described as "fuzzy." Normally, hair color is fairly uniform, although some neonates have a blend of light and dark hair. Sporadic patches of white hair may be a familial trait and is a benign finding, but a white forelock and other pigmentation defects in the eyes or skin may be associated with deafness or mental retardation (Waardenburg, 1951; Fletcher, 1998). The anterior hairline varies, with normal growth of pigmented hair onto the forehead of hirsute babies. The posterior hairline ends at the neck crease. Usually one off-center hair whorl is present in the parietal region (Fletcher, 1998).

Face and Neck

The face should be inspected for shape, symmetry, and the presence of bruising or dysmorphic features. The overall facial configuration should be evaluated; the features should be proportional and symmetric. Unusual facial features may be familial or pathognomonic of a malformation syndrome. Gag, sucking, and rooting reflexes should be evaluated.

The newborn has a relatively short neck that should be palpated or observed for symmetry, appearance of the skin, range of motion, masses, and fistulous openings. The neck should be symmetric with the head, demonstrating full range of motion (Katz & Nishioka, 1998). In utero positioning can cause asymmetry of the neck. Redundant skin or webbing may be evident. The clavicles can be palpated at this time; they should be intact and without crepitus or swelling.

Ears

The ears are evaluated and compared for shape, configuration, position, amount of cartilage, and signs of trauma. The position of the ears at term should be similar bilaterally, approximately 30% of the pinna should lie above a line from the inner and outer canthi of the eye toward the occiput. The rotation of the ears should also be assessed; the long axis of the pinna should lie approximately 15 degrees posterior to the true vertical axis of the head (Figure 20-13). Abnormalities of the external ear may be associated with syndromes, but often they represent minor structural variations and may be within the normal range (Johnson, 1996).

The presence and patency of the auditory canal can be documented by inspection. Otoscopic examination is not usually part of the examination in the newborn period because the ear canals are filled with vernix, amniotic debris, and blood. This

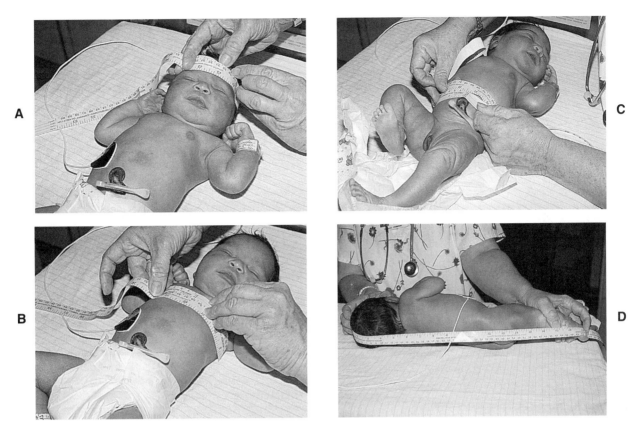

FIGURE **20-8**
Newborn measurements. **A,** Circumference of head. **B,** Circumference of chest. **C,** Circumference of abdomen. **D,** Length, crown to rump. (Total length includes the length of the legs). If the measurements are taken before the infant's first bath, the nurse must wear gloves. From Lowdermilk DL et al (2000). *Maternity and women's health care,* ed 7. Mosby: St Louis. Courtesy Marjorie Pyle, RNC, Lifecircle, Costa Mesa, CA.

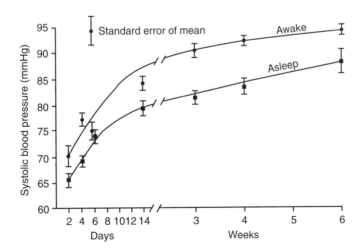

FIGURE **20-9**
Increase in systolic blood pressure between ages 2 days and 6 weeks in infants awake and asleep (values obtained by cuff measurement). From Early A et al (1980). Blood pressure in the first six weeks of life. *Archives of disease in childhood* 55:755-757.

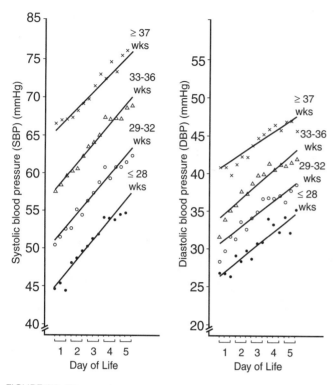

FIGURE **20-10**
Systolic and diastolic blood pressures plotted for the first 5 days of life, with each day subdivided into 8 hour periods. Infants are categorized by gestational age into four groups: 28 weeks or younger (n = 33), 29 to 32 weeks (n = 73), 33 to 36 weeks (n = 100), and 37 weeks or older (n = 110). From Zubrow AB et al (1995). Determinants of blood pressure in infants admitted to neonatal intensive care units: a prospective multicenter study. Philadelphia Neonatal Blood Pressure Study Group. *Journal of perinatology* 15:470.

TABLE **20-9**	Blood Pressure Ranges in Different Weight Groups of Premature Newborns*		
Birth Weight (g)	**BLOOD PRESSURE (mm Hg)**		
	Systolic	**Diastolic**	
501-750 (n = 18)	50-62	26-36	
751-1000 (n = 39)	48-59	23-36	
1001-1250 (n = 30)	49-61	26-35	
1251-1500 (n = 45)	46-56	23-33	
1501-1750 (n = 51)	46-58	23-33	
1751-2000 (n = 61)	48-61	24-35	

From Hegyi T et al (1994). Blood pressure ranges in premature infants. I. The first hours of life. Journal of pediatrics *124:627-633.*
*Measurements were obtained by blood pressure cuff or umbilical artery transducer in the first 3 to 6 hours of life.

TABLE **20-10**	Oscillometric Measurements: Mean Arterial Blood Pressure		
Birth Weight (g)	**MEAN ARTERIAL PRESSURE ± STANDARD DEVIATION**		
	Day 3	**Day 17**	**Day 31**
501-750	38 ± 8	44 ± 8	46 ± 11
751-1000	43 ± 8	45 ± 7	47 ± 9
1001-1250	43 ± 8	46 ± 9	48 ± 8
1251-1500	45 ± 8	47 ± 8	47 ± 9

From Fanaroff AA, Wright E (1990). Profiles of mean arterial blood pressure (MAP) for infants weighing 50 to 1500 grams. Pediatric research *27:205A.*

TABLE **20-8**	Blood Pressure Values According to Site and Age		
Site and Age	**BLOOD PRESSURE (mm Hg)**		
	Systolic	**Diastolic**	**Mean**
Right Arm			
Less than 36 hours old	62.6 ± 6.9	38.9 ± 5.7	48 ± 6.2
Over 36 hours old	68.4 ± 8.8*	43.5 ± 6.2*	53 ± 7.3
Total	64.7 ± 8.1	40.6 ± 6.2	49.8 ± 7
Calf			
Less than 36 hours old	61.9 ± 7	39.6 ± 5.3	47.6 ± 6
Over 36 hours old	66.8 ± 10.1*	42.5 ± 7.3*	51.5 ± 9*
Total	63.6 ± 8.6	40.6 ± 6.3	49 ± 7.5

Values were obtained by blood pressure cuff measurement in 219 healthy term infants, 140 less than 36 hours old and 79 over 36 hours old. Values are given as means ± standard deviation.
*Significantly different from values in infants less than 36 hours old (p < 0.05).

condition clears in approximately 60% of term infants by 1 week of age but may persist for weeks. Less debris is seen in preterm babies, whose canals may clear more quickly.

Because infants frequently remain hospitalized beyond the neonatal period and because evaluation of the middle ear is part of a health maintenance examination, it is appropriate to include otoscopic examination in this section. The otoscope is used differently in young infants than in adults. In a neonate the ear lobe is pulled toward the chin, and the speculum is directed toward the face. The ear canals of preterm babies are prone to collapse because they are more pliable. Positive pressure applied through the pneumatic otoscope prevents the cartilaginous ear canal from obscuring the view (Fletcher, 1998). The neonatal tympanic membrane is thicker, grayer, and more vascular than that of an adult or older child (Figure 20-14).

Infants should also be assessed for behavioral response to noise stimuli. However, routine formal audiologic testing is becoming more common in the newborn period.

Eyes
The eyes should show spontaneous range of motion and conjugate movements. The lids should be symmetric in both horizontal and vertical placement, and the lashes should be directed outward in an orderly fashion. The eyes should be clear and should have an evenly colored iris, which may be dark grey,

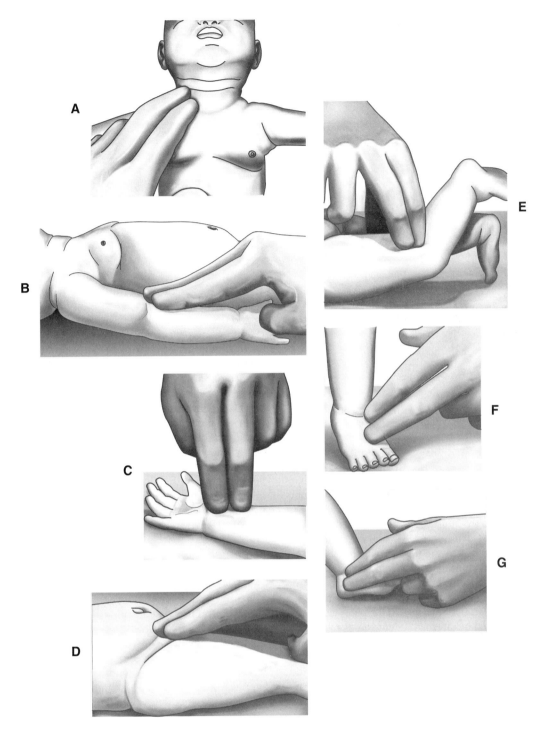

FIGURE **20-11**
Palpation of arterial pulses. **A,** Carotid. **B,** Brachial. **C,** Radial. **D,** Femoral. **E,** Popliteal. **F,** Dorsalis pedis. **G,** Posterial tibial.

blue, or brown, depending on race. Pigmentation should be similar between the two eyes. Permanent eye color is not established for several months, but darker races may show permanent pigmentation in the first week of life. The surface of the conjunctiva should be smooth. During the first few days of life, the cornea may appear slightly hazy as a result of corneal edema, but thereafter the cornea should be clear and shiny. The sclerae normally are white, but a bluish coloration may be noted in premature and other small infants because their sclerae are thinner (Fletcher, 1998; Gupta et al, 2002).

An ophthalmoscope is used to assess the pupillary and red reflexes. The light should be directed on the pupils from a distance of approximately 6 inches. The pupils should be round and equal in diameter and should constrict equally in response to light (pupils equal and reactive to light, or PERL). The beam of light illuminating the retina causes the red reflex. The retina (fundus) appears as a yellowish-white/gray or red background, depending on the amount of melanin in the pigment epithelium. The pigment varies with the complexion of the baby, with dark-skinned infants having pale retinal reflexes (Seidel & Ball, 1999).

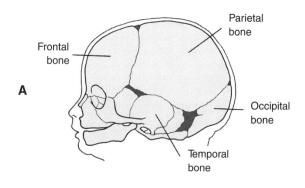

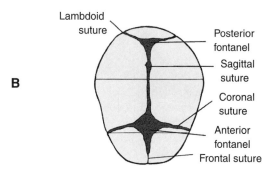

FIGURE **20-12**
Major bones of the head in the newborn with sutures and fontanels. From Lowdermilk DL et al (2000): *Maternity and women's health care,* ed 7. Mosby: St Louis.

Nose

The nose should be evaluated for shape and symmetry, patency of nares, skin lesions, or signs of trauma. The nasal mucosa should be pink and slightly moist; secretions should be thin, clear, and usually scanty (Fletcher, 1998). The nose should be midline. Immediately after birth the nose may be misshapen as a result of compression in utero, but this should correct spontaneously in a few days (Fletcher, 1998; Southgate & Pittard, 2001). Obstructions and deformities may denote anatomic malformations or congenital syndromes. The patency of the nares can be demonstrated by alternate occlusion of each naris using gentle pressure (Fletcher, 1998). Nasal flaring may be indicative of respiratory distress but "the use of ali nasi activation in otherwise healthy premature infants varies with activity and sleep states, so by itself cannot be used as a sign of respiratory distress" (Fletcher, 1998).

Mouth

The mouth is inspected for size, shape, color, and presence of abnormal structures and masses. It should be evaluated both at rest and while the infant is crying. The speed of response and intensity of neonatal reflexes, such as rooting, gag, and suck, are also assessed. The mouth is a midline structure, symmetric in shape and movement. The mouth, chin, and tongue should be in proportion, with the lips fully formed (Katz & Nishioka, 1998).

The mucous membranes should be pink and moist, and oral secretions should be thin and clear. Excessive secretions or drooling suggests inability to swallow or esophageal or pharyngeal obstruction. Both the hard and soft palates should be inspected and palpated to rule out clefts. A high-arched palate may be seen in malformation syndromes, but it generally is insignificant if it appears as an isolated characteristic (Aucott, 1997).

The tongue should be smooth on all surfaces; the lingual frenulum may be short but not so short as to restrict tongue movement. Limitation of movement would be obvious on crying, when the tip of the tongue would form an inverted V (Fletcher, 1998).

Thorax

The chest is evaluated for size, symmetry, musculature, bony structure, number and location of nipples, and ease of respiration (Southgate & Pittard, 2001). It should be symmetric in shape and movements. Because the anteroposterior diameter is approximately equal to the transverse diameter, the chest appears round. The chest circumference of a term infant should be about 2 cm smaller than the head circumference (Askin, 1996). At all gestational ages, the chest measurement normally is smaller than the OFC (Fletcher, 1998).

Occasional mild subcostal retractions may be seen in healthy newborns because of decreased compliance of the ribs (Fletcher, 1998). A paradoxical breathing pattern is typical of newborns, especially during sleep. On inspiration the chest wall is drawn in and the abdomen protrudes; the reverse occurs on expiration (Fletcher, 1998; Katz & Nishioka, 1998).

The amount of breast tissue depends on the gestational age and birth weight, whereas areolar development reflects only gestational age. Two nipples should be present in equal alignment. The internipple distance varies by gestational age and chest circumference, but the ratio of internipple distance to chest circumference should be less that 0.28 (Fletcher, 1998). Widely spaced nipples are associated with a variety of congenital syndromes.

Newborn breast tissue may hypertrophy as a result of the influence of maternal hormones. A milky substance (witches' milk) may appear toward the end of the first week of life, and this discharge may persist for a few weeks to several months (Askin, 1996; Fletcher, 1998).

Abdomen

The abdomen is inspected for contour and size, symmetry, character of skin, and umbilical cord location and anatomy. Palpation yields information about muscle mass and tone of the abdominal wall, location and size of viscera, tenderness, and masses (Fletcher, 1998). Bowel sounds are detected on auscultation; they are relatively quiet in newborns until feedings are established. Compared with term babies, preterm neonates have less active bowel sounds. Evaluating changes in bowel sounds from the infant's baseline is more clinically useful than an isolated assessment (Fletcher, 1998).

The normal abdomen in an infant is round and soft and protrudes slightly. The umbilical cord should be bluish white, shiny, and moist and should have two arteries and one vein. To facilitate palpation, the knees and legs should be flexed toward the hips, which allows the abdominal muscles to relax. The edge of the liver can be palpated 1 to 2 cm below the right costal margin at the midclavicular line; this edge should be smooth, firm, and well defined (Connor, 1996). The tip of the spleen can be felt below the left costal margin in newborn infants. The size of the spleen depends on variables such as circulating blood volume, day of life, method of delivery, and type of therapy, which must be considered when interpreting the significance of mild enlargement (Fletcher, 1998).

The kidneys are located in the flanks. The lower pole of both kidneys should be palpable because of the reduced tone of neonatal abdominal muscles (Vogt & Davis, 2001). The kidneys should be smooth and firm to the touch. Enlarged kidneys

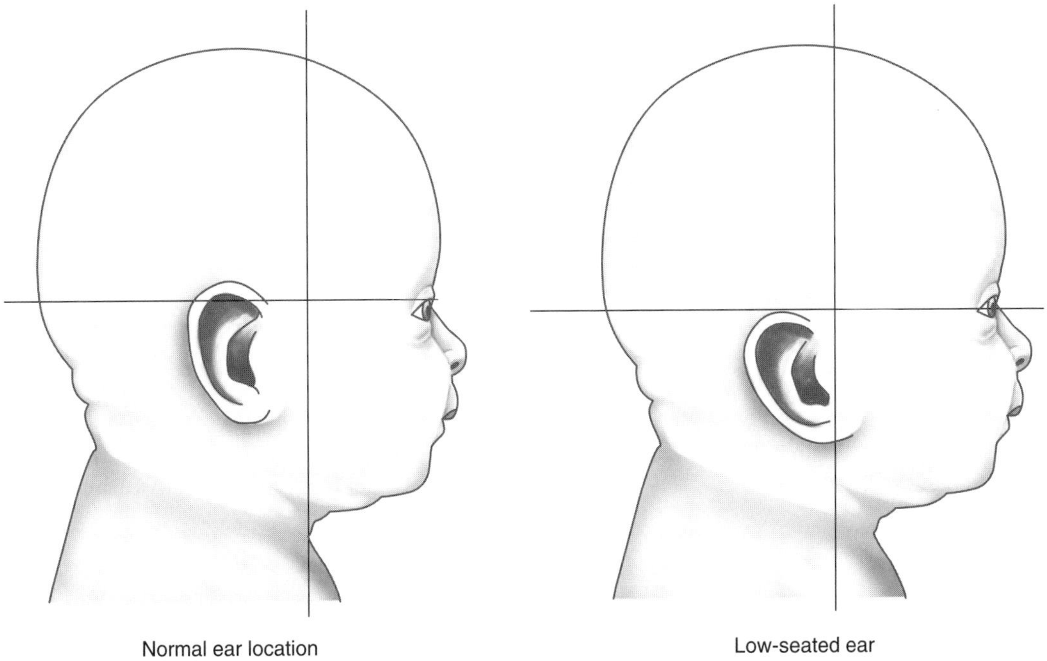

Normal ear location

Low-seated ear

FIGURE **20-13**
Ear position.

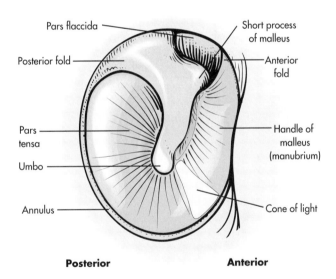

Pars flaccida

Posterior fold

Pars tensa

Umbo

Annulus

Short process of malleus

Anterior fold

Handle of malleus (manubrium)

Cone of light

Posterior   **Anterior**

FIGURE **20-14**
Normal landmarks of the right tympanic membrane as seen through an otoscope. From Lewis SM et al (2000). *Medical-surgical nursing: assessment and management of clinical problems*, ed 5. Mosby: St Louis.

are somewhat easy to detect, but normal-size neonatal kidneys may be somewhat more difficult to find. The fact that voiding has occurred reflects the presence of some renal tissue (Cavaliere, 1996).

Anogenital Area

The anogenital area should be examined with the infant supine. Gestational age affects the appearance of the external genitalia. Maturational changes are described in Figure 20-6 and Table 20-7. The genitalia should be readily identifiable as male or female.

- Males: The normal length of the penis at term is 3.5 cm (plus or minus 0.7 cm) (Fletcher, 1998). Gentle traction is applied on the foreskin to visualize the urethral meatus; the opening should be at the central tip of the glans. Physiologic phimosis, a nonretractable foreskin, normally is seen in newborns. The opening in the prepuce should be large enough to allow urination. The urine stream should be forceful and straight. The inguinal area and scrotum should be palpated for masses, swelling, and the presence of testes. The testes should be firm, smooth, and comparatively equal in size. Testicular descent begins at approximately 27 weeks' gestation. At term both testes should be in the scrotum, which should be fully rugated. The scrotum should be more deeply pigmented than the surrounding skin (Cavaliere, 1996).
- Females: The labial, inguinal, and suprapubic areas are inspected and palpated to detect masses, swelling, or bulges. The clitoris should be located superior to the vaginal opening. Hymenal tags and mucousy/bloody vaginal discharges are benign, transient findings.

Edema of the genitalia is common in both sexes in breech deliveries. It may also be due to the effects of transplacentally acquired maternal hormones. The perineum should be smooth and should have no dimpling, fistulae, or discharges (Cavaliere, 1996; Lepley & Gardner, 1998).

The anus is evaluated for patency and tone. Patency can be documented by gentle insertion of a soft rubber catheter. The passage of meconium does not assure a patent anus, because meconium may be passed through a fistulous tract (Fletcher, 1998). Gentle stroking of the anal area should produce constriction of the sphincter, known as the anal wink (Katz & Nishioka, 1998).

Back

The infant should be placed in the supine position while the back is examined for curvature, patency, and presence of structural abnormalities. Vertebrae are palpated for enlargement and pain. Symmetry should be seen on both sides of the back and between the two scapulae. The spine should be straight and flexible and should have no visible defects, such as pits, hair tufts, or dimples (Katz & Nishioka, 1998).

Extremities and Hips

The extremities are observed for symmetry, degree of flexion, and presence of defects and fractures. Full range of motion should be present, and the extremities should move symmetrically. Although symmetry of gluteal skin folds suggests normal hips, the Ortolani and Barlow maneuvers should be performed to confirm the stability of the hips (Figure 20-15). The Ortolani maneuver reduces a dislocated femoral head into the acetabulum, and the Barlow maneuver reflects the ability of the femoral head to be dislocated (Tappero, 1996; Fletcher, 1998).

The limbs should be equal in length, and they should be in proportion to the body; they also should be straight and should have no edema or crepitus. Palpation or movement of the limbs should not produce a painful response. The digits should be equally spaced and have no webbing. The nails should extend to the end of the nail beds.

Reflexes

The most common neonatal reflexes are presented in Table 20-11.

VARIATIONS AND ABNORMAL FINDINGS ON PHYSICAL EXAMINATION

Minor variations and abnormal findings of the physical examination are presented in Table 20-12.

HEALTH MAINTENANCE IN THE FIRST YEAR OF LIFE

The goal of health maintenance, or primary care, is to provide consistent preventive health care for the infant and education for the parents. In addition to the basic surveillance provided for all infants, high-risk infants have other needs that must be addressed. Primary care for these infants often requires a

Text continued on p. 336

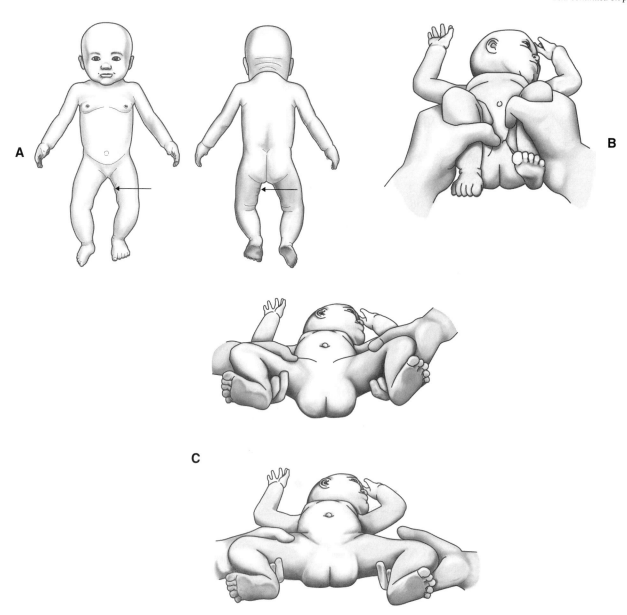

FIGURE **20-15**
Signs of congenital dislocation of hip. **A,** Asymmetry of gluteal and thigh folds. **B,** Barlow maneuver. **C,** Ortolani maneuver. Redrawn from Wong DL (2003). *Wong's nursing care of infants and children,* ed 7, St Louis: Mosby.

TABLE 20-11	Assessment of Neonatal Reflexes		
Reflex	**Technique**	**Response**	**Comments**
Asymmetric tonic neck	With infant supine and in light sleep or quiet awake state, turn head to right until jaw is over shoulder; hold for 15 seconds, then release.	Occipital flexion and mental extension; right arm and leg are extended, left arm and leg are flexed. Premature neonates may lie at rest in this position for extended periods.	Reflex appears at 35 weeks' gestation and disappears by 6 to 7 months of age (Fletcher, 1998).
Babinski	Using thumbnail, scratch sole of foot at lateral side from toes to heel.	Dorsal flexion of great toe with extension of other toes.	Care must be taken not to elicit plantar grasp by stimulating sole of foot. Reflex appears at 34 to 36 weeks' gestation, is well established at 38 weeks, and disappears at 12 months of age.
Doll's eyes	Rotate head from side to side, observing eye movement.	As head is moved to right or left, eyes move in opposite direction.	Lack of eye movement with head rotation or movement of eyes in same direction as head may indicate brainstem or oculomotor nerve dysfunction. Reflex is well established and may even be exaggerated at 24 to 25 weeks' gestation (Vannucci & Yaeger, 2002).
Galant (truncal incurvation)	Place infant prone, either lying on flat surface or in suspension; lightly stroke along either side of spinal column from shoulder to buttocks.	Normal response is strong incurvation of whole vertebral column toward stimulated side.	Reflex is first seen at 28 weeks' gestation (Fletcher, 1998).
Glabellar	Hold head firmly and tap forehead just above nose.	Normal response is tighter closure of both eyes and wrinkling of brow.	Asymmetry, absent or exceptionally strong response (closure longer than 1 second), or generalized startle is abnormal (Fletcher, 1998).
Moro	Hold infant suspended over mattress, supporting head with one hand and body with other hand; rapidly lower both hands 10 to 20 cm without flexing neck but do not allow baby to drop back to mattress.	Symmetric abduction of arms and extension at elbows with hands open completely, followed by adduction of arms and flexion at elbows with curling of fingers; infant cries or grimaces at conclusion.	Response attenuates and ultimately disappears with repetition as habituation occurs. No response is seen at less than 26 weeks' gestation; extension only at 30 weeks; variable adduction at 34 weeks; complete response at 38 weeks. Reflex disappears at 6 months of age (Vannucci & Yaeger, 2002).
Palmar grasp	Stimulate palmar surface of hand with a finger.	Neonate grasps finger; grasp tightens with attempt to remove finger.	Reflex appears at 28 weeks' gestation, is well established after 32 weeks, and disappears at 2 months of age.
Pupillary	Elicit in darkened environment by presenting bright, sharply focused light from periphery.	Pupils constrict equally.	Reflex is sluggish but present between 28 and 32 weeks' gestation in healthy neonates; it is fully present after 34 weeks (Vannucci & Yaeger, 2002).
Rooting	Stroke cheek and corner of mouth.	Mouth opens and head turns toward stimulus.	Reflex appears at 28 weeks' gestation, followed by long latency period beginning at 30 weeks; it is well established at 32 to 34 weeks and disappears by 3 to 4 months of age (Vannucci & Yaeger, 2002).
Stepping	Hold neonate upright and allow feet to touch flat surface.	Alternating stepping movements.	Reflex appears at 35 to 36 weeks' gestation, is well-established at 37 weeks, and disappears at 3 to 4 months of age.
Sucking	Touch or stroke lips.	Mouth opens, and neonate begins to suck.	Reflex appears at 28 weeks' gestation, is well established by 32 to 34 weeks, and disappears at 12 months of age.

TABLE 20-12	Abnormalities and Variations Found on Physical Examination of Newborns and Infants	
Finding	**Definition/Description**	**Comments**
Skin		
Color	Acrocyanosis (blue discoloration of the hands, feet, and perioral area), commonly seen in the first 6 to 24 hours of life.	Occurs when blood flow to an area is sluggish and all available oxygen has been extracted (Fletcher, 1998); exacerbated by cooling and diminished by warming; normal variation but abnormal if persists beyond the first 24 hours of life.
	Cutis marmorata (mottling of the skin in response to cold or other stressful stimuli); caused by dilation of capillaries, usually greatest on the extremities but may be seen on the trunk.	May be suggestive of other conditions (e.g., cardiovascular hypertension, hypothyroidism) if mottling is extensive, shows no improvement with warming, or persists beyond first few months (Fletcher, 1998).
	Cyanosis (blue discoloration of the skin, tongue, and mucous membranes).	Caused by excess of desaturated hemoglobin in the blood (cardiopulmonary disease) or a structural defect in the hemoglobin molecule (methemoglobin); always an abnormal finding.
	Jaundice (yellow coloring of the skin, mucous membranes, and sclerae).	Caused by deposition of bilirubin; may be physiologic.
	Pallor (absence of color or paleness of the skin).	Caused by a decrease in cardiac output, subcutaneous edema, anemia, or asphyxia (Lissauer, 2002).
	Plethora (ruddy skin coloration in the newborn).	Caused by high circulating red blood cell volume (abnormal finding).
Lesions	Café au lait spots (light tan or brown macules with well-defined borders, representing areas of increased epidermal melanosis); except for deeper pigmentation, appearance is not different from that of surrounding skin.	More common in normal infants of color. Six or more macules, regardless of spots' size or infant's race, may be pathologically significant, especially if located in the axilla.
	Cutis aplasia (localized or widespread foci of absence of some or all layers of skin); defect may be covered by a thin, translucent membrane or scar tissue, or area may be raw and ulcerated.	Occurs predominantly on the scalp and less frequently on the limbs and trunk.
	Ecchymosis (nonblanching purple or blue-black macule larger than 2 mm in diameter); represents extravasation of blood into subcutaneous tissue.	Results from trauma to underlying blood vessels or fragility of the vessel walls.
	Erythema toxicum (white or yellow papules on red macular base), commonly found on face, trunk, or proximal extremities but not on hands or feet.	Common, benign finding; vesicles are rare, sterile, and composed primarily of eosinophils. When vesicles are pronounced or coalescent, they may mimic postural infectious rash.
	Harlequin fetus (most severe form of congenital ichthyosis; skin is completely covered with thick, horny scales resembling armor that are divided by deep red fissures).	Most such infants die of dehydration, infection, or respiratory insufficiency within a few hours or days.
	Harlequin sign (vascular phenomenon represented by distinct midline demarcation in side-lying infants; dependent half is deep red, upper half is pale).	Benign finding that lasts a few seconds to 30 minutes, occasionally reverses when position is changed. Usually a single episode; when recurring or persistent, associated cardiac defect should be considered.
	Strawberry hemangioma (red, raised, circumscribed, soft, compressible, lobulated tumor; may occur anywhere on the body).	Benign tumor of the vascular endothelium that has a proliferative and an involutional phase; most involute spontaneously. Treatment is unnecessary unless vital functions are affected.
	Cavernous hemangioma (similar to strawberry hemangioma; involves dermis and subcutaneous tissue and is soft and compressible on palpation; overlying skin is bluish-red in color).	Cavernous lesions may cause thrombocytopenia (Kasabach-Merritt syndrome) or hypertrophy of bone and soft structures of extremities (Klippel-Trenaunay-Weber syndrome).
	Mongolian spot (blue-black macule, lacking a sharp border, most frequently seen on sacrum, buttocks, flanks, or shoulders).	Benign lesion, common in dark-skinned neonates, resulting from delayed disappearance of dermal melanocytes; lesion gradually disappears during the first years of life.
	Milia (1 mm, pearly white or yellow papules without erythema; in the mouth these are called Epstein pearls).	Epidermal inclusion cysts caused by blockage of sebaceous glands; a benign finding that resolves during the first weeks of life.

TABLE 20-12	Abnormalities and Variations Found on Physical Examination of Newborns and Infants—cont'd	
Finding	**Definition/Description**	**Comments**
Skin—cont'd Lesions—*cont'd*	Miliaria crystallina (1 to 2 mm, thin-walled vesicles with nonerythematous and nonpigmented base) Miliaria rubra (small, erythematous, grouped papules [prickly heat]) Miliaria pustulosis (nonerythematous pustules).	Lesions caused by blockage of sweat glands. They are exacerbated by a warm, humid environment and most frequently develop in intertriginous areas and over the face and scalp. They resolve when the environmental factors are eliminated.
	Neonatal pustular melanosis (small, superficial vesiculopustules with little or no surrounding erythema; crusted or scaly collarettes appear after vesicles rupture; lesions eventually resolve into hyperpigmented areas).	Transient and benign; frequently confused with infectious lesions. Smears of pustular material reveal predominantly neutrophils and no bacteria.
	Salmon patch (nevus; dull, pink-red, irregularly shaped macules that blanch on pressure; commonly found on nape of neck (stork bite), glabella, forehead, eyelids, and upper lip).	Benign finding; lesions are composed of distended, dilated capillaries, and most lesions (except those on the neck) disappear by 1 year of age.
	Port wine stain (nevus, macular lesion; present at birth but may be pale and hard to discern; initially pink in color with sharply delineated borders; progresses to dark red/purple; some develop small, angiomatous nodules).	Developmental vascular malformation that occurs mostly on the face; does not increase in size but grows with the infant; may occur alone or with structural anomalies (e.g., Sturge-Weber syndrome) (Fletcher, 1998).
	Petechiae (tiny red or purple, nonblanching macules that range from pinpoint to pinhead size).	Caused by minute hemorrhages in the dermal or submucosal layers; may be benign and self-limiting or pathognomonic of serious underlying conditions. They are benign when found on presenting part and when localized areas appear at the same time; progressive, widespread areas require evaluation (Fletcher, 1998).
Redundant skin	More skin than is necessary or normally present in a particular area.	Seen in the neck after resolution of cystic hygroma or in the abdomen in a neonate with prune belly syndrome.
Subcutaneous fat necrosis	Firm, nonpitting, circumscribed, reddish violet, subcutaneous nodules that appear during the first weeks of life on the face, arms, trunk, thighs, and buttocks.	May occur secondary to cold or trauma.
Head and Neck Acrocephaly	Congenital malformation of the skull caused by premature closure of the coronal and sagittal sutures; accelerated upward growth of the head gives it a long, narrow appearance with a conic shape at the top (also called oxycephaly).	May be associated with premature closure of sutures; found with certain syndromes (e.g., Crouzon, Apert).
Anencephaly	Failed closure of the anterior neural tube without skull formation; the brain is severely malformed, lacking definable structure, although a rudimentary brainstem usually is present. Congenital malformation of the skull caused by premature closure of the coronal suture; excessive lateral growth of the head gives it a short, broad appearance.	Most affected neonates die within 48 hours without intervention (Fletcher, 1998).
Brachycephaly	Congenital malformation of the skull caused by premature closure of the coronal suture; excessive lateral growth of the head gives it a short, broad appearance.	Condition found with certain syndromes (e.g., trisomy 21, Apert).
Bruit	Abnormal murmurlike sound heard on auscultation of an organ or gland that is caused by dilated, tortuous, or constricted vessels. The specific character of the bruit, its location, its association with other clinical findings, and the time of occurrence in a cycle of other sounds is of diagnostic importance.	Bruits heard over the fontanel or lateral skull associated with signs of congestive heart failure may denote intracranial arteriovenous malformation (Johnson, 1996).

Continued

TABLE 20-12	Abnormalities and Variations Found on Physical Examination of Newborns and Infants—cont'd	
Finding	**Definition/Description**	**Comments**
Head and Neck—cont'd		
Caput succedaneum	Vaguely demarcated pitting edema of the scalp that may extend across suture lines and can shift in response to gravity.	Benign finding that appears at birth (from pressure of the maternal cervix on the fetal skull) and resolves in a few days; incidence of infection with this condition may be higher if internal fetal scalp electrodes are used (Mangurten, 2002).
Cephalohematoma	Extradural fluid collection caused by bleeding between the skull and periosteum; generally occurs over one or both parietal bones and does not cross the suture lines; has distinct margins and may be fluctuant or tense.	1. May form during labor and enlarges for the first 12 to 24 hours; most resolve spontaneously over several weeks to months (Johnson, 1996; Katz & Nishioka, 1998). 2. In 5.4% to 25% of cases, a linear skull fracture is present (Fletcher, 1998). 3. May result in hyperbilirubinemia (Mangurten, 2002).
Craniosynostosis	Premature closure of one or more cranial sutures, causing abnormal skull shape and possibly a palpable ridge along the suture line.	Head growth is restricted in the area perpendicular to the stenotic suture and is excessive in unrestricted areas. Most cases are isolated events, but the condition can occur in some syndromes (Southgate & Pittard, 2001).
Craniotabes	Congenital thinness of bone at the top and back of the head. Bones may collapse and recoil upon palpation (Ping-Pong); condition may be due to bone resorption or delay in ossification (Fletcher, 1998).	1. Common finding in preterm babies; in term babies the condition is caused by the pressure of the skull against the maternal pelvic brim; spontaneous resolution usually occurs in a few weeks (Fletcher, 1998). 2. May be seen with congenital syphilis (Southgate & Pittard, 2001).
Dolichocephaly (scaphocephaly)	Congenital malformation of the skull in which premature closure of the sagittal suture results in restricted lateral growth. Skull shape often seen in premature babies as a result of prolonged positioning with head turned to the side.	In both cases the head is long and narrow.
Encephalocele	Protrusion of brain tissue through a congenital defect in the cranium; most often occurs in the occipital midline but may also be seen in the frontal, temporal, or parietal areas (Fletcher, 1998).	Other cranial defects frequently are seen; 50% of cases involve hydrocephalus; 10% to 20% show absence of neural elements (Fletcher, 1998).
Macrocephaly	Excessive head size in relation to weight, length, and gestational age. Facial features usually are normal.	May be familial or may reflect pathologic condition (e.g., hydrocephalus, hydrancephalus); occipitofrontal circumference (OFC) is over 90%.
Microcephaly	Abnormally small head size relative to weight, length, and gestational age.	Small OFC (under 10%) reflects poor brain growth.
Molding	Process by which the head shape is altered as the fetus passes through the birth canal. The biparietal diameter becomes compressed, the head is elongated, and the skull bones may overlap at the suture lines.	Benign finding; condition usually resolves during the first few postnatal days.
Neck masses	May be detected on palpation or inspection. Cystic hygroma (soft, fluctuant mass that easily transilluminates; usually laterally placed or over clavicles) (Johnson, 1996). Goiter (anterior mass caused by hypothyroidism). Thyroglossal duct cyst/branchial cleft cyst (may be found high in the neck).	Most common neck mass; caused by development of sequestered lymph channels, which dilate into cysts. Rare in neonates. Also rare in neonates.
Plagiocephaly	Congenital malformation of the skull caused by premature or irregular closure of the coronal or lambdoidal sutures. The resulting asymmetric growth gives the head a twisted, lopsided appearance.	Condition may also be seen with certain syndromes (e.g., Saethre-Chotzen).

TABLE 20-12	Abnormalities and Variations Found on Physical Examination of Newborns and Infants—cont'd	
Finding	**Definition/Description**	**Comments**
Head and Neck—cont'd		
Subgaleal hemorrhage	Bleeding into the potential space between the epicranial aponeurosis and the periosteum of the skull; manifests as a firm to fluctuant scalp mass with poorly demarcated borders that may extend onto the face, forehead, or neck and may be accompanied by signs of hypovolemia (Fletcher, 1998; Ohls, 2001).	May be a life-threatening condition (Mangurten, 2002); can be caused by coagulopathy, asphyxia, or vacuum extraction.
Hair whorls	Two or more hair whorls, or abnormally placed whorls (other than parietal area).	May indicate brain anomaly; it has been postulated that the pattern of hair development correlates with underlying brain development.
Webbed neck	Redundant skin in neck.	Found with Turner, Noonan, and Down syndromes.
Face		
Asymmetry	Unequal appearance or movement of mouth and lips; unequal closure of eyes; uneven appearance of nasolabial folds.	Often caused by in utero positioning but may be due to facial nerve paresis; in mild cases may be evident only with crying (affected side fails to move or moves less when infant cries).
Ears		
Auricular appendage	Accessory tragi, most commonly in pretragal area; may occur within or behind the ear. These structures contain cartilage and are not truly skin tags.	Primarily of cosmetic significance unless accompanied by other diffuse malformations. Seen in certain congenital syndromes (e.g., Goldenhar, Treacher Collins); hearing assessment is indicated when other anomalies are present (Fletcher, 1998).
Auricular sinus	Narrow, fistulous tract most often located directly anterior to helix.	May be familial or may be associated with microtia, auricular appendage, facial cleft syndromes, and syndromic anomalies of the outer ear (Fletcher, 1998).
Low-set ears	Superior attachment of pinna lies below imaginary line drawn between both inner canthi and extended posteriorly.	May be associated with chromosomal or renal anomalies.
Microtia	Severely misshapen, dysplastic external ear.	Usually associated with other malformations that result in conductive hearing loss (Fletcher, 1998).
Eyes		
Blepharophimosis	Narrow palpebral fissures in the horizontal measurement; also known as short palpebral fissures.	Usually caused by lateral displacement of the inner canthi; seen in certain dysmorphic or chromosomal syndromes (Fletcher, 1998).
Brushfield spots	Pinpoint white or light yellow spots on the iris.	Seen in 75% of neonates with Down syndrome but may also be a normal variant; not always visible at birth.
Coloboma	Cleft-shaped defect in ocular tissue (eyelid, iris, ciliary body, retina, or optic nerve).	Result of incomplete embryologic closure of ocular structures; may be an isolated finding or part of a malformation syndrome.
Ectropion	Eversion of the margin of the eyelid, which leaves the conjunctiva exposed.	Seen in facial nerve paralysis, in certain syndromes, and in harlequin fetus and collodion baby (Fletcher, 1998).
Entropion	Inversion of the eyelid; eyelashes may be in contact with the cornea and conjunctiva.	Congenital condition that usually resolves spontaneously without damage.
Epicanthal folds	Vertical fold of skin at the inner canthus on either side of the nose.	Common in Down syndrome; of no clinical significance in babies of Asian extraction; may also be a physical manifestation of in utero compression (Potter facies) (Cavaliere, 1996).
Exophthalmos	Abnormal displacement of the eye characterized by protrusion of the eyeball.	May be caused by increased volume of the orbit (tumor), swelling secondary to edema or hemorrhage, endocrine disorder (e.g., Graves' disease, hyperthyroidism); known as proptosis when accompanied by shallow orbits (Crouzon disease) (Fletcher, 1998).

Continued

| TABLE 20-12 | Abnormalities and Variations Found on Physical Examination of Newborns and Infants—cont'd |

Finding	Definition/Description	Comments
Eyes—cont'd		
Hypertelorism	Increased distance between the orbits, observed clinically as a large interpupillary distance (see Telecanthus).	Frequently seen in craniofacial syndromes.
Hypotelorism	Decreased distance between the orbits, observed clinically as smaller than normal interpupillary distance (Fletcher, 1998; Gupta, Hamming & Miller, 2002).	Frequently seen in trisomies 13 and 21 and in other syndromes.
Leukocoria	White pupil, denoting an abnormality of the lens, vitreous, or fundus; an indication for further evaluation (Gupta et al, 2002).	May be seen on direct visualization or as absence of a red reflex (Fletcher, 1998); most commonly seen in cataracts; also found in retinoblastoma, retinal detachment, and vitreous hemorrhage.
Microphthalmia	Small eye (diameter measures less than 15 mm at birth).	Associated with multisystem conditions or syndromes (e.g., CHARGE, trisomy 13, fetal rubella effects) (Fletcher, 1998).
Nystagmus	Involuntary, rhythmic movements of the eye; may be horizontal, vertical, rotary, or mixed.	Occasional, intermittent nystagmus in an otherwise healthy newborn may be normal in the neonatal period; however, it must be evaluated if frequent or persistent (or both). Pathologic forms may be due to ocular, neurologic, or vestibular defects (Gupta et al, 2002).
Ptosis (blepharoptosis)	Abnormal drooping of one or both eyelids.	Caused by congenital or acquired weakness in the levator muscle or paralysis of the third cranial nerve; may be difficult to detect in neonates unless unilateral with asymmetry between the eyelids (Fletcher, 1998).
Strabismus	Misalignment of the visual axes. Crossed eyes (esotropia)	Results from inheritance, paralysis of the lateral rectus muscle, or refractive errors; may be due to diseases that reduce visual acuity in one eye.
	Wall eye (exotropia)	Rarely seen in neonates; usually not detected until 1 to 2 years of age or later.
Subconjunctival hemorrhage	Bright red area on sclerae.	Caused by rupture of a capillary in the mucous membrane that lines the conjunctiva; commonly seen after vaginal delivery, does not reflect ocular trauma unless massive and associated with other findings; usually resolves in 7 to 10 days.
Synophrys	Meeting of the eyebrows in the midline.	Seen in multisystem conditions or syndromes (e.g., Cornelia de Lange, congenital hypertrichosis).
Telecanthus	Lateral displacement of the inner canthi (Fletcher, 1998); eyes appear too widely set because of a disproportionate increase between the inner canthi; interorbital distance is appropriate.	Evident in fetal alcohol syndrome and other syndromes; not synonymous with hypertelorism, although its presence can lead to a false impression of hypertelorism.
Nose		
Choanal atresia	Obstruction of posterior nasal passages.	Patency is assessed in the quiet state. If condition is bilateral, neonate is cyanotic at rest and pink when crying; if unilateral, baby is unable to breathe if mouth is held closed and unaffected naris is occluded with examiner's finger. Atresia/stenosis may be confirmed by passing a catheter.
Nasal deformation	May result from pressure in utero. May be due to dislocation of the septal cartilage.	Benign condition that resolves in a few days. Attempts to restore normal anatomy are unsuccessful; nares remain asymmetric when tip of nose is compressed (Johnson, 1996; Fletcher, 1998).
Mouth		
Epstein's pearls	Small, white, pearl-like inclusion cysts that appear on the palate and gums.	Benign finding that disappears spontaneously by a few weeks of age.
Cleft lip/palate	Failure of midline fusion during first trimester.	May occur alone or with other malformations.

TABLE **20-12**	Abnormalities and Variations Found on Physical Examination of Newborns and Infants—cont'd	
Finding	**Definition/Description**	**Comments**
Mouth		
Macroglossia	Abnormally large tongue; failure of tongue to fit inside a closed mouth (Fletcher, 1998).	Seen in certain congenital syndromes (e.g., Beckwith-Wiedemann) and hypothyroidism; protruding tongue may indicate poor neuromuscular tone or a small mouth rather than a large tongue.
Micrognathia	Underdevelopment of the jaw, especially the mandible.	Dysmorphic feature seen in certain malformation syndromes (e.g., Pierre-Robin sequence).
Thorax/Chest		
Auscultation	Adventitious breath sounds	
	Crackles	Discrete, noncontinuous bubbling sounds during inspiration; classified as fine, medium, or coarse. Previously called rales.
	Rhonchi	Continuous, nonmusical, low-pitched sounds occurring on inspiration and expiration; caused by secretions or aspirated matter in large airways.
	Stridor	Rough, harsh sounds caused by narrowing of upper airways; present during both phases of respiratory cycle but worse during inspiration; common with laryngomalacia, subglottic stenosis, and vascular ring.
	Wheezes	Musical, high-pitched sound generated by air passing at high velocity through a narrowed airway; heard most often on expiration but can be noted during both phases of respiratory cycle if airway diameter is restricted and fixed.
	Grunting	Sound produced by forceful expiration against a closed glottis; compensatory mechanism to prevent or reverse alveolar collapse.
	Murmur	Grades I through VI assigned depending on intensity and presence of thrill.
Asymmetry	May be unequal in shape or excursion.	1. Asymmetric shape caused by positioning in utero or presence of air trapping or space-occupying lesions. 2. Unequal excursion caused by diaphragmatic hernia, phrenic nerve damage, or air leakage or trapping.
Barrel chest	Increased anteroposterior diameter of the chest.	Result of air trapping in the pleural space (pneumothorax) or distal airways (aspiration or pneumonia), space-occupying lesions, or overdistention from mechanical ventilation (Fletcher, 1988).
Heave	Diffuse, gradually rising impulse seen in the anterior chest overlying the ventricular area.	Usually indicates volume overload.
Pectus excavatum	Deformation of chest wall caused by depressed sternum; also called funnel chest.	May be associated with Marfan, Noonan and other syndromes (Southgate & Pittard, 2001); may develop after birth in neonates with laryngomalacia.
Pectus carinatum	Deformation of chest wall caused by protuberant sternum; also called pigeon chest.	May be associated with Marfan, Noonan, and other syndromes (Southgate & Pittard, 2001).
Retractions	Drawing in of the soft tissues of the chest between and around the firmer tissue of the cartilaginous and bony ribs; seen in intercostal, subcostal, substernal, and suprasternal areas.	Mild subcostal retractions may be seen in healthy newborns; intercostal, substernal, and suprasternal retractions reflect increased work of breathing and suggest respiratory distress.
Supernumerary nipples (polythelia)	Extra nipples; may appear as slightly pigmented linear dimples or may be more defined, with palpable breast nodules.	Normal variant; nipples appear along the mammary line. Prospective studies have refuted the association with renal anomalies; no indication for further evaluation based solely on the presence of supernumerary nipples.
Abdomen		
Abdominal wall defects	Exstrophy of the bladder (protrusion and eversion of the bladder through an embryologic defect, resulting in absence of muscle and connective tissue on the anterior abdominal wall).	Often associated with other defects of the genitourinary (GU) and musculoskeletal systems and the gastrointestinal (GI) tract.

Continued

Finding	Definition/Description	Comments
Abdomen—cont'd		
Abdominal wall defects—cont'd	Gastroschisis (protrusion of viscera through an abdominal wall defect arising outside the umbilical ring; the cord therefore is not inserted on the defect, and the herniated organs are not covered by peritoneum).	Defect usually is to the right of the umbilicus.
	Omphalocele (herniation of viscera through an abdominal wall defect within the umbilical ring; defect usually is covered by a translucent, avascular sac at the base of the umbilicus).	Umbilical cord always inserts into the sac; occasionally the sac may rupture. Defect usually is larger than 4 cm and may be associated with other congenital defects and chromosomal anomalies (Fletcher, 1998).
	Umbilical hernia (failure of the umbilical ring to contract, allowing protrusion of bowel or omentum through the abdominal wall).	Characterized by a fascial defect smaller than 4 cm and intact umbilical skin (Fletcher, 1998; Ryckman, 2002).
Ascites	Abnormal intraperitoneal accumulation of fluid; ascitic fluid may contain large amounts of protein and electrolytes.	May be due to heart failure/hydrops fetalis; congenital infections; GI, hepatic, or GU disorders; or lysosomal storage diseases.
Bruit	See section under Head and Neck	Persistence after a position change may indicate abnormalities of the umbilical vein or hepatic vascular system, hepatic hemangioma, or renal artery stenosis (Connor, 1996).
Diastasis rectus	Midline bulge from xiphoid to umbilicus, seen when abdominal muscles are flexed.	Caused by separation of the two rectus muscles along the median line of the abdominal wall; a common benign finding in newborns that has no clinical significance (Fletcher, 1998).
Distention	Increase in abdominal girth caused by an increase in the volume of intraperitoneal, thoracic, or pelvic contents (Fletcher, 1998).	May be pathologic or benign. Pathologic causes include GI obstruction, ascites, abdominal mass, organomegaly, and depression of the diaphragm (tension pneumothorax). Benign causes include postprandial state, crying, swallowing of air with feedings, air leakage with mechanical ventilation, and administration of continuous positive airway pressure (CPAP).
Patent urachus	Postnatal persistence of communication between the urinary bladder and the umbilicus; may result in passage of urine from the umbilicus, which otherwise appears normal. Other signs are a large, edematous cord that fails to separate after the normal interval (Cavaliere, 1996) and retraction of the umbilical cord during urination.	Lower urinary tract obstruction should be considered.
Prune belly syndrome	Congenital deficiency of abdominal musculature, characterized by a large, flaccid, wrinkled abdomen, cryptorchidism, and GU malformations.	Almost always seen in males.
Scaphoid abdomen	Abdomen with a sunken anterior wall.	May be present with a diaphragmatic hernia or malnutrition.
Single umbilical artery		Seen in fewer than 1% of neonates; approximately 40% of affected newborns have other major congenital malformations. When condition occurs without other abnormalities, it usually is a benign finding (Lissauer, 2002).
Genitalia/ Perineum		
Ambiguous	Presence of a phallic structure not discretely male or female, abnormally placed urethral meatus, and inability to palpate one or both gonads in a male.	May be associated with serious endocrine disorders; rapid evaluation and diagnosis are critical.
Anal atresia	Absence of an external anal opening; imperforate anus.	May be evident by inspection; infant may fail to pass meconium. However, meconium may be passed through a rectovaginal or rectovestibular fistula in a female or a rectoperineal or rectourethral fistula in a male.

Finding	Definition/Description	Comments
Genitalia/Perineum–cont'd		
Chordee	Ventral or dorsal curvature of the penis; most evident on erection.	May occur alone but often accompanies hypospadias.
Cliteromegaly	The appearance of an enlarged clitoris, with no regard to cause (Dahms & Danish, 2002); it may be swollen, enlarged, widened, or merely prominent, as in premature females.	May be a benign finding or may represent masculinization from exposure to excess androgens during fetal life (Fletcher, 1998).
Cryptorchidism	Testis or testes in extrascrotal location (undescended testis or testes); characterized by empty, hypoplastic scrotal sac.	In most cases descent occurs spontaneously by 3 months of age; descent after 9 months is rare. Corrective surgery is recommended at 1 year of age (AAP, 1997b).
Epispadias	Abnormal location of urethral meatus on the dorsal surface of the penis; abnormal urine stream may be seen.	Varies in severity from mild (glanular) to complete version seen in exstrophy of the bladder; all forms are associated with dorsal chordee; may require evaluation by a urologist before circumcision.
Hydrocele	Nontender scrotal swelling caused by fluid collection; arises from passage of peritoneal fluid through patent processus vaginalis.	May be seen with inguinal hernia but can be distinguished from hernia because hydrocele appears translucent on transillumination; entire circumference of testis may be palpated; and it cannot be reduced (Cavaliere, 1996).
Hydrocolpos/ hydrometrocolpos	Manifests as suprapubic mass or protruding perineal mass as a result of accumulation of secretions in vagina or vagina and uterus.	Caused by excessive intrauterine stimulation by maternal estrogens, with obstruction of the genital tract by an intact hymen, hymenal bands, vaginal membrane, or vaginal atresia (Cavaliere, 1996; Fletcher, 1998).
Hypospadias	Abnormal location of urethral meatus on the ventral surface of the penis; caused by incomplete development of the anterior urethra; abnormal urine stream may be seen.	Urethral opening may be found on the glans, scrotum, or perineum. Infants with penoscrotal or perineal type or with glanular form and other genital anomalies or dysmorphic features should be evaluated to rule out disorders of sexual differentiation. Evaluation by a urologist may be required before circumcision.
Hymenal tag	Redundant tissue manifesting as an annular tag protruding from the vagina.	Benign finding; most disappear during the first year of life.
Inguinal hernia	Scrotal mass caused by the presence of loops of intestines in the scrotal sac; arises from persistence of processus vaginalis, often associated with hydrocele.	On examination, the entire circumference of the testis is not palpable, and the scrotum does not transilluminate. Unless incarcerated, hernias are reducible.
Micropenis/ microphallus	Abnormally short or thin penis.	Penis more than two standard deviations below the mean of length and width for age according to standard charts; frequently requires evaluation by an endocrinologist and a geneticist.
Phimosis	Intractable foreskin.	Must be differentiated from physiologic phimosis, a *nonretractable* foreskin that is a normal finding in neonates.
Priapism	Constantly erect penis.	Abnormal finding in neonate (Kenner, 1998).
Retractile testis	Normally descended testis that recedes into the inguinal canal because of activity of the cremaster muscle.	May not be seen in the newborn period because of lack of cremaster reflex in this age group; however, some newborns do demonstrate this response (Cilento et al, 1994; Fletcher, 1998).
Testicular torsion	Twisting of the testis or testes on the spermatic cord; manifests as a swollen, red or bluish red scrotum; may be painful, but this is not a universal symptom in the neonate.	Urgent evaluation and management are required, because the blood supply to the testis is compromised, which results in irreversible ischemic damage to the testis; condition may occur in utero.
Musculoskeletal System		
Arachnodactyly	Unusually long, spiderlike digits.	
Arthrogryposis	Persistent flexure or contracture of one or more joints.	May be associated with oligohydramnios or an underlying neuromuscular disorder (Hudgins & Cassidy, 2002).

Continued

TABLE 20-12	Abnormalities and Variations Found on Physical Examination of Newborns and Infants—cont'd	
Finding	**Definition/Description**	**Comments**
Musculoskeletal System—cont'd		
Brachydactyly	Shortening of one or more digits as a result of abnormal development of phalanges, metacarpals, or metatarsals.	Benign trait if an isolated finding; may be a component of skeletal dysplasias (achondroplasia) and syndromes (Down syndrome) (Hudgins & Cassidy, 2002).
Calcaneus foot	Abduction of the forefoot with the heel in valgus position (turned outward).	Associated with external tibial torsion; often caused by in utero positioning (Hudgins & Cassidy, 2002).
Camptodactyly	Congenital flexion deformity of the finger; bent finger.	Usually involves the little finger; can be a minor variant or familial trait, or part of a syndrome.
Crepitus	Crackling sensation produced by the presence of air in tissues (subcutaneous emphysema) or the movement of bone fragments (clavicular fracture).	
Clinodactyly	Lateral angulation deformity of a finger with either radial or ulnar deviation.	Usually involves the little finger; may be a benign finding if occurring alone but can be associated with congenital syndromes.
Genu recurvatum	Ability of the knee to bend backward.	May be due to trauma, prolonged intrauterine pressure, or general joint laxity.
Kyphosis	Round shoulder deformity; forward bending of the spine. Caused by congenital failure of formation of all or part of the vertebral body, with preservation of the posterior elements and failure of the anterior segmentation of the spine.	Severe deformities may be apparent at birth; less severe abnormalities may not appear until several years later; a progressive deformity can result in paraplegia (Hudgins & Cassidy, 2002).
Lordosis	Exaggeration of the normal curvature in the cervical and lumbar spine.	Caused by a bony abnormality of the spine.
Lymphedema	Puffiness of the dorsum of the hands or feet.	Characteristic of Noonan or Turner syndrome.
Metatarsus valgus	Congenital deformity of the foot in which the forepart rotates outward away from the midline and the heel remains straight.	Fixed deformity of the foot, which cannot be brought into neutral position; compare with metatarsus adbuctus, a functional deformity in which the foot can be brought into neutral position (Grover, 2000b).
Metatarsus varus	Congenital bony abnormality of the foot in which the forepart rotates inward toward the midline and the heel remains straight.	Fixed deformity; the foot cannot be brought into neutral position. Compare with metatarsus adductus, a functional deformity in which the foot can be brought into neutral position (Grover, 2000b).
Meningocele	Saclike protrusion of the spinal meninges through a congenital defect in the spinal column.	Herniated cyst is filled with cerebrospinal fluid but does not contain neural tissue; affected infants usually do not show neurologic deficits (Sarnat, 2002).
Myelomeningocele	Defect identical to meningocele but with associated abnormalities in the structure and position of the spinal cord.	Affected infants usually show neurologic deficits below the level of the abnormality.
Polydactyly	Presence of more than the normal number of digits; there may be a complete extra digit (preaxial) that is normal in appearance, or a skin tag (postaxial).	May be an isolated finding, inherited as an autosomal dominant trait, or may occur in a variety of syndromes (trisomy 13, Meckel-Gruber syndrome).
Rachischisis	Congenital fissure of the spinal cord in which the incompletely folded cord is splayed apart and exposed along the back.	Caused by incomplete neuralation; often accompanied by anencephaly (Fletcher, 1998).
Rocker bottom feet	Deformity of the foot in which the arch is disrupted, giving a rounded appearance (rocker bottom) to the sole.	Usually seen in conjunction with congenital syndromes (trisomies 13 and 18).
Scoliosis	Failure of formation or segmentation of the vertebrae; manifests as lateral (side to side) curvature of the spine.	May be congenital or acquired; may occur as part of another condition or may be idiopathic (Fletcher, 1998; Cooperman & Thompson, 2002).

multidisciplinary approach, and the health care provider is responsible for coordinating medical, developmental, and social services. Because high-risk infants face the possibility of developmental delays, neurologic sequelae, and nutritional deficits, follow-up must include formal developmental, neurologic, and nutritional assessments in addition to routine screening tests.

The health care provider may need to schedule longer and more frequent visits to evaluate the infant adequately and to assess the family's adjustment to caring for the child. The health care provider also is responsible for giving the parents comprehensive anticipatory guidance (AAP, 1997a; Sifuentes, 2000).

TABLE 20-12	Abnormalities and Variations Found on Physical Examination of Newborns and Infants—cont'd	
Finding	**Definition/Description**	**Comments**
Musculoskeletal System—cont'd		
Simian crease	Single transverse line in the palm.	May be benign, but when accompanied by other dysmorphic features (e.g., incurving fifth finger, epicanthal folds, low-set thumb), it may be a sign of Down syndrome.
Spinal dimple, dermal sinus	Pit or depression that occurs along the midline of the back, often at the base of the spinal cord in the lumbosacral area; may be accompanied by tufts of hair.	May be a benign finding, especially if the base of the defect can be visualized; however defect can extend into the spinal cord, representing a neural tube defect and tethered spinal cord.
Syndactyly	Fusion of two or more digits; may involve only soft tissue (simple) or may include bone or cartilage (complex).	May occur as an isolated defect or as part of a syndrome (e.g., Cornelia de Lange, Smith-Lemli-Opitz) (Fletcher, 1998).
Talipes equinovarus	Clubfoot; congenital deformity of the foot and lower leg marked by adduction of the forefoot (turned inward and pointed medially), varus position of the heel (turned inward), and downward pointing of the toes.	May be congenital (isolated deformity), teratologic (associated with underlying neuromuscular disorder), or positional (normal foot held in equinovarus position in utero) (Cooperman & Thompson, 2002).
Tibial torsion	Abnormal rotation of the feet while the knees are pointing forward; may be internal (toes in) or external (toes out).	Often caused by in utero positioning; resolves spontaneously (Cooperman & Thompson, 2002).
Torticollis	Shortening of the sternocleidomastoid muscle, resulting in head tilt toward the affected muscle and chin rotation toward the unaffected muscle; a palpable mass may appear during the first few weeks of life.	May be due to birth trauma, intrauterine malposition, muscle fibrosis, venous abnormalities in the muscle, or congenital cervical vertebral abnormalities (Cooperman & Thompson, 2002).
Neurologic Examination		
Brachial plexus injuries	Paralysis of all or part of the arm as a result of birth trauma.	
	Erb-Duchenne palsy (upper arm paralysis): Arm is adducted and internally rotated, with elbow extension, flexion of the wrist, and pronation of the forearm. The arm falls to the side of the body when passively abducted, and the Moro reflex is absent on the affected side but the grasp is intact.	Arises from injury to the fifth and sixth cervical roots; most common brachial plexus injury.
	Klumpke palsy (lower arm paralysis): Hand is paralyzed, and voluntary movement of the wrist and grasp reflex are absent.	Rare; results from injury to the eighth cervical and first thoracic roots; usually Horner syndrome (ptosis, miosis, and enophthalmos) is present on the affected side; delayed pigmentation of the iris may be seen.
	Paralysis of the entire arm: Arm is completely motionless, flaccid, and powerless and hangs limply; all reflexes are absent, and sensory deficit may extend to the shoulder.	
Facial nerve palsy	Facial weakness or paralysis arising from compression of the seventh cranial nerve, caused by intrauterine position or forceps delivery; characterized by asymmetry of facial movement (most evident on crying), ptosis, and unequal nasolabial folds.	
Phrenic nerve injury	Cause of respiratory distress secondary to paralysis of the diaphragm; arises from upper brachial plexus injury.	Rarely occurs as an isolated phenomenon; accompanies signs and symptoms of Erb-Duchenne palsy (Cooperman & Thompson, 2002).

The American Academy of Pediatrics has published guidelines for health supervision (AAP, 1997a). These guidelines indicate the elements that can be included in office visits for patients from birth to 21 years of age. The guidelines are intended to be used in the care of infants, children, and adolescents whose "health and adaptation are thought to be within the normal range" (AAP, 1997a). However, the approach has been designed to be flexible and can easily be modified for follow-up of high-risk infants. More frequent visits can be scheduled as needed. Guidelines for health supervision for the first year of life are summarized in Table 20-13.

Text continued on p. 344

TABLE 20-13	Guidelines for Health Supervision of Infants in the First Year of Life*
Age	**Procedures**

Newborn	**Health Assessment**
	This visit may take place while the infant is still in the hospital.
	• Ask welcoming questions (e.g., "How is the baby?" "How are you doing?" "How is the feeding going?")
	
	Examination of the Infant
	Physical Examination
	• Examine the baby with the parents present and demonstrate findings, even normal and minor ones.
	• Observe parent-infant interactions.
	• Take measurements (length, weight, head circumference).
	• Perform a full physical examination.
	Testing
	• Mother's laboratory tests
	• Evidence of blood incompatibility
	• Metabolic screening
	
	Immunizations
	• Hepatitis B (dose 1) may be given.
	
	Anticipatory Guidance
	• Discuss the feeding method the parents have chosen (vitamin and fluoride supplementation as indicated).
	• Discuss the infant's sleep position and environment.
	• Explain the care of the skin, cord, and circumcision.
	• Discuss the reasons for breast engorgement and vaginal discharge.
	• Explain the meaning of jaundice if indicated.
	• Discuss the extent to which family members and friends should visit.
	• Discuss injury prevention:
	  □ Microwave safety (do not use to heat bottles)
	  □ Hot water heater temperature (should be set at 120° F)
	  □ Car safety seat use
	  □ Crib safety
	  □ Siblings
	  □ Pets
	  □ Smoke detectors
	• Explain when and how to call the health care provider.
	• Discuss the postpartum adjustment of the mother, siblings, and family.
	• Discuss the individuality of the infant.
	
	Closing the Visit
	• Ask the parents if they have any questions or concerns.
	• Comment on the parents' strength and capability.
	• Carry out discharge planning.

2 to 4 weeks	**Health Assessment** • Ask welcoming questions. • Ask what issues need to be discussed at this visit. • Inquire about changes in family life and what stressors have arisen. • Review the status of concerns discussed at the newborn visit. **Examination of the Infant** • Review the birth history. • Complete a family history: diabetes, tuberculosis, anemia, emotional problems, other significant conditions, household composition, pets, use of cigarettes, alcohol, or other drugs. *Physical Examination* • Take measurements (length, weight, head circumference). • Perform a general physical examination. • Check for red reflex, heart murmurs, abdominal masses, and hip dislocation. • Check developmental progress. • Perform metabolic screening. • Review results of newborn metabolic screening (tests and reporting vary by state). **Immunizations** • Give hepatitis B (dose 1 if not given at birth; dose 2 if first dose was given at birth).

Age	Procedures

2 to 4 weeks— cont'd

Anticipatory Guidance
Nutrition
- Answer questions about breastfeeding.
- Discuss vitamin and fluoride supplementation if indicated.

Sleep Patterns
- Suggest naps for the mother; advise the parents to share feedings when possible.

Social Interaction with Family
- Suggest ways to encourage interaction with the infant.

Injury Prevention
- Discuss the following:
  - □ Car safety seats
  - □ Smoke detectors
  - □ Hot water heater temperature
  - □ Infant's sleeping position

Closing the Visit
- Review the problems discussed; devise a management plan for each one.
- Ask the parents if they have other questions or concerns.
- Make positive statements about the baby's development.
- Comment encouragingly on the parents' caregiving skills.
- Provide information on where to call if a problem arises.
- Schedule the next visit.

2 months

Health Assessment
- Ask welcoming questions.
- Ask if the parents have any concerns.
- Ask about siblings and about changes and stress in the family.
- Inquire about the mother's return to work.
- Review the status of issues discussed at the previous visit.
- Ask specific questions about the infant's nutrition, elimination, sleep pattern, behavior, and development.

Examination of the Infant
Physical Examination
- Take measurements (height, weight, head circumference).
- Perform a general physical examination.

Observation of Behavior and Development
Note the following:
- Developmental milestones
- Temperament (ability to cuddle and be consoled, excessive crying or irritability)
- Parent-infant interaction

Testing
- Hematocrit/hemoglobin if infant was premature or low birth weight or had significant hemolysis or excessive blood loss

Immunizations
- Provide the family with vaccine information sheets.*
- Give diphtheria-tetanus-pertussis (DTaP or DPT) (dose 1); polio (dose 1); *Haemophilus influenzae* type b (Hib) (dose 1); hepatitis B (dose 1 or dose 2).
- Recommend acetaminophen for fever and irritability.

Anticipatory Guidance
Nutrition
- Discuss supplementation of vitamin D, iron, and fluoride as indicated.
- Advise the parents not to feed the baby honey or corn syrup.
- Recommend that no solids be fed until the baby is 4 to 6 months old.

Elimination
- Discuss normal elimination patterns.

Sleep Patterns

Social and Family Relationships
- Urge the parents to play with, talk to, and cuddle the baby.
- Inquire about alternative care arrangements when both parents work.

Continued

Age	Procedures
2 months— cont'd	**Anticipatory Guidance—cont'd** • Advise the parents to spend time alone with the other children. • Assess for signs of maternal depression. *Injury Prevention* • Discuss the use of car seats. • Emphasize the hazard of the infant falling from the bed or table if left unattended. • Stress the importance of a smoke-free environment. • Discuss gun safety measures. **Closing the Visit** • Review the problems discussed; devise a management plan for each one. • Ask the parents if they have other questions or concerns. • Schedule the next visit.
4 months	**Health Assessment** • Ask welcoming questions. • Ask if parents have any concerns or questions. • Ask about stress in the family. • Inquire about work and child care issues. • Review the status of issues discussed at the previous visit. • Ask specific questions about the infant's nutrition, elimination, sleep pattern, behavior, and development; also about family relationships. **Examination of the Infant** *Physical Examination* • Take measurements (height, weight, head circumference). • Perform a general physical examination. *Observation of Behavior and Development* Note the following: • Developmental milestones • Interactions with caregivers • Temperament (ability to cuddle and to be calmed) *Testing* • Hematocrit/hemoglobin if indicated **Immunizations** • Provide the family with vaccine information sheets.* • Give DTaP or DPT (dose 2); polio (dose 2); Hib (dose 2); hepatitis B (dose 2 if not given yet). • Recommend acetaminophen for fever and irritability. **Anticipatory Guidance** *Infections* • Advise the parents to expect about six upper respiratory tract infections a year; explain that antibiotics usually are ineffective against these infections and that unnecessary antibiotic use may be harmful. *Nutrition* • Recommend the introduction of solid foods (one at a time). • Advise the parents not to feed the baby honey or corn syrup until the infant is 1 year old. • Discuss iron supplementation (in formula or cereal). *Elimination* • Ask family about elimination patterns. *Sleep Patterns* *Developmental Progress* • Consider investigation of persistent "colic." *Social and Family Relationships* • Urge the parents to play with, talk to, and cuddle the baby. • Inquire about sibling rivalry. • Recommend that the parents take "free time" for themselves. *Injury Prevention* • Discuss the use of an appropriate car safety seat. • Explain how to choose safe toys. • Repeat warning about the danger of the infant falling from a bed or table if left unattended. • Discuss appropriate use of a microwave oven to heat the baby's food.

Age	Procedures
4 months— cont'd	**Closing the Visit** • Review the problems discussed; devise a management plan for each one. • Ask the parents if they have other questions or concerns. • Make positive statements about the baby's development and temperament. • Schedule the next appointment.
6 months	**Health Assessment** • Ask welcoming questions. • Ask what issues need to be discussed. • Ask about stress in the family. • Inquire about work and child care issues. • Review the status of issues discussed at the previous visit. • Ask specific questions about the infant's nutrition, elimination, sleep pattern, behavior, and development; also about family relationships. **Examination of the Infant** *Physical Examination* • Take measurements (height, weight, head circumference). • Perform a general physical examination. *Observation of Behavior and Development* Note the following: • Developmental milestones • Interactions with caregivers • Temperament *Testing* • Hematocrit/hemoglobin (at 6 to 12 months) • Sickle cell testing (as indicated) **Immunizations** • Provide vaccine information sheets for the family*; review the benefits and risks of vaccines. • Give DTaP or DPT (dose 3); polio (dose 3); Hib (dose 3); hepatitis B (dose 3 if due). • Recommend acetaminophen for fever and irritability. **Anticipatory Guidance** *Nutrition* • Advise the introduction of solids (if not already done). • Recommend offering the infant sips from a cup. *Elimination* • Ask family about elimination patterns. *Sleep Patterns* • Ask family about sleep patterns. *Observation of Development and Behavior* Note the following: • Stranger anxiety • Language development (advise parents to talk and read to the infant) *Injury Prevention* • Advise the parents on child-proofing the home (e.g., protecting the infant from hot liquids and surfaces). • Provide the local poison control telephone number. • Explain the use of syrup of ipecac. • Discourage the use of infant walkers. • Reinforce the proper use of microwave ovens to heat the baby's food. • Encourage the use of sunscreen. • Explain that swim classes are not recommended at this age. **Closing the Visit** • Review the problems discussed; devise a management plan for each one. • Ask the parents if they have other questions or concerns. • Make positive statements about the baby's development and temperament. • Schedule the next appointment.
9 months	**Health Assessment** • Ask welcoming questions. • Ask what issues need to be discussed at this visit.

Continued

TABLE 20-13	Guidelines for Health Supervision of Infants in the First Year of Life*—cont'd

Age	Procedures
9 months	**Health Assessment—cont'd** • Inquire about changes and stress in the family. • Inquire about the parents' approach to discipline. • Review the status of issues discussed at the previous visit. • Ask specific questions about the infant's nutrition, elimination, sleep pattern, behavior, and development; also about family relationships and injury prevention measures. **Examining the Infant** *Physical Examination* • Take measurements (height, weight, head circumference). • Perform a general physical examination. *Observation of Behavior and Development* Note the following: • Developmental milestones • Interactions with caregivers • Temperament *Testing* • Hematocrit/hemoglobin (at 6 to 12 months) • Lead toxicity screening **Immunizations** • Review immunizations to see if the infant is up-to-date. • Give PPD (this is given now or at 1 year if the infant is at risk of exposure to tuberculosis). • Give hepatitis B (dose 3 if due). **Anticipatory Guidance** *Nutrition* • Encourage the parents to establish regular mealtimes. • Recommend the introduction of table foods and drinking from a cup. *Elimination* • Recommend that parents delay toilet training until about 2 years of age or until the baby seems ready. *Sleep Patterns* • Recommend that the parents establish a regular bedtime routine. *Observation of Development and Behavior* Note the following: • Separation anxiety • Discipline • Language development • Intensified sibling rivalry *Injury Prevention* • Advise the parents on child-proofing the home. • Advise the parents to avoid giving the baby foods that can be aspirated; stress safety while eating. • Provide the local poison control telephone number. • Explain the use of syrup of ipecac. • Discourage the use of infant walkers. • Recommend changing from an infant car seat to a toddler model. **Closing the Visit** • Review the problems discussed; devise a management plan for each one. • Ask the parents if they have other questions or concerns. • Make positive statements about the baby's development and temperament. • Schedule the next appointment.
12 months	**Health Assessment** • Ask welcoming questions. • Ask what issues need to be discussed at this visit. • Inquire about changes or stress in the family. • Ask about the parents' approach to discipline. • Review the status of issues discussed at the previous visit.

TABLE 20-13	Guidelines for Health Supervision of Infants in the First Year of Life*—cont'd

Age	Procedures
12 months— cont'd	**Health Assessment—cont'd** • Ask specific questions about the infant's nutrition, elimination, sleep pattern, behavior, and development; also about family relationships and injury prevention measures. **Examination of the Infant** *Physical Examination* • Take measurements (height, weight, head circumference). • Perform a general physical examination. *Observation of Behavior and Development* Note the following: • Developmental milestones • Interactions with caregivers • Temperament *Testing* • Hematocrit/hemoglobin (at 6 to 12 months) • Lead toxicity screening • Give PPD (if not administered at 9 months, if the infant is at risk of exposure to tuberculosis). **Immunizations** • Provide the family with vaccine information sheets.* • Review immunizations to see if the infant is up-to-date. • Give measles-mumps-rubella (MMR) (per local regulations). • Varicella vaccine may be administered. **Anticipatory Guidance** *Infections* • Advise the parents to expect about six upper respiratory tract infections a year; explain that antibiotics usually are ineffective for these infections and that unnecessary antibiotic use may be harmful. *Nutrition* • Explain that the infant may seem to have less of an appetite; advise the parents not to force food on the child. • Recommend weaning to a cup. • Recommend changing from baby food to all table foods. *Elimination* • Advise the parents to delay toilet training until about 2 years of age or until the baby seems ready. *Sleep Patterns* • Recommend that the parents establish a regular bedtime routine. • Advise the parents not to allow the baby to sleep with them unless it is a cultural practice. *Observation of Development and Behavior* Note the following: • Infant's developing autonomy (explain this to the parents) • Discipline • Language development • Cognitive and motor skills *Injury Prevention* • Recommend ways to child-proof the home; stress window, stair, and bathtub safety. • Advise the parents to avoid giving the baby foods that can be aspirated. • Provide the local poison control telephone number. • Explain the use of syrup of ipecac. • Discourage the use of infant walkers. • Stress the importance of using the appropriate car safety seat. **Closing the Visit** • Review the problems discussed; devise a management plan for each one. • Ask the parents if they have other questions or concerns. • Make positive statements about the baby's development and temperament. • Schedule the next appointment.

Modified from American Academy of Pediatrics Committee on Psychosocial Aspects of Child and Family Health (1997a). Guidelines for health supervision III. The Academy: Elk Grove Village, IL.
*Available from the American Academy of Pediatrics, Publications Department, 141 Northwest Point Boulevard, Elk Grove Village, IL 60001-1098; 847.434.4000 (phone); 847.434.8000 (fax); www.aap.org.

TABLE 20-14	Recommended Childhood Immunization Schedule United States, 2002											
Age ► Vaccine ▼	Birth	1 mo	2 mos	4 mos	6 mos	12 mos	15 mos	18 mos	24 mos	4 to 6 yrs	11 to 12 yrs	13 to 18 yrs
Hepatitis B[1]	Hep B #1	only if mother HBsAg(−)									Hep B series	
		Hep B #2			Hep B #3							
Diphtheria, Tetanus, Pertussis[2]		DTaP	DTaP	DTaP		DTaP				DTaP	Td	
Haemophilus influenzae type b[3]		Hib	Hib	Hib	Hib							
Inactivated Polio[4]		IPV	IPV		IPV					IPV		
Measles, Mumps, Rubella[5]						MMR #1				MMR #2	MMR #2	
Varicella[6]						Varicella				Varicella		
Pneumococcal[7]		PCV	PCV	PCV	PCV					PCV	PPV	
------- Vaccines below this line are for selected populations -------												
Hepatitis A[8]										Hepatitis A series		
Influenza[9]						Influenza (yearly)						

☐ *Range of recommended ages*   ▨ *Catch-up vaccination*   ▩ *Preadolescent assessment*

This schedule indicates the recommended ages for routine administration of currently licensed childhood vaccines, as of December 1, 2001, for children through age 18 years. Any dose not given at the recommended age should be given at any subsequent visit when indicated and feasible. ▨ *Indicates age groups that warrant special effort to administer those vaccines not previously given. Additional vaccines may be licensed and recommended during the year. Licensed combination vaccines may be used whenever any components of the combination are indicated and the vaccine's other components are not contraindicated. Providers should consult the manufacturer's package inserts for detailed recommendations.*

Approved by the Advisory Committee on Immunization Practices (www.cdc.gov/nip/acip), the American Academy of Pediatrics (www.aap.org), and the American Academy of Family Physicians (www.aafp.org).

Immunizations

The AAP has published recommendations for routine childhood immunization through the first 18 years of age. These recommendations are presented in Table 20-14.

HEALTH MAINTENANCE FOR HIGH-RISK INFANTS IN THE FIRST YEAR OF LIFE

History

It is important for the primary care provider to review the infant's medical history, including a complete family history and the record of the hospital course. Pertinent history to be reviewed is shown in Table 20-15. In addition to providing routine health care maintenance and anticipatory guidance to the parents, the primary care provider must monitor the status of associated medical conditions and developmental sequelae.

Growth and Nutrition

Expected increases in weight, length/height, and head circumference in the first year are summarized in Table 20-16. Weight, length/height, and OFC are measured and plotted on the appropriate graphs. The parameters for premature infants must be corrected for preterm birth. Adjustments generally

are made until 2 to 2½ years of age. Premature infants frequently show accelerated ("catch-up") growth, which first manifests in the head circumference. This may begin as early as 36 weeks postconceptual age or as late as 8 months adjusted age (Sifuentes, 2000). Increases in the OFC of more than 2 cm per week are worrisome and should be investigated, because they may signify a pathologic process (hydrocephalus) rather than catch-up growth (Sifuentes, 2000).

Weight gain is evaluated in grams per day. Many high-risk infants are placed on special diets (24 calories/ounce of feeding regimens (feedings every 2 hours or continuous feedings). It is important to review the necessity of continuing or modifying the feeding plan according to the adequacy of growth. The need for dietary supplements (vitamins, minerals, human milk fortifier), medications (ranitidine, metoclopramide), and biochemical monitoring (e.g., for rickets or osteopenia) should also be addressed.

Physical Examination

A complete physical examination should be performed at each visit. Depending on the infant's history and needs, special attention may be required in certain areas, which are listed in Table 20-17.

TABLE 20-15	Recorded Elements of the History, Medical Course, and Current Needs for Neonates

Component	Elements
History	Prenatal and perinatal course
	Hospital course:
	Birth weight, gestation
	Illnesses, surgical procedures
	Radiographic studies
	Discharge examination
	Weight, head circumference, length
Nutrition information	Current diet and feeding schedule
	Feeding problems:
	Gastroesophageal (GE) reflux, feeding intolerance
	Dietary supplements:
	Vitamins, minerals, human milk fortifier
	Current deficiencies:
	Osteopenia/rickets, anemia
Medications	Doses
	Serum levels
	Oxygen requirements
Immunizations	Immunizations given in the hospital
	Respiratory syncytial virus (RSV) prophylaxis
Laboratory data	Most recent values:
	Hemoglobin, hematocrit
	Bilirubin
	Pending laboratory studies
	Need for further testing
	Newborn screening results
Current problems and complications	Retinopathy of prematurity (ROP), ophthalmologic problems (e.g., strabismus)
	Hearing deficits
	Bronchopulmonary dysplasia (BPD)/chronic lung problems
	GE reflux
	Intraventricular hemorrhage (IVH)
	Developmental deficits
	Other

Based on Sifuentes M (2000). Well-child care for preterm infants. In Berkowitz CD, editor. Pediatrics: a primary care approach, ed 2. WB Saunders: Philadelphia.

TABLE 20-16	Expected Increases in Weight, Length/Height, and Head Circumference in the First Year of Life

Parameter	Age (months)	Expected Increase
Weight	Birth to 3	25 to 35 g/day
	3 to 6	12 to 21 g/day
	6 to 12	10 to 13 g/day
Length/height	Birth to 12	25 cm/year
Occipitofrontal circumference (OFC)	Birth to 3	2 cm/month
	4 to 6	1 cm/month
	7 to 12	0.5 cm/month

Based on Grover G (2000a). Nutritional needs. In Berkowitz CD, ed. Pediatrics: a primary care approach, ed 2. WB Saunders: Philadelphia.

Laboratory Tests and Monitoring Examinations

All standard screening tests required for healthy infants should be performed according to AAP recommendations. Other tests may be necessary for high-risk infants, such as periodic electrolyte determinations for babies receiving diuretics. Consideration should be given to measuring serum levels for such drugs as anticonvulsants, methylxanthines, and digoxin.

Repeat ophthalmologic examinations may be required to evaluate the extent and progression or regression of retinopathy of prematurity (ROP). Further follow-up may be indicated, because some infants are at risk for strabismus, myopia, ambly-opia, glaucoma, and other visual deficits. The infant may need serial auditory evaluations (brainstem auditory evoked response [BAER] behavioral audiograms) and other studies, such as electroencephalography, electrocardiography, echocardiography, radiography, pneumography, and neuroradiologic imaging (computed tomography [CT] or magnetic resonance imaging [MRI]). Infants receiving supplemental oxygen often benefit from periodic pulse oximetry (Sifuentes, 2000).

Immunizations

Vaccines are administered according to chronologic (postnatal) age, not gestational age. The standard doses and intervals are followed, as recommended by the AAP (Table 20-13). Former premature infants have adequate serologic responses to immunizations without increased incidence of untoward effects (Sifuentes, 2000). High-risk infants, especially premature infants with a history of respiratory distress syndrome (RDS) or RDS/BPD (RSD with bronchopulmonary dysplasia), benefit from respiratory syncytial virus (RSV) prophylaxis.

Psychosocial Needs

Families of high-risk infants require a great deal of support and anticipatory guidance. Health care providers must seek to understand parental expectations and legitimize their fears while providing support and encouragement. Parents should be given consistent, honest information and realistic appraisals of their infant's status and prognosis (Sifuentes, 2000).

NICU graduates may be at risk for vulnerable child syndrome (VCS) (Box 20-1). Because parents continue to perceive their child as vulnerable and fragile, abnormal parent-infant interactions develop. By assessing for early, subtle signs, health care providers may prevent progression of the disorder.

SUMMARY

The comprehensive history and physical assessment create the framework for identifying problems and planning interventions. Assessment allows the nurse to gather information and to evaluate and integrate that information as care of the newborn proceeds. Although careful attention to the obvious is important, subtle findings detected by an experienced practitioner also may play a crucial role in the continuing care of the infant and family.

TABLE 20-17	Monitoring for Subsequent Conditions in High-Risk Infants	
System	**Condition**	**Comments**
Ocular	Retinopathy of prematurity (ROP), strabismus, visual abnormalities	
Oropharyngeal	Palatal groove, high arched palate, abnormal tooth formation	May develop secondary to intubation or may be due to congenital abnormalities.
	Discolored teeth	Caused by high bilirubin levels.
Thoracic/respiratory	Retractions, wheezing, stridor	Sequelae of chronic lung disease.
	Chest scars	Caused by chest tube placement.
Cardiovascular	Hypertension	Blood pressure monitoring is especially important for an infant who had umbilical artery catheters in place.
Abdominal	Hypoplastic umbilicus	Use of umbilical catheters and suturing frequently are the cause of this condition.
Genitourinary	Hernias	Increased risk in preterm babies.
	Cryptorchidism	
Extremities	Developmental hip dysplasia	
	Scars on heels or extremities	Sequelae of blood sampling, placement of intravenous (IV) lines, or extravasation of IV fluid.
Neuromuscular	Abnormal tone, asymmetric movements and reflexes, persistence of primitive reflexes and fisting, sustained clonus, scissoring	Abnormalities must be identified as soon as possible and the patient and family referred to appropriate intervention services.
	Poor suck-swallow coordination	

Based on Sifuentes M (2000). *Well-child care for preterm infants.* In Berkowitz CD, editor. Pediatrics: a primary care approach, ed 2. WB Saunders: Philadelphia.

BOX 20-1	
Characteristics of Vulnerable Child Syndrome	

Exaggerated separation anxiety (both infant and parent)
Sleep difficulties
Overprotectiveness
Overindulgence
Lack of appropriate discipline
Excessive parental preoccupation with infant's health

REFERENCES

American Academy of Pediatrics Committee on the Fetus and Newborn and the American College of Obstetricians and Gynecologists Committee on Obstetrics (1996). Use and abuse of the Apgar score. *Pediatrics* 98:141-142.

American Academy of Pediatrics Committee on Psychosocial Aspects of Child and Family Health (1997a). *Guidelines for health supervision III.* The Academy: Elk Grove Village, IL.

American Academy of Pediatrics, Urology Section, Action Committee Report (1997b). Timing of elective surgery on the genitalia of male children with particular reference to the risks, benefits, and psychologic effects of surgery and anesthesia. *Pediatrics* 97:590.

Apgar VA (1953). A proposal for a new method of evaluation of the newborn infant. *Current research in anesthesiology analogs* 32:260-267.

Askin D (1996). Chest and lung assessment. In Tapperro EP, Honeyfield ME, editors. *Physical assessment of the newborn,* ed 2. NICU Ink: Petaluma, CA.

Aucott S (1997). Physical examination. In Fanaroff AA, Martin RM, editors. *Neonatal-perinatal medicine: diseases of the fetus and infant,* ed 6. Mosby: St Louis.

Ballard JL et al (1991). New Ballard Score, expanded to include extremely premature infants. *Journal of pediatrics* 119:417-423.

Blake WW, Murray JJ (1998). Heat balance. In Merenstein GB, Gardner SL, editors: *Handbook of neonatal intensive care,* ed 4. Mosby: St Louis.

Cavaliere TA (1996). Genitourinary assessment. In Tapperro EP, Honeyfield ME, editors. *Physical assessment of the newborn,* ed 2. NICU Ink: Petaluma, CA.

Cilento BG et al (1994). Cryptorchidism and testicular torsion. *Pediatric clinics of North America* 40:1133-1149.

Connor GK (1996). Abdomen assessment. In Tapperro EP, Honeyfield ME, editors. *Physical assessment of the newborn,* ed 2. NICU Ink: Petaluma, CA.

Cooperman DR, Thompson GH (2002). Neonatal orthopedics: congenital abnormalities of the upper and lower extremities and spine. In Fanaroff AA, Martin RM, editors. *Neonatal-perinatal medicine: diseases of the fetus and infant,* ed 7. Mosby: St Louis.

Dahms WT, Danish RK (2002). Abnormalities of sexual differentiation. In Fanaroff AA, Martin RM, editors. *Neonatal-perinatal medicine: diseases of the fetus and infant,* ed 7. Mosby: St Louis.

D'Harlingue AE, Durand DJ (2001). Recognition, stabilization, and transport of the high-risk newborn. In Klaus MH, Fanaroff AA, editors. *Care of the high risk neonate,* ed 5. WB Saunders: Philadelphia.

Engel J (1997). *Pocket guide to pediatric assessment,* ed 3. Mosby: St Louis.

Fletcher MA (1998). *Physical diagnosis in neonatology.* Lippincott-Raven: Philadelphia.

Grover G (2000a). Nutritional needs. In Berkowitz CD, editor. *Pediatrics: a primary care approach,* ed 2. WB Saunders: Philadelphia.

Grover G (2000b). Rotational problems of the lower extremities: in-toeing and out-toeing. In Berkowitz CD, editor. *Pediatrics: a primary care approach,* ed 2. WB Saunders: Philadelphia.

Gupta BK et al (2002). The eye: diagnosis and evaluation. In Fanaroff AA, Martin RM, editors. *Neonatal-perinatal medicine: diseases of the fetus and infant,* ed 7. Mosby: St Louis.

Hegyi T et al (1994). Blood pressure ranges in premature infants. I. The first hours of life. *Journal of pediatrics* 124:627-633.

Hudgins L, Cassidy SB (2002). Congenital anomalies. In Fanaroff AA, Martin RM, editors. *Neonatal-perinatal medicine: diseases of the fetus and infant,* ed 7. Mosby: St Louis.

Johnson CB (1996). Head, eyes, ears, nose, mouth, and neck assessment. In Tapperro EP, Honeyfield ME, editors. *Physical assessment of the newborn,* ed 2. NICU Ink: Petaluma, CA.

Katz K, Nishioka E (1998). Neonatal assessment. In Kenner C et al, editors. *Comprehensive neonatal nursing: a physiologic perspective,* ed 2. WB Saunders: Philadelphia.

Kenner C (1998). Assessment and management of genitourinary dysfunction. In Kenner C et al, editors. *Comprehensive neonatal nursing: a physiologic perspective,* ed 2. WB Saunders: Philadelphia.

Kliegman RM, Das US (2002). Intrauterine growth retardation. In Fanaroff AA, Martin RM, editors. *Neonatal-perinatal medicine: diseases of the fetus and infant,* ed 7. Mosby: St Louis.

Lepley CJ et al (1998). Initial nursery care. In Merenstein GB, Gardner SL, editors. *Handbook of neonatal intensive care,* ed 4. Mosby: St Louis.

Lissauer T (2002). Physical examination of the newborn. In Fanaroff AA, Martin RM, editors. *Neonatal-perinatal medicine: diseases of the fetus and infant,* ed 7. Mosby: St Louis.

Mangurten HM (2002). Birth injuries. In Fanaroff AA, Martin RM, editors. *Neonatal-perinatal medicine: diseases of the fetus and infant,* ed 7. Mosby: St Louis.

McLean F, Usher R (1970). Measurements of liveborn fetal malnutrition infants compared with similar gestation and with similar birth weight normal controls. *Biology of the neonate* 16:215-221.

Metcoff J (1994). Clinical assessment of nutritional status at birth. *Pediatric clinics of North America* 41:875-891.

Ohls R (2001). Anemia in the newborn. In Polin RA et al, editors. *Workbook in practical neonatology,* ed 3. WB Saunders: Philadelphia.

Ryckman FC (2002). Selected anomalies and intestinal obstruction. In Fanaroff AA, Martin RM, editors. *Neonatal-perinatal medicine: diseases of the fetus and infant,* ed 7. Mosby: St Louis.

Sarnat HB (2002). Embryology and malformation of the central nervous system. In Fanaroff AA, Martin RM, editors. *Neonatal-perinatal medicine: diseases of the fetus and infant,* ed 7. Mosby: St Louis.

Seidel HM et al (1999). *Mosby's guide to physical examination,* ed 4. Mosby: St Louis.

Sifuentes M (2000). Well-child care for preterm infants. In Berkowitz CD, editor. *Pediatrics: a primary care approach,* ed 2. WB Saunders: Philadelphia.

Southgate WM, Pittard WB (2001). Classification and physical examination of the newborn infant. In Klaus MH, Fanaroff AA, editors. *Care of the high risk neonate,* ed 5. WB Saunders: Philadelphia.

Stanley FJ (1994). Cerebral palsy trends: implications for perinatal care. *Acta obstetricia et gynecologica Scandinavica (Copenhagen)* 73:5-9.

Tappero EP (1996). Musculoskeletal system assessment. In Tapperro EP, Honeyfield ME, editor. *Physical assessment of the newborn,* ed 2. NICU Ink: Petaluma, CA.

Vannucci RC, Yaeger JY (2002). Newborn neurologic assessment. In Fanaroff AA, Martin RM, editor. *Neonatal-perinatal medicine: diseases of the fetus and infant,* ed 7. Mosby: St Louis.

Vargo L (1996). Cardiovascular assessment. In Tapperro EP, Honeyfield ME, editors. *Physical assessment of the newborn,* ed 2. NICU Ink: Petaluma, CA.

Vogt BA et al (2001). The kidney. In Klaus ME, Fanaroff AA, editors. *Care of the high risk neonate,* ed 5. WB Saunders: Philadelphia.

Waardenburg PJ (1951). A new syndrome combining developmental anomalies of the eyelids, eyebrows, and nose root with pigmentary defects of the iris and head hair and with congenital deafness. *American journal of human genetics* 3:195.

CHAPTER 21

RESPIRATORY SYSTEM MANAGEMENT AND COMPLICATIONS

JAVIER CIFUENTES, ASHLEY HODGES SEGARS, WALDEMAR A. CARLO

The mechanisms that bring about normal pulmonary function are complex. The clinician must fully comprehend the physiologic processes associated with respiratory disease of the infant. Only through advanced knowledge can the clinician efficiently assess and evaluate the newborn's respiratory status. Systematic use of these assessment skills allows the clinician, as part of the collaborative team, to positively affect patient outcome.

EMBRYOLOGIC DEVELOPMENT OF THE LUNG

Pulmonary development of the embryo proceeds along a predetermined sequence throughout gestation. Pulmonary development begins with formation of an out pouching of the embryonic foregut during the fourth week of gestation and continues on to form sufficient alveoli to maintain gas exchange in most infants by 32 to 36 weeks of gestational age. Additional alveoli continue to develop in the newborn infant and well into childhood, perhaps as late as the seventh year of life (Table 21-1). Sequential branching of the lung bud, which appears at about 4 weeks and is complete by the sixth week, marks the embryonic phase of lung development. The following 10 weeks are marked by the formation of conducting airways by branching of the aforementioned lung buds. This phase, the pseudoglandular phase, continues through week 16 and ends with completion of the conducting airways. The canalicular phase follows through week 28, when gas exchange units, known as acini, develop. Type II alveolar cells, the surfactant-producing cells, begin to form during the latter part of this phase. Mature, vascularized gas-exchange sites form during the saccular phase, which spans the 29th through 35th weeks. During this phase, the interstitial space between alveoli thins, so respiratory epithelial cells tightly contact developing capillaries. The alveolar development phase, marked by expansion of gas-exchange surface area, begins at 36 weeks and extends into the postnatal period. The alveolar wall and interstitial spaces become very thin, and the single capillary network comes into close proximity to the alveolar membrane. No firm boundaries separate these phases, and gas exchange, albeit inefficient, is possible relatively early in gestation, even before mature, vascularized gas-exchange sites form. Lung development is a continuum that is marked by rapid structural changes. Interference at any time by premature birth or by disease introduces the possibility of inducing iatrogenic disease through intervention (Hodson, 1998).

NEWBORN PULMONARY PHYSIOLOGY AND THE ONSET OF BREATHING

The fetal lung is fluid filled, underperfused, and dormant with regard to gas exchange. The fetal lung receives only approximately 10% of the cardiac output. Because the placenta is the gas-exchange organ in fetal life, a high blood flow is directed toward it rather than to the lungs (Figure 23-1 in Chapter 23). Consequently, most of the right ventricular output is shunted from the pulmonary artery across the ductus arteriosus into the aorta, bypassing the pulmonary circulation.

Within moments after the umbilical cord is clamped, the newborn undergoes an amazing transformation from a fetus floating in amniotic fluid to an air-breathing neonate. When the normal onset of breathing occurs, the ensuing chain of events converts the fetal circulation to the circulation pattern of an adult. The lung fluid is absorbed and replaced with air, thus establishing lung volume and allowing for normal neonatal pulmonary function (Nelson, 1994). The process of fetal lung fluid absorption begins before birth, when the rate of alveolar fluid secretion declines. Reabsorption speeds up during labor. Animal data suggest that as much as two thirds of the total clearance of lung fluid occurs during labor. This clearance probably results from the cessation of active chloride secretion into the alveolar space. Oncotic pressure favors the movement of water from the air space back into the interstitium and into the vascular space. With the onset of breathing and lung expansion, water moves rapidly from the air spaces into the interstitium and is removed from the lung by lymphatic and pulmonary blood vessels. Because a large portion of the clearance of lung fluid occurs during labor, neonates born without labor after cesarean section are at particularly high risk for delayed absorption of fetal lung fluid and thus for transient tachypnea of the newborn (Bland, 1998).

With the onset of breathing, highly negative intrathoracic pressures are generated with inspiratory efforts, filling the alveoli with air. Replacing alveolar fluid with air causes a precipitous decrease in hydrostatic pressure in the lung; therefore pulmonary artery pressure decreases, which lowers pressure in the right atrium and increases pulmonary blood flow. These changes result in an increase in alveolar oxygen tension (PaO_2), which causes constriction of the ductus arteriosus, which normally shunts right ventricular blood away from the

TABLE **21-1**	Stages of Normal Lung Growth	
Phase	**Timing**	**Major Event**
Embryonic	Weeks 4 to 6	Formation of proximal airway
Pseudoglandular	Weeks 7 to 16	Formation of conducting airways
Canalicular	Weeks 17 to 28	Formation of acini
Saccular	Weeks 29 to 35	Development of gas exchange sites
Alveolar	Weeks 36 through postnatal life	Expansion of surface area

lungs. By clamping of the cord, the large, low-resistance, placental surface area is removed from the circulation. This change in resistance causes an abrupt increase in systemic arterial pressure, reflected all the way back to the left atrium. As left atrial pressure rises, its flap valve closes the opening between the atria, known as the foramen ovale. This closure prevents blood from bypassing the lungs by eliminating the shunt across the foramen ovale from the right atrium to the left atrium. As a result of closure of fetal pathways and decreased pulmonary artery pressure, systemic pressure is greater than pulmonary artery pressure. The infant successfully converts from the pattern of fetal circulation to neonatal circulation when blood coming from the right ventricle flows in its new path of least resistance (lower pressure) to the lungs instead of shunting across the foramen ovale to the left atrium or across the ductus arteriosus from the pulmonary artery to the aorta.

Understanding ventilation enables the clinician to assess the infant in respiratory distress and devise strategies for management. The respiratory system is composed of the following: (1) the pumping system (the chest wall muscles, diaphragm, and accessory muscles of respiration), which moves free gas into the lungs; (2) the bony rib cage, which provides structural support for the respiratory muscles and limits lung deflation; (3) the conducting airways, which connect gas-exchanging units with the outside but offer resistance to gas flow; (4) an elastic element, which offers some resistance to gas flow but provides pumping force for moving stale air out of the system; (5) air-liquid interfaces, which generate surface tension that opposes lung expansion on inspiration but supports lung deflation on expiration; and (6) the abdominal muscles, which aid exhalation by active contraction.

Limitations in the respiratory system predispose the newborn to respiratory difficulty. The circular, poorly ossified rib cage, with a flat instead of angular insertion of the diaphragm, is less efficient at generating negative intrathoracic pressure to move air into the system. Small muscles hinder the strength and endurance of respiratory muscles and a relative paucity of type I muscle fibers. The newborn has a relatively low functional residual capacity (lung volume at the end of exhalation) because his or her comparatively floppy chest wall offers little resistance to collapse, even when a normal amount of functional surfactant is present.

An alveolar cell known as the type II pneumocyte produces pulmonary surfactant, surface tension-reducing mixture of phospholipids, and proteins found in mature alveoli. Surfactant coats the alveoli, preventing alveolar collapse and loss of

lung volume during expiration—that is, as expiration ensues and the lung deflates, the alveolar diameter becomes smaller. Surfactant coating of the alveolus reduces surface tension so that collapse is prevented and less pressure is required to reinflate it with the next inspiration. Neonates with respiratory distress syndrome (RDS) have surfactant deficiency. In the absence of surfactant, surface tension is high, and the tendency is toward collapse of alveoli at end expiration.

Surface tension is the force that arises from the interaction among the molecules of a liquid. Molecules in the interior of the liquid bulk are attracted to each other, but molecules on the surface of the liquid are attracted to other molecules in the interior of the liquid, which results in the movement of the surface molecule toward the bulk of the liquid. This explains why a droplet of water over a surface tends to adopt a given size and not continuously expand. If we think of the alveolus as a soap bubble, the molecules of the wall of the bubble are attracted to each other, which tends to collapse the bubble. The pressures across the wall of the bubble act against the surface tension and avoid the collapse of the bubble. The relationship between the surface tension and the distending pressures and the pressure across the wall of the bubble are described by the Laplace's law, as shown in the following equation:

$$P = 2\,ST/r$$

P is pressure; ST is surface tension; and r is radius of the alveolus. It is difficult to inflate a small or collapsed alveolus because it has a very small diameter. As its volume increases, the pressure needed to continue inflation becomes progressively less—that is, compliance of the alveolus and thus compliance of the lung has improved. Coating the alveoli with an agent that decreases surface tension reduces the effort required to inflate the lungs from a low volume. Pulmonary surfactant is a surface tension-reducing mixture of phospholipids and proteins found in mature alveoli. An alveolar cell known as the type II pneumocyte produces surfactant. Surfactant coats the alveoli, which prevents alveolar collapse and loss of lung volume during expiration—that is, as expiration ensues and the lung deflates, the alveolar diameter becomes smaller. Surfactant coating of the alveolus reduces surface tension so that collapse is prevented and less pressure is required to reinflate it with the next inspiration. Neonates with respiratory distress syndrome (RDS) have surfactant deficiency. In the absence of surfactant, surface tension is high, and the tendency is toward collapse of alveoli at end expiration.

Compliance is the elasticity, or distensibility, of the lung. It is expressed as the change in volume caused by a change in pressure as follows:

$$C_L = VP$$

C_L is compliance of the lung; V is volume; and P is pressure. The higher the compliance, the larger the volume delivered to the alveoli per unit of applied inspiratory pressure. Surface tension and compliance are particularly important in the preterm infant with RDS. Surface tension is a force that opposes lung expansion. Surfactant deficiency leads to increased surface tension in the alveoli. Lungs with higher surface tension are more difficult to inflate. During expiration, some alveoli collapse, so lung volume at the end of expiration is decreased (low functional residual capacity). Clinically, the presence of retractions and other signs of respiratory distress manifest the effects of this increased surface tension. Respiratory muscles contract to inflate the lungs against the surface tension that acts in the opposite direction. The negative pleural pressure easily deforms the floppy thoracic wall of the preterm infant. When a preterm infant with RDS is intubated, a high peak inspiratory pressure (PIP) is required to expand the thorax (i.e., tidal volume is obtained only with a high change in pressure). After surfactant is administered, chest expansion increases with the same PIP. This effect (increased compliance) is due to a decrease in surface tension (i.e., a smaller force opposing lung distention). Thus the tidal volume obtained with the same PIP is increased. Before surfactant is administered, it is very difficult to inflate the lung because compliance is low. After surfactant is administered, surface tension decreases, and it becomes easier to inflate the lung (i.e., compliance is improved).

Resistance is a term used to describe characteristics of gas flow through the airways and pulmonary tissues. Resistance can be thought of as the capacity of the lung to resist airflow. The principal component of resistance is determined by the small airways. Pressure is required to force gas through the airways (airway resistance) and to overcome the forces of the lung and chest wall, which work to deflate the respiratory system (tissue resistance). At a specific flow rate, resistance is described by the following equation:

$$R = P_1 - P_2 / \dot{V}$$

P_1 and P_2 are pressures at opposite ends of the airway, and $\dot{V}$ is the flow rate of gas (volume per unit of time). Resistance increases as airway diameter decreases. Because the infant has airways of relatively small radius, the resistance to gas flow through those airways is high. The time constant is the time necessary for airway pressure to partially equilibrate throughout the respiratory system and equals the mathematic product of compliance and resistance. In other words, the time constant is a measure of how quickly the lungs can inhale or exhale. The time constant (Kt) is directly related to both compliance (C) and resistance (R). This relationship is described by the following equation:

$$Kt = C \times R$$

An infant with RDS has decreased compliance, so the time constant of the respiratory system is relatively short. In such an infant, little time is required for pressure to equilibrate between the proximal airway and alveoli, so short inspiratory and expiratory times may be appropriate during mechanical ventilation. When compliance improves (increases), however, the time constant becomes longer. If sufficient time is not allowed for expiration, the alveoli may become over distended, and an air leak may result (Carlo et al, 1994).

Blood Gas Analysis and Acid-Base Balance

Oxygen diffuses across the alveolar-capillary membrane, moved by the difference in oxygen pressure between the alveoli and the blood. In the blood, oxygen dissolves in the plasma and binds to hemoglobin. Thus arterial oxygen content (CaO_2) is the sum of dissolved and hemoglobin-bound oxygen, as is shown by the following equation:

$$CaO_2 = (1.37 \times Hb \times SaO_2) \, (0.003 \times PaO_2)$$

CaO_2 is arterial oxygen content (ml/100 ml of blood); 1.37 is the milliliters of oxygen bound to 1 g of hemoglobin at 100% saturation; Hb is hemoglobin concentration per 100 ml of blood (g/100 ml); SaO_2 is the percentage of hemoglobin bound to oxygen (%); 0.003 is the solubility factor of oxygen in plasma (ml/mm Hg); and PaO_2 is oxygen partial pressure in arterial blood (mm Hg).

In the equation for arterial oxygen content, the first term—($1.37 \times Hb \times SaO_2$)—is the amount of oxygen bound to hemoglobin. The second term—($0.003 \times PaO_2$)—is the amount of oxygen dissolved in plasma. Most of the oxygen in the blood is carried by hemoglobin. For example, if a premature infant has a PaO_2 of 60 mm Hg, an SaO_2 of 92%, and a hemoglobin concentration of 14 g/100 ml, then CaO_2 is the sum of oxygen bound to hemoglobin ($1.37 \times 14 \times 92/100$) = 17.6 ml, plus the oxygen dissolved in plasma (0.003×60) = 0.1 ml. In this typical example, only 1% of oxygen in blood is dissolved in plasma; 99% is carried by hemoglobin. If the infant has an intraventricular hemorrhage and the hemoglobin concentration decreases to 10.5 g/dl but PaO_2 and SaO_2 remain the same, then CaO_2 ($1.37 \times 10.5 \times 92/100$) + ($0.003 \times 60$) equals 13.4 ml/100 ml of blood. Thus, without any change in PaO_2 or SaO_2, a 25% decrease in hemoglobin concentration (from 14 to 10.5 g/dl) reduces the amount of oxygen in arterial blood by 24% (from 17.6 to 13.4 ml/100 ml of blood). This is an important concept for persons who care for patients with respiratory disease. SaO_2 and hemoglobin should be monitored and, if low, corrected to keep an adequate level of tissue oxygenation. Besides SaO_2 and hemoglobin, cardiac output is the other major determination of oxygen delivery to the tissues.

The force that loads hemoglobin with oxygen in the lungs and unloads it in the tissues is the difference in partial pressure of oxygen. In the lungs, alveolar oxygen partial pressure is higher than capillary oxygen partial pressure so that oxygen moves to the capillaries and binds to the hemoglobin. Tissue partial pressure of oxygen is lower than that of the blood, so oxygen moves from hemoglobin to the tissues. The relationship between partial pressure of oxygen and hemoglobin is better understood with the oxyhemoglobin dissociation curve (Figure 21-1). Several factors can affect the affinity of hemoglobin for oxygen. Alkalosis, hypothermia, hypocapnia, and decreased levels of 2,3-diphosphoglycerate (2,3-DPG) increase

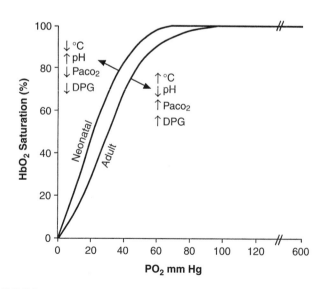

FIGURE **21-1**

Oxyhemoglobin equilibrium curves of blood from term infants at birth and from adults (at pH 7.40).

the affinity of hemoglobin for oxygen (as shown in Figure 21-1 by a left shift of the curve). Acidosis, hyperthermia, hypercapnia, and increased 2,3-DPG have the opposite effect, decreasing the affinity of hemoglobin for oxygen, so that the hemoglobin dissociation curve shifts to the right. This characteristic of hemoglobin facilitates oxygen loading in the lung and unloading in the tissue, where the pH is lower and alveolar carbon dioxide tension ($PaCO_2$) is higher. Fetal hemoglobin, which has a higher affinity for oxygen than adult hemoglobin, is more fully oxygen-saturated at lower PaO_2 values. This is represented by a left shift on the curve of dissociation of hemoglobin.

Once loaded with oxygen, the blood should reach the tissues to transfer oxygen to the cells. Oxygen delivery to the tissue depends on cardiac output (CO) and CaO_2, as described in the following equation:

$$Oxygen\ deliver = CO \times CaO_2$$

In the case of the infant discussed previously, increased CO compensates for the decrease in CaO_2 that results from anemia. The key concept is that when a patient's oxygenation is assessed, more information than just PaO_2 and SaO_2 should be considered. PaO_2 and SaO_2 may be normal, but, if hemoglobin concentration is low or CO is decreased, oxygen delivery to the tissues is decreased. With this approach, the clinician should be able to better plan the interventions needed to improve oxygenation.

As in the adult, the acid-base balance in the neonate is maintained within narrow limits by complex interactions between the pulmonary system (which eliminates carbon dioxide) and the kidneys (which conserve carbon dioxide and eliminate metabolic acids). Carbon dioxide elimination, which is more efficient than oxygenation across the alveolar capillary membrane, is usually not as problematic as oxygenation. Carbon dioxide has a high solubility coefficient, so cellular diffusion is very efficient and no measurable partial pressure gradient exists between venous blood and the tissues. Therefore elevated carbon dioxide tension (PCO_2) values in arterial blood samples nearly always indicate ventilatory dysfunction. Dissolved carbon dioxide moves rapidly across cell membranes of peripheral chemoreceptors, thus making them sensitive to changes in ventilation. Increased intracellular PCO_2 elevates the cellular hydrogen ion concentration as carbon dioxide combines with water to form carbonic acid. This stimulates neural impulses to the medulla, which stimulates respiration. However, excessively high PCO_2 levels can depress ventilation. Acid-base balance is controlled by homeostatic mechanisms and is expressed as follows:

$$pH = 6.1\ log\ HCO_3^-\ 0.03 \times PCO_2$$

It can be seen from this mathematical relationship that acid-base balance depends on the interplay of bicarbonate ion (HCO_3^-) and carbon dioxide. Serum pH is tightly regulated in the normal range. Low pH (acidosis) can contribute to vasoconstriction and result in worsening hypoxemia caused by extrapulmonary shunt across the ductus or foramen ovale. A pH of less than 7.0 is not well tolerated and is associated with a poor survival rate.

If $PaCO_2$ rises above normal, as in hypoventilation, pH declines and the patient suffers from respiratory acidosis. The patient with a chronic respiratory acidosis may retain bicarbonate, thus self-inducing a compensatory metabolic alkalosis. A patient who is hyperventilated with a low $PaCO_2$ has respiratory alkalosis. Depressed bicarbonate ion concentration (less

than approximately 20 mmol/L in plasma) is called metabolic acidosis and can be associated with any cause of anaerobic metabolism, such as poor CO from congenital heart disease—for example, hypoplastic left heart syndrome or severe aortic coarctation—or from myocardial ischemia, myocardiopathy, myocarditis, or septic shock. Metabolic acidosis that results from renal bicarbonate wasting commonly develops in extremely immature infants. Less common causes for prolonged and severe metabolic acidosis are the inborn errors of metabolisms, including urea-cycle defects and amino acidopathies.

The clinician should become proficient at interpreting blood gas data. With knowledge of the accepted normal values and definitions of the simple blood gas disorders and their compensatory mechanisms, the clinician can examine data in light of the disease process and interpret blood gas values in a fairly straightforward manner. Normally, the body does not overcompensate for a pH above or below the normal range. Therefore when presented with an abnormal pH, the clinician rapidly determines whether acidosis (Figure 21-2A) or alkalosis exists (Figure 21-2B). An examination of $PaCO_2$ and HCO_3^- determines whether the process is respiratory, metabolic, or mixed. The clinician should determine which derangement occurred first. For example, an acidotic, acutely ill hypoxemic infant with a high $PaCO_2$ and depressed HCO_3^- is usually hypoventilating and suffering metabolic acidosis secondary to anaerobic metabolism. The infant with a low $PaCO_2$ is hyperventilating, either spontaneously or secondary to overzealous mechanical ventilation. A concomitantly low pH and low $PaCO_2$, indicate that the infant is compensating for metabolic acidosis with hyperventilation in an effort to normalize the pH. A pure metabolic alkalosis with high pH is nearly always caused by bicarbonate administration. Infants with bronchopulmonary dysplasia usually have a compensated respiratory acidosis, with an elevated $PaCO_2$ and concomitantly elevated HCO_3^-. The pH may be in the normal range or slightly acidotic. A severely depressed pH usually indicates acute decompensation.

ASSESSMENT OF THE NEONATE WITH RESPIRATORY DISTRESS

The assessment of a neonate with respiratory distress should always begin with the compilation of a detailed perinatal history. In many cases, the history is difficult to obtain, especially when the infant has been transferred from one center to another, often with incomplete records. Even so, every effort should be made to obtain as much information as possible. The clinician is often able to gain important supplemental information from the father or visiting relatives at the bedside. A review of the maternal-perinatal history and a complete physical examination, combined with a limited laboratory and radiologic evaluation, leads to a timely diagnosis in most circumstances. Many neonatal diseases, including many with nonpulmonary origins, may manifest with signs of respiratory distress. Therefore a comprehensive differential diagnosis must be considered (Figure 21-3).

History

In most situations, data from a patient's history can direct the clinician to the correct diagnosis of neonatal respiratory distress. The prenatal record should be reviewed carefully for possible causes of the infant's difficulties. The mother's age, gravidity, parity, blood type, and Rh status should be recorded. The obste-

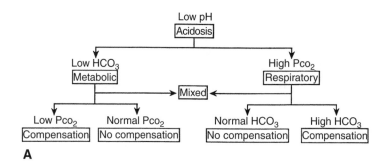

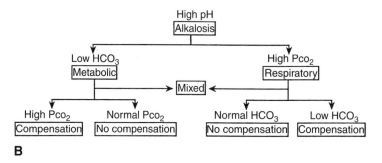

FIGURE **21-2**
Acid-base balance: diagnostic approach.

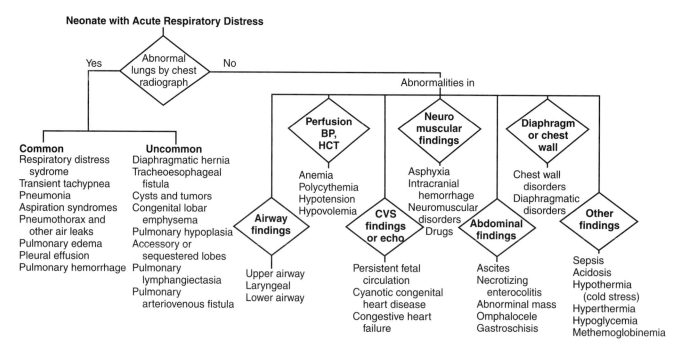

FIGURE **21-3**
Neonate with acute respiratory distress.

trician's best estimate of gestational age should be documented as determined by first trimester ultrasound or last menstrual period. Ultrasonography often provides information related to anomalies, which is useful in the anticipation of required support at birth. Historical information such as previous preterm birth is relevant as it is often associated with an increased risk of premature delivery in subsequent pregnancies. Because excessive maternal weight gain occurs with diabetes, multiple gestation, or polyhydramnios, pre-pregnancy weight and total gain should be noted. The clinician is often alerted to the possibility of gestational diabetes with abnormal glucose tolerance screening results, which will be reflected in the prenatal record.

The duration of rupture of membranes, the presence of maternal fever with or without accompanying amnionitis, and the presence of meconium-stained amniotic fluid are important pieces of information that may help in the differential diagnosis of a newborn with respiratory distress. Additionally, antepartum and intrapartum administration of certain medications may affect diagnosis and management of these infants. Administration of steroids to the mother reduces the likelihood that RDS will develop in the infant; administration of narcotics to the mother close to delivery may result in poor respiratory effort by an otherwise normal infant.

Physical Examination of the Respiratory System

One or more of the major signs of respiratory difficulty (e.g., cyanosis, tachypnea, grunting, retractions, and nasal flaring) are usually present in neonates with both pulmonary and nonpulmonary causes of respiratory distress. Observation of the distressed infant with the unaided eye and ear is the clinician's first step in the physical assessment. Cyanosis may be central, as caused by pulmonary disease and cyanotic heart disease, or peripheral, as occurs in conditions with impaired CO. Tachypnea typically manifests infants with decreased lung compliance such as RDS, whereas patients with high airway resistance (e.g., airway obstruction) usually have deep but slow breathing. Grunting is produced by an adduction of vocal cords during expiration. Grunting holds gas in the lungs throughout expiration, which helps maintain lung volume and avoid alveolar collapse. At the end of expiration the gas is released and rapidly propelled causing an audible grunt. Grunting is more typical of infants with decreased functional residual capacity such as preterm infants with RDS. Chest wall retractions occur more often in very premature infants because of the highly compliant chest wall (Bates & Balisteri, 2002). When the infant is intubated, observation of the chest gives important information. Careful observation of chest wall excursions produced by the ventilator allows the clinician to adjust the magnitude of the ventilator pressure so that optimal gas exchange is achieved while risk of barotrauma is minimized. The chest of an intubated infant should move only slightly than that of a healthy spontaneously breathing infant. The clinician should assess the appropriateness of the magnitude of the chest expansion in ventilated patients. The nurse should assess for and report changes in chest rise in an intubated infant. Abrupt decreases in the chest rise may indicate atelectasis, a plugged endotracheal tube, a pneumothorax, or ventilator failure. Slow decreases in the chest rise over the hours may indicate of a deteriorating lung compliance or gas trapping. An over-inflated thorax, as determined from radiographs, is a sign of gas trapping. In the intubated infant, this observation should prompt the clinician to adjust the positive end-expiratory pressure (PEEP) or expiratory time so that gas trapping and air leakage are prevented. An anguished intubated infant with cyanosis and gasping efforts may have endotracheal tube obstruction.

Careful attention should be given to the sounds that emanate from the respiratory tract, as variations in quality often aids in localization of the source of respiratory distress. Stridor is common in neonates with upper airway and laryngeal lesions. Inspiratory stridor occurs most often with upper airway and laryngeal lesions, whereas expiratory stridor suggests lower airway problems. Hoarseness is a common sign of laryngeal disorders. Forced inspiratory efforts may indicate upper airway or laryngeal involvement, whereas expiratory wheezes suggest a lower airway disease. Congenital airway disorders that may cause respiratory distress in the neonate are included in Figure 21-3.

> ### BOX 21-1
>
> #### Neuromuscular Disorders that May Cause Respiratory Distress in the Neonate
>
> Myopathies
> Myasthenia gravis
> Werdnig-Hoffmann disease
> Spinal cord disorder
> Poliomyelitis
> Others

Adapted from Battista MA, Carlo WA (1992). Differential diagnosis of acute respiratory distress in the neonate. Tufts University School of Medicine and Floating Hospital for Children reports on neonatal respiratory diseases, 2(3), 1-4, 9-11.

Auscultation of the chest further aids the examiner. Because they have low lung volumes, infants with RDS have faint breath sounds, usually without rales. In comparison, the infant with pneumonia may have rales indicative of alveolar filling. Auscultation allows the clinician to detect the presence of secretions in the airway and to evaluate the response to physiotherapy and suctioning. Rhonchi may be heard in neonates with airway disease, such as meconium aspiration syndrome (MAS). Unequal breath sounds may be due to a pneumothorax or to one of the many causes of diminished ventilation to a lung lobe (e.g., atelectasis, main stem bronchial intubation, and pleural effusion). A shift of the apex of the heart can occur with a pneumothorax, diaphragmatic hernia, unilateral pulmonary interstitial emphysema, pleural effusion, or atelectasis, which may be differentiated by transillumination of the chest. Dullness to percussion may be due to a pleural effusion or solid mass. Muffled heart tones suggest a pneumopericardium. Respiratory distress may occur in many chest wall disorders that restrict ribcage movements. Increased oral secretions and choking with feedings are common in neonates with a tracheoesophageal fistula. Because newborns are obligate nasal breathers, those with choanal atresia typically improve with crying and have worsening respiratory distress with rest and feeding. Characteristic Potter facies and other compression deformities and contractures may be present in neonates with hypoplastic lungs secondary to oligohydramnios.

Examination of the cardiovascular system and assessment of peripheral perfusion yield many clues toward a diagnosis. Pallor and poor perfusion may indicate anemia, hypotension, or hypovolemia. Polycythemia with plethora may also cause respiratory distress. Cardiovascular signs of congestive failure (e.g., hyperactive precordium, tachycardia, and hepatomegaly), poor CO, pathologic murmurs, decreased femoral pulses, and nonsinus rhythm suggest a primary cardiac cause for the respiratory distress.

When hypotonia, muscle weakness, or areflexia accompanies respiratory distress, a neuromuscular cause should be considered (Box 21-1). In such cases, an accompanying history of less frequent fetal movement often is involved. Sometimes a history of muscular disease exists in the family. Brachial plexus injury or fracture of a clavicle may accompany phrenic nerve injury and diaphragm paralysis.

Abnormalities found on abdominal examination enlighten the examiner to other causes of respiratory difficulty. Abdominal distention that results from causes such as ascites, necrotizing enterocolitis, abdominal mass, ileus, or tracheoesophageal fistula can cause respiratory distress, whereas a scaphoid configuration of the abdomen suggests a diaphragmatic hernia.

Other nonpulmonary disorders such as sepsis, metabolic acidosis, hypothermia, hyperthermia, hypoglycemia, and methemoglobinemia may also cause respiratory distress in the neonate.

Radiographic and Laboratory Investigation.   Radiographic examination is often the most useful part of the laboratory evaluation and may serve to narrow the differential diagnosis. An anteroposterior view is usually sufficient, but a lateral chest radiograph may be useful when fluid, masses, or free air is suspected. Other diagnostic imaging techniques (ultrasonography, fluoroscopy, computed tomography, or magnetic resonance imaging) may be helpful in selected patients. Bronchoscopy allows direct visualization of the upper airway. This technique, albeit invasive and technically difficult, may in selected cases be a great aid in the differential diagnosis and treatment of patients with a suspected airway lesion.

Much can be learned from a relatively small battery of laboratory tests. In the NICU setting, the clinician is often called upon to collect specimens for and interpret results of physiologic testing. Considerable skill is required in sampling both venous and arterial blood from small patients who are at substantial risk for iatrogenic anemia and vascular damage. Ideally, the hospital laboratory is equipped to do most routine tests on microliter quantities of blood. The clinician must monitor total quantities of blood sampled from the infant and be alert to the development of anemia.

Analysis of arterial blood for pH and gas tensions is perhaps one of the most common tasks of the clinicians caring for the infant with respiratory illness. Noninvasive methods to assess gas exchange, such as transcutaneous blood gas measurements or oxygen saturation, may also be used. Because oxygen delivery to the tissues so intimately depends on circulating red blood cell volume, a hematocrit should be performed.

COMMON DISORDERS OF THE RESPIRATORY SYSTEM

A large variety of disorders may afflict neonates. The most common disorders are discussed here. Figure 21-3 lists both pulmonary and nonpulmonary congenital anomalies that cause respiratory symptoms in the newborn infant. Several diseases may start later in the neonatal period and extend into infancy (Box 21-2). The most common is bronchopulmonary dysplasia (BPD), a chronic lung disease that affects newborns, mainly

---

BOX 21-2

Causes of Late Respiratory Distress in the Neonate

Bronchopulmonary dysplasia
Pneumonia (bacterial, viral, or fungal)
Congestive heart failure
Recurrent pneumonitis or aspiration
Upper airway obstruction
Wilson-Mikity syndrome
Idiopathic pulmonary fibrosis (Hamman-Rich syndrome)
Pulmonary lymphangiectasia
Cystic fibrosis
Immature lungs

---

premature infants exposed to mechanical ventilation and oxygen for RDS or other respiratory problems.

Respiratory Distress Syndrome (RDS)

RDS, or hyaline membrane disease (the term hyaline membrane disease originated from the histological observation of alveolar space lined by an eosinophilic membrane formed by cellular debris), is the most common cause of respiratory distress in premature neonates (Bates & Balisteri, 2002). More than 40,000 cases of RDS are estimated to exist per year in the United States (Moise & Hansen, 1998). Fifty to sixty percent of infants born before 29 weeks' gestation have RDS (Lemons et al, 2001) and account for thousands of patient days in the NICUs and millions of dollars in health care expenditures. In rare cases, RDS develops in full-term infants born to mothers with diabetes or in full-term infants who have experienced asphyxia. RDS is progressively more common the lower the infant's gestational age. The lung is deficient in pulmonary surfactant, a surface tension–reducing agent that prevents alveolar collapse at end expiration and loss of lung volume. Progressive atelectasis leads to intrapulmonary shunting, owing to perfusion of unventilated lung, and subsequent hypoxemia. The radiograph displays a characteristic ground glass, reticulogranular appearance with air bronchograms. When the lung inflation is poor, the arterial blood gas analysis usually reveals respiratory acidemia as well as hypoxemia.

Therapy is directed toward improving oxygenation as well as maintaining optimal lung volume. Continuous positive airway pressure (CPAP) or Positive End Expiratory Pressure (PEEP) is applied to prevent volume loss during expiration. In severe cases, mechanical ventilation via tracheal tube is required. Exogenous surfactants (artificial and natural), which are available for intratracheal instillation, improve survival and reduce some of the associated morbidity of RDS. The earlier surfactant is administered, the better the effect on gas exchange. Clinical trials indicate that prophylactic surfactant administration to extremely premature infants in the delivery room is more effective than waiting for the treatment after development of RDS (Soll & Morley, 2000). Prophylactic high-frequency ventilation for treatment of RDS has mixed results, but these new modes of ventilation should be considered as alternatives to conventional mechanical ventilation in specific circumstances, such as in infants with air leaks as interstitial emphysema or bronchopleural fistula and severe respiratory failure. Infants greater than 34 weeks who have RDS and respiratory failure unresponsive to ventilatory management have responded favorably to extracorporeal membrane oxygenation (ECMO).

Nursing care for infants with RDS is demanding; the most unstable infants often require a 1:1 nurse:patient ratio. The nurse must monitor the quality of respirations and observe the degree of difficulty that the infant is experiencing. Worsening retractions may signal progressive volume loss and impending respiratory failure. Arterial blood gas tensions and pH should be measured frequently, and continuous noninvasive monitoring of oxygenation may allow early identification of gas exchange problems. The risk of pneumothorax and right mainstem intubation is high, and the symmetry of breath sounds must be verified regularly. A crying infant loses airway pressure when the mouth is open and therefore must be kept calm when receiving nasal CPAP. The intubated infant must be monitored for appropriate endotracheal tube position and patency. Suctioning of the airway should be done carefully. The suction catheter should be passed only as far as the end of the endotracheal tube because overzealous suctioning can denude the tracheal epithelium (Cordero et al, 2000). Lung volume can be lost during prolonged disconnection from the ventilator. Rapid loss of lung volume can precipitate hypoxemia, so disconnection time is particularly important when high frequency ventilation is being used. Any sudden decompensation should alert the nurse to investigate for ventilator failure, pneumothorax, or tracheal tube plugging (Figure 21-4). These infants often have invasive catheters, and the nurse should be adept at caring for them.

A common complication of RDS in the tiny premature infant is Bronchopulmonary Dysplasia (BPD). BPD generally refers to a chronic obstructive pulmonary disorder characterized by pulmonary fibrosis, bronchiolar metaplasia, emphysema, and interstitial edema. It is most commonly seen in survivors of extreme prematurity who were diagnosed with RDS, but extremely-low-birth-weight infants may develop BPD without history of RDS (Charafeddine et al, 1999). Infants with mild BPD generally include those who continue to require oxygen supplementation for a total of at least 28 days (Jobe & Bancalari, 2001). The diagnosis of moderate or severe BPD is used for those neonates more than 28 days after birth who require oxygen supplementation and/or ventilatory support at 36 weeks of postmenstrual age. The incidence of BPD increases as gestational age decreases. Approximately 20% to 30% of premature infants with birth weights less than 1500 g have moderate to severe BPD. Moderate to severe BPD develops in about 50% of infants with birth weights less than 750 g (Lee et al, 2000; Lemons et al, 2001).

Air Leaks

Pneumothorax is a frequent complication of RDS and other neonatal respiratory disorders. Pneumothorax is just one of a number of entities that compose the air leak syndromes, which are characterized by air in an ectopic location (Box 21-3). Many air leak syndromes begin with at least some degree of pulmonary interstitial emphysema, which is the result of alveolar rupture from overdistention, usually concomitant with mechanical ventilation or continuous distending airway pressure. Pulmonary interstitial emphysema occurs most commonly in preterm infants but may be seen in infants of any gestational age. Lung compliance is nonuniform, and areas of poor aeration and alveolar collapse exist. Interspersed are alveoli of normal or near-normal compliance, which become overdistended. The more normal lung units (those with better compliance) become overdistended and eventually rupture. Air is forced from the alveolus into the loose tissue of the interstitial space and dissects toward the hilum of the lung, where it may track into the mediastinum—causing a pneumomediastinum—or into the pericardium—causing a pneumopericardium. The astute clinician may notice that an infant's chest becomes barrel-shaped with overdistention and that breath sounds become distant on the affected side. In contrast, the infant who suffers a pneumothorax becomes unstable, with development of cyanosis, oxygen desaturation, and carbon dioxide retention. The infant may become hypotensive and bradycardic because the high intrathoracic pressure impedes CO. A tension pneumothorax, in which the free pleural air compresses the lung, is a medical emergency, and prompt relief by thoracentesis or tube thoracostomy is indicated.

Transient tachypnea of the newborn occurs typically in infants born by cesarean section, particularly in the absence of labor. The cause of the disorder is thought to be transient pulmonary edema that results from the infant's "missed" chance during labor to absorb pulmonary alveolar fluid. The chest radiograph may show increased perihilar interstitial markings and small pleural fluid collections, especially in the minor fissure. In contrast to the infants with RDS, infants with transient tachypnea tend to have a normal or low PCO_2. Oxygenation can usually be maintained by supplementing oxygen with a hood, although some infants benefit from a short course of positive pressure support. The infant usually recovers in 24 to 48 hours.

Pneumonia

Pneumonia may be of bacterial, viral, or of other infectious origin (Table 21-2). Pneumonia may be transmitted transplacentally, as has been shown with group B streptococcus, or via an ascending bacterial invasion associated with maternal amnionitis and prolonged rupture of the membranes. The usual organisms of active postamnionitis pneumonia are group B streptococcus, Escherichia coli, Haemophilus influenzae, and, less commonly, Streptococcus viridans, Listeria, monocytogenes, and anaerobes.

A strong association exists between bacterial pneumonias and premature birth, which may be due to a developmental deficiency of bacteriostatic factors in the amniotic fluid. Alterna-

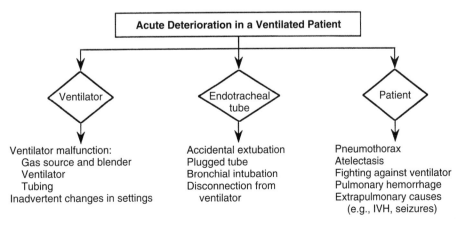

FIGURE **21-4**
Acute deterioration in a ventilated patient.

BOX 21-3

Types of Air Leaks Associated with Respiratory Distress in the Neonate

Pneumothorax
Pulmonary interstitial emphysema
Pneumomediastinum
Pneumopericardium
Pneumoperitoneum
Pulmonary venous air embolism
Subcutaneous emphysema
Pseudocyst

Adapted from Battista MA, Carlo WA (1992). Differential diagnosis of acute respiratory distress in the neonate. Tufts University School of Medicine and Floating Hospital for Children reports on neonatal respiratory diseases, 2(3), 1-4, 9-11.

TABLE 21-2 | **Organisms that May Cause Pneumonia in the Neonate**

Bacterial	Viral	Other
Group B streptococcus	Cytomegalovirus	*Candida* (and other fungi)
Escherichia coli	Adenovirus	*Ureaplasma*
Klebsiella	Rhinovirus	*Chlamydia*
Staphylococcus aureus	Respiratory syncytial virus	Syphilis
Listeria monocytogenes	Parainfluenza	*Pneumocystis carinii*
Enterobacter	Enterovirus	Tuberculosis
Haemophilus influenzae	Rubella	
Pneumococcus		
Pseudomonas		
Bacteroides		
Others		

Adapted from Battista MA, Carlo WA (1992). Differential diagnosis of acute respiratory distress in the neonate. Tufts University School of Medicine and Floating Hospital for Children reports on neonatal respiratory diseases, 2(3), 1-4, 9-11.

tively, the infection may be a precipitating factor in preterm labor. Amnionitis can occur even in the presence of intact membranes. Blood cultures and other diagnostic tests are necessary to help direct specific antimicrobial therapy. The clinician should be attuned to the labor history. Were membranes ruptured for more than 12 to 24 hours? Did the mother have fever before delivery? Did the mother received intrapartum antibiotic if risk factors for group B streptococcus sepsis were present? (CDC, 1996). The full-term infant who exhibits tachypnea, grunting, retractions or temperature instability should be evaluated carefully. Blood counts may be helpful, and the neutropenic infant in particular should be carefully monitored. Infection should be considered in any newborn with respiratory distress or more than transient oxygen requirements. Tracheal aspirates obtained within 8 hours of birth and that show both bacteria and white blood cells on Wright's stain are highly predictive of pneumonia.

Pending culture results, treatment is usually begun with broad-spectrum antibiotics (e.g., a penicillin) and aminoglycoside or cephalosporin. A lumbar puncture may be undertaken or may be postponed until results of blood culture are obtained. When cultures result in the identification of the organism, the study of antibiotic sensitivity allows the clinician to identify the most effective antibiotic or combination of antibiotics for the causative agent. Antibiotic treatment for up to 10 to 14 days may be necessary.

Persistent Pulmonary Hypertension of the Newborn

Persistent pulmonary hypertension of the newborn (PPHN), or persistent fetal circulation, is a term applied to the combination of pulmonary hypertension (high pressure in the pulmonary artery), subsequent right-to-left shunting through fetal channels (the foramen ovale or ductus arteriosus) away from the pulmonary vascular bed, and a structurally normal heart. The syndrome may be idiopathic or, more commonly, secondary to another disorder—such as MAS, congenital diaphragmatic hernia, RDS, asphyxia, sepsis, pneumonia, hyperviscosity of the blood, or hypoglycemia (Walsh-Sukys et al, 2000).

The neonatal pulmonary vasculature is sensitive to changes in PaO_2 and pH and, during stress, can become even hyperreactive and constrict to cause increased pressure against which the neonatal heart cannot force blood flow to the lungs. If the pulmonary artery pressure is higher than systemic pressure, blood flows through the path of least resistance, away from the lungs through the foramen ovale and the ductus arteriosus. The infant becomes progressively hypoxemic and acidemic, and the cycle perpetuates.

Collaborative management of infants with PPHN demands the greatest diligence that the health care professional can summon. Because the pulmonary vasculature is unstable, almost any event can precipitate severe hypoxemia including routine procedures such as endotracheal tube suctioning, weighing, positioning, and diaper changes, etc. Under these circumstances, minimal stimulation is usually practiced.

Occasionally, sedation and even muscle paralysis are necessary to prevent spontaneous episodes of hypoxemia or deterioration associated with procedures (e.g., suctioning and position changes). Alkalosis—either with bicarbonate infusion or by hyperventilation—often relaxes the pulmonary vascular bed and allows better pulmonary perfusion and thus oxygenation. The approach to therapy should be directed toward preventing hypoxemia and acidosis because the infant may be stable with a PaO_2 around 100 mm Hg and a high pH (usually more than 7.55). The critical pH necessary for overcoming pulmonary vasoconstriction seems to be unique to the individual and may be referred to as a "set point." High applied ventilator pressures predispose the lung to air leak syndromes, further increasing the risk of sudden destabilization. Vasopressor therapy with dopamine and dobutamine is often used in conjunction with hyperventilation. Presumably, they act both to improve contractility of the stressed myocardium, which improves CO, and to raise systemic arterial pressure above pulmonary artery pressure to reduce right-to-left shunting.

When conventional therapies fail, high-frequency ventilation may be attempted. Approximately 30% to 60% of patients who fail conventional mechanical ventilation respond to high-frequency ventilation (Clark et al, 1994). However, the exact role of high-frequency ventilation on mortality or in preventing the need for ECMO needs further evaluation. Since the early 1990s, inhalation of nitric oxide—alone and in association with high-frequency ventilation—has been shown to be a promising new therapy for PPHN (The Neonatal Inhaled Nitric Oxide Study Group, 1997; Davidson et al, 1998).

When oxygenation cannot be accomplished despite the use of conventional mechanical ventilation, high-frequency ventilation, or nitric oxide, ECMO has proven to be an effective therapy (UK Collaborative ECMO Trial Group, 1996). Neonatologists disagree about the exact indications for ECMO, and some centers report impressive survival statistics without the use of ECMO (Mok et al, 1999). However, ECMO often is the only treatment that improves the outcome of some infants who fail less invasive therapies.

Meconium Aspiration Syndrome (MAS)

MAS is the most common aspiration syndrome that causes respiratory distress in neonates. The role of meconium in the pathophysiology of aspiration pneumonia has become controversial. It is unclear whether the material itself causes pneumonitis severe enough to lead to hypoxemia, acidosis, and pulmonary hypertension or whether the presence of meconium in the amniotic fluid is merely a marker for other events that may have predisposed the fetus to severe pulmonary disease. The severely ill infant with meconium aspiration syndrome typically comes from a stressed labor and has depressed cord pH from metabolic acidosis. These infants are often postmature and exhibit classic signs of weight loss, skin peeling, and deep staining of the nails and umbilical cord.

Pulmonary disease arises both from chemical pneumonitis, interstitial edema, and small airway obstruction and from concomitant persistent pulmonary hypertension. The infant may have uneven pulmonary ventilation with hyperinflation of some areas and atelectasis of others, leading to ventilation-perfusion mismatching and subsequent hypoxemia. The hypoxemia may then exacerbate pulmonary vasoconstriction, leading to deeper hypoxemia and acidosis. Infants with MAS may have evidence of lung overinflation with a barrel-chested appearance. Auscultation reveals rales and rhonchi. The radiograph shows patchy or streaky areas of atelectasis and other areas of overinflation.

The depressed infant with meconium-stained fluid should receive endotracheal suction at birth. If the infant has absent or depressed respirations, is hypotonic, or has a heart rate of fewer than 100 bpm, then rapid intubation under direct laryngoscopy to allow for suctioning of the airway is recommended (International Guidelines for Neonatal Resuscitation, 2000). Endotracheal suctioning at birth is used to prevent MAS in the newly born with meconium-stained fluid but is not necessary if the infant is vigorous at birth (Wiswell et al, 2000).

As with other cases of pulmonary hypertension, nursing care of infants with MAS centers on maintenance of adequate oxygenation and acid-base balance and on the avoidance of cold stress, which contributes to acidosis. A high incidence of air leaks exists in these infants, and positive pressure ventilation is best avoided if the patient can be adequately oxygenated, even at very high-inspired oxygen concentrations. Use of antibiotics for these infants is also controversial. No studies have shown that infection is causal, but meconium itself may enhance bacterial growth as a culture medium. Antibiotics are often used, however, particularly in desperately ill infants, at least until a bacterial infection is ruled out. The infant is often exquisitely sensitive to environmental stimuli and should be treated in as quiet an environment as possible. Interventions should be preplanned to maximize efficiency of handling the infant. Infants with very severe respiratory failure and MAS improve with the administration of exogenous surfactant (Lotze et al, 1998).

Although aspiration of meconium is most common, the neonate may become symptomatic due to the aspiration of blood, amniotic fluid, or gastrointestinal contents. The history is important in the differential diagnosis because radiographs are nondiagnostic.

Pulmonary Hemorrhage

Pulmonary hemorrhage is rarely an isolated condition and usually occurs in an otherwise sick infant. RDS, asphyxia, congenital heart disease, aspiration of gastric content or maternal blood, and disseminated intravascular coagulation and other bleeding disorders may play a role in the cause of pulmonary hemorrhage. Pulmonary hemorrhage affects approximately 10% of infants receiving either natural or artificial surfactant. Massive bleeding may also occur as a complication of airway suction secondary to direct trauma of the respiratory epithelium.

Pulmonary hemorrhage is manifested by the presence of bloody fluid from the trachea. When massive, it may be heralded by a sudden deterioration with pallor, shock, cyanosis, or bradycardia. Attention must be given to maintenance of a patent airway because an obstructed endotracheal tube requires emergency replacement. Suctioning must be done with great care to avoid precipitation of further bleeding. Clotting factors can be consumed rapidly, and the nurse should be alert to signs of generalized bleeding.

Pleural Effusions

Pleural effusions may be caused by accumulation of fluid between the parietal pleura of the chest wall and the visceral pleura enveloping the lung. A pleural effusion may also be due to chylothorax (lymphatic fluid) or hemothorax (blood). Lymphatics drain fluid that filters into the pleural space. Fluid accumulates in the pleural space as a result of either increased filtration or decreased absorption. An increase in filtration pressure, as seen with increased venous pressure in hydrops fetalis or congestive heart failure, leads to pleural effusion. The rate of filtration into the pleural space also increases if the pleural membrane becomes more permeable to water and protein, as occurs with infection.

Pleural effusion with high glucose content in an infant who is receiving parenteral nutrition via a central venous catheter should raise the suspicion of catheter perforation into the pleural space. If the infant is also receiving lipid infusion, the fluid may appear milky and be confused with chylothorax.

Chylothorax may be congenital or acquired and is associated with obstruction or perforation of the thoracic duct. It may also be a surgical complication of repair of diaphragmatic hernia, tracheoesophageal fistula, and congenital heart defects. Congenital chylothorax may be suspected in the infant who cannot be ventilated in the delivery room. Breath sounds are difficult to hear, and chest movement with ventilation is minimal. Bilateral thoracenteses may be lifesaving. The typical pleural fluid in a chylothorax—opalescent and rich in fat—is present only if the infant has been fed.

Pleural effusions that impede respiratory function typically require drainage, by thoracentesis or tube thoracostomy. It may be necessary for chest tubes placed for chylothorax and thoracic duct injury to remain in place for extended periods while the infant is given total parenteral nutrition, receiving nothing by mouth, thus minimizing thoracic duct flow.

Apnea

Apnea is the common end product of a myriad of neonatal physiologic events. Hypoxemia, infection, anemia, thermal instability, gastroesophageal reflux, metabolic derangement, drugs, and intracranial disease can cause apnea. An infant with visible respiratory excursions but absent air entry should be examined for obstructive causes of apnea. The presence of a cardiac murmur with bounding pulses should alert the nurse to patent ductus arteriosus as a possible contributor to worsening apnea in the small preterm infant. These causes should be ruled out before idiopathic apnea of prematurity is diagnosed.

Apnea is observed in more than half of surviving premature infants who weigh less than 1.5 kg at birth. The respiratory control mechanism and central responsiveness to carbon dioxide is progressively less mature the lower the gestational age. In contrast to adults, infants respond to hypoxemia with only a brief hyperpneic response followed by hypoventilation or apnea. In any infant who has apnea, hypoxemia should always be ruled out before the clinician embarks on any other workup or institutes therapy.

Care of the infant experiencing apneic episodes requires close observation. Obstructive apnea cannot be detected with the impedance respiratory monitor, because normal or pronounced respiratory excursions of the chest wall exist. Prompt tactile stimulation for mild "spells" is often sufficient to abort the episode of apnea, obviating the need for further therapy. Infants with apneic episodes accompanied by cyanosis and profound bradycardia need prompt attention to their immediate needs as well as more aggressive diagnostic and therapeutic intervention.

Sensory stimulation with waterbeds or other means can sometimes be used to manage these infants, particularly those with mild apnea. Many apneic neonates respond to nasal CPAP at low pressures because the apnea may be due to airway obstruction or intermittent hypoxemia. Pressure support may also stimulate pulmonary stretch receptors, thus stimulating respiration. Nursing care that is directed toward promoting a neutral thermal environment, normoxia, optimal airway maintenance, and prevention of aspiration is essential in the care of neonates at risk for apnea.

Use of methylxanthines, such as aminophylline, has markedly simplified the treatment of apnea in some premature infants. Xanthines appear to exert a central stimulatory effect on brainstem respiratory neurons and often markedly decrease the frequency and severity of apneic episodes. The clinician must be attuned to the toxicities of aminophylline, including tachycardia, excessive diuresis, and vomiting, which may precede neurologic toxicity at inadvertently high blood drug levels. Caffeine may be associated with a lower risk of adverse effects and has similar activity (Steer & Henderson-Smart, 2000).

CONGENITAL ANOMALIES THAT AFFECT RESPIRATORY FUNCTION

Diaphragmatic Hernia

Congenital diaphragmatic hernia occurs at a frequency of 1 in 2500 live births and may be unsuspected until birth. Herniation of abdominal contents into the chest cavity early in gestation is accompanied by ipsilateral pulmonary hypoplasia. By mechanisms that are not well understood, there is often some degree of pulmonary hypoplasia on the contralateral side. Most infants are symptomatic at birth, with severe respiratory distress in the delivery room. The affected newborn's abdomen is usually scaphoid, and breath sounds are absent on the side of the defect (a left-sided defect occurs in 90% of cases). Bowel sounds may be heard in the chest, and heart sounds may be heard on the right side because the herniated abdominal contents push the mediastinum to the right.

As soon as the diagnosis is suspected, bag and mask ventilation should be avoided because it fills the hernia contents with air and can compress the lungs and worsen ventilation. When CDH has been diagnosed prenatally, the infant should be intubated and mechanical ventilation should be begun immediately after birth. An orogastric tube should be placed to aid in decompression of the herniated abdominal viscera. Ventilation should be attempted with a rapid rate and low inflation pressure, thus attempting to minimize ventilator-associated lung injury (Bohn et al, 1996). Symptomatic neonates often have pulmonary hypertension and progressive right-to-left shunting. Hypotension is common, and, when adequate intravascular volume is established, dopamine infusion may be helpful. Pulmonary vasodilators have been advocated by some clinicians and have met with variable success, but they should not be used unless adequate systemic blood pressure can be maintained. Although evidence of surfactant deficiency in these newborns exists, surfactant administration is controversial (Bohn et al, 1996).

Survival rate is poor in infants who are symptomatic at birth, and ECMO commonly is required, often to no avail. Surgery to repair the defect is indicated. Controversy regarding the urgency of the procedure exists among pediatric surgeons, and some prefer to stabilize the patient with mechanical ventilation, vasopressors, and correction of acidosis before undertaking surgical intervention; others perform surgical repair while the patient is maintained on ECMO (Chapter 23).

Congenital Heart Disease

Congenital heart disease commonly manifests with signs of respiratory distress. Neonates with congenital heart disease and who demonstrate right-to-left shunting and decreased pulmonary blood flow (e.g., tetralogy of Fallot, pulmonary valve atresia, and tricuspid valve atresia or stenosis) usually present with profound cyanosis unresponsive to oxygen supplementation. Neonates with congenital heart disease and who demonstrate increased pulmonary blood flow or obstruction to the left outflow tract (e.g., transposition of the great vessels, total anomalous pulmonary venous return, atrioventricular canal, hypoplastic left heart syndrome, and critical coarctation of the aorta) may transiently improve with oxygen supplementation. Neonates with noncyanotic lesions such as patent ductus arteriosus and ventricular septal defect may present with signs of congestive heart failure (Chapter 23).

Choanal Atresia

Choanal atresia causes upper airway obstruction in the neonate. The choanae, or nasal passages, are separated from the nasopharynx by a structure known as the bucconasal membrane, which normally perforates during gestation. Failure of this developmental event results in an obstructed airway, occurring bilaterally in 50% of cases. Most affected infants are female and half of affected infants have associated anomalies as CHARGE (coloboma, heart defects, atresia of the choanae, retardation of growth and development, genital and urinary abnormalities, and ear abnormalities and/or hearing loss) association. Because newborns are obligate nasal breathers, they have chest retractions and severe cyanosis (particularly during feeding), and paradoxically turn pink when crying. Emergency treatment consists of tracheal intubation or placement of an oral airway. Surgical correction is indicated (Park et al, 2000).

Cystic Hygroma

A variety of space-occupying lesions can impose on the airway of the newborn (Box 21-4). Most are derived from embryonic tissues. Cystic hygroma, derived from lymphatic tissue, is the most common lateral neck mass in the newborn. It is multilobular, is multicystic, and, when large, obstructs the airway. Surgery is curative, although it is sometimes technically difficult. The clinician must always be mindful of the airway and its patency. Many of these lesions are of great cosmetic concern and cause great distress in the parents. A care plan should address these parental concerns. It is sometimes helpful to facilitate contact with parents of other children with similar problems who can share similar experiences.

Pierre Robin Syndrome or Sequence

The major feature of Pierre Robin syndrome or sequence is micrognathia (a small mandible). The tongue is posteriorly displaced into the oropharynx, thus obstructing the airway. Sixty percent of affected patients also have a cleft palate. Obstructive respiratory distress and cyanosis are common and may be severe. In an emergency, as with all airway obstructions (obstructive apnea), tracheal intubation should be undertaken. Infants with Pierre Robin syndrome or sequence are nursed in the prone position to prevent the tongue from falling backward. Nasogastric tube feedings are usually required in the neonatal period. With good care, the infant has a good prognosis for survival; the mandible usually grows; and the problem resolves by 6 to 12 months of age.

The newer term for this condition, in many cases, is sequence, but syndrome can also be used because the clusters of symptoms can occur in many ways. Sequence refers to a pattern that is a result of a single problem in morphogenesis that leads to this variety of problems. Syndrome is usually used when no one determinant can be identified. For example, it may result from multifactorial inheritance, may be part of other conditions, or may be genetic (whereby one or more genes are responsible). Thus this condition is more than just an explainable, describable syndrome or a sequence of visible defects (Van den Elsen et al, 2001).

COLLABORATIVE MANAGEMENT OF INFANTS WITH RESPIRATORY DISORDERS

Supportive Care

Supportive care of the infant in respiratory distress requires attention to detail. The clinicians' primary goals are to minimize oxygen consumption and carbon dioxide production. These goals are accomplished by maintaining a neutral thermal environment and ensuring normoxia. The nurse must be skilled in physical assessment to interpret signs and symptoms, such as cyanosis, gasping, tachypnea, grunting, nasal flaring, and retractions. By understanding the pathophysiology of breathing, the nurse knows that the infant with retractions has decreased lung compliance and that the cyanotic infant has poor tissue oxygenation.

Excellent communication is needed between the neonatal nurse and the rest of the neonatal team. Acutely ill neonates with respiratory disease are often unstable, and their condition can deteriorate rapidly, so astute observation skills are necessary. Assessment is a continuous process, and effective communication among nurses, respiratory therapists, physicians, and supportive staff is necessary for proper delivery of intensive care. The nurse, who is the primary bedside caregiver, is the gatekeeper for all interactions between the patient and the environment. The nurse who is caring for an unstable patient should be the patient's advocate, whether such a role involves regulating the timing of a physical examination by the physician or venipuncture for laboratory investigation.

Technical competence is an important facet of the nurse's repertoire. The nurse is responsible for maintaining intravenous lines and tracheal tube patency, accurately measuring volumes of intravenous intake as well as urinary output, and operating advanced electronic machinery. Moreover, the nurse must also be adept at interpreting arterial blood gas and laboratory data in order to communicate these to the rest of the care team and to develop a cogent management plan. Many functions are shared to some degree with respiratory therapists. Whether nurses or respiratory therapists make ventilator changes, the nurse should become familiar with the effects of ventilator setting changes on blood gases. $PaCO_2$ is affected briefly by changes in ventilator rate and tidal volume. Tidal volume depends on the difference between PIP and PEEP. Thus, to decrease $PaCO_2$, either rate or inspiratory pressure should be increased. PaO_2 depends on the fraction of inspired oxygen concentration (FiO_2) and mean airway pressure (MAP). MAP depends on PIP, PEEP, inspiratory to expiratory time ratio, and gas flow. To improve PaO_2, the most effective changes are to increase MAP by increasing PIP or PEEP or to increase FiO_2. Table 21-3 shows the effect of ventilator setting changes on blood gases. The nurse should also be familiar with ventilator functioning so that malfunctions can be detected promptly. The nurse should always be prepared to bag-ventilate an intubated neonate in the event that decompensation occurs while the status of the ventilatory

---

BOX 21-4

Thoracic Cysts and Tumors that May Cause Respiratory Distress in the Neonate

Teratoma
Cystic hygroma
Neurogenic tumor
    Neuroblastoma
    Ganglioneuroma
    Neurofibroma
Bronchial or bronchogenic cyst
Intrapulmonary cyst
Gastrogenic cyst
Hemangioma
Angiosarcoma
Mediastinal goiter
Thymoma
Mesenchymoma
Lipoma
Cystic adenomatous malformation

Adapted from Battista MA, Carlo WA (1992). Differential diagnosis of acute respiratory distress in the neonate. Tufts University School of Medicine and Floating Hospital for Children reports on neonatal respiratory diseases, 2(3), 1-4, 9-11.

TABLE **21-3**	Effects of Ventilator Setting Changes on Blood Gases		
Ventilator Setting Changes		**PaCO₂**	**PaO₂**
≠PIP		Ø	≠
≠PEEP		≠	≠
≠Frequency		Ø	±≠
≠I:E ratio		æ	≠
≠FiO₂		æ	≠
≠Flow		±Ø	±≠

≠, increase; Ø, decrease; ±, minimal effect; æ, no consistent effect; FiO_2, fraction of O_2 in dry inspired air; PEEP, positive end-expiratory pressure; PIP, peak inspiratory pressure.
Modified from Carlo WA, et al (1994). Advances in conventional mechanical ventilation. In Boynton BR et al (Eds.), New therapies for neonatal respiratory failure (p. 144). New York: Cambridge University Press.

apparatus is checked. Nurses and therapists often share such functions as airway suctioning, monitoring and recording of inspired oxygen concentration, and delivery of chest physical therapy.

The delivery of oxygen therapy should always be carefully monitored. Desired oxygenation parameters should be recorded in the nurses' notes and followed up with measurement of arterial blood gases or by noninvasive means. The acutely ill infant should have FiO_2 measured continuously and recorded frequently. The goal for oxygenation depends on the patient's diagnosis and condition. For example, in infants with PPHN, an apparently acceptable saturation may occur despite marked right-to-left shunting. In preterm infants oxygen saturation can be kept in the low nineties, thus avoiding the risks associated to hyperoxia in preterm infants (The STOP-ROP Multicenter Study Group, 2000). Procedures such as suctioning, chest physiotherapy, and handling may lead to desaturations and may have to be minimized.

Airway suctioning is a procedure that may be associated with cardiopulmonary derangement, hypoxemia, bradycardia, and hypertension. Different techniques to perform airway suctioning exist—including preoxygenation (increase in FiO_2 before the procedure), normal saline instillation before the suctioning to improve secretion aspiration, and the use of closed system to avoid disconnection from the ventilator. The nurse should become familiar with the techniques used in the NICU and be aware of the associated complications.

The sudden decompensation of a ventilated infant should alert the nurse to assess disconnection of the ventilator, pulmonary air leak, ventilator failure, or obstructed tracheal tube (Figure 21-4). The very small infant who suddenly decompensates may have experienced a severe intracranial hemorrhage.

Care of the infant who is receiving CPAP can be particularly challenging. These infants should be kept calm and swaddled if necessary. Crying releases pressure through the mouth; thus lung volume is lost. Nasal CPAP can be effective, but particular attention must be given to maintaining patency of the nose, the nasal prongs, and the pharynx. The infant's nares and nasal septum should be guarded from pressure necrosis from inappropriately applied prongs. The infant who requires mechanical ventilation must be constantly assessed for airway patency. If the infant is unable to grunt against a closed glottis and to maintain positive airway pressure, the condition may worsen if airway pressure is not maintained properly. Suctioning of the airway should be done only as often as necessary to remove pulmonary secretions that could occlude the airway. The suction catheter should be passed no further than the end of the tracheal tube because epithelium is easily damaged. Vibration and percussion should be used judiciously in the infant with pulmonary secretions to loosen them and allow removal via suction. There is perhaps little need to vigorously suction the intubated infant with RDS in the first 24 hours because secretions are minimal and lung volume is lost with every disconnection of the ventilator circuit.

ASSESSMENT AND MONITORING

The most important aspect in monitoring patients with respiratory disease is the close and continuous observation of signs and symptoms. The color of the patient gives important clues. An infant with pink lips and oral mucosa has good oxygenation and perfusion; a cyanotic patient has poor tissue oxygenation. If the hemoglobin concentration is too low, the patient can be hypoxemic, but because the concentration of deoxyhemoglobin is low, there may be no cyanosis. An infant with tachypnea and retraction usually has decreased lung compliance. A patient with barrel-shaped thorax, taking deep breaths, and with a normal or low respiratory rate probably has an increased airway resistance and gas trapping. Observation of the intubated patient is especially important. An anguished infant, who is cyanotic and breathing deeply, may have an obstructed endotracheal tube. An infant with RDS and increased chest expansion over time, despite no change in ventilatory pressure, is experiencing improvement in lung compliance. The same infant with later asymmetry in chest and sudden deterioration of oxygenation may have a pneumothorax. Cardiac beats, easily seen through the thoracic wall, may be caused by the presence of a symptomatic patent ductus arteriosus. A recently extubated infant, in whom increased retractions and inspiratory stridor develop, probably has upper airway obstruction. Auscultation helps in the diagnosis of increased airway resistance or the presence of secretions. It also allows the clinician to assess the response to different treatment maneuvers, such as suctioning, chest physiotherapy, and bronchodilation. Asymmetries in auscultation suggest mainstream bronchial intubation, atelectasis, pneumothorax, or pleural effusion.

Great progress has been made in noninvasive monitoring of blood gas tensions, but blood sampling is still necessary for pH determination and arterial samples are preferable. Capillary specimens are undependable, especially for PO_2. If peripheral perfusion is adequate, capillary blood approximates arterial values of pH and PCO_2. However, capillary blood PaO_2 values do not reliably reflect arterial oxygenation.

Neonatal care has changed dramatically with the advent and widespread use of transcutaneous monitoring of PaO_2, $PaCO_2$, and SaO_2. The neonatal intensive care team should become familiar with the devices used in noninvasive gas monitoring. Knowing the basis for their functioning as well as how to interpret the information they provide and being aware of clinical situations in which the information provided is not reliable or needs to be complemented before any management decisions are made is essential.

Transcutaneous PO_2 ($TcPO_2$) is measured with an electrode that is applied over the skin and heated to 42° C to 44° C. The electrode measures skin PO_2, not arterial PO_2. Skin PO_2 measurement depends on skin perfusion and on oxygen diffusion across the epidermis. Warming the skin to 42° C to 44° C under the electrode increases skin perfusion so that $TcPO_2$ correlates better with arterial PO_2. For initiation of $TcPO_2$ monitoring, 10 to 15 minutes are needed to obtain a stable reading. After that, $TcPO_2$ reflects changes on FiO_2 with a 10 to 20 second delay. After 4 to 6 hours, the method becomes unreliable because of changes in skin secondary to hyperthermia, so the electrode position should be changed. In premature infants with more labile skin, the electrode placement should be changed even more frequently to avoid skin burns. The nurse should be aware of situations that make $TcPO_2$ lose its reliability. Overestimation of oxygenation occurs when an air bubble or leak between the electrode and the skin occurs or when the calibration is improper. Underestimation occurs with skin hypoperfusion, in older infants (increased thickness of the skin), with insufficient heating of the electrodes, or with improper calibration.

$TcPO_2$ monitoring has been largely supplanted by continuous pulse oximetry. Arterial oxygen saturation is computed from absorption of emitted low-intensity red or infrared light. The probe is attached to a finger or toe in large infants or to a hand or foot in small premature infants. Pulse oximetry offers the following advantages over transcutaneous oxygen monitoring: (1) avoidance of heating the skin and the risk of burns; (2) elimination of a delay period for transducer equilibration; (3) accurate measurement regardless of presence of edema or patient age; (4) in vitro calibration not required; and (5) frequent position changes not required. However, the nurse should be aware that SaO_2 higher than 97% may be associated with PaO_2 higher than 100 mm/Hg. This is important in premature infants who are at risk for retinopathy of prematurity. SaO_2 between 92% and 97% is associated with a safe range of PaO_2—that is, 45 to 100 mm Hg. With SaO_2 over 97%—and especially when it is 100%—the clinician cannot predict a patient's PaO_2. When the saturation is 100%, the PaO_2 can be 100 mm Hg or even higher (Figure 21-1). This situation is particularly important in infants with PPHN because the decision whether to wean ventilator settings depends on PaO_2. In these patients, the simultaneous use of $TcPO_2$ and pulse oximetry is a useful alternative.

A common problem of pulse oximetry is the presence of motion artifact, an altered signal caused by movement of the part of the body where the sensor is applied. Because the pulse waveform is not detected, this movement is recognized by the loss of correlation between the oximeter pulse rate and the electrical monitor heart rate. With new technology the motion artifacts have been minimized (Malviya et al, 2000). Peripheral pulse oximetry may not detect pulse signals in patients with hypotension and poor perfusion. $TcPO_2$ may also give false readings in this situation. The clinician should be aware that pressure of the probe over the skin can produce skin pressure necrosis. This consideration is particularly important in the premature infant. Phototherapy may interfere with accuracy of SaO_2 monitoring, but this problem can be avoided by covering the sensor with an opaque material (e.g., a diaper).

$TcPO_2$ monitoring and pulse oximetry are useful in several clinical situations. They may be used in neonates with mild respiratory distress, such as transient tachypnea, to assess the oxygen requirement, and to allow weaning without placement of an arterial catheter. In infants receiving mechanical ventilation, $TcPO_2$ or pulse oximetry helps to assess the effects of ventilator setting changes, thus reducing the need for arterial blood sampling. Continuous oxygenation monitoring reduces the risk of hyperoxemia or hypoxemia during interventions

such as airway suctioning, position change, lumbar puncture, or venous cannulation. This monitoring is particularly helpful in the care of infants who do not tolerate excessive stimulation, such as those with PPHN. $TcPO_2$ and pulse oximetry monitoring are also useful in caring for patients with PPHN because simultaneous monitoring of preductal (head, right arm, right upper chest) and postductal (left arm, abdomen, legs) $TcPO_2$ or SaO_2 allows assessment of the magnitude of ductal shunting or the response to therapies such as vasodilation or alkalinization.

Transcutaneously measured PCO_2 is accomplished with a glass electrode that is pH-sensitive. Transcutaneous PCO_2 response is slower than that of $TcPO_2$, and the value measured must be corrected for skin production of carbon dioxide. Thus transcutaneously measured values are 1.37 times higher than arterial PCO_2 values. Most modern monitors display an electronically corrected value to $TcPO_2$. This modality is especially useful for monitoring chronically ventilated patients without indwelling catheters. Blood gas values during arterial puncture or vigorous crying during the procedure are often affected by breath holding and shunting and thus may be misleading.

ENVIRONMENTAL CONSIDERATIONS

Maintenance of the therapeutic environment is an important nursing function. Much attention has been given recently to the effects of sensory stimulation on the infant with respiratory distress. The sick newborn often has unstable pulmonary vasculature and may be particularly prone to hypoxic vasoconstriction. This phenomenon may be triggered in some individuals by excess stimulation, such as loud noise, handling, or venipuncture. It has been shown that the agitated neonate has more difficulty with oxygenation and that a quiet, minimally stimulating environment allows for more stable oxygenation (Als, 1996). The nurse should develop a care plan that allows the baby long periods of undisturbed rest by clustering interventions into short periods whenever possible. Positioning the infant in the flexed or fetal position or "nesting" may help in calming some infants.

FAMILY CARE

Neonates with respiratory distress frequently require multiple instrumentation. They may have endotracheal tubes, umbilical catheters, oximeter probes, chest leads, and other paraphernalia attached or applied to the skin. All of these interventions can give parents an unnatural feeling or increased separation from the infant. The nurse should explain the equipment surrounding the bedside as well as the function of invasive catheters, monitoring leads, and tracheal tubes. Terminology appropriate to the parents' level of understanding should be used. Even the most astute parents may be bewildered, and repetition is necessary. Staff should maintain consistent terminology so that the parents do not become confused between "respirators" and "ventilators." Whenever possible, the use of frightening or inaccurate terms should be avoided. Imagine the fear engendered by the phrase, "We paralyzed your baby last night."

Parents should be involved in developing and implementing the plan of care as much as possible. The mother who plans to breastfeed can be assisted in pumping her breasts and freezing the milk, even if enteral feedings are delayed for some time. This pumping may be the only thing that she alone can do for her baby.

Often lost in the bustle of critical care is the need for privacy. The perceptive nurse senses this need and backs away from the bedside when appropriate, allowing the parent some time with the infant.

SUMMARY

Most infants admitted to the NICU have respiratory illness. Nursing care of these infants requires a broad knowledge of newborn physiology and practical skills in the application of therapies that are directed toward solving the many problems that sick infants can have. The nurse often must anticipate these problems. While managing the nursing care for several patients, the neonatal nurse must also care for the sickest of infants. Parents and family of all infants in the NICU require special attention not only to achieve an understanding of the complex issues surrounding the infant's illness but also to calm fears and guilt that are often experienced. The rewards of being part of the accomplishments in the NICU may be overlooked as they are usually slowly achieved. But, when they are recognized, the victories surpass the greatest of expectations.

REFERENCES

Als H (1996). The very immature infant environmental and care issues. Presentation at The Physical and Developmental Environment of the High Risk Neonate. Graven Conference, Graven Study Groups of the Physical and Developmental Environment of the High Risk Neonate, Clearwater Beach, FL.

Bates MD, Balistreri WF (2002). The neonatal gastrointestinal tract: part one: development of the human digestive system. In Fanaroff AA, Martin RJ (eds). *Neonatal-perinatal medicine: diseases of the fetus and infant*, ed 7, St Louis: Mosby.

Bland RD (1998). Formation of fetal lung liquid and its removal near birth. In Polin and Fox, *Fetal and neonatal physiology*, ed 2, Philadelphia: WB Saunders.

Bohn DJ, et al (1996). Postnatal Management of Congenital Diaphragmatic Hernia. *Clinics in perinatology*, 23, 843-872.

Carlo WA, et al (1994). Advances in conventional mechanical ventilation. In Boynton BR, et al (Eds): *New therapies for neonatal respiratory failure*. New York: Cambridge University Press.

Charafeddine L, et al (1999). Atypical Chronic Lung Disease Patterns in Neonates, *Pediatrics*, 103, 759-765.

CDC (1996). Prevention of perinatal group B streptococcal disease: a public health perspective. Centers for Disease Control and Prevention. MMWR *Morbidity & mortality weekly report*. May 31, 45 (RR-7), 1-24.

Clark RH et al (1994). Prospective, randomized comparison of high frequency oscillation and conventional ventilation in candidates for extracorporeal membrane oxygenation. *Journal of pediatrics*, 124 (3), 447-454.

Cordero L et al (2000). Comparison of a closed (trach care MAC) with an open endotracheal Suction System in Small Premature Infants. *Journal of perinatology*, 20, 151-156.

Davidson D, et al (1998). Inhaled nitric oxide for the early treatment of persistent pulmonary hypertension of the term newborn: a randomized, double-masked, placebo-controlled, dose-response. *Multicenter study pediatrics*, 101, 325-334.

Hodson WA (1998). Normal and abnormal structural development of the lung. In Polin and Fox: *Fetal and neonatal physiology*, ed 2, Philadelphia: WB Saunders.

International Guidelines for Neonatal Resuscitation (2000). An Excerpt from the Guidelines 2000 for Cardiopulmonary Resuscitation and Emergency Cardiovascular Care: International Consensus on Science. *Pediatrics*, 106(3). URL: http://www.pediatrics.org/cgi/content/full/106/3/e29

Jobe AH, Bancalari E (2001). Bronchopulmonary dysplasia. *American journal of respiratory critical care medicine*, 163, 1723-1729.

Lee SK et al (2000). Variations in practice and outcomes in the Canadian NICU network: 1996-1997. *Pediatrics*, 106, 1070-1079.

Lemons JA et al (2001). Very low birth weight outcomes of the National Institute of Child Health and Human Development Neonatal Research Network, January 1995 through December 1996, *Pediatrics*, 107: e1.

Lotze A et al (1998). Multicenter study of surfactant (beractant) use in the treatment of term infants with severe respiratory failure, *Journal of Pediatrics*, 132, 40-47.

Malviya S et al (2000). False alarms and sensitivity of conventional pulse oximetry versus the Masimo SET technology in the pediatric postanesthesia care unit. *Anesthesia & Analgesia*, 90(6), 1336-1340.

Moise AA, Hansen TN (1998). Acute, acquire parenchy mal lung disease. In Hansen TN, et al (Eds.), *Contemporary diagnosis and management of neonatal respiratory diseases*. Newton, PA: Handbooks in Health Care.

Mok Q et al (1999). Persistent pulmonary hypertension of the term neonate: a strategy for management. *European journal of pediatrics*, 158, 825-827.

Nelson N (1994). Physiology of transition. In Avery GB, et al (Eds.), *Neonatology, pathophysiology and management of the newborn*, ed 4, Philadelphia: JB Lippincott.

Park AH (2000). Endoscopic versus traditional approaches to choanal atresia. *Otolaryngology Clinics of North America*, 33, 77-90.

Soll RF, Morley CJ (2000). Prophylactic versus selective use of surfactant for preventing morbidity and mortality in preterm infants. *Cochrane database systems review*, 2, CD000510.

Steer PA, Henderson-Smart DJ (2000). Caffeine versus theophylline for apnea in preterm infants. *Cochrane database systems review*, 2, CD000273.

The Neonatal Inhaled Nitric Oxide Study Group (1997). Inhaled nitric oxide in full-term and nearly full-term infants with hypoxic respiratory failure. *New England journal of medicine*, 336(9), 597-604.

The STOP-ROP Multicenter Study Group (2000). Supplemental therapeutic oxygen for prethreshold retinopathy of prematurity (STOP-ROP): a randomized, controlled trial. I: Primary outcomes. *Pediatrics*, 105, 295-310.

UK Collaborative ECMO Trial Group (1996). UK collaborative randomised trial of neonatal extracorporeal membrane oxygenation. *Lancet*, 348(9020), 75-82.

Van den Elsen AP et al (2001). Diagnosis and treatment of the Pierre Robin sequence: results of a retrospective clinical study and review of the literature. *European journal of pediatrics*, 160, 47-53.

Walsh-Sukys MC et al (2000). Persistent pulmonary hypertension of the newborn in the era before nitric oxide: practice variation and outcomes. *Pediatrics*, 105, 14-20.

Wiswell TE et al (2000). Delivery room management of the apparently vigorous meconium-stained neonate: results of the multicenter, international collaborative trial. *Pediatrics*, 105:1-7.

CHAPTER 22

New Technologies Applied to the Management of the Respiratory System

Jonathan E. Schwartz

This chapter focuses on innovative technologies and newer strategies for the management of intractable hypoxemia and respiratory failure in the newborn. These include exogenous surfactant administration, conventional and high frequency ventilation, inhaled nitric oxide, extracorporeal membrane oxygenation, and liquid ventilation. Discussion of these technologies and strategies requires understanding of the pathophysiology of neonatal hypoxemia as well as the standard treatments for hypoxemia in the newborn. Neonatal cardiorespiratory physiology and the physiology of transition are discussed in depth elsewhere in this book and will only briefly be covered in this chapter.

NEONATAL HYPOXEMIA

In the neonate, the transition from complete dependence on the maternal-placental unit for oxygenation to complete respiratory self-reliance must occur rapidly and requires a cascade of immediate responses (Table 22-1). The central nervous system responds to changes in oxygen and carbon dioxide tensions by generating the necessary efferent signals to establish a regular respiratory pattern. The chest wall and its respiratory muscles must have sufficient stiffness and strength to respond to the signals received from the central nervous system. The pulmonary blood flow must be adequate for the delivery of oxygen from the alveolus to the body, and shunting through the ductus arteriosus and foramen ovale must be minimal. Adequate cardiac output is needed to deliver oxygen to the tissues, and the affinity of hemoglobin for oxygen must allow oxygen release to the tissues. All of the above responses need to occur within minutes of birth, and, unsurprisingly, a large proportion of the problems in the neonatal intensive care unit (NICUs) relate to tissue oxygenation.

For numerous reasons outlined in the following sections, preterm newborns are at particular risk for hypoxemia during extrauterine transition. The respiratory control center of the preterm infant often lacks sufficient maturity to sustain regular respiration, as manifested by the frequent occurrence of periodic breathing and apnea. The chest wall may be highly compliant, which leads to inefficient breathing and causes inward or expiratory movement of the rib cage (retractions) during inspiration. The highly compliant chest wall is often confronted with a stiff lung (low compliance) because of surfactant deficiency. This problem causes increased work for the respiratory muscles. The respiratory muscles are also more susceptible to fatigue because they have exercised less *in utero* compared to those of full-term newborns. Surfactant deficiency can lead to airway collapse and intrapulmonary shunting, which severely limit systemic arterial oxygen tension. The preterm ductus arteriosus also may remain patent and shunt blood away from the systemic organs. Furthermore, the preterm newborn's blood hemoglobin concentration is lower than that of the full-term newborn, thereby limiting oxygen-carrying capacity. Finally, there are limits to how much the preterm infant can increase cardiac output to respond to increased oxygen demand or other deficits in oxygen delivery.

Term newborns have different problems that may interfere with the ability to establish adequate tissue oxygenation at birth. Aspiration of meconium, infectious pneumonia, retained fetal lung fluid, and air leak syndromes are some examples of respiratory disorders that can cause intrapulmonary shunting, hypoxemia, and increased the work of breathing for the newborn. Hypoxemia, whether caused by a known respiratory disorder or idiopathic in nature, can result in pulmonary arterioles that remain constricted rather than dilate normally. Constricted pulmonary arterioles elevate pulmonary vascular resistance and lead to a vicious cycle of right to left (pulmonary-to-systemic) shunting, maintenance of pulmonary vasoconstriction, and protracted neonatal hypoxemia. The condition described above is termed persistent pulmonary hypertension of the newborn (PPHN).

Two additional threats to normal tissue oxygenation at birth are anemia and polycythemia. A variety of events may lead to neonatal anemia—including abruptio placenta, placenta previa, fetal-maternal hemorrhage, trauma to the cord or fetal placental vessels, and timing of cord clamping. Anemia results in a diminished oxygen-carrying capacity and thus an increased risk for inadequate tissue oxygenation. Polycythemia may be caused by intrauterine events such as chronic hypoxia and twin to twin transfusion or extrauterine events such as delayed cord clamping. Paradoxically, polycythemia increases blood oxygen-carrying capacity but may decrease tissue oxygen delivery by causing poor tissue blood flow from hyperviscosity or right-to-left ductal shunting.

TABLE 22-1	The Neonatal Respiratory System	
Components	**Functions**
Central and peripheral nervous system	Control of breathing
Chest wall (ribs and respiratory muscles)	Pump
Pulmonary circulation	Oxygen uptake from alveoli
Hemoglobin	Oxygen transport
Systemic cardiac output	Oxygen delivery
Mitochondria	Oxygen-dependent energy production

CONVENTIONAL MANAGEMENT OF NEONATAL HYPOXEMIA

The perinatal caregiver's first line of defense for the prevention or treatment of hypoxemia is an increased inspired oxygen concentration. Although fetal hypoxemia does not respond dramatically to an increase of maternal inspired oxygen concentrations, providing oxygen by mask or nasal cannula to mothers whose fetuses show signs of hypoxia is an accepted mode of therapy in most obstetrical units. Administration of oxygen dramatically increases maternal arterial oxygen tension (PaO_2) but increases fetal PaO_2 by only a few millimeters of mercury. However, because fetal PaO_2 is on the steep portion of the oxygen-hemoglobin dissociation curve, small changes in fetal PaO_2 are associated with relatively large increases in fetal blood-oxygen content.

After birth, the response to an increased inspired oxygen concentration in the hypoxic newborn depends on the cause of the hypoxemia. When hypoxemia is caused by hypoventilation, PaO_2 increases in an approximately one-to-one relationship with alveolar oxygen tension. Thus the PaO_2 increases by approximately 60 mm/Hg in the hypoventilating newborn who is placed in 30% oxygen. On the other hand, when hypoxemia is caused by an intrapulmonary or extrapulmonary right-to-left shunt (pulmonary-to-systemic shunt), the neonatal PaO_2 increases minimally in response to an increased inspired oxygen concentration. For example, a newborn with a 50% right-to-left shunt (i.e., 50% of right ventricular output does not pass through the lungs) has a PaO_2 of approximately 50 to 55 mm/Hg in room air. Placing the newborn in a head hood that contains 100% oxygen may raise the PaO_2 to only 60 to 65 mm/Hg. In infants with right-to-left shunts who are placed on oxygen, blood oxygen content may increase significantly because of the position and shape of the oxygen-hemoglobin dissociation curve, although little is gained in terms of PaO_2. Although increasing the inspired oxygen concentration in the hypoxemic newborn may be essential to prevent permanent cell injury or cell death, this benefit must be weighed against the risk for chronic lung disease due to the toxic effects of pulmonary oxygen.

Another technique used in the newborn at risk for hypoxemia is the maintenance of an adequate oxygen-carrying capacity by intermittent blood transfusion. Although few scientific studies have been published, it is empirically accepted that prevention and treatment of anemia in the newborn with cardiorespiratory disease are important aspects of management. For example, transfusion of infants with bronchopulmonary

dysplasia results in decreased use of oxygen. Some studies support the administration of human erythropoietin combined with iron supplementation to reduce the risk of repeated blood transfusions. In one study, using this treatment study patients received significantly less transfusions (1.0 vs. 2.9) than controls (Carnielli et al, 1998). However, this treatment may not be cost-effective because donor blood is usually split into quad packs, and therefore a small but significant reduction in number of transfusions would not reduce exposure to different blood donors.

Decreasing oxygen demand and thus minimizing the newborn's metabolic rate can achieve reducing the risk for cell injury secondary to tissue hypoxia. Depending on the specific thermal environment, the neonatal energy (and oxygen) expenditure necessary to keep warm may be great or small. This relationship has been recognized for more than 40 years and has led to studies designed to define the thermal environment in which energy expended to keep warm is minimal (neutral thermal environment). Attempts to create a near-neutral thermal environment have shown improved survival of sick premature newborns, presumably by favorably affecting the balance between oxygen demand and oxygen supply.

Another critical factor that affects the delivery of oxygen to the tissues is the adequacy of organ blood flow. Organ blood flow may be globally decreased because of decreased cardiac output, thus increasing the risk for tissue hypoxia. Methods commonly employed for maintenance of adequate cardiac output include volume expansion of the hypovolemic newborn and inotropic drugs to stimulate the poorly contractile myocardium. Clinical evaluation often is used to estimate cardiac output, including determination of the rate of capillary refill; determination of the presence or absence of acrocyanosis, skin mottling, or relative coolness of the extremities; and determination of pulse strength and blood pressure. Laboratory aids, including serial hematocrit determinations to diagnose acute blood loss and echocardiography to evaluate cardiac contractility, are at times helpful. Bedside evaluation of neonatal cardiac output is difficult, remains an inexact science, and has little benefit in the long-term outcome of the infant. Therefore it will not be addressed in this text. Determination of the distribution of organ blood flow is also almost impossible. Even when cardiac output is normal or nearly normal, some organs suffer hypoxic insults because of low blood flow. If, for example, necrotizing enterocolitis results in part from decreased intestinal blood flow and thus decreased intestinal oxygenation, it would be useful to be able to estimate that flow. Similarly, decreased urine output may indicate decreased renal blood flow; however, waiting for changes in blood and urine chemistries, (e.g., elevated creatinine) may mean that an irreversible renal hypoxic injury already has occurred. Rapid determination of the distribution of neonatal organ blood flow awaits the development of new methods.

A discussion of strategies now available in NICUs for the management of hypoxemia would not be complete without at least mentioning the widespread use of techniques for measuring or estimating blood-oxygen tension or blood-oxygen saturation. The direct measurement of PaO_2 and oxygen saturation in small samples of blood (0.1 to 0.2 ml) has been available for several years. Although they are not in widespread use, indwelling vascular catheters for the continuous measurement of blood PaO_2 or oxygen saturation are available. Perhaps the most significant technologic development for aiding the management of potentially hypoxic sick newborns has been noninvasive methods of measuring transcutaneous PaO_2 and transcutaneous oxygen saturation nearly continuously to provide fairly reliable estimations of blood-oxygen levels. These critically important new tools for management of sick newborns are discussed in more detail in Chapter 18.

TREATMENT OF NEONATAL LUNG DISEASE WITH EXOGENOUS SURFACTANT

It has generally been accepted for more than 30 years that respiratory distress syndrome (RDS), or hyaline membrane disease, is associated with an abnormal gas-liquid interface in the lung. Normal airways contain a surface-active substance, now called surfactant, that reduces airway and alveolar surface tension and therefore increases lung compliance. In the late 1950s, studies determined that the liquid found in the airways of premature infants and of infants whose mothers had diabetes and who died with RDS had a diminished ability to decrease surface tension in vitro (Avery & Mead, 1959; Pattle, 1958). Thus the hypothesis that decreased lung compliance in infants with RDS was due to lack of surfactant was developed.

RDS is characterized by diffuse pulmonary microatelectasis. Atelectasis causes tachypnea, low tidal volume breathing, and increased work of breathing. Clinically, infants with RDS have retractions as a consequence of decreased lung compliance, expiratory grunting to prevent further atelectasis, and hypoxemia secondary to intrapulmonary shunting. RDS is therefore defined as the immediate onset after birth of tachypnea, retractions, grunting, and cyanosis in a premature infant or in an infant of a mother with diabetes. The chest radiograph in these patients usually confirms the presence of diffuse microatelectasis with uniform increased opacity of the alveolar portions of the lung and widespread air bronchograms. The arterial carbon dioxide tension ($PaCO_2$) may be either increased or normal, thus reflecting the infant's ability to compensate for decreased lung compliance. When the infant breathes room air, the PaO_2 is always decreased because of intrapulmonary shunting. The arterial hydrogen ion concentration (pH) reflects the presence or absence of an elevated $PaCO_2$ and the adequacy of tissue oxygenation. Infants with RDS often have both a metabolic and a respiratory acidosis.

Surfactant Biochemistry and Physiology

Surfactant is generally defined as the noncellular liquid found in the more distal airways and alveoli of normal lungs. Although surfactant contains a mixture of various phospholipids, proteins, and neutral lipids, the extent to which each of these components contributes to the surface tension–decreasing properties of surfactant is not certain.

Surfactant is produced and secreted by cuboid type II pneumocytes that line the distal airways. Phospholipids and surfactant-specific proteins are packaged within intracellular lamellar bodies. These are secreted by exocytosis into the liquid lining layer of the airway. Within the hypophase of this liquid interface between the pneumocytes and lung gas, surfactant forms a regular microscopic latticework called tubular myelin. It is thought that surfactant exerts its surface tension–decreasing activity by the movement of certain surfactant components from the hypophase to the gas-liquid interface. Surface tension is decreased by molecular interactions as the gas-liquid interface is compressed during expiration. An intrapulmonary conservation of surfactant in which "used surfactant" is reabsorbed by the type II pneumocyte, is repackaged, and is resecreted probably exists.

TABLE 22-2	Exogenous Surfactants
Name	**Source**
Calf lung surfactant extract	Bovine
Human	Amniotic fluid
Curosurf®	Porcine
Survanta®	Bovine
Infasurf®	Bovine
Exosurf®	Artificial

Surfactant Replacement

Exogenous surfactant was first given to premature infants with RDS in the mid 1960s. In these studies, dipalmitoylphosphatidylcholine (DPPC) was administered by nebulized aerosol. Clear benefits were not seen in these studies nor in similar human trials in the mid 1970s. Studies of tracheal instillation of exogenous surfactants in surfactant-deficient premature rabbits and lambs, also performed in the 1970s, showed more promise than the early human studies of aerosolized surfactant. Survival was improved, and decreased ventilator pressures were required after instillation of surfactant.

The first convincing human study that pointed to the possible benefits of exogenous surfactant administration to premature humans with RDS was that of Fujiwara and associates (1980). Ten premature infants with RDS were given surfactant on the first day of life. All showed a decreased oxygen requirement and a decreased ventilator positive-pressure requirement. Since Fujiwara's pioneering work, several different exogenous surfactants have been developed and tested in infants with RDS. These exogenous surfactants can be broadly classified into two types: (1) natural surfactants derived from animal lungs or human amniotic fluid, and (2) artificial surfactants composed of "off-the-shelf" chemical mixtures (Table 22-2).

Natural Surfactants.   The natural surfactants that have been developed and tested in premature infants include those of bovine, porcine, and human origin. At least three different bovine surfactant preparations have been evaluated in premature newborns by use of randomized controlled clinical trials.

An organic solvent extract of fluid obtained by lavage of recently slaughtered calves was developed by Enhorning et al and was first reported in 1985. This procedure resulted in a surfactant that contained approximately 97% phospholipid, mostly phosphatidylcholine. Several controlled trials using this type of surfactant, which is referred to as calf lung surfactant extract (CLSE), have been published.

Given intratracheally in the delivery room to preterm newborns, CLSE resulted in improved oxygenation, decreased respiratory support during the first 72 hours of life, shorter duration of total oxygen therapy, and fewer infants with pulmonary interstitial emphysema (Enhorning et al, 1985). As a preventive therapy, surfactant is given intratracheally in the delivery room in the first minutes of life to premature newborns at risk for developing RDS.

The other bovine surfactant subjected to controlled clinical trial was developed by Fujiwara in Japan and adopted by Abbott Laboratories for testing in the United States. This natural surfactant has also been tested in both the prevention and the rescue modes. Given as a single preventive dose in the first 15 minutes of life to infants between 750 and 1250 g birth weight, this bovine surfactant (Survanta®) was associated with a decreased average fraction of inspired oxygen (FiO₂). No differences in alveolar to arterial oxygen ratio, mean airway pressure, or severity of respiratory disease at age 28 days were noted (Soll et al, & Ross Collaborative Surfactant Prevention Study Group, 1990).

A protein-depleted organic solvent extract of minced porcine lung (Curosurf®) has been evaluated in Europe. In the rescue mode, Curosurf® was administered to infants with RDS with birth weights between 700 and 2000 g between 2 and 15 hours of age. Infants randomized to receive Curosurf® showed improved oxygenation, decreased occurrence of air leaks, decreased frequency of bronchopulmonary dysplasia, and improved survival (51% versus 31%). The relatively high mortality in the control group in this study suggests significant unknown differences between this population and those studied with use of other surfactants (Collaborative European Multicenter Study Group, 1988).

A small multicenter randomized study of infants weighing 700 to 1500g compared Curosurf® with Survanta (Speer et al, 1995). This study found that both drugs rapidly reduced oxygen and ventilatory requirements. Curosurf®-treated infants had significantly higher arterial to alveolar oxygen ratios and significantly lower mean airway pressures. Trends that did not reach statistical significance showed a lower frequency of pneumothorax (6% versus 12.5%), intracranial hemorrhage (3% versus 12.5%), and mortality (3% versus 12.5%) in the Curosurf® group.

Artificial Surfactants. Two artificial surfactants have been tested in newborn infants with RDS. Artificial surfactants is distinguishable from natural surfactants by the absence of the surfactant-associated proteins. Exosurf® Neonatal, an artificial surfactant manufactured by Burroughs Wellcome Company (1990), is composed of DPPC, cetyl alcohol, and tyloxapol. Recent studies that compare Exosurf® and Survanta® have been undertaken. One study retrospectively analyzed infants who had received four doses of either Exosurf® or Survanta® for rescue. Survanta® was found to improve respiratory function more quickly as evidenced by lower FiO₂ and mean airway pressure requirements but ultimately had no impact on eventual respiratory outcome (Modanlou et al, 1997). Infasurf® (also a natural surfactant) was compared to Exosurf® in a large randomized, multicenter, blinded study and was shown to be more effective in decreasing the severity of RDS and air leaks even though no difference in survival without BPD or duration of hospitalization was noted (Hudak et al, 1996). Infasurf® was compared to Survanta® in a prospective, randomized, double-blind, multicenter trial in regards to both treatment and prevention of respiratory distress syndrome (Bloom et al, 1997). The treatment arm enrolled infants with established RDS who weighed less than 2001 g, and the prevention arm enrolled infants of 29 or fewer weeks' gestation and with birth weight less than 1251 g. In the treatment-arm infants who received Infasurf® had lower oxygen requirements and mean airway pressures than infants to received Survanta® but no difference in duration of mechanical ventilation, duration of supplemental oxygen, mortality, or chronic lung disease. In the prevention arm, no differences between the two treatments in terms of adverse events, chronic lung disease, or dosing complications were found. However, in a subset of infants under 600 g, Infasurf® treatment was associated with a much higher mortality rate than Survanta® was (63% as compared to 26% p = 0.007).

The survival rate of this subset treated with Survanta® is higher than reported in other studies and is therefore difficult to interpret. A meta-analysis done to compare natural versus synthetic surfactants demonstrated greater improvement in the need for ventilatory support in infants treated with natural surfactants. A significant decrease in the occurrence of air leaks was also demonstrated (Soll & Cochrane Database, 2000).

Surfactant administration is associated with a number of adverse effects. Because surfactant is expected to reach noncolonized portions of the lung, sterile technique must be used during dosing. Some surfactants are given by bolus during disconnection of the endotracheal tube from the ventilator tubing. Exosurf® is given through a side port on specially designed endotracheal tube adapters. All surfactants produce transient gas-exchange abnormalities during administration of the dose, usually hypoxemia and hypercarbia. Transcutaneous PO₂, PCO₂, and oxygen saturation should be monitored continuously during the dosing procedure. Physiologic instability should be expected during dosing, and close monitoring of blood gases and ventilator settings is warranted for a period of 8 to 12 hours after each dose. Under all but emergency circumstances, the American Academy of Pediatrics recommends that surfactant be administered only in nurseries able to sustain long-term mechanical ventilation.

Although exogenous surfactant is used in most tertiary NICUs in the United States, many questions about surfactant administration remain unanswered. The importance of the surfactant-associated proteins to neonatal outcome is unknown. Determination of the appropriate timing, dose, and method of surfactant administration awaits additional clinical trials. It is generally agreed that exogenous surfactant administration provides a net benefit to sick newborns with RDS, but the mortality rates and frequency of chronic lung disease remain high in surfactant-treated infants.

Nursing Care: Surfactant Therapy

Nurses play an important role in caring for infants who receive surfactant replacement therapy in the NICU. The nursing care of the infants before, during, and after surfactant administration is unique to this treatment modality. It is important for nurses to have a working knowledge of the specific care needs of infants treated with surfactant.

Before administration of surfactant, nurses should consider several factors. Accurate weights of the infants must be determined to ensure the proper doses of surfactant to be given. Confirmation of proper placement of the infants' endotracheal tubes by chest radiographs must be documented. These infants should have continuous cardiac and respiratory monitoring. Cardiac monitoring may include electrocardiograms as well as arterial catheters. Respiratory monitoring may include transcutaneous measurement of PO₂ or PCO₂ and pulse oximetry. Nurses may also suggest sedation or increases in ventilator settings before dosing for infants who do not tolerate handling or who become hypoxic quickly. Endotracheal suctioning is another essential part of nursing care prior to the administration of surfactant. These infants should be suctioned approximately 15 minutes before surfactant dosing to rid the infants of secretions that may inhibit the administration of the surfactant.

The nursing care of infants during surfactant dosing is also unique to this treatment modality. Of utmost importance during dosing is the ongoing nursing assessment and monitoring of the infants. Because dosing with surfactant may be stressful for the infants, nurses must be alert for signs that indicate the need to slow or stop the dosing momentarily to allow the infants to recover. Some signs that the infants may be stressed by dosing include bradycardia, duskiness, and decrease in transcutaneous PO_2 or oxygen saturation. Optimal positioning of infants during surfactant administration is another critical facet of nursing care. Infants receive some surfactants, such as Survanta®, in four aliquots, each in a different body position.

The infants are positioned head down, head turned to the right; head down, head turned to the left; head up, head turned to the right; and head up, head turned to the left. The infants are held in each position for 30 seconds after the dose is administered into the endotracheal tube. Administration of Exosurf® requires only turning the head from midline to the right, then midline to the left.

Lastly, nurses have specific responsibilities after surfactant is administered to infants. Immediately after dosing, the nurse should assess the infant's skin color, respirations, oxygen saturation, and transcutaneous monitoring. Arterial blood gas should be sampled, and the ventilator should be weaned appropriately. Surfactant produces changes in pulmonary compliance that generally require rapid weaning of ventilator settings, but some infants may also experience respiratory distress immediately after dosing. Endotracheal suctioning is delayed after dosing of surfactant for at least 1 to 2 hours to prevent removal of the instilled surfactant. Other side effects of this effective therapy are sudden changes in cerebral blood flow, which makes intraventricular hemorrhage a real possibility, and changes in retinal blood flow, which increases chances for retinopathy of prematurity.

CONVENTIONAL VENTILATORY SUPPORT AND RESPIRATORY CONSIDERATIONS

Although this chapter focuses on new technologies, it is important that standard ventilation therapies be briefly mentioned. Both the use of continuous positive airway pressure (CPAP) and conventional mechanical ventilation (CMV) will be discussed.

Continuous Positive Airway Pressure

Continuous positive airway pressure (CPAP) can be defined as the use of positive pressure continuously throughout the respiratory cycle. The use of CPAP generally implies that the infant is breathing spontaneously without the aid of a ventilator. Three devices are commonly used to administer CPAP (nasal prongs, endotracheal tubes, and nasopharyngeal tubes), each with its own advantages and disadvantages. Nasal prongs are noninvasive but may not always transmit optimal pressure to the airway because they are easily dislodged and may cause damage to the nasal septum with prolonged use. Endotracheal tubes give optimal transmission of pressure and can be converted easily to mechanical ventilation but can cause pharyngeal grooves or subglottic stenosis with prolonged use. Nasopharyngeal CPAP is more stable than prongs but can result in nasopharyngeal irritation and plugging with secretions.

Physiologic effects of CPAP are increased transpulmonary pressure with a resultant increase in functional residual capacity, stabilization of collapsed alveoli, and improvement in ventilation/perfusion matching. These improvements lead to better oxygenation and ventilation. In preterm infants with relatively floppy airways, CPAP can provide increased pressure to the posterior pharynx and prevent airway collapse during inspiration and prevent obstructive apnea (Hansen, 1998). Although CPAP is relatively safe, some complications are associ-

ated with its use. Excessive levels of CPAP can raise intrathoracic pressure and compress the right atrium and vena cava, thus compromising venous return. Excessive CPAP may also overdistend alveoli and result in air leaks.

Conventional Mechanical Ventilation

The two types of conventional ventilators commonly used in neonatal intensive care units are pressure or volume ventilators. Pressure ventilators are used more frequently than volume ventilators. These ventilators are constant-flow, time-cycled, and pressure-limited devices. This means there is a constant flow of gas through the endotracheal tube, breaths are given at fixed intervals, and a pre-set peak inspiratory pressure is maintained through the duration of the inspiration. In a pressure-limited ventilator an increase in ventilation (decrease in pO2) can be achieved by increasing ventilator rate or increasing tidal volume. Oxygenation improvement is achieved by increasing the mean airway pressure (increasing PIP, increasing Ti, increasing PEEP, increasing flow, and increasing rate) or by increasing the FiO2. An increase in ventilation (decrease in pCO2) can be achieved by increasing ventilator rate or increasing tidal volume. If compliance changes in a compression ventilator, no change in pressure is delivered. The disadvantages are decreases in tidal volume if the compliance decreases or over-distention if compliance improves.

Volume ventilators deliver the same tidal volume with each breath, regardless of the pressure needed to achieve the pre-set volume. In a volume-limited ventilator, an increase in ventilation is achieved by increasing the ventilator rate or increasing delivered tidal volume. An increase in oxygenation will occur if the FiO2, PEEP, or tidal volume is increased. The disadvantage to the volume ventilator is that a fixed volume will be delivered regardless of changes in compliance and can lead to the use of very high peak inspiratory pressures.

The newer conventional ventilators can use a variety of different operating modes. In this chapter, intermittent mandatory ventilation (IMV), synchronous IMV, and assist control will be briefly discussed. IMV provides a continuous flow of oxygen/air through the ventilatory circuit; however, the neonate can breathe spontaneously. The term mandatory refers to the number of mandatory breaths per minute that are set by the caregiver. The settings allow PIP, rates, inspiratory time, and flow to be adjusted to individual ventilation. This very simply means giving intermittent breaths at a fixed rate. If the infant is breathing faster than the pre-set rate, then the ventilator does not support those breaths. The disadvantage with this mode is that infants may exhale during the ventilator's inspiratory cycle and thus "fight" against the ventilator. SIMV is similar to IMV except that the ventilator senses the infant's spontaneous respirations and mechanically delivered breaths are synchronized to those efforts. If the infant is breathing faster than the set SIMV rate, those breaths are not supported, which is similar to the IMV mode. SIMV is more flexible than IMV and can be used for primary ventilatory support and weaning. However, in some cases SIMV may fail as a weaning mode because at low set rates the infant must exert a considerable work of breathing. In one study in which SIMV was compared to IMV, SIMV was shown to improve oxygenation, reduce the need for long-term ventilation or sedation, and reduce complications such as barotrauma and intracranial bleeds (Hargett, 1995). In a large randomized trial, SIMV was found as effective as conventional ventilation, but no major advantages were demonstrated over conventional ventilation. Assist/control ventilation (A/C) is also known as patient-triggered ventilation (PTV). This therapy uses the spontaneous respiratory efforts of the infant to "trigger" a mechanical breath by the ventilator. In PTV a sensor is used to detect a variety of stimuli such as airflow, airway pressure, chest wall movement, and esophageal pressure. When the machine detects an inspiration, it delivers a breath with a pre-set PIP, inspiratory time, and airflow. PTV is therefore similar to SIMV and has the theoretical advantage of supporting all breaths by the ventilator, even those above the set rate. A disadvantage of patient-triggered ventilation is that very immature infants have weak respiratory effort that does not trigger this machine (Carlo & Ambalavanan, 1999). Backup respiratory rates may be used to reduce this problem. When compared to CMV in a meta-analysis, PTV demonstrated a benefit over CMV with regard to a reduction in air leak and a shorter overall duration of mechanical ventilation (Greenough & Cochrane Database 2000). Further studies need to determine whether PTV causes a reduction in chronic oxygen dependency in comparison to CMV.

HIGH-FREQUENCY VENTILATION

In contrast to HFV, CMV uses ventilator rates and tidal volumes that correspond to the spontaneous ventilation patterns of newborns. High mean and peak airway pressures may be required during CMV to adequately ventilate noncompliant lungs. Exposure to high inflating pressures may lead to lung and airway injury, including pulmonary interstitial emphysema, pneumothoraces, bronchopleural fistulas, and bronchopulmonary dysplasia. HFV attempts to avoid these complications by delivering low tidal volumes at high frequencies. HFV may be used as a "rescue" technique to prevent further damage in infants who have developed complications secondary to CMV. HFV allows severely ill infants to be adequately ventilated at lower volumes than with CMV while improving gas exchange. HFV may be used perioperatively and postoperatively to reduce movement of the airway and thoracic cavity. HFV may be beneficial to infants who have preexisting pneumothoraces or bronchopleural fistulas. There is no generally accepted ventilator rate, which defines the term high frequency. Accepted definitions generally include ventilator rates at 2 to 4 times the natural breathing frequency and ventilation with tidal volumes smaller than anatomic dead space (Eichenwald & Stark, 1999). Gas transport during high frequency cannot be explained by conventional concepts of ventilation and lung mechanics.

Three types of HFV are approved for use in the United States: the high-frequency oscillatory ventilator (HFOV), the high-frequency jet ventilator (HFJV), and the high-frequency flow interrupter (HFFI) (Table 22-3). The HFOV has a diaphragm or piston that oscillates a flow of gas, thus creating both positive and negative pressure changes. Mean airway pressure is generated by gas flow through a filter, which acts as a resistor. The respiratory therapist or clinician can adjust the

mean airway pressure, frequency, and amplitude. The mean airway pressure affects lung inflation and can be increased by increasing MAP oxygenation. The piston amplitude affects ventilation and increases in ventilation occur when amplitude is increased. The HFOV is the only HFV in which inspiration and exhalation are active.

High-frequency jet ventilation (HFJV) delivers tidal volumes that may be less than or greater than anatomic dead space at frequencies of 60 to 600 breaths per minute. HFJV operates similarly to constant-flow time-cycled ventilation with passive expiration. With a HFJV, a high-pressure gas source is connected to a small airway cannula with use of a high-frequency flow interrupter valve. This valve opens and closes rapidly, thus propelling the pressurized gas into the airway. HFJV requires a specific endotracheal tube with a lumen for the jet gas flow and a lumen for the fresh gas flow. The fresh gas flow allows entrainment of gases and addition of PEEP. There is a port, near the jet gas flow lumen, for the instillation of nebulized saline to prevent tracheal erosion. A conventional ventilator may be used with a jet ventilator to provide "background" ventilation or sighs at a low rate. Background ventilation may decrease the risk for microatelectasis that may occur with long-term HFJV. The operator can adjust the PIP of the jet and the CMV as well as the PEEP and frequency. To increase the pO2 the PIP, the operator adjusts PEEP and FiO2. Elimination of carbon dioxide is dependent on the PIP to PEEP pressure difference.

The HFFIs have both conventional and high-frequency options. A high-pressure source of gas is delivered into a standard ventilator circuit, and this flow of gas is interrupted by a valve mechanism that is operated by a microprocessor. The operator can adjust the PIP, PEEP, and frequency. The conventional ventilator is often used to give intermittent "sigh" breaths. Oxygenation depends primarily on the PEEP that is delivered by the conventional ventilator, whereas ventilation depends primarily on the difference between the PIP and the PEEP.

A trial in premature monkeys examined pathologic lung changes in animals after 6 hours of management with one of four strategies: CMV alone, HFOV alone, CMV plus surfactant, and HFOV plus surfactant (Jackson et al, 1994). The group treated with HFOV and surfactant had significantly less proteinaceous edema than with any other management strategy, which allowed speculation that this treatment strategy might reduce the risk for bronchopulmonary dysplasia. The Provo multicenter trial (n = 125) showed that, in comparison to CMV infants, those infants who were treated with the "high-volume" HFOV strategy for RDS, required fewer doses of surfactants and fewer days of oxygen therapy and demonstrated a lower incidence of CLD (24% versus 44%) (Gertsmann et al, 1996). However, this trial enrolled a very small number (n = 21) of infants who were under 1001 g at birth or those infants at highest risk for CLD. There was no increase in IVH. Meta-analysis of six studies that compare HFOV and CMV reveal no difference in mortality between the two modalities (Henderson-Smart & Cochrane Database, 2000).

Trends toward lower rates of CLD but also trends toward increases in grades 3 and 4 IVH and in periventricular leukomalacia exist. If the two trials in which the low-volume strategy was used are eliminated, the outcomes become much more favorable, and an increase in IVH or PVL no longer occurs. Future trials need to elucidate whether a true benefit to HFOV exists and whether the therapy should still be used with some reservations.

Three randomized trials have compared HFJV to CMV (Carlo, 1990; Keszler, 1997; and Wiswell, 1996). Both the

TABLE 22-3	Classification of High-Frequency Neonatal Ventilators	
Type	**Maximal Rate (breaths/min)**	**Expiration**
Pressure-limited, time-cycled	150	Passive
Jet	250 to 300	Passive
Oscillator	1800	Active

studies of Carlo and Wiswell demonstrated no difference in CLD between the two modalities, whereas Kezsler showed a statistically significant decrease in CLD—from 40% to 20%. Of concern was the increase in PVL in the trial conducted by Wiswell. Meta-analysis of these three studies demonstrates no significant increase in mortality or severe IVH (Bhuta & Henderson-Smart, 2000).

Only one large study has used the HFFI (Thome, 1999). In this study 284 very-low-birth-weight infants were enrolled (mean weight HFFI = 888 g versus mean weight CMV = 870 g) and treated with one of the two ventilators. Unfortunately, this study showed no difference in outcome with respect to CLD. As with HFOV, further studies need to determine safety and efficacy of either HFJV or HFFI versus CMV.

Little data from large, multicenter, randomized trials that examine the use of HFV for lung diseases other than respiratory distress syndrome exist. It is generally accepted that HFV is useful in the management of newborns with severe pulmonary interstitial emphysema because airway pressures may be significantly reduced and thus theoretically decrease the risk for further air leak, other pressure-related airway injury, and decreased cardiac output.

Complications Associated with High-Frequency Ventilation

HFV can provide adequate ventilation to infants, but its use is associated with the possibility of complications. The gases that are used during HFV need to be heated to avoid the delivery of cold gas into the airway. Cold air can lead to fluid overload, hypothermia, and necrotizing tracheobronchitis (NTB). NTB is a lesion of the airway that is caused by epithelial erosion and loss of cells in the airway; it is commonly found near the distal end of the endotracheal tube. It leads to formation of granulation tissue that can cause impaired gas exchange, airway obstruction, or atelectasis. With high ventilatory frequencies, the inspiratory and expiratory times are decreased, which may increase the risk for gas trapping in the lungs. Gas trapping occurs less often during HFOV because it is the only form of HFV in which expiration is active. With some high-frequency ventilators, such as the jet and flow interrupter, expiration occurs by passive recoil of the distended respiratory system (lung and chest).

Nursing Care—High-Frequency Ventilation

Caring for infants who receive HFV presents many challenges to NICU nurses. Nurses must adopt new skills and alter those used in caring for infants who are conventionally ventilated. Specific care needs unique to infants who receive HFV include physical assessment, airway management, and positioning and comfort (Tables 22-4 & 22-5).

One of the most challenging yet critical aspects of caring for these infants is the physical assessment. Recognizing subtle changes in the physical exam is critical because these changes may signify changes in the infants' condition. Of extreme importance is the assessment of chest wall vibration, which is an indicator of tidal volume. Even small changes in the vibrations may indicate a change in the neonate's condition. Decreased chest vibration may indicate pneumothorax, endotracheal secretions, and mechanical malfunction (Avila et al, 1994). The noise of the ventilator and the constant vibration of the infants make auscultation of breath sounds, heart tones, and bowel sounds difficult. If oscillating ventilators are used, this evaluation is best done when the infants are momentarily removed from the ventilator (for routine circuit changes) or

when the ventilator is in standby (interruption of oscillation but not from ventilator mean airway pressure). Disconnection from HFV is discouraged because of possible alveolar collapse. Therefore, when necessary, disconnection from HFV should be limited to short periods. If the infant is receiving HFOV, it is also important to auscultate breath sounds to assess the symmetry of oscillatory intensity while he or she is being oscillated (Avila et al, 1994).

The second specific area of care unique to infants who receive HFV is airway management. Suctioning of these infants requires two people—one person to suction and another to either manually ventilate or return the infants to HFV. Remember that disconnection from HFV may lead to alveolar collapse, so the infants may need to be manually ventilated or the mean airway pressure increased after suctioning. It is generally accepted practice to suction infants while they are disconnected from HFOV and HFJV. Positioning and comfort of infants who are receiving HFV are also important facets of care. Because of the physical restraints of the delivery devices and the importance of disconnecting the infant from the ventilator for only short durations, positioning and repositioning become challenging. Two caregivers should be used for repositioning— one to turn the infant and stabilize the endotracheal tube and another to reposition the circuit and ventilator (Avila et al, 1994). Although water mattresses are not recommended, sheepskins, lamb's wool, and egg-crate mattresses may be used to provide comfort and prevent skin breakdown. However, there is rising concern that infants may inhale fibers from sheepskin so it may not be used in some units.

Sedatives, paralytics, and analgesics may be necessary to facilitate comfort for infants while they are receiving HFV. Interventions such as bundling and soothing music may decrease the need for pharmacologic agents. Whereas some believe that

TABLE 22-4	Nursing Responsibilities and Interventions for Oscillated Infants Before High-Frequency Ventilation
Responsibility	**Intervention**
Obtain and record baseline physiologic data	Record temperature, heart rate, respiratory rate, systolic and diastolic blood pressures, transcutaneous PO_2, and PCO_2
Obtain and record baseline biochemical data	Draw blood samples for arterial gases
Maintain current ventilation	Record ventilator parameters: rate, PIP, PEEP, MAP, inspiratory:expiratory ratio, FiO_2
Assemble and prepare equipment	Ensure that infant is attached to monitoring devices for heart rate, intra-arterial blood pressure, transcutaneous oxygen and carbon dioxide
	Check alarms on all monitors
	Assist with arterial line insertion

PIP, *peak inspiratory pressure;* PEEP, *positive end-expiratory pressure;* MAP, *mean airway pressure.*
From Inwood MS (1991). *High-frequency oscillation. In Nugent J (Ed.),* Acute respiratory care of the neonate, *Petaluma, CA: NICU Ink.*

TABLE 22-5	Nursing Responsibilities and Interventions for Oscillated Infants During Oscillation
Responsibility	**Intervention**
Monitor and document physiologic parameters	Record hourly temperature, heart rate, spontaneous respirations, systolic and diastolic blood pressure
	Measure and record accurate intake and output of fluids every 8 hours
Monitor and document biochemical parameters	Draw arterial blood gas samples as ordered
Maintain patent airway	Monitor for continuous vibration of chest
	Assess transcutaneous PO_2 and PCO_2 hourly
	Perform endotracheal suctioning every 2 hours and prn
	Record amount, color, and consistency of secretions
	Assess bilateral air entry while hand bagging at sigh pressures, before and after suctioning
	Ensure adequate humidification of gas flow
Prevent pneumothorax	Maintain ordered MAP
	Observe for decreased vibrations of the chest
	Assess infant for signs of respiratory difficulty: increase spontaneous respirations, increased chest retraction, diminished air entry, increased FiO_2 requirements, increased transcutaneous PCO_2 readings
	Obtain chest radiograph as required and ensure that oscillator is stopped during filming
Provide pulmonary support	Monitor and record MAP, amplitude, frequency, and FiO_2 hourly
	Perform a sustained inflation after endotracheal suctioning and disconnection at ordered pressure and duration
	Record infant's response to sigh
Provide physical care	Reposition infant from side to side or from prone to supine every 2 hours
Provide emotional support to family	Provide accurate, consistent information
	Promote bonding by encouraging nurse specialist or social worker for assistance with coping skills
	Encourage parents to attend parents' support group

MAP, mean airway pressure.
From Inwood MS (1991). High-frequency oscillation. In Nugent J (Ed.), Acute respiratory care of the neonate. Petaluma, CA: NICU Ink.

the noise and the constant vibration may be disturbing to the infants, others believe them to have a calming effect.

INHALED NITRIC OXIDE

In the past 20 years, it has become apparent that vascular endothelium has an important role in the regulation of blood vessel smooth muscle tone as well as in other important physiologic functions. Relaxation of vascular smooth muscle in response to acetylcholine requires an intact endothelium. Nitric oxide (NO) is thought to be the molecule released from the endothelium that is responsible for vascular smooth muscle relaxation. These findings were the catalyst for additional investigations of the biologic effects of NO.

NO has an unpaired electron and therefore rapidly combines with other free radicals. The biologic half-life of the molecule is estimated to be 110 to 130 msec (Lunn, 1995). In vivo, biologic activity of NO is limited because it is rapidly inactivated within the vessel lumen. Inactivation occurs because NO has a high affinity for hemoglobin and avidly binds to the iron of heme proteins to form a biologically inactive compound, nitrosyl-hemoglobin. Nitrosyl-hemoglobin is then oxidized to form methemoglobin and nitrate.

The NO molecule is synthesized from the amino acid L-arginine in a reaction that is catalyzed by a group of enzymes called the nitric oxide synthases (NOS). The by-product of this reaction is L-citrulline: L-arginine molecular $O_2 >$ NO L-citrulline.

Three major types or isoforms of NOS exist. The first isoform is the endothelial or constitutive type, which is located in vascular endothelial cell wall, endocardium, myocardium, and platelets. Neuronal NOS is the isoform located in both the peripheral and central nervous systems. The third isoform, inducible NOS, is not present under normal physiologic conditions but is produced in response to various inflammatory stimuli. Excitation of the inducible NOS causes production of much greater quantities of NO than activation of other isoforms. Activation of inducible NOS during sepsis plays a major part in producing vasodilation and consequent hypotension.

The biologic actions of NO are mediated through the guanylate cyclase-cyclic guanosine monophosphate (cGMP) system. After formation from L-arginine in the endothelial cell, NO readily diffuses into the cytosol of smooth muscle because it is a small, lipophilic molecule. Once inside the smooth muscle cell, NO binds soluble guanylate cyclase, which in turn catalyzes the formation of cGMP from guanosine triphosphate. Increases in cGMP lead to activation of cGMP-dependent protein kinase, which triggers a reduction in intracellular calcium concentration through extrusion and sequestration. The decreased calcium concentration causes smooth muscle relaxation.

NO is a biologic mediator of a variety of physiologic responses in numerous systems in the body. In the healthy state, the arterial circulation is partially dilated by basal production of NO in the endothelium. At birth, production of endogenous NO in response to rhythmic distention of the lung, shear stress, and acetylcholine release plays a major role in mediating a decrease in pulmonary vascular resistance. In addition to being an important determinant of basal tone in small arteries and arterioles, NO inhibits platelet aggregation and adherence and may alter vascular permeability. In the nervous system, NO may have a role in memory formation, pain perception, and electrocortical activation, but more research is needed to support this hypothesis. In the gastrointestinal and genitourinary tracts, NO participates in control of signals that regulate smooth muscle relaxation. NO is produced in large quantities in response to various immunologic stimuli. It may also have a role in nonspecific immunity because it is generated when macrophages are activated.

A particularly frustrating problem for caregivers in the NICU is the treatment of acute hypoxic respiratory failure due to pulmonary arterial vasoconstriction. Successful adaptation for extrauterine life depends on the ability of the fetus to make a transition from fetal to postnatal circulation. A variety of factors, probably related to adverse intrauterine events, may alter the ability of the newborn to decrease pulmonary vascular resistance at birth and make this adaptation. When pulmonary vascular resistance remains elevated postnatally, blood is shunted right to left across the ductus arteriosus and foramen ovale and away from the lungs, thus causing hypoxemia. This condition, PPHN, is seen either in isolation or in conjunction with various diseases such as meconium aspiration syndrome, severe birth asphyxia, sepsis, congenital diaphragmatic hernia, and RDS. In the past, pharmacologic interventions—such as tolazoline, an alpha-adrenergic blocker with histamine-like properties—have been used to decrease pulmonary vascular resistance. However, the effects of these drugs are unpredictable and inconsistent, and because they are not selective for the pulmonary bed, nearly 50% of patients develop systemic hypotension. Sodium nitroprusside is another drug that causes vasodilation through activation or release of NO, but it is not selective for the pulmonary arterial bed and decreases systemic vascular resistance as well. Other intravenous vasodilators, such as prostaglandin I_2 and adenosine triphosphate-magnesium chloride, may selectively decrease pulmonary vascular resistance. The ideal agent for the treatment of pulmonary hypertension would be one that causes pulmonary vasodilation without decreasing systemic vascular resistance.

The early 1990s saw the development of theories that inhaled NO would diffuse from the alveolar space across the epithelium to directly mediate vascular smooth muscle relaxation. Ultimately, NO would diffuse into the lumen of the pulmonary blood vessels and be inactivated on binding hemoglobin, thus avoiding effects on the systemic circulation. Theoretically, inhaled NO could increase systemic oxygenation by two mechanisms: by global pulmonary arterial vasodilation with increased pulmonary blood flow and cardiac output or by improved matching of ventilation and perfusion in the lung.

Concern grew, however, with potential toxic effects that might be associated with the use of inhaled NO. One potential problem is the formation of excess amounts of methemoglobin, thus causing the clinical condition known as methemoglobinemia. This serious condition is associated with hypoxemia because of the inability of methemoglobin to carry oxygen. The body's defense mechanism against the formation of methemoglobin is the enzyme methemoglobin reductase, which readily converts methemoglobin back to hemoglobin. If the rate of accumulation of methemoglobin is slow, this enzyme will limit increases in methemoglobin. To date, significant methemoglobin levels have not been noted in trials in which low concentrations of inhaled NO have been used in neonates.

Another possible problem is the production of nitrogen dioxide and higher oxides of nitrogen such as peroxynitrite when NO is used with high concentrations of oxygen. Nitrogen dioxide and peroxynitrite in high concentration can directly damage the lung. Using low concentrations of NO and limiting the time of mixing of NO and oxygen minimizes the formation of these toxic molecules.

In a Canadian study, 23 near-term infants who were referred for ECMO and who had oxygen indexes greater than 20 were given randomized doses of 5 to 80 ppm of INO. If less than a 10 torr increase in PaO_2 or 10% increase in saturation after two doses of INO given in a randomized fashion occurred, then ECMO was instituted. Thirteen infants in this study had PPHN that was documented by echocardiography. Eleven of these infants had improvement in PaO_2 and saturation after receiving INO and were not placed on ECMO. Ten had hypoxic respiratory failure without documented PPHN, and only three of these infants improved after INO. The other seven were placed on ECMO. No significant benefit in PaO_2 response with increasing doses of INO was demonstrated. No toxic effects from methemoglobin or dangerously increased levels of nitrogen dioxide were seen in this study (Finer et al, 1994).

A few fairly recent multicenter, double-masked, randomized, placebo-controlled studies have been conducted and determined that INO can decrease the need for ECMO in infants with PPHN. The NINOS study enrolled 235 patients under the age of 2 weeks with PPHN and compared responses to either 20 ppm of INO or placebo gas, which was 100% oxygen. The primary hypothesis was that INO would result in a reduction in the risk of death or need for ECMO by 120 days from 50% in controls to 30% in infants who received INO (Finer, 2000). This study encouraged the use of all other aggressive modalities in the treatment of PPHN and was terminated early by an External Data Safety Monitoring Committee when treated infants where shown to have a statistically significant lower risk of death or need for ECMO. Another well conducted multicenter trial matched control and treatment infants for diagnoses, blood gases, oxygen indices, and ventilator settings (Roberts et al, 1992). The trial was stopped early at interim analysis when it demonstrated a significant increase in systemic oxygenation when INO treated infants were compared to controls. A third multicenter randomized trial compared high-frequency oscillatory ventilation (HFOV) to INO in term and near-term infants with hypoxic respiratory failure (Kinsella & Abman, 1995). This study showed an equivalent response to either modality. In this study if infants failed to respond to either treatment used alone (n = 125), they would then receive treatment with both. Thirty-two percent of infants who failed with a single modality improved with a combination of both treatments, which lead the investigators to speculate that INO works better with maximized lung recruitment. A recent, large randomized study had similar results to the NINOS trial despite the use of lower doses of nitric oxide (Clark, 2000). 248 infants with hypoxemic respiratory failure were randomly assigned to be controls or to receive treatment with 24 hours of INO at 20 ppm followed by another 96 hours of INO at 5 ppm. The two groups were then compared with regards to ECMO requirements. Sixty four percent of controls versus 38% of treated infants (p = 0.001) required ECMO. Mortality was not different in the two groups, but treated infants showed a lower incidence of chronic lung disease. When data on INO is subjected to a meta-analysis, the following conclusion can be drawn (Finer, 2000). INO significantly improves oxygenation and lowers the oxygenation index 30 to 60 minutes after treatment. A significant overall reduction in the combined incidence of need for ECMO and death in infants treated with INO also occurs. Extensive data on long-term outcome of infants treated with INO is not yet available. Some existing data on neurodevelopmental follow-up after the NINOS trial has been gathered (Finer & Barrington, 2001). Of the 173 infants seen at follow-up, no differences exist between control and INO-treated infants with respect to incidence of cerebral palsy, mental or psychomotor development index scores, or hearing loss.

NO gas is supplied in aluminum tanks that contain high concentrations of gaseous NO in equilibrium with inert nitrogen. This gas is added to the inspiratory limb of the ventilator circuit by flowmeters and blenders. Use of high flow rates limits NO mixing time with oxygen and decreases the formation of nitrogen dioxide. Scavenging equipment at the expiratory limb of the ventilator eliminates potentially toxic exhaust gases. In-line monitoring of NO and a chemoluminescence analyzer performs nitrogen dioxide tests to determine levels. Samples of gas in the ventilator circuit are aspirated, and the concentrations of these two molecules are determined. Blood is periodically monitored for methemoglobin levels when patients receive INO.

INO holds promise as a selective pulmonary vasodilator that may soon be added to the clinician's armamentarium. Several small pilot studies suggest that INO may be effective in decreasing pulmonary vascular resistance and improving oxygenation without reducing systemic blood pressure or cardiac output. Extreme care must be taken to monitor blood levels of methemoglobin and the formation of higher oxides of nitrogen when NO is used. Until larger controlled trials are completed, the benefit:risk ratio of INO as a possible treatment for neonatal pulmonary hypertension remains unknown.

Nursing Care: Nitric Oxide

Multicenter trials have shown that INO decreases the chance that some critically ill infants will need ECMO. Future studies are currently underway to determine the most effective and safe doses of INO in the management of newborns with respiratory dysfunction. Over the next several years the use of this treatment modality will slowly increase, and the nursing care of these infants as we know it today will change. Like liquid ventilation, NO therapy would bring with it many new challenges to NICU nurses.

TREATMENT OF NEONATAL HYPOXEMIA WITH EXTRACORPOREAL MEMBRANE OXYGENATION (ECMO)

The use of ECMO is a complex and expensive therapy for infants with severe respiratory failure. Because this therapy has limited applicability to most NICU nurses, it will be discussed only briefly. The first heart-lung machines, designed to serve the function of cardiopulmonary bypass during pediatric cardiac surgery, were developed in the 1950s. Blood was removed from the patient and pumped through an oxygenator before return to the systemic circulation. At the end of the surgical procedure, the patient was disconnected from the machine, and pulmonary and systemic flows were restored with the patient's own heart as the pump. In the mid-1970s, the first attempts at prolonged cardiopulmonary bypass in infants with potentially reversible hypoxemia were made. The differences between these efforts and those employed during cardiac surgery were that the duration of bypass was measured in days rather than hours and that the underlying disease that led to hypoxemia was potentially reversible lung disease rather than primary cardiac disease.

In the last 20 years, prolonged cardiopulmonary bypass, also known as extracorporeal membrane oxygenation (ECMO) or extracorporeal life support, has been used in thousands of newborn infants with hypoxemia that appears to be intractable to aggressive nonsurgical management. A few controlled clinical trials of ECMO have been performed (UK Collaborative Trial Group, 1996). In the absence of such trials, much controversy still exists about the uses of ECMO. Despite its efficacy in improving oxygen delivery in sick newborns, the mortality and morbidity associated with its use remains significant. The long-term morbidity associated with the use ECMO is primarily adverse neurodevelopmental outcomes. The proponents of ECMO argue that mortality and morbidity would actually be greater in these patients if ECMO were not available. The opponents of ECMO argue that without additional trials, we will be unable to distinguish ECMO-related complications from disease-related complications.

A 1995 study examined neurodevelopmental status at age 5 years in ECMO-treated infants compared with a cohort of normal 5-year-olds (Glass et al, 1995). In the group treated with ECMO, 17% of children had major developmental disabilities, similar to rates seen in infants born with birth weights of less than 750 g. The average IQ was also lower for ECMO-treated infants, and they were at significantly higher risk for school failure and behavioral problems. Differences between the two groups may be related to initial severity of illness or to the ECMO process itself or both.

Despite these controversies, ECMO is widely used in the United States as well as in several other industrialized nations. Neonatal ECMO is used in the management of intractable hypoxemia in near-term newborns with meconium aspiration syndrome, RDS, pneumonia/sepsis, and congenital diaphragmatic hernia. Many contraindications to the use of ECMO exist. The most important contraindication is prematurity. Early reports of ECMO use in premature infants revealed alarmingly high rates of intracranial hemorrhage. Whether intracranial hemorrhage in these patients is related to the systemic anticoagulation required with ECMO or to the abnormal cerebrovascular pressures and flows associated with ECMO is unknown. Other contraindications to ECMO include preexisting intracranial hemorrhage and hypoxemia that is not potentially reversible, such as seen in patients with cyanotic congenital heart disease.

ECMO is an expensive and labor-intensive procedure. Two caretakers are required 24 hours per day—one to provide nursing care directly to the patient and one to monitor the functional integrity of the circuit and its various components because a variety of technical malfunctions can occur. During ECMO the circuit must be heparinized, and the most frequently reported ECMO complication is hemorrhage secondary to this. Table 22-6 lists other common complications of ECMO.

Although it is used widely, ECMO is likely to be replaced by less invasive and less risky preventive and therapeutic procedures. However, at this time, referral to an ECMO center is a logical approach when infants with severe hypoxic respiratory failure do not respond to surfactants, conventional or high-frequency ventilation, or inhaled nitric oxide therapy.

LIQUID VENTILATION

The skills, technologies, and resources for managing respiratory compromise in neonates have continued to improve. Despite these advancements, prematurity and respiratory distress are

TABLE 22-6	Complications of Extracorporeal Membrane Oxygenation
Complication	**Rationale and Treatment**
Physiologic	
Electrolyte/glucose/ fluid imbalance	Sodium requirements decrease to 1 to 2 mEq/kg/day; potassium requirements increase to 4 mEq/kg/day secondary to action of aldosterone
	Calcium replacement may be required if citrate is a component of prime blood anticoagulant
	Hyperglycemia may occur if citrate-phosphate-dextrose anticoagulated blood is used; reduce dextrose concentration of maintenance and heparin infusions
	Maintain total fluid intake of 100 to 150 ml/kg/day
	Fluid intake should balance output; furosemide may be required if positive fluid balance occurs
Central nervous system deterioration: cerebral edema, intracranial hemorrhage, seizures	This significant complication of ECMO can be related to pre-ECMO hypoxia, acidosis, hypercapnia, or vessel ligation
	Drug of choice for seizures is phenobarbital
	Serial electroencephalograms and cranial ultrasound examinations may be required
Generalized edema	Extracellular space is enlarged by distribution of crystalloid solution from the prime fluid and action of aldosterone and antidiuretic hormone
	Furosemide or hemofiltration may be indicated if edema causes brain or lung dysfunction
Renal failure	Acute tubular necrosis results from pre-ECMO hypotension and hypoxia
	Monitor output and indicators of renal failure: blood urea nitrogen, creatinine
	Increase renal perfusion by increasing pump flow and use of dopamine (5 µg/kg/min)
	Hemodialysis may be added to the circuit if necessary
Bleeding/thrombocytopenia	Most frequent cause of death
	Large foreign surface of ECMO circuit lowers platelet function and count
	Most common in infants requiring surgery or chest tubes
	Minimize with good control of ACT (180 to 200 seconds) and judicious use of platelets and frozen plasma
	All surgical procedures must be done with electrocautery
Decreased venous return/ hypovolemia	Infant must have adequate circulating volume to obtain adequate flow rates
	Manifested by collapsing silicone bladder triggering bladder box alarm and decrease in extracorporeal flow rate, arterial pressure, and arterial pulse amplitude
	Blood sampling, wound drainage, or peripheral dilatation may account for hypovolemia
	Check for pneumothorax, partial venous catheter occlusion, or malposition, which may decrease venous drainage and return
	Replace volume with packed cells, fresh frozen plasma
	Treat pneumothorax with chest tube placement
	Raise level of bed to enhance gravity drainage of venous blood
Hypervolemia	Caused by overinfusion of blood products, which causes a larger percentage of blood to flow through malfunctioning lungs
	Can also be caused by renal ischemia and excretion of renin/angiotensin
	Manifested by widening pulse amplitude and decreasing systemic oxygenation at an extracorporeal flow rate
	Treat overinfusion by removing blood from the circuit; renal hypertension may dictate use of captopril or labetalol
Patent ductus arteriosus	Left to right shunting may occur, thus causing increased blood flow to the lungs and necessitating high pump flows without expected increase in PaO_2
	Ligation may be indicated because weaning will not be successful
Mechanical	
Tubing rupture, air in oxygenator	Increase ventilator to pre-ECMO parameters; take patient off bypass (repair circuit, aspirate air, replace malfunctioning oxygenator); be prepared to resuscitate infant
Power failure	Always plug pump into hospital's emergency power supply; hand crank until emergency power is available
Decannulation	Apply firm pressure; come off bypass; increase ventilator parameters; repair vessel; replace blood volume; be prepared to resuscitate infant

ACT, *activated coagulation time;* ECMO, *extracorporeal membrane oxygenation.*
From *Nugent J (1997). Extracorporeal membrane oxygenation. In acute respiratory care of the neonate, ed 2, Petaluma, CA: NICU Ink. Adapted from Nugent J (1986). Extracorporeal membrane oxygenation in the neonate. Neonatal network, 4(5), 33. Reprinted with permission of NICU Ink, Santa Rosa, CA.*

still associated with significant morbidity and mortality. Modern therapies can cause lung injury that eventually may lead to a chronic lung disease. To decrease lung injury, efforts have concentrated on decreasing inspired oxygen concentration and decreasing inspiratory pressure. To decrease inspiratory pressure, surface tension in the alveoli must be uniformly decreased. This surface tension arises because of the air-liquid interface at the lining of the alveolar membrane. Surfactant therapy is used to decrease surface tension but is not always successful in improving acute respiratory distress or preventing chronic lung disease. Liquid ventilation has been studied as a therapy that could reduce surface tension in the alveoli. Because this therapy is still considered experimental, it will only briefly be discussed.

As early as the 1920s, Neergaard demonstrated that oxygenated saline could be used to inflate the lung and improve ventilation. However, saline proved to be inadequate because of its low gas-carrying ability and its high viscosity. In 1966, Clark and Gollan demonstrated that perfluorochemical liquids could support the respiration of animals. Perfluorochemical liquids are inert, have high solubility for respiratory gases, and minimize surface tension. They appear to be absorbed only minimally through the mature epithelium. Limited clinical experience and extensive work in animals suggest that these compounds are relatively nontoxic, even when given intravenously.

A liquid gel surfactant that acts to decrease surface tension, enhance alveolar stability, and protect the respiratory epithelium, lines the alveolus. The surface tension forces within the alveolus are the result of the air-fluid interface and are dramatically increased by the absence of surfactant. Surfactant production and function are usually deficient in preterm infants. This deficiency results in noncompliant alveoli that tend to collapse spontaneously. Because surfactant deficiency tends to be nonhomogeneous, alveolar surface tension varies from one portion of the lung to another. Respiratory function in preterm infants is characterized by stiff lungs, increased work of breathing, uneven ventilation, and ventilation-perfusion mismatch. One way to decrease alveolar surface tension is to eliminate the air-liquid interface in the alveolus by filling it with liquid. Elimination of the air-liquid interface can improve alveolar compliance, reverse ventilation-perfusion abnormalities, and—if the liquid contains oxygen—increase oxygen uptake (Shaffer et al, 1999).

Tidal Liquid Ventilation

Efforts were initially made to entirely replace gas breathing with liquid respiration. In tidal liquid ventilation (TLV), a liquid is used to transport dissolved oxygen and carbon dioxide; inhaled liquid brings dissolved oxygen to the lungs, and exhaled liquid carries off carbon dioxide. During TLV, both functional residual capacity and tidal volume are replaced by perfluorocarbon liquid. Technically, TLV is difficult. Clinically, provisions need to be made to mechanically deliver and withdraw liquid from the lung. Equipment is needed for eliminating carbon dioxide from the liquid and for equilibrating it with oxygen. TLV requires new equipment and procedures. Moreover, the high viscosity of the perfluorocarbon liquid limits the number of breaths that can be delivered per minute.

Partial Liquid Ventilation (PLV)

PLV, also known as perfluorocarbon-associated gas exchange (PAGE), is a hybrid method that attempts to overcome some of the limitations of TLV while retaining the advantages of liquid ventilation. During PLV, functional residual capacity is replaced by liquid, but tidal ventilation is conventional, using oxygen-enriched gas and standard ventilator equipment. The lung is filled with perfluorocarbon liquid to a volume equivalent to the normal pulmonary functional residual capacity. This volume of liquid is left in the lung, and gas ventilation is resumed with use of conventional gas ventilators. On inspiration, oxygen is pushed down the airway into the liquid-filled alveoli, where it forms bubbles and where oxygen and carbon dioxide are exchanged in the liquid from bubbles to the alveoli. This process oxygenates the alveolar perfluorocarbon reservoir and purges it of carbon dioxide. On exhalation, the gas is expelled from the lung. Breaths can be delivered at a frequency appropriate for the size and needs of the patient because the viscosity of the liquid does not limit respiratory rate. PLV has been shown to be effective in surfactant-deficient premature lambs. PLV improved oxygenation and carbon dioxide elimination as well as lung compliance. It has also been shown to work in two models of ARDS, oleic acid lung injury, and saline lavage. A small, nonrandomized study treated thirteen preterm infants who failed conventional management of severe respiratory distress with PLV (Leach et al, 1996). In this study when PaO_2 and compliance improved, the oxygen index decreased significantly within one hour of treatment. Six term infants with respiratory failure and no improvement after ECMO were treated with PLV in another study (Greenspan, 1997). The study concluded that PLV appeared to be safe, improved lung function, and recruited lung volume. Three clinical studies have been done in children—none with control groups that suggest PLV may be a safe and effective treatment for pediatric ARDS. A large adult trial is currently underway to evaluate PLV in the treatment of adult ARDS and further studies in neonates and children are on hold while awaiting these results.

Experience suggests that PLV may eventually provide a strong addition to the available strategies for managing respiratory failure in preterm infants. Careful clinical trials remain to be done, but in the absence of unforeseen problems of toxicity or adverse effects, it is likely that liquid ventilation techniques will assume an important role in care of neonates with lung disease.

Nursing Care: Liquid Ventilation. The nursing care of infants with respiratory compromise may be greatly affected if future advances prove liquid ventilation to be safe and effective. Because of the complexity of the delivery systems, a specialized team, similar to an ECMO team, will be required to care for these infants. These specialists will need to be trained in fluid mechanics and liquid breathing techniques.

SUMMARY

Hypoxemia continues to contribute significantly to both morbidity and mortality in NICUs. As our understanding of the pathophysiology of neonatal hypoxemia improves, new approaches to prevention and treatment are suggested. The development of new therapeutic techniques—such as surfactant replacement, ECMO, HFV, NO, and liquid ventilation—holds the promise of improved neonatal outcome. There is a paucity of data regarding long-term outcome with these newer therapies and whether they confer significant benefits over older conventional methods. Therefore caution must be used before we are tempted to readily employ these techniques at the bedside. The evaluation and discovery of newer and safer methods to prevent and treat neonatal hypoxemia requires the collaborative efforts of basic scientific research and ongoing large, multicenter, randomized clinical trials.

REFERENCES

Avery ME, Mead J (1959). Surface properties in relation to atelectasis and hyaline membrane disease. *American journal of diseases of children*, 97, 517-523.

Avila K et al (1994). High-frequency oscillatory ventilation: A nursing approach to bedside care. *Neonatal network*, 13(5), 23-30.

Bhuta T, Henderson-Smart DJ (2000). Elective high frequency jet ventilation versus conventional ventilation for respiratory distress syndrome in preterm infants. *Cochrane database of systematic reviews*. Issue 4, 2000.

Bloom BT et al (1997). Comparison of Infasurf to Survanta in the Treatment and Prevention of Respiratory Distress Syndrome. *Pediatrics*, 100(1), 31-38.

Burroughs Wellcome Company (1990). *Synthetic lung surfactant for the treatment of neonatal respiratory distress syndrome* (Product Monograph). Research Triangle Park, NC: Author.

Carlo WA et al (1990). Early randomized intervention with high-frequency jet ventilation in respiratory distress syndrome. *Journal of pediatrics*, 117(5), 765-770.

Carlo WA, Ambalavanan N (1999). Conventional mechanical ventilation: traditional and new strategies. *Pediatrics in review*, 20, e117-e126.

Carnielli VP et al (1998). Iron supplementation enhances response to high doses of recombinant human erythropoietin in preterm infants. *Archives of disease in childhood, fetal & neonatal*, 79(1), F44-48.

Clark RH et al (2000). Low-does nitric oxide therapy for persistent pulmonary hypertension of the newborn. Clinical inhaled nitric oxide research group. *New England journal of medicine*, 342(7), 469-474.

Collaborative European Multicenter Study Group (1988). Surfactant replacement therapy for severe neonatal respiratory distress syndrome: an international randomized clinical trial. *Pediatrics*, 82(5), 683-691.

Eichenwald EC, Stark AR (1999). High frequency ventilation: current status. *Pediatrics in review*, 20, e127-133.

Enhorning G et al (1985). Prevention of neonatal respiratory distress syndrome by tracheal instillation of surfactant: A randomized clinical trial. *Pediatrics*, 76(2), 145-153.

Finer NN (2000). Inhaled nitric oxide in term and near-term infants: neurodevelopmental follow-up of the neonatal inhaled nitric oxide study group (NINOS). *The journal of pediatrics*, 136(5), 611-617.

Finer NN et al (1994). Inhaled nitric oxide in infants referred for extracorporeal membrane oxygenation: Dose-responses. *Journal of pediatrics*, 124(2), 302-308.

Finer NN, Barrington KJ (2001). Nitric oxide for respiratory failure in infants born at or near term. *Cochrane database of systematic reviews*. Issue 2, 2001.

Fujiwara T et al (1980). Artificial surfactant therapy in hyaline membrane disease. *Lancet* 1(8159), 55-59.

Gertsmann OR et al (1996). The PROVO multicenter early high-frequency oscillatory ventilation trial: Improved pulmonary and clinical outcome in respiratory distress syndrome. *Pediatrics*, 98(6p & 1), 1044-1057.

Glass P et al (1995). Neurodevelopmental status at age five years of neonates treated with extracorporeal membrane oxygenation. *Journal of pediatrics*, 127(3), 447-457.

Greenough A et al (2000). Synchronized mechanical ventilation for respiratory support in newborn infants. *Cochrane database of systematic reviews*. Issue 4, 2000.

Greenspan JS et al (1990). Liquid ventilation of human preterm neonates. *Journal of pediatrics*, 117(1, part 1), 106-111.

Hansen TN (1998). *Contemporary diagnosis and management of neonatal respiratory disease*, ed 2, Newton, PA: Handbooks in Health Care.

Hargett KD (1995). Mechanical ventilation of the neonate. In Barnhart SL, Czervinske MP (Eds.), *Perinatal and pediatric respiratory care*. Philadelphia: WB Saunders.

Hudak ML et al (1996). A multicenter randomized, masked comparison trial of natural versus synthetic surfactant for the treatment of respiratory distress syndrome. *The journal of pediatrics*, 128(3), 396-406.

Jackson JC et al (1994). Reduction in lung injury after combined surfactant and high-frequency ventilation. *American journal of respiratory and critical care medicine*, 150(2), 534-539.

Keszler M et al (1997). Multicenter control clinical trials of high-frequency jet ventilation in preterm infants with uncomplicated respiratory distress syndrome. *Pediatrics*, 100(4), 593-599.

Kinsella JP, Abman SH (1995). Recent developments in the pathophysiology and treatment of persistent pulmonary hypertension of the newborn. *Journal of pediatrics*, 126(6), 853-863.

Leach CL et al (1996). Partial liquid ventilation with perflubron in premature infants with severe respiratory distress syndrome. The liquivent study group. *New England journal of medicine*, 335(11), 761-767.

Lunn RJ (1995). Inhaled nitric oxide therapy. *Mayo clinic proceedings*, 70, 247-255.

Modanlou HD et al (1997). Comparative efficacy of exosurf and survanta on earlt clinical course of respiratory distress syndrome and complications of prematurity. *Journal of perinatology*, 17(6), 455-460.

Pattle RE (1958). Properties, function and origin of alveolar lining layer. *Proceeding of the Royal Society of London*, B148, 217-240.

Roberts JD et al (1992). Inhaled nitric oxide in persistent pulmonary hypertension of the newborn. *Lancet*, 340(8823), 818-819.

Shaffer TH et al (1999). Liquid ventilation: current status. *Pediatrics in review*, 20e, 134-142.

Soll RF (2000). Natural surfactant extract versus synthetic surfactant for neonatal respiratory distress syndrome. *Cochrane database of systematic reviews*, Issue 4, 2000.

Soll RF et al, & Ross Collaborative Surfactant Prevention Study Group (1990). Multicenter trial of single-dose modified bovine surfactant extract (Survanta) for prevention of respiratory distress syndrome. *Pediatrics*, 85(6), 1092-1102.

Speer CP et al (1995). Randomized clinical trial of two treatment regimens of natural surfactant preparations in neonatal respiratory distress syndrome. *Archives of disease in childhood: fetal and neonatal edition*, 72(1), F8-F13.

Thome V et al (1999). Randomized comparison of high frequency ventilation with high-rate intermittent positive pressure ventilation in preterm infants with respiratory failure. *Journal of pediatrics*, 135(1), 9-11.

UK Collaborative Trial Group (1996). UK collaborative randomized trial of neonatal extracorporeal membrane oxygenation. *Lancet*, 348, 75-82.

Wiswell TE et al (1996). High-frequency jet ventilation in the early management of respiratory distress syndrome is associated with a greater risk for adverse outcomes. *Pediatrics*, 98(6 Pt 1), 1035-1043.

CHAPTER 23

ASSESSMENT AND MANAGEMENT OF THE CARDIOVASCULAR SYSTEM

JUDY WRIGHT LOTT

Cardiovascular disease in newborns and infants usually arises from a congenital heart anomaly. The transition from fetal to neonatal circulation often reveals cardiac compromise. To understand the basis of neonatal cardiac problems, nurses must have a solid foundation in the normal physiology of cardiac function. This chapter presents the physiology of normal cardiac function, including fetal circulatory patterns and the changes that occur during transition to extrauterine life. The most common congenital heart defects (CHDs) and cardiac complications are described. Information about incidence, hemodynamics, manifestations, diagnosis, and medical and surgical management is included. Because some CHDs are not identified during the neonatal period, information about the presentation of some defects in older infants is also included. The chapter concludes with a discussion of nursing support for the family of an infant with a congenital heart defect.

CARDIOVASCULAR ADAPTATION

Fetal Circulation

A knowledge of the normal route of fetal blood flow is essential for understanding the circulatory changes that occur in the newborn at delivery. The pattern of fetal circulation is shown in Figure 23-1. Fetal circulation involves four unique anatomic features:

1. The placenta is the exchange organ for oxygen and carbon dioxide and for nutrients and wastes.
2. The ductus venosus allows most of the blood from the placenta to bypass the liver and enter the inferior vena cava.
3. The foramen ovale is an opening in the interatrial septum that permits a portion of the blood to flow from the right atrium directly to the left atrium.
4. The patent ductus arteriosus (PDA) is a tubular communication between the pulmonary artery and the descending aorta that allows blood to flow from the pulmonary artery to the aorta, bypassing the fetal lungs (Park, 1996; Lott, 2003).

Oxygen diffuses into the fetal circulation from the maternal uterine arteries in the placenta. From the placenta, the oxygenated blood flows through the umbilical vein to the fetus. The fetal circulation divides at the liver; about half of the blood enters the liver, and the remainder bypasses the liver through the ductus venosus. Blood from the ductus venosus enters the inferior vena cava. Blood of lower oxygen content coming from the gastrointestinal tract, legs, and liver mixes with the blood of higher oxygen content in the inferior vena cava. The mixed blood then enters the right atrium (Park, 1996; Lott, 2003).

The blood from the right atrium flows directly to the left atrium through the foramen ovale. From the left atrium, the blood goes to the left ventricle and then to the head and neck through the ascending aorta. This circulatory pattern ensures that the fetal brain constantly receives well-oxygenated blood (Park, 1996; Lott, 2003).

The blood returns from the head and neck through the superior vena cava to the right atrium and then flows into the right ventricle. From the right ventricle the blood enters the pulmonary arteries. Only a small portion of this blood enters the pulmonary circuit to perfuse the lungs; most of the blood is shunted through the ductus arteriosus into the aorta to supply oxygen and nutrients to the trunk and lower extremities (Park, 1996; Lott, 2003).

Most of the blood flow from the lower extremities rejoins the fetal circulation through the internal iliac arteries via the umbilical cord to the placenta, where it is reoxygenated and recirculated. A small amount of the blood from the lower extremities passes back into the ascending vena cava, mixes with fresh blood from the umbilical vein, and is recirculated without reoxygenation. Fetal circulation, therefore, can be described as two parallel circuits rather than as the serial circuit present in extrauterine life (Park, 1996; Lott, 2003).

Neonatal Circulation

The cardiac and pulmonary systems undergo drastic changes at birth, and these changes usually occur functionally immediately upon onset of respirations. The most significant change is that the lungs become the primary oxygenation organ, rather than the placenta. Clamping of the umbilical cord and the subsequent removal of the placenta produce immediate circulatory changes in the newborn. With the first breath and occlusion of the umbilical cord, the newborn's systemic resistance rises, reducing blood flow through the ductus arteriosus. Cord occlusion causes a prompt increase in blood pressure and a corresponding stimulation of the aortic baroreceptors and sympathetic nervous system.

The onset of respirations and consequent lung expansion result in a decrease in pulmonary vascular resistance, which

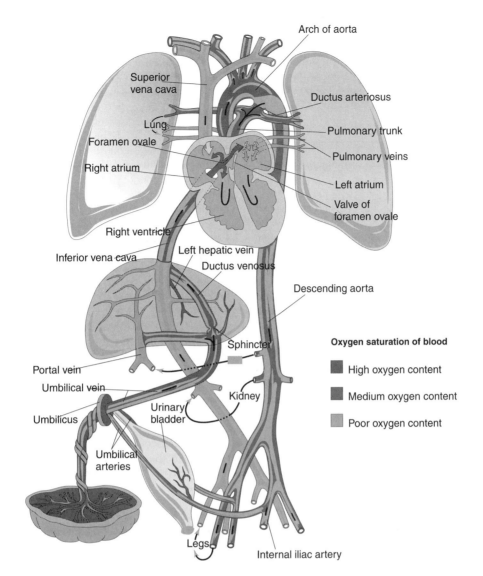

Arch of aorta

Superior
vena cava

Ductus arteriosus

Lung

Pulmonary trunk

Foramen ovale

Pulmonary veins

Right atrium

Left atrium

Valve of
foramen ovale

Right ventricle

Left hepatic vein

Inferior vena cava

Ductus venosus

Descending aorta

Sphincter

Oxygen saturation of blood

Portal vein

High oxygen content

Umbilical vein

Kidney

Medium oxygen content

Umbilicus

Urinary
bladder

Poor oxygen content

Umbilical
arteries

Legs

Internal iliac artery

FIGURE **23-1**
Fetal circulation. From Moore KL, Persaud TVN (1998). *Before we are born: essentials of embryology
and birth defects*, ed 5. WB Saunders: Philadelphia.

occurs secondary to the direct effect of oxygen and carbon dioxide on the blood vessels. Pulmonary vascular resistance declines as arterial oxygen increases and arterial carbon dioxide decreases (Park, 1996; Lott, 2003).

Most of the right ventricular output flows through the lungs and increases the pulmonary venous return to the left atrium. The increase in the amount of blood in the lungs and heart causes pressure in the left atrium of the heart. The increased pressure in the left atrium, combined with the increased systemic vascular resistance, functionally closes the foramen ovale.

The ductus arteriosus normally closes within 15 to 24 hours after birth; this occurs in response to the increase in arterial oxygen caused by pulmonary respiratory effort and the effects of sympathomimetic amines and prostaglandins. The ductus arteriosus is anatomically obliterated by constriction by 3 to 4 weeks of age. Clamping of the umbilical cord causes the cessation of blood flow through the ductus venosus, which is anatomically obliterated by approximately 1 to 2 weeks after birth. Also after birth, the umbilical vein and arteries no longer transport blood and are obliterated.

The term functional closure refers to the cessation of flow through a structure caused by changes in pressure; anatomic closure refers to obliteration of a structure by constriction or tissue growth. Because anatomic closure of the fetal pathways lags behind functional closure, the shunts may open and close intermittently before anatomic closure, resulting in transient functional murmurs.

Pulmonary artery pressure remains high for several hours after birth. As pulmonary vascular resistance diminishes, the direction of blood flow through the ductus arteriosus reverses. Initially bidirectional, the flow becomes entirely left to right; it is functionally insignificant by approximately 15 hours after birth. Intermittent or functional murmurs do not cause any cardiovascular compromise for the newborn and are not clinically significant. Transient cyanosis occurs with conditions that cause transient opening of fetal shunts, which allows unoxygenated blood to shunt from the right side of the heart to the left side, thereby bypassing the pulmonary circuit.

Any murmur or cyanosis in the newborn should be carefully evaluated and monitored to detect cardiovascular abnormalities (Park, 1996; Lott, 2003). Hypoxemia can cause a constricted ductus arteriosus to reopen and may reestablish higher pulmonary vascular resistance, leading to persistent pulmonary hypertension of the newborn (PPHN). The ductus arteriosus responds to hypoxemia by opening, whereas the pulmonary arterioles respond by constricting (Park, 1996; Lott, 2003).

NORMAL CARDIAC FUNCTION

The normal anatomy of the heart is shown in Figure 23-2.

Heart Valves

Blood flow through the heart is directed through two sets of one-way valves. The semilunar valves are the pulmonary valve and the aortic valve. The pulmonary valve connects the right ventricle and the pulmonary artery. The aortic valve connects the left ventricle and the aorta. The two atrioventricular (AV) valves are the tricuspid valve and the mitral valve. The tricuspid valve connects the right atrium and the right ventricle. The mitral valve connects the left atrium and the left ventricle (Lott, 2003).

Cardiac Cycle

Normal cardiac function involves two stages: systole and diastole. During systole, contraction of the ventricle causes the pressure inside the ventricle to rise to approximately 70 mm Hg in newborns (approximately 120 mm Hg in adults). When sufficient pressure has been generated, the aortic and pulmonary valves open and blood is ejected from the ventricles.

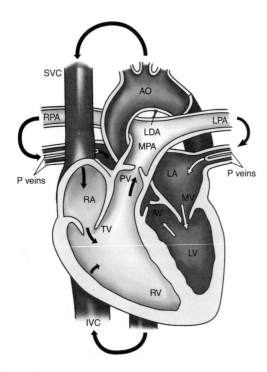

FIGURE **23-2**
Normal cardiac anatomy and circulation. AO, Aorta; AV, aortic valve; IVC, inferior vena cava; LA, left atrium; LDA, ligamentum ductus arteriosus; LPA, left pulmonary artery; LV, left ventricle; MPA, main pulmonary artery; MV, mitral valve; PV, pulmonary valve; P veins, pulmonary veins; RA, right atrium; RPA, right pulmonary artery; RV, right ventricle; SVC, superior vena cava; TV, tricuspid valve.

As the blood flows from the ventricles, the pressure declines, and the aortic and pulmonary valves close.

During diastole, the mitral and tricuspid valves open, and 70% of the blood in the atria flows into the ventricles. A small portion of the blood flows back into the aorta and enters the coronary arteries to perfuse the heart. At the end of diastole, a small atrial contraction occurs (4 to 6 mm Hg on the right side and 7 to 8 mm Hg on the left side), and the mitral and tricuspid valves close. Metabolism of the heart is diminished during diastole. The average newborn's cardiac cycle lasts approximately 0.4 second; 0.2 second for diastole and 0.2 second for systole (based on a heart rate of approximately 150 beats per minute [bpm]) (Opie, 2001).

Cardiac Output

Cardiac output (CO) is the amount of blood pumped by the left ventricle in 1 minute. Cardiac output is equal to the stroke volume (SV) multiplied by the heart rate (HR):

$$CO = SV \times HR$$

The stroke volume is the volume of blood pumped per beat from each ventricle. The higher the stroke volume, the higher the volume of blood found in the systemic circulation.

An increase in cardiac output increases systole and decreases diastole. Cardiac output can be influenced by changes in the heart rate, pulmonary vascular resistance, and systemic resistance to flow.

Cardiac output also is influenced by the amount of blood returned to the heart, as explained by the Frank-Starling law, which states that within physiologic limits, the heart pumps all the blood that enters it without allowing excessive accumulation of blood in the veins. The passive movement of blood through the veins, the thoracic pump, and the venous muscle pump determine venous return. Normally, when a higher volume of blood enters the heart, contractility increases in response to stimulation of stretch receptors in the heart muscle. However, a newborn's heart has fewer fibers and is unable to stretch sufficiently to accommodate greater volume, therefore an increase in the heart rate is the only effective mechanism by it can respond to the increased volume (Colucci & Braunwald, 2001; Opie, 2001; Lott, 2003).

Cardiac failure occurs when the volume of blood exceeds the heart's ability to pump. Local factors that affect venous return to the heart include hypoxia, acidosis, hypercarbia, hyperthermia, increased metabolic demand, and an increase in metabolites (potassium, adenosine triphosphate, and lactic acid).

Other factors that influence cardiac output include vascular pressure and resistance. Pressure and resistance are inversely related; if pressure in the arterial bed increases, resistance decreases, and flow improves. The size (radius) of vessels influences resistance; the greater the radius of a vessel, the lower the resistance. Resistance to vascular flow is greater in vessels obstructed by thromboses or constriction (Colucci & Braunwald, 2001; Opie, 2001; Lott, 2003).

Autonomic Cardiac Control

Cardiovascular function is modulated by the autonomic nervous system. Baroreceptors and chemoreceptors in the aorta and carotid sinus provide feedback to the autonomic nervous system. Feedback from these receptors stimulates the parasympathetic or sympathetic nervous system. The parasympathetic nervous system is less powerful than the sympathetic nervous system.

Stimulation of the parasympathetic and sympathetic nervous systems results in vagal nerve stimulation and a decrease in heart rate. Most parasympathetic and sympathetic nervous system effects affect the atria, but a decrease in ventricular contractility may also occur. Right vagal stimulation affects the sinoatrial (SA) node, and left vagal stimulation affects the AV node. Acetylcholine is the active neurotransmitter for the parasympathetic and sympathetic nervous systems (Colucci & Braunwald, 2001; Opie, 2001; Lott, 2003).

Stimulation of the sympathetic nervous system through the ganglionic chain results in the release of norepinephrine and epinephrine, which act on the SA node, the AV node, the atria, and the ventricles. Maximum stimulation of the sympathetic nervous system can increase the heart rate to 250 to 300 bpm. Contractility can be improved by approximately 100%. Alpha- and beta-adrenergic receptors are stimulated; with alpha receptors, this results in an increase in contractility (inotropic) and heart rate (chronotropic); with beta2 receptors, it causes vasodilation, bronchodilation, and smooth muscle relaxation (Kaplan, 2001).

Term newborns have fewer receptors but are capable of normal cardiovascular system function. A preterm newborn's body is not able to smoothly maintain autonomic function, and more energy is expended in the effort. For this reason, cardiovascular signs, such as color changes and bradycardia, may occur as a result of an excessive demand for autonomic nervous system function.

CARDIAC ASSESSMENT

Early recognition of the signs and symptoms of congenital heart disease leads to earlier diagnosis and treatment and may improve the patient's outcome (Goh, 2000). Careful assessment for these factors, therefore, is a crucial component of newborn care. Cardiac assessment requires history taking, physical assessment, and interpretation of diagnostic tests. Review of the maternal, fetal, and neonatal histories also is helpful.

A number of factors are associated with CHDs, including (1) maternal infections, especially viral and protozoal infections early in the pregnancy; (2) maternal use of tobacco, alcohol, or drugs; and (3) maternal diseases. Table 23-1 lists heart defects commonly associated with the maternal history. Birth weight may also aid in the identification of a CHD. Macrosomia is associated with maternal diabetes and transposition of the great arteries (TGA), whereas infants of mothers with viral diseases frequently are small for gestational age (Park, 1996; Little, 2001).

A family history of hereditary disease, congenital heart disease, or rheumatic fever is significant. For certain hereditary diseases, a CHD is a component of the disorder's expression (Table 23-2). (Hereditary conditions are discussed in Chapter 11.) The overall incidence of CHDs is 8 per 1000 live births, or approximately 1%, excluding persistent patent ductus arteriosus (PDA) in preterm newborns. If the mother had a CHD, however, the incidence in her children rises to approximately 3% to 4% (Park, 1996; Pyeritz, 2001).

A neonatal history of cyanosis, tachypnea without pulmonary disease, sweating, poor feeding, edema or, in older infants, failure to gain weight suggests congenital heart disease. Careful evaluation of the maternal, fetal, and neonatal histories, in conjunction with a thorough physical assessment, identifies infants for whom further diagnostic testing is indicated.

Physical Assessment

The assessment of a newborn suspected of having cardiovascular dysfunction involves inspection, palpation, and auscultation (Park, 1996; Braunwald, 2001).

Inspection. Valuable information about the newborn's cardiovascular system can be obtained by observing the infant's general appearance before the examination. The three states of the newborn that should be observed are sleeping or awake, alert or lethargic, anxious or relaxed. Respiratory effort, including signs of respiratory distress (e.g., nasal flaring, expiratory grunting, stridor, retractions, or paradoxical respirations), should be observed. Tachypnea and tachycardia are early signs

TABLE 23-1	Maternal Conditions and Associated Congenital Heart Defects
Condition	**Defect**
Maternal Disease	
Diabetes mellitus	Cardiomyopathy, transposition of the great arteries ventricular septal defect, patent ductus arteriosus
Lupus erythematosus	Congenital heart block
Collagen disease	Congenital heart block
Congenital heart defect	Increased risk of congenital heart defect (3% to 4%)
Viral Disease	
Rubella	
First trimester	Patent ductus arteriosus, pulmonary artery branch stenosis
Later	Various cardiac and other defects
Cytomegalovirus	Various cardiac and other defects
Herpesvirus	Various cardiac and other defects
Coxsackie virus B	Cardiomyopathy
Drugs	
Amphetamines	Ventricular septal defect, patent ductus arteriosus, atrial septal defect, transposition of the great arteries
Phenytoin	Pulmonary stenosis, aortic stenosis, coarctation of the aorta, patent ductus arteriosus
Trimethadione	Transposition of the great arteries, tetralogy of Fallot, hypoplastic left heart syndrome
Progesterone; estrogen	Ventricular septal defect, tetralogy of Fallot, transposition of the great arteries
Alcohol	Ventricular septal defect, patent ductus arteriosus, atrial septal defect, tetralogy of Fallot

Data from Hazinski MF (1984). Cardiovascular disorders. In Hazinski MF, editor. Nursing care of the critically ill child. Mosby: St Louis; and Park MK (1988). Pediatric cardiology for practitioners. Mosby: St Louis.

TABLE **23-2**	Congenital Heart Defects Associated with Specific Genetic or Chromosomal Abnormalities
Disease or Syndrome	**Defect**
Trisomy 13 or 18	Patent ductus arteriosus, ventral septal defect
Trisomy 21	Endocardial cushion defect, ventral septal defect, patent ductus arteriosus
Turner syndrome	Coarctation of the aorta
Marfan syndrome	Aortic stenosis, mitral valve stenosis, aortic aneurysms, total anomalous pulmonary venous return
Williams syndrome (elfin facies)	Aortic stenosis, peripheral pulmonary artery stenosis
DiGeorge syndrome	Interrupted aortic arch
Neurofibromatosis	Pulmonary valve stenosis

Data from Park M (1988). Pediatric cardiology for practitioners. Mosby: St Louis.

of left ventricular failure. Severe left ventricular failure also causes dyspnea and retractions (Park, 1996; Braunwald, 2001).

The neonate's color also should be observed. Cyanosis is a bluish coloring of the skin, mucous membranes, and nail beds that occurs when the circulation has at least 5 g/dl of deoxygenated hemoglobin. If cyanosis is present, the nurse should note whether it is peripheral or central cyanosis and if it improves with crying, does not change, or becomes worse with crying. In addition to cardiac defects, causes of cyanosis include pulmonary, hematologic, central nervous system, or metabolic diseases. Pulmonary and cardiac defects are the two most common causes of central cyanosis in the newborn.

Pallor may indicate vasoconstriction arising from congestive heart failure (CHF) or circulatory shock caused by severe anemia. Prolonged physiologic jaundice may occur in infants with CHF or congenital hypothyroidism, which is associated with PDA and pulmonary stenosis (PS). A ruddy or plethoric appearance often is seen with polycythemia. Such infants may appear cyanotic without significant arterial desaturation.

Sweating is very suggestive of a CHD in the newborn. Sweating is caused by sympathetic overactivity, a compensatory mechanism for diminished cardiac output.

Precordial activity is a reliable parameter of cardiac dysfunction. Precordial bulging suggests chronic cardiac enlargement. Precordial activity without bulging may be associated with acute onset of cardiac dysfunction.

Pectus excavatum may cause a pulmonary systolic ejection murmur or a large cardiac silhouette on an anteroposterior chest radiograph because of the decreased anteroposterior chest diameter. Pectus excavatum does not cause cardiac dysfunction (Park, 1996).

Palpation.   The precordium and peripheral pulses are palpated. Palpation of the precordium can detect hyperactivity, thrill, and the point of maximum impulse (PMI). Irregularity or inequality of rate or volume can be detected by counting the peripheral pulse rate. Evaluation of the carotid, brachial, femoral, and pedal pulses can detect differences between sides

and upper and lower extremities. If the pulses are unequal, the blood pressure should be measured in each of the four extremities. Weak leg pulses with strong pulses in the arms suggest coarctation of the aorta (COA). If the right brachial pulse is stronger than the left, supravalvular aortic stenosis or coarctation proximal to or near the origin of the left subclavian artery may be present (Park, 1996).

Heart defects that lead to "aortic runoff," including PDA, aortic insufficiency, large arteriovenous fistula, or persistent truncus arteriosus, cause bounding pulses. However, preterm newborns frequently have a bounding pulse, because the subcutaneous tissue is relatively diminished. Also, preterm infants frequently have PDA secondary to prematurity. Cardiac failure or circulatory shock causes weak or thready pulses (Park, 1996).

A hyperactive precordium indicates a heart defect with increased volume, such as a CHD with a large left to right shunt (e.g., PDA, ventricular septal defect [VSD]) or heart disease with valvular regurgitation (e.g., aortic regurgitation or mitral regurgitation). The location of the PMI depends on whether the right or left ventricle is dominant. With right ventricular dominance, the PMI is at the lower left sternal border; with left ventricular dominance, the PMI is at the apex. A diffuse, slow-rising PMI is called a heave, which is associated with volume overload. A sharp, fast-rising PMI is called a tap, which is associated with pressure overload. A normal newborn has right ventricular dominance (Park, 1996).

The apical impulse of the newborn normally is felt in the fourth intercostal space to the left of the midclavicular line. Displacement of the apical impulse downward or laterally may indicate cardiac enlargement (Park, 1996).

The presence and location of a thrill provide important diagnostic information. The palms of the hands, rather than the fingertips, should be used to feel for a thrill, except in the suprasternal notch and carotid arteries. The examiner should palpate for the presence of thrills in the upper left, upper right, and lower left sternal border, in the suprasternal notch, and over the carotid arteries. A thrill in the upper left sternal border derives from the pulmonary valve or pulmonary artery. Thrills in the lower left sternal border suggest pulmonary stenosis, pulmonary artery atresia or, occasionally, PDA. A thrill in the upper right sternal border signifies aortic origin, usually aortic stenosis or, less frequently, pulmonary stenosis (PS), PDA, or COA. A thrill over the carotid arteries along with a thrill in the suprasternal notch suggests COA or aortic stenosis (AS) or other defects of the aorta or aortic valve (Park, 1996).

The abdomen is palpated to determine the size, consistency, and location of the liver and spleen. Increased liver size is a frequent finding with CHF (Park, 1996).

Auscultation.   Careful auscultation by a skilled evaluator is an essential component of any cardiovascular assessment. Auscultation assesses heart rate and regularity, heart sounds, systolic and diastolic sounds, and heart murmurs. Skillful evaluation of cardiac sounds requires systematic auscultation and much practice.

Identification of Heart Sounds.   Individual heart sounds should be identified and evaluated before evaluation of cardiac murmurs is attempted. The four individual heart sounds are S_1, S_2, S_3, and S_4. S_3 and S_4 are rarely heard in the newborn. S_1 is the sound caused by closure of the mitral and tricuspid valves after atrial systole and is best heard at the apex or lower left sternal border. S_1 is the beginning of ventricular systole. Splitting of S_1 is infrequently heard in newborns. Wide splitting of S_1 is heard with right bundle branch block or Ebstein anomaly (Park, 1996).

S_2 is the sound created by closure of the aortic and pulmonary valves, which marks the end of systole and the beginning of ventricular diastole. S_2 is best heard in the upper left sternal border or pulmonic area. Evaluation of the splitting of S_2 is important diagnostically. The volume of blood ejected from the aorta and pulmonary artery and the resistance against which the ventricles must pump determines the timing of the closure of the aortic and pulmonary valves. In the immediate newborn period, there may be no appreciable splitting of S_2. Because the right and left ventricles pump similar quantities of blood and the pulmonary pressure is close to the aortic pressure, these valves close almost simultaneously; thus S_2 is heard as a single sound. As pulmonary vascular resistance declines, pulmonary resistance subsequently drops below the aortic pressure, causing a split of S_2 as the valve leaflets on the left side of the heart (aortic valve) close before those on the right side (pulmonary valve). S_2 should be split by 72 hours of life.

The absence of a split S_2 or the presence of a widely split S_2 usually indicates an abnormality. A fixed, widely split S_2 occurs in conditions that prolong the right ventricular ejection time or that shorten the left ventricular ejection time. Some of these conditions are (1) atrial septal defect (ASD) and partial anomalous pulmonary venous return (PAPVR) (in which an increased amount of blood is ejected by the right ventricle, resulting in volume overload); (2) pulmonary stenosis (stenosis delays right ventricular ejection time, resulting in pressure overload); (3) right bundle branch block (in which electrical activation of the right ventricle is delayed); (4) mitral regurgitation (in which forward output is diminished and left ventricular ejection time is shortened); and (5) idiopathic dilated main pulmonary artery (in which the increased capacity of the main pulmonary artery results in less recoil to close the valves, delaying closure) (Park, 1996).

A narrowly split S_2 occurs with early closure of the pulmonary valve (pulmonary hypertension) or delayed closure of the aortic valve. A single S_2 is significant because it may indicate the presence of only one semilunar valve (such as occurs with aortic or pulmonary atresia and truncus arteriosus). A single S_2 may also occur with a critical pulmonary stenosis, TGA, or tetralogy of Fallot (TOF), in which the pulmonary closure is not audible. Severe aortic stenosis may result in a single S_2 because aortic closure is delayed. Severe pulmonary hypertension may cause early closure of the pulmonary valve, resulting in a single S_2.

The relative intensity of the aortic and pulmonary components of S_2 must be assessed. In the pulmonary area (upper left sternal border), the aortic component usually is louder than the pulmonary component. An increase in the intensity of the pulmonary component, compared with the aortic component, occurs with pulmonary hypertension. Conditions that cause a decrease in the diastolic pressure of the pulmonary artery (e.g., critical pulmonary stenosis, TOF, tricuspid atresia) may result in diminished intensity of the pulmonary component. Evaluation of intensity is difficult and requires frequent practice listening to heart sounds (Park, 1996).

As mentioned previously, S_3 and S_4 are rarely heard in the neonatal period; their presence denotes a pathologic origin. Likewise, a gallop rhythm (the result of a loud S_3 and S_4) and tachycardia are abnormal.

After assessing the individual heart sounds, the examiner evaluates systolic and diastolic sounds. The ejection sound, or click, occurs after S_1 and may sound like splitting of S_1. The ejection click is best heard at the upper left or right sternal border or base. The pulmonary click can best be heard at the second or third left intercostal space and is louder with expiration. The aortic click, best heard at the second right intercostal space, does not change in intensity with a change in respiration. Ejection clicks are associated with pulmonary or aortic stenosis or with the dilated great arteries seen in systemic or pulmonary hypertension, idiopathic dilation of the main pulmonary artery, TOF, or truncus arteriosus (Park, 1996).

CARDIAC MURMURS

Cardiac murmurs should be evaluated for intensity (grades 1 to 6), timing (systolic or diastolic), location, transmission, and quality (musical, vibratory, or blowing). The grade scale for murmurs is as follows:

Grade 1: Barely audible
Grade 2: Soft but easily audible
Grade 3: Moderately loud; no thrill
Grade 4: Loud; thrill present
Grade 5: Loud; audible with stethoscope barely on chest
Grade 6: Loud; audible with stethoscope near chest

The murmur grade is recorded as $\frac{1}{6}$, $\frac{2}{6}$, and so on. Again, practice in auscultation improves the listener's evaluation skills. The intensity of the murmur is affected by cardiac output; anything that increases cardiac output (e.g., anemia, fever, exercise) increases the intensity of the murmur (Park, 1996; Braunwald, 2001).

The next step in evaluating a murmur is classifying it in relation to S_1 and S_2. Murmurs are categorized as systolic, diastolic, or continuous.

Systolic Murmurs

Most heart murmurs are systolic, occurring between S_1 and S_2. Systolic murmurs are either ejection or regurgitation murmurs. Ejection murmurs occur after S_1 and end before S_2. Ejection murmurs are caused by the flow of blood through stenotic or deformed semilunar valves or by increased flow through normal semilunar valves. Systolic ejection murmurs are best heard at the second left or right intercostal space. Regurgitant systolic murmurs begin with S_1, with no interval between S_1 and the beginning of the murmur. Regurgitation murmurs generally continue throughout systole (pansystolic or holosystolic). Regurgitation systolic murmurs are caused by the flow of blood from a chamber at a higher pressure throughout systole than the receiving chamber. Regurgitation systolic murmurs are associated with only three conditions: VSD, mitral regurgitation, and tricuspid regurgitation (Park, 1996).

Location.   Determining the location of the maximum intensity of the murmur aids in the evaluation of a cardiac murmur. Figure 23-3 shows the locations at which various systolic murmurs can be heard.

Transmission of the murmur is related to its location. A knowledge of transmission can assist in determining the origin of the murmur. A systolic ejection murmur that transmits well to the neck usually is aortic in origin, whereas one that transmits to the back usually is pulmonary in origin. An apical systolic murmur that transmits well to the left axilla and lower back is characteristic of mitral regurgitation, but one that

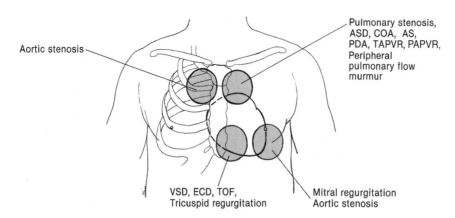

FIGURE **23-3**

Location of systolic murmurs. *AS*, Aortic stenosis; *ASD*, atrial septal defect; *COA*, coarctation of the aorta; *ECD*, endocardial cushion defect; *PAPVR*, partial anomalous pulmonary venous return; *PDA*, patent ductus arteriosus; *TAPVR*, total anomalous pulmonary venous return; *TOF*, tetralogy of Fallot; *VSD*, ventricular septal defect.

transmits to the upper right sternal border and neck is likely to be aortic in nature (Park, 1996).

Quality. Murmurs are described as musical, vibratory, or blowing (Park, 1996). VSD or mitral regurgitation murmurs have a high-pitched, blowing quality. Murmurs associated with aortic stenosis or pulmonary valve stenosis have a rough, grating quality. Determining the quality of a murmur is a subjective judgment, and expertise is gained only after extensive practice.

Diastolic Murmurs

Diastolic murmurs occur between S_1 and S_2. These murmurs are classified according to their timing in relation to heart sounds as early diastolic, mid-diastolic, or presystolic.

Early diastolic (protodiastolic) murmurs occur early in diastole, right after S_2, and are the result of incompetence of the aortic or pulmonary valve. Aortic regurgitation murmurs are high pitched and are best heard with the diaphragm of the stethoscope at the third left intercostal space. Aortic regurgitation murmurs radiate to the apex, and bounding pulses are present with significant regurgitation. Aortic regurgitation murmurs occur with bicuspid aortic valve, subaortic stenosis, and subarterial infundibular VSD. Pulmonary regurgitation murmurs are medium pitched unless pulmonary hypertension is present, in which case they are high pitched. Diastolic regurgitation murmurs, which are heard best at the second left intercostal space, radiate along the left sternal border. Pulmonary regurgitation murmurs occur with postoperative TOF, pulmonary hypertension, or postoperative pulmonary valvotomy for pulmonary stenosis, or with other pulmonary valve deformities (Park, 1996; Braunwald, 2001).

Mid-diastolic murmurs result from abnormal ventricular filling. They are low pitched and can best be heard with the bell of the stethoscope placed lightly on the chest wall. The murmur results from turbulent flow caused by stenosis of the tricuspid or mitral valve. Mitral mid-diastolic murmurs are best heard at the apex and are referred to as apical rumbles. Mitral mid-diastolic murmurs are associated with mitral stenosis or large VSDs with a large left to right shunt or PDA, which produces relative mitral stenosis secondary to increased flow across the normal-size mitral valve. Tricuspid mid-diastolic murmurs can best be heard along the lower left sternal border and are as-

sociated with ASD, total or partial anomalous pulmonary venous return, endocardial cushion defects, or abnormal stenosis of the tricuspid valve.

Presystolic (or late diastolic) murmurs are caused by flow through AV valves during ventricular diastole, which results when active atrial contraction ejects blood into the ventricle. These low-frequency murmurs are found with true mitral or tricuspid valve stenosis (Park, 1996; Braunwald, 2001).

Continuous Murmurs

Continuous murmurs begin in systole and continue throughout S_2 into all or part of diastole. Continuous murmurs are caused by (1) aorticopulmonary or AV connection (e.g., PDA, AV fistula, or persistent truncus arteriosus), (2) disturbances of flow in veins (e.g., venous hum), and (3) disturbances of flow in arteries (e.g., COA or pulmonary artery stenosis) (Park, 1996).

In newborns the most frequently heard continuous murmur is caused by PDA. The PDA murmur is described as a machinery murmur, louder during systole, peaking at S_2, and diminished during diastole. PDA murmurs are loudest in the left infraclavicular area or in the upper left sternal border (Park, 1996; Braunwald, 2001).

Other Murmurs

Functional or innocent cardiac murmurs are common in children and can occur in newborns. Innocent murmurs occur in the absence of abnormal cardiac structures. Functional murmurs are asymptomatic. Any unusual or abnormal finding warrants consultation. Findings such as cyanosis, an enlarged heart size on examination or an enlarged cardiac silhouette on the chest radiograph, an abnormal electrocardiogram (ECG), a diastolic murmur, a grade ⅜ systolic murmur or a less intense murmur with a thrill, weak or bounding pulses, or other abnormal heart sounds have pathologic origins and must be investigated (Park, 1996).

A pulmonary flow murmur is commonly found in low-birth-weight (LBW) infants. Infants with a pulmonary flow murmur have relative hypoplastic right and left pulmonary arteries at birth because of the small amount of blood flow during fetal life. The increased flow after birth creates turbulence in the small vessels, which is transmitted along the smaller branches of the pulmonary arteries. The pulmonary flow murmur is best heard at the upper left sternal border. It has a grade of $\frac{1}{6}$ to $\frac{2}{6}$ intensity and is transmitted to the right and left chest, both axillae, and the back. There are no other significant cardiac findings. This murmur usually disappears by 3 to 6 months after birth. Persistence beyond this period should lead to further evaluation for anatomic pulmonary artery stenosis (Park, 1996).

CONGENITAL HEART DEFECTS

Etiology

Cardiac development takes place during the first 7 weeks of gestation. Major structural defects can arise from interference with the maternal-placental-fetal unit during this critical period. The causes of CHDs are classified as chromosomal (10% to 12%), genetic (1% to 2%), maternal or environmental (1% to 2%), or multifactorial (85%).

Many chromosomal abnormalities are associated with structural heart defects. Among infants with trisomy 21 (Down syndrome), 30% to 50% have a structural heart defect. In one study of 243 children with trisomy 21, 44% had associated congenital heart defects The most common CHDs with trisomy 21 are endocardial cushion defects (ECD), and the most common ECDs were ASD and VSD (Freeman et al, 1998). Specific genetic abnormalities account for only a small percentage of CHDs. Marfan syndrome is associated with defects of the aorta, such as aortic insufficiency or an aortic aneurysm (Park, 1996; Ardinger, 1997; Pyeritz, 2001).

Maternal or environmental factors include maternal illness and drug ingestion. Maternal rubella during the first 7 weeks of pregnancy carries a 50% risk of congenital rubella syndrome (CRS) with major defects of multiple organ systems. Heart defects seen with CRS include PDA and pulmonary artery branch stenosis. Other viral diseases (e.g., cytomegalovirus infection) and protozoal diseases (e.g., toxoplasmosis) are also associated with CHDs. Diagnosis of a CHD calls for a careful maternal history to identify viral-like illnesses that may have gone unrecognized or unreported at the time of occurrence and careful examination of the newborn to rule out other congenital defects (Park, 1996; Ardinger, 1997; Pyeritz, 2001).

Maternal drug use may also cause cardiac malformations. Half of newborns with fetal alcohol syndrome (FAS) have a congenital heart defect. Only a few drugs (e.g., thalidomide) are proven teratogens, but no drug is known to be completely safe. Only recently has it been recognized that environmental hazards pose a threat to fetal development.

Metabolic disease in the mother increases the risk of CHDs. Infants of diabetic mothers have a 10% risk of having a CHD. TGA, VSD, and generalized hypertrophic cardiomyopathy are the defects most often found in infants of diabetic mothers (Park, 1996; Ardinger, 1997).

Most CHDs are considered to be multifactorial in origin; that is, these defects probably arise from the interaction of a number of causes. Research into the genetic causes of cardiac defects may identify a specific genetic origin for some defects currently thought to have a multifactorial origin. Infants with other congenital defects often have associated CHDs. Multiple defects can arise in the structures that are forming at the time of an agent or environmental factor's exposure which leads to an interference with normal development.

Incidence

Estimates of the incidence of congenital heart defects vary from 4.05 to 10.2 per 1000 live births. As mentioned previously, the overall incidence of CHD is slightly less than 1%, or 8 per 1000 live births, excluding PDA in the preterm newborn (Park, 1996; Nouri, 1997). Congenital heart defects are the single most important factor in infant mortality caused by birth defects, and hypoplastic left heart syndrome is the most frequent specific cause of congenital heart defect (Centers for Disease Control, 1998). Recent reviews of the incidence of congenital heart defects have demonstrated an overall increase in CHDs. It is surmised that some of the increase can be attributed to better diagnosis and reporting; however, changes in the distribution of risk factors may account for actual increases. The prevalence of VSDs, TOF, atrioventricular septal defects, and pulmonary stenosis increased from 1968 through 1997. The prevalence of TGA declined during that same time period (Botto & Correa, 2001). Because the overall incidence of CHD is approximately 1% of all live births and because the incidence of individual defects is less than 1%, the incidence of individual defects usually is given as a percentage of total CHDs. The incidence of a specific defect within the overall incidence of CHDs is included in the discussion of that defect. Identification of cardiovascular abnormalities and prompt institution of appropriate therapy is extremely important in the care of newborns, because approximately 95% of congenital heart defects can be partly or fully corrected (Cooley, 1997).

Some CHDs are not detected in the neonatal period; others are identified but initially are managed medically. For these reasons, the following discussion of CHDs extends beyond the neonatal period. Table 23-3 presents an overview of the diagnosis of CHDs.

The discussion of defects is based on the common pathophysiologic features. CHDs can be classified in numerous ways. The simplest classification is based on whether the defect produces cyanosis, a method described by Taussig in 1947. As mentioned previously, cyanosis is the bluish discoloration of the skin that occurs when approximately 5 g/dl of desaturated hemoglobin is present in the circulating volume (Taussig, 1947). The appearance of cyanosis, therefore, depends on the hemoglobin concentration. An infant with low hemoglobin may be hypoxic but may not appear cyanotic, therefore low hemoglobin cannot be the sole criterion for determining pathologic origin. Cyanosis in the extremities, or acrocyanosis, is frequently seen in newborns because of reduced blood flow through the small capillaries. Oxygen is extracted from the hemoglobin in the capillaries, giving the skin a blue appearance. This blue appearance is a normal phenomenon in the newborn. Differentiation of central cyanosis from peripheral or acrocyanosis is essential.

The presence or absence of cyanosis depends on whether deoxygenated blood is oxygenated by passing through the lungs. CHDs that allow the blood to pass through the lungs and then shunt from the left side of the heart and back to the right side of the heart generally are acyanotic defects. Defects that shunt deoxygenated blood directly to the left side of the heart, bypassing the lungs, are cyanotic defects. Some defects have mixed anatomic or functional features and do not fit into this schema, or the classifications overlap. For this discussion, three categories are used: (1) defects that involve communication between the systemic and pulmonary circulations (i.e., those with a left to right shunt, or acyanotic defects); (2) defects that involve obstruction of the vascular or valvular systems, with or without right to left shunt; and (3) defects that involve abnormalities in the origin of the pulmonary arteries or veins.

TABLE 23-3	Diagnosis of Congenital Heart Defects				
Defect	**Chest Radiograph**	**Electrocardiogram**	**Echocardiogram**	**Catheterization**	**Laboratory Values**
Patent ductus arteriosus (PDA)	Increased pulmonary vascularity, cardiac enlargement, left aortic arch	Left atrial and ventricular enlargement, abnormal QRS axis for age	LA:AO ratio over 1.3 (term), 1 (preterm); increased left atrium and ventricle (two dimensional [2-D])	Increased oxygen (O_2) saturation in pulmonary artery, increased right ventricular and pulmonary artery pressure (with pulmonary hypertension)	N/A
Atrial septal defect (ASD)	Mild heart enlargement, prominent main pulmonary artery, increased pulmonary vascularity	Right axis deviation, incomplete right bundle branch block, right ventricular hypertrophy	Dilated right ventricle, paradoxical movement of ventricular septum	Increased O_2 in right atrium, normal right-side atrium, normal right-side pressure, 10% partial anomalous pulmonary venous return	N/A
Aortic stenosis (AS)	Normal heart size, slight prominence of left ventricle and aorta	Normal or mild left ventricular hypertrophy, inverted T waves	Prominent septal thickening, abnormal mitral valve motions	Anatomic and physiologic alterations in cardiac function	N/A
Ventral septal defect (VSD)	Enlarged heart, increased pulmonary markings	Left and right ventricular hypertrophy	Large left atrium (M-mode), presence or absence of other defects (2-D)	Increased O_2 in right ventricle, increased systolic pressure in right ventricle and pulmonary artery	N/A
Endocardial cushion defect (ECD)	Cardiomegaly, increased pulmonary vascularity	Left axis deviation, prolonged P-R interval, right and left atrial enlargement, right ventricular hypertrophy, incomplete right bundle branch block	Ventricular dilation, abnormal mitral and tricuspid valves	Increased O_2 in right atrium, increased right ventricular or pulmonary artery pressure (or both); angiographic evidence of "goose neck" deformity of ventricular outflow area	N/A
Tetralogy of Fallot (TOF)	Normal heart size but boot-shaped contour, decreased pulmonary markings, prominent aorta, right aortic arch in one third of cases	Right axis deviation, right ventricular hypertrophy	Large ventricular septal defect; aortic dextroposition; and pulmonary stenosis; size of main, right, and left pulmonary arteries (2-D)	Demonstrates anatomy of right ventricular outflow region; also shows microcytic anemia	Increased hemoglobin, hematocrit clotting time, and prolonged clotting time

Condition	Chest X-ray	ECG	Echocardiography	Cardiac Catheterization	Laboratory
Pulmonary stenosis (PS)	Normal heart size, normal pulmonary vascularity, enlarged pulmonary artery, right ventricle filling (lateral)	Right axis deviation, right atrial enlargement, right ventricular hypertrophy	Decreased valve leaflet motion, small changes in thickness of right ventricular wall	Elevated right ventricular pressure, normal or slightly diminished pulmonary artery pressure	N/A
Truncus arteriosus (TA)	Cardiomegaly, absence of main pulmonary artery segment, large aorta, increased pulmonary vascularity	Right or left ventricular hypertrophy (or both)	Absence of two semilunar valves	Left to right shunt at level of ventricle, pressure equal in ventricles, truncus, and pulmonary arteries	Increased hemoglobin and hematocrit
Transposition of the great arteries (TGA)	Enlarged heart with narrow base, enlarged ventricles, increased pulmonary vascularity	Right axis deviation, right ventricular hypertrophy	Abnormal origin of great vessels	Increased right ventricular pressure, catheter can enter aorta from right ventricle, pulmonary artery can be entered only through patent ductus arteriosus or atrial septal defect	Increased hemoglobin and hematocrit; polycythemia
Coarctation of the aorta (COA)	Cardiomegaly, postcoarctation dilation (by age 5 years), notching of ribs from collateral vessels	Left ventricular hypertrophy, inverted T waves in left precordial leads, right ventricular hypertrophy (severe)	Visualization of narrowed aorta and location of associated defects; allows evaluation of aortic valve movement, structure, and function and of left ventricular size and function	Performed to determine exact location and for evaluation	N/A
Hypoplastic left heart syndrome (HLHS)	Cardiomegaly, increased pulmonary vascularity, interstitial emphysema	Prominent right ventricular forces, decreased left ventricular forces	Small left ventricle	Performed for evaluation for surgical intervention or if echocardiogram is inconclusive	N/A
Total anomalous pulmonary venous return (TAPVR)	Cardiac enlargement, large pulmonary artery, increased pulmonary flow	Right ventricular hypertrophy, right axis deviation, right atrial hypertrophy (after 1 month)	Right atrial enlargement and patent foramen ovale; inability to demonstrate continuity between pulmonary veins and left atrium (2-D)	Higher O_2 saturation in right atrium; angiographic evidence of opacification of pulmonary artery circulation, pulmonary venous circulation, and abnormal circulation	N/A

LA: AO, *Left atrium to aortic root (ratio)*; N/A, *Not applicable*.

Defects Involving Communication between the Systemic and Pulmonary Circulations with Left to Right Shunt

Typically, defects involving communication between the systemic and pulmonary circulations with left to right shunt, or acyanotic defects, do not produce cyanosis because the circulation has sufficient oxygenated blood. The left to right shunts increase the pulmonary blood flow and the workload of the heart. The acyanotic heart defects discussed here are patent ductus arteriosus, ventricular septal defect, atrial septal defect, endocardial cushion defect, and persistent truncus arteriosus (TA).

Patent Ductus Arteriosus.   The ductus arteriosus is a wide, muscular connection between the pulmonary artery and the aorta. The ductus arteriosus originates from the left pulmonary artery and enters the aorta below the subclavian artery; it allows oxygenated blood from the placenta to bypass the lungs and enter the circulation. The ductus arteriosus closes functionally by about 15 hours after birth. Some shunting of blood may occur during the first 24 hours after birth, but the ductal opening must be larger than 2 mm for significant shunting to occur.

Closure of the ductus arteriosus occurs in response to the increase in arterial oxygen concentration that follows initiation of pulmonary function. Other factors that contribute to closure of the ductus arteriosus include a decrease in prostaglandin E (PGE) and an increase in acetylcholine and bradykinin (Park, 1996). Persistence of the ductus arteriosus beyond 24 hours after birth is considered a PDA in the term newborn. PDA in the preterm newborn presents a different clinical problem and is discussed separately (Park, 1996).

Patent Ductus Arteriosus in the Term Newborn

Incidence.   PDA accounts for approximately 5% to 10% of all congenital heart defects, excluding those in preterm newborns. The incidence is higher in females (about 3:1) (Park, 1996).

Hemodynamics.   In extrauterine life, the flow of blood through the ductus arteriosus is reversed. The PDA allows blood to flow from left to right, thereby reentering the pulmonary circuit and increasing pulmonary blood flow. The amount of blood flowing through the PDA and the effects of the ductal flow depend on the difference between systemic and pulmonary vascular resistance and the diameter and length of the ductus. High pulmonary blood flow causes increased pulmonary vascular resistance, pulmonary hypertension, and right ventricular hypertrophy. Figure 23-4 shows the hemodynamics of PDA.

Manifestations.   A small PDA may be asymptomatic. A large PDA with significant shunting may produce signs of congestive heart failure with tachypnea, dyspnea, and hoarse cry. Frequent lower respiratory tract infections, coughing, and poor weight gain are common in older infants with PDA.

Diagnosis.   The diagnosis of PDA is based on the history and physical examination findings, radiographs, and echocardiograms. Characteristic findings on physical examination include bounding peripheral pulses, widened pulse pressure (over 25), and a hyperactive precordium. A systolic thrill may be felt at the upper left sternal border. A grade ⅙ to ⁴⁄₆ continuous "machinery" murmur is audible at the upper left sternal border or in the left infraclavicular area. The murmur is heard throughout the entire cardiac cycle because of the pressure gradient between the aorta and the pulmonary artery in both systole and diastole. In severe PDA with a large shunt, S_2 may be accentuated because of pulmonary hypertension (Park, 1996).

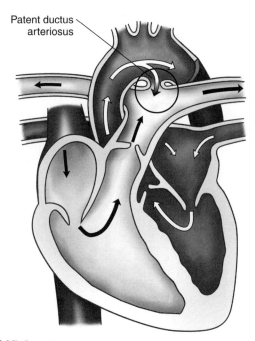

Patent ductus arteriosus

FIGURE 23-4
Patent ductus arteriosus is a communication between the pulmonary artery and the aorta.

A small PDA may not be distinguishable on chest radiographs. With more severe shunting, cardiomegaly and increased pulmonary vascularity may be seen. An ECG may show left atrial and ventricular enlargement and an abnormal QRS axis for age. The definitive diagnosis is made by echocardiogram. With two-dimensional echocardiography, PDA can be visualized directly. A ductus is considered hemodynamically significant if the left atrium to aortic root ratio (LA:AO) is greater than 1:3 in term newborns or greater than 1:0 in preterm newborns (Park, 1996).

Management.   Medical management includes administration of prophylactic antibiotics to prevent bacterial endocarditis. There are no exercise restrictions if pulmonary hypertension is not a factor. Definitive treatment involves surgical ligation through a posterolateral thoracotomy. Corrective surgery is performed in patients between 1 and 2 years of age unless CHF, recurrent pneumonia, or pulmonary hypertension is present. The mortality rate is less than 1% (excluding preterm newborns). The prognosis is excellent, and complications are rare (Park, 1996).

Patent Ductus Arteriosus in the Preterm Newborn

Hemodynamics.   Patent ductus arteriosus is a common complicating factor in the care of preterm newborns. As the newborn recovers from respiratory distress, pulmonary vascular resistance declines as oxygenation improves. In preterm newborns the ductus arteriosus is not as responsive to increased oxygen content as in term newborns, and it does not close. The decrease in pulmonary vascular resistance causes blood to shunt from left to right and reenter the pulmonary circuit, leading to increased pulmonary venous congestion, which reduces lung compliance and results in stiff lungs. Consequences of large shunts include symptoms of CHF, inability to wean from ventilatory support, or an increased oxygen requirement.

Clinical findings indicative of PDA include bounding peripheral pulses, a hyperactive precordium, widened pulse pressures (over 25), and a continuous murmur, best heard at the upper left and middle sternal border. Radiographic findings include increased pulmonary vascularity and cardiomegaly. PDA can be visualized directly by two-dimensional echocardiography and Doppler flow studies (Park, 1996).

Management.   Management of PDA depends on the severity of the symptoms. Conservative management consists of fluid restriction and diuretic therapy. Use of cardiac glycosides is controversial in the preterm newborn. The preterm newborn's myocardium has a greater amount of connective tissue and water, which may reduce the distensibility of the left ventricle; digitalis, therefore, would have no effect. Also, digitalis toxicity may occur because of poor elimination of the drug. If digitalis is used, the dose should be reduce and monitored carefully (Park, 1996).

Indomethacin, a prostaglandin synthetase inhibitor, may be used to close the ductus arteriosus. PGE_2 is produced in the walls of the ductus arteriosus to prevent closure during fetal life. Indomethacin inhibits the production of PGE_2 and promotes ductal closure. Smaller babies may require a higher dose to obtain effective plasma levels. Indomethacin works best if used in newborns younger than 13 days of life; it is not effective after 4 to 6 weeks after birth. The dosage is dependent on age, weight, and renal function. Because indomethacin is highly nephrotoxic, the blood urea nitrogen (BUN) and creatinine levels must be monitored. Contraindications to the use of indomethacin include renal failure, a low platelet count, bleeding disorders, necrotizing enterocolitis, and hyperbilirubinemia (Park, 1996).

Surgical ligation is reserved for cases in which indomethacin fails or is contraindicated. The mortality rate for ligation is slightly less than 2%. The mortality rate is highest in the more preterm, sicker infants, especially if pulmonary hypertension has developed (Park, 1996).

Ventricular Septal Defect.   A VSD is a defect or opening in the ventricular septum caused by imperfect ventricular division during early fetal development. The defect can occur anywhere in the muscular or membranous ventricular septum. The size of the defect and the degree of pulmonary vascular resistance are more important in determining the severity than the location. With a small defect, there is considerable resistance to the left to right shunt at the defect, and the shunt does not depend on the pulmonary vascular resistance. With a large VSD, there is little resistance at the defect, and the amount of left to right shunt depends on the level of pulmonary vascular resistance (Park, 1996; Turner & Hunter, 1999).

Incidence.   VSD is the most common congenital heart defect. It accounts for approximately 20% to 25% of all CHDs.

Hemodynamics.   The hemodynamic consequences of a VSD depend on whether it is a small, moderate, or large defect.

Small Ventricular Septal Defect.   Small VSDs produce minimal shunting and may not be symptomatic. The chest radiograph and the ECG generally are normal. A loud, harsh, pansystolic heart murmur may be best heard in the third and fourth left intercostal spaces at the sternal border (Park, 1996; Turner & Hunter, 1999). Figure 23-5 shows a ventricular septal defect.

Moderate Ventricular Septal Defect.   With moderate-size VSDs, the blood is shunted from the left ventricle to the right ventricle because of higher pressure in the left ventricle and higher systemic vascular resistance. Because this shunting occurs during systole, when the right ventricle contracts, the blood enters the pulmonary artery rather than remaining in

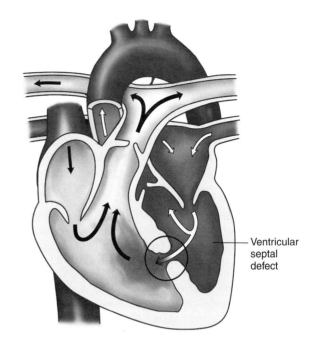

Ventricular septal defect

FIGURE **23-5**
Ventricular septal defect is a communication between the right and left ventricles.

the right ventricle. This prevents the development of right ventricular hypertrophy.

Large Ventricular Septal Defect.   With large VSDs, blood is shunted from the left ventricle to the right ventricle. The larger the VSD, the greater the volume of blood shunted to the right side of the heart. The pressures in the right ventricle and pulmonary artery are higher than normal. If pulmonary artery pressure is significantly increased, the pulmonary arterioles may thicken, and the increased resistance may reduce the left to right shunt. Pulmonary vascular disease can lead to right to left shunting and cyanosis.

Manifestations.   Manifestations of VSD depend on the degree of shunting. Small VSDs may produce no hemodynamic compromise and may be asymptomatic. Larger defects are associated with diminished exertional tolerance, recurrent pulmonary infections, poor growth, and symptoms of CHF. With severe VSD, pulmonary hypertension and cyanosis may be seen.

Diagnosis.   In VSD, a systolic thrill may be palpated at the lower left sternal border. A precordial bulge may be seen with very large VSDs. A grade 2/6 to 5/6 regurgitant systolic murmur is heard at the lower left sternal border. An apical diastolic rumble also may be heard, and the pulmonary heart sound may be loud.

Radiography can aid detection of moderate to large VSDs (Danford et al., 2000). In such cases chest radiographs will show cardiomegaly involving the left atrium, left ventricle, and possibly the right ventricle, as well as increased pulmonary vascularity. An ECG may reveal left ventricular hypertrophy, and right ventricular hypertrophy may also be present in severe cases. An echocardiogram (M-mode) will show a large left atrium. A two-dimensional echocardiogram will show other defects and the size and location of the VSD (Park, 1996).

Physical examination of infants with a large VSD that was not detected in the neonatal period may reveal inadequate weight gain, cyanosis, and clubbing of the digits.

Management.   Treatment of a VSD depends on the severity of the defect and the symptoms. VSDs can close spontaneously, therefore defects that cause no compromise may be observed to allow time for such closure. Small VSDs generally close spontaneously by approximately 6 years of age. Muscular VSDs have a higher spontaneous closure rate (69%) than perimembranous VSDs (29%) (Turner & Hunter, 1999).

Initial management of hemodynamically significant VSDs includes monitoring for signs of CHF and prompt initiation of therapy. Congestive heart failure in the older infant is treated with diuretics and digitalis. Unless pulmonary hypertension is a factor, activities need not be restricted. Prophylaxis against bacterial endocarditis is indicated.

Surgical management involves direct closure of the VSD. Cardiopulmonary bypass is required for surgical correction. The timing of the surgery depends on the severity of the circulatory and pulmonary compromise. Infants with significant left to right shunting with evidence of severe compromise require surgery. Indications for surgical correction include signs of CHF that do not respond to conservative medical management and increasing pulmonary vascular resistance. For asymptomatic children with a moderate VSD, surgical correction usually is performed between 2 and 4 years of age. Thomson, Gibbs, and Van Doorn (2000) reported using a cardiac catheter across a muscular VSD to aid closure, a technique that improved visualization of the defect from the right side of the heart and that minimized the size of the surgical incision in the left ventricle. The mortality rate for VSD correction is approximately 5%. The rate is higher among smaller infants, those with other defects, and those with multiple VSDs.

Atrial Septal Defect.   An ASD is a defect or opening in the atrial septum that develops as a result of improper septal formation early in fetal cardiac development.

The three types of ASDs are ostium secundum, commonly associated with the mitral valve; ostium primum, an ECD associated with anomalies of one or both AV valves; and sinus venosus, often associated with partial anomalous pulmonary venous connection (Park, 1996).

Incidence.   ASDs account for 5% to 10% of all congenital heart defects.

Hemodynamics.   An ASD usually does not produce symptoms until pulmonary vascular resistance begins to decline and the right ventricular end-diastolic and right atrial pressures drop. All types of ASDs produce some changes in blood flow.

With an ASD, blood shunts from left to right across the defect because the right ventricle, which is more compliant than the left, offers less resistance to filling. Any factors that reduce right ventricular distensibility or that obstruct flow into the right ventricle (e.g., pulmonary stenosis or tricuspid stenosis) can reduce the volume or reverse the direction of the shunt (Massin et al, 1998). The left to right shunt increases right ventricular volume, but pulmonary vascular resistance declines, therefore the pulmonary artery pressure is almost normal. The large pulmonary blood flow gradually leads to an increase in pulmonary artery pressures. Figure 23-6 shows an atrial septal defect.

Manifestations.   Newborns with an ASD usually are asymptomatic, although a grade ²/₆ or ³/₆ systolic ejection murmur may be present, which can best be heard at the upper left sternal border. S₂ may be widely split and fixed. With a large ASD,

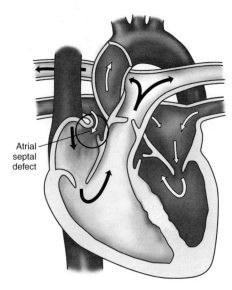

FIGURE **23-6**
Atrial septal defect is a communication between the right and left atria.

a mid-diastolic rumble caused by the relative tricuspid stenosis may be audible at the lower left sternal border (Park, 1996). On the chest radiograph, the heart is enlarged and has a prominent main pulmonary artery segment and increased pulmonary vascularity. An ECG can aid detection of atrial septal defects, showing right axis deviation and mild right ventricular hypertrophy. Incomplete right bundle branch block may be seen (Park, 1996; Danford et al, 2000).

With an ASD, an echocardiogram by M-mode shows increased right ventricular dimension and paradoxical movement of the ventricular septum. The diagnosis can be made with a two-dimensional echocardiogram, which shows the location and size of the defect. Children with ASDs usually are thin and may be easily fatigued. By late infancy, a precordial bulge caused by enlargement of the right side of the heart may be present.

Management.   An untreated ASD can lead to CHF, pulmonary hypertension, and atrial dysrhythmias in adults. Spontaneous closure of ASDs occurs in the first 5 years of age in up to 40% of children (Park, 1996). Medical management of ASD consists of prevention or treatment of CHF. No restrictions on activities are needed. The defect is corrected surgically by placing a simple patch or by direct closure during open heart surgery using cardiopulmonary bypass. The timing of the surgery depends on the severity of the defect. A significant left to right shunt is an indication for surgical correction. Surgery is performed when the patient is between 2 and 5 years of age. The surgery is not performed in infants unless CHF unresponsive to medical management is a factor. The mortality rate for the surgery is less than 1%. The highest risk is for small infants with CHF or increased pulmonary vascular resistance (Park, 1996).

Endocardial Cushion Defects.   ECDs result from inappropriate fusion of the endocardial cushions during fetal development. These defects produce abnormalities of the atrial septum (ostium primum), ventricular septum, and AV valves. ECDs take many forms and are characterized by downward displacement of the AV valves as a result of deficiency in ventricular septal tissue and an elongation of the left ventricular outflow tract. The term complete AV canal describes the large opening

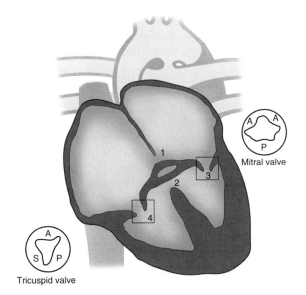

FIGURE **23-7**
Endocardial cushion defect. *1,* Ostium primum atrial septal defect; *2,* ventricular septal defect in the inlet portion of the ventricular septum; *3,* cleft in the anterior mitral valve leaflet; *4,* cleft in the septal leaflet of the tricuspid valve, which produces common anterior and posterior cusps of the atrioventricular valve. *A,* Anterior; *S,* septal; *P,* posterior.

TABLE **23-4**	Four Major Types of Truncus Arteriosus	
Type	**Incidence**	**Description**
I	60%	Main pulmonary artery arises from truncus and divides into left and right pulmonary arteries; pulmonary blood flow is increased.
II	20%	Pulmonary artery arises from posterior portion of truncus arteriosus; pulmonary blood flow is normal.
III	10%	Pulmonary artery arises from sides of truncus arteriosus; pulmonary blood flow is normal.
IV	10%	Bronchial arteries arise from descending aorta to supply lungs; pulmonary blood flow is decreased.

in the center of the heart between the atria and the ventricles. The defects that can occur in the AV canal are (1) an ostium primum ASD, (2) a VSD in the inlet portion of the ventricular septum, (3) a cleft in the anterior mitral valve leaflet, and (4) a cleft in the septal leaflet of the tricuspid valve, which results in common anterior and posterior cusps of the AV valve (Park, 1996).

Incidence. ECDs account for 2% of all congenital heart defects, and 30% of ECDs appear in infants with Down syndrome. Of infants with ECDs, 10% also have PDA, and 10% have TOF (Park, 1996).

Hemodynamics. The hemodynamic consequences of ECDs depend on the type and severity of the defect. Interatrial and interventricular shunts, left ventricle to right atrium shunts, or AV valve regurgitation may be seen. Figure 23-7 shows an endocardial cushion defect.

Manifestations. The manifestations of ECDs arise from the increased pulmonary blood flow caused by the abnormal connection between both ventricles and the atria and by absent or malformed AV valves. The newborn may have respiratory distress, signs of CHF, tachycardia, and a cardiac murmur. The mitral regurgitation may be heard as a grade $\frac{3}{6}$ or $\frac{4}{6}$ holosystolic regurgitant murmur audible at the lower left sternal border, which transmits to the left back and may be audible at the apex. A mid-diastolic rumble is present at the lower left sternal border or at the apex, caused by the relative stenosis of the tricuspid and mitral valves. S_1 is accentuated, and S_2 is narrowly split. The sound of the pulmonary closure is increased in intensity (Park, 1996; Kwiatkowska et al, 2000).

The chest radiograph reveals generalized cardiomegaly with increased pulmonary vascularity and a prominent main pulmonary artery segment. An ECG shows left axis deviation with a prolonged P-R interval, right and left atrial enlargement,

right ventricular hypertrophy, and incomplete right bundle branch block. In an infant with an ECD, signs of CHF, recurrent respiratory infections, and failure to thrive may be noted. Physical examination reveals a poorly nourished infant with signs of respiratory distress and tachycardia (Park, 1996; Kwiatkowska et al, 2000; McElhinney et al, 2000).

Management. Initial medical management is aimed at preventing or treating CHF with diuretics and digitalis. Prophylaxis against bacterial endocarditis is required before and after surgical correction. Definitive management consists of surgical closure of the ASD and VSD, with reconstruction of AV valves under cardiopulmonary bypass, deep hypothermia, or both. In some cases, pulmonary artery banding may be performed as a palliative procedure if significant mitral regurgitation is not a factor. This procedure carries a slightly higher mortality risk than primary surgical repair.

Surgery is indicated with CHF unresponsive to medical therapy, recurrent pneumonia, failure to thrive, or a large shunt with development of pulmonary hypertension and increasing pulmonary vascular resistance. The repair is performed in patients approximately 6 months to 2 years of age. The mortality rate has declined in recent years to approximately 5% to 10%. The mortality rate for patients who undergo pulmonary banding is approximately 15%. Factors that increase the risk of this procedure include (1) very young age, (2) severe AV valve incompetence, (3) hypoplastic left ventricle, and (4) severe symptoms before surgery (Park, 1996).

Persistent Truncus Arteriosus. The truncus arteriosus is a large vessel located in front of the developing fetal heart that gives rise to the coronary and pulmonary arteries and the aorta. Persistent truncus arteriosus (PTA) results from inadequate division of the common great vessel into a separate aorta and pulmonary artery during fetal cardiac development. A single large great vessel arises from the ventricles and gives rise to the systemic, pulmonary, and coronary circulations. Inadequate closure of the conal ventricular septum results in a VSD. Four types of this defect have been described (Table 23-4) (Park, 1996).

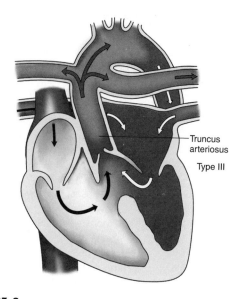

FIGURE 23-8

Persistent truncus arteriosus is a single arterial vessel that gives rise to the coronary arteries, pulmonary arteries, and aorta.

Incidence. PTAs account for less than 1% of all congenital heart defects.

Hemodynamics. Desaturated blood from the right ventricle and oxygenated blood from the left ventricle are received in the truncus arteriosus. The pressures of the two ventricles are equal. The truncus arteriosus supplies blood to the systemic and pulmonary circuits. The amount of flow depends on the resistance of the two circulations. Because pulmonary vascular resistance is high at birth, the pulmonary and systemic flows are relatively equal initially. Pulmonary resistance gradually declines over time, causing an increase in pulmonary blood flow. CHF may develop as a result of the increased pulmonary blood flow. If CHF is not corrected, pulmonary vascular disease develops in response to high pressure and increased pulmonary blood flow, subsequently reducing pulmonary blood flow. These changes, although compensatory initially, complicate the hemodynamics after surgical correction. The volume overload is compounded by incompetent truncal valves, which allow regurgitation of blood into the ventricles. A PTA is shown in Figure 23-8.

Manifestations. The presence of cyanosis depends on the amount of pulmonary blood flow. Signs of CHF may be the first indication of persistent truncus arteriosus. On auscultation, systolic click at the apex and upper left sternal border may be noted. The VSD may produce a harsh, grade 2/6 to 4/6 systolic murmur heard along the lower sternal border. Increased pulmonary blood flow may produce an atrial rumble. Truncal valve insufficiency produces a high-pitched, early diastolic decrescendo murmur. Bounding arterial pulses and a widened pulse pressure may also be seen. S_2 is single. If PTA is not detected in the newborn period, symptoms of poor feeding, failure to thrive, frequent respiratory infections, and signs of CHF appear.

Diagnosis. On chest radiographs the heart is enlarged, and pulmonary blood flow may be increased. Half of PTA cases have a right aortic arch (Park, 1996). An ECG reveals a nor-

mal QRS axis and ventricular hypertrophy. Echocardiography demonstrates the truncus arteriosus overriding a VSD and the absence of the pulmonary valve (Park, 1996).

Management. Medical management consists primarily of treatment of CHF and prophylaxis with antimicrobials. Pulmonary artery banding, instituted as a palliative measure, may be performed in small infants with increased pulmonary blood flow and CHF unresponsive to medical management. The mortality rate for this group of infants is close to 30% (Park, 1996).

The definitive surgical correction is the Rastelli procedure (Table 23-5). Surgery is performed in infants, because the mortality rate for uncorrected PTA is higher than the mortality rate for surgical correction, which ranges from 20% to 60%. Repeated surgery may be required to enlarge the conduit as growth occurs (Park, 1996).

Defects Involving Obstruction of the Vascular or Valvular Systems with or without Right to Left Shunt

Defects involving obstruction of the vascular or valvular systems, with or without right to left shunt, are CHDs that arise from a defect of either the vascular or the valvular system that results in obstruction of blood flow and a right to left shunt with either reduced or increased pulmonary blood flow. The defects described in this section are aortic stenosis (AS), tetralogy of Fallot (TOF), pulmonary valve atresia or stenosis (PVA or PVS), hypoplastic left heart syndrome (HLHS), and coarctation of the aorta (COA).

Aortic Stenosis. Aortic stenosis is one of a group of defects that result in obstruction to ventricular outflow. AS may be valvular, subvalvular, or supravalvular; valvular stenosis is the most common type, and supravalvular is the least common form (Park, 1996).

With valvular stenosis, a bicuspid valve usually is present. Subvalvular stenosis can involve either a simple diaphragm or a long, tunnel-like ventricular outflow tract. Idiopathic hypertrophic subaortic stenosis is a form of subvalvular stenosis that manifests as a cardiomyopathy. Supravalvular stenosis is associated with Williams syndrome (elfin facies), which is characterized by mental retardation, short palpebral fissures, and thick lips (Park, 1996).

Incidence. AS accounts for 5% of all congenital heart defects. It is four times more common in males.

Hemodynamics. Aortic stenosis causes an increase in the pressure load on the left ventricle, leading to left ventricular hypertrophy. The resistance to blood flow through the stenosis gradually causes a pressure gradient between the ventricle and the aorta. Eventually, coronary blood flow decreases. Aortic stenosis is shown in Figure 23-9.

Manifestations. Symptoms depend on the severity of the defect. Mild aortic stenosis may not cause symptoms. With more severe defects, activity intolerance, chest pain, or syncope is seen. With severe defects, CHF develops.

Diagnosis. Physical examination reveals normal development without cyanosis. A narrow pulse pressure and a higher systolic pressure in the right arm may be noted with severe supravalvular aortic stenosis. A systolic murmur of approximately grade 2/6 to 4/6 is present, best heard at the second right

TABLE **23-5**	Common Cardiac Surgical Procedures		
Procedure	**Type**	**Defect**	**Description**
Blalock-Hanlon	Palliative	Transposition of the great arteries (TGA)	Surgical creation of an atrial septal defect; rarely used but still useful for complex TGA or mitral atresia and single ventricle
Blalock-Taussig	Palliative	Tetralogy of Fallot, pulmonary artery defect, pulmonary stenosis, ventricular septal defect	Anastomosis of the subclavian artery and pulmonary artery to improve pulmonary blood flow
Brock	Corrective	Pulmonary valve atresia	Blind pulmonary valvotomy of the pulmonary valve
Damus	Corrective	Single ventricle and narrow aorta (only obstruction)	Pulmonary valve is connected to the aorta to increase outflow
			Pulmonary arteries are connected to aorta in a Y
Fontan	Corrective	HLHS (stage 2 Norwood), tricuspid atresia, tricuspid stenosis	Bypassing the right ventricle by connecting the right atrium to the pulmonary artery
Glenn	Corrective	Used after HLHS (stage 1 Norwood or PABAND). Used for tricuspid atresia or HLHS.	Connects the superior vena cava and the right pulmonary artery. It is detached completely from the right atrium creating a bi-directional shunt.
Gore-Tex shunt	Palliative	Tetralogy of Fallot	Interposition of Gore-Tex between the subclavian artery and the ipsilateral pulmonary artery
Jatene	Corrective	Transposition of the great arteries	Switching of transposed great arteries to their anatomically correct position
Mustard	Corrective	Transposition of the great arteries	Use of a pericardial or synthetic baffle in the atria to shunt venous blood across the right atrium to the left ventricle and into the pulmonary artery; systemic blood is shunted across the left atrium to the right ventricle, which delivers blood to the aorta
Norwood	Palliative	Hypoplastic left heart syndrome (stage 1 Norwood)	1. The main pulmonary artery is divided, and the proximal stump is anastomosed to the descending aorta; the distal main pulmonary artery is closed. 2. Right-sided Gore-Tex shunt is performed to increase pulmonary blood flow. 3. The atrial septum is excised to allow interatrial mixing.
Potts	Palliative	Tetralogy of Fallot	Rarely used; surgical creation of a window between the descending aorta and the left pulmonary artery; difficult to take down
Pulmonary artery banding	Palliative	Ventricular septal defect, single ventricle	Placement of a band around the pulmonary artery to reduce blood flow to the lungs
Rashkind	Corrective	Pulmonary artery defect, transposition of the great arteries	Atrial septostomy created at cardiac catheterization by passing a balloon-tip catheter through the patent foramen ovale, inflating the balloon, and snapping it back through the patent foramen
Rastelli	Corrective	Transposition of the great arteries, tetralogy of Fallot, pulmonary artery defect, truncus arteriosus	Commonly used with all valved conduits from the right ventricle to the pulmonary artery
Senning	Corrective	Transposition of the great arteries	Use of atrial tissue to create an intraatrial baffle to shunt blood from the vena cava to the left ventricle and from the pulmonary veins to the right ventricle
Waterston	Palliative	Tetralogy of Fallot	Creation of a window between the ascending aorta and the pulmonary artery, improving oxygenation of systemic blood; rarely used because of the distortion or obstruction of the pulmonary artery

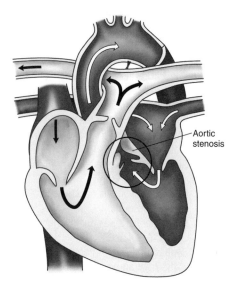

FIGURE **23-9**
Aortic stenosis is a narrowing or thickening of the aortic valvular region.

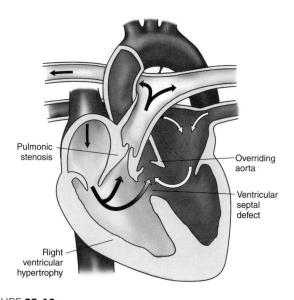

FIGURE **23-10**
Tetralogy of Fallot consists of pulmonary stenosis, ventricular septal defect, overriding aorta, and hypertrophy of the right ventricle.

or left intercostal space with transmission to the neck. With valvular aortic stenosis, an ejection click may be heard. With severe aortic stenosis, paradoxical splitting of S_2 may be noted. With bicuspid aortic valve or subvalvular stenosis, aortic insufficiency may cause a high-pitched, early diastolic decrescendo murmur (Park, 1996).

Chest radiographs may be normal or may show a dilated ascending aorta or, in the case of valvular stenosis, a prominent aortic "knob" caused by post-stenotic dilation (Park, 1996). Cardiomegaly is present if CHF or severe aortic regurgitation is a factor. An ECG may be normal or may show mild left ventricular hypertrophy and inverted T waves. An echocardiogram shows prominent thickening of the septum and abnormal mitral valve motion. A two-dimensional echocardiogram shows the anatomy of the aortic valve (bicuspid, tricuspid, or unicuspid) and that of subvalvular and supravalvular aortic stenosis.

Cardiac catheterization may be performed to identify the exact anatomy and to analyze pressure gradients.

Management.   Management is aimed at preventing or treating the CHF with fluid restriction, diuretics, and digitalis. In children with moderate to severe aortic stenosis, activity is restricted to avoid an increased demand on the heart. Balloon valvuloplasty sometimes is performed when the cardiac catheterization is done to improve circulation. With critical aortic stenosis, the patency of the ductus arteriosus must be maintained with PGE_1 to prevent hypoxia.

The type of surgical correction depends on the exact location and severity of the defect. The procedure may consist of aortic valve commissurotomy or valve replacement with a prosthetic valve or a graft. Placement of prosthetic valves usually is deferred until adult-size prosthetic valves can be inserted. The timing of the surgery depends on the severity of the defect. Infants with critical aortic stenosis with CHF must have corrective surgery. Surgery is performed on children if the peak systolic pressure gradient is above 80 mm Hg or if chest pain is a symptom.

The mortality risk for infants and small children is 15% to 20%. As in all cases, sicker, smaller infants have the highest

mortality rate. The mortality rate in older children is approximately 1% to 2% (Park, 1996).

Tetralogy of Fallot.   Tetralogy of Fallot was first described in 1888. The defect is the result of lack of development of the subpulmonary conus during fetal life. TOF consists of a large VSD, pulmonary stenosis or some other right ventricular outflow tract obstruction, an overriding aorta, and a hypertrophied right ventricle (the right ventricle may not be hypertrophied initially). Pulmonary valve atresia is seen in the most severe form of TOF.

Incidence.   TOF accounts for 10% of all congenital heart defects. Because repair generally is not carried out in the first year of life, TOF is the most common cyanotic heart defect beyond infancy.

Hemodynamics.   In TOF, the ventral septal defect allows equalization of pressure in the ventricles. Unsaturated blood flows through the VSD into the aorta because of the obstruction to blood flow from the right ventricle into the pulmonary artery. TOF is shown in Figure 23-10.

Manifestations.   Cyanosis, hypoxia, and dyspnea are the cardinal signs of TOF. Newborns may have just a loud murmur, or they may be cyanotic. Severe decompensation ("tet") spells are common in infants or children but can also occur in neonates. Children instinctively assume a squatting position, which traps venous blood in the legs and reduces systemic venous return to the heart. Chronic arterial desaturation stimulates erythropoiesis, causing polycythemia. The increased viscosity of the blood, caused by an increase in the number of red blood cells and by microcytic anemia, may lead to cerebrovascular accident (stroke). Brain abscesses may also occur as a result of bacteremia and compromised cerebral flow in the microcirculation. Two primary consequences of the chronic hypoxemia and polycythemia are (1) an increased risk of hemorrhagic diathesis, which arises from the thrombocytopenia caused by a shortened platelet survival time and reduced platelet aggregation, and (2) impaired synthesis of vitamin K—dependent clotting factors.

Diagnosis.   Neonates with TOF show varying degrees of cyanosis, depending on the severity of the obstruction to blood flow through the right ventricular outflow tract. A long, loud, grade ⅗ to ⅚ systolic ejection murmur is heard at the middle and upper left sternal border. A ventricular tap may also be noted along the lower left sternal border, and a systolic thrill may be palpated at the lower and middle left sternal border. With severe tetralogy of Fallot, a PDA murmur may be heard (Park, 1996).

A chest radiograph demonstrates reduced or normal heart size with decreased pulmonary vascularity. The contour of the heart may be a typical boot shape caused by the concave main pulmonary artery segment with upturned apex. Right atrial enlargement and a right aortic arch may also be seen.

An echocardiogram shows a large VSD and an overriding aorta. The anatomy of the right ventricular outflow tract and pulmonary valve can be identified with a two-dimensional echocardiogram.

In addition to the manifestations seen in the neonate, the infant or child with TOF may show clubbing of the fingers.

Management.   The definitive therapy for TOF is surgical repair under cardiopulmonary bypass. The surgical correction sometimes can be delayed with careful medical management. Neonates with only mild cyanosis improve when the pulmonary vascular resistance declines. Medical management is aimed at preventing or treating hypoxemia, polycythemia, infection, and microcytic hypochromic anemia. Careful follow-up is essential to detect signs of clinical deterioration. Parents need adequate education and support for home management (Park, 1996; Dipchand et al, 1999).

Dehydration must be avoided because of the increased risk of cerebral infarcts with hemoconcentration. Polycythemia develops as a compensatory mechanism to increase the oxygen-carrying capacity of the blood. If volume is diminished, however, the increased viscosity of the blood may further impede cerebral circulation.

Parents must be taught to recognize the early signs and symptoms of decompensation. They must also be taught to recognize and treat hypercyanotic, or tet, spells (Table 23-6). Tet spells are precipitated by events that lower the systemic vascular resistance, producing a large right to left ventricular shunt. Increased activity, crying, nursing, or defecation may trigger a hypoxemic episode. The right to left shunt causes a decrease in the partial pressure of oxygen (PO_2), an increase in the partial pressure of carbon dioxide (PCO_2), and a decrease in pH; this stimulates the respiratory center, causing an increase in the rate and depth of respirations (hyperpnea). Hyperpnea causes an increase in systemic venous return by increasing the efficiency of the thoracic pump. Because the right ventricular outflow tract obstruction prevents the increased blood flow from entering the pulmonary artery, the increased flow is shunted through the aorta, which further reduces the arterial PO_2. Severe, uninterrupted hypercyanotic spells lead to loss of consciousness, hypoxemia, seizures, and death.

Surgical treatment is indicated for hypercyanotic (tet) spells that result in increased hypoxemia, metabolic acidosis, inadequate systemic perfusion, increased cyanosis, or polycythemia. Systemic perfusion can be evaluated by observing peripheral

TABLE 23-6	Symptoms and Treatment of Hypercyanotic (Tet) Spells
SYMPTOMS	
Irritability, crying	Loss of consciousness
Hyperpnea	Seizures
Cyanosis	Decreased murmur
Diaphoresis	Metabolic acidosis
Treatment	**Rationale**
Knee to chest or squatting position	Traps blood in the lower extremities to reduce systemic venous return; increases pulmonary blood flow
Oxygen administration	Improves arterial oxygen saturation
Morphine sulfate (0.1 to 0.2 mg/kg/dose)	Suppresses respiratory center to reduce hyperpnea
Bicarbonate	Corrects acidosis and eliminates stimulation of respiratory center
Propranolol (Inderal) (0.15 to 0.25 mg/kg/dose)	May reduce spasms of right ventricular outflow tract or may act peripherally to stabilize the infant's condition

pulse intensity, urine output, capillary filling time, blood pressure, or peripheral vasoconstriction.

Surgical management can be either palliative or corrective (Table 23-5). Palliative procedures are undertaken to improve pulmonary blood flow by creating a pathway between the systemic and pulmonary circulations. These procedures also allow time for the right and left pulmonary arteries to grow. Palliative procedures are indicated for newborns with TOF and pulmonary atresia, severely cyanotic infants younger than 6 months of age, infants with medically unmanageable tet spells, or children with a hypoplastic pulmonary artery, in whom corrective surgery is difficult (Park, 1996).

Surgical correction is performed under cardiopulmonary bypass after the infant is 6 months old. Surgery may be delayed until 2 to 4 years of age in asymptomatic children or in children who undergo palliative procedures. The defect is repaired by patch closure of the VSD and resection and widening of the right ventricular outflow tract. Complications of cardiac surgery are listed in Box 23-1 and Table 23-7. The mortality rate for TOF varies with the severity of the circulatory compromise caused by the defect. The postoperative mortality rate is 5% to 10% in the first 2 years for uncomplicated TOF. More severe cases have a higher mortality rate, show residual pulmonary outflow tract obstruction, and may require further surgery. Because myocardial damage may occur from the restriction of the right ventricular blood flow during the surgery, cardiac support is needed to ensure adequate myocardial perfusion. Some centers use extracorporeal membrane oxygenation (ECMO) to support the cardiovascular perfusion. ECMO is also being attempted after surgical procedures for TGA and total anomalous pulmonary venous return (TAPVR), but infants with tetralogy o Fallot make up the largest group of patients who benefit from its use. Many of these infants experience pulmonary hypertension secondary to the cardiac problem or the

BOX 23-1

Complications of Cardiac Surgery

Low Cardiac Output
Hypovolemia
  Hemorrhage
  Diuresis
  Inadequate fluid volume
Tamponade
  Mediastinal bleeding
  Inadequate mediastinal drainage
Decreased cardiac contractility
  Hypervolemia
  Electrolyte imbalance
  Cardiac dysfunction
Increased systemic vascular resistance
Increased pulmonary vascular resistance
Arrhythmias
Hypothermia

Congestive Heart Failure
Uncorrected congenital heart defect (CHD) (after palliative procedure)
Corrected CHD, resulting in changes in ventricular preload, contractility, and afterload
Hypervolemia
Electrolyte imbalance
Arrhythmias

Respiratory Distress
Atelectasis
Pneumothorax
Hemothorax
Pleural effusion
Chylothorax
Congestive heart failure

Low cardiac output
Pulmonary hypertension
Inadequate ventilatory support
Ineffective pleural drainage
Hypoventilation secondary to pain

Renal Dysfunction or Failure
Poor systemic and renal perfusion
Intravascular hemolysis
Thromboembolus
Nephrotoxic drugs

Electrolyte Imbalance
Effects of cardiopulmonary bypass
Diuretics
Stress response
Fluid administration
Blood administration
Renal failure

Neurologic Abnormalities
Hypoxia
Acidosis
Poor systemic perfusion
Thromboembolism
Electrolyte imbalance

Infection
Surgery
Prosthetic material
Invasive monitoring or procedures
Inadequate nutrition

---

surgical correction. With ECMO, management of cases can focus on reducing pulmonary vascular resistance and diminishing right to left shunting during the immediate postoperative period.

Pulmonary Atresia. Pulmonary atresia results in the absence of communication between the right ventricle and the pulmonary artery. The atresia can be at the level of the main pulmonary artery or the pulmonary valve. Atresia of the pulmonary valve, with a diaphragm-like membrane, is the most common type. The right ventricle usually is hypoplastic and has thickened walls. Less frequently, the right ventricle is normal in size with tricuspid regurgitation. The presence of PDA, ASD, or patent foramen ovale to allow mixing of blood is crucial for survival.

Incidence. Pulmonary atresia accounts for less than 1% of all congenital heart defects (Park, 1996).

Hemodynamics. Pulmonary atresia with ASD results in a small, hypoplastic right heart. The absence of a right ventricular outflow tract results in high right ventricular end-diastolic pressures. Tricuspid insufficiency occurs, and right atrial pressures increase, causing systemic venous blood to shunt from the right to the left atrium through the patent foramen ovale or ASD. Mixed venous blood flows into the left ventricle and aorta. The PDA produces the only pulmonary blood flow. Closure of the PDA causes severe cyanosis, hypoxemia, and acidosis.

With a VSD, the right ventricle usually is adequate in size. Systemic venous blood shunts from the right ventricle through the VSD to the left ventricle and enters the aorta. The PDA still provides the only pulmonary blood flow. Pulmonary atresia is shown in Figure 23-11.

Manifestations. Pulmonary atresia usually is seen with cyanosis at birth. Tachypnea is present, but no obvious respiratory distress is noted. S_2 is single, and a soft systolic PDA murmur can be heard in the upper left sternal border. Tricuspid insufficiency may produce a harsh systolic murmur along the lower right and left sternal border (Park, 1996).

The heart may be normal in size or enlarged on the chest radiograph. The main pulmonary artery segment is concave and similar to the radiographic appearance of tricuspid atresia. Pulmonary vascular markings are decreased and continue to decrease as the PDA closes.

TABLE 23-7	Complications of Cardiac Surgery: Postoperative Syndromes		
Syndrome	**Cause**	**Symptoms**	**Management**
Postcoarctectomy syndrome	Arises from changes in pressure and flow	Severe, intermittent abdominal pain, fever, and leukocytosis; abdominal distention; melena, and ascites with gangrenous bowel; rebound systemic hypertension	Monitor blood pressure; prevent hypertension; delay postoperative feeding.
Postpericardiotomy syndrome	Immunologic syndrome; a response to blood in the pericardial sac	Fever, chest pain, pericardial and pleural effusions, hepatomegaly, leukocytosis, left shift, increased erythrocyte sedimentation rate, persistent changes in ST and T waves on electrocardiogram	
Postperfusion syndrome	Cytomegalovirus	Fever, splenomegaly, atypical lymphocytosis Onset: 3 to 6 weeks after surgery	Self-limiting disease process; only supportive care required
Hemolytic anemia syndrome	Trauma of red blood cells or autoimmune action	Fever, jaundice, hepatomegaly, reticulocytosis Onset: 1 to 2 weeks after surgery	Iron supplementation or blood transfusions, correction of turbulent flow

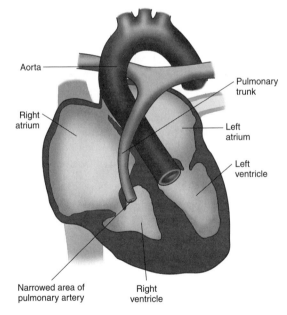

FIGURE **23-11**
Pulmonary atresia.

An ECG may reveal a normal QRS axis, left ventricular hypertrophy (type I), or, less frequently, right ventricular hypertrophy (type II). Right atrial hypertrophy is seen in approximately 70% of cases (Park, 1996). A two-dimensional echocardiogram reveals the atretic pulmonary valve and the hypoplastic right ventricular cavity and tricuspid valve. The location and size of the atrial communication are estimated by echocardiograophy.

Management. Immediate management of pulmonary atresia involves administration of prostaglandin to maintain duc-

tal patency. PGE₁ (Prostin) is given as a continuous intravenous infusion. The initial dose is started at 0.1 μg/kg/minute. When the desired effect has been achieved, the dosage is reduced incrementally to a maintenance dose of 0.01 μg/kg/minute. Careful attention to the site of the infusion is important.

A balloon atrial septostomy is performed at cardiac catheterization to promote better mixing of systemic and pulmonary venous blood in the atria. As soon as the newborn's condition has been stabilized, surgical correction is performed. Initially, a systemic-pulmonary artery shunt is performed, using Gore-Tex between the left subclavian artery and the left pulmonary artery (Blalock-Taussig procedure). If pulmonary valve atresia is present, a closed heart pulmonary valvotomy (Brock procedure) may be performed. The mortality rate for these procedures is 10% to 25%.

If the initial systemic-pulmonary shunt is not effective, a second shunt is attempted in another location. Reconstruction of the right ventricular outflow tract can be attempted if the right ventricle is large enough. This procedure has a mortality rate of 25%. The Fontan procedure is attempted for a hypoplastic right ventricle in late childhood. The mortality rate for this procedure can be as high as 40%.

The prognosis for pulmonary atresia depends on the size of the pulmonary outflow tract established through surgery and the degree of fibrosis of the right ventricle. With severe fibrosis and significant outflow tract obstruction, the risk is greater that dysrhythmias and right ventricular dysfunction will develop (Park, 1996).

Pulmonary Stenosis. Pulmonary stenosis arises from abnormal formation of the pulmonary valve leaflets during fetal cardiac development. Pulmonary stenosis can be valvular, subvalvular (infundibular), or supravalvular. Valvular pulmonary stenosis is the most common type, accounting for 90% of cases. Pulmonary stenosis frequently is seen in Noonan syndrome, and it is one of the four defects found in TOF. Isolated infundibular pulmonary stenosis is uncommon.

Incidence. Pulmonary stenosis accounts for 5% to 8% of all congenital heart defects. It is often associated with other defects.

Hemodynamics. Pulmonary stenosis results in obstruction to blood flow from the right ventricle to the pulmonary artery. The right ventricle hypertrophies because of the increased pressure caused by the obstruction to outflow. Pulmonary blood flow volume is normal in the absence of intracardiac shunting. Pulmonary stenosis is shown in Figure 23-12.

Manifestations. Pulmonary stenosis may be asymptomatic if it is mild. Moderate pulmonary stenosis may cause easy tiring. Severe or critical pulmonary stenosis causes CHF.

Diagnosis. The findings of pulmonary stenosis depend on the severity of the defect. A pulmonary systolic ejection click can be heard at the upper left sternal border. S_2 may be widely split, and the pulmonary component may be soft and delayed. A systolic ejection murmur (grade $\frac{2}{6}$ to $\frac{5}{6}$) is audible at the upper left sternal border and transmits across the back. The severity of the pulmonary stenosis is directly related to the loudness and duration of the murmur. A systolic thrill sometimes can be felt at the upper left sternal border. Hepatosplenomegaly may be present with CHF.

The ECG is normal with mild pulmonary stenosis. With moderate stenosis, right axis deviation and right ventricular hypertrophy may be noted. With severe pulmonary stenosis, right atrial hypertrophy and right ventricular strain occur.

Radiographically, the heart size is normal and has a prominent main pulmonary artery segment. In mild to moderate pulmonary stenosis, pulmonary markings are normal. The critical type of pulmonary stenosis causes decreased pulmonary markings. CHF results in increased heart size. An echocardiogram demonstrates diminished motion of the pulmonary valve leaflets and poststenotic dilation of the main pulmonary artery segment (Park, 1996; Danford et al, 1999).

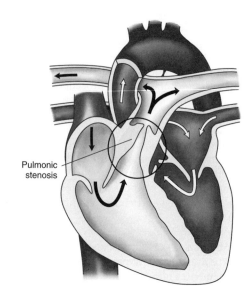

FIGURE **23-12**
Pulmonary stenosis.

Management. Management of pulmonary stenosis is determined by the severity of the obstruction to flow. The mild type generally requires no therapy except antimicrobial prophylaxis against subacute infective endocarditis (SAIE). Moderate pulmonary stenosis is treated through balloon valvuloplasty during cardiac catheterization. Surgical correction is performed in children when the right ventricular pressure measures 80 to 100 mm Hg and balloon valvuloplasty is not successful or when the pulmonary stenosis is infundibular in origin. Infants with critical pulmonary stenosis and CHF require PGE_1 infusion to maintain ductal patency until surgery is performed (Park, 1996). Careful fluid and electrolyte management requires balancing the need for fluids against the prevention of further expansion of the extracellular fluid volume and consequent strain on the heart's ability to pump (Burlet et al, 1999).

The overall prognosis for pulmonary stenosis is excellent. The mortality rate is less than 1% in older infants, although the rate is higher in newborns with critical pulmonary stenosis and CHF (Park, 1996).

Hypoplastic Left Heart Syndrome. Hypoplastic left heart syndrome (HLHS) consists of a group of cardiac defects that includes a small aorta, aortic and mitral valve stenosis or atresia, and a small left atrium and ventricle. The great vessels usually are normally related.

Incidence. HLHS accounts for only 1% to 2% of all congenital heart defects, but it is the leading cause of death from CHD in the first month of life. The disorder also accounts for 7% to 8% of heart defects that cause symptoms in the first year of life. HLHS is not associated with abnormalities in other organ systems.

Hemodynamics. Left ventricular output is greatly reduced or eliminated because of the valvular obstruction and small size of the left ventricle. The left atrial and pulmonary venous pressures are elevated, and pulmonary edema and pulmonary hypertension are present. With a PDA, blood shunts from the pulmonary artery into the aorta. The PDA provides the only cardiac output, because there is little or no flow across the aortic valve. Retrograde flow through the aortic arch supplies the head, upper extremities, and coronary arteries.

Although circulation is abnormal in utero, the high pulmonary vascular resistance and the low systemic vascular resistance make survival possible. The right ventricle maintains normal perfusion pressure in the descending aorta by a right to left ductal shunt. At birth, the onset of pulmonary ventilation causes the pulmonary vascular resistance to decline. The systemic vascular resistance increases because the placenta is eliminated. Closure of the ductus arteriosus further reduces systemic cardiac output and aortic pressure, leading to metabolic acidosis and circulatory shock. The increased pulmonary blood flow increases the left atrial pressure and causes pulmonary edema (Park, 1996). Figure 23-13 shows HLHS.

Manifestations. Progressive cyanosis, pallor, and mottling are presenting symptoms of HLHS. Tachycardia, tachypnea, dyspnea, and pulmonary rales are present. The S_2 is loud and single. Poor peripheral pulses and vasoconstriction of the extremities are noted on examination. Cardiac murmur may be absent, or a grade $\frac{1}{6}$ to $\frac{3}{6}$ nonspecific systolic murmur may be heard (Park, 1996).

Diagnosis. On radiographic studies, HLHS shows mild to moderate heart enlargement and pulmonary venous congestion or pulmonary edema. The metabolic acidosis identified by arterial blood gas studies is a result of diminished cardiac output. Right ventricular hypertrophy is the characteristic finding on an ECG. An echocardiogram usually is diagnostic. The findings demonstrate the components of the small left-sided heart structures and the dilated or hypertrophied right-sided heart structures; these findings include a small left ventricle, small ascending aorta and aortic root, absent or abnormal mitral valve, and enlarged right ventricle. The left ventricle to right ventricle end-diastolic ratio is abnormal (Park, 1996).

Management. Medical management of HLHS is aimed at preventing hypoxemia and correcting metabolic acidosis. PGE_1 is administered through continuous infusion to maintain ductal patency. Balloon atrial septostomy may be performed to decompress the left atrium.

Surgical correction of HLHS is experimental and has a high mortality rate, but this defect once was considered 100% fatal. Surgical correction is performed in stages. The first stage, the modified procedure, is performed in the neonatal period to maintain pulmonary blood flow and create interatrial mixing of blood. The second stage, a modified Fontan procedure, is performed at 6 months to 2 years of age. This procedure closes the Gore-Tex shunt and the atrial communication and forms a direct anastomosis of the right atrium and pulmonary artery (Table 23-5 for a description of these procedures) (Park, 1996).

The first-stage surgical repair has a mortality rate of nearly 75%, and the mortality rate for the second-stage procedure is 50% (Park, 1996). Nursing care is critical after the first-stage repair. During the immediate postoperative period, it focuses on assessment of homeostasis and pulmonary blood flow. Attention to nutritional status is important for long-term recovery.

The following elements should be meticulously assessed:

- Vital signs (for symptoms of blood loss)
- Chest tube output exceeding 10% of the total blood volume per hour over a period of several hours
- Platelet counts that may require treatment with fresh-frozen plasma, platelets, or cryoprecipitate at 10 ml/kg until the patient's condition is stable
- Daily liver function studies (which may indicate vitamin K treatment)
- Guaiac testing of bodily fluids such as stool and gastric drainage
- Ventilatory status (to maintain a mean airway pressure under 10 cm H_2O or a peak inspiratory pressure under 25 cm H_2O)
- Blood gases (for persistent acidosis or systemic hypotension, as evidenced by arterial oxygen pressure over 45 mm Hg or saturation over 85%)

Dopamine (5 to 10 μg/kg/minute) may be required to reduce pulmonary vasoconstriction. Dobutamine and isoproterenol are not used because they dilate the pulmonary arterioles, aggravating the condition. Fentanyl may be used to balance pulmonary vascular resistance. Diuretics or peritoneal dialysis may be necessary to maintain fluid balance. With acidosis and stiffening lungs, high-frequency ventilation sometimes is used to support pulmonary function. ECMO has also been used in those infants with acidosis and stiffening lungs.

Initially, nutritional support is provided through total parenteral nutrition (TPN). Weighing the infant daily; monitoring the urine for ketones, glucose, and protein; and measuring serum levels of electrolytes and trace minerals are necessary to adjust the parenteral fluids. Enteral feedings may be started in the first 2 weeks after surgery if the infant's condition is stable and after the greatest danger of necrotizing enterocolitis has passed.

Pericardial effusion may develop several days or weeks after the Fontan procedure, and changes in tissue perfusion and in systemic blood flow return may arise with this development. Cardiac transplantation, although experimental, may provide an improved prognosis for infants with HLHS. If surgical intervention is an option, it is essential that the parents be informed of all available treatments, including the risks and the prognosis.

Coarctation of the Aorta. Coarctation is a narrowing or constriction of the aorta in the aortic arch segment, most commonly below the origin of the left subclavian artery. Coarctation may occur as a single lesion caused by improper development of the aorta, or it may occur secondary to constriction of the ductus arteriosus. The severity of the circulatory compromise depends on the location and degree of constriction. Coarctation proximal to the ductus arteriosus (preductal COA) has associated defects in 40% of cases, including VSD, TGA, and PDA. The collateral circulation is poorly developed with preductal COA. Postductal COA usually is not associated with other defects, and the collateral circulation is more effective. Infants with postductal COA may not be symptomatic. More than half of infants with COA have a bicuspid aortic valve (Park, 1996).

Incidence. COA accounts for 8% of all congenital heart defects. It occurs twice as often in males and is found in 30% of infants with Turner syndrome (Park, 1996).

Hemodynamics. Coarctation creates an obstruction to flow, which leads to varying pressure across the aortic segment. The portion of the aorta proximal to the constriction has an elevated pressure, which leads to increased left ventricular

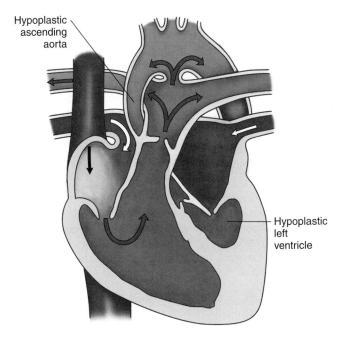

FIGURE **23-13**
Hypoplastic left heart syndrome.

Hypoplastic ascending aorta

Hypoplastic left ventricle

pressure. The increased left ventricular pressure results in left ventricular hypertrophy and dilation. Collateral circulation develops from the proximal to the distal arteries, bypassing the constricted segment of the aorta. This is a compensatory mechanism to increase flow to the lower extremities and abdomen, and the result is lower pulses in the lower extremities. COA is shown in Figure 23-14 (Park, 1996).

Manifestations.   The severity and emergence of symptoms depend on the location and degree of constriction and whether associated cardiac defects are a factor. Symptoms of coarctation include signs of CHF and absent, weak, or delayed pulses in the lower extremities with bounding pulses in the upper extremities. With CHF, however, all pulses may be weak. With severe COA, S_2 is loud and single. A systolic thrill may be felt in the suprasternal notch. An ejection click may be audible at the apex with a bicuspid aortic valve or systemic hypertension. A systolic ejection murmur of grade $\frac{2}{6}$ or $\frac{3}{6}$ may be heard at the upper right and middle or lower left sternal border and at the left interscapular area in the infant's back; however, no murmur is heard in more than half of infants with COA. Correction of CHF may produce the murmur (Park, 1996).

Diagnosis.   Diagnosis of COA is based on the history, physical findings, radiographs, ECGs, and echocardiographic data. In asymptomatic infants and children, chest radiographs may show a normal or slightly enlarged heart, and dilation of the ascending aorta may be evident. The "E" sign on barium swallow is characteristic but usually is not evident until at least 4 months of age. The "E" appearance is due to the large proximal aortic segment or prominent subclavian artery above the constricted segment and the poststenotic dilation of the descending aorta below it (Park, 1996). In symptomatic infants and children, radiographs show cardiomegaly and increased pulmonary venous congestion.

The ECG of an asymptomatic child may show left axis deviation of the QRS and left ventricular hypertrophy. In a symptomatic child, the ECG reveals normal or right axis deviation of the QRS. Right ventricular hypertrophy or right bundle branch block is seen in infants, whereas left ventricular hypertrophy is seen in older children (Park, 1996). A two-dimensional echocardiogram demonstrates the location and degree of the constriction and whether associated defects are present.

Management.   Surgical correction is the definitive treatment for COA. Surgery is delayed until 3 to 5 years of age if the signs and symptoms can be controlled medically. Earlier surgery is indicated if medical management is not successful.

The goals of medical management are to ensure adequate oxygenation, to prevent or treat CHF, and to prevent SAIE. PGE_1 may be needed to maintain ductal patency if the constricted segment is at the level of the ductus arteriosus (Park, 1996).

Surgical correction of COA involves excision of the constricted segment of the aorta and repair with an end-to-end anastomosis or a patch, Dacron, or bypass tube graft (Park, 1996). As an alternative, a subclavian flap aortoplasty may be performed. Surgery is indicated when CHF with or without circulatory shock is a factor. With a large VSD, pulmonary artery banding may be performed at surgery to reduce pulmonary blood flow in an attempt to prevent pulmonary hypertension. The band is removed and the VSD repaired at 6 months to 2 years of age. The mortality rate for surgical correction of COA is less than 5%. Postoperative complications include renal failure and recoarctation.

Defects Involving Abnormalities in the Origin of the Pulmonary Arteries or Veins

These defects arise from a defect in the bending and rotation of the heart as it grows and elongates. The result is abnormal alignment of the heart vessels and resulting cyanosis.

Transposition Defects.   Transposition defects are a group of malformations that have in common an abnormal anatomic relationship between the cardiac chambers and the great arteries.

Complete Transposition of the Great Arteries or Vessels. Transposition of the great arteries or vessels (TGA [or TGV]) is the result of inappropriate septation and migration of the truncus arteriosus during fetal cardiac development. TGA may be dextrotransposition of the great arteries (D-TGA) or levotransposition of the great arteries (L-TGA). With D-TGA, the aorta arises from the right ventricle, and the pulmonary artery arises from the left ventricle. The aorta receives unoxygenated systemic venous blood and returns it to the systemic arterial circuit. The pulmonary artery receives oxygenated pulmonary venous blood and returns it to the pulmonary circulation.

With L-TGA, the great vessels are transposed, with the aorta arising from the right ventricle and the pulmonary artery arising from the left ventricle. The aorta is to the left and anterior to the pulmonary artery. This type of transposition is called congenitally corrected TGA, because functionally the hemodynamics are normal. The oxygenated blood comes into the left atrium, enters the right ventricle, and passes through the aorta to the systemic circulation. However, other cardiac defects often are associated with this condition (Park, 1996).

Incidence.   TGA accounts for 5% of all congenital heart defects. It is more common in males (3:1). D-TGA is the most common cyanotic heart defect in newborns.

Hemodynamics.   Hemodynamically, complete D-TGA gives rise to two separate, parallel circulations. Oxygenated

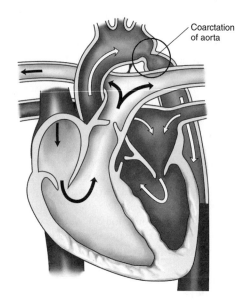

FIGURE **23-14**
Coarctation of the aorta is a narrowing or constriction of the aorta near the ductus arteriosus.

blood from the lungs is returned to the left atrium, enters the left ventricle, and passes through the pulmonary artery to the lungs again. Desaturated blood from the systemic circulation enters the right atrium, passes to the right ventricle, enters the aorta, and is directed back into the systemic circulation. The end result is that the heart, brain, and other vital tissues are perfused with desaturated blood. This defect is incompatible with life. A communication must exist between the two circulations to allow mixing of oxygenated and desaturated blood. This communication can be at the ductal, atrial, or ventricular level. The best mixing occurs with a large VSD. Figure 23-15 shows transposition of the great arteries (Park, 1996).

Manifestations.   Marked cyanosis is the prominent sign of TGA. The degree of cyanosis varies with the amount of communication between the two circulations. Signs of CHF are present. S_2 is loud and single. If a VSD is present, a loud, harsh systolic murmur of varying intensity can be heard. Hypoglycemia, hypocalcemia, and metabolic acidosis often are present.

Diagnosis.   On radiographic studies, the heart is enlarged and has a narrow base because the aorta is over the pulmonary artery. The heart is described as egg shaped (Park, 1996). Pulmonary blood flow is increased. An ECG shows right axis deviation of the QRS and right ventricular hypertrophy; an echocardiogram reveals the abnormal origin of the great arteries from the ventricles. Associated defects can also be visualized by echocardiography.

Management.   TGA is a cardiac emergency. Immediate medical management includes correction of acidosis, hypoglycemia, and hypocalcemia; administration of oxygen; infusion of PGE_1; and treatment of CHF. Cardiac catheterization and a balloon atrial septostomy are performed to promote mixing of oxygenated and desaturated blood in the atria. If the septostomy and PGE_1 infusion do not sufficiently improve oxygenation, surgical excision of the posterior aspect of the atrial

septum (Blalock-Hanlon procedure) is performed without cardiopulmonary bypass as a palliative measure. This procedure has a mortality rate of 10% to 25% (Park, 1996).

Definitive surgical correction involves switching the right- and left-sided structures at the ventricle level (Rastelli procedure), the artery level (Jatene procedure), or the atrium level (Senning or Mustard procedure) (see Table 23-5 for descriptions of these procedures).

The prognosis for TGA without surgical intervention is poor; 90% of patients die within the first year of life. The surgical procedures have high mortality rates and a high rate of postoperative complications (e.g., dysrhythmias, obstruction to systemic or pulmonary venous return, and right ventricular dysfunction). The Jatene procedure is newer but seems to minimize many complications associated with intraatrial repair operations; however, the long-term results of this procedure must be evaluated. The type and timing of surgical correction depend on the patient's condition and the anatomic defect, therefore each case must be decided individually. A typical management approach is presented in the flow diagram in Figure 23-16.

Total Anomalous Pulmonary Venous Return.   With TAPVR, the pulmonary veins drain into the right atrium (rather than the left atrium), either directly or through connection with the systemic veins. No direct connection exists between the pulmonary veins and the left atrium.

Incidence.   TAPVR accounts for 1% of all congenital heart defects. It occurs about equally in males and females.

Hemodynamics.   If an ASD or patent foramen ovale exists with TAPVR, a portion of the mixed blood from the right atrium can cross into the left atrium, the left ventricle, and on into the systemic circulation. The direction of the blood flow and the amount that crosses the atrial communication into the left atrium or that enters the left ventricle are determined by the compliance of the ventricles.

Two clinical hemodynamic states exist with TAPVR. If pulmonary blood flow is unobstructed, this flow is greatly increased. The result is highly saturated blood in the right atrium and mild cyanosis. If pulmonary blood flow is obstructed, the volume of flow is diminished and cyanosis is severe. Pulmonary edema often occurs secondary to elevated pulmonary venous pressure. Obstruction to pulmonary blood flow is a common occurrence when the TAPVR is below the diaphragm (Park, 1996). TAPVR is shown in Figure 23-17.

Manifestations.   The manifestations of TAPVR depend on whether pulmonary venous obstruction (PVO) is a factor. TAPVR without PVO produces a history of mild cyanosis, frequent pulmonary infections, poor growth, and CHF. TAPVR with PVO manifests as severe cyanosis and respiratory distress in the neonatal period, with progressive growth failure. Feeding is associated with increased cyanosis secondary to compression of the common pulmonary vein by the filled esophagus (Park, 1996). Signs and symptoms of CHF are also present.

Diagnosis.   TAPVR without PVO produces a precordial bulge with hyperactive right ventricular impulse. The PMI is at the xiphoid process or lower left sternal border. S_2 is widely split and fixed; the pulmonic sound may be pronounced. A grade $^2/_6$ or $^3/_6$ systolic ejection murmur can be heard at the

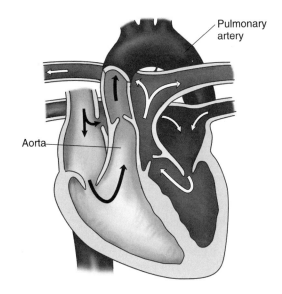

FIGURE **23-15**
With transposition of the great arteries or vessels, the aorta arises from the right ventricle, and the pulmonary artery arises from the left ventricle. The result is two distinct circulatory (parallel) pathways.

Pulmonary artery

Aorta

Surgical Procedures for Transposition of the Great Arteries

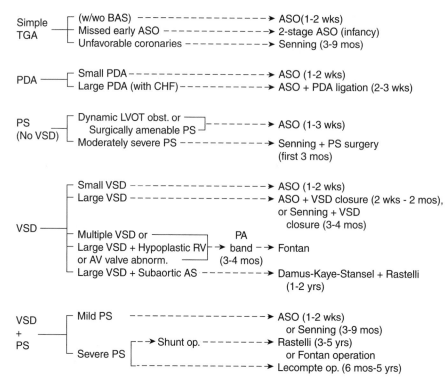

Simple TGA
- (w/wo BAS) ------------------→ ASO(1-2 wks)
- Missed early ASO -----------→ 2-stage ASO (infancy)
- Unfavorable coronaries ---------→ Senning (3-9 mos)

PDA
- Small PDA----------------→ ASO (1-2 wks)
- Large PDA (with CHF)---------→ ASO + PDA ligation (2-3 wks)

PS (No VSD)
- Dynamic LVOT obst. or Surgically amenable PS ------→ ASO (1-3 wks)
- Moderately severe PS ---------→ Senning + PS surgery (first 3 mos)

VSD
- Small VSD ------------------→ ASO (1-2 wks)
- Large VSD ------------------→ ASO + VSD closure (2 wks - 2 mos), or Senning + VSD closure (3-4 mos)
- Multiple VSD or Large VSD + Hypoplastic RV or AV valve abnorm. → PA band (3-4 mos) → Fontan
- Large VSD + Subaortic AS --------→ Damus-Kaye-Stansel + Rastelli (1-2 yrs)

VSD + PS
- Mild PS ------------------→ ASO (1-2 wks) or Senning (3-9 mos)
- Severe PS → Shunt op. ---------→ Rastelli (3-5 yrs) or Fontan operation
  ------------------→ Lecompte op. (6 mos-5 yrs)

FIGURE **23-16**

Flow diagram of surgical management of transposition of the great arteries. "Senning" on the diagram indicates an intraatrial repair, either the Senning or the Mustard operation. From Park MK (1996). *Pediatric cardiology for practitioners, ed 3.* Mosby: St Louis.

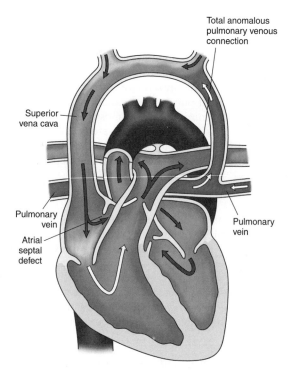

Total anomalous pulmonary venous connection

Superior vena cava

Pulmonary vein

Atrial septal defect

Pulmonary vein

FIGURE **23-17**

With total anomalous pulmonary venous return, all the pulmonary veins empty into the right atrium.

upper left sternal border, and a mid-diastolic rumble is always present at the lower left sternal border. The rhythm is a quadruple or quintuple gallop (Park, 1996).

TAPVR with PVO may produce minimal cardiac findings. S₂ is loud and single, and a gallop rhythm is noted. A faint systolic ejection murmur may be heard at the upper left sternal border, and pulmonary rales may be audible.

Radiographic findings of TAPVR without PVO include mild to moderate cardiomegaly and increased pulmonary markings. The characteristic "snowman" sign occurs because of the anatomic appearance of the left superior vena cava, the left innominate vein, and the right superior vena cava. This sign is seldom visible before 4 months of age. With TAPVR with PVO, the heart size is normal radiographically, and signs of pulmonary edema can be seen (Park, 1996).

On an electrocardiogram, TAPVR without PVO shows right axis deviation of the QRS and sometimes right atrial hypertrophy. TAPVR with PVO shows right axis deviation for age and right ventricular hypertrophy in the form of tall R waves in the right precordial leads.

An echocardiogram of TAPVR without PVO reveals the pulmonary veins draining into a common chamber posterior to the left atrium. The ASD and small left atrium and left ventricle can be seen. When present, a dilated coronary sinus that protrudes into the left atrium or a dilated innominate vein and superior vena cava can be seen. A two-dimensional echocardiogram of TAPVR with PVO shows the small left atrium and left ventricle. Anomalous pulmonary venous return below the diaphragm can be visualized directly. Doppler echocardiography can be used to detect the venous flow pattern (Park, 1996).

Management.   Treatment of TAPVR requires surgery, which is emergent when PVO exists below the diaphragm. Medical management is aimed at preventing or treating CHF and preventing hypoxemia. Diuretics may be required to manage pulmonary edema. Balloon atrial septostomy is performed at the time of cardiac catheterization to enlarge the interatrial communication and promote better mixing of blood. Surgery may be delayed if the response to medical management is good, but it usually is performed during infancy (Park, 1996).

The surgical procedure depends on the site of the anomalous drainage. Cardiopulmonary bypass is required. Surgery involves anastomosis of the pulmonary veins to the left atrium, closure of the ASD, and division of the anomalous connection. The mortality rate for surgery is high, 10% to 25%, but it is lower than that for medical management alone.

Experimental Treatments in the Postoperative Period

As discussed previously, for many of the cardiac defects, the morbidity and mortality rates remain high after surgery. Many centers are attempting treatments aimed at reducing pulmonary vascular resistance and persistent pulmonary hypertension and improving cardiac output. These treatments include ECMO, especially for infants with TOF, and high-frequency jet ventilation for infants who have undergone first-stage repair (Norwood procedure) for HLHS repair (Norwood et al, 1983). Newer treatments include nitric oxide (NO) administration and ultrafiltration.

Inhaled NO acts as a pulmonary dilator; it directly affects pulmonary and systemic vascular resistance. Its use is being investigated for infants who have undergone procedures that require cardiac bypass (e.g., bidirectional Glenn or Fontan procedures).

Ultrafiltration is an experimental procedure undertaken after open-heart surgery. It is similar to peritoneal dialysis in that it removes water and solutes to increase the hematocrit and blood pressure and to reduce the cardiac workload and pulmonary vascular resistance. These effects probably are due to a change in the pressure gradient between the blood and the dialyzing solution. The result is restoration or maintenance of blood volume, which reduces the need for transfusions. The improved perfusion also alleviates edema. As contractility of the heart improves, the cardiac workload declines, possibly because cardiodepressant proteins present after cardiac surgery are removed. Although investigational, this procedure appears to be a possible treatment for capillary leakage syndrome, which is prevalent after cardiac surgery.

Congenital Arrhythmias

Cardiac arrhythmias in infants generally arise from primary cardiac lesions, generally from abnormal conduction pathways. Alternatively, cardiac arrhythmias can develop after corrective cardiac surgery. It is not clear whether the arrhythmia is caused by the surgical procedure or the initial heart defect. Other factors that can contribute to the development of arrhythmias are electrolyte imbalances, neurologic conditions, and infections. Generally, in infants, rhythm disturbances are not the primary manifestation of a cardiac problem; CHF or cyanosis is present before dysrhythmias occur (Sacchetti et al, 1999). However, some conditions manifest with rhythm disturbances in the newborn period. The most common are congenital complete heart block (CCHB) and supraventricular tachycardia (SVT).

Congenital Complete Heart Block.   The AV node and the bundle of His arise as separate structures that join. Congenital heart block is a result of a discontinuity between the atrial musculature and the AV node or the bundle of His and the AV node. In most cases the exact cause of the discontinuity is unknown, and the remainder of the heart anatomy is normal. Certain antibodies passed from mothers with systemic lupus erythematosus (SLE) are associated with the condition. Congenital heart block can be a manifestation of CHDs, including congenitally corrected transposition of the great arteries.

CCHB can be diagnosed by detection of consistent fetal bradycardia (heart rate of 40 to 80 bpm) by auscultation, fetal echocardiography, or electronic monitoring. A newborn with a ventricular rate below 50 bpm and an atrial rate above 150 bpm is at significant risk. If the newborn has an associated heart defect, the risk for mortality is higher.

Treatment.   Asymptomatic infants do not require treatment. If the infant is in congestive heart failure, digitalization generally is the first line of treatment. Insertion of a pacemaker is necessary for infants with CHF that does not respond to digitalization. Children with pacemakers require close follow-up to monitor for complications or adverse effects of the pacemaker (Bevilacqua & Hordof, 1998).

Supraventricular Tachycardia.   SVT can arise in utero or in the neonatal period. The most common arrhythmias that produce signs are paroxysmal SVT with or without ventricular preexcitation, atrial flutter, and junctional tachycardia. If the SVT occurs in utero, it can lead to heart failure and hydrops fetalis. SVT in the fetus is treated through maternal administration of digitalis. If digitalization is not successful, propranolol, quinidine, felcainide, or amiodarone are used. The fetus is delivered if there is evidence of fetal lung maturity.

In most cases of SVT, no cause is found. In other cases, the cause may be long-acting thyroid stimulators and immune gamma$_2$-globulin from hyperthyroid mothers, hypoglycemia, or Ebstein anomaly of the tricuspid valve. Of infants with SVT, 10% to 50% have Wolfe-Parkinson-White syndrome (WPW), in which the atrial impulse activates the whole or some part of the ventricle, or the ventricular impulse activates the whole or some part of the atrium earlier than would be expected if the impulse traveled via the normal pathway. WPW is characterized by a normal QRS, regular rhythm, ventricular rates of 150 to 200 bpm. The onset is usually sudden and it may stop just as quickly. However, if untreated it can be fatal.

Symptoms produced by the SVT after birth are subtle and often go undetected until signs of CHF have been present for 24 to 36 hours. Treatment with digitalis or adenosine, cardioversion, transesophageal atrial pacing, or elicitation of the diving reflex (by covering the infant's face with a cold washcloth for 4 to 5 seconds) generally is successful at establishing normal sinus rhythm. After conversion, digitalis is continued for 9 to 12 months. Therapy is discontinued abruptly, without weaning dosages.

Recurrence is more likely in patients with WPW and is treated with the above drugs, alone or in combination. Recurrence declines between 2 and 10 years of age. The prognosis for SVT is good.

Congestive Heart Failure

CHF is a condition in which the blood supply to the body is insufficient to meet the metabolic requirements of the organs. CHF is a manifestation of an underlying disease or defect rather than a disease itself. Before CHF develops, compensatory mechanisms are activated to maintain adequate cardiac output (Park, 1996). The normal mechanisms that regulate cardiac output are listed in Box 23-2. CHF is classified according to the cause; Box 23-3 shows common causes of CHF in newborns.

Increased volume may be caused by fluid overload or fluid retention. In a normally functioning myocardium, fluid retention does not cause CHF; however, fluid retention complicates CHF arising from other causes. In neonates, increased volume most often is caused by a congenital heart defect or by altered hemodynamics, as in PDA.

CHF caused by obstruction to outflow occurs when the normal myocardium pumps against increased resistance. The increased resistance may be caused by structural defects, such as valvular stenosis or COA, or by pulmonary disease or pulmonary hypertension. CHF caused by pulmonary disease is called *cor pulmonale*. Severe systemic hypertension can also cause increased resistance.

CHF in the neonate usually arises from abnormal stress placed on the heart rather than from an ineffective myocardium. However, electrolyte imbalances, acidosis, and myocardial ischemia affect the heart's ability to function effectively. Conditions such as rheumatic fever, infectious myocarditis, Kawasaki disease, and anomalous origin of the left coronary artery diminish the effectiveness of the heart.

Dysrhythmias that may cause CHF include complete AV block or sustained primary tachycardia. AV block results in a severe bradycardia that prevents adequate circulation of blood. Tachycardia shortens the ventricular filling time, reducing cardiac output.

Severe anemia can cause CHF through an excessive demand for cardiac output. Because the oxygen-carrying capacity of the blood is diminished, the heart must pump more blood per minute to meet tissue oxygenation requirements. If the heart cannot meet the excessive demand, CHF develops (Park, 1996).

Compensatory mechanisms function to meet the body's increased demand for cardiac output. These mechanisms are regulated by the sympathetic nervous system and by mechanical factors. However, the compensatory mechanisms can sustain adequate cardiac output for only a short period; if the underlying condition is not corrected, CHF develops.

Sympathetic Nervous System Compensatory Mechanisms.

A drop in blood pressure stimulates vascular stretch receptors and baroreceptors in the aorta and carotid arteries, which trigger the sympathetic nervous system. A decline in systemic blood pressure inactivates baroreceptors, causing an increase in (1) sympathetic stimulation, (2) heart rate, (3) cardiac contractility, and (4) arterial blood pressure. Catecholamine release and beta-receptor stimulation increase the rate and force of myocardial contraction. Catecholamines also increase venous tone, so that blood is returned to the heart more effectively. Circulation to the skin, kidneys, extremities, and splanchnic bed is diminished, allowing better circulation to the brain, heart, and lungs. A decrease in renal blood flow stimulates the release of renin, angiotensin, and aldosterone; this causes retention of sodium and fluid, resulting in an increased circulating volume. The increased volume increases the workload of the heart.

BOX 23-2

Regulation of Cardiac Output

Sympathetic Nervous System
- Activated by:
  Vasomotor center through peripheral sympathetic fibers
  Secretion of norepinephrine from the adrenal medulla ("fight or flight" response)
- Activation is characterized by tachycardia, increased contractility, peripheral vasoconstriction, and pupil dilation

Parasympathetic Nervous System
- Activated by vagal fibers
  Atria: Stimulation causes decrease in heart rate
  Ventricles: Stimulation causes decrease in contractility

Baroreceptor Reflexes
- Located in the walls of the carotid sinuses and in the aortic arch
- Act as pressure receptors stimulated by blood pressure
- Stimulation results in inhibition of the sympathetic portion of the vasomotor center, stimulation of the parasympathetic (vagal) center, and a decline in arterial blood pressure

---

BOX 23-3

Congestive Heart Failure in the Newborn

Causes of Congestive Heart Failure
Increased volume
Obstruction to flow
Ineffective myocardial function
Arrhythmias
Excessive demand for cardiac output

Congenital Heart Defects
Hypoplastic left heart syndrome
Interrupted aortic arch
Coarctation of the aorta
Total anomalous pulmonary venous return with obstruction
Arteriovenous malformation (cranial or hepatic)
Transposition of the great arteries
Patent ductus arteriosus (preterm infants)

Acquired Heart Defects
Myocardial dysfunction
Anemia
Polycythemia or hyperviscosity
Tachyarrhythmias
Myocarditis

Mechanical Compensatory Mechanisms.

The heart muscle thickens to increase myocardial pressure. This hypertrophy is effective in the early stages, but as soon as the muscle mass increases, compliance decreases. The change in compliance requires greater filling pressure for adequate cardiac output. The hypertrophied heart eventually becomes ischemic because it does not receive circulation adequate to meet its metabolic needs. Ventricular dilation occurs as myocardial fibers stretch to accommodate heart volume. Initially this increases the force of the contraction, but it, too, fails after a point.

Effects of Congestive Heart Failure.

When the right ventricle is unable to pump blood into the pulmonary artery, the lungs oxygenate less blood, pressure in the right atrium and systemic venous circulation increases, and edema occurs in the extremities and viscera. When the left ventricle is unable to pump blood into the systemic circulation, pressure in the left atrium and pulmonary veins increases and the lungs become congested with blood, causing an increase in pulmonary pressures and pulmonary edema. The following conditions are the end effects of CHF:

- *Decreased cardiac output,* which stimulates the sympathetic nervous system, causing tachycardia, increased contractility, increased vasomotor tone, peripheral vasoconstriction, and diaphoresis.
- *Decreased renal perfusion,* which stimulates the renin-angiotensin-aldosterone mechanism, causing sodium and water retention.
- *Systemic venous engorgement,* which results in hepatomegaly, jugular venous distention, periorbital and facial edema and, occasionally, ascites and dependent edema.
- *Pulmonary venous engorgement,* which produces tachypnea, decreased tidal volume, decreased lung compliance, increased airway resistance, early closure of the small airways with air trapping, increased work of breathing, and increased respiratory effort, grunting, and rales; stimulation of the j-receptors in the lung causes the infant to become apprehensive.

Diagnosis.

The diagnosis of CHF is based on clinical signs and symptoms, laboratory data, and chest radiography. In contrast to infants with cyanotic heart disease, infants with CHF usually have significant respiratory distress with tachypnea, grunting, and retractions. They have peripheral pallor, appearing ashen or gray in color, and are irritable. The precordium is active, and loud murmurs usually can be heard throughout systole and diastole. Pulses usually are full, but a difference may be seen between the upper and the lower extremities. Hepatomegaly is common.

In addition to hypoxemia, arterial blood gas studies may reveal a metabolic acidosis arising from the decreased systemic blood flow. With severe acidosis, concurrent respiratory acidosis may be seen because of the pulmonary edema caused by left-sided heart failure. Pulmonary ventilation-perfusion mismatch may cause hypoxemia. Hypocalcemia often is present in infants with CHF because they have an inappropriate response to stress. Infants with DiGeorge syndrome may have hypocalcemia because of absent parathyroids. Aortic arch abnormalities (e.g., interrupted aortic arch, HLHS, and COA) often are associated with DiGeorge syndrome (Park, 1996).

Hypoglycemia may be present in infants with severe CHF. The myocardium depends on glucose; a decline in glucose levels diminishes the heart's ability to compensate for CHF. On the chest radiograph, the heart is enlarged and increased pulmonary congestion can be seen. An ECG generally is not diagnostic unless the CHF is caused by an arrhythmia. Nonspecific changes in the T waves, changes in the ST segment, and a higher P wave may be seen.

Electrolyte imbalances usually include relative hyponatremia, which is due to the increase in free water. Hypo-

chloremia and an increase in bicarbonate may result from respiratory acidemia and the use of loop diuretics. Hyperkalemia results from the release of intracellular cations, which is related to poor tissue perfusion. Elevated lactic acid levels are also indicative of tissue hypoxia. Atrial natriuretic factor (ANF), a peptide hormone, may be important in the regulation of volume and blood pressure. ANF is released from the atria when they are distended. ANF release causes natriuresis, diuresis, and vasodilation. ANF acts with other volume regulators, such as renin, aldosterone, and vasopressin. An increase in ANF may be found with increased pulmonary blood flow, increased left atrial pressure, or pulmonary hypertension.

Children with corrected or uncorrected congenital heart defects often have abnormal homeostasis, suggesting a chronic compensated disseminated intravascular coagulopathy with reduced synthesis of clotting factors or deranged platelet aggregation (or both) (Goel et al, 2000), therefore bleeding problems may be present.

Management.

The goal of management of CHF is to improve cardiac function while identifying and correcting the underlying cause. General measures that reduce the demand on the heart are helpful, but pharmacologic intervention is the most efficacious therapy.

General Measures.

General measures for managing CHF include oxygen administration, ventilation, fluid restriction, and sedation.

Administration of oxygen improves ventilation and perfusion at the alveolar level, and ventilation with positive end-expiratory pressure (PEEP) at 6 to 10 cm H_2O may relieve the effects of CHF by reducing pulmonary edema.

Fluid restriction may reduce the circulating volume. Careful monitoring of serum electrolytes, intake and output, and weight is essential. It is imperative that all fluid be counted in the total daily fluid volume. Infants with CHF do not usually feed well and may require caloric supplementation with hyperalimentation or gavage feedings (Park, 1996).

Infants with CHF are irritable and agitated, which further complicates their status. Sedation with continuous infusions of morphine sulfate or fentanyl may improve the infant's comfort and oxygenation. Other measures that reduce cardiac demand include maintenance of a normal hematocrit, maintenance of the thermoneutral environment, and minimal stimulation. Cautious use of sedation may reduce anxiety and agitation, increasing comfort and reducing the demand for oxygen.

Pharmacologic Interventions.

Table 23-8 lists the medications most often used in the management of cardiac conditions. The mainstay of management of CHF beyond the neonatal period is digitalis (digoxin). Digoxin slows conduction through the AV node, prolongs the refractory period, and slows the heart rate through vagal effects on the SA node.

The use of digoxin in preterm or term neonates is controversial. The preterm newborn is at risk for digitalis toxicity because of the narrow range between the therapeutic and toxic drug levels. Preterm infants require a lower maintenance dose because of their limited renal excretion of the drug (Table 23-9). If digoxin is used, the neonate must be carefully monitored for signs and symptoms of digitalis toxicity. Lead II ECGs should be obtained before each dose for the first 3 days; the dose should be withheld if the P-R interval is longer than 0.16 second or if an arrhythmia is present. The digoxin level should

TABLE 23-8	Drugs Used in the Management of Congenital Heart Defects				
Drug	**Dosage**	**Action**	**Onset**	**Comments**	
Diuretics					
Furosemide (Lasix)	1 mg/kg/dose given intravenously (IV) 1 to 3 mg/kg/dose	Loop diuretic; inhibits sodium and chloride resorption in the proximal tubule	15 to 30 minutes 30 to 60 minutes	Associated with increased patent ductus arteriosus and calcium loss	
Spironolactone (Aldactone)	1.5 to 3 mg/kg/day given orally (PO)	Competitive antagonist of aldosterone	3 to 5 days	Potassium sparing	
Chlorothiazide	20 to 40 mg/kg/day PO	Inhibits sodium and chloride resorption along the distal tubules	1 to 2 hours		
Inotropic Agents					
Dopamine	Low: 2 to 5 μg/kg/minute Moderate: 5 to 10 μg/kg/minute High: 10 to 20 μg/kg/minute	Increases renal blood flow; has beta-adrenergic effects Increases renal blood flow, heart rate, BP, contractility Induces peripheral vasoconstriction; increases heart rate, contractility		Monitor electrocardiogram, blood pressure (BP)	
Dobutamine	2 to 10 μg/kg/minute	Increases renal blood flow, contractility	Rapid	Reduces systemic vascular resistance and increases pulmonary wedge pressure	
Isoproterenol	0.05 to 0.5 mg/kg/minute	Increases venous return to the heart and reduces pulmonary vascular resistance		May produce tachycardia, dysrhythmias, and decreased renal perfusion	
Vasodilator					
Sodium nitroprusside (Nipride)	0.5 to 6 μg/kg/minute	Directly relaxes smooth muscles in arteriolar and venous walls; increases cardiac output if the decrease occurs secondary to myocardial dysfunction	Seconds	Monitor BP, thiocyanate levels, and heart rate; drug is light sensitive	
Prostaglandin					
Prostaglandin E$_1$ (PGE$_1$)	0.05 to 0.1 mg/kg/minute	Causes vasodilation and smooth muscle relaxation of ductus arteriosus and pulmonary and systemic circulations; increases arterial saturation by 25% to 100%	Rapid	Monitor BP; vasopressors may be required; may produce apnea, flush, fever, seizurelike activity, reduced heart rate	
Prostaglandin Synthetase Inhibitor					
Indomethacin	*Initial dosing:* 0.2 mg/kg IV every 24 hours (first dose) 0.1 mg/kg IV (second and third doses) *Infant age over 48 hours but less than 14 days:* 0.3 mg/kg IV and 3 doses every 12 hours *Infant age over 14 days but less than 6 weeks:* 0.2-0.3 mg/kg every 12 hours	Promotes ductal closure by inhibiting PGE$_2$ in the walls of the ductus	12 to 24 hours	Monitor renal function, bilirubin, electrolytes, glucose, platelets, bleeding	

TABLE 23-9	Digoxin Regimens for Preterm and Term Infants	
Total Digitalizing Dose	**Maintenance Dose**
Preterm Infant	
0.025-0.05 mg/kg	0.008-0.012 mg/kg/day
Term Infant	
0.04-0.08 mg/kg	0.005-0.01 mg/kg/day ($\frac{1}{8}$ DD)

To digitalize:
1. Give one half the total digitalizing dose (TDD).
2. Six to 8 hours later, give one fourth the TDD.
3. Six to 8 hours later, obtain a rhythm strip; if normal, give one fourth the TDD.
4. Give the maintenance dose (one eighth the TDD) 12 hours after the last digitalizing dose and then every 12 hours.

Slow digitalization, with less risk of toxicity, can be achieved by starting with the maintenance dose.

be monitored and should be under 2 ng/ml (Park, 1996). Blood samples for measuring this level should be drawn after the drug has achieved equilibrium in the body, approximately 6 to 8 hours after administration.

Other inotropic agents can be used to improve cardiac output. Dopamine, a norepinephrine precursor, has direct and indirect beta-adrenergic effects that are dose dependent. Low doses (2 to 5 μg/kg/minute) increase renal blood flow with minimal effect on the heart rate, blood pressure, or contractility. Moderate doses (5 to 10 μg/kg/minute) increase the renal blood flow, heart rate, blood pressure, and contractility; the pulmonary artery pressure may rise, but peripheral resistance is not affected. High doses (10 to 20 μg/kg/minute) cause alpha effects, resulting in peripheral vasoconstriction, an increased cardiac rate, and increased contractility (Park, 1996).

Dobutamine is a synthetic catecholamine that acts on beta- and alpha-adrenergic receptors. Dobutamine (2 to 10 μg/minute) has diminished effects on the heart rate and rhythm and causes less peripheral vasoconstriction.

Isoproterenol (Isuprel), a synthetic epinephrine-like substance, has beta$_1$- and beta$_2$-adrenergic effects. The usefulness of Isuprel in neonates is limited because the drug increases the heart rate, can cause arrhythmias, and reduces systemic vascular resistance, which may worsen the hypotension (Park, 1996).

Diuretics. Diuretics are useful in the treatment of CHF to reduce sodium and water retention. The primary goal is to increase renal perfusion (with inotropic agents or vasodilators) and to increase sodium delivery to distal diluting sites of the renal tubules. Diuretics increase renal excretion of sodium and other anions by inhibiting tubular resorption of sodium (Park, 1996).

Furosemide (Lasix), a loop diuretic, blocks sodium and chloride resorption in the ascending limb of the loop of Henle. Loop diuretics interfere with the formation of free water and with free water resorption by preventing the transport of sodium, potassium, and chloride into the medullary interstitium. Loop diuretics increase excretion of potassium by delivering higher amounts of sodium to sites in the distal nephron where potassium can be excreted. Furosemide also increases excretion of calcium but does not affect the kidneys' ability to regulate acid-base balance.

Spironolactone (Aldactone), an aldosterone antagonist, may be useful because it is a potassium-sparing diuretic. Spironolactone works by binding to the cytoplasmic receptor sites and blocking the action of aldosterone, thus impairing the resorption of sodium and the secretion of potassium and hydrogen ion. Spironolactone has no effect on free water production and absorption. Thiazide diuretics (chlorothiazide and hydrochlorothiazide) inhibit sodium and chloride resorption along the distal tubules. They are not as effective as the loop diuretics and are used infrequently (Park, 1996).

Complications of Diuretic Therapy. Diuretic therapy can result in severe electrolyte imbalances if not monitored carefully. The complications of diuretic therapy include (1) volume contraction, (2) hyponatremia, (3) metabolic alkalemia or acidemia, and (4) hypokalemia or hyperkalemia. When diuretics are used, the fluid and electrolyte balance must be maintained through administration of water and electrolytes. The adequacy of the volume can be determined by monitoring serum electrolytes, BUN, creatinine, urinary output, weight, specific gravity, and skin turgor.

The increased renal loss of sodium with diuretic therapy can lead to hyponatremia unless adequate amounts of sodium are provided. Increased release of antidiuretic hormone also may be a factor because of changes in the osmoreceptors or inhibition of antidiuretic hormone action. Reducing the amount of total water and improving cardiac output, thereby increasing renal perfusion, can best manage this condition.

Metabolic alkalosis can result from administration of loop diuretics that interfere with sodium- and potassium-dependent chloride reabsorption. Hypochloremia results in increased production of aldosterone and an increase in the bicarbonate concentration. Hypokalemia is a common complication of loop diuretic therapy. An increased ratio of intracellular to extracellular potassium results in the clinical signs and symptoms of hypokalemia. Hypokalemia increases the risk of digoxin toxicity. In contrast, hyperkalemia may result when cardiac output is low and tissue perfusion is severely compromised. Other complications of diuretic therapy include increased calcium excretion, hyperuricemia, and glucose intolerance.

Vasodilators may be used in severe CHF to reduce the right and left ventricular preload and afterload to improve cardiac function. Vasodilators cause arterial and venous dilation, resulting in a decrease in systemic and pulmonary vascular resistance. Sodium nitroprusside (Nipride) is a smooth muscle relaxant that reduces ventricular afterload by reducing pulmonary and systemic vascular resistance, venous return, ventricular preload. This leads to a decreased ventricular end-diastolic volume, an increased ejection fraction, an increased heart rate and cardiac index, and decreased pulmonary and systemic resistance. Sodium nitroprusside is sensitive to light and must be stored in dark containers. Side effects are cyanide toxicity and decreased platelet function (Park, 1996).

The prognosis for CHF depends on the severity of the underlying condition and on the degree of CHF.

Subacute Infective Endocarditis. SAIE can be a complication of CHD. Two factors are important in the development of SAIE: (1) structural abnormalities that create turbulent flow or pressure gradients and (2) bacteremia. All cardiac defects that produce turbulent flow or have a significant pressure gradient predispose the patient to bacterial invasion of the cardiac endothelium. The turbulent flow damages the endothelial lining and encourages platelet-fibrin thrombus formation. Prevention

BOX **23-4**

Antimicrobial Prophylaxis to Prevent Subacute Infective Endocarditis in Children with Cardiac Defects

I. Dental procedures and oral respiratory tract surgery
A. Standard regimen
1. Amoxicillin (50 mg/kg) given IV or IM 1 hour before procedure, followed by 25 mg/kg given 6 hours after procedure.
B. Alternative regimens
1. *Allergy to penicillin and/or amoxicillin:* Erythromycin ethylsuccinate or erythromycin stearate (20 mg/kg) given orally 2 hours before procedure, followed by erythromycin (10 mg/kg) given 6 hours after initial dose.
2. *Inability to take oral medications:* Ampicillin (50 mg/kg) given intravenously (IV) or intramuscularly (IM) 30 minutes before procedure, followed by ampicillin (25 mg/kg) given IV or IM 6 hours after initial dose.
3. *Allergy to penicillin and/or amoxicillin and inability to take oral medications:* Clindamycin (10 mg/kg) given IV 30 minutes before procedure, followed by clindamycin (5 mg/kg) given IV 6 hours after initial dose.
4. *High-risk child not a candidate for standard regimen:* Ampicillin (50 mg/kg) given IV or IM plus gentamicin (2 mg/kg) given IV or IM 30 minutes before procedure, followed by amoxicillin (25 mg/kg) given orally 6 hours after initial dose; or repeat ampicillin plus gentamicin regimen.
5. *High-risk child allergic to ampicillin, amoxicillin, or penicillin:* Vancomycin (20 mg/kg) given IV over 1 hour, starting 1 hour before procedure. No repeat dose is necessary.
II. Gastrointestinal or genitourinary procedure
A. Standard regimen
1. Ampicillin (50 mg/kg) plus gentamicin (2 mg/kg) given IV or IM 30 minutes before procedure, followed by amoxicillin (25 mg/kg) given 6 hours after initial dose; *or* repeat ampicillin plus gentamicin regimen 8 hours after initial dose.
B. Alternative regimens
1. *Child allergic to ampicillin, amoxicillin, or penicillin:* Vancomycin (20 mg/kg) given IV over 1 hour plus gentamicin (2 mg/kg) given IV or IM 1 hour before procedure; repeat vancomycin plus gentamicin regimen 8 hours after initial dose.
2. *Low-risk patient:* Amoxicillin (50 mg/kg) given orally 1 hour before procedure, followed by amoxicillin (25 mg/kg) given 6 hours after initial dose.

From Dajani AS et al (1997). Prevention of bacterial endocarditis: recommendations by the American Heart Association. American Heart Association: Dallas.

of bacterial SAIE requires scrupulous daily oral care, as well as prophylactic antimicrobials for dental procedures (Park, 1996). All congenital heart defects except secundum-type ASDs predispose the patient to SAIE. Ventral septal defects, TOF, and aortic stenosis are the congenital heart defects most often associated with SAIE (Park, 1996).

Vegetation of SAIE usually occurs on the low-pressure side of the defect, whereas endothelial damage is established by the jet effect of the defect. More than 90% of SAIE cases are caused by *Streptococcus viridans, Streptococcus faecalis* (enterococcus), and *Staphylococcus aureus.* Other organisms include *Haemophilus influenzae, Escherichia coli,* and *Pseudomonas, Proteus, Aerobacter,* and *Listeria* spp. *Candida* organisms may infect infants who undergoing long-term antimicrobial or steroid therapy.

Prevention. Procedures for which SAIE prophylaxis is indicated include (1) all dental procedures, (2) tonsillectomy or adenoidectomy, (3) surgical procedures involving the respiratory mucosa, (4) bronchoscopy, (5) incision and drainage of infected tissue, and (6) gastrointestinal or genitourinary procedures. Prophylaxis recommendations for children are listed in Box 23-4; complete information can be obtained from the American Heart Association's Council on Cardiovascular Diseases in the Young, Committee on Rheumatic Fever and Infective Endocarditis (American Heart Association National Center, 7272 Greenville Avenue, Dallas, TX 75231; www. americanheart.org).

SUPPORT OF THE FAMILY OF THE INFANT WITH A CONGENITAL HEART DEFECT

Families with infants with CHDs feel confusion, guilt, anger, and fear. The family needs support to cope with the short- and long-term consequences of the condition. The severity of the defect, the availability of treatment, and the prognosis influence the amount and kind of support required. The parents of infants with even minor defects (by health care professional standards) are overwhelmed by the knowledge of their infant's condition. The nurse can reassure them by pointing out the improvement in cardiac care over the past 60 years. More than 95% of congenital heart defects can be partly or fully corrected by a combination of medical and surgical management (Cooley, 1997). However, it is estimated that approximately 25% of the infants born with CHDs grow into adults with persistent, nonoperated defects, residual defects, or cardiovascular sequelae after surgical intervention (Meberg et al, 2000). Parents must be able to discuss quality of life issues with health care professionals, so that the parents can be sure they are making informed decisions about treatment options (Moyen et al, 1997). The impact of the cardiac defect on other systems of the body must also be discussed, because the parents may not be aware of the associated complications, such as respiratory problems, that often accompany these defects (Lubica, 1996).

Although often overlooked, the neurologic prognosis is a key factor in determining the overall quality of life of a child with a CHD. Pediatric neurologists can be integrated into the health care team to assist parents in assessing the neurologic prognosis of their child and to begin early intervention programs to facilitate the best outcome (Shevell, 1999). Parents need frequent contact with members of the health care team; caretakers should speak with the parents routinely, not just when major changes occur in the infant's condition.

Although most CHDs do not have an identifiable genetic pattern, genetic counseling should be offered to all parents with a newborn with a congenital heart defect. Parents will want answers to questions about the cause of the defect, the likelihood of a recurrence in future pregnancies, and if there may be associated defects (Ardinger, 1997; Welch & Brown, 2000). Recent work on the Human Genome Project and other advances in the study of genetics offer promise of determining specific genetic causes of heart defects (Belmont, 1998). These advances may offer improved specific information to fully answer parents' questions. In addition, future innovation may greatly improve the ability to diagnose CHDs prenatally (De-Vore, 1998), thereby providing greater opportunity for fetal surgery to correct some defects, for improved immediate management at birth or, in some cases, for termination of the pregnancy. Most congenital heart defects can be identified through targeted transvaginal or transabdominal ultrasound examinations; however, these defects evolve in utero at different stages, therefore a single sonogram may not be sufficient to detect all CHDs (Yagel et al, 1997). Health care professionals must be keenly aware of all options to ensure that parents receive the most up-to-date information upon which to base decisions.

Family members should be given an accurate description of the defect; diagrams and models illustrating the defect should be used. Parents need frequent reassurance and repetition of information. Parents of infants who do not require immediate surgery but who eventually will require surgical correction must be educated about all aspects of the infant's care, including signs and symptoms of deterioration, medication administration, activity limitations, and normal development. Because growth failure with a cardiac defect is common, efforts to maximize nutrition are important; extra support is needed if the mother planned to breastfeed her baby (Lambert & Watters, 1998; Varan et al, 1999). Careful follow-up is important to prevent complications.

Identification of support persons for the family is extremely valuable. Parents may be encouraged to talk to other parents of newborns with the same or similar defects. Many neonatal intensive care units have active support groups consisting of parents of patients. Care should be taken in selecting supporters. Parents with a term newborn with a CHD may not be able to relate to parents of a preterm neonate. Other family members or friends should not be overlooked; they can become valuable support persons if they are provided appropriate guidance and education. The needs of siblings should also be assessed. Siblings need support, education, and guidance appropriate for their age and comprehension of the situation. Parents may not recognize their other childrens' needs because of the overwhelming situation. Health care providers can facilitate the parent-child relationship during the initial period and throughout the course of the management.

Financial resources should be addressed because preoperative, operative, and postoperative care is expensive. Many parents need assistance in obtaining aid to which they are entitled. Even the most knowledgeable parents may not be aware of resources available to them. If experimental surgery is contemplated, parents may need assistance in speaking with private insurance companies regarding coverage. Referrals should be made for the parents to appropriate local, state, federal, or private organizations that pertain to the CHD; these include the Department of Family and Children Services, the March of Dimes, and Children's Medical Services. The family may qualify for the Special Supplemental Nutrition Program for Women, Infants, and Children.

Discharge planning must be comprehensive for the newborn infant who will receive medical management for a CHD before corrective surgery. A thorough assessment of the home should be done before discharge. Contact with the primary care provider responsible for routine management of the infant is imperative. Initial contact by telephone should be followed up with a copy of the complete medical record and discharge summary. If the infant requires any special equipment for home care, the equipment should be obtained before discharge so that the parents can be taught how to use it. Practical details must also be addressed, such as whether the infant's room has enough electrical outlets for the equipment. Notification of local emergency medical services, power companies, and other relevant companies should be completed before discharge.

REFERENCES

Ardinger RH (1997). Genetic counseling in congenital heart disease. *Pediatric annals* 26:99-104.

Belmont JW (1998). Recent progress in the molecular genetics of congenital heart defects. *Clinical genetics* 54:11-19.

Bevilacqua L, Hordof A (1998). Cardiac pacing in children. *Current opinion in cardiology* 13:48-55.

Botto LD et al (2001). Racial and temporal variations in the prevalence of heart defects. *Pediatrics* 107:1-8.

Braunwald E, editor (2001). *Heart disease: a textbook of cardiovascular medicine*. WB Saunders: Philadelphia.

Burlet A et al (1999). Renal function in cyanotic congenital heart disease. *Nephron* 81:296-300.

Centers for Disease Control (1998). Trends in infant mortality attributable to birth defects: United States, 1980-1995. *Morbidity and mortality weekly report* 47:773-778.

Colucci WS, Braunwald E (2001). Pathophysiology of heart failure. In Braunwald E, editor. *Heart disease: a textbook of cardiovascular medicine*. WB Saunders: Philadelphia.

Cooley DA (1997). Early development of congenital heart surgery: open heart procedures. *Annals of thoracic surgery* 64:1544-1548.

Danford DA et al (1999). Pulmonary stenosis: defect-specific diagnostic accuracy of heart murmurs in children. *Journal of pediatrics* 134:76-81.

Danford DA et al (2000). Effects of electrocardiography and chest radiography on the accuracy of preliminary diagnosis of common congenital cardiac defects. *Pediatric cardiology* 21:334-340.

DeVore GR (1998). Influence of prenatal diagnosis on congenital heart defects. *Annals of the New York academy of sciences* 847:46-52.

Dipchand AI et al (1999). Tetralogy of Fallot with nonconfluent pulmonary arteries and aortopulmonary septal defect. *Cardiology in the young* 9:75-77.

Freeman SB et al (1998). Population-based study of congenital heart defects in Down Syndrome. *American Journal of Medical Genetics* 80(3), 213-217.

Goel M et al (2000). Haemostatic changes in children with cyanotic and acyanotic congenital heart disease. *International House of Japan*, 559-563.

Goh TH (2000). Common congenital heart defects: the value of early detection. *Australian Family physician* 29:429-435.

Kaplan NM (2001). Systemic hypertension therapy. In Braunwald E, editor. *Heart disease: a textbook of cardiovascular medicine*. WB Saunders: Philadelphia.

Kwiatkowksa J et al (2000). Atrioventricular septal defect: clinical and diagnostic problems in children hospitalized in 1993-1998. *Medical science monitor: international medical journal of experimental and clinical research* 6:1148-1154.

Lambert JM, Watters NE (1998). Breastfeeding the infant/child with a cardiac defect: an informal survey. *Journal of human lactation* 14(2), 151-155.

Little WC (2001). Assessment of normal and abnormal cardiac function. In Braunwald E, editor. *Heart disease: a textbook of cardiovascular medicine.* WB Saunders: Philadelphia.

Lott JW (2003). Fetal development: environmental influences and critical periods. In Kenner CA, Lott JW, editors. *Comprehensive neonatal care: a physiologic perspective.* WB Saunders: Philadelphia.

Lubica H (1996). Pathologic lung function in children and adolescents with congenital heart defects. *Pediatric cardiology* 17:314-315.

Massin MM et al (1998). Heart rate behavior in children with atrial septal defect. *Cardiology* 90:269-270.

McElhinney DB et al (2000). Aortopulmonary window associated with complete atrioventricular septal defect. *Journal of thoracic and cardiovascular surgery* 119:1284-1285.

Meberg A et al (2000). Outcome of congenital heart defects: a population-based study. *Acta paediatrica* 89:1344-1351.

Moyen LK et al (1997). Quality of life in children with congenital heart defects. *Acta paediatrica* 86:975-980.

Norwood WI et al (1983). Physiologic repair of aortic atresia: hypoplastic left heart syndrome. *New England journal of medicine* 308: 23-26.

Nouri S (1997). Congenital heart defects: cyanotic and acyanotic. *Pediatric annals* 26:95-98.

Opie LH (2001). Mechanisms of cardiac contraction and relaxation. In Braunwald E, editor. *Heart disease: a textbook of cardiovascular medicine.* WB Saunders: Philadelphia.

Park MK (1996). *Pediatric cardiology for practitioners,* ed 3. Mosby: St Louis.

Pyeritz RE (2001). Genetics and cardiovascular disease. In Braunwald E, editor. *Heart disease: a textbook of cardiovascular medicine.* WB Saunders: Philadelphia.

Sacchetti A et al (1999). Primary cardiac arrhythmias in children. *Pediatric emergency care* 15:95-98.

Shevell MI (1999). The role of the pediatric neurologist in the management of children with congenital heart defects: a commentary. *Seminars in pediatric neurology* 6:64-66.

Taussig WB (1947). *Cyanosis in congenital malformations of the heart.* Oxford University Press: New York.

Thomson JD et al (2000). Cardiac catheter guided surgical closure of an apical ventricular septal defect. *Annals of thoracic surgery* 70: 1402-1404.

Turner SW et al (1999). The natural history of ventricular septal defects. *Archives of disease in childhood* 81:413-416.

Varan B et al (1999). Malnutrition and growth failure in cyanotic and acyanotic congenital heart disease with and without pulmonary hypertension. *Archives of disease in childhood* 81:49-52.

Welch KK, Brown SA (2000). The role of genetic counseling in the management of prenatally detected congenital heart defects. *Seminars in perinatology* 24:373-379.

Yagel S et al (1997). Congenital heart defects: natural course and in utero development. *Circulation* 96:550-555.

CHAPTER 24

FLUIDS, ELECTROLYTES, VITAMINS, AND TRACE MINERALS

REGINALD TSANG, SERGIO DeMARINI, LINDA L. RATH

Water and electrolytes are vital components of the body at any age. The laws that regulate fluid and electrolyte balance in the newborn are the same as those that control this process in children and adults. However, the newborn's body water distribution is both quantitatively and qualitatively different. Furthermore, rapid changes occur at the time of birth, and sick newborns pose additional challenges. Consequently, special care is required to maintain an appropriate fluid and electrolyte balance, especially in very-low-birth-weight (VLBW) infants.

In this discussion the recommendations of the American Academy of Pediatrics (AAP) have been followed whenever possible. In all other instances the conclusions drawn are based on current medical evidence in the field.

WATER AND ELECTROLYTES

Water

Physiology. Water is the main component of the human body. It is distributed both inside and outside the cells, therefore a practical simplification is to classify total body water (TBW) as intracellular water (ICW) and extracellular water (ECW). ICW is the total amount of water in all the body's cells. ECW is the total amount of water outside the cells; it comprises the water in the interstitial space and in the intravascular space (plasma).

The distribution of TBW between intracellular and extracellular spaces depends on the water's relative content of solutes (electrolytes, proteins); that is, on its relative osmolality. The total number of solute particles in solution determines the osmolality of a solution. Osmolality values are expressed in osmoles or milliosmoles per kilogram of water (Osm/kg or mOsm/kg). Because cell membranes are completely permeable to water but not to most solutes, water shifts from one compartment to the other until equilibrium is established between the osmolalities on both sides of the membrane. The osmolality of intracellular and extracellular spaces, therefore, is equal, although the composition of ICW is different from that of ECW; sodium (Na) is the main extracellular ion, whereas potassium (K) is the main intracellular ion. The size of a compartment depends on the number of osmoles in it, which in turn determines the water content.

In each compartment, a main solute acts to keep water in the compartment:

- The volume of the intracellular compartment is maintained mainly by K salts and is regulated by the Na-K cellular pump.
- The volume of the extracellular compartment is maintained mainly by Na salts and is regulated by the kidneys.
- In the extracellular space, the volume of the intravascular compartment is maintained mainly by the colloidal osmotic pressure of plasma proteins.

Changes in Water Distribution

TBW declines with growth (Figure 24-1). It constitutes more than 90% of the total body weight in the first trimester of gestation, about 80% at 32 weeks' gestation, about 78% at 40 weeks' gestation, and approximately 60% to 65% at the end of the first year of life. The ratio of ECW to ICW also changes with growth. ECW declines from approximately 60% of body weight in the second trimester to about 45% at term. Correspondingly, ICW increases from about 25% of body weight in the second trimester to approximately 33% at term.

At birth an acute expansion of ECW is superimposed on the gradual changes that took place during fetal life. Through an unknown mechanism, water and electrolytes shift from the intracellular space to the extracellular space (Baumgart & Costarino, 2000). The newborn at birth, therefore, is in a state of excess extracellular fluid, a condition that is particularly prominent in preterm infants (TBW and ECW are greater at lower gestational ages). Because the excess ECW is lost through diuresis, some weight loss (5% to 10% in term infants) usually occurs as a consequence of these physiologic changes in body water distribution. Postnatal loss and regaining of weight reflect changes in the interstitial water component of ECW, whereas plasma volume remains essentially unchanged. In preterm infants, the postnatal weight loss is greater (usually 10% to 20%) and occurs more frequently in the smallest infants. As long as the intravascular volume is adequate and serum electrolytes are normal, it appears inappropriate to replace all fluid losses during the first days of life. Administration of large amounts of fluids increases the risk of symptomatic patent ductus arteriosus (PDA) and bronchopulmonary dysplasia (BPD).

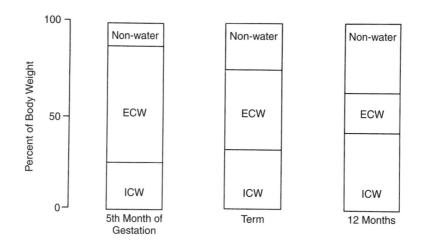

ECW: Extracellular water
ICW: Intracellular water

FIGURE **24-1**
Changes in body water distribution. *ECW,* Extracellular water; *ICW,* intracellular water.

TABLE **24-1**	Approximate Water Requirements of Newborns in the First Week of Life*			
	BIRTH WEIGHT			
Time Period	**Under 1000 g**	**1000-1500 g**	**1501-2000 g**	**Full Term**
First 48 hours	80-140	60-100	60-80	40-60
End of first week	150-200	140-160	110-150	100-150

Amounts are given as ml/kg/day.

Water Balance and Body Metabolism

The human body loses a variable amount of water and electrolytes daily. To maintain body fluid balance, fluid losses must be replaced periodically. Maintenance fluid requirements are calculated to replace water and electrolytes normally lost through urine, stool, skin, and the respiratory tract. Water turnover is part of cellular metabolism and usually is related precisely to the basal metabolic rate. The basal metabolic rate is the amount of energy the body must produce to maintain homeostasis at rest and in a thermally neutral environment. Carbohydrates, lipids, and proteins are the substances used to produce energy. Waste products are heat, nitrogen, carbon dioxide, and water. To excrete waste products, the body normally loses water through the kidneys (to eliminate nitrogen), the skin (to eliminate excess heat), and the respiratory tract (to eliminate carbon dioxide). Therefore a high body energy expenditure means a large amount of waste products and, consequently, large water losses.

The cells generate some water as a byproduct of cell metabolism (i.e., water of oxidation). This amount of water, which must be subtracted from fluid requirements, is approximately equal to water losses in stools, therefore the latter can be omitted from the usual calculations of required water intake.

Water Requirements

Maintaining the overall body water and salt composition ordinarily requires replacement of renal water and electrolyte losses and insensible water losses from the respiratory tract and skin evaporation. An approximate estimate of maintenance fluids is: 100 ml of water is needed for each 100 kilocalories (kcal) of energy expended.

Although this relationship between metabolic rate and water loss holds true in full-term infants, it is not valid in preterm infants. Immature renal function, very high insensible water losses as a result of skin immaturity and a higher body surface area to body mass ratio, and neonatal illnesses significantly affect fluid balance (Baumgart & Costarino, 2000). Although values for fluid requirements are available (Table 24-1), they provide only an approximate guideline for the individual infant.

Fluid requirements may be determined more accurately if factors that influence insensible water loss (IWL) are taken into account (Table 24-2). For example, radiant warmers and phototherapy increase insensible water loss, whereas use of a plastic blanket under a radiant warmer or adequate humidification in an incubator reduces IWL.

Monitoring a newborn's urine output can help to further individualize fluid requirements. According to Lorenz and colleagues (1995), most preterm infants show a definite postnatal pattern of diuresis, which has three phases: the prediuretic phase, the diuretic phase, and the homeostatic phase (Table 24-3). The prediuretic phase occurs in the first 48 hours of life. In this phase, the glomerular filtration rate, urine output, and sodium and potassium excretion are all very low. Water is lost mainly by IWL. Because only water is lost through the skin,

TABLE **24-2**	Factors Affecting Water Loss in Neonates

Increases Water Loss	Reduces Water Loss
WATER LOSS FROM THE SKIN	
Low gestational age	High humidity in incubator
Forced convection in incubator	Double-walled incubator
Radiant warmer	Plastic heat shield
Hyperthermia	Plastic blanket
Activity	Semipermeable skin patches
Phototherapy	
WATER LOSS FROM THE RESPIRATORY TRACT	
Tachypnea	Continuous distending pressure with humidified gas
Inadequate humidification	Artificial ventilation with humidification
RENAL WATER LOSS	
Diuretics	Renal failure
Osmotic diuresis (hyperglycemia, mannitol)	Inappropriate secretion of antidiuretic hormone
Congenital adrenal hyperplasia	Congestive heart failure

TABLE **24-3**	Pattern of Postnatal Diuresis in Preterm Infants during the First Week of Life

	PHASES OF POSTNATAL DIURESIS		
Factors	**Prediuretic**	**Diuretic**	**Homeostatic**
Age	First 2 days	2-5 Days	After 2-5 days
Diuresis	Very low	Sudden increase	Varies with intake
Urine sodium	Very low	Sudden increase	Varies with intake
INTERVENTIONS			
Water	Fluid restriction	Allow physiologic weight loss	Provide calories for growth
Sodium	None	Provide enough to maintain normal serum sodium level	Provide growth allowance

Lorenz JM et al (1995). Phases of fluid and electrolyte homeostasis in the extremely low birth weight infant. Pediatrics 196:484-489.

the appropriate steps in calculating fluid intake during this phase are the following:

- Intake is limited to insensible water losses.
- No sodium, chloride, or potassium is given.
- The standard intravenous solution should provide only glucose at a rate of 4 to 6 mg/kg/minute (with or without amino acids).

The diuretic phase usually begins on day 2 to 5 of life. Urine output and sodium and potassium excretion all increase abruptly. Fluid intake is adjusted as follows:

- Water intake is increased to maintain a normal serum sodium concentration and to obtain a total weight loss (in preterm infants) between 10% and 20%.
- Consideration can be given to adding sodium (to keep the serum Na level normal) and potassium (if the serum K level declines) to the intravenous solution.

In the homeostatic phase, which follows the diuretic phase, diuresis stabilizes. The goal of fluid and electrolyte intake in this phase is to allow an adequate caloric intake without causing fluid overload.

Appropriate administration of fluid is important, because both excessive fluid restriction and fluid overload lead to clinical consequences (Figure 24-2). Excessive fluid restriction may lead to dehydration, hyperosmolality, hypoglycemia, and hyperbilirubinemia. In preterm infants, high volumes of parenteral fluids have been associated with a higher incidence of PDA and BPD. It is important to realize that the occurrence of BPD has been correlated with fluid volume administered during the first 4 days of life. Maintaining the fluid and electrolyte balance, therefore, is extremely important in preterm infants. Close monitoring of clinical hydration, body weight, urine output, and the serum Na concentration should allow the best possible decisions on fluid administration.

Sodium. Sodium is the main extracellular ion, constituting, with its salts, more than 90% of the total amount of solutes in the extracellular space. Sodium is absorbed in both the small intestine and the colon; the largest amount is absorbed in the jejunum. Sodium absorption involves several mechanisms:

- Passive absorption, after glucose absorption, secondary to the flow of water
- Active absorption, stimulated by glucose and amino acids
- Active absorption, uncoupled with glucose, involving the Na-K pump
- Active absorption in exchange with hydrogen ions

The overall process is very efficient. Adults normally absorb 98% of ingested sodium.

The kidneys excrete sodium, which is filtered by glomeruli and reabsorbed throughout the tubules and the collecting ducts. Most of the sodium is absorbed with chloride (Cl), but small amounts are absorbed in exchange with potassium ions (K^+) or hydrogen ions (H^+). Under normal circumstances, 96% to 99% of filtered sodium is reabsorbed. The main factors involved in the regulation of sodium resorption are the oncotic and hydrostatic pressures in the peritubular capillaries and the action of aldosterone, which increases the absorption of sodium in exchange with K^+ or H^+. Although antidiuretic hormone does not affect the excretion of sodium directly, it can influence the serum Na concentration indirectly because it regulates the excretion or resorption of free water.

The Na concentration in human milk is 12 to 20 mEq/L (12 to 20 mmol/L). The current recommendation for standard formulas is 20 to 60 mg/100 kcal (6 to 17 mEq/419 kJ [kilojoules]) (AAP, 1998); the recommendation for growing preterm infants is 38 to 58 mg/100 kcal (1.66 to 2.5 mEq/419 kJ). Because of their high urinary loss of sodium, VLBW infants (those weighing less than 1500 g) temporarily may require up to 4 to 8 mEq/kg/day by the end of the first week of life. Thereafter, urinary losses in these infants are markedly reduced. The nor-

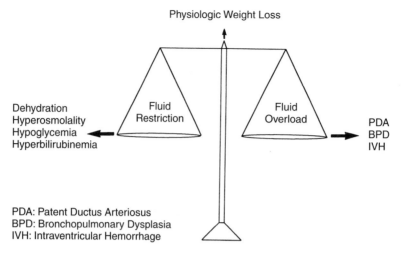

FIGURE **24-2**

Risks of fluid administration. *PDA*, Patent ductus arteriosus; *BPD*, bronchopulmonary dysplasia; *IVH*, intraventricular hemorrhage.

BOX **24-1**

Disorders of Sodium Balance

Hyponatremia
Early
Perinatal asphyxia
Respiratory distress syndrome
Diuretics
Nebulization associated with nasal continuous positive
    airway pressure
Hypotonic fluid administered to mother during labor
Late
VLBW infant fed human milk or standard formula
With overhydration: congestive heart failure, renal failure
With dehydration: adrenal insufficiency, vomiting, diarrhea,
    peritonitis

Hypernatremia
With Dehydration
Vomiting, diarrhea with inadequate fluid replacement
Osmotic diuresis (hyperglycemia, mannitol)
Radiant warmers
"Hyperosmolar state" in infants weighing less than 800 g
With Overhydration
Excessive administration of sodium bicarbonate (NaHCO$_3$)
Errors in administration of sodium chloride (NaCl)

---

mal serum Na concentration ranges from 130 to 150 mEq/L. Disorders of sodium balance are listed in Box 24-1.

Hyponatremia.   Hyponatremia (a serum Na level below 130 mEq/L) is caused by retention of water relative to sodium. When the serum Na concentration and, therefore, serum osmolality decline, water moves into cells. The increased water content in the brain causes the signs and symptoms of hyponatremia. Vomiting, lethargy, and apnea may occur with various degrees of hyponatremia, but seizures and coma usually are not seen unless the serum Na concentration falls below 115

mEq/L. Neonatal hyponatremia usually is classified as early or late, depending on the timing of the occurrence.

Early Hyponatremia.   Early hyponatremia, which often occurs in the first 2 days of life, is caused by extrinsic perinatal factors. It is not influenced by parenteral administration of additional sodium and water.

Early hyponatremia most often is caused by perinatal asphyxia. The mechanism is diminished excretion of free water, which is caused by increased secretion of antidiuretic hormone (syndrome of inappropriate secretion of antidiuretic hormone, or SIADH) and impairment of renal function by hypoxia. Severe respiratory distress syndrome (RDS) also predisposes newborns to hyponatremia, probably for the same reasons, and diuresis precedes the resolution of the acute phase of RDS.

Early hyponatremia can be iatrogenic in origin. Possible causes include administration of large volumes of hypotonic fluid to the mother during labor; nebulization with nasal continuous positive airway pressure (CPAP), resulting in water overload; and use of diuretics with excessive free water replacement. Infants with early hyponatremia usually are in a state of excess water, and fluid restriction is the appropriate treatment.

Late Hyponatremia.   The most common form of late hyponatremia typically is seen after the first week of life in growing VLBW infants fed either human milk or standard formulas. These infants have a negative sodium balance in the first weeks of life because of a combination of factors, including an inadequate sodium intake and temporary unresponsiveness of the renal tubules to aldosterone (Baumgart & Costarino, 2000). Preterm infants weighing more than 1500 g usually require 2 to 3 mEq/kg/day of sodium; VLBW infants initially may require amounts as high as 4 to 8 mEq/kg/day to obtain a positive sodium balance. Spontaneous improvement in sodium balance within weeks is the rule.

At any time, neonatal hyponatremia may occur in association with overhydration (dilutional hyponatremia) or dehydration (true hyponatremia).

Hyponatremia with overhydration may occur in newborns with congestive heart failure (congenital heart disease, PDA), renal failure, or SIADH. Because total body sodium is increased but TBW is even more increased, administration of sodium would only cause additional expansion of the extracellular space, which can aggravate the infant's condition. Fluid restriction is the treatment.

Either renal or extrarenal sodium and water losses can cause hyponatremia with dehydration. Renal losses usually result from adrenal insufficiency (salt-losing type of congenital adrenal hyperplasia, adrenal hemorrhage), although infants with a urinary tract obstruction occasionally may have similar electrolyte disorders. Extrarenal losses may result from disorders such as vomiting, diarrhea, and peritonitis. Treatment is directed both at the underlying disorder and at volume replacement with sodium chloride (NaCl)–containing solutions. The amount of sodium needed to correct a low serum Na level can be calculated according to the standard formula:

Na to be given (mEq/mmol) = 0.6 × Weight (kg) × (Desired serum − Na actual serum Na)

The correction usually is made over several hours, and the target is a serum Na concentration of about 135 mEq/L. However, this general rule has two important exceptions:

- If shock is present or impending, normal saline should be given intravenously (IV) and rapidly at 10 to 20 ml/kg over 20 to 30 minutes; this treatment is repeated until arterial blood pressure is normal.
- With symptomatic hyponatremia, which almost always occurs only when the serum Na level is below 115 mEq/L, hypertonic saline should be infused. However, because either an abrupt or a large increase in osmolality carries the risk of intracranial hemorrhage and congestive heart failure (CHF), the aim of the initial correction in this case should be a lower than normal serum Na concentration, such as 120 to 125 mEq/L.

Hypernatremia.   Hypernatremia (a serum Na level over 150 mEq/L) is an increase in the serum Na concentration. It may be accompanied by dehydration or, in rare cases, by overhydration. Hypernatremia with dehydration is caused by an insufficient water intake, by increased renal or extrarenal water losses, or by a combination of these two factors. Hypernatremia with overhydration usually is iatrogenic in origin.

When hypernatremia and, therefore, hyperosmolality develop, water moves out of the cells into the extracellular space to achieve an osmotic equilibrium between intracellular and extracellular fluid. This attempt to equilibrate intracellular and extracellular fluids results in volume depletion of the intracellular space. Brain cells can protect themselves, maintaining their intracellular volume by generating new solutes, called idiogenic osmoles. Idiogenic osmoles are substances (amino acids, polyols, trimethylamines) synthesized by the brain as a protective response to serum hyperosmolality. Idiogenic osmoles are neither produced nor catabolized rapidly, therefore this mechanism is effective within certain limits and only if hyperosmolality does not develop too rapidly. Similarly, correction of hypernatremia with hypotonic solutions should not be performed rapidly, because idiogenic osmoles cannot be metabolized quickly and cerebral edema can occur as a result of movement of water into brain cells.

In VLBW infants, sodium restriction during the first 3 to 5 days of life (i.e., no sodium other than with transfusions) may prevent hypernatremia and reduce the need for parenteral fluid.

Hypernatremia with Dehydration.   Hypernatremia with dehydration results from water losses for which fluid replacement is inadequate. Water loss may occur from the gastrointestinal tract (vomiting, diarrhea). Inadequate replace-

ment of fluids may include failure to provide the appropriate water intake, especially when this shortcoming is compounded by administration of high-solute fluids. Renal water loss may occur when an increased amount of solute, such as glucose or mannitol, must be excreted (osmotic diuresis). Significant IWL through the skin occurs when infants are placed under radiant warmers; the magnitude of these losses is inversely related to gestational age.

Hypernatremia with dehydration must be corrected slowly, because cerebral edema can easily develop. Intravascular volume should be restored quickly with isotonic fluids, but water deficits should be corrected slowly and with great caution by administration of hypotonic fluids.

A hyperosmolar state can occur in the first days of life in infants of less than 26 weeks' gestation who weigh less than 800 g. These infants' immature skin and large surface allow massive evaporative losses of free water, which results in significant dehydration (weight loss of 20% or more in the first 48 hours) accompanied by hypernatremia, hyperkalemia, and hyperglycemia, without oliguria. Once this hyperosmolar state is fully established, correction involves the risk of volume overload. The suggested strategy for preventing this syndrome is as follows:

- IWL through the skin is reduced by using an incubator with a high relative humidity (instead of an overhead warmer), with or without a plastic shield or Saran wrap blanket.
- The infant's weight, urine output, serum Na level, and glucose concentration are monitored frequently.
- Sodium is restricted, and the smallest volume of fluids is given that allows the serum Na concentration to be maintained within normal limits (the initial rate is 80 to 100 ml/kg/day with subsequent increases, usually without exceeding 150 ml/kg/day).

Hypernatremia with Overhydration.   Hypernatremia with overhydration is almost always iatrogenic in origin. It may occur after administration of sodium bicarbonate during cardiopulmonary resuscitation or for acidosis or RDS, or it may arise from errors in the administration of NaCl with fluids. Because administration of sodium increases serum osmolality, it results in a shift of water into the intravascular space. An acute expansion of plasma volume may result in intracranial bleeding and heart failure with pulmonary edema. Treatment of hypernatremia with overhydration involves restricting sodium intake and providing diuretic therapy.

Potassium.   Potassium is the main intracellular cation. Its concentration in cells is maintained by the membrane sodium-potassium adenosine triphosphatase (Na^+, K^+-ATPase) pump. Because potassium is involved in the regulation of cell membrane potential, variations in the serum K concentration have important effects. Although every cell is susceptible to fluctuations in the serum K concentration, the effects on myocardial cells are the most prominent and severe.

Dietary potassium is mainly absorbed in the small intestine by passive absorption, and it is actively secreted in the colon. The kidneys excrete potassium. Probably all filtered potassium is reabsorbed in the proximal tubule. Potassium is then secreted by the distal tubules in exchange with sodium in a process regulated by aldosterone. The amount of potassium secreted normally is proportional to intake, so that balance is maintained.

The potassium requirement for both preterm and full-term infants is 2 to 3 mEq/kg/day. The current recommendation for standard infant formulas is 80 to 200 mg/100 kcal (14 to

---

BOX 24-2

Disorders of Potassium Balance

Hypokalemia
Inadequate intake
Gastrointestinal losses: vomiting, diarrhea, continuous gastric aspiration
Renal losses: diuretics, steroids, renal tubular acidosis

Hyperkalemia
Excessive intake
Impaired excretion: renal failure, congenital adrenal hyperplasia
Movement of potassium out of cells: catabolic states, acidosis

---

34 mEq/419 kJ) (AAP, 1998). The recommendation for growing preterm infants is 65 to 100 mg/100 kcal (1.66 to 2.5 mEq/419 kJ) (Tsang et al, 1993).

The normal serum concentrations are 3.5 to 5 mEq/L. Disorders of potassium balance are listed in Box 24-2.

Hypokalemia. Hypokalemia (a serum potassium level below 3.5 mEq/L) can be caused by inadequate intake, gastrointestinal losses (diarrhea, vomiting, continuous aspiration, and removal of gastrointestinal contents), and renal losses (diuretics, steroid therapy, renal tubular acidosis, Bartter syndrome).

The consequences of hypokalemia are related to the effects on muscle cells. Although abdominal distention and diminished bowel motility may occur, the cardiac effects are of much greater concern, and an electrocardiogram (ECG) may be a better measure of serious toxicity than the serum K concentration. ECG changes include a depressed ST segment, a flattened T wave, and a higher U wave. A prolonged P-R interval, a widening QRS complex, and various arrhythmias may follow, particularly in newborns treated with digoxin.

Treatment involves potassium replacement. Potassium chloride should be given very slowly (less than 0.3 mEq/kg/hour), and the serum K concentration or ECG, or both, should be checked frequently. Rapid IV administration of potassium may cause fatal arrhythmias.

Hyperkalemia. Hyperkalemia (usually defined as a serum K level over 6.5 mEq/L) can be caused by an excessive intake of potassium, impaired excretion (renal failure, salt-losing congenital adrenal hyperplasia), or increased movement of potassium from intracellular to extracellular space (catabolic states, acidosis of any origin). Spurious hyperkalemia, which is caused by venipuncture (injury to red blood cells), must be ruled out. Hyperkalemia occurs in approximately 50% of infants whose birth weight is less than 1000 g, and it is especially common in infants with low urine output in the first hours of life. The proposed mechanism is an increased potassium flow from the intracellular to the extracellular compartment, caused by a decline in the activity of Na^+, K^+-ATPase; increased catabolism does not seem to play a significant role. Cardiac toxicity is the main issue and is better reflected by ECG changes than by the serum K concentration. The typical ECG sequence is peaked T waves, disappearance of P waves, and a widening QRS complex, which fuses with the T wave to form a sine wave. Ventricular fibrillation may follow.

Treatment is directed at the underlying disorder, but several temporary measures can be taken, including administration of the following:

- 10% calcium gluconate (1 ml/kg, IV), to antagonize the effect of hyperkalemia on the myocardium
- Sodium bicarbonate (1 to 2 mEq/kg, IV), to raise the blood pH and, consequently, increase potassium influx into cells
- Infusion of glucose and insulin at a ratio of 4 g of glucose to 1 unit of insulin, to increase cellular uptake of potassium
- Furosemide (1 mg/kg, IV), to increase renal excretion
- A potassium-binding resin, Kayexalate (1 g/kg, by rectum or by mouth), to increase intestinal excretion

Although experience with the drug in newborns is limited, Salbutamol may be administered by aerosol to try to increase cellular uptake of potassium. All these measures are temporary; if the serum K concentration continues to rise and exceeds 8 mEq/L, peritoneal dialysis or exchange blood transfusions using a mixture of washed red blood cells (RBCs) and fresh-frozen plasma (to avoid a high blood K level) should be instituted.

Chloride. Chloride is the main inorganic anion in the extracellular fluid, and together with sodium, it is essential for maintenance of plasma volume. Chloride is administered as NaCl in the diet. Intestinal absorption is passive in the jejunum and occurs secondary to sodium absorption. In the ileum and colon, chloride is actively absorbed in exchange with bicarbonate. Normally only minimal amounts of chloride are lost in the feces. Chloride is excreted by the kidneys; like sodium, it is filtered by the glomeruli and reabsorbed throughout the tubules and collecting ducts. Normally 99% of the filtered chloride is reabsorbed.

Chloride resorption is inversely related to bicarbonate resorption. The serum concentrations of chloride and bicarbonate are also inversely correlated, which keeps the total anion concentration (Cl^- HCO_3^-) constant. For this reason, although chloride has no buffer effect, it plays an important part in acid-base regulation. When chloride is retained in the body, the serum bicarbonate level declines and metabolic acidosis follows. When chloride is lost from the body, the serum bicarbonate level rises and metabolic alkalosis ensues.

The current chloride recommendation for infant formulas is 55 to 150 mg/100 kcal [10 to 28 mEq/419 kJ] (AAP, 1998). The recommendation for growing preterm infants is 59 to 89 mg/100 kcal [1.66 to 2.5 mEq/419 kJ]. Normal serum Cl concentrations are 90 to 112 mEq/L in full-term infants and 100 to 115 mEq/L in preterm infants. Disorders of chloride balance are listed in Box 24-3.

Hypochloremia. Hypochloremia (a serum Cl level below 90 mEq/L) may be caused by diminished intake or by increased loss of chloride (gastrointestinal or renal). Clinical manifestations include metabolic alkalosis, hypokalemia and, in the case of a chronic disturbance, failure to thrive.

Insufficient intake has occurred with some old soy formulas that had a very low chloride content. The diagnosis of insufficient chloride intake is based on the dietary history and on the absence of urinary chloride, which indicates a normal ability to retain chloride to compensate for the low intake. Prolonged vomiting (pyloric stenosis) or continuous aspiration and removal of gastric contents (e.g., necrotizing enterocolitis, abdominal surgery) can increase gastrointestinal losses of chloride as hydrochloric acid (HCl).

BOX 24-3

Disorders of Chloride Balance

Hypochloremia
Decreased intake: some soy formulas
Increased gastrointestinal losses: vomiting (pyloric stenosis), continuous gastric aspiration, congenital chloridorrhea
Increased renal losses: diuretics, Bartter syndrome

Hyperchloremia
Increased bicarbonate losses: renal tubular acidosis
Excessive administration of NaCl: absolute or relative (renal failure)
Hypertonic dehydration (apparent hyperchloremia)

Congenital chloridorrhea is a rare disorder of severe diarrhea, beginning at birth, caused by impairment of the active Cl transport system in the ileum and colon. Analysis of feces shows an acid pH and a greatly increased Cl concentration. Diarrhea is caused by the osmotic effect of excess chloride, and hypokalemia ensues as a secondary consequence of diarrhea. Treatment involves a diet low in NaCl and potassium supplementation. The most common cause of increased renal loss of chloride is diuretic therapy. Frequent indications for this treatment in infancy are congestive heart failure and, especially, BPD.

Chronic administration of furosemide, which often is part of the treatment for BPD, may cause chloride deficiency with secondary metabolic alkalosis. Alkalosis, in turn, causes hypoventilation and an increase in the arterial carbon dioxide pressure ($PaCO_2$). This clinical picture can simulate pulmonary edema, but in this case the treatment should not be additional diuretic therapy (as in pulmonary edema), but rather correction of the hypochloremia.

Metabolic alkalosis with hypochloremia and hypokalemia caused by increased renal loss of chloride is the characteristic feature of Bartter syndrome, in which the underlying mechanism is a defect in tubular resorption of chloride. Elevated urinary Cl and prostaglandin concentrations are diagnostic. Replacement with NaCl and potassium chloride (KCl) or treatment with indomethacin (a prostaglandin antagonist), or both, usually is effective.

Hyperchloremia.   Hyperchloremia (a serum Cl level over 115 mEq/L) usually is associated with metabolic acidosis and can be caused either by bicarbonate depletion or by an excessive chloride intake. Diarrhea is the most common cause of hyperchloremic metabolic acidosis, because in the intestine chloride is absorbed with sodium, and bicarbonate is excreted with potassium. Increased loss of bicarbonate occurs with renal tubular acidosis. Usually only the proximal type is diagnosed in the neonatal period, and it occurs mainly in male infants. The renal threshold for bicarbonate drops below normal and the acidity of the urine is not diminished in this condition, and the result is a hyperchloremic metabolic acidosis. The condition is self-limited, and the diagnosis is based on the demonstration that the renal bicarbonate threshold is lower than normal; when the serum bicarbonate concentration is lower than the normal threshold, bicarbonate is retained and acid urine is produced.

Hyperchloremia may follow excessive administration of NaCl. Overtreatment with NaCl may be absolute, as in accidental errors in administration, or relative, as in renal failure. In the latter case, excretion is impaired and can be exceeded by an otherwise "normal" intake; NaCl administration, therefore, must be reduced accordingly. Finally, apparent hyperchloremia, together with increased serum concentrations of other electrolytes, can occur with dehydration when there is a water deficit in relation to solute.

Calcium and Phosphorus.   Calcium (Ca) is the most abundant mineral in the human body. It is an essential component of the skeleton and plays an important role in muscle contraction, neural transmission, and blood coagulation. Phosphorus (P) is essential for bone mineralization, erythrocyte function, cell metabolism, and generation and storage of energy.

The calcium content of human milk is about 39 mg/100 kcal (0.97 mmol/419 kJ), and the phosphorus content is about 19 mg/100 kcal (0.61 mmol/419 kJ). The current recommendations for standard formulas are 60 mg/100 kcal (1.5 mmol/419 kJ) for calcium and 30 mg/100 kcal (0.97 mmol/419 kJ) for phosphorus (AAP, 1998). The recommendations for growing preterm infants are 100 to 192 mg/100 kcal (2.5 to 4.69 mmol/419 kJ) for calcium and 50 to 117 mg/100 kcal (1.61 to 3.77 mmol/419 kJ) for phosphorus. With parenteral nutrition, a calcium intake of 60 to 90 mg/kg/day (1.5 to 2.25 mmol/kg/day) and a phosphorus intake of 47 to 70 mg/kg/day (1.5 to 2.25 mmol/kg/day) currently is recommended. To avoid precipitation in the parenteral solution, the Ca concentration should be maintained between 500 to 600 mg/L (12.5 to 15 mmol/L), and the P concentration should be maintained between 390 and 470 mg/L (12.5 to 15 mmol/L).

Calcium.   Calcium transport in the intestine occurs by both passive and active processes. Active intestinal transport involves carriers called calcium-binding proteins. Vitamin D in its active form, 1,25-dihydroxyvitamin D, is essential for the active process. Parathyroid hormone (PTH) is involved only through stimulation of production of 1,25-dihydroxyvitamin D. Vitamin D deficiency and almost any form of intestinal malabsorption can impair calcium transport. Corticosteroids diminish calcium absorption by inhibiting its transfer in the intestinal mucosa. Anticonvulsants can directly inhibit intestinal transfer of calcium (phenytoin) or can interfere with vitamin D metabolism (phenobarbital and phenytoin).

The serum Ca concentration is maintained within narrow limits by the action of parathyroid hormone, 1,25-dihydroxyvitamin D, and calcitonin. PTH and 1,25-dihydroxyvitamin D increase the serum Ca level, and calcitonin reduces it.

The kidneys excrete calcium, and filtered calcium is reabsorbed in most segments of the tubules. Parathyroid hormone increases tubular resorption of calcium, whereas calcitonin is thought to increase calcium excretion. Disorders of calcium balance are listed in Box 24-4.

Hypocalcemia.   Neonatal hypocalcemia is defined as an ionized serum Ca concentration below 4.4 mg/dl (1.1 mmol/L) in full-term infants. For preterm infants, for whom insufficient normative data on ionized calcium are available, a total serum Ca concentration below 7 mg/dl (1.75 mmol/L) continues to be a reasonable definition. Hypocalcemia conventionally is divided into early hypocalcemia, which occurs in the first 2 days of life, and late hypocalcemia, which occurs after the first 2 days, usually at about 1 week of age. Neonatal hypocalcemia may be

---

BOX 24-4

Disorders of Calcium Balance

Hypocalcemia
Early
Preterm infant
Infant of insulin-dependent diabetic mother
Perinatal asphyxia
Late
Cow milk–based formula
Hypomagnesemia
Hypoparathyroidism
Phototherapy
Maternal vitamin D deficiency

Hypercalcemia
Excessive administration of calcium or vitamin D (or both)
Subcutaneous fat necrosis
Williams syndrome
Idiopathic hypercalcemia
Hyperparathyroidism

---

asymptomatic or can cause symptoms such as irritability, tremors, poor feeding, muscle twitching, and seizures.

Early hypocalcemia is relatively common and sometimes is caused by perinatal factors. Approximately 30% of preterm infants (those less than 37 weeks' gestation), 35% of birth-asphyxiated infants, 17% to 32% of infants of insulin-dependent diabetic mothers, and up to 90% of VLBW infants (those weighing less than 1500 g) develop hypocalcemia in the first days of life (DeMarini & Tsang, 2001). Several factors appear to be involved, including abrupt termination of maternal calcium supply, temporary functional hypoparathyroidism (in infants of diabetic mothers), an increased calcitonin concentration (in asphyxiated and preterm infants), and 1,25-dihydroxyvitamin D resistance (in VLBW infants).

Late hypocalcemia typically occurs by the end of the first week of life and is caused by an increase in the dietary phosphate load. It was relatively common with the use of evaporated cow milk formulas, the phosphate content of which greatly exceeded that of human milk. Current formulas have a phosphorus content closer to that of human milk, and late neonatal hypocalcemia is much less common, although it has not disappeared. Maternal vitamin D deficiency may be a predisposing factor. Phototherapy appears to be an another factor associated with neonatal hypocalcemia, especially in preterm infants. The mechanism is not completely understood.

In rare cases late hypocalcemia can occur as a consequence of subclinical maternal hyperparathyroidism; maternal hypercalcemia leads to fetal hypercalcemia, which suppresses the fetal parathyroid glands. After birth, when the maternal source of calcium is no longer available, the suppressed parathyroid glands are unable to maintain a normal serum Ca concentration. Because the maternal hyperparathyroidism often is asymptomatic, neonatal hypocalcemia may provide the initial clue to the maternal disease. Another uncommon but serious condition that can cause symptomatic hypocalcemia is severe hypomagnesemia (see the section on Magnesium later in the chapter).

Several factors complicate the choice of treatment for neonatal hypocalcemia: (1) it may coexist with other perinatal complications, such as asphyxia and hypoglycemia, which can cause similar clinical signs; (2) it may be associated with seizures without being the cause of the seizures; and (3) in most cases, the condition is asymptomatic and self-limited.

If the hypocalcemia is asymptomatic, 10% calcium gluconate (9.4 mg of elemental calcium per milliliter) may be given orally (PO) at a rate of 75 mg/kg/day divided into six equal doses. If hypocalcemia is symptomatic (e.g., seizures), 10% calcium gluconate must be given intravenously at a rate of 2 ml/kg over 10 minutes; the heart rate should be closely monitored and the infusion stopped immediately at the first sign of bradycardia.

Hypercalcemia. Hypercalcemic disorders (a serum Ca level over 11 mg/dl [2.75 mmol/L]), such as subcutaneous fat necrosis, Williams syndrome, congenital hyperparathyroidism, hyperprostaglandin E syndrome, and familial hypocalciuric hypercalcemia, are exceedingly rare among newborns. Hypercalcemia usually is of iatrogenic origin and results from excessive administration of calcium or vitamin D.

The clinical signs, which are nonspecific, include constipation, polyuria, and bradycardia. Nephrocalcinosis and nephrolithiasis caused by hypercalcemia can be aggravated by dehydration and administration of furosemide.

Treatment of hypercalcemia is as follows:
- Calcium and vitamin D supplementation is suspended, and dietary intake of Ca and vitamin D is restricted (human milk or vitamin D–free formula is given).
- Urinary excretion of calcium is promoted by fluid administration (about twice the maintenance requirement).
- In the case of vitamin D excess, glucocorticoids are given to reduce intestinal absorption and bone resorption of calcium.
- With failure of other interventions, biphosphonates (etidronate or pamidronate) can be given, although experience with these drugs in newborns is limited.

Phosphorus. Phosphorus is absorbed mainly in the jejunum by both active and passive diffusion. Absorption depends mainly on the absolute amount of phosphorus in the diet, the relative concentrations of calcium and phosphorus (an excessive amount of either can diminish absorption of the other), and whether substances are present that bind to phosphorus and make it unavailable for absorption (e.g., phytates in soy-based formulas).

The kidneys excrete phosphorus; normally about 10% to 15% of the filtered phosphorus is excreted. Parathyroid hormone directly influences phosphorus excretion through its phosphaturic effect. Disorders of phosphorus balance are listed in Box 24-5.

Hypophosphatemia. Hypophosphatemia (a serum P level below 4 mg/dl [1.29 mmol/L]) is a common feature in preterm infants with rickets of prematurity, which is caused by insufficient intake of calcium and phosphorus. Rickets of prematurity is common in VLBW infants fed regular formulas, especially human milk with a low phosphorus content. Preterm formulas provide a higher concentration of calcium and phosphorus and can produce bone mineralization similar to intrauterine bone mineralization. In very rare cases, hypophosphatemia is caused by neonatal hyperparathyroidism.

In infancy, hypophosphatemia can be caused by diseases of vitamin D metabolism (vitamin D–dependent rickets) or by disorders of renal phosphorus transport (familial hypophosphatemic rickets).

Severe hypophosphatemia (a serum P level below 1 mg/dl [0.32 mmol/L]) is uncommon and may occur only in newborns receiving parenteral alimentation with an inadequate amount of phosphorus. Respiratory failure and decreased myocardial performance have been described as possible consequences of severe hypophosphatemia.

Hyperphosphatemia. Neonatal hyperphosphatemia (a serum P level over 7 mg/dl [2.26 mmol/L]) can be caused by ingestion of milk formulas containing high amounts of phosphorus, by excessive parenteral administration of phosphorus, by impaired phosphorus excretion (renal failure), or by defects in hormonal regulation (hypoparathyroidism). Severe hyperphosphatemia may cause metastatic calcifications and hypocalcemia. Management includes alimentation with human milk or with a low-phosphorus formula (e.g., Similac PM 60/40) and calcium supplementation to increase binding to phosphorus and its fecal excretion. Reducing the parenteral phosphorus intake usually resolves parenteral hyperphosphatemia. In renal failure, 1,25-dihydroxyvitamin D, which exerts its effects independent of functioning renal tissue, can be given to counteract hypocalcemia secondary to hyperphosphatemia.

Supplementation with 1,25-dihydroxyvitamin D and calcium may be used to treat hypoparathyroidism that arises from maternal hyperparathyroidism (transient hypoparathyroidism) or from DiGeorge syndrome (permanent hypoparathyroidism, which includes aplasia of the thymus and parathyroid glands, T cell immunodeficiency, defects of the aortic arch, and peculiar facies).

Magnesium. Magnesium (Mg) is distributed primarily in the skeleton and the intracellular space. It is involved in energy production, cell membrane function, mitochondrial function, and protein synthesis.

Magnesium is absorbed by passive diffusion throughout the small intestine. Absorption is related to intake, and approximately 50% to 70% of dietary magnesium is absorbed. The kidneys primarily regulate the serum Mg concentration; under normal circumstances, less than 5% of the filtered magnesium is excreted. Parathyroid hormone increases the serum Mg concentration, possibly through mobilization from bone. An acute decline in the serum Mg concentration increases secretion of parathyroid hormone, but chronic magnesium deficiency reduces PTH secretion and therefore may cause hypocalcemia.

The magnesium content of human milk is about 5 mg/100 kcal (0.21 mmol/419 kJ). The recommendation for standard formulas is 6 mg/100 kcal (0.25 mmol/419 kJ) (AAP, 1998). The recommendation for growing preterm infants is 6.6 to 12.5 mg/100 kcal (0.275 to 0.53 mmol/419 kJ).

A parenteral intake of 4.3 to 7.2 mg/kg/day (0.18 to 0.3 mmol/kg/day) currently is recommended. The Mg concentration in the parenteral solution should be maintained between 36 and 48 mg/L (1.5 to 2 mmol/L) to avoid precipitation. Disorders of magnesium balance are listed in Box 24-6.

Hypomagnesemia. Theoretically, magnesium transfer from mother to fetus might be impaired with placental malfunction, and placental insufficiency appears to predispose the infant to neonatal hypomagnesemia (a serum Mg level below 1.6 mg/dl [0.66 mmol/L]). In infants of diabetic mothers, hypomagnesemia appears to be a consequence of maternal magnesium depletion. Any severe malabsorption syndrome can cause magnesium deficiency, and an isolated defect in intestinal absorption of magnesium has been described.

Hypomagnesemia in the neonatal period usually is transient (except in malabsorption cases) and asymptomatic, but it can cause hyperexcitability and, occasionally, severe intractable hypocalcemic seizures that are unresponsive to calcium infusion and anticonvulsants. The mechanism of the resultant hypocalcemia is diminished secretion of PTH caused by magnesium depletion. The treatment is 0.2 ml/kg of 50% magnesium sulfate given intramuscularly (IM) or intravenously. This dose can be repeated, with monitoring of the serum Mg concentration every 12 hours, until normomagnesemia is achieved.

Hypermagnesemia. Neonatal hypermagnesemia (a serum Mg level over 2.8 mg/dl [1.15 mmol/L]) is an iatrogenic event caused either by parenteral nutrition or, more commonly, by maternal treatment with magnesium sulfate ($MgSO_4$) for tocolysis or preeclampsia. Other causes are administration of magnesium-containing antacid for treatment of stress ulcers and treatment of persistent pulmonary hypertension of the newborn with $MgSO_4$. Reported clinical signs of hypermagnesemia include hyporeflexia, lethargy, and respiratory depression. Neonatal serum Mg concentrations rarely rise to potentially dangerous levels and often gradually return to normal after several days. Hypermagnesemia does not cause hypocalcemia in the neonatal period and appears to be associated only with hypotonia. Usually no treatment is necessary. In severe cases, exchange blood transfusion has been used to lower the elevated serum concentrations.

WATER-SOLUBLE VITAMINS

Thiamine (Vitamin B₁)

Thiamine is a necessary coenzyme in carbohydrate and amino acid metabolism. Intestinal absorption is both active and passive; transport is active at physiologic concentrations and passive at pharmacologic concentrations. Thiamine is absorbed throughout the small intestine, but mainly in the duodenum, through the active and passive mechanisms. The kidneys excrete thiamine, and urinary excretion varies according to dietary intake.

The thiamine content of human milk is about 30 μg/100 kcal (0.09 μmol/419 kJ). For standard formulas, the AAP (1998) recommends a minimum content of 40 μg/100 kcal (0.12 μmol/419 kJ). The recommendation for growing preterm infants is 150 to 200 μg/100 kcal (0.45 to 0.59 μmol/419 kJ) (Tsang et al, 1993). The recommended parenteral intake for stable preterm infants is 200 to 350 μg/kg/day (0.59 to 1.04 μmol/kg/day).

Deficiency. Thiamine deficiency results in beriberi, but it is almost never seen in the neonatal period. Infantile beriberi occurs only in breastfed infants of thiamine-deficient mothers. The clinical signs, which become apparent after 1 to 4 months, include aphonia, cardiac signs (dyspnea and cyanosis), and neurologic signs (bulging fontanelle and seizures). Thiamine deficiency can be determined from reduced activity of the erythrocyte enzyme transketolase or by measuring the whole blood thiamine concentration.

Toxicity. Thiamine toxicity has not been reported with oral administration and is very rare in parenteral administration. Very large IV doses of thiamine have caused anaphylaxis and respiratory depression.

Riboflavin (Vitamin B₂)

As part of the coenzymes flavin adenine dinucleotide (FAD) and flavin mononucleotide (FMN), riboflavin is involved in electron transport and is essential to glucose, amino acid, and lipid metabolism. Riboflavin is absorbed in the proximal part of the small intestine, and amounts in excess of needs are excreted unchanged in the urine. The average riboflavin content of human milk is approximately 50 to 60 μg/100 kcal (0.13 to 0.16 μmol/419 kJ). The AAP (1998) recommends a concentration of 60 μg/100 kcal (0.16 μmol/419 kJ) for standard formulas and 200 to 300 μg/100 kcal (0.53 to 0.80 μmol/419 kJ) for stable preterm infants. Riboflavin and riboflavin phosphate are degraded by light (both sunlight and phototherapy).

Deficiency. Riboflavin deficiency results in epithelial abnormalities (stomatitis, cheilosis, glossitis, seborrheic dermatitis), normocytic anemia, and vascularization of the cornea. Riboflavin intake does not seem to be sufficient in preterm infants fed human milk, especially if the infant undergoes phototherapy. The clinical significance of this deficiency is unclear, but supplementation may be reasonable. Although the vitamin is inactivated by light, clinical riboflavin deficiency caused by phototherapy has not been reported.

Toxicity. No toxic effects of riboflavin have been reported in newborns.

Vitamin B₆

Vitamin B₆ is the generic term used to describe three substances: pyridoxine, pyridoxal, and pyridoxamine. The metabolic functions of these vitamins include synthesis of neurotransmitters, heme, and prostaglandins and interconversion of amino acids. Absorption occurs in the proximal small intestine by passive diffusion.

The vitamin B₆ content of human milk ranges from 150 to 250 μg/L (0.73 to 1.19 μmol/L), depending on maternal intake of the vitamin (Schanler, 1997). The AAP (1998) recommends a concentration of 60 μg/100 kcal (0.29 μmol/419 kJ) for standard formulas and 125 to 175 μg/100 kcal (0.61 to 0.85 μmol/419 kJ) for preterm infants. Vitamin B₆ is inactivated by light. Pyridoxal and pyridoxamine are heat labile, whereas pyridoxine is heat stable.

Deficiency. Vitamin B₆ deficiency can develop with any severe malabsorption condition and with dietary deprivation (human milk low in vitamin B₆, goat milk). Clinical signs include microcytic anemia, failure to thrive, irritability, and seizures. Isoniazid binds to and inactivates vitamin B₆, therefore infants receiving this drug may need vitamin B₆ supplementation. Neonatal pyridoxine-dependent seizures are caused by a congenital abnormality of vitamin B₆ metabolism, and pharmacologic doses of vitamin B₆ are needed.

Toxicity. There are no reports of vitamin B₆ toxicity in newborns. However, seizures have been reported in adults taking large doses of pyridoxine.

Cyanocobalamin (Vitamin B₁₂)

Vitamin B₁₂ is essential to the synthesis of DNA nucleotides and to carbohydrate and lipid metabolism. It can be synthesized only by microorganisms and is absent in plants. Absorption of vitamin B₁₂ takes place in the distal third of the ileum and requires the presence of intrinsic factor, a glycoprotein secreted by the stomach. The vitamin is transported in plasma by a specific protein (transcobalamin II). Vitamin B₁₂ is stored in the liver.

The average cobalamin concentration in mature human milk is 0.7 μg/L (0.51 nmol/L). The AAP (1998) recommends a cobalamin content of 0.15 μg/100 kcal (0.11 nmol/419 kJ) in standard formulas and 0.25 μg/100 kcal (0.18 nmol/419 kJ) for stable preterm infants.

Deficiency. Vitamin B₁₂ deficiency causes hematologic changes (megaloblastic anemia, thrombocytopenia, leukopenia) and neurologic changes (demyelination of the spinal cord and mental retardation). Neurologic manifestations may precede anemia. Because liver stores at birth are very large and usually sufficient for most of the first year of life, vitamin B₁₂ deficiency rarely develops in infancy.

Nutritional deficiency occurs exclusively in infants fed breast milk from strictly vegetarian (vegan) mothers and has been described as early as 4 months of age. Vegan mothers and their infants have high urinary concentrations of methylmalonic acid. Vitamin B₁₂ deficiency can develop in infants with short bowel syndrome if the terminal ileum (the site of absorption) is resected. The onset of vitamin B₁₂ deficiency from intrinsic factor deficiency occurs at about 6 months of age. Congenital transcobalamin II deficiency is a rare but important cause of vitamin B₁₂ deficiency; signs can occur after only 6 weeks of life, and mental retardation is invariably present. Because both folic acid and vitamin B_{12} deficiency can cause megaloblastic anemia and because folic acid can interfere with vitamin B_{12} metabolism, the differential diagnosis becomes important. A large folate intake may mask the hematologic signs of vitamin B_{12} deficiency and can aggravate the neurologic damage.

Toxicity.   Toxicity from vitamin B_{12} has not been reported.

Folic Acid

Folic acid is essential to the synthesis of nucleic acids and to the metabolism of some amino acids. Maximum absorption of folic acid takes place in the proximal jejunum. Absorption is active with physiologic doses of folic acid and mainly passive with pharmacologic doses. Folic acid is stored in the liver in small amounts, but the half-life is prolonged by enterohepatic recirculation.

The average folic acid concentration in mature human milk is approximately 25 µg/L (56 nmol/L), although heat treatment reduces the folic acid concentration in milk. The current recommendation for standard formulas is 4 µg/100 kcal (9 nmol/419 kJ) (AAP, 1998). For preterm infants, the recommended intake is 21 to 42 µg/100 kcal (48 to 95 nmol/419 kJ).

Deficiency.   Signs of deficiency include hypersegmentation of neutrophils, megaloblastic anemia, poor growth, irritability, and hypotonia. Neurologic disorders, such as seizures and mental retardation, are seen only with the congenital, isolated defect of folic acid absorption. Folic acid deficiency may be associated with prematurity (rapid growth and diminished hepatic stores), hemolytic disease of the newborn (increased erythropoiesis), anticonvulsant therapy (interference with absorption), prolonged antibiotic therapy (diminished production from intestinal bacterial flora), and any malabsorption syndrome. Folic acid and vitamin B_{12} supplementation may ameliorate anemia of prematurity (Worthington-White et al, 1994), although the issue remains controversial.

Toxicity.   There are no reports on toxic effects of folic acid in infancy. However, at least theoretically, very large doses of folic acid may reduce the serum concentration of phenytoin. In preterm infants, folic acid may diminish zinc absorption.

Ascorbic Acid (Vitamin C)

Vitamin C is required for collagen synthesis, for normal function of osteoblasts and fibroblasts, and for metabolism of some amino acids. It also acts as an antioxidant. Ascorbic acid is actively absorbed in the small intestine, and a feedback mechanism apparently regulates absorption of the vitamin. Very large doses of vitamin C appear to diminish the efficiency of intestinal absorption and to leave affected individuals prone to rebound deficiency once intake declines. Vitamin C is excreted by the kidneys either unchanged or as oxalic acid.

The vitamin C concentration in human milk is about 50 mg/L (284 µmol/L) in human milk. The AAP (1998) recommends a concentration of 8 mg/100 kcal (45 µmol/419 kJ) for standard formulas. The recommendations for stable preterm infants is 15 to 20 mg/100 kcal (85 to 114 µmol/419 kJ) (Tsang et al, 1993). Heat treatment significantly reduces the amount of vitamin C in milk; consequently, pasteurization of banked human milk reduces its vitamin C content.

Deficiency.   Vitamin C deficiency is very rare but can occur in infants fed pasteurized, unsupplemented cow milk or vitamin C–deficient breast milk. Vitamin C deficiency is associated with transient tyrosinemia and neonatal scurvy.

Transient tyrosinemia arises from a partial enzymatic deficiency that causes an elevation in the serum concentration of the amino acid tyrosine. The tyrosine concentration declines with administration of vitamin C. Transient tyrosinemia is common, occurring in as many as 10% of full-term infants and 30% of preterm infants during the first week of life. The amount of dietary tyrosine also plays a role, because a high protein intake and casein-predominant formulas can increase the serum tyrosine concentration. Because these transiently elevated concentrations are so common, it seems unlikely that they could be regarded as abnormal.

Neonatal scurvy is very rare. It is characterized by hemorrhages in the skin, subperiosteal spaces, and costochondral cartilage; by anemia resulting from diminished iron absorption; and by failure to thrive. Rebound scurvy, or scurvy that develops after abrupt discontinuation of a large vitamin C intake, has been reported in infants of mothers who took large amounts of vitamin C during their pregnancy (Schanler, 1997).

Toxicity.   Large doses of vitamin C may diminish vitamin B_{12} absorption, increase iron absorption, and increase the incidence of nephrolithiasis in congenital disorders such as oxalosis and cystinuria. Parenteral administration of 100 mg/kg/day (568 µmol/kg/day) to premature infants in the first week of life was not associated with adverse effects (Bass et al, 1998).

Niacin

Niacin includes nicotinic acid and its amide, nicotinamide. As components of the coenzymes nicotinamide adenine dinucleotide (NAD) and nicotinamide adenine dinucleotide phosphate (NADP), niacin is involved in mitochondrial electron transport, lipid synthesis, and glycolysis.

Because niacin can also derive from the amino acid tryptophan, dietary intake of both niacin and tryptophan is evaluated to calculate niacin requirements. For this reason, it is customary to use niacin equivalents (1 mg of niacin = 1 niacin equivalent = 60 mg of tryptophan).

The average concentration of niacin in human milk is 0.8 niacin equivalents/100 kcal, which also is the recommended concentration for standard formulas (AAP, 1998). The recommendation for preterm infants is 3 to 4 mg/100 kcal (25 to 33 µmol/419 kJ) (Tsang et al, 1993). Heating and storage do not significantly affect the niacin content in milk.

Deficiency.   Pellagra (rough skin) is the consequence of niacin deficiency. In adults, signs include dermatitis and inflammation of the mucous membranes, diarrhea, and dementia.

Toxicity.   Toxicity is related to the proportion of nicotinic acid and may manifest as cutaneous vasodilation, arrhythmias, and increases in intestinal motility and gastric acid secretion.

FAT-SOLUBLE VITAMINS

Vitamin A

Vitamin A exists in many isomeric forms; the basic and most active component is all-trans retinol. Vitamin A can be administered in different forms (retinol itself, palmitate esters of retinol, provitamins) and in different units (micrograms, international units [IU]). Vitamin A activity usually is defined as the equivalent weight of retinol (retinol equivalent [RE]). One RE is equal to 1 μg or 3.33 IU of retinol and to 6 μg or 10 IU of the provitamin beta carotene. Placental transfer of the vitamin appears to be limited, and hepatic retinol stores are low at birth. Dietary retinol is absorbed in the proximal intestine, and under normal circumstances, about 50% is absorbed. Retinol is incorporated into chylomicrons and transported to the liver, where it is stored, mainly in the stellate cells. From the liver, retinol is released into the circulation according to need; it is transported in plasma, bound to retinol-binding protein, and delivered to tissues. Retinol facilitates the visual process in the rod cells of the retina and plays a role in regulating and differentiating epithelial cells. Retinol appears to be necessary for normal lung growth.

With parenteral nutrition, a considerable amount of retinol is lost in the delivery set. Loss during infusion can be corrected by adding vitamin A to IV lipids (Werkman et al, 1994) or by infusing the daily dose of multivitamin preparation over 6 hours rather than 24 hours (Inder et al, 1995).

The average vitamin A concentration in mature human milk is approximately 2230 IU/L. The AAP (1998) recommends a concentration of 250 to 750 IU (75 to 225 RE/100 kcal) for standard formulas. The recommendation for preterm infants is 583 to 1250 IU/100 kcal (175 to 375 RE/100 kcal). An intake of 1250 to 2333 IU/100 kcal (375 to 700 RE/100 kcal) is recommended for infants with chronic lung disease.

Deficiency. The classic signs of vitamin A deficiency (night blindness, dryness of the cornea progressing to ulceration, perifollicular dermatitis) are of no value in the neonatal period. In clinical practice, a serum retinol concentration below 10 μg/dl (0.35 μmol/L) is accepted as indicative of unequivocal vitamin A deficiency. In preterm infants, deficiency commonly is defined by a serum retinol concentration below 20 μg/dl (0.7 μmol/L).

Vitamin A deficiency may occur with any form of fat malabsorption (diminished absorption), in preterm infants (low hepatic stores and diminish intake), in infants given parenteral nutrition (adherence of retinol to plastic tubing), and in infants with bronchopulmonary dysplasia. In infants with BPD, vitamin A deficiency is not absolute but relative, possibly owing to an increased requirement for vitamin A. It has been speculated that vitamin A deficiency might result from increased requirements during the healing process for the bronchiolar epithelium. At dosages of 5000 IU given intramuscularly three times a week, vitamin A supplementation was associated with a significant reduction in oxygen use at 36 weeks' postconceptional age (Tyson, 1999). However, there was no difference in other outcome variables, such as days on the ventilator and length of stay. Because chronic lung disease involves several other risk factors and shows marked variations among units, the decision to give the vitamin intramuscularly varies.

Toxicity. Vitamin A toxicity occurs from significant overdosage. The clinical signs are those of increased intracranial pressure: bulging anterior fontanelle, vomiting, and other neurologic symptoms.

Vitamin D

Vitamin D is essential for normal metabolism of calcium and phosphorus. Through the effects of its active form,

1,25-dihydroxyvitamin D, it is necessary for parathyroid hormone action in mobilizing calcium and phosphorus from bone; for intestinal absorption of calcium and phosphorus; and, indirectly, for bone formation.

Vitamin D can be obtained through the diet or can be synthesized by the skin after exposure to sunlight. Regardless of its origin, vitamin D is transported to the liver, where it is converted into 25-hydroxyvitamin D (25-OHD), and subsequently to the kidneys, where it is converted into the final, active metabolite, 1,25-dihydroxyvitamin D. 25-OHD is the major circulating vitamin D metabolite, and it is regarded as an indicator of vitamin D status. It is transferred from mother to fetus, and maternal vitamin D deficiency may be a predisposing factor for late neonatal hypocalcemia.

The serum concentration of 1,25-dihydroxyvitamin D appears to be tightly regulated. The synthesis of 1,25-dihydroxyvitamin D is facilitated by PTH, hypocalcemia, and hypophosphatemia. Placental transfer of 1,25-dihydroxyvitamin D has been demonstrated only after pharmacologic maternal doses. It is not clear if maternal-fetal transfer occurs, at least in significant amounts, under normal circumstances.

The current recommendation is a daily intake of 400 IU for both full-term and preterm infants (AAP, 1998), or 125 to 333 IU/100 kcal (Tsang et al, 1993). Breastfed full-term infants receiving adequate exposure to sunlight ($\frac{1}{2}$ to 2 hours per week average with face and hands exposed) do not appear to require vitamin D supplementation.

Deficiency. Vitamin D deficiency results in bone demineralization or rickets. Clinical signs are craniotabes, frontal bossing, widened ribs with enlargement of the costochondral junctions, and muscle weakness.

Laboratory findings include a low serum 25-OHD concentration (as a result of diminished intake); an increased serum PTH level, stimulated by a transiently low blood calcium level (to maintain a normal serum Ca level); normal or increased 1,25-dihydroxyvitamin D level (as a result of PTH stimulation); and restored serum Ca and low serum P concentrations (as a result of the effects of PTH).

Rickets can be caused by inadequate vitamin D intake, by inadequate exposure to sunlight, and by any form of fat malabsorption. Rickets or osteopenia of prematurity, a common disorder in VLBW infants, is caused neither by dietary vitamin D deficiency nor by abnormality of vitamin D metabolism, but by insufficient intake of calcium and phosphorus. A vitamin D dose of 200 IU/kg/day, up to a maximum of 400 IU/day, maintains a normal vitamin D status in preterm infants (Backström et al, 1999).

Toxicity. Excessive doses of vitamin D can cause hypercalcemia, restlessness, polyuria, and failure to thrive. Calcinosis occurs mainly in the kidneys but may also occur in the cardiovascular system, lungs, and intestine.

Vitamin E

Vitamin E is made up of several compounds, named tocopherols, which are important biologic antioxidants; among these, α-tocopherol is believed to be most active. Vitamin E protects the polyunsaturated fatty acid of biologic membranes from peroxidation.

Oral administration of either α-tocopherol or α-tocopherol acetate results in satisfactory absorption, even in very small preterm infants. However, fixed oral daily doses of vitamin E can produce variable serum concentrations. Moreover, absorption may be diminished in sick infants. Tocopherols are absorbed in the jejunum and transported by either chylomicrons or low-density lipoproteins to body tissues. The serum tocopherol concentration may not reflect the tissue concentration, because tocopherol is carried by plasma lipoproteins, which are diminished in the newborn.

Vitamin E is excreted mainly in feces. Biliary excretion is small, and urine excretion is almost negligible. The half-life of tocopherol is approximately 2 days. Because excretion is minimal, vitamin E is cleared from serum by tissue uptake or metabolic degradation, or both.

The average vitamin E concentration in mature human milk is about 2.3 IU/L. The recommendation of the American Academy of Pediatrics (1998) for standard formulas is based on both caloric intake and dietary content of polyunsaturated fatty acids: 0.7 IU of vitamin E/100 kcal or at least 0.71 IU of vitamin E per gram of linoleic acid. During the first 2 to 3 weeks of life of enterally fed preterm infants, intake usually is too low to achieve vitamin E sufficiency, therefore the vitamin should be supplemented at a dosage of 6 to 12 IU/kg/day (up to a maximum of 25 IU/kg/day).

Pharmacologic doses of vitamin E have shown no benefit for physiologic anemia of prematurity or BPD. The effects on retinopathy of prematurity and on intraventricular hemorrhage are controversial. If pharmacologic doses must be given, a dosage exceeding 25 IU/kg/day may result in tissue concentrations greater than needed for maximum antioxidant effect.

Deficiency. Vitamin E deficiency can occur in two categories of patients. Infants with severe forms of fat malabsorption can develop vitamin E deficiency and neurologic and myopathic abnormalities over several years. Preterm infants fed milk formulas both low in vitamin E and high in polyunsaturated fatty acids may develop, at about 2 months of age, a syndrome consisting of anemia, thrombocytosis, and peripheral edema. This syndrome does not occur with current preterm formulas.

Toxicity. Very large doses of vitamin E can cause calcification at injection sites, creatinuria, inhibition of wound healing, and fibrinolysis. An increased incidence of necrotizing enterocolitis has been associated with high oral doses of a hyperosmolar preparation. An intravenous preparation, tocopherol acetate in polysorbate, has been associated with a fatal syndrome consisting of renal failure, thrombocytopenia, hepatomegaly, cholestasis, and ascites.

Vitamin K

Two forms of vitamin K are naturally available: vitamin K_1, or phylloquinone, which is synthesized by plants, and vitamin K_2, or menaquinone, which is synthesized by animals.

Vitamin K is required for the synthesis of coagulation factors II, VII, IX, and X and for conversion of inactive precursors into active clotting factors. Dietary vitamin K is absorbed in the small intestine and transported with chylomicrons through the lymphatic system. Intestinal bacteria synthesize vitamin K, and this form probably is absorbed in the colon. In adults, about 50% of the total amount of vitamin K in the body comes from intestinal bacteria. The intestine is sterile at birth, and no significant synthesis of vitamin K by the intestinal flora occurs in the first few days of life. Vitamin K is stored in the liver, but storage capacity appears to be limited. Excretion occurs mainly with bile in the feces; urinary excretion is quantitatively less important.

The concentration of phylloquinone in human milk is about 2.1 μg/ml (4.6 μmol/L); it is about 4.9 μg/ml (10.9 μmol/L) in cow milk and 55 to 58 μg/ml (122 to 129 μmol/L) in milk formulas (Greer, 1997). Dietary intake of vitamin K, therefore, depends on both the quality and quantity of ingested milk. A deficiency state is seen almost exclusively in breastfed infants who do not receive vitamin K.

The following recommendations have been made for vitamin K supplementation:

- *At birth:* 0.5 to 1 mg (1.1 to 2.2 μmol) given IM *or* 1 to 2 mg (2.2 to 4.4 μmol) given PO
- *Infants receiving total parenteral nutrition:* Daily supplementation at a dosage of 8 to 10 (μg/kg (18 to 22 nmol/kg) *or* a weekly bolus injection of 0.3 to 1 mg (0.66 to 2.2 μmol)
- *Standard formulas:* A minimum concentration of 4 μg/100 kcal (9 nmol/419 kJ) (AAP, 1998)
- *Preterm infants:* An intake of 6.66 to 8.33 μg/100 kcal (15 to 18.5 nmol/419 kJ)

Deficiency. Vitamin K deficiency may result in hemorrhagic disease of the newborn. Bleeding usually occurs from the umbilical stump or after minor procedures (e.g., circumcision, blood sampling), but serious events such as gastrointestinal and cerebral hemorrhages are also possible.

Three clinical forms of hemorrhagic disease of the newborn, early, classic, and late, have been recognized.

- The early type occurs on the first day of life in infants born to mothers receiving anticonvulsant therapy (phenytoin, phenobarbital). These infants should be given an injection of vitamin K intramuscularly immediately after birth. This form of the disease may be prevented by antepartum maternal vitamin K supplementation.
- The classic type occurs between 2 and 10 days of life in breastfed infants who were not given vitamin K at birth.
- The late type, the most common form of the disease, occurs at a mean age of 6 weeks in infants with fat malabsorption. This type frequently is complicated by intracranial bleeding (83%), and it has a high mortality rate (14%).

A single intramuscular dose of vitamin K at birth effectively prevents the classic form of the disease. No randomized trials have been done to assess the effect of a single oral dose on the classic form of the disease or of a single oral or intramuscular dose on the late form (Puckett & Offringa, 2000). Some evidence indicates that a single intramuscular dose of vitamin K can almost always prevent the late form of the disease and is more effective than a single oral dose (Von Kries, 1999). Multiple daily or weekly oral doses may be as effective as a single dose given intramuscularly (Wariyara et al, 2000).

Toxicity. There is no evidence of vitamin K toxicity, except for RBC hemolysis and hyperbilirubinemia after administration of large doses of the synthetic vitamin K_3 (menadione).

TRACE MINERALS

Zinc

Zinc, as a cofactor, is necessary for the synthesis of nucleic acids and for the metabolism of proteins, lipids, and carbohydrates; it therefore is essential to normal growth and development.

Zinc accumulation in the fetus mainly occurs during the third trimester. Consequently, preterm infants have lower body stores than full-term infants. However, stores are limited in both full-term and preterm infants, and dietary intake is essential for maintaining optimum zinc status in the newborn. Zinc is absorbed in the duodenum and proximal jejunum. Although cases of zinc deficiency in breastfed infants have been reported, zinc absorption is greater from human milk than from formulas. Excretion occurs mainly through feces; urinary excretion is far less important.

The zinc concentration in human milk ranges from 60 to 22 μmol/L (Atkinson & Zolotkin, 1997). This concentration declines over time and is not influenced by maternal zinc supplementation (Krebs et al., 1995). Healthy preterm infants given 23 μmol/kg/day show a retention rate similar to the intrauterine accretion rate (Wastney et al, 1999).

The recommended concentration of zinc for standard formulas is 500 μg/100 kcal (7.5 μmol/419 kJ) (AAP, 1998). The current recommendation for enteral feedings in stable, growing preterm infants is 833 μg/100 kcal (12.7 μmol/419kJ). With parenteral nutrition, a zinc intake of 400 μg/kg/day (6.1 μmol/kg/day) is recommended for stable preterm infants.

Deficiency. Zinc deficiency can arise from inadequate intake, diminished absorption (preterm infant), or increased loss (malabsorption syndromes, ostomies). A serum zinc concentration below 40 μg/dl (6.1 μmol/L) generally is accepted as an indication of deficiency. However, in mild, subclinical zinc deficiency, the serum zinc concentration can be in the low normal range.

Dietary zinc deficiency has been reported only in breastfed preterm infants, owing to the large variations in the zinc concentration of human milk. Signs of deficiency include reduced growth velocity, acro-orificial rash, hypoproteinemia, and generalized edema. Acrodermatitis enteropathica is an autosomal recessive disease that involves a defect in the intestinal absorption of zinc. The disease is characterized by a dermatitis that affects the extremities and perioral/perigenital areas; diarrhea; and failure to thrive, which progresses to thymic atrophy and immunodeficiency.

Toxicity. Zinc toxicity has not been reported in newborns. Overdosage may result in copper deficiency and an increase in the serum cholesterol concentration.

Copper

Copper is necessary for normal functioning of oxidative enzymes (e.g., cytochrome oxydase) and for synthesis of collagen, melanin, and catecholamines. Both full-term and preterm infants are born with significant liver stores (Atkinson & Zlotkin, 1997). Active absorption takes place mainly in the duodenum. Copper absorption appears to be greater with human milk than with formulas. In plasma, approximately two thirds of copper is bound to ceruloplasmin. In newborns, limited ceruloplasmin synthesis results in low plasma ceruloplasmin and, consequently, a low serum copper concentration. Neither the serum copper level nor the ceruloplasmin concentration is an adequate index of copper status in the first weeks of life. Copper excretion occurs almost exclusively through the bile.

Despite wide variation in copper content, human milk appears adequate for both full-term and preterm infants. The recommended copper concentration for standard formulas is 60 μg/100 kcal (0.93 μmol/419 kJ) (AAP, 1998). The recommendation for stable, growing preterm infants is 100 to 125 μg/100 kcal (1.6 to 2 μmol/419 kJ). With parenteral nutrition, a copper intake of 20 μg/kg/day (0.31 μmol/kg/day) is recommended for stable preterm infants.

Deficiency. Copper deficiency can result from inadequate intake (cow milk, total parenteral nutrition) or increased loss (malabsorption syndromes, ostomies).

Clinical signs of copper deficiency include pallor (as a result of anemia and hypopigmentation), hypotonia, psychomotor retardation, hypochromic anemia unresponsive to iron therapy, neutropenia, osteoporosis, pseudoscurvy, and failure to thrive (Atkinson & Zlotkin, 1997; Hoyle et al, 1999).

Toxicity. Copper toxicity has not been reported in newborns. However, IV administration of normal amounts to infants with cholestasis results in liver damage, because excess copper cannot be excreted. Exogenous copper intoxication may be one of the causes of infantile cirrhosis (Dieter et al, 1999).

NURSING MANAGEMENT

Obtaining vascular access in a sick newborn has become as routine a part of the admission procedure as obtaining vital signs and weighing the patient. Nurses are responsible for providing peripheral or central vascular access and ensuring safe delivery of IV fluids. They also must be able to recognize the signs and symptoms of disorders in hydration and prevent complications that may be associated with fluid administration.

Assessment and Evaluation in Fluid and Electrolyte Therapy

The estimation of a patient's fluid and nutritional needs depends on the infant's age and weight and the disease process involved. The fluid and electrolyte needs of a 4-kg infant with perinatal asphyxia and seizures are different from those of a 32-week, 1750-g infant with RDS or a 23-week, 460-g infant with multiple complex needs. These infants represent varying points on the continuum of fetal growth and development, and each represents a different disease process; each also requires careful management of fluid and electrolytes to maintain homeostasis.

Fluid needs can be calculated using body weight, body surface area, or caloric expenditure (Behrman et al, 1995). Caloric expenditure is a easy method in which the infant's caloric needs are calculated, and fluid and electrolyte requirements are related to it. To begin these calculations, it must be remembered that 1 kcal is the amount of heat needed to raise 1 L of water 1° C. Caloric expenditures up to 10 kg = 100 calories/kg/24 hours. For example, a 1700-g infant would expend 170 calories in 24 hours, whereas a 460-g infant would expend 46 calories in 24 hours. As stated by Bakewell-Sachs (1999), this can be expressed as

$$\text{Energy intake} = \text{Energy stored} + \text{Energy expended} + \text{Energy excreted}$$

Caloric expenditures can be modified by an increase or decrease in body temperature and by specific disease states. Caloric expenditure can be used to determine water needs, because for every 100 calories metabolized, 100 ml of fluid is needed (Behrman et al, 1995). Water needs are determined by calculating IWL from the skin and pulmonary system and actual losses from the urine, stool, and sweat (Table 24-4).

TABLE 24-4	Fluid Intake and Output in Neonates	
	Range (ml/100 cal/ 24 hours)	Average* (ml/100 cal/ 24 hours)
Output		
Insensible water losses		
Pulmonary	10-20	15
Skin	25-35	30
Urine	50-70	60
Stool	5-10	7
Sweat	0-20	0
Intake		
All fluids consumed		112
Water of oxidation		−12

Average maintenance requirement is 100 ml/100 cal/day.

TABLE 24-5	Electrolyte Components of Intravenous Fluids	
Solution	mEq Na/1000 ml	mEq Na/100 ml
D$_5$W ½ NS (dextrose 5%, ½ strength, normal saline)	77	7.7
D$_5$W ¼ NS	38.5	3.8

Na, *Sodium.*

Insensible water loss can be affected by a variety of factors, including skin integrity and the degree of that integrity. An example of this is the newborn infant with a large gastroschisis. This midline abdominal wall defect predisposes the infant to large insensible water losses because of the exposed abdominal organs and absent omentum or peritoneum. Another example is a 23-week, 400-g infant with the typical "translucent" skin that has not yet formed a protective keratin layer; this condition predisposes the infant to dehydration secondary to large insensible water loss through the skin. Environmental factors also affect IWL; these factors include the presence or absence of humidity and increased or decreased ambient temperature. The use of radiant warmers has long been understood to affect an infant's fluid status by increasing insensible losses in a relatively open, unprotected environment. Phototherapy has similar effects, with the additional problem of thermoregulation. Increases in the metabolic rate, body temperature, and activity all must be included in the calculation of fluid needs.

Fluids usually are calculated on a daily basis, taking into consideration past losses, projected losses, and maintenance requirements. However, depending on the disease process, fluids may need to be calculated more often, even as often as every 4 hours, to keep up with losses and to make appropriate adjustments in fluid therapy. A general estimate of fluid requirements can be calculated on the basis of the guidelines presented in Table 24-1. Again, these are just guidelines; requirements differ according to gestational age and disease process. The fluid requirement for a premature, low-birth-weight infant may be as high as 150 to 200 ml/kg/day in some cases during the first 24 hours of life; on the other hand, for a full-term, asphyxiated infant, fluids may be restricted to no more than 40 to 50 ml/kg/day for the first 72 hours of life.

Electrolyte requirements usually are calculated on the basis of 100 calories metabolized:

- Sodium: 2 to 3 mEq/100 cal/24 hours (2 to 3 mEq/kg/day)
- Potassium: 1 to 2 mEq/100 cal/24 hours (1 to 2 mEq/kg/day)

Standard IV solutions containing a predetermined amount of sodium are routinely used in neonatal intensive care units (e.g., 5% dextrose in 0.45% NaCl) with potassium chloride and other electrolytes or minerals added as indicated (Table 24-5).

Caloric requirements cannot be met solely by the IV solutions commonly used in NICUs (i.e., 5% or 10% dextrose). These solutions are relatively low in calories; there are only 4 calories per gram of glucose (carbohydrate). The number of calories in intravenous solutions is calculated on a percent solution and based on grams per 100 ml. Therefore 5% dextrose in water (D$_5$W) contains 5 g of dextrose per 100 ml of fluid, 10% dextrose in water (D$_{10}$W) contains 10 g/100 ml, and so on. To carry this calculation further, D$_5$W and D$_{10}$W IV solutions contain 20 and 40 calories, respectively (D$_5$W = 5 g/100 ml at 4 cal/g = 20 cal).

The dextrose concentration used also depends on the infant's gestational age and renal function. The premature kidneys, unable to concentrate urine and conserve electrolytes and glucose, may alter glucose excretion, "spilling sugar" into the urine. An essential test of the infant's response to IV glucose therapy can easily be done at the bedside with a urine dipstick and a few drops of urine. This test can detect glucose, protein, ketones, and blood in the urine and can determine the pH level, an important indicator of acid-base balance.

Determination of the specific gravity is another essential bedside test that requires only a few drops of urine. The specific gravity, which normally is between 1.008 and 1.012, is an early indicator of hydration status. The urine dipstick and specific gravity tests should be performed at least every shift while the infant is receiving IV fluids and more often as the infant's condition warrants.

Fluid intake and output should be strictly monitored to ensure adequate hydration. Giving too much or too little fluid affects urine output (UOP), as do disease processes such as acute renal failure and drug administration (e.g., indomethacin or aminoglycoside antibiotics). UOP is monitored and calculated hourly over a 24-hour period. It should be no less than 1 ml/kg/hour/day. For example, for a 2-kg infant:

UOP = 240 ml/24 hours = 10 ml/2 kg = 5 ml/kg/hour

This is an adequate UOP for an infant of this weight and gestation.

For infants requiring long-term IV therapy, total parenteral nutrition (TPN) is used to improve nutritional status, and it may be started within the first 24 to 72 hours of life. TPN spares protein, increases calories and, when used in conjunction with Intralipid (an IV fat emulsion preparation), further maximizes caloric intake. If the TPN solution is infused through a peripheral vein, the glucose concentration is limited to no more than 12.5% because of the risks of tissue irritation and sloughing with infiltration; however, if the solution is infused through central lines, a higher glucose concentration may be used. With this route, in addition to the increased glucose concentration (which increases calories), higher concentrations of protein, fat, and other essential minerals and trace elements may be infused.

Caloric supplementation with TPN is as follows:

- Glucose: As noted above
- Protein (4 cal/g): 1 to 3 g/kg/day; 4 to 12 cal/kg/day
- Fat (9 cal/g): Up to 4 g/kg/day (10% emulsion, 1.1 cal/ml; 20% emulsion, 2 cal/ml)

The nurse is responsible for monitoring hourly fluid intake and should always double-check fluid orders to ensure that the ordered rate and solution are appropriate for that infant.

Weight is an important indicator of overall fluid status. Infants are usually weighed daily; extremely-low-birth-weight (ELBW) infants and infants with excessive fluid losses and needs may be weighed more often (i.e., every 12 hours or even every 6 hours) with fluid needs recalculated on the basis of weight changes. It is important to weigh infants carefully, because inaccuracies that show extreme weight fluctuations can have a detrimental impact on therapy. For example, an inaccurate weight measurement showing an increase of 100 g in a 12-hour period for an infant with severe RDS may result in an unnecessary dose of furosemide. The infant should be weighed nude, with as much equipment removed as possible (e.g., ECG leads, probes), at the same time each day, and on the same scale. In-bed scales that give a constant weight readout simplify the weighing process and cause the infant minimal stress.

The physical examination can reveal changes in the infant's fluid status and should be used in conjunction with laboratory data to plan interventions in fluid and electrolyte therapy. A general assessment for hydration status includes the infant's color, skin turgor, activity, mucous membranes, fontanelles, vital signs, and UOP, as follows:

- *Color:* Pink and well perfused, rather than pale and mottled (indicates dehydration)
- *Skin turgor:* Good turgor, rather than "tenting" (indicates dehydration) or edematous and shiny (indicates fluid overload)
- *Activity:* Active with good tone, rather than lethargic and hypotonic (indicates dehydration or overhydration)
- *Mucous membranes:* Pink and moist, rather than dry and gray (indicates dehydration)
- *Fontanelles:* Soft and flat, rather than depressed (indicates dehydration) or tense and full (may indicate overhydration)
- *Vital signs:* Bradycardia/tachycardia within normal range rather than slowed, normotensive rather than hypotensive or hypertensive, hypothermia rather than hyperthermia, or temperature instability
- *UOP:* Normal, rather than excessive (indicates overhydration), diminished, or absent (indicating dehydration)

SUMMARY

The care of infants with alterations in fluid and electrolyte balance presents a management challenge for both physicians and nurses. A thorough understanding of the underlying pathophysiology and the rationale for therapy enables the health care team to provide more informed care for these infants and to anticipate and prevent problems.

REFERENCES

American Academy of Pediatrics, Committee on Nutrition (1998). *Pediatric nutrition handbook.* American Academy of Pediatrics: Elk Grove Village, IL.

Atkinson SA, Zlotkin SH (1997). Recognizing deficiencies and excesses of zinc, copper, and other trace elements. In Tsang RC et al, editors. *Nutrition during infancy.* Digital Educational Publishing: Cincinnati.

Backström MC et al (1999). Randomised controlled trial of vitamin D supplementation on bone density and biochemical indices in preterm infants. *Archives of disease in childhood (fetal and neonatal)* 80:F161-F166.

Bakewell-Sachs S (1999). Neonatal nutrition. In Deacon J, O'Neill P, editors. *Core curriculum for neonatal intensive care nursing,* ed 2. WB Saunders: Philadelphia.

Bass WT et al (1998). Evidence for safety of ascorbic acid administration to the premature infant. *American journal of perinatology* 15:133-137.

Baumgart S, Costarino AT (2000). Water and electrolyte metabolism in the micropremie. *Clinics in perinatology* 27:131-146.

Behrman RE et al, editors (1995). *Nelson textbook of pediatrics,* ed 15. WB Saunders: Philadelphia.

DeMarini S, Tsang RC (2001). Disorders of calcium, phosphorus, and magnesium metabolism. In Fanaroff AA, Martin RJ, editors. *Neonatal perinatal medicine.* Mosby: St Louis.

Dieter HH et al (1999). Early childhood cirrhosis in Germany between 1982 and 1994 with special consideration of copper etiology. *European journal of medical research* 4:233-242.

Greer FR (1997). Special needs and dangers of fat-soluble vitamins A, E, and K. In Tsang RC et al, editors. *Nutrition during infancy.* Digital Educational Publishing: Cincinnati.

Hoyle GS et al (1999). Pseudoscurvy caused by copper deficiency. *Journal of pediatrics* 134:379.

Inder TE et al (1995). Vitamin A and E status in very-low-birth-weight infants: development of an improved parenteral delivery system. *Journal of pediatrics* 126:128-131.

Krebs NF et al (1995). Zinc supplementation during lactation: effects on maternal status and milk zinc concentration. *American journal of clinical nutrition* 61:1030-1036.

Lorenz JM et al (1995). Phases of fluid and electrolyte homeostasis in the extremely low birth weight infant. *Pediatrics* 196:484-489.

Neonatal Cochrane Reviews. Available online at www.nichd.nih.gov/cochraneneonatal/puckett/review.htm. Systematic reviews of research studies.

Puckett RM, Offringa M (2000). Prophylactic vitamin K for vitamin K deficiency bleeding in neonates. *Cochrane Database of Systematic Reviews.* 2000; (4); CD002776. Review.

Schanler RJ (1997). Who needs water-soluble vitamins? In Tsang RC et al, editors. *Nutrition during infancy.* Digital Educational Publishing: Cincinnati.

Tsang RC et al (1993). *Nutritional needs of the preterm infant: scientific basis and practical guidelines.* Williams & Wilkins: Baltimore.

Tyson JE et al (1999). Vitamin A supplementation for extremely low birth weight infants. *New England journal of medicine* 340:1962-1968.

Von Kries R (1999). Oral versus intramuscular phytomenadione: safety and efficacy compared. *Drug safety* 21:1-6.

Wariyara U et al (2000). Six years' experience of prophylactic oral vitamin K. *Archives of disease in childhood (fetal and neonatal)* 82:F64-F68.

Wastney ME et al (1999). Zinc absorption, distribution, excretion, and retention by healthy preterm infants. *Pediatric research* 45:191-196.

Werkman SH et al (1994). Effect of vitamin A supplementation of intravenous lipids on early vitamin A intake and status of premature infants. *American journal of clinical nutrition* 59:586-592.

Worthington-White DA et al (1994). Premature infants require additional folate and vitamin B$_{12}$ to reduce the severity of the anemia of prematurity. *American journal of clinical nutrition* 60:930-935.

NUTRITION: PHYSIOLOGIC BASIS OF METABOLISM AND MANAGEMENT OF ENTERAL AND PARENTERAL NUTRITION

MARY MASON WYCKOFF, JACQUELINE M. MCGRATH, TERRY GRIFFIN, JILL MALAN, ROSEMARY WHITE-TRAUT

INTRODUCTION

Maximizing the nutritional needs of premature and sick infants is essential to their healing and survival. This goal may, however, be difficult to accomplish due to the multiple complications experienced by infants born at under 1500 grams (Fletcher, 1998). The gastrointestinal (GI) system is immature, and lags occur in the development of motility, digestion, and the ability to tolerate enteral feedings. They have also immature and uncoordinated suck, swallow, and breathe mechanisms. Sucking behaviors are thought to be an ideal barometer of central nervous system maturation and organization and should be used a measure for neurodevelopment (Medoff-Cooper et al, 1993).

Due to inherent problems, central line access, feeding access, and feeding intolerance, most low-birth-weight and high-risk infants receive only minimal nutrition for the first week of life. Infants may be left NPO for several days because of the old belief in not using an already stressed gut. This timeframe of inadequate nutrition contributes to a weight loss of 10% to 15% below normal weight for the first 2 weeks of life (Heird & Gomez, 1996; Heird & Wu, 1996). Most clinicians accept this initial weight loss as physiological water loss. To compensate for these losses, the infant may receive additional non-nutritional volume. However, excessive volume depletes the nutritional system, which causes compartmental spacing, pulmonary edema, and generalized edema. This causes increased stress to the already compromised system. Hence the infant may develop the initial stages of growth retardation and malnutrition.

Exogenous protein losses in the absence of exogenous protein intake are at least 1 g/kg/day. Depending on energy intake, endogenous glycogen or lipid stores meet the infant's energy requirement. If energy intake is approximately 40 kcal/kg/day when using normal D10W, endogenous glycogen or lipid losses will amount to another 2 to 5 g/kg/day. This will account for a 10 g/k/day difference, which is about half of the intake. Thus the weight loss during the first 5 to 7 days also represents losses of endogenous stores (Heird & Gomez, 1996; Heird & Wu, 1996). This further increases the infant's potential for growth retardation and malnutrition because they are working harder to maintain homeostasis. These changes may not occur if the infants were provided with the appropriate nutrition to meet their metabolic demands. This clinical problem, however, receives only token discussion in many neonatal intensive care units (NICU). Nutritional demands continue to be under-managed by medicine—even in the NICU.

Once born, these infants are under conditions of total starvation unless nutrition is provided to them. They have minimal reserves as compared to their full term counterparts. Daily provision of intravenous (IV) glucose prolongs survival by only about 7 days. Therefore the mandate is to meet the basic nutrient requirements of preterm and high-risk infants. Understanding their metabolic limitations while avoiding physiologic stress and morbidity related to the delivery of enteral and parenteral nutrition is critical to their survival. The need for nutritional and occupational therapists to become active members of the caregiving team in the NICU is rapidly increasing.

This chapter briefly reviews the metabolism of nutrients, minerals, and vitamins in the neonate. The developmental and physiologic disabilities that are unique to the premature and sick infant are examined, and interventions are explored. Finally, an evaluation of current nursing practice in the delivery and monitoring of enteral and parenteral nutrition is included.

GASTROINTESTINAL (GI) FUNCTION

The placenta provides the nutritional needs of the fetus and facilitates function of the fetal gastrointestinal (GI) tract, which is important in amniotic fluid homeostasis. At about 4 weeks' gestation, the stomach develops from the ectoderm (Newell, 1996). The endoderm becomes the epithelium of the intestinal track, which is further supported by the mesoderm. The mesoderm is believed to be responsible for differentiation and expression of the first digestive enzymes. Functionality of the GI tract begins with the development of the digestive and liver enzyme systems, including the absorptive surfaces of the intestine. Intestinal villi begin to develop at 7 weeks and develop throughout the entire intestine by 14 weeks. The GI track has a muscle structure that consists of two layers: an inner circular sheath overlaid by an outer longitudinal coating of muscle tissues. The circular layer develops at about 5 weeks' gestation while the outer layer is not apparent until about 8 weeks' gestation. The layers thicken with increasing gestation age. Both are necessary for contraction and motility within the GI tract. At 25 weeks' gestation gastric motility is about 60% of that of a term infant. At 16 weeks, the fetus swallows 2 to 6 cc of amniotic fluid per day, and meconium begins to form (Fletcher, 1998). By term, the infant swallows 450 cc/day of amniotic fluid, with a gastric emptying time of 20 cc/hr. Intestinal motility and peristalsis develop gradually as the bowel is stimulated and mature during the third trimester. However, by the twentieth week of gestation, the fetal stomach's cellular composition is similar to that of the term infant (Newell, 1996).

In the premature and critically ill child, the provision of adequate nutritional support for growth and development is an ongoing challenge. Limitations of GI function cause the infants to be at risk for dehydration, reflux, malabsorption, electrolyte imbalance, and necrotizing enterocolitis. Because the development of motility and peristalsis occur during the third trimester, premature infants have higher risks. Infants who have cardiorespiratory disease and require assisted ventilation and/or who are physiologically unstable will also have a delay in oral-motor coordination as well as in gastrointestinal function because the gut may be compromised secondary to these other medical conditions.

The child's genetic endowment, intrinsic timing mechanisms, initiation of feeding, and diet composition also influence the development of GI function. The hormonal regulatory mechanisms have a critical role in development of the GI system after birth. Specific peptide hormones, enteroglucagon, gastrin, motilin, and neurotensin stimulate the system. Enteroglucagon promotes growth of the intestinal mucosa. Gastrin promotes growth of gastric mucosa and exocrine pancreas. Motilin and neurotensin are responsible for development of the GI system motor activity. Gastric inhibitory peptide initiates the enteroinsular axis and subsequent glucose tolerance.

A major stimulus for increased secretion of these hormones is initiation of enteral feeding, which induces surges in plasma concentrations of the hormones. This response is often delayed postoperatively in critically ill or preterm infants at birth and in children because they are not orally fed. Minimal enteral feeding as little as 0.5 to 1 cc/kg/hour will trigger surges (Berseth, 1995). This concept is important for maturation or repair of the GI system rather than for providing nutritional support.

Gastrointestinal (GI) function, which is immature at birth, increases the risk of malabsorption and malnutrition. Functional and anatomic maturation includes the suck-swallow reflexes, esophageal motility, function of the lower esophageal sphincter, gastric emptying, intestinal motility, and development of the absorptive surface area. The immature system also has decreased blood flow to GI area, which increases the risk for necrotizing enterocolitis. Most aspects of gastrointestinal functioning can be bypassed by providing gavage or transpyloric feedings; however, delayed gastric emptying frequently presents as feeding intolerance in preterm infants, thus resulting in abdominal distension, vomiting, and feeding residuals (Kelly & Newell, 1994).

Reflexes required for oral intake mature in the fetus during the third trimester. Gestational age at birth and/or exposure to enteral feedings does not influence the development of nutritive sucking and swallowing. Coordination of suck, swallow, and breathing has been considered the most complex task of infancy. All components are present by 28 weeks, but they are not at all mature. The swallow reflex is well developed by 28 to 30 weeks but is easily exhausted. The swallow reflex is completed by 34 weeks. Nonnutritive sucking can be demon-strated in infants by 26 weeks, but a rhythmic pattern is not developed until 32 to 34 weeks. The gag reflex is complete at 34 weeks. Coordination of breath, suck, and swallow occurs at 32 to 34 weeks for short periods; however, these mechanisms are not yet coordinated enough to sustain the infant's nutritional needs. True synchrony of suck, swallow, and breath in a 1:1:1 pattern does not occur until 36 to 38 weeks' post-conceptional age (PCA).

Infants with physiologic disabilities in which the absence or the weakness of the gag and cough reflexes exist should be monitored for an increased risk of aspiration. The assessment for the presence of a gag reflex may be performed by direct observation during the passing of a feeding tube. However, the adequacy of the gag reflex may be more difficult to assess, and the risk of aspiration should be considered for all infants who are being naso/orogastric tube fed.

Esophageal motility is decreased in the newborn during the first 12 hours. The lower esophageal sphincter (LES) is primarily above the diaphragm and subject to intrathoracic pressures, which results in esophageal reflux. Esophageal reflux is common and can be seen on a radiographic film in 38% of normal term infants in the first week of life. The sphincter remains small and inadequate for the first 6 to 12 months. Gastric emptying takes a minimum of 2 to 6 hours.

Intestinal motility has been described and identified by the postconceptional age at which motility dramatically improves (Baker & Berseth, 1997; Berseth, 1996). The investigators examined the frequency of duodenal contractions in newborns, the number of contractions per burst, and the intraluminal peak pressure per burst. The frequency and strength of the bursts increased after delivery regardless of the gestational age at the time of delivery. Considerable improvement occurred at 32 weeks' gestation, and infants whose mothers had received prenatal steroids demonstrated a mature pattern than that of infants of comparable gestations. Other studies of infants with known central nervous system abnormalities or insult had bursts at half the rate expected for their gestational age. Motility is thus a function of gestation, postnatal maturation, and disease state, with a definite link to the central nervous system. A fourfold increase has been noted in gastric motility between 28 and 38 weeks' PCA. If intestinal motility is the limiting factor in the progression of enteral feedings, it should be identified as such before multiple formula changes are tried. Identifying the specific source of the enteral feeding characteristics so that a plan can be devised to eliminate the causative factor is essential.

Incompetence of the ileocecal valve is not plainly assessed by the clinician. This valve acts as a barrier between small and large bowel contents, thus separating bacterial flora as well as regulating the time needed for the small bowel to absorb nutrients before its contents are delivered to the colon for water absorption. When reflux through this valve occurs, the small bowel is colonized with bacteria. With the presence of undigested nutrients in the small bowel, bacteria proliferate and can produce hydrogen gas. This mechanism is part of the sequence of events hypothesized in the process that leads to necrotizing enterocolitis.

Elevated gastrin levels in the newborn delay gastric emptying and are influenced by muscle tone, magnesium, mucus, pyloric sphincter tone, and the presence of amniotic fluid hormones. The type of food also affects gastric emptying time. Carbohydrates increase emptying time. Fats decrease emptying time. Medium chain triglycerides empty faster than long chain triglycerides. Mucous will generally delay emptying especially during the first 24 hours. Delayed gastric emptying appears to be an issue in most infants. Term and preterm infants improve their emptying times within the first 24 to 48 hours of life. Gastric emptying is delayed in disease states. Transpyloric feeding may be a consideration in these situations.

Content of dietary intake is also known to affect gastric emptying. Human milk empties more rapidly than formula or dextrose water. D_5W empties faster than $D_{10}W$. Higher caloric density formulas are retained in the stomach for longer periods. Although these formulas are associated with slower emptying, more of the calories are retained over comparative periods. The stomach empties more quickly if the infant is in a prone or right lateral position. Upright or semi-upright positions decrease the likelihood of air passing from the stomach to the duodenum.

The gastric capacity of an infant is approximately 6 cc/kg of body weight. Increased gastric volumes may compromise respiratory function and interfere with delivery of adequate nutrients. In preterm infants, large residual gastric volumes may develop and lead to gastric distention and vomiting.

Premature infants may have impaired rectosphincteric reflex, which creates a delay in stool evacuation, sometimes to the point of a functional obstruction. Many premature infants require rectal stimulation to evacuate the rectum. Although the passage of the first stool in a premature infant is slightly delayed when compared with term infants, meconium should pass by 72 hours of life. Thereafter rectal evacuation should be evaluated in relation to oral feeding volumes and symptoms of obstruction. Isolated intestinal perforations without the histologic findings of necrotizing enterocolitis may in part be due to the distention of the premature bowel to the point of perforation. Although described in association with IV indomethacin, it has also been described in very-low-birth-weight infants who have had no indomethacin; therefore the mechanism of immature GI function most likely plays a role (Buchheit & Stewart, 1994).

The premature infant has many developmental and mechanical disabilities that make use of the GI tract difficult or impossible. The digestive tract matures more rapidly with postnatal age and physiologic stability and needs to be reassessed regularly so that its use is not delayed. Increasing evidence exists suggesting that small amounts of enteral nutrient delivery enhance maturation of the GI tract (Berseth, 1999). In the future, manometrics (a tool to evaluate intestinal motor activity in response to various feeding techniques) may yield clearer recommendations on the methods of feeding best suited for the premature infant (Koenig et al, 1995).

A randomized controlled trial examining an aggressive GI nutritional regimen in critically ill very-low-birth-weight infants showed that poor nutritional intake compounds the poor energy reserves of infants who weigh 1 kg or less at birth (Wilson et al, 1997). An extremely preterm infant has only 2% of body weight as fat and <0.5 % as glycogen as compared with 15% and 1.2% respectively in the term infant. This study also documented increased metabolic demands in ventilated low-birth-weight infants and in both ventilator dependent and oxygen dependent children with chronic lung injury. The energy expenditure for these groups of high-risk infants is about 25% higher than in fulterm controls. The researchers hypothesized that maximizing nutritional interventions could improve developmental outcome in sick low-birth-weight infants.

Early minimal feeds promote growth in critically ill premature infants (Troche et al, 1995). Early hypocaloric enteral feeds are well tolerated in premature infants with severe respiratory distress syndrome. Troche et al (1995) provided preterm infants with early hypocaloric feedings and found it took fewer days for these infants to reach 120 cc/kg/day of enteral feeds, which subsequently enhanced weight gain by day of life 30. These findings suggest that early hypocaloric feeding improves GI system maturity and function, thus leading to improved absorption of the enteral nutrients and greater weight gain (Troche et al, 1995).

Meetze and associates (1992) found GI priming prior to full enteral nutrition to be a safe procedure for sick and premature infants. No differences were noted in safety or efficacy for infants with patent ductus arteriosus or infants who require mechanical ventilation. GI priming was also evaluated in critically ill infants. Infants were not excluded unless death was considered imminent. The researchers found that GI priming improved early feeding tolerance by increasing the levels of serum gastrin, which maintains function of the GI tract during hyperalimentation. Risk of necrotizing enterocolitis did not increase with mechanical ventilation or umbilical arterial catheterization.

Therefore, according to clinically based research, low-birth-weight infants benefit from early hypocaloric feedings by inducing surges in GI system hormones, improved feeding intolerance, degrease gastric residuals, fewer days with parental nutrition, and fewer feeding disruptions, with better weight gain by day 30. These results suggest that hypocaloric feeding facilitates the development and maturation of the gut. Human milk appears to further enhance this process. Development of the gastrointestinal tract is maturational and full feedings may be best tolerated when a gradual increase in feeding volume and content is provided.

NUTRIENTS

In addition to affecting the maturation of the gut and both short- and long-term growth of the infant and healing, neonatal nutrition also may affect behavioral development (Wauben & Wainwright, 1999). Nutrient deficiencies during early life may affect neurotransmitters, which regulate neurogenesis, neural migration, and synapse formation essential for normal brain development during embryonic and early postnatal life. Thus proper nutrition during infancy cannot be ignored; the effects may be lifelong even with reestablishment of appropriate nutrition later in development.

Protein

The amino acids, which are needed to synthesize the body's proteins, are provided by the many of forms of protein, which are essential constituents of all living cells. Amino acids consist of carbon, hydrogen, oxygen, and nitrogen. Proteins serve as enzymes, antibodies, lubricants, messengers, and carriers (Berdanier, 2000). In the stomach, protein is broken down into polypeptides and amino acids. This occurs through the activity of pepsin and hydrochloric acid. The second mechanism of protein breakdown and absorption is the pancreatic or intraluminal phase, during which the polypeptides are broken down into smaller peptides and amino acids. The last phase of protein absorption, intestinal absorption, is a two-step process during which the small polypeptides continue to break down into amino acids and are subsequently absorbed. This second mechanism is the direct absorption of macromolecules. During the first stages after birth and during critical illness, catabolism erodes the proteins, thus affecting structural and functional roles of the body. Dietary protein alone has an anabolic effect independent of energy. The nitrogen quality is an important determinant of nitrogen balance (Byers & Jeejeebhoy, 1997).

The common practice is to initiate intravenous nutrition with a simple glucose infusion. The preterm infant has a rate of protein synthesis that exceeds what is necessary for net protein gain—10 to 12 g/kg/day for synthesis versus 2 g/kg/day for gain. When administration of protein is below the range of protein synthesis, protein breakdown will exceed synthesis, thus resulting in a catabolic state. Therefore initiation of amino acids within the first hours of life should be a consideration.

Glucose intolerance, which is the more common reason for being unable to provide for energy needs, may be alleviated by careful administration of insulin. Premature infants are unable to tolerate an energy intake that approaches the amount necessary for normal growth. Most premature infants will tolerate a glucose intake of at least 5 g/kg/day and a lipid intake of at least 1 g/kg/d (Heird & Gomez, 1996; Heird & Wu, 1996). This combination will result in nitrogen equilibrium and could provide a slight positive nitrogen balance without causing hyperaminoacidemia or azotemia (Heird & Gomez, 1996; Heird & Wu, 1996).

Protein absorption in the preterm and term infant is inefficient when compared with that of the adult, but it allows adequate use of enteral protein even in the very small premature infant. The intake needs to be adjusted to account for the relative inefficiency of absorption, and then nitrogen balance can be achieved.

Glutamine. Glutamine is a neutral gluconeogenic amino acid that is synthesized by all tissues. Glutamine is a double nitrogen, which functions as a nitrogen shuttle between the various organs. The major site for synthesis is skeletal muscle, where it is released for use throughout the body. Positive outcomes have been documented when supplemental glutamine is provided to infants with disease states, GI disorders, immune function deficiencies, and metabolic stress states. Glutamine is the most abundant amino acid in the human body and is a structural component of protein function in nitrogen transfer between tissues. Glutamine is an important fuel for rapidly dividing cells, eterocytes, lymphocytes, macrophages, and fibroblasts. Glutamine is removed from the circulation and uses its five-carbon chain for energy.

Neu and associates (1997) found that enteral glutamine supplementation for low-birth-weight infants decreased morbidity. Glutamine is described as a "conditionally essential" amino acid for critically ill, metabolically stressed patients. This predominant amino acid is supplied to the fetus through the placenta. Human milk and amniotic fluid has been reported to contain greater quantities of free glutamine than cow's milk or commercial formulas (Neu et al, 1997).

Glutamine is the oxidative fuel for the enterocyte and the colonocyte and is necessary for the maintenance of intestinal structure in both normal and stressed states. Glutamine supplementation has been shown to prevent villous atrophy and bacterial translocation. These conditions are associated with long-term support with parenteral nutrition (Van Der Hulst et al, 1993).

For infants with short bowel syndrome, the administration of glutamine and growth hormone with a modified diet significantly enhanced the absorption of nitrogen, carbohydrates, calories, water, and sodium. This improvement in absorption decreased and eliminated the need for parenteral nutrition (Byren et al, 1995).

Glutamine may be considered the "survanta" for the GI system. Research involving 68 low-birth-weight infants showed the odds of developing sepsis was 3.8 times higher in infants not treated with glutamine (Neu et al, 1997). This study further showed increased tolerance in enteral feedings in infants who received glutamine. The study measured the percentage of days that feedings needed to be held; results were 8.8% versus 23.8%. This study provides evidence for decreased morbidity in low-birth-weight infants who receive enteral glutamine supplementation (Neu et al, 1997).

Fat

Fat absorption can also be divided into three phases: intraluminal, mucosal, and transport or delivery. In the intraluminal phase, triglycerides are converted into free fatty acids and monoglycerides, which are absorbed into mucosal cells. Long-chain fatty acids require bile acids for absorption and, owing to the slow rate of bile acid synthesis and the increased rate of turnover, this process is extremely inefficient in preterm infants. Thus this fat source is avoided when possible. In the mucosal phase of absorption, the free fatty acids are taken through a number of steps, forming phospholipids, cholesterol esters, cholesterol, chylomicrons, and very low-density lipoproteins. Chylomicrons are transported through the lymphatic system to the thoracic duct and eventually into the superior vena cava (SVC). Damage to the thoracic duct, which can occur in chest surgery, can then lead to the collection of chyme in the chest and require that dietary fat be modified or totally avoided until the leak resolves. Although it has been found to occur as early as 22 to 26 weeks' gestation, the entire process of fat absorption remains inefficient in preterm infants. Only about 65 to 75% of dietary fat is absorbed in the 32-week premature infant, as compared with 95% absorption in the adult. This translates into the need to adjust dietary fat in quantity and quality when feeding the premature or sick infant. Dietary fat in infancy is fundamental for the provision of energy for rapid growth, fat-soluble vitamins and essential fatty acids. Fat contributes 35 to 55% of the dietary calories and is therefore an essential nutrient for adequate growth.

Long chain polyunsaturated fatty acid (LCPUFA) such as docosahexaenoic acid (DHA) and arachidonic acid (AA) are found in high proportions in the structural lipids of cell membranes, especially the central nervous system. Associated with the rapid brain growth is the accumulation of LCPUFA, which is necessary for the formation of the neural tissue (Gershwin et al, 2000). During pregnancy, DHA and AA cross the placenta to the fetus. Postnatally these fatty acids are supplied in breast milk, which contains a full complement of polyunsaturated fatty acids including the precursors and metabolites. Supplementation has been researched and suggests that early visual development is better in infants who receive LCPUFA supplementation as compared with those fed standard formula (Uauy et al, 1994).

Carbohydrates

There are three major classifications of carbohydrates: monosaccharides, oligosaccharides, and polysaccharide. Monosaccharides consist of a single polyhydroxy aldehyde or ketone unit. There are two to ten monosaccharide units in an oligosaccharide. Disaccharide is the most common oligosaccharide. Polysaccharides consist of many monosaccharides (Berdanier,

2000). Absorption is a three-phase mechanism. Movement of the partially digested stomach contents (chyme) into the duodenum stimulates pancreozymin release also know as cholecystokinin. The low pH of chyme stimulates the release of secretin a hormone secreted by the epithelial endocrine cells of the small intestine, which in turn stimulates the exocrine pancreas to release bicarbonate and water to raise the pH of the chyme. This process maximizes the activity of the digestive enzymes located on the surface of the luminal cell (Berdanier, 2000).

During the pancreatic or intraluminal phase, the polysaccharides are broken down into mono- and disaccharide. Amylase is the primary enzyme responsible for this process, and the pancreas into the small intestine secretes it. At term, amylase is only at 10% of adult levels. The brush border of the neonate's intestines contains the enzymes that break down the disaccharide. Although maltase, isomaltase, invertase, sucrase, and palatinase are all found at functional levels in the fetus as early as 23 weeks, lactose levels remain low even in a full-term birth in comparison to those of an adult. This fact accounts for the presence of sugars other than lactose in most premature formulas. Lastly, active mucosal transport of monosaccharides or of simple sugars such as glucose is found even in the fetus and continues to provide a simple mechanism for carbohydrate absorption when other mechanisms fail. Infants with intestinal damage following necrotizing enterocolitis or prolonged ileus with atrophy may be disaccharide-intolerant yet absorb glucose or glucose polymers such as Polycose®.

The absorption of carbohydrates is therefore somewhat inefficient in the premature infant. The provision of corn syrup solids in premature formulas is meant to reduce carbohydrate malabsorption because of the relative lactose deficiency. The transient nature of lactose malabsorption when the infant's own mother's milk is used confirms the infant's ability to adapt rapidly once fed an exclusive disaccharide-containing enteral diet.

In summary, the absorption of the three major nutrients is relatively inefficient in the preterm as well as in the term infant. The mechanisms of digestion and absorption are essential for understanding the various dietary adjustments. This will facilitate the realization of risk factors of dietary intolerance and screening for intolerance in individual neonates.

VITAMINS, MACROMINERALS, AND TRACE MINERALS

Vitamins are organic compounds the body requires in small amounts for metabolic processes but cannot produce endogenously (Katz, 2001). Fat soluble vitamins (i.e., A, D, E, and K) are generally stored in the body in sufficient reserves. The absorption of these vitamins in the infant and preterm infant is unclear. Vitamin A functions in the generation of epithelial cells, in the growth of bones and teeth, and in the immune system. Vitamin A deficiency, due to malnutrition or malabsorption may result in extreme cases of severe eye injury and visual impairment (Katz, 2001). Vitamin D promotes intestinal absorption of calcium. Deficiency may manifest in rickets. Vitamin E functions as a lipid antioxidant and protects and preserves the integrity of cellular and subcellular membranes. Intakes of vitamin E will rise with the intake of polyunsaturated fatty acids (PUFA). Deficiency may manifest as muscle weakness, hemolysis, and impaired vision. Vitamin K is essential in the production of prothrombin, clotting factors VII, IX and X and proteins C and S. Vitamin K also appears to have other functions, particularly related to bone and kidney metabolism. Deficiency results in coagulopathy.

Infants are specifically prone to deficiency due to lack of intestinal flora (Katz, 2001).

Water-soluble vitamins, the B complex thiamine (B_1) riboflavin (B_2), niacin (B_3) Pantothenic acid (B_5) pyridoxine (B_6) folate, biotin, cyanocobalamin (B_{12}) and ascorbic acid (Vitamin C), are less likely to create deficiency states owing to their relative availability and method of absorption in infants. Thiamine functions as a cofactor and generates accessible energy, which is released from ingested macronutrients. Riboflavin catalyzes oxidation. The metabolic functions of vitamin B_6 and niacin require adequate riboflavin. Riboflavin deficiency manifests as a skin deficiency. Niacin functions in glycolysis, cellular respiration and fatty acid metabolism. Niacin can be synthesized from amino acid tryptophan, their ingestion is not essential if tryptophan is available in sufficient amounts. Pantothenic acid is essential to the metabolism of an energy release from carbohydrate, protein and fat. Pyridoxine is a fundamental requirement to amino acid metabolism and requirements rise as protein intake rises. Deficiency may manifest as dermatitis, anemia and seizures. Folic acid is essential for the viability of rapidly dividing tissues. Biotin participates in fatty acid synthesis, gluconeogensis and the citric acid cycle. Deficiency may cause vomiting, dermatitis, alopecia and glossitis. Vitamin B_{12} produces the active form of folate and folate metabolism. Deficiency impairs myelin formation and may result in neuropathy. Vitamin C is a cofactor in hydroxylation reaction in the production of collagen. Vitamin C is of importance in wound healing and the production of collagen (Katz, 2001).

To maintain physiological volume and tonicity of the infant's body compartments, sodium and fluid salt homeostasis need to be maintained. Water retention causes secondary retention of sodium and chloride. This imbalance may result in hyponatremia or hypernatremia dependent on whether excess water or excess sodium and chloride are retained. The brain, which is the most sensitive organ, may be damaged. In hyponatremia water is transferred to cells, thus resulting in edema; in hypernatremia fluid is transferred out of the cells, thus resulting in cell constriction with risk of capillary rupture. In VLBW infants these fluctuations are more pronounced than in fullterm infants. With the grave risk of leukomalacia and intraventriular and other bleeding into the brain it is important that fluid and electrolyte homeostasis stays within physiologic limits (Strange, 1993).

Fluid and sodium losses during the first week of life may result in a weight reduction of 5% to 10%. Besides urine, water is lost in stools, expired air, and evaporation through the skin, which—depending upon prematurity—may be quite high. The renal capacity of VLBW infant's concentration of urine is low, which may also result in dehydration. In attempting to hydrate these infants, healthcare professionals may overhydration the patient if fluid intake is managed at a high rate to provide sufficient energy and macronutrients. Severe complications such as chronic lung disease, symptomatic ductus arteriosus, and necrotizing enterocolitis may also occur. (Herin & Zetterstrom, 1994).

Adequate tubular reabsorption of sodium develops during the second and third postnatal weeks in infants of gestation ages 26 to 29 weeks and 31 to 34 weeks, respectively (Herin & Zetterstrom, 1994). With term deliveries the sodium concentration in breast milk may vary between 12 and 20 mmol/l during the first 2 to 3 weeks and then falls to 8 mmol/l. In a preterm birth the sodium concentration may remain high for longer periods of time. During the first 2 to 3 postnatal days, when natriuresis/diuresis occurs as a result of contraction of extracellular compartments when VLBWs have a larger loss of water, extra intake of sodium may be harmful and should be avoided (Herin & Zetterstrom, 1994). Infants may need additional sodium supplementation after the second or third week of life.

Higher doses of sodium may be required when infants receive furosemide; require assisted ventilation; have renal impairment, symptomatic ductus arteriosus, or neonatal polycythemia. Infants who have impaired GI tracts, receive hypertonic feedings, or experience diarrhea have increased intestinal permeability, which leads to large intestinal losses of electrolytes and water (Herin & Zetterstrom, 1994). This causes the infant to experience dehydration and electrolyte imbalance more rapidly than the adult. Basic requirements also vary in the infant because renal absorption and excretion of these minerals are not well regulated, owing to organ immaturity, which is accentuated in the premature infant.

Plasma potassium concentrations increase initially after birth, despite the absence of potassium intake. Plasma potassium then decreases and seems to stabilize by approximately the fourth day of life (Lorenz et al, 1997). With the increasing survival of extremely-low-birth-weight (ELBW) infants, hyperkalemia continues to be a problem despite appropriate fluid management. Potassium shifts from intracellular to extracellular space, even in the absence of exogenous potassium supplementation and despite negative total body potassium balance. This shift occurs in a range of premature neonates in the immediate postnatal period, as is explained by Sato and colleagues (1995). Renal potassium secretory capacity is limited because of the low glomerular filtration rate (GFR). VLBW infants are at risk of hyperkalemia during the first days of life. With the onset of diuresis the increase in GFR facilitates potassium excretion (Sato et al, 1995). Administration of potassium and the choice of formulas should be evaluated to take these concerns into consideration.

Calcium is a vital structural component of the skeleton, is essential for muscular contractions, and participates in the coagulation process (Katz, 2001). Calcium absorption occurs through a carrier-mediated mechanism and passive diffusion. The carrier-mediated mechanism depends on a vitamin D_3 metabolite. Passive diffusion occurs across the intestinal mucosa against a concentration gradient. If bulk water flow through the intestinal tract occurs, as with diarrhea, calcium losses will be exaggerated because of the diffusion mechanism.

Phosphorus functions in the synthesis of nucleic acids and phospholipids and in the formation of high-energy phosphate bonds in ATP. Phosphorus intake should approximate calcium intake (Katz, 2001). Magnesium is vital to the integrity of mitochondrial membrane and functions as a cofactor in diverse metabolic pathways involving more than 300 enzymes. Deficiency may result in irritability, seizures and failure to thrive (Katz, 2001).

The primary function of iron is to transport oxygen as a component of hemoglobin, and the bulk of iron is spread in the red blood cells. Iron deficiency may manifest as a depleted ferritin, impaired erythropoiesis, and then anemia. Iron is absorbed in the upper small intestine. Absorption is enhanced by ascorbic acid and impaired by fiber (Katz, 2001).

Selenium is a constituent of glutathione peroxidase, which is an important antioxidant and enzyme system involved in the synthesis of thyroid hormones (Katz, 2001).

Ingested zinc is absorbed in the proximal small bowel. Absorption varies based on the bioavailability of the source and the presence of other minerals in the diet such as iron and copper, which are known to interfere with absorption. Zinc functions in nearly one hundred enzyme systems and plays prominent roles in CO_2 transport and digestion. Zinc also influences DNA and RNA synthesis, immune function, collagen synthesis, olfaction, and taste. Zinc deficiency manifests as impaired growth, immune system function, and wound healing (Katz, 2001).

PARENTERAL NUTRITION

Basic Needs

By 2 to 3 weeks of age, the resting metabolic rate in preterm infants, when parenterally fed in a thermoneutral environment is 40 kcal/kg/day and is 50 kcal/kg/day when orally fed. Weight gain should be achieved at 50 kcal/kg/day above energy maintenance expenditure (AAP, 1996-1997, 1998). Thus to achieve a steady weight gain a stressed environment, infants should receive greater than 90 to 110 kcal/kg/day during parental feeds and 120 kcal/kg/day when enterally fed. The expenditure of energy is increased by lack of thermoregulation, infection, surgery, increased respiratory and metabolic activity secondary to increased respiratory requirements, and congestive heart failure. Premature infants further expend more energy because of increased metabolic needs and higher energy needs for synthesis of new tissue (Yao et al, 1997).

A study that calculated basic metabolic requirement (BMR) in premature infants who received assisted ventilation and in premature infants with chronic lung disease and growth failure found resting energy expenditure or BMR was 67 kcal/kg/day (Billeaud et al, 1992). This caloric need assumes that infants do not break down any of their own tissue to sustain body functions. Because IV calories are used most efficiently, 50 kcal/kg/day to an infant administered solely by the IV may meet the BMR only in the most stable infants but will not accommodate for growth. If these calories are provided enterally, the loss of calories via inefficient absorption must be considered.

Meeting the BMR translates into an infant receiving 125 ml/kg/day of $D_{10}W$ to obtain 50 kcal/kg/day, using the value of 0.4 kcal/ml of $D_{10}W$. When D_5W is used, the amount is prohibitive (250 ml/kg/day). Once the BMR is met, calories and protein are increased to allow positive nitrogen balance and protein sparing and to meet growth requirements. The birth weight is used for calculations until it is exceeded. After birth weight is achieved, the actual weight of the infant is used (Kuschel & Harding, 2001; Wesley & Bello, 2001). Goal weight gain is 15 to 20 g/kg/day.

Total parenteral kilocalories are less than the enteral needs because of the energy requirement for digestion. A mixed fuel system facilitates energy use. Eight percent to 12% are protein calories, 40% to 55% are carbohydrate calories, and 35% to 50% are fat calories (Kuschel & Harding, 2001; Wesley & Bello, 2001). IV nutrient delivery is balanced and provides maintenance as well as growth needs. Recommended IV protein intake should be 3 g/kg/day. Some preliminary observations have led to recommendations of 3.5 g/kg/day for preterm infants (Pereira, 1995). Although third-trimester accretion is approximately 2 to 3 g/kg/day, certain postnatal events such as surgery, respiratory disease, or necrotizing enterocolitis increase the protein needs and rapidly deplete the protein stores.

Fat needs are minimal to prevent a deficiency state. Fats should make up 40% to 50% of total caloric intake and therefore are a large contributor to total required calories. IV fat intake should not exceed 3 to 4 g/kg/day for all infants and should be monitored at least weekly with triglycerides and cholesterol levels. Providing 3 to 4 g/kg/day may prevent a risk of excess lipid accumulation and the complication of fat overload syndrome. This has a potentially harmful effect on oxygen diffusion. Elevated triglycerides and cholesterol levels present additional concerns. Several authors have shown that the 20% lipid solutions are better tolerated because of the efficiency of triglyceride clearance in the 20% solutions.

Carbohydrate intake should also represent 40% to 50% of the total caloric intake. Excess should be avoided even if the blood glucose level is normal, owing to the potential development of cholestasis and its contribution to carbon dioxide production and oxygen consumption. Maintaining carbohydrate intake at 20 g/kg/day reduces these risks. To summarize, the balance and absolute amount of nutrients needed for TPN are the following:

Protein:

8% to 12% of total caloric intake; 2.5 to 3.5 g/kg/day

Fat:

40% to 50% of total caloric intake; 3 to 4 g/kg/day

Carbohydrate:

40% to 50% of total caloric intake; as tolerated to 20 g/kg/day

Carbohydrates, protein, vitamins, minerals, electrolytes, trace elements, and other additives are combined in the TPN. Intralipids are provided independently.

Caloric needs based on activity consummation are basal needs of 50 kcal/kg/day; activity is 15 kcal/kg/day; cold stress 10 kcal/kg/day; fecal loss 12 kcal/kg/day; growth 25 kcal/kg/day. The recommendations for target calories vary from 90 to 120 kcal/kg/day intravenously (Kuschel & Harding, 2001; Wesley & Bello, 2001). Providing this intake through peripheral IV access is impractical and risky (Pereira, 1995). When TPN is used to supplement inadequate feedings the parenteral component should be decreased when feeds are tolerated at 50% goal and discontinued when feeds at 75% goal. The formula provided should be fortified at 22 kcal/ounce (Kuschel & Harding, 2001; Wesley & Bello, 2001).

In the past it has been common practice to initiate a simple glucose infusion, and studies support initiating amino acids on the first postnatal day. There is loss of protein from 0.5 to 1 g/kg/day, which causes significant growth delay and may cause morbidity in preterm infants. Recommendations are for 2 to 2.5 g/kg/day of amino acids starting on the first day of life and at least within 48 hours of birth. Total energy intake should reach approximately 60 kcal/kg/day as soon as feasible (Hay, 1994).

Cysteine supplementation may increase whole blood glutathione concentration (Mendoza et al, 1993). Supplementation with cysteine at a minimum of 0.5 mmol/kg/day is recommended. Infusate that contains cysteine hydrochloride may result in metabolic acidosis; however, the additive appears to be more beneficial. The metabolic acidosis may be offset by the addition of acetate to the solution.

Enteral fluid and nutrient needs will not be discussed here, but in most cases the total fluid volume that the infant can safely receive, based on organ maturity and disease state, dictates the concentration of all other nutrients to be delivered. The basic principles governing the calculation of fluid to be delivered are no different for total IV nutrition than for IV glucose or volume. Fluid issues focus on providing that which is balanced and adequate in a volume that the infant can safely handle (Chapter 24).

Infants' nutrient needs—protein, carbohydrate, and fat—are essential for the survival of low-birth-weight infants. Research has been described that supports the use of early, small-volume enteral feeding to promote maturation of intestinal motor function in preterm infants (Berseth, 1992; Meetze et al, 1992). A recent research report also described the effect of different volumes and concentrations of gastric and transpyloric feedings on the intestinal motor response to feeding in preterm infants (Koenig et al, 1995). Research in this arena will provide a scientific basis for decisions concerning the initiation of enteral feeding for preterm infants (Lebenthal, 1995).

Balanced IV nutrition to even the smallest premature neonate is essential. Nurses need to understand the rationale of the IV nutrients that they deliver. As with any IV medication, these solutions have the potential to create short- and long-term complications, and the nurse must clearly understand these complications and how to monitor for them. Severe hyperglycemia has resulted from human error in providing inappropriately prepared nutrients and glucose. The most common error is the transposing of the water and the solution of 50% to 70% dextrose. The result is a solution containing a very high concentration of glucose. To prevent this type of error, pharmacists can implement the use of a refractive index measurement. The instrument measures what essentially is the specific gravity of the solution from a known value based on the percent of glucose and amino acid. After solutions are prepared and tested they are sent to the intensive care units. This minimizes the risk of severe central nervous system bleeding, neurologic devastation, and death.

Methods of Delivery and Technical Problems

Parenteral nutrients can be delivered in many ways in today's NICU. Table 25-1 lists the methods and the risks and benefits of each. The clinician must then decide how best to deliver IV nutrients in the face of immaturity and disease.

Premature infants of less than 32 weeks' gestation rarely have a GI tract that will function fully within 2 weeks. In premature infants of all gestations, disease affects the GI tract, rendering it immobile for sometimes days to weeks. GI dysfunction also occurs in many term infants in the NICU. Infants may suffer from asphyxia, severe lung disease, or congenital anomalies. Most infants admitted to NICUs will require approximately 2 to 3 weeks of some form of IV nutrition.

The major constraints to peripheral IV nutrient delivery are the amount of glucose and the amount of protein that can be administered. The maximal carbohydrate (glucose) concentration that can be delivered is 10% to 12.5%, and the amount of protein is 2 g/dl. These values are based on the subsequent osmolality of the solution that is tolerated by peripheral veins. The higher the osmolality, the more likely that infiltration and tissue damage will occur. Most sick infants require fluid limitations, which makes it impossible to administer 80 kcal/kg/day and 3 g of protein/kg/day via peripheral vein. Other major issues of peripheral administration are the adequacy of peripheral veins, pain of intermittent "restarts," hypoxia from crying, cost of personnel time, and poor subsequent growth if nutrient delivery is low or frequently interrupted. The mean dwell time for peripheral IVs is approximately 36 to 49.5 hours (Smith & Wilkinson-Faulk, 1994; Stanley et al, 1992; Treas & Latinis-Bridges, 1992).

TABLE 25-1	Methods of Intravenous Access Techniques and the Risks and Benefits of Each
Pros/Benefits	**Cons/Risks**
Peripheral	
Not an option for low-birth-weight infants	High fluid volumes required to meet energy and protein needs of sick infants (150-200 ml/kg)
Reduced risk of systemic infection	Intermittent pain, hypoxia, cold stress, and hypoglycemia with restarts
Multiple team members have insertion skills	
No central venous access risks	Possible tissue damage with infiltration
Low cost per device	Loss of extremity in severe infiltration
	Higher risk of infiltration due to use of infusion pumps
	Mean dwell time 36-49.5 hours (Smith, Wilkinson-Faulk, 1994; Stanley et al, 1992; Treas, Latinis-Bridges, 1992)
	Restriction of positioning and motion when extremities used
	Limited veins in very small infants and infants with long-term IV needs
	May have increased pain agitation, apnea, and increased oxygen due to multiple attempts and needs for restarts
Central	
Nutrient needs met with limited fluids (high caloric density possible)	Central access risks effusion, thrombus, and infection
Staff time minimal once inserted (no need for restarts)	If surgical access is used, vein loss, cost increased for device and surgeon fee
No positional restraints	Need for radiograph to determine tip and follow-over time
Percutaneous access can be attained with no vein loss, no surgical incision; small size reduces thrombus, embolus, and effusion risks of central access	Increased nursing skill required for patient monitoring and troubleshooting device
	Nurses may be educated to insert PICCs
No intermittent loss of therapy (glucose and fluids) due to infiltration	Decreased pain, agitation, apnea and increased oxygen consumption because of multiple restarts

IV, intravenous.
PICC, peripherally inserted central catheters.

For these reasons the use of peripherally inserted central catheters (PICCs) has become the acceptable norm in this population of sick infants. Several authors describe the procedure and the risks, feasibility, and care of these lines (Baranowski, 1993; Neubauer, 1995; Pettit & Mason Wyckoff, 2001; Stephenson & Khan, 1993; Stringer et al, 1992). Multiple devices on the market can be used for this procedure. PICCs are made of polyurethane and silicone and are usually peripherally inserted (Brown, 1995). There are double-lumen devices and catheters small enough to insert in infants less than 500 grams.

The veins of choice for cannulation are the cephalic or basilic as primary, axilla, external jugular, temporal, posterior auricular, femoral, greater saphenous, lesser saphenous, and popiteal vein (Pettit & Mason Wyckoff, 2001). The arm veins can be cannulated at the hand or the antecubital fossa; they flow directly to the axillary vein, then the innominate vein, and finally the SVC. The veins in the head flow through the jugular into the subclavian then the SVC. The saphenous veins in the leg flow to the femoral vein, the iliac vein, and eventually the inferior vena cava (IVC). In neonatology, this site has the same low risk for insertion, as do the upper extremity veins. The tip placement of the catheter is SVC or IVC to provide the highest flow area, laminar flow—which minimizes the risk of infiltration—and extravasation and reduces the possibility of arrhythmia. The right atrial junction is not an acceptable placement (INS 1997, NAVAN 1998, Pettit & Mason Wyckoff, 2001). Concentrations of glucose and protein

intake can be increased to meet the infant's needs even in the circumstance of conservative fluid restriction. Glucose concentrations of 20% to 25% and protein concentrations as high as 4% may be used, when appropriately placed and clinically indicated to achieve adequate nutrient intake.

The position of the catheter tip must be confirmed by radiography. Many catheters are radiopaque and will not require using contrast injection. The catheters are to be flushed with a minimum syringe size of 5 to 10 cc, which will provide the maximum pressure per catheter manufacturer (INS, 2000). Broviac catheters, which are placed surgically, are reserved for infants who need months of parenteral nutrition, such as those with short bowel syndrome or the rare infant who cannot have a peripheral vein successfully cannulated for a PICC. The success of PICC insertion requires skill and knowledge; staff education is of the utmost importance. The care and maintenance of the catheters—including the commitment of early insertion before peripheral sites are used for other venous punctures—is the mainstay for a successful program. A comprehensive review of maintenance and troubleshooting can be found in the NANN *Guideline for Practice: Peripherally Inserted Central Catheters* (INS, 1997; Pettit & Mason Wyckoff, 2001). The authors of this guideline have contributed greatly to this technology and have supported it as a nursing procedure under standardized protocol (INS, 2000; Pettit & Mason Wyckoff, 2001).

If peripheral access is chosen, it should be reserved for infants who weigh more than 1500 grams and will not require long-term vascular access (i.e., less than 3 days). Peripheral access involves nutritional limitations in all premature and sick infants and is unrealistic for more than a few days. Peripheral access site care must be meticulous to preserve the skin integrity of the neonate and to prevent the solution from infiltration. All NICUs that use peripheral alimentation must have a procedure or protocol for initial treatment of the site.

A factor that contributes to tissue necrosis is the vascular supply to the site of infiltration. If arterial flow is adequate and venous return is unrestricted, damage is reduced. For these reasons, the site for peripheral TPN must be selected carefully. For example, a foot vein should not be considered if the foot previously showed vascular compromise from an umbilical artery line. Although the color of the foot may be normal and the pulse palpable, unexpected tissue damage, probably owing to a clinically undetected decreased arterial flow, may exist.

The technical risks of central access are many (Fioravanti et al, 1998; Klein & Shahrivar, 1992; Ochikubo et al, 1996; Trotter, 1996, 1998). The most common risks are infiltration, infection, and loss of the device resulting from technical difficulties such as occlusion. Infiltration risks can be eliminated when the catheter placement is in the SVC or IVC. When this is not feasible and the catheter is placed in the subclavian vein or when the infant grows and the catheter tip begins to migrate, staff must monitor closely for signs of infiltration. For catheter tips in the innominate, subclavian, auxiliary, or jugular vein, swelling can usually be detected with regular inspection of the neck or chest wall. When the patient has generalized edema, detection becomes more difficult, and an asymmetrical swelling that does not disappear with position change may be detected first. Careful review for the presence of differential edema on a radiograph may be helpful. Infiltration is generally actually rare. To minimize risk, lower glucose solutions may be used in infants when it is not feasible to thread the catheter tip to the SVC/IVC. If the catheter tip can be threaded only to the subclavian vein, the glucose limit may need to remain at 15% until the time a second catheter can be threaded to the SVC.

The infectious risks of the PICC are also reported to be low (Maki, 1994; Raad et al, 1994). All invasive devices increase the risk of infection in sick infants. The PICC is no exception but should not be implicated immediately as the focus of infection in all infants who have positive cultures. It is well known that certain resistant bacterial strains and fungi are present on the skin of these infants within a few days after admission to a NICU. Any losses of skin integrity, tracheal trauma, or skin puncture—such as with a chest tube insertion or arterial puncture—can introduce the flora into the bloodstream. It is imperative that PICC insertions are performed under sterile conditions and that a sterile occlusive dressing is placed and left intact until it is no longer occlusive (INS, 1997; Pettit & Mason Wyckoff, 2001). The PICC line system needs to include a closed end needless device. If absolute sterile technique is maintained and all opening of systems are managed sterilely, the risk of infection is reduced. Fungal infection remains a problem due to the presence of IV fat in the system. This provides an ideal culture medium for *Candida albicans* and all yeasts, including *Malassezia furfur*. This fungus can cause infection and will also occlude the line. An occlusion with fungus, such as *M. furfur*, requires that the line be removed at this time, as there is no pharmacological treatment for this fungus. The modified seldinger technique may be available for the neonate in the near future. Fungal growth requires that fat be

added to the traditional agar plates; recovery of the organism from catheter tips and blood cultures is low.

The technical difficulties of maintaining PICCs can be minimized with staff education and systematic, ongoing monitoring. Clinicians should maintain a record of insertion complications, which should be followed up systematically. Through this process, staff may be informed and educated about how to handle technical problems.

Finally, complications can be related to patient intolerance of the solution components. These complications include metabolic imbalances and clinically significant deficiency states if essential nutrients, minerals, or vitamins are omitted. All NICUs should have system checks in place to aid in the comprehensive ordering of these solutions. Systems include standardized order sheets, computer programs that calculate solution additives based on target orders per kilogram per day, or manual pharmacist checks to determine safety and completeness.

It should be possible to avoid metabolic problems by systematically advancing fluid constituents and regular laboratory monitoring, growth graphs, and daily screens such as bedside serum glucose testing. Hyperglycemia and hypoglycemia are probably the most common ongoing problems associated with the use of TPN. Reduction of these problems is through a system that requires a calculation of grams of glucose per kilogram per day or milligrams per kilogram per minute when the TPN rate is ordered. Traditionally, the percent glucose is ordered incrementally; thus as IV rate changes are made, the glucose load either exceeds that which is tolerated or is inadequate. For example, a 1-kg infant may be receiving a 7.5% glucose solution on day 3 of life. and the blood glucose remains stable. The order for day 4 is for 10% glucose, which is incremental, but at the same time the fluids are liberalized and the ultimate glucose received jumps from 8 to 12 g/kg/day. Most preterm infants cannot adequately metabolize this increased glucose load and experience hyperglycemia, which may require a work-up for sepsis, since hyperglycemia is a symptom of many other complications, including infection. Hyperglycemia sometimes occurs under the best circumstances in very-low-birth-weight infants. With the mandate of providing calories to meet the BMR as soon as possible, it is sometimes necessary to use insulin additives in the TPN solution. It has been shown that this practice is feasible and can improve the glucose tolerance in very-low-birth-weight infants, thus providing better caloric intake early in hospitalization.

TPN is a collaborative therapy; it is ordered by the physician/NNP (Neonatal Nurse Practitioner), checked and mixed by the pharmacist, and monitored by the nurse. Nurses will most likely be the first to observe technical or metabolic complications. If an infant exhibits a dramatic change in serum glucose or electrolyte levels, part of the differential diagnosis includes the possibility of a TPN solution preparation error. A sample from the TPN bag is sent to the laboratory for analysis. The laboratory must be informed of what the concentration is thought to be so that appropriate dilutions can be performed before the sample is analyzed.

An article on Y-site compatibility by Zenk (1992) provides current compatibility information for medications that can be administered with TPN, including IV fat. Of particular importance is the information about the compatibility of dopamine with TPN and fat and the compatibility of vancomycin with TPN. This information assists nurses in the administration of these common medications using only one line for IV access.

For more discussion of the rare metabolic complications, the reader is referred to the references at the end of this chapter and to Chapter 27.

ENTERAL NUTRITION

Growth charts provide clinicians with the ability to plot weight, length, and head circumference of infants as immature as 24 weeks, compare individual infants with standardized norms of infants of similar gestation, and establish the infant's baseline. The appropriate graphs show intrauterine growth curves that demonstrate the infant's full potential, had the gestation been carried to term. Postnatal growth is almost never ideal in this population because of disease states and technical constraints of nutrient delivery. The specific growth chart should be evaluated if it is appropriate to be used for the specific population. The Babson growth charts that were developed in 1976 are probably most amenable to generalization in that they show intrauterine growth curves, allowing an infant to be plotted from 24 weeks to 1 year adjusted age. NICUs located high above sea level should consider other curves, since data for the Babson graph were taken from infants born at sea level. Neonatal specialists in Denver and Arizona have developed modified growth curves for infants born at high altitudes. Once the infants' measurements have been plotted on the birth parameters, caloric adjustments should be made to keep them on this curve. Daily gains should aim for about 15 to 20 g/kg/day. Two studies have demonstrated that when gain is viewed as a per kilogram number, all infants are comparable. For example, although the 600 g infant may gain only 9 g/day, this is equivalent to 14 g/kg/day. Published data on average percent of weight loss by birth weight also exist. Although this information comes from descriptive data, it has been observed in other units that have similar nutritional goals. If weight losses in premature infants are high and time to regain birth weight exceeds 3 weeks, a change in therapy is needed.

Although it is clear that the caloric intake should be higher when enteral nutrition is started, it should be gradually increased as parenteral nutrition is gradually reduced. The ultimate target intake may take time to achieve. Therefore TPN supplementation is essential until full enteral feedings are tolerated. This transition must be monitored closely for adequacy and balance of nutrients. IV calories should not be withdrawn until infants are receiving target calories of 120 kcal/kg/day for at least a day or two. Because this is when a great deal of intolerance to enteral nutrients tends to develop—including necrotizing enterocolitis—consideration of maintaining the central access for several days is indicated in case enteral feedings need to be reduced.

Fluid intake should be considered between 60 to 100 ml/kg/day, depending on the infant's diagnosis, to provide basic hydration. Infants with lung disease may need moderate restriction, with increased caloric density of the formula for the target caloric goal.

Fortified human milk or premature formulas provide the premature infant with the additional protein, vitamins, and minerals needed when target caloric intake is achieved. Standard infant formulas should not be used in the premature infant population because they are too low in protein and have an inadequate vitamin and mineral content for the growing preterm infant. Since the early 1980's discussions among health professionals have suggested that pooled mature human milk may be inadequate in protein and minerals and that

growth rate and quality are poor when it is used in premature infants. When an elemental diet is needed, such as with infants who have had bowel resection for necrotizing enterocolitis, the most commonly prepared diet currently available is protein hydrosylate formula (Pregestimil®). It contains protein in an enzymatically hydrolyzed casein mixed with three amino acids. The carbohydrate consists of glucose polymers, which are easily digestible. The fat content is 60% medium chain triglycerides, 20% oleic safflower oil, and 20% corn oil. It is almost isotonic. Some practitioners use a soy protein formula (Alimentum®) because they believe that this substance is more easily digested. Its protein is casein hydrolysate, with amino acids cysteine, tyrosine, and tryptophan. The carbohydrate is sucrose and modified tapioca starch, with the fat being medium chain triglycerides, safflower, and soy oils with linoleic acid. Its osmolarity is 330 mOsm/L per 100 kcal. Adjustments when possible may be necessary in calcium, phosphorus, and protein content. Table 25-2 presents a comparison of formulas.

Methods of Enteral Feeding

Gavage feedings, either by the orogastric or the nasogastric route, are indicated for preterm infants who are unable to feed orally. Generally, infants are transitioned gradually from parenteral nutrition to gavage feedings, receiving them until sucking and swallowing reflexes are coordinated sufficiently to prevent aspiration of milk during oral feedings. A major controversy in the administration of gavage feedings for preterm infants is whether continuous or intermittent feedings, or some combination of these routes, should be used. A secondary consideration is whether selected nursing interventions might minimize the physiologic and biochemical alterations that have been noted during and after intermittent gavage or bolus feedings.

Trophic Feedings

Trophic or minimal enteral feedings (MEF) are subnutritional feedings that are administered by tube and are intended to prime the gut for future feedings. These feedings are usually small (a few ccs), dilute (often half-strength formula), and frequent (every 2 to 3 hours) and are provided by gravity via a gavage tube. Results from research are varied; however, greater evidence from both retrospective analysis and controlled trials seems to suggest increased feeding tolerance, fewer residuals, and fewer days to full feeding with a decreased incidence of ecrotizing enterocolitis. More research is needed in the area of MEF and minimal enteral nutrient delivery in relationship to the development of NEC and also to the development of biliary cholesistasis, a complication of long-term TPN.

Continuous Versus Intermittent Gavage or Bolus Feedings

Before the 1970s, preterm infants received gavage or bolus feedings intermittently, at 1 to 4 hour intervals. Clinical distress and regurgitation during and after feedings were managed by administering milk in smaller volumes, at slower rates, and at more frequent intervals. In the 1970s, an alternative to intermittent gavage or bolus feedings was introduced and was referred to as transpyloric continuous nasojejunal (CNJ) alimentation. This technique became widely used, especially for small, ill preterm infants. CNJ feedings involved insertion of a small feeding tube through the nose into the stomach; GI peristalsis moved the tube into the jejunum within a 24-hour

TABLE 25-2	Comparison of Formulas		
	FORMULA TYPE		
	Premature	**Standard**	**Soy**
Energy*	24 kcal/oz	20 kcal/oz	20 kcal/oz
Protein	Whey-to-casein (60:40)	Whey-to-casein (60:40 or 18:82)	Soy protein isolate
	22-24 g protein/L	15 g protein/L	18 g protein /L
Fat	MCT and LCT	LCT	LCT
Carbohydrate	Glucose polymers	Lactose	Sucrose and/or glucose
	Lactose polymers		
Calcium (Ca) and phosphorus (P)	Fortified to meet needs of preterm infant	Not fortified to meet needs of preterm infant	Not fortified to meet needs of preterm infant
	Ca-to-P ratio 1.8-2:1	Ca-to-P ratio 1.3-1.5:1	Ca-to-P ratio 1.3-1.4:1
Iron	Available with or without iron fortification	Available with or without iron fortification	Available with iron fortification only

*Premature formula is available as ready-to-feed 20 kcal/oz or 24 kcal/oz. Standard cow's milk-based and soy protein-based formulas are available commercially as ready-to-feed, powder, or liquid concentrate. The powdered and liquid concentrates are less expensive and can be prepared with less water to increase the caloric concentration not to exceed 30 kcal/oz.
MCT, medium-chain triglycerides; LCT, long-chain triglycerides.
From Klaus MH, Fanaroff AA (2001). Care of the high-risk neonate, ed 5, Philadelphia: WB Saunders.

period. Once correct tube placement was documented, milk feedings were connected to an infusion pump and allowed to flow continuously at a prescribed rate (milliliters per hour). Theoretically, preterm infants could receive larger daily volumes of milk with minimal physiologic and biochemical alterations. The continuous milk flow minimized gastric distention and consequent circulatory and respiratory changes. Additionally, the milk was delivered into the jejunum, bypassing both the cardiac and the pyloric sphincters, so the probability of regurgitation and aspiration was reduced. Transpyloric tubes were often difficult to pass and required verification of placement by radiograph. Recent research has not demonstrated significant advantages of transpyloric feeding over gastric feeding, and transpyloric feeding may increase risks for tube misplacement, necrotizing entercolitis, and malabsorption. This feeding regimen is no longer recommended for routine use (Newell, 2000).

CNJ feedings were gradually replaced with continuous nasogastric (CNG) feedings. CNG feedings were administered by slow infusion rates into the stomach so that rapid distention of the stomach was avoided. The CNG route was used to avoid the adverse physiologic and biochemical responses—tachycardia, tachypnea, bradycardia, apnea, cyanosis, and hypoxemia—associated with intermittent gavage or bolus feedings.

Current Clinical Practices

Neither the literature nor clinicians agree about whether gavage feedings for small preterm infants should be administered continuously by infusion pump (CNG) or intermittently by gavage or bolus into the infant stomach. Whether feeding tubes should be replaced before each feeding or left indwelling is another debated issue. Also controversial is whether tubes should be placed orally or nasally.

Proponents of CNG feedings cite the previously mentioned adverse physiologic and biochemical responses to intermittent feedings and emphasize that these responses do not occur with CNG feedings. Proponents of intermittent gavage or bolus feedings have expressed concern that CNG feedings permit

bacterial growth and that infusion pumps and disposable infusion tubing, which must be used with CNG feedings, represent an additional, perhaps unnecessary patient expense.

CNG feedings have been associated with improved weight gain when compared with bolus feedings. Although this study demonstrated minor differences in mean infant weight gain for the two feeding methods, numerous methodological limitations compromise the study results. In a separate study, patterns of enteroinsular hormone secretion were noted to differ for preterm infants, depending on whether feedings were administered by the intermittent or CNG route. Interestingly, in this research no differences in weight gain were noted for the two groups of infants. Another study reported adverse effects on pulmonary function for preterm infants after intermittent gavage feedings when compared with infants who received continuous feedings. After a bolus feeding administered over a 15 to 20 minute period, infants demonstrated significant decreases in tidal volume, minute ventilation and dynamic compliance and a significant increase in pulmonary resistance. Infants who were studied after receiving the same volume per body weight by continuous feedings given over a 3-hour period demonstrated no significant changes in pulmonary function data.

In a study to evaluate the effects of different feeding strategies on time to oral feeds, on growth, bone mineralization, nutrient retention, biochemical measures of nutritional status, feeding tolerance and morbidity, researchers concluded that bolus feeds resulted in improved feeding tolerance and growth. An additional benefit was decreased cost of infusion pumps and supportive care for infants on CNG feeds (Schanler et al, 1999). A prospective, randomized trial comparing continuous and bolus feeding methods suggested that very-low-birth-weight infants (<1500 grams) achieved similar growth and macronutrient retention rates and had comparable lengths of hospitalization in both the continuous and bolus feeding groups (Silvestre et al, 1996). In another study of feeding tolerance in very-low-birth-weight (<1250 grams) infants, the researchers concluded that feeding tolerance was improved in infants fed by the bolus method (Dollberg et al, 2000). The infants in the bolus-feeding group reached full feeds sooner and with less delay compared with those in the continuous feeding group.

A recent analysis of randomized and quasi-randomized clinical trials examining the risks and benefits of bolus or continuous feedings in infants who weighed less than 1500 grams at birth revealed that more studies are needed before universal recommendations could be made (Premji & Chessell, 2001). The authors cited small sample sizes, methodological limitations, conflicting results and inconsistencies in controlling variables that could affect results of the studies reviewed. Either method of milk delivery may be acceptable in individual situations (Newell, 2000).

Gavage Feedings of Expressed Mother's Milk

Milk expressed by mothers of preterm infants can be fed to the infants by gavage until the infant is able to suckle at the breast provided that certain safeguards are observed. Two outcomes preclude administration of expressed mother's milk by the CNG route when traditional infusion tubing is used: (1) nutrient loss and (2) bacterial growth in expressed mother's milk that has been colonized previously.

Studies since the 1970s have documented that milk lipid losses during CNG infusion are significant. These nutrient losses are especially significant for very-low-birth-weight preterm infants, and it is this population that usually receives CNG feedings. In one study, investigators compared lipid losses for two types of infusion tubing: one with a lumen capacity of 5 ml and the other with a lumen capacity of 0.6 ml. The CNG feedings were simulated, and expressed mother's milk was infused at a rate of 2 ml/hour. The findings revealed that statistically and clinically significant lipid losses occurred for both types of tubing; however, the mean difference between lipid values before and after feeding was greatest for the larger lumen tubing.

It has been suggested that elevating the tip of the infusion syringe to an angle between 25 and 40 degrees could reduce lipid losses during CNG feedings. However, there are no studies that support this hypothesis. Nutrient loss—especially milk lipids—may be unavoidable when the CNG route administers expressed mother's milk.

The potential for bacterial growth in already colonized expressed mother's milk has been widely recognized in recent years. Contrary to widespread opinion, expressed mother's milk is seldom sterile and may contain a variety of potentially pathogenic organisms. The particular concern with respect to CNG feedings is that expressed mother's milk is allowed to remain at room temperature, often for several hours, before reaching the infant's stomach. The warm temperature permits further bacterial growth; so the infant may receive a sizable inoculate of bacteria. Although term infants can apparently consume a variety of bacteria during breastfeeding without adverse effects, this principle cannot be generalized to small preterm infants, who have immature immune systems and do not receive milk directly from the breast.

Continuous infusion of expressed mother's milk by syringe pump may circumvent problems with bacterial growth in that the syringe pump and infusion tubing can be changed frequently (e.g., every 2 hours), with minimal wasting of expressed mother's milk. There is also theoretical support—but no empirical evidence—for feeding infants fresh rather than frozen expressed mother's milk. The antiinfective properties of expressed mother's milk are optimally preserved if the expressed mother's milk is not frozen or heat processed. Thus the preterm infant

would receive maximal protection from expressed mother's milk contaminants if (1) the expressed mother's milk has only small concentrations of skin flora; (2) the expressed mother's milk is administered within 24 hours of expression; and (3) the tubing is changed every 2 to 3 hours. However, there is no indication that these management strategies minimize the nutrient losses that occur with CNG feeding.

Orogastric and Nasogastric Routes for Intermittent Gavage or Bolus Feedings

A clinical dilemma concerning intermittent gavage or bolus feedings is whether orogastric or nasogastric intubation should be used for milk administration. Clinically, nasogastric tubes are simpler to insert and maintain in position than orogastric tubes; determining the correct insertion length is essential for both methods (Gallagher et al, 1993). However, reports have suggested that the use of indwelling nasogastric tubes may compromise respiration for smaller preterm infants. In one study, pulmonary function was studied in preterm infants with nasogastric and orogastric tubes in place, but not during infusion of milk. Infants who weighed less than 2 kg demonstrated diminished minute ventilation and respiratory rate, increased pulmonary resistance and work of breathing, and peak transpulmonary pressure change with nasogastric but not orogastric intubation. The investigators proposed that the nasogastric tube partially occluded the nares, especially in smaller infants, causing acute pulmonary compromise, for which smaller, less mature infants may be unable to compensate.

Some health professionals feel that there is less periodic breathing and apnea and higher transcutaneous partial pressure of oxygen ($tcPO_2$) values when preterm infants have orogastric rather than nasogastric tubes in place. It has been hypothesized that the infant works harder with a nasogastric tube in place. Use of a palatal stabilizer for the orogastric may also help with the stability of the tube and to decrease the energy expenditure. However, little systematic research to support this assertion has appeared since this was first proposed in the early 1980s.

With proper tube placement into the stomach and not into the lower end of the esophagus Symington and her associates (1995) found no difference in weight gain, apnea, or bradycardia between matched groups of preterm infants who received either indwelling NG or intermittent OG feedings. However, it has been hypothesized that indwelling feeding with an NG may be less optimal because of the increased airway resistance in the nares and the continuous inhibition of the esophageal sphincter, increasing the risk of reflux. Symington suggests that indwelling tubes may be more economical (changed less often) and cited this as the only clinically significant difference in the two methods of enteral feedings.

Tube Placement. For placement, the tube is first measured by extending it from the xyphloid process to the ear of the infant and than to mouth or nares and adding one centimeter. The tube may be quickly and smoothly inserted into the nares while the infant is offered a pacifier. Insertion orally can be slightly more difficult; however, the same technique can decrease the stress of insertion. The tube is secured to the side of mouth or nares with tape or other clear adhesive dressing. Many of the clear adhesive dressings are kinder and gentler to the delicate skin of the preterm infant. The tube may be removed after each feeding or left indwelling for 1 to 3 days. However, some of the softer silastic tubes may be left in place for a month or more. In the past, checking for placement was done by inserting air into the tube and listening for a gastric bubble; recently, however, this technique has been found to be somewhat inaccurate. Checking the aspirate from the tube for gastric pH maybe a more reliable technique for assessing tube placement into the stomach of infants.

Type of Gavage Tube. Two decisions with respect to selection of a tube for gavage feedings are tube size and tube material. Ideally, the tube used for gavage feedings should have the smallest bore to deliver the feeding, especially for nasogastric intubation in which the nare will be partially occluded. For nasally placed tubes, a 5 French size is desirable. However, the 5 French has a very small end hole and may become occluded during feeding. An 8 French may be used for orogastric intubation because occlusion of the nare is not a consideration.

Available materials for gavage tubes are polyvinyl chloride and polyurethane. The majority of gavage tubes are constructed of polyvinyl chloride, a stiff plastic that hardens over time, with potential for perforating the GI tract during or after insertion. Tubes made of polyvinyl chloride should be used for a single feeding or left in place for no more than 1 day. Thus if these tubes are used routinely, nurses need to develop a mechanism whereby the tubes are changed on a daily basis. For gavage tubes that will remain in place for longer than 1 day, a tube made of a softer, more biocompatible plastic, such as polymeric silicone or polyurethane, should be used. Several types of polyurethane feeding tubes are available commercially in sizes 5, 6, and 8 French. Small-bore polyurethane feeding tubes with weighted tips are also available and should be considered for infants with reflux.

Nursing Interventions

Routine nursing care during gavage feedings should include abdominal assessments consisting of palpation, auscultation, and abdominal girths at least every four hours with more close assessment when *any* one parameter has changed in the past four hours. Aspirates/residuals should be checked before feeding and should not exceed either the hourly rate (if continuous) or what would have been given if the bolus feedings were hourly. These parameters may be altered by the infant's intolerance for stress from the NICU environment, handling and/or procedures. Thus the infant's behavioral cues also need to be a part of this routine assessment. Always consider what has been happening to and around the infant during examination of the infant.

Research is limited related to checking for feeding residuals or what to do with them if found. Most nurses routinely check for residuals but the protocols for what to do when found vary greatly from unit to unit. Some refeed at each feeding. Some refeed at most feedings, depending on the consistency and content of the residual. Some never refeed. It has been suggested that gastric aspirates contain gastric acids, enzymes, electrolytes, and fluids that the infant requires. Consequently, if residuals are discarded, electrolyte imbalances and metabolic complications could ensue. Thus if residuals are discarded infants must be more closely monitored for issues related to these concerns.

Selected Nursing Interventions During Intermittent Gavage or Bolus Feedings

Selected nursing interventions have been proposed to ameliorate the adverse physiologic and biochemical responses during intermittent gavage or bolus feedings. These interventions can be categorized as follows: (1) controlling the rate of milk flow;

(2) warming the milk to body temperature; (3) optimizing infant position, including skin-to-skin holding; (4) using intermittently placed gavage tubes rather than indwelling gavage tubes; and (5) providing nonnutritive sucking opportunities. At present, well-controlled clinical trials in which these interventions have been tested either singly or in combination have not been conducted. Additionally, these interventions, because of their potential to influence a variety of other outcome measures, should be controlled when other feeding-related interventions are under investigation. For example, a study that focuses on the effect of milk temperatures should include controls for infusion rate, infant position, and nonnutritive sucking. However, these variables have not been well controlled in previous published research, so conclusions from this body of literature are not optimal.

Administration Rate. As previously mentioned, concerns about distending the infant's stomach with rapid infusion rates have created a major controversy exists as to whether gavage or bolus feedings should be administered continuously or intermittently. However, continuous usually refers to milliliters per hour, whereas intermittent usually refers to numbers of minutes to complete the infusion, regardless of volume to be administered. Thus allowing 10 minutes for infusion of a gavage or bolus feeding may be a relatively rapid or slow rate, depending on the volume to be infused. Thus clinical protocols for intermittent gavage or bolus feedings should reflect an infusion rate (in milliliters per kilogram of body weight per minute) rather than an infusion time.

Milk Temperature. Although early feeding techniques for preterm infants included warming milk to approximately body temperature prior to feeding, this procedure was abandoned with the advent of commercially prepared "ready-to-feed" formula. Thus in clinical practice, preterm infants receive formula that may be as much as −3.88 degrees C to −1.11 degrees C (25 degrees F to 30 degrees F) lower than body temperature. Studies in the late 1980s suggested that milk temperature might influence the body temperature response of preterm infants; one study was conducted with gavage feedings, whereas other studies were conducted with oral feedings. A recent study found significant improvement in feeding tolerance, as measured by volume of gastric residual, for preterm infants who received gavage-fed milk warmed to body temperature in comparison to infants who received milk warmed to room temperature (24 degrees C) or cool milk (10 degrees C) (Gonzales et al, 1995). Additionally, no significant differences were found in body temperature for infants in any of the three milk temperature groups in this study. However, it is important to generalize this finding cautiously, as the infants in this study were maintained in a neutral thermal environment, with heating equipment keeping the body temperature within set parameters during data collection. A study in which infants are allowed to self-regulate body temperature in an incubator or open crib may produce different findings regarding the effect of milk temperature on infant body temperature.

Infant Position. Studies since the 1970s have looked at infant position and feedings. Mizuno and Aizawa (1999) compared supine and prone positioning during gavage feeding in preterm infants with chronic lung disease. All infants were ventilated at the time of the study. The prone position resulted in a significant increase in arterial oxygen saturation during feeding.

The work of breathing during feeding appeared to be increase in the supine position. However, this is only one study with a small sample size of only seven infants. In the absence of definitive data concerning an optimal infant position, the nurse should recognize that infant position may influence oxygenation during gavage feeding. For infants who demonstrate hypoxemia, modification of position may promote improved oxygenation. Infants who are held in skin-to-skin holding during gavage feeding have been found to experience increased sleep, decreased stress and increased opportunities for social interaction.

Intermittent versus Indwelling Tube Placement. Gavage tube placement may result in adverse effects for the infant. These effects may include bradycardia as a result of vagal stimulation, reflux, and aspiration. To minimize these effects, some nurseries prefer to secure gavage tubes in place between feedings, decreasing the frequency with which infants are subjected to the procedure. In contrast, other clinicians feel that because nasogastric tubes compromise breathing, and orogastric tubes are prone to accidental removal, gavage tubes should be placed for every feeding and removed when the feeding is completed. One research report measured the incidence of apneic and bradycardic episodes and the amount of weight gain for preterm infants with indwelling versus intermittently placed gavage tubes (Symington et al, 1995). Although no significant differences were found in the incidence of apneic and bradycardic episodes between the two groups, the percentage of infants who exhibited such episodes was smaller for the indwelling group than for the intermittent group, despite the fact that all indwelling tubes were placed via the nasogastric route and all intermittent tubes were placed via the orogastric route. This study suggests that indwelling tubes could be used safely for this population, thus resulting in an economic advantage. Although this study has clinical merit, a study controlling for the feeding route while comparing infant response to indwelling and intermittent feeding tubes would help further understanding in this controversy.

Nonnutritive Sucking. The beneficial long-term effects of providing nonnutritive sucking with a pacifier during intermittent gavage feeding have been described for preterm infants and include fewer gavage feedings; accelerated maturation of the sucking reflex, with earlier initiation of bottlefeedings; greater daily weight gain; shorter hospital stay; and hospital cost savings. However, in a well-controlled prospective study, nonnutritive sucking was not associated with improved growth outcome for very-low-birth-weight preterm infants. Thus the data on long-term outcome measures with respect to offering nonnutritive sucking during gavage feeding are inconclusive, and further study is needed. However, no published studies have reported adverse outcomes associated with nonnutritive sucking provided when safe pacifiers are used.

Although studies for the past two decades have demonstrated that nonnutritive sucking in preterm infants is accompanied by the more immediate benefit of increased oxygenation, as measured by tcPO$_2$, these infants were studied while at rest, not during gavage feeding. More research is needed before conclusive conclusions can be drawn.

Transition from Gavage to Oral Feedings

Although all preterm infants who require gavage feedings undergo a "transition" period in which gavage feedings are discontinued and oral feedings are initiated, few research-based guidelines have been developed for managing this process. However, most NICUs have written policies concerning when oral feedings can be introduced to preterm infants; criteria usually include a minimal weight and postconceptional age. Kinneer and Beachy (1994) reported factors that nurses ranked as the most important indicators of an infant's readiness to initiate oral feeding. These factors included nonnutritive sucking, a strong gag reflex, demanding feedings, and a postconceptional age greater than or equal to 34 weeks' gestation. The authors suggested that further research was needed to determine the predictive validity of nonnutritive sucking and other infant behaviors for nutritive sucking ability.

Pickler and associates (1997) examined the medical records of 40 preterm infants to describe the bottlefeeding histories of preterm infants. Records were examined for physical indices related to and predictive of bottlefeeding initiation and progression. Infant morbidity ratings were closely correlated with postconceptional age at first bottlefeeding, full bottlefeeding, and discharge. Thus prematurity and disease status as well as instability were related to initiation and transition time. Pridam and associates (1998) also examined medial records for similar indications of feeding progression and found that individual infant characteristics as well as environmental and historical characteristics contributed significantly to shortening or lengthening transition time. However, Kliethermes and associates (1999) found that infants receiving gavage feedings supplementation rather than bottlefeeding supplementation during the transition to breastfeeding were 4.5 times more likely to be breastfeeding at discharge and 9.4 times more likely to be fully breastfed than infants who received supplemental with bottles. These findings suggest that an infant's transition from gavage feeding to breastfeeding may affect his or her long-term ability to breastfeed and that bottlefeeding should be avoided if full breastfeeding is the goal. This practice is contrary to most feeding practices in NICUs in the United States.

The development of competent oral feeding skills is a requisite for physiologic adaptation and survival during infancy (Medoff-Cooper & Ray, 1995). Oral feeding is a highly organized and intricate behavior that encompasses the activities of food seeking/obtaining, ingestion, and swallowing. Physiologically, oral feeding involves complex interaction of the brain and central nervous system, oral-motor reflexes, and multiple muscles of the mouth, pharynx, esophagus and face (Tuchman, 1994). Infant oral feeding requires the rhythmic coordination of sucking and swallowing a bolus of fluid while at the same time balancing the demands for breathing (Mathew et al, 1992). Oral feeding has been regarded as the most highly organized behavioral activity of early infancy (Conway, 1994). For term infants, oral feeding is a "natural physiologic process" that proceeds with minimal difficulty during the first days of life. However, the transition to oral or nipplefeedings in preterm infants may be significantly delayed as a result of anatomic and functional immaturity of the GI system, anesthesia or analgesia, acute and/or chronic illness, neurobehavioral maturation, oral-motor dysfunction, and behavioral aversion.

Another issue to consider is that during transition to oral nipplefeeding the infant may be also receiving intermittent gavage feeding requiring the use of a nasogastric feeding tube. Most nurses choose a nasogastric because it can be inserted prior to oral feeding and does not appear to interfere with the oral feeding process. However, Shiao and associates (1995) found that desaturation events during the feeding are increased in duration by the presence of the nasogastric tube. They also found that the presence of the tube lengthened the transition to full nipplefeedings. They suggest that starting oral feedings with higher baseline saturations (95% or greater) may benefit these infants.

Feeding orally requires the integration of three functions: sucking, swallowing, and breathing. According to the classic study by Gryboski (1969), sucking movements precede swallowing, which, in turn, inhibits respiration. Initially, preterm infants demonstrate an "immature sucking pattern," which is characterized by short sucking bursts, which, in turn, are preceded or followed by swallows. As preterm infants mature, sucking bursts become more prolonged, with multiple swallows occurring during these bursts (Gryboski, 1969). The integration of sucking, swallowing, and breathing is apparently related to both the maturity and the general health status of the preterm infant.

The problem with most NICU feeding protocols is that they do not incorporate individual infant differences with respect to oral feeding. Some preterm infants may be able to feed orally as early as 32 weeks' postconceptional age, whereas other infants may demonstrate difficulty in the coordination of sucking, swallowing, and breathing until near term or even beyond. At present, no universally accepted clinical tools for assessing readiness to feed orally or for quantitatively measuring an infant's ability to feed exist. A tool developed for either purpose should include noninvasive measures of oxygenation because a primary goal of early oral feeding is the avoidance of hypoxemia. Thus oximetry or $tcPO_2$ measures should be a part of management protocols for the transition of preterm infants from gavage to oral feedings.

Scheduled versus Cue-Based Feedings

Cue-based, or self-regulatory, feedings for clinically stable preterm infants have been used since the 1950s. Self-regulatory feedings involve feeding the infant based on caregiver interpretation of infant hunger versus feeding the infant every 3 or 4 hours, independent of the presence or absence of behaviors that suggest hunger. Demand feedings generally refer to an infant's being fed when crying commences, whereas cue-based feedings refer to an infant's being fed based on demonstrated hunger cues—that is, alert state, hand-to-mouth movement, and rooting reflex, which precede the onset of crying. Hunger cues for term infants are recognized as real. Some health professionals have suggested a cluster pattern of state or activity changes (orally directed behaviors, such as mouthing, sucking, and rooting as well as clinical indices, such as cough, yawn, or sneeze) that occurred before feeding for preterm infants at 32 to 33 weeks of gestation (Cagan, 1995). This study suggests that cue-based feeding would be feasible for young preterm infants.

Infants fed on demand generally require fewer gavage feedings and fewer feedings per day. They also tend to be discharged a few days earlier than other infants. Pridham and associates (1999) found that infants who were initially fed ad lib took smaller volumes and fewer calories but with experience fed nearly the same as those on a prescribed intake, thus suggesting that weight gain would be adequate over time. Although these data support the practice of establishing self-regulatory feeding protocols for clinically stable preterm infants and suggest potential advantages for infants, parents, nurses, and third-party payers, this study should be replicated with a larger sample of preterm infants.

Health professionals, although supportive of self-regulatory feedings in theory, have raised legitimate questions about how to institute such a policy in the NICU. One major unanswered question is whether preterm infants demonstrate the same early hunger cues as term infants and, if so, whether the busy NICU nurse will be able to identify those cues before the onset of crying. An additional concern evolves from the reality that each NICU nurse may be caring for three to four clinically stable preterm infants, all of whom may awake to feed at the same time. Clearly, self-regulatory feedings would be implemented most successfully in a NICU in which parents were present to recognize and respond to their infants's hunger cues.

BREASTFEEDING

Breast milk is the recommended source of nutrition for all infants, including premature and high-risk infants (American Academy of Pediatrics Policy Statement, 1996-1997). A series of recent research reports has indicated that preterm infants receive specific health benefits from human milk in comparison to commercial formula (Meier & Brown, 1996; Schanler, 2001). Despite these recommendations, mothers who deliver preterm or high-risk infants are less likely to initiate breastfeeding than mothers of fullterm infants (Griffin et al, 2000; Meier, 2001). It has been demonstrated that a combination of professional and peer support is an effective and powerful motivator for mothers to provide breast milk to their hospitalized infants (Meier, 2001). When given scientific information describing the importance of breast milk, most mothers will choose to temporarily provide milk for their infants even if they have no intention of nursing their infants later (Griffin et al, 2000; Meier, 2001).

Preterm infants are seldom allowed to breastfeed until bottlefeedings have been well established and an arbitrary weight criterion is achieved. However, delay in initial breastfeeding is associated with undesirable outcomes for mothers and preterm infants. The most important of these is breastfeeding failure, defined as the cessation of breastfeeding during the infant's hospitalization or in the early period after discharge, before the mother's intended weaning. The breastfeeding failure rate for mothers of preterm infants may exceed 50% of those mothers who try to breastfeed by the time infants are discharged from the hospital nursery.

Significance of Breastfeeding for Preterm Infants and Mothers

Successful breastfeeding has numerous advantages for preterm infants and their mothers. Breastfeeding provides infants with specific advantages with regard to general health, growth, and development. Breastfeeding has also been demonstrated to significantly decrease the risk for many acute and chronic illnesses in infants and young children (Schanler, 2001; American Academy of Pediatrics Policy Statement, 1996-1997). Breastfeeding is associated with lower rates of postneonatal morbidity than is formula feeding in the United States and with lower rates of postneonatal mortality and morbidity in developing countries. Also, preterm infants subjected to painful procedures and separation from their mothers after birth experience the pleasurable sensations and closeness of breastfeeding.

Physiologically, a series of research reports have demonstrated that breastfeeding is less stressful than bottlefeeding for preterm, term, and cardiac disordered infants (Dowling, 1999; Meier & Brown, 1996). This greater physiologic stability among breastfed infants may be a result of being able to control the flow of milk during breastfeeding so that breathing is not interrupted (Meier & Brown, 1996).

For mothers, breastfeeding may facilitate mother-infant attachment and provide a sense that they are contributing something to the care of their infant that no one else can. Mothers have stated that providing breast milk is their "only tangible claim" to their infants because the NICU staff provides all other caretaking (Kavanaugh et al, 1997). Providing milk for infant feeding helps mothers cope with the emotional stresses of the NICU experience by giving them control over an aspect of their infant's care, such as in early tolerance of enteral feeds where their milk "made the difference" (Meier, 2001).

Model for Providing Breastfeeding Support in the Neonatal Intensive Care Unit

In one study, investigators reported that 72% of mothers of high-risk infants who began milk expression were still breastfeeding at the time of the infant's discharge from the NICU (Meier & Mangurten, 1993). These investigators proposed a five-phase temporal model for supporting lactation in the NICU: (1) assisting the mother in the collection and storage of milk; (2) gavage feeding of expressed mother's milk; (3) managing in-hospital breastfeeding sessions; (4) breastfeeding support after discharge; and (5) consultation with the family or nursery personnel, or both. Investigators proposed two additional recommendations based on the data generated by this study. First, the amount of time required to provide breastfeeding interventions for mothers of infants in the NICU probably necessitates retaining a fulltime nurse to coordinate support if more than 100 mothers per year elect to breastfeed. Second, the nurse who coordinates such a program should have experience not only in lactation management but also in the clinical care of high-risk infants.

Assisting with Milk Collection and Storage

Within the proposed model of lactation support the nurse should contact each mother who expresses an interest in breastfeeding, and a suitable breast pump should be obtained before the mother's discharge from the hospital. Mothers should be encouraged to rent a hospital-grade, electric breast pump with a double collection kit so that both breasts may be emptied simultaneously. A double-pump collecting device results in a higher prolactin concentration and greater milk yield than does sequential pumping (Hill et al, 1996). The double collection pump is necessary after delivery and after discharge from the hospital (Meier, 2001). Mothers should be instructed to initiate milk expression as soon as possible after delivery and to express their milk 8 to 10 times in a 24-hour period, a schedule that corresponds to breastfeeding patterns of low-risk term infants. In the first 24 to 48 hours, mothers can anticipate obtaining drops of milk, and by 72 hours, most mothers produce measurable amounts of milk. While mothers are expressing drops of milk, they should pump 8 to 10 times per day for 10 to 15 minutes each session. Once milk flows, it is important for mothers to pump for 2 consecutive minutes after final droplets of milk are expressed. Although this process may take 20 to 30 minutes, it is of paramount importance because it ensures that the breasts are completely emptied. If emptying is incomplete, the milk will be low-fat and low-calorie, and overall milk volume will be diminished (Griffin et al, 2000; Meier, 2001). It has been recommended that mothers keep a written milk expression record that indicates the frequency and amount of

pumping; this is useful information for managing lactation problems (Meier, 2001).

Nonpharmacologic Support of Milk Volume

Milk supply may be enhanced when mothers pump at their infant's bedside where they can see and touch their infant (Griffin et al, 2000; Meier, 2001). These mothers can pump discreetly, if needed, with the use of screens or by positioning themselves toward the wall (Meier, 2001). Milk supply may be also be enhanced when mothers pump after Kangaroo Care (Meier, 2001). Infant suckling at an emptied breast may be initiated once the infant is extubated (Griffin et al, 2000; Meier, 2001). This nonnutritive sucking (NNS) provides breast stimulation that differs from the pump and can have beneficial effects (Meier, 2001). This type of NNS can be successful with nasal ventilation (Meier, 2001).

Management of In-Hospital Breastfeeding Sessions

Research since the 1980s has suggested that, contrary to popular opinion, breastfeeding may be less stressful than bottlefeeding for small preterm infants. In a study in which preterm infants served as their own controls for 32 bottlefeedings and 39 breastfeedings, the $tcPO_2$ declined during bottlefeedings but not during breastfeedings. Additionally, at young gestational ages, infants demonstrated different suck-breathe patterns during breastfeedings and bottlefeedings. During breastfeeding, infants breathed within sucking bursts. However, during bottlefeeding, bouts of breathing were alternated with sucking bursts, rather than being integrated into the sucking bursts (deMonterice, 1993). These different patterns of suck-swallow-breathe coordination for small preterm infants result in less ventilatory disruption during breastfeeding.

In a study by Meier and Mangurten (1993), preterm infants as small as 1200 g and as immature as 32 weeks' gestation were permitted to breastfeed. Most infants had not attempted bottlefeeding at the time of initial breastfeeding. During initial breastfeedings, these infants organized sucking into bursts of three to five sucks, with audible swallowing. These data support the results of previously published research that suggest that preterm infants can breastfeed earlier in the hospital stay than currently thought.

For clinical purposes, breastfeeding may be initiated for preterm infants as early as 32 weeks' gestation. Additionally, a preterm infant does not need to demonstrate the ability to feed by bottle prior to the initiation of breastfeeding. Other components of breastfeeding protocols should include (1) noninvasive monitoring of cardiorespiratory and oxygenation responses to feeding, as recommended previously for bottlefeeding; (2) test weighing with electronic scales to estimate volume of intake during breastfeeding; and (3) observation and recording characteristics of infant sucking and maternal milk flow. According to the model of lactation support described previously (Meier & Mangurten, 1993), the mean amount of time spent in assisting mothers with in-hospital breastfeeding sessions was 1 hour per feeding session. This phase of lactation support is extremely time-consuming and should be managed by a nurse who is knowledgeable about lactation and high-risk preterm infants.

The use of a nipple shield may be beneficial for the small preterm infant who is unable to successfully nurse at the breast (Griffin et al, 2000; Meier et al, 2000; Meier, 2001). Nipple shields may be used for preterm infants that experience difficulty latching on or sustaining a sucking response and may temporarily facilitate milk transfer and ease the work of feeding (Griffin et al, 2000; Meier et al, 2000; Meier, 2001).

Pharmacologic Support of Milk Volume

Mothers who express milk for their preterm infants frequently experience a diminishing milk supply within 6 weeks after birth (Hill et al, 1996; Hill et al, 1997). Decreasing milk volume must be detected and treated early to preserve lactation. Metoclopromide (Reglan) has been used on a short-term basis (12 to 14 days) with this population to stimulate prolactin production and increase milk yield. The use of metoclopramide therapy may be most effective if initiated within 3 days after a mother reports a decrease in milk volume that does not improve with nonpharmacologic intervention (Meier, 2001).

Breastfeeding Consultation After Discharge

Anecdotal responses of mothers who participated in the model of lactation support study suggest that a different set of concerns originates during the period after discharge with respect to breastfeeding a preterm infant. One report indicates that paramount among these concerns is the mother's fear that the infant will not consume enough milk during breastfeeding (Kavanaugh et al, 1995). This concern is not the same as the concern of mothers of fullterm infants that their milk supply is inadequate; mothers of these preterm infants were able to observe the adequacy of their milk supply with milk expression for complementary or supplemental feedings. Their concern, instead, was related to the adequacy of milk transfer, which involves the synchrony of maternal milk ejection and infant sucking. Mothers managed this concern with the use of complementary or supplemental bottles until they felt infant intake was adequate, approximately 2 weeks after discharge. Another appropriate method for mothers breastfeeding preterm infants in the early period after discharge is test weighing, using a scale designed for this purpose (Meier et al, 1994). The BabyWeigh (Medela, Inc., McHenry, Illinois) was found to give an accurate estimate of intake when used by mothers and investigators, whereas evaluation of infant cues, such as infant latching onto the breast and infant sucking, were not accurate for estimating the volume of intake.

Previously, most consumer-oriented information has focused on generalizing recommendations for term, healthy infants to smaller, less stable preterm infants. For example, mothers of preterm infants were frequently told just to "trust" lactation and to feed their infants on demand or to wake their infants frequently (i.e., every 1 to 2 hours) so that they can feed small volumes from the breast. These recommendations are not research-based and can be potentially dangerous for preterm infants.

Until the knowledge base has been developed in this area, neonatal nurses need to use in-hospital breastfeeding information to help mothers prepare for discharge. For example, an evaluation of serial test weighings during breastfeedings will provide the nurse with information about an individual infant's pattern of milk intake, and interventions can be planned to meet the breastfeeding needs of a particular mother-infant pair. An additional helpful intervention is to prepare the mother for the types of advice that she is likely to receive from family members, friends, and even primary care providers. This intervention will help the mother identify information that is erroneous so that she will know to question it and to contact the nurse concerning appropriate management strategies.

As a component of the lactation model, the nurse coordinator should telephone the mother within 48 hours after infant discharge and again 48 hours after the first telephone call. Mothers should be encouraged to telephone the nurse following the visit to the pediatrician at 1 week after discharge to share information and recommendations from the pediatrician. Even though mothers have access to the nurse coordinator in the period after discharge, they often hesitate to call, thinking that the call will be a disturbance. Thus when the nurse initiates the call, the mother is likely to have at least one major question concerning breastfeeding management strategies.

ORAL FEEDINGS

Oral feeding is considered the most highly organized behavior of the young infant (Conway, 1994). Successful oral feeding requires the interaction of intact cranial nerves, adequate sucking and swallowing reflexes, functional interaction of the lips, jaw, tongue, palate, pharynx, larynx, and esophagus, and integration of the autonomic and central nervous systems (Conway, 1994; White-Traut et al, 2002). Associated problems of prematurity include difficulty organizing behavioral state and coordinating feeding. Preterm infants during nipple feeding often develop physiologic instability that is manifested by apnea, bradycardia, and decreased oxygen saturation (desaturation). These physiologic and biochemical changes are due to a variety of reasons, such as inadequate sucking-swallowing-and breathing coordination, poor autonomic control, inadequate neurobehavioral organization, and inadequate central nervous system (CNS) integration (White-Traut et al, 2002). The preterm infant faces many challenges that are likely to jeopardize or delay the development of healthy, normal feeding patterns. These include medical factors that interfere with normal infant development; environmental factors such as intense visual, auditory, and tactile stimuli that interfere with the ability to organize behavioral state and coordinate efficient feeding; and care giving factors such as inconsistent caregivers (Pinnington et al, 2000). Regulation of respiration and heart rate develops just before the initiation of oral feeding. This regulation must occur for successful oral feeding, otherwise transition to complete oral feeding will be delayed (Mandich et al, 1996).

Feeding ability is influenced by many factors, including gestational age; postconceptional age; current behavioral state; physiologic status; neurologic status; neurobehavioral organization; health status; muscle strength; and the coordination of sucking, swallowing, and breathing (Conway, 1994; White-Traut et al, 1994).

The sucking reflex is an essential component of feeding (Conway, 1994) and develops during early fetal development. Sucking later integrates with breathe-suck-swallow (BSS) to develop a functional feeding pattern. Initially, sucking bursts are short in duration and become longer in duration as the premature infant matures. Sucking precedes swallowing and also inhibits respiration (Gyrboski, 1969). The sucking reflex is one of the earliest integrated behaviors observed in the human fetus and begins as early as 18 weeks of gestation (Conway, 1994). Swallowing is noted in fetuses by 10 to 14 weeks' gestation (Conway, 1994). Despite the early appearance of these reflexes, they are not well developed until 32 to 34 weeks of gestation. Nonnutritive sucking patterns, number of sucks, and the time required per sucking burst in healthy preterm infants show changes as gestational age increases and oral feeding progresses (Medoff-Cooper, 1991; Medoff-Cooper et al, 1993,

Medoff-Cooper et al, 2000). Oral feeding may require a large amount of effort for the premature infant and reduce the infant's strength and endurance for full feedings. By 34 weeks, endurance during oral feeding is developing, and the infant may tolerate full oral feeding (Gron-Wargo et al, 1994).

A preterm infant's feeding ability and weight gain are the major parameters used to decide the infant's readiness for discharge from the special care nursery (Conway, 1994). Feeding difficulties put the preterm infant at higher risk for failure to thrive and long-term hospitalization (Conway, 1994). When infants are hospitalized longer, their families run physical, psychological, and financial risks, and the nation spends more on health care. Adequate assessments of the infant's ability to tolerate nipplefeeding and appropriate interventions to promote safe and effective feeding will help the infant's progress successfully. Once the infant's health status has been stabilized and the infant has reached a certain age and weight, introduction of oral feeding becomes the next step toward full recovery and discharge.

Current clinical practice during the initiation of oral feeding involves placing the infant on a structured feeding schedule and wakening the infant during vital signs and diaper change before feeding. Feeding often follows this nursing care, and the infant may not be alert at the initiation of feeding. If the infant appears to be having difficulty coordinating breathing, sucking, and swallowing or if the infant becomes fatigued, the nurse will discontinue the feeding and insert an oral-gastric tube to complete the feeding. The preferred mode of feeding of term infants may be the synchronized coordination of sucking, swallowing, and breathing to produce a ratio of 1:1:1. For preterm infants, periods of apnea during vigorous feeding have been documented with periods of rapid breathing unaccompanied by sucks. Often the nipple is blocked with the tongue, suggesting that lack of feeding coordination in preterm infants is caused more by neuromuscular immaturity than by lack of experience.

Several researchers studied physiologic stability of preterm infants during feeding. Most recently Dowling (1999) looked at physiologic stability. Several changes in physiologic stability during nipplefeeding have been reported over the years. These changes include decreased oxygenation as measured by transcutaneous oxygen tension ($tcPO_2$), oxygen saturation (SaO_2) (Dowling, 1999; Hill, 1992), changes in respiratory patterns (Dowling, 1999; Hill, 1992), and changes in heart rate (Hill, 1992). However, these studies did not address interventions to facilitate physiologic stability during nipplefeeding preterm infants.

Traditionally, nurses have not identified bottlefeeding as an intervention that requires professional attention. Consequently, convalescing preterm infants have been referred to as "feeders" or "growers," suggesting that staff other than professional nurses can provide their care. Given the documented frequency of hypoxemia during bottlefeeding, nurses should refocus professional care on the assessment and management of feeding-related hypoxemia as well as behavioral indicators.

The assessment of hypoxemia should include routine noninvasive monitoring of small preterm infants as bottlefeedings are initiated. Numerous studies have emphasized that clinical indices alone are inadequate in the identification of hypoxemia. For initial bottlefeedings, a preterm infant should be fed while attached to a cardiorespiratory monitor and either an oximeter or a $tcPO_2$ monitor, preferably with a trend recorder to document the oxygenation pattern throughout the feeding.

Parameters on the oxygenation tracing that should be evaluated include: (1) percentage of decline from baseline during sucking, (2) extent of recovery of oxygenation during rest periods and in the period after feeding, and (3) which phases of the tracing, if any, were accompanied by tachycardia, bradycardia, or apnea. Noninvasive monitoring of oxygenation can be discontinued for an individual infant based on the nurse's decision that the infant does not demonstrate significant hypoxemia.

A second intervention is to select the appropriate nipple for the infant. In a simulated study of sucking, a variety of nipple units routinely recommended for term and preterm infants were compared. Results of this study revealed marked variation in rates of flow for different nipple units; variations were noted not only for different types of nipples but also for different nipple units of the same type. In particular, the Nuk-type nipple, often recommended for use with breastfed infants, was characterized by higher flow than comparable standard nipple units. The investigator raised the consideration that feeding-related apnea and bradycardia in preterm infants might be related, in part to nipple units that permit high flow.

Milk that flows rapidly from the nipple necessitates more frequent swallowing on the part of the infant. Because swallowing interrupts respiration, more frequent swallowing might compromise ventilatory function for the preterm infant. However, Dowling (1999) reported that selected preterm infants were able to maintain regular breathing patterns, and consequently oxygenation, during bottlefeeding with Nuk-type nipples. Therefore, each infant should be evaluated individually to determine the infant's ability to regulate milk flow from a particular nipple unit.

Infants should first be fed with a low flow nipple and then progressed to higher flow if well tolerated. Milk flow is considered to be ideal if the infant tolerates it without excessive drooling and choking (Mathew et al, 1992). Hill & Rath (1999) found that drooling was correlated with the infant's postnatal age, physiological status and sucking abilities. Drooling decreased with postnatal age but was associated with gestational age or post conceptional age suggesting that experience may be an additional factor in drooling and feeding competence. Oral support has been suggested as an intervention to improve oral feeding competence (Einarsson-Backes et al, 1994; Hill et al, 2000).

A third nursing intervention, related to controlling the rate of milk flow, is to allow the infant to set the pace of the feeding (Jordon, 1998). Preterm infants tend to suck at a slower rate than term infants and therefore consume less volume per suck. Preterm infants may require more time to complete a feeding than do term infants and that the ability to pace the bottlefeeding may be a protective mechanism, allowing the infant to expend less energy while feeding.

A related intervention is the avoidance of force-feeding for preterm infants. In the non-research literature, a frequent recommendation for feeding preterm infants is to stimulate the infant in order to complete a bottlefeeding. Consequently, in the clinical setting it is not unusual to see nurses manipulating infants' faces, mouths, and the bottle, forcing an already fatigued infant to complete the remainder of a feeding. One research report described apnea, documented on a polygraph tracing, associated with nurse-induced sucks (Dowling, 1999). Thus stimulating an infant to suck has the potential for interfering with the infant's self-regulation of sucking and breathing, which, especially for a fatigued infant, may precipitate hypoxemia.

The preceding is an example of a situation in which non-invasive monitoring would alert the nurse to an infant who is hypoxemic and fatigued and who should be allowed to rest while the remainder of a feeding is infused by gavage. In one study in which tcPO$_2$ was compared during bottlefeedings and breastfeedings for preterm infants, the investigator noted that clinical indices of fatigue during bottlefeeding were manifested when tcPO$_2$ values were between 40 and 50 mm Hg, a finding that is clearly suggestive of hypoxemia.

A difficult or immature feeder may display more incoordination of sucking, swallowing and breathing requiring more intensive intervention and attention. These infants are often easily overstimulated, and tired with nipple-feeding. Careful attention to their individualized needs is required for these infants to become successful with nipple-feeding.

Lastly, infant-caregiver interaction, co-regulation and caregiver commitment to feeding must be considered. Feeding success for the infant is largely dependent on the care-providers attention to the individualized needs of the infant. The infant and care provider must have reciprocity for successful nipple-feeding to occur (Wood, 1991). This reciprocity may be difficult to achieve if there is no consistency in care provider thus consistency of care is an issue of concern when promoting feeding success. Documentation of feeding readiness cues, and stress behaviors during the feeding as well as interventions used to support the infant can promote feeding success when multiple care providers feed the preterm infant.

Research Evaluating Feeding Interventions

Successful oral feeding is a major determinant of readiness for discharge to home and therefore, it is essential to identify effective interventions for infants experiencing inefficient feeding or difficulty organizing behavioral state. Difficulty with feeding increases length of hospital stay thus adding to the high cost of health care. Nursing care should include the assessment of prefeeding behaviors and behavioral states prior to and during feeding, minimize the length of oral feeding episodes, provide prefeeding stimulation and/or oral support, and consider age, maturation and behavioral ability (Daley & Kennedy, 2000; White-Traut et al, 2002).

In light of the importance of feeding interventions for at risk infants, it is unfortunate that few research studies have been conducted identifying effective interventions that facilitate physiologic stability during nipplefeeding. Two studies suggest that a reduced flow feeding apparatus (or nipple) is most optimal for the preterm infant (Lau & Schanler, 2000; Mathew et al, 1992). NNS sucking immediately prior to bottlefeeding was shown in one study to improve oxygen saturation (Pickler et al, 1996). NNS during gavage feeding may also improve GI motility and improve patterns of weight gain.

Nurses are responsible for feeding hospitalized preterm infants, and, to date, little research provides nurses with clinical protocols for assessing and organizing behavior before feeding. Kinneer & Beachy (1994) identified common behavioral indicators of hunger cues. These included vigorous sucking, rooting, and crying. Cagan (1995) identified prefeeding behaviors in the premature infant, which include hand to mouth, hand swipes at mouth, sucking on hand, sucking on tongue, and empty sucking. Equally important is the presence of alert behavioral states immediately before and during feeding (Holditch-Davis et al, 2000, McCain, 1997; White-Traut et al, 2002).

Several researchers (Conway, 1994; Gaebler & Hanzlik, 1996; Hill, 1992; McCain, 1997; Pickler et al, 1996; White-Traut et al, 1997, 2002) conducted studies on interventions to facilitate feeding preterm infants. These interventions include sensory stimulation modalities such as visual, auditory, kinesthetic, tactile stimulation; NNS; and perioral and intraoral simulation (Pinelli & Symington, 2001). Sensory stimuli are administered both individually (unimodal) and in various combinations (multimodal) (White-Traut et al, 1997). These interventions were found to be beneficial for preterm infants in terms of growth, motor activity, neurobehavioral function, autonomic stability, oral feeding, parent-infant interaction, and decreased hospital stay (Mueller, 1996; Pinelli & Symingon, 2001). Despite these studies, data are inconclusive on optimal type, patterning, sequencing, and timing of stimulation (Mueller, 1996).

Pickler et al (1996) studied the effects of NNS on behavioral organization and feeding performance in preterm infants. This study found that NNS had a positive effect on behavioral state. When infants received NNS, they were more likely to be alert and more organized to start bottlefeeding. This result was consistent with the findings of McCain (1992), which indicated that the optimal state before feeding included awake and quiet behaviors. Anderson et al (1990) showed that preterm infants who were given a self-regulatory feeding protocol exhibited regular quiet sleep between feeding and improved weight gain.

Gaebler & Hanzlik (1996) studied the effects of stroking and a perioral and intraoral prefeeding stimulation program on healthy, growing, preterm infants. These stimulation techniques enhanced the infants' oral motor skills and provided pleasurable perioral and intraoral experiences that facilitated the maintenance of normal sensory interpretation for preterm infants.

Research by White-Traut and colleagues (1997) examined the immediate response of homogeneous groups of preterm infants to two forms of unimodal sensory stimulation and two forms of multimodal stimulation. Their findings suggest that vestibular stimulation may be used together with auditory, tactile, and visual stimulation to help preterm infants organize behavior, especially before feeding. Subsequent research by White-Traut and colleagues demonstrated that a multisensory (auditory, tactile, visual, and vestibular [ATVV]) intervention administered just before feeding facilitated alert behavior, increased the frequency of prefeeding behaviors, and improved feeding efficiency of preterm infants (White-Traut et al, 2002). Their findings support the use of ATVV intervention before feeding as a means of enhancing alert behavioral states and increasing the frequency of prefeeding behaviors to improve feeding efficiency.

Nursing Interventions

Traditionally, nurses have not identified bottlefeeding as an intervention that requires professional attention. Consequently, convalescing preterm infants have been referred to as "feeders" or "growers," suggesting that staff other than professional nurses can provide their care. Given the documented frequency of hypoxemia during bottlefeeding, nurses should refocus professional care on the assessment and management of feeding-related hypoxemia.

The assessment of hypoxemia, the first intervention, should include routine noninvasive monitoring of small preterm infants as bottlefeedings are initiated. Numerous studies have emphasized that clinical indices alone are inadequate in the identification of hypoxemia. For initial bottlefeedings, a preterm infant should be fed while attached to a cardiorespiratory monitor and either an oximeter or a tcPO$_2$ monitor, preferably with a trend recorder to document the oxygenation pattern throughout the feeding. Parameters on the oxygenation tracing that should be evaluated include (1) percentage of decline from baseline during sucking; (2) extent of recovery of oxygenation during rest periods and in the period after feeding; and (3) which phases of the tracing, if any, were accompanied by tachycardia, bradycardia, or apnea. Noninvasive monitoring of oxygenation can be discontinued for an individual infant based on the nurse's decision that the infant does not demonstrate significant hypoxemia.

A second intervention is to select the appropriate nipple for the infant. In a simulated study of sucking, a variety of nipple units routinely recommended for term and preterm infants were compared. Variations have been noted not only for different types of nipples but also for different nipple units of the same type. In particular, the Nuk-type nipple, often recommended for use with breastfed infants, was characterized by higher flow than comparable standard nipple units. The investigator raised the consideration that feeding-related apnea and bradycardia in preterm infants might be related, in part, to nipple units that permit high flow.

Milk that flows rapidly from the nipple necessitates more frequent swallowing on the part of the infant. Because swallowing interrupts respiration, more frequent swallowing might compromise ventilatory function for the preterm infant. However, Dowling (1995) reported that selected preterm infants were able to maintain regular breathing patterns—and consequently oxygenation—during bottlefeeding with Nuk-type nipples. Therefore each infant should be evaluated individually to determine his or her ability to regulate milk flow from a particular nipple unit. Infants should be offered a low flow nipple first and progressed to a higher flow nipple when they have demonstrated tolerance. Use of high flow nipples during the transition to nipplefeeding should be avoided, as this is a time the infant is acquiring new skills and it is difficult to evaluate suck swallow coordination when flow is also an issue.

A third nursing intervention, related to controlling the rate of milk flow is to allow the infant to set the pace of the feeding (Jordon, 1998). As stated earlier in the chapter, preterm infants generally generate lower sucking pressures and expend less energy than term infants to obtain the same total volume of milk. Additionally, preterm infants suck at a slower rate than term infants and consume less volume per suck. Preterm infants may require more time to complete a feeding than do term infants, and the ability to pace the bottlefeeding may be a protective mechanism that allows the infant to expend less energy while feeding.

A related intervention is the avoidance of force-feeding for preterm infants. As noted above, force-feeding is not recommended by research findings yet is an acceptable practice in most NICUs. It is not unusual for nurses to stimulate the preterm infant to complete a bottlefeeding. Nurses manipulate infants' faces, mouths, and the bottle, forcing an already fatigued infant to complete the remainder of a feeding. One research report described apnea, documented on a polygraph tracing, associated with nurse-induced sucks (Dowling, 1995). Thus stimulating an infant to suck has the potential for interfering with the infant's self-regulation of sucking and breathing, which, especially for a fatigued infant, may precipitate hypoxemia.

The preceding is an example of a situation in which noninvasive monitoring would alert the nurse to an infant who is hypoxemic and fatigued and who should be allowed to rest while the remainder of a feeding is infused by gavage. Clinical indices of fatigue during bottlefeeding are manifested when tcPO$_2$ values were between 40 and 50 mm Hg, a finding that is clearly suggestive of hypoxemia.

Lastly, taste cannot be ignored. Knowledge of flavor perception in human infants has expanded substantially over the past few decades (Mennella, 1993). The sense of taste is well developed in the preterm infant. In fact the preterm infant's sense of taste may be stronger than an adult's. Mature taste cells begin appearing at about 14 weeks' gestation. The ability to detect sweet tastes is present by about 32 weeks' gestation, and infants prefer sweet over sour; however no evidence suggests that providing sweet or sour solutions at an early age will influence the child's preference at a later time. Little research has been done on this matter. Studies with breast milk have shown that different flavors of milk within different cultures are probably related to maternal diet and that these different flavors might lead to preferences in later life, but the research is inconclusive at this time. Given that we have much to learn in this area, it would be better to err on the side of caution and refrain from mixing flavors or providing noxious tastes with routine feedings such as mixing vitamins or medications with the feeding.

Gastroesophageal Reflux (GER) and Feeding Intolerance

Gastroesophageal reflux (GER) is abnormal frequent passage of gastric contents into the esophagus. Reflux is experienced by most preterm infants and may detract from feeding success as well as delay growth and development. Nursing interventions that can facilitate infants who have reflux include elevating the head of the bed at least 30 degrees, positioning the infant in prone or sidelying, and providing frequent feedings of small volumes to decreases gastric distension. Many care providers choose to thickened feedings with cereal; however, this practice must be done with consistency to be successful. The research that suggests thickening of feedings found that prethickened infant formulas (by the manufacturer) worked best. However, since these are seldom available, a consistent approach that guarantees uniformity is required (Vanderplas et al, 1998). Do not add cereal to formula until just before feeding; cereal left in formula for extended periods becomes very thick and chunky in nature, thus diminishing the infant's ability to extract it from the nipple. Cross-cut nipples or large single hole nipples are suggested. Nipples that are cut by nursing staff at each feeding are inappropriate because the inconsistent size of the cut detracts from the infant's ability to regulate his or her own feeding. Sometimes the flow is too fast (large cuts in nipples increases chances for reflux) and sometimes is too slow (small cuts in nipple hole tire the infant quickly).

Pharmacologic interventions should be reserved for times when all other interventions have failed and should be monitored closely; they are not without their own issues and concerns.

SUMMARY

This chapter has reviewed the principles of digestion, absorption, and metabolic processes. It included developmental and physiologic considerations of the premature or sick neonate. Practical issues were addressed regarding neonatal nutrition.

REFERENCES

American Academy of Pediatrics (1996-1997). Work group on breast-feeding: breastfeeding and the use of human milk. *Pediatrics,* 100(6), December, 1035-1039.

American Academy of Pediatrics (1998). Nutritional needs of preterm infants. *Pediatric nutrition handbook,* ed 4, Elk Grove Village, IL: Author.

Anderson G et al (1990). Self-regulatory gavage-to-bottlefeeding for preterm infants: effects on behavioral state, energy expenditure, and weight gain. In Funk SG et al (Eds.), *Key aspects of recovery: improving nutrition, rest, and mobility,* New York: Springer.

Baker JH, Berseth CL (1997). Duodenal motor responses in preterm infants fed formula with varying concentrations and rates of infusion. *Pediatric research,* 42(5), 618-622.

Baranowski L (1993). Central venous access devices—current technologies, uses, and management strategies. *Journal of intravenous nursing,* 16, 167-194.

Berdanier C (2000). *Advanced nutrition: macronutrients.* Boca Raton, Florida: CRC Press.

Berseth CL (1992). Effect of early feeding on maturation of the preterm infant's small intestine. *Journal of pediatrics,* June, 947-953.

Berseth CL (1995). Minimal enteral feedings. *Clinics in perinatology,* 22(1) March, 195-204.

Berseth CL (1996). Gastrointestinal motility in the neonate. *Clinics in perinatology,* 23(2), 179-190.

Berseth CL (1999). Assessment in intestinal motility as a guide in feeding management of the newborn. *Clinics in perinatology,* 26(4), 1007-1015.

Billeaud C et al (1992). Energy expenditure and severity of respiratory disease in very-low-birth-weight infants receiving long-term ventilatory support. *Journal of pediatrics,* 120(3), 461-464.

Brown JM (1995). Polyurethane and silicone: Myths and misconceptions. *Journal of intravenous nursing,* 18, 120-122.

Buchheit JQ, Stewart DL (1994). Clinical comparison of localized intestinal perforation and necrotizing enterocolitis in neonates. *Pediatrics,* 93(1), 32-36.

Byers P, Jeejeebhoy K (1997). *Enteral and parenteral nutrition: critical care,* Philadelphia: Lippincott-Raven.

Byren T et al (1995). A new treatment for patients with short bowel syndrome: growth hormone, glutamine and the preservation of gut integrity. *Annals of surgery,* 222:243-255.

Cagan J (1995). Feeding readiness behavior in preterm infants. *Neonatal network,* 14(2), 82.

Conway A (1994). Instruments in neonatal research: measuring preterm infant feeding ability, part I: bottlefeeding. *Neonatal network,* 13(4), 71-73.

Daley HK, Kennedy CM (2000). Meta analysis: Effects of interventions on premature infants feeding. *The journal of perinatal and neonatal nursing,* 14, 62-77.

deMonterice D (1993). *Differences in Coordination of Sucking and Breathing During Breast and Bottlefeeding.* Paper presented at the Perinatal Nursing Research Forum, January 1993, Santa Fe, NM: Mead Johnson Nutritionals.

Dollberg S et al (2000). Feeding tolerance in preterm infants: randomized trial of bolus and continuous feeding. *Journal of the American college of nutrition,* 19(6), 797-800.

Dowling D (1995). *Responses of preterm infants to enteral feeding.* Unpublished doctoral dissertation. Chicago: University of Illinois.

Dowling D (1999). Physiological responses of preterm infants to breastfeeding and bottlefeeding with the orthodontic nipple. *Nursing research,* 48(2), 78-85.

Einarsson-Backes LM et al (1994). The effect of oral support on sucking efficiency in preterm infants. *The American journal of occupational therapy,* 48(6), 490-498.

Fioravanti J et al (1998). Pericardial effusion and tamponade as a result of percutaneous silastic catheter use. *Neonatal network* 17, 39-42.

Fletcher M (1998). *Physical diagnosis in neonatology,* Philadelphia: Lippincott-Raven.

Gaebler C, Hanzlik R (1996). The effects of a prefeeding stimulation program on preterm infants. *The American journal of occupational therapy,* 50(3), 184-192.

Gallagher KJ et al (1993). Orogastric tube insertion length in very-low-birth-weight infants. *Journal of Perinataology,* 13(2), 128-131.

Gershwin M et al (2000). *Nutrition and Immunology.* Totowa, NJ: Humana Press.

Gonzales I et al (1995). Effect of enteral feeding temperature on feeding tolerance in preterm infants. *Neonatal network,* 14(3), 39-43.

Griffin TL et al (2000). Mothers' performing creamatocrit measures in the NICU: accuracy, reactions, cost. *Journal of obstetric, gynecologic, and neonatal nursing,* 29(3), 249-257.

Gron-Wargo S et al (1994). *Nutritional care for high-risk newborns.* Chicago: Precept Press, Inc.

Gryboski JD (1969). Suck and swallow to the premature infant. *Pediatrics,* 43(1), 96-102.

Hay W (1994). *Neonatal nutrition and metabolism,* Volume 2. Denver: University of Colorado Health and Sciences Center, Ross Pediatrics.

Heird WC, Wu C (1996). *Nutrition growth and body composition.* Houston: USDA/ARS Children's Nutrition Research Center, Department of Pediatrics, Baylor College of Medicine.

Heird W, Gomez M (1996). Parental nutrition in low-birth-weight infants. *Annual reviews of nutrition,* 16, Houston: Baylor College of Medicine.

Herin P, Zetterstrom R (1994). Sodium, potassium, and chloride needs in low-birth-weight infants. *Acta paediatric supplement,* 405, 43-48.

Hill A (1992). Preliminary findings: a maximum oral feeding time for premature infants, the relationship to physiological indicators. *Maternal-child nursing journal,* 20(2), 81-91.

Hill AS et al (2000). Oral support measures used in feeding the preterm infant. *Nursing research,* 49(1), 2-10.

Hill AS, Rath LS (1999). The relationship between drooling, age, sucking pattern characteristics, and physiological parameters of preterm infants during bottlefeeding. *Research and nursing practice.* www.graduateresearch.com.

Hill PD et al (1996). The effect of sequential and simultaneous breast pumping on milk volume and prolactin levels: a pilot study. *Journal of human lactation,* 12(3), 193-199.

Hill PD et al (1997). Breastfeeding patterns of low-birth-weight infants after hospital discharge. *Journal of obstetrics, gynecology and neonatal nursing,* 26(2), 189-197.

Holditch-Davis D et al (2000). Feeding and nonfeeding interactions of mothers and prematures. *Western journal of nursing research,* 22, 320-334.

Intravenous Nursing Society (1997). Position paper: peripheral inserted central catheters. *Journal of intravenous nursing,* 20(4), 172-174.

Intravenous Nurses Society (2000). Infusion nursing standards of practice. *Journal of intravenous nursing,* 23(Suppl. 6), S1-S88.

Jordon S (1998). The controlled or paced bottlefeeding. *Mother baby journal,* 3(2), 21-24.

Katz D (2001). *Nutrition in clinical practice.* Philadelphia. Lippincott Williams and Wilkins.

Kavanaugh K et al (1995). Getting enough: mothers' concerns about breastfeeding a preterm infant after discharge. *Journal of obstetric, gynecologic, and neonatal nursing,* 24(1), 23-32.

Kavanaugh K et al (1997). The rewards outweigh the efforts: breastfeeding outcomes for mothers of preterm infants. *Journal of human lactation,* 13(1), 15-21.

Kelly EJ, Newell SJ (1994). Gastric ontogeny: clinical applications. *Archives of diseases in childhood,* 71(2), F136-F141.

Kinnear MD, Beachy P (1994). Nipple feeding premature infants in the neonatal intensive-care unit: factors and decisions. *Journal of obstetric, gynecologic, and neonatal nursing,* 23, 105-112.

Klein JF, Shahrivar F (1992). Use of percutaneous silastic central venous catheters in neonates and the management of infectious complications. *American journal of perinatology,* 9, 261-264.

Kliethermes PA et al (1999). Transitioning preterm infants with nasogastric tube supplementation: increasing likelihood of breastfeeding. *Journal of obstetric, gynecologic, and neonatal nursing*, 28(3), 264-273.

Koenig WJ et al (1995). Manometrics for preterm and term infants: a new tool for old questions. *Pediatrics*, 95(2), 203-206.

Kuschel CA, Harding JE (2001). Protein supplementation of human milk for promoting growth in preterm infants. http://www.nichd.nih.gov/cochrane/cochrane.htm#N

Lau C, Schanler RJ (2000). Oral feeding in premature infants: advantage of a self-paced milk flow. *Acta paediatrica*, 89, 453-459.

Lebenthal E (1995). Gastrointestinal maturation and motility patterns as indicators for feeding the premature infant. *Pediatrics*, 95(2), 207-209.

Lorenz J et al (1997). Potassium metabolism in extremely-low-birth-weight infants in the first week of life. *Journal of pediatrics*, 131, 81-86.

Maki DG (1994). Yes, Virginia, aseptic technique is very important: maximal barrier precautions during insertion reduce the risk of central venous catheter-related bacteremia. *Infection control and hospital epidemiology* 15, 227-230.

Mandich M et al (1996). Transition time to oral feeding in premature infants with and without apnea. *Journal of obstetric, gynecologic, and neonatal nursing*, 25, 771-776.

Mathew OP et al (1992). Sucking patterns of neonates during bottle-feeding: comparison of different nipple units. *American journal of perinatology*, 9, 265-269.

McCain G (1992). Facilitating inactive awake states in preterm infants: a study of three interventions. *Nursing research*, 41(3), 157-160.

McCain GC (1997). Behavioral state activity during nipplefeedings for preterm infants. *Neonatal network*, 16(5), 43-47.

Medoff-Cooper B (1991). Changes in nutritive sucking patterns with increasing gestational age. *Nursing research*, 40, 245-247.

Medoff-Cooper B (2000). Nutritive sucking and neurobehavioral development in preterm infants from 34 weeks PCA to term. *MCN: The journal of maternal child nursing*, 25(2), 64-70.

Medoff-Cooper B et al (1993). The development of sucking patterns and physiologic correlates in very-low-birth-weight infants. *Nursing research*, 42(2), 100-105.

Medoff-Cooper B, Ray W (1995). Neonatal sucking behaviors. *Image: journal of nursing scholarship*, 27(3), 195-200.

Meetze WH et al (1992). Gastrointestinal priming prior to full enteral nutrition in very-low-birth-weight infants. *Journal of pediatric gastroenterology and nutrition*, 15(2), 163-170.

Meier PP et al (1994). A new scale for in-home test-weighing for mothers of preterm and high risk infants. *Journal of human lactation*, 10(3), 163-168.

Meier PP (2001). Breastfeeding in the special care nursery: crematures and infants with medical problems. *Pediatric clinics of North America*, 48(2), 425-442.

Meier PP et al (2000). Nipple shields for preterm infants: effects on milk transfer and duration of breastfeeding. *Journal of human lactation*, 16(2), 106-114.

Meier P, Brown LP (1996). State of the science: breastfeeding for mothers and low-birth-weight infants. *Nursing clinics of North America*, 31(2), 351-365.

Meier PP, Mangurten HH (1993). Breastfeeding the preterm infant. In J Riordan, K Auerbach (Eds.), *Breastfeeding and human lactation*, Boston: Jones, Bartlett.

Mendoza M et al (1993). Cysteine supplementation increases whole blood glutathione concentration in parenterally fed preterm infants. *Pediatric resuscitation*, 33, 307A.

Mennella JA (1993). Early flavor experiences: when do they start? *Zero to three*, 14(20), 1-7.

Mizuno K, Aizawa M (1999). Effects of body position on blood gases and lung mechanics of infants with chronic lung disease during tube feeding. *Pediatrics international*, 41, 609-614.

Mueller C (1996). Multidisciplinary research of multimodal stimulation of premature infants: an integrated review of literature. *Maternal child nursing journal*, 24(1), 18-31.

National Association of Vascular Access Networks (NAVAN) (1998). Tip location of peripherally inserted central catheters: NAVAN position statement. *Journal of vascular access devices*, 3, 8-10.

Neu J et al (1997). Enteral glutamine supplementation for very-low-birth-weight infants decreases morbidity. *Journal of pediatrics*, 131(5), 691-698.

Neubauer AP (1995). Percutaneous central IV access in the neonate: experience with 535 silastic catheters. *Acta paediatrica*, 84, 756-760.

Newell SJ (1996). Gastrointestinal function and ontogeny: how should we feed the preterm infant? *Seminar in neonatology*, 1, 59-66.

Newell SJ (2000). Enteral feeding of the micropremie. *Clinics in perinatology*, 27(1), 221-233.

Ochikubo CG (1996). Silicone-rubber catheter fracture and embolization in a very-low-birth-weight infant. *Journal of perinatology*, 16, 50-52.

Pereira GR (1995). Nutritional care of the extremely premature infant [Review]. *Clinics in perinatology*, 22(1), 61-75.

Pettit JD, Hughes K (1993). Intravenous extravasation: mechanisms, management, and prevention. *Journal of perinatal and neonatal nursing*, 6(4), 74-85.

Pettit J, Mason Wyckoff M (2001). *Peripherally inserted central catheters: guideline for practice*. Glenview, IL: National Association of Neonatal Nurses.

Pickler RH et al (1996). Effects of nonnutritive sucking on behavioral organization and feeding performance in preterm infants. *Nursing research*, 45(3), 132-135.

Pickler RH et al (1997). Bottle-feeding histories of preterm infants. *Journal of obstetric, gynecologic, and neonatal nursing*, 26(4), 414-420.

Pinelli J, Symington A (2001). Nonnutritive sucking for promoting physiologic stability and nutrition in preterm infants. *The Cochrane library*, Issue 4.

Pinnington LL et al (2000). Feeding efficiency and respiratory integration in infants with acute viral bronchiolitis. *The journal of pediatrics*, 137, 523-526.

Premji S, Chessell L (2001). Continuous nasogastric milk feeding versus intermittent bolus milk feeding for premature infants less than 1500 grams. *The Cochrane library*, Issue 4.

Pridham K et al (1998). Transition time to full nipplefeeding for premature infants with a history of lung disease. *Journal of obstetric, gynecologic, and neonatal nursing*, 27, 533-545.

Pridham K et al (1999). The effects of prescribed versus ad libitum feedings and formula caloric density on premature infant dietary intake and weight gain. *Nursing research*, 48(2), 86-93.

Raad II et al (1994). Prevention of central venous catheter-related infections by using maximal sterile barrier precautions during insertion. *Infection control and hospital epidemiology*, 15, 231-238.

Sato K et al (1995). Internal potassium shift in premature infants: cause of nonoliguric hyperkalemia. *Journal of pediatrics*, 126, 109-113.

Schanler RJ (2001). The use of human milk for premature infants. *Pediatric clinics of North America*, 48(1), 207-219.

Schanler RJ et al (1999). Feeding strategies for premature infants: randomized trial of gastrointestinal priming and tube-feeding method. *Pediatrics*, 103(2), 434-439.

Shiao SPK et al (1995). Nasogastric tube placement: effects on breathing and sucking in very-low-birth-weight infants. *Nursing research*, 44(2), 82-88.

Silvestre MA et al (1996). A prospective randomized trial comparing continuous versus intermittent feeding methods in very low birth weigh neonates. *Journal of pediatrics*, 128(6), 748-752.

Smith AB, Wilkinson-Faulk D (1994). Factors affecting the life span of peripheral intravenous lines in hospitalized infants. *Pediatric nursing*, 20, 543-547.

Stanley MD et al (1992). Infiltration during intravenous therapy in neonates: comparison of teflon and vialon catheters. *Southern medical journal*, 85, 883-886.

Stephenson T, Khan J (1993). A new technique for placement of central venous catheters in small infants. *Journal of parenteral and enteral nutrition*, 17, 479-480.

Strange K (1993). Maintenance of cell volume in the central nervous system. *Pediatric nephrology*, 1, 689-697.

Stringer MD et al (1992). Performance of percutaneous silastic central venous feeding catheters in surgical neonates. *Pediatric surgery international*, 7, 79-81.

Symington A et al (1995). Indwelling versus intermittent feeding tubes in premature neonates. *Journal of obstetric, gynecologic, and neonatal nursing*, 24, 321-326.

Treas LS, Latinis-Bridges B (1992). Efficacy of heparin in peripheral venous infusion in neonates. *Journal of obstetric, gynecologic, and neonatal nursing*, 21, 214-219.

Troche B et al (1995). Early minimal feedings promote growth in critically ill premature infants. *Biological neonate*, 67, 172-181.

Trotter CW (1996). Percutaneous central venous catheter-related sepsis in the neonate: an analysis of the literature from 1990-1994. *Neonatal network*, 15, 15-28.

Trotter CW (1998). A national survey of percutaneous central venous catheter practices in neonates. *Neonatal network*, 17, 31-38.

Tuchman DN (1994). Physiology of the swallowing apparatus. In DN Tuchman, RS Walter (Eds.), *Disorders of feeding and swallowing in infants and children: pathophysiology, diagnosis, and treatment*, San Diego, CA: Singular Publishing Group, Inc.

Uauy R et al (1994). Safety and efficacy of N-3 fatty acids in the nutrition of very-low-birth-weight infants: soy oil and marine oil supplementation of formula. *Journal of pediatrics*, 124, 612-620.

Van Der Hulst R et al (1993). Glutamine and the preservation of gut integrity. *Lancet*, 341, 13, 663-665.

Vanderplas Y et al (1998). Nutritional management of regurgitation in infants. *Journal of the American college of nutrition*, 17(4), 308-316.

Wauben IPM, Wainwright PE (1999). The influence of neonatal nutrition on behavioral development: a critical appraisal. *Nutrition reviews*, 57(2), 35-44.

Wesley JR, Bello DK (2001). Parenteral nutrition in the neonatal and pediatric patient. http://allnurses.com/

White-Traut R et al (2002). Feeding readiness behaviors and feeding efficiency in response to ATVV intervention. *Neonatal and infant nursing review*.

White-Traut R et al (1994). Environmental influences on the developing premature infant: theoretical issues and applications to practice. *Journal of obstetric, gynecologic, and neonatal nursing*, 23(5), 393-401.

White-Traut R et al (1997). Responses of preterm infants to unimodal and multimodal sensory intervention. *Pediatric nursing*, 23(2), 169-193.

Wilson DC et al (1997). Randomized controlled trial of an aggressive nutritional regimen in sick very-low-birth-weight infants: archives of disease in childhood. *Journal of the British paediatric association*, 77, F4-F11.

Wood AF (1991). Factors affecting reciprocity between nurses and preterm infants during feeding. *Journal of perinatal and neonatal nursing*, 4(4), 62-70.

Yao S et al (1997). *Manual of neonatal care: nutrition*. Philadelphia: Lippincott-Raven.

Zenk K (1992). Y-site compatibility of drugs commonly used in the NICU. *Neonatal pharmacology quarterly*, 1(2), 13-22.

CHAPTER 26

ASSESSMENT AND MANAGEMENT OF THE GASTROINTESTINAL SYSTEM

Janet L. Thigpen, Carole Kenner

The intake and digestion of foodstuffs and the elimination of waste products are critical to long-term survival. Although many complex metabolic processes are involved, the ability to maintain adequate nutrition ultimately requires that the gastrointestinal (GI) tract be patent and structurally intact. With only a few exceptions, the vast majority of conditions that cause GI dysfunction are the result of congenital anatomic malformations. The discovery and management of GI dysfunction thus require knowledge of both embryogenesis and normal anatomy. Although some anomalies involve external defects and are immediately apparent, most causes of dysfunction are hidden from view and may initially cause few symptoms unless allowed to progress to the point at which serious pathophysiologic changes present a major threat to life. The input and support of a variety of nursing, medical, and other specialists are required for optimal outcomes—that is, the infant's physiologic well-being and the parents' psychosocial stability. The emotional needs of parents and their work through the process of grief over the loss of the expected "perfect" child cannot be underestimated. Visible defects, especially those involving the face, appear to be particularly difficult for parents to accept. The frequent GI malformations are associated with other congenital anomalies and prematurity, and the possible need for transport to a distant center where corrective surgery can be accomplished places additional demands on parental coping.

The GI tract is the site of the many complex transport and enzymatic mechanisms required for the biologic absorption and digestion of nutrients. The successful intake and assimilation of these nutrients, however, rests on the capability of the gut to act as a conduit for ingestion, digestion, and elimination. Congenital malformations, particularly those involving anatomic or functional obstruction, clearly hinder this process. Even when structurally intact, however, the supporting gastric and intestinal musculature of the newborn is relatively deficient, making peristaltic movements more infrequent and irregular when compared with those of adults, thus increasing the tendency toward distention. Transport of materials through the tract is further diminished in premature infants, who are characterized by poor sucking and swallowing abilities, small gastric capacity, and incompetent cardioesophageal sphincter (Fletcher, 1994). Debilitated, hypotonic infants may similarly exhibit poor sucking and swallowing and decreased motility. In addition, the bowel seems particularly susceptible to ischemic conditions in which blood flow is preferentially directed away from the GI tract (as well as the kidneys and peripheral vascular bed) toward the brain and heart. Untoward effects of drugs commonly used in the nursery may further compromise intestinal function or integrity. For example, morphine, in addition to its desired analgesic effect, also slows gastric emptying and reduces propulsive peristalsis. Conversely, the antibiotic erythromycin has been shown to accelerate gastric emptying. Ulceration of the GI tract with possible bleeding and perforation are reported side effects of tolazoline, dexamethasone, and indomethacin (Kubota et al, 1994; Young & Mangum, 2001).

The basics of ingestion, digestion, elimination, and metabolism are discussed in Chapters 24 and 25. The major purposes of this chapter are to discuss the embryologic development of the GI tract and resultant normal anatomic structure and to describe common causes of neonatal dysfunction with their implications for care.

EMBRYOLOGIC DEVELOPMENT OF THE GASTROINTESTINAL TRACT

The formation of the GI tract depends largely on the folding that the embryo undergoes at the end of the first month of development. Initially, the embryo is shaped like a flat, circular plate. However, in the third week, with the beginning development of the nervous system, the area that becomes the cranial region expands, and the neural plate elongates so that the flat disk assumes a shape more closely resembling a pear, with a broad cephalic and very narrow caudal end. The continued longitudinal growth of the primitive central nervous system causes the embryonic disk to bend so that the cranial and caudal portions fold ventrally toward one another. Simultaneously, the rapid proliferation of cells alongside the primitive neural tube causes the disk to fold laterally so that the sides also move ventrally toward each other. By 4 weeks' gestation, the head-to-toe and side-to-side folding is complete, and the embryo more closely resembles a horseshoe-shaped cylinder. The hollow internal cavity, lined by what once was the dorsal portion of the yolk sac that was invaginated during the folding process, forms the basis of the primitive GI tract. The ventral flexure partitions the tube-like cavity into three regions: (1) the foregut, (2) the midgut, and (3) the hindgut. The cephalic area is called the foregut and gives rise to the esophagus, stomach, proximal duodenum (above the bile duct), liver, pancreas, and biliary apparatus as well as the lower respiratory system. The mouth develops from a surface depression in the ectoderm called the stomodeum, or primitive mouth, and involves the most cranial part of the foregut, which is referred to by some as the pharyngeal gut. The middle region is the midgut, from which the distal duodenum, the remainder of the small intestine, the ascending colon, and most of the transverse colon are formed. The hindgut, the most distal portion of the cavity, gives rise to the rest of the colon, rectum, and upper anal canal as well as the genitourinary structures. The anus originates from an ectodermal depression called the proctodeum, or anal pit, and involves the most caudal part of the hindgut, which is referred to as the cloaca. For the purposes of discussion, further review of embryogenesis correlates with these major regions.

Pharyngeal Gut

Early in the fourth week of fetal life, a depression appears on the ventral surface of the head and is called the stomodeum. Oval thickenings, the nasal placodes, develop above and on either side of this primitive mouth. Subsequently, C-shaped elevations, called simply the nasal elevations, develop at the margins of the nasal placodes. As this development continues, the nasal placodes deepen and sink to form the nasal pits that become the nostrils. The medial nasal elevations and the area above the stomodeum continue to grow and eventually merge with each other to form the future philtrum, the vertical groove in the middle of the upper lip. Maxillary processes on either side of the stomodeum grow forward and fuse first with the lower edge of the lateral nasal elevations and then extend below the nasal pits to reach and merge with the primitive philtrum to form a continuous ridge above the stomodeum during the eighth embryonic week. It is from this ridge that the upper lip develops. Similarly, two mandibular processes below the stomodeum meet and fuse to form the lower lip and jaw.

The palate is formed between the 5th and 12th weeks of embryonic development. A wedge-shaped extension of the maxillary processes grows beneath the olfactory pits, separating the future nostrils from the upper lip to form the median palatine process or primary palate. The maxillary process also gives rise to a shelf-like projection called the lateral palatine process. Initially, the palatine process projects downward on each side of the tongue, but as the tongue descends, the processes gradually grow toward each other in a horizontal plane. The free edges of these lateral processes fuse first with the posterior portion of the primary palate and then with each other in the midline, starting from the front and progressing posteriorly until the fusion is complete. The palate formed by the fusion of these two lateral palatine processes is called the secondary palate; this palate subsequently merges with the free edge of the nasal septum.

Foregut

Between 4 and 5 weeks' gestation, a small diverticulum or outpouching appears on the ventral wall of the newly established foregut. As this diverticulum grows, folds develop along its length and eventually grow together in a zipper-like fashion to form an esophagotracheal septum. When completed, this septum divides what was once the proximal foregut into a ventral portion, the primitive respiratory system with its set of lung buds, and a dorsal portion, the esophagus. Initially very short, the esophagus rapidly lengthens over the next 2 to 3 weeks to accommodate the development of the lungs, heart, and neck.

During this same interval, at about 4 weeks, a more distal area along the foregut begins to dilate and gradually develops into the stomach. At first this primitive stomach is located in the neck, but it gradually descends during the next 8 weeks to its final abdominal position as the esophagus lengthens, whereas descending, differential growth rates along the sides of the primitive stomach result in the formation of the greater and lesser curvatures. Around 11 weeks, differentiated glandular epithelial cells (primitive parietal cells) begin to appear and have the potential to produce hydrochloric acid as early as 13 weeks' gestation. However, actual acid secretion is not significant until after 33 weeks' gestation (Kelly & Newell, 1994).

The most terminal portion of the foregut, the part that eventually becomes the duodenum, undergoes both external and internal changes during the remainder of the first trimester. Internally, the duodenum begins to generate villi between 5 and 6 weeks' gestation. Interestingly, these villi grow so profusely that the lumen of the duodenum is filled and becomes temporarily occluded by these prolific cells. Not until about 1 month later, between 9 and 10 weeks' gestation, does the duodenum recanalize, thus opening the lumen. Externally, by the beginning of the fourth week, the primitive liver appears as a small bud formed from the lining of the foregut. Shortly thereafter, another outgrowth begins along the stalk that connects the liver to the duodenum, giving rise to the gallbladder and bile ducts. Although initially a hollow organ, the gallbladder and its ducts also experience temporary occlusion as a result of the proliferation of the lining, subsequently recanalizing to allow formation and secretion of bile by the 12th week of gestation. The pancreas also begins with the protrusion of two buds at about 5 weeks' gestation. These buds fuse 1 week later to form a single, definitive pancreas.

Midgut

Initially, the tube-like gut lengthens in tandem with the overall elongation of the embryo. However, by the sixth week of gestation, the rate of growth of the intestinal tube outpaces the elongation of the body, thus causing the tube to bend ventrally. With the simultaneously rapid growth of the liver, the space within the abdominal cavity quickly becomes limited. Consequently, at about 7 weeks' gestation, loops of intestine begin to protrude into the umbilical cord. As the midgut literally herniates, it rotates in a counterclockwise fashion (approximately 90 degrees) around an axis formed by the superior mesenteric artery. At around 10 weeks, when the abdominal cavity has expanded sufficiently and the growth of the liver has slowed, the loops of intestine are retracted into the abdomen (undergoing counterclockwise rotation an additional 180 degrees). Thus during the processes of herniation and return, the intestine has rotated a full 270 degrees. This counterclockwise rotation allows the transverse colon to pass in front of the duodenum and places the cecum and appendix in the right lower quadrant of the abdomen.

Hindgut

The major embryologic process occurring in this third region of the gut involves the formation of the anus. This process takes place in the most terminal part of the hindgut, the cloaca, which is separated from the caudal ectoderm by only a thin barrier called the cloacal membrane. When the embryo is 4 weeks old, a ridge of tissue referred to as the urorectal septum develops in the area that becomes the umbilicus. As this septum grows caudally, the cloaca is divided into a ventral portion, the primitive urogenital sinus, and a dorsal portion, the anorectal canal. By the end of the sixth week of gestation, the septum has reached the cloacal membrane, dividing it into smaller membranes as well: the urogenital membrane, which bounds the ventral urogenital sinus, and the anal membrane, which bounds the dorsal anorectal canal. In the meantime, the tissues around the anal membrane swell so that by the eighth week of gestation this anal membrane is found at the bottom of a depression known as the proctodeum or anal pit. In the ninth week, the anal membrane ruptures and an open pathway is established between the rectum and the outside.

Relationship to Nervous System

Before concluding the discussion of GI embryogenesis, it is necessary to review briefly the concurrent development of the nervous system. The primitive neural tube and the neural crest cells proliferating along its side, which were responsible for the initial folding of the embryo (transforming it from a flat disk into a hollow cylinder), continue their own growth and differentiation while the gut is undergoing its transformation. The primitive neural tube ultimately gives rise to the brain, spinal cord, and central nervous system; the neural crest cells give rise to the peripheral nervous system. The relationship between the peripheral nervous system and the GI system begins immediately on completion of the folding process, at about 5 weeks' gestation, when primitive nerve cells begin migrating along the intestinal tube in a cephalocaudal direction. By 12 weeks, the muscular layers of the intestine have appeared, and the primitive nerve cells, or neuroblasts, have completed their head-to-toe migration so that the entire length of the GI tract is innervated. Thus by the end of the first trimester, the main structures of the intestinal system have all been established. The last two trimesters are characterized by maturation of the tissues and organs and the rapid growth of the body.

PHYSIOLOGY OF THE GASTROINTESTINAL (GI) TRACT

The major function of the GI tract is to transfer food and water from the external to the internal environment, where they can be digested, absorbed, and distributed to the cells of the body by the circulatory system. While these processes are occurring, contractions of the smooth muscle lining the walls of the intestine move the contents through the lumen, releasing any material not digested and absorbed during transit back into the external environment. Technically speaking, this released material is composed of very few "waste products." Although some end products, such as the breakdown products of hemoglobin, are contained in the stool, most metabolic end products are actually eliminated from the body by the kidneys and lungs.

Structure

The GI tract consists of a tube of variable diameter with the same general structure throughout most of its length. Moving from the outside inward toward the lumen, six concentric layers in the wall of the intestine can be identified (Figure 26-1). The first, outermost layer is composed of connective tissue. In the esophagus, where the connective layer is continuous with the deep fascia, it is called the adventitia; in all other portions of the gut, the connective tissue layer is covered with peritoneal epithelial cells and is called the serosa. The next two layers are both made up of smooth muscle—but with each exhibiting a different orientation of its muscle fibers. The outer layer of muscle has its fibers running longitudinally along the gut; the fibers in the inner muscle layer circle the gut. The fourth layer, the submucosa, is composed primarily of connective tissue as well as a few exocrine gland cells, blood vessels, and lymphatics. The fifth layer is again composed of smooth muscle but is of mixed orientation with both longitudinal and circular fibers. The last layer, which actually lines the lumen of the gut, is known as the mucosa and contains most of the exocrine gland cells as well as epithelial cells. The mucosal surface is highly convoluted in the small intestine, with many ridges and valleys giving it a larger surface area for absorption. Elsewhere, the mucosa has a smoother surface (Guyton & Hall, 2000). In addition to these six structural layers, two major nerve plexuses are found in the gut wall; they regulate the contraction of the smooth muscles. The myenteric plexus lies between the longitudinal and circular layers of muscle and is largely motor in function. The submucosal plexus, as its name implies, is located in the submucosa and is mainly sensory. Synaptic connections between the two nerve networks allow one plexus to stimulate activity in the other and vice versa, leading to activity that is conducted both up and down the length of the gut (Guyton & Hall, 2000).

Motility

Once food enters the esophagus, it is moved along by peristaltic waves initiated by impulses from autonomic nerves—more specifically, the enteric nervous system (ENS)—and coordinated by the swallowing center in the medulla. The ENS is regulated by a series of genes that influence receptor sites, transciption, and translation of neuronal signals (Bates & Balistreri, 2002). As the wave of contraction begins, the gastroesophageal sphincter temporarily relaxes to allow the bolus to enter the stomach. Although this sphincter is anatomically indistinct from the remainder of the esophagus, it normally remains tonically contracted so that the contents of the stomach, which are under relatively higher internal pressure in relation to that experienced in the esophagus, do not reflux (Guyton & Hall, 2000).

When filled with food, the peristaltic waves spread across the stomach toward the small intestine. However, the contractions are no longer mediated by the medulla but rather by the nerve plexuses and the effect of smooth muscle stretching. Because the muscle layers are thicker in the distal portion of the stomach (antrum) in comparison with the relatively thin layer surrounding the upper portion of the stomach (fundus), the contractions are most powerful and intense in the antrum. These strong antral contractions fulfill two functions. First, they are the primary force acting to break up the gastric contents and mix them with enzymes to form a semi-fluid mixture called chyme. Second, they force the chyme past the pyloric sphincter into the duodenum. Normally the rate of gastric emptying is controlled by the chemical composition and amount of chyme, but when the stomach is distended or subjected to increased calorific density or high loads of carbohydrate, fat, or acid, the gastric motility may actually decrease so that more time can be devoted to digestion and absorption in the small intestine. In general, formula empties more slowly than breast milk. The effect of infant positioning and the temperature of the feed on gastric emptying are less clear (Ewer et al, 1994; Guyton & Hall, 2000).

The contractions that sweep strongly over the stomach become more oscillatory in nature in the small intestine, promoting the digestive and absorptive processes that occur there. Assisting in the process are pancreatic secretions and bile secreted

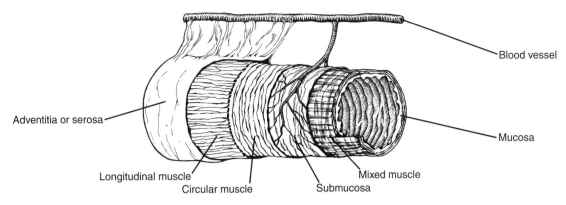

FIGURE **26-1**
Anatomy of the intestinal wall.

by the liver into the duodenum just below the stomach. Although contractions become progressively slower in the small intestine as chyme passes from the duodenum to the jejunum to the ileum, the muscular activity is sufficient to move the contents slowly downward toward the colon. However, distention and luminal injury may bring muscular activity to a halt.

The colon functions primarily as a storage area. Consequently its structure differs from that of the small intestine in several major ways. Because only a minuscule amount (approximately 4%) of the total intestinal contents is absorbed here, no digestive enzymes are secreted, the lumen is no longer convoluted, and it lacks villi. In addition, the longitudinal smooth muscle layer is incomplete. The contractions of the remaining circular smooth muscle layer therefore produce only segmental, not propulsive, movement. Consequently, when the luminal contents enter the colon through the ileocecal sphincter, they are merely concentrated (through the reabsorption of water) until distention of the rectum initiates the defecation reflex and the fecal matter is expelled.

Other Cells

Other tissues or cells are found within the GI system. These are related to immune function. They are described in detail in Chapter 29. These cells are referred to as gut-associated lymphoid tissue or GALT. They are stem cells derived from the hematopoietic system that migrate to the GI tract (Bates & Balistreri, 2002). These are Peyer patches, lymphoid cells of the lamina propria, and intraepithelial lymphocytes (Bates & Balistreri, 2002). They serve to enhance the neonate's immune response.

MATURATION OF GASTROINTESTINAL FUNCTION

The gross anatomy of the supporting musculature and the functional development of GI motility have not been as well studied as has the development of the secretory and absorptive capabilities of the bowel. In general, however, it appears that these supporting structures are relatively thinner in the newborn, especially in the premature newborn, than in the adult. The muscular layers of the stomach are somewhat deficient, with the longitudinal muscle layer being especially thin over the greater curvature. Similarly, the musculature of the intestine is also relatively thin, constituting approximately 50% of the bowel wall in the newborn, as compared with approximately 60% in the adult.

The presence of lanugo and squamous cells in meconium in the newborn bowel indicates that at least some movement of materials from swallowed amniotic fluid occurs. Under normal circumstances, however, little propulsive peristaltic muscle activity appears to occur until late in gestation, and even at term such activity is somewhat irregular and slowed in comparison with that occurring in the adult. Measurable duodenal contractions have been demonstrated by indwelling intraluminal manometry to be present in the infant born as early as the 26th week of gestation, although they occur infrequently (mean of 1.9 contractions per minute) and are relatively weak (mean of 6.3 mm Hg at peak pressure). Between 29 and 32 weeks of gestation, motility spontaneously and significantly improves, with contractions occurring at an average rate of 6.5 per minute and with an average force of 17.1 mm Hg. Neither postnatal age nor type of enteral feed given (breast milk versus formula) nor mode of feeding (instillation by orogastric versus transpyloric tube) appears to affect the timing of this narrow maturational window.

Evidence does point to a somewhat enhanced maturation in infants who receive early enteral feedings with volumes as small as 4 ml/g/hour. Use of diluted formula for these early feedings is, however, controversial because the onset, strength, and duration of motor activity appear to be inversely related to the concentration formula. Manometric studies, in fact, indicate that the routine use of diluted formula (even one-third strength) may not provide an optimal stimulus for gut motility (Koenig et al, 1995). Antenatal corticosteroid treatment to initiate production of pulmonary surfactant does appear to promote gut maturation, but maturation appears to be delayed in infants affected with significant central nervous system insult or abnormality such as asphyxia and hydrocephalus. After 32 weeks' gestation, duodenal function steadily improves and by term reaches a contraction frequency of approximately 10 per minute. Thus the duodenal contraction rate at term approaches but is less than that found in fasting adults of roughly 11 per minute. Furthermore, the number of contractions that occur in a burst or rapid sequence is often fewer than that measured in adults.

The motor mechanism of the colon also appears to be affected by maturation and illness. Although virtually all healthy, full-term newborns (99.8%) pass meconium within 48 hours of delivery, the first passage of stool is frequently delayed in premature infants. Over 90% of infants with birth weight less than 2500 g, 80% of infants weighing less than 1500 g at birth), and 43% of infants with birth weight less than

1000 g, have passed their first stool by the end of 48 hours. Low-birth-weight infants who are ill, especially those with severe respiratory distress syndrome, in whom enteral feedings are consequently delayed, may experience further delay. Data for such infants with birth weights less than 1500 g reveal a mean time of passage of the first stool at 91 hours for those receiving early feedings versus an average of 168 hours for those receiving delayed feedings. Thus even in the absence of congenital GI problems, very-low-birth-weight infants might not be expected to pass their first stool until as late as 7 to 12 days of age.

Bacterial Colonization

As the gut matures postnatally; bacteria is introduced to the GI tract through feedings and invasive procedures. The once sterile gut rapidly changes depending on whether the infant is being fed and what feeding is received. Lactobacillus is passed on to the infant through breast milk and assists with lactose reduction. Secretory IgA and bactericidal enzymes are also passed on to breastfed infants, thus affecting the bacterial growth in the gut. All infants are colonized with Costridium difficile as well as with other anaerobes and facilitated anaerobes (Bates & Balistreri, 2002). The colonization is disrupted by the introduction of medications, especially antibiotics that change the normal flora.

In summary, even when structurally intact, the relatively deficient supporting musculature and immature motor mechanisms of the newborn, particularly the premature newborn, at best allow only irregular peristaltic activity that occurs in somewhat disorganized patterns. This infrequent and irregular activity increases the tendency toward distention in the infant and in the ill or premature infant, thus increasing the likelihood of delayed transit and stooling. Complete and thorough assessment of the GI tract therefore becomes essential to distinguish the expected physiologic deficiencies of the newborn from pathologic causes of dysfunction.

ASSESSMENT OF THE GASTROINTESTINAL TRACT

History

Assessment of the newborn infant ideally begins during the prenatal period. Although newly born, each infant has a history dating to the time of conception. Consequently, historical antecedents to birth may serve as an indicator of increased likelihood of dysfunction of a specific organ system such as the GI tract (Tappero & Honeyfield, 1996). Although most cases of isolated abdominal and GI defects occur sporadically, some (such as cleft lip or palate, or both, and pyloric stenosis) may exhibit familial recurrence patterns, thus suggesting at least some degree of genetic influence mediated by environmental factors. Therefore any initial history taking should include a screen to identify parents who have had a previous child with related genetic or congenital anomaly or other positive family history. Major syndromes that have frequently associated GI anomalies are listed in Table 26-1.

Although a certain degree of risk may be established through genetic screening, the best evidence of fetal GI anomalies is obtained through prenatal ultrasonography. The fetal abdomen can be identified as early as 10 weeks from the last menstrual period, and the stomach can be visualized at 13 weeks' gestation. The transient herniation of the intestine into the umbilical cord has even been documented by ultrasonography. However, because embryogenesis is still underway at this time, first-trimester diagnosis of defects, particularly small ones, is

TABLE **26-1**	Major Syndromes Associated with Gastrointestinal Dysfunction
Syndrome	**Gastrointestinal Component**
Apert's syndrome	Narrow palate with or without cleft palate or bifid uvula
	Pyloric stenosis
	Ectopic anus
Beckwith-Wiedemann syndrome	Omphalocele
Fetal hydantoin syndrome	Cleft lip and palate
	Pyloric stenosis
	Duodenal atresia
	Anal atresia
Meckel-Gruber syndrome	Cleft palate with or without cleft lip
	Bile duct proliferation fibrosis, cysts
	Omphalocele
	Malrotation
	Imperforate anus
Sirenomelia (mermaid syndrome)	Imperforate anus
	Esophageal atresia with tracheoesophageal fistula
Trisomy 13	Cleft lip with or without cleft palate
	Omphalocele
	Incomplete rotation of colon
Trisomy 18	Cleft lip with or without cleft palate
	Pyloric stenosis
	Biliary atresia
	Omphalocele
	Incomplete rotation of colon
	Imperforate anus
Trisomy 21	Short palate
	Tracheoesophageal fistula
	Duodenal atresia
VATER association	Imperforate anus with or without fistula
	Esophageal atresia with tracheoesophageal fistula

Data from Jones KL (1988). Smith's recognizable patterns of human malformation: genetic, embryologic and clinical aspects, ed 4, Philadelphia: WB Saunders.

exceptionally difficult. It is generally not until the second and third trimesters, when the GI structures are established, that reliable visualization becomes possible. Scanning at that point would include a survey of the abdominal wall and insertion of the umbilical cord, visualization of the fluid-filled stomach, and a search for bowel dilation or abnormal echolucencies that resemble cysts and that might indicate collection of fluid within the bowel owing to obstruction. Abnormal facial features such as clefting may even be identified if fetal position allows and if examination is targeted for that area. The presence of polyhydramnios may provide an additional clue to defects high in the GI tract. Normally, in utero the fetus swallows, absorbs, and metabolizes amniotic fluid. However, if the fetus is unable to swallow effectively owing to a GI obstruction, polyhydramnios results.

Postnatally, three cardinal signs point to the possibility of GI obstruction, whether structural or functional: (1) persistent vomiting, especially if it is bile stained; (2) abdominal distention; and (3) failure to pass meconium within the first 48 hours of birth.

Vomiting, as differentiated from reflux, indicates an attempt by an irritated or over-distended bowel to rid itself of its contents. Although vomiting may be initiated by distention or irritative stimuli at any point along the length of the gut, the stomach and duodenum appear to be the most sensitive to these stimuli (Guyton & Hall, 2000). Consequently, vomiting is most often considered an indicator of defects high in the GI tract. The presence of bile further indicates that the point of obstruction is distal to the ampulla of Vater, where bile is emptied from the common bile duct into the duodenum. Conversely, nonbilious vomiting would be noted if obstruction were proximal to the ampulla. Because the mechanism for vomiting requires expulsion of the offending contents up through the esophagus, a patent esophagus is required for true vomiting to occur.

Abdominal distention occurs when large amounts of swallowed air and fluid collect in the bowel and because of obstruction can pass through the gut no further. The situation is compounded as digestive fluids and electrolytes continue to be secreted and proteins are lost from the circulation into the lumen of bowel that becomes progressively edematous as the result of distention (Guyton & Hall, 2000). Because the stomach is shielded by the rib cage, such distention is generally observed when obstruction occurs in the lower small intestine or colon.

Most normal full-term infants pass their first stool by 48 hours of age. Failure to pass meconium within the first 2 days of life therefore generally indicates obstruction of the large intestine, unless such delay can be attributed to the case of an oversedated, debilitated, or premature infant.

Physical Assessment

A systematic approach to assessment of the newborn GI tract includes inspection, auscultation, and palpation. Percussion, although useful in the examination of adults, is unreliable and difficult to perform in the infant because the internal abdominal organs are so small and close together. Consequently, the examiner tends to rely on radiography and other diagnostic procedures instead of percussion.

Inspection

Because many of the GI defects are grossly apparent even to the untrained eye, inspection is a fundamental part of assessment. The mouth is observed for its position, shape, size, and symmetry, and the lips, palate, and uvula are evaluated for clefts. Although complete separation of the lip extending up into the nasal area is obvious, close attention must also be paid for any niche in the lip that might easily be overlooked. Abundant oral secretions or saliva provides an early clue to esophageal atresia, particularly when a history of polyhydramnios has been reported.

The abdomen is next inspected for contour, symmetry, and integrity. Distention of the abdomen, which is normally slightly rounded, serves as a hallmark of obstruction. Although the decreased muscle tone in a premature infant may allow visualization of peristalsis, such movement is not normally observed, and when noted in the presence of vomiting or disten-

tion, it again suggests the possibility of obstruction. The character of the umbilical cord and site of insertion are checked. Although most cases of omphalocele are obvious, an abnormal thickness to the stump or cord itself should raise suspicion of a single herniated loop of intestine. Any such enlargement must be differentiated from a Wharton's jelly cyst or umbilical hernia through the lax rectus muscles. The anus is examined for position, and the perineal area is inspected for fistulas. The muscle tone of the anal sphincter can be determined by stroking the anal area with a gloved finger and observing for the contraction "wink" that normally occurs around the anal opening. If clinically indicated, the examiner can assess for anal patency by digital examination using the gloved little finger. Insertion of a rectal thermometer presents the risk of perforating the rectum and should not be performed for assessment purposes.

Auscultation

Although initially absent, bowel sounds generally become audible within the first 15 to 30 minutes of life, as the bowel fills with swallowed air and peristaltic activity is activated by the parasympathetic nervous system. Normally these sounds should be of a metallic tinkling quality and occur approximately two to five times per minute. Although often helpful in the assessment of the adult sounds may be hyperactive, absent, or even normal in the case of neonatal obstruction. Therefore the presence and intensity of bowel sounds must be interpreted in relation to other pertinent historical and clinical findings. Hyperdynamic sounds in a recently fed infant with a benign history and otherwise insignificant examination should be considered normal; however, marked concern should be raised if hyperdynamic sounds are found in an infant with concurrent findings of distention and vomiting. More often than not, however, the abdomen is misleadingly silent.

Palpation

Abdominal palpation is performed with the infant in a supine position and is best carried out when the infant is quiet and preferably during the first 24 hours of life, when the abdominal musculature is lax. Holding the infant's knees and hips in a flexed position also helps to relax the abdominal musculature. The liver, spleen, and kidneys should be felt with a warm hand using slow, gentle pressure, using the pads of the fingers. Care to perform abdominal palpation in as gentle a manner as possible cannot be overemphasized. The multiple maneuvers involved are often distressing to the newborn, and the pressure applied even during a routine examination may result in significant, although transient, elevations in both systolic and diastolic blood pressures.

The liver is found by placing the index finger just above and to the right of the groin and slowly advancing upward until the edge of the liver can be felt to slip beneath the pad of the finger. Normally the organ is firm (but not hard) with a sharp edge that extends 1 to 2 cm below the right costal margin and can be followed across the abdomen into the left upper quadrant. The spleen is found on the left side in a similar manner, but generally only the tip of the organ is felt at the left costal margin—or it may be entirely unpalpable. The kidneys are located in the flank areas above the level of the umbilicus and are normally 4.5 to 5 cm in length in the term infant. Palpation may be performed bimanually (with one hand supporting and stabilizing the flanks posteriorly while the thumb or a finger of the free hand is moved anteriorly over the same area), or

TABLE **26-2**	Risk Factors Associated with Gastrointestinal Dysfunction
Risk Factor	**Gastrointestinal Dysfunction**
Maternal	
Cigarette smoking	Cleft lip with or without cleft palate
Diabetes	Small left colon syndrome
Hypovitaminosis	Cleft lip with or without cleft palate
Influenza with fever	Cleft lip with or without cleft palate
Ionizing radiation exposure	Biliary atresia
Polyhydraminos	Esophageal atresia with or without TE fistula, duodenal atresia, meconium ileus
Stress and anxiety	Pyloric stenosis
Medications	
Doxylamine succinate-pyridoxine hydrochloride	Pyloric stenosis
Benzodiazepines	Cleft lip with or without cleft palate
Cortisone	Cleft lip with or without cleft palate
Phenytoin	Cleft lip with or without cleft palate
Magnesium sulfate	Meconium plug syndrome
Opiates	Cleft lip with or without cleft palate
Penicillin	Cleft lip with or without cleft palate
Salicylates	Cleft lip with or without cleft palate
Positive Family History	
"Apple peel" type of jejunoileal atresia	Similar anomaly
Cleft lip with or without cleft palate	Similar anomaly
Cystic fibrosis	Meconium ileus
Hirschsprung disease	Similar anomaly
Neonatal	
Apnea	Necrotizing enterocolitis
Aseptic environment	Necrotizing enterocolitis
Asphyxia or ischemic episodes	Biliary atresia, necrotizing enterocolitis
Cyanotic spells	Necrotizing enterocolitis
Exchange transfusion	Necrotizing enterocolitis
Feeding practices	Pyloric stenosis, necrotizing enterocolitis
Hyperbilirubinemia	Duodenal atresia, jejunoileal atresia
Polycythemia	Necrotizing enterocolitis
Respiratory distress	Necrotizing enterocolitis
Vascular catheterization	Necrotizing enterocolitis

a single hand may be used (with the fingers of the hand supporting the flank posteriorly while the free thumb of the same hand explores the flank anteriorly). Although the overlying liver may obscure the upper position of the right kidney, the entire left kidney should be felt easily. The remainder of the abdominal examination consists of a gentle search for pathologic masses. Although most masses found are of renal origin, it may be possible to detect stool-filled bowel, particularly in the case of meconium ileus.

Related Findings

Prenatal ultrasonography and direct postnatal visualization of external defects are diagnostic of GI anomalies. In the absence of these obvious signs, a history of maternal polyhydramnios, vomiting, distention, and failure to pass stool are most indicative of GI dysfunction. Other relatively subtle—and oftentimes nonspecific—signs may also be noted.

Respiratory difficulty may arise as the result of an inability to handle the abundant oral secretions commonly found in esophageal atresia or may develop as a result of aspiration of gastric contents by way of an associated tracheoesophageal fistula. Abdominal distention may impede diaphragmatic excursions and therefore decrease ventilation. Frank airway obstruction may even occur in the case of cleft palate, if the negative inspiratory pressure pulls the tongue into the hypopharynx.

Jaundice may occur if the removal of bilirubin is hampered. In the case of biliary atresia, the conjugated bilirubin, which is a normal component of bile, is unable to pass into the duodenum for excretion in the stool. In cases of intestinal atresias, meconium ileus, and Hirschsprung disease, the enterohepatic circulation becomes exaggerated as stasis of the luminal contents promotes intestinal reabsorption of the bilirubin that is present.

Systemic hypertension may be an additional—although rarely noted—subtle sign. This increase in blood pressure may be appreciated in situations in which masses or distention significantly increases intraabdominal pressure.

Risk Factors

Maternal, neonatal, and other risk factors associated with GI dysfunction may be found in Table 26-2. These factors are dis-

TABLE 26-2	Risk Factors Associated with Gastrointestinal Dysfunction—cont'd
Risk Factor	**Gastrointestinal Dysfunction**
Infections	
Cytomegalovirus	Biliary atresia
Gastroenteritis	Intussusception
Hepatitis A and B	Biliary atresia
Reovirus type 3	Biliary atresia
Respiratory infection	Intussusception
Rubella	Biliary atresia
Viral infection	Pyloric stenosis
Medications	
Hyperosmolar medications	Necrotizing enterocolitis
Xanthines	Gastroesophageal reflux
Other	
Congenital deafness	Hirschsprung disease
Congenital heart disease	Esophageal atresia with or without TE fistula, duodenal atresia, biliary atresia, omphalocele, anorectal atresia
Diaphragmatic hernia	Malrotation
Genitourinary anomalies	Esophageal atresia with or without TE fistula, duodenal atresia, biliary atresia, omphalocele, Hirschsprung disease, malrotation, anorectal atresia
Imperforate anus	Esophageal atresia with or without TE fistula, duodenal atresia
Intestinal atresia or obstruction	Gastroesophageal reflux, esophageal atresia with or without TE fistula, biliary atresia, omphalocele gastroschisis, malrotation
Malrotation	Duodenal atresia, jejunoileal atresia
Meckel's diverticulum	Malrotation, intussusception
Meconium ileus	Jejunoileal atresia
Neurologic abnormalities	Hirschsprung disease, meconium plug syndrome
Ocular neurocristopathies	Hirschsprung disease
Pancreatic defects	Meconium ileus
Tracheoesophageal anomalies	Duodenal atresia, anorectal atresia
Vertebral malformations	Esophageal atresia with or without TE fistula

TE, tracheoesophageal.

cussed in the sections outlining the management of specific problems.

Genetic Consultation

Once the family history has been obtained, it may be clear that a genetic history is important. Some GI disorders are related to chromosomal and single-gene defects. Omphalocele, duodenal atresia, and stenosis have a high association with trisomy disorders. At least 95% of cases of meconium ileus occur in infants with cystic fibrosis (Merenstein & Gardner, 2002). Because cystic fibrosis is inherited as an autosomal recessive disease, a family history of the disease may exist. There is a familiar association with pyloric stenosis. Five percent of infants of affected men have pyloric stenosis, and approximately 20% of infants of affected women are also affected by the disease. Genetic consultation is suggested for infants with these disorders to provide additional counseling to parents on the risk of recurrence (Lincoln-Boyea & Cefalo, 1996). Chromosomal studies should be performed if additional physical findings associated with GI anomaly are found.

Diagnostic Procedures

Radiologic Examination. Air in the GI tract serves as a naturally occurring contrast medium that makes radiologic evaluation of the abdomen a useful tool in the diagnosis of obstruction. At birth, the gut is fluid-filled, but as the infant swallows air after delivery, the radiolucent gas may be followed radiographically as it passes through the bowel. Within the first 30 minutes of life, air should be present in the stomach. By 3 to 4 hours, gas should be seen in the small bowel. After 6 to 8 hours, the entire gut including the colon and rectum should be filled with air. However, this normal progression of gas through the GI tract cannot occur if obstruction is present. No air is able to pass beyond the point of obstruction, so the portion of the intestine distal to the obstruction is generally airless. Nevertheless, air continues to be swallowed so that the part of the alimentary tract that lies above the obstruction can become quite distended and is demonstrated on radiography by often-dramatic radiolucent (black) bubbles. Flat and upright radiographic studies of the chest and abdomen may suffice for identifying esophageal or intestinal atresias. Cross-table lateral radiographs may be helpful by identifying air in the rectum of infants suspected of having intestinal obstruction. A left lateral decubitus film may determine the presence of free air in the intestinal wall or the peritoneal cavity.

Upper gastrointestinal series is often used GE reflux, pyloric stenosis, and malrotation. Contrast material, barium or gastrograffin is swallowed or administered by nasogastric tube and observed by fluoroscopy as it passes through the digestive tract. Gastrograffin, meglumine diatrizoate, is preferred if perforation is suspected because it is a water-soluble solution (Kee, 2001). The procedure may last 30 minutes to 4 hours, depending on the rate of small intestine motility. The patient need not be placed on a nothing-by-mouth status before the examination and may continue feedings after the examination.

Barium or gastrograffin enema is used for examination of the large intestine after contrast solution is instilled through the rectum. It may be diagnostic in cases of malrotation, suspected Hirschsprung's disease, meconium ileus, and meconium plug syndrome. The procedure should be performed prior to any planned upper GI examination because contrast material from the upper GI tract may take several days to clear. The rationale for this is that barium from the upper GI tract may take several days to clear and may interfere with the lower GI study. No special preparation is made other than placing the infant on a nothing by mouth status 4 to 6 hours before the study. Gentle saline enemas may be helpful in clearing barium and trapped air after the contrast procedure. If barium is allowed to harden and form concretions that can become impacted, more aggressive procedures may be required for evacuation.

Ultrasonography

Ultrasonography may be diagnostic in cases of pyloric stenosis, enteric duplication, GE reflux, or biliary atresia if the intrahepatic or proximal extrahepatic tracts are dilated. Conducting gel is placed on the abdomen, and the transducer is placed against the gel on the abdomen. The computer transforms reflected sound waves from tissues into scans, graphs, or audible sound (Kee, 2001).

Gastric Aspirate

A gastric aspirate may be obtained to measure the pH of the gastric contents. A premeasured feeding tube is passed into the stomach. At least 1 ml of gastric contents is gently aspirated into a syringe, and the feeding tube is withdrawn. The syringe is capped, labeled, and sent for testing.

Apt Testing

The Apt test may be used to determine the origin of blood in vomitus or stool by differentiating neonatal GI blood loss from swallowed maternal blood. Bloody aspirate or bloody stool is centrifuged in 5 ml water. One part 0.25% sodium hydroxide is added to five parts supernatant. The fluid remains pink in the presence of fetal blood but turns brown in the presence of maternal blood.

Stool Culture

A stool culture may differentiate between an intestinal lining insult and an infection as the cause of bloody diarrhea. A stool sample is taken from a diaper, placed in a specimen container, labeled, and sent for testing.

Stool Hematest

A stool Hematest is a rapid and convenient method for detection of fecal occult blood—a possible indication GI disease. The test is based on the oxidation of guaiac by hydrogen peroxide, thus resulting in a blue compound. A thin smear of stool is placed on guaiac paper. Developer is applied over the smear. Results are read in 60 seconds. Any blue colorization on or at the edge of the smear indicates a positive occult blood result. Fecal samples need not be tested if hematuria or obvious rectal bleeding is present. Drugs that influence positive results include iron preparations, indomethacin, potassium preparations, salicylates, and steroids. Large amounts of ascorbic acid may cause a false-negative result (Kee, 2001).

Stool-Reducing Substances

Carbohydrate intolerance is detected by the presence of reducing substances in the stool. To perform this test, the liquid portion of stool, which can be collected in a diaper, is aspirated into a syringe. A 1:2 ratio of stool to water is obtained. Fifteen drops of this supernatant are placed in a clean test tube, and a Clinitest (test for urinary glucose) tablet is added. After 15 seconds, the test tube is shaken gently, and the color of the liquid is compared with the color chart provided with the Clinitest tablets. More than 0.5% glucose in the stool indicates an abnormal amount of sugar.

pH Probe Test

The 24-hour pH probe test is considered the gold standard for the diagnosis of GE reflux. A thin flexible pH sensitive electrode is placed into the distal esophagus. The study is scored by determining the amount of time the esophagus is exposed to an acid pH level, which is usually less than 4. Scoring for abnormal results is based on frequency of reflux, number of episodes greater than 4 minutes duration, time of longest episode, and the percentage of time in reflux. A dual sensor may be used, which places an electrode in the distal esophagus and another in the pharyngeal area of the esophagus.

The use of formula feedings may obscure episodes of reflux by buffering the gastric acid. Many clinicians use acid feeding, such as apple juice, to better estimate the true amount of gastric reflux in the esophagus. Interpretation of the data is complex due to confounding factors such as position, activity, frequency and composition of feeding, and medication. Nursing responsibilities include recording the time of feedings and describing the activity level of the infant throughout the test.

Scintigraphy

Gastroesophageal scintigraphy, by feeding radionucleotide tagged formula to the infant, may be used to measure gastric emptying, aspiration with swallowing, and reflux with aspiration. A technitium radioisotope is used because it has relatively low radiation and is easily added to formula.

Endoscopy

Flexible endoscopy with biopsy of the distal esophagus is used to diagnose esophagitis. Biopsy findings suggestive of esophagitis include basal cell hyperplasia, increased stromal papillary length, and demonstration of intraepithelial eosinophils.

Fecal Fat

A fecal fat test may be helpful to screen for malabsorption. Fecal fat content of >6 g/24 h is predictive of malabsorption syndrome. A very small stool sample can cause false test results.

NURSING MANAGEMENT

General Principles

Early recognition accompanied by medical or surgical intervention for infants with GI obstructions or alterations is necessary to decrease the likelihood of a poor outcome. The general considerations that guide nursing care in alterations of the GI system include GI decompression, fluid and electrolyte balance, thermoregulation, positioning, prevention of infection, and nutrition.

Gastric Decompression.   Gastric decompression is extremely important to prevent aspiration, respiratory compromise, or gastric perforation. If the intestinal obstruction is not relieved, abdominal distention may become severe and the upward pressure on the diaphragm may compromise respirations. Connection of an orogastric tube to low intermittent suction minimizes the risk of aspiration and prevents distention from swallowed air. Tube patency is essential if gastric decompression is to be maintained. A 10 French soft vinyl, double-lumen gastric sump tube provides sufficient decompression for most infants. Irrigating the tube every 2 hours with 2 ml air ensures that the tube remains open and functioning.

Fluid and Electrolyte Balance.   Large amounts of extracellular fluid pass into and out of the GI tract as part of the normal digestive process. In intestinal obstruction, the fluids that are normally reabsorbed by the intestine become trapped. Additionally, infants with obstruction often experience "third-spacing," with a shift of fluid from the vascular into the interstitial compartment. This third-spacing is also referred to as capillary leak syndrome. If severe, this loss of intravascular volume can result in relative hypovolemia and hypoperfusion with all their attendant risks. Furthermore, vomiting, diarrhea, and gastric suction can cause excessive volume depletion and electrolyte abnormalities, especially losses of sodium, potassium, and chloride.

The goal of nursing management is to maintain fluid and electrolyte balance. Maintenance fluids are usually run at 60 to 80 ml/kg for the first 24 hours of life and are increased by 10 cc/kg/d or as needed to 120 to 160 cc/kg/d (Zenk, 1999). A rate should be maintained at which urine output is at least 1 to 2 ml/kg/hr and maintains a specific gravity of 1.005 to 1.012. Sodium is provided at a rate of 2 to 3 mEq/kg/d and potassium at 2 mEq/kg/d, as serum electrolytes indicate.

For the infant who is receiving gastric suction, the amount of gastric loss is determined by measuring drainage every 4 to 8 hours. The total volume of gastric output should be replaced every 4 to 8 hours with ½ normal saline with 10 to 20 mEq KCl/L. The replacement fluids are given in addition to maintenance fluids. Fluid volume deficit and electrolyte imbalances may occur if replacement therapy is inadequate. The adequacy for fluid replacement is assessed by changes in vital signs, amount of urinary output, urine specific gravity, levels of electrolytes and blood urea nitrogen, and hematocrit readings.

Metabolic alkalosis may occur with pyloric stenosis or high jejunal obstruction because of loss of acidic gastric juice. In obstructions in the distal segment of the small intestine, larger quantities of alkaline fluids than acidic fluids may be lost, thus resulting in metabolic acidosis. If the obstruction is below the proximal colon, acid-base balance may be maintained because most of the GI fluids are absorbed before reaching the obstruction. Respiratory acidosis may develop in patients with abdominal distention because of carbon dioxide retention from hypoventilation. Correction of acid-base imbalances would be made in the instance of a pH less than 7.35 or greater than 7.45 or for base excess below −4 or above +4 (Merenstein & Gardner, 2002).

Thermoregulation.   Thermoregulation is vital in the care of all newborns and becomes more critical for the stressed neonate. Cold stress dramatically increases oxygen requirements and predisposes the infant to hypoglycemia and metabolic acidosis. An appropriate heat source and monitoring must be ensured for any infant with GI dysfunction. Gastroschisis and omphalocele in particular cause profound heat loss from exposed bowel. Preoperative nursing intervention includes provision of an external heat source and head covering, hourly monitoring of temperature, and, in the case of exposed bowel, use of warm soaks with bowel bag from the feet to the axillae. The use of the plastic wrap also helps decrease evaporative losses.

Positioning.   Head-up positioning accomplishes two management goals in the infant with GI dysfunction. In suspected GER, a 30-degree prone position or left lateral position has been shown to be the most effective position to decrease reflux. For the infant with tracheal esophageal fistula, elevating the head of the bed 30 to 40 degrees helps to avoid reflux of gastric contents into the trachea via a distal fistula. In the case of an isolated esophageal atresia, a flat or head down position may avoid gravity drainage from an overflowing esophageal pouch.

Prevention of Infection.   Newborn infants are uniquely at risk for infections acquired prenatally, intrapartally, and postnatally. Infants who require specialized care as the result of medical or surgical problems have an increased susceptibility for infection. Broad-spectrum antibiotics are administered immediately in presumed neonatal infections. Many institutions administer antibiotics preoperatively to prevent infection.

Nutrition.   Meeting the caloric and metabolic needs postoperatively in the infant with GI dysfunction is challenging. Enteral feeding is delayed owing to surgery of the alimentary tract. Hyperalimentation is indicated to supply these needs. When the infant is ready to begin enteral feedings, clear liquids are begun and progress to elemental feedings such as Pregestimil (protein hydosylate formula), gradually increasing from one-quarter to one-half to full strength. Bowel loss or severity of the defect influences the infant's tolerance to feedings. Initial feedings are small, frequent or continuous-drip, are supplemented with intravenous hyperalimentation, and are gradually advanced. Advancement of feeding should be stopped if signs of intolerance, such as diarrhea, vomiting, abdominal distention, or presence of reducing substances in stool, appear (Zenk, 1999).

General Preoperative Management.   In an infant already afflicted by GI dysfunction, surgery presents an additional stress that the baby is often ill-equipped to tolerate. The principles of preoperative management revolve around the prevention or minimization of identified stressors by replacing all fluid losses, decompressing the distended bowel, and supporting failing organ systems by means of assisted ventilation, radiant heating, parenteral nutrition, and other interventions as needed. Appropriate fluid and electrolyte balance is challenging due to third space losses in the infant with bowel obstruction or necrotizing enterocolitis. The third space fluid losses are isotonic and have an electrolyte composition like serum. Fluid losses from the GI tract due to vomiting or nasogastric suction additionally contribute to negative fluid balance and electrolyte depletion. Nasogastric fluid losses need to be replaced at full volume using one-half normal saline with potassium chloride at 10 to 20 mEq/L. Careful monitoring of the clinical status, including heart rate, blood pressure, perfusion, capillary refill, and urine output, can help guide the rate of fluid replacement.

Laboratory monitoring for potential derangements is essential. Antibiotics should be started early in the neonate with bowel dysfunction, until the etiology is clear. Antibiotic regimens usually include combining a penicillin and an aminoglycoside, such as ampicillin and gentamicin. Clindamycin may be added to cover anaerobes.

General Postoperative Management.

Hydration, maintenance of electrolyte balance, gastric decompression, and fluid loss replacement are continued postoperatively, along with respiratory and other therapy that the individual case warrants. Most patients will have extraneous tubes or devices such as gastrostomy tubes, chest tubes, or drains as well as incision sites. Meticulous care is needed to maintain skin integrity. Skin must be kept dry as much as possible. When tape or adhesive has been placed directly on the skin, gentle and careful removal is mandatory. Pectin-based skin barriers can be used to protect the skin from tape. If enteral feedings are expected to be delayed beyond 3 to 5 days, total parenteral nutrition should be instituted to prevent excessive catabolism. Otherwise, feedings may generally start when bowel sounds are present, stools are being passed normally, and the gastric drainage clears and lessens in amount (Zenk, 1999).

Ostomy Care.

Infants with ostomies require special management. The primary diagnoses leading to fecal diversion in infants are necrotizing enterocolitis, imperforate anus, and Hirschsprung's disease. A colostomy/ileostomy/jejunostomy is formed surgically by opening part of bowel to the outside of the abdomen for the evacuation of feces. It may be temporary or permanent, depending on the indication for surgery. The opening is called a stoma, which is made from the innermost lining of the intestine. Stomas are insensate (no sensory nerves) and incontinent (no sphincter control) and usually shrink for the first 6 to 8 weeks after surgery. If there is more than one stoma, the proximal stoma is the functioning one and the distal stoma(s) are called mucous fistula(s). If two stomas are close together, they may both be in the same pouch. If not, the distal stomas can be covered with dry gauze.

The primary goal in ostomy care is to keep stool off of the skin. Pouching of the stomas is necessary when drainage begins, usually 1 to 2 days post-op. The area around the stoma is washed with warm water, rinsed well, and dried. Soap is not used because it may irritate the skin. The skin and stomas are observed for swelling, change in color, or bleeding. A pattern is drawn for the pectin-based skin barrier wafer and pouch and is used to further pouch changes. The opening of the pouch is cut out so it fits up close to the stoma with no peristomal skin exposed to stool. If the hole is cut too large, stool will leak out and irritate skin or cause the wafer to lose its seal. If the pattern size is too small, the pouch's wafer will sit on the wet stoma, and the pouch will not stick. The hole in the wafer should not be more than 1/8 inch larger than the stoma and the hole in

the pouch should be about 1/4 inch larger than the hole in the wafer. The wafer is applied to the skin and the pouch is applied to the top of the wafer. The bottom of the pouch is folded and tied with a rubber band.

The length of time that the pouch stays on depends on how active the baby is, how liquid the stool is, and how "budded" the stoma is. Usually an infant pouch will stay on 2 to 4 days. To improve the pouch's seal, the peristomal skin needs to be dry before applying the pouch and the pouch held in place for 5 minutes after applying. The bag is emptied as needed, usually when it is a third to half full. If it gets too full, it may break the seal for the wafer and cause the pouch to come off.

Complications.

The short bowel (short gut) syndrome is an unfortunate complication of many neonatal surgeries that involve extensive resection of the GI tract. The loss of considerable absorptive surface results in a complex malabsorptive problem with episodic diarrhea, steatorrhea, and dehydration, which, if allowed to progress, may cause metabolic derangements and ultimately poor growth and development. In the presence of short bowel syndrome, a 1 to 2 year hospitalization may not be unusual. The duration of initial hospitalization and length of dependence on parenteral nutrition are both inversely related to the length of remaining bowel (Chaet et al, 1994). Most infants eventually experience progressive small bowel adaptation, and the surgically shortened intestine grows; the mucosal wall hypertrophies; and the villi become hyperplastic so that the absorptive area is increased. Blood flow to the residual intestine and the proportion of the villus that is enzymatically active are both initially increased but gradually decline as the surface area and length continue to increase with time (Swaniker et al, 1995). However, completely normal absorption may never be achieved in cases of extensive resection in which less than 75 cm of the bowel remains (the approximate length of the small intestine in the normal newborn is 200 cm), particularly when the ileocecal valve has also been removed. General survival is considered possible with as little as 11 cm of residual jejunoileum if the ileocecal valve is intact and with as little as 25 cm when the valve is removed. Perhaps owing to improved techniques and advances in enteral nutrition to stimulate the adaptation response, one case has recently been reported of a survivor with 12 cm of jejunum without an ileocecal valve (Surana et al, 1994). Infants with massive resection and those who demonstrate no spontaneous adaptation after 6 to 12 months (refractory short bowel syndrome) may require radical surgery to slow intestinal transit (e.g., intestinal valves, reversed segment, colon interposition, intestinal pacing or even intestinal transplantation) or increase mucosal surface area (e.g., intestinal lengthening, tapering enteroplasty, neomucosa, small bowel transplantation) and thus increase absorption. Whatever the means, until the intestine adapts and full oral feedings have been achieved, the nurse should work collaboratively with others to monitor fluid and electrolyte status and the calories and nutrients taken in. Prevention of skin breakdown (due to diarrhea) and infection are critical. Parents must be involved in their infant's care, and every effort must be made to stimulate normal growth and development.

Support of Parents.

The birth of an infant with a congenital anomaly or the birth of an infant who is acutely ill elicits feelings of loss, guilt, and confusion for parents. Nurses must expect grief reactions and help the family cope with the crisis. Strategies to help parents cope include support for early contact between parents and infant and explanation with factual information of the infant's condition and plan of care. The lines of communication must be kept open to reinforce information that the family has not been able to process and to assist the family in responding to their grief. Understanding of the disease process is essential for parents to deal later with the prognosis and ongoing health care needs.

CONSIDERATION OF ETHICAL ISSUES

Congenital malformations rarely occur in isolation. When another defect or organ system dysfunction places a major threat on life, decisions regarding the timing of surgical intervention must be made. For example, repair of a serious heart lesion may necessarily precede repair of esophageal atresia, but the resection of necrotic bowel must precede both conditions. Such scheduling decisions are made difficult when it is recognized that some conditions may be improved only at the expense of others. Even when surgical correction of GI dysfunction can be achieved successfully, in the face of multiple malformations (which may not be equally amenable to operative treatment or may result in early demise), the appropriateness of intervention must be reevaluated. Each affected newborn deserves individual consideration. The wishes of the parents and the opinion of each member of the management team must be considered.

MANAGEMENT OF PROBLEMS WITH INGESTION

Cleft Palate and Cleft Lip
Pathophysiology. Although cleft lip and cleft palate are often associated, these defects are embryologically distinct disorders. Cleft lip occurs when the maxillary process fails to merge with the medial nasal elevation on one or both sides. Cleft palate occurs when the lateral palatine processes fail to meet and fuse with each other, the primary palate, or the nasal septum. When both cleft lip and cleft palate occur together, studies indicate that the failure of the secondary palate to close may be a developmental consequence of the abnormalities in the primary palate associated with the cleft lip rather than an intrinsic defect in the secondary palate. It is possible, therefore, that isolated cleft lip and cleft lip with an associated cleft palate represent varying degrees of the same embryologic defect.

Risk Factors
Cleft lip with or without an associated cleft palate affects 14 of every 10,000 newborns, with rates higher in males than in females and in Asians than in whites. In contrast, isolated cleft palate has a lower incidence rate of 4 in 10,000 infants, occurs more frequently in females, and has no clear racial variation. Although rates of recurrence risks indicate that genetic factors are often involved, environmental factors also appear to contribute in some way, thus indicating a multifactorial mode of inheritance.

Maternal medication during the first trimester—especially benzodiazepines, phenytoin, opiates, penicillin, salicylates, and cortisone, including high doses of vitamin A—has been associated with clefting. Occurrence of fever and influenza during the first trimester has also been demonstrated as a possible factor; however, it is questionable as to whether the viral agent or the therapeutic drugs are the causative factors. Threatened abortion in the first and second trimesters and premature delivery of neonates with clefts has also been reported, but it is un-

certain whether this indicates an unfavorable intrauterine environment or simply a symptom of an already malformed fetus (e.g., Pierre Robin syndrome or sequence). An association between clefting and variables such as maternal smoking, maternal diabetes, hypovitaminosis, and hypervitaminosis—especially of vitamin A—has also been supported. Maternal age, however, does not appear to be a factor, although there may be a small but nonsignificant increase in the incidence of clefting with increasing paternal age (Ryckman & Balistreri, 2002; Spilson et al, 2001).

Clearly, cleft lip or cleft palate—or both—can have multiple causes and consequently may represent a malformation, a disruption, or a deformation. When the defect is the result of an inherently abnormal developmental process, as in the case of genetic derangement, it is appropriately called a malformation. An example is pits within the lower lip that lead to a cleft associated with Van der Woude syndrome, autosomal dominant condition. Holoprosencephaly is associated with a median cleft lip. Smith-Lemli-Opitz syndrome is another condition that has deviations along the palatal ridges and can result in a cleft palate. When the developmental process is originally normal but goes awry because of extrinsic factors, as in the case of teratogenic exposure, it is called a disruption. Lastly, when mechanical forces interfere with normal development, as in the case of Pierre Robin syndrome or sequence—in which mandibular hypoplasia causes the tongue to be posteriorly displaced, thus interfering with the fusion of the lateral palatine shelves—the result is called a deformation.

Clinical Manifestations. Generally defined, cleft lip is the term that signifies a congenital fissure in the upper lip, whereas cleft palate indicates a congenital fissure in either the soft palate alone or in both the hard and soft palates. The two conditions may occur in isolation or together. Isolated cleft lip may be either unilateral or bilateral and may range in severity from a slight notch in the lip to a complete cleft into the nostril. Isolated cleft palate may also be unilateral or bilateral and may be as mild as a submucous cleft characterized by a notch at the posterior edge of the hard palate, an imperfect muscle union across the palate, a thin mucosal surface, and a bifid uvula. In this mild form, the diagnosis may never be made. Combined clefts of the lip and palate are the most severe form of the defect, particularly if they are bilateral.

Differential Diagnosis. The major condition that requires differential diagnosis is van der Woude's syndrome, which is inherited as an autosomal dominant trait. This syndrome ranges in appearance from a single, barely visible lower lip depression to frank pits or fistulas usually occurring in pairs on the vermilion of the lower lips, with clefting of the lip with or without palate involvement (Jones & Fletcher, 1996).

Prognosis. Although an excellent prognosis for survival can be expected, an individual born with a cleft defect is faced with more than just a cosmetic problem. Language and speech tend to be retarded in affected individuals. This retardation is further compounded by the fact that hearing impairment is more frequent in these individuals. Olfactory defects have also been demonstrated in males with cleft palate; however, females appear to be affected less frequently. Dental problems, such as malocclusion, irregularity of the teeth, and increased frequency of caries, may also be encountered in affected individuals. Although the majority of cases of cleft lip or palate, or both, are not associated with any recognizable syndrome, there are more than 154 syndromes that include cleft lip or palate, or both, as a feature. Obviously, the prognosis in such cases varies with the associated anomalies involved.

Collaborative Management.

The management of an individual born with a cleft defect is beyond the capabilities of any one professional. Rather, effective care requires the services of a team of individuals: pediatrician, plastic surgeon, audiologist, speech pathologist, dental specialist, geneticist, social worker, and nursing personnel at various levels.

Surgical repair is a priority—not only to achieve closure of the defect but also to minimize maxillary growth retardation, to limit dental deformity, and to allow normal speech development. If the infant is healthy and no complications are expected, a cleft lip can be repaired at about 3 months of age. Repair of an associated cleft palate is generally postponed until a later time to allow medial movement of the palatal shelves, which appears to be initiated by lip closure. Depending on the involvement, palate closure may occur as a two-step process, with the hard palate being corrected at 14 to 16 months of age, followed by soft palate repair at 18 to 20 months of age. If additional repair of the lip or nose is required for aesthetic purposes, it is postponed until sufficient structural growth has been achieved, generally after 12 years of age. Emotional preparation of the parents is frequently the most immediate and demanding nursing problem encountered. The birth of a defective child comes as both a shock and a disappointment to the parents. Information and reassurance are desperately needed at this critical time. Nurses can also provide a role model to influence the parents' attitude toward the child positively and to provide guidance and support as the family copes with the reactions of others.

Feeding is another important aspect in the care of an infant with cleft lip or palate and is one that requires a great deal of patience and attention to technique. In the presence of cleft lip, the infant may have difficulty not only in holding the nipple in the mouth but also in creating the vacuum necessary for adequate sucking. The bottle should be held securely and the cheeks grasped so that the cleft is pushed closed. Even then, large amounts of air may be swallowed; therefore frequent burping should be performed. The infant with cleft palate should be held in an upright or semi-upright position to avoid choking, and the flow of milk should be directed to the side of the mouth. Use of a "preemie" nipple or a special cleft palate nipple may also be helpful. Frequent, small feedings help in preventing fatigue and frustration. Breastfeeding is certainly possible, although considerable creativity may be required. A pillow placed between the infant's back and the mother's arm can maintain the infant in an upright position. Because the clefted areas easily become encrusted with milk and are therefore prone to excoriation and infection, a small amount of sterile water should be offered after each feeding.

Esophageal Atresia and Tracheoesophageal Fistula

Pathophysiology. Esophageal atresia and tracheoesophageal (TE) fistula occur when the trachea fails to differentiate and separate from the esophagus. The atresia appears most likely to be the result of either a spontaneous posterior deviation of the esophagotracheal septum or some mechanical force that pushes the dorsal wall of the foregut in an anterior direction. A fistula occurs when the lateral ridges of the septum fail to close completely in their normal zipper-like fashion so that a communication is left between the foregut and the primitive respiratory tree.

Risk Factors. Esophageal atresia with or without TE fistula occurs approximately once in every 4500 live births (Ryckman & Balistreri, 2002). Although rare cases of familial occurrence have been reported, most cases represent an accident of embryology. A history of maternal polyhydramnios is reported in 14% to 90% of cases. The higher rates are found with an isolated esophageal atresia; the lower rates are found when a fistula allows passage of swallowed amniotic fluid around the obstruction. Associated malformations are present in 30% to 70% of infants. Congenital heart disease is reported most frequently (25% to 40%), with ventricular and atrial septal defects being the most common lesions. Other associated anomalies include vertebral malformations (25% to 30%), atresias of the small intestine (5%), imperforate anus (10% to 20%), and genitourinary anomalies (10% to 21%). Approximately 15% present as part of the VATER association. This acronym represents a complex of V-vertebral and ventricular septal defects, anal A-atresia, TE-tracheoesophageal fistula with E-esophageal atresia, and radial and renal anomalies. Some experts describe the same cluster of symptoms but use VACTERL association. The C stands for congenital heart defects, and the L is for limb deformities. Overall, 20% to 30% of these infants are premature or small for gestational age, but in the case of isolated esophageal atresia, the incidence of prematurity approaches 50%.

Clinical Manifestations. Although the infant may appear well at birth, oral secretions and saliva collect in the upper esophageal pouch and appear in the mouth and around the lips because effective swallowing is not possible. The typical description of "excessive" secretions, however, is a misnomer. The body does not produce greater amounts of secretions; they simply cannot be handled properly and thus become more visible. Respiratory difficulty may be encountered if the secretions and mucus fill the esophageal pouch and overflow into the upper airway or find their way into the trachea through a proximal fistula. Any attempts at feeding are generally accompanied by coughing, choking, and cyanosis. If a distal fistula is present, crying may force air into the stomach, where it collects and causes progressive distention. This gastric distention may impede diaphragmatic excursions, thus leading to worsening respiratory status or a reflux of gastric contents back up through the fistula into the trachea. If there is no distal fistula, the abdomen is more likely to appear scaphoid owing to the lack of swallowed air. True vomiting is not possible (except in the case of an isolated TE fistula) because the esophagus and stomach are not connected. This triad of "excessive" secretions, reflux, and respiratory distress, particularly in association with a maternal history of polyhydramnios, indicates esophageal atresia until proved otherwise (Ryckman & Balistreri, 2002). However, the clinical presentation may vary slightly, depending on the specific type of anomaly found (Figure 26-2). Although there are five major pathologic types of esophageal atresia with or without TE fistula, approximately 100 subtypes have been described (Lambrecht & Kluth, 1994).

Differential Diagnosis. Diagnosis of esophageal atresia is confirmed by attempting to pass a radiopaque catheter from the nares through the esophagus into the stomach. If the esophagus is atretic, the catheter cannot be advanced further than a depth of approximately 9 to 12 cm before meeting re-

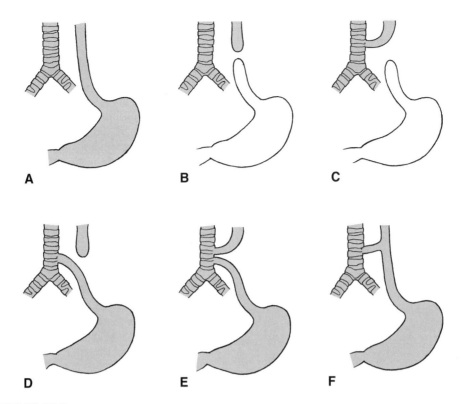

FIGURE **26-2**
Esophageal atresia and transesophageal (TE) fistula. Shading represents areas of lucency typically found on radiographs. Percentages reflect relative occurrence. A, Normal. B, Isolated esophageal atresia (8%), characterized by excessive salivation. C, Esophageal atresia with proximal TE fistula (1%), characterized by respiratory distress, especially with feeding. D, Esophageal atresia with distal TE fistula (86%), characterized by excessive salivation, respiratory distress, and reflux. E, Esophageal atresia with both proximal and distal TE fistulas (1%), characterized by respiratory distress, especially with feeding, and reflux. F, Isolated (H-type) TE fistula (4%), characterized by respiratory distress, especially with feeding, and reflux. Data from Cassani VL (1984). Tracheoesophageal anomalies. *Neonatal network, 3*(2), 20-27; Desjardins JG (1987). Esophageal atresia. In L Stern, P Vert (Eds.), *Neonatal medicine,* New York: Masson Publishing; Sunshine P et al (1983). The gastrointestinal system. In AA Faranoff, RJ Martin (Eds.), *Behrman's neonatal-perinatal medicine: diseases of the fetus and infant,* ed 3, St Louis: Mosby.

sistance, and any contents that are aspirated are alkaline rather than acidic. A chest radiograph shows the tube ending or coiling in the upper esophageal pouch (Figure 26-3). Air in the bowel indicates the presence of a distal TE fistula. If the abdomen is airless, no such fistula is present. Contrast studies are generally contraindicated owing to the danger of aspiration but may become necessary in the diagnosis of an isolated or H-type TE fistula. In these cases, which are more difficult to diagnose, bronchoscopy or endoscopy may be required to allow direct visualization of the fistulous site.

Prognosis.   With early diagnosis and efforts to prevent aspiration pneumonia, most fullterm infants do well, with a survival rate of 97%. However, mortality dramatically increases in the presence of prematurity or associated major anomalies, particularly cardiac disease. When birth weight is less than 1500 g or when major cardiac disease is present, survival is approximately 60%. When both conditions are present, survival falls to 22%. Morbidity and mortality rates depend very much on coexisting conditions such as syndromes or associations. In premature infants with coexisting conditions, mortality is about 50% (Ryckman & Balistreri, 2002).

Collaborative Management.   Surgical correction involves esophageal anastomosis (esophagoesophagostomy) and obliteration of any fistula that is present. The exact technique varies with the type of defect present, but if a great distance separates the two ends of the esophagus, the repair is made more difficult and must often be staged. In this case, the ends may be brought into closer approximation either preoperatively by stretching the upper esophageal pouch daily with a bougie to produce progressive elongation or intraoperatively by performing multiple circular myotomies so that the upper esophageal segment can be lengthened in a telescoping fashion. Alternatively, a combination of the two methods may be used. If these procedures are not effective or if the gap is particularly large, a segment of the small or large intestine or an inverted tube of gastric tissue may be used for esophageal replacement. Such a dramatic procedure is generally delayed until 1 year of age. When the gap makes primary repair impossible, the upper esophageal pouch can be brought to the surface as a cervical esophagostomy ("spit fistula") to allow the drainage of saliva, with gastrostomy performed for feeding. In these protracted cases, sham feeding may be attempted, wherein orally fed milk is collected with saliva in the ostomy bag attached to the

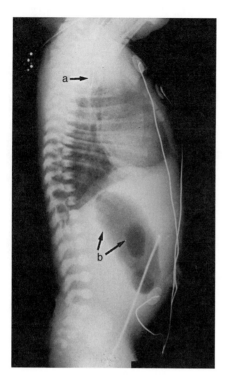

FIGURE 26-3
Coexisting atresia with TE fistula and duodenal atresia. Catheter (A) is seen curled in the upper esophageal pouch. Air in abdomen indicates presence of a distal TE fistula. The "double bubbles" (B) characteristic of duodenal atresia appear to overlie one another on this lateral film. This infant survived surgical repair but later died as a result of multiple congenital anomalies.

esophagostomy stoma and refed through the gastrostomy tube into the stomach (Kimura & Soper, 1994).

Generally, repair is performed through an incision at the base of the neck, but if the lesion is exceptionally low within the chest, a thoracic approach may be used, thus necessitating chest tube placement. A gastrostomy may also be performed to allow feeding during healing (Kemmotsu et al, 1995).

Preoperative care is focused primarily on the reduction of symptoms. To prevent overflow of secretions, a sump catheter (Replogle's tube) is placed in the upper esophageal pouch and connected to low intermittent suction. The tube lumen becomes easily occluded by tenacious secretions and should therefore be changed daily. Catheter irrigation is potentially dangerous and is not recommended. If the secretions are particularly thick, humidified air may assist in liquefying them for easier removal. Elevating the head 30 to 40 degrees helps avoid reflux of gastric secretions into the trachea via a distal fistula. Comfort measures to prevent crying reduce the amount of air swallowed through the fistula, thus limiting gastric distention and further reducing the risk of reflux. If no TE fistula is present, a flat or head-down position may be preferable to avoid gravity drainage of saliva from an overflowing esophageal pouch. The intravenous route should give fluids and electrolytes. Supplemental oxygen and intubation may be needed if respiratory distress occurs. However, use of positive-pressure ventilation increases the propensity for gastric distention and may even necessitate preoperative gastrostomy for decompression.

Postoperatively, vital signs are monitored closely, and frequent assessment is made to look for potential leaking at the anastomotic site. If a chest tube has been placed, such leakage presents as persistent or increased drainage. The endotracheal

tube is generally left in place for at least 24 hours to allow full recovery from anesthesia and relaxants. For suctioning of the airway, the catheter should be well marked and inserted to a predetermined depth above the site to avoid disruption or trauma. The quantity and appearance of secretions and any respiratory difficulties are reported. Feeding by gastrostomy may be started within 48 hours, with oral feedings generally withheld for 5 to 10 days to ensure healing. Gastroesophageal reflux is a common complication because of the upward pull on the lower esophageal pouch and stomach and generally poor peristalsis, occurring in 50 to 75% of infants, and should be managed as described in the next section. Postoperative complications that are frequently seen arising over time include stricture of the anastomosis (40% to 50%) and recurrence of the fistula (5% to 12%). Support and communication are the cornerstones of parental care throughout hospitalization (Ein & Shandling, 1994; Gutierrez et al, 1994; Ravelli et al, 1994).

Gastroesophageal Reflux (GER)
Pathophysiology. Gastroesophageal (GE) reflux is the effortless retrograde passage of acidic gastric contents from the stomach into the esophagus. The term chalasia, refers to an abnormal relaxation of the gastroesophageal junction.

The distal esophagus possesses a physiologic sphincter, which is approximately 0.5 cm long in the infant, called the esophageal vestibule. In adults, the upper portion of the esophagus lies in the thorax, the middle section at the diaphragm, and the lower segment in the abdomen. This segment of terminal esophagus has a higher pressure than that of the stomach below or the esophagus above and helps prevent retrograde flow of gastric contents into the esophagus. LES tone normally increases in response to abdominal pressure, thus protecting against reflux. In infants, this protective mechanism is less effective because the LES is primarily above the diaphragm and subjected to intrathoracic pressure. Immature LES in the preterm infant may not allow effective pressure to be generated and may cause inappropriate relaxation of the muscle. LES pressure remains low for the first 2 weeks of life and increases markedly between 2 to 4 weeks. Adult LES pressures are achieved usually between 12 to 15 months of life. By 18 to 24 months, the esophagus has grown such that the LES is below the diaphragm. Any condition delaying or altering the maturation of this valve may cause reflux of stomach contents in the infant.

Infants are at greater risk for GER because of altered esophageal motility and peristalsis; LES position and immaturity; limited gastric volume and delayed gastric emptying; and impaired intestinal motility.

Risk Factors. Premature infants are at risk for junction may not mature normally, and reflux into the esophagus may continue. Approximately 50% of healthy infants at the age of 2 months may have symptomatic reflux. Regurgitation peaks at 3 months of age and usually resolves by 6 to 12 months of age (Khalaf et al, 2001; Orenstein et al, 1999). The incidence of GE reflux in preterm infants is believed to be higher than term healthy infants recorded at 63% by Khalaf et al (2001). Symptomatic GE reflux has been reported in 3% to 10% of very-low-birth-weight infants (VLBW) (<1500 grams). Comparing outcomes at one year of age in 375 VLBW infants with GE reflux and 345 matched controls, Fuloria et al (2000) found no increased risk of delayed growth or development. Few studies have looked at long-term outcomes of VLBW infants with GE reflux. Researchers need to examine the increased risk of growth or development of these infants.

Infants with high bowel obstructions have delayed maturation of the valve mechanism and are at risk for chalasia resulting from structural weakness. Most infants with congenital diaphragmatic hernia experience reflux after repair—most likely caused by deviation of the esophagus to the affected side, malposition of the stomach, increased intraabdominal pressure, gastric dysmotility, or a combination of these factors. Additionally, infants who have undergone operative repair of tracheoesophageal fistula and/or esophageal atresia have extremely high incidence of GER; as do infants with congenital abdominal wall defects. A high percentage of infants with neurologic damage exhibit GE reflux, possibly due to reduced swallowing frequency and weaker esophageal sphincter control.

Some medications such as diazepam, calcium-channel blockers, theophylline, caffeine, and anticholinergics may worsen GE reflux. (Khalaf et al, 2001).

Clinical Manifestations.

GER may be asymptomatic; present with nonspecific symptoms such as inconsolability, irritability, sleep distrubance, food refusal, and failure to thrive; or present with more obvious symptoms of postprandial regurgitation or vomiting. It has also been implicated in the pathogenesis of apnea, hoarse cry, stridor, reactive airway disease, recurrent bronchopulmonary infections, BPD, chronic lung disease, and ventilator dependence (Ng & Quak, 1998). Persistent vomiting due to GE reflux often leads to failure to thrive. Such infants tend to be pale, thin, hypoactive, listless, and underweight and may be misdiagnosed with a nutritional deficiency.

The most commonly recognized pulmonary symptom associated with GE reflux is recurrent aspiration pneumonia. It is characterized by fever, cough, poor appetite, and typical findings on radiography.

Apneic spells, most commonly seen in the early weeks of life, may be caused by reflux. Gastroesophageal reflux is capable of causing laryngospasm, with cardiac slowing or arrest. Acid in the esophagus can lead to apnea or bronchospasm with wheezing or stridor. Worsening of chronic lung disease or BPD has also been associated with GER. Near Sudden Infant Death Syndrome (SIDS) episodes have been linked with GER, although the associated is unclear. Well-documented recurrent apneic spells have been completely eliminated in many cases after antireflux surgery. Asthma or asthma-like symptoms related to reflux are rare during the first year of life but have been seen occasionally in infants.

Esophagitis is generally not seen in the early months of life. Infants who suffer from esophagitis caused by GE reflux are usually fussy, irritable, and colicky. Frank bleeding is rare but may be present with anemia and guaiac-positive stools.

Healthy premature infants often demonstrate behavior that in symptomatic older infants is associated with acid reflux but in the preterm infant is not reflux (Snel et al, 2000). Reflux specific behavior such as irritability, crying, or grimacing that is established in older term infants may be inappropriate as diagnostic criteria for GER in preterm infants and may lead to unnecessary use of antireflux medications.

Differential Diagnosis.

Differential diagnosis includes ruling out other causes of vomiting, such as distal outlet obstruction as in pyloric stenosis or antral web; vovulus; intussusception; meconium ileus/plug; Hirchsprung disease; sepsis; abnormalities of amino acid metabolism such as urea cycle defects, galactosemia, congenital adrenal hyperplasia; increased intracranial pressure; necrotizing enterocolitis; gastroenteritis; formula intolerance; pancreatitis; cholecystitis; pyelonephritis; hydronephrosis; rumination; and drug toxicity.

Prognosis.

Most infants can be safely treated medically for 3 months before it may be judged that conservative therapy has failed. Seventy-five percent recover when treated medically; 10% to 15% require prolonged medical management; and 10% to 15% require surgery. When symptoms are controlled by medical means, reflux ceases by 15 months of age and therapy can be discontinued. Surgical long-term results are good, with reported 95% total clinical cures assessed at check-ups after 10 years or more. Adverse side effects, including mild gas bloating, slow eating, and inability to burp or vomit, are seen in approximately one third of surgically treated patients.

Collaborative Management.

A multidisciplinary approach in the assessment of the infant with GER and its related problems is important in the diagnostic process. The history, physical examination, and test results of upper GE series or pH probe testing confirm or deny the diagnosis. Nursing and medical collaboration is necessary to assess the effectiveness of conservative treatment modalities. These methods include position, thickening of feedings, monitoring for apnea, pharmacologic management, and parental support.

A 30-degree prone or left lateral position after feedings is better than the upright and supine positions, when the infant is both awake and asleep. Contrary to popular thinking, infants placed in infant seats have 50% more reflux episodes that last twice as long as those that occur in the prone position. Slouching increases pressure on the stomach and the risk of reflux. When infants are positioned in infant seats or car seats, their trunks must be supported to minimize abdominal compression. Kangaroo care has been antecdotally reported to offer benefit by holding the infant in a prone elevated position (Roller, 1999). Positioning the infant at a 45 to 60 degree angle during feedings has been shown to reduce reflux.

Thickened feedings with 1 tablespoon of rice cereal added to 1 to 2 ounces formula may reduce vomiting and crying and increase sleep time after feedings for some infants. Thickened feedings have not been shown to reduce reflux during concurrent pH probe studies unless the infants were also in an elevated prone position. For some infants, thickened feedings increases the length of reflux episodes, thus causing increased coughing and pulmonary complications.

Apneic episodes and recurrent aspiration pneumonia have been associated with GER. Infants suspected of and documented as having clinically significant reflux should therefore undergo continuous respiratory monitoring. This monitoring is particularly important when xanthines are used to treat the apnea. Although xanthines are used to improve respiratory function and reduce apnea, they also increase gastric acid secretion and decrease lower esophageal sphincter pressure, which may further increase GER (Young & Mangum, 2001).

Antacids and H2 antagonists (cimetidine, famotidine, or ranitidine) are used to reduce acidity and associated esophageal pain and damage from acid reflux. Omeprazole, a proton pump antagonist, blocks acid production. It has been used in infants with severe esophagitis who do not respond to other agents. The pharmacologic mainstay of treatment for GER is metoclopramide, a dopamine receptor antagonist, which decreases gastric emptying time and enhances LES pressure. It has a narrow therapeutic range with onset of 30 to 34 minutes. Extrapyradimal side effects sometimes include restlessness, lethargy, and abnormal posturing. Cisapride, a prokinetic agent that enhances gastric motility was widely used in the 1980s and 1990s to manage GE reflux in infants. Concern about its use in preterm infants due to prolonged QT intervals prompted warning from the Federal Drug Administration and to the subsequent discontinuance of use. Once medication is begun, the infant must still be monitored carefully for apnea and regurgitation. Cisapride has not effectively decreased the incidence of apnea (Kimball & Carlton, 2001).

If medical management fails to control life-threatening complications, surgical intervention is indicated. Although many procedures have been devised, the Nissen fundoplication is most widely used in the neonate. In this procedure, the proximal stomach is wrapped around the distal esophagus, creating a junction that is effective in preventing reflux. Infants may have a temporary gastrostomy placed to vent swallowed air and decreased bloating. The tube is usually removed after 3 to 6 weeks. Rate of revision of the fundoplication has been reported to be as high as 24%; the highest failure occurs in infants with associated anomalies such as TEF, lung abnormalities, CDH, and neurologic disorders.

Parental support is essential in nursing management of the infant with GER. The nurse can help parents to identify feeding and position and soothing techniques. Parents need to learn the etiology of GER and its usual course as well as interventions, including medication administration. Parents can also be referred to local support groups or PAGER (Pediatric and Adolescent Gastroesophageal Reflux) at http://www. reflux.org/, for additional information and support.

Pyloric Stenosis

Pathophysiology. Although many cases of pyloric stenosis may be acquired postnatally, this disorder is properly referred to as congenital hypertrophic pyloric stenosis. The pathologic picture consists of marked hypertrophy of the pylorus with spasm of the muscular coat, creating a tumor-like nodule constricting the lumen of the pyloric canal. The cause is poorly understood but probably has a genetic basis with a polygenic mode of inheritance, modified by gender. The prevalence rate typically ranges from 1.5 to 4 per 1000, with higher rates in whites than in blacks. More males, specifically first-born males, have the disease than do females, and approximately 5% of affected infants are born to women who themselves have the disease (Merenstein & Gardner, 2002).

Risk Factors. Associated factors include maternal stress and anxiety, feeding practices, and antenatal exposure to doxylamine succinate-pyridoxine hydrochloride (Bendectin). Seasonal factors, such as infection, have also been reported.

Clinical Manifestations. The infant typically appears healthy for the first 2 weeks of life and then begins vomiting (nonbilious), which worsens to frequent projectile vomiting. The infant may be anxious, irritable, and excessively hungry; have decreased frequency of stool; and lose weight. Vomiting may cause dehydration, metabolic alkalosis, hypochloremia, and hypokalemia. The level of indirect bilirubin is significantly elevated in 5% of affected infants but resolves when stenosis is corrected.

Differential Diagnosis. Most cases (almost 90%) of pyloric stenosis may be clinically diagnosed by palpation of a small, olive-sized mass below the liver. However, if the mass cannot be felt, a barium swallow or ultrasound examination is indicated. The differential diagnosis of nonbilious vomiting includes sepsis, withdrawal syndromes, GER, and metabolic diseases such as organic acidemias, hyperammonemia, galactosemias, and adrenogenital syndrome.

Prognosis. Once it is diagnosed and surgically treated, the prognosis is excellent, with complete relief of symptoms. The mortality rate is less than 1%, provided that the infant has not become too dehydrated and malnourished.

Collaborative Management. Medical and nursing assessment and management of the infant are critical throughout the process of management. Diagnosis of pyloric stenosis may be made by palpation of the hypertrophied pylorus, an olive-like mass in the deep right upper quadrant of the abdomen. Most surgeons are not comfortable with palpatory findings alone and request confirmatory ultrasound before surgical intervention (Jona et al, 1998).

There is no effective medical treatment. The repair is by pyloromyotomy. A simple incision is made in the hypertrophied longitudinal and circular muscles of the pylorus, thus releasing the obstruction. Laparoscopic pyloromyotomy is an alternative, but resolution of ileus and time to discharge is not a major factor. The major advantage is in a smaller incision and cosmetically more appealing (Jona et al, 1998).

Preoperatively, as with any vomiting infant, fluid and electrolyte management is paramount. A nasogastric tube connected to low continuous suction is maintained to prevent distention and vomiting and to decrease the risk of aspiration. Vital signs are monitored every 2 to 4 hours. Thermoregulation is maintained to prevent exacerbation of symptoms.

Postoperatively, intravenous hydration and electrolyte balance must be maintained. Nasogastric suction is continued for 4 to 24 hours. The tube may be disconnected when the infant is fully awake and bowel sounds are present. Assessment of the suture line is made for signs of infection or skin breakdown. Feedings are begun when the baby is fully awake. Most babies leave the hospital within 24 hours.

MANAGEMENT OF PROBLEMS WITH DIGESTION

Biliary Atresia

Pathophysiology. Biliary atresia is the complete obstruction of bile flow due to fibrosis of the extrahepatic ducts. It is the most common form of ductal cholestasis and occurs in approximately 1 in every 10,000 births, with a female predominance. The cause remains unclear. Some clinicians theorize that the obstruction is due to injured bile ducts leading to atresia; others describe the disease as an inflammatory process, whereas still others propose an intrauterine insult from environmental factors or failure of ducts to recanalize. Pathologically, the obstruction of the common bile duct prevents bile from entering the duodenum. Consequently, digestion and absorption of fat are impaired, thus leading to deficiencies in fat-soluble vitamins and vitamin K, which impact bleeding tendencies. Owing to the obstruction, bile accumulates in the ducts and gallbladder and causes distention of these structures. The atresia appears to progress to the intrahepatic ducts, thus leading to biliary cirrhosis and ultimately death if the bile flow is not established.

Risk Factors. Associated congenital defects, found in 15% of reported cases, include congenital heart disease, polysplenic syndrome, small bowel atresia, bronchobiliary atresia, and trisomies 17 and 18. Teratogenic factors include ionizing radiation, drugs, ischemic episode, and viruses such as reovirus type 3, cytomegalovirus, rubella, and hepatitis A and B.

Clinical Manifestations.   Infants appear normal at birth and pass stools with appropriate pigmentation. Clinical signs are subtle, with jaundice persisting after the first week of life. The direct bilirubin level slowly increases and results in a greenish bronze appearance of the skin. Gradually stools become clay-colored to pale to yellowish tan, and the urine becomes dark as the result of bile excretion.

Over a 2 to 3-month period, the liver becomes cirrhotic. Portal hypertension is a major complication. The reverse blood flow results in enlargement of esophageal, umbilical, and rectal veins, which is manifested as splenomegaly, hemorrhoids, enlarged abdominal veins, ascites, and blood in the stools. Additional complications include decreased clotting ability, anemia, and ineffective metabolism of nutrients. End-stage liver disease may lead to rupture of veins in the esophagus and stomach or hepatic coma with eventual death from liver failure.

Differential Diagnosis.   Multiple causes of cholestasis in the infant exist. All causes must be considered in the presence of conjugated hyperbilirubinemia, other causes excluded, and proper therapy instituted. The differential diagnosis includes neonatal hepatitis, choledochal cyst, errors of metabolism, trisomies 18 and 21, α_1-antitrypsin deficiency, neonatal hypopituitarism, cystic fibrosis, TORCH infectious agents (the acronym representing toxoplasma, rubella, cytomegalovirus, and herpes virus, with the O standing for other agents such as syphilis), bacterial sepsis, drug-induced cholestasis, and cholestasis associated with parenteral nutrition.

Prognosis.   Survival in untreated cases of biliary atresia is less than 2 years. Approximately 25% to 35% of patients with a Kasai portoenterostomy will survive more than 10 years without liver transplantation. One third of the patients drain bile but develop complications of cirrhosis and require liver transplantation before the age of 10. The remaining third of patients have bile flow that is inadequate after the Kasai procedure and develop fibrosis and cirrhosis. The overall survival rate after the Kasai procedure and transplantation is >73%. (Bates et al, 1998). Sequential surgical treatment of Kasai portoenterostomy in infancy followed by selective liver transplantation for children with progressive hepatic deterioration yield improved overall survival. Limited donor availability and increased complications after liver transplantation in infants less than 1 year of age mitigate against the use of primary liver transplantation without prior Kasai procedure in infants with biliary atresia (Ryckman et al, 1998).

Predictors of poor outcome after portoenterostomy include operative age >2 months of age, presence of cirrhosis at first biopsy, total nonpatency of extrahepatic ducts, absence of bile ducts at transected liver hilus, and subsequent development of varices or ascites.

Collaborative Management.   Medical, surgical, and nursing staff must strive diligently in the diagnostic work-up and ultimate treatment. Consultation and follow-up care by a gastroenterologist provides guidance for feeding and drug therapy modalities. Parents of these infants can profit from ongoing

support from social services, chaplains, or support counseling sources.

Surgical intervention involves a hepatic portoenterostomy, called the Kasai procedure, which consists of dissection and resection of the extrahepatic bile duct. The porta hepatis, where the ducts normally occur, is cut, and a loop of bowel is brought up to permit bile drainage from the liver surface to the GI tract. If the Kasai procedure is unsuccessful, the only alternative for treatment is transplantation (Chapter 38).

Nurses take an active role in the complex task of diagnosis and treatment of the infant with biliary atresia. Because of the portal hypertension and bleeding tendencies, careful monitoring of vital signs and blood pressure is important. Efficient collection of multiple blood samples is required for tests, including bilirubin, aspartate transaminase (AST), alanine transaminase (ALT), alkaline phosphatase, albumin, protein, and cholesterol determinations; prothrombin time; complete blood count; reticulocyte count; Coombs' test; measurement of platelets and red blood cell morphologic features, thyroxine, thyroid-stimulating hormone, and glucose determinations; cultures; and TORCH titers. Urine is collected for urinalysis, culture, and metabolic screens. Radiography, ultrasonography, liver biopsy, and Heptaobiliary Scan (using hydroxyiminodiacetic acid) or HIDA scan may be performed. The latter is used to determine adequacy of the liver function.

Meeting nutritional requirements is difficult because the infant needs one and one-half to two times the normal caloric requirements owing to affected metabolism, yet ascites and pressure on the stomach make it difficult for the child to eat. Formulas must contain medium-chain triglycerides for easier absorption. Supplementation with fat-soluble vitamins is required because of impaired absorption. Parenteral nutrition is given to provide adequate calories. Phenobarbital, actigall, and cholestyramine may be an ongoing therapy to stimulate bile flow. Vitamin K may be given for coagulopathy.

The whole family requires comprehensive psychosocial support. Family and work life are disrupted by lengthy, repeated hospitalizations. The emotional and physical toll is high because of complex care demands, and dealing with the suffering of the child places further stress on the parents. Social support systems need to be explored to assist families in dealing with the long-term health crisis of an infant with biliary atresia.

Duodenal Atresia
Pathophysiology.   Duodenal atresia occurs as the result of incomplete recanalization of the lumen. The mechanism by which recanalization is prevented is not known but most likely occurs when the proliferative villi adhere abnormally to one another. The result is the formation of a transverse diaphragm of tissue that completely obstructs the lumen). Almost half of all duodenal or postampullary obstructions are due to duodenal atresia (Ryckman, 2002). Overall occurrence is approximately 1 in every 6,000 to 10,000 live births. Over one quarter of these cases are related to Trisomy 21 or Down Syndrome (Ryckman, 2002).

Risk Factors.   Polyhydramnios has been identified as a significant risk factor that occurs in one quarter to one half of women who deliver affected infants. Associated anomalies, present in 60% to 70% of patients, are numerous and include trisomy 21, malrotation, TE anomalies, imperforate anus, congenital heart disease, VATER or VACTERL association, and renal anomalies. An annular pancreas—resulting from the failure of the two-pancreatic buds to fuse normally, allowing the deformed pancreas to encircle the duodenum—is found in approximately 20% of patients. Nearly half of all infants are premature or of low birth weight, and 40% acquire hyperbilirubinemia (Bates & Balistreri, 2002; Ryckman, 2002).

Clinical Manifestations. The significance of polyhydramnios has been noted previously, but in its absence a large amount of gastric aspirate may be obtained on routine delivery room screening. Normally, only small amounts of aspirate are expected (4 to 7 ml), but if more than 10 to 15 ml is obtained, atresia should be suspected (Bloom, 2002).

Although atresia may be located at any point along the duodenum, most obstructions (80% to 90%) are situated below the ampulla of Vater. Consequently, bilious vomiting is a common presenting sign. Failure to pass meconium is noted in approximately 70% of patients. Both the onset of vomiting and the ability to pass stool are related to the site of obstruction. Proximal duodenal obstructions tend to present with vomiting within a few hours of birth, although stool may be passed normally. Distal obstructions tend to present with a later onset of vomiting and failure to pass stool. Abdominal distention is generally not noted, but when present is confined to the upper abdomen, thus giving the lower abdomen an almost scaphoid appearance in contrast.

Differential Diagnosis. Radiographic examination provides confirmation of duodenal atresia with the classic finding of a "double bubble" (Figure 26-3). These bubbles reflect the localization of swallowed air in the stomach and in the distended portion of the duodenum lying above the obstruction; the remainder of the bowel is totally airless. If gas is present elsewhere, other anomalies causing partial obstruction must be presumed. An upper GI series may be helpful in identifying incomplete obstructions such as duodenal stenosis, duodenal web, or annular pancreas or in ruling out associated malrotation.

Prognosis. A 65% to 84% survival rate is reported, with deaths attributed to associated cardiac or renal anomalies or to infectious or respiratory complications.

Collaborative Management. Surgical treatment involves excision of the atretic site (unless the area so closely approximates the pancreatic and bile ducts that injury to these structures is risked) and side-to-side anastomosis of the free ends. The level of the obstruction determines whether a duodenoduodenostomy or a duodenojejunostomy is carried out. A gastrostomy also is performed for decompression to avoid trauma to the anastomotic site. A combined nursing and medical approach facilitates both preoperative stabilization and postoperative recuperation.

Preoperative care is directed toward decompression and hydration. Intermittent gastric suction by use of a sump tube reduces the risk of aspiration or perforation due to over-distention. Vital signs, fluid intake and output, urine specific gravity, and serum electrolytes must be closely monitored, and fluids, electrolytes, and crystalloid must be provided as needed. Antibiotics may be instituted for preoperative prophylaxis or when perforation or sepsis is suspected.

Continued decompression and nutrition are the major postoperative concerns. Total parenteral nutrition is given initially. Oral feedings are generally begun at 10 to 14 days with an oral electrolyte solution and advance to low-osmolality formulas such as Nutramigen or Pregestimil (protein hydrosylate formulas) before moving to regular formula. Often enteral feedings will be given as jejunal ones so that it is introduced distal to the surgical site (Ryckman, 2002).

Jejunoileal Atresia

Pathophysiology. Atresias of the jejunum and ileum are thought to result from mesenteric vascular compromise with necrosis and eventual resorption of the involved area. The presence of bile, meconium, epithelial cells, and lanugo distal to the atresia indicates that this ischemic injury occurs relatively late in utero, possibly as late as 3 to 6 months' gestation (Ryckman, 2002). The occurrence rate is 1 in 20,000 live births, with an apparently equal distribution of atresias between the jejunum and the ileum. There is no linkage to gender and the development of this form of atresia (Ryckman, 2002).

Risk Factors. Owing to the surface area available for absorption proximal to the obstruction, maternal polyhydramnios does not generally present as a risk factor, as it does in the higher atresias of the esophagus and duodenum. Polyhydramnios is reported in only one third of those with jejunal atresia; ileal atresias rarely present with polyhydramnios. Because this group of defects arises after embryogenesis is complete, associated anomalies are rare. When they do occur, they are primarily restricted to the GI tract, with malrotation and meconium ileus being most common. Between 25% and 30% of patients experience hyperbilirubinemia, and 25% to 38% are born prematurely. Of the four types of jejunoileal atresia that have been identified (Figure 26-4), only the "apple peel" or "Christmas tree" type is typically familial, thus indicating that this one form alone may involve some autosomal recessive or multifactorial type of inheritance. Although it is the most rare form of jejunoileal atresia, it carries the highest mortality rate (54%) and higher rates of prematurity and malrotation in comparison with the more conventional types.

Clinical Manifestations. Signs and symptoms generally present at 1 or 2 days of age and are virtually the same for all four types of jejunoileal atresia. Presentation includes bilious vomiting, failure to pass stool, and generalized abdominal distention.

Differential Diagnosis. Abdominal radiographs show multiple bubbles that reflect dilation and collection of swallowed air proximal to the obstruction. Intraperitoneal calcifications are present in 10% of patients, which indicates antenatal intestinal perforation with resultant meconium peritonitis. The peritonitis in this case is due to chemical irritation (there is no infection because the bowel and meconium are sterile before birth), thus causing fibrosis, granuloma formation, and ultimately calcifications. The perforated site usually heals spontaneously before delivery and leaves no evidence of what occurred other than the residual calcifications. The airless, unused distal portion of the gut is generally contracted and of a much smaller caliber than normal. Visualization of this distal "microcolon" by barium or meglumine diatrizoate (Gastrografin) enema may be necessary to rule out malrotation and meconium ileus (Bates & Balistreri, 2002).

Prognosis. With the availability of parenteral alimentation, survival rates have risen to as high as 84% to 96%. Deaths

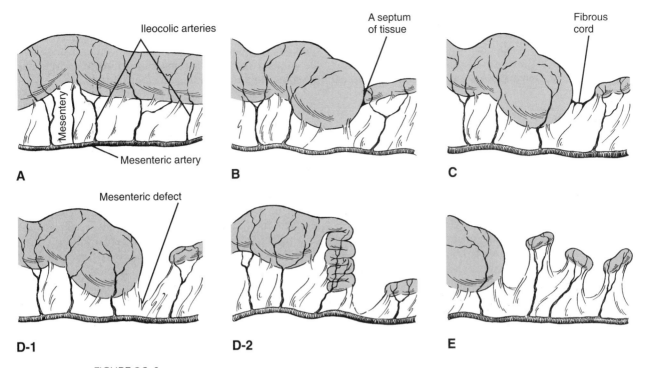

FIGURE **26-4**
Jejunoileal obstruction. Percentages reflect relative occurrence. A, Normal anatomy. B, Type I or di-aphragmatic form (20%): single atresia in which the integrity of the bowel wall is preserved, but its lumen is obstructed by a septum of tissue; the mesentery is intact. C, Type II or cord anomaly (30% to 35%): single but discontinuous atresia with opposing ends connected by a long, fibrous cord; the mesentery is intact. D-1, Type IIIa or mesenteric defect (35% to 45%): single but discontinuous atresia with a V-shaped defect in the intervening mesentery. D-2, Type IIIb or "apple peel" (<1%): single but discontinuous atresia with a V-shaped defect in the intervening mesentery; the intestine coils around a single ileocolic artery, which is its sole source of circulation. E, Type IV or multiple atresias (5% to 10%): multiple discontinuous atresias with intervening V-shaped mesenteric defects, giving it the appearance of sausage links. Data from Gryboski & Walker, 1983; Touloukian, 1978.

are generally the result of prematurity, postoperative short gut or bowel syndrome, or infectious complications.

Collaborative Management.   Surgical management begins with resection of the dilated proximal gut and atretic, bulbous ending and a search for multiple distal atresias. Primary closure by end-to-end or side-to-end anastomosis generally follows, but preliminary tapering of the distended distal segment may be required; as a third alternative, an end-to-oblique closure may be performed. However, if there is considerable discrepancy (more than 2:1) between the dilated proximal portion and the distal microcolon, an ostomy (either double-barrel or single) is created. Once surgical correction is complete, collaboration with the nutritional support team and enterostomal therapist is essential.

The principles of preoperative care involve bowel decompression and intravenous hydration with the correction of any electrolyte imbalance that may occur as the result of vomiting or third-spacing-capillary leak syndrome. Antibiotics may be given prophylactically but certainly should be used in the case of peritonitis.

Recovery of bowel peristalsis and enzymatic integrity may be delayed, thus necessitating parenteral nutrition. When started, initial feedings are of a clear electrolyte solution and progress serially to elemental formulas such as Nutramigen® or Pregestimil® (protein hydrosylate formulas) until standard formula can be tolerated. The nurses should assess diligently for

evidence of short bowel syndrome, commonly seen with atresias that are multiple or of the "apple peel" variety, which necessitate excision of an extensive length of bowel.

Omphalocele
Pathophysiology.   Omphalocele results from the failure of the intestines to return from the umbilical cord into the abdominal cavity. Because some defects can be sufficiently large that they also contain the liver and other organs that do not normally participate in the migratory process, it has been further proposed that their passage can be accommodated only when there is incomplete folding of the embryonic disk so that the future abdominal wall cannot close completely, thus resulting in an unusually large umbilical ring.

Risk Factors.   Omphalocele occurs in roughly 1 of every 5,000 to 6,000 live births, with a male predominance. Multiple and often life-threatening syndromes and anomalies occur with an unusually high frequency (50% to 77%) and include trisomy 13, trisomy 18, Beckwith-Wiedemann syndrome, pentalogy syndrome, congenital heart defects, diaphragmatic and upper midline defects, malrotation, intestinal atresia, and genitourinary anomalies. Additionally, 30% to 33% of affected infants are premature, and approximately 19% are small for gestational age (Seashore, 1978). Of the infants with a central omphalocele, about one quarter will have cardiac anomalies, especially Cantrell pentalogy (cleft sternum, anterior midline diaphragmatic defects, a pericardial defect, congenital cardiac abnormalities which may include ectopia cordis, and an upper abdominal omphalocele) (Ryckman, 2002). Lower omphaloceles are associated in some cases with Beckwith-Wiedemann syndrome (omphalocele, macroglossia, macrosomia, and hypoglycemia) (Ryckman, 2002).

Clinical Manifestations. Omphalocele is generally an immediately apparent anomaly and ranges between 2 and 15 cm in size. However, the small defects that involve perhaps a single loop of intestine may be easily overlooked unless the physical examination is carried out in an unhurried fashion and the umbilical ring is clearly absent on palpation. The larger defects generally contain the intestine and possibly the liver, spleen, stomach, bladder, ovaries and tubes, or testicles. These two extremes most likely reflect the difference in the time at which normal embryogenesis is interrupted. If the interruption is early, around the 3 to 4 week window when infolding is in its last stages, the defect is large. If the interruption occurs later, at about 9 to 10 weeks when migration is generally completed, the defect is smaller. However, in both cases, the intestine—and possibly other abdominal organs—herniate into the umbilical cord. A thin, transparent membrane composed of peritoneum and amnion covers the viscera, and the visible bowel has a normal appearance. The abdominal cavity is often relatively small and underdeveloped, having never held the growing intestine.

Differential Diagnosis. Although a membrane generally covers omphaloceles, intrauterine rupture of that membrane occurs in 11% to 23% of patients. As a consequence of prolonged exposure to the amniotic fluid, the bowel becomes matted and edematous in appearance and difficult to differentiate from gastroschisis. Closer examination may reveal the sac remnants, but if none is noted, one need only look to the base of the cord. In gastroschisis, the umbilical cord is intact, inserted normally at the abdominal wall, and separated from the defect by a small amount of skin.

Prognosis. Prenatal diagnosis has become so sophisticated that most incidences of abdominal wall defects are known well in advance of delivery. This knowledge allows preparation of the family and of the fetus. Ideally, maternal transport to a tertiary center saves the emergency situation of transporting an infant with such a defect. With the improved diagnostics, karyotyping can also be done to determine whether life-threatening chromosomal conditions exist, with the abdominal problem only being one part of the condition.

The overall mortality rate is reported as less than 5% in some cases and up to 30% in others. The mortality rate primarily depends on the size of the defect, associated chromosomal and other anomalies, early detection, and coincidental prematurity or low birth weight (Ryckman, 2002). Malrotation with the resultant danger of volvulus, ischemia, and necrosis is common. Antenatal membrane rupture may also add the dimension of potential sepsis.

Collaborative Management. If surgery is contraindicated because of coexisting chromosomal or other syndromes, the defect may be treated medically by repeatedly painting the sac with silver nitrate solution, silver sulfadiazine mercurochrome, thimerosal (Merthiolate), polymer substances, or alcohol (Ryckman, 2002). These topical agents promote eschar forma-

tion and epithelization with complete coverage by skin within 6 to 8 weeks. Should the patient survive, a later repair of the muscle wall becomes necessary. Biologic dressings have also been used to provide temporary protection. In some cases porcine and human skin grafts are also used.

The definitive surgical treatment is return of the viscera into the abdominal cavity and closure of the defect. This can be done via skin-flapp closure or staged reduction. The procedure employed varies with the size of the defect. Primary closure is preferred, but larger defects (>5 cm) may require a staged repair with a polymeric silicone (Silastic) pouch or chimney (silo) used to suspend the viscera above the patient. Reduction maneuvers are carried out daily to return the suspended organs into the relatively small abdominal cavity. A forceful return and closure under pressure would risk compression of the inferior vena cava, with reduced filling of the heart and decreased cardiac output and impedance of the diaphragmatic excursions, thus resulting in respiratory compromise. A gastrostomy to provide decompression and an appendectomy to avoid atypically presenting appendicitis in later life may be carried out with both primary and staged procedures, depending on the preferences of the surgical team. If a staged repair is performed, complete return of the organs into the abdominal cavity is generally achieved over a period of 7 to 10 days. At that time, the infant is returned to surgery for final closure of the abdominal wall.

These children often require aggressive postoperative respiratory management followed by prolonged total parenteral nutrition. Early psychosocial support of parents must be provided to promote their involvement in what is commonly an extended hospital stay. Genetic counseling may also be required.

The cornerstones of preoperative management include protection of the eviscerated organs, decompression of the gut, and hydration. Thermoregulation is a particular concern because massive evaporative and radiant heat losses may occur through the exposed defect. One researcher has reported that 44% of infants in one patient survey experienced temperatures of less than 35 degrees C (95 degrees F). Care directed in these four areas may overlap, but all are necessary. The first step is to loosely apply sterile, warmed, saline-soaked gauze in a turban style around the defect, wrapping the ends around the body. Great care must be taken to prevent tight application, which might create pressure; two fingers should fit easily between the trunk and the encircling gauze. Some clinicians suggest that an outer, dry sterile dressing also be applied. The dressing is then covered with plastic wrap. As an alternative, sterile bowel bags may be used. Both wrapping and bag techniques provide protection to the defect from trauma and infection and help limit the loss of fluids and body heat. Clearly, sterile gloves must be worn during the necessary manipulation of the bowel. If the defect is small, the infant may be positioned on the back, but if the defect is large, it may be best to place the infant on the side. In the side-lying position, a small blanket or diaper may be slipped between the covered viscera and the bed surface so that no traction is placed on the bowel, which might cause physical injury to the gut or impede circulation. A gastric tube should be passed and set to low intermittent suction for decompression. Appropriate comfort measures to reduce or prevent crying with concomitant air swallowing should also be employed. Intravenous fluids should be started immediately to counteract direct fluid losses from exposure and the loss of fluids from the circulation caused by inflammation and third-spacing. Poor venous return from the lower extremities is also a concern owing to the ever-present potential for vena cava compression. Hydration status, fluid intake and output, and vital signs should be monitored closely for any evidence of hypovolemia, such as tachycardia, thready pulses, hypotension, poor perfusion, and decreased output of urine with increased specific gravity. Umbilical catheterization for venous access is contraindicated because of the nature and site of the defect. Prophylactic antibiotic administration should also be started. Postoperative support varies slightly according to the repair procedure used, but both methods should generally include measures of hydration, decompression, and a search for evidence of increased intraabdominal pressure. Third-spacing, or capillary leak syndrome, may continue to be a problem and may actually be exacerbated by the trauma of surgical manipulation of the bowel. Assessment for signs of hypovolemia should be documented. Serum electrolytes, albumin, and total serum protein values should also be followed, with fluid and other replacements as necessary. Decompression by gastric tube or gastrostomy is generally required for a considerable time until peristaltic activity returns. Ileus and cholestasis are common following repair, so enteral feedings may be considerably delayed, and parenteral alimentation is provided during the interval. When feedings are begun, an elemental formula is used initially. Respiratory support with increased pressures may be required to achieve adequate ventilation if diaphragmatic movements are hampered. Inspection of the lower extremities and palpation of pedal pulses are helpful in assessing for impaired circulation. Elevating the extremities may promote venous return to the heart. In addition to these measures, if a staged repair is undertaken, particular attention must be paid to the infant's tolerance of daily reduction attempts. Furthermore, the silo provides an open port for bacterial invasion. Povidone-iodine or silver sulfadiazine (Silvadene) ointment may be applied with dressing changes, and most certainly antibiotic therapy is continued postoperatively.

Gastroschisis

Pathophysiology.   Gastroschisis is a full-thickness defect in the abdominal wall through which the uncovered intestines protrude. The defect is generally thought to arise as the result of incomplete lateral infolding of the embryonic disk. As a result of this primary failure, the abdominal wall is incompletely formed, allowing herniation of the gut. Three other accepted theories have also been offered. The first suggests that the umbilical coelom (cavity) fails to form, so normal herniation of the midgut into the cord cannot occur. Consequently, during its rapid growth phase the intestine ruptures through the embryonic body wall. Another view considers that a vascular accident occurring in utero leads to occlusion of the omphalomesenteric artery. With its circulation removed, the base of the cord becomes necrotic, leaving an opening through which the intestine can eviscerate. The last theory proposes that gastroschisis may simply be a variant of omphalocele, with early intrauterine rupture of its membranous covering. The membrane remnants are subsequently reabsorbed, and the umbilical cord is reformed around the offset umbilical vessels. For the last two theories, the gap between the evisceration and cord base is presumably filled in by skin.

Risk Factors.   Prematurity (58%) and low birth weight (92%); are extremely common. Malrotation is found in all affected infants, and a few may exhibit intestinal atresia, but anomalies of systems other than the GI tract are infrequent

and relatively minor. The overall incidence is approximately 1 per 30,000 to 50,000 live births. It appears to be more common in younger mothers than is omphaloceles. Nutritional alterations are noted in some mothers who give birth to an infant with gastrochisis. These changes are: α-carotine, total glutathione, and high nitrosamine intakes (Ryckman, 2002).

Clinical Manifestations.   Gastroschisis is an immediately apparent defect in the abdominal wall through which the intestine and possibly portions of the colon protrude. The liver and other solid organs generally remain in the abdominal cavity, although evisceration is possible. The defect is usually small (2 to 5 cm) and located to the right of the umbilicus, from which it is separated by a narrow margin of skin. The bowel is uncovered and, as a consequence of chemical peritonitis caused by long exposure to the amniotic fluid, appears as an edematous and matted mass with no identifiable loops. The abdominal cavity is small and underdeveloped.

Differential Diagnosis.   Although it is often confused with a ruptured omphalocele, in gastroschisis the umbilical cord is inserted normally. The defect is next to rather than in the umbilical cord, and there is no protective sac nor remnants thereof.

Prognosis.   A less than 5% mortality rate is reported for gastroschisis, with all deaths directly related to the defect. Early deaths are largely attributable to a combination of shock, sepsis (associated with perforation or contamination of the exposed bowel), and hypothermia. Profound hypothermia (temperature lower than 35 degrees C [95 degrees F]) is reported to occur in 67% of affected infants. Late deaths come as a result of sepsis, respiratory failure, and the inability of the bowel to sustain nutrition.

Collaborative Management.   Although a primary closure may be possible in gastroschisis, the majority of defects are closed by staged repair using the polymeric silicone pouch as described for omphalocele. Although gastroschisis is a smaller defect than omphalocele, the distortion of the viscera with typical thickening and edema of the bowel make primary closure more difficult. Often the defect must be surgically enlarged to allow thorough inspection of the entire length of the GI tract and to avoid restricting the passage of the eviscerated intestine back into the abdominal cavity. All display some degree of malrotation, predisposing them to both intestinal atresias and infarction. Bowel resection and anastomosis are often necessary; however, primary anastomosis is contraindicated in the face of peritonitis or inflammation. In such situations, an enterostomy is performed away from the defect, with anastomosis delayed until final closure of the abdominal wall. The visceral mass is returned to the abdominal cavity as a whole. Because of the potential for bowel injury and blood loss, no attempt is made to unravel the adherent loops of bowel.

Postoperative nutritional and respiratory support is essential. Consultation with social services is helpful in providing parental support and establishing healthy parent-child relationships. The care of patients with gastroschisis is much like that for omphalocele. The intestines should be covered to protect them from injury and to reduce the loss of fluids and heat. Gastric decompression, fluid resuscitation, and antibiotic prophylaxis round out preoperative care.

Following surgery, the major concerns are venous stasis, respiratory compromise, infection, and nutrition. Edema and cyanosis of the lower extremities and evidence of decreased cardiac output should be reported immediately. Intensive respiratory support is provided, and oxygenation and ventilation are monitored closely. Infection is prevented by careful aseptic dressing changes, daily applications of bacteriostatic solutions or ointments, and systemic administration of antibiotics. Total parenteral nutrition is generally continued for several weeks until intestinal function returns. Feedings are begun with elemental formula, eventually progressing to standard formula, with diligent assessment for evidence of intestinal obstruction during the process.

MANAGEMENT OF PROBLEMS WITH ELIMINATION

Hirschsprung Disease

Pathophysiology. Hirschsprung disease (also known as congenital megacolon or aganglionic megacolon) is an abnormality of the colon marked by the congenital absence of ganglion cells (aganglionosis). Failure of the neural crest cells to migrate in their usual craniocaudal fashion results in aberrant bowel innervation and interrupted neuromuscular conduction of the messages that promote peristalsis of the anal sphincters. This local failure of relaxation results in functional intestinal obstruction. Fecal matter accumulates in the normally innervated proximal bowel, producing dilation (megacolon) and hypertrophy of the muscular wall as normal peristaltic activity works against the obstruction. The distal, aganglionic segment is unused and may appear narrowed in relation to the proximal dilation, but it is in fact of normal caliber. Between the ganglionic proximal section and the distal aganglionic section is a "transition zone" of tapered bowel (Ryckman, 2002).

The rectum is always involved, and most cases (85%) involve the sigmoid colon as well. Rarely, aganglionosis may also be found in the upper portion of the colon or throughout the entire intestine (Stringer et al, 1994). Atypical forms of Hirschsprung disease, in which areas of normal innervation are found between aganglionic areas have also been described, but the presence of such "skip areas" is extremely rare.

The cause of the interrupted migration of ganglion cells is not known, but anoxia is often cited. The theory is that local anoxemia, because of an interference with the source of oxygen to the site, may lead to ischemia, atrophy, and regression of the cells.

Risk Factors. The incidence of Hirschsprung disease is 1 in 5,000 live births, with males predominating. Associated anomalies are relatively infrequent but include trisomy 21 and asymptomatic urologic anomalies. The ganglionic plexuses of the bowel are derived from the same craniocervical neural crest, as are the oral, facial, and cranial ganglia. Consequently, a limited number of infants may also exhibit congenital deafness and ocular neurocristopathies, most commonly in association with Waardenburg's syndrome. Approximately 5% have associated neurologic abnormalities ranging from developmental delay to mental retardation or cerebral palsy. Overall, a positive family history is found in 17% to 30% of cases but rises to 50% when total colonic aganglionosis is present (Marty et al, 1995a). The fact that more males than females are affected has caused some to theorize that a form of X-linked recessive transmission is occurring (Reyna, 1994). More recently, however, a gene has been identified on chromosome 10 that may be involved in the differentiation or proliferation, or both, of neural crest cells (Martucciello et al, 1995).

Clinical Manifestations. The signs and symptoms of Hirschsprung disease in the newborn are primarily those of intestinal obstruction, including bilious vomiting, distention, and failure to pass meconium. The rectum is empty of stool unless the aganglionic segment is very short, in which case rectal examination with the gloved little finger may cause explosive release of gas and evacuation of meconium. If the disease goes undiagnosed, fecal stagnation may lead to increased intraluminal pressures, reduced colonic blood flow, and bacterial overgrowth with resultant enterocolitis. This severe bowel irritation and inflammation may cause "overflow" diarrhea, with complicating dehydration, hypoproteinemia, electrolyte imbalance, and sometimes perforation and shock.

Differential Diagnosis. Hirschsprung disease may be clinically indistinguishable from jejunoileal atresia, meconium ileus, meconium plug syndrome, and small left colon syndrome (Stringer et al, 1994). Plain radiographic examination offers little or no help in differentiation. All conditions show large gas-filled loops of bowel consistent with intestinal obstruction. The rectum may or may not contain air, but when air is present, it generally is of a reduced amount consistent with partial or functional obstruction.

Barium contrast studies are therefore indicated to determine the caliber of the distal colon. Microcolon is typically found with jejunoileal atresia and meconium ileus, but if the colon is of normal size or somewhat enlarged, the obstruction may be the result of Hirschsprung disease, meconium plug syndrome, or small left colon syndrome. Occasionally, barium enema demonstrates the "pigtail" or "funnel" sign characteristic of Hirschsprung disease. This sign is simply a demonstration of the tapering transition zone lying between the dilated, innervated proximal segment and the normal-caliber, aganglionic distal bowel. Unfortunately, in most newborns (75%) the dilation of the proximal colon may not yet be sufficiently dramatic for visualization. When the sign is present, usually in infants older than 2 months of age, it highly suggests Hirschsprung disease, but it may also be found in small left colon syndrome; in its absence, no judgment can be made. However, the margins of the distal colon generally have a saw-toothed appearance in Hirschsprung disease, whereas smooth margins are typically described with small left colon syndrome. Retention of contrast material or barium noted by follow-up film 24 hours later is suggestive of Hirschsprung disease but may also be noted in its absence.

Anorectal manometry is often discussed in the literature as an alternative diagnostic tool. The test is performed to determine the ability of the internal sphincter to relax. Findings should not be considered conclusive but only suggestive in neonates (Ryckman, 2002). Further tests must be done to confirm the diagnosis.

Final diagnosis can be made only by suction or punch rectal biopsy through the anus and histologic examination of the specimen obtained. No anesthesia is required but sedation and pain management is use. The procedure can easily be performed in the nursery. If ganglionic bowel is obtained, either meconium plug syndrome or small left colon syndrome is possible. However, the absence of ganglionic cells in the submucosal plexus firmly establishes the diagnosis of Hirschsprung disease. Should questions regarding diagnosis persist, a full-thickness operative biopsy under general anesthesia may be performed to collect deeper nerve plexuses, but this is rarely needed.

Prognosis. The mortality rate for Hirschsprung disease is generally less than 5% but may be as high as 15% to 20% in the neonatal period, when diagnosis is often delayed and enterocolitis develops. Good surgical results can be expected in the vast majority of patients (90%), but diarrhea, constipation with distention, and intermittent colitis may occur in 2% to 34% of patients as the result of residual aganglionosis, postoperative stricture formation, overactivity of the sphincter, or motility disorders. Delayed toilet training is frequently reported, and 14% to 44% of patients experience problems with soiling, with the actual rate varying in direct proportion to the length of the aganglionic segment (Elhalaby et al, 1995; Heij et al, 1995; Marty et al, 1995b; Moore et al, 1994).

Collaborative Management. Although older children with mild symptoms of Hirschsprung disease may be managed medically with a daily colonic lavage of normal saline to evacuate the bowel, such conservative therapy is inappropriate in the neonatal period owing to the risk of fatal enterocolitis with perforation, peritonitis, and septicemia. In the newborn, the immediate treatment is a temporary colostomy, placed proximal to the aganglionic segment, to decompress the bowel and divert the fecal contents. The definitive repair is carried out between 6 and 12 months of age and involves resection of the affected, aganglionic bowel and anastomosis of the normal bowel to the anus. The enterostomal therapist is clearly an important member of the patient care team.

The surgical procedure may be one of several—Swenson procedure: abdominoperineal sphincter-saving proctectomy and end-to-end anastomosis in the rectal area; Duhamel: oblique end-to-side anastomosis between the proximal ganglionic colon and the anterior aganglionic anorectal wall, thus forming a new rectum, with the posterior portion pulled through the intestine and making a sleeve of good tissue; and Soave procedure: an endorectal mucosal dissecton in the area of the rectum where the muscular tissue is preserved and a sleeve of good, innervated tissue is pulled through to create a viable bowel surface (Ryckman, 2002).

No matter what the surgical procedure, the initial nursing care is directed toward abdominal decompression, return of fluid and electrolyte balance, and the treatment of sepsis. A gastric tube is set to low intermittent suction, and all drainage is measured. Fluids with appropriate electrolytes for the maintenance and replacement of gastric losses should be provided. Actions to combat the fluid shifts that are common following contrast studies with hyperosmolar media may also be necessary. Prophylactic antibiotic therapy is initiated because of the high risk of enterocolitis. If enterocolitis is present, aggressive therapy with fluids, blood, or plasma may be required. The infant should be monitored closely after rectal biopsy. Any bleeding can be controlled with digital pressure.

Colostomy is possible when the diagnosis of Hirschsprung disease is confirmed by rectal biopsy. A preoperative colonic lavage or enema is given to evacuate and prepare the bowel for surgery. Only isotonic solutions such as normal saline should be used to avoid water intoxication and resultant hyponatremia. Following colostomy, the infant must be assessed frequently for respiratory compromise, abdominal distention, hemorrhage, wound dehiscence, and infection. The stomal perfusion and appearance should also be noted and appropriate skin care provided. Intravenous fluids are continued until oral feedings can be started. Routine rectal irrigations with normal saline may reduce the incidence of postoperative enterocolitis.

As the infant becomes ready for discharge, the focus of nursing care shifts to readying the parents for home management of the colostomy. Family teaching should include skin care, normal stomal appearance and stool output, and the construction or application of appliances. Because the definitive repair is generally delayed until the end of the first year, the neonatal nurse most likely is not involved in patient care at that time.

Small Left Colon Syndrome

Pathophysiology. Neonatal small left colon syndrome is a condition of functional immaturity of the large bowel in which the left colon is uniformly narrowed from the anus to the splenic flexure. The proximal colon above the flexure is dilated and distended with meconium. A cone-shaped transition zone lies between the dilated and narrowed distal segments. The cause is unclear but is generally thought to involve the myenteric plexuses that innervate the GI tract in a cephalocaudal direction between 5 and 12 weeks' gestation. Once the plexuses are in position, their maturation and function are largely determined by gestational age. The impression that this condition results from intramural immaturity is supported by histologic findings of increased numbers of small, immature neuronal elements in contrast to the larger, multipolar ganglion cells that normally predominate at term. The neuronal plexuses are present but immature; morphologically they resemble the structure expected at approximately 32 weeks' gestation. The syndrome might therefore be best described as a disease of decreased intestinal motility.

Risk Factors. Approximately 40% of those with small left colon syndrome are the infants of mothers with diabetes. Furthermore, a survey of asymptomatic infants of mothers with diabetes has shown that 50% have a demonstrable narrowed colonic configuration in the absence of frank symptoms. Variable degrees of hypoglycemia, hypocalcemia, and hyperbilirubinemia have also been reported, but these findings may simply reflect the predisposition for hyperinsulinemia and polycythemia in the general population of infants of mothers with diabetes.

Clinical Manifestations. Presenting signs and symptoms are those associated with low intestinal obstruction. These manifestations include bile-stained vomitus, abdominal distention, and failure to pass meconium spontaneously. However, rectal examination may be followed by the passage of very small amounts of meconium in approximately a third of patients.

Differential Diagnosis. On clinical presentation and with plain radiographic studies, this condition is indistinguishable from Hirschsprung disease and meconium plug syndrome. Multiple gas-filled loops of bowel are seen proximally, with decreased air noted distally.

Barium enema shows the uniformly small left colon with a zone of transition at the splenic flexure. Although a zone of transition may also be noted with Hirschsprung disease, the margins of the distal colon generally appear smooth with small left colon syndrome rather than jagged or serrated as described in Hirschsprung disease. Perhaps more distinguishing from Hirschsprung disease is the incidental finding that following contrast studies, the majority (71%) of infants with small left colon syndrome promptly evacuate the barium and begin passing stools spontaneously. As a consequence, the signs and symptoms of low intestinal obstruction disappear. The meconium rarely (5%) contains a significant rubbery plug.

Rectal biopsy for the presence of ganglion cells, although they may appear atypically immature in small left colon syndrome, may ultimately be required to differentiate this syndrome from Hirschsprung disease. If the possibility of meconium plug persists, a follow-up contrast examination should be performed. Despite the passage of meconium, the transition zone persists in infants suffering from small left colon syndrome.

Prognosis. Although the initial presentation may be dramatic, many cases are apparently asymptomatic and go undiagnosed. In either case, the condition spontaneously resolves within the neonatal period with no subsequent stooling problems encountered. Late intermittent obstruction with or without cecal perforation is reported rarely.

Collaborative Management. Management is of a conservative nature. The diagnostic barium enema is generally curative. Only in the rare case of significant intermittent obstruction or cecal perforation is a colostomy required. If the diagnosis of small left colon syndrome is made in the face of a negative maternal history, the suggestion of maternal diabetes may be made to the obstetric team.

As with all intestinal obstructions, initial management involves decompression, intravenous fluids for hydration, and the treatment of electrolyte imbalance. Symptoms generally resolve following barium enema, and oral feeding may be instituted gradually. The nurse must be diligent, however, for evidence of persistent or recurrent obstruction and report abnormal findings accordingly.

Meconium Ileus

Pathophysiology. Meconium ileus is an obstruction of the distal ileum due to an accumulation of abnormally thick, tarry meconium. The condition is a result of pancreatic insufficiency. Pancreatic hydrolytic enzymes are normally responsible for the metabolism of fat and protein. Consequently, if these enzymes are absent, the meconium has an unusually high protein content and abnormal mucous glycoprotein, which makes it more viscid than usual. The resultant thick, tenacious material literally becomes impacted within the ileal lumen, thus producing a functional obstruction.

Risk Factors. Virtually all children (95%) with meconium ileus have cystic fibrosis, although only a small proportion (10% to 15%) of infants with cystic fibrosis present with meconium ileus. Cystic fibrosis, also known as mucoviscidosis, is a genetic disorder with an autosomal recessive inheritance pattern that occurs in 1 of every 2,000 live births. All exocrine glands are affected and produce tenacious mucus that causes not only GI dysfunction but also ultimate respiratory malfunction.

Rarely (5%) meconium ileus occurs in the absence of cystic fibrosis, but pancreatic duct stenosis or partial pancreatic aplasia generally can be demonstrated. The cause of these isolated findings is not known.

Additional findings associated with meconium ileus include maternal polyhydramnios (5% to 10%) and prematurity (10% to 33%).

Clinical Manifestations. Meconium ileus generally presents first with progressive abdominal distention (within 12 to 24 hours of birth), followed by bilious vomiting and failure to pass meconium. On physical examination the meconium mass may be palpated as a movable, doughy or putty-like ball; smaller pellet-like concretions of inspissated meconium may be felt distally. Rectal examination should produce no meconium, but normal sphincter tone should be felt.

Differential Diagnosis. Plain abdominal films show distended loops proximal to the point of obstruction, but unlike the uniformly lucent areas seen in jejunoileal atresia, the dilated areas typical of meconium ileus are of varying sizes and have a "soap-bubble" or "ground-glass" appearance. This appearance reflects the mixture of trapped air and meconium. Calcifications that are the result of antenatal intestinal perforation and consequent meconium peritonitis may also benoted. Barium enema demonstrates a distally unused microcolon, thus differentiating this condition from Hirschsprung disease. The smaller pellet-like masses of meconium may also be noted in the distal segment. A history of cystic fibrosis in siblings virtually ensures the diagnosis of meconium ileus. An immunoreactive trypsin test using a dry blood spot provides a screen for cystic fibrosis, with confirmation by sweat test.

Prognosis. Cystic fibrosis is a condition of delayed mortality, with a mean survival of 22 years. At this age, death comes as a result of obstructive pulmonary disease and infection. The intervening period is marked by poor growth and chronic respiratory and GI dysfunction. The infant mortality rate in cystic fibrosis is 13%, with these early deaths attributed to malabsorption and malnutrition. For a complete discussion of cystic fibrosis, see Chapter 28.

Collaborative Management. In the case of uncomplicated meconium ileus, the bowel can generally be evacuated using a hyperosmolar contrast enema such as meglumine diatrizoate. Because of its hyperosmolarity, fluid is drawn from the interstitial and intravascular spaces into the intestinal lumen, softening the impacted meconium and allowing it to pull away from the intestinal wall. The mass can then be evacuated by normal peristalsis. This nonoperative treatment is generally successful in 15% to 20% of patients.

If repeated enemas are not productive, or if meconium ileus is complicated by bowel ischemia, sepsis, or hypovolemic shock, the obstructing meconium may be surgically removed. A temporary ileostomy may be established. Such an ileostomy is irrigated daily with dilute acetylcysteine until any residual meconium is softened and evacuated. Chest physiotherapy, acetylcysteine sodium aerosols (Mucomyst®), and extra humidity may be helpful in preventing postoperative pulmonary complications (such as atelectasis and pneumonia), to which infants with cystic fibrosis are particularly prone.

Genetic counseling should be provided to parents of affected children, with appropriate referral to a geneticist or genetic counselor. A social worker or other mental health professional may help parents explore their feelings concerning their child's prognosis and their future reproductive plans. Extensive parent teaching of pulmonary toilet and enzyme supplementation is needed. Respiratory therapy personnel and the nutritional support team should consequently be included in parent teaching. Many larger communities have special follow-up clinics for cystic fibrosis patients that may be used to ensure continuity and coordination of care after discharge.

Immediate stabilization of the child with meconium ileus requires decompression with gastric suction and the correction of fluid and electrolyte imbalances. Hydration is particularly important in patients being treated medically with hyperosmolar enemas. Fluids drawn into the intestinal lumen to allow softening and evacuation of the meconium are by default removed from the effective circulation, thus placing the infant at risk for severe hypovolemia and vascular collapse. The extracted fluids should be replaced accordingly. Generally 4 ml of one-half normal saline solution is given for every 1 ml of retained enema. Fluids and suction are continued until the meconium is evacuated and the clinical manifestations of obstruction resolve. When intestinal function is deemed adequate, protein hydrosylate formula feedings may be started, together with the pancreatic enzyme supplement pancrilipase (Viokase®).

If the obstruction is not relieved, decompression, fluids, and electrolytes are continued until surgical treatment can be carried out. Postoperatively, ostomy care becomes a part of nursing management, along with assistance in providing pulmonary toilet. The infant's respiratory status should be monitored closely. If adhesions secondary to meconium peritonitis or surgical manipulation are noted or if the meconium is incompletely removed, signs of obstruction may recur. These signs of persistent or recurrent obstruction must be reported immediately to allow early intervention and reoperation as needed. Feedings are delayed until the obstruction is relieved, the ileostomy is functioning, and bowel activity has returned. Protein hydrosylate formula with added pancrilipase is given initially. Many of these infants feed quite poorly, however, and total parenteral nutrition may be required for these special patients.

Meconium Plug Syndrome

Pathophysiology.   Meconium plug syndrome is a condition in which intestinal obstruction (generally of the lower colon and rectum) occurs as the result of unusually thick meconium in the absence of demonstrable enzymatic deficiency. The syndrome is most likely the result of abnormal gut motility associated with immaturity or hypotonia; ganglion deficiency is not found. The plug is formed primarily from mucus and secretions and therefore appears yellowish white and is gelatinous in consistency, lacking the usual flow properties of normal meconium.

Risk Factors.   Premature infants are especially prone to meconium plug syndrome; however, the condition may also be found in hypotonic infants with central nervous system damage, and some infants of mothers with diabetes are also affected. In the latter case, meconium plug syndrome is considered to be a variant of small left colon syndrome. Treatment of the mother with magnesium sulfate is an additional risk factor that has been noted by some clinicians (Bates & Balistreri, 2002). Meconium plugs are found in about 1 of every 100 newborns, but only a quarter of these infants are unable to evacuate the plug spontaneously and thus experience intestinal obstruction.

Clinical Manifestations.   The signs are those of low intestinal obstruction with failure to stool, followed by abdominal distention and bilious vomiting. Hyperactive bowel sounds are often noted on auscultation, and normal sphincter tone is generally felt on rectal examination. The meconium plug and flatus are often passed after digital examination (Bates & Balistreri, 2002).

Differential Diagnosis.   Plain radiographs indicate a low intestinal obstruction with multiply distended loops of proximal bowel, thus bringing to mind a number of possible conditions, including jejunoileal atresia, meconium ileus, Hirschsprung

disease, small left colon syndrome, or meconium plug syndrome. On barium enema the colon is generally described as being of normal caliber with no evidence of microcolon, thus eliminating the diagnosis of jejunoileal atresia or meconium ileus. The presence of normal ganglion cells on rectal biopsy removes Hirschsprung disease from the differential diagnosis. In the absence of a history of maternal diabetes, meconium plug syndrome becomes the most logical cause for the symptoms presented (Bates & Balistreri, 2002).

Prognosis.   Once the meconium plug is expelled, complete recovery should follow.

Collaborative Management.   Small enemas of warm saline, meglumine diatrizoate, or acetylcysteine are usually all that are needed to dislodge the obstructing meconium plug if it has not already been expelled following rectal examination. Normal stooling patterns should follow. Surgical intervention is rarely needed (Bates & Balistreri, 2002).

Decompression, hydration, and electrolyte balance are the immediate concerns. The special care required following meglumine diatrizoate enema and rectal biopsy has already been discussed. Once the plug is evacuated, symptoms have resolved, and normal intestinal function has returned, feedings can be started.

Anorectal Agenesis

Pathophysiology.   Anorectal agenesis (imperforate anus) refers to a group of congenital malformations that involve the anus or rectum or the junction between the two structures. If the urorectal septum deviates during its growth, the cloaca is abnormally or incompletely partitioned, thus resulting in rectal stenosis or atresia. Rectourethral and rectovaginal fistulas frequently occur in association with these defects. If the anal membrane fails to rupture, the result is a membranous anal atresia.

A whole spectrum of defects is possible, but they are generally classified into four major types (Figure 26-5). The cause of deviated or arrested anorectal development is not known.

Risk Factors.   Anorectal agenesis occurs in 1 of every 1,500 to 5,000 live births. Between 20% and 75% of all affected infants have an associated anomaly. Considering its common origin from the cloaca, it is not surprising that genitourinary tract abnormalities are found most frequently (25% to 50%); approximately 4% of affected infants have the lethal defects of bilateral renal agenesis or dysplasia. Cryptorchidism is noted in 3% to 19% of affected males. Congenital heart disease and esophageal atresia are also reported occasionally, and when the latter is found, the VATER and VACTERL associations should be considered. Approximately half of affected patients have spinal dysraphism, ranging from occult spina bifida (2.2%) to myelomeningocele (2% to 4.4%)—including scoliosis (13.3%), hemivertebra (6.7%), extra segments (8.9%), tethered cord (4% to 13.3%), and fibrolipoma of the cord (8.9% to 38%) (Cortes et al, 1995; Ryckman, 2002; Rivosecchi et al, 1995; Tsakayannis & Shamberger, 1995).

Clinical Manifestations   Presenting signs and symptoms vary slightly with the particular type of defect present. For the majority (those with type III agenesis), the anus is clearly imperforate. Owing to the high incidence of fistulas, meconium may be passed in the urine (in males), or its presence may be noted at the vaginal outlet (in females). With anal stenosis (type I), the anus and rectal vaults are patent but narrowed so

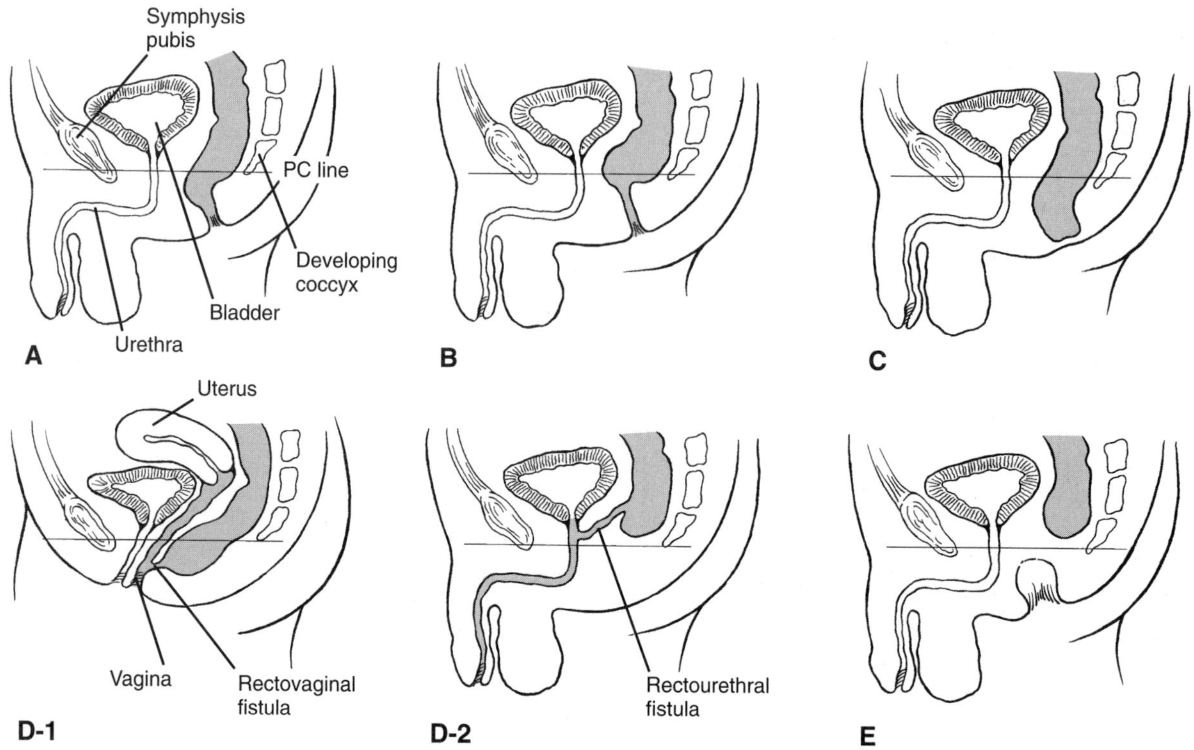

FIGURE **26-5**

Anorectal agenesis. Shading represents areas of lucency typically found on radiograph. Percentages reflect relative occurrence. A, Normal anatomy. B, Type I or anal stenosis (5% to 6%): anus or lower rectum is narrowed but patent. C, Type II or anal membrane (5% to 7%): anal opening covered by a membranous diaphragm. D, Type III or anal agenesis (85%): anus is clearly imperforate; fistulas are present in three quarters of cases. D-1, Type IIIA or low agenesis: bowel ends as a blind pouch below the pubococcygeal (PC) line; most common in females. D-2, Type IIIB or high agenesis: bowel ends as a blind pouch above the pubococcygeal line; most common in males. E, Type IV or anal atresia (3%): rectum and anus are present as blind pouches but are separated by a variable distance. Data from Avery & Taeusch, 1984; Chang, 1980b; deVries & Cox, 1985; Gryboski & Walker, 1983; Moore & Persaud, 1993; Sadler, 1985.

that the pasty stools of the newborn may be passed. The stenosis is generally suspected by the microscopic appearance of the anus and is confirmed on rectal examination. With the remaining two types, the anus may appear misleadingly normal on first inspection. In the membranous type (type II), the anal membrane may become visible within 24 to 48 hours as meconium bulges from beneath the thin epithelial covering, but by then the signs of low intestinal obstruction (distention, bilious vomiting, and failure to pass stool) are also becoming apparent. The atretic type (type IV), which is fortunately rare, generally first presents with the full-blown manifestations of obstruction.

Differential Diagnosis.   Visual and digital rectal examinations are generally diagnostic. In the presence of a fistula, the urine may also be examined for meconium epithelial cells.

An inverted lateral radiograph (upside-down Wangensteen-Rice technique) may demonstrate air collected in the blind-ending upper rectal pouch but is generally unreliable for determining the level of obstruction, owing to the considerable time required for swallowed air to reach this portion of the gut. Even when sufficient time is given, air may be prevented by meconium from reaching the end of the pouch. Nevertheless, if a fistula is present, air may be seen in the bladder or vagina on the plain film.

Contrast studies with barium injected into the blind rectum confirm obstruction but provide no indication of the distance that separates the distal and proximal pouches. Barium injected through the urethra or vagina confirms the presence of a fistula and through retrograde filling indicates the level of the rectal pouch. In those rare situations in which a fistula is not present and the level of the obstruction has still not been determined, a perineal puncture contrast rectogram or needle aspiration may be required. For the rectogram, a needle is inserted through the perineum and guided (by sonography) into the rectal pouch to inject the barium. The needle aspiration is a more conservative alternative and involves advancement of the needle while attempting to aspirate. If the needle has been advanced to a depth of 1.5 cm and no meconium has been obtained, the defect is assumed to be of a high type.

Prognosis.   The outcome for infants with anorectal anomalies largely depends on the type of defect and on the level of the upper rectal pouch in relation to the puborectal muscle, which is the main muscle of sphincter function and continence. This muscle is a central component of the levator ani muscle, which spans the pelvis much like a sling to support the lower end of the rectum. On radiography, the position of this muscle can be estimated by drawing an imaginary line between the symphysis pubis and the developing coccyx (Figure 26-5).

Based on the relation of the pouch to this pubococcygeal line, anorectal anomalies can be classified into three groups that indicate low, high, or intermediate level defect. In low (translevator) types, the rectum descends through and is surrounded by the puborectalis and levator ani muscles so that the sensorimotor mechanisms are generally intact. With high (supralevator) defects, the rectal pouch ends above the puborectalis and levator ani muscles so that the neurologic and muscular mechanisms of continence may be impaired. In intermediate types (supralevator), the rectum again ends above the puborectalis, but the pouch is cradled in the muscular hammock formed by the levator ani so that neuromuscular function is variable and repair more complicated.

The overall mortality rate is approximately 20%, with death largely a reflection of the nature of the defect and the presence of associated anomalies. In general, the supralevator types of defects carry the highest mortality (31%), with intermediate supralevator lesions having the highest death rate of all (45%), followed by high supralevator lesions (29%), and low translevator defects (7%). As a group, the cause of death for most defects is due to the presence of associated anomalies.

For survivors, the main criterion for outcome is fecal continence. When anorectal anomalies are reviewed as a whole, 74% of patients can be expected to have good results, with normal anal function and control of defecation; 14% have fair results, with only occasional soiling or straining; and 12% have poor results, being nearly or completely incontinent or requiring permanent colostomy. Here again, however, the level of the defect largely determines outcome. Most low translevator (92%) and intermediate supralevator (83%) types have good outcomes. Far fewer (51%) of the high supralevator defects has good postoperative results, and a large proportion (23%) has frankly poor results.

Collaborative Management. As might be expected, the treatment of anorectal anomalies varies with the nature of the defect. The higher the lesion, the more technically complicated its repair becomes.

The treatment of anal stenosis (type I defect) consists of repeated dilation using Hegar dilators. When the anus is sufficiently enlarged, and if the infant is otherwise stable, the patient is discharged, with daily digital dilation (using the little finger) to be performed by the parents. Membranous defects (type II) require minimal surgical therapy. The membrane is simply punctured with a hemostat or excised using a scalpel. Repeated dilation is performed as needed.

Low agenesis (translevator, type III lesion) is corrected by perineal anoplasty. After locating the position of the superficial external sphincter using a nerve stimulator, the rectal pouch is brought down through the sphincter to the opening on the anal skin. The fistulous connection, if present, is removed. Gentle irrigations help facilitate stooling and keep the anastomotic site clean until daily dilations can be started, generally between 10 and 14 days postoperatively.

High agenesis (intermediate or high supralevator, type III lesions) and atresia (supralevator, type IV lesions) generally are treated in two phases. The first step is immediate placement of a colostomy for decompression and diversion of fecal contents. If present, the urethrorectal fistula is generally closed or excised to avoid "spill-over" fecal contamination with resultant urinary tract infection. The definitive repair is generally delayed 3 to 12 months to allow growth and pelvic enlargement. At that time, an abdominal-perineal pull-through procedure is performed in which the rectal pouch is literally pulled through the levator sling and anchored to the skin. The colostomy is left intact until healing is complete.

Nonemergent cases (typically stenosis) usually require little in the way of stabilization other than replacement and correction of fluid and electrolyte imbalance. If a fistula is present, these infants are at risk for the development of hyperchloremic acidosis owing to the absorption of urine from the colon. Gastric suction for decompression is instituted prophylactically (in the case of agenesis when the defect is obvious on inspection) or therapeutically (when membranous and atretic types begin to display symptoms of obstruction).

Postoperatively, wound care and monitoring for postoperative complications are added to the regimen. If anoplasty is performed, the site should be inspected (as allowed by the surgical team) for mucosal prolapse, which may occur if there is inadequate sphincter preservation. A colostomy placed for higher defects should receive the standard care and monitoring. The surgeon initially carries out dilatory procedures, but when digital dilation becomes possible, the nurse may assume this task, making sure to provide bedside parent teaching. Throughout recuperation, the urine (or vaginal outlet) should be closely observed for the presence of meconium, which would indicate a recurrent fistula. If such a fistula is suspected, electrolyte and acid-base status should also be monitored for hyperchloremic acidosis. Otherwise, feeding may begin when the colostomy or anoplasty is sufficiently healed and intestinal function resumes. Stool-softening agents may be required.

As children age, psychosocial counseling should become an integral part of continuing care. Longitudinal data indicate that 29% of affected children experience some behavioral problem, ranging from mild (10%) to levels severe enough to influence their daily lives (19%). These maladjustments generally involve social withdrawal, depression, anxiety, and other internalizing behavior and are most apparent in those who achieve continence late or who suffer frequent accidents (Ludman & Spitz, 1995). Adults similarly report social problems related to fecal continence (83%) in addition to problems with sexual function (30%) (Rintala et al, 1994).

Malrotation with Volvulus

Pathophysiology. Malrotation is an anomaly of intestinal rotation and fixation. Although alternative theories have been offered (Kluth et al, 1995), the abnormality most likely arises as the intestine rotates around the axis of the superior mesenteric artery during its entry into and movement from the umbilical cord. Once returned to the abdominal cavity, the intestinal mesentery lies along and eventually adheres to the posterior abdominal wall, thus fixing the intestine in place. The normal 270-degree counterclockwise rotation can be interrupted or deviated at any time, and consequently a variety of rotation and fixation anomalies are possible (Figure 26-6).

The major danger with malrotation is that the intestinal loops may become kinked, knotted, or otherwise obstructed. This knotting and twisting of the bowel is called a volvulus. The resultant occlusion of the intestinal tract or its blood supply can lead to widespread ischemia and necrosis. Nearly two thirds of all cases of malrotation are complicated by volvulus, with the incidence varying with age at the onset of symptoms. Eighty-five percent of patients less than 1 month of age have volvulus, compared with 43% of older children (Seashore & Touloukian, 1994).

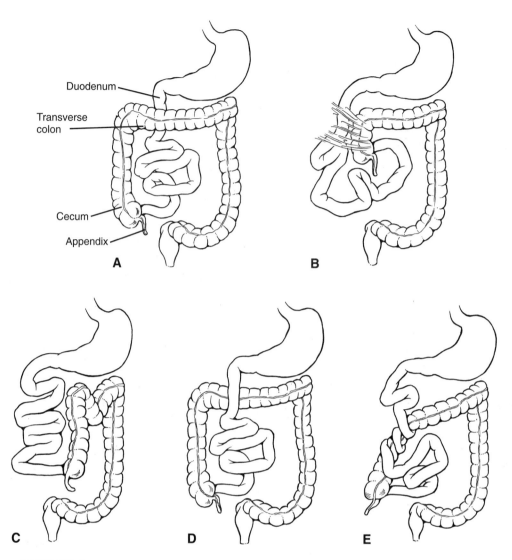

FIGURE **26-6**

Anomalies of rotation and fixation. A, Normal anatomy: cecum lies in right lower quadrant; transverse colon overlies duodenum. B, Incomplete rotation (Ladd bands): cecum lies just below and anterior to the duodenum, where it becomes fixed to the posterior wall by abnormal peritoneal bands; the bands cross over, compress, and obstruct the duodenum. C, Nonrotation ("left-sided colon"): entire small intestine lies in the right side of the abdominal cavity, whereas all of the large intestine lies on the left; volvulus may occur, but the condition is more frequently asymptomatic. D, Reverse (clockwise) rotation: duodenum overlies and may obstruct the transverse colon. E, Nonfixation ("midgut volvulus"): mesentery fails to adhere to the posterior abdominal wall so that the small intestine hangs loosely from the superior mesenteric artery and is free to twist around it or on itself to create a volvulus, typically involving the duodenum. Data from Chang, 1980a; Moore & Persaud, 1993; Sadler, 1985.

Risk Factors. Owing to the rarity of rotational anomalies, their incidence is not known. However, the busiest surgical referral services typically see only two to four cases a year (Seashore & Touloukian, 1994). The anomaly does appear to predominate in males; however, no specific cause has been identified.

Because of the nature of these defects, almost all cases of omphalocele, gastroschisis, and diaphragmatic hernia entail some component of malrotation. The frequency is in fact so high that many clinicians do not consider malrotation an anomaly associated with these conditions but rather an expected component of them. In addition to these defects, associated anomalies such as intestinal atresias, annular pancreas,

Meckel's diverticulum, and urinary tract malformation as well as congenital heart disease are found in 8% to 24% of patients (Seashore & Touloukian, 1994).

Clinical Manifestations. Of all the affected infants only about half of them will present with symptoms in the first week of life. In those who do, the symptoms are generally intermittent or recurrent, indicating that most of these obstructions are partial rather than complete. Most infants demonstrate progressive bilious vomiting and little else. However, when a previously well infant presents with sudden bilious vomiting, a malrotation with volvulus should be the clinician's first thought. In the case of volvulus, the abdomen may become distended, and the stools may be bloody. Bleeding occurs when twisting is severe enough to interfere with venous return from the bowel, thus causing the vessels to become engorged and leak blood into the gut.

Differential Diagnosis.   The differential diagnosis generally includes pyloric stenosis, duodenal atresia, and jejunoileal atresia. The possibility of pyloric stenosis is generally considered because of vomiting in the absence of any other typical signs of GI obstruction. However, the emesis of pyloric stenosis is seldom bile-stained, and this condition is quickly dropped from further consideration.

On plain radiograph, the stomach and upper small intestine are generally distended with air and may mimic the characteristic "double-bubble" of duodenal atresia. However, the presence of small amounts of gas in the distal positions of the gut is more reflective of a partial obstruction by malrotation than of an atresia in the jejunum or ileum. In adults, the gas-filled loops may appear to converge to a point ("convergency sign"). A "spoke wheel" sign of mucosal folds radiating from the center has also been described. However, these radiographic signs have not been reported in neonates (Lee et al, 1995). If doubt persists, a barium enema can be given to locate the position of the cecum under fluoroscopy. If a misplaced colon is seen, the diagnosis of malrotation is confirmed. However, some malrotations (notably reverse rotation) may not be demonstrated. An upper GI series is diagnostic in all cases and allows the exact position of the duodenum to be seen. When volvulus is present, the barium column is noted to end with a peculiar "beaking" effect. This beaking appearance is pathognomonic of a volvulus and is caused by the twisting of the bowel into a sharp point that resembles the beak of a bird. Suspected malrotation is the only situation that warrants an upper GI series; otherwise the procedure should not be carried out in infants.

Prognosis.   When the condition is uncomplicated by infarction or associated anomalies, the survival rate is excellent and may be as high as 99%. However, in the presence of necrosis, survival falls to 35%. An increased risk of dying is also noted with younger age (<3 months) at the time of surgery.

Collaborative Management.   The goals for surgical management are the release of obstruction and counterclockwise rotational reduction of the bowel. If a volvulus is present, it is immediately apparent on opening the abdomen. Normally, the transverse colon is the first structure that is seen. In the case of volvulus, however, the small bowel typically lies anterior to the colon, thus making it the first structure that is encountered. The volvulus is relieved by counterclockwise rotation, and the viability of the bowel is determined with necrotic sections removed. If the necrosis is extensive, rather than perform massive bowel resection, the abdomen is closed. A return "second look" surgery is performed in 24 to 48 hours, at which time it becomes mandatory to remove any unrecovered, infarcted bowel. If the bowel appears viable, the Ladd bands (if present) are divided, and the entrapped duodenum is freed. The entire length of the bowel is then inspected for patency and associated defects and returned to the abdominal cavity; the small intestine is placed on the right and the colon on the left side of the abdominal cavity. Suture fixation of the replaced bowel generally is not necessary. Appendectomy and gastrostomy are generally performed as well.

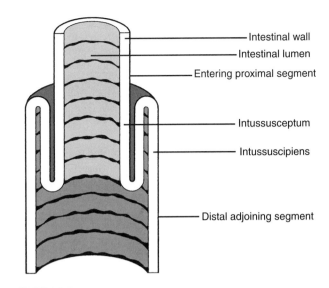

FIGURE **26-7**
Schematic representation of intussusception. The proximal intestinal segment has prolapsed into the lumen of an adjacent distal intestinal segment.

The major postoperative complication is short bowel syndrome, which results from the excision of major portions of the gut. The complex malabsorption problems and prolonged hospitalization with total parenteral nutrition call for consultation and close collaboration with members of the nutritional support team and social services. Wound problems and prolonged ileus may also be noted (Seashore & Touloukian, 1994).

The principles of preoperative stabilization include gastric decompression and correction of fluid and electrolyte deficits. The presence of volvulus places the infant at particular risk for both hypovolemia and metabolic acidosis. Hypovolemia occurs as a result of fluid accumulation in the bowel wall, which effectively reduces the circulating blood volume. Clinically, as the infant worsens, the abdomen becomes distended, erythematous, and tender, and blood is passed into the stool. The heart rate quickens in an attempt to maintain cardiac output, and the infant's color may become ashen. This state constitutes a true surgical emergency.

The same principles of decompression and fluid and electrolyte resuscitation apply postoperatively. Total parenteral nutrition is instituted and continued, often for months in the case of short bowel syndrome, until the intestine has had an opportunity to recover and grow. When feedings are begun, very dilute formula (one-quarter strength protein hydrosylate formula) is given initially; the volume and then the concentration are gradually increased until a normal amount of full-strength formula can be tolerated. This feeding progression is often a tedious process fraught with many setbacks that are frustrating to both the nurse and the parents.

Intussusception
Pathophysiology.   Intussusception is an acquired obstruction in which a part of the intestine prolapses into the lumen of an adjoining distal intestinal segment (Figure 26-7). This luminal prolapse may occur at any site in the GI tract, but typically there are four varieties: (1) enteric intussusception, in which the small intestine prolapses into itself; (2) colic intussusception, in which the large intestine prolapses into itself; (3) ileocecal intussusception, in which the ileocecal valve is

inverted and pushed into the cecum, pulling a segment of ileum with it; and (4) ileocolic intussusception, in which the ileocecal valve remains in place but the ileum prolapses through it into the colon. Rarely, a retrograde intussusception may occur in which a distal intestinal segment prolapses upward into a proximal part. In the neonate, the majority of cases are of the enteric (most often involving the terminal ileum) or ileocecal type.

Risk Factors. Intussusception is an acquired condition and therefore not easily explained by any one causative factor. A small proportion of cases (5% to 13%) appear to have a "lead point," a demonstrable anatomic lesion or defect that may have been the cause of intussusception. Such lead points may include Meckel's diverticula, duplication defects, polyps, hematomas, and lymphomas. The viscid stool common in cystic fibrosis may even be a potential cause. In most situations, the cause is not known (idiopathic intussusception). However, there is often a history of preceding upper respiratory infection or gastroenteritis. Nearly half of all patients demonstrate infection with adenovirus on stool culture. The role played by infection in the phenomenon of intussusception has not yet been determined. The inflammatory response of the intestine to infection may possibly cause an abnormal hyperplasia of lymphoid tissue. The hyperplastic site might then serve as a lead point for intussusception (Lipschitz et al, 1995).

Intussusception is extremely rare in the newborn period; consequently, an overall incidence rate is not known. Even if one could be involved in the care of each affected newborn, one might expect to encounter only one case every 5 years (Rachelson et al, 1955). The usual age for intussusception is between 3 and 24 months, with males predominating.

Clinical Manifestations. Regardless of the site, the intussusception gives rise to two problems. First, it causes a simple mechanical obstruction as the result of the blockage of the distal intestinal lumen by the prolapsed proximal segment. Second, as the intestinal walls are telescoped into one another, the mucosal blood vessels become compressed, congested, and prone to ischemia or infarction. Thus the symptoms of intussusception typically include vomiting, colicky pain, and bloody stools or red "currant jelly" stools (Shanbhogue et al, 1994).

Differential Diagnosis. Plain radiographs may not be helpful in the diagnosis, with 20% to 30% showing only a general picture of intestinal obstruction with dilated proximal loops and an airless distal bowel. On ultrasonography, the affected area often appears as a "doughnut sign" on cross-section. Definitive diagnosis is by barium enema, with the contrast media outlining the gut and end proximally in a characteristic "coiled spring" pattern. This pattern is caused by barium trickling into the transverse folds of the luminal mucosa between the intussusceptum and the intussuscipiens (Shanbhogue et al, 1994).

Prognosis. The prognosis for intussusception in newborns is not good, basically because they present with so few of the signs that classically appear in infants and older children. Consequently, intussusception is rarely considered in the differential diagnosis of intestinal obstruction. When diagnosed, the mortality rate is approximately 41%.

Collaborative Management. Intussusception is so rare that little medical research has been undertaken to determine the best approach for treatment. In older children and adults, an attempt is first made to reduce the intussusception by using the hydrostatic pressure produced by a barium enema. Barium is injected into the rectum and allowed to flow distally until the "coiled-spring" pattern appears. A balloon-tipped catheter is then inserted into the rectum. The balloon is inflated with air, and gentle traction is applied until the balloon is pulled back against the muscular sling of the levatores, thus preventing any outflow of barium. The administration of barium is restarted, which causes the intraluminal pressure to rise slowly as more and more contrast medium is added without an avenue for escape. The pressure is maintained until the intussusception is pushed distally and freed. The procedure can be likened to taking a surgical glove in which one fingertip has been pulled inward, closing the cuff around the mouth, and slowly exhaling until the fingertip of the glove is blown outward. If the intussusception is fully reduced, the barium is seen suddenly to flow freely into the proximal bowel, and the clinical status of the patient should immediately improve. Unfortunately, in infants, full reduction is generally not accomplished, and surgical reduction is required. Recently, an alternate approach of rectal insufflation of air has been reported. Pneumatic reduction, however, generally is not performed in infants less than 3 months of age because of the risk of bowel perforation and rapid tension pneumoperitoneum (Lipschitz et al, 1995; Shiels, 1995).

Surgical intervention involves a manual reduction of the intussusception using a "milking" motion on the proximal bowel. The pressure and squeezing are continued until the loop is freed; traction and pulling should never be applied. The bowel is carefully inspected; any necrotic tissue is removed; and lead points are resected.

The major concerns before reduction are sepsis and shock. In light of the strong association with adenovirus and the frequent history of gastroenteritis or respiratory infection, sepsis should be expected and the appropriate blood work carried out. Antibiotic therapy is initiated pending culture results. Fluid lost into the wall of the trapped intestine or blood lost from congested vessels into the lumen of the intestine, or a combination of both, predisposes to shock and should be appropriately managed with fluid resuscitation and volume expansion. Decompression by gastric suction is also recommended.

Postoperative care is fairly routine; fluids, electrolytes, and decompression are provided as needed. However, the nurse must be aware that intussusception may recur. The recurrence risk is 2% to 20% and is more common following hydrostatic reduction (8% to 13%) than after surgical reduction (0% to 4%). Consequently, even though the intussusception has presumably been resolved, the nurse must be alert for the return of associated signs and symptoms. Increasing gastric drainage may be a particularly helpful clue (Champous et al, 1994).

Necrotizing Enterocolitis

Pathophysiology. Necrotizing enterocolitis (NEC) is an acquired disorder characterized by necrosis of the mucosal and submucosal layers of the GI tract. Any portion of the bowel can be affected, but the ileocecal area predominates (66%), with the antimesenteric side most typically being involved (Lemelle et al, 1994). To the naked eye, the affected intestine appears irregularly dilated with patchy areas of discoloration ranging from pale to dark purple. The pale color indicates areas of ischemic necrosis where the tissues have been deprived of their blood supply; the purple color indicates areas of hemorrhagic necrosis where blood has leaked into the tissues from

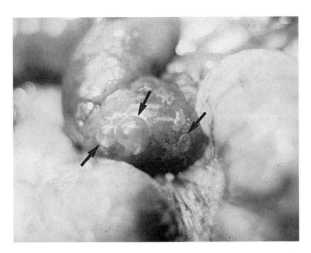

FIGURE **26-8**
Gross operative findings in necrotizing enterocolitis. The gas-filled intramural cysts (*arrows*) are typical of pneumatosis intestinalis. Courtesy Drs. David A. Clark and Jeffery E. Thompson and Wyeth-Ayerst Laboratories, Philadelphia, PA. Copyright© Wyeth.

capillary hemorrhage. Gas-containing cysts (pneumatosis) may be seen in the wall of the intestine as the result of gas dissecting beneath the serosa or submucosa (Figure 26-8). If perforation has occurred, it is usually found in the ileocecal area.

On microscopic examination, the mucosa appears edematous, and the necrotic areas may extend beyond the mucosa and submucosa into the muscular layers. Microthrombi may also be noted in the tiny arterioles and venules of the mesentery, but frank thrombosis of the larger arteries or veins rarely occurs. Contrary to what the name NEC implies, there is really little inflammation in the acute stages of the disease.

The etiology and pathogenesis of NEC have been the focus of extensive debate and research for the past 30 years. Many theories have been offered concerning the factors that cause the disease and their method of introduction to the neonate, but few absolute answers have been found. At present the sum of knowledge indicates that three major pathologic mechanisms occur in combination that lead to the development of NEC. These three mechanisms involve selective ischemia of the bowel, establishment of bacterial flora, and the effect of feeding.

The selective bowel ischemia is really an asphyxial defense mechanism that serves to protect the brain and heart from hypoxia by shunting blood away from the mesenteric, renal, and peripheral vascular bed. This redistribution of blood flow is similar to the "diving reflex" typical of aquatic birds and mammals. Unfortunately, in human infants this relative circulatory insufficiency to the bowel may result in intestinal ischemia. Asphyxiated infants and those suffering respiratory distress syndrome, apneic episodes, or cyanosis are most commonly affected. Although these conditions undoubtedly affect intestinal perfusion, such compromise may be intermittent in nature and of insufficient magnitude alone to induce necrosis without some additional factor. Any condition or procedure that holds potential for causing hemodynamic change may also be at fault. Polycythemia, umbilical artery catheterization, and exchange transfusion as well as maternal cocaine abuse have been implicated in bowel ischemia (Buyukunal et al, 1994; Kosloske, 1994a; Nowicki & Nankervis, 1994).

Colonization of the intestine with bacteria that normally reside within its lumen is a postnatal process. In utero the intestines are sterile, but during the process of delivery and subsequent contact with the surrounding environment, the gut becomes seeded with a wide variety of aerobic and anaerobic bacteria, which then multiply and spread with enteral feedings. In healthy newborn infants, the intestinal flora is established by about 10 days of age; however, in premature and sick infants, the colonization may be delayed, with fewer species of bacteria than are normally present. Attempts at controlling infectious disease within the special care nursery and skill at employing aseptic technique may in large part be responsible. Nevertheless, the result is a newborn with a GI tract that is both structurally and immunologically immature and susceptible to injury from bacterial toxins—that is, the passage of bacteria or bacterial products (such as endotoxins) across the mucosal wall (Deitch, 1994; Israel, 1994). This decreased immunity and lack of resistance may explain the fact that most of the bacteria cultured from affected infants are of species that are otherwise considered a part of the normal intestinal flora. The organisms that are typically isolated include *Escherichia coli* and *Enterobacter, Klebsiella,* and *Clostridium* species. These enteric bacilli do not usually invade normal tissue but are opportunistic pathogens (Chan et al, 1994; Kosloske, 1994a). Based on these observations, several research groups are currently working to develop a means of prophylaxis. Although the administration of oral antibiotics to modify intestinal flora has provided mixed results, oral administration of an immunoglobulin preparation (IgA or IgG, or both) appears promising (Fast & Rosegger, 1994; Maxson et al, 1995; Wolf & Eibl, 1994). The administration of glucocorticoids to accelerate maturation of the GI system may also be potentially beneficial (Faix & Adams, 1994; Vasan & Gotoff, 1994).

Formula feedings have also been cited as an important factor in making the gut susceptible to NEC. In fact, virtually all infants in whom the disease develops (98%) have previously been fed either formula or dextrose solution. It is believed that such intake may simply provide a substance on which bacteria can feed and flourish. In comparison, infants who receive fresh breast milk are rarely affected with NEC, presumably being protected by the secretory immunoglobulin (IgA) and anti-inflammatory components it provides (Buescher, 1994; Kosloske, 1994a).

Hyperosmolar loads of formula or medications may further compound the situation. In response to the osmotic gradient and in a futile attempt to reduce the osmolarity, intestinal secretions are increased and fluid moves into the lumen of the GI tract. As a result of this fluid shift, blood volume is decreased; GI blood flow is reduced; and the intestinal mucosa becomes relatively ischemic, thus increasing the risk of NEC. Furthermore, in vitro studies have demonstrated that the tissue fluid content of the bowel wall itself is also decreased as fluid moves into the lumen. This dehydration of the epithelium causes both morphologic and functional alterations in the mucosal lining of the intestine. The height and width of the villi decrease; the intercellular spaces close; and, as a result, the overall absorptive capacity of the bowel is decreased. Malabsorption with varying degrees of stasis and ileus in turn allows the development of abnormal flora, which further increases the risk of NEC. The complex mechanism of vascular and cellular changes that occur in response to hyperosmolar loads is believed to be responsible for the increased incidence of NEC historically reported for low-birth-weight infants who receive hyperosmolar feedings and certain oral medications, particularly high-dose vitamin E (100 to 200 mg/kg/day, producing tocopherol levels in excess of 3.5 mg/dl) given to impede the development of retinopathy of prematurity. Although vitamin E is no longer given at such high doses, other medications often used in neonatal therapy also possess high osmolality and must be considered potentially damaging to the gut. Even when diluted in formula, a medication such as phenobarbital elixir can increase the osmolality of a feeding by more than twofold. In many cases it may be preferable to give the intravenous preparation of the drug by the oral route to avoid such hypertonic feedings.

The development of NEC apparently occurs as a result of the three pathologic mechanisms—mesenteric ischemia, bacteria, and feeding (particularly hyperosmolar feeding)—operating in concert. Injured by ischemia, the mucosal cells lining the gut stop secreting protective enzymes. Digestive enzymes present autodigest the unprotected luminal cells. Enteric bacteria proliferate in the substrate-rich but immunologically deficient environment and invade the intestinal wall, where they release toxins and produce hydrogen gas. The gas is formed as a result of the catalytic activity of bacterial enzymes acting on formula as a substrate. The gas initially dissects beneath the serosal and submucosal layers of the intestine (pneumatosis intestinalis), but if this gas ruptures into the mesenteric vascular bed, it can be distributed through the systemic vessels into the venous system of the liver (portal venous gas). The bacterial toxins together with ischemia result in necrosis. If the full thickness of the intestinal wall is damaged, perforation can result, releasing free air into the peritoneal cavity (pneumoperitoneum) and producing a true surgical emergency.

Risk Factors. NEC is the most common GI disorder seen in the intensive care nursery and affects approximately 5% of all admissions, although wide differences are reported from center to center (from a low of 1% to a high of 8%). Any condition or situation that leads to ischemia and bacterial overgrowth in the presence of formula feedings can logically be considered a risk factor. However, prematurity is probably the greatest risk factor of all. Although cases in term infants are noted, NEC is almost exclusively a disease of the prematurely born. Of all infants affected, 62% to 94% are premature, with the highest rates in those with lowest birth weight and gestational age. No consistent associations between NEC and sex, race, socioeconomic status, or season of the year have been found (Kosloske, 1994a; Stoll, 1994).

Clinical Manifestations. Symptoms generally present on an overall average (mean) at 12 days of age, although the most common age at onset (mode) is 3 days. However, cases have been reported to occur in infants as old as 90 days. Patients with early-onset NEC (those 21 days of age or younger) typically have less severe respiratory disease and require shorter periods of mechanical ventilation and oxygen supplementation than do patients with late-onset NEC (those older than 21 days). As a consequence, those with early-onset NEC are generally fed early (beginning at an average of 4 days of life) and advanced quickly to full feedings (over a 9-day period on average). Patients with late-onset NEC typically are not fed until 9 days of age and advance to full feedings more slowly, over a 22-day period. When these subgroups are reviewed separately, the early cases typically present with symptoms at 12 days of age; the late cases typically present at 35 days. Regardless of age at onset, no significant difference seems to exist between the groups in terms of symptoms, severity, or sequelae of NEC.

Early signs are highly variable but generally include nonspecific signs of GI compromise (abdominal distention, gastric residuals, vomiting that may or may not be bilious, and bloody stools) or nonspecific signs of infection (lethargy, temperature instability, apnea, and bradycardia), or both. Laboratory findings include abnormal blood gases caused by apnea and acidosis, abnormal blood counts resulting from sepsis, thrombocytopenia resulting from consumption by the necrotic process and infection, and reducing substances in the stool caused by carbohydrate malabsorption. As the disease progresses, hypovolemia occurs as the result of the third-spacing of fluids in the interstitial compartments of the damaged intestine; blood pressure falls; urinary output decreases; and the poorly perfused, often septic infant appears gray, pale, or mottled. Peritonitis is evident by erythema, edema, and tenderness of the abdominal wall. If clotting factors continue to be consumed, disseminated intravascular coagulation may even occur (Gupta et al, 1994; Kanto et al, 1994; Schober & Nassiri, 1994).

Differential Diagnosis. Radiographic findings change as the disease progresses (Figure 26-9). Radiographs taken early in the course of the disease generally exhibit little more than fixed, dilated bowel loops with thickened walls, all due to local edema. The invasion of gas-forming bacteria into the intestinal wall produces the diagnostic picture of pneumatosis intestinalis. This intraluminal air, found in 85% of affected infants, generally appears as tiny, lucent bubbles that may come so close together in some places that they coalesce to form curvilinear or crescent-shaped streaks. If extensive disease is present, air may enter the venous system and outline the hepatic veins. Portal venous gas, found in 15% to 30% of patients, is also diagnostic of NEC. Ultimately, perforation may occur, thus presenting the characteristic appearance of pneumoperitoneum with a layer of free air lying immediately inferior to the abdominal wall. This free air is best seen by a lateral view, but on anteroposterior view it may be noted by the characteristic "football sign" due to air outlining the falciform ligament (Fotter & Sorantin, 1994; Morrison & Jacobson, 1994).

Other diagnostic studies are used sporadically but may be of diagnostic benefit, particularly in the early stages of NEC. These studies include assays of hydrogen in expired breath (which may be increased owing to the fermentative activity of bacteria), hepatic vein ultrasonography (which may detect microbubbles in the portal vein before air can be identified on the plain radiograph), and metrizamide upper GI series (to detect pneumatosis unappreciated radiographically) (Fotter & Sorantin, 1994).

Prognosis. Mortality rates have dramatically decreased over time with improved medical-surgical care and the use of total parenteral nutrition, falling from a rate of 24% to 65% in the 1960s and 1970s to a rate of 9% to 28% in the 1990s. Within groups, mortality varies with treatment. Lower rates occur in those who are managed medically as opposed to those requiring surgical intervention. Persistent acidosis, severe pneumatosis, and the presence of portal venous air are poor prognostic indicators (Kosloske, 1994b; Stoll, 1994).

Of those who survive, approximately 31% experience strictures (mostly colonic) as the result of structural changes in nonperforated, healed ischemic sites. Somewhat fewer patients suffer from short bowel syndrome (9% to 23%) and sepsis (9%). More than 80% of infants with NEC demonstrate evidence of failure of organ systems other than the GI tract.

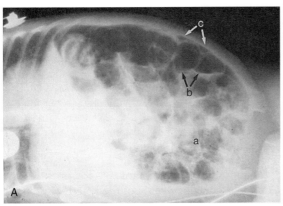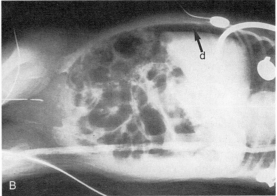

FIGURE **26-9**

Extensive necrotizing enterocolitis in a premature infant. The infant died after a "second look" operation. A, Right lateral decubitus view of the abdomen demonstrates the widespread bubbly lucencies of pneumatosis intestinalis (a), particularly in the right lower quadrant. In comparison, note the few uniformly dark air-filled loops of normal appearing bowel (b). The small triangular lucencies (c) inferior to the left abdominal wall are formed by free air filling in the spaces between bowel loops and are seen only in the very early stages of pneumoperitoneum immediately following perforation. B, Left lateral decubitus view of the abdomen taken 20 minutes later. The lucency overlying the liver (d) demonstrates continued collection of free air in the peritoneal cavity and worsening pneumoperitoneum.

Respiratory failure (91%), renal failure (85%), cardiovascular failure (33%), and hepatic failure (15%) are reported most frequently. The number of systems involved increases with the severity of disease and is highest in nonsurvivors. Neurologic, psychomotor, and psychosocial impairment of a moderate to severe nature may be exhibited, but the rate is not significantly different from the rate that appears in the general premature and very-low-birth-weight population (Horwitz et al, 1995; Mayr et al, 1994; Morecroft et al, 1994).

Recurrent NEC has been reported in 4% to 6% of patients, with an average onset of symptoms approximately 5 weeks after the original episode. Neither the type nor timing of enteral feedings nor the anatomic site or method of management of the initial episode appears to be an influencing factor. Those affected tend to be recovering premature infants (63%), although recurrence is also seen in mature infants with major congenital anomalies (31%), primarily cyanotic congenital heart disease. The mortality rate is similar to that seen with primary NEC (Ricketts, 1994).

Collaborative Management.   Aggressive medical management may be successful in approximately half of all affected neonates (Ricketts, 1994). Such management is based on three traditional principles: (1) bowel rest, (2) prevention of progressive injury, and (3) normalization of systemic responses. Enteral nutrition is discontinued; the stomach is decompressed by low intermittent suction through a large-bore orogastric tube; and fluids and electrolytes are closely monitored and adjusted. Antibiotic therapy (after blood for cultures is drawn), early intubation and ventilation, management of acid-base derangements, and efforts to support blood pressure and blood flow to the gut are undertaken both to prevent continuing injury and to correct systemic responses. Serial abdominal films are made at 6 to 8 hour intervals during acute illness to monitor progression of the disease and to detect perforation (Kanto et al, 1994).

Criteria for surgery are somewhat controversial and may vary slightly from institution to institution. However, expedient laparotomy is ideally performed after the advent of intestinal gangrene but prior to perforation. Absolute indications are pneumoperitoneum or confirmation of intestinal gangrene by positive paracentesis (peritoneal tap producing ≥0.5 ml of fluid that is yellowish brown or brown or contains bacteria that is demonstrated on Gram stain, or both). Nonspecific but supportive findings include clinical deterioration in spite of vigorous clinical management (metabolic acidosis, ventilatory failure, thrombocytopenia, leukopenia or leukocytosis with shift to the left, oliguria, and so on), portal venous air, erythema of the abdominal wall, or persistently dilated and fixed bowel loop (Kosloske, 1994b; Parigi et al, 1994; Ricketts, 1994).

The principles of surgical management include careful examination of the bowel with resection of all grossly necrotic intestine or perforated sites. If the viability of extensive portions of the gut is in question, resection is deferred, with a follow-up second look operation carried out in 24 to 48 hours. Otherwise the bowel ends are brought to the surface to create an ostomy (Ricketts, 1994).

Extensive respiratory therapy may be required throughout hospitalization, especially when marked abdominal distention may interfere with ventilation. Long-term parenteral nutrition can be anticipated, thus making collaboration with the nutritional support team essential.

Because of the high incidence of NEC in the intensive care nursery, a premature infant who experiences any of the early signs of obstruction (vomiting, distention, increased gastric aspirates), one who demonstrates increased episodes of apnea and bradycardia, or one who passes bloody stools should be regarded with a high index of suspicion. Should two or more of the early signs appear together, one should presume NEC until other diagnostic studies can be performed. Feedings are immediately stopped and venous access obtained. A gastric tube is set to intermittent suction for decompression. Vigorous hydration and antibiotic therapy are provided, and total parenteral nutrition is initiated as soon as possible. Circulatory status must be evaluated frequently by monitoring perfusion, vital signs—including blood pressure—and urinary output. All stools are routinely checked for blood. Hematologic studies are performed to look for anemia, thrombocytopenia, and disordered coagulation. Furthermore, blood, platelets, or fresh frozen plasma is given as needed. Oxygenation and acid-base status are also monitored, with respiratory support provided accordingly. Careful, gentle reexamination of the abdomen should be carried out every 8 hours.

Ventilatory and circulatory support are maintained in the postoperative period, and antibiotic therapy is continued for 10 to 14 days past resolution of pneumatosis. Ostomy care is performed as previously described. When stabilized GI function has resumed (generally in 7 to 14 days), feedings are cautiously and slowly begun with small amounts of dilute elemental formula. The amount and concentration of feedings are advanced as tolerated, but these attempts are frequently frustrated by malabsorption associated with short bowel syndrome or the development of strictures. Recurrent distention, residuals, vomiting, intractable constipation, or bloody stools may be noted with partial or complete obstruction due to such strictures.

Short Gut Syndrome

Pathophysiology. The median length of newborn small intestine is approximately 250 cm. Infants with as little as 15 cm and an intact ileocecal valve have survived. The ileocecal valve delays transit time and allows for increased digestion and absorption. Additionally it acts as a barrier to prevent overgrowth of colonic bacteria in the small intestine.

If the ileocecal valve is removed, 30 to 45 cm of bowel is probably needed for survival. The loss of considerable absorptive surface results in a complex malabsorptive problem with episodic diarrhea, steatorrhea, and dehydration, which, if allowed to progress, may cause metabolic derangements and ultimately poor growth and development and possibly death.

Risk Factors. The short bowel (short gut) syndrome is an unfortunate complication of many neonatal surgeries that involve extensive resection of the GI tract, such as necrotizing enterocolitis, gastroschisis, megacystic microcolon, intestinal atresia, Hirschsprung, and vovulus. The removal of even a small section of intestine can result is severe diarrhea and failure to thrive.

Clinical Manifestations. Infants postoperatively fail to tolerate even small amounts of enteral nutrition and exhibit diarrhea and malabsorption. In the presence of short bowel syndrome, months to years of hospitalization may not be unusual (Vennarecci et al, 2000). The duration of initial hospitalization and length of dependence on parenteral nutrition are both inversely related to the length of remaining bowel (Chaet et al, 1994). Most infants eventually experience progressive small bowel adaptation, and the surgically shortened intestine grows; the mucosal wall hypertrophies; and the villi become hyperplastic so that the absorptive area is increased. Blood flow to the residual intestine and the proportion of the villus that is enzymatically active are both initially increased but gradually decline as the surface area and length continue to increase with time (Swaniker et al, 1995).

Prognosis. Infant survival after massive bowel resection is related to the maturity of the infant at the time of resection,

length of the remaining intestine, presence of distal small intestine, presence of the ileocecal valve, presence of an intact colon, intactness of pancreatic and liver function, and absence of other complicating congenital anomalies. Patients with short gut syndrome with chronic dependence on TPN usually have poor quality of life and numerous readmissions for abdominal surgeries, central venous catheter-related infections, dislodgement of central line catheters and/or feeding tubes, wound infections and dehiscence, developmental delay, and TPN associated liver failure.

Collaborative Management. Treatment of short gut syndrome is difficult because of the length of time it takes for intestinal adaptation to take place. Parenteral nutrition is initiated soon after surgery and continued through out the period of refeeding. Elemental formula (casein hydrolysate, glucose, Medium Chain Triglyceride or MCT) is required usually by continuous infusion and is very gradually increased. Medications such as loperamide, diphenoxylate, and phenothiazines have been used in individual patients to help control diarrhea. Cholestyramine may be used to help bind bile acid and thereby decrease diarrhea. Trimethoprim-sulfamethoxazole and metronidazole are used in the treatment of bacterial overgrowth. Infants who show no adaptive response after months of feeding attempts may have radical surgery to slow intestinal transit (e.g., intestinal valves, reversed segment, colon interposition, intestinal pacing, intestinal lengthening, tapering enteroplasty, or neomucosa). Small bowel transplantation presents a life-saving option for these patients. Results of intestinal transplantation continue to improve, with survivial rates of 53% to 72% (Vennarecci et al, 2000). Higher survival rates may be achieved with improved operative technique and postoperative management as well as better patient selection and timing of transplant.

Nursing care of the infant with short gut syndrome includes collaborative management with team members to monitor fluid, electrolyte, and nutritional status. Prevention of skin breakdown due to diarrhea and infection are critical. Parents must be involved in their infants' care, and every effort must be made to stimulate normal growth and development.

Spontaneous Bowel or Gastric Perforations

Pathophysiology. Spontaneous bowel or gastric perforations can be caused by a variety of factors. NEC or ischemia of the bowel are two of the more common problems. Iatrogenic trauma that is secondary to an invasive procedure such as gastric intubation or hyperinflation of the stomach is another potential causative factor. Spontaneous bowel or gastric perforations can also be secondary to mechanical ventilation or distal bowel obstruction that leads to ischemia (Ryckman, 2002).

Risk Factors. Invasive procedures, mechanical ventilation, and history of NEC or intestinal obstructions are all risk factors. Prematurity and perinatal stress has some association with spontaneous perforations. Steroid therapy, especially long-term therapy, has been linked to such perforations (Ryckman, 2002).

Clinical Manifestations. The infant is usually several days old at the time symptoms appear. The third or fourth day is the most common time. There is marked abdominal distention that is tender to the touch and respiratory distress that worsens as the distension increases. There may or may not be vomiting. If the perforation has progressed, hypovolemic shock is possible. This condition is considered a neonatal surgical emergency.

Prognosis. The prognosis is directly related to how quickly the situation is recognized, the age of the infant (maturity), and the severity of the perforation.

Differential Diagnosis. Radiographic studies will confirm perforations. They will usually be in the form of pneumoperitoneum. Contrast studies can confirm but are not suggested (Ryckman, 2002).

Collaborative Management. This situation is an emergency, and the initial treatment is bedside paracentesis with a large IV. A peripheral IV should be inserted for resuscitative measures before this procedure. Insertion of a nasogastric tube for decompression is done simultaneously. If the infant does not respond favorably to this treatment, invasive surgery may be warranted. Surgery is performed to remove any torn tissue and to close the perforation.

Postoperative care centers on maintenance of fluids and electrolytes, blood volume, and broad-spectrum antibiotics (Ryckman, 2002).

Lactobezoars
Pathophysiology. Lactobezoars are an adverse effect of high-caloric feedings. They are firm balls of fat that form in the infant's intestinal tract about 3 to 12 days after enteral feedings have started (Ryckman, 2002). Infants who have received antacids have also been known to form these bezoars (Ryckman, 2002). They are an iatrogenic complication. They may be secondary to delayed gastric emptying, but in most cases there is no known etiology.

Clinical Manifestations. The most common symptoms are those associated with an intestinal obstruction; they include abdominal distention, vomiting, diarrhea, and increasing gastric aspirates (Ryckman, 2002). The infant may or may not have guaiac positive stools, depending on how long the bezoar has been pressured or the amount of pressure it is exerting on the intestinal wall. Some infants exhibit no symptoms.

Differential Diagnosis. The diagnosis can be made either by palpation of a firm ball or mass usually in the upper left quadrant or by radiographic studies (Ryckman, 2002). Contrast studies following injection of a small amount of air into the gastic area can also help with the diagnostic evaluation, as the mass will appear on x-ray.

Prognosis. The prognosis is good and in most cases with minimal complications.

Collaborative Management. The treatment is aimed at relief of the intestinal obstruction. Gastric decompression may or may not be needed to relieve the distention. Gastric perforation, while rare, is always a possibility, and evaluation of the infant for this complication is wise. Ryckman (2002) advocates the prevention as the best treatment by delaying the introduction of high caloric feedings until 2 to 3 weeks of age.

Risk Factors. Prematurity, low birth weight, and the introduction of high-calorie, highly dense formulas are the most common risk factors.

SUMMARY

The present management of infants with GI disorders aims for early recognition with relief of symptoms and eventual resumption of normal function to support nutritional needs. Diligent nursing assessment allows early intervention, and appropriate research-based care ensures the best possible long-term results.

REFERENCES

Bates MD et al, (1998). Biliary atresia: Pathogenesis and treatment. *Seminars in liver disease*, 18(3), 281-293.

Bates MD, Balistreri WF (2002). The neonatal gastrointestinal tract: part one: development of the human digestive system. In Fanaroff AA, Martin RJ (eds). *Neonatal-perinatal medicine: diseases of the fetus and infant*, ed. 7, St Louis: Mosby.

Bloom RS (2002). Delivery room resuscitation of newborn. In Fanaroff AA, Martin RJ (Eds.), *Neonatal-perinatal medicine: diseases of the fetus and infant*, ed. 7, St Louis: Mosby.

Buescher ES (1994). Host defense mechanisms of human milk and their relations to enteric infections and necrotizing enterocolitis. *Clinics in perinatology*, 21(2), 247-262.

Buyukunal C et al (1994). Maternal cocaine abuse resulting in necrotizing enterocolitis: an experimental study in a rat model. *Acta paediatrica*, 83(Suppl. 396), 91-93.

Chaet MS et al (1994). Intensive nutritional support and remedial surgical intervention for extreme short bowel syndrome. *Journal of pediatric gastroenterology and nutrition*, 19(3), 295-298.

Champous AN et al (1994). Recurrent intussusception. *Archives of pediatric and adolescent medicine*, 148(5), 474-478.

Chan KL et al (1994). A study of pre-antibiotic bacteriology in 125 patients with necrotizing enterocolitis. *Acta paediatrica*, 83(Suppl. 396), 45-48.

Cortes D et al (1995). Cryptorchidism in boys with imperforate anus. *Journal of pediatric surgery*, 30(4), 631-635.

Deitch EA (1994). Role of bacterial translocation in necrotizing enterocolitis. *Acta paediatrica*, 83(Suppl. 296), 33-36.

Ein SH, Shandling B (1994). Pure esophageal atresia: a 50-year review. *Journal of pediatric surgery*, 29(9), 1208-1211.

Elhalaby EA et al (1995). Enterocolitis associated with Hirschsprung's disease: A clinical-radiological characterization based on 168 patients. *Journal of pediatric surgery*, 30(1), 76-83.

Ewer AK et al (1994). Gastric emptying in preterm infants. *Archives of disease in childhood*, 71(1), F24-F27.

Faix RG, Adams JT (1994). Neonatal necrotizing enterocolitis: Current concepts and controversies. [Review]. *Advances in pediatric infectious disease*, 9, 1-36.

Fast C, Rosegger H (1994). Necrotizing enterocolitis prophylaxis: oral antibiotics and lyophilized enterobacteria vs. oral immunoglobulins. *Acta paediatrica*, 83(Suppl. 396), 86-90.

Fletcher MA (1994). Nutrition. In Avery GB et al (Eds.), *Neonatology: pathophysiology and management of the newborn*, ed. 4, Philadelphia: JB Lippincott.

Fotter R, Sorantin E (1994). Diagnostic imaging in necrotizing enterocolitis. [Review]. *Acta paediatrica*, 83(Suppl. 396), 41-44.

Fuloria M et al (2000). Gastroesophageal reflux in very-low-birth-weight infants: association with chronic lung disease and outcomes through 1 year of age. *Journal of perinatology*, 20(4), 235-239.

Gupta SK et al (1994). Necrotizing enterocolitis: laboratory indicators of surgical disease. *Journal of pediatric surgery*, 29(110), 1472-1475.

Gutierrez C et al (1994). Recurrent tracheoesophageal fistula treated with fibrin glue. *Journal of pediatric surgery*, 29(120), 1567-1569.

Guyton AC, Hall JE (2000). *Textbook of medical physiology*, ed 11, Philadelphia: WB Saunders.

Heij HA et al (1995). Long-term anorectal function after Duhamel operation for Hirschsprung's disease. *Journal of pediatric surgery,* 30(3), 430-432.

Horwitz JR et al (1995). Complications after surgical interventions for necrotizing enterocolitis: a multicenter review. *Journal of pediatric surgery,* 30(7), 994-999.

Israel EJ (1994). Neonatal necrotizing enterocolitis: a disease of the immature intestinal mucosal barrier. *Acta paediatrica,* 83(Suppl. 396), 27-32.

Jona et al (1998). Laparoscopic pull-through procedure for Hirschsprung's disease. *Seminars in pediatric surgery,* 7(4), 228-231.

Jones KL, Fletcher J (1996). *Smith's recognizable patterns of human malformation: genetic, embryologic and clinical aspects,* ed 5, Philadelphia: WB Saunders.

Kanto WP et al (1994). Recognition and medical management of necrotizing enterocolitis. *Clinics in perinatology,* 21(2), 335-346.

Kee JL (2001). *Laboratory and diagnostic tests with nursing implications,* ed 4, Upper Saddle River, NJ: Prentice-Hall.

Kelly EJ, Newell SJ (1994). Gastric ontogeny: clinical implications. *Archives of disease in childhood,* 71(2), F136-F141.

Kemmotsu H et al (1995). Cervical approach for the repair of esophageal atresia. *Journal of pediatric surgery,* 30(4), 549-552.

Khalaf MN et al (2001). Clinical correlations in infants in the neonatal intensive care unit with varying severity of gastroesophageal reflux. *Journal of pediatrics and gastroenterology and nutrition,* 32(1), 45-49.

Kimball AL, Carlton DP (2001). Gastroesophageal reflux medications in the treatment of apnea in premature infants. *Journal of pediatrics,* 138(3), 355-360.

Kimura K, Soper RT (1994). Multistaged extrathoracic esophageal elongation for long gap esophageal atresia. *Journal of pediatric surgery,* 29(4), 566-568.

Kluth D et al (1995). Rotation of the gut: fact or fantasy? *Journal of pediatric surgery* 30(3), 448-453.

Koenig WJ et al (1995). Manometrics for preterm and term infants: a new tool for old questions. *Pediatrics,* 95(2), 203-206.

Kosloske AM (1994a). Epidemiology of necrotizing enterocolitis. *Acta paediatrica,* 83(Suppl. 396), 2-7.

Kosloske AM (1994b). Indications for operation in necrotizing enterocolitis revisited. *Journal of pediatric surgery,* 29(5), 663-666.

Kubota M et al (1994). Erythromycin improves gastrointestinal motility in extremely low birthweight infants. *Acta paediatrica japonica,* 36(2), 198-201.

Lambrecht W, Kluth D (1994). Esophageal atresia: a new anatomic variant with gasless abdomen. *Journal of pediatric surgery,* 29(4), 564-565.

Lee TY et al (1995). "Spoke wheel" sign of small intestinal volvulus. *American journal of emergency medicine,* 13(4), 477-478.

Lemelle JL et al (1994). Neonatal necrotizing enterocolitis: a retrospective and multicenter review of 331 cases. *Acta paediatrica,* 83(Suppl. 396), 70-73.

Lincoln-Boyea B & Cefalo RC (1996). Principles of Genetic Counseling. In JA Kuller et al (Eds.), *Prenatal diagnosis & reproductive genetics,* St Louis: Mosby.

Lipschitz B et al (1995). Endoscopic pneumatic reduction of an intussusception with simultaneous polypectomy in a child. *Journal of pediatric gastroenterology and nutrition,* 21(1), 91-94.

Ludman L, Spitz L (1995). Psychosocial adjustment of children treated for anorectal anomalies. *Journal of pediatric surgery,* 30(3), 495-499.

Martucciello G et al (1995). Immunohistochemical localization of RET protein in Hirschsprung's disease. *Journal of pediatric surgery,* 309(3), 433-436.

Marty TL et al (1995a). Gastrointestinal function after surgical correction of Hirschsprung's disease: long-term follow-up in 135 patients. *Journal of pediatric surgery,* 30(5), 655-658.

Marty TL et al (1995b). Rectal irrigations for the prevention of postoperative enterocolitis in Hirschsprung's disease. *Journal of pediatric surgery,* 30(5), 652-654.

Maxson RT et al (1995). The protective role of enteral IgA supplementation in neonatal gut origin sepsis. *Journal of pediatric surgery,* 30(2), 231-234.

Mayr J et al (1994). Psychosocial and psychomotoric development of very low birthweight infants with necrotizing enterocolitis. *Acta paediatrica,* 83(Suppl. 396), 96-100.

Merenstein GB, Gardner SL (2002). *Handbook of neonatal intensive care,* ed. 5, St Louis: Mosby.

Moore SW et al (1994). Long-term clinical, manometric, and histological evaluation of obstructive symptoms in the postoperative Hirschsprung's patient. *Journal of pediatric surgery,* 29(1), 106-111.

Morecroft JA et al (1994). Necrotizing enterocolitis—multisystem organ failure of the newborn? *Acta paediatrica,* 83(Suppl. 296), 21-23.

Morrison SC, Jacobson JM (1994). The radiology of necrotizing enterocolitis. *Clinics in perinatology,* 21(2), 347-363.

Ng SC, Quak SH (1998). Gastroesophageal reflux in preterm infants: norms for extended esophageal pH monitoring. *Pediatric gastroenterology and nutrition,* 27(4), 411-414.

Nowicki PT, Nankervis CA (1994). The role of the circulation in the pathogenesis of necrotizing enterocolitis. *Clinics in perinatology,* 21(2), 219-234.

Orenstein SR et al (1999). Gastroesophageal reflux disease in children. *Gastroenterology clinics of North America,* 28(4), 947-969.

Parigi GB et al (1994). Surgical treatment of necrotizing enterocolitis: when? how? *Acta paediatrica,* 83(Suppl. 296), 58-61.

Rachelson MH et al (1955). Intussusception in the newborn infant with spontaneous expulsion of the intussusception. *Journal of pediatrics,* 47(1), 87-94.

Ravelli AM et al (1994). Gastric emptying in children with gastric transposition. *Journal of pediatric gastroenterology and nutrition,* 19(4), 403-409.

Reyna TM (1994). Familial Hirschsprung's disease: study of a Texas cohort. *Pediatrics,* 94(3), 347-349.

Ricketts RR (1994). Surgical treatment of necrotizing enterocolitis and the short bowel syndrome. *Clinics in perinatology,* 21(2), 365-387.

Rintala R et al (1994). Fecal continence and quality of life for adult patients with an operated high or intermediate anorectal malformation. *Journal of pediatric surgery,* 29(6), 777-780.

Rivosecchi M et al (1995). Spinal dysraphism detected by magnetic resonance imaging in patients with anorectal anomalies: incidence and clinical significance. *Journal of pediatric surgery,* 30(3), 488-490.

Roller CG et al (1999). Birth kangaroo (skin-to-skin) care and breastfeeding: an eclamptic woman's story. *MCN: American journal of maternal child nursing,* 24(6), 294-295.

Ryckman FC (2002). The neonatal gastrointestinal tract: part iv: selected anomalies and intestinal obstructions. In AA Fanaroff, RJ Martin (Eds.), *Neonatal-perinatal medicine: diseases of the fetus and infant,* ed 7, St Louis: Mosby.

Ryckman FC, Balistreri WF (2002). The neonatal gastrointestinal tract: part two: upper gastrointestinal disorders. In AA Fanaroff, RJ Martin (Eds.), *Neonatal-perinatal medicine: diseases of the fetus and infant,* ed 7, St Louis: Mosby.

Ryckman FC et al (1998). Biliary atresia—surgical management and treatment options as they relate to outcomes. *Liver transplant surgery,* 4(5, Suppl 1), S24-F33.

Schober PH, Nassiri J (1994). Risk factors and severity indices in necrotizing enterocolitis. *Acta paediatrica,* 83(Suppl. 396), 49-52.

Seashore JH (1978). Congenital abdominal wall defects. *Clinics in perinatology,* 5(1), 61-77.

Seashore JH, Touloukian RJ (1994). Midgut volvulus: an ever-present threat. *Archives of pediatrics and adolescent medicine,* 148(1), 43-46.

Shanbhogue RLK et al (1994). Ultrasonography is accurate enough for the diagnosis of intussusception. *Journal of pediatric surgery,* 29(2), 324-328.

Shiels WE (1995). Childhood intussusception: management perspectives in 1995. *Journal of pediatric gastroenterology and nutrition,* 21(1), 15-17.

Snel A et al (2000). Behavior and gastroesophageal reflux in the preterm neonate. *Journal of gastroenterology and nutrition,* 30(1), 18-21.

Spilson SV et al (2001). Association between maternal diabetes mellitus and newborn oral cleft. *Annals of plastic surgery,* 47(5), 477-481.

Stoll BJ (1994). Epidemiology of necrotizing enterocolitis. *Clinics in perinatology,* 21(2), 205-218.

Stringer MD et al (1994). Meconium ileus due to extensive intestinal aganglionosis. *Journal of pediatric surgery,* 29(4), 501-503.

Surana R et al (1994). Short-gut syndrome: intestinal adaptation in a patient with 12 cm of jejunum. *Journal of pediatric gastroenterology and nutrition,* 19(2), 246-249.

Swaniker F et al (1995). Adaptation of rabbit small intestinal brush-border membrane enzymes after extensive bowel resection. *Journal of pediatric surgery,* 30(7), 1000-1003.

Tappero EP, Honeyfield ME (1996). *Physical assessment of the newborn: a comprehensive approach to the art of physical examination,* ed 2, Petaluma, CA: NICU Ink.

Tsakayannis DE, Shamberger RC (1995). Association of imperforate anus with occult spinal dysraphism. *Journal of pediatric surgery,* 30(7), 1010-1012.

Vasan U, Gotoff SP (1994). Prevention of neonatal necrotizing enterocolitis. *Clinics in perinatology,* 21(2), 425-435.

Vennarecci G et al (2000). Intestinal transplation for short-gut syndrome attributable to necrotizing enterocolitis. *Pediatrics,* 105 (2), E25.

Wolf HM, Eibl MM (1994). The anti-inflammatory effect of an oral immunoglobulin (IgA-IgG) preparation and its possible relevance for the prevention of necrotizing enterocolitis. *Acta paediatrica,* 83(Suppl. 396), 37-40.

Young TE, Mangum OB (2001). *Neofax 2001.* Chapel Hill, NC: University of North Carolina.

Zenk K (1999). *Neonatal medications and nutrition: a comprehensive guide.* Santa Rosa, CA: NICU, Ink.

ASSESSMENT AND MANAGEMENT OF THE METABOLIC SYSTEM

CATHERINE THEORELL, MARGUERITE DEGENHARDT

The human genome is estimated to be composed of 50,000 to 100,000 individual genes, each one capable of regulating specific biochemical cellular processes. A disruption in the function of a single gene causes disturbances in cellular function and metabolic errors. In addition, combinations of genes can also cause metabolic errors that result in diseases. Therefore at least the same numbers of genetic errors of metabolism are possible, and an undetermined percentage of these may cause significant disease (Gilbert-Barness & Barness, 2000; Beaudet et al, 2001).

Discoveries in molecular biology that derived from the Human Genome Project have given researchers a more complete picture of the incidence of genetic disease. It is estimated that 1% of live-born infants have monogenic disease, 6% to 8% of hospitalized children have monogenic disease; 29% to 41% of hospitalized children have genetically influenced disease; 20% to 30% of infant deaths are due to genetic causes; and 30% to 50% of postneonatal deaths are the result of congenital malformations. It is also estimated that the genetic makeup of each human being includes six to eight lethal genes (Gilbert-Barness & Barness, 2000).

Incidence varies widely among ethnic groups for some disorders, such as sickle cell anemia (1 in 655 in U.S. African Americans), cystic fibrosis (1 in 2500 in Europeans), Gaucher disease type 1 (1 in 600 in Ashkenazim), and phenylketonuria (1 in 12,000 in U.S. newborns primarily of Northern European descent). However, it is less variant for other diseases, such as achondroplasia (1 in 50,000), Duchenne muscular dystrophy (1 in 3000 males), and hemophilia A (1 in 10,000 males) (Beaudet et al, 2001; Green, 2001).

Identification of the genetic causes of errors in metabolism provides the foundation for the prognosis, genetic counseling, and treatment of affected families. Many of these infants require life-sustaining treatment before a definitive diagnosis can be derived from laboratory tests. It is important that the diagnosis be made accurately and promptly. Often, metabolic disease is suspected only after the routine causes of diseases have been eliminated. The likelihood of metabolic disease is greater in infants with a history of consanguinity or in those whose families have a history of unexplained neonatal death; multiple spontaneous abortion; sudden, unexplained death of a sibling; or previously undiagnosed metabolic diseases (Burton, 2000).

Infants with metabolic disease often become critically ill with nonspecific findings. Symptoms such as vomiting, lethargy, or poor feeding may mimic sepsis in a newborn. However, with errors of metabolism, aggressive management and correction of biochemical abnormalities are required to relieve the symptoms. When the infant's response to emergency treatment is not as predicted, an error in metabolism should be suspected, and appropriate blood and urine specimens should be obtained. Once the diagnosis is strongly suspected or confirmed, and as soon as possible, the multifaceted, complex diagnostic methods and treatment for the disorder must be explained in detail to the family (Burton, 2000; Gilbert-Barness & Barness, 2000).

Emergency treatment and stabilization of infants suspected of having an error of metabolism involves minimizing intake and endogenous production of toxic metabolites by eliminating enteral feedings and supplying high-carbohydrate parenteral fluids such as 10% dextrose in 0.2% sodium chloride (NaCl) at one and one half times the maintenance rate. Potassium chloride (KCl) should be added to parenteral fluids only after renal output has been established. Acidosis, if present, should be corrected using sodium bicarbonate. If the plasma bicarbonate level is under 10 mmol/L, sodium bicarbonate should be administered cautiously. Any intercurrent illness should be treated (Burton, 2000). Many metabolic disorders are exacerbated by infection or catabolic states (Burton, 2000; Gilbert-Barness & Barness, 2000). If intractable seizures are present without hyperammonemia or metabolic acidosis, the infant may require pyridoxine therapy (Gilbert-Barness & Barness, 2000). If a urea cycle defect is suspected, the toxic metabolites should be eliminated as quickly as possible to minimize the neurologic damage associated with these disorders. For these infants, immediate transfer to an institution capable of neonatal hemodialysis is of paramount importance (Falk et al, 1994; Burton, 2000; Gilbert-Barness & Barness, 2000).

Fortunately, metabolic dysfunction in the neonate is a relatively rare occurrence. Although these problems are not always identified until after discharge from the neonatal intensive care unit (NICU), they must be detected as soon as possible to avoid long-term complications, such as developmental delays and mental retardation. This chapter describes prenatal and postnatal detection, biochemical defects, and the clinical manifestations of some of the more common metabolic disorders, as well as their collaborative management.

ROUTINE NEONATAL SCREENING TESTS

The purpose of routine neonatal screening for metabolic disease, which involves nonselective testing of large numbers of newborns, is to identify individuals with a certain genotype or change in the gene structure that is associated with a particular disease or that predisposes the carrier to the disease. Implicit in the concept of neonatal screening are four important elements: (1) accurate identification of affected individuals, (2) availability of specific treatment, (3) earlier implementation of medical management, (3) hope of an improved outcome, and (4) availability of informative genetic counseling (Duran et al, 1994; Gilbert-Barness & Barness, 2000; Green, 2001).

Routine neonatal screening for metabolic disorders emerged after Bickel demonstrated the effectiveness of phenylalanine-restricted diets for individuals with phenylketonuria (PKU) (Bickel et al, 1954). Before this time, no treatment existed for newborns with PKU, and survivors suffered severe neurologic and mental impairment. The method used at that time to screen urine for phenylpyruvic acid failed to detect this disorder in newborns because urinary levels of phenylpyruvic acid may not become elevated for weeks despite markedly high plasma levels of phenylalanine (Paul et al, 1980). By the time the urine test detected PKU, severe neurologic impairment had already occurred. Affected newborns had to be identified earlier to ensure maximum effectiveness of phenylalanine restriction on neurologic outcome.

It was not until 1962 that Guthrie developed a bacterial inhibition assay for phenylalanine measured from whole blood; this provided a reliable, specific screening measure for identifying newborns with PKU (Bickel et al, 1980). Guthrie's test is based on inhibition of the growth of the bacterium *Bacillus subtilis* by biochemical compounds abnormally present in whole blood disk specimens. The elevated blood phenylalanine levels in newborns with PKU resulted in more suppressed bacterial growth around the blood specimen in direct proportion to the elevation of phenylalanine (Bickel et al, 1980). In this way, elevated blood phenylalanine levels could be identified and quantified.

The ingenuity of this method was not the microbiologic test per se but the use of a capillary whole blood specimen impregnated on filter paper. This technique allowed for the widespread implementation of newborn screening programs because it simplified and standardized the process. Guthrie's bacterial inhibition assay is considered a vital contribution to the process of screening for metabolic diseases.

The research conducted on PKU demonstrated that neonatal screening programs were feasible and practical and that defects with a fixed genotype do respond to therapeutic intervention (Burton, 2000; Scriver et al, 2001). By using different inhibitors and bacterial strains, Guthrie adapted his inhibition assay to detect other disorders, including defects in the metabolism of leucine, methionine, histidine, lysine, tyrosine, and galactose.

Since the discoveries related to PKU, research on inherited metabolic disorders has intensified. As a result of this explosion of knowledge, affected individuals can be identified as early as the first trimester of pregnancy; the biochemical complexities of metabolic disease have been defined; and new treatments have been proposed and evaluated (Ploos van Amstel et al, 1994; Burton, 2000). Despite these rapid advances, our understanding of metabolism and metabolic disorders is not yet complete.

The success of widespread screening for PKU in newborns led to the belief that all metabolic disorders could be identified in a similar manner. Although theoretically possible in numerous cases, mass screening for all metabolic disorders is not yet justifiable. A screening test to detect a metabolic disorder is readily justifiable when the same blood sample can be used as that drawn for PKU testing and when the corresponding disorder is relatively common in the population tested and effectively treatable (Burton, 2000; Gilbert-Barness & Barness, 2000; Beaudet et al, 2001; Scriver et al, 2001). For example, screening for congenital hypothyroidism by thyroid-stimulating hormone (TSH) analysis is justifiable, because the disorder occurs in 1 in 3500 births; a sensitive, specific measure is available; and early initiation of treatment limits the severity of the resulting mental disorders (Beaudet et al, 2001; Scriver et al, 2001).

In 1978 the International Symposium on Newborn Screening for Inborn Errors of Metabolism met in Heidelberg, and the National Academy of Sciences defined the initial criteria for selecting diseases amenable to neonatal screening (Gilbert-Barness & Barness, 2000; Scriver et al, 2001):

1. The disease presents a significant problem when the diagnosis is delayed (i.e., high rates of mortality and morbidity).
2. The condition has a high incidence in a population.
3. The condition is amenable to treatment.
4. A simple, inexpensive screening test is available.
5. The test is sensitive and specific, and quality control is maintained.
6. A mechanism exists for collecting samples and delivering them to the laboratory.
7. A reliable means of reporting results exists.
8. Resources for treatment or counseling are available.
9. The cost of screening, diagnosis, and treatment during the asymptomatic phase is outweighed by savings in human misery and fiscal expenditure.

Using these criteria, the symposium members identified four diseases for which reliable tests for large-scale screening of infants are available and that should receive priority in detection: PKU, congenital hypothyroidism, galactosemia, and maple syrup urine disease (MSUD) (Scriver et al, 2001). The symposium identified three other diseases—tyrosinemia, homocystinuria, and histidinemia—that cannot be considered for priority screening because they have important clinical variants that escape detection on testing (homocystinuria, tyrosinemia) or because treatment has not proved effective (histidinemia) (Scriver et al, 2001). Four years after the Heidelberg symposium, a fifth disorder, congenital adrenal hyperplasia, was added to the priority diseases amenable to routine neonatal screening (Burton, 2000; Scriver et al, 2001). Some states, such as Ohio, require the test for homocystinuria.

Other amino acid disorders, the organic acidurias, the transport disorders, and cystic fibrosis are not routinely screened in all states. Screening tests for hyperlipidemias or hemoglobin disorders and hemolytic anemias resulting from erythrocyte abnormalities can be proposed only for high-risk groups. However, in 1989 Ohio mandated routine neonatal screening for the hemoglobinopathies sickle cell anemia and beta-thalassemia. Since then other states have expanded testing to include sickle cell disease and many other disorders.

The purpose of neonatal screening is to diagnose, shortly after birth, infants with genetic diseases in which early treatment prevents or minimizes serious, irreversible complications or even death. However, neonatal screening is not mandated by the federal government. Each state is responsible for setting up a program that selects which newborn screening tests are conducted, the technology for analyzing the specimen, the process of reporting results, and the method of informing the pediatrician of the results. The first mandatory screening law for the detection of PKU was passed in 1963 in Massachusetts (Bickel et al, 1980). Since then each state has defined which tests are to be included in the routine newborn screen. As the genetic complexities of more metabolic disorders are understood, the neonatal screening tests change over time and from state to state. The most common metabolic errors tested in newborn screens nationwide include PKU, congenital hypothyroidism, galactosemia, MSUD, homocystinuria, biotinidase deficiency, sickle cell disease, congenital adrenal hyperplasia, and cystic fibrosis.

Most newborn screening tests are performed on dried filter paper blood spots obtained in the first few days of life. The blood spots should be obtained before 72 hours of life and after 24 hours of consuming at least 1 g% of protein feeding. If the infant is discharged before 24 hours of age, a newborn screen should be obtained before discharge and repeated after discharge. All newborns should be screened before 7 days of age, regardless of gestational age at birth. Because the normal values for newborn screens are based on findings for full-term infants, the results of screens from extremely immature infants may be outside the normal range. When possible, newborn screens should be obtained before any blood transfusions are given because donor blood may invalidate the screening test (Bickel, 1954; Burton, 2000; Gilbert-Barness & Barness, 2000; Beaudet et al, 2001; Scriver & Kaufman, 2001).

Recent advances in molecular genetics have given rise to the possibility that metabolic disorders one day may be screened through DNA mutation analysis. Over the next several years, the states' newborn screening programs will be expanded to include many other genetic metabolic disorders.

The Department of Health Resources and Services Administration, an agency of the Department of Health and Human Services (DHHS), has produced a manual, *Newborn Screening: An Overview of Newborn Screening Programs in the United States and Canada*, that describes for each state and province the current parameters for neonatal screening programs, the testing methods used, and the follow-up resources available for affected families. The manual is updated every 3 years, and copies can be obtained through a medical center library or a state Department of Public Health.

PRENATAL AND NEONATAL DIAGNOSIS OF INHERITED METABOLIC DISORDERS

Prenatal diagnosis of inherited metabolic disorders developed concurrently with advances in chromosomal analysis, molecular genetics, and fetal cell culture. Successful growth of fetal cells in culture soon had researchers interested in investigating the enzymatic machinery of these tissues, which ultimately allowed prenatal diagnosis of a substantial number of inherited metabolic disorders. Each year additional information is discovered that facilitates prenatal diagnosis of an increasing number of metabolic disorders.

Despite the widespread success in prenatal diagnosis of inherited metabolic disorders, such testing is not often indicated (Bickel et al, 1980; Burton, 2000; Gilbert-Barness & Barness, 2000; Beaudet et al, 2001; Scriver et al, 2001). Because most inherited metabolic disorders are rare, and some extremely so,

prenatal diagnosis involves a delicate balance that demands a thorough understanding of the technical, biochemical, ethical, and psychologic difficulties experienced by those involved.

Prenatal screening by means of amniocentesis, chorionic villus sampling, or cordocentesis can be carried out for a considerable number of metabolic disorders (Ploos van Amstel et al, 1994; Gilbert-Barness & Barness, 2000; Beaudet et al, 2001; Scriver et al, 2001). However, these are sophisticated procedures that should be performed only by laboratories experienced in such techniques. Some metabolic conditions are not amenable to prenatal investigation, and postnatal screening for these disorders must be done at the earliest opportunity. Also, prenatal screening is not justifiable when satisfactory treatment is available after early postnatal diagnosis (Burton, 2000; Gilbert-Barness & Barness, 2000; Beaudet et al, 2001; Scriver et al, 2001).

Newborns are not screened for all inherited metabolic disorders. Only newborns suspected of having an inherited metabolic disorder should undergo the rigorous investigation of metabolism. If a neonatal screening test result is positive for an inherited metabolic disorder (e.g., PKU), the diagnostic investigation is not complete. It is important not to make a diagnosis of inherited metabolic disorder too quickly. Ancillary tests often are needed to confirm the diagnosis and to avoid errors in management. For example, galactosuria can be seen in newborns without galactosemia or galactokinase deficiency (Burton, 2000; Gilbert-Barness & Barness, 2000; Beaudet et al, 2001; Green, 2001). Also, an increase in serum phenylalanine, tyrosine, and methionine levels may be seen with various hepatic disorders or in immature newborns receiving an excessive protein intake (Burton, 2000; Gilbert-Barness & Barness, 2000; Scriver & Kaufman, 2001). Severe hyperammonemia is not always caused by a specific enzyme deficiency but may be due to hepatic dysfunction arising from other causes (Burton, 2000; Gilbert-Barness & Barness, 2000). With severe hypoglycemia, hyperinsulinemia first should be ruled out, especially in the absence of ketosis (Burton, 2000; Gilbert-Barness & Barness, 2000; Scriver et al, 2001).

In the analysis and investigation of metabolic disorders, a positive screening test result must be followed up with complementary determinations of compounds. For example, a positive test result for PKU must be followed up by determining the levels of phenylalanine, tyrosine, orthohydroxyphenylacetic acid, phenylpyruvic acid, and urinary biopterins to confirm the diagnosis and identify the exact type of hyperphenylalaninemia (Burton, 2000; Gilbert-Barness & Barness, 2000; Scriver & Kaufman, 2001). This confirmational stage is critical, because moderate, transient hyperphenylalaninemias and immaturity tyrosinemias are common and do not require treatment; biopterin deficiency as a cause of hyperphenylalaninemia does not respond to dietary restrictions and requires different treatment (Bickel et al, 1954; Burton, 2000; Gilbert-Barness & Barness, 2000; Scriver & Kaufman, 2001).

Clinical manifestations of inherited metabolic disorders may be general or specific (Burton, 2000). Often the nurse has the first opportunity to take a detailed history from the parents. Frequently the history shows recurrent spontaneous abortions (Burton, 2000), unexplained neonatal deaths, or psychomotor deficiencies in the family and warrants a precise study of genealogy (Gilbert-Barness & Barness, 2000; Beaudet et al, 2001). Specific investigation of consanguinity should be performed to analyze for the presence of an autosomal recessive disorder. An X-linked disorder might be suspected if male siblings, cousins, and uncles are affected. The medical histories of siblings should be analyzed for the occurrence of neonatal deaths or abnormalities, even if these supposedly were caused by acquired disorders such as septicemia, anoxia, or subarachnoid hemorrhage. Previous children with a history of hypoglycemia, acute encephalopathy, ataxia, metabolic acidosis, hepatomegaly, or acute episodes of "intoxication" or vomiting should increase suspicion that an inherited metabolic disorder may exist (Gilbert-Barness & Barness, 2000; Beaudet et al, 2001).

Circumstances leading to the onset of symptoms are very important in the investigation of inherited metabolic disorders. An important negative finding is the absence of fetal or perinatal distress that may explain the abnormalities. Metabolic disorders often are characterized by an interval of variable duration during which the newborn apparently is normal. For example, in Tay-Sachs disease, the clinical manifestations may take months to appear; in MSUD, the symptoms appear after 5 to 6 days; and in pyruvate carboxylase deficiency, symptoms begin several hours after birth (Gilbert-Barness & Barness, 2000; Beaudet et al, 2001; Scriver et al, 2001). Clinical manifestations may also take on an intermittent or cyclic character, brought about by increases in protein intake or tissue catabolism (Burton, 2000; Gilbert-Barness & Barness, 2000).

Often the neonate with an inherited metabolic disorder shows neurologic manifestations such as hypotonia, hypertonia, lethargy, alternating hyperexcitability and somnolence, myoclonia, abnormal eye movements, alteration in levels of consciousness, coma, and seizures (Gilbert-Barness & Barness, 2000; Scriver et al, 2001). Additional clinical manifestations that would lead to the suspicion of an inherited metabolic disorder include vomiting, diarrhea, poor feeding, weight loss, dehydration, and failure to thrive. Hepatomegaly with hyperbilirubinemia may be present (Burton, 2000; Gilbert-Barness & Barness, 2000). The infant may appear to have a hemorrhagic syndrome and splenomegaly (Burton, 2000; Gilbert-Barness & Barness, 2000; Scriver et al, 2001). The infant's breath or sweat may have an unusual odor, or the urine may have an unusual odor or color (Burton, 2000; Gilbert-Barness & Barness, 2000).

Clinical manifestations in an infant with an undiagnosed inherited metabolic disorder usually occur in the absence of infection, central nervous system (CNS) hemorrhage, or congenital defects (Burton, 2000; Gilbert-Barness & Barness, 2000). Despite institution of conventional therapy, no relief exists for these symptoms, although some transient improvement in clinical manifestations may occur after elimination of enteral intake, an exchange transfusion, venovenous hemofiltration, or hemodialysis/peritoneal dialysis (Falk et al, 1994; Burton, 2000; Gilbert-Barness & Barness, 2000).

The initial laboratory investigation of an infant suspected of having a metabolic disorder should include blood determinations for the glucose level, acid-base equilibrium, and ammonia levels. In addition, a complete blood count, coagulation studies, and electrolyte, calcium, magnesium, blood urea nitrogen, and creatinine measurements should be performed to rule out other possible causes of the symptoms (Burton, 2000). The urine should be tested for ketones (Acetest), reducing sugars (Clinitest), glucose (Clinistix), phenylpyruvic acid (Phenistix), and toxic substances (Burton, 2000; Gilbert-Barness & Barness, 2000). When an inherited metabolic disorder is suspected, it is important that a sample or a series of samples of blood and urine be set aside for later testing (Duran et al, 1994; Burton, 2000; Gilbert-Barness & Barness, 2000; Beaudet

et al, 2001), preferably before administration of any blood products.

Certain clinical manifestations may be found alone or in association with abnormal laboratory findings. For example, neurologic symptoms may occur alone or in association with metabolic acidosis or alkalosis, ketosis, hypoglycemia, or hyperammonemia; hypoglycemia may be associated with ketosis; and severe acidosis may be associated with hematologic symptoms, pancytopenia, or hepatic insufficiency (Burton, 2000; Gilbert-Barness & Barness, 2000; Scriver et al, 2001). Depending on the suspected etiology, more sophisticated testing can be undertaken, such as ion exchange or gas chromatography of blood and urine for amino acid quantification, gas chromatography of urinary organic acids coupled with mass spectrometry, and determinations of pyruvemia, erythrocyte galactose-1-phosphate, and urinary oligosaccharides and mucopolysaccharides (de Franchis et al, 1994; Duran et al, 1994; Burton, 2000; Gilbert-Barness & Barness, 2000; Beaudet et al, 2001). Enzyme and complex DNA analysis can also be done on blood cells, hepatocytes, or cultured skin fibroblasts to assist in the diagnosis of the metabolic disorder (Burton, 2000; Gilbert-Barness & Barness, 2000; Beaudet et al, 2001). A positive response to treatment is an additional diagnostic finding. For example, the symptoms associated with galactosemia rapidly improve when galactose is removed from the diet (Burton, 2000; Gilbert-Barness & Barness, 2000; Luzzatto et al, 2001).

Because metabolic disorders may be inherited, an accurate diagnosis must be made even if the infant has died. With all infants suspected of having had a metabolic disorder, skin samples should be obtained after death for fibroblast cultures and enzyme analysis. If possible, blood and urine samples should be obtained for biochemical analysis. Needle biopsy specimens of the liver, kidneys, brain, and muscle tissue should be obtained as soon as possible after death for ultrastructural studies. Delay in obtaining these tissue specimens makes ultrastructural studies difficult and enzyme analysis impossible (Duran et al, 1994; Burton, 2000; Gilbert-Barness & Barness, 2000; Beaudet et al, 2001; Scriver et al, 2001).

To facilitate an understanding of the ways metabolism disorders affect the neonate, a brief description of normal metabolism is presented, followed by a description of some of the metabolic disturbances encountered in clinical practice.

CARBOHYDRATE METABOLISM

Circulating glucose plays an essential role in the provision of fuel for many tissues. Glucose occupies a unique position in intermediary metabolism for two reasons:

1. Glucose is the substrate of glycolysis that is the sole pathway for the production of adenosine triphosphate (ATP) in anaerobic life. Although human beings as a whole do not exist in an anaerobic condition, erythrocytes, which are devoid of mitochondria, are completely dependent on glycolysis for their supply of ATP.

2. Glucose is the major substrate of brain metabolism. Ketone bodies are easily used by brain tissue, but the normal concentrations of these substances are low and increase only during fasting. Fatty acids are bound to albumin in the blood and cannot penetrate the blood-brain barrier. A decline in the blood glucose level, therefore, may result in neurologic injury; this in itself justifies the development of rather elaborate mechanisms of hepatic control over blood glucose.

Figure 27-1 presents a brief summary of carbohydrate metabolism. The main dietary carbohydrates are starch, sucrose, and lactose, which are hydrolytically degraded into the free sugars, glucose, fructose, and galactose. Hydrolysis of the oligosaccharides occurs through the action of oligosaccharidases located in the wall of the intestine.

Fructose is rapidly used by the liver and converted to glucose and lactate. Intravenous administration of fructose results in the development of lactic acidemia from the intense usage of that sugar. In addition, fructose-1-phosphate accumulates in the liver, causing depletion of inorganic phosphate and ATP; this is followed by the conversion of adenine nucleotides to uric acid, resulting in hyperuricemia (Ali et al, 1998).

The liver also rapidly uses galactose, and its metabolism normally causes no problem; only in congenital galactosemia does the galactose concentration in the blood increase. Galactosemia is discussed in greater detail later in this chapter. Unlike the metabolism of glucose, the metabolism of fructose and galactose is not subject to tight regulation.

All tissues of the body use glucose, and its penetration into muscle and adipose tissue is controlled by insulin. As the primary regulator of blood glucose, the liver takes up glucose during times of abundance after meals and converts it mostly to glycogen. The liver uses very little of this glucose for its own energy needs, instead consuming mostly fatty acids. By the breakdown of glycogen and by gluconeogenesis during times of fasting, the liver delivers a large amount of glucose to the blood for use by the brain, erythrocytes, and other tissues. The concentration of glucose in the blood is the primary stimulus that elicits glucose uptake or glucose output by the liver. The hepatic threshold of glucose is the glucose concentration at which the liver is converted from an organ of glucose output to an organ of glucose uptake (Sunehag et al, 1999).

Glucose transport across the hepatic membrane is an efficient carrier-mediated process that is not influenced by insulin. The primary action of glucose in the hepatocyte is to bind to phosphorylase *a*, an active hepatic enzyme. The activity of phosphorylase *a* is inhibited by glucose, and the glucose-bound phosphorylase *a* is rapidly converted to phosphorylase *b* by phosphorylase phosphatase. Thus the first effect of an elevated blood glucose level is to diminish and eventually arrest glycogen degradation in the liver (Saudubray et al, 2000).

An elevated blood glucose level also stimulates glycogen synthesis by allowing the activation of glycogen synthetase. The enzyme responsible for glycogen synthesis, synthetase phosphatase, is strongly inhibited by phosphorylase *a*. This mechanism thus prevents glycogen synthesis when blood glucose levels are low (Chakrapani et al, 2001).

Gluconeogenesis is the mechanism by which lactate and amino acids are converted to glucose. Gluconeogenesis occurs in the liver and the kidneys; it plays a major role in glucose control under fasting conditions and allows the removal of

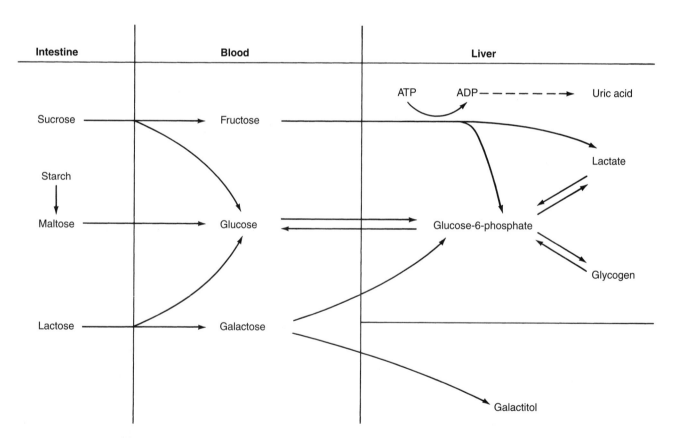

FIGURE **27-1**

Summary of carbohydrate metabolism. The primary dietary carbohydrates are starch, sucrose, and lactose, which are hydrolytically degraded into the free sugars glucose, fructose, and galactose. Hydrolysis of the oligosaccharides occurs through the action of oligosaccharidases located in the intestinal wall. This specific location of the enzymes prevents the accumulation of free sugars in the intestine and their utilization by microorganisms. *ADP*, Adenosine diphosphate; *ATP*, adenosine triphosphate.

large amounts of lactic acid from the blood. Gluconeogenesis seems to operate continuously in the liver even in fed states. The rate of gluconeogenesis is increased by the release of glucagon and also during fasting states.

Most of the enzymes involved in gluconeogenesis are freely reversible and are common to glycolysis (Figure 27-2). However, there are three exceptions: (1) at the level of interconversion of pyruvate and phosphoenolpyruvate, at which the glycolytic enzyme pyruvate kinase is reversed by a two-step conversion involving pyruvate carboxylase and pyruvate carboxykinase; (2) at the level of the interconversion between fructose diphosphate and fructose-6-phosphate, at which phosphofructokinase is reversed by hexose diphosphatase; and (3) at the level of interconversion of glucose and glucose-6-phosphate, at which glucokinase is reversed by glucose-6-phosphate (Moukil et al, 2000).

The main advantage of the interconversion recycling system is that it allows very large changes in glucose uptake and output to be controlled only by substrate concentration. An increase in the glucose concentration influences the phosphorylase syn-

thetase system, and the recycling of glucose and glucose-6-phosphate allows the second system to keep pace with the first (Saudubray et al, 2000).

DISORDERS OF CARBOHYDRATE METABOLISM

Carbohydrates are important components of diets throughout the world; after intestinal hydrolysis and absorption, they serve as a critical source of metabolic energy. Defects in hydrolysis or absorption result in retention of residues in the intestinal tract and, ultimately, gastrointestinal (GI) symptoms. Carbohydrate intolerance is a common clinical problem that may have serious consequences, particularly when it occurs early in life.

The predominant symptoms of an infant with carbohydrate intolerance are intestinal. They are the result of the osmotic effects of unabsorbed carbohydrate in the lumen of the small intestine and of the products of bacterial fermentation in the large intestine. The osmotic pressure of the unabsorbed carbohydrate in the small intestine leads to secretion of water and electrolytes into the lumen until osmotic equilibrium is

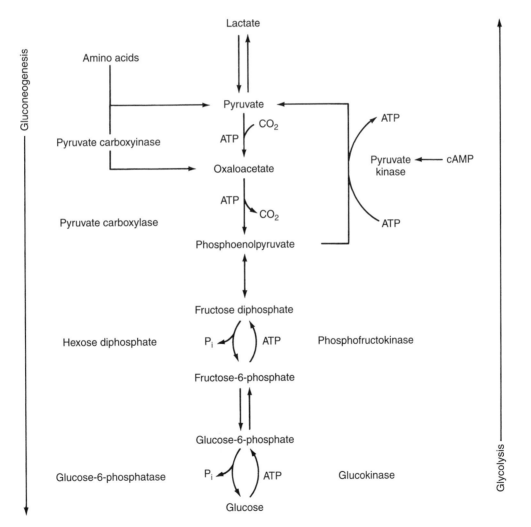

FIGURE **27-2**
Pathway of glycolysis and gluconeogenesis. Most of the enzymes responsible for gluconeogenesis are freely reversible and are common to glycolysis. The three exceptions are at the level of interconversion of pyruvate to phosphoenolpyruvate, the interconversion between fructose diphosphate and fructose-6-phosphate, and the interconversion of glucose and glucose-6-phosphate. *ADP,* Adenosine diphosphate; *ATP,* adenosine triphosphate; *cAMP,* cyclic adenosine monophosphate; CO_2, carbon dioxide; P_i, inorganic phosphate.

reached. A proportion of the carbohydrate may be excreted unchanged in the stool, but most of it is hydrolyzed (reduced). Ideal and colonic bacteria hydrolyze the carbohydrate into small molecules, short-chain organic acids, hydrogen, carbon dioxide, and other fermentative products. The organic acids lower the stool pH, inhibit water absorption from the colon, and contribute to the increased mobility (Castro-Rodriguez et al, 1997; Desjeux, 2000). The severity of the symptoms varies with age, the extent of the enzyme deficiency, the load of the offending carbohydrate, and the colon's ability to reabsorb the excessive fluid delivered to it by the small intestine.

Watery, acidic diarrhea and excoriated buttocks are the hallmarks of carbohydrate intolerance in infants; however, fluid losses can be profound and life-threatening. Abdominal distention may be prominent, along with recurrent vomiting. Weight loss is common in affected infants (Scriver et al, 2001). Older children may have mild or intermittent loose stools, with cramping abdominal pain and bloating.

The risk of further sequelae is high, especially in infants. Dehydration may be complicated by metabolic acidosis. Large amounts of bicarbonate are secreted into the intestinal lumen to neutralize the contents and hydrogen ions produced by bacterial fermentation of the carbohydrate. Untreated lactose intolerance in infancy can lead to a more generalized malabsorption of other sugars, nitrogen compounds, and fats, with further impairment of nutrition (Lee & Boey, 1999; Desjeux, 2000).

In the diagnosis of carbohydrate disorders, a positive family history of symptoms may emerge, suggesting a primary carbohydrate malabsorption. The most important information is obtained from a detailed dietary history that links the symptoms to carbohydrate ingestion. For infants, this requires full knowledge of the composition of infant formulas and weaning foods. The nurse has a pivotal role in obtaining a detailed dietary history from the parents and in relating these findings to the clinical presentation.

The clinical response to dietary restriction is at times the last confirmatory evidence of carbohydrate intolerance. Clinically, many infants with carbohydrate intolerance are too ill to justify formal challenges or to undergo detailed invasive investigations. An empiric diagnosis is made based on the history, clinical manifestations, and stool examination. Then a prescription for lactose-free, disaccharide-free, or even carbohydrate-free diets is given. The diagnosis is confirmed later, after the infant has recovered and the baby's condition has been stabilized. The nurse often is a key player in the investigation, diagnosis, evaluation, and management of these disorders.

Examination of the stools of infants suspected of having carbohydrate disorders involves measurement of reducing substances, glucose, pH, and organic acid content, in addition to carbohydrate chromatography. The indices for carbohydrate intolerance in infants with diarrhea are: concentrations of the reducing substances above 0.25%; 1+ glucose level; and stool pH under 6. All tests must be performed on the liquid portion of fresh stool specimens, preferably collected on nonabsorbent material, because formed stools are unlikely to contain significant amounts of sugars. The tests must be performed immediately, because fecal bacteria hydrolyze sugars very rapidly at room temperature, and pH declines while lactic acid content increases quickly (Castro-Rodriguez et al, 1997; Calvo et al, 2000). All stools must be tested, because some specimens may be carbohydrate free even in infants with severe intolerance.

Tests for reducing substances of stool are very useful but can yield false-positive or false-negative results. Antibiotic therapy and the type of sugar in the diet must be considered when interpreting the results of the pH and sugar measurements in stool. Fecal pH is influenced by the degree of colonic fermentation of unabsorbed carbohydrate. A pH under 6 frequently is found in infants with fermentative diarrhea, but higher values do not exclude the diagnosis. The fecal pH depends on the bacterial fermentation of carbohydrates; any factor that modifies this relationship may alter the stool pH without influencing the capacity to tolerate carbohydrates. False-positive results can be due to nonabsorbable sugars such as lactulose or plant hexoses, oligosaccharides of bacterial origin, or noncarbohydrate substances that may be present without any sugar intolerance. Sugars such as lactose, sucrose, glucose, and galactose may be found in healthy neonates. For these reasons, carbohydrate chromatography may be necessary to test the significance of the stool reducing substances. Carbohydrate malabsorption can be accurately determined when the detailed dietary description is compared with the results of this test.

The observed response to an oral sugar load is one of the standard tests of carbohydrate malabsorption. The shape of the blood sugar curve after ingestion is a measure of absorption, whereas the symptoms after ingestion (coupled with stool examination) indicate clinical intolerance. The nurse often is responsible for assessing the infant throughout the carbohydrate oral challenge test, obtaining frequent blood and stool specimens, and evaluating the infant's clinical response.

Breath tests have also been used in the diagnosis of carbohydrate malabsorption. Hydrogen breath tests do not require the use of radiolabeled compounds. The amount of hydrogen excreted in the breath correlates well with the amount produced in the intestine by fermentation of carbohydrates. The proximal small intestine, the site of carbohydrate absorption, is not normally colonized by H_2-producing bacteria. Therefore the breath concentration of hydrogen after an oral load of sugar is a measure of the degree of malabsorption. Breath hydrogen measurement is the most accurate, sensitive, and specific indirect test for detecting lactose deficiency, and its results are not affected by gastric emptying and intermediary glucose metabolism. In premature infants, the results of laboratory tests of carbohydrate absorption, such as the breath hydrogen level, frequently are "abnormal" and therefore are of limited usefulness in the clinical management of these infants. Breath analysis is used for full-term neonates and older infants.

DISORDERS OF GALACTOSE METABOLISM

There are three known inherited abnormalities of galactose metabolism, which are transmitted by autosomal recessive inheritance. The metabolic disorders result from a deficiency of galactokinase, galactose-1-phosphate uridyltransferase, or uridine diphosphate galactose 4-epimerase, the enzymes of the pathway that converts galactose to glucose.

Galactokinase deficiency has mild clinical symptoms, resulting mainly in cataracts. Galactose-1-phosphate uridyltransferase deficiency manifests as failure to thrive, vomiting, liver disease, cataracts, and developmental delay. Even when a lactose-free diet is followed, transferase-deficient patients may develop long-term complications, including poor growth, speech abnormality, mental deficiency, neurologic syndromes and, in females, ovarian failure. The pathophysiology of both the acute toxicity syndromes and the long-term complications is uncertain (Ning et al, 2000).

Two forms of uridine diphosphate galactose 4-epimerase deficiency have been identified. One form is benign and can be detected using screening procedures that assay red blood cell galactose-1-phosphate. The other form is clinically similar to transferase deficiency and responds to restriction of dietary galactose (Walter et al, 1999; Riva et al, 2001). In this condition, some dietary galactose is necessary for the formation of uridine diphosphate galactose, which is essential in various metabolic processes.

Most galactose in the diet is in the form of the disaccharide lactose, which is synthesized in the mammary gland from glucose. Lactose is the primary carbohydrate source for nursing mammals; it provides approximately 40% of the energy in human milk. Lactose digestion is initiated by hydrolysis of the disaccharide into absorbable monosaccharides glucose and galactose. Lactose is hydrolyzed by the galactosidase lactase in the brush border of the small intestine.

The main pathway of galactose metabolism is the conversion of galactose to glucose, which requires several enzymatic steps. In the normal pathway of galactose metabolism, galactose is phosphorylated with ATP to form galactose-1-phosphate (Ning et al, 2000). The galactose-1-phosphate reacts with uridine diphosphate glucose (UDP-glucose), which is catalyzed by galactose-1-phosphate uridyltransferase, to produce two products: glucose-1-phosphate and UDP-galactose. Classic galactosemia results from a block in this step (Moukil et al, 2000; Saudubray et al, 2000). The UDP-galactose formed is converted to UDP-glucose by UDP-galactose 4-epimerase. The UDP-glucose formed can then serve as a substrate for the transferase reaction. These reactions function in a cyclic manner until all of the galactose-1-phosphate entering the pathway from galactose is converted to glucose-1-phosphate and subsequently to glucose (Ning et al, 2000; Scriver et al, 2001).

When no galactose is introduced to the pathway from an external source, protective processes act to produce galactose and its metabolites, which are critical to the formation of complex lipids and glycoprotein. Glucose-1-phosphate reacts with uridine triphosphate (UTP) by means of UDP-glucose pyrophosphorylase activity to form UDP-glucose, which can then be epimerized to form UDP-galactose. Epimerase maintains equilibrium between UDP-glucose and UDP-galactose in nearly all cells. The UDP-galactose formed can also serve as a source of cellular galactose-1-phosphate and galactose. Free galactose is produced by turnover of glycolipids and glycoproteins (Scriver et al, 2001).

If galactose cannot be metabolized because of a deficiency or because of inefficiency of galactokinase, transferase, or epimerase, two alternative pathways are available. Galactose can be reduced to galactitol by aldolase reductase or oxidized to galactonate by an oxidase or dehydrogenase (Scriver et al, 2001).

Hereditary Galactokinase Deficiency

Hereditary galactokinase deficiency is an autosomal recessive disorder of galactose metabolism. The incidence of galactokinase deficiency varies from 1 in 40,000 to 1 in 155,000 across European populations (Abdullah et al, 1996; Scriver et al, 2001). The difference in occurrence has not yet been explained, although genetic heterogeneity may be one factor. Racially determined galactokinase polymorphism has been de-

tected in North American blacks, in whom the red blood cells are less active than in Caucasians.

The absence of clinical symptoms in the newborn period and the appearance of cataracts in older patients on unrestricted diets differentiate this disorder from transferase deficiency. Because galactokinase-deficient newborns are asymptomatic or develop cataracts as the first and only abnormality, diagnosis in early infancy depends on the routine screening of blood and urine for galactose.

The diagnosis of galactokinase deficiency can be made by finding normal amounts of galactose-1-phosphate uridyltransferase and an absence of galactokinase in the red blood cells (Chakrapani et al, 2001; Scriver et al, 2001). High blood galactose levels are best detected after milk feedings. Reducing substances in the urine may be identified as galactose. The urine of any newborn with cataracts should be examined for sugar by means of a method that does not use glucose oxidase. An assay of the blood for the defect should also be done (Calvo et al, 2000).

Galactokinase-deficient adults are not mentally deficient, although the visual deprivation caused by the cataract formation may affect psychomotor development. Galactokinase-deficient individuals have no aversion to milk and experience no discomfort from drinking it. They are asymptomatic except for the cataracts that appear in infancy. If the milk intake is high, these individuals excrete substantial amounts of galactose and galactitol, and after an oral galactose load, the blood galactose level rises excessively (Ning et al, 2000; Scriver et al, 2001).

The nuclear cataracts seen with this disorder develop as a result of an accumulation of galactitol in the lens. The trapped galactitol causes swelling and disruption of lens fibers. Formation of the cataracts is caused by a complex sequence of events, including disturbances in the balance of water, electrolytes, amino acids, proteins, energy-rich phosphates, and reduced glutathione (Scriver et al, 2001). Treatment of galactokinase deficiency with a galactose exclusion diet must be continued throughout life. These patients may tolerate minute amounts of galactose; however, in infants with galactose-1-phosphate uridyltransferase deficiency, no amount of galactose is tolerated (Ning et al, 2000).

Hereditary Galactose-1-Phosphate Uridyltransferase Deficiency

Hereditary galactose-1-phosphate uridyltransferase deficiency is an autosomal recessive disorder involving a deficiency of galactose-1-phosphate uridyltransferase, which catalyzes the metabolism of galactose-1-phosphate to galactose to uridine diphosphate (Ning et al, 2000). Incidence rates vary widely but are estimated at approximately 1 in 155,000 (Desjeux, 2000). The absence of transferase activity of erythrocytes is the basis for diagnosing galactosemia (Scriver et al, 2001). The enzyme deficiency can also be demonstrated in many other tissues, such as cultured skin fibroblasts, and in cultured amniotic fluid. Heterozygotes have approximately one half of normal enzyme activity in their red blood cells (Scriver et al, 2001).

Infants with galactosemia have a normal birth weight but fail to gain weight after they begin ingesting milk. Symptoms, which usually appear in the second half of the first week of life, include jaundice, vomiting, and diarrhea (Lee & Boey, 1999). The jaundice and unconjugated hyperbilirubinemia often are associated with severe hemolysis, mimicking erythroblastosis fetalis. Many affected newborns receive exchange transfusions before diagnosis. Nuclear cataracts appear within days or weeks and become irreversible within weeks of their appearance (Scriver et al, 2001). If milk feedings continue, the disease usually progresses, resulting in abnormal liver function, hepatomegaly, cirrhosis, and death. Occasionally a patient does not show failure to thrive, but rather motor retardation, hepatomegaly, and cataracts several months after birth. The incidence of *Escherichia coli* sepsis and neonatal death is high in infants with transferase deficiency galactosemia, probably because leukocyte bactericidal activity is inhibited. For this reason, neonates with *E. coli* sepsis and older infants with cataracts should be suspected of having galactosemia and should be tested for the enzyme deficiency (Calvo et al, 2000; Scriver et al, 2001).

A presumptive diagnosis of galactosemia may be made with identification of galactose in the urine and blood. The presence of reducing substance in the urine that does not react with glucose oxidase reagents (e.g., Clinistix) is consistent with the presence of galactose (Castro-Rodriguez et al, 1997; Calvo et al, 2000). However, lactose, fructose, and pentose may also yield a positive result. Although this test is a useful, noninvasive method of screening, it is important to note that normal newborns may excrete galactose up to 60 mg/dl in the first 5 days of life, and this level may be detected for up to 2 weeks in premature infants.

Thirty-eight states require screening for galactosemia in newborns (Saudubray et al, 2000; Scriver et al, 2001). The disorder can be diagnosed with a simple filter paper blood specimen in a manner similar to that used to detect PKU. A complete protocol for the detection of all disorders of galactose metabolism has been described. As the result of widespread screening of newborns, many patients have been diagnosed early in the course of the disease and with proper diet management have avoided the acute toxic effects of galactosemia.

The outcome for infants with galactosemia depends on early diagnosis and treatment. In general, the clinical manifestations of the disorder are reversed a few weeks after initiation of appropriate treatment, but the long-term outcome and intellectual development are uncertain. Follow-up of galactosemic individuals has shown that many have developed very well, whereas others have had more severe problems involving growth, development, brain function and, in females, ovarian dysfunction (Scriver et al, 2001).

The causes of variability in response to treatment require further study. Family differences related to genetic or sociologic factors may account for some of these findings. Another determinant is the age at which the diagnosis is made; the outcome is more favorable if the infant is treated early. Furthermore, galactose-1-phosphate accumulates in the cord blood of an infant born to a galactosemic mother, even if the mother follows a restricted lactose intake throughout pregnancy (Abdullah et al, 1996; Scriver et al, 2001). It can be inferred, then, that the intrauterine environment is unfavorable to the homozygous fetus, resulting in irreversible prenatal damage to the brain or ovaries or both.

Hereditary Uridine Diphosphate Galactose 4-Epimerase Deficiency

Hereditary uridine diphosphate galactose 4-epimerase deficiency, which is inherited as a recessive trait, is caused by the absence of UDP-galactose 4-epimerase in the blood. The incidence has been estimated at 1 in 23,000 in Japan, where screening programs were established. This error of metabolism

is not very common in the United States. (More information can be found on the CD.)

DISORDERS OF FRUCTOSE METABOLISM

Fructose is an important source of carbohydrate in the human diet. It is metabolized predominantly in the liver, kidneys, and small intestine and to a lesser extent in adipose tissue. The three known inherited abnormalities of fructose metabolism are essential fructosuria, hereditary fructose intolerance, and hereditary fructose-1,6-diphosphatase deficiency (Ali et al, 1998; Hillebrand et al, 2000).

Essential fructosuria is a benign, asymptomatic disorder caused by the absence of fructokinase, resulting in hyperfructosemia and fructosuria.

Hereditary fructose intolerance is characterized by hypoglycemia and vomiting after ingestion of fructose. In infants, prolonged fructose ingestion leads to poor feeding, vomiting, jaundice, hepatomegaly, hemorrhage, and possibly hepatic failure and death (Stormon et al, 2001). The disorder results from a deficiency of fructose-1-phosphate aldolase in the liver, kidney cortex, and small intestine. Hypoglycemia occurs after fructose ingestion because fructose-1-phosphate inhibits glycogenolysis and gluconeogenesis. Patients remain healthy on a diet free of fructose and sucrose.

Hereditary fructose-1,6-diphosphatase deficiency is characterized by episodes of hyperventilation, apnea, hypoglycemia, ketosis, and lactic acidosis (Lund & Leonard, 2000). The enzyme defect severely impairs gluconeogenesis, leading to accumulation of amino acids, lactate, and ketones (gluconeogenic precursors) as liver glycogen stores are depleted. Beyond early childhood, patients develop normally and become more tolerant of fasting.

Fructose is a major food constituent in human nutrition, occurring in some fruits and vegetables and honey. It is also a component of the disaccharide sucrose, which is used extensively as a sweetening additive for food, medications, and even infant formulas.

Fructose is metabolized in two ways in the human body. After ingestion, it is partly assimilated into glucose in the intestine through phosphorylation by fructokinase to fructose-1-phosphate (Ali et al, 1998; Scriver et al, 2001). The greater part reaches the liver, where it is extracted and rapidly phosphorylated to fructose-1-phosphate. Fructaldolase then splits fructose-1-phosphate into two triodes, which may be used for energy by entering the tricarboxylic acid (TCA) cycle or may be condensed to fructose-1,6-diphosphate and used for glucose or glycogen formation (Scriver et al, 2001). A small part of fructose passes through the liver and is transported to other tissues, such as adipose or muscle tissue, where it is metabolized to fructose-6-phosphate by the enzyme hexokinase (Scriver et al, 2001). In the kidneys, fructose is metabolized in the same way as in the intestine and the liver. As mentioned before, the three known inherited enzyme defects in the fructose pathway are (1) deficiency of fructokinase, or essential fructosuria; (2) deficiency of fructaldolase B, or hereditary fructose intolerance; and (3) deficiency of fructose-1,6-diphosphatase (Hillebrand et al, 2000).

Hereditary Fructose Intolerance

Hereditary fructose intolerance is inherited as an autosomal recessive trait and has an estimated incidence of 1 in 20,000 (Corpe et al, 1999; Hillebrand et al, 2000; Lund & Leonard,

2000). The disorder once was thought to be very rare, but it has become evident that hereditary fructose intolerance is more common. It occurs as a result of a deficiency in fructose-1-phosphate aldolase activity in homozygotes. With fructose intake, fructose-1-phosphate accumulates in the liver, kidneys, and small intestine because the defective aldolase B is unable to split it. In heterozygotes, fructose-1-phosphate aldolase activity is reported to be normal (Ali et al, 1998; Scriver et al, 2001).

In infants with hereditary fructose intolerance, the appearance and severity of symptoms depend on the intake of fructose. In the absence of fructose (e.g., with breastfeeding), no metabolic derangement occurs. With the intake of sucrose in the form of fruits and vegetables at weaning, the first symptoms are seen. The younger the child, the more severe the reaction to dietary fructose, and this reaction may be life-threatening.

Older children and infants develop an aversion to sweets and protect themselves from most or all exposure to the noxious sugar. If they consume fructose repeatedly in small amounts, a milder but chronic form of hereditary fructose intolerance is observed. The clinical manifestations of an acute ingestion include sweating, trembling, dizziness, nausea, vomiting, apathy, lethargy, coma, and convulsions. Clinical manifestations of chronic exposure include failure to thrive, vomiting, poor feeding, jaundice, hepatomegaly, cirrhosis, edema, ascites, and hemorrhages (Ali et al, 1998; Scriver et al, 2001). The organs most involved are those with a considerable pathway for metabolizing fructose: the liver and the kidneys.

Laboratory findings in infants with hereditary fructose intolerance include signs of liver dysfunction (Stormon et al, 2001). Test results are abnormal for the serum transaminase level, prothrombin time, serum protein level, plasma methionine level, and/or tyrosine level. Disturbed renal function may also be present and is manifested by melituria, proteinuria, hyperaminoaciduria, and acidosis. Diminished levels of serum phosphorus and potassium, fructosuria, organic aciduria, and metabolic acidosis mirror derangements of intermediate metabolism and are symptoms of the disorder. Morphologic study of liver tissue in infants with hereditary fructose intolerance has revealed fatty changes with vacuolization, fibrosis, and formation of bile ductules (Scriver et al, 2001).

The diagnosis of hereditary fructose intolerance is suspected from a detailed nutritional history and from clinical manifestations. Because of the nonspecific nature of the clinical manifestations, other metabolic disorders (e.g., tyrosinosis, glycogenosis), hepatitis, liver cirrhosis, or liver tumor must be ruled out. Pyloric stenosis may be suggested if vomiting is the primary symptom. Septicemia or intrauterine infection may clinically manifest in the same way as hereditary fructose intolerance, especially if clotting disturbances and hematologic changes are obvious (Calvo et al, 2000).

The diagnosis is confirmed by a fructose tolerance test or by enzyme assay of liver tissue or intestinal mucosa (Lund & Leonard, 2000). The fructose tolerance test requires a single intravenous dose of fructose. This challenge results in a rapid decline in fructose, which is associated with an increase in the serum magnesium and uric acid levels and a decline in the serum phosphorus and glucose levels. Maximum effects are seen 40 minutes after the fructose injection (Scriver et al, 2001). Once the diagnosis is established, treatment must be started immediately with a fructose-free diet. This results in nearly immediate clearance of symptoms except for hepatomegaly, which may persist for many months. Fatty changes of hepatocytes occasionally have been seen many months after initiation of

treatment. In young infants with severe liver damage, immediate withdrawal of fructose from the diet does not guarantee survival. Severe liver dysfunction may lead to hemorrhagic diastases and fatal liver failure (Scriver et al, 2001; Stormon et al, 2001).

Hereditary Fructose-1,6-Diphosphate Deficiency. Fructose-1,6-diphosphate deficiency is an extremely rare disease that is inherited as an autosomal recessive trait (Leonard & Morris, 2000; Scriver et al, 2001). (More information can be found on the CD.)

Carbohydrate Malabsorption in the Intestinal Brush Border

The three inherited disorders of the intestinal membrane, congenital lactase deficiency, sucrase-isomaltase deficiency, and congenital glucose-galactose malabsorption, are rare, autosomal recessive abnormalities. Clinical manifestation includes severe, watery diarrhea and dehydration after birth, after weaning, or after starch dextrins have been added to the diet. (For more information please consult the CD.)

Congenital Glucose-Galactose Malabsorption. In the neonatal period, congenital glucose-galactose malabsorption results in severe GI symptoms after ingestion of milk. Renal tubular resorption of glucose is also impaired, resulting in glycosuria. Unless foods containing glucose or galactose are withdrawn from the diet, the condition can be fatal. In vivo and in vitro studies have demonstrated a defect in or complete absence of sodium-coupled mucosal uptake of glucose in affected infants (Abdullah et al, 1996). The defect is thought to lie at the brush border level of the cell, but the precise molecular disarrangement has not yet been defined. Absorption of fructose, xylose, and the amino acids leucine and alanine is intact. An artificial milk with fructose as the only carbohydrate provides a satisfactory basis for early dietary treatment (Desjeux, 2000). As in some other congenital disorders of carbohydrate intolerance, a limited dietary tolerance to offending carbohydrates develops with increasing age, but some form of lifelong dietary restriction is required (Scriver et al, 2001).

AMINO ACID METABOLISM

Amino acids play a major role as constituents of intracellular and extracellular proteins. Some amino acids cannot be synthesized at rates sufficient to enable normal development, and these essential amino acids (isoleucine, leucine, lysine, methionine, phenylalanine, threonine, tryptophan, and valine) must be derived from exogenous sources such as dietary protein and nonprotein nitrogen. Estimates of the daily requirement for the essential amino acids have been established. Although histidine is not an essential amino acid, its presence is essential for normal infant growth.

The amino acids alanine, arginine, asparagine, aspartic acid, cysteine, glutamic acid, glutamine, glycine, histidine, proline, serine, and tyrosine can be synthesized from a reduced form of nitrogen and a carbon skeleton. Major sources of the carbon chain are f-alpha-ketoglutarate, pyruvate, and oxaloacetate; the reduced form of nitrogen becomes available from recycling of other compounds.

The detailed pathways of amino acid metabolism are beyond the scope of this discussion. For the purpose of this chapter, two facts are important: (1) the fetus is a rapidly growing organism supplied by the mother with all the necessary amino acids, which it uses to build up body tissues; and (2) probably only minor amounts of amino acids are used by the fetus for purposes other than growth.

The deposition of nitrogen is greater during the perinatal period than at any other time of life. The magnitude of protein synthesis can be demonstrated by the nitrogen content of the fetus, which at 6 weeks' gestation is 0.4 g, by 20 weeks is 15 g, and by full-term gestation is 500 g (Scriver & Kaufman, 2001). In the early postnatal months, this trend of nitrogen deposition continues.

The synthesis of any protein is a complex, multistep process that results in macromolecule formation from the 20 individual amino acids in a specific sequence that is under genetic control. All protein synthesis has two basic steps: (1) DNA that has the genetic code for the protein makes RNA; and (2) RNA makes the protein from cytosolic amino acids. All cellular constituents are continuously degraded and replaced. In the perinatal period, marked accumulation of protein occurs because synthesis is accomplished by placental transport of amino acids and the rate of synthesis exceeds that of degradation. The process of birth temporarily interrupts the high rate of protein synthesis in the fetus, regardless of maturity. This disruption in protein synthesis, which is caused by a shift in the constant nutrient supply of the placenta to the inadequate and sporadic intake of the first days of life, results in a negative nitrogen balance.

Gastrointestinal digestion and absorption of released amino acids are well developed in neonates. This is evidenced even in small preterm infants by the total stool nitrogen content, which does not exceed 15% of intake. Nitrogen is retained with avidity, and the amount retained is proportional to the intake (Scriver & Kaufman, 2001). In contrast to adults, in whom the effect is only transient, a high-protein intake results in high protein retention in neonates. Amino acid levels in infants, therefore, represent a net balance between a number of different processes, including (1) the amount available from the diet; (2) the amount used for tissue repair and growth; (3) the amount used for specific purposes; (4) the amount excreted in the urine; and (5) the amount remaining that must be metabolized. When an error of protein metabolism is investigated, all these processes merit consideration (Scriver & Kaufman, 2001).

Disorders of Amino Acid Metabolism

Disorders of amino acid metabolism may involve a specific enzyme disorder that affects the metabolism of a single amino acid or a group of amino acids; specific deficiencies in one of the intestinal absorption or renal tubular resorption systems; or intralysosomal accumulation of an amino acid (Burton, 2000; Gilbert-Barness & Barness, 2000; Beaudet et al, 2001; Scriver et al, 2001). Although there are only 20 amino acids, they undergo a multitude of reactions (e.g., hydroxylation, oxidation, transamination, methylation, and coupling), and a metabolic disorder can result when one of these processes is disrupted. Examples of select types of amino acid disorders are discussed in the following section. The diagnostic methods used in a suspected case of PKU establishes the rigorous investigation required in the evaluation of these disorders.

Hyperphenylalaninemias. The hyperphenylalaninemias are disorders of phenylalanine hydroxylation. The minimum requirements for a normal reaction are phenylalanine hydroxy-

lase (PAH), oxygen, L-phenylalanine, and tetrahydrobiopterin (BH_4) cofactor. For the pterin cofactor to function as a catalyst, dihydropterin reductase (DHPR) and reduced pyridine nucleotide are required. Other enzymes are also involved in recycling BH_4, which is an obligatory component of hydrolase function (Scriver & Kaufman, 2001).

Hyperphenylalaninemia, defined as a plasma phenylalanine level over 2 mg/dl (120 μmol), is a heterogeneous disease caused by mutations at the genetic sites that encode components of the hydroxylation reaction. The known and putative forms involve (1) primary deficiency in PAH activity (PKU and nonphenylketonuria [non-PKU]); (2) impaired synthesis of BH_4 as a result of enzyme deficiency; and, (3) impaired recycling of BH_4 as a result of deficient activity of DHPR or other putative enzyme systems (Scriver & Kaufman, 2001).

Two conditions are necessary to cause clinical manifestations: the genetic mutation and exposure to L-phenylalanine. In the BH_4-deficient forms, mutation alone is the principal cause of the disease. Patients with PKU have a plasma phenylalanine level above 1000 μmol; patients with non-PKU hyperphenylalaninemia have a lower phenylalanine level than those of PKU-affected infants. PKU is a disease with impaired cognitive and neurophysiologic consequences; non-PKU hyperphenylalaninemia signifies less clinical harm, and it may be a benign condition. The BH_4-deficient forms of the hyperphenylalaninemias have no categoric degree of hyperphenylalanine; they impair two other hydroxylation reactions involving tyrosine and tryptophan and the synthesis of the corresponding neurotransmitter derivatives (L-dopa and 5-hydroxytryptophan). The pathogenesis of the brain disorder in the different hyperphenylalaninemias involves the effects of phenylalanine on essential cellular processes in the brain, notably myelination, protein synthesis, and the consequences of deficient neurotransmitter supply (Burton, 2000; Gilbert-Barness & Barness, 2000; Scriver & Kaufman, 2001).

The genes that encode the components of the hydroxylation reaction are at various stages of analysis in normal and mutant genomes. Loci on chromosomes 4, 10, 11, 12, and 14 have been identified as playing a role in the hydroxylation reactions associated with hyperphenylalaninemia (Blau et al, 2001; Scriver & Kaufman, 2001).

Treatment requires restoration of blood phenylalanine levels to values as near normal as possible for as long as possible throughout life. Available data indicate that any deviation from this policy may incur a cost in neurophysiologic function and brain myelination in classic PKU-affected individuals. Whether it also applies to non-PKU hyperphenylalaninemia is unclear, but current opinion is shifting toward prudent (pretreatment) options, contrary to the past policy of no treatment. The BH_4-deficient forms of hyperphenylalaninemia require adjunct therapy that includes the supplements L-dopa and 5-hydroxytryptophan, BH_4 (with disorders of the cofactor synthesis), and folinic acid (with DHPR deficiency).*

Neonatal screening is the best method of screening for hyperphenylalaninemia. Both classification of the phenotype or disease (diagnosis) and case finding of BH_4 deficiency require measurement of phenylalanine, pterins (neopterin, biopterin, and BH_4), and neurotransmitter derivatives in

---

*Cleary et al, 1994; Costello et al, 1994; Potocnik & Widhalm, 1994; Ris et al, 1994; Beaudet et al, 2001; Blau et al, 2001; and Scriver & Kaufman, 2001.

plasma and urine (Burton, 2000; Gilbert-Barness & Barness, 2000; Scriver & Kaufman, 2001). In all forms of hyperphenylalaninemia, the activity of the mutant enzyme can be assessed either directly (by measurement in a population of cells, such as hepatocytes) or indirectly (by DNA analysis, enzymatic assay, and measurement of metabolites in amniotic fluid) (Scriver & Kaufman, 2001).

Maternal hyperphenylalaninemia has pathologic effects on the fetus that compromise growth and cause congenital malformations, including microcephaly and mental retardation in non-PKU infants. Fetal neuropathologic effects occur as a result of excessive intrauterine phenylalanine exposure from the positive transplacental gradient. Women with hyperphenylalaninemia require preconception reproductive counseling and should receive treatment for and be in strict control of phenylalanine levels before conception and throughout pregnancy. With meticulous care, a normal neurologic outcome is possible for the fetus (Gilbert-Barness & Barness, 2000; Scriver & Kaufman, 2001).

Hyperphenylalaninemia is a generic term for a disease distinguished by a phenylalanine level persistently above its normal plasma values. The metabolic dysfunction can have clinical consequences, depending on its pathogenesis and degree. The deficient enzyme names the associated diseases; for example, PKU is hyperphenylalaninemia resulting from total or nearly total deficiency of PAH activity. Different mutations at the PAH site can cause a lesser degree of hyperphenylalaninemia (non-PKU hyperphenylalaninemia). The distinction between these two hyperphenylalaninemias is arbitrary and rests with the plasma phenylalanine values over 16.5 mg/dl (1000 μmol) and lower tolerance for dietary phenylalanine (less than 500 mg/dl in classic PKU).

The disorders associated with the synthesis or maintenance of BH$_4$ are important in two additional hydroxylation reactions involving L-tryptophan and L-tyrosine, notably in the brain. The hydroxylated derivatives of these substrates, 5-hydroxytryptophan and L-dopa, are the precursors to serotonin and catecholamines and are neurotransmitters that influence brain development and function. Therefore the diagnosis of these variants is relevant to the prognosis and treatment of every infant with hyperphenylalaninemia (Burton, 2000; Gilbert-Barness & Barness, 2000; Scriver & Kaufman, 2001).

Phenylketonuria and Non-Phenylketonuric Forms of Hyperphenylalaninemia.   PKU is perhaps the best-known specific enzyme deficiency that results in a metabolic encephalopathy (Scriver & Kaufman, 2001). The incidence of PKU varies; it is 1 in 4500 live births in Northern Ireland, 1 in 10,000 live births among Caucasians, and 1 in 61,000 live births in Japan (Gilbert-Barness & Barness, 2000; Scriver & Kaufman, 2001). The average incidence of PKU in the United States ranges from 100 to 120 per 1 million live births (Gilbert-Barness & Barness, 2000; Beaudet et al, 2001; Scriver & Kaufman, 2001). The disease affects primarily people of western and central European descent; it is rare in blacks and in non-European populations (Bickel et al, 1980; Beaudet et al, 2001; Scriver & Kaufman, 2001).

PKU is an autosomal recessive trait with equal sex distribution. The chromosomal region involved in the classic form is 12q22-q24.1; a defect in this region results in a deficiency of the enzyme PAH, which is found primarily in the liver (Scriver & Kaufman, 2001). PAH is a participant, along with DHPR, in the complex conversion of phenylalanine to tyrosine (Bur-

ton, 2000; Gilbert-Barness & Barness, 2000; Scriver & Kaufman, 2001) (Figure 27-3). Although PAH deficiency is a hepatic disease, the major clinical effect of the associated metabolic hyperphenylalaninemia is seen in brain function. The variant metabolic disease thus is the cause of the neurotoxicity of disorders of PAH activity. Disorders of BH$_4$ synthesis and maintenance have both indirect and direct effects on brain development and function; the indirect effects are exerted through abnormal phenylalanine metabolism, and the direct effects arise from impairment of tryptophan and tyrosine hydroxylation.

PKU is characterized by (1) serum phenylalanine levels above 25 mg/dl (1500 μmol) (the normal level is under 2 mg/dl [120 μmol]); (2) normal serum tyrosine levels; and (3) urinary excretion of phenylpyruvic acid and orthohydroxyphenylacetic acid under normal protein dietary conditions (Burton, 2000; Gilbert-Barness & Barness, 2000; Scriver & Kaufman, 2001). PAH deficiency may be expressed in greater or lesser (to completely absent) amounts (Svensson et al, 1994; Gilbert-Barness & Barness, 2000; Scriver & Kaufman, 2001). In classic PKU, PAH is itself inactive, with less than 1% normal activity (Scriver & Kaufman, 2001). In the absence of PAH, the enzymes that convert phenylalanine into phenylethylamine and phenylpyruvic acid are present, causing increasing concentrations of these compounds in the urine (Svensson et al, 1994; Scriver & Kaufman, 2001).

There are no abnormal metabolites in PKU, only normal metabolites in abnormal amounts. With regard to neurotoxicity, phenylalanine is itself the villain. Induced high plasma values are associated with measurable acute impairment of higher integrative functions and with abnormal electroencephalographic (EEG) results. Both urine dopamine excretion and plasma L-dopa levels correlate inversely with plasma phenylalanine levels and positively with measures of brain dysfunction. Magnetic resonance imaging (MRI) and spectroscopy studies have demonstrated that plasma phenylalanine levels alter brain chemistry when the level exceeds 22.5 mg/dl (1300 μmol) (Cleary et al, 1994; Ris et al, 1994).

Chronic phenylalanine levels above 20 mg/dl (1200 μmol) result in central nervous system damage, and some experts believe that individuals with phenylalanine levels chronically above 12 to 15 mg/dl (720 to 900 μmol) are also at risk for CNS damage (Cleary et al, 1994; Scriver & Kaufman, 2001).

The threshold value for neurotoxicity in the acute effect may not correspond to the value associated with chronic neurotoxicity. Chronic neurotoxicity can manifest itself in at least two ways. First, it may occur in the brain white matter, where changes visible on MRI are more prevalent than the overt neurologic dysfunction. These findings are emerging in patients presumed to be well treated who have only modest chronic elevations of plasma phenylalanine (i.e., levels under 10 mg/dl [600 μmol]) (Cleary et al, 1994). Second, the intelligence quotient (IQ) scores of treated PKU patients are distributed below the normal range despite good long-term control of plasma phenylalanine in the range of 1 to 5 mg/dl (60 to 300 μmol). The relationship between the morphologic and biochemical alterations in PKU is still being determined. Etiologic factors include metabolites that act as toxins to the brain; inhibition of inhibitory neurotransmitters (e.g., gamma-aminobutyric acid [GABA]); impaired synthesis of serotonin; impaired transport of essential amino acids into brain cells; chronic insufficiency of glutamine; or inhibition of brain pyruvate kinase (Gilbert-Barness & Barness, 2000; Scriver & Kaufman, 2001).

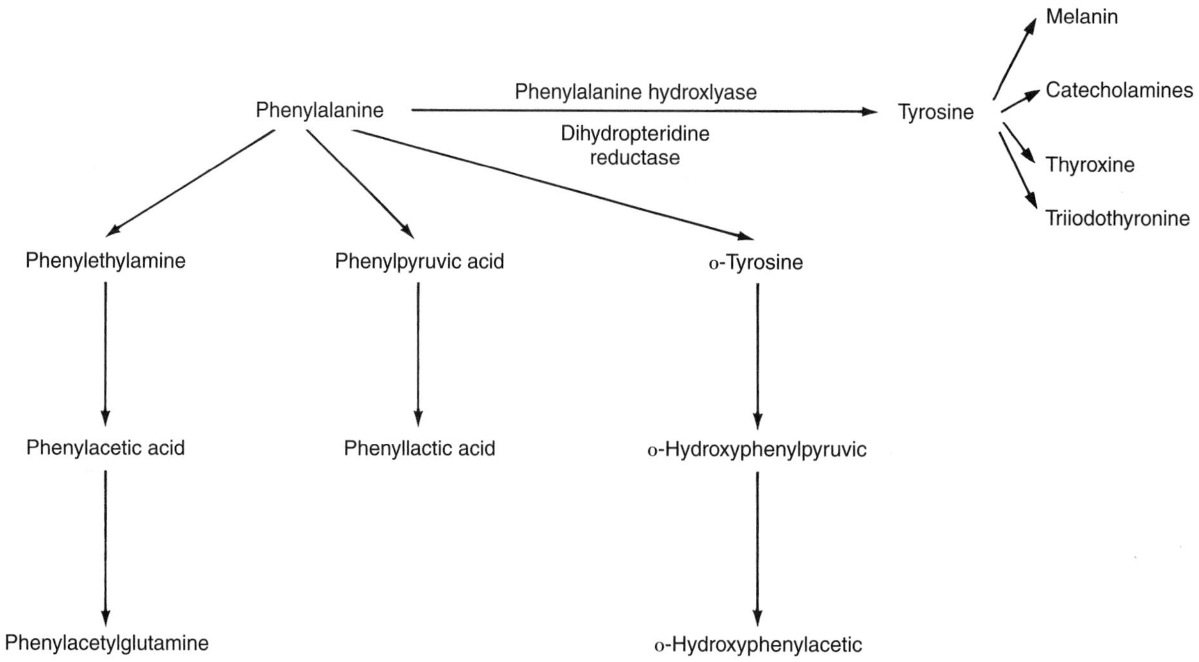

FIGURE **27-3**
Conversion of phenylalanine to tyrosine. Phenylalanine hydroxylase, an enzyme found primarily in the liver, is one participant in the complex conversion of phenylalanine to tyrosine. A second enzyme, dihydropteridine reductase, also participates in the reaction but requires the reduced pteridine cofactor tetrahydrobiopterin.

These findings are disturbing and significant. The data suggest that the neurotoxic threshold value for phenylalanine is different for the acute and chronic effects on the brain. The degree of any postnatal (or fetal) hyperphenylalaninemia could cause irreversible changes in brain structure (myelin) and function (cognition). If hyperphenylalaninemia recurs later in life, such as when treatment is terminated after satisfactory brain development has been achieved in the early-treated PKU patient or during bouts of intercurrent illness, reversible chemical changes again appear. If the neurotoxic effect persists, irreversible changes in the white matter, with deterioration in cognitive function, could then follow (Cleary et al, 1994; Scriver & Kaufman, 2001).

Overt clinical manifestations occur in untreated PKU-affected infants. Symptoms are virtually absent in untreated non-PKU infants. Early diagnosis and treatment of newborns with hyperphenylalaninemia has made the classic PKU disease manifestations a matter of historical rather than common occurrence. However, symptoms of classic PKU are still occasionally reported, and they assume greater relevance as patients terminate treatment for one reason or another.

Clinical manifestations vary, depending on the expression of enzyme activity (Svensson et al, 1994). In the first weeks of life, digestive problems and vomiting may lead to the false diagnosis of pyloric stenosis. In untreated infants, mentation is normal at birth but over time progressively deteriorates. Delay in psychomotor development or a regression in development occurs after several months. After the first year, the IQ of an untreated infant may be below 20; fewer than 4% have an IQ above 50 (90 to 110 is the normal range for this age) (Costello et al, 1994; Scriver & Kaufman, 2001). After the first few months, approximately 25% of patients have myoclonic or grand mal seizures, and 80% have EEG abnormalities (Scriver & Kaufman, 2001). In a study that described the natural

history of symptoms over 22 years in 51 patients with untreated PKU, 25% developed epilepsy; 50% were profoundly retarded (IQ below 35); approximately 50% were moderately retarded (IQ of 37 to 67); and 5% had an IQ above 68. The mean phenylalanine level in this group fell from 29 to 20 mg/dl (1694 to 1180 μmol) despite similar dietary intakes (Gilbert-Barness & Barness, 2000).

Other clinical manifestations are cited in the literature. A direct cause and effect relationship may be difficult to determine because of the relatively small number of PKU individuals, although some degree of agoraphobia seems to be a newly recognized and prevalent symptom. Individuals affected by PKU have hypopigmentation of the hair, skin, and irises as a result of the diminished production of melanin. Eczema in early childhood is common (Burton, 2000; Gilbert-Barness & Barness, 2000; Scriver & Kaufman, 2001). The urine has a musty odor caused by the excretion of phenylacetic acid (Burton, 2000; Gilbert-Barness & Barness, 2000; Scriver & Kaufman, 2001).

In behavior these children may be hyperactive and aggressive, which may be indistinguishable from the behavior of children with autism or various childhood psychoses (Scriver & Kaufman, 2001). Children with PKU show constant agitation and abnormal movements. Unceasing movement of the hands and fingers is seen, and violent anteroposterior contortions of the trunk may be noted. Neurologic examination reveals hypertonia, exaggerated tendon reflexes, and trembling with a clumsy, rigid walk (Scriver & Kaufman, 2001).

On pathologic examination, the weight of the brain is low and myelin content is diminished (Gilbert-Barness & Barness, 2000; Scriver & Kaufman, 2001). MRI changes in patients with PKU are compatible with disturbances in the water content of the white matter; the severity of the abnormality strongly correlates with the phenylalanine level at the time of imaging (Cleary et al, 1994; Gilbert-Barness & Barness, 2000; Scriver & Kaufman, 2001). The abnormal MRI changes are reversible if they are of recent onset and reflect greater turnover of myelin during states of hyperphenylalaninemia. In the context of cognitive development and brain function, hyperphenylalaninemia may alter the patterns of neuronal connections and result in fewer permanent synaptic connections (Gilbert-Barness & Barness, 2000). Neuropsychologic studies show prolonged central motor conduction time, prolonged visual evoked potentials, and impaired peripheral sensory nerve conduction. MRI changes have not been strongly correlated to IQ scores (Cleary et al, 1994; Costello et al, 1994; Gilbert-Barness & Barness, 2000).

Many comparison studies of intellectual and neuropsychologic measures have been performed with adults affected by PKU and with their unaffected control siblings. Adults who were diagnosed and treated early in life had normal intelligence, attention, and complex visual constructional ability (Costello et al, 1994; Ris et al, 1994). Intellectual outcome is best predicted by the degree of early neurologic insult, whereas performance on novel problem solving was best predicted by the current phenylalanine level. These results provide further convincing evidence that treatment should be continued well into adulthood (Ris et al, 1994) and perhaps for life (Gilbert-Barness & Barness, 2000; Scriver & Kaufman, 2001).

The goal of screening for hyperphenylalaninemia is early medical intervention; the goal of diagnosis is correct medical intervention. To screen for PKU, the infant's blood is collected as dried spots on filter paper and tested by means of bacterial inhibition; chromatographic, fluorometric, or enzymatic assay; or tandem mass spectrometry (Gilbert-Barness & Barness, 2000; Scriver & Kaufman, 2001). If the specimen is properly stored, phenylalanine in dried blood spots on filter paper is stable for years. The microbiologic and chromatographic methods are semiquantitative, with limitations in accuracy at lower phenylalanine concentrations. The fluorometric assay is fully quantitative down to and into the normal range.

A crucial characteristic of a screening test is its sensitivity; that is, the ability to minimize the frequency of false-negative test results. The timing of the sample collection and the threshold value are critical to the accuracy of a screening test. The PKU screening test is done after birth, and the capillary blood phenylalanine level in affected cases is lower the closer the day of testing is to the day of birth. Because of this, the sensitivity of the test could be impaired if screening is done on the first or second day of life rather than on day three or four. The greatest risk of false-negative results exists if testing is performed before 24 hours of age (Gilbert-Barness & Barness, 2000; Scriver & Kaufman, 2001).

New birthing practices and early discharge from birthing units have created challenges for neonatal screening programs. Routine follow-up or repeat testing of infants discharged early who had negative first results would be financially prohibitive and inefficient. Conversion of the test methodology from microbiologic or chromatographic (semiquantitative) to fluorometric (fully quantitative) has technical merits but currently would require a massive reorganization of most screening programs in the United States. The threshold value to signify hyperphenylalaninemia has been lowered to improve sensitivity. If the critical value of 2 mg/dl is used for screening, few infants with true PKU will be missed (Scriver & Kaufman, 2001). While accepting a tolerable increase in the rate of false-positive results, the lower threshold prevents many false-negative results that

occurred with early discharge of normal newborns. Currently only one case of PKU is missed for every 70 detected in the United States (Scriver & Kaufman, 2001). The cause for this can be errors of compliance and procedure as well as biologic variation in the postnatal rise of phenylalanine (Beaudet et al, 2001; Scriver & Kaufman, 2001).

False results, whether positive or negative, may also arise from technical factors, such as ampicillin contamination of the sample, administration of total parenteral nutrition with some amino acid solutions, and even the lot variability of the filter paper. In affected newborns, the plasma level of phenylalanine increases after normal feedings begin. By the fourth or fifth day, infants with classic PKU have phenylalanine levels 10 to 20 times normal (Gilbert-Barness & Barness, 2000; Scriver & Kaufman, 2001). Most of these newborns are detected after 1 day of adequate protein intake, even if the screening method used detects at least 4 mg/dl of phenylalanine (Scriver & Kaufman, 2001).

Enhanced urinary excretion of phenylpyruvic acid (indicative of PKU) produces a blue-green color when urine is mixed (1:1) with 5% ferric chloride solution. Phenistix testing (Ames Laboratories, Elkhart, Indiana) was an early method of PKU screening (Paul et al, 1980). However, in many infants with PKU, the urine test does not show a positive result for at least several weeks after birth despite markedly elevated serum phenylalanine levels. This occurs because the enzyme that converts phenylalanine to phenylpyruvic acid often is delayed in its appearance. PKU screening, therefore, should not depend on the urine test for phenylpyruvic acid (Gilbert-Barness & Barness, 2000; Scriver & Kaufman, 2001).

A positive result on the neonatal screening test only identifies an infant with hyperphenylalaninemia; the diagnostic test identifies the cause of the condition. Some infants who show a positive first result on the screening test have brief, transient hyperphenylalaninemia of no further clinical significance; most, however, have persistent hyperphenylalaninemia. Among the latter group, hyperphenylalaninemia is caused predominantly (in more than 97% of cases) by a deficiency of PAH. Approximately 1% to 3% of infants with hyperphenylalaninemia have impaired synthesis or recycling of BH_4; these cases require specific treatment to offset the BH_4 deficiency. Because plasma phenylalanine levels alone do not distinguish between the BH_4-impaired and BH_4-sufficient forms of hyperphenylalaninemia, every case of persistent hyperphenylalaninemia must be investigated further to assess metabolism of BH_4 (Gilbert-Barness & Barness, 2000; Blau et al, 2001; Scriver & Kaufman, 2001) (Figure 27-4).

Diagnostic tests in the newborn include direct measurement of the plasma phenylalanine level and the plasma phenylalanine response to BH_4. There are no reliable phenylalanine metabolites, and phenylalanine-loading tests are not recommended in the newborn. A program of 3 days of protein feeding at normal volumes has been used in older subjects to classify the type of PKU. Tests for pterin metabolites are reliably done only in laboratories with expertise in this assay. The pterin tests are measured from dried blood spots on filter paper. Total activity formerly was assayed by its cofactor effect on phenylalanine hydroxylation in vitro. "Activity" of these two assays is high in untreated cases with ambient hyperphenylalaninemia and intact BH_4 synthesis; it is low in disorders of BH_4 homeostasis. Normal phenylalanine values are under 150 μmol in neonates and under 120 μmol in older subjects. In the phenylalanine response to BH_4 test, BH_4 is given orally when

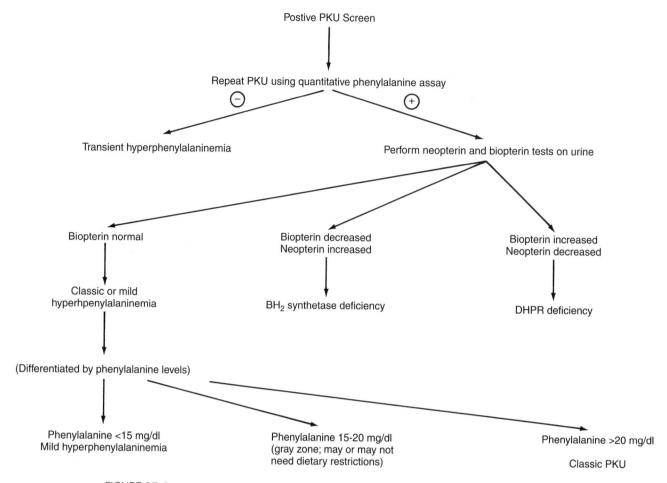

FIGURE **27-4**
Verification of phenylketonuria (PKU) diagnosis. *BH₂*, Dihydropteridine; *DHPR*, dihydropteridine reductase.

the phenylalanine level is elevated; a fall in the phenylalanine level indicates BH₄ deficiency.

Diagnostic tests can also be performed at the enzyme level. Direct measurement of PAH activity requires a liver biopsy (Burton, 2000; Gilbert-Barness & Barness, 2000; Scriver & Kaufman, 2001). DHPR activity is measured in many tissues, including the liver, skin fibroblasts, amniocytes, erythrocytes, leukocytes, platelets, and dried blood on filter paper (Gilbert-Barness & Barness, 2000; Blau et al, 2001; Scriver & Kaufman, 2001). Complex DNA studies using venous blood, dried blood spots, buccal cells, and cultures of skin fibroblasts can be performed to analyze the mutation. The indications for prenatal diagnosis are not trivial in hyperphenylalaninemia. Treatment under some conditions may be difficult to obtain or administer, and the prognosis for a normal outcome is not certain in all cases. Amniocytes, chorionic villus samples, amniotic fluid, and fetal erythrocytes have been analyzed to diagnose and classify the type of PKU prenatally (Gilbert-Barness & Barness, 2000; Scriver & Kaufman, 2001).

Once the diagnosis has been established, the treatment consists of early and competent management of a low-phenylalanine diet, which has been feasible since the 1950s (Gilbert-Barness & Barness, 2000; Scriver & Kaufman, 2001). Optimally, treatment of PKU requires (1) an early start for treatment (i.e., within the first month after birth); (2) continuous treatment throughout childhood, adolescence, and adulthood, and

certainly preconceptionally and gestationally in PKU-affected women; and (3) restriction of phenylalanine intake to amounts sufficient to hold plasma phenylalanine values as close as possible to the normal range (4 to 8 mg/dl, or 250 to 500 μmol).

Phenylalanine tolerance varies according to the infant and the severity of the enzyme deficiency (Svensson et al, 1994; Gilbert-Barness & Barness, 2000; Scriver & Kaufman, 2001). Atypical forms of PKU result in a variable amount of PAH activity and thus a higher tolerance for phenylalanine in the diet; these forms are associated with less severe mental retardation. The atypical forms are also autosomal recessive and may require dietary restriction of phenylalanine (Costello et al, 1994; Gilbert-Barness & Barness, 2000; Scriver & Kaufman, 2001).

Protein intake cannot be reduced sufficiently to prevent the hyperphenylalaninemia without causing deficiencies of other essential amino acids. PKU infants are consumers with special needs, and they need selective restriction of phenylalanine intake. The tolerance for dietary phenylalanine to maintain "nontoxic" phenylalanine levels in young PKU patients is 25% of normal or less (approximately 250 to 500 mg of phenylalanine per day) (Burton, 2000; Gilbert-Barness & Barness, 2000; Scriver & Kaufman, 2001). A semisynthetic diet low in phenylalanine and adequate in other nutrients is used to treat PKU patients. Several commercial products consisting of modified protein hydrolysates or mixtures of free amino acids provide the essential amino acids in suitable proportions. The nutritional composition of these products is vastly different from that of human milk.

Because phenylalanine is an essential amino acid, small amounts of this natural protein source must be added to the diet to ensure minimal phenylalanine levels (Gilbert-Barness & Barness, 2000). Complete restriction of all phenylalanine from the diet results in phenylalanine deficiency, manifested by anemia, growth retardation, cutaneous lesions, and mental deficiency. Phenylalanine deficiency is as detrimental as elevated levels of the amino acid (Gilbert-Barness & Barness, 2000; Scriver & Kaufman, 2001).

The dietary mode of treatment has pitfalls. Transient hyperphenylalaninemia, followed by hypophenylalaninemia, is a hazard during overtreatment of PKU. This occurs when phenylalanine is used for anabolic needs when the normal protein synthesis is impaired by a deficiency of other essential nutrients. Adjustments of phenylalanine and protein intake are a challenge during bouts of intercurrent illness or in the growing preterm infant with PKU. Breast milk has been given safely as a supplement to the low-phenylalanine formula used in infancy. Both the long-term hypophenylalaninemia during excessive treatment and the persistent hyperphenylalaninemia during treatment have adverse consequences. The poor gustatory properties of the commercial diets are likely to affect compliance adversely. Close follow-up is essential for these infants because phenylalanine levels can become elevated when tissue catabolism releases amino acids into the blood (Falk et al, 1994; Scriver & Kaufman, 2001). Parents therefore must be aware of the first signs of illness in their infant and reduce the phenylalanine in the diet even further to prevent toxic accumulation. In addition, during periods of anabolism and growth, dietary phenylalanine must be increased to prevent hypophenylalaninemia (Scriver & Kaufman, 2001).

Aspartame is a popular artificial sweetener that, upon hydrolysis in the intestines, releases free L-phenylalanine, L-aspartic acid, and methanol. It accounts for approximately 12% of the total sweeteners consumed. The wide availability of aspartame makes it a relevant hazard in the dietary management of PKU patients. For example, a quart of aspartame-sweetened flavored drink contains 280 mg, or half the daily allowance, of phenylalanine. PKU homozygote patients and their families must be meticulously careful about reading product labels and adjusting the diet accordingly (Trefz et al, 1994).

The aspartame hazard for pregnant PKU heterozygotes is still debated. Newer studies have compared large-bolus ingestion of aspartame in normal subjects and heterozygotes. No significant disturbance of blood phenylalanine, tyrosine, or large amino acid levels were noted in response to the load in either group. An aspartame intake above the 90th percentile (the equivalent of drinking 24 12-ounce servings of aspartame-sweetened beverage over 8 hours) increased the blood phenylalanine level by less than 1 mg/dl (40 μmol) in the heterozygotes 30 minutes after ingestion, a trivial change (Trefz et al, 1994).

Controlled trials of treatment by selective restriction of phenylalanine intake have never been attempted with infants. Information about the effectiveness of this therapy is empirically derived from case reports of alternative dietary regimens in which the infant developed classic PKU symptoms and in never-treated PKU patients who still have the neuropsychologic manifestations of the disease. In contrast, patients treated meticulously after neonatal diagnosis are essentially free of the classic IQ deterioration. Retrospective evidence to support these findings is substantial (Ris et al, 1994; Gilbert-Barness &

Barness, 2000; Scriver & Kaufman, 2001). One study compared the IQ scores of 28 PKU-affected, late-treated and early-treated sibling pairs. The study demonstrated a significant difference in IQ scores between the early-treated individuals (all IQs were above 80) and their late-treated siblings (mean IQ, 45; range, 30 to 81). A comparison of the IQ scores of the early-treated individuals and their unaffected siblings revealed that the mean IQ scores were 94 and 99, respectively.

The Northern American Collaborative Study has been evaluating the outcome of early-treated PKU cases. The study has found that early treatment is compatible with attainment of a normal IQ score, a finding confirmed by several other investigators (Costello et al, 1994; Scriver & Kaufman, 2001). IQ score correlates positively with the age at which dietary treatment was stopped and the mean parental IQ score and negatively with the age at which treatment had begun and on the plasma values during treatment. The patients treated earliest and longest and whose plasma phenylalanine levels were kept under 15 mg/dl (900 μmol) throughout life had the best IQ and psychologic test scores.

In addition to changes in IQ scores, treated PKU patients have measurable deficits in the performance of conceptual, visuospatial, and language-related tasks and in reading and arithmetic skills. Despite these deficits, early-treated PKU-affected individuals function well in daily life. The response to early treatment for PKU has established that (1) early treatment can ameliorate the clinical impact of the disease; (2) early-treated children have a mean IQ score approximately 0.5 standard deviation below the scores of unaffected siblings and population norms; (3) a high proportion of early-treated subjects (not just those of poorly treated cases) showed some degree of intellectual impairment attributable to events in early childhood rather than to later relaxation or termination of treatment; and (4) most early-treated PKU-affected children function within the broad range of ability and attend regular schools.

There has been a long-term concern that premature termination of treatment might impair later neurologic function. Early comparative studies (performed in the 1950s) of the effects of continued versus terminated dietary treatment showed a decline in IQ scores after treatment was discontinued. Subsequent studies clearly confirmed these initial results, more in some patients than in others (Potocnik & Widhalm, 1994; Scriver & Kaufman, 2001). The effects of treatment termination are apparent in more than IQ scores. They can also appear as deviant EEG findings, reduced neurotransmitter levels, impaired vigilance, and impaired reaction times. Behavioral problems have been reported as occurring more frequently with termination than with relaxation of treatment (Potocnik & Widhalm, 1994; Scriver & Kaufman, 2001).

Although IQ and cognitive function have been the foci of past research, much of the current research focuses on the abnormalities of brain white matter revealed by MRI. The changes reflect abnormal myelin synthesis or demyelination (Cleary et al, 1994; Gilbert-Barness & Barness, 2000; Scriver & Kaufman, 2001). The significance of the MRI changes is unclear, because they have been demonstrated in continuously well-treated individuals and seems to be more severe in patients with a history of poor control of phenylalanine levels. Evidence indicates that MRI changes and overt neurologic deterioration can improve both when dietary treatment is reinstated and when plasma phenylalanine levels return to normal (Ris et al, 1994). Although MRI changes seem to be much more common than overt neurologic changes and more prevalent than measurable psychologic deficits in treated and post-treated PKU patients, the association with long-term hyperphenylalaninemia seems undeniable. It may no longer be possible to cite non-PKU hyperphenylalaninemia to illustrate normal cognitive function in the presence of modest increases in phenylalanine. In reality, there may be no threshold value for blood phenylalanine at which the brain escapes some effect of persistent elevations in the amino acid. The outcome correlates with the quality of treatment and its success in normalizing the blood phenylalanine level.

The Maternal PKU Collaborative Study investigated the effects of nutrient intake on pregnancy outcome. The study found that 80% of fetuses could be adversely affected and demonstrated that women with PKU who reach childbearing age should adhere strictly to dietary restrictions on phenylalanine. The normal transplacental gradient favors the fetus from early pregnancy onward, with the fetal to maternal ratio of phenylalanine in the range of 1.5:1 to 2.9:1 (Scriver & Kaufman, 2001). The fetal phenylalanine level, therefore, cannot be accurately predicted from the corresponding maternal level, except that it is at least as high as or perhaps nearly three times higher than the maternal level. The goal is to keep the maternal plasma phenylalanine level as near normal as possible, as early as possible in the pregnancy. If an affected woman has stopped following the low-phenylalanine diet, it is essential that preconceptional teaching help her to understand the need to resume dietary restrictions before pregnancy.

Maternal phenylalanine levels above 15 mg/dl (900 μmol) have been associated with an increased risk of cardiac defects, prenatal and postnatal growth retardation, microcephaly, and permanently impaired mentality in heterozygous infants (Gilbert-Barness & Barness, 2000; Scriver & Kaufman, 2001). The degree of impaired mentality in infants is in proportion to the degree of elevation in the maternal phenylalanine level. Thus a genetically normal infant is affected if the maternal diet is not closely followed. When these heterozygous infants are tested for PKU with normal neonatal screening tests, the excess serum phenylalanine has already been cleared from the infant's blood and the test result is normal (Gilbert-Barness & Barness, 2000; Scriver & Kaufman, 2001). In such cases, the cause of the infant's impairment may be difficult to isolate if the mother's PKU status is unknown. Routine screening of infant cord blood for phenylalanine identifies some PKU-affected mothers who did not resume dietary restrictions; however, the neurologic damage to the infants has already occurred. Some authors advocate routine screening of maternal urine for phenylpyruvic acid early in pregnancy to detect PKU-affected women; however, even early identification and subsequent control of elevated maternal serum phenylalanine levels may not be enough to prevent mental impairment of the infant (Gilbert-Barness & Barness, 2000; Scriver & Kaufman, 2001).

Every PKU-affected woman of childbearing years should follow a low-phenylalanine diet and should have low serum phenylalanine levels before conception (Gilbert-Barness & Barness, 2000; Scriver & Kaufman, 2001). During pregnancy, the serum phenylalanine level should be under 8 mg/dl (500 μmol) to maximize neonatal outcome (Gilbert-Barness & Barness, 2000; Scriver & Kaufman, 2001). At least one investigator has advocated the use of maternal surrogates or "gestational carriers" for some women affected by PKU to minimize fetal exposure to any elevation in phenylalanine in utero.

In addition to dietary therapy, alternative modes of treatment theoretically are possible in PKU. Enzyme "replacement" is possible through the use of heterologous partial liver transplantation or implantation of normal hepatocytes. This could replace the deviant or missing PAH activity and would constitute "multigene" therapy. Investigation into this treatment remains experimental.

The most promising surrogate enzyme replacement is bacterial phenylalanine ammonia lyase. After ingestion, it converts phenylalanine to a nontoxic derivative and an equivalent amount of ammonia. It does not require a cofactor. In animal research, this enzyme replacement was much more effective at lowering elevated phenylalanine levels than was a low-phenylalanine diet. Further research in this area may be limited by the extremely high cost of this enzyme.

The limitations and inadequacies of conventional diet therapy and the absence of any significant steps in enzyme replacement therapy or new knowledge about the molecular basis of PKU mutations have prompted investigators to consider specific gene therapy. Promise lies in implanting a normal PAH gene in place of or in addition to the mutant cells of a PKU patient. An expressible PKU gene is available, as is the method for delivering the incoming normal gene into the cell. Integration of the gene into the nuclear genome of the target cell is likely, and there is assurance that it will be expressed and transmitted to daughter cells. This research is being conducted on animal models, but no human research has been attempted as yet (Scriver & Kaufman, 2001).

Hyperphenylalaninemia Caused by Defects of BH₄ Recycling. Hyperphenylalaninemia arising from defects of BH_4 recycling is a rare condition. (For more information please see the CD.)

Three enzymes, each pterin dependent, catalyze the hydroxylation of phenylalanine, tyrosine, and tryptophan. Accordingly, it was expected that some patients would have a persistent elevation of phenylalanine with neurologic deficits related to diminished neurotransmitter derivatives of tyrosine and tryptophan. Careful investigation of the progressive neurologic disorders in these patients with hyperphenylalaninemia, whose condition seemingly was well controlled by diet therapy, revealed two etiologies. In some cases the cause was attributed to impaired recycling of BH_4 as a result of DHPR deficiency; in other cases the cause was attributed to impaired BH_4 cofactor synthesis. The incidence among all cases of hyperphenylalaninemia is 1 to 3 cases per 1 million births with worldwide occurrence and no evidence of regional or ethnic clusters (Burton, 2000; Beaudet et al, 2001; Scriver & Kaufman, 2001).

Procedures for early identification of BH_4-deficient patients have become an integral part of all neonatal screening programs for three reasons: (1) cases of BH_4 deficiency cannot be distinguished from other forms of neonatal hyperphenylalaninemia by blood values alone; (2) conventional treatment of PKU is inadequate for BH_4 deficiency; and (3) until BH_4-deficient forms of hyperphenylalaninemia have been excluded, there is uncertainty about the cause of the elevated phenylalanine level, the choice of treatment, and the prognosis (Gilbert-Barness & Barness, 2000; Blau et al, 2001; Scriver & Kaufman, 2001).

Since the first reports of BH_4-deficient forms of hyperphenylalaninemia were published in 1975, the DHPR gene has been cloned; the mutations are found on chromosome 4, whereas genes for the corresponding enzymes are found on chromosomes 14, 11, and 10. The loci for all the enzymes have been characterized, and heterogeneity at the levels of the genotype and phenotype has been established. BH_4 deficiency is an autosomal recessive disorder (Gilbert-Barness & Barness, 2000; Beaudet et al, 2001; Blau et al, 2001; Scriver & Kaufman, 2001).

The treatment goals for this condition are to minimize the hyperphenylalaninemia, correct the neurotransmitter deficiency, and maintain folate homeostasis. A low-phenylalanine diet is recommended to maintain plasma phenylalanine levels in the near normal range. This diet avoids interruption of neurotransmitter synthesis by the excessive phenylalanine in vivo and prevents the other effects of phenylalanine on the brain (Gilbert-Barness & Barness, 2000; Blau et al, 2001). Because DHPR is necessary to maintain amounts of cofactor for synthesis of amines from tyrosine and tryptophan, replacement of these neurotransmitters is likely to be effective in DHPR deficiency. L-dopa and 5-hydroxytryptophan are given around the clock to restore normal circadian metabolism. The effectiveness of treatment is inversely related to the age at which it begins. Treatment with BH₄ is not practical because in the absence of DHPR to recycle it, catalytic amounts of BH₄ cannot be maintained by the body. It is thought that BH₄ also plays a role in folate metabolism, which is also deficient in these patients. Thus supplementation with folinic acid is part of the normal treatment. The objective is to achieve cerebrospinal fluid (CSF) concentrations of tetrahydrofolate in the high normal range and to prevent demyelination and other signs of cortical dysgenesis (Gilbert-Barness & Barness, 2000; Blau et al, 2001; Scriver & Kaufman, 2001).

Hyperphenylalaninemia Caused by Defects of BH₄ Synthesis.

An inadequate supply of endogenous BH₄ cofactor impairs the hydrolase function. This factor was recognized early as the cause of hyperphenylalaninemia in "atypical PKU." The clinical signs and symptoms are parkinsonian in nature; they include characteristic truncal hypotonia and increased limb tone with pronated hand postures. Difficulty swallowing, ocular spasms, somnolence, irritability, hyperthermia, seizures, and impaired neuropsychologic development are all clinically evident (Costello et al, 1994; Gilbert-Barness & Barness, 2000; Blau et al, 2001). (For more information please see the CD.)

Replacement of BH₄ abolishes the hyperphenylalaninemia, and daily treatment with BH₄ is required. Because the enzyme dihydrobiopterin is present in adequate amounts, the replaced BH₄ can be "recycled" more effectively and adequate BH₄ levels can be achieved. BH₄ replacement is expensive, and its availability is very limited. Replacement of dopamine and serotonin is necessary to abolish the CNS symptoms because BH₄ does not penetrate the blood-brain barrier. L-Dopa and 5-hydroxytryptophan are given to restore the neurotransmitter levels, and fine adjustments of dosage and schedule are needed to restore circadian rhythms. For reasons yet unknown, the response to treatment varies. Postnatal treatment may be too late if the fetal phenotype has already affected CNS development (Blau et al, 2001; Gilbert-Barness & Barness, 2000; Scriver & Kaufman, 2001).

Hypertyrosinemias.

In human beings, tyrosine, an essential amino acid, is obtained from two sources: hydrolysis of dietary intake or tissue protein and hydroxylation of phenylalanine. Tyrosine is the starting point of the synthetic pathway leading to the synthesis of catecholamines, thyroid hormone, and the melanin pigment. The major fate of tyrosine is to be incorporated into proteins or degraded for its component molecules. Degradation of tyrosine occurs primarily in the cytosol of the hepatocytes that produces glucose and ketones. For the most part, the rate of tyrosine degradation is determined by the activity of tyrosine aminotransferase (TAT) (Gilbert-Barness & Barness, 2000; Mitchell et al, 2001; Scriver et al, 2001). Most errors of tyrosine catabolism produce hypertyrosinemia. Hypertyrosinemia may also occur in various acquired conditions, including severe hepatocellular disease (Burton, 2000).

Hepatorenal hypertyrosinemia, or type I tyrosinemia, is an autosomal recessive disease caused by a deficiency of fumarylacetoacetate hydrolase (FAH). Symptoms, which vary considerably, include acute liver failure, cirrhosis, hepatocellular carcinoma, renal Fanconi syndrome, glomerulosclerosis, and crises of peripheral neuropathy. In untreated patients, the tyrosine levels are elevated. Elevated plasma or urinary levels of succinylacetone are diagnostic for this condition. Dietary restriction of tyrosine and phenylalanine may elicit a partial response in many patients. Hepatic transplantation cures the liver manifestations and prevents further neurologic crises. Treatment with 2-(2-nitro-4-trifluoromethylbenzoyl)-1,3 cyclohexanedione (NTBC), an inhibitor of 4-hydroxyphenylpyruvate dioxygenase (pHPPD), has been reported to produce marked improvement in hepatic and renal function. The mutant gene responsible for the FAH deficiency has been mapped to chromosome 15 q23-q25 (Burton, 2000; Gilbert-Barness & Barness, 2000; Mitchell et al, 2001). Mutational heterogeneity in FAH activity has been found among patients from the French Canadian province of Quebec and among the Scandinavian populations, both of which have a higher incidence of this disease than the general world population.

Type II tyrosinemia is a deficiency of the enzyme TAT, which results in oculocutaneous tyrosinemia. The ocular and cutaneous symptoms are characterized by palmoplantar keratosis and painful corneal erosions associated with photophobia. Half of reported patients have mental retardation. The ocular and cutaneous symptoms respond to dietary restriction of tyrosine and phenylalanine. This disorder has been mapped to chromosome 16 q22.1-q22.3 (Gilbert-Barness & Barness, 2000; Mitchell et al, 2001).

Type III tyrosinemia results in three different conditions associated with dysfunction of the enzyme 4-hydroxyphenylpyruvate dioxygenase (pHPPD): primary pHPPD deficiency, hawkinsinuria, and transient tyrosinemia of the newborn (Burton, 2000; Gilbert-Barness & Barness, 2000; Mitchell et al, 2001).

Primary pHPPD deficiency has been described rarely in the literature. The three case reports were neurologically abnormal. Biochemically, the patients demonstrated hypertyrosinemia and elevated urinary excretion of 4-hydroxyphenyl derivatives. This disorder has been mapped to chromosome 12 q14-qter (Mitchell et al, 2001).

Hawkinsinuria is an autosomal dominant condition putatively caused by dysfunction of pHPPD. It results in acidosis and failure to thrive in infancy. Hypertyrosinemia is minimal or absent. An amino acid thought to be an intermediate of the pHPPD reaction, hawkinsin, is excreted in the urine and is diagnostic for this condition. Symptoms may respond to dietary protein restriction and to administration of ascorbate. This disorder has not yet been linked to a chromosome (Burton, 2000; Mitchell et al, 2001).

Transient tyrosinemia of the newborn results from a combination of pHPPD immaturity, elevated tyrosine and phenylalanine intake, and a relative ascorbate deficiency. Improvement is spontaneous but can be accelerated by administration of ascorbate and by dietary protein restriction, especially of tyrosine and phenylalanine. Most children with transient tyrosinemia are asymptomatic and recover without adverse effects on development. However, the adverse consequences of this disorder have not been eliminated in all cases.

Typical plasma tyrosine levels in normal subjects range from 25 to 103 μmol in newborns and 35 to 90 μmol in adults. Urinary levels are 6 to 55 μmol per millimole of creatinine in the newborn and 2 to 23 μmol in the adult. A fetal to maternal gradient is present, the fetal plasma tyrosine level being approximately twice as high as the maternal level. In adults, tyrosine is efficiently (97% to 99%) reabsorbed by the renal tubules. The transamination product of tyrosine, 4-hydroxyphenylpyruvate (pHPP), is found in low concentration in the plasma and is actively cleared by the renal tubules. As pHPP accumulates, related products are excreted that form part of the basis for diagnostic testing for this disorder (Gilbert-Barness & Barness, 2000; Mitchell et al, 2001).

The enzymes that mediate the metabolism of tyrosine are still being investigated. Normal activity of the first enzyme, TAT, usually is one half to one third that of the second enzyme, pHPP, which, in turn, is one half to one tenth that of the last enzymes of tyrosine catabolism, maleylacetoacetate (MAA) isomerase and FAH (Gilbert-Barness & Barness, 2000; Mitchell et al, 2001).

Hypertyrosinemia can arise from several inherited and acquired conditions, including transient tyrosinemia of the newborn, errors of tyrosine catabolism, severe hepatocellular disease, hyperthyroidism, and scurvy. Most of these causes can be diagnosed by the clinical history, physical examination, and readily available laboratory tests. Transient tyrosinemia of the newborn, severe hepatocellular disease, and errors of tyrosine catabolism are the most common causes.

The most difficult clinical problem with the group of metabolic disorders resulting in hypertyrosinemia is in the context of hepatic dysfunction. It must be determined whether the elevated tyrosine levels are caused by primary hepatorenal tyrosinemia or whether the tyrosine level is elevated as a result of secondary hepatocellular dysfunction. The determination of plasma amino acids is not diagnostic in these patients because both tyrosine and methionine can be nonspecifically elevated with cirrhosis and acute liver failure (Burton, 2000; Gilbert-Barness & Barness, 2000; Mitchell et al, 2001).

The presence of renal tubular dysfunction in patients with hepatocellular failure is consistent with hepatorenal tyrosinemia but is also seen in other inherited metabolic diseases, such as galactosemia, hereditary fructose intolerance, certain lactic acidoses, and glycogen storage diseases (Figure 27-5). The presence of a family history suggestive of tyrosinemia is helpful in the diagnosis. The presence of high levels of succinylacetone in blood or urine establishes the diagnosis (Bur-

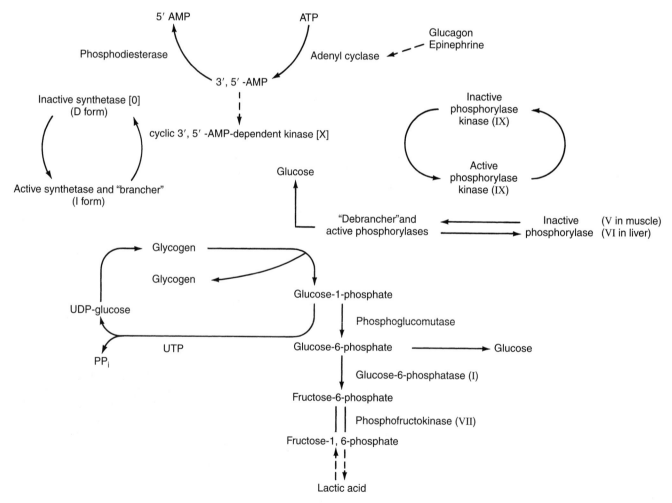

FIGURE 27-5

Summary of glycogen metabolism. Enzymes responsible for the various disorders of glycogen metabolism are noted with parentheses. *AMP,* Adenosine monophosphate; *ATP,* adenosine triphosphate; *PP$_i$,* inorganic pyrophosphate; *UTP,* uridine triphosphate.

ton, 2000; Gilbert-Barness & Barness, 2000; Mitchell et al, 2001).

A practical consideration is that plasma levels of tyrosine and of several other amino acids can be mildly elevated in nonfasting subjects. Repeated amino acid analyses by chromatography should be obtained before investigation for hypertyrosinemia, especially if the patient has none of the other symptoms associated with the metabolic disorders of tyrosine catabolism. Some disorders of tyrosine catabolism and its branch pathways are not associated with hypertyrosinemia, and 4-hydroxy-phenylic derivatives of tyrosine can be found in increasing amounts in patients with primary liver disease. Urinary 4-hydroxyphenylacetate is commonly of gut bacterial origin and may be increased in malabsorption. Lastly, patients receiving certain parenteral nutritional solutions containing N-acetyltyrosine may excrete large amounts of this compound (Burton, 2000; Gilbert-Barness & Barness, 2000; Mitchell et al, 2001).

Hepatorenal Tyrosinemia: Fumarylacetoacetate Hydrolase Deficiency (Type I Tyrosinemia).

Hepatorenal tyrosinemia is a clinically severe error of metabolism that affects principally the liver, kidneys, and peripheral nerves; it arises from a deficiency of FAH. The mechanism by which the hepatic and renal symptoms of tyrosinemia are produced is unknown, and many questions in the areas of pathophysiology and treatment remain unanswered. Advances in the confirmation of the enzymatic deficiency, cloning of the human FAH gene, new medical and surgical therapies, and development of an animal model of the disease no doubt will have an explosive impact on this disease in the future.

In contrast to other errors of amino acid metabolism in which the metabolites preceding the enzymatic-blocked enzyme are excreted in high levels, in FAH deficiency, the preceding compounds upstream from the block, MAA and fumarylacetoacetate (FAA), have not been isolated as circulating or excreted metabolites. It therefore is speculated that these reactive metabolites may be compartmentalized in tyrosinemia, causing damage within single cells (Gilbert-Barness & Barness, 2000; Mitchell et al, 2001).

A secondary deficiency of hepatic pHPPD activity (usually from 0 to 30% of normal activity) is an important factor in hepatorenal tyrosinemia and at first was thought to be the etiology of the disease. The mechanism of pHPPD inactivation is unknown, but it may occur as a result of the abnormal sulfhydryl metabolism observed in hepatorenal tyrosinemia. Research has indicated that inactivation of pHPPD may serve a protective function in this disorder by reducing the production of FAA and other tyrosine derivatives downstream. Lindstedt and colleagues (1992) found a correlation between the severity of the clinical manifestations of the disease and the degree of residual hepatic pHPPD activity. Administration of 2-(2-nitro-4-trifluoromethylbenzoyl)-1,3-cyclohexanedion (NTBC), a potent inhibitor of pHPPD, has been associated with improvement in the hepatic and renal function of these patients (Mitchell et al, 2001). However, use of this drug is limited, and it is not known if it prevents the development of hepatocellular carcinoma (Mitchell et al, 2001). Gene therapy trials are currently being investigated.

A deficiency of methionine adenosyltransferase (MAT) explains the hypermethioninemia seen in many tyrosinemic children. This sulfhydryl-containing enzyme, which has multiple distinct forms, mediates the major pathway of methionine catabolism. FAA inhibits one form of this enzyme, but the clinical relevance of this observation has yet to be explored (Mitchell et al, 2001). The significance of hypermethioninemia in hepatorenal tyrosinemia, other than as an approximate index of hepatic function, is uncertain. Patients with an isolated deficiency of MAT show normal development and no liver dysfunction despite elevated methionine levels (Burton, 2000; Gilbert-Barness & Barness, 2000; Mitchell et al, 2001), which suggests that the hypermethionine levels in hepatorenal tyrosinemia may be well tolerated.

The best-established pathophysiologic mechanism in hepatorenal tyrosinemia is the role of succinylacetone in the acute episodes of porphyria-like peripheral neuropathy. Succinylacetone is the most potent known inhibitor of the porphyrin synthetic enzyme delta-aminolevulinic acid (delta-ALA) dehydratase (Mitchell et al, 2001). This compound is excreted in very high levels in children with hepatorenal tyrosinemia and has been shown to be neurotoxic (Mitchell et al, 2001). Evidence supports the theory that delta-ALA is responsible for the neurologic crises of hepatorenal tyrosinemia.

Succinylacetone has other effects at high concentrations, including inhibition of renal tubular transport and heme synthesis and inhibition of cell growth and immune function (Mitchell et al, 2001). The way in which these effects influence the clinical symptoms is unknown.

Hepatorenal tyrosinemia is an autosomal recessive trait. Obligatory heterozygotes (parents of the affected offspring) have approximately 50% of normal enzyme activity and yet are asymptomatic and have normal levels of tyrosine-related metabolites (Mitchell et al, 2001).

There are two population clusters of hepatorenal hypertyrosinemia: in a small French Canadian province of Quebec and in Scandinavia. The population genetics suggest that the mutant gene was introduced into Canada by founder couples settling the region who may have emigrated from northern France and were related to one another. The overall incidence of hepatorenal tyrosinemia in Quebec is 1 in 16,786 live births. The incidence in Scandinavia is approximately 1 in 100,000 live births, an incidence higher than elsewhere in the world (approximately 1 in 150,000 live births). Lack of French Canadian or Scandinavian ancestry does not exclude the diagnosis (Burton, 2000; Gilbert-Barness & Barness, 2000; Mitchell et al, 2001).

Neonatal screening for hepatorenal tyrosinemia has been available since the 1970s. Initially screening was done to check tyrosine levels; however, elevated tyrosine levels overlapped with those found in transient neonatal tyrosinemia. Currently screening measures other values that are abnormal with hepatorenal tyrosinemia, such as the levels of methionine, succinylacetone, or delta-ALA dehydratase (Mitchell et al, 2001). Antenatal screening for tyrosinemia is available (Gilbert-Barness & Barness, 2000; Mitchell et al, 2001).

In Quebec the blood succinylacetone level has been screened, along with tyrosine, since the 1980s. A threshold of 248 μmol (4.5 mg/dl) has been selected as the cutoff level for tyrosine, and approximately 2.4% of neonates born in Quebec currently have levels that exceed this amount. The low cutoff value and the high specificity of the succinylacetone marker are believed to have allowed complete detection of all affected newborns while eliminating false-negative results. In Quebec, the average age at follow-up for affected newborns is 20 days (Mitchell et al, 2001).

In the United States, when screening for neonatal tyrosinemia is performed, the initial threshold value for the blood tyrosine level is 331 μmol (6 mg/dl); at this level, 10% of newborns are recalled for further testing. Currently the threshold value has been raised to 663 μmol (12 mg/dl), for which the recall rate is 0.1%. In Georgia, neonatal screening has not identified any patients with hepatorenal tyrosinemia, although one case of oculocutaneous tyrosinemia and five cases of prolonged severe transient neonatal hypertyrosinemia have been detected since 1978. Several children were identified as having secondary hypertyrosinemia arising from unrecognized hepatocellular disease or feeding errors (Mitchell et al, 2001). In the other states, the proportion of newborns with tyrosine levels above the threshold value of 331 μmol (6 mg/dl) is approximately 0.12%.

A new screening method using delta-ALA dehydratase is under investigation; this technique should detect FAH deficiency, succinylacetone accumulation, and inhibition of delta-ALA dehydratase deficiency. The decision to initiate neonatal screening for hepatorenal tyrosinemia involves many factors, including the impact of presymptomatic detection on the family, the incidence of the disease, and the marginal increase in cost of the procedure.

Hepatorenal tyrosinemia should be suspected in any newborn with evidence of hepatocellular disease, cirrhosis, or diminished synthetic function (especially perturbed coagulation) for which the cause is not evident. The presence of hypophosphatemic rickets and other renal tubular diseases or of typical neurologic crises also suggests the diagnosis (Burton, 2000; Gilbert-Barness & Barness, 2000; Mitchell et al, 2001).

In symptomatic patients, the plasma tyrosine level usually is elevated to a variable degree, but it may be affected by a low-protein diet, and an elevated tyrosine level is found in many other disorders of amino acids metabolism. An increased amount of succinylacetone in the blood or urine is pathognomonic for hepatorenal tyrosinemia. FAH enzymatic analysis should be performed using lymphocytes, erythrocytes, or hepatocytes. Enzyme analysis must be interpreted in the context of the patient's clinical and biochemical findings (Burton, 2000; Mitchell et al, 2001).

Prenatal diagnosis is available through three methods: determination of succinylacetone in amniotic fluid, FAH assay, and molecular analysis in amniocytes. In general, the assay of succinylacetone in amniotic fluid has been an excellent means of prenatal diagnosis in 36 pregnancies at risk among French Canadians (Ploos van Amstel et al, 1994).

The hepatic manifestations of hepatorenal tyrosinemia include acute decompensation, chronic cirrhosis, and hepatocellular carcinoma. Approximately 69% of deaths were attributed to liver failure and coagulopathy, and 16% to 37% were attributable to hepatocellular carcinoma. It is important to remember that these conditions are not exclusive and may coexist (Pitkanen et al, 1994; Gilbert-Barness & Barness, 2000; Mitchell et al, 2001).

The liver profile of a patient with hepatorenal tyrosinemia is characterized by a marked decline in synthetic function and significantly reduced clotting factors compared with other parameters of hepatic function. The prothrombin and partial thromboplastin times may be markedly prolonged, and administration of vitamin K does not correct this abnormality. Serum transaminase levels vary and may be normal or only slightly elevated. Of the commonly used hepatic function tests, the serum bilirubin value is the least sensitive indicator of dysfunc-

tion, and jaundice is rare in the early phases of this disease (Burton, 2000; Gilbert-Barness & Barness, 2000; Mitchell et al, 2001).

A hepatic crisis may be precipitated by infections or other catabolic conditions. Ascites and GI bleeding are common. Hepatomegaly is present in varying degrees. A "boiled cabbage" odor may be detectable (Burton, 2000; Mitchell et al, 2001). Elevated levels of plasma tyrosine, methionine, and other amino acids may be observed during hepatic crises. Renal tubular function may deteriorate during these episodes. Although some crises spontaneously resolve, some progress to complete liver failure and hepatic encephalopathy. Between crises mild hepatomegaly, normal or mildly elevated transaminases, and a normal bilirubin level are noted. In severe episodes, transaminases rapidly and markedly increase, hyperbilirubinemia may develop, and the alpha-fetoprotein level is elevated (100,000 to 400,000 ng/ml) (Pitkanen et al, 1994; Gilbert-Barness & Barness, 2000; Mitchell et al, 2001).

Cirrhosis eventually develops in all patients, and the risk of hepatocellular carcinoma is extremely high with hepatorenal tyrosinemia. The incidence of hepatocellular carcinoma has been reported to range from approximately 17% to 37% (Pitkanen et al, 1994; Mitchell et al, 2001). Hepatocellular carcinoma has been reported to develop in infants as young as 21 months. Hepatic nodules develop with cirrhosis, and there is no reliable, noninvasive way to determine whether they are malignant. Although their presence is worrisome, most nodules are benign. However, a high degree of suspicion should be maintained if transaminase levels rise significantly from baseline in the absence of a liver crisis.

The neurologic crises of hepatorenal tyrosinemia are acute episodes of peripheral neuropathy followed by a recovery phase. Painful paresthesias, autonomic signs (tachycardia, hypertension, and ileus), and sometimes-progressive paralysis dominate the acute period (Gilbert-Barness & Barness, 2000; Mitchell et al, 2001). Recovery follows. The painful crises are preceded by a minor infection and associated with irritability, decreased activity, and often vomiting. The infant shows extreme hyperextension of the trunk and neck, which can be mistaken for opisthotonos or meningitis and for tonic convulsions, but the patient is conscious. It is important to note that the mental development of these children is normal and that during these crises, their mental function is not diminished. The excruciating pain, the abnormal, striking postures, and frequent self-mutilation make these crises very dramatic and disturbing for all involved. The active phase usually lasts from 1 to 7 days. Weakness and paralysis may develop, and mechanical ventilation may be required for respiratory muscle weakness. Recovery is possible, even after prolonged ventilation for respiratory insufficiency. Patients with repetitive severe crises may have some degree of chronic muscle weakness. The neurologic crises are not associated with exacerbation of liver dysfunction. Plasma transaminase levels, prothrombin times, and plasma bilirubin level are unchanged from baseline values between crises (Mitchell et al, 2001).

Several other complications may occur during this time. Tongue lacerations, severe bruxism, vomiting, and ileus complicate the nutritional management of these patients. Marked hyponatremia, hypophosphatemia, and hypokalemia occur, especially in children with renal tubular dysfunction. Neurologic crises are a major cause of morbidity. An appreciable risk of death from respiratory insufficiency exists. All tyrosinemic patients who are ill must be closely monitored for signs of neurologic deterioration. Respiratory insufficiency occurs rapidly, therefore children with impending neurologic crisis should be hospitalized for continuous monitoring of respiratory function during the acute phase (Gilbert-Barness & Barness, 2000; Mitchell et al, 2001).

Children with hepatorenal tyrosinemia always have some degree of renal involvement, with signs ranging from mild tubular dysfunction to overt renal failure. Both tubular function and glomerular function may be affected. The severity of tubular dysfunction varies and is exacerbated during episodes of decompensation. Clinically, hypophosphatemic rickets develops with hepatorenal tyrosinemia, caused principally by tubular losses of phosphorus. Renal tubular acidosis, aminoaciduria, and glycosuria may also be seen. Nephromegaly and nephrocalcinosis may occur frequently (Gilbert-Barness & Barness, 2000; Mitchell et al, 2001).

Pancreatic islet cell hypertrophy associated with hypoglycemia has been reported. The relationship between pancreatic function and acute liver failure is uncertain. Hypertrophic cardiomyopathy, macrosomia, and ataxia have also been reported (Mitchell et al, 2001).

Management of hepatorenal tyrosinemia is difficult because of the lack of reliable biologic parameters of good metabolic control. Although medical management can slow the progression of the disease, patients are at risk for liver failure, hepatocellular carcinoma, and neurologic crises.

Diet therapy has long been used in the early management of this disorder. Dietary restriction of phenylalanine and tyrosine has been demonstrated to improve renal dysfunction (Gilbert-Barness & Barness, 2000; Mitchell et al, 2001). Any acute increase in tyrosine or phenylalanine intake results in increased tyrosine metabolites downstream and places the patient at risk for acute liver decompensation. When the diagnosis of hypertyrosinemia is made in the newborn, tyrosine levels are elevated, but they decline after 24 to 48 hours of feeding with tyrosine-free formula. After the tyrosine levels decline sufficiently, tyrosine and phenylalanine are added in the form of breast milk or formula. The rate of reintroduction depends on the child's clinical state and the plasma levels of tyrosine. After the acute phase, the intake of phenylalanine and tyrosine is titrated according to the infant's growth and metabolic needs. Treatment is individualized according to the evaluation of the child's metabolic state and individual requirements for tyrosine and phenylalanine. Maintaining the plasma tyrosine level within the normal range ensures adequate growth. An important goal of therapy is to avoid catabolic stress and to stimulate anabolism with adequate dietary intake of energy and nutrients. When catabolic stress occurs, the tyrosine and phenylalanine levels are reduced early in the course of the event, but they return to normal when anabolism resumes (Gilbert-Barness & Barness, 2000).

The renal tubular disease usually improves to some extent with dietary therapy. Vitamin D-resistant rickets is the primary dysfunction in tyrosinemia. Nephrocalcinosis may develop, and some children may require alkali for renal tubular acidosis. No specific therapy is available for the deterioration in glomerular function seen in some patients (Mitchell et al, 2001).

The management of liver disease in hepatorenal tyrosinemia has followed the traditional regimens of reducing the offending protein during periods of crisis and providing adequate sustenance for growth. Despite seemingly good control of diet, hepatic symptoms often progress to cirrhosis and liver failure or to the development of hepatocellular carcinoma. Early liver transplantation has completely changed the therapeutic approach to this disease. Liver transplantation is performed on younger and smaller infants and preferably should be performed before the development of acute liver failure and hepatocellular carcinoma. Liver transplantation still carries a 10% to 15% mortality rate, and the child faces a lifetime of immunosuppressive therapy with cyclosporine. For the patient in stable condition, elective transplantation should be timed in light of the current quality of life, the liver status, the risk of acute hepatic or neurologic decompensation, and the experience of the local pediatric liver transplantation team.

In early studies NTBC, a potent inhibitor of pHPPD, has shown promise that it may diminish or eliminate the neurologic crises of hepatorenal tyrosinemia and slow the progression of the hepatic and renal disease (Gilbert-Barness & Barness, 2000; Mitchell et al, 2001).

Oculocutaneous Tyrosinemia: Tyrosine Aminotransferase Deficiency (Type II Tyrosinemia). Oculocutaneous tyrosinemia is caused by the autosomal recessive deficiency of tyrosine aminotransferase. Males and females are equally affected. Consanguinity of the parents has been present in at least 20 cases. The disease affects the skin, ocular cornea, and central nervous system. Ocular and cutaneous lesions may manifest individually or together, and symptoms can vary among members of a family. The disorder is also known as Richner-Hart syndrome and keratosis palmoplantaris with corneal dystrophy. (For more information please consult the CD.)

Deficiency of 4-Hydroxyphenylpyruvate Dioxygenase (Type III Tyrosinemia). At least three conditions are caused by a dysfunction of pHPPD: primary deficiency of pHPPD, hawkinsinuria of the newborn, and transient tyrosinemia of the newborn. In most cases, dysfunction of pHPPD apparently is compatible with normal development and function. The biochemical abnormalities respond well to therapy. (Please see the CD for more information.)

Disorders of Histidine Metabolism

The two known disorders of histidine metabolism are histidinemia and urocanic aciduria. Histidinemia, an autosomal recessive trait mapped to a location on chromosome 12, is caused by a defect in histidase, which catalyzes the conversion of histidine to urocanic acid. This enzyme is most readily identified in the stratum corneum of the skin. As a result of the metabolic block, the concentration of histidine in the blood, urine, and CSF increases and the concentration of urocanic acid in the blood and the skin decreases. The amount of histidine metabolites in the urine also increases. Histidinemia seems to be benign in most individuals, although neurologic dysfunction has been reported in some cases. Urocanic aciduria arises from a defect in the enzyme urocanase that prevents the enzyme from catalyzing the conversion of urocanic acid to imidazolonepropionic acid. In this apparently benign disorder, an increase in the urinary level of urocanic acid is the only known metabolic aberration (Levy et al, 2001).

Initially described in 1961, histidinemia has been found to be the one of the most common and well-known disorders of histidine metabolism. In various world locations where neonatal screening is performed routinely, the incidence is 1 in 12,000 live births among more than 20 million screened infants. The incidence is particularly high in Japan, with reports of 1 in 9600 live births (Levy et al, 2001). The prominence of this disorder prompted a study of histidase, which is found primarily in the liver and skin. The deficiency of urocanic acid in histidinemia may have implications for the putative functions of urocanic acid as a natural sunscreen against ultraviolet light and as a mediator of ultraviolet light-induced immunosuppression (Levy et al, 2001).

The primary disorder of histidine metabolism is histidase deficiency resulting in an increased serum level of histidine. This error of metabolism blocks the conversion of histidine to urocanic acid, resulting in accumulation of histidine and histidine metabolites and a deficiency of urocanic acid. Whether histidine is an essential amino acid has been the subject of debate, although it seems clear that histidine is essential for human infants. Withdrawal of histidine from the diet of young infants results in a reduced rate of weight gain and a drop in nitrogen retention (Levy et al, 2001). In addition, a rash resembling infantile eczema develops (Burton, 2000; Gilbert-Barness & Barness, 2000).

When these patients are treated with a low-histidine diet, the blood histidine level declines in direct response to the dietary changes. The effect of a low dietary histidine intake on older children and adults remains uncertain, given the apparent lack of consequences with this disorder. If histidine biosynthesis occurs, it may be sufficient only for basic physiologic needs and may be insufficient for needs of growth or physiologic stress (Levy et al, 2001). Thus it appears that histidine would be an essential amino acid for infants, growing children, and perhaps adults.

The major pathway is through urocanic acid to glutamic acid through a sequence of reactions catalyzed by four enzymes (Figure 27-6). The first step in this pathway is the nonoxidative deamination of L-histidine to trans-urocanic acid by histidase (histidine ammonia-lyase). This enzyme is found primarily in the liver and skin (Levy et al, 2001). In the liver, urocanic acid is an intermediate in the conversion of histidine to glutamic acid, whereas in the skin, it accumulates and may function as an ultraviolet protectant and immunoregulator (Levy et al, 2001). The second step in the sequential reaction requires the cytosolic enzyme urocanase, which catalyzes the nonoxidative conversion of trans-urocanic acid to imidazolonepropionic acid. Urocanase is deficient in patients with urocanic aciduria. Urocanase activity has been found only in the liver; there is no detectable activity in the skin, and this accounts for the accumulation of urocanic acid in the skin. The third step in the enzymatic sequence is the conversion of imidazolonepropionic acid to formiminoglutamic acid, an important step that links histidine catabolism to folate metabolism. The enzyme responsible for this conversion is imidazolonepropionic acid hydrolase. The fourth step in the

enzymatic conversion is the formation of formiminotetrahydrofolic acid from formiminoglutamic acid catalyzed by the enzyme formiminotransferase. Tetrahydrofolic acid is required for this reaction, and glutamic acid is liberated (Levy et al, 2001).

Histidinemia is an autosomal recessive trait. The human histidase gene has been mapped to a location on chromosome 12. The characteristic finding in histidinemia is an increased serum concentration of histidine, which varies from 290 to 1420 μmol (normal range is 70 to 120 μmol) (Levy et al, 2001). The highest values are seen at 1 year of age, and slightly lower values are seen in older children and adults. The variation of levels also reflects dietary protein (histidine) intake and the degree of metabolic block (Levy et al, 2001). The urinary histidine level is elevated in affected individuals, probably reflecting overflow from the blood (Levy et al, 2001). In contrast to errors of metabolism with devastating neurologic consequences in which the CSF to plasma ratio is markedly elevated (e.g., nonketotic hyperglycinemia), histidine is found in the CSF in a normal CSF to plasma ratio. However, the CSF to plasma ratio also is normal in some other neurologically devastating errors of metabolism, such as PKU (Scriver & Kaufman, 2001).

The children identified during the first decade after the discovery of histidinemia showed speech disorders and mental retardation. However, since selective screening of impaired individuals was replaced with widespread population screening for this disorder, quite a few individuals were found to have histidinemia and normal intelligence and normal speech, which suggests that histidinemia might actually be benign and that the clinical abnormalities reported initially were coincidental with rather than caused by the genetic disorder. Several prospective follow-up studies of neonates screened for histidinemia in Massachusetts, Japan, and Los Angeles support the view that histidinemia does not cause disease (Levy et al, 2001).

The diagnosis of histidinemia is based on an elevated blood histidine level and increased excretion of histidine in the urine. The urinary metabolite imidazolepyruvic acid usually can be detected using the ferric chloride method. The green color is very similar to that seen with urine from an individual with PKU.

Because 99% of histidinemic patients apparently do not require treatment and only 1% might benefit, treatment is rarely a consideration. Histidase has been encapsulated for potential use as enzyme replacement therapy.

Before routine neonatal screening, histidinemia was thought to be a very rare disorder. Neonatal screening dramatically altered this view and demonstrated that histidinemia is one of the more common metabolic disorders (Levy et al, 2001). In phenylketonuric infants, false-positive results in the bacterial assay for histidine can occur as a result of the elevated phenyl-

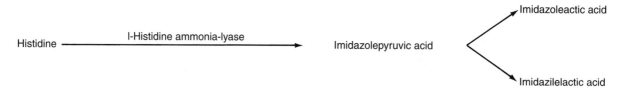

FIGURE **27-6**
Metabolism of histidine. In histidinemia, the enzyme histidine ammonia-lyase is deficient. The normally minor degradative pathway by which imidazolepyruvic acid is converted to imidazoleacetic acid and imidazolelactic acid is enhanced in this disorder.

alanine level. The wide incidence range for histidinemia may reflect differing sensitivities of screening methods rather than true population differences.

Recognition that maternal hyperphenylalaninemia causes fetal damage has increased interest in other maternal errors and fetal consequences. Because maternal histidinemia is such a common metabolic disorder, it has generated considerable interest. Various reports in the literature have examined the children of histidinemic mothers (Levy et al, 2001). These children generally have been normal and have not shown microcephaly, mental retardation, or congenital anomalies, as are seen in the children of mothers with PKU. There is no conclusive evidence, therefore, that an adverse fetal effect derives from maternal histidinemia.

Urocanic Aciduria. Urocanic aciduria is a rare disorder of histidine metabolism. Autosomal recessive transmission is the most likely mode of inheritance. (Please see the CD for more information.) Of the children with urocanic aciduria reported in the literature, all have been mentally retarded and 75% have shown growth retardation. Biochemical studies are consistent with a defect in urocanase. The level of urocanic acid in the urine was up to 50 times the normal amount. Histidine loading aggravated the condition and increased urinary excretion of urocanic acid. The patients were proved to have urocanase deficiency, and all had abnormalities after histidine loading (Levy et al, 2001).

The mental retardation seen in early reports of urocanic aciduria may not be related to the disorder. In all the early reports of the disease, patients were referred as a result of investigation into their mental retardation. Four other infants with urocanic aciduria have been identified through neonatal screening, and they have maintained normal development without diet or other therapy. It therefore is likely that urocanic aciduria is benign and that the mental retardation described in reported cases is coincidental rather than causal. The incidence likely is higher than the reports indicate, because the disorder may escape detection by the conventional investigative methods. Urocanic acid is ninhydrin negative and therefore cannot be identified by amino acid analysis. It also is not soluble in ethyl acetate, the solvent normally used in organic acid extraction of urine.

Nonketotic Hyperglycinemia. Nonketotic hyperglycinemia is an autosomal recessive error of glycine degradation in which large amounts of glycine accumulate in all tissues, including the central nervous system. The diagnosis is established by calculating the CSF to plasma ratio of glycine. A value greater than 0.08 is diagnostic. The diagnosis is confirmed by measuring the activity of the glycine cleavage enzyme system in liver tissue (Gilbert-Barness & Barness, 2000; Hamosh & Johnston, 2001). (Please see the CD for more information.)

Neonatal Nonketotic Hyperglycinemia. Neonatal nonketotic hyperglycinemia is the most common form of nonketotic hyperglycinemia, and patients manifest strikingly similar symptoms. These infants typically are products of normal, uncomplicated pregnancies with appropriate growth in all parameters at birth. No external congenital anomalies are present. The symptom-free interval ranges from 6 hours to 8 days, although 66% of patients become symptomatic by 48 hours (Gilbert-Barness & Barness, 2000; Hamosh & Johnston,

2001). Progressive development of hypotonia, lethargy, and refusal to feed ensues. Wandering eye movements and increased deep tendon reflexes are present. As the encephalopathy progresses to coma, frequent segmental myoclonic jerks, apneic episodes, and hiccups develop. Most infants require assisted ventilation in the first weeks of life (Gilbert-Barness & Barness, 2000; Hamosh & Johnston, 2001). (Please see the CD for more information.)

Cystathionine Beta-Synthase Deficiency. Deficiency cystathionine beta-synthase (CBS) is inherited as an autosomal recessive trait with considerable genetic heterogeneity. Obligate heterozygous individuals have had 22% to 47% of mean control values for CBS activity in liver cells, skin fibroblasts, and lymphocytes (Mudd et al, 2001). (Please consult the CD for more information.)

Homocystinuria caused by CBS deficiency is accompanied by an abundance of clinical manifestations in which four organ systems show major involvement: the eye and the vascular, skeletal, and central nervous systems. Other organ systems, including the liver, skin, and hair, may also be involved. The risk that a manifestation of the disease will develop increases with age. If the individual is pyridoxine responsive, the manifestations usually are milder.

The most consistent finding in CBS deficiency is ectopia lentis, or dislocation of the ocular lens. The dislocation usually is in a downward direction and rarely occurs before age 2 (Mudd et al, 2001). After 2 years of age, the incidence of lens dislocation increases, so that by age 38, only 3% of untreated patients have intact lenses (Mudd et al, 2001). Along with the dislocation, a marked myopia develops when the lens begins to loosen, and the myopia worsens as the subluxation progresses. Acute pupillary block glaucoma, optic atrophy, retinal degeneration and detachment, cataracts, and corneal abnormalities are also highly prevalent in this disorder (Mudd et al, 2001).

The most consistent skeletal manifestation, osteoporosis, occurs in the spine, followed by the long bones. In at least 50% of untreated patients, osteoporosis is detectable by the end of the second decade of life (Gilbert-Barness & Barness, 2000). As a result of the spinal osteoporosis, vertebral collapse and scoliosis are common. Additional skeletal manifestations include increased length of the long bones; irregular, widened metaphyses; growth arrest lines; pes cavus; and high, arched palate (Mudd et al, 2001).

The primary vascular clinical manifestation, thromboembolism, is the major cause of morbidity and death in patients with CBS deficiency. Vascular occlusion can occur in any vessel at any age. In an international survey, 158 patients were reported to have had 253 thromboembolic events (Mudd et al, 2001). Among these events, 51% occurred in peripheral veins (32 of these cases involved pulmonary embolism); 32% were cerebrovascular accidents; 11% affected peripheral arteries; 4% resulted in myocardial infarctions; and 2% were nonspecific. Complications of thromboembolism include optic atrophy, hemiparesis, cor pulmonale, renal hypertension, seizures, and focal neurologic damage (Gilbert-Barness & Barness, 2000; Mudd et al, 2001). The manifestation of vascular thromboembolism depends on age and pyridoxine responsiveness. Untreated pyridoxine-responsive patients are at little risk until about 12 years of age; the risk increases thereafter, so that by 20 years of age, the cumulative risk for a thromboembolic event is about 25%. Untreated pyridoxine-nonresponsive patient have a cumulative risk of 25% by 15 years of age (Mudd et al, 2001). The risk factors are based on the clinically apparent thromboembolic events. Efforts at ultrasonic detection of vascular disease have documented early vascular disease even without symptoms of ischemia (Gilbert-Barness & Barness, 2000; Mudd et al, 2001).

The most frequent clinical manifestation of CNS disturbance in CBS deficiency is mental retardation, often manifesting as developmental delay during the first and second years of life. The IQ scores of untreated patients vary widely, ranging from 10 to 138, the median being approximately 64. The distribution of pyridoxine-responsive patients shifted toward the higher IQ scores (median, 78) compared with the distribution for pyridoxine-unresponsive patients (median, 56). Among infants with CBS deficiency who go untreated from early infancy, 21% have seizures, most often the grand mal type (Mudd et al, 2001). Abnormal EEGs have been reported. Signs of focal neurologic signs and hemiparesis suggest a cerebrovascular event (Mudd et al, 2001).

The presence of one or more of the typical signs and symptoms may lead to a suspicion of CBS deficiency, but definitive diagnosis is based on the presence of certain biochemical abnormalities. The most consistent biochemical abnormality is homocystinuria (Mudd et al, 2001). The presence of homocystine is suspected when the result of the urinary cyanide-nitroprusside reaction is positive. Because this test also detects other disulfide compounds, homocystine must be specifically identified.

False-negative results can occur in tests for homocystinuria. With pyridoxine-responsive forms of CBS deficiency, a marked response may be seen with even very small amounts of supplemental folate therapy (as little as one vitamin tablet daily), and thus the homocystinuria may escape detection. Before testing, any supplemental vitamins should be discontinued for 2 to 4 weeks, and the amount of folate intake should be calculated based on the dietary history.

Homocystinuria alone is not sufficient to establish the diagnosis of CBS deficiency. Homocystinuria is a nonspecific symptom, because homocystine is excreted in other errors of metabolism; for this reason, a serum amino acid analysis should be performed. In CBS deficiency, amino acid analysis should reveal hyperhomocystinemia and a markedly reduced concentration of cystine. Often an elevated level of methionine also is found. Direct enzyme analysis assayed from liver biopsy samples, cultured skin fibroblasts, or lymphocytes confirms the diagnosis (Burton, 2000; Mudd et al, 2001).

The goals of medical management of CBS deficiency are (1) to control or eliminate biochemical abnormalities so as to prevent clinical disease, halt the progression of existing clinical defects, and ameliorate clinical manifestations that may be reversible; and (2) to provide supportive treatment of complications. Whenever possible, treatment should begin before the onset of complications, many of which may cause irreversible damage. The maximum benefit of therapy is obtained when the disorder is detected in the neonatal period either through neonatal screening or from the family history (Mudd et al, 2001).

Administration of pyridoxine has proved effective at reducing or eliminating the biochemical abnormalities in many patients with pyridoxine-responsive CBS deficiency (Mudd et al, 2001). The doses of pyridoxine have varied widely, and some patients have a dose-response correlation (Mudd et al, 2001). The effectiveness of pyridoxine in preventing initial clinically detectable thromboembolic events has been established (Mudd et al, 2001). For prevention of thromboembolism alone, pyridoxine treatment is strongly indicated for pyridoxine-responsive patients at any age. A similar analysis documented a decreased frequency of lens dislocation among pyridoxine-responsive patients who were treated with pyridoxine (Mudd et al, 2001). In addition, there is evidence that behavior and IQ scores improved in several late-treated pyridoxine-responsive patients (Gilbert-Barness & Barness, 2000; Mudd et al, 2001).

Folate deficiency is a factor in this disorder, and folate may have to be replenished to effect a pyridoxine response. In other patients, folate therapy alone may be enough or may be used in combination with vitamin B_{12} and pyridoxine to achieve the lower concentrations of homocystine (Gilbert-Barness & Barness, 2000; Mudd et al, 2001).

Vitamin therapy alone for CBS-deficient patients responsive to pyridoxine may not be as effective at reducing the biochemical abnormalities as vitamin therapy combined with a methionine-restricted diet. Even patients with maximum pyridoxine responsiveness have a reduced tolerance to methionine, and these patients may show episodic increases in methionine or homocystine concentrations after protein intake (Mudd et al, 2001). For these reasons, a methionine-restricted diet or small, frequent feedings may be prudent.

Most CBS-deficient patients detected by neonatal screening have been treated with diets low in methionine to reduce the accumulation of methionine and homocystine and have been given supplemental L-cystine to provide at least some of this amino acid. Current commercially available diets are based on a methionine-free synthetic mixture supplemented with L-cystine. The methionine requirement is met with the addition of small amounts of milk and later by the addition of low-protein foods in carefully controlled amounts (Mudd et al, 2001). The amount of dietary protein is regulated by keeping the blood methionine level in the normal range and by the absence of homocystine in the urine and blood. Methionine restriction, started from early infancy, has been shown to prevent or delay a number of serious complications of this disorder. Most patients detected by neonatal screening have been pyridoxine unresponsive, therefore the data are more convincing. In an international survey, the mean IQ score for early-treated pyridoxine-nonresponsive patients was 94 ± 4, approximately 35 points above the mean IQ of late-treated pyridoxine-nonresponsive patients (Mudd et al, 2001). Early dietary treatment also tends to delay or prevent lens dislocation in some patients and may prevent seizures (Mudd et al, 2001). Early-treated patients tend to have lower incidences of thromboembolism and osteoporosis (Mudd et al, 2001). Treatment may be indicated for newborns who are responsive to pyridoxine, along with a methionine-restricted diet.

Patients detected after the newborn period who are unresponsive to pyridoxine therapy represent the greatest challenge to treatment. Compliance with a methionine-restricted diet is difficult to achieve in older children. When accepted and maintained, there is evidence of improvement in the biochemical abnormalities (Mudd et al, 2001), and results appear promising in terms of preventing thromboembolic events (Mudd et al, 2001).

To date, most screening of newborns for CBS deficiency have relied on the detection of hypermethioninemia. Current data on prevalence rates for this disorder vary widely, from 1 in

58,000 live births in Ireland to 1 in 889,000 live births in Japan. The current cumulative rate of detection is 1 in 344,000 live births worldwide, which may be an underestimate of the frequency of the disorder. Hypermethioninemia may not be detected during the time newborn blood is obtained for screening, because since the 1970s, feeding practices have provided a lower protein intake (Mudd et al, 2001).

An alternative to screening newborns for hypermethioninemia to identify CBS deficiency is to attempt to detect abnormal levels of homocystine in the blood or urine. To date, no specific or reliable test has been firmly established as a tool for routine neonatal screening (Mudd et al, 2001). Prenatal diagnosis of CBS deficiency is feasible in the first and second trimesters of pregnancy using extracts of cells cultured from amniotic fluid to detect the activity of CBS (Mudd et al, 2001).

Gamma-Cystathionase Deficiency.   Deficient activity of gamma-cystathionase has been reported in several patients with cystathioninuria. In these cases, urinary excretion of cystathionine was increased, and the amino acid accumulated and was present in elevated concentrations in body fluids and tissues. (Please see the CD for more information.)

Urea Cycle Enzymes and the Congenital Hyperammonemias.   The urea cycle, which consists of a series of biochemical reactions, has two roles in metabolism. To prevent accumulation of toxic nitrogenous compounds, the urea cycle incorporates nitrogen not used for net biosynthetic purposes into urea, which is the waste nitrogen product in human beings. The urea cycle also encompasses several of the biochemical reactions required for de novo synthesis of arginine (Brusilow & Horwich, 2001). (Please see the CD for more information.)

Disorders of Branched-Chain Amino and Keto Acids: Maple Syrup Urine Disease

MSUD, or branched-chain ketoaciduria, is caused by a deficiency in the activity of the branched-chain alpha-keto acid dehydrogenase (BCKAD) complex. This metabolic block results in the accumulation of the branched-chain amino acids (BCAAs) leucine, isoleucine, and valine and the corresponding branched-chain alpha-keto acids (BCKAs). Like many metabolic disorders, MSUD has five different phenotypic classes, based on clinical manifestations and biochemical responses to thiamine administration. The five forms are classic, intermediate, intermittent, thiamine responsive, and dihydrolipoyl dehydrogenase (E3) deficient (Chuang & Shih, 2001).

MSUD is an autosomal recessive disorder of panethnic distribution. The worldwide incidence is 1 per 185,000 live births, according to routine screening of 26.8 million newborns. In countries where consanguineous marriage is common (Saudi Arabia, Spain, Turkey, and India), the frequency is higher. In the Old Order Mennonite population of Lancaster and Lebanon counties in Pennsylvania, MSUD occurs in approximately 1 in 176 newborns (Burton, 2000; Beaudet et al, 2001; Chuang & Shih, 2001).

The BCAAs constitute about 35% of the indispensable amino acids in muscle and 40% of the preformed amino acids required by human beings. The catabolic pathways for BCAAs begin with the transport of these amino acids into cells, where they undergo reversible transamination by isoforms of the branched-chain aminotransferase to produce BCKAs. Leucine

is catabolized to alpha-ketoisocaproate; isoleucine is catabolized to alpha-keto-beta-methylvalerate, and valine is catabolized to alpha-ketoisovalerate. Oxidative decarboxylation of the BCKAs is catalyzed by the single BCKAD multienzyme complex, generating the respective branched-chain acyl coenzyme A (acyl-CoA), which is further metabolized into separate pathways. The end products of leucine catabolism are acetyl-CoA and acetoacetate. Valine yields succinyl-CoA, and isoleucine produces acetyl-CoA and succinyl-CoA. BCAAs are the precursors for fatty acids and cholesterol synthesis through acetyl-CoA. These amino acids are also substrates for energy production through succinyl-CoA and acetoacetate (Chuang & Shih, 2001).

Oxidation of the BCAAs occurs primarily in the liver, kidneys, heart, and adipose tissue. There is evidence that transamination is the rate-limiting step in the catabolism of BCAAs in the liver, where aminotransferase activity is low. In extrahepatic tissues, oxidative decarboxylation of the alpha-keto acids is the rate-limiting step. A significant portion of the BCKAs appears to originate from the skeletal muscle and circulates to the liver, where it is oxidized (Gilbert-Barness & Barness, 2000; Chuang & Shih, 2001).

The human BCKAD genes have been located on different chromosomes, including chromosomes 1 p31, 6 p21-p22, 7 q31-q32, and 19 q13.1-13.2. The genomic structure also has been characterized, including the regulatory and promoter regions of the genes of the BCKAD complex (Gilbert-Barness & Barness, 2000; Chuang & Shih, 2001).

Most untreated patients with the classic form of MSUD die in the early months of life from recurrent metabolic crises and neurologic deterioration. Treatment involves both long-term dietary management and aggressive intervention during acute metabolic decompensation. Advances in both aspects of treatment since the mid-1980s have considerably reduced morbidity and mortality, as well as the length of hospitalization. The age at diagnosis and the subsequent metabolic control are the most important determinants of long-term outcome. Patients in whom treatment is initiated after 10 days of age rarely achieve normal intellect (Sweetman & Williams, 2001).

Successful pregnancies have occurred in classic MSUD patients. The major concerns are the stress of pregnancy on metabolic homeostasis and the rapidly changing nutritional requirements in the course of a pregnancy. These factors require intensive monitoring.

Three essential amino acids—leucine, isoleucine, and valine—are classified as BCAAs. The carbon skeletons of BCAAs are incorporated into proteins and undergo oxidative degradation in mitochondria. The catabolism of BCAAs has nutritional, biochemical, and clinical significance. After protein is ingested, the BCAAs contribute to more than 60% of the increase in amino acid concentration in human blood (Sweetman & Williams, 2001). BCAAs are metabolized in skeletal muscle as an alternative fuel source and are also actively metabolized in the kidneys, heart, adipose tissue, and brain (Sweetman & Williams, 2001). In the liver, the BCKAs derived from BCAAs are rapidly catabolized to yield ketone bodies and succinyl-CoA. Adipose tissue and muscle use the acetyl-CoA produced from leucine for the synthesis of long-chain fatty acids and cholesterol. Leucine also appears to play an important role in promoting protein synthesis, inhibiting its degradation, and stimulating insulin secretion (Chuang & Shih, 2001). Clinically, BCAA infusions counteract the catabolic state observed in sepsis and severe trauma. In patients with liver cirrhosis, hepatic encephalopathy, and chronic renal failure, plasma BCAA levels are diminished. Dietary supplementation with BCAAs or BCKAs restores nitrogen balance and ameliorates the pathophysiologic disturbances.

MSUD is caused by greatly elevated levels of leucine, isoleucine, and valine (Gilbert-Barness & Barness, 2000; Chuang & Shih, 2001; Sweetman & Williams, 2001). The disorder was first described in the mid-1950s as four cases of familial cerebral degenerative disease characterized by onset within the first week of life, urine with an odor resembling maple syrup, and death within 3 months. Later reports described variant forms of MSUD that had milder clinical manifestations and episodic symptoms that were related to infection, increases in dietary protein, and stress (Chuang & Shih, 2001). Attempts at dietary therapy were largely unsuccessful. In 1964 a more rigorous and successful dietary therapy involving restriction of BCAAs was proposed (Chuang & Shih, 2001). In 1971, a new thiamine-responsive form of MSUD was identified in which the hyperaminoacidemia was completely corrected by administration of thiamine in pharmacologic doses without recourse to dietary restrictions (Scriver et al, 2001). This early phase of the history of MSUD defined the phenotypes, identified the metabolic block, and devised dietary treatment. Subsequently, genetic control of this metabolic disease has been intensively investigated.

Classic Maple Syrup Urine Disease.   MSUD with a neonatal onset of encephalopathy is now considered the most severe and most common form of this disease. The levels of the BCAAs, especially leucine, are greatly increased in the blood, CSF, and urine; the presence of alloisoleucine is diagnostic of MSUD. In classic MSUD, 50% or more of the BCKAs are derived from leucine. The activity of the BCKAD complex in skin fibroblasts or lymphocytes usually is less than 2% of normal. Affected newborns appear normal at birth, with symptoms usually developing between 4 and 7 days of age. Breast-feeding may delay onset to the second week of life. Lethargy and poor sucking with little interest in feeding are usually the first signs. These signs are followed by weight loss and progressive neurologic signs of altering hypotonia and hypertonia with dystonic extension of the arms resembling decerebrate posturing. Ketosis and the maple syrup or burnt-sugar odor become obvious at this time. Seizures and coma ensue, leading to death if the disease goes untreated.

Most patients die within the first months of life from recurrent metabolic crises or neurologic deterioration, often precipitated by infection or other stressors such as vaccination or surgery. Sudden death has been reported in the first week of life (Chuang & Shih, 2001). Surviving patients suffer from severe neurologic damage, including mental retardation, spasticity, or hypotonia, and occasionally cortical blindness. Although early treatment has greatly improved the outlook for these infants, complications can occur. Sudden onset of transient ataxia lasting 30 minutes to 1 hour has been seen even in patients with good metabolic control. During ketonemia, older patients have experienced visual hallucinations. Even with treatment, some patients have died from uncontrollable brain edema (Chuang & Shih, 2001).

Intermediate Maple Syrup Urine Disease.   Patients with the intermediate form of MSUD have persistently elevated levels of BCAAs and neurologic impairment, but they have no catastrophic illness in the neonatal period. Many do not have

episodes of acute metabolic decompensation. The residual enzyme activity ranges from 3% to 30% of normal. About 20 patients have been reported to have intermediate MSUD. Diagnosis is most common between 5 months and 7 years of age, during evaluation for developmental delay and seizures. Several patients have had episodes of ketoacidosis, but acute encephalopathy was rare (Chuang & Shih, 2001).

Intermittent Maple Syrup Urine Disease.   Patients with the intermittent form of MSUD show normal early development, with normal growth and intelligence. However, they are at risk for acute metabolic decompensation during stressful situations. While they are asymptomatic, the laboratory data, including the plasma BCAA levels, are normal. The activity of the BCKAD complex in these patients ranges from 5% to 20% of normal. Many cases of intermittent MSUD have been reported. The initial symptoms generally appear between 5 months and 2 years of age in association with otitis media or some other infection, but they may appear as late as the fifth decade of life (Chuang & Shih, 2001). Episodes of acute behavioral change and unsteady gait may progress to seizures and stupor or coma. The amino acid and organic acid profiles at these times are characteristic of MSUD. Death has occurred during these episodes of metabolic decompensation.

Thiamine-Responsive Maple Syrup Urine Disease.   A number of putative thiamine-responsive patients have been reported (Scriver et al, 2001). In general, these patients do not have acute neonatal illness, and the early clinical course has been similar to that of intermediate MSUD. Scriver described the first case, which involved a girl who had developmental delay at 11 months of age. Her plasma BCAA concentrations were found to be five times higher than normal, and alloisoleucine was detected. These levels fell abruptly to normal with a constant protein-restricted diet and after thiamine administration; they rebounded during the two trials of thiamine withdrawal (Scriver et al, 2001). The combined treatment of protein restriction and thiamine supplementation was continued, and the girl's BCAA levels were maintained over the years. The skin fibroblast BCKAD complex activity was 30% to 40% of normal. Other reports of patients with thiamine-responsive MSUD can be found in the literature (Chuang & Shih, 2001). Thiamine-responsive patients are heterogeneous in their response to treatment, and a wide range of dosages has been administered with limited success. No patients have been treated with thiamine alone; all have been treated with a combination of low (BCAA) protein diet and thiamine for metabolic control (Scriver et al, 2001).

Dihydrolipoyl Dehydrogenase (E3)–Deficient Maple Syrup Urine Disease.   E3 deficiency is a rare disorder, and only a handful of patients have been described. (Please see the CD for more information.)

Screening for MSUD is done in many U.S. states and in at least 18 countries (Chuang & Shih, 2001). The Guthrie bacterial inhibition assay detects the elevated leucine level in blood spots. In states that screen for MSUD, a blood leucine level above 4 mg/dl or a level of 3 to 4 mg/dl (305 μmol) in the first 24 hours of life mandates immediate telephone contact with the infant's pediatrician. Infants with classic MSUD, the intermediate form, and E3 deficiency usually can be identified in the newborn period. Infants with the intermediate variety tend to have lower leucine levels than those with classic MSUD and may be missed. It is unlikely that infants with the intermittent form can be identified, because their blood BCAA levels are normal when the child is asymptomatic. No cases of thiamine-responsive MSUD have been detected by neonatal screening (Chuang & Shih, 2001).

If a newborn shows symptoms, the diagnosis can be made easily by amino acid analysis or organic acid profiling. The BCAA levels are greatly elevated in blood, CSF, and urine, and the presence of alloisoleucine is pathognomonic. Alloisoleucine, a metabolite of leucine, has delayed clearance, remains elevated in the plasma for several days after an episode of metabolic decompensation, and is detectable in classic MSUD at all times. The plasma alanine level is low, and the ratios of blood to CSF BCAAs and BCKAs are reduced in encephalopathic infants (Chuang & Shih, 2001). The urine 2,4-dinitrophenylhydrazine (DNPH) test is a simple test for alpha-keto acids and is useful in screening. Acidification of the urine enhances its maple syrup odor (Burton, 2000; Chuang & Shih, 2001; Gilbert-Barness & Barness, 2000).

Gas chromatography–mass spectroscopy analysis of urine or plasma organic acids produces characteristic profiles when the infant is symptomatic. The metabolic profile of an infant with the intermittent form of MSUD is normal during remission. In older patients, transient elevation of BCAA levels without the appearance of alloisoleucine may occur after several days of fasting and should not be mistaken for a form of MSUD. Mild to moderate elevation of the BCAA levels in association with increases in lactate, pyruvate, alpha-ketoglutarate, and the BCKAs and their hydroxy derivatives is diagnostic for E3 deficiency (Chuang & Shih, 2001).

A close linear relationship exists between elevated plasma BCAA and BCKA levels in MSUD patients, and adequate monitoring may be accomplished by determining the plasma BCAA levels (Chuang & Shih, 2001). Early detection is possible in patients at high risk for the disorder (e.g., siblings of affected patients) by using quantitative analysis of amino acids from plasma. The characteristic elevation of the leucine level and the appearance of alloisoleucine can be seen as early as 24 hours of life, regardless of the type of feeding.

Urine metabolic screening is less sensitive than plasma amino acid analysis for early detection of MSUD. Changes in the urinary amino acid levels may be minimal even when the plasma amino acid levels are two to four times normal. With young affected infants, a distinctive odor of maple syrup or burnt sugar is detectable on a wet diaper. It is important to note that the urine of normal infants may be mistaken for having unusual odors, depending on the use of spices and curry in the diet of breastfeeding mothers (Burton, 2000).

Obtaining cells for culture allows enzymatic analysis and direct determination of activity. Postmortem material is largely unsatisfactory in this disorder because of the instability of the BCKAD complex. Currently only skin fibroblasts and lymphoblasts are suitable for diagnostic studies because they are relatively homogeneous cell populations (Burton, 2000; Sweetman & Williams, 2001).

A prenatal diagnosis is made using cultured amniotic fluid cells, direct analysis of tissue from chorionic sampling, and cultured chorionic cells (Gilbert-Barness & Barness, 2000; Sweetman & Williams, 2001). The activity of the BCKAD complex in cultured amniocytes and chorionic villi is in the same range as that seen in skin fibroblasts. In the future, with the development of DNA diagnostic techniques, detection of known mutations in fetuses at risk should be possible. Attempts at prena-

tal diagnosis of MSUD by determining the concentrations of BCAAs and alpha-keto acids and their corresponding alpha-hydroxy acids in amniotic fluid were unsuccessful.

The neuropathology of MSUD involves the white matter. However, the spongy changes in the white matter and delayed myelination are not specific to MSUD and are seen in other metabolic disorders (Burton, 2000; Gilbert-Barness & Barness, 2000; Brusilow & Horwich, 2001; Scriver et al, 2001). Patients who die during an acute metabolic crisis show severe cerebral edema. In untreated cases, myelin deficiency and striking spongy degeneration of the white matter are prominent findings. A delay in myelination occurs mainly in the tracts normally myelinated after birth. The pyramidal tracts of the spinal cord, the myelin around the dentate nuclei, the corpus callosum, and the cerebral hemispheres are most affected. In treated patients, the neuropathologic effects may be similar but of a lesser degree, or the examination may yield normal findings.

Management of MSUD requires restriction of the specific amino acids to the levels required for growth and development. This minimizes accumulation of intermediates that damage organs, particularly the nervous system. In MSUD patients, an increase in the plasma leucine level is associated with the appearance of neurologic symptoms, whereas an increase in the isoleucine level is associated with an intensified odor of maple syrup in the urine. An increase in the valine level does not seem to have any clinical effects. Leucine and its keto acid, therefore, are considered the neurotoxic metabolites in MSUD, and the plasma leucine concentration is an important parameter in monitoring treatment.

The two aspects of MSUD treatment are long-term dietary management and therapy during acute metabolic crisis (Chuang & Shih, 2001). The principles of dietary management are to normalize the concentrations of blood BCAAs by limiting the intake of the three amino acids while providing nutrition adequate to maintain growth and development. A trial of thiamine therapy is advised for every patient to determine thiamine responsiveness (Scriver et al, 2001). Dietary therapy must be continued throughout life. Commercial diets are available, consisting of BCAA-free formula with an amino acid intake of 2 to 3 g/kg/day (Gilbert-Barness & Barness, 2000). The requirement for leucine is met by the addition of a calculated amount of standard formula for infants or of dietary protein for older children and adults. The isoleucine and valine concentrations in natural food are low in relation to leucine, and supplementation of these free amino acids is necessary to maintain normal plasma levels. Plasma BCAA levels should be kept as close to normal as possible to minimize neurotoxic effects. These levels may need to be monitored weekly during the first 6 months of life, and the monitoring may be extended if good metabolic control is achieved and the infant is thriving (Chuang & Shih, 2001).

It is well known that infection has particularly deleterious effects on the metabolic status of patients with MSUD. It often precipitates acute decompensation. During the infection, and occasionally during the incubation period, tolerance of protein is lower, and endogenous BCAAs from protein catabolism are increased. The plasma BCAA and BCKA concentrations rise to toxic levels. Behavioral changes and loss of appetite often are the first signs of metabolic disturbance. Immediate reduction of dietary protein and substitution of BCAA-free synthetic formulas and protein-free foods are instituted to ensure an adequate calorie intake. Nutritional changes are intended to promote anabolism and to prevent the BCAA and BCKA concentrations from reaching toxic levels. Prompt treatment of the infection prevents further deterioration (Chuang & Shih, 2001).

Acute metabolic decompensation associated with infections leads to acute deterioration in cerebral function. This is a life-threatening condition, and aggressive therapy is imperative. Clinical improvement is not possible until tissue catabolism is reversed.

The three aspects of treatment of an acute metabolic crisis are (1) rapid removal of the toxic metabolite, (2) nutritional support, and (3) minimization of the catabolic state and promotion of anabolism.

Toxic metabolites initially were removed by exchange transfusion, with limited success. The effects were transient, and rebound was common. Peritoneal dialysis can be performed to initially remove toxic metabolites. The advantages of peritoneal dialysis are that it is relatively simple to perform, and neurologic status improves significantly in a few hours. A needle can be inserted into the peritoneum to initiate dialysis while a comatose patient is transported from an outlying hospital to a medical center. Studies have suggested that hemodialysis may be more effective than peritoneal dialysis at lowering the BCAA and BCKA levels (Chuang & Shih, 2001). The disadvantage of hemodialysis is that it requires specialized equipment and a specially trained team. Continuous arteriovenous filtration has also been used in the treatment of acute metabolic crisis in MSUD. This technique has technical limitations, however, and not all medical centers have personnel with the expertise to perform the procedure. All these procedures are invasive, and they can reduce the plasma leucine level to approximately 1 mmol, but they are minimally effective below that level. They are useful in the initial treatment of severe metabolic decompensation. The choice of procedure depends on the availability and expertise of personnel at an institution.

Parenteral nutrition therapy has been developed for MSUD. The preparation consists of a BCAA-free L–amino acid mixture combined with glucose, lipid, electrolytes, and vitamins to provide balanced nutrition. The plasma concentrations of isoleucine and valine decline faster than leucine during treatment and must be supplemented after 1 to 2 days of therapy. An alternative nutritional approach is the stimulation of anabolism with insulin and growth hormone or the prevention of catabolism with high-calorie continuous nasogastric feeding (Gilbert-Barness & Barness, 2000; Chuang & Shih, 2001; Scriver et al, 2001).

Liver transplantation has been successfully performed in a well-controlled patient with hepatic insufficiency and metabolic decompensation caused by fulminant hepatitis A infection. The plasma BCAA levels fell to normal dramatically and remained stable on a normal diet. Alloisoleucine was still detectable, most likely produced by skeletal muscle (Chuang & Shih, 2001).

MSUD is a suitable disease for attempting gene therapy, because increasing the enzyme activity by even a small percentage may alter the phenotype from the classic form to the intermittent form of the disease. A stable gene transfer into MSUD cells has been reported. Stable chromosomal integration and persistent restoration of BCKAD complex activity were achieved. This may represent the first step in developing gene therapy in animal models and subsequently in human beings with MSUD.

The team approach to management and parental understanding and cooperation are essential for successful metabolic control. The outcome of treatment in more than 150 patients with classic MSUD and more than 25 patients with the variant forms of MSUD have now been reported (Gilbert-Barness & Barness, 2000; Chuang & Shih, 2001). Most patients were diagnosed by neonatal screening or by laboratory testing based on clinical suspicion. A small number were prospectively treated because of affected siblings. Approximately one third of the classic MSUD patients had IQ scores above 90, and one third had scores between 70 and 90. These patients scored higher on the verbal aspects of the examination than on the performance aspects. Short attention span and minor learning disabilities were observed even in patients treated soon after birth. Poor intellectual outcome was often associated with neurologic sequelae, such as spasticity and quadriplegia (Chuang & Shih, 2001). Approximately one fifth of the classic MSUD patients died, most during acute metabolic decompensation precipitated by infection. The cerebral edema that develops during these crises and the recovery phases can be fatal, especially in preschool-age patients. Acute metabolic encephalopathy is less likely to occur after 5 or 6 years of age. Older patients tolerate stress better, particularly if effective biochemical control is maintained (Chuang & Shih, 2001).

The most important determinants of long-term outcome for patients with MSUD are the age at diagnosis and the subsequent course of the disease. Treatment initiated before 10 days of age yields the best results; only a few patients treated after 14 days of age achieved normal intelligence. Diagnosis during infancy usually is associated with a milder neonatal course. Unfortunately, the impact and severity of the acute neonatal form of the disease and the subsequent metabolic complications are difficult to quantify and predict.

ORGANIC ACIDEMIAS: DISORDERS OF PROPIONATE AND METHYLMALONATE METABOLISM

Propionyl-CoA is formed by the catabolism of several essential amino acids, odd-chain fatty acids, and cholesterol. It is metabolized primarily by enzymatic conversion to methylmalonyl-CoA, which is subsequently converted to succinyl-CoA. This metabolic sequence depends on the activity of several enzymes: propionyl-CoA carboxylase, methylmalonic-CoA racemase, and methylmalonic-CoA mutase. Propionyl-CoA requires biotin as a cofactor, and methylmalonyl-CoA mutase requires adenosylcobalamin, a cobalamin (vitamin B_{12}) coenzyme (Fenton et al, 2001). Problems with errors of metabolism occur infrequently but are important. (Please see the CD for more complete information.)

Propionic Acidemias

Propionic acidemia refers to a heterogenous group of inborn metabolic disorders that result in the accumulation of propionic acid in the blood. The disorder may arise from a primary deficiency of propionyl-CoA carboxylase or from abnormalities of biotin metabolism that lead to a deficiency of the several biotin-dependent carboxylases (Gilbert-Barness & Barness, 2000; Fenton et al, 2001). (Please see the CD for more information.)

Methylmalonic Acidemias

The inherited forms of methylmalonic acidemia have several different biochemical bases: two distinct defects in the mutase enzyme, two distinct defects of adenosylcobalamin synthesis, and three distinct defects of both adenosylcobalamin and methylcobalamin synthesis (Gilbert-Barness & Barness, 2000; Fenton et al, 2001). This discussion is limited to the disorders associated with a deficiency of methylmalonyl-CoA mutase. (Please see the CD for more information.)

DISORDERS OF THE PYRUVATE DEHYDROGENASE COMPLEX

Defects in five enzyme components of the pyruvate dehydrogenase (PDH) complex have been documented as leading to a PDH deficiency. A profile of enzymatic activity for each of the five components can be developed for a patient suspected of having the deficiency. Patients have been described with defects in the E1 PDH, E2 transacetylase, and the E3 lipoyl dehydrogenase enzymes, as well as in the X-component and in PDH phosphatase (Robinson, 2001). (Please see the CD for more information.)

DISORDERS OF THE PYRUVATE CARBOXYLASE COMPLEX

Pyruvate carboxylase is the first enzyme in the gluconeogenic pathway; it is activated under conditions in which fatty acids are mobilized and acetyl-CoA is generated. It has binding sites for ATP, bicarbonate (HCO_3^-), and acetyl-CoA and is almost totally dependent on the presence of acetyl-CoA for activity. Pyruvate carboxylase is the major regulatory enzyme in the pathway of gluconeogenesis; it is regulated by the acetyl-CoA to CoA and ATP to adenosine diphosphate (ADP) ratios in liver mitochondria. The liver and kidneys have the highest concentrations of pyruvate carboxylase, but it is also found in lesser amounts in other tissues such as the brain, muscles, adipocytes, and fibroblasts, in which it helps maintain intermediates for the citric acid cycle (Scriver et al, 2001). (For more information please see the CD.)

METABOLIC ERRORS THAT AFFECT BLOOD AND BLOOD-FORMING TISSUE: PYRUVATE KINASE AND GLUCOSE-6-PHOSPHATASE DEFICIENCIES

Human red blood cells are devoid of nuclei and cytoplasmic organelles. This structure simplifies their physiology but also restricts their metabolic capacities and their ability to adapt to changing environmental conditions. The unique properties of hemoglobin allow it to mediate gas transport and exchange without expending energy. However, maintenance of membrane plasticity depends on an adequate source of high-energy phosphate, specifically ATP, which is also necessary for a number of other essential cell functions, such as maintenance of ionic fluxes in opposition to the electrochemical gradient, preservation or generation of membrane components and intracellular nucleotides, synthesis of glutathione, and initiation and maintenance of glycolysis itself. In addition, reducing energy is required for preserving the functional valance of hemoglobin iron and for protecting enzyme and structural proteins from irreversible oxidative denaturation (Hirono et al, 2001).

Energy requirements of the red blood cells are fulfilled almost entirely by the metabolism of glucose, with the consequent generation and storage of high-energy phosphates, principally ATP, or as reducing equivalents in the form of glutathione (GSH) and the pyridine nucleotides reduced nicotinamide adenine dinucleotide (NADH) and reduced nicotinamide adenine dinucleotide phosphate (NADPH). Glucose is assimilated by facilitated transport and phosphorylated by hexokinase, providing a common substrate for anaerobic glycolysis through the Embden-Meyerhof pathway or for oxidative glycolysis via the hexose monophosphate (HMP) shunt. Normally, the anaerobic pathway predominates by a factor of 10, but oxidant stimulation of HMP shunt activity can reverse the ratio (Gilbert-Barness & Barness, 2000; Hirono et al, 2001).

Anaerobic glycolysis in the red blood cell is regulated by the kinase-mediated enzymatic reactions, principally phosphofructokinase, hexokinase, and pyruvate kinase. These enzymes are sensitive to numerous feedback regulators, including substrates, products, cofactors, intermediates, and electrolyte and hydrogen ion concentrations. Fixation of inorganic phosphate occurs at the glyceraldehyde-3-phosphate dehydrogenase step, allowing generation and subsequent transfer of high-energy phosphate to ADP. This results in a net gain of two molecules of ATP for every one of catabolized glucose. The 1,3-phosphodiester can revert to a low-energy state by a mutation to 2,3-diphosphoglycerate, which comprises one half to two thirds of all organic phosphates in the erythrocyte and has an important regulatory influence on hemoglobin affinity (Gilbert-Barness & Barness, 2000; Hirono et al, 2001). Diversion through this pathway bypasses an ATP-generating step but simultaneously contributes to a large reservoir of potential substrate for pyruvate kinase, thus providing a sensitive regulator to optimize the ATP to ADP ratios. The pyridine nucleotide ($NAD^+/NADH$) cycled by anaerobic glycolysis is an essential cofactor in methemoglobin reduction via cytochrome b5 reductase (Hirono et al, 2001).

During oxidative glycolysis, HMP shunt activity maintains high concentrations of reduced GSH, a cysteine-containing compound with a very low oxidation potential, allowing it to protect other cellular proteins from oxidant damage by serving as a sacrificial reductant. The oxidized form of nicotinamide adenine dinucleotide phosphate ($NADP^+$) is the obligate cofactor for each dehydrogenase reaction in the shunt, and the $NADP^+$ to NADPH ratio is the principal regulator of glucose catabolism via this pathway. HMP shunt activity can be stimulated twentyfold to thirtyfold or more in response to oxidant challenge (Hirono et al, 2001).

Glucose is oxidized at the 1-carbon position, generating carbon dioxide (CO_2) and ribulose 5-phosphate, which can be modified and recombined into two intermediates of anaerobic glycolysis. One of the intermediates, fructose-6-phosphate, can undergo isomerization back to glucose-6-phosphate, providing additional substrate for recycling back through the HMP shunt if the $NADP^+$ to NADPH ratio compels it to do so (Hirono et al, 2001).

On the basis of the known physiologic functions of these two major pathways, defective enzymes in either can be expected to interfere with erythrocyte metabolism with predictable results. Enzyme defects of anaerobic glycolysis result in increased concentrations of glycolytic intermediates proximal to the defective enzyme, impaired production of ATP, and chronic hemolysis with its characteristic clinical sequelae (Burton, 2000). In contrast, enzyme defects of the HMP shunt more often are characterized by susceptibility to oxidant stresses, including acute episodic hemolysis in otherwise hematologically normal individuals. Glucose-6-phosphate dehydrogenase (G6 PD) deficiency is the model of the latter group of disorders, and pyruvate kinase deficiency is the model for the former group.

Pyruvate Kinase Deficiency

Pyruvate kinase deficiency is the most common enzyme defect of anaerobic glycolysis that results in a hereditary hemolytic anemia. This disorder has been documented to occur worldwide and is characterized by lifelong chronic hemolysis of variable severity. In more severely affected patients, splenectomy often results in amelioration of the hemolytic process. The defective pyruvate kinase enzyme in affected erythrocytes results in increased concentrations of 2,3-diphosphoglycerate and diminished levels of ATP in relation to cells of comparable age (Gilbert-Barness & Barness, 2000; Hirono et al, 2001).

Pyruvate kinase deficiency is inherited as an autosomal recessive trait. Heterozygous carriers usually have 40% to 60% of the normal red blood cell pyruvate kinase activity, and they do not have any significant hematologic or clinical abnormalities. In the absence of consanguinity, clinically affected patients usually are compound heterozygotes with two mutant alleles. Thus they have two intracellular mixtures of defective pyruvate kinase enzymes, which complicate the interpretation of the biochemical data. Genes encoding the principal natural pyruvate kinase enzymes have been identified, as have several mutations that result in hemolytic anemia (Hirono et al, 2001).

Pyruvate kinase deficiency and G6PD deficiency are the two most common red blood cell enzyme defects associated with chronic hemolytic anemia and are equally prevalent in the population (Hirono et al, 2001). In contrast, all the other enzyme defects combined account for fewer than 20% of such cases and thus are not discussed in this chapter.

Pyruvate kinase deficiency occurs equally in males and females. It has been most commonly reported in the kindreds of northern Europe, but it is also found throughout the United States, Canada, Japan, Western Europe, Southeast Asia, Australia, and New Zealand. Pyruvate kinase deficiency has also been reported in Mexicans, Arabs, Filipinos, Africans, African Americans, and those of partial Native American ancestry. The Amish in western Pennsylvania have a particularly high prevalence of a severe form of the disease (Burton, 2000; Beaudet et al, 2001; Hirono et al, 2001).

Pyruvate kinase deficiency is transmitted as an autosomal recessive trait, with clinical consequences occurring in only homozygotes or compound heterozygotes. In rare instances, however, heterozygotes are hematologically normal. In affected patients, the primary clinical manifestation is chronic hemolytic anemia that varies in severity from asymptomatic and fully compensated to life-threatening with a lifelong requirement for transfusions (Hirono et al, 2001). The latter cases often manifest as neonatal anemia and jaundice that require exchange transfusions.

Pyruvate kinase deficiency has no distinguishing or pathognomonic features. Affected individuals usually manifest the hallmarks of a chronic hemolytic process: variable degrees of jaundice, slight to moderate splenomegaly, and an increased number of gallstones. In most cases the anemia and jaundice are apparent in infancy or early childhood, if not in the neonatal period. In rare instances, cases escape detection until adulthood (Hirono et al, 2001).

Early onset of symptoms is characteristic of more severe forms of the disorder, and late onset is typical of milder cases. Milder cases may be asymptomatic, and the diagnosis may emerge during evaluation of pregnancy or acute illness. Thus there is a full spectrum of clinical severity. The most severe cases require multiple transfusions or even splenectomy in early childhood to maintain acceptable hemoglobin levels. Beyond early childhood or after splenectomy, transfusion requirements often diminish, and hemoglobin concentrations tend to stabilize 1 to 3 g/dl higher than normal. Lower hemoglobin levels are

better tolerated because of the diminished oxygen affinity induced by characteristically elevated concentrations of red blood cell 2,3-diphosphoglycerate activity (Hirono et al, 2001).

Chronic hemolysis is exacerbated by pregnancy or acute illness, especially viral infections (Hirono et al, 2001). Pregnancy may be well tolerated but may necessitate transfusions in some patients who previously required few or no transfusions. Parvolike viruses have been reported in association with aplastic crisis in pyruvate kinase deficiency (Hirono et al, 2001). Other clinical effects of pyruvate kinase deficiency include growth retardation and frontal bossing, although general neurodevelopment is not impaired. After splenectomy, growth and development may be enhanced in severely affected children. Rare complications include kernicterus, hydrops fetalis, chronic leg ulcers, acute pancreatitis secondary to biliary tract disease, iron overload, splenic abscess, and spinal cord compression from extramedullary hematopoiesis (Hirono et al, 2001).

Red blood cell morphologic abnormalities are not a prominent feature of pyruvate kinase deficiency. Milder cases may show only macrocytosis and a few smaller, irregularly contracted or spiculated cells. All these findings are more prevalent when the disease is severe, particularly after splenectomy, when siderocytes, target cells, and Howell-Jolly bodies become more prominent (Hirono et al, 2001). These findings, however, are nonspecific. The anemia varies in severity but usually is normochromic and macrocytic. Splenectomy often results in a paradoxic rise in the reticulocyte count, frequently as high as 40% to 70%, but this is not a pathognomonic finding. Hemoglobin concentrations range from 6 to 12 g/dl, and the hematocrit ranges from 17% to 37%. Hemoglobin is of the adult type (AA), and hemoglobins F and A_2 are within normal limits. The leukocyte and platelet counts are normal to slightly increased (Hirono et al, 2001).

In pyruvate kinase deficiency, the erythrocyte osmotic fragility test results are normal, and the antiglobulin (Coombs') test result is negative. The erythrocyte life span is moderately to severely shortened. The spleen sequesters and destroys many pyruvate kinase–deficient reticulocytes as a result of the diminished deformability (Hirono et al, 2001). Although reticulocytes have the advantage of highly efficient ATP generation through mitochondrial oxidative phosphorylation, that process is greatly suppressed in the acidotic and hypoxemic environment of the spleen. Splenectomy permits longer survival of these newly formed cells, therefore the reticulocyte count may paradoxically rise after splenectomy even though the anemia is less severe. The liver is also a major site of pyruvate kinase–deficient red blood cell destruction. Because leukocytes and platelets do not share the enzyme defect, their cell counts are unaffected (Hirono et al, 2001).

Pyruvate kinase deficiency is not associated with any other organ dysfunction. Indirect hyperbilirubinemia occurs in proportion to the severity of hemolysis, and fecal urobilinogen excretion is accordingly increased. Although the liver shares the abnormality, its function is not impaired sufficiently to alter standard hepatic function tests. Liver function is not significantly impaired because hepatocytes can synthesize the enzyme, a process not available to the red blood cell. Compensatory erythrocyte hyperplasia may expand marrow spaces to produce radiographic changes characteristic of more severe anemia (Hirono et al, 2001).

Definitive diagnosis of pyruvate kinase deficiency requires demonstration of specific red blood cell enzyme abnormalities.

Erythrocyte enzyme deficiency may range from 5% to 25% of normal in affected patients and 40% to 60% in heterozygous carriers, who remain hematologically normal. Care must be taken with laboratory assays to ensure that erythrocyte preparations are free of leukocytes, because white blood cells have 300 times more pyruvate kinase activity per cell than do erythrocytes. Reticulocytes and young erythrocytes have disproportionately more pyruvate kinase activity than older red blood cell populations, which must be considered in the interpretation of in vitro assays (Hirono et al, 2001).

Glucose-6-Phosphate Dehydrogenase Deficiency

G6PD, an enzyme found in all cells, is the first step in the intermediary metabolism of glucose-6-phosphate to pentose phosphate in the HMP pathway. It produces NADPH, the coenzyme that is the main hydrogen donor for the numerous enzymatic reactions involved in various biosynthetic pathways and for preservation and regeneration of the reduced form of glutathione. Because catalase and glutathione are essential for detoxification of hydrogen peroxide, the defense of cells against this compound depends ultimately and heavily on G6PD. This is especially true of red blood cells, which are exquisitely sensitive to oxidative damage and which lack other NADPH-producing enzymes.

The gene that encodes the protein for G6PD has been mapped to the long arm of the X chromosome, therefore one of the two G6PD alleles is subject to inactivation in females.

G6PD deficiency is the most common known red blood cell enzyme deficit. It is estimated to affect more than 400 million people worldwide. The highest incidences are found in tropical Africa, in the Middle East, in tropical and subtropical Asia, in some areas of the Mediterranean, and in Papua New Guinea. The prevalence rates vary in these geographic regions from 5% to 25% (Burton, 2000; Beaudet et al, 2001).

The most common clinical manifestations are neonatal jaundice and acute hemolytic anemia. In some cases the hyperbilirubinemia is severe enough to cause permanent neurologic sequelae or death. The active hemolytic anemia is triggered by a number of drugs, by infections, or by the ingestion of fava beans. In a proportion of cases, the hemolysis can be life-threatening. The mechanism of hemolysis is thought to occur as a result of the inability of red blood cells to withstand the oxidative damage produced, directly or indirectly, by the triggering agent. Red blood cell destruction is largely intravascular, therefore hemoglobinuria is present. Between episodes of hemolytic anemia, most of those with G6PD deficiency are asymptomatic. A very small proportion of G6PD-deficient individuals have a chronic hemolytic disorder, which might be quite severe (Luzzatto et al, 2001).

G6PD deficiency is genetically heterogeneous. Numerous different variants have been reported on the basis of diverse biochemical characteristics. This diversity suggests that these variants result from many allelic mutations in the G6PD gene seen in the different parts of the world where this abnormality is prevalent. Genetic heterogeneity also explains the diversity of clinical manifestations.

Clinical manifestations of G6PD deficiency have been known for centuries. Pythagoras, the Greek mathematician, warned his followers against the dangers of eating fava beans; at the turn of the twentieth century, Italian physicians described the clinical manifestations of favism (Luzzatto et al, 2001). Because of the erratic response to the consumption of fava beans, the genetic inheritance pattern was difficult to es-tablish, and the disorder was first attributed to allergies or a toxic reaction. The fact that certain drugs caused a hemolytic reaction in susceptible persons was not recognized until the 1950s. Observant practitioners during this time noticed that the condition tended to run in families. In 1956, the discovery of the low levels of G6PD in the red blood cells of these affected patients began the biochemical investigation into this disorder. Since the 1960s, the biochemical basis and clinical manifestations of G6PD deficiency have been established. More recently, the molecular structure of the normal gene and various mutations has been defined.

Most individuals with G6PD deficiency are asymptomatic and go through life unaware of the genetic abnormality. The only common clinical manifestation is acute hemolysis, which may be rapidly compensated and often remains undetected. Clinical manifestations of the disorder result from an interaction of the molecular properties of each G6PD molecular variant, exogenous factors, and genetic factors for the population. G6PD deficiency can cause clinical pathologic conditions, including drug-induced hemolysis, infection-induced hemolysis, favism, neonatal jaundice, and chronic nonspherocytic hemolytic anemia.

G6PD deficiency was discovered as a direct consequence of investigations into the development of hemolysis in patients who had received primaquine (Luzzatto et al, 2001), which in other individuals causes no red blood cell destruction. Subsequently, G6PD deficiency has become the prototype of hemolytic episodes arising from a unique interaction between genetic and exogenous factors. Clinical hemolysis and jaundice typically begin within 1 to 2 days of exposure to the drug (Luzzatto et al, 2001). The hemolysis is largely intravascular and is associated with hemoglobinuria. The anemia worsens until the seventh or eighth day. Heinz bodies are characteristically found in peripheral blood. The reticulocyte count begins to rise and the hemoglobin level begins to recover on the eighth to tenth day. A self-limited course is characteristic with some G6PD variants because the newly produced cells have a higher amount of G6PD activity and therefore are less susceptible than the older cells, which are selectively destroyed (Luzzatto et al, 2001). A more protracted hemolysis occurs with a high drug dosage or in patients with severe G6PD deficiency.

Data were analyzed for drug interactions and hemolysis in G6PD-deficient individuals. There is strong evidence that a relatively short list of drugs can trigger hemolysis, including antimalarials (primaquine, pamaquine, pentaquine), sulfonamides (sulfanilamide, sulfacetamide, sulfapyridine, sulfamethoxazole), sulfones (thiazosulfone, dapsone), nitrofurans (nitrofurantoin), antipyretics (acetanilid), and other drugs and chemicals (naphthalene, trinitrotoluene, toluidine blue). Drugs that have a possible association with hemolytic episodes include chloroquine, sulfamethoxypyridazine, sulfadimetine, sulfamerazine, aspirin, ciprofloxacin, norfloxacin, chloramphenicol, and vitamin K analogs. Drugs that have a doubtful association with hemolytic episodes include quinine, sulfadiazine, acetaminophen, probenecid, phenacetin, para aminosalicylate (PAS), levodopa, and dimercaprol (Burton, 2000; Luzzatto et al, 2001).

A number of inherited and acquired factors influence an individual's susceptibility to and the severity of drug-induced hemolysis. Inherited factors include the metabolic integrity of the erythrocyte, the precise nature of the enzyme defect, and genetic differences in pharmacodynamics. Acquired factors include the drug dose and the absorption, metabolism, and excretion of the drug; the presence of additional oxidative stress, such as infection; the effect of the drug on enzyme activity; the preexisting hemoglobin level; and the age distribution of the red blood cell population (Luzzatto et al, 2001).

Infection is the most common cause of hemolysis in G6PD-deficient individuals who live outside the areas where favism is prevalent. The severity and clinical consequences of hemolysis are influenced by a number of factors, including concurrent administration of oxidant drugs, the preexisting level of hemoglobin, hepatic function, and age. Various bacterial, viral, and rickettsial infections have been reported as precipitants, but most important are infectious hepatitis, pneumonia, and typhoid fever (Luzzatto et al, 2001). Gastrointestinal and respiratory viral infections are reported to cause more severe hemolysis in children. Hemolysis is more common in children with G6PD deficiency who develop hepatitis than in normal children, but the degree and the duration of jaundice is out of proportion to the degree of hemolysis. This suggests that the jaundice is of hepatocellular origin (Luzzatto et al, 2001).

Favism is a condition described as an episode of acute hemolysis after ingestion of broad (fava) beans. It has occurred on an epidemic scale in areas now known to have an increased prevalence of G6PD deficiency (the Mediterranean, Middle East, Far East, and North Africa). This geographic region correlates to the area where fava beans are customary in the diet. Not all G6PD-deficient individuals are sensitive to fava beans, and even those who are show remarkable variability from one exposure to the next. It is thought that an additional, as yet unidentified factor is responsible for the variable hemolytic response to fava beans (Luzzatto et al, 2001). Clinically, favism manifests as a sudden onset of acute hemolysis within 24 to 48 hours after ingesting the beans. Pallor and hemoglobinuria are hallmarks of this disorder. Jaundice is always present, but because not all the hemolysis is intravascular, the bilirubin level is less than in hemolytic attacks triggered by drugs or infection. The hemolysis is severe, and the amount of hemoglobinuria is greater, therefore hemoglobin catabolism is reduced, leaving less hemoglobin to be recycled by the liver. The mainstay of prevention is avoidance of fava beans. Neonatal screening and health education are essential in communities with a high prevalence of G6PD deficiency. Severe cases require supportive treatment of red blood cell transfusions. The administration of desferrioxamine, which reduces the iron-dependent formation of damaging oxygen radicals, is being investigated (Luzzatto et al, 2001).

G6PD deficiency is the most common red blood cell enzyme deficiency that results in neonatal jaundice. Jaundice appears by 1 to 4 days of age, at about the same time as or slightly earlier than physiologic jaundice and later than blood group isoimmunization. Reports of abnormal red blood cell morphology, mild anemia, and reticulocytosis suggest an element of hemolysis, but impaired hepatic function, similar to that seen in normal neonates, may well be the major cause in both premature and full-term G6PD-deficient infants (Luzzatto et al, 2001).

The jaundice seen in G6PD-deficient infants shows wide variation in frequency and severity in different populations. In endemic areas where G6PD deficiency is prevalent, it is the major cause of neonatal jaundice. Although kernicterus is a rare complication, the most common cause of it in Africa and Southeast Asia is G6PD deficiency (Luzzatto et al, 2001). The reasons for this variability are not completely understood, and both genetic and environmental factors are likely to be important. The severity of neonatal jaundice does not correlate with the G6PD activity of the red blood cells. Management of

neonatal jaundice generally involves avoidance of oxidant drugs and prompt treatment of hypoxia, sepsis, and acidosis in newborns. Specific measures include elimination of mothball use in the home, prophylactic administration of phenobarbital, and exchange transfusion. Phototherapy once was contraindicated in infants with G6PD deficiency because it was thought to reduce the level of riboflavin and diminish its antioxidant activity. Several studies have shown that phototherapy is indeed effective at reducing the level of unconjugated bilirubin and should remain as the mainstay of treatment for neonatal jaundice whenever the bilirubin level is not high enough to warrant an exchange transfusion (Burton, 2000; Luzzatto et al, 2001).

Although a slight degree of chronic hemolysis accompanies G6PD deficiency, most affected individuals experience significant hemolysis and anemia only under conditions of oxidant stress. The degree of chronic hemolysis varies, depending on the type of G6PD variant. Such variants have been described in many parts of the world (almost always in males), regardless of the type of G6PD endemic to the area. The degree of enzyme deficiency may be severe, and detailed biochemical characterization of the residual enzyme often is complicated by the enzyme's instability. In rare cases associated with granulocytic dysfunction, hemolysis may be aggravated by the increased susceptibility to infections (Luzzatto et al, 2001). Sometimes the chronic hemolysis may arise from an association of mild G6PD deficiency with an unrelated, genetically transmitted erythrocyte abnormality such as pyruvate kinase deficiency or congenital spherocytosis (Luzzatto et al, 2001).

Clinically, affected individuals have a history of neonatal jaundice, often requiring an exchange transfusion. A history of infection or drug-induced hemolysis is also common. Gallstones may be a prominent feature. Splenomegaly is usually but not always present. Although occasionally the hemoglobin level is normal and the hemolysis is well compensated, oxidant stress can lead to a dramatic fall in the hemoglobin level. The red blood cell half-life is shortened to 2 to 17 days, and all patients have a reticulocytosis of 4% to 34% (Luzzatto et al, 2001). Occasionally the degree of reticulocytosis is out of proportion to the length of red blood cell half-life. Red blood cells usually do not show abnormal osmotic fragility. In contrast to the acute hemolysis, the hemolysis in chronic hemolytic anemia is only partly intravascular, and studies have shown increased sequestration of red blood cells in the liver and spleen (Luzzatto et al, 2001). Management of these patients has included the use of vitamin E (an antioxidant) and splenectomy. There are conflicting reports on the efficacy of both these therapies (Luzzatto et al, 2001).

The diagnosis of G6PD deficiency is relatively easy. Careful attention must be paid to the method and interpretation of test results. Prenatal diagnosis has been reported (Luzzatto et al, 2001). The wide geographic distribution of the disorder and high prevalence among developing countries make it important to adopt simple, inexpensive tests. The actual enzyme activity of G6PD, not the amount of G6PD protein, should be measured. G6PD activity is greater in younger erythrocytes than in older ones, therefore reticulocytosis may lead to a false-normal result. Because of red blood cell mosaicism arising from random X chromosome inactivation in females, heterozygotes have a mixture of normal and G6PD-deficient cells. The proportion of the two cell types can vary enormously, ranging from completely normal activity to complete deficiency. In this case, microscopic evaluation of the individual cells on a slide is necessary. All of the existing methods for determining G6PD activity depend essentially on the production of NADPH. The direct enzyme assay gives a quantitative measurement, and a number of other procedures provide convenient screening tests that classify individuals only as G6PD normal or G6PD deficient (Luzzatto et al, 2001).

LIPID METABOLISM

Lipids are a heterogeneous group of substances that can be extracted from tissues. The three main classes of lipids—fatty acids, triglycerides, and phospholipids—function as insulation and as an energy source, in addition to providing structure to cell membranes. Fat insulation consists mainly of triglycerides packed densely into adipocytes. Triglycerides are hydrolyzed into fatty acids and glycerol, which serve as an energy source. Phospholipids provide an important component of all cellular membranes.

Fatty Acids

The sources of fatty acids in the blood are the supply of fat in the diet and the release of fatty acids from adipose tissue. Suckling infants have a high level of fatty acids in the blood, and fatty acid use at this time is greater than at any time before birth or after weaning (Havel & Kane, 2001). Fatty acids are synthesized in two metabolic pathways: malonyl-CoA and reversal of beta-oxidation. The rate of fatty acid synthesis is greater in the fetus than in the adult. This rate of fatty acid synthesis declines rapidly after birth, possibly in relation to the accumulation of some metabolites (glycerol, fatty acids, and acyl-CoA) and the increased rate of gluconeogenesis, which reduces the availability of citrate (Havel & Kane, 2001). Fatty acid oxidation occurs in the mitochondria. As opposed to passive, gradient-dependent transport across cell membranes, fatty acids must be converted from acyl-CoA to acylcarnitine to be transported across the mitochondrial membrane. Once inside the mitochondrion, the acylcarnitine is reassembled into acyl-CoA and oxidized (Havel & Kane, 2001).

Oxidation of fatty acids requires more oxygen than does oxidation of carbohydrates. After birth, fatty acid oxidation is greatly enhanced. In brown fat, fatty acid oxidation is completely dependent on the presence of carnitine and ATP. Carnitine is also important for acetate oxidation and for optimum ketone production by liver mitochondria. Lysine is the precursor of carnitine, and when protein ingestion is severely limited, a carnitine deficiency may also exist (Havel & Kane, 2001).

Because the liver lacks the enzyme needed to transfer CoA from succinyl-CoA to acetoacetate, the final products of fatty acid oxidation in the liver are the ketone bodies: acetoacetic acid, beta-hydroxybutyric acid, and acetone. The rate of ketone body production depends on the supply of fatty acids to the liver. After birth, large amounts of fatty acids from the blood enter the liver. The fatty acids are broken down into ketone bodies, which are then transported to other tissues and organs, where they serve as a source of energy (Havel & Kane, 2001).

Triglycerides

The blood triglyceride level depends on fat absorption from the intestines, the release of triglycerides from the liver, and the removal of triglycerides from the blood. Triglycerides cannot serve as an immediate energy source because they must first be hy-

drolyzed into fatty acids and glycerol. In the blood, triglycerides are transported as lipoproteins and are removed from the blood by many tissues. After birth, chylomicrons appear in the blood 1 to 3 days after feedings have been initiated (Havel & Kane, 2001). The major storage site of triglycerides is adipose tissue.

Lipogenesis is the process by which fatty acids combine with CoA to form acyl-CoA. Three molecules of acyl-CoA and glycerol-3-phosphate combine to form a triglyceride molecule. Lipolysis is not a reversal of the synthetic process. The rate of fatty acid synthesis depends on a sufficient supply of glycerol-3-phosphate. If fatty acids accumulate, the excess acyl-CoA inhibits further fatty acid synthesis and glycolytic reactions. In lipolysis, triglycerides are hydrolyzed by tissue lipases into fatty acids and glycerol. Glycerol-3-phosphate is produced by phosphorylation of glycerol by glycerol kinase. The glycerol released from adipose tissue during lipolysis can be used for energy only after being phosphorylated (Havel & Kane, 2001).

Phospholipids

Phospholipids are any lipid molecules that contain a radical derived from phosphoric acid. Phospholipids are an important part of cell walls and cell particle membranes, myelin sheaths, and lung secretions. Age changes the composition of fatty acids in phospholipids. The composition also changes in various organs. The fatty acid composition of phospholipids is less dependent on dietary changes than is that of triglycerides.

The metabolism of fatty acids cannot be discussed without an understanding of the relationships between glucose and fatty acid metabolism. Several control points exist at which it is determined whether glucose or fatty acids will be predominantly synthesized or oxidized. For example, glucose synthesis is promoted by fatty acid oxidation. A high-fat diet enhances gluconeogenesis and fatty acid oxidation and results in a decline in lipid synthesis. The elevated level of fatty acids supplied to the newborn after birth is responsible for the decreased rate of glycolysis in the liver and the brain, the increased rate of acetoacetate formation, the decreased rate of fatty acid synthesis in the liver, and the postnatal increase in the rate of gluconeogenesis (Havel & Kane, 2001). After birth, the rate of fatty acid oxidation and ketone body formation increases dramatically as a result of sympathetic stimulation of lipolysis in adipose tissue and the resulting increased delivery of fatty acids to the liver (Havel & Kane, 2001).

Disorders of Lipid Metabolism

Disorders of lipid metabolism may affect any component of fatty acid, triglyceride, or phospholipid synthesis or degradation. Disorders of lipid metabolism may also affect beta-oxidation of fatty acids in the mitochondria. General clinical manifestations of a lipid metabolic disorder include vomiting, changes in level of consciousness, metabolic acidosis, odor of sweaty feet, severe hypoglycemia without ketosis, hyperammonemia, and hepatic and/or muscular lipid accumulation. These clinical manifestations may occur acutely after birth or intermittently. The fulminant neonatal course is rapidly fatal.

Lipoprotein Disorders: Abetalipoproteinemia, Familial Combined Hyperlipidemia, and Tangier Disease.   Very-low-density lipoproteins (VLDLs) and chylomicrons, which transport triglycerides to the peripheral tissues in the blood, are major lipoprotein secretory products of the liver and intestine. Each class of these lipoproteins contains a protein of high molecular weight (a beta-lipoprotein) that is essential for the secretion of the lipoprotein particle and that has a high affinity for lipids, remaining with the lipoprotein complex throughout its metabolic processing in plasma or lymph. Familial beta-lipoprotein deficiencies represent one of several classes of lipoproteins that are absent or are present in abnormally low concentrations in the plasma. The three most common types of disorders are abetalipoproteinemia, familial combined hyperlipidemia, and Tangier disease.

The single structural gene for beta-lipoproteins is responsible for the synthesis of the two types of lipoproteins found in human beings. The predominant beta-lipoprotein of VLDLs and low-density lipoproteins (LDLs) is apo B-100. The predominant type of apo B in chylomicrons is apo B-48. Several disorders result from the abnormal secretion of apo B–containing lipoproteins (Kane & Havel, 2001).

Abetalipoproteinemia is an autosomal recessive disorder characterized by the virtual absence of VLDLs and LDLs from plasma. Fat malabsorption is severe, and triglycerides accumulate in erythrocytes and in the liver. Acanthocytosis of erythrocytes is common. Spinocerebellar ataxia, peripheral neuropathy, degenerative pigmentary retinopathy, and ceroid myopathy all appear to occur secondary to defects of transport of tocopherol in the blood. Intracellular accumulation of beta-lipoprotein results from an impairment in the assembly or secretion of triglyceride-rich proteins. The absence of activity of microsomal triglyceride transfer protein, a factor critical to the lipidation of B proteins, was the first recognized defect in lipoprotein deficiencies. Treatment involves restriction of dietary fat to prevent steatorrhea and supplementation with tocopherol to prevent progression of the neuromuscular and retinal degenerative disease (Kane & Havel, 2001).

The clinical manifestations of hypobetalipoproteinemia are indistinguishable from those of abetalipoproteinemia in the homozygous state: acanthocytosis, neuromuscular disability, and malabsorption. Clinically, this disorder is distinguished from recessive abetalipoproteinemia by the appearance of hypolipidemia in heterozygotes. The defects that underlie this disorder involve the gene for apo B. A number of mutations have been identified that involve secretion of a truncated form of the apo B protein, an abnormal rate of apo B protein synthesis, or removal of apo B from the blood (Kane & Havel, 2001).

Chylomicron retention disease is characterized by fat malabsorption and the absence of chylomicrons in plasma after fat ingestion. Some patients show acanthocytosis and neurologic manifestations. Large numbers of nascent chylomicrons crowd the enterocyte as a result of a specific defect in the secretion of chylomicrons. High levels of apo B-100 have been found in the cytoplasm and endoplasmic reticulum of the enterocyte (Kane & Havel, 2001).

Familial combined hyperlipidemia is probably the most prevalent genetically determined disorder of lipoproteins. It significantly increases the risk of coronary atherosclerosis. It is recognized as an autosomal dominant trait with high penetrance that leads to high levels of apo B-100 and elevated levels of VLDLs, LDLs, or both in plasma.

Abetalipoproteinemia.   This autosomal disorder occurs as a result of the absence of apolipoprotein B and is characterized by very low plasma cholesterol and triglyceride levels. It has a higher incidence among Ashkenazic Jews, who constitute 25% of those affected (Burton, 2000; Gilbert-Barness & Barness, 2000; Kane & Havel, 2001). It affects males more often than

females, and heterozygotes are in good health. The clinical manifestations, which develop shortly after birth, include fat malabsorption, acanthocytosis, pigmented retinitis, and ataxia (Kane & Havel, 2001).

Malabsorption of fat is a central pathologic feature of abetalipoproteinemia. Steatorrhea occurs after birth and is associated with malabsorption of the fat-soluble vitamins A, D, E, and K. Affected infants are poor feeders and have frequent vomiting and voluminous steatorrheic stools; the result is somatic underdevelopment and failure to thrive. Hepatic steatosis occurs with severe disturbances in plasma lipid levels, which are less than 50% of normal. Triglyceride levels often are undetectable, phospholipid levels are reduced by 75%, and the cholesterol level often is below 0.025 g/L. Unlike vitamins A and K, in which modest supplementation achieves normal plasma levels, the transport of tocopherol is severely limited in this disorder. The abnormal lipoproteins of abetalipoproteinemia appear incapable of incorporating normal amounts of vitamin E even in the presence of relatively large supplements. Massive supplementation, however, somehow increases the flux into the body, eventually increasing the vitamin E levels in adipose tissue appreciably (Kane & Havel, 2001). The intestinal villi are normal, but the mucosa has a yellow discoloration from the greatly increased lipid content. Electron microscopy has demonstrated an increase in lipid droplets in the cells, even if no fat has been ingested for days (Kane & Havel, 2001). Despite the inability of the liver to secrete VLDLs, abnormalities of liver function are uncommon.

Severe anemia develops because of the abnormally shaped erythrocytes. Red blood cell survival frequently is shortened, and hyperbilirubinemia has been described. Reticulocytosis and erythroid hyperplasia occur in many patients, which suggests that erythropoiesis is not notably impaired. Acanthocytosis is not found in the bone marrow, which suggests that the membrane changes leading to the malformation are acquired by contact with the plasma (Kane & Havel, 2001).

Ocular involvement manifests as retinitis pigmentosa, diminished visual acuity, nystagmus, and ophthalmoplegia. The more severe cases of retinopathy occur in patients with the more severe neurologic impairment, which suggests a common mechanism. Major pathologic features are the loss of photoreceptors, loss of pigmented epithelium, and relative preservation of submacular pigmented epithelium (Kane & Havel, 2001). These retinal changes closely resemble the retinopathy of vitamin E deficiency. Deficiency of vitamin A may also contribute to the retinopathy, and some patients benefit from additional supplementation. The onset of symptoms varies. Compromise of visual acuity may occur during the first decade, although many patients are asymptomatic until adulthood. Loss of night or color vision frequently is a presenting sign. Patients often are unaware of the slow progression of the ophthalmologic disease. Nystagmus and complete loss of vision can occur. Neuropathy affects the oculomotor nerve and results in ophthalmoplegia (Kane & Havel, 2001).

The most characteristic degenerative sites in the nervous system are the large sensory neurons of the spinal ganglia and their heavily myelinated axons. A progressive neuropathy and extensive demyelination of these areas occurs. The first neurologic signs are a diminution in the intensity of the deep tendon reflexes, which may occur in the first few years of life. Vibratory sense and proprioception tend to be lost progressively, and an ataxic gait develops. Neurologic problems are evident in 35% of the children by 10 years of age. By 20 years of age, mild to severe ataxia and intellectual deficits are present (Kane & Havel, 2001). Untreated patients are unable to stand by the third decade. Muscle contractions are common, leading to pes cavus, pes equinovarus, and kyphoscoliosis. Muscle weakness is a frequent feature of this disorder. The clinical determination that myopathy is present tends to be obscured by the frequent presence of degenerative peripheral neuropathy. Cardiomyopathy may lead to death early in the second decade of life (Kane & Havel, 2001). Slow neuromuscular development has been recorded in a number of cases. Attributing the developmental delay to this disorder is difficult because specific neuropathologic cerebral disease is lacking. In addition, slow neurologic development is common in infants who have steatorrhea and fail to thrive and may reflect nutritional deficiencies. Furthermore, because many patients with this disorder are products of consanguineous matings, other rare inborn errors may be responsible for the mental retardation (Kane & Havel, 2001).

The diagnosis of this disorder is suggested by the absence of apolipoprotein B, low serum cholesterol levels, low triglyceride levels, and plasma devoid of chylomicrons (Kane & Havel, 2001). Levels of vitamins A, E, and K, folic acid, and iron also are low (Kane & Havel, 2001).

Treatment involves early dietary restriction of long-chain triglycerides to control the gastrointestinal symptoms. Fatty acids derived from medium-chain triglycerides do not require the formation of chylomicrons for absorption; they are transported mainly by albumin as free fatty acids via the hepatic portal system and serve as energy substrate for the liver but are not necessary nutrients. Hepatic function should be monitored in affected patients receiving medium-chain triglyceride supplements. Infant formula should contain medium-chain triglycerides (Kane & Havel, 2001).

Prolonged observation of vitamin E supplementation has concluded that such supplementation does inhibit the progression of the neurologic disease and probably leads to regression of symptoms even if supplementation is started in adulthood (Kane & Havel, 2001). The retinopathy may be prevented if therapy is started early, or it may be stabilized if the disease is already present when therapy begins. The myopathy is also reversed with vitamin E therapy (Kane & Havel, 2001). Treatment requires large doses (1000 to 10,000 mg/day) of oral vitamin E until the reliability and safety of parenteral preparations have been established. Vitamin E therapy can prevent neurologic symptoms if treatment is started before these symptoms appear. If vitamin A and carotene levels are low, additional supplementation may be beneficial. Because vitamin D has its own transport mechanism and because the symptoms of vitamin D deficiency are not associated with this disorder, no specific supplementation is necessary. Supplementation with vitamin K should be given if bruising, bleeding, or hypoprothrombinemia is present (Kane & Havel, 2001).

Familial Combined Hyperlipidemia.   Familial combined hyperlipidemia was identified as a disease in studies of the survivors of myocardial infarction and their relatives. Three patterns of lipoprotein distribution were recognized: elevated plasma levels of VLDLs, of LDLs, or of a combination of the two. The pattern may change over time in an affected individual or within a family. Family pedigrees are compatible with an autosomal dominant pattern. Although seen in childhood, the manifestations are limited until about the third decade of life.

Plasma triglyceride levels tend to remain between 200 to 400 mg/dl but may be much higher. LDL levels usually exceed 100 mg/dl. Most affected family members have apo B levels above 85 mg/dl. Xanthoma formation is less common than in heterozygous familial hypercholesterolemia at similar LDL levels. The prevalence of familial combined hyperlipidemia is estimated to be 1% to 2% of the population in North America and Europe (Kane & Havel, 2001). Treatment goals include achievement of ideal body weight and restriction of cholesterol and saturated fats. Hypercholesterolemia appears to respond well to treatment with hydroxymethylglutaryl (HMG)—CoA reductase inhibitors. Triglyceride levels respond to a lesser extent. The addition of nicotinic acid often reduces the VLDL levels dramatically and appears to have a synergistic effect on LDL levels. The use of bile acid–binding resins alone frequently increases the triglyceride level. A combined regimen of bile acid–binding resins and nicotinic acid often is very effective (Kane & Havel, 2001).

Tangier Disease.   Tangier disease is an extremely rare, autosomal recessive disorder characterized by a severe deficiency or absence of normal high-density lipoproteins (HDLs) in plasma, resulting in the accumulation of cholesterol esters in many tissues of the body (Assmann et al, 2001).

Tangier disease involves abnormal metabolism of apolipoprotein A, which results in hypercatabolism of HDL constituents. Clinical manifestations include tonsillar hypertrophy with yellow-orange bands. Other organs such as the spleen, thymus, intestinal mucosa, skin, liver, and lymphatic ganglia also hypertrophy (Assmann et al, 2001). Hemolysis and hemolytic anemia have been reported. HDL deficiency and a low plasma cholesterol concentration accompanied by normal or elevated triglyceride levels in combination with hyperplastic adenoidal tissue are pathognomonic.

In patients with Tangier disease, the plasma apo-I concentration is less than 3% that of controls, and the small amount of HDL in the plasma of affected individuals differs from that in normal plasma. Levels of chylomicron remnants and VLDLs are very abnormal. Heterozygotes are asymptomatic and have half-normal concentrations of HDLs, apo-I, and apo-II (Assmann et al, 2001).

The altered erythrocyte morphology is caused by the decrease in cholesterol and increase in phosphatidylcholine in the red blood cell membranes. Ocular abnormalities include corneal opacifications, ectropion, retinal pigment mottling, and diplopia. Peripheral neuropathy occurs and is thought to result from abnormal lipid deposition in Schwann cells. Although the disease may be asymptomatic, relapses are common and occasionally devastating. Weakness, paresthesias, increased sweating, diplopia, ocular nerve palsies, diminished or absent deep tendon reflexes, muscle atrophy, and loss of pain and temperature sensation may occur. Most patients have some degree of neuromuscular dysfunction, although symptoms may be subtle and transient (Assmann et al, 2001).

Despite the HDL deficiency and the very elevated cholesterol ester accumulation in tissues, the risk of atherosclerosis does not appear to be higher for these patients. No evidence of coronary artery disease or vascular disease has been reported in patients under 40 years of age. Documented evidence of cardiovascular and cerebrovascular disease has been reported in patients over 40 years of age, but these patients also had additional risk factors such as obesity, smoking, and hypertension (Assmann et al, 2001).

The molecular basis of the disorder is still unknown but likely is related to a defect in the pathway of intracellular lipid transfer processes (Assmann et al, 2001). No specific treatment exists for Tangier disease.

Familial Hyperlipoproteinemia: Familial Lipoprotein Lipase Deficiency. These disorders are characterized by a marked elevation of cholesterol, triglycerides, or both and of LDLs, which may increase the risk of accelerating atherosclerosis.

Familial lipoprotein lipase deficiency is one of three disorders in which chylomicrons accumulate in the plasma. Chylomicronemia can also occur in individuals with common familial forms of hypertriglyceridemia who also have an acquired cause of hypertriglyceridemia, such as untreated diabetes mellitus, estrogen or antihypertensive drug therapy, or alcohol use.

Familial lipoprotein lipase deficiency is a rare autosomal recessive disorder characterized by massive accumulation of chylomicrons in plasma and a corresponding increase in the plasma triglyceride concentration. The concentration of VLDLs may be normal (Brunzell & Deeb, 2001; Utermann, 2001). More than 30 structural defects in the lipoprotein lipase gene are associated with lipoprotein lipase defects. This lipolytic enzyme is present on the vascular endothelial cells of extrahepatic tissues and is essential for hydrolysis of chylomicron and VLDL triglycerides to provide free fatty acids to tissues for energy.

The disease usually is detected in childhood on the basis of repeated episodes of abdominal pain, recurrent attacks of pancreatitis, eruptive cutaneous xanthomatosis, and hepatosplenomegaly. The severity of the symptoms is directly related to the degree of hyperchylomicronemia, which in turn is related to dietary fat intake (Brunzell & Deeb, 2001).

The diagnosis is based on a finding of low or absent enzyme activity and is confirmed by demonstration of the defect in the structure of the lipoprotein lipase gene. The disorder is not associated with atherosclerotic vascular disease, but recurrent pancreatitis may threaten the patient's life. Heterozygotes have a 50% decrease in lipoprotein lipase but normal or only slightly abnormal plasma lipid levels (Brunzell & Deeb, 2001).

Restricting dietary fat to less than 20 g/day usually is sufficient to reduce plasma triglyceride levels and to keep the patient free of symptoms. The available lipid-lowering drugs are not effective (Brunzell & Deeb, 2001).

Familial lipoprotein lipase deficiency occurs as a result of diminished extrahepatic activity of lipoprotein lipase, which catalyzes the removal of triglyceride-rich lipoprotein from the blood. It is associated with an elevation of levels of chylomicrons, cholesterol, and triglycerides in the serum. Heterozygotes have elevated serum triglyceride levels (Brunzell & Deeb, 2001). The clinical manifestations usually are detected late in the first decade, but some are detected as early as infancy or as late as the fourth decade of life.

In infancy, splenomegaly, anorexia, colicky pain, failure to thrive, and malaise are common. At all ages the most common symptom is episodic abdominal pain. Young patients learn to prevent abdominal pain by avoiding foods with high fat content. In older individuals, abdominal pain from pancreatitis is common and may be life-threatening. The pancreatitis usually is acute in onset and often recurrent and occasionally leads to total pancreatic necrosis and death. Mild fat malabsorption can occur. The pain varies from mild to incapacitating. Serum and urine amylase levels may be normal or elevated in pancreatitis from hyperchylomicronemia. Hepatomegaly is common; splenomegaly is less commonly documented. The hard, enlarged spleen can return to normal size within 1 week of lowering the triglyceride levels in patients with lipoprotein lipase deficiency who are placed on a very low fat diet (Brunzell & Deeb, 2001).

Painless yellow xanthomas develop in skin creases and other pressure areas when the serum cholesterol is above 2000 mg/dl (Brunzell & Deeb, 2001). The lesions result from extravascular phagocytosis of chylomicrons by macrophages in the skin and reflect the chronic hyperchylomicronemia. The xanthomas are localized over the buttocks, knees, and extensor surfaces of the arms. They may become generalized and usually are not tender except when they are continually traumatized. When the plasma triglyceride levels are lowered, the xanthomas clear over the course of several months. Recurrent or persistent xanthomas indicate that therapy to lower triglyceride levels is ineffective (Brunzell & Deeb, 2001).

The diagnosis of this disorder can be made when there is a marked increase in chylomicrons; normal or decreased levels of HDLs, LDLs, and VLDLs; and increased serum cholesterol and triglyceride levels. In the chylomicron fraction of blood, triglyceride levels may rise to 2500 to 29,000 mg/dl, and serum cholesterol may not increase until triglyceride levels are over 3000 mg/dl (Brunzell & Deeb, 2001). The diagnosis is confirmed when the removal of dietary fat results in a dramatic fall in the triglyceride and cholesterol levels (Brunzell & Deeb, 2001). Despite a markedly elevated serum cholesterol level in this disorder, there is no increased risk for atherosclerosis (Brunzell & Deeb, 2001). In the past, many affected patients died of pancreatitis at an early age. However, with the improved recognition of the disease, patients can lead a fairly normal life by avoiding unnecessary surgery and maintaining a low-fat diet.

Familial Cholesterolemia

Familial hypercholesterolemia is characterized by an elevated concentration of LDLs, deposition of LDL-derived cholesterol in tendons and skin, and autosomal dominant inheritance (Goldstein et al, 2001).

Heterozygotes number approximately 1 in 500 people, making familial hypercholesterolemia among the most common errors of metabolism. Heterozygotes have twofold elevations in plasma cholesterol (350 to 550 mg/dl) from birth. Tendon xanthomas and coronary atherosclerosis develop after ages 20 and 30, respectively (Goldstein et al, 2001).

Homozygotes are more severely affected and number about 1 in 1 million people. They have severe hypercholesterolemia (650 to 1000 mg/dl). Cutaneous xanthomas appear in the first 4 years of life. Coronary heart disease begins in childhood and frequently causes death from myocardial infarction before age 20 (Goldstein et al, 2001).

The primary defect is an inability of the LDL receptors to bind with circulating LDLs. When LDL receptors are deficient, the rate of removal of LDLs from plasma declines, and the level of LDLs rises in inverse proportion to the receptor number. The excess plasma LDLs are deposited in scavenger cells and other cell types, producing xanthomas and atheromas.

The LDL receptor gene has been mapped to chromosome 19. Five classes of mutations at the LDL receptor locus have been identified. Each class has been subdivided into multiple alleles, and more than 150 different mutant alleles have been described (Goldstein et al, 2001).

Heterozygotes have one normal and one mutant allele; their cells are able to take up LDLs at approximately half the normal rate. Homozygotes show a total or near total absence of LDL binding (Goldstein et al, 2001).

Treatment is directed at lowering the plasma LDL level. In heterozygotes, the most effective therapy is administration of drugs that stimulate the single normal gene to produce additional messenger RNA for the LDL receptor, such as through the combined administration of a bile acid–binding resin and an inhibitor of HMG-CoA reductase. These drugs enhance LDL receptor activity in the liver, which in turn increases LDL catabolism and decreases LDL production. Homozygotes with two nonfunctional genes are resistant to drugs that work by stimulating LDL receptors. Effective treatment can lead to a reduced rate or slower progression of coronary artery disease (Goldstein et al, 2001).

Familial hypercholesterolemia is an autosomal dominant disorder that occurs as a result of a complete lack of LDL cell membrane receptors. It is characterized clinically by a lifelong elevation in the concentration of LDL cholesterol in the blood, leading to premature coronary heart disease. The disorder was the first genetic disease recognized to cause myocardial infarctions (Goldstein et al, 2001).

Normally, LDL cholesterol binds to cell surface membrane receptors, and only cholesterol is taken into the cell. Once inside the cell, cholesterol inhibits an enzyme that is essential for further cholesterol synthesis. Thus, in this disorder, cholesterol production is not inhibited, and serum LDL cholesterol levels rise. Clinical manifestations of xanthomas are present in all homozygotes by 4 years of age and may be present at birth. There is early, generalized atherosclerosis and cardiovascular death as early as 5 to 20 years of age. In heterozygotes, symptoms of coronary artery disease occur by 30 years of age and may be associated with joint pain, polyarthritis, and cardiac murmurs (Goldstein et al, 2001). Diagnosis of this disorder is suggested by serum cholesterol levels over 650 ml/dl in homozygotes and 300 ml/dl in heterozygotes, with an elevation in levels of LDL (Goldstein et al, 2001). The definitive diagnosis occurs when LDL receptor function is measured in cultured skin fibroblasts (Goldstein et al, 2001). Treatment of this disorder with drugs and a diet low in saturated fat and cholesterol has met with very limited success to date. Drastic surgery to create a portacaval shunt or sustained plasmapheresis has not been successful in long-term studies (Goldstein et al, 2001). Cholestyramine and other bile acid sequestrants have had some success with nicotinic acid and fenofibrate (Goldstein et al, 2001).

Prenatal diagnosis can be accomplished by functional assays for quantitative assessment of LDL receptor activity in cultured amniotic fluid cells, by measurement of the cholesterol level in fetal cord blood obtained at 24 weeks' gestation, or by chorionic villi samples taken at 8 weeks of gestation. The diagnosis is confirmed by skin fibroblast cultures of aborted fetuses. Measuring the cord blood LDL cholesterol level in infants born to a parent known to carry the familial hypercholesterolemia gene defect makes the neonatal diagnosis. Neonatal cord blood screening is not a reliable means of screening heterozygotes in the general population because, as with adults, most infants with elevated LDL cholesterol levels do not have familial hypercholesterolemia (Goldstein et al, 2001).

Treatment of heterozygotes exploits the feedback regulatory system that controls the transcription of the single normal LDL gene. When the demand for cholesterol is increased, normal and heterozygote cells produce an increased number of LDL receptors as a result of enhanced transcription. The acid-binding resins (cholestyramine and cholestipol) were the first class of drugs to exploit this mechanism. These agents have been used since the mid-1960s to lower LDL cholesterol by 15% to 20% percent in heterozygous hypercholesterolemic states. The liver compensates for the cholesterol deficiency by increasing the synthesis of cholesterol. Currently, bile acid sequestrants are used, along with pharmacologic agents that reduce hepatic cholesterol synthesis. Lovastatin and chemically modified versions have become available for human therapy. In animal models, these drugs block cholesterol synthesis and elicit two compensatory mechanisms: hepatocytes (1) synthesize increased amounts of HMG-CoA reductase and (2) synthesize increased numbers of LDL receptors via transcriptional induction. The plasma levels fall as a result of the increased number of LDL receptors. Combined therapy of cholestyramine and lovastatin has reduce the plasma LDL levels by 50% percent (Goldstein et al, 2001).

Surgically created partial ileal bypass prevents bile salt resorption and produces essentially the same therapeutic effect in heterozygotes as does cholestyramine (Goldstein et al, 2001). The major drawbacks are frequent bowel movements, overt diarrhea, kidney stones, gallstones, and symptomatic bowel obstruction.

Dietary restriction of cholesterol to 150 mg/day is recommended for every person with hypercholesterolemia. Total fat intake should also be limited, and intake of saturated fats should be severely restricted. An important consideration in the treatment of familial hypercholesterolemia is the need to identify and treat affected family members. All first- and second-degree relatives should have plasma cholesterol determinations, followed by drug or diet therapy as indicated (Goldstein et al, 2001).

Therapy for familial hypercholesterolemia homozygotes differs from that of heterozygotes in that the former are resistant to the therapies just discussed. Because homozygotes do not have LDL receptors, the number of these receptors cannot be enhanced by messenger RNA transcription induction, dietary changes, ileal bypass, or bile acid sequestrants. If the LDL receptor is partly functional, the patient should be aggressively treated with a combination of bile acid–binding agent, an HMG-CoA reductase inhibitor, and nicotinic acid in addition to strict dietary measures (Goldstein et al, 2001).

Surgical portacaval shunts have been used on a limited number of patients from 2½ to 5 years of age, resulting in a reduction in cholesterol from 25% to 50%. Regression of xanthomas commonly occurs as the cholesterol level declines, and regression of aortic stenotic lesions and stabilization and regression of coronary artery disease have been documented (Goldstein et al, 2001). Portacaval shunt surgery is not associated with a significant enough reduction in LDL cholesterol to be used as the sole therapy for these patients.

The most successful approach for homozygotes is direct removal of LDL cholesterol by use of a continuous-flow blood cell separator that exchanges the patient's plasma with normal plasma or albumin. If the procedure is repeated every 1 to 2 weeks and combined with oral nicotinic acid, the mean plasma cholesterol level can be reduced by about 50% percent on a long-term basis (Goldstein et al, 2001). This therapy produces regression of xanthomas and some amelioration of coronary artery disease and has been reported to extend the life span of affected individuals by 5½ years. More recently, plasma exchange has been replaced with LDL pheresis. In this method, the plasma is passed in a continuous manner extracorporally over columns that remove VLDLs, LDLs, and intermediate-density lipoproteins but do not absorb HDLs or other plasma proteins. After the procedure, the fall in the LDL cholesterol level is about 70%, and this concentration rises to prepheresis levels in 1 week. Angiographic regression of coronary artery disease has been reported in about 50% of patients treated long term (Goldstein et al, 2001).

Liver transplantation has been performed on a limited number of homozygotes. The first was a 6-year-old girl with a cholesterol level of 1000 mg/dl who had had repeated myocardial infarctions. After liver transplantation, her cholesterol level fell to 200 to 300 mg/dl. Thirteen months after transplantation, she started lovastatin treatment, and her LDL cholesterol fell even farther, to 150 mg/dl. Thus liver transplantation not only lowered her cholesterol level but also restored responsiveness to lovastatin, the action of which requires an LDL receptor gene (Goldstein et al, 2001). Liver transplantation has been performed in five patients, four of whom recovered from transplant surgery. In all the survivors, the transplanted liver reduced the LDL cholesterol level significantly. These results underscore the importance of hepatic LDL receptors and emphasize the potential value of a direct gene therapy approach in which a normal LDL receptor gene is delivered to hepatocytes in vivo (Goldstein et al, 2001).

DISORDERS OF LYSOSOMAL ENZYMES

Gangliosidoses

Several types of gangliosidoses manifest in infancy with progressive encephalopathies and psychomotor deterioration, retinal lesions, and a particular neuronal alteration.

GM$_1$ Gangliosidosis.   GM$_1$ gangliosidosis is an autosomal recessive disorder that results from a deficiency of hydrolase ganglioside GM$_1$ beta-galactosidase (acid beta-galactosidase), which normally uses ganglioside GM$_1$ and galactose-containing glycoproteins as substrates (Gravel et al, 2001). As a result of this enzyme deficiency, ganglioside GM$_1$ that is normal in composition accumulates in the gray matter of the brain and in lesser amounts in the liver (Gilbert-Barness & Barness, 2000; Gravel et al, 2001). Galactose-containing glycoprotein also accumulates in the liver (Gravel et al, 2001). The clinical manifestations often are evident at birth, with edema affecting the face and extremities and occasionally with ascites. A poor appetite, weak sucking, ineffective swallowing, and subnormal weight gain also are seen. After several months, facial dysmorphism is apparent, with an enlarged skull, large forehead, coarse facial features, flattened nose, low-set ears, macroglossia, and hypertelorism. Psychomotor deterioration is progressive. The infant has a dull expression, is hypoactive and hypotonic, and never learns to sit independently. Tonic-clonic seizures may develop. Hepatomegaly is present (Gilbert-Barness & Barness, 2000; Gravel et al, 2001). Ophthalmologic examination reveals a cherry-red macular spot in 50% percent of these patients (Gravel et al, 2001). Affected patients who survive beyond the first year manifest decerebrate rigidity, blindness, deafness, spastic quadriplegia, and poor responsiveness to all external stimuli. Death usually occurs by 3 years of age. The disorder can be diagnosed by examining bone marrow, liver, or spleen tissue for foamy histiocytes (Gravel et al, 2001). Prenatal diagnosis is possible. No treatment is available.

GM$_2$ Gangliosidoses.   The GM$_2$ gangliosidoses are a group of inherited disorders caused by excessive intralysosomal accumulation of ganglioside GM$_2$, particularly in neuronal cells. Enzymatic hydrolysis of ganglioside GM$_2$ requires a substrate-specific cofactor. There are two isoenzymes of beta-hexosaminidase. Defects in any of the three genes that regulate the synthesis of these proteins result in the accumulation of gangliosides in the cell (Gravel et al, 2001). Only Tay-Sachs disease is discussed here.

Clinical phenotypes in the GM$_2$ gangliosidoses vary widely, ranging from an infantile-onset form with rapidly progressive, neurodegenerative disease that culminates in death before 4 years of age (Tay-Sachs disease) to later-onset, subacute or chronic forms with more slowly progressive neurologic conditions compatible with survival into childhood or adolescence or with long-term survival. Chronic forms include several manifestations, including progressive dystonia, spinocellular degeneration, motor neuron disease, and psychosis (Gravel et al, 2001).

At least 54 genetic mutations have been described. Most mutations are associated with the severe, infantile-onset disease. The subacute and chronic forms of the disease are associated with variable low levels of residual enzyme activity, and the level of activity correlates with the severity of the disease (Gravel et al, 2001). Specific therapy for GM$_2$ gangliosidoses is not available.

All GM$_2$ gangliosidoses exhibit an autosomal recessive inheritance pattern. Two hexosaminidase enzymes (HEX A and HEX B) are present in all normal tissues except red blood cells. The defective genes for HEX A have been mapped to chromosome 15 and those for HEX B and GM$_2$ activator/cofactor to chromosome 5. Heterozygotes for any of the defects are completely asymptomatic. The availability of rapid and inexpensive methods for identifying heterozygotes for HEX A defects has made large-scale screening programs for family and population carriers possible. When these tests are combined with DNA-based diagnostics, the type of mu-tation (acute, subacute, or chronic) can be identified (Gravel et al, 2001).

In the non-Jewish population, the incidence is approximately 6 in 1000 for HEX A mutations and 36 in 10,000 for HEX B mutations. Of these mutations, the acute, infantile type of disease characterizes about 35%, and the chronic form accounts for about 5%. Among Ashkenazic Jews of North America and in Israel, a heterozygote frequency of 33 in 1000 was found for HEX A mutations, 95% of which were characterized as the infantile or acute form of the disease. Extensive genetic counseling and monitoring of at-risk pregnancies has reduced the incidence of Tay-Sachs disease in the Ashkenazic population by 90% (Beaudet et al, 2001; Gravel et al, 2001).

All HEX A deficiency disorders can be diagnosed prenatally from amniotic fluid, cultured amniotic fluid cells, or chorionic villus biopsy specimens (Gravel et al, 2001). Tay-Sachs disease results from a deficiency of HEX A, which results in the accumulation of its substrate, ganglioside GM$_2$, in enormous amounts in the cerebrum. The amount of ganglioside GM$_2$ in the visceral organs is not significantly increased (Gravel et al, 2001). Tay-Sachs disease is most prevalent among Ashkenazic Jews, with an incidence of 1 in 3600 live births, compared with an incidence in the non-Jewish population of 1 in 360,000 live births (Burton, 2000; Beaudet et al, 2001; Gravel et al, 2001).

The clinical manifestations of Tay-Sachs disease appear shortly after birth, with an exaggerated startle reaction to sharp sounds. Audiogenic myoclonia is very characteristic of this disorder. By 3 months of age, evidence is seen of motor weakness, which progresses. Although affected infants may learn to sit and crawl, they never learn to walk. After the first year, these infants have poor muscle tone, rapid mental and motor deterioration, ineffective swallowing, and generalized paresis. Ophthalmologic examination reveals an infiltrated, cream-colored macula with a central cherry-red spot. By 16 months macrocephaly develops from the cerebral gliosis, and the ventricles are enlarged. By 18 months there is evidence of progressive sensory deficits leading to blindness and deafness. Subsequently, seizures, spasticity, and decerebrate rigidity develop. The infant's facial appearance is "doll-like," with pale pink translucent skin, long eyelashes, and fine hair. Deglutitional complications and infections lead to death by 2 to 5 years of age (Burton, 2000; Gilbert-Barness & Barness, 2000; Gravel et al, 2001).

The diagnosis of Tay-Sachs disease can be made by determining the levels of HEX A and HEX B in cord blood (Gravel et al, 2001). To identify carriers of the mutation, the enzyme can be assayed from venous blood. However, this enzyme increases after the eighth week of pregnancy in general, therefore screening should be done before pregnancy. In addition, the carrier test is not reliable in women who are taking oral contraceptives or who have diabetes, hepatitis, an acute myocardial infarction, pancreatitis, or rheumatoid arthritis (Gravel et al, 2001). Definitive diagnosis of carrier state or true disorder is made by enzyme assay from blood leukocytes (Gravel et al, 2001) or by DNA diagnostics. The only treatment for this disorder is prevention by carrier identification.

Sphingomyelin Lipidoses: Niemann-Pick Disease (Types A and B)

Niemann-Pick disease (NPD) types A and B are lysosomal storage disorders that result from deficient activity of acid sphingomyelinase (ASM). NPD type A is a fatal disorder of infancy characterized by failure to thrive, hepatomegaly, and a rapidly progressive neurodegenerative course that leads to death by 2 to 3 years of age. In contrast, NPD type B is a variable disorder usually diagnosed in childhood by the presence of hepatomegaly. Most type B patients have little or no neurologic impairment and survive into adulthood. In severely affected type B patients, progressive pulmonary infiltration causes pulmonary insufficiency and lifestyle changes (Burton, 2000; Gilbert-Barness & Barness, 2000; Schuchman & Desnick, 2001).

The pathologic hallmark of both types of NPD is the lipid-laden foam cell often referred to as the "Niemann-Pick cell." These cells arise from the accumulation of sphingomyelin and other lipids in the monocyte–macrophage system, which is the primary pathologic site of the disease (Gilbert-Barness & Barness, 2000; Schuchman & Desnick, 2001).

Patients with type A have less than 5% of normal ASM activity in their cells and tissues. Patients with type B, who have milder disease, may have residual enzyme activity that ranges from 5% to 10% of normal. Both type A and type B are inherited as autosomal recessive traits. NPD type A has a high incidence among Ashkenazic Jews compared with the general population. The incidence among the Ashkenazic population is approximately 1 in 120 live births, with a carrier frequency of 1 in 60 (Burton, 2000; Gilbert-Barness & Barness, 2000; Schuchman & Desnick, 2001).

The ASM gene has been mapped to chromosome 11, and 12 mutations that result in NPD types A and B have been identified in that gene. Diagnosis of types A and B disease can be made by enzymatic determination of ASM activity in cell or tissue extracts. Heterozygote detection requires molecular studies. Prenatal diagnosis by enzymatic or molecular analysis (or both) has been done through chorionic villi sampling and cultured amniocytes (Burton, 2000; Gilbert-Barness & Barness, 2000; Schuchman & Desnick, 2001).

No specific therapy exists for either type of Niemann-Pick disease. Current research is directed at enzyme replacement and gene transfer in the type B form.

NPD types A and B are diseases of cellular sphingomyelin metabolism, and they vary in onset, rate of progression, and neurologic symptoms. Sphingomyelin is a constituent of cellular membranes and also occurs in extracellular lipoproteins. In visceral organs, it constitutes 5% to 10% of the total phospholipid content; in erythrocytes, plasma, and the white matter of the brain, the proportion exceeds 20%. Because of the wide distribution of sphingomyelin in the body, a defect in the catabolism of this substance results in severe visceral and neuronal abnormalities. The increase in sphingomyelin content in visceral organs is more pronounced in patients with type A disease than in those with the type B form. Accumulation of sphingomyelin in the nervous system has not been demonstrated in patients with type B disease (Burton, 2000; Gilbert-Barness & Barness, 2000; Schuchman & Desnick, 2001).

NPD is an autosomal recessive disorder that occurs as a result of diminished activity (0 to 9% of normal) of ASM, an enzyme that catalyzes the breakdown of sphingomyelin (Burton, 2000; Gilbert-Barness & Barness, 2000; Schuchman & Desnick, 2001). Sphingomyelin accumulates progressively in the central nervous system and visceral organs. Clinical manifestations of this disorder include jaundice, generalized edema, progressive developmental delay, failure to thrive, hepatosplenomegaly, and feeding difficulties, which lead to emaciation. Often the abdomen is protuberant and the extremities are osteoporotic and thin. In 50% of affected infants, a cherry-red spot in the macular region is evident on ophthalmologic examination. Progressive neurologic deterioration with progressive loss of motor and intellectual function interferes with feeding, swallowing, and breathing. General muscular –hypotonia, weak tendon reflexes, progressive deterioration, and recurrent respiratory infections are observed after the first months. Subsequently, seizures develop, and death occurs by 3 years of age (Burton, 2000; Gilbert-Barness & Barness, 2000; Schuchman & Desnick, 2001). In some instances, the onset of symptoms may occur after a period of relatively normal development. The diagnosis is made by means of a bone marrow aspiration to evaluate for large, foamy histiocytes; a specific enzyme assay for acid sphingomyelinase; and molecular studies of tissue to determine heterozygotes (Burton, 2000; Gilbert-Barness & Barness, 2000; Schuchman & Desnick, 2001). Like Tay-Sachs disease, NPD has a higher frequency among Ashkenazic Jews. No specific treatment is available (Burton, 2000; Gilbert-Barness & Barness, 2000; Schuchman & Desnick, 2001).

NPD type B does not involve the central nervous system but does entail abnormal accumulation of sphingomyelin in the viscera and 5% to 10% of normal activity of acid sphingomyelinase (Burton, 2000; Gilbert-Barness & Barness, 2000; Schuchman & Desnick, 2001). The visceral manifestations include hepatosplenomegaly, interstitial pulmonary infiltrates, and a predisposition to respiratory infections and repeated pneumothoraces. Children with NPD type B may develop normally during several years before the hepatosplenomegaly is detected. No neurologic abnormalities are found, the fundi are normal, and intellectual development is undisturbed. Marked hepatosplenomegaly persists, and the prothrombin time is prolonged (Burton, 2000; Gilbert-Barness & Barness, 2000; Schuchman & Desnick, 2001).

Cellular Cholesterol Lipidoses: Niemann-Pick Disease (Type C)

NPD type C, an autosomal recessive lipidosis that results from an error in cellular trafficking of exogenous cholesterol, is associated with the lysosomal accumulation of unesterified cholesterol. This disorder is biochemically distinct from NPD types A and B. Most patients with NPD type C have progressive neurologic disease and hepatic damage (Patterson et al, 2001).

The clinical manifestations of NPD type C vary. Symptoms most commonly manifest in late childhood with variable degrees of hepatosplenomegaly, ophthalmoplegia, progressive ataxia, dystonia, and dementia. Death occurs in the second decade. This disorder may also manifest in the neonatal period with fatal liver disease or in the infantile period with hypotonia and developmental delay. The clinical manifestations may also appear as late as adulthood, in which psychosis and dementia predominate as symptoms (Burton, 2000; Gilbert-Barness & Barness, 2000; Patterson et al, 2001).

NPD type C has a panethnic distribution. Genetic isolates have been described in Nova Scotia (formerly called NPD type D) and southern Colorado. Despite the variable clinical manifestations, studies have not shown genetic heterogeneity (Patterson et al, 2001). NPD type C is as least as common as types A and B combined. The true prevalence of the disease is underestimated because of the lack of a definitive diagnostic test before the discovery of the abnormalities of cellular cholesterol processing.

Foam cells are present in many tissues with NPD type C but are not specific for this form of NPD. Foam cells may be absent in patients lacking visceromegaly. The primary molecular defect in NPD type C is unknown. Unesterified cholesterol, sphingomyelin, phospholipids, and glycolipids are stored in excess in the liver and spleen. Glycolipids are elevated in the brain (Patterson et al, 2001). The diagnosis of NPD type C requires both measurement of cellular cholesterol esterification and documentation of filipin-cholesterol staining in cultured fibroblasts during LDL uptake.

Symptomatic treatment of seizures, dystonia, and cataplexy is effective in many patients with NPD type C. Various drug protocols have been used to lower hepatic cholesterol levels, but it is not known whether this therapy influences the neurologic progression of the disease (Patterson et al, 2001).

The onset of neurologic manifestations arrives later in NPD type C than in types A and B, occurring at 3 to 4 years of age. The initial manifestations include spasticity, ataxia, loss of speech, grand mal seizures, and moderate visceromegaly. In the following years, intellectual functions are lost, and neurologic abnormalities become more pronounced. Urinary incontinence develops, as do seizures and inability to walk; after a period of vegetative existence, the patient dies. The accumulation of sphingomyelin is less severe than in other types of NPD, and ASM activity in tissues often is paradoxically normal. Death occurs by 5 to 15 years of age (Burton, 2000; Gilbert-Barness & Barness, 2000; Patterson et al, 2001).

PURINE METABOLIC DISORDERS

Hypoxanthine-Guanine Phosphoribosyltransferase Deficiency: Lesch-Nyhan Syndrome

Lesch-Nyhan syndrome is caused by a complete deficiency of hypoxanthine-guanine phosphoribosyltransferase (HPRT), a purine salvage enzyme. The disease is characterized by hyperuricemia, choreoathetosis, spasticity, mental retardation, and compulsive self-mutilation. Patients with a partial deficiency of HPRT have hyperuricemia and gouty arthritis but generally are spared the neurologic consequences of Lesch-Nyhan syndrome (Jinnah & Friedmann, 2001).

Patients with Lesch-Nyhan syndrome are clinically normal at birth. By 6 months of age, developmental delay is evident. Choreoathetoid movements begin within the first year. Self-mutilation is present in most patients and may begin as early as 6 months or as late as 16 years. Gouty arthritis in patients with partial HPRT deficiency develops during adulthood (Burton, 2000; Gilbert-Barness & Barness, 2000).

The HPRT enzyme is expressed in all tissues at low levels except in the basal ganglia, in which the levels are higher, presumably because the rate of de novo purine synthesis is low. The human HPRT gene lies on the X chromosome. The genetic lesions that lead to HPRT deficiency are heterogeneous. DNA mutation techniques are used in the diagnosis of affected males and to determine the carrier status of asymptomatic females. Tissues can be analyzed for the presence or absence of HPRT activity (Jinnah & Friedmann, 2001).

Treatment with allopurinol, an inhibitor of xanthine oxidase, reduces serum uric acid levels and prevents most of the symptoms associated with hyperuricemia. There is no effective therapy for the neurologic complications of Lesch-Nyhan syndrome (Gilbert-Barness & Barness, 2000; Jinnah & Friedmann, 2001).

Lesch-Nyhan syndrome is an X-linked recessive disorder that occurs as a result of a deficiency of hypoxanthine–guanine phosphoribosyltransferase, an enzyme necessary for purine metabolism. Hypoxanthine deficiency prevents the conversion of hypoxanthine into nucleotide inosinic acid, and guanine phosphoribosyltransferase deficiency prevents the conversion of guanine into the nucleotide guanylic acid (Jinnah & Friedmann, 2001). These two enzyme deficiencies result in an enhanced rate of conversion to uric acid. The hyperuricemia causes hyperuricuria, uric acid lithiasis, and uric acid tophi.

Clinical manifestations at birth may include clubfeet and congenital hip dislocation caused by spasticity in utero. Occasionally, the first clinical sign is the presence of sandy orange crystals in the infant's diapers. When this disorder is present, the uric acid level usually exceeds 9 mg/dl. Uric acid crystalluria leads to symptomatic nephrolithiasis and azotemia. Renal complications may lead to renal insufficiency and renal failure. Bony demineralization and partial osteopenia occur. An increased in the blood uric acid level causes urate stones to develop in the urinary tract and produces urate tophi in subcutaneous tissues and joints (Burton, 2000; Gilbert-Barness & Barness, 2000; Jinnah & Friedmann, 2001).

The clinical course of neurologic impairment is fairly well defined in Lesch-Nyhan syndrome. After unremarkable prenatal and birth histories, delayed motor development becomes evident by 3 to 4 months (Burton, 2000; Jinnah & Friedmann, 2001). Frequent vomiting, hypotonia, and respiratory difficulty develop. Pyramidal signs appear, including hyperreflexia, extensor plantar reflexes, sustained ankle clonus, and scissoring.

Extrapyramidal signs develop between 8 and 12 months of age, as evidenced by dystonia, chorea, and fine athetoid movements of the head and feet. The electromyogram is normal. During the second and third years of life, finger-chewing, lip-biting, tooth-grinding, and increased spasticity are easily recognized. Growth retardation occurs in all cases. IQ scores have been reported in the range of 40 to 80 on conventional testing. The EEG may be normal or may show diffuse slowing. More than 50% of affected patients have seizures and bilateral cortical atrophy with developmental delay. Compulsive self-mutilation, such as biting associated with tissue loss, is seen between 2 and 16 years of age and is aggravated by stress. Patients begin by biting their lips, buccal mucosa, or fingers, and the destructive urge often is so severe that arm restraints or dental extraction is necessary to prevent serious injury (Jinnah & Friedmann, 2001). The mutilation differs from that seen occasionally in other mentally retarded individuals. Lesch-Nyhan patients show a loss of tissue around the mouth or hands, as opposed to hypertrophy or callous formation. These patients display aggression toward other people, such as hitting and spitting, and opisthotonic posturing. Aggression towards others usually is followed by remorse. Death usually occurs in the second or third decade from pneumonia, aspiration, or chronic renal failure (Jinnah & Friedmann, 2001).

The diagnosis can be made by enzymatic assay from leukocytes or cultured skin fibroblasts or with DNA-based mutation detection techniques (Gilbert-Barness & Barness, 2000; Jinnah & Friedmann, 2001). Variable activity of these enzymes alters the severity of the disorder. Treatment with allopurinol, a xanthine oxidase inhibitor, can prevent the nephropathy by reducing uric acid levels to within the normal range. Treatment with allopurinol results in the excretion of large amounts of xanthine and hypoxanthine, which are relatively insoluble. Thus the dose must be titrated carefully, and fluid intake must be greatly increased to minimize the likelihood of xanthine stone formation. Allopurinol does not reverse the CNS dysfunction. Although diazepam, phenobarbital, levodopa, and haloperidol have shown some benefit in some patients, no therapy has proved to be universally effective (Gilbert-Barness & Barness, 2000; Jinnah & Friedmann, 2001). To prevent self-mutilation and aggression, the use of restraints and behavior modification have had some success. Currently, gene therapy is being investigated as a possible treatment for Lesch-Nyhan patients. The devastating nature of the disease, the lack of therapeutic options, and the development of efficient gene transfer techniques have made this disease a candidate for gene therapy. The HPRT gene has been transferred into HPRT-deficient cells in animal models. This therapy has not yet been used in human beings (Gilbert-Barness & Barness, 2000; Jinnah & Friedmann, 2001).

Hereditary Xanthinuria

A deficiency of the enzyme xanthine dehydrogenase results in the inability to degrade the purine bases hypoxanthine and xanthine to uric acid, the normal end product of purine metabolism in human beings. Xanthine and hypoxanthine accumulate in place of uric acid in plasma and urine. Xanthine is excreted; a salvage pathway recycles hypoxanthine. Excess xanthine in the defect is derived from guanine nucleotide catabolism; guanine is converted to xanthine via the enzyme guanase (Raivio et al, 2001).

The clinical manifestations of classical xanthinuria relate to the extreme insolubility of the purine base xanthine and its high renal clearance. The disease may manifest in the neonatal period as renal damage caused by xanthine calculi. The renal damage may be severe, leading to renal failure and death.

Whereas classical xanthinuria results from a deficiency of xanthine dehydrogenase, a second type of xanthinuria results from a deficiency of three enzymes—xanthine dehydrogenase, sulfite oxidase, and aldehyde oxidase—which have a common (and, in this case, deficient) molybdenum cofactor. This disorder manifests in the neonatal period with intractable seizures and is not discussed further.

Xanthine dehydrogenase is concentrated predominantly in the liver and intestinal mucosa. This mutant enzyme has not yet been studied on the molecular level; however, complementary DNA for the human enzyme has been cloned. The gene locus for xanthine dehydrogenase has been linked to chromosome 2 (Raivio et al, 2001). The genetic defect in classic xanthinuria and the cofactor deficiency is inherited as an autosomal recessive trait. Heterozygotes for the classical defect have 50% of the normal enzyme activity with normal uric acid levels. No specific treatments have proved successful for these patients; however, a high fluid intake and avoidance of purine-rich foods may be beneficial.

Hereditary xanthinuria is an autosomal recessive disorder that occurs as a result of a deficiency of xanthine dehydrogenase, an enzyme that catalyzes the oxidation of hypoxanthine to xanthine and of xanthine into uric acid (Raivio et al, 2001). It is characterized by excessive urinary excretion of xanthine, which is extremely insoluble. The clinical manifestations of this disorder vary. Approximately 20% of affected individuals are asymptomatic, whereas others have xanthine urinary tract calculi, myopathy, and arthropathy; males represent two thirds of the cases. The symptoms, which may begin at birth, include persistent emesis, poor weight gain, irritability, hematuria, urinary tract infection, renal colic, crystalluria, urolithiasis, and acute renal failure. The severity of the disease may lead to nephrectomy or terminal uremia. There may be cramping after exercise, and myopathy and polyarthritis may be present (Raivio et al, 2001); these features are presumably caused by deposition of xanthine crystals in skeletal muscle. The renal symptoms tend to occur in childhood, and the myopathy and arthropathy tend to occur later in life.

In the absence of urolithiasis, diagnosis of this disorder is difficult in the newborn who that exhibits acute renal failure. Renal ultrasonography can detect crystal urolithiasis and should be performed in all infants with hematuria and acute renal failure not attributable to perfusion injury. Very low serum uric acid levels (usually under 1 mg/dl) are indicative of the diagnosis (Raivio et al, 2001). The ratio of xanthine to hypoxanthine is significantly elevated, and in the urine, uric acid excretion is decreased and xanthine is increased (Raivio et al, 2001). Because the enzyme is not expressed in all tissues, the enzyme deficiency is confirmed through liver or intestinal mucosal biopsy. Prenatal diagnosis is available, although not required for classic xanthinuria, and chorionic villus or amniotic fluid sampling detects cofactor deficiency.

Treatment of classic xanthinuria includes a high fluid intake and restriction of dietary purine to prevent stone formation (Raivio et al, 2001). Because of the poor solubility of xanthine at any pH, alkalization of the urine is relatively ineffective at preventing stone formation. Vigorous exercise should be avoided. Lithotripsy or lithotomy may be required if obstructive nephropathy develops.

Pyrimidine Metabolic Disorders

Hereditary Orotic Aciduria.   Pyrimidines, along with purines, are the building blocks of DNA and RNA. Like purines, pyrimidines have two routes of nucleotide formation: the de novo pathway, which begins with ribose phosphate, amino acids, CO_2, and ammonia, and the salvage pathway, which scavenges free bases and nucleosides back to nucleotides. The de novo and salvage pathways are balanced and connected through the enzymes that degrade the nucleotides (Webster et al, 2001).

The four defects of pyrimidine metabolism are hereditary orotic aciduria, pyrimidine 5'-nucleotase deficiency, dihydropyrimidine dehydrogenase deficiency, and dihydropyrimidinuria (Webster et al, 2001). Only hereditary orotic aciduria is discussed in this section.

The end product of purine metabolism is uric acid, which is easily recognized and quantified. No equivalent end product derives from pyrimidine metabolism. Hereditary orotic aciduria results from a defect in the de novo pathway. It is an autosomal recessive disorder that caused by a severe deficiency of the last two enzyme activities of the pathway. Although two enzymes are affected in this disorder, they are regulated by a single polypeptide encoded by a single gene localized to chromosome 3 (Webster et al, 2001).

Only a few dozen cases of hereditary orotic aciduria have been reported in the literature. All patients have had macrocytic hypochromic megaloblastic anemia and orotic acid crystalluria. Treatment with uridine has produced clinical improvement in most patients. Other clinical manifestations of the disorder include crystal lithiasis, cardiac malformations, and strabismus (Webster et al, 2001). Infections are a problem in some patients with various alterations of immune function. Mild intellectual impairment has not been a constant feature before treatment.

Hereditary orotic aciduria is an extremely rare autosomal recessive disorder that occurs as a result of the deficiency of the last two sequential enzymes in the pyrimidine pathway: orotate phosphoribosyltransferase and orotidine-5'-phosphate decarboxylase. Orotate phosphoribosyltransferase converts orotic acid into orotidine-5'-phosphate, and orotidine-5'-phosphate converts orotidine-5'-phosphate into uridine-5'-phosphate (Webster et al, 2001). Affected individuals are totally dependent on exogenous sources of pyrimidines for survival. The clinical manifestations, which appear in infancy, are failure to thrive and retarded growth and development. Bilateral strabismus is seen, and the hair is fine and dry. Splenomegaly and megaloblastic anemia may be present. Orotic acid crystals in the urine may cause urinary tract obstruction (Webster et al, 2001).

Screening the urine for orotic acids can confirm the diagnosis (Webster et al, 2001). In this disorder, orotic acid excretion is 1000 times higher than normal (Gilbert-Barness & Barness, 2000; Webster et al, 2001). Hematologically, hypochromia, anisocytosis, poikilocytosis, erythroid hyperplasia, and atypical megaloblastic changes in the bone marrow are seen (Burton, 2000; Webster et al, 2001). The definitive diagnosis is made by enzymatic assay of red blood cells, white blood cells, or cultured skin fibroblasts (Webster et al, 2001).

Treatment with glucocorticoids leads to hematologic improvement in a few patients, although no changes occur in the bone marrow (Webster et al, 2001). Pyrimidine replacement with the nucleotide uridine is the treatment of choice and leads to hematologic remission and normal growth and development if initiated early (Webster et al, 2001). Several women with hereditary orotic aciduria have had a number of pregnancies. The reports in the literature suggest that uridine is not teratogenic and that pregnancy is well tolerated. The dose of uridine must be adjusted to maintain an affected woman's normal nonpregnant hemoglobin level and amount of orotic acid excretion (Webster et al, 2001).

Treatment with uridine reverses the megaloblastic anemia and reduces the amount of orotic acid excreted; however, it is not necessarily an indication that the effects of the metabolic defect have been eliminated in other tissues. The long-term prognosis of survival into early adult life is excellent in most treated individuals and even in some in whom treatment was delayed (Webster et al, 2001).

SUMMARY

Because many metabolic disorders can be identified in the prenatal and postnatal periods, the demand has grown for early screening for these disorders. It is extremely important, therefore, that both the general public and the medical community intelligently evaluate each disorder in terms of the need for and desirability of screening. Such an evaluation must be based on both humanistic and economic considerations.

Neonatal screening programs must be revised to reflect the importance of screening for a particular disease in a given population. Such an evaluation is necessary to eliminate screening for disorders with less severe consequences or for those that occur very rarely; disorders with more severe consequences and those that occur more often should be included in the screening program. Expanded and revised neonatal screening can provide the tools for improved preventive health measures and for genetic counseling in the areas of greatest need in each specific population. The use of gene therapy to replace or augment the missing substrate or enzyme offers hope in the future. Currently, however, early neonatal detection is the best weapon against iatrogenic or long-term sequelae from correctable metabolic dysfunctions. Unquestionably, the management of newborns with inborn errors of metabolism requires collaboration among the physician, nurse, family, geneticist, neurologist, ophthalmologist, endocrinologist, teacher, nutritionist, and social worker.

REFERENCES

Abdullah A et al (1996). Congenital glucose-galactose malabsorption in Arab children. *Journal of pediatric gastroenterology & nutrition* 23:561-564.

Ali M et al (1998). Hereditary fructose intolerance. *Journal of medical genetics* 35:353-365.

Assmann G et al (2001). Familial analphalipoproteinemia: Tangier disease. In Scriver CR et al, editors. *The metabolic and molecular bases of inherited disease,* ed 8. McGraw-Hill: New York.

Beaudet AL et al (2001). Genetics, biochemistry, and molecular bases of variant human phenotypes. In Scriver CR et al, editors. *The metabolic and molecular bases of inherited disease,* ed 8. McGraw-Hill: New York.

Bickel H et al (1954). Influence of phenylalanine intake on the chemistry and behaviour of a phenylketonuric child. *Acta paediatrica* 43:64-77.

Bickel H et al (1980). *Neonatal screening for inborn errors of metabolism*. Springer-Verlag: New York.

Blau N et al (2001). Disorders of tetrahydrobiopterin and related biogenic amines. In Scriver CR et al, editors. *The metabolic and molecular bases of inherited disease*, ed 8. McGraw-Hill: New York.

Brunzell JD, Deeb SS (2001). Familial lipoprotein lipase deficiency, Apo C-II deficiency and hepatic lipase deficiency. In Scriver CR et al, editors. *The metabolic and molecular bases of inherited disease*, ed 8. McGraw-Hill: New York.

Brusilow SW, Horwich AL (2001). Urea cycle enzymes. In Scriver CR et al, editors. *The metabolic and molecular bases of inherited disease*, ed 8. McGraw-Hill: New York.

Burton BK (2000). Inborn errors of metabolism in infancy: a guide to diagnosis. *Pediatrics* 102:e69.

Calvo M et al (2000). Diagnostic approach to inborn errors of metabolism in an emergency unit. *Pediatric emergency care* 16:405-408.

Castro-Rodriguez JA et al (1997). Differentiation of osmotic and secretory diarrhoea by stool carbohydrate and osmolar gap measurements. *Archives of disease in childhood* 77:201-205.

Chakrapani A et al (2001). Detection of inborn errors of metabolism in the newborn *Archives of disease in childhood (fetal & neonatal)* 84:F205-F210.

Chuang DT, Shih VE (2001). Maple syrup urine disease (branched-chain ketoaciduria). In Scriver CR et al, editors. *The metabolic and molecular bases of inherited disease*, ed 8. McGraw-Hill: New York.

Cleary MA et al (1994). Magnetic resonance imaging of the brain in phenylketonuria. *Lancet* 344:87-90.

Corpe CP et al (1999). Intestinal fructose absorption: clinical and molecular aspects. *Journal of pediatric gastroenterology & nutrition* 28:364-374.

Costello PM et al (1994). Intelligence in mild atypical phenylketonuria. *European journal of pediatrics* 153:260-263.

de Franchis R et al (1994). Identical genotypes in siblings with different homocystinuric phenotypes: identification of three mutations in cystathionine beta-synthase using an improved bacterial expression system. *Human molecular genetics* 3:1103.

Desjeux JF (2000). Can malabsorbed carbohydrates be useful in the treatment of acute diarrhea? *Journal of pediatric gastroenterology & nutrition* 31:499-502.

Duran M et al (1994). Selective screening for amino acid disorders. *European journal of pediatrics* 153(suppl 1):S33-S37.

Falk MC et al (1994). Continuous venovenous hemofiltration in the acute treatment of inborn errors of metabolism. *Pediatric nephrology* 8:330-333.

Fenton WA et al (2001). Disorders of propionate and methylmalonate metabolism. In Scriver CR et al, editors. *The metabolic and molecular bases of inherited disease*, ed 8. McGraw-Hill: New York.

Gilbert-Barness E, Barness LA (2000). *Metabolic diseases: foundations of clinical management, genetics and pathology*. Eaton Publishing: Natick, MA.

Goldstein JL et al (2001). Familial hypercholesterolemia. In Scriver CR et al, editors. *The metabolic and molecular bases of inherited disease*, ed 8. McGraw-Hill: New York.

Gravel RA et al (2001). The GM$_2$ gangliosidoses. In Scriver CR et al, editors. *The metabolic and molecular bases of inherited disease*, ed 8. McGraw-Hill: New York.

Green ED (2001). The human genome project and its impact on the study of human disease. In Scriver CR et al, editors. *The metabolic and molecular bases of inherited disease*, ed 8. McGraw-Hill: New York.

Hamosh A, Johnston MV (2001). Nonketotic hyperglycinemia. In Scriver CR et al, editors. *The metabolic and molecular bases of inherited disease*, ed 8. McGraw-Hill: New York.

Havel RJ, Kane JP (2001). Introduction: the structure and metabolism of plasma lipoproteins. In Scriver CR et al, editors. *The metabolic and molecular bases of inherited disease*, ed 8. McGraw-Hill: New York.

Hillebrand G et al (2000). Hereditary fructose intolerance and alpha-1-antitrypsin deficiency. *Archives of disease in childhood* 83:72-73.

Hirono A et al (2001). Pyruvate kinase and other enzymopathies of the erythrocyte. In Scriver CR et al, editors. *The metabolic and molecular bases of inherited disease*, ed 8. McGraw-Hill: New York.

Jinnah HA, Friedmann T (2001). Lesch-Nyhan syndrome and its variants. In Scriver CR et al, editors. *The metabolic and molecular bases of inherited disease*, ed 8. McGraw-Hill: New York.

Kane JP, Havel RJ (2001). Disorders of the biogenesis and secretion of lipoproteins containing the b apolipoproteins. In Scriver CR et al, editors. *The metabolic and molecular bases of inherited disease*, ed 8. McGraw-Hill: New York.

Lee WS, Boey CM (1999). Chronic diarrhea in infants and young children: causes, clinical features and outcome. *Journal of pediatrics & child health* 35:260-263.

Leonard JV, Morris AM (2000). Inborn errors of metabolism around time of birth. *Lancet* 356:583-587.

Levy HL et al (2001). Disorders of histidine metabolism. In Scriver CR et al, editors. *The metabolic and molecular bases of inherited disease*, ed 8. McGraw-Hill: New York.

Lindstedt S et al (1992). Treatment of hereditary tyrosinemia type I by inhibition of 4-hydroxyphenylpyruvate-dioxygenase. *Lancet* 340(8823), 813-817.

Lund AM, Leonard JV (2000). False positive fructose loading: a pitfall in the diagnosis of fructose-1,6-bisphosphatase deficiency. *Journal of inherited metabolic disease* 23:634-635.

Luzzatto L et al (2001). Glucose-6-phosphate dehydrogenase. In Scriver CR et al, editors. *The metabolic and molecular bases of inherited disease*, ed 8. McGraw-Hill: New York.

Mitchell GA et al (2001). Hypertyrosinemia. In Scriver CR et al, editors. *The metabolic and molecular bases of inherited disease*, ed 8. McGraw-Hill: New York.

Moukil MA et al (2000). Study of the regulatory properties of glucokinase by site-directed mutagenesis: conversion of glucokinase to an enzyme with high affinity for glucose. *Diabetes* 49:195-201.

Mudd SH et al (2001). Disorders of transsulfuration. In Scriver CR et al, editors. *The metabolic and molecular bases of inherited disease*, ed 8. McGraw-Hill: New York.

Ning C et al (2000). Galactose metabolism by the mouse with galactose-1-phosphate uridyltransferase deficiency. *Pediatric research* 48:211-217.

Patterson MC et al (2001). Niemann-Pick disease type C: a lipid trafficking disorder. In Scriver CR et al, editors. *The metabolic and molecular bases of inherited disease*, ed 8. McGraw-Hill: New York.

Paul TD et al (1980). Urine screening for metabolic disease in newborn infants. *Journal of pediatrics* 96:653-656.

Pitkanen S et al (1994). Serum levels of oncofetal markers CA 125, CA 19-9 and alpha-fetoprotein in children with hereditary tyrosinemia type I. *Pediatric research* 35:205.

Ploos van Amstel JK et al (1994). Prenatal diagnosis of type I hereditary tyrosinemia. *Lancet* 344 (8918), 336.

Potocnik U, Widhalm K (1994). Long-term follow-up of children with classical phenylketonuria after diet discontinuation: a review. *Journal of the American college of nutrition* 13:232-236.

Raivio KO et al (2001). Xanthine oxidoreductases: a role in human pathophysiology and in hereditary xanthinuria. In Scriver CR et al, editors. *The metabolic and molecular bases of inherited disease*, ed 8. McGraw-Hill: New York.

Ris MD et al (1994). Early treated phenylketonuria: adult neuropsychologic outcome. *Journal of pediatrics* 124:388-392.

Riva E et al (2001). Prevention and treatment of cow's milk allergy. *Archives of disease in childhood* 84:91.

Robinson BH (2001). Lactic acidemia: disorders of pyruvate carboxylase and pyruvate dehydrogenase. In Scriver CR et al, editors. *The metabolic and molecular bases of inherited disease*, ed 8. McGraw-Hill: New York.

Saudubray JM et al (2000). Genetic hypoglycaemia in infancy and childhood: pathophysiology and diagnosis. *Journal of inherited metabolic disease* 23:197-214.

Schuchman EH, Desnick RJ (2001). Niemann-Pick disease types A and B: acid sphingomyelinase deficiencies. In Scriver CR et al, editors. *The metabolic and molecular bases of inherited disease*, ed 8. McGraw-Hill: New York.

Scriver CR et al, editors (2001). *The metabolic and molecular bases of inherited disease*, ed 8. McGraw-Hill: New York.

Scriver CR, Kaufman S (2001). The hyperphenylalaninemias: phenylalanine hydroxylase deficiency. In Scriver CR et al, editors. *The metabolic and molecular bases of inherited disease*, ed 8. McGraw-Hill: New York.

Stormon M et al (2001). The changing pattern of diagnosis of infantile cholestasis. *Journal of pediatric & child health* 37:47-50.

Sunehag AL et al (1999). Gluconeogenesis in very low birth weight infants receiving total parenteral nutrition. *Diabetes* 48:791-800.

Svensson E et al (1994). Severity of mutation in the phenylalanine hydrolase gene influences phenylalanine metabolism in phenylketonuria and hyperphenylalaninemia heterozygotes. *Journal of inherited metabolic disease* 17:215-222.

Sweetman L, Williams JC (2001). Branched-chain organic acidurias. In Scriver CR et al, editors. *The metabolic and molecular bases of inherited disease*, ed 8. McGraw-Hill: New York.

Trefz F et al (1994). Neuropsychological and biochemical investigations in heterozygotes for phenylketonuria during ingestion of high dose aspartame. *Human genetics* 93:369-374.

Utermann G (2001). Familial lipoprotein lipase deficiency, Apo C-II deficiency, and hepatic lipase deficiency. In Scriver CR et al, editors. *The metabolic and molecular bases of inherited disease*, ed 8. McGraw-Hill: New York.

Walter JH et al (1999). Generalized uridine diphosphate galactose-4-epimerase deficiency. *Archives of disease in childhood* 80:374-376.

Webster DR et al (2001). Hereditary orotic aciduria and other disorders of pyrimidine metabolism. In Scriver CR et al, editors. *The metabolic and molecular bases of inherited disease*, ed 8. McGraw-Hill: New York.

CHAPTER 28

ASSESSMENT AND MANAGEMENT OF THE ENDOCRINE SYSTEM

VIVIAN W. GAMBLIAN, JEANNE WEILAND, NANCY C. PARK

Alterations in the endocrine system are common during the neonatal period. Unfortunately, these dysfunctions are normally complex and affect other or all body systems. This chapter highlights the most common endocrine problems: (1) growth hormone (GH) deficiency or excess; (2) syndrome of inappropriate antidiuretic hormone (SIADH); (3) hypothyroidism; (4) hyperthyroidism; (5) maternal diabetes; (6) ambiguous genitalia; and (7) cystic fibrosis. The discussion begins with a review of the endocrine system, its organs, and the hormones it produces that regulate endocrine function.

PHYSIOLOGY OF THE ENDOCRINE SYSTEM

In utero the placenta acts as the major endocrine organ, producing precursors for hormones, allowing movement of hormones across the membrane from maternal circulation to fetal circulation, and promoting steroid synthesis. Human chorionic gonadotropin (hCG), human chorionic somatomammotropin, human placental lactogen, and progesterone are the main hormones that the placenta produces. Early in fetal development, the organs of the endocrine system begin to take shape.

The endocrine system comprises several organs: the hypothalamus; the pituitary, pineal, thyroid, parathyroid, and adrenal glands; the gonads; and the pancreatic islet cells. The pituitary gland is composed of two main parts: the adenohypophysis (anterior pituitary) and the neurohypophysis (posterior pituitary). The pituitary begins to function at 8 to 9 weeks' gestation. The thyroid gland and its accompanying cells begin to secrete triiodothyronine (T_3) and thyroxine (T_4) and trap iodine by 11 to 12 weeks' gestation (Dorton, 2000). T_3 and T_4 regulate thyrotropin-releasing hormone (TRH) by blocking its synthesis and the fetal secretion of thyroid-stimulating hormone (TSH). TSH cannot cross the placenta, but TRH can. The presence of HCG also effectively reduces TSH action. During the second half of gestation, the parathyroid gland and the chief and oxyphil cells form. The adrenal glands arise because of the migration of neural crest cells. These cells are also responsible for innervation of the bowel and formation of the midline fusion. The adrenal medulla develops primarily from the neural cells. The cells in this region differentiate to produce norepinephrine- and epinephrine-secreting cells. The adrenal cortex's growth peaks at 16 weeks' gestation, with a gradual regression over the remainder of gestation and the first

6 months of postnatal life. At 16 weeks' gestation, the adrenal gland is actually larger than the metanephric kidney. The adrenal glands are capable of steroid synthesis by 8 weeks' gestation, even though the peak growth period extends over another 8 weeks.

The pancreas is one of the major endocrine organs; the islets of Langerhans constitute its endocrine portion. The islets of Langerhans contain alpha, beta, C, and delta cells. The alpha cells, which are present at 10 weeks' gestation, produce glucagon. The precursors of the beta cells, present by 13 weeks' gestation, produce insulin. The beta cells are fully functional by 14 to 16 weeks' gestation. The ability of the fetus to produce insulin is important because maternal insulin does not cross the placental barrier. The C cells and delta cells of the pancreas are derived from neural crest cells. Their function is not well delineated.

In addition to the major endocrine organs, other cells aid endocrine regulation. Endocrine cells are present throughout the gastrointestinal and respiratory systems and the brain; they are called amine precursor uptake and decarboxylation cells or gastroenteropancreatic cells. These cells are responsible for the secretion of peptide hormones. Gastrin cells, which are found in the regions of the pylorus and duodenum, secrete the hormone gastrin. Enterochromaffin cells, located in the gastric area, secrete serotonin. The delta cells—in the islets of Langerhans, the gastric area, and the small intestines—are responsible for the secretion of somatostatin. These hormones, along with the hormones produced in the hypothalamus, serve as the principal controls for a variety of metabolic activities within the human body. Hormone actions vary widely in type of action and rapidity of effect, with some effects occurring in seconds and others over a period of hours, weeks, or years.

The endocrine, or hormonal, system uses chemical substances (hormones) that are produced and secreted by a cell or group of cells into body fluids. The result is physiologic control of other cells and cell function. Local hormones, thus named because of their specific local effects, include acetylcholine, secretin, cholecystokinin, and many others. In contrast, general hormones are secreted by specific endocrine glands and are transported via the systemic circulation to distant points at which the physiologic action occurs. Some general hormones affect many body tissues, as do GH, which is secreted by the adenohypophysis, and thyroid hormone, which is secreted by the thyroid gland. The majority of general hormones, however, exert their effect only on specific target tissues.

Chemistry of Hormones

Chemically, endocrine hormones may be described as proteins, derivatives of amino acids, peptides, or steroids (Table 28-1). Most protein hormones link directly with nuclear DNA. They have long, complex chains, unlike the short chains of the peptides. Generally, peptide and protein hormones act rapidly, within seconds to minutes. Thyroid hormone and epinephrine and norepinephrine from the adrenal medulla are amino acids derived from tyrosine. They enter the cell membrane by combining with a specific receptor; their purpose is protein synthesis.

The gonads and the adrenal cortex secrete steroids, which are derived from the mesenchymal layer of the embryo. Typically, the action of steroid hormones occurs slowly, over a period of hours or days. The action of steroid hormones causes protein synthesis in target cells, which then act as enzymes or carrier proteins to activate other cells.

Hormonal Control by Negative Feedback

The phenomenon by which endocrine hormones maintain appropriate levels of secretion is known as negative feedback. The hypothalamus is responsible for releasing hormones that move to the anterior pituitary by way of a hypothalamic-hypophyseal (pituitary) portal system. This system is not fully functional until about 15 weeks' gestation.

The releasing hormones act as stimulants on the adenohypophysis (anterior pituitary) to produce a specific trophic hormone. This hormone, in turn, acts as an inductor to stimulate a specific endocrine gland to produce yet another hormone that acts on a specific target organ. This mechanism produces a cascade effect. In general, the specific hormone is secreted until the physiologic effect is achieved. At that point, information is transmitted that causes the producing gland to stop secretion. A critical blood level of a specific hormone is the determining factor that tells the hypothalamus to stop secreting releasing factors. Conversely, under-secretion results in decreased physiologic effects of the hormone. This feedback mechanism signals the need to secrete a greater amount of hormone to produce the appropriate physiologic response.

Mechanisms of Hormonal Action

Hormones affect the function of target tissues in a number of ways. They may alter the cellular chemistry, adjust the cell membrane permeability, or act on the cell as a whole. Some hormones stimulate adenosine 3', 5'-cyclic monophosphate

(cAMP) to be formed in the cell. cAMP then triggers hormonal effects within the cell, acting as a "second messenger" for hormone mediation. Box 28-1 lists hormones affected by cAMP.

Another intracellular hormonal mediator (or second messenger) is cyclic guanosine monophosphate (cGMP), which is similar to cAMP in structure and action, except that it contains the base guanine rather than adenine. Prostaglandins may also act as a type of intracellular hormonal mediator.

Hormone interaction with target tissues is dependent on the cell's recognition of specific hormones via receptor sites. This recognition is related to hormone receptor binding. The receptors may be membrane-bound, cytoplasmic, or intranuclear. A receptor, by definition, is a cellular molecule that is highly selective in its affinity for a particular hormone. The hormone regulates the result of the receptor's binding with a given hormone. Thus the hormone acts as a catalyst, or initiator, in the process but not as a participant per se.

Membrane receptors for hormones are specific in that the hormone binds with high affinity. However, other agonists and antagonists may also bind with the receptors. Numerous chemical and pharmacologic agents act as agonists or antagonists at the membrane receptor level. Hormone membrane receptors act to trigger the "first" message. The hormone itself triggers the "second" message, which culminates in the desired specific cellular event.

As mentioned, two types of second messengers are cAMP and cGMP. The action of cAMP is cell-specific. Both cAMP and cGMP act on cell protein kinases. Some hormone actions appear to attain their desired effects by reducing cAMP. The ratio of cAMP to cGMP appears to produce a metabolic balance. Hormones may also alter cell membrane permeability for certain substances. For example, insulin facilitates glucose entry into certain cells.

Intracellular Receptors

Some hormones (e.g., thyroid hormone) have receptors in the cell nucleus or within the cytosol. Many factors determine the intracellular binding of hormones. Only cells with specific receptors respond to the hormone. Additionally, intracellular hormone–receptor interactions are concentration-dependent, have a limited period of effectiveness, and are reversible. It is believed that the hormone-receptor interaction triggers a regulatory protein that induces a specific change in the cell's DNA, ultimately causing a change in the genetic transcription that is necessary for protein synthesis.

TABLE **28-1**	Chemistry of Hormones				
Hormone Origin	**Protein**	**Peptides**	**Amino Acid Derivatives**	**Steroids**
Pancreas	X			
Anterior pituitary	X			
Thyroid			X	
Adrenal medulla			X	
Posterior pituitary		X		
Adrenal cortex				X
Ovary				X
Testis				X

BOX **28-1**

Hormones Affected by Cyclic Adenosine Monophosphate

Adrenocorticotropic hormone
Thyroid-stimulating hormone
Luteinizing hormone
Follicle-stimulating hormone
Parathyroid hormone
Glucagon
Vasopressin
Secretin
Catecholamines
Hypothalamic-releasing factors

GROWTH FACTORS

Growth factors have become increasingly important in understanding the physiology of the endocrine system. These substances are made up of peptides or polypeptides and are divided into three subgroups. Although they are named "growth factors," each of these substances plays an important role in cell proliferation and/or cell function specific to its messenger and receptor functions.

The first subgroup comprises growth factors that stimulate multiplication of different types of cells. Examples of this subgroup include Insulin-like Growth Factor-1 (IGF-1), nerve growth factor, and epidermal growth factor (EGF). Each of these factors is necessary for proliferation of its special cells or regulating function of its special cells. More than 20 types of growth factors have been identified within this subgroup.

The second subgroup, known as cytokines, also comprises many different types. These cytokines are produced by macrophages and lymphocytes and play a significant role in immune system function.

The third subgroup is known as colony-stimulating factors. These regulate the maturation and proliferation of red blood cells (RBC) and white blood cells (WBC).

ALTERATIONS IN THE ENDOCRINE SYSTEM

Growth Hormone

Human growth hormone (hGH) is a protein that consists of 191 amino acid residues. A gene located on the long arm of chromosome 17 encodes for GH. GH (somatotropin) is secreted from somatotroph cells in the anterior portion of the pituitary gland (Dorton, 2000). GH is secreted in pulses rather than in a continuous manner. Secretion is under the control of two hypothalamic peptides: growth hormone–releasing factor (GHRF) and somatostatin. GHRF stimulates the release of GH from the anterior pituitary gland. GHRF is thought to play a significant role in the magnitude of GH secretion. Somatostatin, in contrast, inhibits GH release and is thought to be the primary cause for the timing and duration of GH pulsatile release (Argente & Chowen, 1994).

The actions of GH influence growth rate. GH affects proliferation and differentiation of various cells. Uptake of GH by liver and skeletal muscle cells improves amino acid transport and protein synthesis. Liver cells increase glucose output and produce insulin-like growth factors called somatomedins. The insulin-like growth factors—specifically IGF-1—which are in synergy with GH, appear to stimulate skeletal growth. An anti-insulin effect occurs in muscle (Ganong, 2000). In fact, GH has been used in the treatment of hyperinsulinemia. Metabolism of carbohydrates is improved, and circulating free fatty acid lipids are increased in the presence of GH (Ganong, 2000).

As early as 10 weeks after conception, GH can be detected in the fetal anterior pituitary gland. High levels of GH in the cord blood of neonates have a fetal origin because GH does not cross the placental barrier. Concentrations of GH in full-term and premature newborns have not been statistically different (Bona et al, 1994). Despite high levels, GH seems to have little effect on gestational size. Rather, somatomedins appear to play a bigger role in fetal tissue growth and differentiation (Bona et al, 1994). Certain tactile-kinesthetic stimulation may encourage GH release and protein synthesis in very small preterm neonates. Weight gain and awake, active periods appear to improve when preterm infants are given appropriate stimulation.

In all infants, a rapid decline of GH occurs 1 to 2 weeks postnatally; however, throughout the first 8 weeks of life, these levels are persistently higher than those in adults.

Growth Hormone Deficiency

Pathophysiology.   GH deficiency is not thought to be the root cause of the majority of short stature cases in humans. Familial and hereditary factors are often the basis for such occurrences. When GH and related hormones are involved, the cause of deficiency is variable. Various defects produce low levels or the absence of GH. For example, a defect of the hypothalamus limits stimulation of the pituitary to release GH. Primary pituitary tumors may exist. Developmental or degenerative lesions of the pituitary also prohibit GH secretion. Certain congenital defects, such as mid-line abnormalities (i.e., cleft palate and septo-optic dysplasia) may contribute to alterations in the function and/or structure of the pituitary gland (Dorton, 2000). Septo-optic dysplasia is a sporadic condition in which dwarfism with documented GH deficiency occurs. This developmental anomaly can involve defects in the brain, optic tract, and pituitary gland. The somatotrophs may be unable to produce GH if the gene response for its production is defective. Under such circumstances, target organs may be unable to respond to hormonal stimulation. Lastly, the hormone itself may be abnormal and rendered useless.

Clinical Manifestations.   Deficiency of growth hormone may not be apparent until months or years when growth falls below the third percentile or is 6 cm/yr before age 4 years (Beers & Berkow, 2002). To remain within the scope of this text, only clinical manifestations of neonatal and early infancy GH deficiency are described. Although GH deficiency can, in some cases, lead to short stature in childhood and beyond, it is not necessarily responsible for intrauterine growth restiction or small-for-gestational-age neonates. Comparison of levels measured directly on cord and venous blood in neonates who were average-for-gestational-age and those who were small-for-gestational-age indicates that GH can be higher in small for gestational age neonates during the first 3 days of life. This higher level may be due to a resistance at the level of the hGH receptor or a insulin-like growth factor-1 synthesis defect (Varvarigou et al, 1994).

Neonates.   Neonates with isolated GH deficiency can have height and birth weight within normal range. The neonate with isolated GH deficiency often presents with persistent hypoglycemia, the mechanism of which is not clearly defined but which may be related to the production of insulin-like growth factors (somatomedins). Micropenis in the male is also a characteristic sometimes associated with GH deficiency.

Infants.   Infants younger than 6 months of age often present with failure to thrive, poor feeding, and subnormal height velocity. Hypoglycemia may also be present in this age group. A thorough history and physical examination includes assessing the infant for pallor, lethargy, and excessive perspiration, which are also signs of GH deficiency.

GH deficiency can be a part of many different disorders. Any condition that disrupts GH production, stimulation, secretion, or tissue response can result in deficiency. For example, a neonate with congenital absence of the anterior pituitary gland manifests signs and symptoms similar to those in isolated GH deficiency. In addition, many other glands and hormones are affected because the pituitary is the master endocrine gland. Clinical features include early lethargy, hyperbilirubinemia, a minute penis in males, hypoplastic gonads and thyroid, hypoglycemia, cyanosis, convulsions, and circulatory collapse.

Septo-optic dysplasia is a sporadic condition in which dwarfism with documented GH deficiency occurs. This developmental anomaly can involve defects in the brain, optic tract, and pituitary gland. An association of optic disk hypoplasia with an absent septum pellucidum was first described. Neonates with severe disease may present with hypoglycemia, hypotonia, prolonged jaundice, microphallus, and seizures. The young infant may present with defective vision, hypotonia, behavioral delay, and seizures.

Risk Factors. The incidence of GH deficiency has been quoted to be as high as 1 in 4,000 and as low as 1 in 30,000 live births. This discrepancy has been thought to be due to missed diagnoses that result from professional oversight rather than lack of parental concern. GH deficiency appears to be more prevalent in boys than in girls, with an incidence of 2:1 to as much as 4:1. However, these ratios reflect GH deficiency diagnosed throughout childhood and adolescence. Researchers propose that the ratios reflect the probability that boys are more likely than girls to seek medical attention for short stature.

There have been conflicting reports about whether perinatal trauma (septo-optic dysplasia) is a significant risk factor for GH deficiency. It is postulated that perinatal trauma or difficulty compromises the blood supply to the pituitary gland, which can result in deficient GH secretion. In circumstances of therapeutic radiation for malignant tumors, impaired growth may occur as a result of the radiologic impact on the CNS and/or spine.

Differential Diagnosis. GH deficiency can be diagnosed in several ways. Direct measurement of GH is the first; however, the pulsatile nature of the hormone makes random measurements of little value. Maximal secretory levels must be stimulated either physiologically or pharmacologically and then measured. The response of an individual's GH to pharmacologic stimuli may confirm the diagnosis. Attempts to characterize GH secretion in premature infants by quantifying urinary GH excretion also are inadequate. Immature renal proximal tubular function in both preterm and full-term neonates does not allow urine GH levels to adequately depict endogenous GH secretion. It has been observed that the level of insulin-like growth factors is constant throughout the day, and low levels are seen in the majority of children with GH deficiency. However, many other factors influence circulating insulin-like growth factors; consequently, they have limited screening and diagnostic value for deficient GH. Measurement of IGF-1 is of minimal value because levels are normally very low in infancy and because variations in normal to subnormal values are indistinguishable. Generally, testing remains subject to laboratory error and arbitrary conclusions by the interpreter. Work has also been done with GHRF. It is used to evaluate the GH-releasing capacity of the anterior pituitary gland. L-dopa, glucagon, or propranolol combined with GHRF can also be used to evaluate hypothalamic function. An associated short-stature GH disorder involves a deft either at the GH receptor site or in IGF-1 synthesis. Laron syndrome is such a disorder and has a distinct phenotype (Beers & Berkow, 2002).

Collaborative Management. Nurses caring for neonates with isolated GH deficiency manifested by persistent hypoglycemia should monitor vital signs and laboratory values closely. The nurse is an ideal person to ensure coordinated care from multiple disciplines. Parents need to be kept well informed throughout hospitalization. They may require encouragement and education about how to ask questions, assert their needs, and be their children's advocates. Current support systems for parents should be evaluated, and any necessary alterations should be suggested. If genetic cause of the deficiency is suspected, the family needs referral to a genetic center for evaluation and counseling.

The use of biosynthetic GH, prepared by recombinant DNA technology, may be indicated. Parents need to be taught how to administer GH subcutaneously and how to give other hormonal supplements as ordered. Treatment with biosynthetic human GH is associated with a transient decrease in the percentage of B lymphocytes and T lymphocytes. For this reason, the primary caretakers must be instructed to notify the physician in charge of GH replacement therapy if the child has significant problems with recurring infections. Such teaching includes not only how and when to give medication but also how to recognize adverse side effects and signs and symptoms of toxicity. They also need telephone numbers of the local poison control center and health care professionals.

The patient's response to this therapy is typically reevaluated at the end of six to twelve months. Desired growth is a doubling of or an increase of 3 cm/year beyond the pretreatment growth pattern. GH is usually not reimbursed by insurance. Caution is advised as to its arbitrary use in short but otherwise healthy children.

Hormone replacement is often a long-term need. The importance of compliance with medication therapy may need to be stressed repeatedly. Often support groups are a significant benefit to the therapeutic regime, family adaptation, and awareness of research efforts. MAGIC (Major Aspects of Growth in Children) Foundation is a national, nonprofit organization specific to growth disorders.

Syndrome of Inappropriate Antidiuretic Hormone (SIADH)

The survival rate of infants at high risk has greatly increased; the need for optimal management has increased concurrently. Infants with Respiratory Distress Syndrome (RDS) and pulmonary disease, periventricular or intraventricular hemorrhage, meningitis, or perinatal asphyxia are at greatest risk for the development of problems associated with antidiuretic hormone (ADH) and renal function, affecting fluid and electrolyte imbalances. Fluid and electrolyte balance is one of the most critical and challenging issues faced in the neonatal intensive care unit environment. The goal of homeostasis of all physiologic functions requires a strong understanding of the neonate's complex body systems in order that supportive therapy may be successful.

The endocrine system, along with the autonomic nervous system, functions to maintain metabolic stability by compensating during times of stress, such as in the case of asphyxia. The kidney carries out the role of maintaining fluid and electrolyte balance by means of hormonal feedback mechanisms in response to osmoreceptors.

Physiology of Antidiuretic Hormone. ADH, or vasopressin (arginine vasopressin), is a hormone produced by the hypothalamus and stored in the anterior pituitary gland. It is normally secreted in physiologic states when there is an increase in serum osmolality. The primary function of ADH is to control fluid and electrolyte balance. It contributes to the adaptation to changes in intravascular (extracellular) volume by regulating renal clearance of free water. ADH allows the renal distal tubules to absorb water from the collecting ducts and consequently decrease urine output. Specialized osmoreceptors in the anterior hypothalamus control the release of ADH in response to plasma osmolality. ADH also exerts a modest vasopressor effect on baroreceptors in the left atrium and carotid sinus, thus causing vasoconstriction in response to hypotension. Under normal conditions, the response of the kidney to plasma hypo-osmolality is to concentrate the urine maximally (Table 28-2; Figure 28-1). Hence, disorders that affect the release and actions of ADH are indicative of ineffective maintenance and balance of fluid and electrolytes.

Clinical Manifestations. SIADH is a condition in which there is increased secretion of ADH, which leads to water retention when there is already a low serum osmolar state or relative fluid overload. In this situation, the continued reabsorption of free water leads to plasma hypo-osmolality, hyponatremia, and expanded intravascular volume. Increased plasma volume results in an increased glomerular filtration rate and increased fractional excretion of sodium, further decreasing the sodium concentration. Signs and symptoms associated with SIADH secretion indicate water retention or edema. The most classic signs are low serum osmolality and hyponatremia accompanied by high urine osmolality.

Risk Factors. In the newborn population, the most frequent cause of inappropriate ADH secretion is asphyxia, with signs that include low serum osmolality; low serum potassium, chloride, and calcium levels; high urinary sodium levels in the face of severe hyponatremia; decreased free water clearance; and elevated urine specific gravity. SIADH has been reported in both full-term and preterm infants in association with meningitis, pneumonia, hypoplasia of the anterior pituitary and idiopathic vasopressin secretion, surgical repair of a patent ductus arteriosus, pneumothorax, pain, positive pressure ventilation,

periventricular-intraventricular hemorrhage, and, as mentioned, perinatal asphyxia (Figure 28-2).

Differential Diagnosis. The diagnosis of SIADH assumes normal cardiac output as well as normal renal, adrenal, and thyroid function. Therefore these systems must first be evaluated for normal function before a diagnosis of SIADH can be made. It is based on laboratory findings and the clinical manifestations listed previously.

Collaborative Management. SIADH can mimic and be confused with clinical symptoms of other disorders and is often difficult to diagnose. Collaborative management of the clinical manifestations through early recognition and detection is essential in promoting recovery. The nurse must be familiar with the various conditions that place the neonate at risk for the development of SIADH. Interventions are therefore related to finely tuned assessment skills, with close attention to perinatal history, physical examination, and evaluation of laboratory and clinical data.

A vicious cycle ensues if attempts are made to treat the hyponatremia and fluid imbalance with administration of sodium chloride infusions, because this intervention not only can exacerbate the hypervolemia but also can correct the hyponatremia only briefly because the sodium is quickly lost in the urine. The treatment of choice is fluid restriction, which decreases the availability of free water. Exceptions are if the serum sodium level is less than approximately 120 mEq/L or if neurologic signs such as seizures are present. More rapid elevation of serum tonicity may be achieved with furosemide (Lasix),

TABLE 28-2	Permeability in Presence of Antidiuretic Hormone			
	PERMEABILITY			**Active Transport of Na**
	H$_2$O	**Urea**	**NaCl**	
Loop of Henle				
Thin descending limb	4+	+	±	0
Thin ascending limb	0	3+	4+	0
Thick ascending limb	0	±	±	4+
Distal convoluted tubule	±	±	±	3+
Collecting tubule				
Cortical portion	3+*	0	±	2+
Outer medullary portion	3+*	0	±	1+
Intermedullary portion	3+	3+	±	1+

Values indicated by asterisks are in the presence of vasopressin. These values are 1+ in absence of vasopressin.
Adapted from Kokko, JP (1979, February). Renal concentrating and diluting mechanisms. Hospital practice, 14(2), 113.

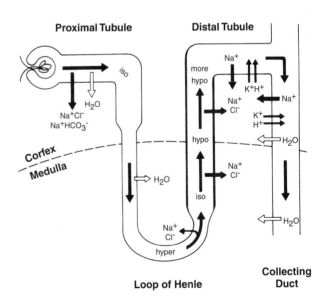

FIGURE **28-1**
Tubular reabsorption and secretion. Summary of changes in the osmolality of tubular fluid in various parts of the nephron. The thickened wall of the ascending limb of the loop of Henle indicates relative impermeability of the tubular epithelium to water. In the presence of vasopressin, the fluid in the collecting ducts becomes hypertonic, whereas in the absence of this hormone, the fluid remains hypotonic throughout the collecting duct. Aldosterone promotes reabsorption of Na$^+$ and secretion of H$^+$ and K$^+$ in the distal convoluted tubule. From Cannon PJ (1977). The kidney in heart failure. *New England journal of medicine*, 296(1), 26-32. Copyright © 1977, Massachusetts Medical Society.

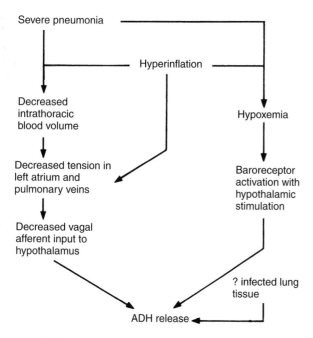

FIGURE **28-2**
Possible mechanism of origin for syndrome of inappropriate antidiuretic hormone, ruling out pneumonia. From Rivers RPA et al (1981). Inappropriate secretion of ADH in infants with respiratory infections. *Archives of disease in childhood,* 56(5), 361.

1 mg/kg intravenously every 6 hours, whereas urinary sodium is replaced milliequivalent for milliequivalent with hypertonic saline (3% solution). This therapy results in accelerated loss of free water with no net change in total body sodium. Fluid restriction alone should be relied on only after the serum sodium level exceeds 120 mEq/L.

Overall responsibility involves a high degree of sensitivity to infants at risk. The signs of SIADH include the following (values vary according to institution):

Hyponatremia	Serum sodium levels <135 mEq
Serum hypo-osmolality	Serum osmolality <275 mOsm
Urine hyperosmolality	Urine osmolality >1000 mOsm
High urine sodium	Urine sodium levels >220 mEq/ 24 hours

Appropriate collaborative actions or interventions include (1) monitoring urine output; (2) maintaining intravenous fluids; (3) monitoring urine specific gravity and dipsticks with every void every 4 hours; (4) monitoring laboratory data and documenting the results of the renal panel serum and urine osmolarity and urine electrolytes; (5) notifying the physician or nurse practitioner of urine volumes that exceed the fluid intake and adjusting the intravenous fluids accordingly; and (6) monitoring for signs and symptoms of water intoxication. The signs and symptoms of water intoxication include irritability, lethargy, seizure activity, or a change in neurologic examination results or reflex activity. Bringing the delicate fluid and electrolyte balance of the infant with water intoxication back into control presents a challenge. It requires a diligent effort at collaborative care.

Thyroid Gland
Development. The first endocrine gland to appear during embryologic development is the thyroid gland. It begins to de-

velop about 25 days after conception. The thyroid evolves from a thickening of epithelial cells at the base of the tongue. As the embryo grows and elongates, the thyroid gland grows a downward duct called a diverticulum. The diverticulum divides into the right and left lobes, which are connected by an isthmus that lies anterior to the developing second and third tracheal ring. By 7 weeks' gestation, the thyroid gland has reached its anatomic position in the neck.

The thyroid gland is an H-shaped structure located below the larynx in the anterior middle portion of the neck. It is composed of many sac-like structures called follicles. These follicles are filled with a secretory substance called colloid, which consists largely of thyroglobulin, a glycoprotein-iodine complex.

Function. Thyroid function is apparent by 11 to 12 weeks' gestation. The thyroid has the ability at this time to accumulate and concentrate the iodine that is being produced. Synthesis of T_4 and iodine occur by 14 weeks' gestation. Secretion of the thyroid hormones is under hypothalamic pituitary control. The hypothalamus secretes thyrotropin-releasing factor (TRF), which promotes release of thyroid-stimulating hormone (TSH) from the pituitary gland. TSH, in turn, stimulates the production of the actual thyroid hormones. The placenta is permeable to limited but significant levels of maternal thyroid hormones. The integrity of the maternal-placental-fetal circulation is critical to the transport of iodine, the substrate for thyroid hormone synthesis in the fetus (Deacon & O'Neill, 1999).

Physiologic Action of Thyroid Hormones. The principal functions of the thyroid gland are to synthesize, store, and release the thyroid hormones triiodothyronine (T_3) and thyroxine (T_4) into the circulating blood. T_3 and T_4 can be studied together because T_4 is the prohormone (stimulating hormone) for T_3. T_3, however, accounts for only 20% of the thyroid hormones in the blood, yet it is the more potent of the two (Deacon & O'Neill, 1999).

The thyroid hormones stimulate the rate of cellular oxidation, which leads to a higher oxygen consumption and production of heat. The thyroid hormones affect protein, carbohydrate, and calcium metabolism. They also incorporate creatinine into the phosphocreatine cycle. Of major influence is sufficient levels of thyroid hormones for normal brain development and for the growth and differentiation of the skeletal and pulmonary tissues.

Transport of Hormones. Nearly all thyroid hormones bind to three major proteins that transport them through the bloodstream: (1) thyroxine-binding globulin (TBG); (2) thyroxine-binding prealbumin; and (3) albumin. The binding of thyroid hormones by serum proteins is important for both physiologic and clinical reasons. Changes in binding protein concentrations or binding affinity can drastically change the total concentration of T_3 and T_4 measured in the serum. When TBG, thyroxine-binding prealbumin, and albumin are normally present in the blood, they reduce the unbound (free) thyroid hormones. Because the free hormone fraction is metabolically active, these binding proteins can exert a major influence on the thyroid gland. However, increases or decreases in serum T_3 or T_4 cannot be said to reflect an alteration in thyroid function until both the T_4-binding capacity and the level of free hormones have been estimated. These binding proteins appear to be involved in the transport of the thyroid hormones but not in facilitating transfer of these hormones into the cell.

Factors Altering Thyroid Hormone–Binding Capacity. In humans, TBG may be congenitally absent, reduced, or even elevated. Alterations in TBG levels can be sporadic or familial. Pedigree studies have shown that the TBG resides on the X chromosome. There is no male-to-male transmission; female offspring or affected males are carriers of this trait, and affected males show full expression of this defect.

Thyroid Hormone Levels in Newborns. The delivery process in the healthy, full-term infant creates a transient increase in TSH, which is believed to be mediated by TRH secretion in response to the cold extrauterine environment and ligation of the umbilical cord. This is accompanied by a sudden rise in T_3 and T_4 levels, followed by a decline over the next several days.

Neonatal serum TSH increases from mean cord serum values of 9 mU/ml to a mean peak of 85 mU/ml within 30 minutes after delivery. The placenta is impermeable to the passage of thyroid hormones from mother to fetus. Thus the fetal hypothalamic pituitary–thyroid system appears to be independent of the maternal system. However, TRH is capable of crossing the placental barrier, thus producing some effects on the fetus. One of these effects is suppression of the fetal thyroid hormone production. With this knowledge, mass screening programs for recognition of neonatal hypothyroidism have been established and used on cord blood or neonatal heel blood.

Thyroid Screening. T_3 levels have been found to be increased in amniotic fluid early in pregnancy and to decrease gradually to cord serum concentrations, which are still higher than maternal values at term. The possible use of amniotic fluid T_3 or cord serum as a diagnostic tool has been proposed. Premature infants often have low levels of T_4 in comparison to the normal range for full-term infants. This condition is referred to as transient hypothyroidism. Serious illness is also associated with low T_4 values. In infants with gestations of fewer than 30 weeks, low levels of TBG may be present. After 30 weeks, TBG has reached the level present at term and therefore does not account for low levels of T_4. Cord blood levels of T_4 range from 6 to 15 mg/dl.

Thyroid Function Tests. Total T_4 ranges from 7.1 to 22.7 mg/dl during the first few months of life. Values vary in infants and children. Values accepted as within normal limits also vary by institution.

Congenital Hypothyroidism
Pathophysiology. Abnormal embryologic development of the thyroid gland is the most common cause of congenital hypothyroidism, which includes the absence of the thyroid gland or the lack of development of the thyroid (ectopic). Other factors that may resent a clinical picture of hypothyroidism include errors of metabolism or synthesis of thyroid hormone, defects of the hypothalamus or pituitary gland, maternal autoimmune thyroid disorders, and interference from certain maternal medications. Transient hypothyroidism may also occur in preterm infants in response to certain therapeutic agents, such as topical disinfectants, ointments, and contrast media. Occurrence of congenital or neonatal hypothyroidism is reported to be 1 in 4000 live births, with a 2:1 female/male ratio (Deacon & O'Neill, 1999).

Clinical Manifestations. The infant is usually more than 42 weeks' gestational age with a birth weight greater than 4000 g and may have a large posterior fontanel because of delayed ossification. There may also be respiratory difficulty from goiter compression. Hypothermia is another concern because thyroid hormones assist in thermoregulation. The infant may appear lethargic and hypotonic and have difficulty feeding as well as delayed passage of meconium. Abdominal distention may be present because of slowed gastric and intestinal motility, thus contributing to prolonged hyperbilirubinemia and constipation. If associated with hypopituitarism, midline defects—such as cleft lip and palate, micropenis, and hypoglycemia—may be present. Gland enlargement (goiter) may occur if thyroid tissue is present but synthesis or metabolism defects exist (Deacon & O'Neill, 1999). There may be an elongated nasal bridge, enlarged tongue, and hoarse cry. These symptoms are directly related to the function of the thyroid and its effect, along with GH, on bone maturation, calcium regulation, temperature regulation, and metabolic rate. A general slowdown of body functions, including a shutdown or slowdown in terms of temperature, occurs. Symptoms of transient hypothyroidism are often absent of the classical features.

Differential Diagnosis. To make a diagnosis of congenital hypothyroidism, blood is drawn for determination of serum T_3, T_4, and TSH levels. Such measurements have become part of comprehensive metabolic screening that is now law in many states and follows recommendations of the American Academy of Pediatrics. Most institutions use the filter paper spot technique, whereby a capillary blood sample from the heel is taken and placed on round filter paper to measure T_4 levels. Abnormal results often occur if blood is drawn within the first 24 hours of life, thus necessitating repeat testing at a later date—usually the first or second week of life. Further testing to confirm abnormal screening values include determination of serum T_4 and TSH as well as free T_4 and T_3, neck ultrasonography, and thyroid radionuclide imaging (Deacon & O'Neill, 1999). Long bone radiographs aid in diagnosis by determining whether the characteristic pattern of scattered bone growth centers are visible; if so, this finding indicates hypothyroidism. This picture is in contrast to one central location of growth normally found at the epiphyseal plate.

Collaborative Management. The goal of treatment is to establish a euthyroid state as soon as possible. Two types of thyroid hormones are available. One type, derived from the extracts of pork and beef, is not used as often as the other type, synthetic thyroid hormones. Thyroid extracts contain 0.21% iodide. Synthetic hormones are available as a sodium salt of L-thyroxine (levothyroxine sodium) and L-triiodothyronine (liothyronine sodium). The latter is more potent than the former, and its intestinal absorption is more complete. In the long run, it is preferable to use levothyroxine because the effects last long (blood TSH levels remain constant); thus it need be given orally only twice a day. The cost of the synthetic hormone, which was once high, is now much reduced. The dose of thyroid hormone prescribed should be adequate to regulate metabolic functions. The T_4 level should increase rapidly to ensure a euthyroid level of this hormone. The dose of levothyroxine during the newborn period is 8 to 10 mg/kg/day for most full-term infants. The goal of treatment is to maintain serum T_4 at 10 to 16 micrograms per deciliter (Fisher & Polk, 1995). The prognosis for mental development has been correlated with the onset of hormone replacement therapy. Delay in instituting hormone replacement therapy or noncompliance with its administration leads to moderate to severe developmental delays. Parents and caregivers need to be informed of the dire consequences associated with the infants not receiving their medication.

Over the first few days after the initiation of replacement therapy, observations must be made for overtreatment problems. Among those are tachycardia, arrhythmias, irritability, hyperactivity, diarrhea, poor weight gain, and long-term premature ossification and thyrotoxicosis. The desired clinical picture is of an infant who becomes more active with normalization of body temperature as therapeutic levels are reached. Monitoring of growth parameters is crucial because this may be the only indication that treatment is truly successful.

Congenital Hyperthyroidism

Neonatal hyperthyroidism is serious and potentially life-threatening. The infant may be born with a very small goiter or even a small thyroid gland. Serum T_4 levels may be low, normal, or even high at birth, depending on the degree of in utero thyroid suppression. Most often, this neonatal thyrotoxicosis is due to maternal Graves' disease. The condition may be temporary in the neonatal period.

Infant of a Hyperthyroid Mother. Maternal hyperthyroidism is present in 1 in 500 pregnancies. This hyperthyroidism creates a great threat to the unborn fetus because of an increase in spontaneous abortions as well as premature births. After the first trimester, the maternal-fetal pituitary–thyroid axes are independent. T_3, T_4, and TSH do not cross the placenta, but antibodies in the form of immunoglobulin G do cross the placental barrier. These antibodies act on the thyroid gland of the fetus, thus increasing thyroid function and GH. The hyperthyroid state occurs as the passage of these antibodies increases during the second and third trimesters of pregnancy. Maternal antithyroid medications and stable iodine can also affect the fetus and neonate. These substances are very effective therapies for both mother and fetus. Nonetheless, they can also result in adverse fetal effects. Therefore the use of stable iodine in pregnant women is contraindicated because of the blockage of fetal thyroid hormone release, which, in turn, leads to hypothyroidism and goiter. Excess dosage of maternal antithyroid medications is also likely to cause fetal and neonatal hypothyroidism.

Differential Diagnosis. The diagnosis of fetal and neonatal hyperthyroidism is determined by the presence of maternal thyroid-stimulating antibodies and clinical manifestations. Elevations of calcium, free T_4 and T_3 are noted unless the mother's Graves disease is treated.

Clinical Manifestations. Heart rates of 160 bpm or greater, goiter, intrauterine growth retardation, mature bone growth greater than expected for gestational age, and craniosynostosis are the common signs and symptoms of hyperthyroidism. Hyperactivity, hyperthermia and increased GI motility may also be observed. Ocular signs may include exophthalmos, eye staring, and lid retractions.

These neonates also experience fatigue and exhaustion owing to the hypermetabolic state and use of energy stores. Diarrhea may result because of increased peristalsis, thus leading to even more loss of nutrients as well as fluids. Heat intolerance and profound diaphoresis are side effects of the increased basal metabolic rate. Another feature of these infants is an eye malformation called exophthalmos. This condition is a concern

because of the inability of the infant's eyelid to close completely. The cornea dries, and abrasions are possible from normal eye and lid movements.

Treatment. The overall objective of therapy is to restore and maintain a euthyroid state. This can be achieved in a variety of ways. No single therapy is ideal. One technique is to use medications that interfere with thyroid hormone synthesis. Methimazole and carbimazole are used throughout the United States. These drugs decrease the active transport of iodine into the thyroid gland. Propranolol is given to the severely hyperthyroid infant to reduce heart rate and lessen tremors. This drug is generally used in the first week of replacement therapy. In some cases digitalization and sedation may be necessary to treat neurologic symptoms.

If medical treatment is not chosen as a mode to restore the infant to a euthyroid state or if the treatment is not effective, surgical removal of part or all of the thyroid gland is possible. However, hypothyroidism may result even if only a small portion of the thyroid is removed.

Radioiodine treatment is another alternative treatment. Beta emissions cause local tissue damage. The radiation dose given is dependent on the individual mass and geometry of the thyroid gland. Reservations about the use of radioiodine therapy in children relate to concerns about the development of thyroid carcinoma or leukemia during adulthood. Damage to the thymus gland, a major immune organ in the neonate, is possible, which leaves the neonate vulnerable to infections.

Collaborative Management. The disease process of hyperthyroidism results in increased metabolic demands (Avery et al, 1999). These infants need a higher caloric intake, often greater than 180 kcal/kg/day (up from about 100 to 120 kcal/kg/day) to maintain positive growth. Providing adequate nutrition with sufficient caloric intake is essential to the well being of these infants. Propranolol may be used to decrease the heart rate and to combat the occurrence of heart failure (Avery et al, 1999).

Lubricating drops or ointment should be used to protect the eye from damage. Head positioning to protect and maintain a patent airway is critical when an enlarged thyroid is present. It is essential that accurate intake and output be documented every 4 hours and that weights be obtained daily in these infants. Head circumference and growth curve determinations should be performed at least weekly. The parents need to understand that thyroid therapy for either hypothyroidism or hyperthyroidism is a lifelong commitment.

Diabetes

Infant of a Diabetic Mother

Maternal Considerations. During pregnancy, a woman experiences increasing levels of estrogen and progesterone. This hormonal increase stimulates pancreatic beta cell hyperplasia and increases the secretion of insulin. This pancreatic beta cell hyperplasia continues as the pregnancy progresses. Pregnant women with diabetes also experience these hormonal changes that make managing their glucose levels more difficult (Gilbert & Harmon, 2003).

Gestational diabetes occurs during pregnancy and is usually self-limited to the pregnancy. It occurs in 2% to 3% of pregnancies (Sills & Rapaport, 1994). Proper screening during pregnancy is essential for all women to monitor accurately for glucose intolerance. One must be aware of certain risk factors that may predispose a woman to gestational diabetes. These risk factors include a previous pregnancy with gestational diabetes, obesity, or a previous infant macrosomatia seen by ultrasonography, maternal glycosuria, or uterine size larger than normal for gestational date.

The severity of maternal diabetes and the duration of the disease contribute to how the infant may be affected. The severity of maternal diabetes can be determined by using White's Classification of the Diabetic Disease Process. (See the White Classification on page 27, in Chapter 12.)

Class A: Gestational diabetic; controlled by diet

Class B: Onset after age 20; duration >10 years

Class C: Onset age 10 to 19; duration 10 to 19 years

Class D: Onset before age 10; duration <20 years; retinitis; hypertension; calcification in the lower extremities

Class F: Nephropathy

Class R: Malignant retinitis

Class H: Heart complications, often over age 35 with early age onset of diabetes, 50% obstetrical maternal mortality; necessitates insulin therapy

Class T: Postrenal transplantation; necessitates insulin therapy

No matter what the maternal class, the fetus is at risk for many problems. These problems include spontaneous abortion, stillbirth, cephalopelvic disproportion (CPD), asphyxia, respiratory distress, hypoglycemia, macrosomatia, congenital anomalies, hypocalcemia, hypomagnesemia, hyperbilirubinemia, and polycythemia. The morbidity of these problems can be diminished with good prenatal care and proper glucose regulation during the antenatal and intrapartum periods. Maintaining glucose control before conception or early in the pregnancy is essential for the woman with insulin-dependent diabetes mellitus. This control offers the infant a better chance for a positive outcome. One of the major neonatal problems is a labile glucose level.

Fetal and Neonatal Risks

Hypoglycemia.   Hypoglycemia is signified by a blood glucose level less than 35 mg/dl for the full-term infant and less than 25 mg/dl for the preterm infant. (McKenna, 2000). The fetus is exposed to large amounts of glucose, as maternal glucose readily crosses the placenta. Glucose content of the amniotic fluid in diabetic women is higher than normal. The reason for this increase is that insulin is a larger molecule than glucose, and it does not cross the placenta easily, so maternal glucose levels are mirrored with the neonatal system and amniotic fluid.

This maternal hyperglycemia leads to fetal hyperglycemia. Because maternal insulin does not cross the placenta, elevated glucose levels stimulate the fetal pancreas to secrete insulin. This stimulation also leads to hyperplasia of the beta cells and increased production of insulin, which continues after delivery. Insulin is the main growth hormone for the fetus, so this hyperinsulinemia leads to fat accumulation and macrosomatia.

Because of this hyperinsulinism and then the loss of maternal glucose at delivery, the infant can become hypoglycemic within a few hours after delivery and must be monitored closely. Common signs of hypoglycemia are jitteriness, cyanosis, irritability, seizures, and apnea. Serum glucose levels need to be monitored frequently. Giving the infant early feedings or intravenous fluids to maintain a proper glucose level may be necessary.

Macrosomatia.   According to Schwartz and associates (1994), despite better control of glucose levels in the pregnant woman with diabetes, macrosomatia (birth weight >4 kg for a full-term infant) continues to occur at a high rate. It is felt that this is a result of fetal hyperinsulinemia.

The infant of a diabetic mother has a characteristic appearance. These infants are large-for-gestational-age with increased adipose tissue, have a full face liberally covered with vernix, and are plethoric. The placenta and umbilical cord are also large.

Growth acceleration is especially apparent in infants of mothers with poorly controlled diabetes. These infants have a smaller head circumference to weight ratio and a larger weight to length ratio. Infants of diabetic mothers can experience CPD, leading to difficult deliveries secondary to their size. Birth trauma includes brachial plexus trauma, fractured clavicle, facial palsy, shoulder dystocia, asphyxia, and subdural hemorrhage. One must also be prepared for birth asphyxia resulting from CPD. The mother's ability to deliver vaginally must be assessed, and cesarean sections must be performed for CPD to avert complications.

Respiratory Distress Syndrome (RDS).   Also known as hyaline membrane disease, RDS is a disease in which there is a decreased amount of surfactant. This lack of surfactant leads to alveolar collapse and an inability to ventilate adequately. Pulmonary surfactant is a lipoprotein produced by alveolar type II epithelial cells. After formation, it is secreted into the alveolar space, where it forms a film that covers the alveolar surface and creates the needed surface tension to maintain alveolar expansion.

Recent research has shown that the pregnant diabetic woman may have a disorder in the production of the lipoprotein. Lung development in the infant of a diabetic mother is related to the pregnant woman's glucose control during the pregnancy (Zapata et al, 1994). Hyperinsulinemia influences the fetal lung maturity in infants of diabetic mothers by inhibiting the fetal lung synthesis of surfactant.

Zapata and associates (1994) conducted a study that observed the association between the presence of hypoglycemic episodes and fetal lung maturity. They found a significant association between episodes of hypoglycemia during the pregnancy and improved fetal lung maturity. The hypoglycemia acts as a stressor and accelerates the maturation of the fetal lung.

Studies have shown that with advances and proper management of diabetic mothers and their infants, RDS is not as much a problem as it once was. One still must be aware of the chance for respiratory distress. Some women with poor diabetes control or poor prenatal care are at risk for having infants with RDS secondary to surfactant deficiency and not gestational age.

Hypocalcemia and Hypomagnesemia.   Hypocalcemia and hypomagnesemia are major metabolic problems exhibited by infants of diabetic mothers. The incidence is related to the severity of the maternal diabetes; both problems must be followed closely. The symptoms are similar to those seen with hypoglycemia.

Hypocalcemia develops within the first 3 days of life and is seen primarily in the infant of the insulin-dependent diabetic mother. It is thought that hypocalcemia may be secondary to decreased hypoparathyroid functioning that results from hypomagnesemia. The infant should be observed for hypocalcemia and hypomagnesemia and treated as needed.

Hyperbilirubinemia and Polycythemia.   Hyperbilirubinemia is a common occurrence in the infant of a diabetic mother. Most infants of diabetic mothers have the unconjugated form of bilirubin circulating in their systems. This finding suggests an impairment of the glucuronidation system. Hyperbilirubinemia may also be related to decreased albumin levels, thus leaving less albumin available for binding bilirubin.

Polycythemia is also often observed in infants of diabetic mothers. The infant with polycythemia may exhibit signs and symptoms such as jitteriness, tachypnea, cyanosis, priapism, and oliguria. Treatment is usually a partial exchange transfusion using normal saline, plasma protein fraction (Plasmanate), or 5% albumin.

A complication of polycythemia that occurs frequently in infants of diabetic mothers is renal vein thrombosis. Signs include hematuria and a palpable renal mass. Renal vein thrombosis is usually treated medically, but on rare occasions a nephrectomy may be required.

Congenital Anomalies.   The most significant source of morbidity and mortality in the infant of a diabetic mother is major congenital anomalies. It is thought that hyperglucosemia that occurs early in pregnancy is teratogenic. Preconceptual glucose control is essential because anomalies may occur before the woman knows she is pregnant. Many of these defects occur before the seventh week of gestation as a result of maternal hyperglycemia, which inhibits cellular mitosis, thus resulting in anomalies (Hitti et al, 1994; Novak & Robinson, 1994).

A correlation exists between the occurrence of congenital anomalies and high glycosylated hemoglobin levels. The most common anomalies involve the cardiac, musculoskeletal, and central nervous systems. The occurrence of congenital heart disease in the infant of a diabetic mother can be as high as five times that of normal infants. Atrial or ventricular septal defects, transposition of the great vessels, and coarctation of the aorta are the most common heart lesions seen.

Hitti and associates (1994) found an increase in the frequency of skeletal malformations. These infants are at risk for delayed ossification and osseous defects. Caudal regression syndrome is a common malformation, as is agenesis or hypoplasia of the femur. Central nervous system anomalies include hydrocephalus, meningomyelocele, and anencephaly. These areas of development are usually completed by the seventh week after conception.

Another congenital defect is the small left colon syndrome. This syndrome does not occur very often, and there is not much known about it. A possible cause is a spasm of the ileum as a result of high glucagon levels. It usually resolves spontaneously early in the neonate's life without the need for surgical intervention. Maintaining hydration and gastric decompression is necessary, as is monitoring for infection. Once feedings are initiated, the infant should be observed closely for bowel obstruction.

Collaborative Management.   The nurse, in collaboration with the health care team, needs to observe the infant of a diabetic mother closely after delivery to provide quick intervention if problems arise. The infant of a diabetic mother must be monitored for signs and symptoms of hypoglycemia to prevent adverse effects on the central nervous system. These include jitteriness, extreme hunger (sucking vigorously on hands and fingers), diaphoresis, cyanosis, tachypnea, lethargy, seizures, and apnea. Serum glucose levels must be monitored frequently until they are stable at 80 to 120 mg/dl. After delivery, the glucose level must be monitored at least every hour until it has stabilized. Hypoglycemia is classified as glucose levels less than 30 mg/dl for the term infant, 20 mg/dl for the preterm infant, and 40 mg/dl for any infant who is showing signs and symptoms of hypoglycemia. If the infant's condition is stable, early feedings should be given. Intravenous fluids of 10% dextrose in water at 6 to 8 mg/kg/minute should be started for the infant un-

able to take oral feedings. If the glucose levels remain low, administering an intravenous bolus of dextrose may be necessary with a concentration no greater than $D_{10}W$. Administration of more concentrated dextrose solutions may cause rebound hypoglycemia. Failure to achieve stable glucose levels may require pharmacologic and/or surgical intervention.

Diazoxide has become a first line drug for treatment of hyperinsulinemia. The drug inhibits secretion of insulin and promotes mobilization of glycogen stores. Diazoxide has met with high clinical success with stabilization of serum glucose levels achieved within 24 to 48 hours. Dosage is started at 10 to 15 mg/kg/day in two to three divided doses and then is titrated to achieve the desired serum level of glucose. Fluid imbalance is a significant adverse effect but is usually manageable with chlorothiazide (Kistler & Spiering, 1998; Stanley, 1997).

Glucagon may be administered IM, IV, or SQ. Rebound hyperglycemia is a significant side effect; thus its use is discouraged except for emergency situations when IV access is denied (McKenna, 2000). Octreotide, which inhibits release of pancreatic hormones from islet cells and of growth hormone, is another alternative medication. When pharmacologic interventions fail, removal of the organ (partial or near total, up to 95% of the organ) may be necessary. Following surgical intervention, medications are needed to manage glucose levels for the patient's lifetime.

The infant should be monitored for any signs of birth trauma, such as brachial plexus damage or a fractured clavicle, especially in the macrosomic infant. If decreased movement is noted in an arm or if the infant cries when an extremity is moved, a radiograph should be obtained to look for a fracture. If a fracture is present, the affected extremity should be stabilized and an orthopedic consultation obtained. Bottle-feeding may be difficult for the macrosomic infant. These infants have weaker reflex functioning and poor motor behavior during the first 2 days of life.

When caring for an infant of a diabetic mother in whom there was poor glucose control during pregnancy, the nurse should be observant for the possibility of respiratory distress. Treatment should be the same as for other infants with RDS. No special considerations for treatment are needed.

The infant also needs to be monitored for hypocalcemia and hypomagnesemia. The signs, such as jitteriness or lethargy, usually appear within the first 3 days of life and are similar to those seen in hypoglycemia (Chapter 24). If these signs persist after glucose levels are stabilized, blood levels of calcium and magnesium should be obtained and supplementation given as needed.

A spun hematocrit should be carried out to assess for polycythemia. A partial exchange transfusion may need to be performed for a central hematocrit greater than 65%. The infant may need to be given phototherapy for treatment of hyperbilirubinemia. The infant also needs to be monitored for any congenital anomalies. Appropriate actions should be taken depending on the type of anomaly.

Many of the problems that occur are transient and resolve within a few days. For infants who are affected more severely, it is imperative that the parents be given the support and education needed for these problems. Counseling on further pregnancies may also be required.

Many problems can occur with infants of diabetic mothers. Proper screening, good prenatal care, and aggressive management of maternal diabetes decrease morbidity and mortality in these infants.

Ambiguous Genitalia

When the sperm fertilizes the ovum at conception, the genetic sex of the embryo is determined. However, during the first 7 weeks of gestation, the primitive gonads contain both ovarian (cortical) and testicular (medullary) components (Avery et al, 1999), thus creating a "bipotential environment" in which either gender's characteristics may emerge. This initial stage of "sexual indifference" lasts until the seventh week of gestation, when the gonads, which are the future testes or ovaries, begin to acquire sexual characteristics. The determining factor in sexual differentiation involves not only genetic information contained within the original X and Y sex chromosome combination but also a number of additional components, including hormonal and environmental influences. Failure to achieve sexual differentiation owing to defective gene expression or abnormal external influences, or both, may result in the congenital anomaly of ambiguous genitalia. This anomaly may occur as a single manifestation or as part of a larger syndrome.

Although most conditions that result in ambiguous genitalia are not life-threatening (with the exception of the salt-wasting form of congenital adrenal hyperplasia), it is vitally important that early diagnosis be made and treatment instituted to minimize any negative sequelae and maximize outcome. Prolonged delay in intervention can lead to serious consequences for both patient and family. To gain a better understanding of ambiguous genitalia, it is helpful to know the normal development and sexual differentiation of the embryo.

Normal Embryologic Development and Sexual Differentiation.   Normal sexual differentiation is contingent on the successful development of the genital system. Development and differentiation occur at three levels: the gonads, the internal genital ducts, and the external genitalia (Figure 28-3). This orderly sequence of events takes place early in fetal development.

Near the fifth week of gestation, the gonads begin to develop with primordial germ cell migration to the urogenital ridge. The indifferent gonad consists of both male germ cells at the inner medullary position and female germ cells at the outer cortical position. The chromosomal sex determined at fertilization directs the development of the gonad into either a testis or an ovary. The medulla differentiates into a testis, whereas the cortex regresses in an embryo with XY chromosomal makeup; the cortex differentiates into an ovary, whereas the medulla regresses in an XX chromosomal embryo.

At 7 to 8 weeks of gestation, the fetus possesses two pairs of genital ducts: the mesonephric (or wolffian) ducts and the paramesonephric (or mullerian) ducts. Development of these ducts into male or female internal structures depends on the release or nonrelease of specific hormones, respectively. At this time, the male testes produce and release two hormones: a masculinizing androgen hormone (testosterone) and a müllerian-inhibiting substance (MIS). Testosterone stimulates the development of the mesonephric ducts to form the male genital tract, including the epididymis, vas deferens, seminal vesicles, and ejaculatory ducts. The MIS causes regression of the paramesonephric ducts, which would have developed into female reproductive structures. In the absence of these hormones, the female fetus develops the paramesonephric ducts into female internal genitalia, including fallopian tubes, uterus, cervix, and upper vagina. In addition, the mesonephric ducts regress in the female fetus. Thus the male testis is active in producing hormones for sexual differentiation, whereas the female ovary has a passive role in sexual differentiation.

During the 7th through 16th weeks of gestation, the external genitalia differentiate. In the presence of testosterone in the male fetus, virilization of the genital tubercle occurs, producing a penis. The ureteral folds fuse and form the anterior urethra while the genital swellings fuse and form the scrotum. The urogenital sinus develops to form the prostate. In the absence of testosterone in the female fetus, the genital swellings form the labia minora and labia majora, respectively. The urogenital sinus develops to form the lower vagina.

It is important to emphasize that sexual differentiation of both internal and external genitalia occurs in a fixed sequence at specific critical periods of development. If there are abnormal circulating androgens during the differentiation period of the female external genitalia, varying degrees of virilization may occur, thus resulting in urogenital sinus fusion and clitoral enlargement. In addition, lack of substantial MIS hormone in the male fetus may not adequately suppress the paramesonephric ducts, and subsequent female internal structures may develop. It is evident that a wide variety of sexual differentiation abnormalities may occur in the fetus. Some conditions result in evident ambiguous genitalia at birth, whereas others may not be detected until puberty. Basic knowledge of

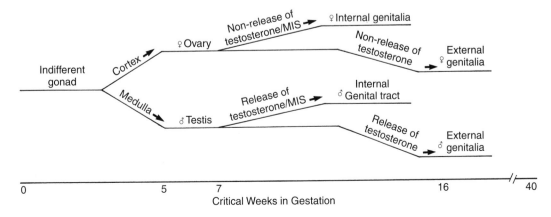

FIGURE **28-3**
Sexual differentiation in the developing fetus.

these categories aids the nurse in the assessment and management of these individuals.

Abnormal Sexual Differentiation.

The more common disorders of sexual differentiation can be categorized into two generalized groups: congenital adrenal hyperplasia (CAH) and disorders of gonadal differentiation (Box 28-2). The most common cause of ambiguous genitalia in the newborn is CAH, but not all patients with the disorder show sexual ambiguity. The same is true for disorders of gonadal differentiation.

Congenital Adrenal Hyperplasia.

CAH is an autosomal recessive inborn error of metabolism that affects male and female fetuses equally. It is estimated that from 1 in 5,000 to 1 in 15,000 births result in CAH. Affected female infants often present with some degree of virilization of the external genitalia, but the internal female structures remain normal. Conversely, few male infants show any genital anomalies and the condition may go unrecognized until later infancy or childhood.

Pathophysiology. The adrenal cortex consists of three regions: the outer zona glomerulosa, the middle fasciculata, and the inner zona reticularis, which adjoins the adrenal medulla. The reticularis, however, does not complete differentiation until about 3 years of age. There are three classes of hormones produced by the adrenal gland: mineralocorticoids, glucocorticoids, and sex steroids. Specific enzymes are necessary for the biosynthesis of these hormones. Adrenocorticotropic hormone (ACTH) stimulates the adrenal gland to produce the steroids. When sufficient quantities are released into the bloodstream, ACTH is turned off by a negative feedback mechanism.

Many forms of CAH exist. Abnormally high ACTH levels with low plasma cortisol levels are pathognomonic of all forms of CAH. Each type is the result of a separate enzyme deficiency necessary for production of a particular steroid. No matter which form of CAH is operating, a deficiency in cortisol results. This deficiency, in turn, prohibits the natural negative feedback loop necessary to turn off pituitary secretion of ACTH. Thus ACTH continues to stimulate the adrenal gland to synthesize and secrete deficient steroids, and adrenal hyperplasia ensues.

BOX 28-2

Sexual Differentiation

I. Congenital adrenal hyperplasia
  A. Rare enzyme defects
  B. Nonclassic forms
    1. Nonclassic 21-hydroxylase deficiency
  C. Classic 21-hydroxylase deficiency
II. Disorders of gonadal differentiation
  A. Phenotypic females with abnormal differentiation
    1. Turner's syndrome
    2. Swyer's syndrome
  B. Phenotypic males with abnormal differentiation
    1. Klinefelter's syndrome
    2. XX males
  C. Sexual ambiguity with gonadal dysgenesis
    1. Male pseudohermaphroditism
    2. True hermaphroditism
    3. Leydig cell hypoplasia
    4. Testicular regression syndrome

The types and symptoms of CAH depend on which steroids are deficient and which are produced in excess. To remain within the scope of this text, only the types of CAH typically detected in the neonatal period or early infancy are discussed.

CAH may be separated into three categories: rare enzyme defects, nonclassic forms, and classic forms. The rare enzyme defects may be incompatible with life and are thus rarely seen clinically. The nonclassic forms are usually hidden at birth, with no major developmental abnormalities noted. If signs of the disorder appear at all, they are typically seen later in life. One of the classic forms of CAH, 21-hydroxylase deficiency, is the most common autosomal recessive disorder in humans. Although the nonclassic forms of CAH are more prevalent in the general population, the classic forms are expressed most commonly in the neonatal population.

Clinical Manifestations and Risk Factors in 21-Hydroxylase Deficiency

CAH due to 21-hydroxylase deficiency accounts for 90% to 95% of all cases of CAH. The severe form occurs in 1 in 5,000 to 1 in 14,000 births. A milder form is present in 0.3% of whites and in 1% to 3% of European Jews. The mutated gene responsible for 21-hydroxylase deficiency is located within the HLA complex of genes on the short arm of chromosome 6. Many of the gene deletions that result in 21-hydroxylase deficiency are associated with the haplotype HLA-B47;DR7.

CAH due to 21-hydroxylase deficiency results in a buildup of 17-hydroxyprogesterone that is not converted to 11-deoxycortisol. Without sufficient circulating cortisol, the negative feedback loop to the hypothalamus and pituitary does not operate. Increasing amounts of ACTH continue to be secreted, thus resulting in high levels of circulating androgens. Excess circulating androgens lead to progressive virilism, which begins during prenatal development. Female neonates can present with mild clitoral enlargement with or without labioscrotal folds or, in severe cases, with a penile urethra. Premature female neonates are at risk for delayed diagnosis because prominent clitoris and electrolyte imbalance caused by renal immaturity are not uncommon (Cruz et al, 1995). The increased testosterone does not, however, interfere with normal development of internal genitalia, uterus, or fallopian tubes. Consequently, virilized females have the potential for a normal female reproductive life, complete with childbearing. Androgen excess also contributes to initial rapid skeletal growth with early closure of the epiphyses and consequent short adult stature.

Males with 21-hydroxylase deficiency often appear normal at birth. An enlarged penis with small testicles may be present. The disorder may go unrecognized until precocious puberty develops during later infancy or early childhood. This condition may be seen in the development of early pubic hair, advanced muscular development, and rapid growth. Infertility may result if the condition is not treated.

The classic form of 21-hydroxylase deficiency is the most common presenting CAH disorder. Twenty-five percent of affected newborns have a simple virilizing form. Seventy-five percent of patients with classic 21-hydroxylase deficiency are unable to synthesize adequate aldosterone, which is a necessary component for the transport of sodium ions across cell membranes. A defect in aldosterone biosynthesis results in the inability of the distal and collecting tubules of the kidney to reabsorb sodium. Salt wasting creates high urinary sodium levels. Serum sodium levels drop while serum potassium levels rise. In an effort to increase levels of aldosterone, large amounts of renin are released into the plasma. As a result, circulating angiotensin II is also increased. Despite high levels of the natural vasoconstrictor, blood pressure falls, presumably owing to down-regulation of angiotensin receptors in vascular smooth muscle. Patients with this form of CAH may die in the neonatal period as a result of hyponatremic shock. Rapid diagnosis with accurate treatment is clearly an important goal for these newborns.

Blood spots routinely collected for newborn screening can be used to detect the 17-hydroxyprogesterone concentration. Benefits to earlier diagnosis and treatment include premature pubarche, and prevention of severe adrenal crisis postnatal growth acceleration. Although false-positive results in preterm, sick, or low-birth-weight infants have been reported, it is interesting to note that the male:female ratio of affected individuals detected by screening programs was 1:1. Published case surveys of CAH detected because of symptoms repeatedly report a higher prevalence in females than in males. Male infants with the salt-wasting form of CAH may die early in infancy without the cause being identified. Also, in male patients with the simple virilizing form of CAH, the disorder may be diagnosed later in life or not at all.

Treatment involves replacing deficient cortisol with hydrocortisone or a similar synthetic substitute, such as dexamethasone. In addition, mineralocorticoid replacement is necessary in the salt-wasting form. The goal of hormone replacement therapy is to prevent adrenal crisis, achieve normal growth and development, and suppress excessive androgen production. Supplemental medication must be taken for the duration of the patient's life. Surgical repair of ambiguous genitalia may also be indicated.

3-HYDROXYSTEROID DEHYDROGENASE DEFICIENCY OF CONGENITAL ADRENAL HYPERPLASIA

3-Hydroxysteroid dehydrogenase deficiency is also due to recessive genes that have been mapped to the short arm of chromosome 1. Testosterone, aldosterone, and cortisol levels are all reduced. Males have incomplete prenatal genital development that results from decreased androgen synthesis in the testes as well as in the adrenal gland. Females can experience mild masculinization because of the increased production of a weak androgen that is produced before the deficient enzyme in the hormone biosynthesis pathway of the adrenal gland. The majority of patients with 3-hydroxysteroid dehydrogenase deficiency have varying degrees of salt wasting owing to insufficient aldosterone levels.

11-Hydroxylase Deficiency
The second most common form of CAH is 11-hydroxylase deficiency. The recessive genes involved in this disorder are located on the long arm of chromosome 8. Unlike the other two forms of CAH described, 11-hydroxylase deficiency is distinguished by hypertension, hypokalemia, and sodium retention in the majority of patients. 11-Deoxycortisol is not converted to cortisol, and deoxycorticosterone is usually not converted to corticosterone. Again, because there is deficient cortisol, which acts as a negative feedback to turn off adrenal production of steroids, excess prenatal androgen secretion results in female virilization with normal internal female reproductive organs.

17-Hydroxylase and 17,20-Lyase Deficiency
A defect in the microsomal enzyme $P450_{c17}$, which catalyzes both 17-hydroxylase and 17,20-lyase, is present in both the adrenals and gonads. Consequently, a reduction in all androgens and estrogens results. Males present with pseudohermaph-roditism and gynecomastia. Females express infantile genitalia. Neither male nor female adolescents experience pubertal changes. Hypertension and hypokalemia may develop because of elevated concentrations of deoxycorticosterone. The recessive gene for the $P450_{c17}$ enzyme has been mapped to chromosome 10.

Collaborative Management
Newborns. The degree of female virilization does not indicate the degree of adrenal insufficiency. An endocrinologist and geneticist must evaluate a newborn with ambiguous genitalia. Serum hormone concentrations must be determined, and blood for chromosomal analysis must be drawn. The neonate with confirmed CAH needs to be closely monitored during the first few weeks of life for signs of acute adrenal insufficiency. Replacement hormone therapy may be started when CAH is suspected. At the latest, it needs to be started once a diagnosis is made. Eventually, virilized females can undergo surgical correction.

Emphasis is now placed on prenatal diagnosis and treatment of CAH resulting from 21-hydroxylase deficiency. The goal is to avoid corrective genital surgery after birth by preventing virilization of females. Oral dexamethasone or hydrocortisone is administered to the pregnant mother as early as possible during the first trimester. A chorionic villus sampling, performed between 8 and 12 weeks' gestation, or amniocentesis, performed between 14 and 18 weeks' gestation, can be used for DNA analysis and gender determination (Kuller et al, 1996).

If the fetus is a male or an unaffected female, the mother can discontinue treatment. Therapy is continued to term if the fetus is an affected female. It is thought that the extra glucocorticoid in the maternal circulation crosses the placenta and thus provides negative feedback for fetal ACTH secretion. Hyperplasia of the adrenal gland along with oversecretion of androgens can then be circumvented. Reported maternal side effects have typically been mild and reversible and include weight gain, hypertension, edema, and mood swings. However, with higher doses of 1 to 1.5 mg/day, maternal side effects have been more severe and include excessive weight gain, glucose intolerance, facial hirsutism, marked cushingoid features, hypertension, and mood swings.

The effectiveness of prenatal treatment has been variable. Several explanations have been postulated. The dosage of glucocorticoids may have been inadequate or the onset of treatment may have been late. Exogenous cortisol appears to have a high affinity for serum corticosteroid-binding globulin. The placenta catalyzes a portion of exogenous dexamethasone. The amount of exogenous glucocorticoids that reaches the fetus is influenced by maternal metabolism. Another factor that limits the success of exogenous glucocorticoid administration is that fetal adrenal function is regulated by other factors in addition to ACTH. Lastly, the fetal ACTH–glucocorticoid feedback mechanism may not be sufficiently developed during early gestation.

Parents. The parents of a newborn with CAH-induced ambiguous genitalia require immediate information about questionable sex assignment. Naming their child is postponed until the sex can be genetically determined. Explanations about the cause and treatment must be simple and concise and require repeated reinforcement as the child grows. Health care providers should refer to the neonate as "baby," "infant," or "child." It must be emphasized that virilized females possess normal internal reproductive organs and that external genitalia can be surgically corrected.

Parents need time to verbalize their feelings. Because CAH is recessively inherited, parents often feel guilt for having given their child "bad genes" and "causing" their infant's condition. The nurse needs to emphasize that the parents have no control over the genes their newborn received. Parents need to know that every person has some altered genes that can cause genetic anomalies. Every person has a background risk of 2% to 3% for having a child with a birth defect. Therefore the parents are not somehow different or "defective" because they transmitted an altered gene to their offspring.

Parents may experience anger and disappointment over the loss of their prenatal ideas and dreams of a perfect child. Their child's "normal features" need to be emphasized. Any concerns about their child growing up as a masculine female, feminine male, or homosexual owing to the ambiguous genitalia should be discussed openly to allow parents an opportunity for catharsis. Nurses need to encourage parent-infant activities that promote bonding. Parents may also require help accessing current support systems and obtaining new support persons or agencies as needed.

The parents must be taught medication administration and schedules. Compliance must be stressed and the need for lifelong hormone replacement therapy emphasized. Parents also need to be familiarized with signs and symptoms of dehydration. Frequent and regular evaluation of affected infants is necessary to monitor and adjust the dosage of cortisone when ACTH suppression may be inadequate. Certain stressors, such as illness, trauma, and surgery, may trigger an adrenal crisis that requires medication adjustment.

Disorders of Gonadal Differentiation.

Disorders of gonadal differentiation involve abnormal combinations of the sex chromosomes X and Y. Basic descriptions of these disorders can be classified into three separate categories based on phenotypic expression or the observable characteristics of the individual.

The first general category involves phenotypic females with abnormal gonadal differentiation. Two specific types include Turner's syndrome and Swyer's syndrome. Individuals with Turner's syndrome have a 45,X genotype with characteristic congenital anomalies that include skeletal defects, webbing of the neck, lymphedema of the hands and feet at birth, and shortened stature in adulthood. The gonads are eventually reduced to fibrous streaks; that leads to primary amenorrhea, sexual infantilism, and infertility. Recognition of the syndrome before puberty may be accomplished by obtaining a karyotype of the chromosomal set. The incidence of Turner's syndrome is 1 in 2,200 female births. Treatment involves sex hormone (estrogen) replacement therapy at puberty and subsequent low-dose maintenance estrogen administration.

Swyer's syndrome, like Turner's syndrome, often presents at puberty with primary amenorrhea. Streak gonads are seen but without the congenital anomalies that accompany Turner's syndrome. The karyotype may reveal a 46,XX or 46,XY genotype. Treatment involves hormone replacement therapy and exploratory surgery to remove streak gonads.

The second general category consists of phenotypic males with abnormal gonadal differentiation. Two types include Klinefelter's syndrome and XX male phenotypes. The karyotype of individuals with Klinefelter's syndrome shows one additional X chromosome. Mosaic combinations (usually 46,XY, 47,XXY) may also be possible. Adult XXY males present with small testes, sterile seminiferous tubules, and gynecomastia owing to lowered testosterone levels. Mental retardation may also

be seen. Diagnosis is made through Barr screening to determine the sex chromosomal arrangement. Treatment includes testosterone replacement therapy in individuals with postpuberal hypogonadism.

XX male phenotypes have testicular development in the absence of a Y chromosome. Individuals usually present with infertility problems. Either dominant or recessive autosomal genes may result in genetic inheritance of the disorder.

The third general category comprises sexually ambiguous individuals with gonadal dysgenesis. Identifiable types include (1) male pseudohermaphroditism; (2) true hermaphroditism, (3) Leydig cell hypoplasia; and (4) testicular regression syndrome.

Individuals with pseudohermaphroditism with mixed gonadal dysgenesis have impaired testicular function, which leads to early fetal testicular dysgenesis. Sexual ambiguity is seen with the presence of one or two testes, hypospadias, cryptorchidism, and an intact uterus. There is an increased risk of gonadal tumors. In addition, Turner's syndrome–like characteristics may be seen. The sex of rearing is preferably female if the syndrome is diagnosed in infancy and treated at an early age, usually younger than 2 years. If the child is older, sex reassignment may psychologically impair the individual. Thus it is better to correct the hypospadias and cryptorchidism surgically, remove gonadal streaks, and monitor for tumor development. Testosterone hormone replacement should be provided at puberty, and the individual should retain his male gender.

True hermaphrodites possess both testicular and ovarian tissue, often combined in the same gonad, called an ovotestis. The newborn presents with ambiguous genitalia and abnormal internal anatomic structures. Although internal testicular tissue usually degenerates, the ovarian tissue remains functional, and thus fertility may be possible in the female sex. For this reason, female is the desired sex of rearing. Treatment involves surgical removal of internal organs contradictory to the desired sex.

Leydig cell hypoplasia and embryonic testicular regression syndrome are both rare occurrences. Sexual ambiguity is often seen, and these disorders may be genetically transmitted.

Additional Causes of Ambiguous Genitalia

In addition to the causes of ambiguous genitalia previously discussed, certain forms may be caused by other, less common factors. They include maternal exposure to androgens, 5a-reductase deficiency, and end-organ androgen insensitivity. Maternal exposure to androgens may be either exogenous (through the use of certain prescribed oral contraceptives) or endogenous (by increased circulating androgens resulting from a maternal tumor).

Strategies in Assessment.

Any neonate who presents with ambiguous genitalia, regardless of the severity, should be thoroughly evaluated. It is a critical problem that needs both medical and social intervention. Assessment of the newborn with ambiguous genitalia includes a complete family history and physical examination, followed by a thorough diagnostic evaluation.

Family History.

A complete history begins with the construction of a family pedigree. A pedigree is a diagram that identifies all family members, their relationship to the affected individual, and their personal health history with emphasis on specific hereditary conditions. Genetics plays an important part in individuals with ambiguous genitalia and should be investigated carefully. In addition, special attention should be directed to the mother and her prenatal and reproductive history. Maternal ingestion of potentially androgenic substances (including certain forms of oral contraception) during pregnancy; a family history of maternal aunts with sterility, amenorrhea, or an inguinal hernia containing a gonad or an unexplained infant death in the neonatal period may assist in establishing a diagnosis.

Physical Examination.   Specific physical findings that are seen with sexual ambiguity include: (1) a structure that resembles an enlarged clitoris or a micropenis with hypospadias; (2) partial fusion of the labioscrotal folds; and (3) absence of gonads or one palpable gonad in the incomplete scrotum of a term infant. Downward bowing of the penile-clitoral structure, called chordee, can also be present. Varying degrees of ambiguity may be seen, depending on the severity of the disorder.

Whenever a physical examination reveals ambiguous genitalia, further diagnostic evaluation is essential. Major medical centers often have a comprehensive team to conduct a diagnostic evaluation of these infants.

Diagnostic Evaluation.   The goals of the diagnostic evaluation in the infant presenting with sexual ambiguity are to determine the cause of the abnormality and to develop an appropriate plan of care. It should be explained to the parents that although their infant was born with sexual organs that appear underdeveloped or unfinished, a thorough evaluation can help define the extent of the condition and can determine the most effective strategy to complete the unfinished sex organs.

A comprehensive diagnostic evaluation involves three areas of testing: (1) measurement of the circulating hormones; (2) analysis of the chromosomes; and (3) visualization of the internal organs.

First, measurement of the circulating hormones identifies the presence of abnormal levels. Evaluating specific hormone levels can be accomplished through measurement of urinary 17-ketosteroids and blood pregnanetriol levels. Elevation of these hormonal levels may indicate CAH. These levels may also be assessed prenatally via the amniotic fluid to identify an affected fetus. However, it should be noted that affected males may not have abnormal amniotic fluid levels.

Infants with ambiguous genitalia in which CAH has been ruled out may be further evaluated with serum testosterone measurement and an hCG stimulation test. Performed when the infant is between 2 and 9 weeks of age, these tests can help determine the integrity of the hypothalamic-pituitary axis in male infants and can identify the presence of testicular tissue in infants with ambiguous genitalia.

Second, analysis of the chromosomes determines the chromosomal or genetic sex of the infant. Complete chromosomal analysis can be performed through the establishment of a karyotype. In the past, attempts were made to identify the chromosomal sex of the infant immediately through analysis of buccal smears, which is currently considered ineffective because no information is provided about the structure or possible mosaicism of the chromosomes.

Advances in genetics have provided information about the sex-determining gene, zinc finger Y, which can be identified on part of the Y chromosome with the use of a probe. The probe can determine the integrity of the gene and can be useful in the diagnosis for an infant with ambiguous genitalia.

Third, visualization of the internal organs provides a comprehensive picture of the anatomic structures involved in an infant with abnormal sexual differentiation. Pelvic ultrasonography is an important diagnostic tool for determining the presence of a uterus or urogenital sinus, or both. Contrast studies (genitography) may further clarify the presence of a urogenital sinus. Magnetic resonance imaging can be useful in identifying the presence of undescended testes. Endoscopy of the urogenital sinus may determine the presence of a small or abnormal vagina. Laparotomy or laparoscopy and gonadal biopsy in the infant is controversial because of the limited availability of smaller-sized instruments. These procedures should be performed only in infants who require removal of the gonads, such as true hermaphrodites and infants with mixed gonadal dysgenesis. After the infant with ambiguous genitalia has been thoroughly assessed and a diagnosis has been made, a collaborative team approach to managing the infant must be established to optimize successful intervention.

Collaborative Management.   The focus of management for an infant who presents with ambiguous genitalia involves assessment and diagnosis of the disorder as well as physical stabilization of the neonate who is experiencing a salt-wasting adrenal crisis from CAH. Explanations and support for the family are critical. A comprehensive plan of care should be established by the primary physician and should be conveyed clearly to all persons involved with the infant's care. Inclusion of specialists from pediatric endocrinology, urology, psychiatry and genetics is highly recommended (Deacon & O'Neill, 1999).

A determination as to the desired sex of rearing is made only after extensive diagnostic testing and in-depth discussions among the team members and family. The traditional approach to basing gender assignment on the infant's anatomy with less emphasis on the chromosomal sex has recently been challenged. Newer studies show that the brain may be programmed by the genetic influence, thus making psychological adjustment to the opposing sex futile (Reiner, 1997a, b). Consideration must be given to a full host of additional factors, including the pathology of the cause for the ambiguity, the choice for future sexual function and fertility, and societal and cultural factors. (Deacon & O'Neill, 1999; Diamond & Sigmundson, 1997; Reiner, 1997a, b). Contributing to the dilemma are questions of immediate and complete surgery versus staged intervention that delays assignment until the patient is able to participate in the decision-making process. The trauma of undetermined gender assignment versus multiple genital reconstructive surgeries is also in question (Deacon & O'Neill, 1999).

Trial testing with either human chorionic gonadatropin or testosterone and evaluating the infant's genital tissue response may be useful to sex assignment. Once the determination of gender is made, a surgical plan is devised. Complete or staged reconstruction of the externala genitalia is determined by degree of the defect and considerations with the medical team and family. Most often, gonads of the unassigned sex are removed to reduce future risk of malignancy (Deacon & O'Neill, 1999). Follow-up includes hormonal therapy at puberty to elicit secondary sexual development, and psychological counseling at critical developmental stages may be appropriate.

Nursing care for the infant who presents with ambiguous genitalia can be challenging. To develop an effective plan of care, the nurse must establish three levels of concern on which to focus. These levels include immediate, midrange, and long-term needs and goals (see section on CAH for details of management).

The immediate needs and goals of the newborn with ambiguous genitalia involve the potential for a life-threatening adrenal crisis, as may be seen in the neonate with salt-wasting CAH. The primary goal is directed toward achieving an elevation of circulating cortisol and replacement of sodium and water deficits. Fluid and electrolyte status and circulating cortisol levels should be monitored carefully (Chapter 24).

Parents often wonder about the risk of recurrence, which, in fact, depends on the actual diagnosis of their affected child. In the more common classic 21-hydroxylase deficiency of CAH, there is a 25% risk of a subsequent affected sibling. Thus involvement of genetics specialists as active members of the patient care team is important for parents to determine the risk in subsequent childbearing.

Families may benefit from referrals to social services to assist them with available community resources. Support groups may be established so that families and affected individuals can gain confidence in knowing that they are not alone in dealing with the disorder.

CYSTIC FIBROSIS

Cystic fibrosis (CF), formerly known as mucoviscidosis or CF of the pancreas, is an inherited, chronic, progressive, metabolic disorder that affects the exocrine glands, or the mucus-secreting glands, of the body. Classic CF is characterized by chronic pulmonary infection, pancreatic insufficiency, and increased salt loss through the sweat glands.

Pathophysiology

The gene responsible for CF is the cystic fibrosis transmembrane conductance regulator (CFTR) gene and is a mutation on the long arm of human chromosome 7. Mutation of the CFTR gene leads to an abnormality in chloride conductance by epithelial cells in mucosal membranes. This leads to excessive salt content within the sweat and to the production of thick mucus secretions in the intestinal and respiratory tracts. Approximately 75% of individuals with CF have at least one gene with the DF508 deletion. In some individuals, both genes are affected, whereas others (approximately 50%) have a second gene with a different mutation. To date, more than 850 mutations in the CFTR gene have been identified (Zeitlin, 2000). These mutations have been grouped into five classes according to the specific defect that results in the CFTR protein. The fact that there are many mutations that cause CF may partially explain the large patient-to-patient variability seen in the presentation, manifestations, and degree of severity of the disease. Currently, researchers are working on the correlation between specific mutations (genotype) and clinical characteristics (phenotype) (Rosenstein & Zeitlin, 1998). For example, DF508 homozygosity is strongly associated with pancreatic insufficiency (Cystic Fibrosis Genotype-Phenotype Consortium, 1993), whereas some other mutations are associated with normal pancreatic function.

Pulmonary disease probably begins with the development of mucus plugging or obstruction of small airways. Eventually, the patient experiences chronic inflammation and obstruction of larger airways. As the patient is colonized with bacteria, infection sets in. Repeated infection and inflammation leads to structural changes in the airway, consisting of damage to respiratory epithelium, supporting structures' airway wall, and pulmonary

vasculature. Repeated exacerbations can result in bronchiectasis and pulmonary fibrosis. Pulmonary parenchymal changes cause an increase in pulmonary vascular resistance, thus leading to pulmonary hypertension, cor pulmonale, and cardiorespiratory failure.

The course of CF is chronic and progressive, characterized by frequent respiratory infections with *Haemophilus influenzae*, *Staphylococcus aureus*, and *Pseudomonas aeruginosa*. *Burkholderia cepacia* (formerly *Pseudomonas cepacia*) is seen less commonly but may be associated with greater morbidity and mortality than *P. aeruginosa* colonization.

Hyperinflation or emphysema due to partial airway obstruction and patchy areas of atelectasis due to complete airway obstruction are early radiographic findings. Characteristically, patients exhibit generalized nodulocystic shadowing and increased bronchial markings. Destructive changes within the airways eventually lead to severe bronchiectasis with a "honeycomb" appearance of the lung on radiograph.

Risk Factors

CF is the most common fatal genetic disorder affecting Caucasians. It is inherited as a recessive condition with a carrier frequency of 1 in 30. The incidence of CF in the United States is approximately 1 in 2,500 individuals of European ancestry. The incidence in the African-American population is 1 in 15,000; it is estimated to be much less common in Asians and Native Americans.

Clinical Manifestations

A combination of symptoms is the usual presentation for CF; these include respiratory infections, abnormal stools, and failure to thrive. Less common presentations are intestinal obstruction (such as meconium ileus), rectal prolapse, nasal polyps/sinus disease, prolonged neonatal jaundice, hyponatremic-hypochloremic dehydration, and hypoproteinemia.

Pulmonary disease is usually a major clinical problem for the patient with CF later in life, but it can also present in the neonatal period. Recent studies using bronchoscopy in infants with CF indicate that inflammation and air trapping may be present at birth, especially in infants colonized with *P. aeruginosa* (Rosenfeld et al, 1994). The most constant symptom of pulmonary involvement is a cough that is initially dry and later becomes productive and increased at night. Decreased exercise tolerance, tachypnea, retractions, nasal flaring, and an increased anteroposterior diameter of the chest are common signs. Crackles and wheezes may be heard on auscultation. Digital clubbing may be apparent, depending on the severity of the pulmonary disease. As the disease progresses, pulmonary exacerbations caused by viral and bacterial infections are common and may develop into pneumonia. Once generalized bronchiectasis is evident, the clinical course steadily progresses with frequent exacerbations and eventually respiratory failure, cor pulmonale, and death.

Pancreatic insufficiency dominates the clinical picture in the majority of neonates and infants with CF. Between 80% and 90% of patients suffer from pancreatic insufficiency, which is apparent at birth. The pancreas produces enzymes for digestion that pass through the pancreatic duct to the small intestine. In CF, the pancreatic duct becomes obstructed with thick mucus, which does not allow the passage of enzymes. This obstruction leads to fibrosis and destruction of the pancreas.

Consequently, food (predominantly proteins and fats) cannot be digested and absorbed normally, thus leading to signs and symptoms of malnutrition. Absorption of the fat-soluble vitamins—A, D, E, and K—is therefore impaired. Clinical manifestations include frequent, bulky, loose, greasy, malodorous stools (steatorrhea) and poor growth.

Approximately 10% to 20% of newborns with CF present with meconium ileus that is a functional bowel obstruction due to large quantities of thick meconium in the small and large intestine. This obstruction presents between 24 and 48 hours of age with abdominal distention, vomiting, and failure to pass meconium. Occasionally, meconium may escape into the peritoneum through a perforation and cause meconium peritonitis. The patient with CF may have many other complications that need to be assessed (Box 28-3).

Differential Diagnosis

The diagnosis of CF is based on a combination of typical clinical signs and symptoms as well as a positive sweat test. The accepted method to confirm the diagnosis of CF is the Gibson-Cooke sweat test. This method uses pilocarpine iontophoresis with quantitative analysis of chloride (Gibson & Cooke, 1959), and it is more than 90% sensitive. A sweat chloride concentration of greater than 60 mEq/L is diagnostic in children; 75 mg

---

BOX 28-3

Complications of Cystic Fibrosis

Respiratory
Recurrent pneumonia
Recurrent bronchiolitis
Atelectasis/emphysema
Pansinusitis
Haemophilus influenzae, Staphylococcus aureus, Pseudomonas aeruginosa, and *Burkholderia cepacia* (formerly *Pseudomonas cepacia*) infection
Pneumothorax
Hemoptysis (usually self-limiting and associated with pulmonary exacerbation)

Gastrointestinal
Meconium ileus (10% to 20%)
Malabsorption/steatorrhea due to pancreatic insufficiency (80%)
Failure to thrive with a weight and/or height less than fifth percentile
Rectal prolapse (5%)
Biliary cirrhosis (3% to 5%)
Distal Intestinal Obstructive Syndrome (seen in the older child and associated with a partial bowel obstruction from thick stool and secretions)
Intussusception
Fat-soluble vitamin deficiencies
Hypoproteinemia/edema

Miscellaneous
Nasal polyps (20%)
Heat prostration with hyponatremia/hypochloremia dehydration
Azoospermia
Digital clubbing/hypertrophic pulmonary osteoarthropathy
Diabetes mellitus (3% to 5%)

---

of sweat is needed to obtain an accurate result. Sweat testing in the newborn period is difficult, as infants may not produce sufficient quantities of sweat. If a sufficient quantity is collected, the results are as valid as in older individuals.

The most common cause of a false-positive sweat test is laboratory error. False-positive results can also be found in malnutrition, adrenal insufficiency, ectodermal dysplasia, nephrogenic diabetes insipidus, hypothyroidism, and mucopolysaccharidosis. False-negative results can occur in the presence of edema and hypoproteinemia.

DNA analysis can be performed on buccal smears (cheek cell smears) or blood tests of infants when sufficient sweat is unobtainable. This test is 90% sensitive for the North American white population. Two recognized CFTR mutations are acceptable as diagnostic (Rosenstein & Cutting, 1998).

Prenatal testing for CF includes DNA analysis of chorionic villus samples during the first trimester (8 to 10 weeks) or amniotic fluid samples collected after 14 weeks. If a positive family history of CF exists, the risk can usually be assessed in the fetus by testing through mutation analysis or restriction fragment length polymorphism markers to determine haplotype. The most appropriate test depends on each individual's situation. Thus the patient or family is referred to a geneticist for assessment.

Limited newborn screening programs are available in the United States. Newborn screening for CF uses the immunoreactive trypsin (IRT) assay, which is performed on a dried blood spot. A newborn with CF can have extremely high levels of plasma trypsinogen in comparison to normal infants. This elevation is presumed to occur because of pancreatic duct obstruction. Newborns with an elevated IRT will have CF mutational analysis performed. The rationale for newborn screening is that early diagnosis may lead to earlier treatment, thereby reducing the morbidity and mortality associated with CF. However, screening is not accepted worldwide because an improvement in outcome is not clearly demonstrated in relationship to earlier diagnosis and because there is no screening method available that detects at least 90% of affected individuals.

Collaborative Management

There is still no cure for CF. Care revolves around preventing the progression of the disease and treating the symptoms. The comprehensive management of CF requires input from an interdisciplinary team within a CF center that follows the standards and guidelines recommended by the Cystic Fibrosis Foundation.

Team members usually include a pulmonologist, gastroenterologist, nurse, social worker, nutritionist, respiratory therapist, and physical therapist. Practitioners of other disciplines, such as psychology, genetics, and internal medicine, may be required. The first goal of therapy is to minimize pulmonary infections and prevent the progression of disease. This goal is accomplished by using airway clearance techniques such as chest physiotherapy and postural drainage. In older children, other methods, such as flutter devices, therapy vests, and positive expiratory pressure valves, are used. Occasionally, bronchodilators are used in combination with airway clearance. rhDNase (Pulmozyme) is used as an aerosol to reduce the viscosity of mucus secretions by breaking down the DNA. Oral, aerosolized, or intravenous antibiotics are used during respiratory exacerbations to help decrease bacterial colonization and minimize inflammation. High-dose ibuprofen, used in children between 5 and 13 years of age, acts to reduce inflammation of the lung tissue to slow the progression of lung disease (Konstan et al, 1995). Supplemental oxygen becomes necessary when hypoxemia occurs.

Double lung transplantation may be an option in end-stage disease. It has been performed successfully in a relatively small number of CF patients. Survival is 75% at 1 year and 55% at 3 years (UNOS, 2001).

A second goal of therapy is to assure adequate nutrition. The aim of nutritional therapy is to foster normal growth and development while contributing to the general health of the individual. Data suggest that lung function and exercise capacity may improve with optimal nutritional management.

Pancreatic enzyme therapy is used to replace the enzymes that normally reach the intestine via the pancreatic duct. A diet high in calories (120% to 150% of the recommended daily allowance) and protein (200% of the recommended daily allowance) is needed, along with vitamin supplementation, with emphasis on the fat-soluble vitamins (A, D, E, and K) in a water-soluble form. The diet prescription varies among individuals. With appropriate enzyme replacement, neonates are successfully fed popular infant formulas or breast milk. At times, infants are often prescribed an elemental or predigested formula such as Pregestimil, especially if the infant is nutritionally deprived at the time of diagnosis. To meet an individual's nutritional goals, an increased calorie per ounce of formula may be given (e.g., 24 or 27 kcal/oz).

Individuals may also receive feedings via nasogastric, gastrostomy, or jejunostomy tubes if oral intake is poor. Salt is added liberally to the diet to replace salt loss via sweat. CF-related diabetes that requires insulin is found in 5% to 6% of individuals with CF, seen mostly in adolescents and adults. A thorough nutritional assessment is an important component of a patient's treatment.

A third goal of treatment is to facilitate family coping skills and adaptation to a lifelong condition. Families are confronted by enormous psychological stresses, financial obligations, and time burdens. The nurse can assist in the adjustment process, and referral to the social worker or psychologist may be indicated. Families can be referred to a genetic specialist for genetic counseling and future planning.

In the majority of cases, a diagnosis of CF is made in the first year of life. Therefore the neonatal nurse must be alert to the signs and symptoms of respiratory and nutritional problems that are associated with CF. (For nursing management of meconium ileus, see Chapter 26.)

If an infant is suspected of having CF, the nurse assists in making a referral to the CF clinic and collaborates with the nurse on the CF team to help coordinate efforts and avoid confusing the family with conflicting information. He or she can allay parents' fears about the sweat test or genetic testing by explaining how the test is performed and letting the parents know when the results will be available. After the diagnosis is confirmed and the team physician or nurse initiates the educational process, the nurse provides support and facilitates the adaptation process. He or she provides written and verbal information and assesses the family's understanding of the diagnosis. The nurse also provides clarification regarding the diagnosis, genetic issues, therapy, home management, medications, equipment, normal growth and development, and follow-up routine. As a patient advocate, the nurse refers a family to their local Cystic Fibrosis Foundation and parent support group and assists the family in locating community information, service, and support resources as well as funding sources. The nurse enables and empowers the family of a child newly diagnosed with CF by providing opportunities for the family to acquire the necessary knowledge and skills so that they can become competent and independent. A nurse sensitive to family needs helps a family understand what CF means to them and how to incorporate it into their lifestyles. The nurse portrays a hopeful and positive outlook so that parents feel encouraged and able to help their child lead a full and happy life.

Prognosis

Since CF was first recognized as a clinical syndrome in the mid-1940s, treatment has improved considerably and has resulted in greater longevity and quality of life for individuals with CF. Survival statistics are improving steadily, and the median age of survival is now approaching 32 years of age (Cystic Fibrosis Genotype-Phenotype Consortium, 1993; Cystic Fibrosis Foundation, 1997). It is estimated that the life expectancy of children with CF diagnosed today is 40 to 50 years. Therefore it is important for a family to treat children with CF as normally as possible and to plan for education, career, marriage, and other long-term goals as with any other child.

SUMMARY

The endocrine system is a highly complex structure, and its function touches on every other body system. It is not surprising that neonates with alterations in endocrine function require an accurate and thorough head-to-toe assessment.

REFERENCES

Argente J, Chowen JA (1994). Neuroendocrinology of growth hormone secretion. Growth genetics & hormones, 10(2), 1-5.

Avery GB et al (Eds.) (1999). Neonatology: pathophysiology and management of the newborn, ed 5, Philadelphia: JB Lippincott.

Beers M, Berkow R (2002). Merck manual diagnosis & therapy. (Includes facsimile of first edition of the Merck Manual.) Whitehouse Station, NJ: Merck Co. Inc.

Bona G et al (1994). Growth hormone, insulin-like growth factor-I and somatostatin in human fetus, newborn, mother plasma and amniotic fluid. Panminerva medica, 36(1), 5-12.

Cruz TVD et al (1995). Delayed diagnosis of congenital adrenal hyperplasia in a premature female infant. Journal of Kentucky medical association, 93(1), 19-21.

Cystic Fibrosis Foundation. (1997). Patient Registry 1996, Annual Data Report, Bethesda, MD.

Cystic Fibrosis Genotype-Phenotype Consortium (1993). Correlation between genotype and phenotype in patients with cystic fibrosis. New England journal of medicine, 329(18), 1308-1313.

Deacon J, O'Neill P (1999). Core curriculum for neonatal intensive care nursing, ed 2, Philadelphia: WB Saunders.

Diamond M, Sigmundson HK (1997). Management of intersexuality: Guidelines for dealing with persons with ambiguous genitalia. Archives of pediatric adolescent medicine 151, 1046-1050.

Dorton AM (2000). The Pituitary gland: embryology, physiology, and pathophysiology. Neonatal network, 19(2), 9-17.

Fisher DA, Polk DH (1995). Thyroid disease in the fetus, neonate and child. In DeGroot LJ (Ed.). Endocrinology, ed 3, Philadelphia: WB Saunders.

Ganong WF (2000). Circumventricular organs: definition and role in the regulation of endocrine and autonomic function. Clin Exp Pharmacol Physiol, 27(5-6):422-427.

Gilbert E, Harmon J (2003). Manual of high risk pregnancy and delivery, ed 3, St Louis: Mosby.

Hitti IF et al (1994). Bilateral femoral hypoplasia and maternal diabetes mellitus. *Pediatric Pathology*, 14(4), 567-574.

Kistler CH, Spiering K (1998). Nesidioblastosis: a case study. *Journal of perinatal & neonatal nursing*, 11(4), 65-74.

Konstan M et al (1995). Effect of high-dose ibuprofen in patients with cystic fibrosis. *New England journal of medicine*, 332(13), 848-854.

Kuller JA et al (Eds.). (1996). *Prenatal diagnosis & reproductive genetics*. Philadelphia: JB Lippincott.

McKenna LL (2000). Pancreatic disorders in the newborn. *Neonatal network*. 19(4), 13-20.

Novak RW, Robinson HB (1994). Coincident DiGeorge anomaly and renal agenesis and its relation to maternal diabetes. *American journal of medicine genetics*, 50(4), 311-312.

Reiner W (1997a). Sex assignment in the neonated with intersex or inadequate genitalia. *Archives of pediatric adolescent medicine*, 151, 1044-1045.

Reiner W (1997b). To be male or female—that is the question. *Archives of pediatric adolescent medicine*, 151, 224-225.

Rosenfeld M et al (1994). Changes in pulmonary function associated with pseudomonal respiratory colonization in infants with cystic fibrosis. *Pediatric pulmonology*, 10 (Suppl.), 262. [Poster abstract 298 presented at 8th annual North American Cystic Fibrosis Conference. Orlando, FL, October 20-23.]

Rosenstein BJ, Cutting GR (1998). The diagnosis of cystic fibrosis: a consensus statement. *Journal of pediatrics*, 132, 589-595.

Rosenstein BJ, Zeitlin PL (1998). Cystic fibrosis. *Lancet*, 351(9098), 277-282.

Schwartz R et al (1994). Hyperinsulinemia and macrosomia in the fetus of the diabetic mother. *Diabetes care*, 17(7), 640-648.

Sills IN, Rapaport R (1994). New-onset IDDM presenting with diabetic ketoacidosis in a pregnant adolescent. *Diabetes care*, 17(8), 904-905.

Stanley CA (1997). Hyperinsulinism in infants and children. *Pediatric clinics of North America*, 44(2), 363-74.

UNOS Transplant Patient Data Source (2001) www.patients.unos.org.

Varvarigou A et al (1994). Growth hormone, insulin-like growth factor-1 and prolactin in small for gestational age neonates. *Biology of the neonate*, 65(2), 94-102.

Zapata A et al (1994). Influence of metabolic control of pregnant diabetics on fetal lung maturity. *Scandinavian journal of clinical & laboratory investigation*, 54(16), 431-434.

Zeitlin PL (2000). Future pharmalogical treatment of cystic fibrosis. *Respiration*, 67, 351-357.

ASSESSMENT AND MANAGEMENT OF THE IMMUNE SYSTEM

JUDY WRIGHT LOTT, CAROLE KENNER

The primary function of the immune system is to protect the body from invading microorganisms such as bacteria, viruses, fungi, protozoa, and parasites. During gestation, the healthy fetus grows and develops within the protective environment of the mother's uterus. During and after birth, however, the newborn is exposed to a wide variety of microorganisms. The newborn's host defense mechanisms must combat hostile microorganisms in its environment. Even though the host defense mechanisms begin to develop early in gestation, many of these mechanisms do not function as efficiently at the time of birth—even in the term newborn—as they function in older infants, children, or adults. The immaturity of the complex immune system becomes apparent in light of the relatively high prevalence of infectious disease that occurs during the neonatal period as well as the increased prevalence of neonatal infection caused by agents considered to be of low pathogenicity in older individuals (Kapur et al, 2002). Although the cells of the fetal and neonatal immune system are not fully developed, they show a remarkable ability to respond to the environment. Nonetheless, humans at these early stages of development are susceptible to injury caused directly by immunologic mechanisms or imposed by infectious microorganisms that overwhelm the relatively immature and inexperienced immune system These immune system processes form the foundation for the prevention, diagnosis, and treatment of neonatal infectious diseases. This chapter will describe the basic components of the immune system, physiologic processes involved in an immune response, and common neonatal and infant alterations in the immune system including human immunodeficiency virus (HIV).

GENERAL DEVELOPMENT OF THE IMMUNE SYSTEM

The immune response is characterized as a sequence of adaptive cellular responses to threats from a dynamic and potentially hostile environment. Although the cells and functions that make up the immune system appear early in gestation, the majority of them are not activated until the newborn interacts with the external environment. In intrauterine infections, however, the environment of the fetus may be so changed that activation of some of these cells and functions may begin prior to birth.

EMBRYOLOGIC DEVELOPMENT OF THE IMMUNE SYSTEM

Host defense mechanisms may be separated into two major categories: nonspecific or innate mechanisms and specific or adaptive mechanisms, described as follows:

1. The nonspecific innate mechanisms, which include physical barriers—the skin, chemical barriers—gastric acid for one, phagocytic components-neutrophils, monocytes (blood), macrophages-lung, liver sinusoids or Kupffer cells, synovial cells, perivascular microglial cells and mesangial or kidney tissue, natural killer (NK) cells, the inflammatory response, and amplification systems—including complement proteins, acute phase reactants, and cytokines. All these mechanisms function effectively without necessitating prior exposure to a microorganism or its antigens. Every living organism has an innate ability to defend itself against invasion.

2. The specific or adaptive mechanisms, consisting of the lymphocytes, which include thymus-derived or cell-mediated (T cell) and humoral or antibody-mediated (B cell) immune responses, operate most effectively with prior exposure to the infective agent or its antigens. The other component of the adaptive immune system is the antibody or immunoglobulin (Ig). There are receptor sites on the lymphocytes that rely on Ag receptor genes to regulate their responses. For the B cells the regulators are surface immunoglobulins, or sIgs. T cells have T-cell receptor (TCR) regions. Genes in this area have the ability to clone themselves and belong to what is referred to as the Ig-gene family. The TCR is comprised of an alpha and beta chain associated with the CD3 molecule. The combination of the TCR/CD3 is called the TCR/CD3 complex (http://www.merck.com/pubs/mmanual/section12/chapter146/146a.htm). Approximately 166 clusters of differentiation (CD) or surface markers are known (http://www.ncbi.nlm.nih.gov/prow). These responses are learned responses. They rely on prior exposure and memories of this exposure within the cells—thus the response is called adaptive.

Both the innate and adaptive mechanisms are interrelated and interdependent. The body defends against infection by preventing access to pathogenic microorganisms by mechanical barriers, including intact skin and mucus and other body fluids, such as tears, saliva, and urine, which protect the epithelial surfaces.

Phagocytes, which arise from the bone marrow stem cells, engulf particles—including infectious agents—and internalize and destroy them. Chemotaxis is the process by which phagocytes are attracted to the site of infection. Phagocytosis, or cell-eating, is the most primitive of the host defense mechanisms. Although the most important phagocytic cells are the polymorphonuclear leukocytes, other cells, including monocytes and the nonmobile phagocytic cells of the reticuloendothelial system, are also involved in phagocytosis (Lewis & Wilson, 2001; Kapur et al, 2002). Specific phase defects in some areas of phagocytic function have been recognized in normal newborns, which suggests that the newborn may be compromised because of its deficiencies in both cellular and humoral factors involved in the process of phagocytosis. Under certain conditions, both in vitro and in vivo, neonatal polymorphonuclear leukocytes demonstrate less phagocytic capability than those of adults.

Inflammatory Response

Inflammation is the body's response to injury; it consists of the following three reactions:

- Increased blood supply to the area
- Increased capillary permeability
- Migration of leukocytes (polymorphonuclear neutrophils or PMNs) and macrophages out of the capillaries into surrounding tissues

A spectrum of cellular and systemic events are activated upon invasion by microorganisms as tissue injury occurs. The host attempts to restore and maintain homeostasis, and this produces the inflammatory response. The acute inflammatory response is characterized by blood vessel dilation and the accumulation of white blood cells (WBCs) and fluid. Shortly thereafter, neutrophilic granulocytes, which phagocytize and kill pathogenic microorganisms, appear. The ensuing febrile reaction, which results from increased metabolic activity probably precipitated by the release of endogenous pyrogens from the host's WBCs, is underdeveloped in the newborn; thus fever is not always present in infection during the neonatal period. Likewise, an increase in WBCs and sedimentation rate, which is often associated with bacterial infection in older infants, children, and adults, is infrequent in neonates. However, some signs of inflammatory responses are seen in newborns, including an increase in total numbers of band (immature neutrophil) forms as well as activation of the coagulation system with disseminated intravascular coagulation (DIC). The deficiency of complement components as well as the deficiency of some coagulation factors (i.e., vitamin K-dependent factors), contributes to the diminished inflammatory response of neonates.

Humoral Immunity

Complement System. The complement system consists of approximately more than 34 serum proteins, many of which are enzymes that interact with each other and with other components of the immune system. If they are in the inactive state or precursors they are called zymogens. Others are active and exist on the surface of the cell. The complement system assists the immunologically specific effects of antibody by the opsonization and lysis of red blood cells and bacteria. There are three pathways: classical, alternative, and mannan-binding lectin (MBL) pathway. These three lead into a final pathway call the terminal pathway or membrane attack complex (MAC) (http://www.merck.com/pubs/mmanual/section12/chapter146/146d.htm). The functions of the complement sys-

tem are (1) cell activation, (2) cytolysis of target cells, and (3) opsonization of cells to facilitate phagocytosis of bacteria. In the classical pathway the antibody and antigen combine in a complex referred to as C1 molecules or complexes. The C1 esterase inhibitor or C1INH is the regulator. Heparin and protamine-a heparin antagonist also activate this pathway. A C-reactive protein directly activates the pathway without antibodies being present. The alternative pathway is activated by a variety of substances. These include yeast, endotoxins, and other innate immune responses. The result is a cleavage of C3 molecules; which are regulated by properdin. Its' decay will accelerate substances such as factor H. (http://www.merck.co/pubs/mmanual/section12/chapter146/146e.htm). The Mannan Binding Lectin pathway is related to innate immunity and foreign substance invasion. C3 cleavage is affected. One of the examples of this activity is anaphylatoxin activity leading to anaphylaxis. Whatever the mechanism of activation; the MAC pathway is regulated by S proteins or vitronectin.

When activated, the complement system creates a cascade effect with amplification that works to "complement" antibody activity in destroying bacteria and to rid the body of antigen-antibody complexes. In so doing, the complement system induces an inflammatory response. Synthesis of most complement components begins early in fetal development—as early as 5 weeks' gestation—and is not related to the presence of antigen. Reasonable quantities appear in the serum at 12 to 14 weeks' gestation, remain at these somewhat low levels until about 26 to 28 weeks' gestation, and then markedly increase, so that, at term, total complement titers are at least half of the corresponding levels in adults. The concentration of complement decreases slightly after birth and recovers by 3 weeks of age; this may indicate that antigen stimulation may be involved in the induction of complement synthesis (Lewis & Wilson, 2001). Little is known regarding the biologic activities of this system in the newborn despite its significant role in the natural resistance to infection.

Levels of complement can be measured by total hemolytic complement assays or CH50 or complement fixation tests, or CFTs.

Immunoglobulins (Igs). Immunoglobulins (antibodies) are a group of glycoproteins in the serum and tissue fluids of all mammals. They comprise four chains—two light and two heavy ones. There are four distinct regions that contain regional genes. These are C, V, D, and J regional genes. Where these regions join, the likelihood of somatic point mutations in the genes increases. More genetic research is examining these areas to determine what, if any, role they play in immune function.

Immunoglobulins are produced when the host's lymphoid system comes into contact with immunogenic foreign molecules (antigens); they bind specifically to the antigen that induced their formation. The five classes of immunoglobulins are the following:

1. Immunoglobulin G (IgG) is the major immunoglobulin in normal human serum. It makes up approximately 70% to 75% of the total immunoglobulin pool and is distributed evenly between the intravascular and extravascular pools. IgG is the major antibody of secondary immune responses and the exclusive antitoxin class. Maternal IgG is transported across the placenta only during the last trimester.
2. Immunoglobulin M (IgM) makes up approximately 10% of the immunoglobulin pool and is confined primarily to the intravascu-

lar pool. IgM is the predominant early antibody; it is frequently directed against antigenically complex infectious organisms. The fetus in response to intrauterine infection produces IgM.

3. Immunoglobulin A (IgA) makes up approximately 15% to 20% of the immunoglobulin pool. It is the predominant immunoglobulin in seromucous secretions such as saliva, tracheobronchial secretions, colostrum, milk, and genitourinary secretions. Secretory IgA is abundant in seromucous secretions and is protected from proteolysis by combination with another protein (the secretory component).

4. Immunoglobulin D (IgD) makes up less than 1% of the total plasma immunoglobulins, but it is present in large quantities on the membrane of many circulating B-lymphocytes. The precise biologic function of IgD is not known; it may be involved in antigen-triggered lymphocyte differentiation.

5. Immunoglobulin E (IgE) is a trace serum immunoglobulin found on the surface membrane of basophils and mast cells in all individuals. It may function in active immunity to helminths; more commonly, it is associated with immediate hypersensitivity diseases such as asthma and fever (Lewis & Wilson, 2001).

Much concern is raised today about autoimmune diseases. One such concern is the ability of the body to recognize self from non-self. When this function fails, the body turns on itself and attacks tissue and organs. The regulation of this function is related to major histocompatibility complexes or MHC. MHC is regulated by genes found on chromosome 6. HLA-D, HLA-DR, HLA-DP, and HLA-DQ are the most common products related to these complexes. These complexes are responsible for tissue rejection of organ transplants for example. T cells primarily recognize MHCs.

Cellular Immunity

Leukocytes. Leukocytes, or white blood cells (WBCs), are nucleated cells that protect the body against infection. There are three types of leukocytes: (1) granulocytes, which include neutrophils, eosinophils, and basophils; (2) monocytes; and (3) lymphocytes.

Granulocytes. Granulocytes, or polymorphonuclear leukocytes, are produced in the bone marrow. They evolve from myeloblasts into myelocytes and, finally, into mature granulocytes. The types of granulocytes are differentiated by cell-staining techniques. Neutrophils can leave the blood circulation and enter the tissues, where they ingest foreign substances and bacteria through phagocytosis. These cells are called phagocytes. Eosinophils are also phagocytes because they ingest and destroy antigen-antibody complexes. The function of the basophils is not fully known. Basophils appear to act similarly to the mast cells found in connective tissue, releasing histamine (bronchoconstrictor) and heparin (anticoagulant). Monocytes arise from the bone marrow and develop into phagocytic macrophages. Monocytes ingest foreign particles and fragmented cells. Lymphocytes originate in lymphogenous sites including bone marrow, lymph nodes, spleen, liver, thymus, subepithelial lymphoid tissue, and connective tissue. Lymphocytes develop from lymphoblasts or other lymphocytes and are involved in cellular immunity and antibody formation. There are two different types of lymphocytes: T-lymphocytes and B-lymphocytes. T-lymphocytes (T cells) are involved in cell-mediated immunity, and B-lymphocytes (B cells) produce antibodies. Infections stimulate the increased production and maturation of lymphocytes. T cells have one of two functions: positive or negative. Those that recognize MHCs are positive,

and those that result in attacks on self are negative. T cells also have helper or suppressor functions. CD4s are T-helper (T_H) lymphocytes. These produce other cells that are referred to as cytotoxic T cells or T_C that act on specific MHCs. These can originate from either CD4 or CD8 cells (http://www.merck.com/pubs/mmanual/section12/chapter146/146b.htm). Generally, the number of WBCs produced depends upon the body's need for them. Infection, tissue damage, or presence of viral agents stimulates increased production and circulation of leukocytes.

Granulocytes and monocytes arise from a common stem cell, or colony-forming unit (G-CSF and M-CSF, respectively). The eosinophil has a separate stem cell (CFU-Eo). The three types of granulocytes develop through the following similar stages: myeloblast, promyelocyte, myelocyte, metamyelocyte, band, and polymorphonuclear neutrophil or mature segmented neutrophil. In the routine differential count, the different stages of the eosinophils and basophils are not identified; they are just counted as eosinophils and basophils. The neutrophil stages are always identified (Lewis & Wilson, 2001).

Neutrophil Kinetics. As the myeloblast develops into the mature, segmented neutrophil, the myeloblast, promyelocyte, and myelocyte undergo cell division. These cells constitute the mitotic pool and generally undergo a total of three to five cell divisions over 6 to 7 days. During the promyelocyte stage, the cell produces nonspecific granules. The number of granules per cell decreases with each cell division. At the myelocyte stage, the cell produces specific granules. In the metamyelocyte stage, mitosis is not possible. The metamyelocyte matures for approximately 7 to 8 days in the storage pool. The number of bands and segmented neutrophils in the storage pool is approximately 15 times the number in the peripheral blood, and the mitotic pool is approximately one third the size of the storage pool.

The release of mature segmented neutrophils into the peripheral blood is not completely understood but appears to be a selective release. It is thought that substances such as colony-stimulating factor and granulopoietin regulate granulocyte production and control the movement of granulocytes from the bone marrow to the blood. When the mature segmented neutrophils leave the storage pool, approximately 50% of the neutrophils circulate freely in the circulating pool. The other 50% adhere to the walls of the vessels and constitute the marginal pool. The cells in the marginal pool are not included in the WBC count, so the differential represents only half the number present. The cells constantly change between the circulating and marginal pools. The mature segmented neutrophils are released first, along with a small percentage of bands. When the demand for neutrophils increases, more mature segmented neutrophils are released. If the demand is still not met, increased numbers of bands are released from the storage pool into the peripheral blood, reflecting an increased percentage of bands. Because the presence of infection creates a greater demand for release of neutrophils and consequently the release of immature neutrophils, a ratio of bands to segmented neutrophils greater than 0:3 or of immature neutrophils to total neutrophils equal to or greater than 0:2 should create suspicion of infection. The neutrophils in the peripheral blood are replaced approximately every 9 hours. Neutrophils do not return to the bone marrow. From the marginal pool, neutrophils randomly enter tissues and body cavities, where they carry out their major function of stopping or retarding the action of foreign material or infectious agents by doing the following:

- Moving into the area of inflammation or infection
- Phagocytizing foreign material
- Killing and digesting foreign material. The neutrophils are generally the first phagocytic cell to reach infected areas, followed by monocytes.

Eosinophils.   Eosinophils are primarily tissue cells; they leave the blood and move into the tissues, where they localize in areas exposed to the external environment (e.g., skin, lungs, and gastrointestinal tract). Once in the tissues, eosinophils do not return to the blood. Eosinophils are metabolically more active than neutrophils, although their function is not clearly known. Eosinophils are capable of phagocytizing foreign material and antigen-antibody complexes, but this is not thought to be their primary function. Eosinophils are thought to be anti-inflammatory cells because they modulate reactions in which basophils and mast cells are active. Eosinophils also help defend against helminths (parasites) by attaching to the parasite and releasing toxic substances.

Basophils.   Basophils develop from a cell similar to the myeloblast, although the specific stem cell has not been identified. The function of basophils is not fully understood; they exhibit chemotaxis and some phagocytosis. Basophil granules contain peroxidase, histamine, and heparin. Basophils synthesize an eosinophil chemotactic factor, a slow-reacting substance of anaphylaxis, and platelet-activating factor. Basophils appear to participate in immediate hypersensitivity reactions and are involved in some delayed hypersensitivity reactions. Basophil membranes bind IgE. When specific antigens react with the membrane-bound IgE, degranulation occurs, and the contents of the basophil granules are released into the surrounding area. This response releases the eosinophil chemotactic factor and causes accumulation of eosinophils in the area.

Mast Cells.   Mast cells are similar to basophils; they are found in the thymus, spleen, and bone marrow. Mast cells are of mesenchymal origin. The mast cell is slightly larger than the basophil and contains serotonin and some proteolytic enzymes in addition to the contents of the basophil.

Monocytes.   Monocytes originate from the same committed stem cell as the neutrophil. The precursor of the monocyte is the promonocyte (sometimes called the myelomonoblast). The monocyte is considered an immature cell. The promonocyte is less phagocytic and less motile than the monocyte. After formation, the promonocyte undergoes 2 to 2 ½ mitotic divisions over 2 days. The monocyte differentiates in the tissues into macrophages. Monocytes and macrophages are motile, capable of chemotaxis, able to move through blood vessel walls, and able to migrate to areas of inflammation. They respond to migration-inhibiting factor, which is produced by the T-lymphocytes to immobilize macrophages, and to chemotactic inhibitors. The monocyte and macrophage are capable of phagocytosis and pinocytosis. Monocyte production (hence, circulation) is increased in inflammation.

The functions of the monocyte in providing immunity are the following:

- Acts as a defense mechanism against intracellular parasites, including certain bacteria, fungi, and protozoa

- Removes damaged and old cells, plasma protein, and plasma lipids
- Participates in iron metabolism
- Processes antigen information for lymphocytes
- Produces and secretes various substances, including lysosomal enzymes, acid phosphatase, proteinase, collagenase, plasminogen activator, thromboplastin, platelet-activating factors, complement factors, and interferons.

Colony-Stimulating Factors.   Stem cells that are found in the fetal and neonatal immune tissue, primarily in the bone marrow, differentiate during development into myeloid and lymphoid stem cells. These pluripotent cells can form any type cell needed by the body up until the time they are committed to a certain developmental pathway. These are the cells that are undergoing so much scrutiny in relationship to their potential to treat immune dysfunctions, tissue rejection, and forms of cancer.

These colony-forming units or cells then become committed to a specific pathway of further maturation and development. Further development is a result of stimulating factors that cause colonies of cells to divide rapidly. These factors, then, are referred to as colony-stimulating factors. The colony-stimulating factors regulate hematopoiesis. Granulocyte-monocyte colony-stimulating factors (GM-CSFs) and granulocyte colony-stimulating factors (G-CSFs) are the two main types currently identified. Under their influence, the neutrophil storage pool is induced to release neutrophils and then enhance chemotaxis and bacteria-killing actions of the neutrophils. Thus they contribute to phagocytosis of the nonspecific immune system. GM-CSF and G-CSF are produced naturally by fetal and neonatal tissue, but each can be administered postnatally in recombinant forms.

The environment plays a key role in the continued production of effective phagocytes and granulocytes. The site of granulopoiesis requires either a stimulating factor by itself or contact with another cell that may act as a regulator or receptor of other cells. Many authors refer to the need for an adherent layer of cells, consisting of "fibroblast-like cells, macrophages, reticular adventitial cells, adipocytes, and endothelial cells," which, in turn, synthesize proteins in the form of "collagen, fibronectin, thrombonectin, hemonectin, and glycosaminoglycans." A major component of interest in neonatal immunocompetency is fibronectin. Fibronectin is a glycoprotein whose action is not completely understood. One known action is as an opsonin that coats bacteria and enhances phagocytosis. Located within the neutrophils and neutrophil storage pools, fibronectin is carried by the polymorphonuclear leukocytes to the site of invasion by a foreign substance. Fibronectin appears to have a role in the regulation of vascular permeability of the surrounding tissue. The implication is that microvascular integrity and permeability are also regulated by its presence. This action of fibronectin may have adverse effects, such as development of capillary leak syndrome, which is often associated with overwhelming sepsis as well as respiratory distress syndrome. It is theorized that fibronectin may also be responsible for the build-up of fibrinous tissue in the pulmonary tree, often associated with chronic lung changes in the neonate. Thus alveolar macrophages most likely produce fibronectin. The locus for fibronectin is chromosome 2. Fibronectin levels continue to increase over the first few weeks of postnatal life, thus increasing the newborn's ability to fight bacterial infections. Plasma concentration in term infants is approximately 220 mg/ml. Levels are reduced in the premature infant as they are in the presence of respiratory distress syndrome, sepsis, malnutrition, or asphyxia. Fibronectin contains binding sites for *Staphylococcus aureus, Streptococcus pyogenes,* and *Treponema pallidum.* Fibronectin may also facilitate binding of *Escherichia coli.* After an infection, fibronectin levels reduce to normal in approximately 5 days (Klein, 2001).

Lymphocytes. Lymphocytes are produced by the lymph nodes, spleen, thymus, and bone marrow and are a vital part of the immune system. Mature lymphocytes appear in the peripheral blood in varying sizes. The lymphocytes are classified as small, medium, or large. Lymphocytes function in the production of circulating antibodies and in the expression of cellular immunity. Antibodies are a class of molecules produced by B-lymphocytes, which act as flexible adaptors between the infectious agent and phagocytes. Any particular antibody molecule can bind to only one type of infectious agent. Antibodies attach to antigens. The mature lymphocyte has little or no endoplasmic reticulum, has only a small Golgi apparatus, possesses only a few mitochondria, and has ribosomes that are free and in clusters. Peripherally circulating lymphocytes include B, T, and null lymphocytes. The distinction is based on function and immunologic (cell surface) criteria; they are not morphologically distinguishable on peripheral blood smear. There are two main classes of lymphocytes: B-lymphocytes and T-lymphocytes (Lewis & Wilson, 2001).

B-lymphocytes. The B-lymphocytes, derived from the bone marrow, were first discovered in birds (in the bursa of Fabricius). The B-lymphocytes migrate from the bone marrow to the peripheral lymphatic tissues, where they interact with antigens and differentiate into a plasma cell that secretes immunoglobulins for defense against infection (humoral immunity).

B-lymphocytes are programmed to produce a specific antibody in response to an encounter with an antigen, after which they can interlock and mark the antigen for destruction. B-lymphocytes originate from hematopoietic stem cells, and their development occurs in a progression of stages that are based on morphology and functional criteria. B-lymphocyte differentiation begins in the fetal liver around the eighth week of gestation, when pre-B-lymphocytes appear. Soon thereafter, the cells migrate from the liver and are maintained in the bone marrow. At this point, the B-lymphocytes are immature; they express surface IgM but are extremely susceptible to inactivation by antigen binding. At 13 weeks' gestation, most B-lymphocytes can produce both IgM and IgD. B-lymphocytes are first observed in the peripheral blood at 12 weeks' gestation and are essentially at the level of term neonates by 15 weeks' gestation. IgG that is passively transferred from the mother's circulation is seen as early as the fourth week of gestation, but no other immunoglobulin is able to cross the placenta. Term newborns probably have a full complement of B-lymphocytes that are capable of synthesizing each type of immunoglobulin. Yet, newborns fail to respond effectively to all antigens, and their response to protein antigens is mainly through IgM production and a slow response as compared with the IgG response in adults. Most of these B-lymphocytes remain fixed in lymph nodes and spleen, although some seem to recirculate.

The primary response results when the immune system first encounters something foreign. This encounter creates a memory within the cells or the cell's surface receptors. Upon a second encounter an anamnestic or booster response occurs that is more rapid and stronger than the primary response. This response is the basis for booster vaccinations.

T-lymphocytes. T-lymphocytes are crucial in regulating the elaborate immune system, and, in particular, cytotoxic T-lymphocytes can directly attack body cells that are infected. Most of the lymphocytes that appear in the thymus originate from hematopoietic stem cells; they enter the thymus about the eighth week of gestation and are induced into lymphoid differentiation. During cellular maturation, many lymphocytes die, whereas others migrate to the thymic medulla. Mature T-lymphocytes migrate from the thymus and circulate through the lymphatics and vasculature. These circulating T-lymphocytes are long-lived, perhaps up to 10 years, explaining the phenomenon of no immediate immunologic deficit upon removal of the thymus. After birth, the thymus plays an ever-changing role in proportion to body size. It is largest during fetal development and continues to grow during childhood; involution begins at the time of puberty.

Generally, T-lymphocytes acquire immunocompetence early in fetal development, although T-lymphocyte-mediated suppression of immune responsiveness is slightly higher in newborns as compared with adults. Neonatal T-lymphocytes invoke increased spontaneous suppressor activity and suppressor effects for natural killer (NK) cell activity (Lewis & Wilson, 2001). The killer cells activity is further differentiated into MHC-restricted killer cells: cytotoxic T-lymphocytes (CTL), allogeneic cytotoxi T-lymphocytes (CTL), syngeneic CTL; MHC–non-restricted killer cells: natural killer cells-innate; and lymphokine-activated killers or LAK. In addition, T-lymphocyte cytotoxicity in the newborn is less than that in adults. This relatively decreased cytotoxicity may increase the severity of viral infections during the newborn period and may prevent graft-versus-host disease in response to maternal cells transferred to the fetus. A low T-lymphocyte function may occur as a result of neonatal viral infection, hyperbilirubinemia, steroid therapy, or maternal medications.

T-lymphocytes mature in the thymus and then travel to the peripheral tissues, where they interact with antigens to form specific effector cells, which act in delayed hypersensitivity reactions, suppression of tumors, graft rejection, and against some intracellular organisms (cellular immunity). The T-lymphocytes may also assist in regulating both humoral and cellular immune responses.

T-lymphocytes secrete interleukins that stimulate further production of T- and B-lymphocytes. Interleukin-2 (IL-2) is considered a T-cell growth factor. IL-2 is one type of cytokine. Cytokines include tumor necrosis factor (TNF), IL-2, interleukin-6 (IL-6) and interleukin-8 (IL-8) and hematopoietic colony-stimulating factors (CSF). These are produced by monocytes and macrophages. Infants who have sepsis have high plasma levels of TNF and IL-6, indicating that interleukin production has been stimulated. Cytokines are being researched for their potential role in treatment of sepsis. Interferon is a related factor that is released by T-lymphocytes, which, in turn, stimulate B-lymphocyte growth and release of other cytokines. The importance of interferon is its role in viral inhibition. IL-2 mutations are related to X-linked severe combined immunodeficiency (SCID).

Cytokines also make up chemokines or substances that result in chemotaxis and leukocyte migration (http://www.merck.com/pubs/mmanula/section12/chapter146/146a.htm). One form of these chemokines are believed to be responsible for allowing HIV to enter into monocytes and macrophages.

A third population of lymphocytes, null lymphocytes, lacks the characteristics of the mature T- and B-lymphocytes and are termed null lymphocytes. The natural killer (NK) lymphocytes are thought to be in this group of cells. NK cells are leukocytes capable of recognizing cell-surface changes on virally infected cells; NK cells bind to these infected cells and kill them. Interferon, produced by virally infected cells and by lymphocytes, activates NK cells to induce a state of viral resistance in unaffected tissue cells. This state is the first line of resistance against many viruses. Acute phase proteins are serum proteins that increase rapidly in concentration (up to 100 times) following infection. C-reactive protein is an acute phase protein that binds to the C protein of pneumococci. C-reactive protein promotes the binding of complement, which facilitates its uptake by phagocytes; this process is known as opsonization.

Lymphocytes first appear in fetal tissue at approximately 40 days of gestation; there is a rapid increase in the blood level until 25 weeks of gestation (175 days). By birth, both term and preterm neonates have lymphocyte counts ranging from 3,700 to 10,000/mm^3, reflecting the absolute lymphocytosis during the newborn period. The majority of lymphocytes are long-lived, with a life span of approximately 4 years. Some may live up to 10 years. About 15% of the total number live for only 3 to 4 days (Lewis & Wilson, 2001).

MATERNAL-FETAL-NEONATAL RELATIONSHIPS

The development of the immune system in the fetus and newborn cannot be studied in isolation from maternal influences. The ability of the mother's body to tolerate the fetus during pregnancy, rather than rejecting it as a foreign body, is not well understood. It is well documented that maternal blood with immunocompetent T-lymphocytes circulates in contact with fetal cells, that both fetal and maternal cells are exchanged through the placenta, and that humoral and cellular immunity to fetal antigens develops in the mother. The predominant transfer of antibody occurs by way of passage of IgG from the maternal to the fetal circulation by an active transport process. Such immunity is transient; nevertheless, it may provide protection during a vulnerable time of life. Although this passive antibody may protect the newborn, this process may interfere with active antibody synthesis after immunization. Secretory IgA in breast milk may also interfere with successful immunization, particularly with live polio virus, by neutralization of virus by antibody in the gastrointestinal tract (Lewis & Wilson, 2001).

Inherited Newborn Immunodeficiencies
Phagocytic Disorders. Neutropenia (low neutrophil count) is the most common sign of phagocytic dysfunction and is easily detected by a simple complete blood count (CBC) with differential. The cause of neutropenia can be further evaluated by bone marrow examination, blood smear examination, and other specific tests such as the dye test for chronic granulomatous disease. Defects in neutrophil chemotaxis, described in patients with recurrent abscesses, can be evaluated by special tests.

Disorders of Antibody Formation. Evaluation of antibody-mediated immunity begins with quantitative immunoglobulins; however, because most of the neonate's immunoglobulin is maternal, this test is not particularly helpful during the first 3 months of life. IgM elevation in the cord blood may indicate intrauterine infection, however, and elevations of both IgM and IgA suggest maternal-fetal bleeding (Kapur et al, 2002). Studies of circulating B-lymphocytes should be performed in infants with immunoglobulin deficiency. Some infants who cannot make immunoglobulins do have circulating B-lymphocytes, but these cannot differentiate into plasma cells and secrete immunoglobulins or antibodies, as is common in patients with acquired agammaglobulinemia (called common variable immunodeficiency) (Kapur et al, 2002).

T-Lymphocyte Immunodeficiency. Because T-lymphocytes constitute the vast majority of the circulating peripheral lymphocyte population, lymphopenia is seen when the number of T-lymphocytes is decreased. Delayed hypersensitivity skin reactions are not elicited in patients with cell-mediated immunodeficiency, but because such positive reactions require both a competent T-lymphocyte immunity and exposure to the specific antigens used, few neonates can mount a response in the first 6 months of life. Therefore other tests of lymphocyte responses are necessary to diagnose those infants with T-lymphocyte abnormalities, such as DiGeorge syndrome and severe combined immunodeficiency disease (SCID).

Severe Combined Immunodeficiency Disease (SCID).
SCID refers to a group of disorders characterized by the absence of both T-lymphocyte and B-lymphocyte immunity. This congenital absence of cell-mediated and antibody-mediated immunity causes a profound susceptibility to a broad range of bacterial, viral, protozoal, and fungal infections. In infants with this disorder, symptoms of life-threatening infection usually develop during the first 3 months of life, and the infants often die quickly without immunologic reconstitution. The Human Genome Project has created some speculation that at least one form of SCID may be an error of metabolism that can potentially be successfully treated in utero. Another form of X-linked SCIDS is related to genes found on chromosome 6.

Complement Disorder. Both persistent and transient deficiencies of components of serum complement have been reported. The usual serum screening for complement levels of serum proteins detects defects in the classic pathway but does not ascertain deficiencies in the alternative pathways.

ASSESSMENT OF THE IMMUNE SYSTEM

Evaluation of the neonatal immune system is challenging, encompassing the dynamic, rapidly evolving, adaptive, and changing boundaries of the newborn in response to its modifications in relation to the internal and external environment.

Subjective Data
A carefully detailed history, with particular emphasis on the family background and the pregnancy, is imperative. Areas to be included in the history are family history of immune diseases, previous stillbirths or newborn deaths in the family, infections during pregnancy, maternal medications, previous illnesses in the mother, and prior isoimmunization of the mother.

Objective Data
A comprehensive physical examination of the newborn, in conjunction with the history is the first step in evaluation. It

should provide a solid basis for interpretation of further objective data, including laboratory data. All diagnostic test results should be evaluated in relation to the clinical picture of the newborn.

Diagnostic Work-up

Because of the differences in the developmental status of the newborn's host defense mechanisms and the lack of exposure to antigens, the laboratory and clinical evaluation of the function of these mechanisms is slightly different from that performed for older children and adults. All host defense systems, including phagocytic, complement, antibody, and cell-mediated immunity, should be thoroughly evaluated. Initial screening tests should be performed, moving on to more definitive testing to establish a specific diagnosis.

INFECTION IN THE NEONATE

Identifying and caring for the infected newborn can be one of the greatest challenges in nursing. Nurses are often the first to recognize that there is something wrong with an infant, leading to investigation of the symptoms. Usually, treatment is begun once a presumptive diagnosis of infection is made. Outcome of neonatal sepsis is improved with early diagnosis and implementation of therapy. It is imperative that early signs of infection be recognized so that the infection can be diagnosed and appropriate therapy started.

Clinical Manifestations

Some of the signs and symptoms that are identified in an infected newborn are listed in Table 29-1. Temperature instability or hypothermia, the inability of the neonate to maintain temperature in the neutral thermal zone (usually between 97.7° F and 99° F) (36.5° to 37° axillary), may be an indication of serious infection. Newborns traditionally do not have well-developed febrile mechanisms; thus the absence of fever does not indicate the absence of infection in a newborn. Premature infants often present with a low body temperature. Hyperthermia can occur in term newborns, with temperatures of more than 100.1° F or 38° C, but it is relatively rare in preterm infants.

An infected infant often presents with lethargy, poor feeding, and decreased reflexes. The newborn may eat well in the morning but by evening may suck on nipples poorly or have residuals if being gavage fed. A newborn with infection may have abdominal distention, delayed gastric emptying time, and perhaps diarrhea or loose green or brown stools. Over a longer period, it may be identified that a particular infant has poor weight gain. Hypoglycemia or hyperglycemia, as well as glycosuria, may be present in an infected newborn who is unable to maintain normal metabolic processes in the face of an invasion of infectious microorganisms. Infected preterm infants often exhibit problems handling glucose loads.

Vascular perfusion is typically decreased when an infant is infected. Often, a sick neonate appears gray, mottled, or ashen in color. A sick infant may have poor perfusion, prolonged capillary filling time, and hypotension. Doppler ultrasound, have shown skin blood flow changes as early indicators of neonatal sepsis (Lott, personal communication, 2001). Skin changes can also include cyanosis and petechiae. Thrombocytopenia may also be present. Infections can cause DIC, thereby affecting the prothrombin time, partial thromboplastin time, and split fibrin product laboratory values of the newborn.

TABLE 29-1	Signs and Symptoms of Neonatal Infection

Clinical
General
Poor feeding
Irritability
Lethargy
Temperature instability

Skin
Petechiae
Pustulosis
Sclerema
Edema
Jaundice

Respiratory
Grunting
Nasal flaring
Intercostal retractions
Tachypnea/apnea

Gastrointestinal
Diarrhea
Hematochezia
Abdominal distention
Emesis
Aspirates
CNS
Hypotonia
Seizures
Poor spontaneous movement

Circulatory
Bradycardia/tachycardia
Hypotension
Cyanosis
Decreased perfusion

Laboratory Values
White blood cell count
Neutrophils	<5000 cells/mm^3, neutropenia
	>25,000 cells/mm^3, neutrophilia
Absolute neutrophil count (neutrophil and bands)	<1800 cells/mm^3 (during first week)
Immature: total neutrophil ratio	0:2
Platelet count	<100,000, thrombocytopenia
Cerebrospinal fluid	
Protein	150 to 200 mg/L (term)
	300 mg/L (preterm)
Glucose	50% to 60% or more of blood glucose level

Adapted with permission from Lott JW, Kilb JR (1992). The selection of antibacterial agents for treatment of neonatal sepsis, or which drug kills which bug? Neonatal pharmacology quarterly, 1(1), 19-29.

Newborns may exhibit hemolytic anemia, thereby significantly decreasing oxygen-carrying capacity, especially in the preterm infant.

Apnea in a term newborn in the first few hours of life can be a serious sign of inability to regulate the brain's respiratory center. Respiratory distress can be an early sign of pneumonia and must be considered carefully. Apnea in the first 24 hours of life in a preterm newborn is a common sign of infection. Cardiovascular shock can be a sudden clinical sign of fulminate sepsis and necessitates immediate and aggressive intervention to restore adequate circulation. Unexplained bradycardia may also be caused by infection. Sclerema (hardening of the skin) and sudden purpura, rash, or petechiae are signs of systemic infection.

A complete blood count can provide initial clues for diagnosis of infection. An infected infant may demonstrate leukopenia, especially neutropenia with a cell count of polymorphonuclear leukocytes less than 5000/mm^3, or the infant may have a large number of immature leukocytes (>25,000 cells/mm^3)—in particular, bands, with the band to leukocyte ratio greater than 0:2.

Indications of bacterial infection include the following:

- Increased total neutrophils—neutrophilia
- Decreased total neutrophils—neutropenia
- Increased immature forms (bands, metamyelocytes, sometimes promyelocytes, and myeloblasts)
- Increased band to segmented neutrophil ratio equal to or greater than 0:3 or immature neutrophils to total neutrophils greater than or equal to 0:2
- Presence of Dohle bodies (aggregates of reticuloendothelial system)
- Presence of vacuoles in nucleus
- Toxic granules in cell
- CD11b found on neutrophils
- Increased interleukin 8 (IL-8) levels

Other symptoms of sepsis in the newborn include jaundice, hepatosplenomegaly, and irritability. The diagnosis of sepsis in a newborn is very difficult to make and is most often based on clinical findings.

Risk Factors

Prematurity is the primary risk factor for infection. Premature infants are far more susceptible to the invasion of foreign microorganisms. Because of being born prematurely, these infants have decreased transmission maternal antibodies (passive immunity). The maternal antibodies, developed by exposure to antigens and subsequent creation of an antibody defense system, provide temporary protection to the newborn, but preterm newborns are born before the majority of maternal antibodies are transferred from the maternal circulation. Also, the cellular immune system is not well developed in the preterm newborn, thus there is decreased phagocytic cellular defenses.

Prolonged rupture of the fetal membranes (PROM) is a well-known risk factor for the development of infection. The fetus is at increased risk because the break in the amniotic sac provides a pathway for the migration of microorganisms up the vaginal vault to the fetus. The Delaying delivery in a pregnancy in a mother with PROM and a preterm fetus until pulmonary maturity is achieved creates the potential environment for bacterial proliferation and subsequent newborn infection. The benefit in promoting maturity of the immature lungs is weighed against the risk of overwhelming infection in the baby. PROM lasting longer than 24 hours is considered a risk factor in the evaluation of infants for potential for infection (Marlowe et al, 1997).

A mother with a fever or illness before or during delivery can pass the infection on to her infant. If maternal temperature is 101° F at delivery, evaluation for infection in the newborn is warranted. Maternal cervical or amniotic fluid cultures may be helpful to determine the causative microorganism. If the maternal illness suggests viral infection, newborn viral cultures should be obtained. Early identification of causative agents in the mother may help in the management of the newborn by allowing faster identification of the microorganism and initiation of appropriate antimicrobial therapy.

The presence of foul-smelling amniotic fluid is indicates newborn antimicrobial therapy in symptomatic infants. Routine blood cultures and a CBC with differential are indicated for identification of newborn infection. Under these circumstances, the placenta should be sent for pathologic evaluation.

Other risk factors associated with newborn infection are antenatal or intrapartal asphyxia, iatrogenic complications of treatment modalities, and postnatal invasive procedures. A predisposition for infection of very-low-birth-weight babies placed on indomethacin therapy for treatment of patent ductus arteriosus has been reported.

Stress in any form inhibits the newborn's ability to fight infection by increasing the metabolic rate, thus requiring more oxygen and energy to support or sustain the body's vital functions. If the newborn is severely compromised and the oxygen levels remain low, regional tissue damage can result. Ischemic or necrotic areas in the lungs, heart, brain, or gastrointestinal system provide a receptive environment for colonization and overgrowth of normal bacterial flora. This overgrowth of bacteria is one of the most common sources of newborn sepsis. Damaged tissue can be repaired only if the infectious process is reversed and adequate tissue perfusion is restored.

Several known maternal factors are associated with newborn infection: low socioeconomic status, malnutrition, inadequate prenatal care, substance abuse, PROM (before 37 weeks of gestation or at the start of labor), presence of a urinary tract infection at delivery, peripartum infection, clinical amnionitis, and general bacterial colonization. Newborn risk factors include antenatal stress, intrapartal stress (perinatal asphyxia), congenital anomalies, male sex, multiple gestations, concurrent neonatal disease processes, prematurity, immaturity of the immune system, invasive admission procedures, and antimicrobial therapies.

Differential Diagnosis

The microorganisms responsible for newborn infection have changed over the past 60 years, and there are marked regional variations. Microorganisms commonly responsible for early-onset infection include Streptococci, *Listeria monocytogenes*, and the gram-negative enteric rods. Late-onset infections are most often caused by Staphylococci, *Pseudomonas*, or *Bacteroides fragilis* (anaerobes) (Table 29-2). After day 7, nosocomial microorganisms should be considered. These microorganisms include *Staphylococcus epidermidis*, particularly when invasive medical devices, such as endotracheal tubes and arterial lines, have been used; *S. aureus* (common skin contaminant); and the spectrum of gram-negative enteric rods, including *Klebsiella, Pseudomonas, Serratia*, and *E. coli*. Hospitalized preterm newborns are often affected by repeated episodes of infection. Many of these episodes are termed presumed, sus-

TABLE **29-2**	Microorganisms Causing Neonatal Sepsis	
Gram-positive	**Gram-negative**
Cocci	
Streptococcus	Neisseria meningitidis
Group A	Neisseria gonorrhoeae
Group B	Branhamella catarrhalis
Group D	
Pneumococci	
Staphylococcus aureus (coagulase positive)	
Staphylococcus epidermidis (coagulase negative)	
Rods	
Listeria monocytogenes	Enterobacteriaceae*
Corynebacterium diphtheriae	Escherichia coli
Bacillus cereus	Klebsiella
Anaerobes	Shigella
Clostridium difficile	Proteus
Clostridium perfringens	Salmonella
Clostridium botulinum	Serratia
Clostridium tetani	Citrobacter
	Haemophilus influenzae
	Pseudomonas
	Anaerobes
	Bacteroides fragilis

Also called coliforms.
Used with permission from Lott JW, Kilb JR (1992). The selection of antibacterial agents for treatment of neonatal sepsis, or which drug kills which bug? Neonatal pharmacology quarterly, 1(1), 19-29.

pected, or clinical infection because no microorganism is recovered and cultured, despite clinical evidence of infection that responds to antimicrobial agent therapy.

A high index of suspicion of infection, resulting in early identification of the microorganism and institution of appropriate therapy provide the best outcome. Early and accurate diagnosis of infection in the newborn is a difficult task, complicated by the non-specificity of the signs of sepsis exhibited by the newborn (Gerdes & Polin, 1998). The evaluation for infection generally includes a CBC with differential, platelet count, and blood, urine, and cerebrospinal fluid (CSF) cultures. Gram stain of the CSF or urine can give an early indication of the type of microorganism responsible for the infection. Cell count and protein and glucose levels of the CSF may also indicate the presence of infection. A chest radiograph can identify the presence of pneumonia. Other tests that may be useful include latex agglutination (LA) or counterimmunoelectrophoresis (CIE) of urine or CSF or other body cavity fluids, erythrocyte sedimentation rate (ESR), and acute phase proteins (Anwer & Mustafa, 2000). Other nonspecific findings, such as hypoglycemia, hypocalcemia, thrombocytopenia, hyponatremia, and metabolic acidosis may also be present. Definitive diagnosis is based on recovery of a microorganism in blood, CSF, urine, or other body fluids.

Newer methods to detect sepsis before the appearance of the common signs of infection occur would improve outcome

by providing a window of opportunity to eliminate the microorganism before the cascade of events that occur in sepsis have begun. Successful surveillance methods such as PCR measurement of first oropharynx aspirate, heart rate analysis, measurement of C-reactive protein, or skin blood flow velocity may provide mechanisms to offer early treatment to some infants with infection and prevent infants who are not infected from receiving unnecessary treatment (Chan & Ly, 1997; Griffin & Moorman, 2001; Pedreira et al, 1997).

Prognosis
The introduction of broad-spectrum antimicrobial agents dramatically improved the prognosis for infection, and there has been a decline in sepsis-associated neonatal and infant deaths in the U.S. (Stoll et al 1998; Yurdakok, 1998). However, infection still accounts for significant morbidity and mortality in the neonatal period. Consequences of bacterial sepsis include prolonged hospitalization, increased hospital costs, and increased mortality. Sepsis case fatality rates range from less than 10% to greater than 50%, with the highest mortality rates for preterm infants and infants with early onset disease. Improved knowledge and technology to care for younger gestational age and smaller newborns has led to an increased population of newborns at higher risk for bacterial sepsis. The overall reported incidence of neonatal sepsis in the U.S. is approximately 1 to 8 cases/1,000 live births, with a mortality rate of about 25% (Gerdes & Polin, 1998; Stoll et al, 1998). However, neonatal sepsis rates are much higher in developing countries. As many as 30 million newborns (20%) born in developing countries contract sepsis in the neonatal period, and more than 1.5 million of them die (Stoll, 2001). Half of all neonatal deaths that occur on the first day of life are caused by infection. Even with aggressive therapy, the mortality rate for early-onset group B Streptococcal infection is high. Major complications of sepsis include respiratory distress, shock, acidosis, DIC, and meningitis.

Collaborative Management
Collaborative management for a newborn with sepsis is aimed at the traditional "ABCs": airway, breathing, circulation, which includes the following:

- Oxygen therapy
- Ventilatory support
- Correction of acidosis
- Volume expanders
- Extracorporeal membrane oxygenation (ECMO) if persistent pulmonary hypertension (PPHN) is present
- Antimicrobial agents and immune therapy

The exact management plan is based upon an assessment of clinical signs, careful history, and appropriate laboratory findings.

Antimicrobial Agents. The selection of antimicrobial agents is based on the identification of the microorganism present and the infant's response to therapy. Infectious microorganisms are divided into two broad classes, based upon gram-stain results: gram-positive and gram-negative. The shape of the microorganism categorizes it as either a coccus or a rod. Generally, the gram-positive organisms respond to broad-spectrum antibiotics, such as penicillin analogues, first-generation cephalosporins (beta-lactamases), and the beta-lactamase penicillins. The gram-negative microorganisms are most often susceptible to aminoglycosides and cephalosporins. Tests must be run to determine the specific sensitivity of a microorganism to the antimicrobial agent selected to ensure that the appropriate agent is prescribed. Indiscriminant use of antimicrobial agents increases the risk of resistance to routinely prescribed antimicrobial agents, thus complicating effective therapy (Kaushik et al, 1998).

Gram-positive cocci generally respond to penicillin, unless the microorganism produces beta-lactamase (or penicillinase). The beta-lactamase destroys the penicillin. S. aureus is a beta-lactamase-producing microorganism and is therefore not responsive to penicillin. A group of semisynthetic penicillins with added side chains are used for treatment of S. aureus sepsis. Of this group, nafcillin and oxacillin are most often used. Other similar drugs are methicillin, dicloxacillin, and cloxacillin. First-generation cephalosporins, such as cefazolin, cephalexin, and cephalothin, are also resistant to beta-lactamase.

S. epidermidis and S. aureus strains may be resistant to penicillin, semisynthetic penicillins, and cephalosporins. Methicillin-resistant S. aureus is unresponsive to the semisynthetic penicillins. In this case, vancomycin is the drug of choice. It may also be used for S. epidermidis and sepsis related to foreign bodies or invasive procedures. The emergence of resistant strains to available antimicrobial agents is an increasing problem due to the lack of other safe and effective antimicrobial agents to treat the infection.

Third-generation cephalosporins are used to treat gram-negative cocci that are penicillin- and methicillin-resistant. Listeria monocytogenes, a gram-positive rod, generally responds to ampicillin therapy. Aminoglycosides or third-generation cephalosporins are the drugs of choice for gram-negative enteric rods. Some gram-negative rods are classified according to their lactose-fermentation ability. The lactose-fermenters, E. coli and Klebsiella, are sensitive to aminoglycosides and third-generation cephalosporins. Shigella and Salmonella are non-lactose-fermenters, which respond well to ampicillin and third-generation cephalosporins.

Haemophilus influenzae is usually sensitive to ampicillin and third-generation cephalosporins, although some strains are ampicillin-resistant. Pseudomonas requires the following combination therapy: aminoglycoside and an anti-pseudomonas penicillin such as azlocillin, carbenicillin, imipenem, mezlocillin, piperacillin, and ticarcillin.

Two anaerobics microorganisms, Bacteroides fragilis (gram-negative) and Clostridium (gram-positive) are sometimes the cause of newborn infections. B. fragilis is susceptible to metronidazole (Flagyl), clindamycin, chloramphenicol, and some of the newer beta-lactamases, such as imipenem and ampicillin with sulbactam. Clostridium is usually susceptible to penicillin. A combination of ampicillin or penicillin and gentamicin is useful for antibacterial action against Streptococci, L. monocytogenes, and gram-negative enteric rods. This combination of antimicrobial agents has a synergistic effect (in vitro), increasing the efficacy of either drug therapy used alone. Additional therapy or selection of other agents is necessary if Staphylococcal infection is suspected, if Pseudomonas or Bacteroides (most often iatrogenically acquired) is present, if there is an outbreak of resistant organisms, or if prolonged ampicillin and gentamicin therapy has been used. Antimicrobial agents must be reevaluated after completion of cultures and sensitivity testing. See Table 29-3 for common antimicrobial agents.

The use of intravenous immune globulin (IVIG) for the prevention and treatment of neonatal infection has been proposed (Jensen & Pollock, 1997, 1998). Jensen and Pollock

Antimicrobial Agent	Dosage
Penicillin G	Sepsis
	25,000 to 50,000 IU/kg/dose
	q 12 hours <7 days
	q 8 hours >7 days
	q 6 hours >7 days
	Group B streptococcus
	Higher dose aminoglycoside
Ampicillin	Sepsis
	100 to 200 mg/kg/dose
	q 8 to 12 hours <7 days
	q 6 to 8 hours >7 days
	Meningitis
	200 to 400 mg/kg/dose
	q 8 to 12 hours <7 days
	q 6 to 8 hours >7 days
Methicillin	25 to 50 mg/kg/dose IV
	q 8 to 12 hours <7 days
	q 6 to 8 hours >7 days
Gentamicin	<7 days postnatal age
	≤29 weeks: 2.5 mg/kg/dose q 24 hours
	30-34 weeks: 3 mg/kg/dose q 24 hours
	≥35 weeks: 2.5 mg/kg/dose q 12 hours
	>7 days postnatal age
	≤29 weeks: 3.0 mg/kg/dose q 24 hours
	30 to 34 weeks: 2.5 mg/kg/dose q 12 hours
	≥35 weeks: 2.5 mg/kg/dose q 8 hours
Vancomycin	≤29 weeks: 18 mg/kg/dose q 24 hours
	30 to 36 weeks: 15 mg/kg/dose q 12 hours
	37 to 44 weeks: 10 mg/kg/dose q 8 hours
	≥45 weeks: 10 mg/kg/dose q 6 hours

q, every.
Used with permission from Lott JW, Kilb JR (1992). The selection of antibacterial agents for treatment of neonatal sepsis, or which drug kills which bug? Neonatal pharmacology quarterly, 1(1), 19-29.

(1997) conducted a meta-analysis of the available published data. A total of 4933 newborns enrolled in 12 studies comprised the sample for the meta-analyses. Results of this meta-analyses showed that IVIG administration offered minimal benefit for prevention of sepsis in low-birth-weight infants, but mortality decreased when IVIG was administered to infected newborns. Infected newborns that did not receive IVIG had 6 times the risk of dying than infants who did receive the IVIG.

TYPES OF NEONATAL INFECTION

This section briefly describes the types of microorganisms that typically cause neonatal infection and their clinical manifestations, diagnoses, and collaborative management. The discussion includes both congenitally acquired and nosocomially acquired infections caused by bacterial, viral, fungal, and protozoal organisms.

Congenital Infections

The microorganisms most often responsible for congenitally acquired infections have been grouped together as the TORCH infections. These include *toxoplasmosis*, *others*, *rubella*, *cytomegalovirus* (CMV), and *herpes*. The "others" category includes various microorganisms that have been responsible for congenital infections. However, the list of microorganisms implicated in congenital infections has grown, so the acronym is no longer inclusive. It is common for this acronym to include S on the end for syphilis. It is still used when discussing infections acquired by the fetus in utero. These conditions may mimic neonatal hemochromatosis that results from iron deposits in the liver, skin, and heart. The symptoms are similar to TORCHS infections.

Toxoplasmosis.   Perinatal healthcare workers discovered the importance of the parasite *Toxoplasma gondii* in the 1980s. *Toxoplasma gondii* is a pathogen that is ever-present in nature. Perinatal transmission takes place when the mother contracts the protozoa and the subsequent protozoemia transmits the organism transplacentally to the fetus. The microorganisms then invade and multiply within the placenta and eventually enter the fetal circulation. The life cycle of *Toxoplasma* is complicated. The predominant host of this organism is the ordinary house cat; however, other animals can serve as hosts. There are significant differences in the prevalence rates of this microorganism throughout the world (Remington et al, 2001). The tissue cyst form of the microorganism persists in the flesh of animals, such as cattle and sheep. The oocyte form of the parasite persists in soil contaminated by cat feces. Thus congenital toxoplasmosis is known to be transmitted from undercooked meat or food or from fomites in cat feces. In the United States, approximately 20% to 70% of the population has been exposed to this protozoa. There is wide variability in the prevalence of seropositive women of childbearing age among countries, geographic regions of the same country, and ethnic origin; different cultural practices regarding food are probably the major cause of this difference. Because meat is the main vector for transmission, areas where there is less *T. gondii* present in meat due to improved methods for processing or cooking meat have lower prevalence rates. The greatest risk is when a nonimmune pregnant woman is exposed to this *T. gondii* during fetal organogenesis (weeks 4 to 8 of gestation), when the risk for congenital anomalies is high (Remington et al, 2001).

Clinical Manifestations.   Acute toxoplasmosis in a pregnant woman often goes undetected and undiagnosed. Clinical questioning after the identification of an infected newborn or infant often leads to reflection and memories of a period of enlarged lymph nodes and fatigue without fever. Women sometimes report a mononucleosis-like or flu-like syndrome that may have a febrile course, with malaise, headache, fatigue, sore throat, and sore muscles. These symptoms may persist up to 6 months; however, that duration is unusual. A newborn with congenital toxoplasmosis can present with hydrocephalus, chorioretinitis, and intracranial calcifications (Box 29-1). There is a wide variety of clinical signs in the scope of the disease. The newborn can appear normal at birth or exhibit severe erythroblastosis, hydrops fetalis, and other clinical signs (Remington et al, 2001).

Neurologic signs similar to encephalitis (e.g., convulsions, bulging fontanelles, nystagmus, and increased head circumference) may be the only significant presentation of this clinical

---

BOX 29-1

Guidelines for Evaluation of Newborn of Mother Who Acquired Her Infection during Gestation to Determine Whether Infant Has Congenital *Toxoplasma* Infection and to Assess Degree of Involvement

History and physical examination
Pediatric neurologic evaluation
Pediatric ophthalmologist examination of retinae
Complete blood cell count with differential, platelet count
Liver function tests (bilirubin, GGTP)
Urinalysis, serum creatinine
Serum quantitative immunoglobulins
Serum Sabin-Feldman dye test (IgG), IgM ISAGA, IgA ELISA, IgE ISAGA/ELISA* (with maternal serum, perform same tests as for infant except substitute IgM ELISA for the IgM ISAGA and also obtain AC/HS*)
Cerebrospinal fluid cell count, protein, glucose and *T. gondii*-specific IgG and IgM antibodies as well as quantitative IgG to calculate antibody load
Subinoculate into mice or tissue culture 1 ml peripheral blood buffy coat or clot and digest of 100 g placenta (see Diagnosis for method of digestion). Consider PCR of buffy coat from approximately 1 ml blood, cell pellet from approximately 1 ml cerebrospinal fluid, and cell pellet from 10 to 20 ml amniotic fluid (see Diagnosis)
Brain computed tomography scan with and without contrast medium enhancement
Auditory brainstem response to 20 dB

GGTP, *Gamma-glutamyltranspeptidase*; PCR, *polymerase chain reaction.*
When performed in combination in laboratories, these tests have demonstrated a high degree of specificity and sensitivity in establishing the diagnosis of acute infection in the pregnant woman and congenital infection in the fetus and newborn.
From Remington JS, Klein JO: Infectious diseases of the fetus and newborn infant, ed 5, Philadelphia: WB Saunders.

---

problem. If the newborn receives treatment, signs may disappear, allowing normal cerebral growth and development if there was no permanent neurological damage.

Mild cases of the disease can easily go unrecognized in the newborn. Signs of delayed onset of disease in premature newborns include severe central nervous system or eye lesions appearing at 3 months of age. In term newborns, delayed disease may occur in the first 2 months of life and is usually mild. Clinical signs include generalized infection, enlarged liver and spleen, late-onset jaundice, enlarged lymph nodes, or late-onset central nervous system problems, including hydrocephalus and eye lesions. Infants with congenital toxoplasmosis may have new lesions that appear until age 5 (Remington et al, 2001).

Collaborative Management.   The best and most effective treatment is prevention and early recognition. The cost effectiveness of pregnancy serology screening depends on the costs of the tests and the estimated cost of treating the infection, if identified early. At present in the United States, screening is done erratically and there are no particular screening standards. Counseling education for the prevention of toxoplasmosis should focus on avoidance of raw meat and use of gloves during feline litter box handling and during gardening in what may be contaminated soil. Pregnant women who are sero-negative should exercise caution to avoid the risk of contracting *T. gondii* during pregnancy through avoiding cat litter, digging in the soil, and handling or eating undercooked meat. They should inform their health care providers if they experience any signs that could be attributed to *T. gondii* infection.

Treatment for congenital toxoplasmosis is pyrimethamine plus sulfonamides (Table 29-4). The suggested dose is 2 mg/kg/day orally for 2 days followed by 1 mg/kg/day for 2 or 6 months, then 1 mg/kg/day every Monday, Wednesday, and Friday for one year, given in doses of 100 mg/kg/day in two divided oral doses for one year. Leucovorin 10 mg is given three times weekly during pyrimethamine therapy and for one week after therapy. These drugs are potentially toxic and need close monitoring.

Corticosteroids are given in the form of prednisone at 1 mg/kg per day in two divided doses elevated protein in cerebrospinal fluid (CSF) or active chorioretinitis resolve. (Remington et al, 2001).

Toxoplasmosis is one of the most common causes of deafness. The Collaborative Perinatal Project found a doubling in the frequency of deafness in infants of mothers with the antibody for toxoplasmosis. There was a 60% increase in microcephaly and a 30% increase in low intelligence quotients (less than 70) in relation to high antibody levels in mothers (Remington et al, 2001).

Nursing Management. Nursing management is supportive and depends on the severity of the infection. Neurologic impairment at birth can be significant and require ventilation and seizure control. Non-pregnant personnel should care for documented positive infants to prevent risk of transmission.

Rubella. In 1941, N. McAlister Gregg described 78 patients with congenital cataracts. These patients were small-for-gestational-age and had feeding difficulties and congenital heart problems. A history of German measles during pregnancy was found in 68 of the cases (87%). Much of the current knowledge about the effects of congenital rubella was established by Gregg's report on these patients (Gregg, 1941). It has been further established that the rubella virus can be responsible for other abnormalities. The most important consequences of rubella are the miscarriages, stillbirths, fetal anomalies, and therapeutic abortions that result when rubella infection occurs during early pregnancy, especially during the first trimester. An estimated 20,000 cases of CRS occurred during 1964 to 1965 during the last U.S. rubella epidemic before rubella vaccine became available.

The largest number of cases of rubella occurred in 1969, with 57,686 reported cases. With the advent of vaccination in 1969, the number of cases began to decline rapidly; since 1992, fewer than 500 cases were reported annually. The majority of these cases occurred in populations that do not accept conventional medicine and do not immunize their children. However, the proportion of cases of adults over 20 years old has increased from 29% in 1991 to 74% in 1999. Since 1992, about 6 cases of congenital rubella syndrome have been reported annually; these cases were seen in infants whose mothers were from countries where rubella vaccine is not normally given (CDC, 2001).

Since 1992, reported indigenous rubella and CRS have continued to occur at a low but relatively constant endemic level with an annual average of less than 200 rubella cases (128 cases in 1995 and 213 cases in 1996). However, in the United States, surveillance for CRS relies on a passive system. Consequently, the reported annual totals of CRS are regarded as minimum figures, representing an estimated 40% to 70% of all cases. Failure to immunize many young children has resulted in an increase in rubella incidence. Therefore, despite a national immunization program, at least 10% of women of childbearing age are vulnerable to the virus, particularly the wild virus, because either they have not been immunized or have not acquired immunity from the infection themselves. Small rubella outbreaks have been reported all over the United States. Although the epidemiology of the infection over the past 25 years has changed and the incidence has significantly decreased, rubella has not been eradicated. Prevention of rubella in post-pubertal women and CRS continues to be a major goal of the CDC.

Clinical Manifestations. The anomalies most commonly associated with CRS are auditory (e.g., sensorineural deafness), ophthalmic (e.g., cataracts, microphthalmia, glaucoma, chorioretinitis), cardiac (e.g., patent ductus arteriosus, peripheral pulmonary artery stenosis, atrial or ventricular septal defects), and neurologic (e.g., microcephaly, meningoencephalitis, mental retardation). In addition, infants with CRS frequently exhibit both intrauterine and postnatal growth restriction. Other conditions sometimes observed among babies who have CRS include radiolucent bone defects, hepatosplenomegaly, thrombocytopenia, and purpuric skin lesions. Newborns who are moderately or severely affected by CRS are readily recognizable at birth, but mild CRS (e.g., slight cardiac involvement or deafness) may be detected months or years after birth—or not at all.

Although CRS has been estimated to occur among 20% to 25% of infants born to women who acquire rubella during the first 20 weeks of pregnancy, this figure may underestimate the risk for fetal infection and birth defects. When infants born to mothers who were infected during the first 8 weeks of gestation were followed for 4 years, 85% were affected. When infections occur between weeks 9 to 12 of gestation, the risk drops to about 52%. Infection after the twentieth week of gestation rarely causes defects. Unapparent (subclinical) maternal rubella infection can also cause congenital malformations. Fetal infection without clinical signs of CRS can occur during any stage of pregnancy.

The typical presentation of the rubella virus is mild, with malaise, low-grade fever, headache, and conjunctivitis. In 1 to 5 days, a macular rash appears on the face and usually disappears after 3 to 4 days. Natural viremia is necessary for placental and fetal rubella infection. Most cases occur following primary disease. Frequently, skin rashes that resemble rubella may occur as a result of adenovirus, enterovirus, or other respiratory virus infections. Laboratory titers are recommended to confirm the diagnosis of rubella infection.

A fetus infected with rubella often has cardiac defects and deafness. The central nervous system seems particularly vulnerable to the rubella virus, especially if the virus is acquired before the first 16 weeks of gestation. Hearing loss, mental retardation, cardiac malformations, and eye defects characterize congenital rubella syndrome.

The rubella virus can slow cell replication. This causes intrauterine growth retardation and a failure of cell differentia-

TABLE 29-4	Guidelines for Treatment of *Toxoplasma gondii* Infection in the Pregnant Woman and Congenital *Toxoplasma* Infection in the Fetus, Infant, and Older Child.		

Manifestation of Infection	Medication	Dosage	Duration of Therapy
In pregnant women with acute toxoplasmosis First 21 weeks of gestation or until term if fetus not infected	Spiramycin[a]	1 g every 8 hr without food	A = until fetal infection documented or excluded at 21 wk; if documented, in alternate months with pyrimethamine, leucovorin, and sulfadiazine[b]
If fetal infection confirmed after 18th week of gestation	Pyrimethamine *plus*	Loading dose: 100 mg per day in two divided doses for 2 days then 50 mg per day	As in A[b]
	Sulfadiazine *plus*	Loading dose: 75 mg/kg per day in two divided doses (maximum 4 g per day) for 2 days, then 100 mg/kg per day in two divided doses (maximum 4 g per day)	As in A[b]
	Leucovorin (folinic acid)	10-20 mg daily[c]	During and for 1 wk after pyrimethamine therapy
Congenital *Toxoplasma* infection in the infant[d]	Pyrimethamine[d] *plus*	Loading dose: 2 mg/kg per day for 2 days, then 1 mg/kg per day for 2 or 6 mo,[e] then this dose every Monday, Wednesday, Friday[d]	1 yr[f]
	Sulfadiazine[d] *plus*	100 mg/kg per day in two divided doses	1 yr[f]
	Leucovorin[d]	10 mg three times weekly[c]	During and for 1 wk after pyrimethamine therapy
	Corticosteroids[g] (prednisone) have been used when cerebrospinal fluid protein is ≥1 g/dl and when active chorioretinitis threatens vision	B = 1 mg/kg per day in two divided doses	C = Until resolution of elevated (≥1 g/dl) cerebrospinal fluid protein level or active chorioretinitis that threatens vision
Active chorioretinitis in older children	Pyrimethamine *plus*	Loading dose: 2 mg/kg per day (maximum 50 mg) for 2 days, then maintenance, 1 mg/kg per day (maximum 25 mg)	D = Usually 1-2 wk beyond the time that signs and symptoms have resolved
	Sulfadiazine *plus*	Loading dose: 75 mg/kg, then maintenance, 50 mg/kg every 12 hr	As in D
	Leucovorin	10-20 mg three times weekly[c]	During and for 1 wk after pyrimethamine therapy
	Corticosteroids[g]	As in B	As in C

[a] Available only on request from the U.S. Food and Drug Administration, telephone number 301-443-5680.

[b] The only studies are those of Daffos et al. However, because Daffos and colleagues found pyrimethamine-sulfadiazine therapy to be superior to spiramycin for treatment of the fetus, continuous therapy with pyrimethamine, sulfadiazine, and leucovorin should be considered in the third trimester. This regimen has been used extensively in France and appears to be safe and feasible. Alternatively, in the United States, daily administration of pyrimethamine (50 mg per day) and sulfadiazine (1 g each 6 hr) plus leucovorin (10 mg) administered every other day to the mother has been used in the treatment of a limited number of fetuses in utero. This treatment was begun after the eighteenth week of gestation and continued until birth of the infant. Subsequent treatment of the infant is the same as that described under treatment of congenital infection. This appears to have been feasible and safe treatment for a small number of patients. When the diagnosis of infection in the fetus is established earlier, we suggest that sulfadiazine be used alone until approximately 20 weeks of gestation, at which time pyrimethamine should be added to the regimen.

[c] Adjusted for megaloblastic anemia, granulocytopenia, or thrombocytopenia; blood cell counts, including platelets, should be monitored as described in text.

[d] Optimal dosage, feasibility, and toxicity currently being evaluated or planned in ongoing Chicago-based National Collaborative Treatment Trial, telephone number 773-834-4152.

[e] These two regimens are currently being compared in a randomized manner in the National Collaborative Treatment Trial. Data are not yet available to determine which, if either, is superior. Both regimens appear to be feasible and relatively safe.

[f] The duration of therapy is unknown for infants and children, especially those with AIDS. See discussion in the Congenital Toxoplasma Infection and AIDS section.

[g] Corticosteroids should be used only in conjunction with pyrimethamine, sulfadiazine, and leucovorin treatment and should be continued until signs of inflammation (high cerebrospinal fluid protein >1 g/dl) or active chorioretinitis that threatens vision have subsided—dosage can then be tapered and discontinued; use only with pyrimethamine, sulfadiazine, and leucovorin.

Adapted from information appearing in The New England Journal of Medicine, Daffos F, Forestier F, Capella-Pavlovsky M, et al. Prenatal management of 746 pregnancies at risk for congenital toxoplasmosis. N Engl J Med 31:271-275, 1988.

From Remington JS, Klein JO: Infectious diseases of the fetus and newborn infant, ed 5, Philadelphia: WB Saunders.

tion during fetal organ formation. Tissue damage also seems to occur from the inflammatory response to the infection or is even possibly an autoimmune reaction. Myocarditis, pneumonitis, hepatosplenomegaly, and vascular stenosis can also be present because of these processes. As is seen with other severe congenital infections, signs and symptoms may continue to develop until the patient is 10 to 20 years of age. Late clinical signs of this disease include insulin-dependent diabetes, thyroid abnormalities, hypoadrenalism, hearing loss, and eye damage.

Differential Diagnosis. The possibility of subclinical infection with rubella highlights the need for laboratory confirmation. Clinical confirmation of rubella isolation is obtainable in approximately 4 to 6 weeks. The detection of rubella antibody confirms the presence of the infection. Rubella-specific IgG persists for life and can be detected by enzyme immunoassay. With confirmed serologic results, the risk of fetal damage after 16 weeks' gestation appears to be small.

Demonstration of rubella-specific IgM in fetal blood obtained by cordocentesis has been used to establish diagnosis in utero. Chorionic villus sampling has also demonstrated recovery of the virus during the first trimester.

Collaborative Management. All infants should be vaccinated against rubella at 15 months of age and again just before school entry. Also, women who do not have detectable IgG rubella antibody and are of childbearing age (and not pregnant) should be immunized. After immunization, they should avoid pregnancy for at least 3 months to decrease the risk for development of rubella syndrome in the fetus. Health care workers who may be inadvertently exposed to rubella should be immunized if they do not have immune titers. If a woman receives rubella vaccine and has recently received blood products or RhoGAM (RhIG), the vaccine may not trigger an immune response because blood products and RhoGAM have pooled sera that may contain antibodies against rubella. Thus the woman's body does not produce antibodies. These women should have titers drawn 6 weeks after vaccination or at most 3 months after vaccination (CDC, 2001; Cooper & Alford, 2001).

In more than 500 women who were accidentally immunized against rubella while pregnant, there were no cases of congenital rubella syndrome. Rubella vaccination is not recommended during pregnancy, yet the risks to the fetus have been determined to be negligible, and an inadvertent rubella vaccination by itself is not considered an indication for termination of pregnancy.

Currently, treatment in the nursery of the rubella-infected infant is rare. Therapy for identified problems, such as respiratory, cardiac, or neurologic deficits, is supportive, and there is no specific recommended therapy. Caretakers should have known immune titers and not be pregnant. Rubella-specific IgM can usually accurately identify these infants. Persistent shedding of the virus may last until 1 year of life; thus pregnant women should avoid contact with these patients. Follow-up care for surgical corrections of heart defects and cataracts as well as special schooling may be needed for these infants.

Cytomegalovirus. Infection with CMV, a member of the herpes family, is common. CMV is a DNA virus covered with a glycoprotein coat that closely resembles the herpes and varicella-zoster viruses. By adulthood, most people have been exposed to CMV, and antibodies have developed to it. CMV

infection is more prevalent in lower socioeconomic groups and is especially common in developing countries. In the United States, women of childbearing age from lower socioeconomic groups have an incidence of infection of approximately 6%, whereas those from higher socioeconomic groups have an incidence of approximately 2%. CMV may lie dormant, with periods of exacerbation followed by remission. During remission, the patient is asymptomatic, but the virus is shed (Nelson & Demmier, 1997). The virus is usually transmitted person to person through body fluids and secretions. Blood, urine, breast milk, cervical mucus, semen, and saliva harbor CMV. The virus can cause an infectious mononucleosis-like syndrome, with general malaise, liver complications, fever, and general fatigue. Perinatal transmission can occur within 2 to 3 days of infection by transplacental crossing of the organism. The fetus can also contract the virus intrapartally while descending through the birth canal from infected maternal cervical secretions. CMV can also be transmitted through infected breast milk (Stagno, 2001).

Clinical Manifestations. More damage occurs to the fetus when the exposure to and acquisition of CMV occur from a primary lesion. Congenital CMV occurs in approximately 0.2% to 2.2% of all newborn infants. Primary lesions cause intrauterine growth restriction, microcephaly, periventricular calcifications, deafness, blindness, congenital cataracts, profound mental retardation, hepatosplenomegaly, and jaundice. A characteristic pattern of petechiae, called "blueberry muffin" syndrome, is associated with congenital CMV. Approximately 26% of severely infected infants die. Severe complications at birth are seen in approximately 5% of congenital infections. Sequelae develop in 5% to 15% of asymptomatic infected infants and in 90% of symptomatic infected infants (Stagno, 2001). Recurrent CMV infections are not as severe because of partial antibody protection from previous exposure. The incidence of neonatal complications is reported to be from 5% to 10% for hearing loss, 2% for chorioretinitis, and less than 1% for mental retardation.

Diagnosis. Suspicious clinical findings or obstetric history warrant further investigation for CMV infection. Urine culture for CMV is the most rapid and sensitive indicator of infection. IgG and IgM antibody titers should also be measured. Elevated IgM levels alone denote exposure to CMV but are not diagnostic because there is no method to determine the timing of the exposure. Elevated neonatal IgG titers indicate perinatally acquired CMV infection. A negative maternal IgG titer and a positive neonatal IgG titer indicate postnatal transmission. Experimentally, elevated rheumatoid factors may provide evidence to support the diagnosis of CMV in subclinical cases (Stagno, 2001).

Prevention. Transmission of CMV via infected blood products has been significantly decreased through the use of CMV-negative donors or irradiation of blood products. Premature and low-birth-weight infants are especially vulnerable to the infusion of this virus in blood products. The best method of prevention is the institution of standard precautions, including good hand-washing techniques.

Collaborative Management. Newborns with CMV infection exhibit a wide range of symptoms. General supportive therapy is based on the presence of these clinical manifestations. Specific therapy for CMV is still in the experimental stage but includes immunoglobulin therapy, vaccines, and chemotherapy. Intravenous immunoglobulin therapy provides passive immunity to at-risk infants but not to those already infected. Two live attenuated vaccines for CMV have been developed and tested on renal transplant patients. Theoretically, these vaccines would be useful preconceptually or perinatally to prevent vertical transmission; however, only limited research has been done with this population. Chemotherapy offers the most promise for treatment of neonatal CMV infection; however, it has not been shown to be clinically effective in improving outcome.

Chemotherapeutic agents under investigation include idoxuridine, cytosine arabinoside, adenine arabinoside, acyclovir, leukocyte interferon, interferon stimulators, and ganciclovir. Toxicity and immunosuppression associated with these agents raise concern about widespread neonatal use (Stagno, 2001).

Syphilis. The microorganism *Treponema pallidum* has persisted as a threat to perinatal patients over the past 400 years. Despite available therapy for the past 40 years, many women do not receive adequate treatment for primary or secondary infections. In addition, the virus is known to lie dormant, much like the herpes family of viruses. Currently, the incidence of syphilis is increasing, owing to an increase in substance abuse, sexual practices involving multiple partners, and human immunodeficiency virus (HIV)-positive immunocompromised individuals, who act as reservoirs for *T. pallidum*. Consequently, there has been a resurgence of congenital infections. Recent worldwide concern regarding the role of genital ulcers in conjunction with HIV infection has created great concern for eradication of sexually transmitted diseases (Ingall & Sanchez, 2001).

Screening at the first prenatal visit most often makes the diagnosis of antepartum syphilis. Screening usually involves the use of the venereal disease research laboratory (VDRL) test or rapid plasma reagin (RPR) test, each of which measures anticardiolipin antibody. These tests are reactive in almost 80% of patients with secondary or early latent (less than 1 year duration) primary syphilis. A definitive diagnosis can be made with an elevated VDRL or RPR accompanied by a positive *T. pallidum* fluoroantibody test or a reactive serologic test for *T. pallidum* in the CSF. Condylomata lata, bony changes, or snuffles in the presence of a positive serologic test are diagnostic (Ingall & Sanchez, 2001).

Untreated syphilis adversely affects pregnancy outcome. Vertical transmission of treponemas can occur at any time during pregnancy. The microorganisms can cause preterm labor, PROM, stillbirth, congenital infection, or neonatal death.

The rate of syphilis has changed undergone changes due to the changes in treatment and changes in the control program. An effective control program that included provision of penicillin and adequate personnel dedicated to the eradication of syphilis led to a decline after World War II, to an all time low in 1956. The success of the control program led to decreased resources being allocated to the program, and there was a significant increase in the 1960s that resulted in increased resources and a consequent decline in the rate, which in turn generated another decrease in funding, followed by another increase in the rate in the 1980s. There has been an 86% decline in the incidence of primary and secondary syphilis since 1990s. This improvement has been attributed to improved education, adequate allocation of resources, wider screening practices and better identification of infected individuals, and

improved counseling and patient education services (Ingall & Sanchez, 2001).

Despite the decline, syphilis is endemic in the U.S. Syphilis is more prevalent in racial and ethnic minorities who live in poverty and receive inadequate medical care (Ingall & Sanchez, 2001). Current, untreated secondary infection causes the greatest risk of damage to the fetus, particularly if infection occurs during the period of organogenesis. Late untreated syphilis in the mother usually results in delivery of an unsymptomatic infant who needs treatment in the newborn nursery. Congenital syphilis primarily affects young, unmarried women from low socioeconomic backgrounds who receive inadequate or no prenatal care. The recent decline in syphilis has led to a decrease of congenital syphilis, although a change in the criteria for making the diagnosis may account for some of the decline.

Clinical Manifestations. When newborns acquire syphilis from hematogenous spread across the placenta, the effects are on the major organ systems of the fetus, especially the central nervous system. Common presentations of the infected infant are hepatosplenomegaly, jaundice, low birth weight, intrauterine growth retardation, anemia, and osteochondritis. There is often a bilateral superficial peeling of the skin (desquamation) on the neonatal palms and soles. Nonimmune hydrops is a common presentation in congenital syphilis. The symptoms of perinatal syphilis are similar to those of any other viral infection that spreads hematogenously from the mother to the placenta and on to the developing fetus (Ingall & Sanchez, 2001).

Differential Diagnosis. A lumbar puncture for CSF analysis and radiographs of the long bones facilitate the definitive diagnosis of syphilis in the neonate. Congenital neurosyphilis is always a consideration, and the CSF should be examined for the presence of spirochetes. Radiologic changes such as osteochondritis (a blurring of the epiphyseal borders) demonstrate recent fetal infection (within 5 weeks' gestation), and periostitis represents prolonged involvement, probably within 16 weeks or second-trimester infection.

Stillborn infants should be examined by whole-body radiographic study and autopsy if possible. Spirochetes can be visualized by special staining techniques (Ingall & Sanchez, 2001). Interpretation of serologic tests for syphilis on serum obtained from cord blood is complicated because of the transplacental transfer of maternal IgG antibody. VDRL titers at least two dilutions higher than maternal VDRL titers indicate probable fetal infection.

Prognosis. Infants with syphilis should receive the same amount of follow-up as normal infants. Serologic measurements can be made at follow-up visits at 1, 2, 3, 6, and 12 months of age. The infection can be effectively treated, but the physiologic and developmental prognosis depends on the degree of organ damage sustained during fetal development.

Collaborative Management. Newborns with a reactive serologic test for syphilis require treatment if the following are relevant:

1. The infant has clinical, laboratory, or radiographic findings, or a combination of these
2. No documented therapy before delivery from an infected mom
3. Inadequate or unknown maternal treatment status

4. Maternal treatment with drugs other than penicillin
5. Maternal treatment within 4 weeks of delivery
6. Maternal nontreponemal antibody titers did not decrease at least fourfold, despite adequate therapy
7 Maternal serologic evidence of relapse or re-infection after therapy
8. Follow-up of infant is uncertain (Ingall & Sanchez, 2001).

The recommended treatment for a newborn infected with congenital syphilis is penicillin. Treatment of proven congenital syphilis should consist of aqueous crystalline penicillin G, 50,000 units/kg every 12 hours for the first week of life and every 8 hours beyond the first week of life for 10 days, or aqueous procaine penicillin G 50,000 units/kg IM once daily for 10 days. If more than one day of therapy is missed, the regimen should be restarted. For infants in whom the status of congenital syphilis is not proven but for whom a high risk exists, treatment as above or with a single dose of benzathine penicillin G 50,000 units/kg IM with close serologic follow-up is recommended. Isolation of an infant with suspicious symptoms may be necessary until appropriate treatment is given. There is a definite role for nursing education and support in the treatment of an infant exposed to syphilis. The 10-day course of penicillin treatment may lead to the establishment of a trusting relationship between the nurse and family, thus providing opportunity to give more information regarding sexual risk factors. Families often need encouragement and support to get treatment for other sexual partners and to obtain other necessary medical evaluations (such as HIV screening or drug counseling).

Herpes Simplex Virus.   Herpes simplex virus (HSV) is a member of a family of large DNA viruses. They contain linear, double strands of DNA. The herpes family also includes CMV, varicella-zoster, and Epstein-Barr virus. HSV possesses the quality of "latency," whereby the virus can persist in a latent state for a period of time and then be reactivated by certain stimuli. A strand of the viral DNA persists in an infected individual for a lifetime; thus the virus maintains a "foothold" in its host. Clinical experiences demonstrate that, after primary HSV infection, at the site of the infection (perhaps an oral or genital site), the microorganism invades the sensory nerve endings and remains there. The more severe the primary infection, as determined by the size and extent of the skin lesion, the more likely are frequent recurrences.

Potential stimuli for HSV reactivation include periods of stress, emotional trauma, and prolonged exposure to the sun. Maintenance of the latency state and recurrence of the virus are topics of intense current research. There are many unanswered questions about what triggers latency and about the cofactors for reactivation of the virus.

Maternal HSV is usually the source of neonatal infection. The risk of neonatal infection is estimated to be 5% if it is recurrent herpes and higher if it is a primary infection (Arvin & Whitley, 2001; Mogami, 1997). Recurrent infections are the most common problem in pregnancy. Transmission of the infection to the fetus can be caused by passage through infected genital secretions in the intrapartum period or by ascending infection from the vaginal vault via ruptured (or not) membranes. Many women can be asymptomatic and still be shedding HSV. Although primary infection is less common, it causes the most severe neonatal disease, most likely including central nervous system problems, disseminated disease into other organ systems, and probable death. The incidence of

intrapartum transmission with a primary infection is approximately 40% to 50%. Many neonatal complications such as prematurity, intrauterine growth restriction, and respiratory distress syndrome can potentiate the neonate's illness, thus limiting the ability to fight off HSV. The severity of neonatal infection ranges broadly from severe to benign and asymptomatic, but the incidence of neonatal herpes is approximately 1,500 to 2,000 cases per year (D'Andrea & Ferrera, 1998). Susceptibility of the newborn to HSV is increased because there is a lack of passively acquired maternal antibody in some infants. The failure of newborns to control HSV may also be related to decreased production of or response to interferon or perhaps to decreased production of cellular cytotoxic immune mechanisms (Arvin & Whitley, 2001).

Clinical Manifestations.   Acquisition of HSV in utero can result in spontaneous abortion, preterm birth, or a normal baby. Manifestations of the disease are broad; the clinical presentation of the congenital acquisition of the infection includes skin vesicles or scarring, hypopigmentation, chorioretinitis, microcephaly, and hydranencephaly. There are three categories of neonatal patients. The first category includes patients with localized infections of the skin, eyes, or mouth. The second category includes patients with encephalitis. In this group, neurologic sequelae occur in approximately 50%. Approximately one third of these patients do not have skin vesicles, and they are identified by history alone. CSF is positive for the virus in 25% to 40% of these cases. Presence of cells and increased protein are very common in the CSF of patients with encephalitis, and they die if not treated. The third category of neonatal patients includes those with disseminated disease characterized by irritability, seizures, respiratory distress, jaundice, DIC, shock, and other symptoms of viral and bacterial sepsis. All major neonatal organs may be involved. Liver and the adrenals are the most common reservoirs for the virus. The central nervous system is involved in 70% to 90% of affected neonates. In more than 20% of the newborns with disseminated disease, skin vesicles do not develop, making identification of positive infants more difficult (Arvin & Whitley, 2001). It should be noted that it is possible for a newborn to present with Herpes zoster infection, although it is not common (Mogami, 1997).

Differential Diagnosis.   Laboratory tests are the most common way to differentiate HSV infection from other bacterial and viral infections. The most rapid method includes a cytologic examination. Routine cultures should be obtained from any vesicle on the skin, oropharyngeal or eye secretions, or stool. Viral typing is done for epidemiologic purposes only. HSV types I and II are the most commonly known. Type I has been most closely associated with any herpes found outside the genital area; type II is commonly referred to as genital herpes. However, either type can occur almost anywhere in the body. Treatment does not differ for these different viral types.

Risk Factors.   Intrapartal transmission is more likely to occur in the presence of ruptured membranes. Other risk factors include intrauterine fetal monitoring and fetal scalp sampling. It is not recommended that women infected with HSV be monitored by these methods. Transmission from mother to infant from an infected breast lesion has been reported. Transmission has also been documented from oral lesions (Arvin & Whitley, 2001).

Prevention. Presence of maternal active HSV genital lesions is a contraindication to vaginal delivery. If the membranes have been ruptured 4 hours or longer, cesarean section may or may not prevent transmission to the neonate. Postnatal nosocomial transmission is greatly reduced with good hand-washing techniques and universal precautions.

Collaborative Management. Acyclovir has become the drug of choice for treating HSV infections. Acyclovir appears to be very helpful in decreasing the frequency of the reactivation of the virus, particularly in the treatment of herpes simplex encephalitis. Acyclovir is a selective inhibitor of viral replication and thus has few side effects. The recommended dosage is 30 mg/kg/day intravenously divided over 8 hours. Duration of therapy is 14 to 21 days.

Early identification and intervention are essential, because early institution of antiviral therapy has been shown to improve outcome and decrease sequelae (Arvin & Whitley, 2001). Acyclovir is a potent drug with potential for toxicity; neonatal therapeutic ranges have not been established. Monitoring of the infant's physiologic status is necessary to detect potential side effects. Adequate hydration is necessary to minimize the risk of nephrotoxicity, and dosage adjustments are necessary if renal clearance is impaired. Infected infants must be isolated, because viral shedding provides a reservoir for infecting other infants in the nursery.

HSV continues to be a life-threatening neonatal infection in the United States. There is growing concern about transmission of the virus to unborn children with the concomitant increase in genital herpes as a sexually transmitted disease. It is important for all health care providers in the perinatal arena to maintain a high index of suspicion in infants whose symptoms may be compatible with HSV infection. Early identification allows prompt treatment or necessary continued observation or both. Continued research may produce a more rapid method of virus identification and perhaps a safe and effective vaccine. Prevention of neonatal HSV depends on improved knowledge regarding the factors of virus transmission between mother and infant. Cesarean section in women with active genital herpes is still recommended; however, there is no benefit of cesarean section unless there are active herpetic lesions at the time of delivery (Arvin & Whitley, 2001).

Primary nursing responsibilities in the management of a family with HSV infection are education and support. Mothers should be educated as to the mode, methods, and possible origins of the HSV, and concerns should be addressed regarding potential transmission to newborns. Nurses are often the first to document a mother's comment that she "had a small bump or blister and fever" right before her infant was born. Careful history taking and thorough questioning can often identify potentially infected patients early. With the diagnosis of genital herpes and subsequent monitoring procedures, families often feel stigmatized as well as anxious. Parents and responsible family members need education and support. Mothers with a history of genital HSV should be investigated for findings of active infection during the prepartum period. The definition of an active lesion includes one of the following at birth:

1. Positive viral culture of a lesion
2. Positive fluorescent antibody test
3. Presence of skin vesicles or lesions
4. Cytologic screen with identified HSV markers

All family members with active lesions anywhere on the body should be taught careful hand washing techniques to use before handling the baby. Any person with an oral HSV infection who handles the infant must wash well, wear a mask, and not kiss the infant anywhere until the lesions are completely crusted over and healed.

A common nursing concern is whether a mother with active genital herpes should be isolated. Transmission occurs with direct contact with the infected lesion. There must be thorough hand washing before handling the infant and after touching the genital area. The risks for transmission are unknown, but they are low. Hospital personnel usually gown and glove until viral status is known. Positive cultures at birth may just reflect colonization, and cultures should be repeated at 24 to 48 hours. If these are positive, the infant is considered to be positive for infection. Breastfeeding is contraindicated if the mother has a lesion on her breast. Infants are not isolated unless they themselves are infected. Many nurseries have guidelines regarding a 24- to 48-hour observation period to check cultures on an infant who was delivered vaginally through an infected genital area. An uninfected child does not require prolonged hospitalization, and upon discharge the family needs information and education. Families should be informed that immediate medical consultation should be obtained with the development of major findings, including malaise, irritability, fever, temperature instability, respiratory distress, apnea, large abdomen or liver, sudden changes in skin color, new skin vesicles, lesions on the mucous membranes, or conjunctivitis. Sudden onset of systemic disease in a small recovering preterm infant can include DIC and shock. Skin lesions are often absent in these severe cases, which may delay diagnosis.

Varicella. Varicella is the member of the herpes virus family that commonly causes chickenpox as well as varicella-zoster. Most women of childbearing age in the United States have been exposed to or have contracted this virus, yet women from other parts of the world may not be seropositive. Incidence of this virus in pregnant women is very low, probably around 0.4 to 0.6 in 10,000 pregnancies (Gershon, 2001).

Symptoms of varicella are usually present 10 to 21 days after exposure, with an average onset of symptoms around 15 days. Signs and symptoms include fever, malaise, and an itchy rash. The maculopapular rash eventually forms vesicles and crusts over. Potential complications include pneumonia, encephalitis, arthritis, and bacterial cellulitis. If the virus is contracted early in pregnancy, the damage is likely to be cutaneous, musculoskeletal, neurologic, and ocular. Infants can have intrauterine growth retardation, microcephaly, cerebellar and cortical atrophy, cataracts, and chorioretinitis. If the mother contracts varicella infection in the last 3 weeks of pregnancy, the risks for congenital infection are one in four. The severity of neonatal disease is determined by the timing of the exposure. Infections are generally severe if contracted within 4 days before and 2 days after delivery. Severe viral respiratory distress with significantly depleted maternal passive antibody transmission puts the infant at an even greater risk for other complications. When maternal varicella infection occurs 5 to 21 days before delivery, the newborn has a much milder course of the disease and appears more capable of fighting the infection. This milder course is probably due to passive immunity transmitted to the infant via maternally derived antibodies.

The diagnosis of varicella is made by isolation of HSV. Strict isolation of identified infants or of those whose symptoms are highly suspicious for infection is necessary. Acyclovir can be used for treatment of severe disease in newborns. Varicella-zoster immune globulin (VZIG) can be given to newborns to decrease the severity of infection in those exposed or prolong the incubation period (Arvin & Whitley, 2001). It is recommended that VZIG (125 units or 1.25 ml) IM be administered to infants whose mothers have the onset of varicella 5 days or less before delivery or in the first 48 hours after delivery (Arvin & Whitley, 2001).

Prevention. Typically, if a mother has contracted varicella infection late in pregnancy, other persons—such as health care workers, family members, or other newborns—may have been exposed. Exposed susceptible persons should be protected with VZIG. A live attenuated varicella vaccine is available. Despite initial skepticism, the vaccine has proven to be safe and highly effective; it prevents varicella in about 90% of those vaccinated and decreases the incidence of varicella zoster in immunocompromised and healthy individuals (Arvin & Whitley, 2001).

Gonorrhea. *Neisseria gonorrhoeae* is a species of small gram-negative diploid bacteria. They are diploid because they grow in pairs. Infection with this organism is seen most frequently in young adults, aged 15 to 24 years. There are approximately 120 cases per 100,000 population in the U.S.; it is estimated that many cases—perhaps as many as 50% of cases—are not reported (Gutman, 2001). In females, infection is asymptomatic, which compromises detection of the disease. Infected tissue and secretions from the cervix, pharynx, urethra, or rectum easily transmit the organism. The incubation period is approximately 2 to 7 days. Pelvic inflammatory disease results from infection by this organism (Gutman, 2001).

Clinical Manifestations. Gonorrhea infections are often mild but often cause blockage of the fallopian tubes. Perhaps 50% of women are asymptomatic with an infected cervix. In a pregnant woman, gonorrheal colonization of the cervix can cause inflammation and weakening of the fetal membranes and early rupture. Chorioamnionitis with *N. gonorrhoeae* as the causative organism can occur in the antepartum period and during labor and delivery; it is also related to increased risk of postpartum endometritis.

Disseminated gonococcal infection may present during pregnancy, causing arthritis, tendinitis, general aching, fever, and malaise. A previous history of gonorrhea presents a strong possibility that it may recur during pregnancy. Sexual partners should be screened and given treatment, because reinfection after treatment is common.

Gonococcal conjunctivitis in the newborn has historically been a risk from transmission via the birth canal. In the United States, prophylaxis is mandated by law and silver nitrate 1% solution, erythromycin drops (0.5%), or tetracycline (1%) drops are administered in both eyes of the neonate at birth. Fetal scalp electrodes have been identified as a potential method of organism transmission to the fetus. *N. gonorrhoeae* has been isolated from scalp abscesses, gastric and pharyngeal aspirates, conjunctival aspirates, and other blood and body fluids. Maternal and neonatal risks from exposure to the gonorrheal microorganism are significant and make it particularly important to screen for gonorrhea during pregnancy. Infected women have a higher incidence of premature labor, PROM, and infectious complications (Gutman, 2001).

Prevention. Use of silver nitrate solution, erythromycin, or tetracycline for prevention of gonococcal ophthalmia neonatorum is one of the early achievements in preventive medicine. Routine prophylaxis is mandated by law in the United States and has made a significant difference in the treatment of ocular disease. Chlamydia conjunctivitis has become far more common than gonococcal conjunctivitis in the neonate because of the continual screening for gonorrhea and the routine use of silver nitrate. Erythromycin ointment in both eyes is a more common prophylactic practice, because it covers both gonococcal and chlamydial organisms and causes less chemical conjunctivitis than silver nitrate (Gutman, 2001).

Collaborative Management: Mother. The appropriate treatment for a pregnant woman includes ceftriaxone, 125 mg intramuscularly once or spectromycin 2 g IM once, plus erythromycin, 500 mg orally three times a day for 7 days (Gutman, 2001). Follow-up, per the CDC, requires cervical and rectal cultures for *N. gonorrhoeae* be obtained 4 to 7 days after treatment. Ideally, pregnant women should also receive treatment for chlamydia infection. In the nonpregnant woman, treatment with doxycycline, ofloxacin, and azithromycin is effective, but their use in pregnancy is not advised.

Collaborative Management: Neonate. Infants who are delivered by an infected, untreated mother are usually given a complete sepsis work-up, including a lumbar puncture, and are placed on ampicillin and gentamicin therapy. If cultures confirm the presence of the microorganism and resistance is an issue, then infants should be treated with ceftriaxone, 25 to 50 mg/kg/day intravenously or intramuscularly in single doses, or cefotaxime, 25 mg/kg intravenously or intramuscularly every 12 hours for a total of 7 to 14 days (Gutman, 2001). Education and support regarding the origin of the infectious agent are important in the treatment of gonorrhea. Sexual partners of infected persons should be encouraged to seek testing and appropriate antibiotic treatment for chlamydia as well as gonorrhea (Gutman, 2001).

Hepatitis B Virus. The hepatitis B virus (HBV) is fairly large, (approximately 42 mm in diameter) double-stranded DNA-containing virus. Exposure to infected blood and body fluids, percutaneous introduction of blood, and administration of infected blood products are the principal routes of transmission. Contamination or infection of wounds can easily transmit the disease. The virus is fairly strong and is able to live on inanimate objects or fomites. Deactivation requires at least 1 minute in boiling water and extended autoclaving time.

In the adult, HBV infection produces systemic illness with general malaise, jaundice, anorexia, and nausea. Early stages of the disease may include fever, rash, and sore joints. Health care workers have historically been particularly vulnerable to this virus because of their repeated exposures to contaminated blood and body fluids and needle sticks. A carrier state of HBV can precipitate chronic liver disease (Crumpacker, 2001). In certain areas of the world, such as Africa, Southeast Asia, and the Pacific Rim, the virus is considered endemic. In these areas, carrier rates are estimated to be 35%. Approximately 40% of these carriers have been identified as having been perinatally infected (Crumpacker, 2001).

Hepatitis B surface antigen (HB$_s$Ag) is an important test in assessing a woman's risk of transmitting HBV to her unborn child. The presence of HB$_s$Ag and hepatitis B$_e$ antigen (HB$_e$Ag) is the best indication of infectiousness. It is currently recommended that all pregnant women be screened at their first prenatal visit for HB_sAg and HB_eAg to prevent prenatal transmission (Crumpacker, 2001).

Infection early in pregnancy with HBV causes a 50% risk of neonatal HBV infection. Ninety percent of infants born to women who are positive for both HB_sAg and HB_eAg are at risk for development of HBV infection by their first birthdays if they are not given treatment. Infants born to women who are positive for HB_sAg but negative for HB_eAg have lower rates of perinatal infection (20%). Infants who do not receive treatment are likely to become carriers, which may eventually lead to primary hepatocellular carcinoma (Crumpacker, 2001).

Treatment for these infants should be HBV vaccine along with hepatitis B immunoglobulin. For neonates whose mothers are HB_sAg-positive or -exposed, 0.5 ml of HBV vaccine should be given intramuscularly in the anterolateral thigh at or within 24 hours of delivery. Vaccination of 0.5 ml should be repeated at 1 and 6 months, and booster injections are suggested at 12 months and may need to be repeated at 5-year intervals. The vaccine can be used in infants who have been exposed to HIV. There is usually an immune response in these infants despite an altered CD_4 count. The response appears somewhat diminished. If HBIG is not available, standard immune serum globulin (ISG) should be given at birth (2.0 ml) and at age 1 month (Crumpacker, 2001).

Vertical transmission of HBV may occur during vaginal delivery. The sharing of bodily secretions during sexual intercourse can result in disease transmission also. HBV has a long incubation period: 50 to 190 days, averaging 90 days. Current recommendations are for all pregnant women to be screened initially and again before delivery. Screening is essential to identify potential risk for perinatal transmission and for protection of those who are exposed to antigen-positive blood. Family clustering of HBV has been identified through spread via household contact (Crumpacker, 2001).

Clinical Manifestations. Prematurity, low birth weight, and hyperbilirubinemia are clinical signs of HBV infection. Hepatosplenomegaly is also a common presenting symptom in an infant infected with a virus. An infant infected with HBV can be asymptomatic or present with a picture of fulminant sepsis.

Risk Factors. Pregnant women in high-risk categories (i.e., those known to have sexual contact with HBV-infected persons) should be screened so that appropriate follow-up can be provided. Persons in certain ethnic groups, such as Asians (Taiwanese especially) and Australian aborigines; intravenous drug users; and health professionals are especially at risk for the development of HBV. Individuals living in poor sanitary conditions are also at risk (Crumpacker, 2001).

Collaborative Management and Prevention. Vaccination is recommended for individuals who are at risk for exposure to HBV, including health care workers, family members of chronic carriers, persons with large numbers of heterosexual partners, and intravenous drug users. Hb_sAg protein is administered to the deltoid muscle once and then again 1 month and 6 months later. If the mother's antigen status is unknown at delivery, titers should be drawn, and the woman should be vaccinated if the result is Hb_sAg-positive. If the test results are unavailable or cannot be obtained, the neonate should be treated as if the mother were positive.

Proper and prompt identification of women in high-risk groups and knowledge of HBV status are important in the delivery room to determine whether the infant is at risk for infection. In accordance with universal infection control measures, appropriate barriers are used to protect health care workers from blood and body secretions. Delivery room and nursery personnel should always wear gloves when handling any new infant. The infant of a mother with confirmed HBV infection should be bathed with soap and water immediately, with special attention to removing all blood and secretions present on the skin and hair. The infant may be breastfed (unless the mother's nipples are cracked) and may receive routine care.

Human Papillomavirus. Genital warts, or condylomata acuminata, are caused by human papillomavirus (HPV). HPV is a double-stranded DNA virus. Two specific strains of HPV have been identified as causing venereal warts and thus are of concern as sexually transmitted viruses. The incidence of this disease has increased rapidly since the 1980s, along with that of other sexually transmitted diseases. The time lag between exposure and infection can be up to 6 months (Arvin & Maldonado, 2001). Symptoms of HPV infection include warty growths on the vagina, cervix, vulva, perineum, buttocks, or inner thigh. The presence of these warts can be extremely uncomfortable during vaginal delivery. Intrapartal transmission is possible if genital warts are visible. Current maternal treatment to prevent transmission includes carbon dioxide laser therapy and 85% trichloroacetic acid. Condyloma in 31 of 32 women (97%) was controlled with this combination therapy. The incidence of maternal-to-newborn transmission is approximately 2% with this treatment (Arvin & Maldonado, 2001). Newborns can contract a respiratory or laryngeal papillomatosis from infection with this virus.

Prenatal treatment is associated with low complication and recurrence rate. The treatment alleviates the need for a cesarean delivery. Examination, treatment, and follow-up of sexual partners are important aspects of treatment, because 50% of partners are infected.

Clinical Manifestations. Laryngeal papillomatosis causes newborns to have a "weak cry" or hoarseness. The expected incidence of laryngeal papilloma in an infant born to a woman with untreated HPV is approximately 78% (Arvin & Maldonado, 2001). The newborn may have stridor or other respiratory symptoms.

Collaborative Management. Education and counseling of mothers and their partners are the primary concerns in the treatment of condyloma. Patients are instructed about methods of transmission and methods to decrease transmission. Emotional support is important, because venereal disease is extremely painful and demoralizing. Condyloma lesions have a high recurrence rate (70%). Early identification of newborns at risk for laryngeal papillomas is important to prevent respiratory complications. Newborns who experience respiratory distress and stridor should be evaluated for laryngeal papillomas. Supportive ventilatory therapy may be needed.

There may be long-term complications from perinatal transmission of HPV; for example, one area of research is the study of increased risk of cervical cancer in females who were exposed in utero (Arvin & Maldonado, 2001). The relationship between HPV and cancer of the cervix and vulva has been studied (Arvin & Maldonado, 2001).

Chlamydia.   *Chlamydia* is a genus of bacteria that grows between cells. Chlamydial infection is one of the most common sexually transmitted diseases. Probably 50% of infected women of childbearing age are asymptomatic. Studies have shown that the infected population primarily comprises sexually active women between 18 and 35 years of age who have a high school education or less and three or more sexual partners in the previous 3 months (Schachter & Grossman, 2001). The infection can present as cervicitis, salpingitis, urethritis, or pelvic inflammatory disease.

Chlamydia trachomatis infection has been identified as causing a significant increase in the incidence of PROM, the number of low-birth-weight babies, and the rate of infant mortality (Arvin & Maldonado, 2001). Thus screening pregnant women for chlamydia is important because of its frequency and the fact that treatment with erythromycin or clindamycin may prevent transmission to the newborn.

Clinical Manifestations.   Chlamydia conjunctivitis can present in the newborn with a very watery discharge that may progress to purulent exudate. Application of erythromycin ointment at birth for ocular prophylaxis successfully treats both chlamydial and gonococcal conjunctivitis. Pneumonia can occur in newborns who have contracted chlamydia from their mothers' genital tracts. The incubation period is anywhere from 5 days to 3 to 4 months. Typical presentation is tachypnea, barrel chest, and an increased oxygen requirement. The infant may have interstitial infiltrations, hepatosplenomegaly, and increased eosinophils. In a prospective study of chlamydia, there was a 16% incidence of pneumonia in infants identified as being at risk for chlamydial infection (Arvin & Maldonado, 2001).

Diagnosis of chlamydial infections is based on physical and laboratory examination; in cases of conjunctivitis, Giemsa-stained conjunctival scrapings provide a method of direct fluorescent antibody testing. The definitive diagnosis for chlamydial pneumonia is made by culture of the respiratory tract or identification of high levels of IgM antibodies to chlamydia.

Collaborative Management and Prevention.   Treatment of chlamydia infection in the newborn is usually with ampicillin and gentamicin if the infant's work-up is for generic sepsis. Once the chlamydia organism is identified, more specific treatment is with erythromycin for 10 to 14 days.

If chlamydia is confirmed in a pregnant woman and is treated, her sexual partners also require treatment. Rapid screening and diagnosis can be made using monoclonal antibodies, and some laboratories offer a chlamydia test called Chlamydiazyme, which gives results very quickly, thus allowing appropriate treatment to be initiated early. Positive results indicate the need for treatment, but negative results indicate that repeated screening is needed.

Education and counseling regarding the method of transmission of chlamydia are important. This organism may be present for many years in the female genital tract and produce no symptoms. The organism does not respond to partial treatment; an infected woman and all her sexual partners must receive full treatment as soon as possible. Men should wear condoms to prevent transmission during sexual relations. Without treatment, the severe complications for the woman include pelvic inflammatory disease, ectopic pregnancy, and endometritis. The common newborn complication is pneumonia. Supportive ventilation in the newborn is usually necessary.

Bacterial Infections

Group B Streptococcus.   Group B beta-hemolytic streptococci were unknown to the perinatal scene until the early 1970s when they replaced *E. coli* as the single most common agent associated with bacterial meningitis during the first 2 months of life. Implementation of a preventative strategy led to a 65% decline in the incidence of early-onset infection from 1993 to 1998, to an incidence of about 1.7 to 0.6 per 1,000 live births (Edwards & Baker, 2001; Logsdon & Casto, 1997). Surveillance programs estimate that 3,900 early-onset infections and 200 neonatal deaths were prevented in 1998 by the use of intrapartum antibiotics (Edwards & Baker, 2001).

Group B streptococcus infections present as an early or late onset illness. Estimates of early onset rates vary from 0.7 to 3.7 per 1,000 live births; late onset rates vary from 0.5 to 1.8 per 1,000. The number of newborn deaths associated with either early onset (before the first week of life) or late onset continues to be high, particularly in high-risk urban centers. The mortality rate of infected newborns varies according to birth weight, with the smaller, less mature infants having the highest mortality rates. The mortality rate for newborns with meningitis is greater than 20%, and there is significant risk for permanent neurologic sequelae of survivors of meningeal infections.

Pathophysiology.   *Streptococcus* is a gram-positive diplococcus with an ultrastructure similar to that of other gram-positive cocci. It was classified as hemolytic because of its double zone of hemolysis surrounding colonies on blood agar plates. Culture of body fluids, such as blood, urine, CSF, and other secretions, is the most common method of identifying group B streptococci.

Counterelectrophoresis and latex agglutination are rapid assays that enable a presumptive diagnosis before cultures are returned. Rapid identification of the group B streptococcus organism is important in treating colonized pregnant women and in the early diagnosis and treatment of infection in the sick, unstable septic infant. To accurately predict maternal colonization with group B streptococci, both vaginal and rectal areas should be cultured on more than one occasion (AAP, 1997; Beri & Lourwood, 1997; Edwards & Baker, 2001).

Clinical Manifestations.   Group B streptococcus has been identified as a relatively common cause of mid-gestational fetal loss in women who experience vaginal hemorrhage, PROM, fetal membrane infection, and spontaneous abortion. The rate of stillbirth is reported to be as high as 61% in association with these bacteria. Early-onset neonatal infections with group B streptococcus can be asymptomatic or can manifest with severe symptoms of respiratory distress and shock, which can rapidly progress to death (Edwards & Baker, 2001).

Early-onset group B streptococcus infection usually appears within the first 24 hours of life and is most common in premature infants. Congenital pneumonia is a common presenting symptom in infants who weigh 1,000 g or less. The most common presentations are pneumonia and meningitis. Signs of respiratory distress, apnea, grunting, tachypnea, and cyanosis are common. Hypotension is found in 25% of newborns with group B streptococcus infection; these infants are at risk for cardiopulmonary collapse. Nonspecific signs of sepsis include lethargy, poor feeding, temperature instability, abdominal distention, pallor, tachycardia, and jaundice. Experienced health care professionals may observe that the neonate "just doesn't look right," which is sometimes a critical point for early detection and implementation of therapy.

Overwhelming group B streptococcal septicemia is often compounded by meningitis. Lumbar puncture and examination of the CSF is the only way to exclude meningeal involvement and therefore is an important part of the workup. Seizures may occur in infants with group B streptococcal meningitis. Low-birth-weight infants have been identified as particularly vulnerable, but term infants are also susceptible.

Late-Onset Infection. Late-onset infection with group B streptococcus usually occurs in term newborns 7 days to 12 weeks of age. The fatality rate is less than that with early-onset infection, but meningitis is a common complication. Of the survivors, 25% to 50% suffer permanent neurologic damage of varying from mild handicaps to severe impairment (Edwards & Baker, 2001).

Complications include global or profound mental retardation, spastic quadriplegia, cortical blindness, deafness, uncontrolled seizures, hydrocephalus, and diabetes insipidus. Thus early treatment is an important part of the prevention of long-term serious sequelae. An infant with a positive blood culture can often be asymptomatic initially. The diagnosis of group B streptococcal infection is complicated because signs and symptoms of neonatal infection are not specific and symptoms may represent other conditions of the neonate. For example, apnea may be a symptom of central nervous system immaturity in the preterm neonate, but it is also associated with infection. The health care professional must maintain a high index of suspicion for infection in all conditions involving the neonate. Therefore infection must be considered in the differential diagnosis of many problems found. Screening tests such as complete blood count with differential are often used to identify the need for further evaluation for sepsis. Abnormal results indicate the necessity for definitive testing and implementation of antimicrobial therapy.

Collaborative Management. Regional and institutional differences in infectious agents must be considered in the selection of antimicrobial therapy. Before culture results are returned, a broad-spectrum penicillin and an aminoglycoside are started to provide coverage for the most prevalent microorganisms that cause infection. Generally, ampicillin and gentamicin are selected until culture results and sensitivities are available. Group B streptococcus is generally very sensitive to penicillin G, and, in many institutions, it is substituted for ampicillin once the diagnosis is made. See Table 29-3 for drugs.

Therapy is maintained for 7 to 10 days for sepsis and 14 to 21 days for meningitis. The lumbar puncture may be repeated midway or at the end of therapy to ensure that no microorganisms remain in the CSF.

Fluid management, volume expansion, and appropriate antimicrobial therapy are the key components of nursing care. Infants with group B streptococcal infection are often very labile and do not tolerate frequent interventions. Minimal handling is sometimes required for their care.

Edwards and Baker (2001) recommended active immunization of all women of childbearing age, either before pregnancy or late in pregnancy (at approximately 7 months' gestation). They estimate that a successful vaccination program of pregnant women in the third trimester could prevent up to 95% of GBS neonatal infection. They point out that the cost of developing a suitable vaccine, although considerable, would probably be less than the cost of the care required by the critically ill newborn and the chronically ill, debilitated, severely handicapped newborn—consequences of GBS neonatal infection.

Staphylococcus. From the 1950s to the 1970s, coagulase-positive S. aureus was the main organism identified as a pathogen in hospitals (Shinefield & St. Geme, 2001). In the 1980s, coagulase-negative organisms, in particular S. epidermidis, were discovered to be equally important. These organisms have caused many serious and even fatal infections in newborns.

Ill neonates and premature infants who are already immunocompromised are particularly vulnerable to Staphylococcal infections. Any open skin lesions, surgical incisions, or puncture wounds secondary to diagnostic tests or procedures are conducive to bacterial growth, especially S. aureus or S. epidermidis (Shinefield & St. Geme, 2001). Nosocomial infections may also be transmitted to the neonate via contaminated articles or on the hands of health professionals. Overgrowth of S. epidermidis may occur in nurseries where an attempt has been made to reduce colonization of S. aureus. Resistant organisms pose a threat to preterm infants who require extensive invasive treatments. They are particularly susceptible to colonization with coagulase-negative staphylococci or even methicillin-resistant S. aureus (Shinefield & St. Geme, 2001).

Staphylococci release endotoxins that have systemic effects. One of these effects is alteration of the skin's protective layer. Scalded skin syndrome is one of the most dramatic results of these endotoxins. Integumentary dysfunction secondary to staphylococcal infection is discussed in Chapter 34.

Other clinical presentations of Staphylococcal infection include pneumonia; toxic shock syndrome (TSS); eye, ear, nose, and throat infections; septicemia; osteomyelitis; septic arthritis; meningitis; endocarditis; and enteric infections.

Collaborative Management. Management and supportive therapy for staphylococcal infection are initially the same as for infection with group B Streptococci. Antimicrobial therapy begins with ampicillin and gentamicin. Once definitive cultures and sensitivities are available and the organism is ampicillin-resistant, the drug of choice is one of the synthetic penicillins: oxacillin, methicillin, cloxacillin, dicloxacillin, or nafcillin. If the organism is methicillin-resistant, the best available drug is vancomycin. Some infections, such as endocarditis or ventriculo-peritoneal (VP) shunt infections, combination therapy may be indicated with the addition of rifampin, gentamicin, or cephalothin. However there is a high incidence of resistance to aminoglycosides and the Beta lactams; thus a combination of vancomycin and rifampin is generally the best regimen. Rifampin is not used alone, despite its good antistaphylococcal activity, because resistance to rifampin occurs rapidly when it is used as a sole therapeutic agent (Shinefield & St. Geme, 2001).

Efforts to control of Staphylococcal infection in nurseries have been aimed at three areas that lead to colonization of infants with Staphylococcal bacteria: environment, personnel, and the infants themselves. Adequate space between infants, adequate personnel to care for the infants, decreased exposure to other infants through rooming-in or small nursery cohorts, and good skin care of the infants are considered important in the prevention of colonization. The most important factor in reducing colonization is adequate hand washing by all personnel before and after handling each infant (Shinefield & St. Geme, 2001).

Escherichia coli.   *Escherichia coli* or *E. coli* is a gram-negative, non-spore-forming motile rod. It is a normal inhabitant of the gastrointestinal tract in adults and the newborn's gastrointestinal tract is colonized within the first few days after birth through environmental exposure and enteral feedings. Eschericihia coli is the most frequent cause of gram-negative infection in the newborn. Presentations of *E. coli* infection include: sepsis, pneumonia, diarrhea, necrotizing enterocolitis (NEC), omphalitis, urinary tract infections (UTI), organ or bone abscesses, and spinal adhesions (Klein, 2001; Steinlen & Knecht, 1999). E. coli has multiple strains, but only a few are associated with neonatal infections. One particular is the K1 capsular antigen, which is associated with neonatal meningitis (Klein, 2001). Several strains of *E. coli* have been identified with outbreaks of inflammatory or noninflammatory diarrhea. These strains are known as enterotoxigenic *E. coli* (ETEC), enteroinvasive *E. coli* (EIEC), enteropathogenic *E. coli* (EPEC), enterohemorrhagic *E. coli* (EHEC), and enteroaggregative *E. coli* (EaggEC). There is also a higher risk of *E. coli* meningitis or sepsis in newborns with galactosemia (Bingen et al, 1997; Klein, 2001).

Collaborative Management.   Therapy for *E. coli* infection is appropriate antimicrobial therapy and supportive therapy. *E. coli* is generally sensitive to aminoglycosides and third-generation cephalosporins; however, it is important that sensitivity testing be monitored closely to ensure that the appropriate antimicrobial agent is prescribed. Gram-negative infection is frequently severe and rapidly progressive. Supportive therapy is aimed at promoting adequate oxygenation, ventilation, and cardiovascular support while providing antimicrobial therapy to combat the microorganism. Other management depends upon the clinical presentation of the disease.

Listeria monocytogenes.   *L. monocytogenes* has been recognized as a cause of perinatal complications since the early 1900s. It is a gram-positive, motile bacterium found in birds and mammals, including domestic and farm animals. It is found in soil, fecal material, and unpasteurized milk. *Listeria* infection appears to be an underdiagnosed and underreported cause of congenital sepsis. Human infection is primarily foodborne.

Recent data suggest that the incidence is 0.7 cases per 100,000 population in the United States and 0.4 cases per 100,000 in Canada (Bortolussi & Schlechi, 2001). This amounts to approximately 1,700 cases of Listeriosis in the U.S., with a 40% mortality rate. Neonatal listeriosis is about 13 per 100,000 live births, about 30% of the total listeriosis cases. Neonatal listeriosis presents as either early-onset or late-onset patterns. The mortality rate for early-onset infection is about 25%, whereas the mortality rate for late-onset infection is about 15%. Long-term morbidity of survivors has not been adequately studied (Bortolussi & Schlechi, 2001).

Clinical Manifestations.   A mother infected with *Listeria* commonly has flu-like symptoms, including malaise, fever, chills, diarrhea, and back pain. It is also possible to contract the infection and remain asymptomatic or have only minor symptoms. This organism has been identified as a cause of spontaneous abortion. If contracted between 17 and 28 weeks' gestation, *Listeria* can cause fetal death or premature birth of an acutely ill newborn; who may die hours later. However, early maternal treatment with intravenous ampicillin and gentamicin has been associated with normal newborn outcome (Bortolussi & Schlechi, 2001). Infection late in pregnancy may cause the infant to be born with a congenital infection, usually pneumonia. Mortality rates are high but are usually related to the amount of prematurity. Late-onset listeriosis, which can occur up to 4 weeks after delivery, can easily result in meningitis. A term newborn with listeriosis has less chance of dying but often suffers complications of hydrocephalus and mental retardation (Visintine et al, 1977). However, in either preterm or term neonates in whom meningitis develops, there is a 70% mortality rate if treatment is delayed (Bortolussi & Schlechi, 2001).

Newborns infected with *Listeria* may be born prematurely and be meconium-stained, exhibit apnea and flaccidity, have a papular erythematous skin rash and hepatosplenomegaly, and be poor feeders (Visintine et al, 1977). Preterm birth associated with meconium staining should raise the index of suspicion for neonatal listeriosis.

Collaborative Management.   Intrapartum administration of antibiotics may decrease fetal morbidity and mortality rates. Ampicillin in combination with an aminoglycoside is the most common treatment. Investigators have shown that newborn survival rates are significantly different if the mother as well as the infant receives treatment (71% versus 29%) (Bortolussi & Schlechi, 2001).

Careful hand washing is a very important aspect of caring for the infant infected with *Listeria*. Institutional policy may require that the infant be isolated for the first 24 hours of life, until the antibiotics are on board. The mother's urine, stool, and lochia should be cultured, and, if positive, she should be given ampicillin. Early detection and institution of therapy lead to the best outcome. Listeriosis often presents suddenly in the last trimester of pregnancy, thus precipitating an unexpected preterm delivery. Extensive emotional support may be necessary for the mother and family.

Neonatal Meningitis

Pathophysiology.   Meningitis can be a sequela of newborn sepsis. The incidence of neonatal sepsis is reported to be 1 to 8.1 in 1,000 live births (Klein, 2001). The incidence of meningitis associated with newborn sepsis is thought to be approximately 25% of those presenting with sepsis. The prevalence of meningitis is higher during the first month after birth than at any other time period. Meningitis is a more common complication of late-onset sepsis. The morbidity rate is higher for preterm infants than for term infants. Morbidity of survivors of infection with gram-negative bacilli or group B streptococci approaches 20% to 50%. Group B streptococcus has taken over *E. coli* as the leading cause of neonatal bacterial meningitis (Chang Chien et al, 2000).

Complications of meningitis include mental and motor problems, seizure disorders, hydrocephalus, hearing loss, blindness, and abnormal speech patterns. Infants with seizures that last 72 hours or longer, have coma, need inotropic support, and have leukopenia have the worst outcomes (Klinger et al, 2000).

In most cases, meningitis results from bacteremia caused by the most commonly occurring pathogens in the newborn. However, recovery of the specific microorganism must be attempted due to the potential for other microorganisms. An inoculation of organisms may pass the blood-brain barrier and infect the CSF. Cytologic tests on the CSF can identify the presence of an inflammatory response. A Gram stain of the CSF fluid should be prepared, and other appropriate cultures should be obtained. High CSF protein and low glucose levels are also indicators of meningitis. See Table 29-1 for additional information.

Clinical Manifestations. Initially, the infant with meningitis presents with signs and symptoms of generalized sepsis. In addition, the meningeal irritation results in increased irritability, crying, increased intracranial pressure leading to bulging fontanelles, lethargy, tremors or twitching, seizure activity, vomiting, alterations in consciousness, and diminished muscle tone. Focal signs include hemiparesis, horizontal deviation of the eyes, and some cranial nerve involvement (Klein, 2001).

Risk Factors. The National Institutes of Health (NIH) sponsored a collaborative perinatal project study, which found that low-birth-weight infants are three times more likely to acquire meningitis than full-term infants (Klein, 2001). In one study, meningitis was 17 times more frequent in the low-birth-weight groups. It seems that the smaller the baby, the more frequent the signs and symptoms of sepsis and meningitis. Very-low-birth-weight infants who weigh less than 750 g have been identified as having high rates of sepsis and other complications (Klein, 2001).

It appears that male infants are more vulnerable to sepsis and meningitis. There has been a suggestion regarding a sex-linked factor—that is, that a particular gene located on the X chromosome is involved with the function of the thymus or with synthesis of immunoglobulin to defend the newborn host. Female infants have lower rates of respiratory distress syndrome and lower rates of most congenital infections.

Geography and socioeconomic factors are influential in patterns of neonatal disease. These differences probably reflect populations served, including unique cultural activities and sexual practices, as well as local customs. It probably also reflects different treatment patterns in local nurseries and variations of antimicrobial selections.

Prognosis. Brain abscess is associated with a poor prognosis; approximately 50% of affected patients die. Destruction of brain tissues, hemorrhages, and infarcts causing necrosis to vital brain cells may cause extensive brain damage, leading to death or poor neurologic outcomes. With the introduction of ultrasonography and computerized tomography, brain abscesses are being identified earlier (Klein, 2001).

Collaborative Management. The selection of antimicrobial therapy for meningitis is based on the causative microorganism. Supportive therapy is necessary for the newborn with meningitis. Acute observation and monitoring of vital signs and activity level are crucial. Infants who become critically ill with meningitis may deteriorate quickly and need rapid, acute interventions. Infants often require long-term antibiotic therapy, and venous access is often a problem. Placement of a percutaneous line for parenteral nutrition may be necessary. Families need educational and emotional support during the long-term hospitalizations, particularly if complications develop.

Viral Agents

Respiratory Syncytial Virus. Respiratory syncytial virus (RSV) is an infection usually found in older infants. It is thought that maternal antibodies protect infants for the first few weeks of life but that as passive immunity diminishes, these infants become more vulnerable. Premature infants, already immunocompromised, are more susceptible to the virus during their long-term hospitalizations. The mortality rate for infants who acquire RSV infections during the first few weeks after birth is high (Arvin & Maldonado, 2001; Kang & Kim, 1997).

Clinical Manifestations. An infant who is infected with RSV before 4 weeks of age may be asymptomatic or may have an upper respiratory infection with fever, bronchiolitis, apnea, or pneumonia. There may be a definite need for assisted ventilation, and deaths have occurred in rapidly fulminating disease, for which there is little available treatment. Small preterm infants who are already in significant pulmonary and cardiac jeopardy with respiratory distress syndrome or bronchopulmonary dysplasia are especially susceptible to development of severe infections. Nosocomial transmission of the virus between caretakers is possible; such transmission appears to result in less severe infection. The first clinical signs of transmission include a clear nasal discharge at approximately 10 to 52 days of life, followed by cough and wheezing. Radiologic changes compatible with pneumonia may also be found. (Arvin & Maldonado, 2001).

Treatment and Prevention. Good hand washing is extremely important in the prevention of transmission of RSV between critically ill patients. RSV-infected secretions can remain viable for up to 6 hours on countertops, 45 minutes on cloth gowns and paper tissues, and 20 minutes on skin. Thus all infected infants should be cared for in cohort. Caretakers should be consistently assigned to decrease transmission rates. Gown and glove precautions can significantly reduce nosocomial transmission of RSV.

Any infant with a runny nose, nasal congestion, or unexplained apnea should be considered for isolation and be investigated for RSV infection. Attention should be specific for those infants older than 4 weeks of corrected age. Specific cultures and screens should be performed because specific treatment is available if RSV is found.

Collaborative Management. There is no consensus regarding the benefit of ribaviran treatment for identified RSV infection in infants. Aerosolized ribaviran therapy has been shown in some studies to have some benefit for infants with lower respiratory infection with RSV, although other studies have not demonstrated a clear improved outcome (Arvin & Maldonado, 2001). Infants who are at increased risk for complications of RSV due to congenital heart disease, chronic lung disease, or immunodeficiency and infants with severe illness or respiratory failure should be evaluated for ribaviran therapy. In addition, administration of RSV-IVIG may offer some benefit to these infants. The administration of a monoclonal antibody preparation, palivizumab, has been shown to reduce hospitalizations due to RSV by 55% in certain high-risk children. Criteria for consideration for palibizumab include infants who are younger than two years of age, have chronic lung disease, have required medical therapy for lung disease within 6 months of RSV season, or were born at 32 to 35 weeks' gestation. RSV-IVIG is contraindicated, and palivizumab is not recommended for children with congenital heart disease (Arvin & Maldonado, 2001).

If Ribavirin is prescribed, those who have been trained appropriately should closely monitor administration. Ribavirin can be administered safely to infants receiving mechanical ventilation and to infants in an oxygen hood. Specific safety precautions should be taken to protect the caretaker, because ribavirin has been identified as being potentially teratogenic. Protective measures include wearing a gown, gloves, and mask when in direct contact with the particles or mist that contains ribavirin. Ideally, no pregnant woman would take care of an infant with RSV who is receiving ribavirin. Close monitoring of the pulmonary status, including the use of oxygen and mechanical ventilation, may be necessary. Isolation of the infected infant from other infants who could potentially be infected is important; the usual method for isolation is to minimize risk of the spread of the airborne virus and ribavirin particles.

Adenovirus and Rotavirus.

Adenoviruses and rotavirus are considered medically important because of their ability to cause neonatal diarrhea. Adenoviruses are very small; rotaviruses are approximately 70 nm in size. Both these categories of organisms can cause significant viral gastroenteritis in the newborn population (Cleary et al, 2001). Breastfeeding, with the transmission of secretory IgA, is thought to be one of the best protections against illness caused by adenovirus or rotavirus. Animal data support the theory that breast milk provides immunologic protection from sepsis when the gastrointestinal system is involved, as long as there is no existent endotoxemia. This protection may be related to the presence of secretory IgA or the presence of naturally occurring lactobacilli and *E. coli* in greater numbers in the gut when breast milk rather than commercial formula is given. In addition to IgA, human milk contains lactoferrin macrophages and lymphocytes that may be involved in the protective effect of human milk for prevention of infection (Yau, 2000).

Rotavirus is a double-stranded RNA virus that has a wheel-like appearance under electron microscope. Rotavirus, like other acute diarrhea diseases in general, is uncommon in newborns. Infants are usually at greater risk at 3 or 4 months of age; risk increases with age with a peak incidence between 6 and 24 months. However, with prolonged length of stay in a neonatal intensive care unit (NICU), nosocomial transmission is possible. In newborn nurseries, attack rates are unpredictable; however, a seasonal pattern is seen (Cleary et al, 2001). Within the same city, attack rates among infants may show dramatic variations in different hospitals and different years.

Once introduced, the virus is able to spread steadily until changes in admission policies or nursing practices stop the cycle. Exactly how the virus is introduced and transmitted is uncertain. Some of the ways a newborn could acquire infection include the following:

- Ingestion of viral particles at or shortly before the time of delivery
- Transfer of virus from infants or toddlers excreting the virus, via hands of nursery personnel or parents
- Transmission by direct contact with adults or older children excreting the virus
- Infection by airborne or droplet particles
- Infection by fomites
- Ingestion of contaminated foods or formula (Cleary et al, 2001)

Transfer of particles from infant to infant on the hands of nursery and medical staff is probably the most common means of viral spread.

Clinical Manifestations.

An infected newborn may be asymptomatic or may have severe gastrointestinal problems. Early signs of illness include lethargy, irritability, and poor feeding, usually followed by the passage of watery yellow or green stools that are free of blood but contain mucus. Vomiting and slight fever may accompany the diarrhea for a time. Rotavirus has been identified as a potential cause of necrotizing enterocolitis. Specific methods of virus detection include radioimmunoassay, immunofluorescence, latex agglutination, and enzyme-linked immunosorbent assay. Some nurseries use the commercially available product Rotazyme II, which is quick and effective (Cleary et al, 2001).

Collaborative Management.

The primary goal of treatment is to provide supportive electrolytes and fluid management. Minimizing the fluid and electrolyte losses that result from diarrhea is the key component of care. Persistent or recurrent diarrhea with the use of milk-based formulas or breast milk demands further investigation of carbohydrate intolerance or cow's milk intolerance. Some critically ill infants who may have reduced gastrointestinal absorptive surface (short bowel syndrome) or severe mucosal damage may require an elemental diet or parenteral nutrition.

Hand washing after each contact with the affected infant remains the single most important method of preventing the spread of the infection. Rotaviruses and adenoviruses are often excreted in an infant's stool 2 or 3 days before the illness is recognized. The isolation of an infant with diarrhea is often too late to prevent cross-contamination. Infants in whom gastroenteritis develops should be moved out of the nursery area if there are adequate facilities. The use of an incubator is helpful, because it may be a reminder that appropriate gowning and gloving are necessary before the infant can be handled. Encouraging the rooming of infants with their mothers can be helpful in containing nursery epidemics (Cleary et al, 2001).

Several live orally administered rotavirus vaccines are being tested for their effectiveness in young infants. Also, milk-containing concentrates of immunoglobulin prepared from rotavirus-hyperimmunized cows have been fed to infants hospitalized for acute rotavirus gastroenteritis. This practice appears to reduce excretion of the virus significantly and has prevented rotavirus diarrhea outbreaks in nurseries. This vaccine may prove useful in HIV-infected infants. Research has demonstrated that they have the ability to attach a rotavirus even without a vaccine. Thus its use may decrease the risk of infectious compromise in these infants.

Human Immunodeficiency Virus (HIV).

Human immunodeficiency virus (HIV) continues to be a very real part of neonatal care. Despite new methods of treatment for childbearing women that have decreased vertical transmission of HIV, newborns and infants are still being infected. CDC (2001) reported approximately 6,812 cases of HIV/AIDS in children under 5 years old in the United States. Approximately 1.4 million children under 15 have AIDS, with 500,000 deaths reported in 2000 to this same age group. Worldwide women are increasingly affected by HIV/AIDS, with 16.4 million reported. The most significant increases have been among African Americans and Hispanics. New York, California, Florida, and Texas are the four highest states reporting HIV cases. The top five cities are New York City, Los Angeles, San Francisco, Miami, and Washington DC.

Vertical transmission from a mother to a fetus has been positively impacted by use of zidovudine or ZDV or AZT during pregnancy and the intrapartum period. Sometimes other antiviral agents are added to ZDV.

What is HIV? In the literature, the virus is known by three names: (1) HIV, human immunodeficiency virus; (2) LAV, lymphadenopathy-associated virus; and (3) HTLV-III, human T-cell lymphotropic virus type III. The term AIDS is a generic label referring to individuals who may be infected but are asymptomatic or individuals who are symptomatic. Therefore because of the generic use of the label, it is more appropriate to use the term HIV infection, which covers the entire range from asymptomatic to the terminally ill individual.

Etiology and Pathophysiology. HIV-1 is part of the lentivirus subfamily of human retroviruses and requires a cell surface receptor for attachment and penetration into the cell. The current theory is that HIV is an RNA virus that has a gp120 surface molecule that attaches to the CD4 receptor sites on the cell's surface. The gp120 surface molecule acts as a key to open the lock on the surface of the CD4 (T-helper cell), thus allowing the HIV to move inside the cell easily. In older HIV literature, the CD4 cells were referred to as T-helper lymphocytes or T4 cells. The term retrovirus refers to the ability of the virus to enter the target cell via the receptor site; then during cell division, the virus's RNA material is copied into the DNA. By using the enzyme reverse transcriptase, the new cell continues to replicate the virus throughout the infected individual's life. Other cells that have CD4 receptor sites include B-lymphocytes, monocytes, macrophages, and glial cells of the brain. Any of these cells may also become infected with the retrovirus through the process previously described for the CD4 cells, which explains the variety of symptoms a person infected with HIV may manifest. In addition, HIV may also attack other cells that do not have the CD4 receptor sites that are readily detectable on the surface membrane. Other receptor sites in certain cells, such as those of the central nervous system, may allow the lock-and-key mechanism with the HIV gp120 on the cell's surface. Once HIV has entered a cell, it results in immunodeficiency that renders the cell incapable of combating infections. The reason is that the CD4 cells that normally assist in an immune response are rendered useless. At this point, not only does the HIV infection result in immunodeficiency, but the infected cells can also readily pass into the peripheral and central nervous system, gastrointestinal (GI) tract, heart, lungs, and kidney of the infected individual.

The premature or full-term infant has an immature immune system. The T-cell or cell-mediated immune system is mature. However, the B-cell or humoral system is physiologically immature. The B cells are involved in the formation of functional antibodies. T cells are differentiated into CD4 cells (previously referred to as T-helper cells) and CD8 cells (previously referred to as T-suppressor cells). In the noninfected infant, CD4 cells enhance an immune response to infection, and CD8 cells dampen a response. In the case of HIV in the adult, the ratio of CD4 cells to CD8 cells is reversed, thus leaving the individual vulnerable to bacterial and opportunistic infections. It is unclear whether the CD4:CD8 ratio in the infant follows the same pattern as in the adult.

Infants exposed to HIV may manifest signs and symptoms at an earlier stage because of the inability of the humoral system to manufacture antibodies. Hence bacterial infections and other types of opportunistic infections are more likely to occur in the infant infected with HIV than in the adult infected with HIV, in whom a mature immune system exists.

Transmission. Another concept addressed in the literature is the degree of infectiousness. The infectiousness increases as HIV progresses. The degree of infectiousness may correlate with CD4 cell counts. Thus the longer an individual has been seropositive for HIV and the lower the CD4 cell counts, the more correlation there is with the risk of transmission. Therefore there is an increased frequency of the viremia and secretion of HIV.

Risk Factors. The major risk factors are the following:
- Multiple sexual partners
- Unsafe sex
- Intravenous drug use
- Sexually transmitted infections
- Gay and bisexual activity
- Lack of prenatal care

With the increase in international HIV/AIDS cases, the United States has entered into the International Partnership Against HIV/AIDS in Africa (IPAA). Part of this initiative is the Leadership and Investment in Fighting an Epidemic (LIFE). This program addresses HIV in Africa and India with emphasis on HIV/AIDS prevention and health care (CDC, 1998). The major objectives to address these risk factors are the following:
- Reducing mother-to-child (perinatal) HIV transmission in developing countries
- Developing effective interventions for high-risk populations
- Identifying possible factors that may confer immunity to HIV
- Working to reduce the impact of HIV/AIDS in developing countries through practical treatment regimens

Clinical Manifestations. Most newborns show no physical signs of infection. As the infant ages, the symptoms of recurrent respiratory infections, opportunistic infections such as pneumocystis carinii, cytomegalovirus, or mycobacterium tuberculosis, poor feeding, poor weight gain, failure to thrive-organic, developmental delays or loss of previously acquired milestones, and irritability may be noted. Unfortunately these manifestations are not specific to HIV.

Diagnosis. The diagnosis can be made even in the neonate via viral cultures, polymerase chain reactions (PCR), or viral load testing (Baley & Goldbarb, 2001). Viral assays include HIV DNA PCR-93% accurate by 14 days of life or HIV RNA PCR. These tests should be done within 48 hours of birth, at 1-2 months, and 3-6 months (Anderson, 2001). If IgG is tested, this level is considered inaccurate until 18 months of age or older because it reflects maternal antibodies. P24 antigen test often results in false-positive findings.

Collaborative Management. Wortley et al (2001) reported that when good prenatal surveillance for HIV was implemented along with use of ZDV, only 8% of children exposed to HIV in utero were infected, in comparison to 16% when no ZDV was given. Brocklehurst (2001) found that the addition of immunoglobulin to ZDV did not significantly change the neonatal infection rate. (See Table 29-5 and Box 29-2 for more information about prophylaxis and treatment.)

CDC suggests the following:
- All HIV-exposed infants receive ZDV prophylaxis (2 mg/kg every 6 hours for first 6 weeks of life).
- If no ZDV has been received before delivery, start the medication in the first 12 to 24 hours of life.

BOX 29-2

CDC Guidelines for Perinatal Transmission Prophylaxis

- Antepartum: Initiation at 14 to 34 weeks' gestation and continued throughout pregnancy
  - PACTG 076 Regimen: ZDV 100 mg 5 times daily
  - Acceptable Alternative Regimen:
    - ZDV 200 mg 3 times daily or
    - ZDV 300 mg 2 times daily
- Intrapartum: During labor, ZDV 2 mg/kg intravenously over 1 hr, followed by a continuous infusion of 1 mg/kg intravenously until delivery
- Postpartum: Oral administration of ZDV to the newborn (ZDV syrup, 2 mg/kg every 6 hr) for the first 6 weeks of life, beginning at 8 to 12 hours after birth

---

Source: Anderson JR (2001). HIV and reproduction. In JR Anderson (Ed.). A guide to the clinical care of women with HIV. Atlanta: CDC.

- If there is concern about the compliance for 6 weeks with ZDV, a one-time dose of Nevirapine can be given. The dose is 2 mg/kg. However, the usefulness of this therapy needs further testing.
- If the infant is HIV-positive then Antiretroviral Treatment (ART) is given
- All HIV-exposed infants should receive *P. carnii* pneumonia prophylaxis (trimethoprim-sulfamethoxazole-150/750 mg/m^2/ day in two divided doses po on consecutive days), starting at 4-6 weeks of age and continuing for the first year of life. (Anderson, 2001, 262-263).

Unless no safer method of feeding exists, an infant born to a HIV positive mother should not be breastfed. Breast milk is a vehicle for transmission of the virus between the mother and her infant. Follow-up care is needed for both the mother and her infant, especially during the infant's first year of life. Immunizations should be given on schedule to provide the most comprehensive coverage for prophylaxis against infection. See the American Academy of Pediatrics (AAP) guidelines for the Immunization Schedule in Chapter 20.

Isolation.   Isolation is not necessary for the neonate who has been exposed to HIV. If, however, enteritis, draining wounds, congenital syphilis, cytomegalovirus, herpes, rubella, or other viral infections are present, the neonate should be placed in isolation for these disease entities, not the HIV itself.

If none of the reasons to isolate the infant is present, the nursing staff should promote early contact between the neonate and the mother. Nursing staff should instruct the mother to wash her hands and change soiled gowns and linen before handling her infant. During this period, the mother or care provider should be educated regarding signs and symptoms of infections and ways to minimize them.

Three "Cs" of Care.   In provision of care to the HIV patient, three "Cs" can be applied to the situation: comprehensive, consistent, and compassionate. Comprehensive care includes an alliance of mental health and medical professionals to provide both emotional and physical supportive care. Consistent care refers to building a sense of trust and rapport between parents and care providers. Lastly, compassionate care refers to supportive education, stressing the importance of empathy, including human touch, when dealing with the individual with HIV.

Closely aligned to the three Cs of care are the basic principles of nursing care. Four important points must be kept in mind to provide high-quality comprehensive care to newborns infected with HIV. The first point is that the infant and family are the unit of treatment, not the disease itself. To carry out this principle, the aspects of infant development and psychosocial concerns need to be taken into consideration. The second principle is that care should be community-based and family-centered. Every effort should be made to devise and support outpatient and family-centered treatment. One of the primary reasons is that community-based care is less costly than in-hospital care. In addition, community-based care attempts to improve the quality of life of the infant and family.

Third, culturally appropriate and sensitive questions must be asked to determine the psychosocial dimensions of the illness and the milieu in which it occurs. The health care providers need to be nonjudgmental of the parents, who may be from culturally diverse backgrounds or have a history that may involve previous or current drug abuse. These are just two examples of modifying ways that nursing care needs to be culturally appropriate.

Lastly, another factor to take into consideration is the quality of the infant's and family's life and the family's right to a dignified death. Dignity in all stages of care and impending death must be an underlying theme in the care of an infant or child infected with HIV. The fact that HIV is currently fatal does not lessen the infant's and family's need for love, physical intimacy, and social and cognitive stimulation.

Fungal Agents

Candida albicans.   *Candida* species is a fungus that is frequently found in humans, and *C. albicans* is the most prevalent form in newborns. *Candida* organisms are oval yeast-like cells that can bud to reproduce. *C. albicans* produces endotoxins, hemolysis, pyrogens, and proteolytic enzymes that are damaging to tissues. Early recognition and treatment of fungal sepsis are imperative to prevent severe central nervous system complications and death. Prolonged broad-spectrum antibiotic treatment for small premature infants may predispose infants to *Candida* overgrowth in the gastrointestinal tract. This overgrowth may predispose the infant to disseminated fungemia. Administration of hyperalimentation, frequent use of indwelling venous lines, and invasive procedures may also predispose the infant to *C. albicans* infection. One study has identified previous antibiotic therapy and assisted ventilation as the major factors that correlated to *Candida* sepsis (Khoory & Vino et al, 1999; Miller, 2001).

Clinical Manifestations.   The newborn infected with systemic *C. albicans* presents a picture similar to that of any infected infant, such as serious clinical signs of sepsis, often worsening with no presence of positive cultures. The infant is typically 20 to 30 days of age, has difficulties with oral feeds, depends on hyperalimentation, and has been given multiple courses of antibiotics. The infant may have respiratory distress, abdominal distention, guaiac-positive stools, carbohydrate intolerance, candiduria, temperature instability, and hypotension (Khoory et al, 1999).

TABLE 29-5 Comparison of Intrapartum/Postpartum Regimens for HIV-Infected Women at Labor Who Have Had No Prior Antiretroviral Therapy

Drug Regiment	Source of Evidence	Maternal Intrapartum	Infant Postpartum	Data on Transmission	Advantages	Disadvantages
Nevirapine	Clinical trial, Africa; compared with oral ZDV given intrapartum and for 1 week to the infant	Single 200 mg oral dose at onset of labor	Single 2 mg/kg oral dose at age 48 to 72 hr*	Transmission at 12 mo 16% with nevirapine compared to 24% with ZDV, a 35% reduction**	Inexpensive Oral regimen Simple, easy to administer Can give directly observed treatment	Unknown efficacy if mother has nevirapine-resistant virus
ZDV/3TC	Clinical trial, Africa; compared with placebo	ZDV 600 mg orally at onset of labor, followed by 300 mg orally every 3 hr until delivery AND 3TC 150 mg orally at onset of labor, followed by 150 mg orally every 12 hr until delivery	ZDV 4 mg/kg orally every 12 hr AND 3TC 2 mg/kg orally every 12 hr for 7 days	Transmission at 6 wk 10% with ZDV/3TC compared to 17% with placebo, a 38% reduction.	Oral regimen Compliance easier than 6 weeks of ZDV alone as infant regimen is only 1 week	Potential toxicity of multiple drug exposure
ADV	Epidemiologic data, U.S.; compared with no ZDV treatment	2 mg/kg intravenous bolus, followed by continuous infusion of 1 mg/kg/hr until delivery	2 mg/kg orally every 6 hr for 6 weeks	Transmission 10% with ZDV compared with 27% with no ZDV treatment, a 62% (95% CI, 19% to 82%) reduction.	Has been standard recommendation based on clinical trial results.	Requires intravenous administration and availability of ADV intravenous formulation Compliance with 6 weeks infant regimen
ZDV and nevirapine	Theoretical	ZDV 2 mg/kg intravenous bolus, followed by continuous infusion of 1 mg/kg/hr until delivery AND Nevirapine single 200 mg oral dose at onset of labor	ADV 2 mg/kg orally every 6 hr for 6 weeks AND Nevirapine single 2 mg/kg oral dose at age 48 to 72 hr	No data	Potential benefit if maternal virus is resistant to either nevirapine or ADV Synergistic inhibition of HIV replication with combination in vitro	Requires intravenous administration and availability of ADV intravenous formulation Compliance with 6 weeks infant ZDV regimen Unknown efficacy and limited toxicity data

*If the mother received nevirapine less than 1 hr before delivery, the infant was given 2 mg/kg oral nevirapine as soon as possible after birth and again at 48 to 72 hr.
**Owor M et al (2000). The one-year safety and efficacy data of the HIVNET 012 trial. XIII International AIDS Conference, Durban, South Africa (Abst LibOr1), July 9-14, 2000.
Adapted from Perinatal HIV Guidelines, 2000.
Source: Anderson JR (2001). HIV and reproduction. In JR Anderson (Ed.). A guide to the clinical care of women with HIV. Atlanta: CDC.

Differential Diagnosis.   A positive *Candida* culture should never be considered a contaminated specimen. Intermittently positive cultures may reflect transient candidemia, and usually, removal of any indwelling catheters and lines and changing of antibiotic therapy may be indicated. In symptomatic low-birth-weight infants with positive systemic cultures, treatment should begin pending culture results. Mortality rates are high in newborns with systemic candidiasis, especially in the presence of other debilitating disease; survival is increased with better recognition of infection and institution of specific therapy (Khoory et al, 1999; Miller, 2001).

Collaborative Management.   The most effective drug for treatment of *C. albicans* infection is amphotericin B. This toxic, potent antifungal agent must be used cautiously. The initial dose is 0.1 to 0.3 mg/kg given intravenously over a period of 2 to 6 hours. The maintenance dosage is 0.5 to 1.0 mg/kg/day over 2 to 6 hours. Lower doses are started until higher doses can be tolerated. Increments of 0.1 mg/kg/day are used to increase the daily dose slowly. Many infants tolerate a total dose of 25 to 30 mg/kg if titrated over approximately 1 month (Khoory et al, 1999; Miller, 2001). Often, if organ involvement is minimal, infants can be successfully given lower doses. If meningitis is suspected, 5-fluorouracil (5-FU) may be used. This antifungal agent acts to inhibit DNA synthesis so that *Candida* replication cannot occur. Dosage recommendations for this drug are based on extrapolated data from adults; there is no clearly established recommendation. Average daily dosage is 100 mg/kg/day in 4 divided doses, in conjunction with amphotericin B.

Miconazole has also been used to treat systemic candidiasis in newborns. Dosage guidelines for this drug have not been established; however, 10 mg/kg/day in two divided doses, followed by oral therapy. Safety and efficacy of these drugs in the treatment of newborns have not been established.

Renal toxicity is a major side effect of amphotericin B therapy because it causes renal vasoconstriction and decreases both renal blood flow and glomerular filtration rate. This damage can result in hyponatremia, hypokalemia, increased blood urea nitrogen, and increased creatinine as well as acidosis. If the medication makes the patient oliguric, most physicians recommend stopping the drug until the next day. Thrombocytopenia, granulocytopenia, fever, nausea, and vomiting are the common side effects associated with amphotericin B. One major side effect of 5-FU is bone marrow depression, resulting in a decreased platelet count.

Because of the insidious onset of candidiasis, the septic infant who is not responding to traditional antibiotic treatment may have *Candida*. Catheter tips at intravenous sites and percutaneous lines should be changed and cultured. Urine can easily be cultured for the presence of *Candida*. Thrush and monilial rashes are indicative of candidiasis. These can easily be treated with oral and local antifungal agents.

Monitoring of infants receiving amphotericin B is challenging because infants may have reactions to this medication. Blood pressure should be monitored every half hour, and urine output should be followed up closely. Vital signs and laboratory work, including liver enzyme tests, should be followed up daily to detect early signs of neonatal toxicity (Khoory et al, 1999; Miller, 2001).

Nosocomial Infections.   Both colonization and infection are nosocomial events, meaning "of or related to a hospital." The common meaning of the term nosocomial is "hospital-acquired." Nursery-acquired infections are reported to the Centers for Disease Control, which has a National Nosocomial Infections Surveillance System. The incidence of nosocomial infections in NICUs is 5 to 25%. Infants who are critically ill and remain in a pathogen-filled environment are often in jeopardy because of their prolonged length of stay in the hospital. The mortality rate associated with these infections is between 5% and 20%, depending on the geographic area and specific birth weight groups (Harris & Goldman, 2001).

Coagulase-negative staphylococcus has been identified as a major cause of nosocomial infections. Low birth weight, multiple gestation, and prolonged hospitalization are significant factors for nosocomial infection. Yeast infections often occur if previous antibiotic therapy has been given. This infection is also associated with colonization of vascular catheters, assisted ventilation, and necrotizing enterocolitis.

Nursery epidemics can be caused by gram-negative and gram-positive or viral organisms because they have the following:

- The ability to colonize or infect human skin or the gastrointestinal tract
- The ability to be carried from person to person by hand contact
- Characteristics that allow existence on hands of personnel or in fluids or on inanimate objects, including intravenous fluids, respiratory support equipment, solutions used for medications, disinfectants, and banked breast milk.

Resistance to antibiotics is a serious problem in many NICUs, particularly with gram-negative enteric pathogens. Aminoglycoside resistance is a problem in many urban nurseries, as is colonization and infection with methicillin-resistant *S. aureus*. Respiratory infections with RSV, influenza virus, parainfluenza virus, rhinovirus, and echovirus occur in many nurseries. These are more difficult to identify and thus more difficult to report. CMV infection has been reported as a transfusion-related problem in low-birth-weight infants, thus prompting the current policy of using CMV-screened blood donors. Hepatitis A infection has also been reported as a transfusion-related problem that may develop in infants and staff in NICUs. Hepatitis C is sometimes linked to use of immunoglobulins, such as Gammagard by Baxter. Almost any organism—given the right environment and support—can become a nosocomially transmitted infection.

Infection Control Policies

Policies and procedures in nurseries should be set up by the hospital infection control committee based on the recommendations of the American Academy of Pediatrics and the CDC. The significance of these policies to newborns should be detailed in a hospital policy book. The following topics should be covered:

- Ocular prophylaxis
- Skin and cord care
- Nursery staff
- Nursery design and environment
- Hand washing
- Staff apparel
- Isolation
- Visitors
- Employee health
- Epidemic control

SUMMARY

This chapter presents an overview of the function and development of the components of the neonatal immune system.

Many factors place the neonate at high risk for infection. The nurse is in a unique role to implement methods for prevention of infection in nurseries, to detect early signs and symptoms of infection, and to participate in infection control. A better understanding of the neonatal immune system, methods of perinatal acquisition of organisms, common microorganisms, signs and symptoms of infections, and appropriate therapy provides the nurse with a sound basis for management of care as well as the development of hospital infection control policies for the NICU.

REFERENCES

American Academy of Pediatrics (1997). *Report of the Committee on Infectious Diseases and Committee on Fetus and Newborn.* Revised guidelines for prevention of early-onset Group B Streptococcal (GBS) infection. *Pediatrics,* 99(3), 489-496.

Anderson JR (2001). HIV and reproduction. In JR Anderson (Ed.). *A guide to the clinical care of women with HIV.* Atlanta: CDC.

Anwer SK, Mustafa S (2000). Rapid identification of neonatal sepsis, *Journal of the Pakistan Medical Association,* 50(3), 94-98.

Arvin AM, Maldonado YA (2001). Other viral infections of the fetus and newborn. In JS Remington, JO Klein (Eds.), *Infectious diseases of the fetus and newborn infant,* ed 5, Philadelphia: WB Saunders.

Arvin AM, Whitley RJ (2001). Herpes Simplex virus infections. In JS Remington, JO Klein (Eds.), *Infectious diseases of the fetus and newborn infant,* ed 5, Philadelphia: WB Saunders.

Baley JE, Goldbarb J (2001). Neonatal infections. In MH Klaus, AA Fanaroff (Eds.). *Care of the high-risk neonate,* ed 5, Philadelphia: WB Saunders.

Beri R, Lourwood DL (1997). Chemoprophylaxis for group B Streptococcus transmission. *The annals of pharmcotheraphy,* 31(1), 110-112.

Bingen E et al (1997). Virulence patterns of Escherichia coli K1 strains associated with neonatal meningitis, *Journal of clinical microbiology,* 35(11), 2981-2982.

Bortolussi R, Schlechi WF (2001). Listeriosis. In JS Remington, JO Klein (Eds.), *Infectious diseases of the fetus and newborn infant,* ed 5, Philadelphia: WB Saunders.

Brocklehurst P (2001). Interventions aimed at decreasing the risk of mother-to-child transmission of HIV infection (Cochrane Review). *The Cochrane Library,* 3, 1-3. http://www.update-software.com/ccweb/cochrane/revabstr/ab000102.htm

CDC (1998). *Trends in the HIV & AIDS epidemic.* Atlanta, GA: CDC.

CDC (2001). www.cdc.gov.

Centers for Disease Control (2001). Health information for international travel 2001-2002.

Chan DK, Ly H (1997). Usefulness of C-reactive protein in the diagnosis of neonatal sepsis. *Singapore medicine journal,* 38(6), 252-255.

Chang Chien HY et al (2000). Characteristics of neonatal bacterial meningitis in a teaching hospital in Taiwan from 1984-1997. *Journal of microbiology, immunology, and infection,* 33(2), 100-104.

Cleary TG et al (2001). Microorganisms responsible for neonatal diarrhea. In JS Remington, JO Klein (Eds.), *Infectious diseases of the fetus and newborn infant,* ed 5, Philadelphia: WB Saunders.

Cooper LZ, Alford CA (2001). Rubella. In JS Remington, JO Klein (Eds.), *Infectious diseases of the fetus and newborn infant,* ed 5, Philadelphia: WB Saunders.

Crumpacker CS (2001). Hepatitis. In JS Remington, JO Klein (Eds.), *Infectious diseases of the fetus and newborn infant,* ed 5, Philadelphia: WB Saunders.

D'Andrea CC, Ferrera PC (1998). Disseminated herpes simplex virus infection in a neonate. *The American journal of emergency medicine,* 16(4), 376-378.

Edwards ME, Baker CJ (2001). Group B Streptococcal Infections. In JS Remington, JO Klein (Eds.), *Infectious diseases of the fetus and newborn infant,* ed 5, Philadelphia: WB Saunders.

Gerdes JS, Polin R (1998). Early diagnosis and treatment of neonatal sepsis. *Indian journal of pediatrics,* 65, 63-78.

Gershon AA (2001). Chickenpox, measles, and mumps. In JS Remington, JO Klein (Eds.), *Infectious diseases of the fetus and newborn infant,* ed 5, Philadelphia: WB Saunders.

Griffin MP, Moorman JR (2001). Toward the early diagnosis of neonatal sepsis and sepsis-like illness using novel heart rate analysis. *Pediatrics,* 107(1), 97-104.

Gregg NM (1941). Congenital cataract following German measles in the mother. *Transactions of the ophthalmological society of Australia,* 3, 35.

Gutman LT (2001). Gonococcal infections. In JS Remington, JO Klein (Eds.), *Infectious diseases of the fetus and newborn infant,* ed 5, Philadelphia: WB Saunders.

Harris JS, Goldmann DA (2001). Infections acquired in the nursery: epidemiology and control. In JS Remington, JO Klein (Eds.), *Infectious diseases of the fetus and newborn infant,* ed 5, Philadelphia: WB Saunders.

http://www.merck.com/pubs/mmanual/section12/chapter146/146a.htm
http://www.merck.com/pubs/mmanual/section12/chapter146/146b.htm
http://www.merck.com/pubs/mmanual/section12/chapter146/146d.htm
http://www.merck.com/pubs/mmanual/section12/chapter146/146e.htm

Ingall E, Sanchez PJ (2001). Syphilis. In JS Remington, JO Klein (Eds.), *Infectious diseases of the fetus and newborn infant,* ed 5, Philadelphia: WB Saunders.

Jensen HB, Pollock BH (1997). Meta-analyses of the effectiveness of intravenous immune globulin for prevention and treatment of neonatal sepsis. *Pediatrics,* 99(2), E2, 1-11.

Jensen HB, Pollock BH (1998). The role of intravenous immunoglobulin for the prevention and treatment of neonatal sepsis. *Seminars in perinatology,* 22(1), 50-63.

Kang JO, Kim CR (1997). Nosocomial Respiratory Syncytial Virus infection in a newborn nursery, *Journal of Korean medical science,* 12(6), 489-491.

Kapur R et al (2002). Developmental Immunology. In AA Fanaroff, RJ Martin (Eds.), *Neonatal-perinatal medicine: diseases of the fetus and infant,* ed 7, St Louis: Mosby.

Kaushik SL et al (1998). Neonatal sepsis in hospital born babies. *Journal of communicable diseases,* 30(3), 147-152.

Khoory BJ et al (1999). Candida infections in newborns: a review, *Journal of chemotherapy,* 11(5), 367-378.

Klein RO (2001). Bacterial sepsis and meningitis. In JS Remington, JO Klein (Eds.), *Infectious diseases of the fetus and newborn infant,* ed 5, Philadelphia: WB Saunders.

Klinger G et al (2000). Predicting the outcome of neonatal bacterial meningitis. *Pediatrics,* 106(3), 477-482.

Lewis DB, Wilson CB (2001). Developmental immunology and role of host defenses in fetal and neonatal susceptibility to infection. In JS Remington, JO Klein (Eds.), *Infectious diseases of the fetus and newborn infant,* ed 5, Philadelphia: WB Saunders.

Logsdon BA, Casto DT (1997). Prevention of Group B Streptococcus infection in neonates. *The annals of pharmacotherapy,* 31(7-8), 897-906.

Lott JW (2001). Personnal communication.

Marlowe SE et al (1997). Prolonged rupture of membranes in the term newborn. *American journal of perinatology/neonatology,* 14(8), 483-486.

Miller MJ (2001). Fungal infections. In JS Remington, JO Klein (Eds.), *Infectious diseases of the fetus and newborn infant,* ed 5, Philadelphia: WB Saunders.

Mogami S (1997). Congenitally-acquired Herpes zoster infection in a newborn, *Dermatology,* 194, 276-277.

Nelson CT, Demmier GJ (1997). Cytomegalovirus infection in the pregnant mother, fetus, and newborn infant. *Infections in perinatology,* 24(1), 151-160.

Pedreira DA et al (1997). PCR in the first oropharynx aspirate of the newborn: a possible source for identification of congenital infection agents. *Revista do Instuto de Medicina Tropical de Sao Paulo,* 39(6), 363-364.

Remington JS et al (2001). Toxoplasmosis. In JS Remington, JO Klein (Eds.), *Infectious diseases of the fetus and newborn infant*, ed 5, Philadelphia: WB Saunders.

Schachter J, Grossman M (2001). Chlamydia. In JS Remington, JO Klein (Eds.), *Infectious diseases of the fetus and newborn infant*, ed 5, Philadelphia: WB Saunders.

Shinefield HR, St. Geme JW III (2001). Staphylococcal infections. In JS Remington, JO Klein (Eds.), *Infectious diseases of the fetus and newborn infant*, ed 5, Philadelphia: WB Saunders.

Stagno, S (2001). Cytomegalovirus. In JS Remington, JO Klein (Eds.), *Infectious diseases of the fetus and newborn infant*, ed 5, Philadelphia: WB Saunders.

Steinlen M et al (1999). Neonatal Escherichia coli meningitis: Spinal adhesions as a late complication. *European journal of pediatrics*, 158(12), 968-970.

Stoll BJ (2001). Neonatal infections: a global perspective. In JS Remington, JO Klein (Eds.), *Infectious diseases of the fetus and newborn infant*, ed 5, Philadelphia: WB Saunders.

Stoll BJ et al (1998). Decline in sepsis-associated neonatal and infant deaths in the United States, 1979-1994. *Pediatrics*, 102(2), e18.

Visintine AM et al (1977). Infection in infants and children. *American journal of diseases of children*, 131(4), 393-397.

Wortley PM et al (2001). Successful implementation of perinatal HIV prevention guidelines. *Morbidity and mortality weekly review*, 50(RR06), 15-28.

Yau KIT (2000). Prevention and control of neonatal sepsis. Editorial. *Acta paediatrica taiwanica*, 41(3), 117-118.

Yurdakok M (1998). Antibiotic use in neonatal sepsis. *The Turkish journal of pediatrics*, 40, 17-33.

CHAPTER 30

ASSESSMENT AND MANAGEMENT OF THE HEMATOLOGIC SYSTEM

NANCY M. SHAW

Invasion of the endometrium by the primitive placenta permits simple diffusion of nutrients, which provides the initial nutritional support for the newly fertilized ovum. The developing embryo requires a large and consistent source of sustenance, and it quickly outgrows both the nutrients available in the surface lining of the endometrium and the rate at which simple diffusion can supply its needs. Consequently, the development of an efficient form of nutrient transport, such as that provided by circulating blood, is of utmost importance for continued growth of the embryo; this explains the early embryologic appearance of the hematologic and cardiovascular systems. Through the activation of these two systems, nutrition for the embryo and fetal membranes is provided at the interface between the fetal and maternal circulations by means of passive and active diffusion, active transport, and pinocytosis. Although blood begins to circulate by the third to fifth week of gestation, the cardiovascular and hematologic systems undergo refinement in the following months.

This chapter outlines the embryologic development of the hematopoietic system. It also describes the more common neonatal hematologic problems and associated high-risk factors, along with collaborative management strategies.

EMBRYOLOGIC DEVELOPMENT OF THE HEMATOPOIETIC SYSTEM

The hematopoietic system is characterized by the presence of pluripotent stem cells that differentiate into the three types of circulating blood cells: red blood cells (RBCs), white blood cells (WBCs), and platelets. Hematopoiesis is a continuous process that involves cell maturation and destruction concurrent with new cell production. Gestational age and postnatal age influence this maturational process and govern individual cell components, the level of activity, and the site of production.

The characteristics of the neonatal erythrocyte predispose both preterm and term infants to problems associated with hemolysis and immature hepatic response to erythrocyte destruction, as well as to the effects of shortened erythrocyte life span (as is seen in physiologic neonatal anemia and anemia of the premature infant). In addition to maturational influences, pre-existing maternal diseases and intrauterine abnormalities can impair RBC function and production, resulting in increased oxygen and nutritional requirements for the growing fetus.

The production of platelets and clotting factors is also a function of gestational age. Although some factors are deficient at birth, several clotting factors and platelets are present in concentrations similar to adult levels. However, many of these components are functionally different from those of adults, possibly because of impaired activity or limited ability to respond to heightened needs. Coagulation dysfunction in the newborn may also be the result of genetic abnormalities (e.g., X-linked hemophilia), pre-existing maternal illness (e.g., immune thrombocytopenic purpura), or infection (e.g., disseminated intravascular coagulation).

The production and function of WBCs are also affected by gestational age; this subject is covered in more detail in Chapter 29.

Primitive Vascular Formation

Vasculogenesis, the development of blood vessels, begins in the yolk sac of the fertilized ovum during the third week of gestation. This development starts in response to the relative paucity of nutrition available to the rapidly growing embryo. It is initially observed between the two cell layers of the yolk sac, the extraembryonic mesoderm and the extraembryonic endoderm. The extraembryonic mesoderm originates from one of the two initial layers of the primitive embryo, the intraembryonic ectoderm, and the extraembryonic endoderm originates from the intraembryonic endoderm. The cells that form the two layers of the yolk sac also give rise to the placenta and fetal membranes.

Mesenchymal cells, or loose embryonic connective tissue in the extraembryonic mesoderm, can differentiate into various types of tissue. Some mesenchymal cells aggregate to form blood islands in the mesodermal tissue beneath the endoderm. The cells forming the blood islands quickly segregate into two specific cell lines, endothelial cells and hemoblasts (hemocytoblasts). The endothelial cells assemble around an inner cavity that develops in the blood island, forming the primitive endothelial lining of the newly formed vessels. These vessels fuse and extend to create the vascular system for the yolk sac that eventually is incorporated into the primitive gut.

Blood cell formation, or hematopoiesis, can be identified in the yolk sac during the third week of gestation with the appearance of hemoblasts (Moore & Persaud, 1998). It is theorized that hemoblasts arise from stem cells that migrated into

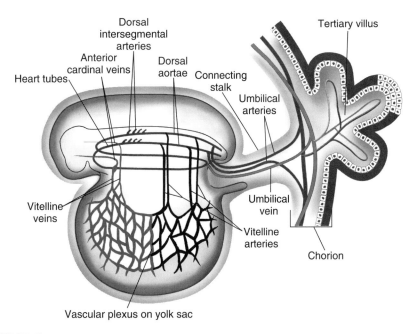

FIGURE **30-1**
The developing vasculature of the yolk sac, connecting stalk, chorion, and embryo eventually fuse and connect the circulations of the embryo and fetal membranes. This union provides for delivery of nutrients and removal of waste products in the embryo and its supporting structures. Redrawn from Moore K, Persaud T [1993]. *The developing human: clinically oriented embryology*, ed 5. WB Saunders: Philadelphia.

the yolk sac from the primitive ectoderm. Hemoblasts, surrounded by the flattened endothelial cells, are the precursors of primitive plasma and blood cells (Larsen, 1997).

Blood vessel formation in the connecting stalk and chorion occurs concurrently with vasculogenesis in the yolk sac, and vascular formation in all three areas is complete by the third week. The vessels in the connecting stalk become the umbilical vessels that indirectly link the embryo to maternal circulation through the placenta; vessels in the chorion give rise to the vasculature of fetal membranes and the villi of the placenta; and vessels in the yolk sac become the vitelline vessels, which contribute to the abdominal vasculature that will be incorporated into the body of the embryo. The formation of blood cells in the yolk sac regresses at the end of the second month of gestation, at which time hematopoiesis primarily becomes the function of the liver (Larsen, 1997).

Vasculogenesis in the embryo lags behind that of the yolk sac by approximately 1 to 2 days and evolves through a different process (Larsen, 1997). Vascular development starts in the middle layer of the embryo, which is now trilaminar (three-layered: endoderm, mesoderm, and ectoderm). The middle layer, the intraembryonic mesoderm, differentiates into three paired portions (paraxial, intermediate, and lateral mesoderm) that align themselves along the vertical axis of the embryo. The lateral mesoderm splits into two layers, the dorsal layer, or somatopleuric mesoderm, and the ventral layer, the splanchnopleuric mesoderm. It is the splanchnopleuric mesoderm that gives rise to the embryonic vasculature. Substances from the endoderm layer of the trilaminar embryo initiate vasculogenesis by inducing specific cells of the splanchnopleuric mesoderm to differentiate into angioblasts. Angioblasts flatten and unite to form angiocysts, vesicular structures that eventually fuse to form angioblastic cords. Angioblastic cords develop into the primitive vasculature that invades the embryo to form the circulatory system. Through the process of angiogenesis, new

vessels arise from the angioblastic cords. This vascular complex eventually fuses with the vasculature developing in the yolk sac and connecting stalk at approximately the fourth week of gestation (Figure 30-1).

Unlike vasculogenesis in the yolk sac, vasculogenesis in the embryo does not involve differentiation of mesodermal cells into blood cells. Blood cells initially produced in the yolk sac from primitive hematopoietic stem cells begin to circulate through the embryo after fusion of all vasculature. Plasma and blood cell production in the embryo does not begin until the fifth week of gestation and involves either migration of stem cells from the yolk sac to the liver and other organs of the embryo or independent production of hematopoietic stem cells at these sites (Moore & Persaud, 1998). When fusion of vasculature throughout the embryo and fetal structures occurs and blood circulation is established, primitive erythropoiesis becomes noticeable in the hepatic vascular spaces.

DEVELOPMENT OF HEMATOPOIETIC FUNCTION

Blood cell production in the embryo and fetus progresses through three phases: the megaloblastic (or mesoblastic) period, the hepatic period, and the myeloid period (Figure 30-2). Each phase is marked by changes in cell composition and in the major site of production. The megaloblastic period is characterized by blood cell production in the yolk sac; the hepatic period defines the liver as the major site of hematopoiesis; and the myeloid period defines the bone marrow as the hematopoietic center.

Megaloblastic Period
Vasculature and blood cells are formed from mesenchymal tissue during the first stage of hematopoiesis, known as the megaloblastic (mesoblastic) period. Primitive hematopoietic tissue consists

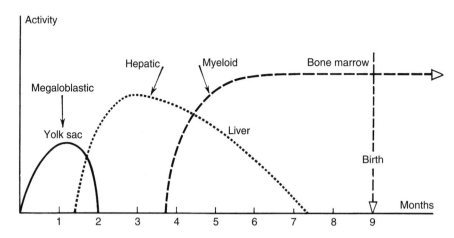

FIGURE **30-2**
Hematopoiesis progresses through three phases during embryonic and fetal life, with each new production period overlapping the previous phase. The initial phase is the megaloblastic (mesoblastic) period, which begins in the yolk sac of the developing embryo. It is quickly replaced by the hepatic period, which marks the emergence of the liver as the major site of hematopoiesis until the bone marrow takes over production during the myeloid period. From Rothstein G (1993). Origin and development of blood and blood-forming tissues. In Lee G et al, editors. *Wintrobe's clinical hematology,* ed 9. Lea & Febiger: Philadelphia.

of cells called hemoblasts, which are derived from the extraembryonic mesodermal tissue of the yolk sac. Although most of these cells differentiate into primitive erythrocytes, they also can give rise to WBCs and megakaryocytes. In contrast, the splanchnopleuric mesoderm of the embryo does not differentiate into hematopoietic stem cells. The embryo relies on circulating blood cells formed in the yolk sac until hepatic production begins during the fifth week. As previously discussed, the source of hepatic stem cells is still a subject of embryonic research.

Primitive erythrocytes produced by the embryo form two distinct generations of cells, primitive megaloblasts and definitive normoblasts (Brugnara & Platt, 1998). These two cell lines arise from similar hemoblasts but are morphologically divergent. Megaloblasts are large cells with a nucleus that give rise to irregularly shaped erythrocytes, which are found in the circulation at 4 to 5 weeks' gestation. Normoblasts are smaller, enucleated cells that arise during the sixth week of gestation and begin to circulate within the next 2 weeks. By 10 weeks' gestation, normoblasts are the predominant form of circulating RBCs.

Hepatic Period

At approximately the fifth to sixth week of gestation, the megaloblastic period ends and the hepatic period begins. This period marks the beginning of the embryonic liver as the major source of blood cells, with concurrent cell formation occurring in the spleen and lymph nodes. Hepatic hematopoiesis involves the production of blood cells from multipotent stem cells that migrated from the yolk sac through the blood into the liver or that arose independently from another line of stem cells (Larsen, 1997). The multipotent stem cells have three significant characteristics: (1) a variable capacity for self-renewal, (2) the potential to differentiate into different cell lines, and (3) the ability to repopulate. As they produce and divide in the liver parenchyma, these cells undergo a process of maturation that diminishes their ability to self-replicate and forces commitment to a specific cell line. Hematopoietic stem cells are considered the common progenitors of erythrocytes, lymphocytes, granulocytes, monocytes,

and megakaryocytes. Hematopoietic stem cells continue to reproduce throughout a person's life, but the available number of stem cells declines with age. These stem cells are the basis for cord banks and stem cell research, which are creating some controversy in the United States. Umbilical cords can be saved and stored for future use in the case of childhood cancers or other immune problems (McMillan, 1996). The importance of stem cells in the development of treatment for a wide variety of diseases, including hematologic disorders, remains to be seen.

The hepatic phase marks the onset of production of specific blood cell lines. During this stage, a portion of the stem cells begins to form erythrocytes (normoblasts), which develop into more mature forms with increasing gestational age. Another line of stem cells differentiates into leukocytes, which can be identified in the embryo at 5 to 7 weeks' gestation. Leukocytes, however, have several sites of production besides the liver parenchyma, including various connective tissues such as the meninges, mesentery, and stromal cells of the lymph plexus. Between the seventh and tenth weeks of gestation, lymphopoiesis is also observed in the gut, thymus, and associated lymphoid tissue. Megakaryocytes, the precursors of platelets, are present in the yolk sac and liver at 5 to 6 weeks' gestation, and platelets can be identified in the blood at approximately 11 weeks.

Myeloid Period

The liver remains the chief organ of hematopoiesis until it is gradually replaced by the bone marrow during the myeloid period of hematopoiesis. This process begins at the fourth month of gestation and becomes quantitatively important by the sixth month. During the last 3 months of gestation, the liver gradually ceases its hematopoietic function as the bone marrow evolves into the chief source of blood cell production. Extramedullary sources of hematopoiesis generally cease by the first postnatal month. The bone marrow is composed primarily of blood vessels occupying cartilaginous lacunae that become invested with hematopoietic stem cells. Theoretically these cells either migrated from the liver to the bone marrow through the

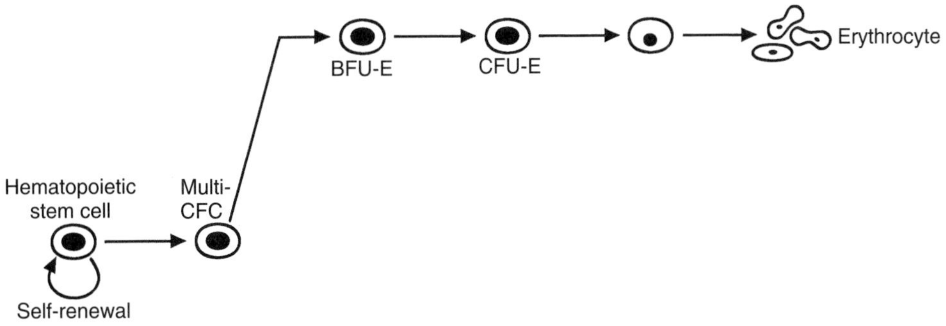

FIGURE **30-3**
Hematopoietic stem cells stimulated to become erythrocytes initially develop into multipotent colony-forming cells (Multi-CFC). A portion of the Multi-CFC become erythroid progenitor cells, the early and late erythroid burst-forming units (BFU-E), which eventually differentiate into erythroid colony-forming units (CFU-E). These progenitor cells progress to form the normoblast, the erythrocyte precursor. Multiple divisions and alterations of the normoblast lead to the development of the reticulocyte. When the reticulocyte extrudes its nucleus, it normally moves out of the predominant production sites (i.e., the liver or bone marrow) and into the blood. Modified from Luchtman-Jones L et al (2002). The blood and hematopoietic system. In Fanaroff A, Martin R, editors. *Neonatal-perinatal medicine: diseases of the fetus and infant*, ed 7. Mosby: St Louis.

blood or arose from an independent source of stem cells. The volume of marrow occupied by hematopoietic tissue increases until term.

The production of all blood cells escalates during the myeloid period. Mature RBCs produced by the marrow appear about 1 week after marrow development and are present in significant numbers at 17 weeks' gestation. In the final 2 months of gestation, RBC production per kilogram of body weight in the fetus is three to four times greater than that in the adult. Concurrent with myeloid RBC production, leukocyte production begins in the bone marrow of the clavicle. Stem cells in the clavicular marrow differentiate to form two separate populations of lymphocytes, T (thymus) cells and B (bone marrow) cells. Other forms of leukocytes (granulocytes and monocytes) develop after the lymphocyte. Although relatively few granulocytes are present during the first half of gestation, their concentration rapidly increases during the last trimester; monocytes are apparent during the fifth fetal month. The increase in bone marrow production of megakaryocytes parallels increasing gestational age. However, after 27 weeks' gestation, platelet counts are similar regardless of gestational age.

ERYTHROCYTE MATURATION

Red blood cells undergo specific changes in composition and concentration during the three stages of hematopoiesis. The production of a mature red blood cell is a complex process that involves initial differentiation of hematopoietic stem cells into RBC precursors and further transition through multiple stages of maturation.

Megaloblastic Period

Hemoblasts, which arise from the extraembryonic mesoderm of the yolk sac during the megaloblastic period, give rise to primitive nucleated RBCs called megaloblasts or megalocytes. The megalocytic form of erythrocyte contains an embryonic form of hemoglobin, the first of three sequential embryonic forms. Megalocytes remain primitive blood cells and do not progress into more mature forms.

Hepatic and Myeloid Periods

The initial form of the erythrocyte that arises from the stem cells, the megaloblast, gradually is replaced by the normoblast (erythroblast) when blood cell formation begins in the liver. Stem cells in the liver and eventually the bone marrow begin to differentiate into multipotent colony-forming cells (Multi-CFC) (Figure 30-3). These cells can differentiate into the various blood cell components when activated by various stimulants, such as erythropoietin, interleukin, and granulocyte-macrophage colony-stimulating factor (GM-CSF). Some Multi-CFCs differentiate into committed progenitors of the erythrocyte, early and late erythroid burst-forming units (BFU-E) that progress to erythroid colony-forming units (CFU-E). BFU-E and CFU-E cells are the precursors of the normoblast, which becomes the dominant cell type at 10 weeks' gestation (Brugnara & Platt, 1998).

When the liver becomes the predominant source of erythrocyte production, a definitive line of RBCs is formed from the normoblasts, which progress through several phases of refinement and accrue hemoglobin before reaching maturation. When the hemoglobin concentration of the normoblast reaches 34%, the nucleus is extruded and the cell becomes a reticulocyte. About 1 to 2 days later, the reticulocyte becomes a mature RBC. The progression is identical in the bone marrow when it assumes erythrocyte production. Control over erythropoiesis during early fetal life is not clearly understood, and the role of erythropoietin is uncertain.

At 10 weeks' gestation, hemoglobin synthesis changes from the embryonic to the fetal form (hemoglobin F). The mechanism by which stem cells and progenitor cells perform this changeover remains unclear. Although low levels of a third form of hemoglobin, adult hemoglobin (hemoglobin A), are detectable at this time, hemoglobin F remains the predominant form during fetal development. At 30 weeks' gestation, 90% to 100% of hemoglobin is the fetal form; the remainder is hemoglobin A. Between 30 and 32 weeks, the percentage of hemoglobin F starts to decline. At 40 weeks, 50% to 75% of RBCs contain fetal hemoglobin; at 6 months of age, 5% to 8%; and at 1 year of age, 1%.

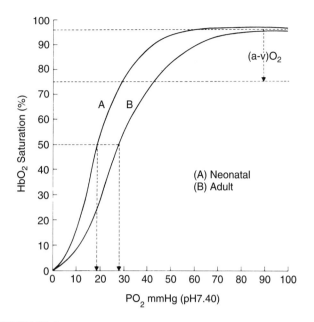

FIGURE **30-4**
The affinity for oxygen (i.e., the ability of the hemoglobin molecule to bind and hold the oxygen molecule) is markedly different between fetal and adult hemoglobin. Fetal hemoglobin has a greater affinity for oxygen. It is able to bind to oxygen more readily at the intervillous spaces of the placenta, a property that is useful in the low partial pressure of oxygen (PO_2) environment of the fetus. Adult hemoglobin has a diminished affinity for oxygen, which allows easier release of oxygen to the tissue when metabolic needs are higher than those that arise in the fetus. From Sacks L, Delivoria-Papadopoulos M (1984). Hemoglobin-oxygen interactions. *Seminars in perinatology* 8:168-183.

Each type of hemoglobin has properties that make it valuable at the time of its synthesis. Each has a different affinity for oxygen that varies its uptake and release to the tissue (Figure 30-4). Fetal hemoglobin has a high affinity for oxygen, binding it more readily at the intervillous spaces in the placenta when the fetal partial pressure of oxygen (PO_2) averages between 25 and 30 mm Hg. Adult hemoglobin has a decreased affinity for oxygen, which allows easier release of oxygen to the tissues when metabolic needs are high and the lungs are functional.

Erythropoietin

The factors that affect RBC production are still unclear, but erythropoietin appears to exert great control over erythropoiesis during late gestation. This circulating glycoprotein hormone, the gene of which is located on the seventh chromosome, is an obligate growth factor that stimulates stem cells to become committed progenitors of the erythrocyte (Figure 30-3). In adults the kidneys produce 90% to 95% of erythropoietin, but in the fetus the liver is considered the predominant site of production throughout most of gestation.

The major stimulus for erythropoietin release is diminished tissue oxygenation. In the absence of erythropoietin, hypoxia has no effect on the production of RBCs. However, if erythropoietin production is intact, hypoxia stimulates a rapid increase in erythropoietin levels, which remain elevated until hypoxia no longer exists. Although the liver is less responsive to hypoxia than the kidneys, production of erythropoietin in the fetus and newborn increases within minutes to hours after a precipitating event such as hypoxia. Erythropoietin acts by directly stimulating the RBC precursors, accelerating their

passage through the various maturational stages. Although erythropoietin levels increase rapidly, no change in the number of erythrocytes is noted for approximately 5 days after a hypoxic stress. When erythropoietin stimulates production of excess RBCs, the red blood cells are released into the circulation before they have reached maturity (i.e., as reticulocytes); this is reflected in an elevated reticulocyte count.

Factors besides hypoxia that increase erythropoietin production in the newborn are maternal hypoxemia, smallness for gestational age, and poor placental function. Erythropoietin levels are also increased by testosterone, estrogen, thyroid hormone, prostaglandins, and lipoproteins. Cord blood levels normally are elevated compared with adult values but drop dramatically to almost undetectable levels in the newborn. The healthy newborn, therefore, produces few RBCs in the first few weeks of life because the hypoxic stimuli of low fetal PO_2 levels are no longer present. Erythropoietin levels do not increase in the term infant until 8 to 10 weeks of age, when tissue hypoxia caused by anemia is sensed by the kidneys.

NORMAL HEMATOLOGIC VALUES IN THE NEWBORN

Factors Affecting Laboratory Values

Normal blood values found shortly after birth reflect a time of maximum change. Blood values at birth depend on (1) the timing of cord clamping, (2) the infant's gestational age, (3) the blood sampling site, and (4) the technique used to obtain adequate blood flow.

The timing of cord clamping and the positional differences between the infant and the placenta can significantly influence newborn blood volume. Complete emptying of placental vessels before clamping can increase blood volume by 61%; one quarter of the placental transfusion occurs within the first 15 seconds, and half of the transfusion is complete by 1 minute.

The average blood volume is approximately 85 ml/kg of body weight in the term infant; it can rise to 90 to 105 ml/kg in the preterm infant. The younger the infant's gestational age, the greater the blood volume per kilogram of body weight. The hemoglobin concentration and hematocrit are also functions of gestational age, especially in infants born before 32 weeks' gestation. The average mean hemoglobin concentration at 26 to 30 weeks is 13.4 g/dl, with an average mean hematocrit of 41.5% (Siberry & Iannone, 2000). In the term infant, mean hemoglobin values range from 16.5 to 18.5 g/dl, with mean hematocrit values between 51% and 56%. Mean hemoglobin values in postmature infants are higher than in the term infant, possibly as a result of progressive placental dysfunction and of oxygen deficit, which stimulates the release of erythropoietin. Table 30-1 summarizes the differences in hematologic values as a function of increasing gestational and postnatal age.

It is important to consider the sampling site and the quality of blood flow when interpreting laboratory values. The hemoglobin levels of capillary blood are 10% to 20% higher than those of venous and arterial blood. This discrepancy can be minimized by warming the extremity before drawing blood to enhance peripheral perfusion, allowing better spontaneous blood flow. Discarding the first few drops obtained on a capillary draw also improves the accuracy of the sample. Sampling by the venous route also requires care; poor blood flow through small-bore needles increases the chance of hemolysis, which can lead to sampling errors. Greater accuracy can be obtained by using the largest possible bore needle and removing the

TABLE 30-1	Age-Specific Normal Blood Cell Values in Fetal Samples (26 to 30 Weeks' Gestation) and Neonatal Samples (28 to 44 Weeks' Gestation)						
Age	Hb (g%)*	HCT (%)*	MCV (fL)*	MCHC (g/% RBC)*	Reticulocytes	WBCs (×10³/mm³)†	Platelets (10³/mm³)†
26 to 30 wk gestation‡	13.4 (11)	41.5 (34.9)	118.2 (106.7)	37.9 (30.6)	—	4.4 (2.7)	254 (180 to 271)
28 wk	14.5	45	120	31.0	(5-10)	—	275
32 wk	15.0	47	118	32.0	(3-10)	—	290
Term§ (cord)	16.5 (13.5)	51 (42)	108 (98)	33.0 (30.0)	(3-7)	18.1 (9 to 30)§	290
1 to 3 dy	18.5 (14.5)	56 (45)	108 (95)	33.0 (29.0)	(1.8 to 4.6)	18.9 (9.4 to 34)	192
2 wk	16.6 (13.4)	53 (41)	105 (88)	31.4 (28.1)		11.4 (5 to 20)	262
1 mo	13.9 (10.7)	44 (33)	101 (91)	31.8 (28.1)	(0.1 to 1.7)	108 (4 to 19.5)	

Modified from Siberry G & Iannone R (2000). Harriet Lane handbook, ed 15. St Louis: Mosby.
Hb, Hemoglobin; Hct, hematocrit; MCV, mean corpuscular volume; MCHC, mean corpuscular hemoglobin concentration; WBCs, white blood cells.
*Data are mean (number in parenthesis is −2 standard deviations [SD]).
†Data are mean (number in parenthesis is −2 SD).
‡In infants younger than 1 month, capillary Hb exceeds venous Hb: at 1 hour old, the difference is 3.6 g; at 5 days, 2.2 g; at 3 weeks, 1.1 g.
§Mean (95% confidence limits).

needle from the syringe before placing the sample in the specimen container. Gestational age also affects the discrepancy between reported capillary and venous results: the younger the gestational age, the larger the discrepancy. The key to accuracy in hematologic laboratory values lies in the use of a consistent sampling site.

FETAL AND NEONATAL BLOOD COMPONENTS

The fetal and newborn RBC life span is much shorter than the adult erythrocyte life span of 120 days. The term newborn's erythrocyte can last 60 to 70 days; that of the preterm infant, 35 to 50 days. One theoretic reason for this difference in RBC life spans is the diminished deformability of the neonatal erythrocyte. Because of its larger size and cylindric shape, the neonatal erythrocyte is more prone to destruction in the narrow sinusoids of the spleen.

The mean RBC count in the term newborn is in the range of 5.1 million to 5.3 million per milliliter, with an elevated reticulocyte count of 3% to 7% during the first 24 to 48 hours of life (Siberry & Iaonne, 2000). Mean RBC counts in the premature infant range from 4.6 million to 5.3 million per milliliter, with a greater number of circulating immature RBCs reflected in a higher reticulocyte count (3% to 10%). In both groups of infants, the reticulocyte count falls abruptly to about 1% and the erythropoietin level drops to low, often undetectable, levels by the first week of life.

WBC counts depend on gestational and postnatal age, and newborn infants show a wide range of leukocyte counts, predominantly neutrophils (bands, segmented neutrophils, and metamyelocytes). The normal mean WBC count at birth is 4400/mm³ in the preterm infant and 18,000/mm³ in the term infant. During the first 12 hours of life, the WBC count rises, reaches a plateau, and then slowly declines. Neutrophil counts in the term infant average about 11,000/mm³ at this time, remaining constant from day 3 to the end of the first month of life (Figure 30-5). In well newborns, the average number of bands, a form of immature neutrophil, is 10% of the total WBC count. The neutrophil count averages about 8000/mm³ in infants of less than 37 weeks' gestation and about 6000/mm³ in

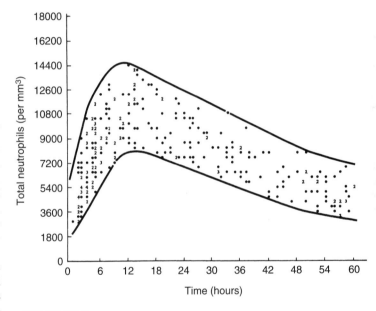

FIGURE 30-5
The normal range of the neutrophil count changes dramatically during the first 3 days of life. The range then stabilizes and remains constant for a short time. The neutrophil count rises during the first 12 hours of life, reaches a plateau, and then slowly begins to decline. From Manroe B et al (1979). The neonatal blood count in health and disease. I. Reference values for neutrophilic cells. Journal of pediatrics 95:89.

infants of less than 32 weeks. Mouzinho and colleagues (1994) studied the neutrophil counts in very-low birth-weight (VLBW) infants and noted a substantially lower range of the absolute neutrophil count (ANC) in the first few days of life compared with the predominantly term infants studied by Manroe and colleagues (1979). This led to a modification of the ANC graph for the VLBW infant during the first 3 days of life (Figure 30-6). By day 4 of life, no difference is noted between the various gestational age groups. Neutrophil counts can be lowered by conditions such as maternal hypertension,

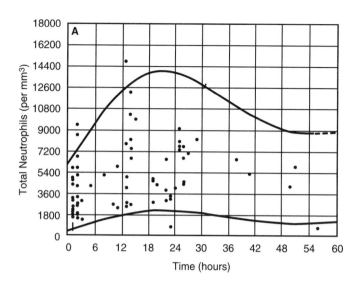

FIGURE **30-6**

The normal range of the neutrophil count is modified by gestational age; the number of neutrophils present in the blood of newborns is inversely related to gestational age. Although the upper limits of normal are maintained in the very-low-birth-weight (VLBW) infant, the lower limits of normal are significantly decreased compared with term or near term infants. From Mouzinho A et al (1994). Revised reference ranges for circulating neutrophils in very-low-birth-weight neonates. *Pediatrics* 94:76.

intraventricular hemorrhage, hemolytic disease, and infection; they can be raised by factors such as surgery, stress, and infection. As the newborn becomes older, WBC composition changes. The number of lymphocytes increases, but the monocyte count remains low.

The sampling site must be taken into consideration in evaluating the WBC count at birth. When peripheral venous and arterial samples are compared with capillary samples, venous samples have an 82% correlation with the values obtained by capillary sampling, and arterial samples have a 77% correlation with capillary sample results.

Because immature RBCs retain their nuclei and are relatively high in number for the first 4 days of life, they can be incorrectly counted in the total WBC count; therefore the WBC count must be corrected for any nucleated RBCs (NRBCs). This correction usually is done by the laboratory when the blood slide is read. If the count is not automatically adjusted, it can easily be done by multiplying the total WBC count by the percentage of NRBCs observed and subtracting this number from the total WBC count:

Adjusted WBC count 5 Total WBC count 2 (Total WBC count 3 NRBCs)

Platelet counts in the newborn do not vary much in relation to gestational age. Counts are similar from 27 to 40 weeks' gestation, with the range of normal falling between 215,000/mm^3 and 378,000/mm^3. Platelet counts under 150,000/mm^3 are considered thrombocytopenic.

ASSESSMENT OF HEMATOLOGIC FUNCTION

Because infants respond to a variety of problems in a similar manner, many clinical findings (e.g., hypoglycemia, hypocalcemia, hypothermia, apnea, bradycardia, cyanosis, lethargy,

---

> ### BOX **30-1**
>
> **Physical Findings Helpful in Evaluating the Integrity of the Hematologic System**
>
> Obvious blood loss—hemorrhage
> Pallor
> Plethora
> Petechiae
> Ecchymosis
> Jaundice
> Hepatosplenomegaly
> Hematomas

poor feeding) warrant at least a complete blood count (CBC) to determine if a hematologic reason exists for these symptoms. With active bleeding, platelet counts, clotting studies, fibrinogen levels, and measurements of products of fibrinolysis (e.g., d-dimer, fibrin split products or fibrin degradation products) can shed light on the type of blood dyscrasia present and can direct the caregiver to the appropriate therapeutic response. These studies also provide a way to monitor and evaluate treatments. However, laboratory data are most helpful when they are used in conjunction with astute observation and physical assessment skills.

Several physical findings can help determine the well-being and homeostasis of the hematologic system (Box 30-1). Cutaneous abnormalities such as hematomas, abrasions, petechiae, and bleeding should alert the nurse to the possibility of a hematologic abnormality. Hepatosplenomegaly also can indicate abnormal breakdown of RBCs. Hepatosplenomegaly concurrent with hyperbilirubinemia and hemolysis can signal alloimmune problems (e.g., Rh and ABO incompatibilities) or acquired, congenital, or postnatal infection (e.g., cytomegalovirus infection, toxoplasmosis, herpes simplex infection, or hepatitis).

HEMATOLOGIC DYSFUNCTION IN THE NEONATE

Blood Group Incompatibilities

Blood group incompatibilities were first recognized in the 1940s with the discovery of the Rh grouping and the first test for detection of antibody-coated RBCs, devised by Coombs in 1946. Before the introduction of Rh immune globulin (RhIgG, RhIG or RhoGAM) in 1964 and its release for general use in 1968, Rh incompatibility accounted for one third of all blood group incompatibilities. With the use of RhIgG, the frequency of Rh incompatibility has dropped significantly, and ABO has become the main blood group incompatibility, with sensitization occurring in 3% of all infants. Both incompatibilities involve maternal antibody response to fetal antigen, leading to RBC destruction by hemolysis. Rh antibody response is elicited on exposure to antigen and does not exist spontaneously, whereas anti-A and anti-B antibodies occur naturally. These entities also differ in the severity of the effect on the fetus and newborn and in the method of treatment.

Other minor blood groupings (e.g., Kell, C, E, Duffy, and Kidd) may also be involved in incompatibilities that result in hyperbilirubinemia, but Rh and ABO incompatibilities are the most common, accounting for 98% of all cases. There are 400 known RBC antigens that can induce antibody production.

Some of these antibodies are induced after transfusion therapy with incompatible blood; others occur in response to the transfer of incompatible fetal blood cells into the maternal circulation during pregnancy. The Rh system alone has 40 discrete antigens, but only five (C, D, E, and c, e) are important.

ABO Incompatibility

Antigens or agglutinogens, present on the RBC surface of each blood type, react with antibodies or agglutinins found in the plasma of opposing blood types. Of the 30 common antigens involved in antigen-antibody reactions, the ABO antigens are one of two groups most likely to be a problem, the other being the Rh group (Guyton & Hall, 1996a). The four major blood types are A, B, O, and AB. Antigens A and B occur on the surface of RBCs in most of the population, making A and B the most common blood types. Antibodies to the antigens of different blood types occur naturally in the plasma (Table 30-2). For example, type A blood has A antigens on the cell surface but has circulating anti-B antibodies in the plasma. Type B blood has just the opposite, B antigens on the cell surface and anti-A antibodies in the plasma. Type AB blood has A and B antigens on the cell surface and neither antibody in the plasma, and type O blood has neither antigen on the cell surface and both anti-A and anti-B antibodies in the plasma. Antigens usually are polypeptides and complex proteins; antibodies are immunoglobulins (mostly IgG and IgM).

With antigen and antibody in harmony, no RBC destruction occurs, but when a conflicting antibody is introduced into the circulation, RBC destruction may occur. RBCs have multiple binding sites to which opposing antibodies can attach. An antibody is capable of simultaneously attaching to several RBCs, thus creating a clump of cells. This clumping of cells, known as agglutination, can cause occlusion of small vessels and impair local circulation and tissue oxygenation. Fetal RBCs coated with antibodies attract phagocytes and macrophages that eventually destroy these agglutinated RBCs, usually through hemolysis by the reticuloendothelial cells in the spleen. Hemolysis can occur without preliminary agglutination, but it is a more delayed process because the body must first activate its complement system. High antibody titers (hemolysins) are required to stimulate this system, which causes the release of proteolytic enzymes that rupture the cell membrane.

In a transfusion reaction, when opposing blood types are mixed, the donor's RBCs are agglutinated, and the recipient's blood cells tend to be protected. The plasma portion of donor blood that contains antibodies becomes diluted by the recipient's blood volume, thus reducing donor antibody titers in the recipient's circulation. However, recipient antibody titers are adequate to destroy the donor RBCs by agglutination and hemolysis or by hemolysis alone. This is the situation in ABO incompatibility. In such cases, the maternal blood type usually is O, containing anti-A and anti-B antibodies in the serum, whereas the fetus or newborn is type A or B. Although incompatibility can occur between A and B types, it is not seen as frequently as AO or BO because of the globulin composition of the antibodies. In the O-type mother, the antibodies are usually IgG and can cross the placenta, whereas the antibodies of the type A or B mother frequently are IgM, which are too large to cross the placenta.

When transplacental hemorrhage (TPH) occurs between ABO-incompatible mother and fetus, fetal blood entering the maternal circulation undergoes agglutination and hemolysis by maternal antibodies. This rapid response prevents the

TABLE 30-2	Blood Groups and Their Constituent Antigens (Agglutinogens) and Antibodies (Agglutinins)		
Genotype	**Blood Group**	**Agglutinogens**	**Agglutinins**
OO	O	---	Anti-A and anti-B
OA or AA	A	A	Anti-B
OB or BB	B	B	Anti-A
AB	AB	A and B	---

From Guyton AC, Hall JE (1996). Blood groups, transfusion, tissue and organ transplantation. In Guyton AC, Hall JE, editors. Textbook of medical physiology, ed 9. WB Saunders: Philadelphia.

development of antibodies to other antigens present on fetal RBCs, because a time lapse is required for activation of the immune system. Consequently, fetal RBCs that are Rh positive in addition to being type A or type B are destroyed by naturally occurring anti-A or anti-B antibodies before any maternal antibodies to Rh factor (anti-D) can be produced. This naturally occurring phenomenon is the basis for the use of RhIgG, in which extrinsic anti-D destroys fetal cells before the maternal immune system can be activated to produce antibodies.

Despite this destruction of fetal RBCs, maternal anti-A or anti-B antibodies of the IgG form can freely cross the placenta and adhere to RBCs in the fetal circulation. For this reason, ABO incompatibility can occur in the first pregnancy (40% to 50% of total occurrences involve primigravidas) because TPH and inoculation of the mother with fetal blood are not necessary for the development of these naturally occurring antibodies. Because the A and B antigens on the fetal and neonatal RBCs are not well developed, only a small amount of maternal antibody actually attaches to the antigen. Other body tissues also have antigen sites to which some of the circulating antibodies can adhere, thereby decreasing the potential for RBC destruction. The resulting small amounts of IgG in the plasma do not stimulate activation of the complement system, therefore hemolysis is minimal. This lack of stimulation of the complement system and the above factors may explain why only 3% to 20% of infants of the 15% to 22% who are ABO incompatible with their mothers become symptomatic (Ozolek et al, 1994).

Erythrocyte antibodies are not usually present in the circulating blood until 2 to 8 months of postnatal age, which prevents maternal inoculation with fetal anti-A or anti-B antibodies. Antibody production then increases, reaching a maximum titer at 8 to 10 years of age (Guyton & Hall, 1996a). The newborn becomes inoculated with A and B antigens after birth through ingestion of food and the resulting bacterial colonization. This initiates production of anti-A or anti-B antibodies that circulate in the plasma, depending on the antigens present on the RBCs.

Clinical Manifestations.   The chief symptom of ABO incompatibility is jaundice within the first 24 hours of life; 90% of all affected infants are female. Hemolysis and anemia are minimal, although signs of a mildly compensated hemolytic state are reflected in certain CBC values. The peripheral blood smear may show evidence of spherocytes, or RBCs lacking the normal central pallor and biconcave, disklike shape of the normal RBC. Because they are smaller than normal RBCs, spherocytes appear thicker. These physical characteristics result in abnormal fragility under osmotic stress. Spherocytes are not distensible or compressible because they lack the normal amount of loose cell membrane, making them more susceptible to destruction in the splenic sinusoids.

Additional laboratory findings include a positive direct Coombs' test result in 3% to 32% of cases (Ozolek et al, 1994) and positive results on both direct and indirect Coombs' tests in 80% of cases when microtechniques are used. The direct Coombs' test is a measurement of the presence of antibody on the RBC surface; the indirect Coombs' test is a measurement of antibody in the serum. ABO incompatibility can also be identified by the performance of an eluate test, which involves washing the RBCs of the newborn and testing the wash for anti-A or anti-B antibodies.

On physical examination, hepatosplenomegaly can be observed, a reflection of extramedullary erythropoiesis generated by the fetus in response to significant hemolysis. In an effort to compensate for increased cell destruction, the liver and spleen manufacture RBCs for a longer period than usually is seen in the fetus and newborn. Engorgement of the splenic sinusoids by hemolyzed RBCs contributes to splenomegaly.

Treatment. Because the antibodies involved in ABO incompatibility occur naturally, elimination of this type of incompatibility is virtually impossible. However, its effects on the fetus and newborn are much less dramatic and life-threatening than those of Rh incompatibility; therefore amniocentesis and monitoring of amniotic fluid bilirubin levels, intrauterine transfusions, and early delivery usually are not necessary. Nevertheless, problems associated with postnatal bilirubin clearance do arise, and phototherapy and possible exchange transfusion become part of the repertoire of care. These two treatment methods are discussed in further detail later in the chapter.

Rh Incompatibility

Incompatibilities involving the Rh system are the second most common alloimmune problem, but the severity of complications far surpasses that of ABO incompatibility. Chromosome 1 stores the genetic material governing Rh antigens, but the number of genes involved in their synthesis has not been fully determined (Scott & Branch, 1999). There are three presumed Rh gene loci with the capability of producing five recognized antigens in the Rh complex: C, D, E, c, and e. The d antigen is considered an absence of antigen D because it cannot be isolated at present. Each individual has a paired set of these factors, having inherited a single set of C or c, D or d, and E or e from each parent. A predilection exits toward three particular combinations, two Rh positive (CDe and cDE) and one Rh negative (cde). Of these six factors, the two involved in Rh determination are D and d. The D antigen is most prevalent; its presence on the RBC indicates an Rh-positive cell, whereas its absence indicates an Rh-negative cell. Because of single-set inheritance from each parent, the potential exists for three different combinations of paired antigens: one pair being both d (Rh negative, homozygous), another pair being both D (Rh positive, homozygous), and the third pair being a combination of d and D (Rh positive, heterozygous). The end product is the production or absence of Rh antigen positioned on the surface of the RBC.

The Rh antigen can be detected as early as 38 days' gestation on the fetal RBC and attains complete development during fetal life. This antigen is necessary for normal function of the RBC membrane and, unlike A and B antigens, which can be found in other tissues, it is confined exclusively to the RBC. Antibodies never occur naturally in the Rh system; exposure to the antigen is necessary to produce antibodies. Such exposure is thought to occur through maternal inoculation with fetal RBCs by transplacental hemorrhage or through undetectable hemorrhage during labor, abortion, ectopic pregnancy, or amniocentesis.

Spontaneous TPH occurs in 50% to 75% of all pregnancies, with the greatest and most severe occurrence at the time of delivery. Fetal RBCs can be found in 6.7% of all pregnancies during the first trimester, 15% in the second trimester, and 28.9% in the third trimester (Scott & Branch, 1999). Spontaneous TPH allows fetal RBCs to pass into the maternal circulation, where antibodies develop in response to any foreign RBC antigen the mother does not possess. The risk of immunization depends on the ABO status of both mother and fetus and the size of the hemorrhage. On the basis of blood type, the risk for maternal Rh immunization in an ABO-compatible Rh-negative mother and Rh-positive fetus is 16%, whereas an ABO-incompatible pregnancy with an Rh-negative mother and Rh-positive fetus runs a 1.5% to 2% risk with each pregnancy. On the basis of the volume of TPH, if the hemorrhage is less than 0.1 ml RBCs, the overall risk for immunization is 3%; if the hemorrhage is greater than 5 ml, the risk increases to 50% to 65%.

The maternal Rh antibody is slow to develop and initially may consist exclusively of IgM, which cannot cross the placenta because of its molecular size. This is followed by the production of IgG, which can cross the placenta into the fetal circulation. The maximum concentration of the IgG form of antibody occurs within 2 to 4 months after termination of the first sensitizing pregnancy (Guyton & Hall, 1996a). If initial immunization occurs shortly before or at the time of delivery, the first Rh-positive infant born to such a mother may trigger the initial antibody response, but the infant will not be affected. However, subsequent exposure to RBCs of Rh-positive fetuses produces a rapid antibody response that consists mostly of IgG. This response results in antibody attachment to antigen sites on the fetal RBCs of these fetuses. The antibody coating of the RBCs forms the basis for a positive result on the direct Coombs' test. The affected RBCs undergo agglutination, phagocytosis, and eventually extravascular hemolysis in the spleen. The byproducts of hemolysis, especially bilirubin, pass through the placenta into the maternal circulation to be metabolized and conjugated by the maternal liver. The rate of destruction of fetal RBCs depends on the amount of anti-D antibodies on the cells, the effectiveness of anti-D antibodies in promoting phagocytosis, and the capability of the spleen's reticuloendothelial system to remove antibody-coated cells.

Erythroblastosis Fetalis

Hemolysis in the fetus caused by Rh incompatibility results in the disease known as erythroblastosis fetalis (EBF); the major consequences are anemia and hyperbilirubinemia. The name is derived from the presence of immature circulating RBCs (erythroblasts), which are forced into the circulation of affected fetuses to compensate for rapid destruction of fetal blood cells. The severity of the disease depends on the degree of hemolysis and the ability of the fetus's erythropoietic system to counteract the ensuing anemia. In an attempt to compensate for rapid destruction, the fetus continues to use extramedullary organs, such as the liver and spleen, which normally would have ceased RBC production after the seventh month of gestation.

Clinical Manifestations.   The clinical manifestations of EBF are similar to those of ABO incompatibility but often are more intense (Table 30-3). Jaundice results from an exaggerated rise in bilirubin, with the premature infant exhibiting an earlier rise and a more prolonged period of elevation. Hepatosplenomegaly may be found on physical examination, along with varying degrees of hydrops. Hydrops fetalis is a severe, total body edema often accompanied by ascites and pleural effusions. Although the pathogenesis is unclear, it is thought to be the result of congestive heart failure and intrauterine hypoxia from severe anemia, portal and umbilical venous hypertension caused by hepatic hematopoiesis, and low plasma colloid osmotic pressure induced by hypoalbuminemia. Low serum albumin levels are a consequence of altered hepatic synthesis, which may be due to local cellular necrosis and compromised intrahepatic circulation. All these factors can lead to portal and venous hypertension and edema. The severity of the anemia and hypoalbuminemia affects the degree of extravasation of fluid into the tissue.

Altered hepatic synthesis can impair production of vitamin K and vitamin K-dependent clotting factors, which can lead to hemorrhage in these infants. Petechiae and prolonged bleeding from cord and blood sampling sites may be initial signs of clotting abnormalities. Hypoglycemia that occurs secondary to hyperplasia of the pancreatic islet cells also is associated with EBF. Products of RBC hemolysis are thought to inactivate circulating insulin, promoting increased insulin release and subsequent pancreatic beta cell hyperplasia. Another theory suggests that potassium or amino acids released from hemolyzed cells may directly stimulate insulin production or indirectly produce this effect by increasing glucagon secretion. Approximately one third of surviving erythroblastotic infants have low blood glucose levels and elevated plasma insulin levels.

Antenatal Therapy

Antenatal Screening.   Adequate antenatal care is important in safeguarding the fetus that may be affected by EBF. Proper screening of any pregnant woman at her first prenatal visit is essential and should include blood type and Rh factor. If the mother is Rh negative, the father's blood type should also be ascertained. If the father is Rh positive, it is essential to determine Rh immunization of the mother by Coombs' testing, specifically the indirect Coombs' test. In addition to blood typing, a concise obstetrical history regarding any previous spontaneous or therapeutic abortions or delivery of an affected infant is important to ensure appropriate management of the current pregnancy. Women who are sensitized require more surveillance throughout the pregnancy than their unsensitized counterparts, and women who have previously given birth to affected infants require the greatest degree of care. Women with anti-D titers of 1:8 or 1:16 need careful surveillance; women with titers of 1:128 may require the first invasive procedure by 20 to 24 weeks.

TABLE 30-3	Comparison of Features Seen in Rh and ABO Incompatibility	
	Rh Incompatibility	**ABO Incompatibility**
Blood Group Setup		
Mother	Negative	O
Infant	Positive	A or B
Type of Antibody	Incomplete (IgG)	Immune (IgG)
Clinical Aspects		
Occurrence in firstborn	5%	40% to 50%
Predictable severity in subsequent pregnancies	Usually	No
Stillbirth or hydrops	Frequent	Rare
Severe anemia	Frequent	Rare
Degree of jaundice	+++	+
Hepatosplenomegaly	+++	+
Laboratory Findings		
Direct Coombs' test (infant)	+	(+) or 0
Maternal antibodies	Always present	Not clear-cut
Spherocytes	0	+
Treatment		
Need for antenatal measures	Yes	No
Value of phototherapy	Limited	Considerable
Exchange transfusion		
Frequency	Approximately 67% of cases	Approximately 10% of cases
Donor blood type	Rh negative	Rh same as infant
	Group-specific when possible	Group O only
Incidence of late anemia	Common	Rare

From Ohls R (2001). Anemia in the newborn. In Polin R et al, editors. Workbook in practical neonatology, ed 3. WB Saunders: Philadelphia; modified from Naiman J (1982). Erythroblastosis fetalis. In Oski F, Naiman J, editors. Hematologic problems in the newborn, ed 3. WB Saunders: Philadelphia.

Investigational studies have been done using polymerase chain reaction (PCR) and fluorescent in situ hybridization (FISH) on maternal blood samples in which fetal nucleated RBCs are present to determine Rh D genotype (Sekizawa et al, 1999). This technique is less invasive than direct fetal blood sampling and consequently less problematic, but its benefits are still under investigation.

RhIgG Therapy. Unsensitized Rh-negative mothers can benefit from antenatal and postpartum administration of RhIgG. The Kleihauer-Betke test for fetal cells in the maternal circulation and the erythrocyte rosetting test that detects Rh-positive fetal cells may be useful screens for determining maternal candidates for RhIgG. Before the inception of RhIgG in 1964, when the first clinical trials were conducted, the frequency of Rh immunization was 7% to 8% in ABO-compatible pregnancies and 1% in ABO-incompatible pregnancies, with close to 50% of all perinatal deaths attributable to EBF. With the use of RhIgG after delivery, the incidence of Rh immunization was dramatically reduced to 1% to 1.8%. Because sensitization was known to occur without evidence of TPH at the time of delivery, the question was raised whether antenatal sensitization occurred in response to frequent, small, and undetectable hemorrhage before or during labor. For this reason, antenatal administration of RhIgG was initiated to eliminate such cases of alloimmunization. Antenatal administration has further reduced the incidence, to as low as 0.1%. However, there will always be pregnancies in which RhIgG fails to suppress the formation of antibodies or in which administration is not feasible. Immunization is not effective if sensitization occurs before the initial antenatal screening or if the RhIgG dosage is inadequate to neutralize a massive TPH. For these reasons, it is estimated that the incidence cannot be reduced beyond 4 in 10,000 pregnancies even with the use of RhIgG.

RhIgG is assumed to adhere to any Rh-positive fetal RBCs that have invaded the maternal circulation. Agglutination, hemolysis, and removal of these foreign RBCs occur before the maternal immune system can recognize the invasion and develop antibodies that would transplacentally cross into the fetus. In the initial preclinical trials in 1963, rapid clearing of invading fetal RBCs was noted after the injection of anti-D antibodies, indicating that this form of immunosuppression involves the entire blood cell and not merely the Rh antigen present on the cell. It is theorized that RhIgG may also suppress the antigen-induced response of B cells to produce antibodies by increasing the production of suppressor T cells. The anti-D from RhIgG enters the fetal circulation, but it does not seem to cause significant hemolysis. Another theory suggests that RhIgG directs the Rh antigen away from the reticuloendothelial system, preventing antibody formation.

Because it is common practice to administer RhIgG and rubella vaccine together, one caution stated in the manufacturer's insert for rubella vaccine should be noted. When a mother receives RhIgG or blood products along with the rubella vaccine, the vaccine may be inactivated by antibodies against rubella present in the donor sera. Donor sera antibodies provide passive immunity and can block the response of the mother's own immune system to the vaccine. As with any type of passive immunity, the mother's protection tends to be transient, and she may remain vulnerable to rubella. To verify protection, rubella titers should be repeated 6 to 8 weeks after simultaneous administration of RhIgG and rubella vaccine.

Several obstetrical conditions can increase the risk of sensitization by increasing the chances of TPH. Some of these problems, which require RhIgG prophylaxis, include the following:

- Therapeutic or spontaneous abortion of any type; the incidence of TPH is higher with therapeutic abortion (three women in 30 may be sensitized)
- Amniocentesis, which has a 10% chance of causing TPH
- Ectopic pregnancies or hydatidiform moles
- Abdominal trauma
- Antepartum bleeding, as with placental abruption or placenta previa

Failure to administer RhIgG after such occurrences may leave these women at risk for sensitization. The American College of Obstetricians and Gynecologists recommends a dose of 50 μg for high-risk situations that arise before 13 weeks' gestation and 300 μg after 13 weeks' gestation, with the 300-μg dose repeated at 28 weeks' gestation.

For an at-risk, Rh-negative mother with low antibody titers on the initial prenatal screen, repeat titers are recommended at 28 weeks' gestation (Scott & Branch, 1999). If titers remain low at this time, an injection of RhIgG (300 μg) is recommended. A single dose given at 28 weeks' gestation is 94% effective in preventing maternal sensitization. Titers need not be repeated until delivery, at which time a second dose of 300 μg is given if titers are low. Some caregivers test earlier (18 to 20 weeks' gestation) and repeat titers monthly (Bowman, 1994).

RhIgG has a half-life of 25 to 27 days and is effective for approximately 2 weeks after antigen exposure. The timing of the dose after delivery is important; administration within 72 hours of delivery is recommended. The dose after delivery allows a maximum estimated fetal transfusion of 30 ml of whole blood or 15 ml of packed RBCs, which leaves 1% of postpartum mothers without full coverage. If massive TPH is suspected, the dose of RhIgG may need to be increased to provide adequate amounts of anti-D antibodies. After administration of RhIgG, the Kleihauer-Betke test can be performed on the mother's blood to check for RBCs with fetal hemoglobin and to help determine the need for additional RhIgG.

Because TPH has the greatest chance of occurring at the time of delivery, maximum antibody titers may not be reached for several months after termination of a pregnancy. All unsensitized Rh-negative mothers should be monitored carefully after delivery for elevated antibody titers, especially those who experienced cesarean section, breech delivery, twin pregnancy, toxemia, placental abruption, placenta previa, or transverse lie.

By reducing the incidence of EBF, use of RhIgG has also reduced the number of available immunized donors that supply the polyclonal anti-D antibodies. The recent development of prophylaxis in the form of monoclonal antibodies against Rh D antigen has reached the stage of clinical trials and may afford an alternate source of RhIgG.

Ultrasonography. In addition to facilitating more accurate instrumentation during amniocentesis and cordocentesis by identifying placental and fetal structures, ultrasonography is very useful in determining the severity and progression of hemolysis in the erythroblastotic infant. Serial sonograms can provide valuable information about fetal well-being, such as the anatomy of the fetus and placenta, amniotic fluid volumes, and whether hydrops is present. Certain findings related to the severity of hemolysis (e.g., hepatosplenomegaly, cardiomegaly, ascites, and oligohydramnios) can help the clinician determine the plan of care.

Ultrasound screening usually begins at 14 to 16 weeks' gestation and is done every 2 weeks. It should include serial biophysical profiles, a series of fetal indices (e.g., nonstress test, fetal movement, breathing effort, fetal musculoskeletal tone, and amniotic fluid volume) that are used to evaluate fetal well-being. The presence of hydrops and ascites on the sonogram determines the timing of the first amniocentesis. Accumulation of 30 ml of peritoneal fluid is used as a marker to identify a severely affected fetus in need of intervention. Hydropic changes in the fetus correlate with a hematocrit below 15%, and the aim of therapy is to keep the hematocrit above 25% and prevent hydropic changes.

Flow Doppler studies are proving beneficial in determining fetal hemoglobin and the status of the fetus before hepatic changes. Serial measurement of the maximum velocity of umbilical vein blood flow and its correlation to the fetal hematocrit may prove beneficial in antenatal prediction of infants who will need postnatal exchange transfusion (Iskaros et al, 1998). The use of blood velocity measurements in the fetal spleen (Bahado-Singh et al, 1999) and the middle cerebral artery (Mari, 2000) as indices of fetal anemia may prove beneficial as noninvasive methods of determining fetal well-being.

Amniocentesis. Elevation of maternal anti-D antibody titers during a pregnancy indicates alloimmunization and excludes further use of RhIgG. In a first-sensitized gestation, the impact on the fetus tends to be mild. These pregnancies can be managed with monthly titers and serial ultrasound examinations to evaluate the fetus for signs of ascites and soft tissue edema. If titers remain low and ultrasound findings are normal, the pregnancy can continue to near term without further testing. Subsequent pregnancies with Rh-incompatible fetuses, however, lead to more adverse fetal effects, and maternal antibody titers become less predictive of fetal well-being.

Amniocentesis becomes a consideration when antenatal maternal blood titers indicate significant sensitization. The procedure is done to extract amniotic fluid samples for evaluation of bilirubin levels. Amniotic fluid develops a xanthochromic appearance as bilirubin is released during RBC destruction and is an indirect reflection of the degree of fetal anemia. Bilirubin is thought to find its way into amniotic fluid by passing from the fetal plasma through the skin and the membrane covering the umbilical cord. The bilirubin levels of amniotic fluid are determined by measuring the optical density (OD), or absorbance, of amniotic fluid at 450 nm, because actual levels are minuscule and difficult to measure. As determined by spectrophotometry, the OD of amniotic fluid normally forms a straight line between 350 and 700 nm and gradually declines as pregnancy progresses. When bilirubin is present, a large bulge appears at 450 nm. The difference between the height of the bulge and the normal curve (OD) indicates the amount of bilirubin in the amniotic fluid. Results are expressed as levels, which are divided into zones of severity based on a modified Liley curve (Figure 30-7). Zone 1 indicates a normal or mildly affected infant; lower zone 2 indicates moderate Rh hemolytic disease with a 20% risk of exchange transfusion; upper zone 2 indicates moderate disease with an 80% risk of exchange transfusion; and zone 3 indicates imminent fetal demise within 7 to 10 days (Gruslin & Moore, 2002). If zone 3 is reached in an advanced pregnancy (i.e., 31 to 33 weeks) and reasonable lung maturation is present, preterm delivery may be indicated after an attempt to enhance lung maturation with maternal steroid therapy. If high zone 2 to zone 3 is reached between 23 and 31 weeks' gestation, intrauterine transfusion may be necessary to maintain the fetus until further maturation occurs.

The reliability of spectrophotometry and the Liley curve still pose a dilemma, although the Liley curve has undergone several modifications since its inception. The original bilirubin

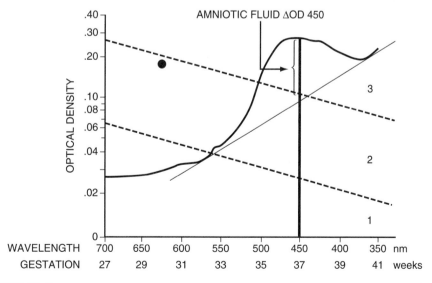

FIGURE **30-7**

The spectral absorption curve of amniotic fluid obtained by amniocentesis is plotted against a graph that depicts the normal optical density (OD), or absorbance, of amniotic fluid. The presence of indirect bilirubin in the amniotic fluid increases the optical density at the 450 nm point of the wavelength. Results are expressed as levels, which are divided into zones of severity; values that fall into zone 1 are considered normal. The amount of bilirubin present can be measured indirectly by calculating the increase in optical density compared with normal values. The severity of hemolysis is classified as moderate (zone 2) or severe (zone 3). From Bowman J (1986). Haemolytic disease of the newborn. In Roberton N, editor. *A textbook of neonatology.* Churchill Livingstone: Edinburgh.

OD graphs were based on gestational ages older than 27 weeks. Because the bilirubin levels of amniotic fluid rise with increasing gestational age, peak at 23 to 24 weeks' gestation, and then decline, the original Liley curves cannot simply be extrapolated downward. Poor correlation between the bilirubin levels of amniotic fluid obtained during the second trimester and actual fetal hematocrits has been reported. Investigators have further modified the Liley curve (Figure 30-8) in an effort to use amniotic fluid OD in pregnancies as early as 14 weeks' gestation (Gruslin & Moore, 2002). Modifications of the original Liley curve tend to embellish the original three zones to more accurately predict fetal well-being. The modified Liley curve remains a valuable assessment tool, even though it is considered more reliable in identifying severely affected fetuses and overestimation of the risk of severity during the early second trimester continues to be a problem (Spinnato et al, 1991).

Amniocentesis is also beneficial in determining the fetal blood type and can be performed at an earlier gestational age than direct fetal sampling. Clinical use of PCR on amniocytes obtained during amniocentesis has been investigated and appears successful in accurately determining fetal blood type (Fisk et al, 1994).

The timing of the initial amniocentesis depends on the previous obstetrical history, maternal titers, and ultrasound evidence of fetal distress. An indirect Coombs' titer of 1:16 or more is considered a critical level and warrants performance of this procedure as early as 16 to 18 weeks' gestation. The fetus of less than 16 weeks' gestation is rarely affected, possibly because antibodies do not cross the placenta before this time. In high-risk pregnancies with severely affected fetuses, amniocentesis usually is performed every 1 to 3 weeks. Amniotic fluid OD is 95% accurate in predicting the severity of hemolysis if serial measurements are done and the last measurement is performed after 26 to 27 weeks' gestation (Bowman, 1994).

The risks involved in amniocentesis are fetal demise, premature rupture of membranes, and an increase in the incidence of TPH by 8.4%. Mothers undergoing amniocentesis in midtrimester or later should receive 300 µg of RhIgG after each procedure.

Cordocentesis.   Introduced in the 1980s, cordocentesis involves cannulation of an umbilical vessel to obtain fetal blood samples and to perform intravenous fetal transfusions. Cordocentesis has better predictive abilities than amniocentesis for determining the severity of fetal hemolytic disease and is useful when fetal sampling and immediate transfusion are necessary to preserve fetal well-being. However, the risks are higher than with amniocentesis, and the procedure usually is not feasible before 18 weeks' gestation. Although fetal loss for both procedures is low, the risk of TPH accompanied by increased antibody titers is higher in mothers undergoing cordocentesis. Titers can exceed 50% when the transplacental approach is used (Kuller et al, 1996; Scott & Branch, 1999). In addition to fetal loss and TPH, adverse effects of cordocentesis include amnionitis and premature rupture of membranes.

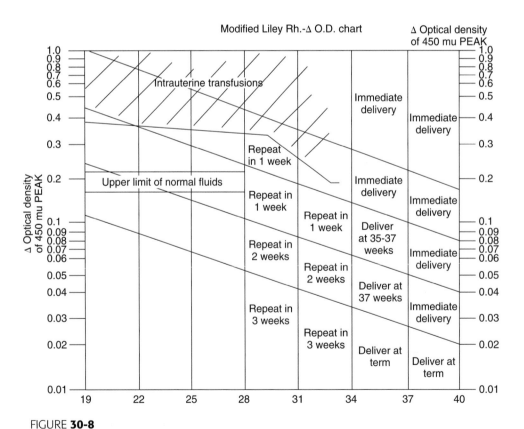

FIGURE **30-8**

Further modification of the original Liley optical density graph allows more accurate interpretation of amniotic fluid bilirubin levels in premature infants of less than 26 weeks' gestation. This modification compensates for the natural increase in the bilirubin levels of amniotic fluid during the second trimester and a natural decrease in amniotic fluid at approximately 24 weeks' gestation. From Gruslin A, Moore T (2002). Erythroblastosis fetalis. In Fanaroff A, Martin R, editors. *Neonatal-perinatal medicine: diseases of the fetus and infant*, ed 7. Mosby: St Louis.

Intrauterine Transfusions. Intrauterine transfusions usually are deemed necessary to salvage an immature fetus so compromised by EBF that death may occur secondary to circulatory collapse before 34 weeks' gestation. The fetus is capable of compensating for anemia with adequate acid-base balance until the hematocrit drops below 50% of normal. With improved techniques and the advent of ultrasonography, survival rates have improved dramatically. The overall survival rate of 34% in 1969 had risen to 60% to 70% by the late 1970s. In the 1980s, survival rates increased to 89% in cases without hydrops and 54% when hydrops was present. In the 1990s, the overall survival rate was 88% to 96%, with survival of hydropic infants ranging from 66% to 85%. The potential risks of intrauterine transfusion include maternal and fetal complications inherent in the performance of an amniocentesis, as well as graft-versus-host phenomenon in the fetus from transfusion of lymphocytes (use of irradiated blood can modify this risk). Graft-versus-host phenomenon may be a potential problem rather than a real issue; no difficulties were seen on follow-up of 275 survivors of intrauterine transfusion using nonirradiated blood (Bowman, 1994).

Intrauterine transfusion involves the instillation of packed RBCs with a hematocrit of approximately 90% into the fetal peritoneal cavity (intraperitoneal transfusion [PT]) or the umbilical vein or artery (intravascular transfusion [IVT]). Type O-negative, irradiated, leukocyte-poor RBCs are used to achieve a hematocrit of 80% are used. The blood is maternally crossmatched and deglycerolized (Scott & Branch, 1999). Maternal RBCs have been used successfully as a source of donor blood in some centers.

In IPT, 80% of the cells injected into the fetal peritoneal cavity are absorbed into the venous circulation through the right lymphatic duct and into the subdiaphragmatic lymph vessels. Approximately 10% to 13% of the blood cells are absorbed every 24 hours in a nonhydropic infant, with complete absorption taking 8 to 10 days. IPT is ineffective in the presence of ascites, and absorption of blood may be too lengthy a process to prevent fetal demise if a fetus is severely hydropic, moribund, or not breathing. IPT is the procedure of choice if the caliber of the umbilical vessel is too small to cannulate or if the position of the fetus does not allow access to the umbilical cord for IVT. If IPT must be done in a hydropic fetus, 20 to 30 ml of ascitic fluid in excess of the planned infusion may need to be removed from the peritoneal cavity before infusion. Because the fetal hematocrit is not usually raised to the desired level with one transfusion, another transfusion is given within 9 to 14 days and then every 3 to 4 weeks until delivery. The volume of blood infused depends on gestational age, and the dosage can be calculated in the following manner:

$$\text{(Gestational age in weeks} - 20) \times 10 = \text{Milliliters of blood}$$

Instillation of RBCs into the fetal peritoneal cavity consists of the following steps, which are accompanied by constant monitoring of fetal heart tones:

1. The placenta and fetal peritoneal cavity are located ultrasonographically.
2. A needle (usually 16 gauge) is inserted into the fetal peritoneal cavity, and an epidural catheter is threaded through the needle.
3. A contrast medium is instilled through the catheter, and placement of the catheter in the peritoneal cavity is verified radiographically.
4. RBCs are infused into the peritoneal cavity at a rate of 10 ml every 3 to 5 minutes.

Ultrasonography is used to perform direct IVT using the umbilical vein and artery (Figure 30-9). Following the first two steps for IPT and amniocentesis, the fetal umbilical vessels are located by ultrasonography. After a contrast study has shown that the catheter tip is positioned intravascularly, fetal blood samples for laboratory analysis are drawn and donor blood is infused directly into the fetal circulation. The umbilical vein is preferred over the umbilical artery because there is less occurrence of fetal bradycardia during the transfusion with this site. Blood is infused at a rate of 10 ml every 1 to 2 minutes, the total volume usually reaching 50 ml/kg. Fewer complications are reported when the increase in umbilical venous pressure during and after the transfusion is held to a maximum of 10 mm Hg. This procedure may need to be repeated every 2 to 3 days to achieve the desired hematocrit of 40% to 55%. When this hematocrit level has been achieved, subsequent transfusions are timed to keep the hematocrit above 25% to 30%. This may require an IVT every 2 to 4 weeks. Survival rates after IVT have improved over the past several years, increasing to an overall survival rate of 84% (94% in nonhydropic infants and 74% in hydropic infants) (Schumacher & Moise, 1996; Janssens, 1997; Grab et al, 1999).

In a comparison of IPT and IVT by Harman and associates (1990), IVT seemed to have less associated mortality and

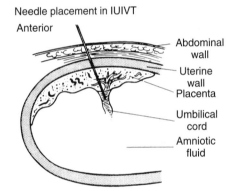

Needle placement in IUIVT

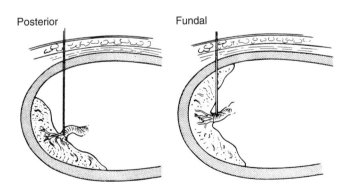

FIGURE **30-9**
Needle placement for intrauterine intravascular transfusion. Direct intravascular transfusion (IVT) involves cannulation of the umbilical cord and placement of the needle in either the vein or the artery. Ultrasonography is used to locate the placenta and to verify appropriate needle placement. Packed red blood cells (PRBCs) are transfused directly into the fetal intravascular compartment. From Scott J, Branch D (1994). Immunologic disorders in pregnancy. In Scott J et al, editors. *Danforth's obstetrics and gynecology*, ed 7. JB Lippincott: Philadelphia.

morbidity. In a group of fetuses who underwent either IVT or IPT, the survival rate was higher (91% versus 66%); the 5-minute Apgar scores were higher (38% versus 14%); and vaginal deliveries were more often accomplished (83% versus 50%) in the IVT group. In a comparison of sensorineural outcome, fetuses who had IVT also fared better than their counterparts who had IPT (Doyle et al, 1993). For these reasons, IVT is the preferred choice of transfusion site in severely affected infants.

Although IPT is technically easier and has longer lasting effects on the fetal hematocrit, it is not very successful in hydropic infants nor does it allow access to fetal blood values. Also, IPT increases the incidence of spontaneous labor. IVT allows for rapid correction of low hematocrit and hydrops, but the fetal hematocrit falls rapidly and the incidence of TPH is high. Fewer IPTs are required compared with IVTs during management of an infant with EBF. Bowman and colleagues (1994) noted that, in the treatment of a fetus from 21 to 34 weeks' gestation, fewer than four IPTs were required, compared with seven to eight IVTs. Using a combination of the two methods may prove helpful in reducing the number of invasive procedures.

IVT also causes bone marrow suppression in the fetus and newborn that affects RBC production. These infants often require follow-up transfusions at 3 to 4 months of age because of delayed erythropoiesis. All infants who have received intrauterine transfusions should have a follow-up hematocrit determination at 8 to 10 weeks. Erythropoietin has shown some promise in the prophylactic treatment of anemia in these infants (Dallacasa et al, 1996).

Prenatal Pharmacologic Agents to Control Hemolysis

Attempts to suppress antibody action on fetal RBCs or to improve bilirubin conjugation and elimination through antenatal use of medications in the Rh-sensitized mother have not proved beneficial. Some of these pharmacologic agents are phenobarbital, promethazine, corticosteroids, and D-positive erythrocyte membrane (EMOT). None of these are currently routinely in use.

One form of antenatal suppressive therapy that appears promising is administration of intravenous immunoglobulin (IVIG) to the mother. Although the mechanism by which IVIG works is unclear, it is theorized that it may affect maternal antibody synthesis, block antibody receptors in the reticuloendothelial system, or prevent antibody transport across the placenta.

Collaborative Postnatal Management of the Infant with Erythroblastosis Fetalis

On delivery of an infant with EBF, assessment of the newborn's cardiorespiratory status is of utmost importance. Because of ascites, pleural effusions, and circulatory collapse, these infants often require stabilization of the airway by intubation and mechanical ventilation. If peritoneal or pleural fluid prevents adequate chest excursion, paracentesis may be required to remove fluid from the abdominal cavity, or thoracentesis (chest tube insertion) may be needed to drain excess pleural fluid.

Delivery of an infant shortly after intraperitoneal transfusion may not allow adequate time for absorption of blood from the peritoneal cavity. The unabsorbed portion could lead to diminished lung expansion, resulting in respiratory failure or restricted mechanical ventilation. Such infants may require paracentesis for removal of blood from the peritoneal cavity.

After initiation of respiratory support, the infant should be assessed for adequacy of circulating blood volume. If the infant is severely hydropic, the inevitable anemia must be corrected with transfusions of packed RBCs, because an exchange transfusion may not be tolerated until the intravascular RBC volume is replenished. Transfusion is accomplished with O-negative or type-specific Rh-negative blood crossmatched against maternal blood. Initial use of a single-volume or partial exchange may offer a degree of cardiovascular stability before a double-volume exchange is attempted. Congestive heart failure, not present at the time of intravascular volume depletion, may become apparent as the infant is transfused. At times a severely affected infant may benefit from digitalization and diuretic therapy.

Prenatal damage to the liver can adversely affect the production of coagulation factors in such infants, making them prone to bleeding disorders. Hepatic damage can intensify any hyperbilirubinemia present, because the hepatic substances required for conjugation may also be impaired. Laboratory evaluation of the infant affected by EBF should consist of liver function studies, hematocrit determinations, and evaluation of coagulation status.

Nursing care of the infant affected by EBF involves scrupulous attention to the infant's cardiorespiratory status and vital signs. Positioning the infant so as to reduce abdominal pressure on the diaphragm permits better chest expansion. Maintaining a normal PO_2 and avoiding overventilation may prevent barotrauma to lungs already compromised by pleural effusions. The lungs may be hypoplastic if their growth has been sufficiently compromised by hydrops in utero, making ventilation difficult and predisposing the infant to extraventilatory air. Vital signs usually are assessed every hour until the infant's condition has stabilized. Hematocrit and bilirubin levels should be checked frequently during the first few hours and days of life to maintain adequate circulating blood volumes and to prevent toxic levels of bilirubin by timely initiation of therapy. If the cord bilirubin levels are significantly elevated, exchange transfusion may be necessary shortly after birth.

If bilirubin levels do not require immediate exchange, blood levels should be checked every 4 to 8 hours, depending on the initial cord blood levels and subsequent rate of rise. In Rh incompatibility, exchange is imminent if the rate of rise exceeds 1 mg/hour for the first 6 hours of life. The interval of blood sampling for bilirubin may be increased to 6 to 12 hours after the first 48 hours of life.

The major therapies used to control excessive unconjugated bilirubin levels are similar for all problems resulting in elevated unconjugated bilirubin levels. Phototherapy and exchange transfusion, the most frequently used therapies, are discussed later in the chapter.

Analysis of Laboratory Data.   The following laboratory data can be helpful in the diagnosis and treatment of EBF:
- The mother's and infant's blood and Rh types.
- Coombs' reactivity: The infant's RBCs are coated with anti-D antibodies, resulting in a positive direct Coombs' test result; on occasion, the heavy coating of neonatal RBCs with antibody can lead to a false Rh typing (Rh negative); if the direct Coombs' test result is positive, the infant should be considered Rh positive.
- The infant's hematocrit, reticulocyte count, and RBC morphologic characteristics: The presence of immature cells or spherocytes helps distinguish Rh incompatibility from ABO incompatibility.

- Plasma bilirubin levels: The initial cord blood bilirubin level and the rate of rise determine the appropriate timing of any exchange transfusion needed to control bilirubin levels. Cord bilirubin levels are closely associated with the severity of disease and the mortality rate.

Bilirubin Metabolism and Hyperbilirubinemia.

Bilirubin production begins as early as 12 weeks' gestation. It is the primary degradation product of hemoglobin, although 20% to 30% is derived from nonerythroid sources such as tissue heme. Bilirubin is produced after completion of the natural life span of the RBC, but ineffective erythropoiesis or premature destruction of blood cells can increase its production. In RBC destruction, the aging or hemolyzed RBC membrane ruptures, releasing hemoglobin that is phagocytosed by macrophages. The hemoglobin molecule then splits into a heme portion and a globin portion. Bilirubin is derived from the degradation of the heme ring in the heme portion that binds to heme oxygenase. The ferric heme breaks down to the ferrous form and then is cleaved to form carbon monoxide and biliverdin. Biliverdin is further reduced to form bilirubin, and carbon monoxide joins with heme to form carboxyhemoglobin.

The four forms of circulating bilirubin are (1) conjugated bilirubin (which is excretable through the kidneys and intestines), (2) conjugated covalently bound bilirubin (which is attached to serum albumin and not found in neonates younger than 2 weeks of age), (3) unconjugated bilirubin (which is reversibly bound to albumin), and (4) free bilirubin (which is unconjugated and unbound). Measurement of conjugated (direct) bilirubin identifies the amount of bilirubin that reacts directly with van den Bergh's reagent. The portion of bilirubin reversibly bound to albumin is lipid soluble. It does not react with van den Bergh's reagent until it is combined with alcohol, thus the term unconjugated (indirect) bilirubin. Free bilirubin is not attached to albumin and can easily cross the blood-brain barrier, causing the damage seen in kernicterus. Measurements of conjugated and unconjugated bilirubin are important in the evaluation of the hyperbilirubinemic infant and provide valuable information for the diagnosis and method of treatment.

Although bilirubin is found in stool and amniotic fluid, the major route of elimination in the fetus is through the placenta. For this reason, bilirubin must be retained in the form that allows its passage into the maternal circulation. Consequently, the enzyme systems found in the fetus enhance the retention of bilirubin in the unconjugated form. Persistence of some of these fetal mechanisms during the newborn period can contribute to jaundice. Plasma concentrations of bilirubin usually are low in the fetus, except in cases of severe hemolytic disease. All bilirubin in the cord blood of the fetus is the unconjugated variety, which is effectively metabolized, conjugated, and excreted by the maternal liver and gallbladder. The mean cord blood bilirubin concentration in an infant unaffected by hemolytic disease is 1.8 mg/dl, regardless of the infant's gestational age or weight.

In the newborn, the major routes of bilirubin excretion are through the intestine and the kidneys. As the production of bilirubin exceeds the newborn liver's capacity to conjugate and eliminate it, plasma levels begin to rise rapidly. Jaundice becomes noticeable when the serum concentration reaches three times the amount normally present in the serum. The conjunctivae become visibly jaundiced at serum levels exceeding 2.5 mg/dl. In the full-term infant, jaundice usually becomes apparent within 2 to 4 days after birth and lasts until the sixth day, reaching a peak concentration of 6 to 7 mg/dl. Although infants born at 37 weeks' gestation or later are considered term, they are more likely to reach or exceed serum bilirubin levels of 13 mg/dl or higher than are infants born at 40 weeks' gestation. The preterm infant has cord blood levels similar to those of the term infant, but peak levels are higher, jaundice lasts longer, and levels peak later, at 5 to 7 days. Among preterm infants, 63% reach levels of 10 to 19 mg/dl, and 22% reach levels above 15 mg/dl.

Although the neonatal liver's conjugating mechanisms are reduced during the first few days of life, the liver is able to metabolize and excrete two thirds to three quarters of the bilirubin circulating throughout the body. Initially bilirubin is transported in the plasma, bound to albumin at two sites—a primary binding site that has a strong bond and a secondary site that has a weak bond. When available albumin binding sites are saturated, bilirubin circulates freely in the plasma. It is this portion of unconjugated bilirubin that can migrate into brain cells, causing damage known as kernicterus. The occurrence of kernicterus is related to the amount of diffusible, loosely bound bilirubin and the availability of albumin binding sites.

When bilirubin reaches the liver, it is transferred from plasma albumin, across the cell membrane of the liver, and into the liver cell. Two proteins, Y and Z, also called ligands, affect bilirubin transfer from plasma to liver. Here the bilirubin is either stored in the cell cytoplasm or removed from the ligands and conjugated in the hepatic endoplasmic reticulum. Conjugation is essential for the excretion of bilirubin into bile. Eighty percent of bilirubin is conjugated with glucuronic acid, becoming bilirubin glucuronide. Glucuronosyltransferase is the important hepatic enzyme required for the production of bilirubin glucuronide. Ninety-five percent of bilirubin glucuronide is excreted into bile and subsequently into the intestine.

Effective excretion of bilirubin from the intestine depends on the length of time needed for the passage of stool and on the presence of substances that break down conjugated bilirubin. The newborn may have diminished bowel motility and delayed meconium passage, which allow longer exposure of stool to bilirubin glucuronidase, the enzyme responsible for breaking down conjugated bilirubin. The action of this enzyme, in conjunction with the newborn's lack of the intestinal flora required to reduce bilirubin to urobilinogen, converts the conjugated form to the unconjugated form, which is then reabsorbed by the intestine.

Kernicterus.

When albumin binding sites are filled, increased amounts of free bilirubin are available for passage into the central nervous system (CNS). Free bilirubin easily crosses the blood-brain barrier and is transferred into the brain cells, causing obvious yellow staining of the brain tissue (kernicterus) that is similar to the effect on the skin. The areas of the brain usually affected by the staining are the hypothalamus, dentate nucleus, and cerebellum. Kernicterus is associated with varying degrees of neurologic damage, but a direct correlation cannot be drawn between serum bilirubin levels and the severity of involvement.

Many factors can influence the bilirubin binding capacity and increase the risk of kernicterus at lower bilirubin levels, including the following:

- The total amount of available serum albumin: Premature infants normally experience a relative hypoproteinemia and have fewer albumin binding sites available for free bilirubin.

- The presence of other substances competing for available binding sites: Certain drugs (e.g., sulfasoxazole, salicylates, sodium benzoate) compete with bilirubin for binding sites or replace bilirubin loosely attached to binding sites.
- Acidosis and hypoxia: Increased production of hydrogen ions and implementation of anaerobic metabolism can impede bilirubin binding. Albumin's ability to bind bilirubin drops to half its potential at a serum pH of 7.1, with free fatty acids produced during anaerobic metabolism competing for albumin binding sites. The simultaneous presence of acidosis and hypoxia, which can open the blood-brain barrier, can expose a sick infant to kernicterus at much lower serum bilirubin levels. Evidence also suggests that tests evaluating bilirubin binding capacity, rather than serum bilirubin concentrations, are better correlated with the appearance of subsequent CNS abnormalities

Clinical Manifestations.   Kernicterus usually becomes evident during the first 5 days of life. Its signs include lethargy or irritability, hypotonia, paralysis of upward gaze, high-pitched cry, poor eating, opisthotonic posturing, and spasticity. It is also associated with deafness, cerebral palsy, and tooth enamel abnormalities. The overall risk for kernicterus is 50% if serum bilirubin levels are 30 mg/dl or higher and 10% if levels are between 20 and 25 mg/dl. Preventing elevated levels of free bilirubin is the primary means of eliminating kernicterus. Prevention may require phototherapy for slowly rising levels but almost certainly demands exchange transfusion if the rise is rapid and marked.

COMMON NONIMMUNE CAUSES OF HYPERBILIRUBINEMIA

Elevated bilirubin levels within the first 24 hours of life or levels exceeding 12 mg/dl are not considered physiologic and deserve investigation. Many conditions other than blood group incompatibilities can cause jaundice in the newborn. Most of the commonly seen disorders result in elevated levels of unconjugated rather than conjugated bilirubin. These pathologic conditions can be classified as (1) those that cause increased breakdown of RBCs (e.g., sepsis, drug reactions, and extravascular blood); (2) those that interfere with bilirubin conjugation (e.g., breast milk jaundice, drug interactions, hypothyroidism, acidosis, and hypoxia); and (3) those that cause abnormal bilirubin excretion (e.g., hypoxia or asphyxia, bowel obstruction, ileus, and congestive heart failure). The single factor most implicated in hyperbilirubinemia is prematurity, with the severity of jaundice directly correlated to declining gestational age. The premature infant is thought to be subject to a combination of increased RBC breakdown secondary to reduced RBC life span and impaired bilirubin conjugation as a result of liver immaturity.

Increased Red Blood Cell Breakdown

Several problems that arise in the perinatal period are associated with excessive and premature destruction of the RBCs by hemolysis. Neonatal bacterial and viral infections and intrauterine viral infections, especially those of the TORCH complex (toxoplasmosis, other agents, rubella, cytomegalovirus, and herpes simplex), have been implicated in the hemolytic destruction of RBCs. Certain medications, such as the synthetic analogs of vitamin K or large doses of natural vitamin K, also induce RBC destruction. Other conditions prevalent in the premature and term newborn can result in the extravasation of large amounts of blood (e.g., cephalhematoma and pulmonary or intracerebral hemorrhages). These extravascular collections of blood cells must undergo hemolysis to be resorbed by the body. Significant hemolysis, regardless of the cause, increases the bilirubin load on a metabolically immature neonatal liver. This increased load often results in hyperbilirubinemia in the newborn.

Interference with Bilirubin Conjugation

Breast Milk Jaundice.   Breast milk jaundice affects approximately 2% to 4% of all breastfed babies and can be divided into two phases, early and late, each with a different time of onset and a different underlying cause. In early onset breast milk jaundice, the infant is affected within the first few days of life. This condition is thought to be due to a combination of maternal and infant factors that lead to diminished fluid intake and dehydration. Predisposing maternal factors include limited maternal milk supply, engorgement, cracked nipples, poor feeding technique, and maternal illness or fatigue; neonatal factors include poor suck, illness, lethargy that accompanies hyperbilirubinemia, and dehydration. Poor intake leads to poor stool output and increased enterohepatic resorption of bilirubin. The recommended treatment is phototherapy and alleviation of dehydration. Frequent breast feedings with avoidance of supplementation, in addition to lactation counseling, are advised.

Late onset breast milk jaundice is a separate entity that is attributed to a change in the chemical or physical composition of breast milk; it usually occurs after the first 3 to 5 days of life (Halamak & Stevenson, 2001). Bilirubin levels can reach 12 to 20 mg/dl between 8 and 15 days and may remain elevated for as long as 2 months. The infant appears healthy, and no evidence of RBC hemolysis is seen. This jaundice is believed to be caused by substances in breast milk that interfere with bilirubin conjugation or increase enterohepatic circulation, resulting in resorption of bilirubin from the intestine. Two substances found in breast milk, pregnanediol and nonesterified fatty acids, are thought to inhibit glucuronyl transferase, the enzyme necessary for bilirubin conjugation in the liver. However, the role of these two substances in the interference with glucuronyl transferase remains questionable.

Recent studies suggest the presence of an unknown substance in breast milk that enhances the breakdown of conjugated bilirubin deposited in the intestine before it can be eliminated in the stool. Conjugated bilirubin is broken down to the unconjugated form and reabsorbed by the small and large bowel. Unconjugated bilirubin diffuses easily into the blood supply of the bowel, where it is redistributed into the circulation.

When breastfeeding is discontinued, the bilirubin level falls within 24 to 48 hours, dropping to half its previous peak level by 48 hours. With resumption of breastfeeding, the bilirubin level starts to rise but at a much slower pace. Interruption of breastfeeding is not recommended; instead, continued and frequent breastfeeding is encouraged. However, the health care provider has the option to supplement nursing with formula or to interrupt breastfeeding and substitute formula, depending on the degree of bilirubin elevation. Supplementation of nursing with water or glucose water does not appear to have any effect on bilirubin levels in healthy term infants.

Drugs that Interfere with Bilirubin Conjugation.   Certain medications ingested by the mother and passed transplacentally to the fetus (e.g., salicylates, sulfa preparations) can interfere with the ability of albumin to bind bilirubin. Administration of these drugs to the newborn can produce the same effect. Other medications, such as sodium benzoate, a commonly used preservative, compete with bilirubin for albumin binding sites.

Hypothyroidism.   Hypothyroidism is one of the more common metabolic disorders associated with hyperbilirubinemia. 20% of all infants with hypothyroidism have elevated bilirubin levels lasting 3 to 4 weeks, with normalization of levels requiring up to 4 months. The suspected mechanism for jaundice is theorized to be a delay in glucuronosyltransferase synthesis or impairment of hepatic proteins that bind bilirubin and remove it from the plasma. The plasma membrane of liver cells may also be altered, resulting in decreased bilirubin influx into the hepatic cells.

Acidosis and Hypoxia.   As previously stated in the discussion of kernicterus, a drop in serum pH alters albumin's ability to bind bilirubin. The accompanying increase in the production of free fatty acids promotes competition between fatty acids and bilirubin for binding sites. In animal models, respiratory acidosis but not metabolic acidosis increases movement of bilirubin across the blood-brain barrier.

Abnormal Bilirubin Excretion

Any disease state resulting in abnormal bilirubin excretion can raise serum bilirubin levels significantly. This is seen in hepatic dysfunction secondary to such entities as hypoxia or asphyxia, bowel obstruction, ileus, and congestive heart failure. However, these conditions have a tendency to elevate both the conjugated and unconjugated bilirubin levels. The diminished bowel motility associated with these conditions lengthens the time during which beta-glucuronidase, which is naturally present in the gut, can act on conjugated bilirubin in the stool. This enzymatic reaction converts conjugated bilirubin into the unconjugated form, which is reabsorbed into the intravascular compartment through the enterohepatic circulation. Direct hepatocellular damage associated with cholestasis and bacterial and viral infections can further impair the liver's ability to metabolize bilirubin.

Treatment of Hyperbilirubinemia
Phototherapy.   The actual mechanisms by which phototherapy reduces unconjugated bilirubin and the exact mode of bilirubin excretion are not clearly understood. Photo-oxidation and photoisomerization are the two mechanisms thought to change bilirubin into water-soluble and excretable forms. Photo-oxidation involves the oxidation of bilirubin pigment deposited in the skin and its conversion into colorless products that can be excreted into the urine. Of the total body bilirubin concentration, 15% can undergo photodegradation through oxidation. Photoisomerization involves the conversion of bilirubin polymers present in the skin into excretable isomers. When the natural form of bilirubin is exposed to blue light at certain wavelengths, it undergoes photoisomerization. This changes it from a tetrapyrrole, a lipid-soluble substance, into five water-soluble isomers. Four of these isomers are excreted into bile without undergoing conjugation. Two are unstable isomers that are incorporated into bile and must be promptly eliminated from the gastrointestinal tract as a component of stool or they revert back to their natural forms, resulting in resorption of bilirubin from the gut and recirculation into the plasma. Two other isomers remain relatively stable and account for most of the bilirubin found in bile. The fifth isomer, lumi-

bilirubin, is a stable, water-soluble form of bilirubin that is eliminated through urine and bile.

Phototherapy is also thought to enhance hepatic excretion of unconjugated bilirubin and to increase bowel transit time. When phototherapy is begun early, a 20% to 35% reduction in the serum bilirubin concentrations is noted by day 2 of life and a reduction of 41% to 55% by day 4. This reduction is more significant than the naturally occurring drop in the untreated infant.

Although no significant adverse effects are attributed to the use of phototherapy, it is not without associated side effects. Some of these problems include dermal rash, lethargy, abdominal distention, possible eye damage, dehydration caused by increased insensible water loss through the skin and digestive tract, thrombocytopenia, hypocalcemia, and secretory diarrhea possibly as a result of a temporary intestinal lactose deficiency. Another effect of phototherapy seen in infants with a significant direct bilirubin component is "bronze baby" syndrome. This syndrome is thought to be due to skin deposition of a photoproduct of bilirubin decomposition, possibly copper porphyrins, which cause bronzing of the skin and urine. Although no harmful effects can be attributed to the bronzing, it can last for several weeks to several months and is somewhat alarming to parents.

Phototherapy is not adequate therapy for a rapidly rising bilirubin level, but it is effective in the treatment of moderate hyperbilirubinemia that has not reached or exceeded levels known to be associated with kernicterus and in reducing the need for exchange transfusions after the first 12 hours of life. Intensive phototherapy can produce a decline of 1 to 2 mg/dl of total serum bilirubin within 4 to 6 hours (Bergman et al, 1994). This is a reflection of the length of exposure necessary for phototherapy to exhibit its effectiveness. The American Academy of Pediatrics (AAP) adopted a set of guidelines for the initiation of phototherapy and exchange transfusion in the term, healthy newborn (Bergman et al, 1994) (Table 30-4). Suggested bilirubin levels for initiation of therapy based on birth weight, including very low birth weight, are found on a chart devised by King and Jung (1990) (Figure 30-10). Recommended levels for the use of phototherapy or exchange transfusion must be adjusted downward for prematurity, acidosis, hypoxia, respiratory distress, asphyxia, and neurologic decompensation (Figure 30-11). Diminished bilirubin-binding capacity of albumin, decreased amounts of circulating albumin, and increased permeability of the CNS expose these infants to increased amounts of free bilirubin, which can easily cross the blood-brain barrier.

Although administration of IVIG to the mother has produced contradictory results, its administration to infants with Rh hemolytic disease may be beneficial. Administration of IVIG to a group of infants with Rh incompatibility was associated with a reduction in the rate of exchange transfusion to 12.5%, compared with 69% in the control group. It is hypothesized that IVIG may interfere with receptors in the reticuloendothelium that are required to induce hemolysis. The optimum dosage has yet to be determined.

However, administration of albumin to an infant undergoing phototherapy may reduce the amount of bilirubin available in the skin for photoisomerization. In an attempt to saturate the increased available albumin binding sites, free bilirubin is drawn into the vascular compartment from the skin, where phototherapy exerts its effect. For this reason, use of albumin in the infant undergoing phototherapy should be carefully weighed.

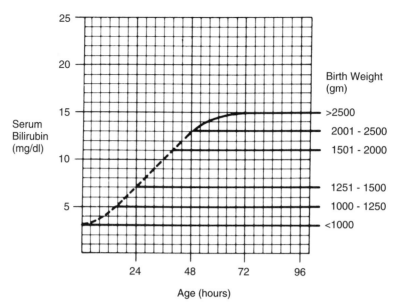

FIGURE **30-10**
Suggested bilirubin levels for initiation of phototherapy in infants of various birth weights and postnatal ages. From King J, Jung A (1990). Phototherapy. In Nelson N, editor. *Current therapy in neonatal-perinatal medicine*. BC Decker: Philadelphia.

TABLE **30-4**	Total Serum Bilirubin Levels and Recommended Therapy in Healthy Term Newborns			
	TOTAL SERUM BILIRUBIN (mg/dl [μmol/L])			
Age (Hours)	**Consider Phototherapy**	**Phototherapy**	**Exchange Transfusion if Intensive Phototherapy Fails**	**Exchange Transfusion and Intensive Phototherapy**
24 or less	---	---	---	---
25 to 48	≥12 (170 total)	≥15 (260)	≥20 (340)	≥25 (430)
49 to 72	≥15 (260)	≥18 (310)	≥25 (430)	≥30 (510)
Over 72	≥17 (290)	≥20 (340)	≥25 (430)	≥30 (510)

Modified from Bergman D et al (1994). American Academy of Pediatrics: practice parameter: management of hyperbilirubinemia in the healthy term newborn. Pediatrics 94:558-561.

Collaborative Management. Infants who require phototherapy benefit most from blue light in the wavelength range at which photoisomerization occurs most efficiently; that is, 420 to 460 nm. In addition to the appropriate wavelength, effective illumination must be maintained. Spectroradiometric readings of 4 to 6 μW/cm^2/nm are considered in the effective therapeutic range. For optimum therapy, phototherapy units should be checked for adequacy of light levels by nursing or bioengineering staff. Prolonged exposure to phototherapy lights may cause retinal damage, which can be minimized with adequate eye protection. Phototherapy units and eye protection should be removed for short periods throughout the day to provide the infant with visual stimulation and interaction with parents and caregivers. Nurses should also be aware that they may experience headaches from prolonged exposure to phototherapy lights.

Infants undergoing phototherapy require temperature stabilization appropriate for their size and overall condition. A larger infant who is basically well can be nursed in an open crib, but

the sick term, premature, or low-birth-weight (LBW) infant requires temperature control through the use of open warmers or closed incubators. Adequate fluid intake and compensatory fluid adjustments for increased insensible water and stool loss may be required to prevent dehydration in these infants. While the infant is receiving phototherapy, bilirubin levels must be monitored frequently to assess the effectiveness of therapy and the need for exchange transfusion. Because phototherapy lights can alter blood bilirubin results, the lights should be turned off when drawing blood for serum bilirubin determinations.

Many hyperbilirubinemic infants who are healthy and not in need of thermoregulation or exchange transfusion can be cared for at home, so long as the AAP guidelines are met. The parents of these infants must have access to home phototherapy equipment and a medical supply company to service the equipment, as well as the support of their medical caregiver. If the infant can remain normothermic in an open crib without clothing, home phototherapy may be considered a cost-effective alternative to hospitalization. The same precautions

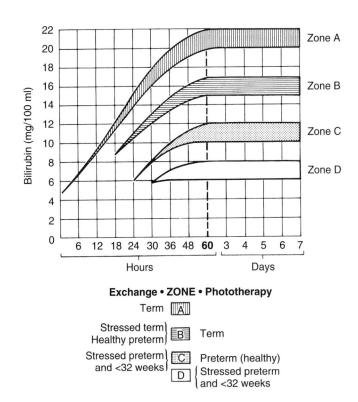

FIGURE **30-11**
The rate of increase in bilirubin levels, gestational age, and the newborn's general condition determine the type of treatment for hyperbilirubinemia and the rapidity of its initiation. This chart is a useful guideline for initiating phototherapy or exchange transfusion in hyperbilirubinemic infants. From Pernoll M et al (1986). Neonatal hyperbilirubinemia and prevention of kernicterus. In Pernoll M et al, editors. *Diagnosis and management of the fetus and neonate at risk*, ed 5. Mosby: St Louis.

| TABLE **30-5** | Maximum Total Serum Bilirubin Concentration Allowed before Exchange Transfusion |

Birth Weight (g)	MAXIMUM CONCENTRATION (mg/dl)	
	Uncomplicated Course	**Complicated Course**
Under 1000	10	10
1000 to 1249	13	10
1250 to 1499	15	13
1500 to 1999	17	15
2000 to 2500	18	17
2500 or over	25	20

From Behrman R et al (2000). The fetus and the neonatal infant. In Behrman R et al, editors. Nelson textbook of pediatrics, *ed 16. WB Saunders: Philadelphia.*

regarding protective eye covering and adequate fluid intake must be observed in these infants. Frequent determination of bilirubin levels is required to ensure adequate treatment, and blood may be drawn daily for this purpose at the physician's office or the neighborhood hospital laboratory or by a home health care worker.

Pharmacologic Agents.   Phenobarbital is thought to accelerate bilirubin excretion by increasing its uptake and conjugation by the liver and by increasing its excretion by enhancing bile flow. However, no increased benefit is noted that cannot be achieved with phototherapy alone. No medications have been approved in the United States as therapy for inhibition of bilirubin synthesis, but clinical trials have preliminarily shown that metalloporphyrins may be effective in controlling hyperbilirubinemia in the term and preterm infant. Metalloporphyrins are inhibitors of heme oxygenase, the enzyme involved in the degradation of heme to biliverdin, an intermediate in the synthesis of bilirubin. Tin-mesoporphyrin and tin-protoporphyrin are the two heme oxygenase inhibitors used in clinical trials as a prophylaxis and as treatment. Although these studies have shown beneficial effects, they are still in the initial stages of investigation.

Exchange Transfusion.   If bilirubin levels start to approach those associated with kernicterus despite phototherapy, exchange transfusion may be necessary to protect the CNS status

of the jaundiced infant. The object of this procedure is to remove bilirubin and the antibody-coated RBCs from the newborn's circulation. In addition, exchange transfusion removes some of the circulating maternal antibodies and Rh-positive fetal RBCs while potentially normalizing the hematocrit. After a single-volume exchange, 75% of the newborn's RBC mass is removed; a double-volume exchange removes 85% to 90% of the cells. However, bilirubin removal is much less effective; only 25% of the infant's total body bilirubin is removed during a double-volume exchange. This probably occurs because the major portion of bilirubin is in the extravascular compartment, an area not affected by the exchange of blood volume. Rebound in bilirubin levels occurs within 1 hour of the exchange, with post-transfusion levels rising as high as 55% of pre-exchange values.

Although EBF remains the primary condition requiring exchange transfusion, the procedure also can be used to reduce levels of circulating metabolic toxins or exogenous drugs and to re-establish a normal hematocrit without further volume overload in anemia-induced congestive heart failure. The mortality rate for exchange transfusions is 1%. This rate includes death during the procedure or within 6 hours after its completion but excludes hydropic, kernicteric, or moribund infants.

The following criteria are used to determine the need for and timing of exchange transfusions, particularly in infants with EBF (Bowman, 1994; Bergman et al, 1994):

- A cord blood bilirubin level over 4.5 mg/dl in term infants and 3.5 mg/dl in preterm infants
- A hemoglobin level under 8 g/dl and a bilirubin level over 6 mg/dl within 1 hour of delivery in a term infant
- A hemoglobin level under 11.5 g/dl and a bilirubin level over 3.5 mg/dl within 1 hour of delivery in a preterm infant
- An increase in bilirubin levels by 0.5 mg/dl/hour despite phototherapy
- A bilirubin level over 20 to 25 mg/dl in an uncompromised term infant (see Table 30-4), 18 mg/dl in the high-risk term newborn, and 10 to 18 mg/dl in the preterm infant, depending on gestational age and condition (Table 30-5)
- A bilirubin level over 10 to 17 mg/dl in a stressed or very immature preterm infant, over 10 to 12 mg/dl if hypoxia and acidosis are present

Identical criteria are used to determine the need for repeated exchange transfusion.

Preparation of an Infant for an Exchange Transfusion.
The infant undergoing an exchange transfusion should be prepared in a manner that produces the most benefit from the procedure while minimizing unnecessary risks. A double-volume exchange usually is done as soon as the need arises and the infant's condition permits. An exchange can be done in several ways. The most common methods use umbilical artery catheters and umbilical vein catheters, although central venous and peripheral arterial lines also can be used. One procedure uses the intermittent push-pull method, in which an aliquot of the infant's blood is withdrawn and replaced with an aliquot of donor blood. This can be done using one or two indwelling lines. Another method is the constant infusion of donor blood through the umbilical or peripheral vein and the constant withdrawal of the infant's blood through an umbilical artery; this method provides for a more consistent arterial blood pressure. When peripheral arterial lines are used, blood can be withdrawn from them but should be returned by a central or peripheral venous line to prevent arterial spasm and clotting of the line.

The placement of the umbilical vein catheter is important to the provision of adequate splanchnic blood flow to the bowel. Infusion of large amounts of blood containing desaturated hemoglobin could result in ischemic injury to the bowel wall mucosa, with subsequent necrosis and sloughing of the mucosa. Such injury can predispose the infant to bowel wall ischemia, necrotizing enterocolitis, and perforation. Proper placement of the umbilical vein catheter above the diaphragm would reduce the potential risk for ischemic injury, but passing the catheter beyond the liver still creates the risk of liver damage and cardiac arrhythmias.

Before and during an exchange, albumin can be administered to infants considered to have low reserves of albumin binding sites. Its administration is thought to provide more available binding sites for circulating free bilirubin and bilirubin deposited in the extravascular compartment. Theoretically, albumin should implement movement of bilirubin into the intravascular space, where it can be removed during an exchange transfusion. The recommended dosage is 1 g/kg of 25% albumin administered 1 to 2 hours before the exchange. Because intravascular albumin rapidly equilibrates with the extravascular compartment, its administration potentially could increase the amount of bilirubin pulled out of the plasma and into the tissue. For this reason, albumin administration before or during an exchange remains controversial. The use of albumin is contraindicated with severe anemia, hydrops, or congestive heart failure.

Selection of Blood Products. The selection and preparation of blood products are aimed at (1) reducing the antigen-antibody reaction, thus preventing hemolysis and additional bilirubin production; (2) removing toxic substances or endotoxins; (3) substituting a higher, more efficient circulating RBC volume for a low RBC mass; and (4) preventing biochemical imbalances caused by blood products during the exchange transfusion.

When exchange is imperative shortly after birth, O-negative blood crossmatched against the mother usually is used. The cells may need to be partly packed if anemia is significant and congestive heart failure is present. If exchange is not urgent, the blood used in Rh incompatibility can be type specific and Rh negative. If the exchange is done for ABO incompatibility, O-type Rh-specific or low-titer (low anti-A and anti-B) O-type cells suspended in AB plasma can be used. Infants who are immunocompromised or who have received intrauterine transfusions and are at risk for graft-versus-host disease should be exchanged with irradiated blood; this eliminates the possibility of giving WBCs, particularly lymphocytes, in the transfused blood. For infants born in areas where the incidence of cytomegalovirus (CMV) infection is high, donor blood that is CMV negative should be used. Frozen, deglycerolized RBCs or blood filtered with leukodepletion filters are other alternatives.

Blood used for exchange transfusion should be as fresh as possible, preferably less than 48 hours old, to prevent problems associated with elevated potassium levels. When blood is older than 72 hours, the membrane of the RBC becomes more permeable, allowing intracellular potassium to leak out of the cell. This time-related phenomenon, coupled with normal RBC hemolysis, increases the amount of potassium in banked blood. Problems with arrhythmias and sudden cardiac death have been attributed to elevated potassium levels in transfused blood. If blood less than 48 hours old is not available, reconstituting RBC concentrates less than 7 days old with fresh-frozen plasma is an alternative. This preparation not only ensures adequate oxygen-carrying capacity of the RBCs but also provides a greater measure of safety with regard to potassium levels than does whole blood older than 48 hours. It is also recommended that RBC concentrates older than 4 days be washed to further remove excess potassium.

Stored whole blood and reconstituted blood are low in platelets, which predisposes the infant undergoing exchange transfusion to bleeding. Platelet transfusion may be necessary after this procedure.

Because of the unpredictable nature of potassium levels in banked blood, it is advisable to measure the level in the donor blood before using it. In one study measuring banked blood preserved with citrate-phosphate-dextrose (CPD), 21% of 28 units less than 4 days old had potassium levels of 11 mEq/L or higher. However, receiving blood with a high potassium content may not necessarily increase the serum potassium levels of these infants from pretransfusion levels.

Physiologic Effects of Exchange Transfusion. Exchange transfusion has a marked effect on the cardiovascular status and the intravascular compartment, which is reflected in pressure changes, volume fluctuations, and biochemical balance.

Intravascular Pressure and Volume Changes. Significant fluctuation in blood pressure and heart rate can occur during an exchange transfusion, with rapid blood withdrawal causing greater pressure drops. With slow blood exchange (3 minutes for one exchange cycle consisting of withdrawal and replacement of an aliquot of blood), the blood pressure drops but returns to baseline during the infusion cycle. However, in a rapid exchange cycle lasting 45 to 60 seconds, the pressure drops, then rises, but does not return to baseline. At aliquots of 5 ml/kg every 3 minutes, an average exchange should take approximately 100 to 110 minutes.

Because cardiac return and output drop during hypotension, an exchange transfusion carries the risk of diminished ileocolonic blood flow caused by sustained arterial hypotension. When an umbilical vein catheter is used for blood infusion, a rise in portal venous pressure during the injection phase can also result in diminished colonic blood flow at the end of injection. Regardless of the cause of gut hypoperfusion, ischemic damage of the intestinal mucosa can occur, resulting in necrotizing enterocolitis and perforation. Difficult or traumatic insertion or prolonged placement of the umbilical vein catheter can also lead to thrombosis of the portal vein and infection.

Because changes in the mean arterial and intracranial pressures seem to parallel each other, exchange transfusion can also affect cerebral blood flow. When arterial pressure declines in response to blood withdrawal and increases in response to infusion, intracranial pressure changes accordingly, a reflection of the immature autoregulatory mechanisms of neonatal cerebral blood flow. Marked fluctuations in intracranial pressure, especially in the preterm infant, can predispose these infants to intraventricular and intracerebral hemorrhage.

Electrocardiographic Changes.   Cardiac conduction abnormalities can occur during exchange transfusion. The precise reasons for these electrocardiographic changes are unclear, because several causative factors are present concurrently. Placement of the umbilical vein catheter, changes in blood volume caused by removal and infusion of blood, and fluctuations in blood pressure can contribute to the occurrence of arrhythmias or electrocardiographic changes. The problems most commonly encountered are P wave elevation, tachycardia, bradycardia, ST segment changes, and abnormal QRS complex.

Metabolic Disturbances.   The common anticoagulants used to preserve banked blood are ACD (acid-citrate-dextrose), CPD, CPD-adenine, and heparin. Heparin is not widely used because it has a limited shelf life and predisposes its receiver to a state of hypocoagulability. However, it does not cause the rebound hypoglycemia, acidosis, and hypocalcemia seen with the other three preparations. The citrate found in blood preserved with ACD and CPD binds calcium, and if it is not metabolized quickly (as is the case in preterm and seriously ill infants), it can lead to acidosis and hypocalcemia. Blood preserved with CPD and CPD-adenine is used more often because it contains half the acid load of ACD-preserved blood. Blood preserved with CPD-adenine has the longest shelf life.

Controversy still exists over the use of calcium supplementation and correction of acidosis during an exchange. Although the total serum calcium level may be lowered, the ionized calcium level does not change during an exchange transfusion. If the initial ionized calcium level is low or drops during the exchange or if electrocardiographic symptoms of hypocalcemia occur, administration of 100 to 200 mg of calcium gluconate is recommended. Blood calcium levels are only transiently raised by administration of calcium supplements (Figure 30-12).

Excessive heating of blood during an exchange produces hemolysis, resulting in elevated serum potassium levels. If the hemolysis is severe, it may produce effects similar to a transfusion reaction and could lead to death. High serum potassium levels can also cause arrhythmias and cardiac arrest. Potassium levels should be monitored closely before, during, and after exchange. With infants who are already hyperkalemic, it may be beneficial to screen the donor blood for its potassium level before the transfusion is started.

Rebound hypoglycemia can occur shortly after completion of an exchange transfusion because the dextrose concentration used in blood preservation is equivalent to 300 mg of glucose per liter of blood. The compensatory insulin release requires adequate supplemental glucose if hypoglycemia is to be avoided. Blood glucose levels should be monitored during and after the exchange.

Alteration of Pharmacokinetics.   Exchange transfusion alters blood levels of certain medications. The two determining

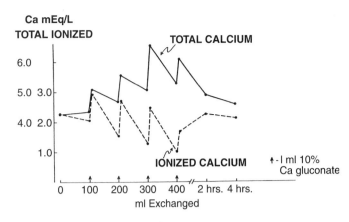

FIGURE **30-12**
Administration of calcium gluconate during exchange transfusion temporarily increases the ionized calcium level, but this response is not sustained. From Maisels M et al (1974). The effect of exchange transfusion on serum ionized calcium. *Pediatrics* 53:683.

factors are the timing of doses in relation to the start of the exchange and the rate of metabolism of the medication. The following medications were evaluated for the percentage of decrease after single-volume and double-volume exchanges (Lackner, 1982):

Drug	Single-Volume Exchange (% Drug Loss)	Double-Volume Exchange (% Drug Loss)
Ampicillin	7.7	14.2
Gentamicin	5.2	10.1
Digoxin	1.2	2.4
Phenobarbital	6.4	12.3
Vancomycin	5.7	11

If the blood levels of a medication would be altered by exchange transfusion, the medication should be given after completion of the exchange. Measuring blood drug levels may prove helpful in determining the need for supplemental doses of medication.

Hematologic Changes.   In the term newborn, the neutrophil count drops during the early phase of exchange transfusion but rises rapidly within hours after completion of the procedure. This phenomenon also occurs in the preterm infant, but the subsequent rise is more gradual. The neutrophil increase does not seem to be bone marrow mediated in either group, because no increase occurs in the immature forms of neutrophils. The increase is suspected to occur through the release of neutrophils from storage pools or from demargination of cells from the vascular walls.

Collaborative Management of the Infant Undergoing an Exchange Transfusion.   In addition to the general nursing care required by a sick infant, specific stabilization procedures are necessary for a successful exchange transfusion. A sample protocol for required care during an exchange is presented in Figure 30-13; the salient points are summarized here.

1. The infant should be in the most stable cardiorespiratory status possible; this includes maintenance of an adequate airway, stable blood gas values reflecting adequate ventilation, and continuous monitoring of vital signs.

PROCEDURE	Page 1 of 2

Section: Unit 7 - Specialized Care	
Title: 7.7 PROCEDURE FOR EXCHANGE TRANSFUSION	
Origination Date: April 1978	Author: Protocol Committee
Review Dates: 3/80, 12/82, 3/83, 5/86, 4/89, 11/91, 4/95, 2/98	Reviewer: Protocol Committee
OSHA Classification: I	

I. PURPOSE:

To outline the nursing responsibilities during an exchange transfusion.

II. SUPPORTIVE DATA:

A. Objective: to provide safe and effective care of a baby receiving an exchange transfusion.
B. Indications: any baby:
   1. Needing regulation of antibody-antigen levels.
   2. Removal to toxins significantly concentrated in the blood and not otherwise removable.
   3. Correction of life-threatening electrolyte and fluid imbalance.
   4. Regulation of the level and type of hemoglobin.
   5. Treatment of coagulation defects not remedied by single component replacement.
C. Contraindications: none.
D. Definitions: none.
E. Information:
   1. The infant should be NPO at least 3 hours prior to procedure with hydration by separate IV. If the patient has not been NPO for 3 hours, an oral-gastric tube must be placed and any stomach contents aspirated back.
   2. A type and cross match for one unit of whole blood should be ready.
   3. The MD/NNP will insert a line for the exchange transfusion.
   4. The first aliquot of blood withdrawn is usually sent for bilirubin and miscellaneous labs. The volume exchanged is usually 160cc/kg in full-term infants, and 180cc/kg in premature infants in passes of 5-10cc's (double volume exchange). The final aliquot of blood out can be used for bilirubin, Hct, and other labs as ordered.

III. EQUIPMENT LIST:

A. Open warmer & ISC temperature probe.
B. 1 unit whole blood typed and cross-matched to the patient.
C. Blood warmer and tubing (from Central Supply).
D. Exchange transfusion tray (from NCCS or Central Supply).
E. Equipment for UAC/UVC insertion.
F. Cardiac monitor.

IV. CONTENT:

A. Follow BSI precautions.
B. Place NGT if needed.
C. Immobilized extremities during the procedure.
D. Set up blood warmer as outlined in PCMC procedure 2.15, Blood/fluid warmers.
E. Monitor vital signs every 15 minutes for the first hour, then every 30 minutes for the next 3 hours. These are recorded on the transfusion record. The infant's general condition is monitored continuously during the procedure by the nurse.
F. Notify the MD/NNP performing the exchange transfusion when each 100cc's of blood has been exchanged.

FIGURE **30-13**
Outline of the nursing procedure for care of an infant during an exchange transfusion. From Fletcher MA, MacDonald MG (1993). *Atlas of procedures in neonatology.* JB Lippincott: Philadelphia; Goetzman BW, Wennberg RP (1991). *Neonatal intensive care handbook,* ed 2. Mosby: St Louis; Sherman-Streeter N (1986). *High-risk neonatal care.* Aspen: Rockville, MD; modified from Primary Children's Medical Center (1995). *Nursing procedure manual.* The Center: Salt Lake City.

V. DOCUMENTATION:

A. Document the following on the transfusion record sheet:
   1. Vital signs.
   2. Aliquots of blood in and out.
   3. Lab specimens.
B. Document the following in nursing notes and flow sheet.
   1. Preparations prior to the exchange.
   2. How the patient tolerated the procedure.
   3. Presence/absence of complications.

VI. EXCEPTIONS/COMPLICATIONS:

The possibilities of complications during exchange transfusions are numerous; therefore, the following is a list of possibile complications and possible reasons for them.

A. Heart failure - Due to transfusion overload if blood volume is miscalculated.
B. Cardiac arrest - Due to hyperkalemia or hypocalcemia. Citrate added to donor blood as an anticoagulant combines with ionized calcium to produce hypocalcemia. After 100cc of blood has been exchanged, calcium gluconate (96 mg/cc) may be given to counteract the effects of calcium binding by the preservative.
C. Irregular cardiac rhythm - Due to contact of catheter tip with myocardium or by rapid injection of blood directly into the heart when catheter is in too deeply, infusion with unwarmed blood, or electrolyte imbalance.
D. Air embolus - Due to large amounts of air sucked into the catheter if the infant gasps deeply when UVC is used and catheter is placed within the thorax or air bubbles are injected during the procedure.
E. Perforation of umbilical vein or artery - During attempts to force catheter passage.
F. Bacterial Infection - Due to poor techique or contaminated from donor blood.
G. Acidemia - Due to the fact that pH of donor blood is often 6.8 or less.
H. Hyperglycemia - followed by hypoglycemia - Donor blood contains dextrose, which may lead to hyperglycemia, followed by hypoglycemia when dextrose is used up by infant's system. Implications would be to check dextrose frequently and observe for signs and symptoms of hyper-hypo-glycemia. A peripheral IV may be needed throughout the procedure to prevent drop in blood glucose during exchange. Follow glucose every hour for 4 hours post-exchange as ordered. Feedings may be resumed 4 hours after transfusion if infant is stable.
I. Transfusion reaction - Especially when giving untyped and unmatched blood. Rare in newborns. Watch for temperature elevation, skin rash, and dark urine.

FIGURE **30-13, cont'd**

2. The infant should be placed in an open warmer with continuous monitoring of temperature to ensure adequate thermoregulation during the procedure. The infant's extremities should be restrained to prevent dislodgement of catheters and intravenous lines or contamination of the sterile field. Drapes should be placed in a manner that permits observation of the infant without compromising warmth or sterility.
3. Pre-exchange laboratory data should include blood type and crossmatch; direct and indirect Coombs' tests; electrolyte determinations; bilirubin, calcium, and glucose levels; and hematocrit level. All blood work except type, crossmatch, and Coombs' tests should be repeated midway through and at the completion of the exchange.
4. Necessary catheters and lines should be placed and kept patent with appropriate intravenous fluids until the procedure begins. Most central venous, umbilical artery catheter, and umbilical vein catheter lines can be kept open with 5% or 10% dextrose solutions. Normal saline or 0.45% saline solutions can be infused through peripheral arterial lines. The addition of calcium and electrolytes should be dictated by the infant's metabolic status.
5. Blood administration sets should be assembled and placed on a blood warmer set at the manufacturer's recommended temperature. If a blood warmer is not used, donor blood should be allowed to reach room temperature before use. Parental consent for blood transfusion and exchange transfusion should be obtained beforehand.

6. Vital signs should be taken before the procedure begins and at 15-minute intervals thereafter. Cardiorespiratory status and blood pressure should be monitored continuously throughout the procedure. If the infant is on a ventilator or receiving oxygen, transcutaneous carbon dioxide and saturation monitors should be used, with blood gas sampling done before, during, and after the procedure. The infant should be carefully observed for any signs of congestive failure, respiratory or circulatory deterioration, or adverse blood reactions.
7. An accurate tally should be kept of blood withdrawal, blood infusion, and medication administration during the procedure. Blood usually is exchanged in aliquots of 10 to 20 ml for a term infant and 5 to 10 ml for a severely anemic, hydropic, or preterm infant.
8. Medication schedules may be need to be adjusted, based on the completion time of the exchange. Measurement of drug levels can help in evaluating the need for adjustment.
9. After the procedure, phototherapy must be resumed, and postprocedural vital signs must be taken every 15 minutes for approximately 2 hours or until the infant's condition is stable.

ANEMIA

Pathophysiology

An infant is considered anemic if the hemoglobin or hematocrit value is more than two standard deviations below normal for the gestational age group (Luchtman-Jones et al, 2002). During the neonatal period, several abnormalities can evoke states of both acute and chronic anemia in the newborn. These forms of anemia often precede and occur independently of the natural propensity for physiologic anemia that exists as a common entity among all infants, both term and preterm. The conditions that most commonly trigger these pathologic anemias are acute or chronic episodes of hemorrhage, acute or chronic RBC destruction and hemolysis, and blood sampling for laboratory analysis.

Clinical Manifestations

Acute Anemia. The physical presentation of acute anemia is more intense than that seen in the chronic form, because the causes of acute anemia are more emergent, life-threatening, and disruptive to the homeostasis of the infant (Box 30-2). The resulting cardiovascular collapse, followed closely by respiratory failure, can overwhelm the neonate with only marginal reserves. Immediate intervention and replacement of lost intravascular volume often are required to achieve stabilization. An infant experiencing an acute anemic episode (hemorrhage being the most common cause) has symptoms reflecting compromise of the cardiorespiratory system: shock, poor peripheral perfusion, poor respiratory effort or respiratory distress, tachycardia, pallor, lethargy, and hypotension. Before signs of acute anemia become apparent, the hemoglobin level must fall precipitously below 12 g/dl.

Acute blood loss results in a recognizable sequence of symptoms based on the volume loss:

- 7.5% to 15% volume loss: Little change is noted in heart rate and blood pressure, but stroke volume and subsequent cardiac output are reduced. Peripheral vasoconstriction occurs, resulting in diminished blood flow to the skeletal muscles, gut, and carcass.
- 20% to 25% volume loss: Hypotension and shock become apparent. Cardiac output is reduced, and peripheral vasoconstriction is present. Low tissue oxygen levels and acidosis become apparent.

Chronic Anemia. Prolonged, or chronic, anemia may not require rapid intravascular volume expansion, but it is by no means completely benign, as is seen with EBF or chronic twin to twin transfusion (Box 30-3). In both of these conditions, infants may require removal of intravascular volume and replacement with volume of a higher hematocrit before stabilization is achieved. Because these infants have had considerable time to adjust to chronic blood loss or hemolysis, the changes in vital signs may reflect poor oxygen-carrying capacity rather than hypovolemia. On physical examination, pallor usually is accompanied by hepatosplenomegaly, a reflection of the body's attempt to compensate for blood loss through extramedullary hematopoiesis. The blood smear may also reflect the long-standing nature of the problem; RBCs appear hypochromic and small, and a greater number of immature RBCs is seen.

Common Causes of Pathologic Anemia in the Newborn

Hemorrhage

Fetal-Maternal Transfusion Caused by Transplacental Hemorrhage. This phenomenon occurs in approximately 50% to 75% of all pregnancies and can be an acute or chronic process. An estimated 5.6% of pregnancies involve a fetal-maternal transfusion in the range of 11 to 30 ml of blood; another 1% involve an exchange of more than 30 ml. Fetal-

---

> **BOX 30-2**
>
> ### Causes of Acute Anemia in the Newborn
>
> **Obstetric Accidents, Malformations of the Placenta and Cord**
> Rupture of a normal umbilical cord
>   Precipitous delivery
>   Entanglement
> Hematoma of the cord or placenta
> Rupture of an abnormal umbilical cord
>   Varices
>   Aneurysm
> Rupture of anomalous vessels
>   Aberrant vessel
>   Velamentous insertion
>   Communicating vessels in multilobed placenta
> Incision of placenta during cesarean section
> Placenta previa
> Abruptio placentae
>
> **Occult Hemorrhage Before Birth**
> Fetoplacental
>   Tight nuchal cord
> Cesarean section
> Placental hematoma
> Fetomaternal
>   Traumatic amniocentesis
>   After external cephalic version, manual removal of placenta, use of oxytocin
>   Spontaneous
>   Chorioangioma of the placenta
>   Choriocarcinoma
> Twin to twin
>   Chronic
>   Acute
>
> **Internal Hemorrhage**
> Intracranial
> Giant cephalhematoma, subgaleal, caput succedaneum
> Adrenal
> Retroperitoneal
> Ruptured liver, ruptured spleen
> Pulmonary
>
> **Iatrogenic Blood Loss**

From Oski F & Naiman J (1982). Anemia in the neonatal period. In Oski F & Naiman J, editors. Hematologic problems in the newborn. WB Saunders: Philadelphia.

maternal transfusions can be verified by the presence of fetal cells in the maternal circulation, which can be detected with the erythrocyte rosette test and the Kleihauer-Betke acid elution test for fetal hemoglobin in maternal blood. The erythrocyte rosette test specifically detects fetal RBCs. The Kleihauer-Betke test consists of an acid wash of a maternal blood smear followed by staining. Fetal hemoglobin resists elution from intact RBCs in an acid solution. Intact cells containing fetal hemoglobin can be distinguished microscopically, when stained, from adult erythrocytes. The presence of stained erythrocytes suggests contamination of maternal blood by fetal blood. This

BOX 30-3

Causes of Chronic Anemia in the Newborn

Immunity disorders
  Rh incompatibility
  ABO incompatibility
  Minor blood group incompatibility
  Maternal autoimmune hemolytic anemia
  Drug-induced hemolytic anemia
Infection
  Bacterial sepsis
  Congenital infections
    Syphilis
    Malaria
    Cytomegalovirus
    Rubella
    Toxoplasmosis
    Disseminated herpes
Disseminated intravascular coagulation
Macroangiopathic and microangiopathic hemolytic anemias
  Cavernous hemangioma
  Large-vessel thrombi
  Renal artery stenosis
  Severe coarctation of aorta
Galactosemia
Prolonged or recurrent acidosis of a metabolic or respiratory nature
Hereditary disorders of the red cell membrane
  Hereditary spherocytosis
  Hereditary elliptocytosis
  Hereditary stomatocytosis
  Other rare membrane disorders
Pyknocytosis
Red cell enzyme deficiencies
  Most commonly glucose-6-phosphate dehydrogenase deficiency, pyruvate kinase deficiency, 5'-nucleotidase deficiency, and glucose-6-phosphate isomerase deficiency
Alpha-thalassemia syndrome
Alpha chain structural abnormalities
Gamma-thalassemia syndromes
Gamma chain structural abnormalities

From Oski F & Naiman J (1982). Anemia in the neonatal period. In Oski F & Naiman J, editors. Hematologic problems in the newborn. WB Saunders: Philadelphia.

test is useful in identifying fetal RBCs in the mother's blood so long as no underlying condition increases the amount of fetal hemoglobin in the mother's blood.

Twin to Twin Transfusion.   This phenomenon, which can be both acute and chronic, occurs in 15% to 33% of all monochorionic (monozygotic) twins, in which the placentas tend to be fused. The anastomosis usually is between an artery of one placenta and the vein of the other, although vascular connections may be artery to artery or vein to vein. In the chronic form of twin to twin transfusion, the size difference between twins can be helpful in determining the donor and the recipient. When the weight difference exceeds 20%, the smaller twin is always the donor. When the weight difference is less than 20%, either twin may be the donor. In such cases, hemat-

ocrit values prove useful in determining the donor and the recipient. The donor twin is anemic, and the blood count reflects increased hematopoiesis, as evidenced by an elevated reticulocyte count and increased numbers of immature RBCs. The recipient develops polycythemia but can exhibit signs of congestive heart failure and pulmonary or systemic hypertension. Laboratory data usually show a difference of 5 g/dl between donor and recipient hemoglobin values. Stillbirths are common in twin to twin transfusion, and both twins are at risk.

Obstetrical Accidents.   Many obstetrical problems, especially those that occur before labor and delivery, can result in chronic as well as acute blood loss. Long-standing problems, such as placenta previa or partial abruption, usually result in anemia. However, acute hemorrhage rather than anemia is the case in problems that occur at the time of delivery. Examples are severe abruption, severing of the placenta during cesarean section, or umbilical cord rupture as a result of sudden tension on a short or tangled cord. A tight nuchal cord can reduce blood volume in a newborn by approximately 20%. Holding a newly delivered infant above the placenta can also reduce the hematocrit and blood volume because of the gravitational drainage of blood from the newborn into the placenta.

Internal Hemorrhage.   A drop in the hematocrit during the first 24 to 72 hours that is not associated with hyperbilirubinemia usually is attributed to internal hemorrhage. Bleeding can occur in various parts of the body secondary to birth trauma or pre-existing anomalies. The areas of potential hemorrhage in the head include the subdural, subarachnoid, intraventricular, intracranial, and subperiosteal spaces. Infants can lose an estimated 10% to 15% of their blood during an intraventricular or intracranial hemorrhage. In cases of traumatic delivery or vacuum extraction, extensive scalp bleeding can result in significant blood loss, which can be estimated by measuring the increase in the head circumference. Each centimeter of increase represents an estimated 38 ml of blood lost from the intravascular compartment. Hemorrhage into the liver, kidneys, spleen, or retroperitoneal space can also occur in association with traumatic and breech deliveries.

Hepatic rupture occurs in approximately 1.2% to 5.6% of stillbirths and neonatal deaths; half of the hemorrhages are subcapsular. Infants with this disorder tend to be stable for 24 to 48 hours and then suddenly deteriorate. This deterioration seems to coincide with rupture of the capsule and hemoperitoneum. Hepatic rupture carries a poor prognosis, but rapid surgery preceded by multiple transfusions can save the infant. Splenic rupture is associated with severe EBF and should be suspected at the time of exchange transfusion if the central venous pressure is low rather than elevated. Signs of splenic rupture include scrotal swelling and peritoneal effusion without free air. Adrenal hemorrhage is seen more often in the infant of a diabetic or prediabetic mother and is characterized by a flank mass with bluish discoloration of the overlying skin.

Red Blood Cell Destruction and Hemolysis

Maternal-Fetal Blood Group Incompatibilities.   Isoimmunization, as in ABO and Rh incompatibility, accounts for most cases of neonatal hemolysis. A reduced RBC life span caused by hemolysis usually is associated with a rise in the bilirubin level, 1 g of hemoglobin yielding 35 mg of bilirubin. Infants who have received intrauterine transfusions or exchange transfusions for blood group incompatibilities are predisposed to a hyporegenerative anemia that develops within the first few months of life.

The pathophysiology is considered to be bone marrow suppression, possibly as a result of the increased amount of hemoglobin A received during the blood transfusions.

Acquired Defects of the Red Blood Cells.   This hemolytic problem is seen in bacterial sepsis and viral infections, especially of the TORCH variety. Drug-induced RBC destruction, caused by either maternal ingestion or direct administration of the drug to the newborn, is another common cause of hemolysis. An example of this would be the hemolysis that could occur with administration of iron supplements to an infant with vitamin E deficiency.

Congenital Defects of the Red Blood Cells.   Defects resulting in destruction of the RBCs can involve the cell membrane, enzymatic system, or hemoglobin component, as in glucose-6-phosphate dehydrogenase deficiency, thalassemia, and hereditary spherocytosis. Although these conditions can cause hemolysis in the newborn period, they are rare diseases.

Blood Sampling.   Blood loss that occurs secondary to sampling is one of the two most frequently causes of chronic anemia in infants, the other being physiologic anemia of the newborn and premature infant. Among two groups of preterm infants admitted to neonatal intensive care units, the average blood loss from sampling during the first 4 to 6 weeks of life was 46 to 50 ml/kg; the severity of illness correlated with the amount of blood removed for sampling. Prudent blood sampling may eliminate unnecessary blood volume depletion and reduce the need for replacement transfusion therapy. Accurate recording of blood lost to sampling can prove beneficial in the assessment of a sick infant's circulatory status and volume needs. However, perfusion status and hematocrit values may be a better determinants of the need for volume expansion or blood transfusions.

Differential Diagnosis

History.   Acute and chronic anemia often can be distinguished from each other and from other problems by analyzing the family history for anemia or jaundice. The maternal history should be carefully examined for evidence of drug ingestion that may affect RBC life span or production, bleeding during the pregnancy or labor, or other incidents surrounding the delivery that may contribute to blood loss in the newborn.

Laboratory Findings.   The type of anemia often can be identified on the basis of laboratory studies that evaluate RBC content and form.

- Hematocrit and hemoglobin levels can define the type as well as the degree of anemia. Blood loss during acute hemorrhage is rapid, with little evidence of the compensatory hematopoiesis seen in chronic anemia. RBCs are of normal size and have a normal hemoglobin mass, and no significant increase is seen in the number of immature RBCs. Hemoglobin values initially may not reflect hemorrhage because the intravascular volume contracts and masks volume loss. It may take several hours for intravascular equilibration to occur before the hemoglobin accurately reflects the extent of the hemorrhage. The site of hemoglobin or hematocrit sampling is important for obtaining accurate information, because capillary sticks on an infant in shock reflect venous stasis. A more accurate sample at this time would be from an arterial or venous source.

- Reticulocyte counts are useful in differentiating chronic and acute forms of anemia. Increased numbers of immature RBCs reflect the degree of hematopoietic activity in response to anemia. Increased hematopoiesis requires a time lapse between the occurrence of anemia and stimulation of the hematopoietic centers.

- Peripheral blood smears are helpful in evaluating iron content and the size and shape of the RBC, which vary in different forms of anemia.

- Blood typing, Rh determination, and Coombs' testing can help identify blood group incompatibilities as causes of anemia.

Treatment

Collaborative Management of the Infant with Acute Anemia. The following measures are used to stabilize the condition of an infant with acute anemia:

- Basic resuscitation of the infant experiencing precipitous blood loss often includes stabilization of the airway by means of intubation and ventilation.

- Rapid line placement for fluid replacement, volume expansion, and blood sampling may require use of the umbilical vein or artery. Central venous pressure measurements can be helpful in assessing the degree of volume loss and the amount of replacement needed.

- If acute volume expansion is required, low-titer, type O-negative blood, plasma, albumin, or saline initially can be used in increments of 10 to 20 ml/kg until a type and crossmatch replacement is available. Failure to respond may indicate continuing internal hemorrhage.

- After the infant's condition has been stabilized, laboratory tests and a physical examination should be performed to determine the cause of the anemia and to rectify the problem.

- Examination of the placenta and maternal blood sample testing for fetal hemoglobin may prove useful in determining the cause of the blood loss.

As with all newborns, the principles of care (provision of warmth, monitoring of vital signs, ongoing assessment and accurate determination of intake and output) are essential to the well-being of the infant who has suffered acute blood loss. After initial stabilization, nursing care must include modifications that either eliminate recurrence of precipitous events or prevent further blood loss. Providing safe care to such infants requires adequate knowledge of the principles and procedures involved in volume expansion and the use of blood products. A review of the use of blood products can be found at the conclusion of this chapter.

Collaborative Management of the Infant with Chronic Anemia.   The major focus of therapy for the infant with chronic anemia is control or elimination of the cause of the anemia. Several forms of chronic anemia in term and preterm infants are linked to dietary deficiencies that can be eradicated by replacement therapy. Chronic forms of anemia requiring symptomatic therapy can also be treated with transfusion therapy and erythropoietin.

Dietary Supplementation.   The three major dietary factors that affect RBC production are iron, folate, and vitamin E. Because all three increase in amount with increasing gestational age, premature birth predisposes the immature infant to anemia as a result of insufficient stores.

Without benefit of iron supplementation, the hematopoiesis necessary to maintain a normal hemoglobin level depletes the infant's iron reserves by the time birth weight is doubled. Various factors can further contribute to iron deficiency anemia, such as low birth weight, low initial hemoglobin levels, and blood loss through trauma, hemorrhage, or sampling. In the term infant, exhaustion of iron reserves normally occurs by 20 to 24 weeks' postnatal age, but this happens much earlier in the preterm infant. Iron stores needed for hemoglobin production are present in insufficient quantities at birth in the premature infant, making supplementation necessary during the first 2 to 4 months to prevent iron deficiency anemia.

In any gestational age group, iron depletion first becomes evident in reduced serum ferritin levels (serum ferritin being a measure of accumulated iron stores) and in the disappearance of stainable iron from the bone marrow. A subsequent reduction in the mean corpuscular volume (i.e., the size) of the RBC is followed by a drop in the hemoglobin level. Although prophylactic iron supplementation does not prevent the initial fall in hemoglobin, administration of 1 to 2 mg/kg/day of supplemental iron should supply term and preterm infants with adequate reserves; 3 to 6 mg/kg/day is recommended in iron-deficient infants or those receiving erythropoietin.

The relationship between serum ferritin levels and the administration of multiple transfusions to a population of newborn infants was evaluated to determine iron supplementation needs in this group. In a study by Arad and associates (1988), serum ferritin levels were measured in four groups of infants: (1) preterm infants transfused with more than 100 ml of packed cells, (2) preterm infants transfused with less than 100 ml, (3) nontransfused preterm infants, and (4) nontransfused term infants. At 4 to 5 months of age, the preterm infants receiving more than 100 ml of RBCs had the highest ferritin levels of all four groups. This would suggest that LBW infants receiving large volumes of RBCs could amass iron stores sufficient for new RBC production during the first 4 to 5 months without the need for additional iron supplementation.

Folate is the generic description for folic acid and its related compounds. Folate is a component of the B-complex vitamins involved in the maturation of RBCs, particularly the synthesis of DNA, which controls nuclear maturation and division. Because bone marrow is one of the body's faster growing and proliferative tissue, folic acid deficiency diminishes its ability to produce RBCs, resulting in a megaloblastic anemia.

High amounts of folate are present at birth in both term and preterm infants, but these levels drop rapidly, especially in LBW infants. It is estimated that approximately 68% of infants weighing less than 1700 g have subnormal levels of folate at 1 to 3 months of age. However, only a few infants actually develop anemia. Human milk and soy-based products contain an adequate amount of natural folate, but commonly used commercial products must be artificially enriched. Premature infant formulas are adequately enriched to satisfy a premature infant's folate needs provided that intake is sufficient. Because folate is absorbed in the duodenum and jejunum, any disease or medication that affects the absorptive surface of these areas can impair folate absorption.

Vitamin E, an antioxidant, is valuable in protecting the RBC membrane from destruction due to lipid peroxidation. Deficiency of this nutrient shortens the life span of the cell by exposing the unprotected, unsaturated membrane lipids to peroxidation and hemolysis. Infants are born in a state of relative vitamin E deficiency that is more intense in the smaller and more premature infants. Vitamin E is required in increasing amounts as the intake of polyunsaturated fatty acids increases.

Deficiency becomes apparent in infants of birth weights less than 1500 g at approximately 4 to 6 weeks of age, resulting in decreased hemoglobin levels ranging from 7 to 10 g/dl. Administration of iron supplementation in the presence of this deficiency intensifies the hemolytic response. Signs and symptoms, as with many neonatal diseases, mimic those of other disease entities that occur in the neonatal period. One of the more obvious symptoms is edema of the feet, lower extremities, and scrotal area. The appearance of the RBC may vary, but abnormalities usually include fragmented or irregularly shaped cells, presence of spherocytes, and thrombocytopenia. Infant formulas are now enriched with adequate amounts of vitamin E, provided formula intake is sufficient.

Transfusion Therapy.   Of all preterm infants admitted to an NICU, approximately 90% receive one transfusion in the first 6 weeks of life; 50% receive cumulative transfusions in excess of their total circulating RBC mass. In determining which infants may need subsequent transfusions after the first 2 weeks of life, gestational age of less than 30 weeks is the best predictor, regardless of severity of illness, number of transfusions during the first week, complications, or hematocrit level at birth. Only 14% of infants of more than 30 weeks' gestation require transfusions after 2 weeks of age.

Although a critically ill infant generally is maintained with a hematocrit above 40%, the benefits of transfusion therapy in the convalescent infant remain controversial. When the effects of transfusion therapy in the convalescent infant were studied, the elimination of symptoms attributed to anemia was not a consistent finding. In premature infants with hematocrits below 30%, apnea, bradycardia, dyspnea, feeding difficulties, poor weight gain despite good calorie intake, lethargy, tachypnea, tachycardia, and increased cardiac output and oxygen consumption appear to be relieved by transfusion therapy in some studies. There appears to be no overall relationship between hematocrit values and physiologic symptoms such as apnea, bradycardia, or changes in heart and respiratory rates, nor does abatement of these symptoms follow transfusion therapy.

In light of the controversy surrounding transfusions, evidence of impaired tissue oxygenation remains the ultimate criterion for the use of blood products. Measurement of lactic acid levels may prove helpful in determining which infants may benefit from transfusion therapy. When the oxygen-carrying capacity of hemoglobin is insufficient for tissue needs, anaerobic metabolism occurs, leading to excess production of lactic acid. Monitoring of lactic acid levels and transfusing only those infants with elevated levels may aid in establishing more sound criteria for transfusion therapy.

Several methods of blood preparation and use have been evaluated to minimize donor exposure and reduce the potential for transmitted disease. Studies suggest that packed RBCs with a shelf life of more than 5 days, and up to 42 days, are safe for use in neonatal transfusions (Liu et al, 1994; Lee et al, 1995). This finding, combined with use of a sterile connection device that allows multiple aseptic entries into a unit of blood, would permit use of a designated unit for each infant at risk for multiple transfusions, thereby significantly reducing donor exposure (Liu et al, 1994; Lee et al, 1995). The desire to limit donor exposure must inevitably be balanced by the limited availability of banked blood. Multiple users on a blood unit may reduce wastage but may possibly expose an infant to multiple donors.

Blood administered to the newborn is often irradiated, which causes cell membrane disruption and potassium leakage

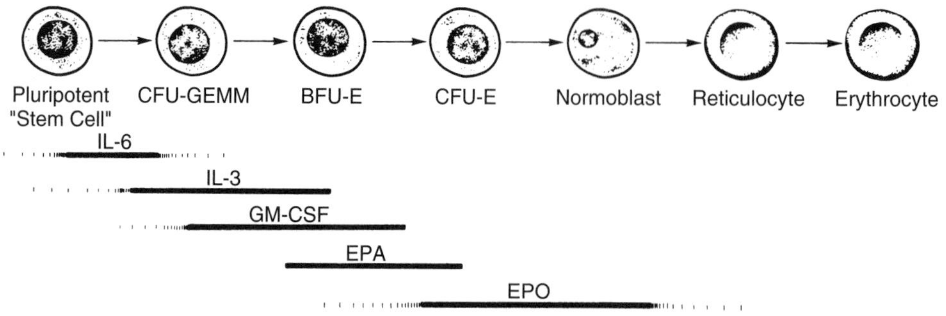

FIGURE **30-14**

The principal action of human recombinant erythropoietin is on the derivatives of the hematopoietic stem cells in the bone marrow that have been designated erythrocyte colony-forming units (CFU-E), the precursors of the red blood cell (RBC). *CFU-GEMM,* Colony-forming units-granulocytes, erythroid cells, macrophages, and megakaryocytes; *BFU-E,* erythrocyte burst-forming units; *IL-6,* interleukin-6; *IL-3,* interleukin-3; *GM-CSF,* granulocyte-macrophage colony-stimulating factor; *EPA,* erythroid potentiating activity; *EPO,* erythropoietin. From Christensen R (1989). Recombinant erythropoietic growth factors as an alternative to erythrocyte transfusion for patients with anemia of prematurity. *Pediatrics* 83:793-796.

from the cell. The decision by the U.S. Food and Drug Administration to change its recommendations for the maximum storage time of irradiated blood from 42 to 28 days affects the length of use of a designated unit (Quinnan, 1993). Although older blood appears to be safe to administer, it is not recommended for rapid transfusions, administration of large aliquots, exchange transfusions, or treatment of coagulopathies.

The establishment of transfusion criteria can effectively minimize donor exposure. These guidelines help determine which infants would benefit from transfusion on the basis of symptoms, hematocrit value, and severity of illness.

Recombinant Human Erythropoietin Therapy.   Cloning of the human erythropoietin (HuEPO) gene in 1985 resulted in the production of large amounts of HuEPO for use as an exogenous stimulant of erythroid progenitor cells in patients with anemia. HuEPO acts primarily on CFU-E, derivatives of the hematopoietic stem cells in the bone marrow and the precursors of the RBCs (Figure 30-14). Studies from the United States and England have shown the use of recombinant erythropoietin to be an effective replacement for transfusion therapy in raising the hemoglobin level in hyporegenerative anemia and end-stage renal disease. Further studies of preterm infants have demonstrated that HuEPO maintains the hematocrit level during the phase of normal anemia of the premature infant, with good proliferation of erythroid progenitor cells in response to HuEPO.

HuEPO has attained recognition as a standard of care for anemia of prematurity, because several clinical trials have established its effectiveness in reducing both the number of transfusions and the cumulative volume of transfused blood needed in treated patients (Messer et al, 1993; Ohls et al, 1993; Maier et al, 1994; Meyer et al, 1994; Ohls et al, 1995). Donato and associates (2000) noted increased reticulocytosis in infants started early on erythropoietin but failed to see a reduction in transfusion requirements in those infants.

The usual response in preterm infants given HuEPO is an increase in blood levels of erythropoietin and reticulocytes, as well as RBC volume, 2 to 3 weeks after initiation of therapy. The accepted dosage of erythropoietin is 200 to 250 U/kg

given subcutaneously three times a week for 2 weeks, although definitive therapeutic dosages have yet to be determined.

HuEPO has been evaluated for its effectiveness as an alternative to transfusion therapy for treatment of anemia in premature infants caused by (1) blood sampling, with administration beginning within the first 2 days of life (Maier et al, 1994; Ohls et al, 1995); (2) physiologic anemia of prematurity, with therapy starting at 1 to 4 weeks of age (Emmerson et al, 1993; Messer et al, 1993; Meyer et al, 1994; Shannon et al, 1995); and (3) anemia of bronchopulmonary dysplasia, with treatment starting at 3 months of age (Ohls et al, 1993).

Serum ferritin levels decline rapidly after initiation of HuEPO therapy in infants with normal pretreatment ferritin levels, despite prophylactic iron supplementation of 2 mg/kg/day. This predisposition to the development of iron deficiency anemia underlines the need for increased iron supplementation in infants treated with HuEPO. Transient thrombocytosis shortly after initiation of therapy and transient neutropenia, lasting as long as 2 months after discontinuation of therapy, have also been documented. It has been postulated that this phenomenon is due to a stimulant effect of HuEPO on megakaryocyte progenitors and a negative effect on granulocyte-monocyte progenitor cells. Before HuEPO was proven effective in raising hematocrit levels, its use was projected to eliminate the need for one third of all transfusions in premature infants.

Physiologic Anemia of the Newborn and Anemia of the Premature Infant

Shortly after birth, the physiologic regulator of RBC production, erythropoietin, falls to barely perceptible levels because the relative intrauterine hypoxia that stimulated its release in utero is no longer present. Erythropoietin levels remain low until another hypoxic stimulus occurs, one created by the normal drop in the hemoglobin level that marks physiologic anemia of the newborn. This drop in the hemoglobin level is due to decreased marrow production of RBCs secondary to diminished circulating erythropoietin levels, a shorter life span of the neonatal RBC with destruction of fetal hemoglobin, and hemodilution caused by growth.

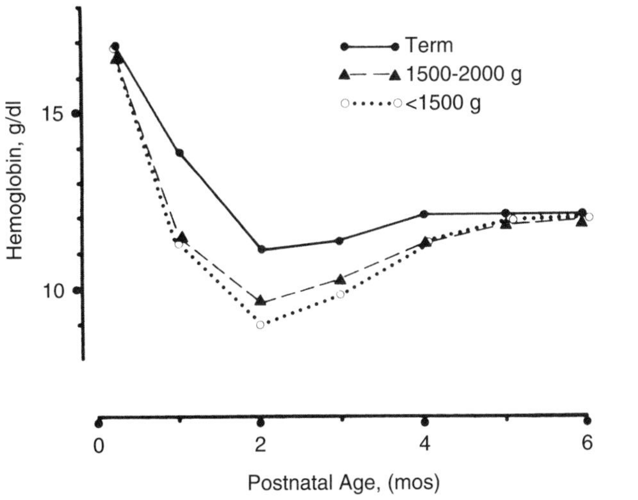

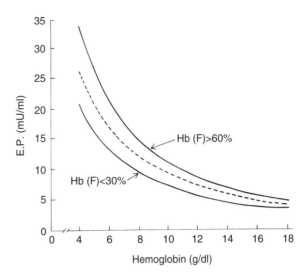

FIGURE **30-15**
Gestational age and birth weight are directly correlated with the timing of the postnatal drop in hemoglobin and with the nadir of the drop. Shown here are the differences between term infants and two groups of preterm infants, one weighing 1500 to 2000 g and the other less than 1500 g. From Brown M (1988). Physiologic anemia of infancy: normal red cell values and physiology of neonatal erythropoiesis. In Stockman J, Pochedly C, editors. *Developmental and neonatal hematology.* Raven Press: New York.

FIGURE **30-16**
Because of the differences in oxygen affinity between adult and fetal hemoglobin, variations in the percentage of available fetal hemoglobin (hemoglobin F) affect erythropoietin levels. Improved oxygen uptake but decreased unloading at the tissue level is associated with hemoglobin F. Therefore the stimulus for erythropoietin production is diminished with lower concentrations of hemoglobin F (<30%). With higher concentrations (60%) of hemoglobin F, the stimulus response is an increase in erythropoietin production. At identical total hemoglobin levels, the stimulus for erythropoietin production is increased whenever the percentage of hemoglobin F exceeds the adult norm. From Stockman J et al (1977). The anemia of infancy and the anemia of prematurity: factors governing the erythropoietin response. *New England journal of medicine* 296:647. Copyright©1977 Massachusetts Medical Society.

The drop in hemoglobin that prompts the postnatal rise in erythropoietin directly correlates with the infant's gestational age and birth weight (Figure 30-15). The smaller and more immature infant reaches a lower nadir at an earlier postnatal age. The hemoglobin level in the term newborn reaches a nadir of 11.4 g/dl ± 0.9 in the first 2 to 3 months of life and plateaus at this level for approximately 2 more months before it gradually increases. Although there is no significant difference in cord blood hemoglobin levels between term infants and preterm infants born after 32 weeks' gestation, the drop in hemoglobin occurs earlier in the preterm infant, is more precipitous, and reaches a lower nadir. Starting at 2 weeks of age, the preterm infant has a drop in hemoglobin of 1 g/dl/week for the first several weeks; the nadir at 6 to 8 weeks of age is 2 to 3 g/dl lower than that of the term infant. An infant weighing 1000 to 1500 g at birth will have a mean hemoglobin nadir of 8 g/dl at 4 to 6 weeks of age.

Infants who have undergone exchange transfusion or multiple transfusions also have a greater fall in the hemoglobin level in the first 3 months of life. This phenomenon theoretically may be due to improved oxygen delivery to tissue associated with the replacement of fetal with adult hemoglobin. Adult hemoglobin has less affinity for oxygen because of the structural difference of the globin portion of the hemoglobin molecule. This, coupled with the increased amount of 2,3-disphosphoglycerate present in the blood, allows adult hemoglobin to release oxygen to the tissue more easily. Improved tissue oxygenation effectively lowers serum erythropoietin levels (Figure 30-16), resulting in decreased RBC production. Consequently, an infant undergoing intrauterine transfusion, exchange transfusion, or frequent postnatal transfusions has improved tissue oxygenation and a decreased erythropoietin level.

The switch in the predominant site of erythropoietin production during fetal life from the liver to the kidneys occurs concurrently with the change in hemoglobin to a more mature form. Hepatic production of erythropoietin in response to hypoxia is not as rapid as the kidneys' response, an adjustment that actually spares the fetus from polycythemia in utero. However, persistence of this hepatic pathway after premature birth may explain why the premature infant's hematocrit values reach a lower nadir that persists longer compared with the term infant. Although erythropoietin levels are reduced in the early newborn period, the erythroid progenitor cells in the bone marrow are exceedingly sensitive to erythropoietin and respond rapidly as blood levels increase. The normal erythropoietin level in infants beyond the newborn period is 10 to 20 mU/ml.

Physiologic anemia does not usually require any form of treatment. With good nutrition, the hemoglobin level in the term infant should start to rise by 3 months of age. With adequate nutrition and iron supplementation, the hemoglobin level in the preterm infant should start to increase by 5 months of age, eventually attaining hemoglobin values comparable to those of the term infant. It is the preterm infant with symptomatic anemia of prematurity who poses the question of transfusion versus HuEPO therapy, a question that has not yet been answered conclusively.

POLYCYTHEMIA

Pathophysiology
Polycythemia, defined as a peripheral venous hematocrit over 65%, occurs in 4% to 5% of the total population of newborns, in 2% to 4% of term infants appropriate for gestational age, and in 10% to 15% of infants either small or large for gesta-

tional age. It has not been observed in infants of less than 34 weeks' gestation. Although the fetus lives in a low PO_2 environment that should induce a polycythemic response, it protects itself by keeping hematocrit levels below 60%. This may be a function of slower fetal hepatic response to hypoxia compared with rapid renal response after birth. The average hematocrit on the first day of life is approximately 50% in the term infant and the preterm infant of more than 32 weeks' gestation and 45% in the preterm infant of less than 32 weeks' gestation. During the first 4 to 12 hours of life, hemoglobin and hematocrit values tend to rise and then equilibrate, especially in infants receiving large placental transfusions.

The choice of sampling site can affect hematocrit values considerably, particularly during the early newborn period when peripheral circulation may be somewhat sluggish. Infants younger than 1 day of age either lack or have diminished cutaneous vasoregulatory mechanisms that reduce peripheral perfusion. Polycythemia further impairs peripheral circulation by increasing blood viscosity and reducing the flow rate. As blood viscosity increases, vascular resistance increases in the peripheral circulation and the microcirculation of the capillaries throughout the body. Compared with venous samples, the hematocrit levels of capillary samples are 5% to 15% higher, and those of umbilical vessel or arterial samples are 6% to 8% lower.

Three major factors determine blood viscosity: hematocrit, plasma viscosity (osmolality), and deformability of the RBCs. With hematocrit levels below 60% to 65%, blood viscosity increases in a linear fashion, but viscosity exponentially increases at higher hematocrit levels.

Variations in the components of plasma affect blood viscosity independent of the hematocrit. Abnormal composition of plasma protein, electrolytes, and other metabolites can either decrease or increase plasma viscosity. Such an increase in the presence of a high hematocrit further increases blood viscosity and reduces the blood flow rate. The ability of cells to modify their shape to successfully traverse the peripheral vascular bed and microcirculation also affects the blood flow rate. The degree of deformability of the cell determines its ability to pass through small vascular spaces; the greater the deformability of the cell, the quicker its passage. Less deformable cells can increase blood viscosity by occluding small vessels, causing sludging in the microcirculation that can lead to thrombosis and tissue ischemia.

The two major types of polycythemia are (1) the active form, which is caused by the production of an excess number of RBCs in response to hypoxia and other poorly defined stimuli; and (2) the passive form, which is caused by RBC transfusion to an infant secondary to maternal-fetal transfusion, twin to twin transfusion, or delayed cord clamping.

Active Polycythemia

Tissue hypoxia, regardless of the cause, elicits an increase in erythropoietin that stimulates RBC production. In the fetus, erythropoietin is produced initially by the liver and then by the kidneys, the adult production site. The kidneys' potential to release erythropoietin is active by 34 weeks' gestation. At this time, a renal erythropoietic factor reacts with a substance in the plasma to produce erythropoietin, the RBC stimulating factor. Hypoxia of the tissues adjacent to the renal tubules, where erythropoietin is thought to be produced, is the potent stimulator of this factor's release.

Many factors can lead to tissue hypoxia associated with the active form of polycythemia. These factors include the following:

1. Maternal factors that result in reduced placental blood flow
   - Pregnancy-induced hypertension
   - Older maternal age
   - Maternal renal or heart disease
   - Severe maternal diabetes (hematocrit values of 64% or higher are found in 42% of infants of a diabetic mother and 30% of gestational infants of a diabetic mother)
   - Oligohydramnios
   - Maternal smoking (the mechanism is thought to be production of carbon monoxide that crosses the placenta and induces a state of tissue hypoxia in the fetus)
2. Placental factors
   - Placental infarction
   - Placenta previa
   - Viral infections, especially TORCH
   - Postmaturity
   - Placental dysfunction that results in a small-for-gestational-age (SGA) infant
3. Fetal syndromes
   - Trisomies 13, 18, and 21
   - Beckwith-Wiedemann syndrome

Passive Polycythemia

Passive polycythemia is a result of increased fetal blood volume caused by maternal-fetal transfusion; twin to twin transfusion, with one twin being polycythemic and the other anemic; or delayed cord clamping. A diagnosis of maternal-fetal transfusion can be considered when (1) the infant's blood is found to contain larger amounts than expected of adult hemoglobin, IgA, or IgM; (2) RBCs in the infant's blood have maternal blood group antigens, if the mother's and the infant's blood groups are different; or (3) XX cells are found in an XY infant. In twin to twin transfusion, morbidity and mortality are comparable in both groups of affected infants, with one twin being anemic and the other polycythemic. By far, however, the most common cause of fetal transfusion is delayed cord clamping with positioning of the newborn below the level of the placenta. Delayed cord clamping can increase the circulating volume by as much as 60% and can raise the hematocrit value by 10%.

Clinical Manifestations

Symptoms of polycythemic hyperviscosity, which usually are evident within the first few days after birth, reflect compromise of various organ systems. The most commonly seen findings include the following:

1. Neurologic symptoms
   - Lethargy
   - Hypotonia
   - Tremulousness
   - Exaggerated startle
   - Poor suck
   - Vomiting
   - Seizures
   - Apnea
2. Cardiovascular symptoms
   - Plethora
   - Cardiomegaly
   - Electrocardiographic changes (right and left atrial hypertrophy, right ventricular hypertrophy)

3. Respiratory symptoms
   - Respiratory distress
   - Central cyanosis
   - Pleural effusions
   - Pulmonary congestion and edema
4. Hematologic symptoms
   - Thrombocytopenia
   - Elevated reticulocyte level
   - Hepatosplenomegaly
5. Metabolic symptoms
   - Hypocalcemia
   - Hyperbilirubinemia
   - Hypoglycemia

Hypoglycemia found in conjunction with polycythemia can be a reflection of (1) increased glucose consumption by an overabundant number of RBCs; (2) increased cerebral extraction of glucose secondary to hypoxia; (3) a state of hyperinsulinemia caused by increased erythropoietin levels; or (4) decreased hepatic glucose production as a result of sluggish hepatic circulation. Hyperbilirubinemia associated with polycythemia is a reflection of increased byproducts of RBC destruction.

The complications of polycythemia center around the increased resistance to blood flow related to hyperviscosity; blood flow to all organ systems is impaired by sluggish circulation. Pulmonary blood flow can be dramatically compromised, resulting in pulmonary hypertension, retained lung fluid, and respiratory distress syndrome. Taxation of the heart by an increased vascular load can lead to congestive heart failure and left to right shunting across the foramen ovale or ductus arteriosus. Sludging of blood in the microcirculation of the kidneys can lead to renal vein thrombosis and renal failure. Impairment of blood flow to the bowel can lead to necrotizing enterocolitis.

Treatment

Although most infants with polycythemia are asymptomatic or minimally symptomatic, the hematocrit level and the presence of symptoms, even if minimal, should form the basis of treatment. Because hematocrit levels of 65% can lead to neurologic abnormalities and levels of 75% or higher are always associated with neurologic changes, an infant with a venous hematocrit of 65% or higher should be considered for partial exchange transfusion.

Partial exchange results in dramatic improvement in symptomatic infants, relieving congestive failure and improving CNS function. It also corrects hypoglycemia, relieves respiratory distress and cyanosis, and improves renal function.

Partial exchange transfusion should be done as the venous hematocrit (Hct) approaches 65% and as symptoms appear; 5% albumin or crystalloid is suggested as replacement for the removed aliquot of blood. With the advent of stricter precautions for prevention of viral transmission by blood products, use of fresh-frozen plasma would not seem advisable. The formula for calculating the partial replacement of blood volume is

$$\text{Replacement volume} = \frac{\text{Observed Hct} - \text{Desired Hct}}{\text{Observed Hct}} \times \text{Blood volume}$$

Collaborative Management of the Infant with Polycythemia.

The care of any newborn infant should include a screening hematocrit determination for polycythemia by 12 hours of age.

This allows both detection of any infant with polycythemia and adequate observation before symptoms become apparent. Because the initial sample usually is obtained by heel stick or finger stick, detection of a high value should be followed by venipuncture confirmation. The infant should be kept adequately hydrated and closely monitored for hypoglycemia and hypocalcemia. A hematocrit value over 65% should prompt careful observation of the infant for any symptoms associated with hyperviscosity. If symptoms appear, the infant should undergo partial exchange transfusion. During the partial exchange, the same care should be provided as that given during a single-volume or double-volume exchange transfusion.

COAGULOPATHIES IN THE NEWBORN PERIOD

Coagulation disorders are present in approximately 1% of all infants admitted to newborn nurseries, the incidence being much higher in sick term or preterm infants. In one study, at autopsy 40% of all infant deaths in the NICU were associated with hemorrhage or thrombosis (Hathaway & Bonnar, 1978). Bleeding disorders affecting the newborn can be classified as (1) intensification of existing transient deficiencies of the coagulation mechanism, (2) disturbances of coagulation associated with certain disease states, (3) inherited deficiencies, or (4) abnormalities of platelets or vascular structures.

Development of Hemostasis and Coagulation

Embryologic Development of Coagulation Factors and Platelets.   The components involved in blood coagulation and fibrinolysis (dissolution of a formed clot) are produced in the liver, vascular wall, and tissue during early fetal life. Many of the clotting factors (procoagulants) and anticoagulants (inhibitors) can be identified during the eighth to twelfth weeks of gestation. However, procoagulants, anticoagulants, and the substances responsible for dissolution of a clot, fibrinolytics, do not increase in number and function or reach adult levels simultaneously (Tables 30-6, 30-7, and 30-8). Some components increase with increasing gestational age, whereas others achieve normal adult levels several weeks to months before the fetus reaches term. Still other components do not achieve normal adult levels until several weeks to months after birth. Although the function of coagulation factors and anticoagulants in the fetus is not identical to that in an older child or adult, initial vascular response to injury by release of tissue thromboplastin is functional in the fetus as early as 8 weeks.

Another major coagulation component, the megakaryocyte, which develops from pluripotent hematopoietic stem cells, can be identified in the embryonic yolk sac at 5 to 6 weeks' gestation. The site of megakaryocyte production changes with either migration of stem cells from the yolk sac or formation of a new colony of stem cells in the fetal liver, spleen and, subsequently, bone marrow. These platelet precursors are identifiable in the fetal liver by 6 weeks' gestation. Two distinct phases of hepatic thrombopoiesis produce two different types of megakaryocytes; those produced during the early phase are less differentiated and smaller than the adult form, whereas those produced during the late phase more closely resemble the adult form in size and nuclear characteristics. True adult-size megakaryocytes do not develop until the end of the first year of life.

Megakaryocytes develop thin cytoplasmic projections that can penetrate and cross the endothelium of the organ in which

TABLE **30-6**	Normal Coagulation Test Results and Blood Levels of Coagulation Factors in the Fetus (19 to 27 Weeks' Gestation) and Newborn (28 Weeks' Gestation to Term)					
Test/Factors	19 to 27 Weeks (Mean ± SD)	28 to 31 Weeks Mean (Boundary)	30 to 36 Weeks, Day 1 Mean (Boundary)	30 to 36 Weeks, Day 5 Mean (Boundary)	Full Term, Day 1 Mean (Boundary)	Full Term, Day 5 Mean (Boundary)
Tests						
Prothrombin time (PT) (seconds)	—	15.4 (14.6 to 16.9)	13 (10.6 to 16.2)	12.5 (10 to 15.3)	13 (10.1 to 15.9)	12.4 (10 to 15.3)
Activated partial thromboplastin time (AAPTT) (seconds)	—	108 (80 to 168)	53.6 (27.5 to 79.4)	50.5 (26.9 to 74.1)	42.9 (31.3 to 54.5)	42.6 (25.4 to 59.8)
Thrombin clotting time (TCT) (seconds)	—	—	24.8 (19.2 to 30.4)	24.1 (18.8 to 29.4)	23.5 (19 to 28.3)	23.1 (18 to 29.2)
Factor						
Fibrinogen (g/L)	1 ± 0.4	2.56 (1.6 to 5.5)	2.43 (1.5 to 3.73)	2.8 (1.6 to 4.18)	2.83 (1.67 to 3.99)	3.12 (1.62 to 4.62)
Factor II (U/ml)	0.12 ± 0.02	0.31 (0.19 to 0.54)	0.45 (0.2 to 0.77)	0.57 (0.29 to 0.85)	0.48 (0.26 to 0.7)	0.63 (0.33 to 0.93)
Factor V (U/ml)	0.41 ± 0.1	0.65 (0.43 to 0.8)	0.88 (0.41 to 1.44)	1 (0.46 to 1.54)	0.72 (0.34 to 1.08)	0.95 (0.45 to 1.45)
Factor VII (U/ml)	0.28 ± 0.04	0.37 (0.24 to 0.76)	0.67 (0.21 to 1.13)	0.84 (0.3 to 1.38)	0.66 (0.28 to 1.04)	0.89 (0.35 to 1.43)
Factor VIII (U/ml)	0.39 ± 0.14	0.79 (0.37 to 1.26)	1.11 (0.5 to 2.13)	1.15 (0.53 to 2.05)	1 (0.5 to 1.78)	0.88 (0.5 to 1.54)
von Willebrand factor (vWF) (U/ml)	0.64 ± 0.13	1.41 (0.83 to 2.23)	1.36 (0.78 to 2.1)	1.33 (0.72 to 2.19)	1.53 (0.5 to 2.87)	1.4 (0.5 to 2.54)
Factor IX (U/ml)	0.1 ± 0.01	0.18 (0.17 to 0.2)	0.35 (0.19 to 0.65)	0.42 (0.14 to 0.74)	0.53 (0.15 to 0.91)	0.53 (0.15 to 0.91)
Factor X (U/ml)	0.21 ± 0.03	0.36 (0.25 to 0.64)	0.41 (0.11 to 0.71)	0.51 (0.19 to 0.83)	0.4 (0.12 to 0.68)	0.49 (0.19 to 0.79)
Factor XI (U/ml)		0.23 (0.11 to 0.33)	0.3 (0.08 to 0.52)	0.41 (0.13 to 0.69)	0.38 (0.1 to 0.66)	0.55 (0.23 to 0.87)
Factor XII (U/ml)	0.22 ± 0.03	0.25 (0.05 to 0.35)	0.38 (0.1 to 0.66)	0.39 (0.09 to 0.69)	0.53 (0.13 to 0.93)	0.47 (0.11 to 0.83)
Prekallikrein (PK) (U/ml)		0.26 (0.15 to 0.32)	0.33 (0.09 to 0.57)	0.45 (0.26 to 0.75)	0.37 (0.18 to 0.69)	0.48 (0.2 to 0.76)
High-molecular-weight kininogen (HMWK) (U/ml)		0.32 (0.19 to 0.52)	0.49 (0.09 to 0.89)	0.62 (0.24 to 1)	0.54 (0.06 to 1.02)	0.74 (0.16 to 1.32)
Factor XIIIa (U/ml)		—	0.7 (0.32 to 1.08)	1.01 (0.57 to 1.45)	0.79 (0.27 to 1.31)	0.94 (0.44 to 1.44)
Factor XIIIb (U/ml)		—	0.81 (0.35 to 1.27)	1.1 (0.68 to 1.58)	0.76 (0.3 to 1.22)	1.06 (0.32 to 1.8)
Plasminogen (U/ml)		—	1.7 (1.12 to 2.48)	1.91 (1.21 to 2.61)	1.95 ± 0.35 (44)	2.17 ± 0.38 (60)

Modified from Andrew M et al (1990). Development of the hemostatic system in the neonate and young infant. American journal of pediatric hematology/oncology 12:97-98; Andrew M et al (1987). Development of the human coagulation system in the full-term infant. Blood 70:166; and Andrew M et al (1988). Development of the human coagulation system in the healthy premature infant. Blood 72:1653.

TABLE **30-7**   Normal Blood Levels of Coagulation Inhibitors in Newborns (30 Weeks' Gestation to Term)

Coagulation Inhibitors	30 TO 36 WEEKS' GESTATION		FULL TERM	
	Day 1 Mean (Boundary)	Day 5 Mean (Boundary)	Day 1 Mean (Boundary)	Day 5 Mean (Boundary)
Antithrombin III (ATIII) (U/ml)	0.38 (0.14 to 0.62)	0.56 (0.3 to 0.82)	0.63 (0.39 to 0.87)	0.67 (0.41 to 0.93)
Alpha$_2$-macroglobulin (α_2-M) (U/ml)	1.1 (0.56 to 1.82)	1.25 (0.71 to 1.77)	1.39 (0.95 to 1.83)	1.48 (0.98 to 1.98)
C1 esterase inhibitor (C1E-NH) (U/ml)	0.65 (0.31 to 0.99)	0.83 (0.45 to 1.21)	0.72 (0.36 to 1.08)	0.90 (0.6 to 1.2)
Alpha$_1$-antitrypsin (α_1-AT) (U/ml)	0.9 (0.36 to 1.44)	0.94 (0.42 to 1.46)	0.93 (0.49 to 1.37)	0.89 (0.49 to 1.29)
Heparin cofactor II (HCII) (U/ml)	0.32 (0.1 to 0.6)	0.34 (0.1 to 0.69)	0.43 (0.1 to 0.93)	0.48 (0.1 to 0.96)
Protein C (U/ml)	0.28 (0.12 to 0.44)	0.31 (0.11 to 0.51)	0.35 (0.17 to 0.53)	0.42 (0.2 to 0.64)
Protein S (U/ml)	0.26 (0.14 to 0.38)	0.37 (0.13 to 0.61)	0.36 (0.12 to 0.6)	0.5 (0.22 to 0.78)

Modified from Andrew M et al (1990). Development of the hemostatic system in the neonate and young infant. American journal of pediatric hematology/oncology 12:98-99; Andrew M et al (1987). Development of the human coagulation system in the full-term infant. Blood 70:167; and Andrew M et al (1988). Development of the human coagulation system in the healthy premature infant. Blood 72:1653.

TABLE **30-8**   Normal Blood Levels of Fibrinolytic Components in Premature and Term Newborns

Fibrinolytic Component	PREMATURE INFANTS		FULL-TERM INFANTS	
	Day 1 Mean (Boundary)	Day 5 Mean (Boundary)	Day 1 Mean (Boundary)	Day 5 Mean (Boundary)
Plasminogen (U/ml)	1.7 (1.12 to 2.48)	1.91 (1.21 to 2.61)	1.95 (1.25 to 2.65)	2.17 (1.41 to 2.93)
Tissue plasminogen activator (TPA) (ng/ml)	8.48 (3 to 16.7)	3.97 (2 to 6.93)	9.6 (5 to 18.9)	5.6 (4 to 10)
Alpha$_2$-antiplasmin (α_2-AP) (U/ml)	0.78 (0.4 to 1.16)	0.81 (0.49 to 1.13)	0.85 (0.55 to 1.15)	1 (0.7 to 1.3)
Plasminogen activator inhibitor (PAI) (U/ml)	5.4 (0 to 12.2)	2.5 (0 to 7.1)	6.4 (2 to 15.1)	2.3 (0 to 8.1)

Modified from Andrew M et al (1990). Development of the hemostatic system in the neonate and young infant. American journal of pediatric hematology/oncology 12:102-103.

they are produced, eventually coming into contact with a blood vessel. These cytoplasmic projections then develop constrictions that pinch off the distal ends, resulting in fragments called platelets. Although erythropoietin and thrombopoietin are involved in the initial stem cell differentiation, the actual inducer of megakaryocyte fragmentation and platelet production is unknown. At 32 weeks' gestation, platelet levels are comparable to those of an adult, but platelet function is not.

Hemostasis

Hemostasis consists of a delicate and dynamic balance between factors that prevent exsanguination and those that keep the blood in a fluid form. The balanced interrelationship among four distinct components ensures orderly hemostasis and fibrinolysis when vascular integrity is destroyed or interrupted. The four constituents are:

- Vascular components: The components of the vascular wall affect the structure and function of damaged blood vessels. Vascular spasm is the first mechanism by which hemostasis is achieved in a damaged vessel.
- Platelets and their activating substances: Formation of a platelet plug is the second mechanism of hemostasis after vascular injury has occurred.
- Coagulation or plasma factors: These factors consist of procoagulants and anticoagulants (inhibitors). Coagulation completes the hemostatic mechanism by strengthening the platelet plug.
- The fibrinolytic pathway: This pathway contributes to disintegration of the clot and re-establishment of normal circulatory flow. It consists of fibrinolytics (substances that lyse a fibrin clot) and inhibitors.

Initial Steps in Hemostasis

Vascular Spasm.   Initial hemostasis in a ruptured blood vessel consists of vascular spasm, a consequence of multiple mediator interactions, nervous reflexes, and localized muscle spasm. Although nervous reflexes are a response to pain, most of the vascular spasm is due to muscle contraction in the vessel wall secondary to direct injury. This vascular response to injury is present in an 8-week fetus and at term is the equivalent of adult norms in regard to capillary fragility and bleeding time. This component is gestational age dependent, as is evident in the increased capillary fragility shown by the preterm infant.

Platelet Plug Formation.   Platelets coming into contact with an injured vascular wall adhere to the wall and form a platelet plug. This hemostatic plug is the primary means of closing small vascular holes at the capillary and small vessel level. The platelets' ability to adhere on contact to a denuded vascular wall requires a glycoprotein, von Willebrand factor, which is synthesized by vascular endothelial cells and megakaryocytes. von Willebrand factor complexes with Factor VIII (antihemophilic factor), and both circulate jointly.

Platelets also have the ability to aggregate (stick to other platelets), forming large clumps. Aggregation is made possible by the platelet's ability to modify its shape and to secrete many biochemical substances (platelet release reaction) that enhance cohesion. When platelets and associated glycoproteins are activated by excess release of these biochemical substances during times of stress, fibrinogen receptors appear on the surface of the platelet. These receptors enhance the platelet's ability to bind fibrinogen, which in turn cross-links the platelets, allowing them to aggregate. This provides a tight mesh of clot

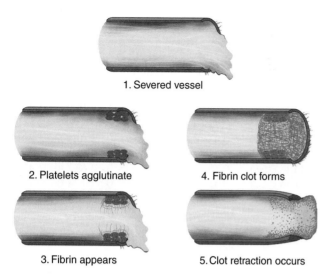

1. Severed vessel

2. Platelets agglutinate

4. Fibrin clot forms

3. Fibrin appears

5. Clot retraction occurs

FIGURE **30-17**

When vessel wall injury occurs, the initial clotting process begins with the formation of a platelet plug. Platelet activation stimulates fibrinogen receptors found on the surface of the platelets, which enhance their aggregation with other platelets and fibrinogen. The fibrin clot that forms retracts and occludes the damaged vascular wall. Redrawn from Guyton AC, Hall JE (2000). Hemostasis and blood coagulation. In Guyton AC, Hall JE, editors. *Textbook of medical physiology*, ed 10. WB Saunders: Philadelphia. From Seegers Witt (1948). *Hemostatic agents*. Courtesy of Charles C. Thomas, Springfield, Il.

around an injured vessel that controls bleeding (Figure 30-17). After 32 weeks' gestation, average platelet counts are comparable to those of term infants and adults, but the ability of platelets to aggregate is diminished.

Coagulation

When bleeding cannot be controlled with merely a platelet plug, circulating plasma coagulation factors are triggered to form a network of fibrin that turns the existing plug into a hemostatic seal. Fibrin threads, necessary to clot formation, can develop within 15 to 20 seconds in the presence of normal coagulation factors. Within 3 to 6 minutes after vascular rupture, the entire opening is occluded by clot; within 30 to 60 minutes, the clot begins to retract, pulling the injured vascular portions together and further sealing the vascular end. This coagulation reaction involves several plasma proteins and three distinct phases. The first phase involves the formation of prothrombin activator, the second involves the activation of prothrombin to thrombin (formation of thrombin), and the third involves the conversion of soluble fibrinogen to fibrin (fibrin clot formation) (Guyton & Hall, 1996b).

Phase I: Formation of Prothrombin Activator. According to the earliest theories on coagulation (cascade theory), prothrombin activator can be generated by two separate pathways, the intrinsic and extrinsic pathways. The intrinsic pathway is triggered by trauma or damage that occurs inside

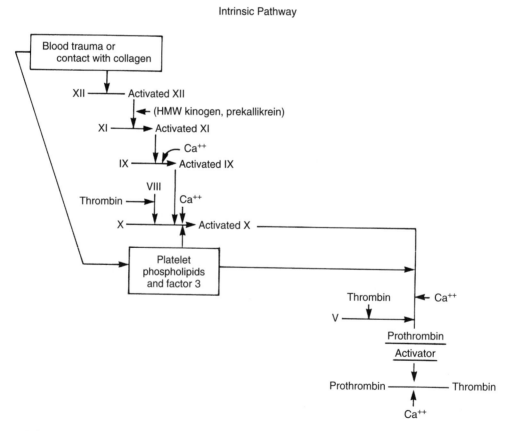

FIGURE **30-18**

The intrinsic pathway for initiating the clotting cascade is activated by trauma to the blood, injury within the vessel, or contact with collagen. *HMW*, High molecular weight. From Guyton AC, Hall JE (2000). Hemostasis and blood coagulation. In Guyton AC, Hall JE, editors. *Textbook of medical physiology*, ed 10. WB Saunders: Philadelphia.

the vessel or to the blood itself, and the extrinsic pathway is triggered by the production of tissue thromboplastin that is generated by vessel wall damage. This bimodal pathway can be interrupted or negated by a deficiency in platelets or any of the plasma coagulation factors or by the presence of inhibitors (anticoagulants) in the plasma. Selective activation of one of these pathways depends on the site and severity of injury.

Activation of the intrinsic pathway is slower because it lacks the major stimulus of the extrinsic pathway, tissue thromboplastin generated by vessel wall damage. The intrinsic pathway relies on blood trauma or injury within the vessel to alter platelets and plasma proteins and to convert dormant factors (zymogens), naturally found in circulating blood, into active proteolytic enzymes (Figure 30-18). Each activated enzyme subsequently reacts with the succeeding factor, changing it into its activated form. The steps of intrinsic activation of coagulation are as follows:

1. An activator (blood trauma, injury within the vessel, or contact with collagen) activates Factor XII, converting it to Factor XIIa, while simultaneously damaging platelets, which causes a release of platelet phospholipids.
2. Factor XIIa, in conjunction with prekallikrein and high-molar-weight kininogen, activates Factor XI, converting it to Factor XIa.
3. Factor XIa activates Factor IX, converting it to Factor IXa.
4. Factor IXa, platelet phospholipid, and Factor VIII combine to activate Factor X, converting it to Factor Xa.
5. Factor Xa combines with Factor V and platelet phospholipids to form prothrombin activator (prothrombinase), which releases

thrombin from prothrombin. Calcium is required for this and the preceding two steps.

The extrinsic pathway can generate thrombin in a matter of seconds when injury occurs outside the vascular space (Figure 30-19). Tissue thromboplastin (tissue factor), composed of glycoproteins and phospholipids, is produced when tissue is injured. When plasma comes in contact with this substance, the initial intrinsic phases are bypassed and the following responses occur:

1. Tissue thromboplastin or tissue factor (Factor III) activates Factor VII to Factor VIIa. These two factors form a complex with glycoprotein in the presence of ionized calcium (tissue factor-Factor VIIa complex) that activates Factor X, converting it to Factor Xa.
2. In the presence of calcium, Factor Xa forms complexes with phospholipids and Factor V to form prothrombin activator.

From this point on, the intrinsic and extrinsic pathways are identical, with both proceeding to phase II.

In an effort to explain discrepancies in factor deficiencies that do not follow the premises of the clotting cascade, Gailani and associates (1991) proposed an alternate (Figure 30-20) that abandons the strict delineation between the intrinsic and extrinsic pathways. Gailani's hypothesis of coagulation modifies the traditional clotting cascade by proposing that the tissue factor-Factor VIIa complex of the extrinsic pathway can directly activate Factor IX. The hypothesis also proposes that Factor VII can be activated by Factors XIIa, IXa, Xa, and thrombin. If the activity of Factor VIIa does indeed modify the clotting cascade by directly activating Factor IX, which directly converts Factor X to Factor Xa, it bypasses several steps

Extrinsic Pathway

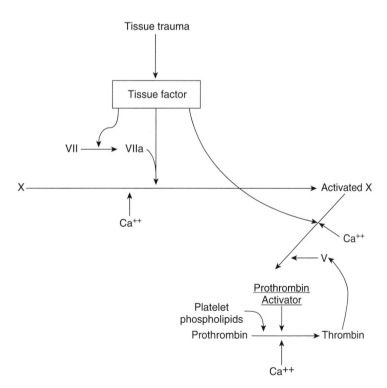

FIGURE **30-19**
The extrinsic pathway for initiating the clotting cascade can generate thrombin rapidly as a result of thromboplastin release from injured tissue. From Guyton AC, Hall JE (2000). Hemostasis and blood coagulation. In Guyton AC, Hall JE, editors. *Textbook of medical physiology*, ed 10. WB Saunders: Philadelphia.

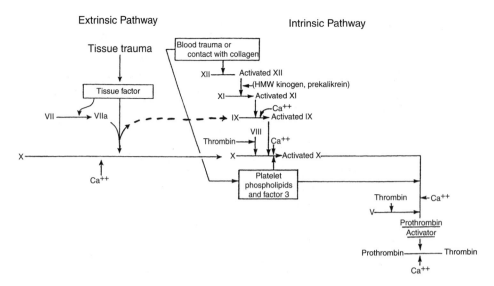

FIGURE **30-20**

The modified cascade theory of coagulation, as postulated by Gailini and associates, blurs the strict separation of intrinsic and extrinsic pathways. It proposes that the tissue factor-Factor VIIa complex enters the intrinsic pathway and activates both Factor VIII and Factor X via the extrinsic pathway. Factor VII can also be activated by Factors XIIa, IXa, Xa, and thrombin. From Guyton AC, Hall JE (2000). Hemostastis and blood coagulation. In Guyton AC, Hall JE, editors. *Textbook of medical physiology*, ed 10. WB Saunders: Philadelphia.

of the extrinsic pathway and could be the principle initiator of coagulation.

Phase II: Formation of Thrombin.

Prothrombin activator from either of the two pathways continues the clotting cascade by further influencing the break down of the unstable plasma protein prothrombin. Prothrombin (Factor II) is synthesized by the liver under the influence of vitamin K, along with the other factors that form the prothrombin complex (Factors VII, IX, and X). When acted on by prothrombin activator, prothrombin forms the potent coagulant thrombin. The newly formed thrombin stimulates completion of the third and final phase of coagulation.

Phase III: Fibrin Clot Formation

Procoagulants. Thrombin promotes the conversion of fibrinogen (Factor I), a protein produced by the liver, into fibrin by splitting off two peptides from the soluble fibrinogen molecule. This exposes two sites, to which other split fibrin molecules can cross-link, forming an insoluble fibrin chain. Fibrin stabilizing factor (Factor XIII) further strengthens the tight bond of this developing fibrin mesh. Fibrin stabilizing factor is naturally found in the plasma and is also secreted by entrapped platelets. The forming fibrin clot begins to contract and retract with the help of platelets that have actin-myosin action, the same action by which a muscle works. Extension of the clot into the surrounding circulating blood promotes further thrombosis. Thrombin from the clot has the ability to cleave prothrombin into more thrombin and enhances the production of prothrombin activator, thus acting as a potent biofeedback system for perpetuation of the clotting cascade.

Anticoagulants. Throughout the entire coagulation pathway, the action of the activated enzymes is modulated at each stage by multiple and specific inhibitors (anticoagulants). Consequently, coagulation is a process of balance between coagulation factors and naturally occurring inhibitors. Some of these anticoagulants are endothelial surface factors that prevent coagulation until the vessel's endothelial wall is damaged. One such factor is the smoothness of the wall, which prevents any adherence and subsequent activation; another is the monomolecular layer of protein covering the wall, which repels plasma clotting factors and platelets.

Two inhibitors, alpha$_1$-antitrypsin and C1 esterase inhibitor, interfere with the coagulation factors involved in the initial activation of the intrinsic pathway, as does Factor Xa despite its role in cleaving prothrombin into thrombin. Factor Xa rapidly binds with a tissue factor pathway inhibitor (TFPI) found in the plasma. This complex, TFPI-Factor Xa, joins with the tissue factor-Factor VIIa complex to form a quaternary complex that inhibits further activation of Factor X by tissue factor (Edstrom et al, 2000).

Thrombin also acts as its own inhibitor by stimulating activation of protein C, which inactivates Factors V and VIII in the presence of another vitamin K-dependent inhibitor, protein S. A deficiency of these two proteins has been implicated in cases of neonatal thrombosis.

Other inhibitors of thrombin formation are (1) fibrin threads created during clot formation, which absorb thrombin, thus removing it from circulation and eliminating its potential for further coagulation; (2) thrombomodulin, found on the endothelial surfaces of the body and in the plasma complexes with thrombin, which eliminates thrombin's ability to cleave fibrinogen; (3) alpha$_2$-macroglobulin, which inhibits proteases, including thrombin; (4) antithrombin III, which combines with thrombin, blocking the conversion of fibrinogen into fibrin; and (5) heparin cofactor II, which removes several activated procoagulants. Both antithrombin III and heparin are

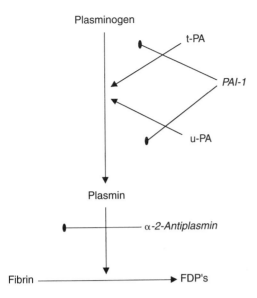

FIGURE **30-21**
The components of the fibrinolytic system involved in the lysis of a fibrin clot. *t-PA*, Tissue plasminogen activator; *PAI-1*, plasminogen activator inhibitor; *u-PA*, urokinase plasminogen activator; *FDPs*, fibrin degradation products. Modified from Edstrom C et al (2000). Developmental aspects of blood hemostasis and disorders of coagulation and fibrinolysis in the neonatal period. In Christensen R, editors. *Hematologic problems of the neonate*. WB Saunders: Philadelphia.

produced in the precapillary connective tissue of the lungs and liver.

Fibrinolysis.   Once a clot develops, it can be invaded by fibroblasts that lay down connective tissue throughout the clot or it can be dissolved. The process of dissolution occurs by activation of naturally occurring factors that lyse the clot. Fibrinolysis is activated simultaneously with stimulation of the coagulation system, with powerful but inactivated anticoagulants built right into the clot (Figure 30-21). One of these anticoagulants, plasminogen, is manufactured by the liver, kidneys, and eosinophils. Under the influence of thrombin, activated Factor XII, tissue plasminogen activator (t-PA; located on the vascular endothelium) and urokinase plasminogen activator (u-PA; found in the urine), plasminogen is converted into plasmin, a proteolytic enzyme that breaks down fibrin into fibrin split products. Plasmin not only digests the fibrin chains but also deactivates fibrinogen; Factors V, VII, and XII; and prothrombin. Plasmin can be inactivated by its inhibitor, alpha$_2$-antiplasmin; tissue plasminogen activator can be inactivated by its inhibitor, plasminogen activator inhibitor-1.

Overall Development of Hemostasis

In summary, both term and preterm newborns have the ability to create a balance between transitory deficiencies in the amount and function of a variety of clotting factors, platelets, and anticoagulant factors. The homeostasis between clotting factors and anticoagulants places the newborn in a mildly hypercoagulable state at birth. Compared with older children and adults, therefore, the newborn has no greater tendency to bleed but does have several differences in regard to coagulation components and reserves, including (1) gestational age-dependent variations in the concentrations of coagulation fac-

tors, anticoagulants, and fibrinolytics; (2) a faster turnover rate of components; (3) a slower rate of synthesis of components; and (4) limited ability to supply necessary components during times of increased need.

COMMON COAGULATION DISORDERS IN THE NEWBORN

Hemorrhagic Disease of the Newborn

The liver produces most of the clotting factors, including those of the prothrombin complex. Adequate function of this complex requires the specific action of vitamin K, which is continuously synthesized by bacteria in the bowel. Vitamin K is not directly involved in the synthesis of these factors but is required for the conversion of precursor proteins produced by the liver into active factors having coagulant capabilities. Vitamin K is especially necessary for conversion of prothrombin binding sites into forms that can bind calcium, which is required for the completion of many steps in the clotting cascade.

Vitamin K–dependent factors reach approximately 30% to 70% of adult levels in the cord blood of term infants but quickly drop to half that amount if the infant is not given vitamin K. Because these factors are gestational age dependent, the more premature the infant, the lower the levels at birth. The exaggerated drop after birth may be due to poor placental transfer of maternal vitamin K, immature liver function, and delayed synthesis of vitamin K by the bowel. Vitamin K-dependent factors slowly rise but do not reach normal adult levels until approximately 9 months of age. Administration of approximately 25 μg (0.025 mg) of vitamin K can prevent this decline and normalize the prothrombin time.

Hemorrhage during the early neonatal period that can be attributed to a deficiency of vitamin K-dependent factors is classified as hemorrhagic disease of the newborn, of which there are three identified forms. The early form, the least common type, is characterized by bleeding within the first 24 hours of life, usually associated with maternal anticonvulsant therapy. It is theorized that anticonvulsants may induce fetal hepatic enzymes involved in the degradation of already low levels of fetal vitamin K. Early neonatal bleeding cannot be prevented by postnatal administration of vitamin K. Daily antenatal administration of large doses of oral vitamin K (10 mg) to mothers receiving anticonvulsant therapy for at least 10 days before delivery was found to be beneficial to the newborn. Vitamin K crosses the placenta, elevating newborn levels of vitamin K for 10 days after birth, with the increase in levels correlating with the timing of the last prenatal dose.

The classic form of hemorrhagic disease usually occurs during the first 2 to 5 days of life and manifests as generalized and, occasionally, dramatic bleeding. The most common sites are the gastrointestinal tract, umbilicus, circumcision site, skin, and internal organs. The usual cause is inadequate intake of breast milk in an infant who has not received prophylactic vitamin K. Breast milk provides adequate vitamin K to prevent this disorder if it is taken in sufficient quantities.

The late form of hemorrhagic disease, which occurs after the first week of life, is more devastating than the early form because of the higher incidence of intracranial hemorrhage (the risk approaches 63%). Permanent neurologic sequelae are seen in 24% of affected infants, and the mortality rate can be as high as 14%. This form of hemorrhagic disease is associated with chronic disease states that interfere with fat absorption or the performance of intestinal flora. Both early and late hemorrhagic disease of the newborn are intensified in breastfed infants.

Definitive diagnosis rests on a history of lack of vitamin K prophylaxis at birth and a prolonged prothrombin time (Figure 30-22), which measures the prothrombin complex clotting factors (Factors II, VII, IX, and X). One test, the protein induced by vitamin K absence or antagonist-II (PIVKA-II) test, is useful in identifying proteins induced by vitamin K deficiency that appear in the plasma of vitamin K-deficient infants. These proteins consist of the inert and functionally defective precursors of prothrombin that are produced when vitamin K levels are deficient.

Several factors can predispose an infant to hemorrhagic disease of the newborn. Almost all these factors involve some form of hepatic dysfunction. The most obvious predisposing factor is failure of an infant to receive prophylactic vitamin K postnatally. Other risk factors include maternal ingestion of anticonvulsants and coumarin anticoagulants (which interfere with the action of the prothrombin complex factors), birth asphyxia, prolonged labor, and breastfeeding. Human milk has a lower vitamin K content than cow's milk. Infants receiving a commercial formula for 24 hours have prothrombin times similar to those of infants receiving vitamin K after birth. Infants with hepatic dysfunction or bowel malabsorption, although not found strictly in the early neonatal period, can develop vitamin K deficiency despite having received prophylaxis at birth. Such disorders as chronic diarrhea, biliary atresia, hepatitis, cystic fibrosis, and prolonged parenteral nutrition do not allow adequate vitamin K production and can result in low prothrombin complex factors. These infants benefit from weekly vitamin K supplementation (1 mg given intramuscularly), the dose recommended by the AAP (1998) for postnatal newborn prophylaxis. The suggested preparation for adminis-

tration to the newborn is the natural aqueous solution of vitamin K rather than the synthetic preparation, which can cause hemolysis. Because of preterm infants' hepatic immaturity and inability to effectively synthesize clotting factors, these infants' response to vitamin K is not as predictable as that of term infants.

Controversy continues over whether intramuscular or oral prophylaxis should be used. At one time, intramuscular administration of vitamin K was linked to the occurrence of childhood cancers; however, this charge has not been substantiated by research. The use of one or two oral doses of vitamin K as an effective treatment is also disputed, and research is needed to determine its efficacy. Research continues in an effort to determine the appropriate timing and number of oral doses of vitamin K and to develop a better oral preparation. Alternative therapies are also being investigated, including antenatal maternal dosing to prevent antenatal intraventricular hemorrhage and postnatal maternal dosing as prophylaxis in the breastfed infant.

Kumar and colleagues (2001) reported that premature infants have high plasma vitamin K levels in the first 2 weeks of life as a result of intramuscular and parenteral supplementation. These researchers measured vitamin K levels in infants who were given 1 mg of vitamin K intramuscularly at birth and who then were given vitamin K parenterally at a dosage of 60 μg/day for those weighing less than 1000 g and 130 μg/day for those weighing more than 1000 g. This research suggests that further studies need to focus on vitamin K levels in the premature infant and attempts need to be made to determine the adequate dose.

Active bleeding caused by hemorrhagic disease of the newborn may require blood replacement or the use of fresh-frozen plasma for immediate clotting factor replacement.

Hemophilia

Classic hemophilia (hemophilia A) is the most frequently inherited coagulation abnormality, accounting for 90% of all genetically linked coagulopathies and 85% of all hemophilias. It is passed from mother to son as an X-linked trait and is caused by Factor VIII deficiency. Factor VIII has two components, a large glycoprotein, known as von Willebrand factor (vWF), which is required for proper platelet adhesion, and a small procoagulant protein, the antihemophilic factor (AHF), which is defective in hemophilia A. Hemophilia A involves the production of structurally and functionally ineffective clotting factors rather than a deficiency in quantity.

The concentration of circulating AHF in the serum determines the severity of the disease. Levels of 1% to 2% are associated with severe disease, 2% to 5% with moderate disease, and over 5% with mild disease, a level at which active bleeding rarely occurs. In a retrospective study of hemophiliacs, approximately 44% of a group of severe hemophiliacs were symptomatic during the first week of life, whereas only 14% of a mildly affected group displayed any bleeding during the first 7 days of life.

Infants affected with hemophilia have a prolonged partial thromboplastin time, but the prothrombin time, thrombin time, and platelet count are relatively normal. The major symptom of hemophilia is bleeding, most often from the circumcision site, scalp, umbilicus, and brain. Not all severe hemophiliacs bleed after circumcision in the early newborn period. The reason for this is unknown, but it has been suggested that tissue thromboplastin release, caused by the cir-

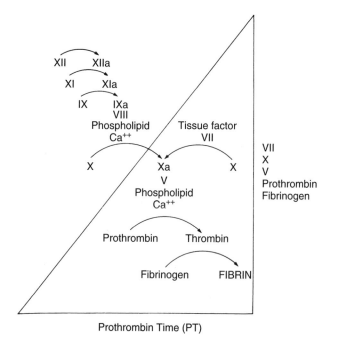

FIGURE 30-22
Prothrombin time (PT) measures the prothrombin complex, which consists of Factors II (prothrombin), VII, IX, and X. These factors depend on vitamin K for synthesis. PT is also a measurement of the extrinsic pathway of coagulation. *Ca,* Calcium. From Lusher J (1987). Diseases of coagulation: the fluid phase. In Nathan D, Oski F, editors. *Hematology of infancy and childhood,* ed 3. WB Saunders: Philadelphia.

cumcision clamp on the foreskin, may initiate the extrinsic pathway and clotting cascade, preventing excessive bleeding.

Diagnosis. Prenatal diagnosis is possible, but the results are not always accurate. Diagnosis involves measurement of the ratio of factor antigen to coagulant antigen on blood samples of fetuses of more than 20 weeks' gestation. If diagnosed with Factor VIII deficiency, the infant should also be evaluated for von Willebrand disease.

Treatment. The ultimate goal of treatment for hemophilia A is to raise the defective or deficient factor to a level that will prevent bleeding; that is, to raise the concentration of AHF to a level of 20%. It is suggested that multiple donor factor concentrates be avoided, but if they are necessary, a pasteurized form should be used. This reduces the risk of transmittable viral diseases such as hepatitis and human immunodeficiency virus (HIV) infection. Acquired immunodeficiency syndrome (AIDS) is now the second most frequent cause of death in those with hemophilia.

Another mode of therapy is the use of cryoprecipitate, obtained by the single donor method, at a dosage of 10 U/kg. Each unit per kilogram raises the AHF level by 1.5% to 2%; a bag of cryoprecipitate contains 80 U. Fresh-frozen plasma, also from a single donor, can be used, but it replenishes multiple factor deficiencies rather than being a specific factor therapy.

Two alternative methods of treatment for mild hemophilia that raise both components of Factor VIII twofold to threefold are 1-desamino-8-D-arginine-vasopressin (DDAVP) as an injection and desmopressin acetate as a nasal spray. The effectiveness and applicability of these two therapies in the newborn are still unknown, but currently they are not recommended for treatment if the AHF level is below 5% or if the infant is younger than 11 months of age. Amicar, an antifibrinolytic agent, has also shown some benefit.

Clinical trials are underway to test the applicability and effectiveness of recombinant Factor VIII in the treatment of hemophilia A. Recombinant Factor VIII would eliminate the transmission of potentially dangerous viral diseases from donor to recipient.

Thrombocytopenia

The normal range of platelets is 150,000 to 450,000/mm^3; the average count in the newborn is approximately 250,000/mm^3. Platelet counts below 150,000/mm^3 are considered abnormal and should be subject to investigation for a possible pathologic process. Platelet function in the neonate reaches normal adult levels between the fifth to ninth postnatal days. Although 14% of all preterm infants and 4% of all term infants are thrombocytopenic, with platelet counts below 150,000/mm^3, not all of these infants are ill.

Thrombocytopenia is the most common bleeding disorder in the newborn; 20% of all NICU admissions have platelet counts below 50,000/mm^3, and 80% of sick infants have counts below 100,000/mm^3. However, the pathogenesis of the thrombocytopenia can be determined in only 60% of these infants. Abnormalities of the platelet count are due to increased destruction or decreased production, and the underlying cause is mediated by maternal, placental, neonatal, or iatrogenic factors. In most thrombocytopenic newborns, platelet counts are low as a result of increased destruction rather than bone marrow depression. The overall mortality rate for infants with thrombocytopenia is 34%; 22% of these infants exhibit a bleed-ing diathesis. Infants with a platelet count below 20,000/mm^3 are at particularly high risk for bleeding.

Maternal Factors. Thrombocytopenia is the most common form of hemostatic problem present during pregnancy; 5% to 7% of healthy mothers have platelet counts below 150,000/mm^3. Some of the maternal factors associated with thrombocytopenia are maternal drug ingestion (e.g., chloramphenicol, hydralazine, tolbutamide, and thiazides), maternal eclampsia and hypertension, placental infarction, and immune-mediated maternal platelet antibodies.

Immune-Mediated Maternal Platelet Antibodies.

Idiopathic Thrombocytopenia. With immune-mediated thrombocytopenia, in which maternal antibodies destroy platelets, 80% of cases are caused by the autoimmune form, or maternal idiopathic thrombocytopenic purpura (ITP), which strikes women during the second to third decade of life. ITP, now also referred to as autoimmune thrombocytopenia, is a pre-existing condition in which maternal lymphocytes produce IgG antiplatelet antibodies (PAIgG) that attack maternal platelets, usually reducing the platelet count to below 150,000/mm^3. These antibodies are specifically directed at platelet antigen and bind to platelets, which are then phagocytosed by cells carrying a specific receptor, the Fc receptor. The greatest number of cells with this receptor are found in the reticuloendothelial system of the spleen, which is also the major site of PAIgG production. ITP is often confused with HELLP syndrome, which, in addition to a low platelet count, involves hemolysis and elevated liver enzymes.

Because IgG can cross the placenta, fetal platelets can also be destroyed by the transplacental passage of platelet antibodies, resulting in thrombocytopenia in the fetus and newborn. The mortality rate is 1% to 10% in these affected infants, and the condition can persist postnatally for as long as 4 months.

Neonatal Alloimmune Thrombocytopenia. The remaining 20% of immune-mediated thrombocytopenias are caused by an alloimmune (isoimmune) reaction in which maternal antibodies are produced against foreign fetal platelets (paternally inherited), whereas maternal platelet levels remain normal. This reaction occurs when fetal platelets, which have an antigen not found on maternal platelets, pass into the maternal circulation. The resultant generation of maternal antibodies in response to the fetal platelets is similar to the mechanism behind Rh incompatibility. Unlike Rh incompatibility, alloimmune thrombocytopenia affects 33% to 50% of first pregnancies. The mother develops IgG antibodies that eventually cross into the fetal circulation, resulting in platelet destruction. The Pl^{A1} alloantibodies are responsible for 50% to 80% of neonates with alloimmune thrombocytopenia. This phenomenon occurs in approximately 1 in 2000 to 1 in 5000 live births. The mortality rate of 10% to 15% in alloimmune thrombocytopenia is higher than that in ITP, because bleeding tends to be more severe. The incidence of intracranial hemorrhage in utero is reported to be as high as 10% to 15%, with most cases occurring between 30 and 35 weeks' gestation. Treatment consists of transfusion of maternal platelets, exchange transfusion, and use of IVIG. Platelets usually normalize in the newborn by 4 weeks of age.

Antenatal Treatment. Antenatal treatment is not universally agreed on, but several sources suggest administration of corticosteroids 1 to 2 weeks before delivery and administration of multiple aliquots of IVIG within 7 to 9 days of delivery.

Steroids and IVIG are theorized to work in similar fashion by (1) diminishing the production of antiplatelet antibodies, (2) interfering with antibody attachment to the surface of the platelets, and (3) reducing platelet destruction by interfering with phagocytic receptors in the reticuloendothelial system. Suggested steroid therapy consists of prednisone (1 to 2 mg/kg/day, orally) for 2 to 3 weeks. When the desired increase in platelet count occurs, usually within 3 weeks, the dose is tapered to a level that will maintain a platelet count over 50,000/mm³. IVIG can be administered in several different doses and for different lengths of time, but the regimen most often used is 400 mg/kg/day given intravenously for 5 days, with an increase in the platelet count expected within 7 to 9 days. In patients who are unresponsive to these two therapies, splenectomy may be necessary to remove the major site of antibody production and platelet destruction.

Serious bleeding during labor and delivery occurs only in infants with platelet counts below 50,000/mm³. Scalp sampling in fetuses of mothers with ITP and delivery by cesarean section of infants with platelet levels below 50,000/mm³ are recommended.

Postnatal Treatment. Postnatal treatment consists of platelet transfusion, exchange transfusion with blood less than 2 days old, steroid therapy (prednisone, 1 to 5 mg/kg/day), and IVIG. The major difference in therapy between ITP and alloimmune thrombocytopenia is the use of washed, irradiated, maternal platelets in infants with alloimmune thrombocytopenia.

Neonatal Factors. Neonatal factors associated with thrombocytopenia include asphyxia, an Apgar score of less than 7, disseminated intravascular coagulation, exchange transfusion, infection, smallness for gestational age, necrotizing enterocolitis, hyperbilirubinemia and phototherapy, meconium aspiration, cold injury, polycythemia, pulmonary hypertension, and cardiopulmonary bypass procedure. Treatment of thrombocytopenia caused by neonatal factors consists initially of amelioration of the underlying problem, followed by symptomatic treatment with platelet transfusion. Transfusion therapy should be considered if platelet counts are in the range of 50,000/mm³ to 100,000/mm³ and active bleeding is present. Platelet transfusion should be considered when the level is below 50,000/mm³ even if active bleeding is not present.

A helpful formula for estimating the rise in platelets after transfusion is: one tenth the volume (in milliliters) of a unit of platelets per kilogram of weight raises the platelet count by 50,000/mm³.

Disseminated Intravascular Coagulopathy

Disseminated intravascular coagulation (DIC) is marked by a generalized deficiency of coagulation factors and platelets, which leaves the infant predisposed to hemorrhage. Because this condition is triggered by a pre-existing illness and does not occur independently, treatment consists of identification and resolution of the underlying problem. Release of tissue factor and substantial injury to endothelial cells are the two major mechanisms that precipitate DIC (Mitchell & Cotran, 1999). The factors most often associated with bleeding that occurs secondary to DIC are obstetrical complications, respiratory distress syndrome, hypoxia, hypotension, necrotizing enterocolitis, and sepsis. Occasionally thrombosis of large vessels can trap platelets and consume an amount of clotting factors sufficient to cause DIC. Mortality rates reach 60% to 80% in infants with DIC who experience severe bleeding.

The hematologic picture of DIC (Table 30-9) reflects a depletion of platelets, prothrombin, fibrinogen, angiotensin III (AT III), protein C, and Factors V, VIII, and XIII. The prothrombin time and partial thromboplastin time are prolonged and are not corrected by the addition of fresh-frozen plasma to the blood sample. The fibrinolytic system is also stimulated, as evidenced by the presence of degradation products of fibrinolysis (i.e., fibrin degradation products or fibrinolytic split products). A commonly used test, measurement of d-dimer, serves as an evaluation of the activation of the fibrinolytic system in that it measures degradation of cross-linked fibrin. However, the d-dimer test may not be very helpful in the newborn because the result commonly is positive in infants who do not have a consumptive coagulopathy.

Successful treatment of DIC depends on alleviation of the underlying cause. Palliative treatment consists of replacement of deficient clotting factors with fresh-frozen plasma and cryoprecipitate, platelet transfusions, and exchange transfusion. Heparin is used infrequently because it carries a higher risk of hemorrhage; it is used only when large-vessel thrombosis occurs.

Differential Diagnosis of Newborn Coagulopathies

Analysis of a number of factors often can aid in the identification of the specific coagulopathy affecting an infant. Careful evaluation of the following factors can pinpoint the correct diagnosis and influence the choice of therapy or intervention:

- A familial history of a bleeding disorder, such as hemophilia
- A maternal history of a bleeding disorder, as in autoimmune thrombocytopenia
- An obstetrical history that suggests a possible abnormality, as in maternal alloimmunization or hypofibrinogenemia
- An adverse neonatal history, such as with hypoxia or asphyxia
- Failure to administer prophylactic vitamin K at birth

TABLE 30-9	Hematologic Findings in Disseminated Intravascular Coagulation
Hematologic Feature	**Finding**
Uniformity of clotting defect	Variable
Capillary fragility	Usually abnormal
Bleeding time	Often prolonged
Clotting time	Variable
One-stage prothrombin time	Moderately prolonged
Partial thromboplastin time	Prolonged
Fibrin degradation products	Present
Factor V	Diminished
Fibrinogen	Often diminished
Platelets	Often diminished
Red cell fragmentation	Usually present
Response to vitamin K	Diminished or absent
Associated disease	Severe; may include sepsis, hypoxia, acidosis, or obstetrical accident
Previous history	Associated diseases; administration of vitamin K

From Oski F (1976). Hematological problems. In Avery G, editor. Neonatology. JB Lippincott: Philadelphia.

- Physical manifestations of a bleeding disorder (e.g., obvious bleeding, the presence or absence of petechiae or ecchymosis) and the infant's overall condition
- Laboratory data that identify specific abnormalities, such as specific coagulation factor deficiencies, thrombocytopenia, and prolonged prothrombin time, partial thromboplastin time, and clotting times

Collaborative Management of a Coagulopathy

Care of an infant with a bleeding diathesis should be aimed at prevention of further injury or bleeding. Supportive care of fragile tissue and limiting the number of blood draws from sites other than central catheters are of great importance in the infant who lacks adequate clotting factors to control bleeding. Appropriate administration of platelets, clotting factors, or blood products requires the correct equipment, the correct method of administration, and conscientious monitoring of vital signs to ensure effective therapy without causing further harm to the infant. Wise decisions regarding replacement blood products are now important in light of the severe and potentially lethal sequelae of acquired infection. Adopting guidelines for transfusion therapy may safeguard infants and eliminate unnecessary exposure to blood products (Table 30-10). Monitoring of laboratory tests to determine continuing needs and the efficacy of therapy is important throughout the infant's course of therapy.

When blood or blood products are administered, the infant must be evaluated continuously for signs of fluid overload and untoward reaction. Although blood reactions are rare in the newborn, they tend to occur within the first 15 minutes of blood or blood product administration. Signs of such reactions include rashes, tachycardia, hypertension, hematuria, cyanosis, and hyperthermia. Throughout the acute course of illness, the hematocrit values and the state of perfusion, rather than the percentage of the infant's blood volume removed, should govern the decision on whether to transfuse. Symptoms of hypovolemia include metabolic acidosis, hypotension, poor perfusion, tachycardia, cyanosis, and shock.

BLOOD AND BLOOD COMPONENT THERAPY

Commonly Used Products

Whole Blood. This product is not used for routine volume expansion because of the hematocrit dilution that occurs. It is used in surgical procedures that require large volumes of blood for replacement; for exchange transfusions; and for priming heart-lung oxygenators for extracorporeal membrane oxygenation.

Packed Red Blood Cells. Blood is "hard spun" to concentrate cells and allow the supernatant to be removed. Because of this form of preparation, less volume can be administered.

TABLE 30-10	Example of Transfusion Guidelines for Preterm Infants	
Hematocrit (%)/ Hemoglobin (g/dl)	**Ventilator Requirements or Symptoms**	**Transfusion Volume**
Hct ≤35/Hb ≤11	Infants requiring moderate or significant mechanical ventilation (mean airway pressure over 8 cm H_2O and fractional concentration of oxygen in inspired gas [FiO_2] over 40%)	15 ml/kg of packed red blood cells (PRBCs) over 2 to 4 hours
Hct ≤30/Hb ≤10	Infants requiring minimal mechanical ventilation (any mechanical ventilation or continuous positive airway pressure [CPAP] under 6 cm H_2O and FiO_2 over 40%)	15 ml/kg PRBCs over 2 to 4 hours
Hct ≤25/Hb ≤8	Infants receiving supplemental oxygen who do not require mechanical ventilation, but for whom one or more of the following is a factor: • Tachycardia (heart rate over 180) or tachypnea (respiratory rate over 80) for 24 hours or longer • Increased oxygen requirement from the previous 48 hours; specifically, a fourfold or greater increase in nasal cannula flow (e.g., 0.25 to 1 L/minute) or an increase in nasal CPAP of 20% or more from the previous 48 hours (e.g., 10 to 12 cm H_2O) • Elevated lactate concentration (2.5 mEq/L or higher) • Weight gain of less than 10 g/kg/day over the previous 4 days while receiving at least 100 kcal/kg/day • Increase in episodes of apnea and bradycardia (more than nine episodes in a 24-hour period or two or more episodes in 24 hours requiring bag and mask ventilation) while receiving therapeutic doses of methylxanthines • Surgery	20 ml/kg PRBCs over 2 to 4 hours (if infant is fluid sensitive, divide into two 10 ml/kg volumes)
Hct ≤20/Hb ≤7	Infants without any symptoms who have an absolute reticulocyte count under 100,000 μl*	20 ml/kg PRBCs over 2 to 4 hours (if infant is fluid sensitive, divide into two 10 ml/kg volumes)

Modified from Ohls R (2001). Anemia in the newborn. In Polin R et al, editors. Workbook in practical neonatology, ed 3. WB Saunders: Philadelphia.
The absolute reticulocyte count is determined by multiplying the number of red blood cells by the percentage of uncorrected reticulocytes.

Packed RBCs can be reconstituted with normal saline, 5% albumin, or fresh-frozen plasma. Packed RBCs can be used in exchange transfusions or in the treatment of anemia in the acutely ill or symptomatic convalescent infant.

Washed Red Blood Cells. For additional protection, RBCs can be washed to remove as much of the plasma, nonviable RBCs, WBCs, and metabolic wastes as possible. To further eliminate the possibility of a graft-versus-host reaction, cells can be irradiated with 5000 rad; this prevents T-lymphocyte proliferation and, when done in conjunction with washing, can remove up to 95% of T lymphocytes.

Frozen Deglycerolized Red Cells. Frozen storage of deglycerolized RBCs allows preservation of rare units of blood, but the cost of preparation increases considerably. In addition, this product tends to have a higher potassium content and hemoglobin concentration. Centrifuging it, removing the supernatant, and diluting it to the desired hematocrit tend to control these problems.

Fresh-Frozen Plasma. A whole unit of fresh-frozen plasma can be thawed, but once entered, it is good for only 6 hours. If, however, it is packaged in aliquots, such as a quad pack, before freezing and then thawed, the quad pack unit is good for 24 hours once it has thawed. Fresh-frozen plasma provides a rich source of coagulation factors; 10 to 15 ml/kg, which contains 1 IU/ml of all clotting factors, raises the overall level of clotting factor activity by 20% to 30%. Fresh-frozen plasma often can normalize prolonged prothrombin and partial thromboplastin times in the newborn who has a generalized deficiency in quantity and activity of available clotting factors.

Platelets. The number of platelets available for circulation after transfusion depends on the storage time. In transfusions using platelet bags less than 7 days old, the rise in platelet levels is comparable to the rise seen with the use of fresh platelets. Use of packs older than 7 days achieves only 70% of the rise seen with the use of fresh platelets. Platelets also can be concentrated by centrifuge if smaller volumes are required. An important caveat: platelets require a special administration set for proper infusion.

Granulocytes. Granulocytes, which are used for infusion in septic infants with severe neutropenia, are prepared from fresh donor blood through the process of plasmapheresis. WBCs are removed from the unit of blood, but a large number of RBCs remain. For this reason, the donor unit must be typed and crossmatched to the infant for blood type and Rh compatibility. WBCs usually are irradiated to eliminate donor T cells in an effort to prevent graft-versus-host responses. The use of granulocyte transfusions remains controversial.

Cryoprecipitate. This form of plasma preparation is rich in Factors VIII and XIII and fibrinogen and is useful in the treatment of hemophilia. Because it is a single donor collection, the risk for infection is lower than with pooled substances. Each unit of cryoprecipitate transfused raises fibrinogen levels by 200 mg/dl per 100 ml of the infant's blood volume.

Factor Concentrates. Factor concentrates are used as specific therapy for identified factor deficiencies. They are obtained from pooled plasma and expose the recipient to multiple donors, thereby increasing the potential for infection, especially with hepatitis B, CMV, and AIDS. Eighty percent of cases of hepatitis B–infected blood can be identified by the third-generation screening tests, and blood screening is also available for CMV. Because the risk for transmission of HIV is increased by pooled concentrates, it is now recommended that concentrates be treated with heat, solvent, steam, detergent, or ultraviolet light to kill any virus that may be present. Currently it is unclear whether such treatment alters or inactivates the clotting activity of factor concentrates.

SUMMARY

The development of the blood cells formed from the pluripotent stem cells begins early in fetal development and becomes more sophisticated as the human organism matures. This maturation continues after birth and throughout adult life. Both term and premature infants have substantial hematologic capabilities, but they are hampered by their inability to compensate as well as the older child and adult on exposure to significant stress. The ability of these infants to maintain themselves adequately during a steady state, however, must be acknowledged.

Many abnormalities in the hematologic system can result from congenital, acquired, perinatal, and postnatal factors. Some of these disturbances occur because of maturational deficiencies, congenital defects, or acquired disease states. The newborn has a limited repertoire with which to respond to and compensate for any such abnormalities. Treatment of these abnormalities depends on the abnormality itself, but symptomatic treatment often plays a major role in therapy. Because of the potentially lethal outcome of some of the illnesses contracted from contaminated blood sources, the appropriateness of the use of blood and blood products must be carefully assessed.

REFERENCES

American Academic of Pediatrics (AAP) and the American College of Obstetrics and Gynecology (ACOG) (1998). *Guidelines for perinatal care*, ed 4. AAP: Elk Grove Village, IL.

Arad I et al (1988). Serum ferritin levels in preterm infants after multiple blood transfusions. *American journal of perinatology* 5(1):40-43.

Bahado-Singh R et al (1999). A new splenic artery Doppler velocimetric index for prediction of severe anemia associated with Rh alloimmunization. *American journal of obstetrical gynecology* 181:49-54.

Bergman D et al (1994). American Academy of Pediatrics: practice parameter: management of hyperbilirubinemia in the healthy term newborn. *Pediatrics* 94:558-561.

Bowman J (1994). Maternal blood group immunization. In Creasy R, Resni R, editors. *Maternal-fetal medicine: principles and practice*, ed 3. WB Saunders: Philadelphia.

Brugnara C, Platt O (1998). The neonatal erythrocyte and its disorders. In Nathan D, Orkin S, editors. *Nathan and Oski's hematology of infancy and childhood*, ed 5. WB Saunders: Philadelphia.

Dallacasa P et al (1996). Erythropoietin course in newborns with Rh hemolytic disease transfused and not transfused in utero. *Pediatric research* 40:357-360.

Donato H et al (2000). Effect of early versus late administration of human recombinant erythropoietin on transfusion requirements in premature infants: results of randomized, placebo-controlled, multicenter trial. *Pediatrics* 105:1066.

Doyle LW et al (1993). Sensorineural outcome at 2 years for survivors of erythroblastosis treated with fetal intravascular transfusions. *Obstetrics and gynecology* 81:931-935.

Edstrom C et al (2000). Developmental aspects of blood hemostasis and disorders of coagulation and fibrinolysis in the neonatal period. In Christensen R, ed. *Hematologic problems of the neonate*. WB Saunders: Philadelphia.

Emmerson AJ et al (1993). Double-blind trial of recombinant human erythropoietin in preterm infants. *Archives of disease in childhood* 68:291-296.

Fisk NM et al (1994). Clinical utility of fetal RhD typing in alloimmunized pregnancies by means of polymerase chain reaction on amniocytes or chorionic villi. *Journal of American obstetrics and gynecology* 171:50-54.

Gailani D, Broze G (1991). Factor IX activation in a revised model of blood coagulation. *Science* 253:909-912.

Grab D et al (1999). Treatment of fetal erythroblastosis by intravascular transfusions: outcome at 6 years. *Obstetrics and gynecology* 93:165-168.

Gruslin A, Moore T (2002). Erythroblastosis fetalis. In Fanaroff A, Martin R, editors. *Neonatal-perinatal medicine*, ed 7. Mosby: St Louis.

Guyton AC, Hall JE (1996a). Blood groups, transfusion, tissue and organ transplantation. In Guyton AC, Hall JE, editors. *Textbook of medical physiology*, ed 9. WB Saunders: Philadelphia.

Guyton A, Hall JE (1996b). Hemostasis and blood coagulation. In Guyton AC, Hall JE, editors. *Textbook of medical physiology*, ed 9. WB Saunders: Philadelphia.

Halamek L, Stevenson D (2001). Neonatal jaundice and liver disease. In Fanaroff A, Martin R, editors. *Neonatal-perinatal medicine*, ed 7. Mosby: St Louis.

Harman CR et al (1990). Intrauterine transfusion: intraperitoneal versus intravascular approach: a case-control comparison. *American journal of obstetrics and gynecology* 162:1053-1059.

Hathaway W, Bonnar J (1978). Coagulation and hemostasis: general considerations. In Hathaway W, Bonnar J, editors. *Perinatal coagulation*. New York: Grune & Stratton.

Iskaros J et al (1998). Prospective noninvasive monitoring of pregnancies complicated by red cell alloimmunization. *Ultrasound obstetrical gynecology* 11:432-443.

Janssens H et al (1997). Outcome for children treated with fetal intravascular transfusion because of severe blood group antagonism. *Journal of pediatrics* 131:373-380.

King J, Jung A (1990). Phototherapy. In Nelson N, editor. *Current therapy in neonatal-perinatal medicine*. BC Decker: Philadelphia.

Kuller JA et al, editors (1996). *Prenatal diagnosis and reproductive genetics*. JB Lippincott: Philadelphia.

Kumar D et al (2001). Vitamin K status of premature infants: implications for current recommendations. *Pediatrics* 108:117-122.

Lackner T (1982). Drug replacement following exchange transfusion. *Journal of pediatrics* 100:811-814.

Larsen W (1997). *Human embryology*, ed 2. Churchill Livingstone: New York.

Lee DA et al (1995). Reducing blood donor exposures in low-birth-weight infants by the use of older, unwashed packed red blood cells. *Journal of pediatrics* 126:280-286.

Liley A (1961). Liquor amnii analysis in management of pregnancy complicated by rhesus immunization. *American journal of obstetrics and gynecology* 82:1359-1371.

Liu EA et al (1994). Prospective, randomized trial of the safety and efficacy of a limited donor exposure transfusions program for premature neonates. *Journal of pediatrics* 125:92-96.

Luchtman-Jones L et al (2002). The blood and hematopoietic system. In Fanaroff A, Martin R, editors. *Neonatal-perinatal medicine*, ed 7. Mosby: St Louis.

Maier RF et al (1994). The effect of epoetin-beta (recombinant human erythropoietin) on the need for transfusion in very-low-birth-weight infants. *New England journal of medicine* 330:1173-1178.

Manroe B et al (1979). The neonatal blood count in health and disease. I. Reference values for neutrophilic cells. *Journal of pediatrics* 95:89.

Mari G (2000). Noninvasive diagnosis by Doppler ultrasonography of fetal anemia due to maternal red cell alloimmunization. *New England journal of medicine* 342:9-12.

McMillan MP (1996). Banking on cord blood. *Journal of obstetric, gynecologic, and neonatal nursing* 25:115.

Messer J et al (1993). Early treatment of premature infants with recombinant human erythropoietin. *Pediatrics* 92:519-523.

Meyer MP et al (1994). Recombinant human erythropoietin in the treatment of anemia of prematurity: results of a double-blind, placebo-controlled study. *Pediatrics* 93:918-923.

Mitchell R, Cotran R (1999). Hemodynamic disorders, thrombosis and shock. In Cotran R et al, editors. *Robbins pathologic basis of disease*, ed 9. WB Saunders: Philadelphia.

Moore K, Persaud T (1998). Formation of germ layers and early tissue and organ differentiation: the third week. In Moore K, Persaud T, editors. *The developing human*, ed 6. WB Saunders: Philadelphia.

Mouzinho A et al (1994). Revised reference ranges for circulating neutrophils in very-low-birth-weight neonates. *Pediatrics* 94:76.

Ohls RK et al (1993). A randomized, double-blind, placebo-controlled trial of recombinant erythropoietin in treatment of the anemia of bronchopulmonary dysplasia. *Journal of pediatrics* 123:996-1000.

Ohls RK et al (1995). Efficacy and cost analysis of treating very-low-birth-weight infants with erythropoietin during their first 2 weeks of life: a randomized, placebo-controlled trial. *Journal of pediatrics* 126:421-426.

Ozolek JA et al (1994). Prevalence and lack of clinical significance of blood group incompatibility in mothers with blood type A or B. *Journal of pediatrics* 125:87-91.

Quinnan G (1993). Recommendations regarding license amendments and procedures for gamma irradiation of blood products. US Department of Health and Human Services, Center for Biologics Evaluation and Research, Food and Drug Administration: Washington DC.

Schumacher B, Moise K (1996). Fetal transfusion for red cell alloimmunization in pregnancy. *Obstetrics and gynecology* 88:137-150.

Scott J, Branch D (1999). Immunologic disorders in pregnancy. In Scott J et al, editors. *Danforth's obstetrics and gynecology*, ed 8. JB Lippincott: Philadelphia.

Sekizawa A et al (1999). Fetal cell recycling: diagnosis of gender and RhD genotype in the same fetal cell retrieved from maternal blood. *American journal of obstetrics and gynecology* 181:1237-1242.

Shannon KM et al (1995). Recombinant human erythropoietin stimulates erythropoiesis and reduces erythrocyte transfusions in very-low-birth-weight preterm infants. *Pediatrics* 95:1-8.

Siberry G, Iannone R (2000). *Harriet Lane handbook*, ed 15. Mosby: St Louis.

Spinnato JA et al (1991). Amniotic fluid bilirubin and fetal hemolytic disease. *American journal of obstetrics and gynecology* 165:1030-1035.

ASSESSMENT AND MANAGEMENT OF THE NEUROLOGIC SYSTEM

SUSAN TUCKER BLACKBURN

The central nervous system (CNS) is one of the extraordinarily complex systems of the human body. Normal function of the CNS is critical to the functioning of every organ in the body and to the integration of organ systems for coordinated physiologic and neurobehavioral processes. Neurologic dysfunction during the neonatal period can arise from insults before, during, or after birth. Such insults can affect the infant's ability to survive the perinatal and neonatal periods and can have implications for later developmental and cognitive outcome. For these reasons, alterations in neurologic function in the neonate have significant immediate and long-term consequences for the infant and family. Early recognition of infants at risk for neurologic dysfunction and prompt implementation of appropriate interventions are crucial for the survival of these infants and for the reduction of long-term morbidity.

This chapter examines the structural and functional development of the CNS in the embryo, fetus, and neonate and the basis for common congenital and developmental anomalies. Neurologic assessment of the neonate and related diagnostic techniques are also presented, as are selected pathophysiologic problems that affect the central and peripheral nervous systems. The neurologic problems examined include neonatal seizures, intracranial hemorrhage, hypoxic-ischemic encephalopathy (HIE), structural alterations, and birth injuries. Nursing management and collaborative management are described for each of these problems. Figure 31-1 shows the general structure of the central nervous system.

EMBRYOLOGIC DEVELOPMENT OF THE CENTRAL NERVOUS SYSTEM

The development of the CNS can be divided into six stages: (1) neurulation, (2) prosencephalic development, (3) neuronal proliferation, (4) neuronal migration, (5) organization, and (6) myelinization. These stages overlap, and development progresses at different rates in various sections of the CNS. Embryologic development of the CNS begins shortly after fertilization, and maturation continues after birth until adulthood. The CNS therefore is one of the earliest systems to begin development and one of the last systems to mature completely. The stages and timing of CNS development are summarized in Table 31-1.

Neurulation

Primary neurulation, or dorsal induction, occurs during the first 3 to 4 weeks of gestation. Formation of the primitive brain and spinal cord occurs during this period. The notochord acts as an inducer for formation of the CNS. The CNS arises as a thickening of the ectoderm on the dorsal portion of the embryo at about 18 days' gestation. This neuroectodermal thickening, known as the neural plate, lies cranial to the primitive streak and extends to the oropharyngeal membrane. The brain and spinal cord develop from the neural plate. The neural plate invaginates, forming the midline neural groove along the dorsal surface of the embryo. The parallel folds of tissue on either side of this groove are called the neural folds. The neural folds eventually form the forebrain, midbrain, and hindbrain and the spinal cord. By the end of the third postconceptional week, the neural folds move together and fuse to form the neural tube. The cranial portion of the lumen of the neural tube forms the ventricles; the caudal portion forms the central canal of the spinal cord. The tissues of the neural tube interact with surrounding mesoderm tissue (somites) to stimulate development of the bony structures of the CNS (i.e., the skull and vertebrae).

In the fusion of the neural folds, some of the neuroectodermal cells on the upper margins are not incorporated into the neural tube. These cells form the neural crest, which lies between the neural tube and the surface ectodermal layer. The neural crest tissue forms the peripheral nervous system, which includes the cranial, spinal, and autonomic system ganglia and nerves, Schwann cells, melanocyte (pigment) cells, meninges, and skeletal and muscular components of the head (Moore & Persaud, 1998). The neural crest cells migrate away from the neural tube in a ventral and lateral direction. These cells migrate and grow anteriorly to form the spinal and cranial nerves and posteriorly to form the ganglia of the cranial nerves and autonomic nervous system.

The neural folds do not fuse simultaneously. Closure of the neural tube begins in the occipitocervical region at about 22 days' gestation. Fusion proceeds in cephalic and caudal directions from this site. For several days the neural tube is fused toward the central area but is open at both ends. The end areas are known as the rostral (anterior) and the caudal (posterior) neuropores. These openings communicate with the amniotic

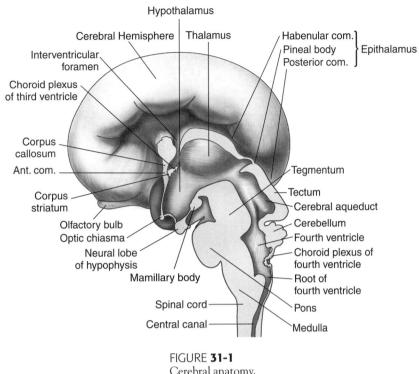

FIGURE **31-1**
Cerebral anatomy.

fluid. The cranial end of the neural tube closes at 24 days' gestation. Fusion of the cranial portion forms the forebrain. Failure of closure leads to anencephaly. The caudal neuropore, which is in the future lumbosacral area, closes in a rostrocaudal direction at 26 days' gestation (Goddard-Finegold, 1998). Once both neuropores are closed, the neural tube is a closed, fluid-filled system that has no further connection to the amniotic cavity unless a defect is present. Failure of these neuropores to close gives rise to neural tube defects (NTDs). Because differentiation of the surrounding mesodermal tissue (somites) into vertebrae, cranium, and dura depends on interaction with the neural tube, NTDs involve not only the neural elements but also the bony structures and meninges.

Secondary neurulation involves two phases, canalization and regressive differentiation. These processes form the spinal cord caudal to the upper lumbar area. Development of the lower lumbar, sacral, and coccygeal areas begins at 28 to 32 days' gestation. These areas arise from a group of undifferentiated cells (caudal cell mass) at the caudal end of the neural tube. Vacuoles develop that gradually coalesce, enlarge, and contact the caudal end of the neural tube. This period of canalization is followed by a period of regressive differentiation, which lasts until after birth and is characterized by regression of much of the caudal cell mass (Goddard-Finegold, 1998; Volpe, 2001b).

Disorders of Neurulation

Congenital anomalies that arise during the period of neurulation result from failure of neural tube closure. Neural tube defects usually are accompanied by alterations in vertebral, meningeal, vascular, and dermal structures; these anomalies include anencephaly, encephalocele, spina bifida occulta, and myelomeningocele. Neural tube defects arise from genetic factors or environmental factors, or both. Most embryos with NTDs are lost early in pregnancy. The incidence is significantly higher in mothers whose diet is poor, especially when folate deficiency is a factor.

Folic acid supplementation at conception reduces the rate of neural tube defects by up to 70% (Ali & Economides, 2000). Folate is a cofactor for enzymes needed in DNA and RNA synthesis that is important to a cell's ability to methylate proteins, lipids, and myelin and to the actions of other B vitamins. Folic acid may reduce the incidence of NTDs by correcting a deficiency or by overcoming a genetically induced metabolic block (Ali & Economides, 2000; Northrup & Volcik, 2000). The American Academy of Pediatrics (AAP) currently recommends that women of childbearing age consume 0.4 mg of folate daily; for women who previously have had an infant with a neural tube defect, the recommendation is 4 mg daily (AAP, 1999). A neural tube defect can be identified prenatally through maternal serum screening, ultrasound examination, and measurement of the alpha-fetoprotein level of the amniotic fluid.

Anencephaly. Anencephaly is caused by failure of the anterior neural tube to fuse in the cranial area. Since the advent of perinatal diagnosis and folic acid therapy, the incidence of anencephaly has declined. Because fusion of the neural tube in this area forms the forebrain, anencephalic infants have minimal development of brain tissue. The more common forms of this anomaly involve the forebrain and the upper brainstem. The brain tissue that does develop is poorly differentiated and becomes necrotic with exposure to amniotic fluid; this results in a mass of vascular tissue with neuronal and glial elements and a choroid plexus marked by partial absence of the skull bones (Volpe, 2001b). The mother may have hydramnios secondary to leakage of large amounts of cerebrospinal fluid (CSF) directly into the amniotic sac. Because anencephaly is caused by failure of the neural tube to close cranially, the alterations in development occur before 23 to 26 days' gestation (around the period of rostral neuropore closure).

Genetic and environmental factors appear to be involved in the development of anencephaly. Many anencephalic infants have other anomalies, the most consistent being adrenal hy-

TABLE 31-1	Stages in the Development of the Central Nervous System and Related Developmental Defects	
Stage	**Peak Period of Occurrence**	**Developmental Defects**
Neurulation	3 to 4 weeks' gestation	Neural tube defects, anencephaly, encephalocele, spina bifida cystica (meningocele, meningomyelocele, myeloschisis), dermal sinus
Prosencephalic development	2 to 3 months' gestation	Holoprosencephaly, holotelencephaly
Neuronal proliferation	3 to 4 months' gestation	Microcephaly vera, macrocephaly, neurofibromatosis, other neurocutaneous disorders
Neuronal migration	3 to 5 months' gestation	Hypoplasia or agenesis of the corpus callosum, schizencephaly, lissencephaly, pachygyria, polymicrogyria
Organization	6 months' gestation to 1 year of age	Alterations in brain development secondary to the effects of Down syndrome and trisomies 13, 14, and 15; behavioral alterations; mental retardation
Myelinization	8 months' gestation to 1 year of age	Brain hypoplasia, neurologic deficits

Modified from Scher MS (2001). Brain disorders of the fetus and neonate. In Klaus MH, Fanaroff AA, editors. Care of the high-risk neonate, ed 5. WB Saunders: Philadelphia; Hill A, Volpe JJ (1989). Fetal neurology. Raven Press: New York; and Volpe JJ (2001). Neurology of the newborn, ed 4. WB Saunders: Philadelphia.

poplasia secondary to pituitary dysfunction. Three fourths of these infants are stillborn; the remainder die during the neonatal period, and fewer than 20% are still alive at 1 week (Volpe, 2001b). Nursing management of infants with anencephaly is supportive, involving provision of warmth and comfort until the infant dies. Families require emotional support and assistance in coping with their grief over the birth of an infant with a defect and the death of their infant. Anencephalic infants have been considered to be candidates for organ donation and have been kept alive for this purpose. This practice has raised many ethical issues involving keeping one infant alive for the good of another and the criteria for determining brain death.

Encephalocele. The incidence of encephalocele is 0.1 to 0.5 per 1000 live births (Fieggen, 1999). Encephaloceles, including craniomeningomyelocele, encephalomyelocele, and other forms of cranium bifida, arise from failure of closure of a portion of the neural tube in the anterior region. Although this defect can occur in any region, approximately three fourths occur in the occipital region. The sac protrudes from the back of the head or the base of the neck. The next most common area is the frontal region, and the orbit, nose, and/or nasopharynx is involved (Goddard-Finegold, 1998; Volpe, 2001b). Hydrocephalus occurs with 50% of occipital encephaloceles because of alterations in the posterior fossa. Hydrocephalus may be present at birth or may develop after repair of the encephalocele (Fieggen, 1999). Encephaloceles may occur in association with meningomyelocele.

The protruding sac varies considerably in size, and the size of the external sac does not correlate with the presence of neural elements. For example, a large occipital sac may contain minimal neural tissue, whereas a small sac may contain parts of the cerebellum or accessory lobes; some occipital lesions have no neural elements in the sac (Fieggen, 1999; Volpe, 2001b). If the sac is leaking CSF at birth, immediate repair is necessary. If the defect is covered by skin, surgery may be delayed until a complete workup, including skull radiography, computed tomography (CT) or cranial ultrasonography, magnetic resonance imaging (MRI) and electroencephalography (EEG), could be performed. Surgical closure helps prevent infection and helps facilitate feeding and other care. If the infant is also hydrocephalic, a shunt usually is inserted. The prognosis for these infants generally is poor if the sac contains significant brain tissue. The mortality rate and later outcome are significantly better for infants with anterior defects than for those with posterior defects (Fieggen, 1999).

Collaborative Management. Collaborative management includes prevention of infection and trauma and positioning to avoid pressure on the defect. Promotion of normothermia is essential, especially in infants with CSF leakage, because these infants are at risk for thermoregulatory problems caused by evaporative losses. Postoperative management includes assessment of ventilation and perfusion, comfort measures, monitoring of neurologic and motor function, promotion of normothermia, prevention of infection, positioning to prevent pressure on the operative site, and monitoring of the site for CSF leakage.

The families of infants with an encephalocele need initial and continuing support and counseling. Initial parental care involves assisting parents with the shock of the defect and its appearance and with their grief over having an infant with an anomaly, as well as helping the parents deal with the outcome implications of this defect. Nursing care also involves enhancing parent-infant interaction and involving the parents in the infant's care when they are ready. Teaching before discharge includes skin care, positioning, exercises, handling and feeding techniques, and activities to promote growth and development.

Spina Bifida. Spina bifida is a general term used to describe defects in closure of the neural tube that are associated with malformations of the spinal cord and vertebrae. Spina bifida arises from defects in closure of the caudal neuropore (open defects) or during secondary neurulation (closed defects). Defects range from minor malformations of minimal clinical significance to major disorders that result in paraplegia or quadriplegia and loss of bladder and bowel control. The degree of sensory and motor neurologic deficit depends on the level and severity of the defect. The two major forms of spina bifida are spina bifida occulta and spina bifida cystica. The treatment of infants with spina bifida is discussed later in this chapter.

Spina bifida occulta occurs in 5% of the normal population (Goddard-Finegold, 1998). This disorder is a vertebral defect at L5 or S1, or both, that arises from failure of the vertebral arch to grow and fuse between 5 weeks' gestation and the early fetal period (Moore & Persaud, 1998). Spina bifida occulta is a defect in the formation of the caudal portion of the spinal cord (secondary neurulation). Most of those with condition have no problems, and the defect may go unrecognized. A few individuals have underlying abnormalities of the spinal cord or the nerve roots, or both; diastematomyelia (division of the spinal cord or nerve roots in an anteroposterior direction by a bony spicule or cartilaginous band); or dermoids or dermal sinuses (Goddard-Finegold, 1998). These abnormalities usually are manifested externally by a hemangioma, dimple, tuft of hair, or lipoma in the lower lumbar or sacral area. A dermal sinus is a tract of squamous epithelium that connects to the dura mater; this defect is found in the midline, usually in the lumbosacral area corresponding to the location of the caudal neuropore. A dermal sinus occasionally is recognized at birth, but more often it is diagnosed later, after repeated episodes of meningitis.

Spina bifida cystica is a generic term for NTDs characterized by a cystic sac containing meninges or spinal cord elements, or both, along with vertebral defects. Epithelium or a thin membrane covers the sac. This defect occurs in approximately 1 in 1000 live births, and, as with anencephaly, the incidence has declined in recent years. The three main forms of spina bifida cystica are meningocele, myelomeningocele, and myeloschisis. Spina bifida cystica can occur anywhere along the spinal column but is seen most often in the lumbar or lumbosacral area. A meningocele involves a sac that contains meninges and CSF, but the spinal cord and nerve roots are in their normal position. These infants usually have minimal residual neurologic deficit if the defect is covered with skin and if appropriate management is instituted early.

Myelomeningocele accounts for 80% of spina bifida cystica. The sac contains spinal cord or nerve roots, or both, in addition to meninges and CSF. During development the nerve tissues become incorporated into the wall of the sac, impairing differentiation of nerve fibers (Moore & Persaud, 1998). Infants with myelomeningocele have neurologic deficit below the level of the sac. Approximately 80% of these malformations occur in the lumbar area, which is the final area of neural tube fusion. This defect occurs at 26 to 30 days' gestation, around the time of caudal neuropore closure.

Myeloschisis is a severe defect in which no cystic covering exists, leaving the spinal cord open and exposed. Myeloschisis is thought to arise from a local overgrowth of the neural plate, which prevents neural tube closure. This defect probably occurs between 18 and 23 days' gestation. The spinal cord in affected patients is a flattened mass of neural tissue. These infants have significant neurologic deficits and are at great risk for infection. This defect can involve the entire length of the spinal cord and can occur in association with anencephaly (Moore & Persaud, 1998). Most infants with this defect are stillborn.

Prosencephalic Development

Prosencephalic development, or ventral induction, involves early development of the brain and ventricular system, which occurs during the second to third month of gestation (peaking at 5 to 6 weeks). The brain develops from the cranial end of the neural tube beginning at the end of the fourth week. The peak period for prosencephalic development is 5 to 6 weeks' gestation. During this period, the three primary brain bulges (or vesicles) and cavities are formed, after fusion of the neural folds in the cranial area. Development of the face is associated with prosencephalic development of the CNS; consequently, alterations in brain development often result in facial malformations (Goddard-Finegold, 1998; Moore & Persaud, 1998).

The primary brain bulges are the forebrain (prosencephalon), the midbrain (mesencephalon), and the hindbrain (rhombencephalon). During the fifth week, the forebrain divides into two secondary vesicles, the telencephalon and the diencephalon, and the hindbrain divides into the metencephalon and the myelencephalon. The derivatives of each of these structures form the structures of the definitive brain. The third and fourth ventricles are formed from cavities within the rhombencephalon and diencephalon; the aqueduct of Sylvius links these two ventricles. The lateral ventricles arise from cavities in the cerebral hemispheres and are connected to the third ventricle by the foramen of Monro (Figure 31-1). Early growth of the neural tube is most rapid in the forebrain region. To give these structures space to grow, the neural tube bends at several points, forming the mesencephalic (midbrain area), cervical (junction of the hindbrain and spinal cord), and pontine flexures.

Disorders of Prosencephalic Development

Malformations that occur during this period generally are thought to arise around the fifth to sixth weeks of gestation. Infants with these anomalies have a poor prognosis, and many are lost in early pregnancy or are stillborn. Malformations of the forebrain include holoprosencephaly and holotelencephaly. Holoprosencephaly is an abnormality in cleavage of the hemispheres that arises from genetic or possibly environmental alterations. Failure of horizontal, transverse, and sagittal cleavage of the prosencephalon disrupts formation of the telencephalon and the diencephalon and their derivatives. The resultant brain has a single monoventricular cerebral mass enclosed by a membrane; aplasia of the optic tract, with absence of the olfactory tracts and bulbs, corpus callosum, and supralimbic cortex, also is characteristic. Partial fusion of the basal ganglia, microcephaly, hydrocephaly, and facial anomalies also may be seen (Goddard-Finegold, 1998; Volpe, 2001b). With holotelencephaly, the parts of the brain that develop from the telencephalon form a single spheroid structure; the diencephalon and its derivatives are less affected.

Congenital hydrocephalus can also arise during this period. At about 6 weeks' gestation, three critical events occur that are related to the formation and circulation of CSF: (1) development of secretory epithelium in the choroid plexus, (2) perforation of the roof of the fourth ventricle, and (3) formation of the subarachnoid space. Alterations in the second and third events give rise to a communicating form of hydrocephalus (Volpe, 2001b).

Neuronal Proliferation

The development of neurons and glial cells involves proliferation in the germinal matrix; migration (to their final destination) in the next stage of CNS development; differentiation of glial cells (during the period of organization) into specific cell types; alignment of neurons; and the development of interneuron and glial-neuron relationships. The peak period of neuronal proliferation lasts from 2 to 4 months' gestation.

During this stage, further development occurs in the subventricular and ventricular zones, where neurons and glial cells are derived from stem cells in the germinal matrix. Initial proliferation involves primarily neurons and radial glia, which are needed for neuron migration. Proliferation of other glia and their derivatives (astrocytes and oligodendrocytes) occurs intensively during the stage of organization, at 5 to 8 months' gestation. During the most intense period of proliferation, before 32 to 34 weeks' gestation, the periventricular area receives a large proportion of the cerebral blood flow. This area is vulnerable to intraventricular hemorrhage in preterm infants.

Disorders of Neuronal Proliferation

Disorders of proliferation arise from inadequate or excessive proliferation of neuronal derivatives, glial derivatives, or glial cell derivatives. Because mature neurons cannot divide, the eventual number of neurons is determined early in gestation. Insults may alter the neuronal-glial stem cells (reducing the number of neurons or glial cells) or may alter cell growth (resulting in smaller cells) (Volpe, 2001b). The resulting disorders include micrencephaly, macrencephaly, and neurofibromatosis. Micrencephaly may be due to a reduction in either the size (micrencephaly vera) or number (radial microbrain) of stem cells.

Micrencephaly vera is associated with a small brain size (caused by a decrease in the size of the proliferating units) that occurs at 2 to 4 months' gestation. These infants often do not have marked neurologic deficits or seizures during the neonatal period, but later they are severely retarded. Micrencephaly vera may be caused by genetic factors (autosomal recessive or dominant trait, X-linked recessive trait, or translocation) or by environmental factors (irradiation, metabolic alteration, or infection). Micrencephaly vera is found with maternal rubella, fetal alcohol syndrome, maternal cocaine use, and maternal phenylketonuria with elevated phenylalanine levels during pregnancy (Goddard-Finegold, 1998; Volpe, 2001b).

Macrencephaly results in a large brain size because of excessive proliferation of neuronal elements or nonneuronal elements, or both. Macrencephaly is associated with genetic disorders (including Beckwith syndrome, Sturge-Weber syndrome, and achondroplasia), chromosomal disorders (e.g., Kleinfelter and fragile X syndromes), and neurocutaneous disorders, such as neurofibromatosis. Neurofibromatosis involves excessive proliferation of nonneuronal elements in the CNS and mesodermal structures of the body, with cutaneous stigmata (Volpe, 2001b). The onset occurs after neuronal proliferation, at the time of glial cell proliferation during organization. Infants with more than five café au lait cells larger than 5 mm in diameter at birth should be further evaluated for neurofibromatosis.

Neuronal Migration

The peak period for the neuronal migration stage is 3 to 5 months' gestation. This stage is characterized by the movement of millions of cells from their point of origin in the subependymal germinal matrix of the periventricular region (Figure 31-1) to their eventual loci in the cerebral cortex and cerebellum. The process of neuronal migration is critical to the formation of the cortex, gyri, and deep nuclear structures. Development of the gyri and sulci follows a predictable pattern that is linked to gestational age. At 21 to 25 weeks' gestation, the central ventricles are large and the brain agyric; gyral development begins by the end of this period.

The mechanisms that guide neuronal migration are not completely understood, but they are mediated by signaling proteins, surface molecules, and receptors on both the neurons and the radial glia (Ikonomidou et al, 2001). Radial glia act as guides for migrating cells. These glia later transform into astrocytes (Volpe, 2001b). The cerebral cortex has essentially achieved its full complement of neurons by 20 weeks' gestation. Later, migration predominantly involves glial cells. The migration of the neurons to both the cortex and the cerebellum is assisted by the radial glia.

Disorders of Neuronal Migration

Errors or exogenous insults before or after birth can alter migration of neurons and glial cells. Alterations in migration can result in hypoplasia or agenesis of the corpus callosum, agenesis of a part of the cerebral wall (schizencephaly), or gyral anomalies (pachygyria, lissencephaly, and polymicrogyria). The preterm infant may be especially vulnerable to gyral alterations. Rapid development of the gyri begins at 26 to 28 weeks' gestation and continues through the third trimester into the postbirth period. Development of gyri results in a marked increase in cerebral surface area (Goddard-Finegold, 1998; Volpe, 2001b).

Organization

The peak period for organization is about the fifth month of gestation to 1 year after birth. However, organizational processes continue for many years after birth, especially in the cerebellum. Some processes, such as synaptogenesis, continue until death. Organizational processes allow the nervous system to act as an integrated whole. These processes include (1) establishment of subplate neurons, which serve as transient "way stations" by providing a place of synaptic contact for axons that ascend from the thalamus and other areas in which connecting cortical neurons are not yet in place; (2) attainment of the proper alignment, orientation, and layering of cortical neurons; (3) arborization or differentiation and branching of axons and dendrites; (4) differentiation of the glial cells; (5) development of synaptic connections ("wiring" of the brain); (6) balancing of excitatory and inhibitory synapses; and (7) cell death and selective elimination of neuronal processes (Volpe, 2001b).

The process of cell death and selective elimination of neuronal processes is important in adjusting the size of individual neurons to their anticipated need and also is an important component of brain plasticity in infants. In the developing brain, neuronal processes targeted for elimination can be saved if they are needed because of damage to other processes; by this means, functional ability is preserved. Excitatory neurotransmitters, such as glutamate, mediate neural development and organization by acting on N-methyl-D-asparate (NMDA) receptors. This action enhances neuronal proliferation, migration, and synaptogenesis (Fox et al, 1996).

Disorders of Organization

Organization of the brain is susceptible to insults from errors of metabolism, abnormal chromosomes, and perinatal insults. Organizational processes are particularly vulnerable in the preterm infant being cared for in an intensive care unit during this period. Alterations in arborization and wiring of the brain can lead to hypersensitivity, poorly modulated behavior, and all-or-nothing responses Alterations in organization are seen in infants with Down syndrome, who have abnormal development of the axons and dendrites and altered synaptic formation, fragile X syndrome (the most common cause of inherited mental retardation in males), Angelman syndrome (microdeletion of long arm of maternal chromosome 15), phenylketonuria, congenital rubella, and trisomies 13, 14, and 15. NMDA receptors are hypersensitive during development. In animal models, blockade of NMDA receptors by substances such as ethanol leads to cell death (Ikonomidou et al, 2001;. Sanchez & Jensen, 2001).

Myelinization

Myelinization begins during the second trimester of pregnancy, at about 20 weeks' gestation, and continues to adulthood. The peak time for myelinization is 8 months' gestation to 1 year of age. The rate of myelinization varies in different parts of the nervous system. This process begins before birth in the peripheral areas, first in the peripheral motor nerves and then in the peripheral sensory nerves. Myelinization also begins before birth in the CNS, moving upward from the brainstem. In the CNS, myelinization occurs first in the sensory areas and then in the motor areas. Myelinization of ascending pathways in the spinal cord, brainstem, and thalamus is completed by about 30 weeks' gestation, and myelinization from the thalamus to the cortex is completed by 37 weeks (Volpe, 2001b). This has implications for neonatal pain management. From birth to adulthood, myelinization proceeds within the cerebral hemispheres in conjunction with development of higher associative and sensory functions. Myelinization is important in most nerve tracts in the CNS because it insulates individual fibers to enhance specificity of connections, increases the number of alternative pathways, and markedly increases the speed of transmission (Volpe, 2001b).

The myelinization stage involves development of myelin sheaths around nerve fibers in the nervous system. Oligodendrocytes or Schwann cells (peripheral nerves) form sheaths. The lipoprotein plasma membranes of these cells wrap themselves around the nerve fibers for several layers. Myelinization of fiber tracts tends to occur before maturation of functional ability (Moore & Persaud, 1998).

Disorders of Myelinization

Myelinization is susceptible to damage from exogenous influences, particularly malnutrition, which can lead to a range of neurologic deficits in which hypoplasia of the cerebral white matter occurs. Primary hypoplasia of the white matter with vacuolization of the myelin occurs in postnatal malnutrition, congenital hypothyroidism, and amino and organic acidopathies such as maple syrup urine disease, homocystinuria, and phenylketonuria. This defect in myelinization can lead to severe neurologic deficits in these infants (Volpe, 2001b).

ASSESSMENT OF NEUROLOGIC FUNCTION

Assessment of neurologic function is a collaborative process involving nurses and other health care professionals. It is an initial step in evaluating an infant's response to the transition to extrauterine life and the impact of perinatal events and pathophysiologic problems on the central and peripheral nervous systems. Assessment of neurologic function and identification of dysfunction encompass several components, including the history, physical examination, neurologic examination, laboratory tests, and other diagnostic techniques.

History

Risk factors noted in the maternal, obstetrical, and neonatal histories can be useful in identifying infants at risk for neurologic dysfunction and specific pathophysiologic factors. Specific risk factors for each problem discussed here are identified later in individual sections. General maternal or family historical factors that must be examined include a family history of NTDs; chromosomal or genetic abnormalities or other malformations; maternal substance abuse; chronic maternal health problems; maternal age, nutritional status, and exposure to teratogens; and the outcome of previous pregnancies.

Obstetrical risk factors include prematurity, postmaturity, placental problems (e.g., abruptio placentae and placenta previa), use of analgesia or anesthesia, and maternal problems (e.g., infection, hypertension, and substance abuse). A large-for-gestational-age (LGA) infant, prolonged or precipitate labor, forceps delivery, and abnormal presentation increase the risk of birth trauma and hemorrhage. Alterations in intrauterine growth and polyhydramnios may be present with an infant who has a CNS malformation. Fetal distress, perinatal asphyxia, and low Apgar scores are associated with intracranial hemorrhage and HIE.

Because neurologic dysfunction also can arise from postnatal problems, the infant's postbirth history is evaluated for status at birth and resuscitation required, asphyxia or hypoxic episodes, shock, hypoperfusion, hemorrhage, infection, and metabolic or electrolyte aberrations. The infant's record is also reviewed for clinical signs, such as seizures or alterations in activity, tone, and state, that are associated with neurologic dysfunction.

Physical Examination

A comprehensive physical examination is an important component of the nursing assessment of any infant at risk for or showing evidence of neurologic dysfunction. Infants are examined especially for evidence of infection and birth trauma, such as ecchymosis, edema, lacerations, and fractures. Temperature, blood pressure, color, and respiratory pattern also are assessed. The infant is examined for signs of vascular alterations, such as a port wine stain along trigeminal nerve branches, which may indicate Sturge-Weber syndrome. The characteristics of the infant's cry (e.g., robustness, presence in response to aversive stimuli, and pitch) may also be useful. Funduscopic examination may be performed to assess for chorioretinitis (associated with intrauterine viral infection), papilledema (seen with cerebral edema, although less reliably in neonates), and congenital anomalies (Amiel-Tison, 1995).

Specific parameters that are particularly important for the nurse to assess in infants with neurologic problems are (1) the head size, shape, and rate of growth; (2) the sutures and fontanels; (3) whether major and minor anomalies are present; and (4) the vertebral column. The first two elements are discussed below. Because CNS anomalies often are associated with other anomalies and syndromes, the infant also is examined for major anomalies of body systems and for isolated or clustered minor malformations, such as low-set or abnormally shaped ears, micrognathia, and hypertelorism of the eyes. The vertebral column is inspected and palpated for evidence of NTDs. Signs that may indicate an underlying defect include hair tufts, dimples, and fistulae.

Head Size, Shape, and Rate of Growth.   The monitoring and plotting of head circumference are basic components of health care for all infants, regardless of gestation or health status. The largest circumference is measured, which usually is the occipitofrontal circumference, about 1 cm above the eyes. The measurement is plotted on the appropriate growth grid for the infant's gender and gestation. The most accurate measurements are made with a metal or plastic tape marked in centimeters. Paper tapes tend to stretch and are less accurate but can be used for initial screening and for infants whose head size raises no concern. The occipitofrontal circumference generally ranges from 32.6 to 37.2 cm in term infants. Infants with caput succedaneum or overriding sutures may need to be remeasured after 3 days to obtain a more accurate measurement (Amiel-Tison, 1995). The head usually grows a maximum of 0.5 cm per week in term infants. Head growth in preterm infants usually is 0.5 cm in the first and second weeks, 0.75 cm during the third week, and 1 cm per week thereafter (Scher, 2001).

Serial measurements must be made to identify changes in the rate of growth as well as in size. Changes in the growth rate are important because an infant may have a significant increase or decrease in head growth but remain within the 10th to 90th percentiles on standard head growth grids. The occipitofrontal circumference should be measured several times over the first days after birth to obtain an accurate baseline after molding and edema from birth have resolved. Head circumference is measured weekly on preterm or ill infants. More frequent measurements may be made if the infant is at risk of developing progressive ventricular dilation.

Head shape can also reflect perinatal events and specific anomalies. The forces of labor and delivery may deform the head, but these changes are transient and disappear within a few days. Infants with craniosynostosis (premature closure of one or more sutures) and hydrocephalus have abnormal head configurations.

Sutures and Fontanels. The entire head is inspected and palpated, and each suture and fontanel is assessed. The anterior fontanel is assessed while the infant is in a quiet state and in a semiupright or sitting position. The fontanel should be open, soft, and flat. Pulsation may be felt normally in a newborn but can be associated with elevated blood pressure. A sunken or depressed fontanel is seen with dehydration, and a bulging fontanel is noted with increased intracranial pressure (ICP). The anterior fontanel usually is diamond shaped and may be small at birth if molding and overriding of the sutures are present; the size increases within a few days to the usual dimensions seen in term infants (i.e., 3 to 4 cm long by 1 to 3 cm wide). The anterior fontanel closes at 8 to 16 months of age. The anterior fontanel may bulge slightly with increased tension when the infant cries and may be slightly depressed when the infant is placed in an upright position. The posterior fontanel closes any time from 8 months' gestation to 2 months after birth. If open at birth, it is 1 to 3 cm wide and has a triangular shape. In rare cases a "third fontanel" may be palpated along the sagittal suture between the anterior and posterior fontanels; this is not a true fontanel but a defect in the parietal bone. It can be palpated in normal infants, but it is also seen in infants with Down syndrome or hypothyroidism.

A 4- to 5-mm separation of all the sutures (Figure 31-2) except the squamosal (temporoparietal) suture is normal in the newborn. The squamosal suture should not be separated more than 2 to 3 mm. Overriding of the bones and molding from delivery may modify this finding in the first few days after birth. Abnormal findings include persistence of suture separation over time, increased separation of the sutures, and separation of the squamosal suture by more than 2 to 3 mm. With increased ICP, separation of the sutures occurs in a specific order: sagittal, coronal, metopic and lambdoidal, and squamosal; therefore

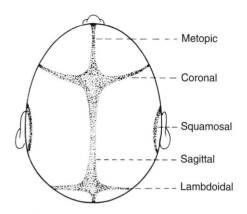

FIGURE **31-2**
Cranial sutures. From Scher M (2001). Brain disorders of the fetus and neonate. In Klaus MH, Fanaroff AA, editors. *Care of the high-risk neonate*, ed 5. WB Saunders: Philadelphia.

separation of the squamosal suture is the most clinically significant (Amiel-Tison, 1995). The cranial bones are inspected and palpated so that fractures, extradural hemorrhage, edema, and areas of uneven ossification of the cranial bones or craniotabes can be identified.

Neurologic Examination
The neurologic examination is useful for evaluating for the presence and determining the extent of neurologic dysfunction in the neonate, for monitoring recovery, and as a prognostic indicator. Factors such as gestational age, health status, the infant's state, medications, and timing of feedings must be considered in the interpretation of neurologic findings. Parameters examined in the assessment of neurologic status include level of consciousness, activity, tone, posture, reflexes, and evaluation of selected cranial nerves (Amiel-Tison, 1995; Volpe, 1998a; Volpe, 2001a). The optimum state of the infant during a neurologic examination is quiet and alert.

Level of Consciousness. Neurologic insults frequently alter the infant's level of consciousness. The level of consciousness may range from normal states of consciousness for gestation to hyperexcitability, irritability, lethargy, hyperalertness, and stupor or coma. The three clinical levels of consciousness that best correlate with outcome are hyperalertness, lethargy, and stupor or coma. In the hyperalert state, the infant has an increased sensitivity to sensory stimulation, with wide open eyes but with a diminished blink response and ability to fixate and follow (Amiel-Tison, 1995; Goddard-Finegold et al, 1998). A lethargic infant responds to tactile and noxious stimuli, but the responses are delayed. A stuporous or obtunded infant's response is limited to noxious stimuli, and a comatose infant shows no response to tactile or noxious stimuli (Volpe, 2001a). Hyperexcitability and irritability can be assessed by noting an infant's response to caregiving actions and medical procedures, as well as the baby's state during intercaregiving intervals and ability to use self-consoling maneuvers or to be soothed by others.

Activity, Tone, and Posture. Infant activity, tone, and general position are assessed, along with spontaneous positioning of the extremities and hands. The infant first is assessed while lying in a resting position. A frog-leg position while supine is seen in immature infants, after breech delivery, and in infants who have experienced severe asphyxia or who have major health problems or neuromuscular disorders (Amiel-Tison, 1995). The quality and symmetry of activity with spontaneous and elicited movement are assessed. Alterations in symmetry of the trunk, face, and extremities at rest or with spontaneous movement suggest congenital anomalies, birth injury, or neurologic insult. Tight fisting is an abnormal sign. A cortical thumb (inside thumb on closure of the hand) may be normal, but it is abnormal if persistent. Opisthotonos and decerebrate or decorticate posturing (Table 31-2) may also occur.

Abnormal movements include seizure activity (described later), jitteriness, and tremors, although the last two findings often are normal. The characteristic movements seen with tremors in the neonate vary, depending on the underlying disorder. For example, tremors associated with metabolic problems usually are low-amplitude, high-frequency movements, whereas tremors associated with CNS problems usually are high-amplitude, low-frequency movements. Jitteriness is a common finding in infants because of the lack of myelinization of the pyramidal tracts. A major function of these tracts is to inhibit spinal reflexes. In the neonate, these unmyelinated tracts respond in a mass way to central arousal with peripheral hyperexcitability. Spontaneous or elicited movement can set off tremors. Tremors can also be associated with metabolic abnormalities, asphyxia, or drug withdrawal. Tremors and jitteriness must be differentiated from seizures. Jitteriness is stimulus sensitive and is not marked by gaze or eye deviations. The predominant movement in jitteriness is tremulousness (rather than the clonic movement seen in seizures), which ceases with passive flexion.

Resting, passive, and active tone is assessed. Resting tone is evaluated by observing the infant at rest in a supine position. Passive tone is evaluated by examining extensibility, which involves maneuvers used in the neuromuscular component of gestational age assessment. The parameters usually examined include posture, dorsiflexion of the foot, scarf sign, passive movements of the arms, popliteal angle, and heel to ear maneuver (Figure 31-3).

Assessment of active tone involves altering the infant's posture to obtain directed motor responses (Amiel-Tison, 1995). Common maneuvers are righting reactions of the legs and trunk and examination of neck flexors and extensors (Figure 31-4). Righting reactions are elicited by holding the infant upright with the feet on a firm surface. The infant's ability to straighten the legs and trunk is assessed. Neck flexors and extensors are assessed using the pull-to-sit maneuver. For the examination of the neck flexors, the infant is pulled to a sitting position, and the tone and position of the head and neck are observed. Neck extensors are examined using a reverse pull-to-sit maneuver; that is, the infant is placed in a sitting position and moved backward toward the bed or the surface of the examination table.

Strength may also be assessed. This parameter is difficult to evaluate in the newborn, therefore only a gross assessment can be obtained. Strength is affected by state, immaturity, and neuromuscular and neurologic problems. Eliciting the grasp reflex and pulling the infant to a sitting position allow assessment of the strength of the upper extremities and neck. The righting reaction can be used to assess strength in the legs. Infants with peripheral nerve injuries, neuromuscular disorders, alterations at the neuromuscular junction, and spinal cord injuries tend to be hypotonic and have muscle weakness. Infants with CNS disturbances secondary to asphyxia, intracranial hemorrhage, Down syndrome, or metabolic disturbances tend to be hypotonic without muscle weakness (Amiel-Tison, 1995; Scher, 2001). Hypertonia is seen less often than hypotonia in neonates with neurologic problems. Marked extensor hypotonia may be seen in association with severe hypoxic-ischemic injury, bacterial meningitis, or massive intraventricular hemorrhage (Scher, 2001; Volpe, 2001a).

Reflexes.   Primary and tendon reflexes are assessed. In infants with neurologic dysfunction, these reflexes may be diminished, absent, or accentuated. The primary reflexes include sucking, grasping, crossed extension, automatic walking (stepping), and the Moro reflex. The primary reflexes are stereotypic responses for the first few months after birth. They should be present, symmetric, and reproducible in the neonatal period and should gradually disappear during infancy (Volpe, 1998a). The primary reflexes are affected by gestational age, but all are present to some degree by 28 to 32 weeks' gestation (Figure 31-5). The tendon reflexes assessed in the neonate are the biceps, knee, and ankle jerk. All should be present and brisk. Ankle clonus generally is not a significant finding in the neonate.

Examination of Selected Cranial Nerves.   Full cranial nerve assessment generally is not performed on the neonate. However, function of these nerves can be evaluated using several relatively simple maneuvers: fixation and following, pupillary responses, doll's eye response, hearing, vestibular response, and suck and swallow. These assessments and the usual findings are summarized in Table 31-3.

Clinical Signs Associated with Neurologic Dysfunction.   Clinical manifestations of neurologic dysfunction can be specific, nonspecific, or subtle. Five types of clinical signs are commonly seen in infants with neurologic problems: (1) CNS depression, (2) hyperirritability, (3) increased ICP, (4) seizures, and (5) movement alterations. Seizures are discussed later. Signs and symptoms of CNS depression, hyperirritability, increased ICP, and movement alterations are listed in Table 31-4.

Diagnostic Techniques

Diagnostic techniques that may be used with infants suspected of neurologic problems include neurophysiologic studies, radiographic assessment, structural brain imaging, measurement of cerebral blood flow, measurement of ICP, cerebral blood flow determination, radionucleotide assessment, cerebral angiography, brainstem-evoked responses, EEG, and lumbar puncture. The three types of brain structural imaging most often used are ultrasonography, CT, and MRI.

Head ultrasound (HUS) examination is used most often to evaluate intracranial structures. HUS is portable, fast, and done at the bedside and involves nonionizing radiation. Cranial and sagittal images can be evaluated by means of the anterior fontanel and periventricular leukomalacia by means of the posterior fontanel. Scans can be real time and multiplanar. Doppler sonography can be used to evaluate cerebral blood flow. HUS is limited in evaluating the posterior fossa and is not useful for interparenchymal and meningeal areas (Barnes & Taylor, 1998; Scher, 2001; Papile, 2002).

CT, which uses ionizing radiation, and MRI, which uses nonionizing radiation, are useful for examinations in the axial

TABLE **31-2** Clinical and Laboratory Features Useful in Differentiation of Tonic Seizures, Decorticate Posturing, Decerebrate Posturing, and Opisthotonos								
Clinical Event	**Duration**	**Provoked by External Stimuli**	**Leg Posture**	**Arm Posture**	**Trunk Posture**	**Change in Respiration**	**Ocular Position**	**Epileptic EEG Changes**
Tonic seizure	Brief, intermittent	No	Extension	Flexed or extended	Usually arched (extended)	Apnea occasionally	Blinking, verticle or horizontal deviation, pupillary changes	Yes
Decorticate posturing	Brief, intermittent	Yes	Extension	Flexed, adducted, internal rotation; fisted	Extended	Typically none	Typically no change	No
Decerebrate posturing	Brief, intermittent	Yes	Extension	Extended, adducted, hyperpronated; fisted	Extended	Tachypnea, irregular breathing, apnea	Pupils enlarged, downward eye deviation; mydriasis	No
Opisthotonos	Prolonged, sustained posture	May or may not	Extension	Variable; often extended	Prolonged arching	Typically none	Typically no change	No
Myoclonic seizures	Brief, intermittent	May or may not	Rapid*	Rapid*	Rapid*	None	None	Yes
Pathologic myoclonus	Brief, intermittent	May or may not	Rapid*	Rapid*	Rapid*	None	None	No
Benign myoclonus	Brief, intermittent during sleep only	No	Rapid*	Rapid*	Rapid*	None	None	No

Modified from Scher MS (2001). Neonatal seizures. In Polin RA & Burg FD: Workbook in practical neonatology, ed 3. WB Saunders: Philadelphia.
Brief, sudden jerk of axial or appendicular musculature.
EEG, Electroencephalographic.

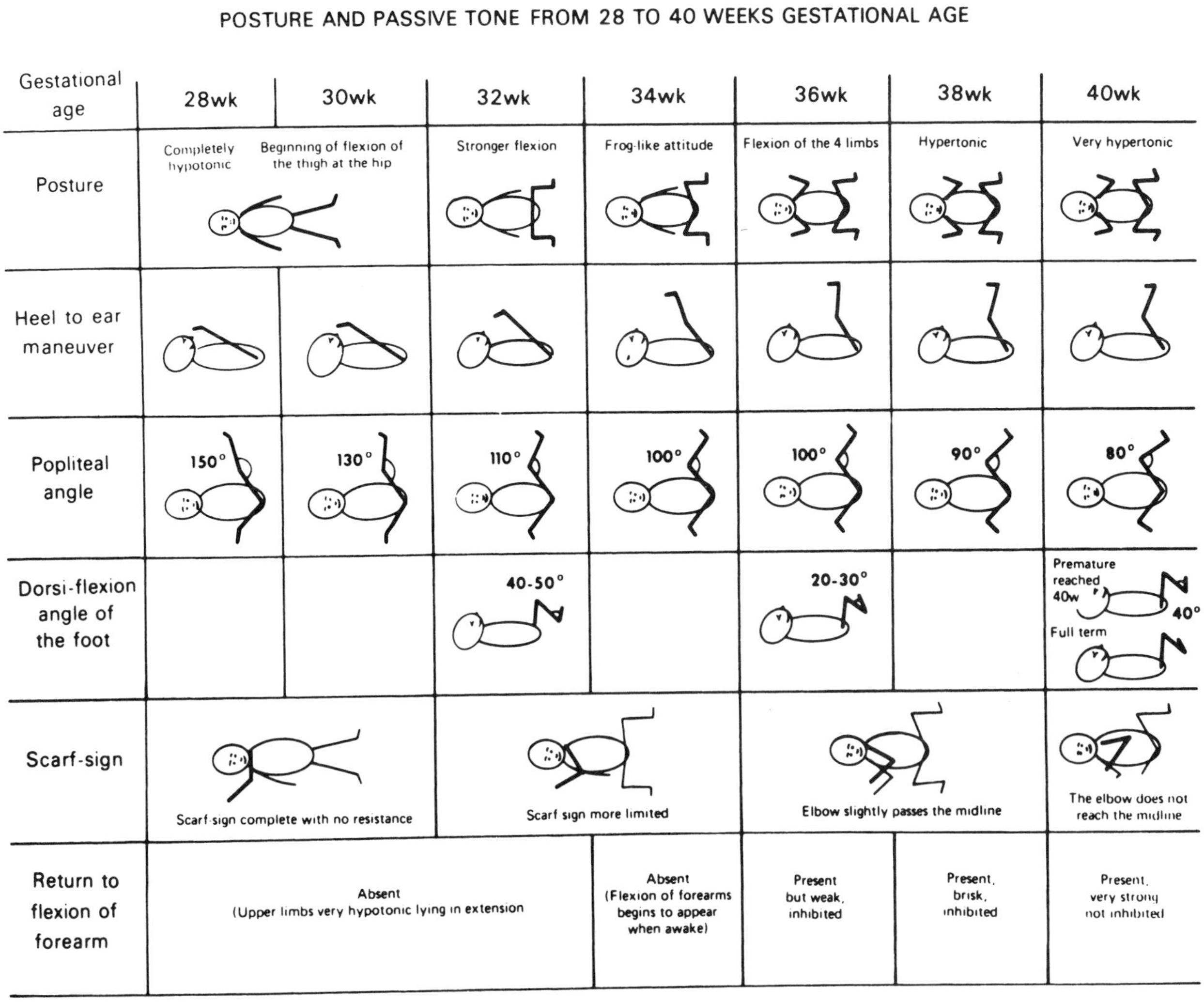

POSTURE AND PASSIVE TONE FROM 28 TO 40 WEEKS GESTATIONAL AGE

Gestational age	28wk	30wk	32wk	34wk	36wk	38wk	40wk
Posture	Completely hypotonic	Beginning of flexion of the thigh at the hip	Stronger flexion	Frog-like attitude	Flexion of the 4 limbs	Hypertonic	Very hypertonic
Heel to ear maneuver							
Popliteal angle	150°	130°	110°	100°	100°	90°	80°
Dorsi-flexion angle of the foot			40-50°		20-30°		Premature reached 40w 40° Full term
Scarf-sign	Scarf-sign complete with no resistance		Scarf sign more limited		Elbow slightly passes the midline		The elbow does not reach the midline
Return to flexion of forearm	Absent (Upper limbs very hypotonic lying in extension			Absent (Flexion of forearms begins to appear when awake)	Present but weak, inhibited	Present, brisk, inhibited	Present, very strong, not inhibited

FIGURE **31-3**
Posture and passive tone from 28 to 40 weeks' gestation. From Rudolph AM, Hoffman J, editors (1991). *Rudolph's pediatrics*, ed 19. Appleton & Lange: Norwalk, CT.

or coronal plane; they also can be helpful if HUS is unsatisfactory. MRI, although not always available, generally is preferable to CT except in cases involving calcifications or acute hemorrhage (Scher, 2001). MRI is slower and usually requires sedation or anesthesia. CT may also require sedation but has greater sensitivity and specificity, especially in infants with unexplained neurologic signs (Barnes & Taylor, 1998).

Laboratory tests are performed to assist in the diagnosis of specific neurologic disorders and to identify underlying causes. The CSF is examined for signs of hemorrhage (increased red blood cells, increased protein, decreased glucose, and xanthochromia) and to rule out infection. Xanthochromia often is a late sign and may reflect an elevated protein level rather than the presence of blood. If the ICP is increased, the pressure of the CSF on needle insertion may reflect this. Other laboratory evaluations include the hematocrit value, serum glucose level, electrolyte levels, blood gases, and acid-base status. A sepsis workup or screening for toxoplasmosis, rubella, cytomegalovirus, and herpes simplex (TORCH) is performed if intrauterine infection or neonatal sepsis and meningitis are suspected. A genetic workup and other metabolic studies are performed if errors of metabolism or other inherited disorders are thought to be present.

Collaborative Management

Collaborative and nursing management specific to each type of neurologic dysfunction is described in later sections. However, in the nursing care of infants with neurologic dysfunction, common nursing diagnoses and management techniques that must be considered with all infants and their families can be identified, including the following:

1. Alteration in level of consciousness
   - Monitor infant's state, activity level, responsiveness, eye movements, head circumference, and vital signs; also monitor for seizure activity and signs of increased ICP.
   - Position infant so as to promote skin integrity, prevent contractures, and reduce ICP (i.e., head in midline and slightly elevated).
   - Monitor fluid and electrolyte status.
   - Maintain adequate ventilation and perfusion.
   - Implement comfort measures.
   - Maintain an appropriate thermal environment.

ACTIVE TONE FROM 32 TO 40 WEEKS GESTATIONAL AGE

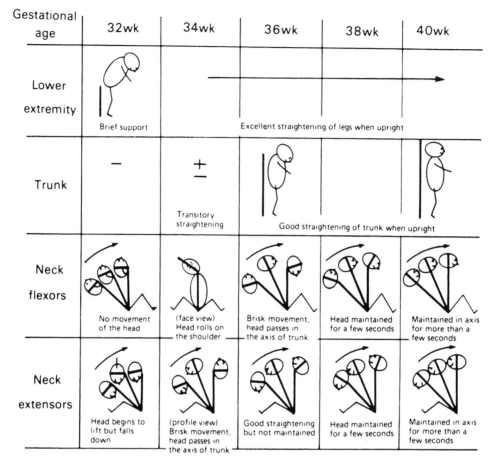

FIGURE **31-4**
Active tone from 32 to 40 weeks' gestation. From Rudolph AM, Hoffman J, editors (1991). *Rudolph's pediatrics*, ed 19. Appleton & Lange: Norwalk, CT.

- Reduce environmental stressors.
- Promote neurobehavioral stability.
2. Potential for injury related to trauma or infection
   - Use aseptic technique.
   - Use sterile technique when appropriate.
   - Position infant to prevent contamination of defects or operative sites.
   - Monitor for signs of localized infection or neonatal sepsis.
   - Handle infant gently.
   - Position infant to reduce potential of trauma or contamination.
3. Impairment of skin integrity
   - Position infant in alignment and change position regularly.
   - Use foam, sheepskin, lambskin, or waterbeds.
   - Massage skin gently to stimulate circulation.
   - Use appropriate skin care measures.
4. Alteration in comfort*
5. Impaired mobility
   - Position infant in alignment and change position regularly.
   - Promote skin integrity.
   - Use gentle range-of-motion exercises.
6. Alteration in thermoregulation*

7. Alteration in nutrition*
8. Promote neurobehavioral organization and development*
9. Altered family processes*
10. Grieving (family)*

TYPES OF NEUROLOGIC DYSFUNCTION

Seizures

Seizures are the most common neurologic sign during the neonatal period. They are not a disease in themselves but a sign of underlying disease processes that have resulted in an acute disturbance within the brain (Volpe, 2001b). If left untreated, these disorders can lead to permanent damage of the CNS or other tissues. Disease processes associated with seizures in the neonate include primary CNS disorders, asphyxia, systemic diseases, and metabolic insults. The reported incidence of neonatal seizures ranges from 1.8 to 3.5 per 1000 live births (Mizrahi, 2001). Seizures are seen more often in preterm infants (22.7%) than in term infants (0.15%) (Scher, 1997). Seizure activity

---

*Specific interventions are discussed in other chapters.

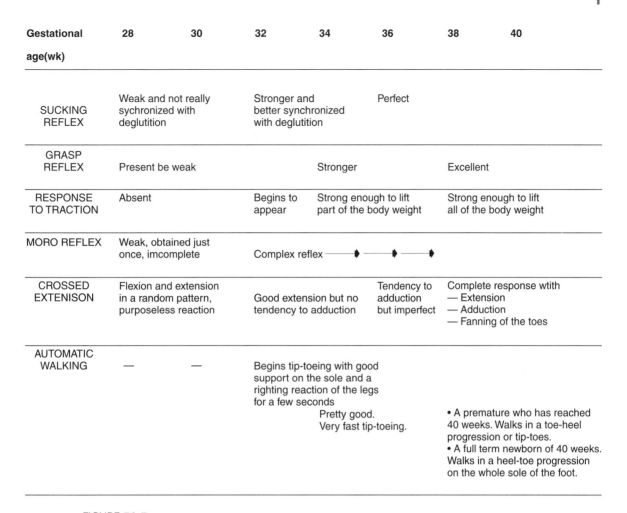

Gestational age(wk)	28	30	32	34	36	38	40
SUCKING REFLEX	Weak and not really sychronized with deglutition		Stronger and better synchronized with deglutition		Perfect		
GRASP REFLEX	Present be weak			Stronger		Excellent	
RESPONSE TO TRACTION	Absent		Begins to appear	Strong enough to lift part of the body weight		Strong enough to lift all of the body weight	
MORO REFLEX	Weak, obtained just once, imcomplete		Complex reflex ⬧——⬧——⬧				
CROSSED EXTENISON	Flexion and extension in a random pattern, purposeless reaction		Good extension but no tendency to adduction		Tendency to adduction but imperfect	Complete response wtith — Extension — Adduction — Fanning of the toes	
AUTOMATIC WALKING	—	—	Begins tip-toeing with good support on the sole and a righting reaction of the legs for a few seconds Pretty good. Very fast tip-toeing.			• A premature who has reached 40 weeks. Walks in a toe-heel progression or tip-toes. • A full term newborn of 40 weeks. Walks in a heel-toe progression on the whole sole of the foot.	

FIGURE **31-5**
Development of selected reflexes from 28 to 40 weeks' gestation. From Rudolph AM, Hoffman J, editors (1991). *Rudolph's pediatrics*, ed 19. Appleton & Lange: Norwalk, CT.

may be an acute, recurrent, or chronic phenomenon. Neonatal seizures usually are acute and disappear within the first few weeks after birth. Recurrent or continuous seizures increase the risk of neurologic damage from the seizure activity itself (Mizrahi, 2001).

Pathophysiology. Seizures are the result of excessive, synchronous electrical discharge or depolarization in the brain that produces stereotypic, repetitive behaviors. Depolarization and repolarization of the nerves are caused by the movement of sodium and potassium across the cell membrane. The inward migration of sodium ions (Na^+) results in depolarization; repolarization is produced by the outward migration of potassium ions (K^+). These processes require an energy-dependent pump and energy in the form of adenosine triphosphate (ATP).

The specific mechanism that causes neonatal seizures is unknown. Such seizures might be the result of one or more of these mechanisms: (1) disturbances in energy production and the Na^+-K^+ pump, (2) altered neuronal membrane permeability to sodium, and (3) imbalances in excitatory and inhibitory neurotransmitters (Volpe, 2001a).

A disturbance in energy production, with changes in the movement of Na^+ and K^+ across the neuronal membrane, can lead to an imbalance between depolarization and repolarization.

The movement of K^+ (repolarization) unbalances the movement of Na^+ (depolarization). Changes in energy production occur secondary to hypoxemia, ischemia, and hypoglycemia. Alterations in the permeability of the neuronal membrane to sodium can occur with hypocalcemia. Calcium normally binds with proteins in the cell membrane to inhibit Na^+ movement. A decrease in the availability of calcium would increase inward movement of Na^+ and lead to depolarization. Hypomagnesemia also increases membrane permeability to Na^+, and alkalosis or hyponatremia, as well, can lead to seizures through this mechanism.

Imbalances in neurotransmitters, resulting in a relative excess of excitatory neurotransmitter (glutamate or acetylcholine) over inhibitory neurotransmitter (gamma-aminobutyric acid [GABA]), increase the rate of depolarization. This can occur as a result of an excess of excitatory substance (associated with hypoxemia, ischemia, and hypoglycemia) or a deficiency of inhibitory substance. Pyridoxine deficiency leads to an inhibitory neurotransmitter deficiency by depressing activity of the enzyme responsible for synthesis of gamma-aminobutyric acid. Elevated levels of excitatory inhibitors derived from ammonia are seen in preterm infants who have an excessive protein intake or in infants who have liver dysfunction after severe asphyxia (Volpe, 2001a).

TABLE **31-3**	Nursing Assessment of Selected Cranial Nerves in the Newborn	
Nerve	**Assessment**	**Implications**
Optic (II)	Blink in response to light (consistent by 28 weeks' gestation)	Visual system intact to the level of the superior colliculi (does not indicate visual cortex function)
	Fixation on object placed approximately 19 cm in front of infant's face (consistent by 32 weeks' gestation)	Presence of vision
	Follows object with eyes and by turning head (consistent by 37 weeks' gestation)	
	Examination of external eye	Evaluation of abnormalities (e.g., cataracts, irregularities of size or shape, microphthalmos, or scleral hemangiomas)
	Funduscopic examination (ophthalmoscope set at −2 to −4 diopters)	Normal newborn optic disc is pale or grayish-white; observe for abnormalities (e.g., retinal hemorrhage or lesion)
Oculomotor (III), trochlear (IV), and abducens (VI)	Pupillary reactivity (equal and responsive to light; appears by 28 weeks' gestation and is consistent by 32 weeks)	Intact cranial nerve III; unequal or nonresponsive pupils in infants over 32 weeks' gestation are associated with increased intracranial pressure or hemorrhage
	Doll's eye maneuver (vestibular response; present by 25 weeks' gestation): hold infant in an upright position at arm's length and rotate in both directions	Stimulation of semicircular canals with impulses sent to the brainstem via nerves III, VI, and VII. Normal response is isotonic deviation of the eyes away from the direction of movement; lack of response is associated with brainstem dysfunction or excessive administration of sedatives such as phenobarbital; disconjugate eye movements and some nystagmoid movement occasionally are seen normally during the first 3 weeks
Trigeminal (V)	Elicit the corneal reflex (may not be reliable in newborn) or observe for a grimace on pinprick	Facial sensation (not usually done routinely but may be useful with an infant with facial paralysis)
	Elicit sucking and ability of infant to bite down on examiner's finger	Masticatory power
Facial (VII)	Observe appearance and symmetry of face at rest and during spontaneous and elicited movement	Abnormalities associated with birth injury and cerebral insults
Acoustic (VIII)	Evaluate auditory function by noting response (blink or startle) to sudden loud noise (seen by 28 weeks' gestation) or (in more mature infants) by cessation of movement and turning to sound while in a quiet, alert state	A gross assessment of auditory function; failure of the infant to respond while in a quiet, alert state in a quiet environment on repeated examinations indicates the need for examination of auditory function
Trigeminal (V), facial (VII), glossopharyngeal (IX), vagus (X), and hypoglossal (XII)	Evaluate sucking (V, VII, XII), swallowing (IX and X), and gag reflex (IX and X)	Impairment interferes with feeding and may indicate or be associated with cerebral insult

Data from Amiel-Tison C (1995). Clinical assessment of the nervous system. In Levene MI, Lilford RJ, editors. Fetal and neonatal neurology and neurosurgery, ed 2. Churchill Livingstone: Edinburgh; Goddard-Finegold J et al (1998). The newborn nervous system. In Taeusch HW, Ballard RA, editors. Avery's diseases of the newborn, ed 7. WB Saunders: Philadelphia; Scher M (2001). Brain disorders of the fetus and neonate. In Klaus MH, Fanaroff AA, editors. Care of the high-risk neonate, ed 5. WB Saunders: Philadelphia; and Volpe JJ (2001). Neurology of the newborn, ed 4. WB Saunders: Philadelphia.

Biochemical Effects of Seizures. Seizures result in increased energy expenditure by the organism, which leads to the following sequence of biochemical events (Figure 31-6): (1) breakdown of ATP to adenosine diphosphate with release of energy; (2) increased glycolysis, stimulated by adenosine diphosphate, with conversion of glycogen to glucose; (3) increased production of pyruvate, which is used by the mitochondria in ATP production; (4) increased oxygen and glucose consumption; (5) increased production of lactate from pyruvate, stimulated by increased adenosine diphosphate; and

TABLE **31-4**	Clinical Manifestations of Central Nervous System Dysfunction
Alteration	**Clinical Manifestations**
Central nervous system depression	Altered level of consciousness
	Weak, absent cry
	Weak, absent primary reflexes
	Poor feeding
	Decreased activity
	Decreased passive tone
	Decreased active tone
	Altered respirations
Hyperirritability	Sharp, excessive crying
	Hyperactivity
	Exaggerated passive tone
	Hypertonia
	Difficult to console
	Low sensory threshold
Increased intracranial pressure	Irritability
	Lethargy
	Increased head circumference
	Palpable sutures, especially squamous
	Bulging, tense fontanel
	Increased extensor tone of neck
	Downward deviation of eyes
	Vomiting (late)
	Dilated head veins (late)
Seizures	See Table 31-6.
Movement alterations	Jitteriness, tremors
	Decerebrate posturing (Table 31-2)
	Decorticate posturing (Table 31-2)
	Opisthotonos (Table 31-2)

Data from Amiel-Tison C, Larroche JC (1988). Brain development and neurological survey during the neonatal period. In Stern L, Vert P, editors. Neonatal medicine, New York: Masson Publishing: New York; Amiel-Tison C (1995). Clinical assessment of the nervous system. In Levene MI, Lilford RJ, editors. Fetal and neonatal neurology and neurosurgery, ed 2. Churchill Livingstone: Edinburgh; and Goddard-Finegold J et al (1998). The newborn nervous system. In Taeusch HW, Ballard RA, editors. Avery's diseases of the newborn, ed 7. WB Saunders: Philadelphia.

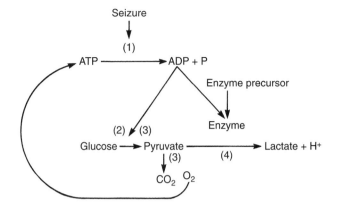

FIGURE **31-6**
Biochemical effects of seizures. *ATP*, Adenosine triphosphate; *ADP*, adenosine diphosphate; *P*, phosphorus; *H$^+$*, hydrogen ion; *CO$_2$*, carbon dioxide; *O$_2$*, oxygen. Modified from Volpe JJ (1987). *Neurology of the newborn*, ed 2. WB Saunders: Philadelphia.

structural and functional differences in the neonatal brain. The peak time for organizational processes in the brain is the sixth month of gestation to 1 year after birth, therefore term and especially preterm infants have relatively immature brain organization at birth. This lack of organization results in an inability to propagate and sustain generalized seizures. For example, the neonate's brain lacks the arborization and synaptic connections (wiring) necessary for a firing neuron to recruit adjacent neurons to fire synchronously. Inadequate organization also leads to a slower response to stimuli (Volpe, 2001b). The lower rate of nerve conduction, limited myelinization, and smaller number of connections between neurons alter the threshold for neuron firing and ability to propagate seizures (Holmes & Ben-Ari, 2001; Volpe, 2001b).

The neonate has more inhibitory than excitatory synapses; this is actually a protective mechanism because it reduces the chance that a generalized seizure will be propagated in the cerebral cortex. As a result, cortical seizures are rare in neonates (Volpe, 2001b). The newborn has more excitatory (glutamate) than inhibitory (GABA) neurotransmitter. The glutamate level is increased (it is needed by the brain for neuronal development and organization); maturation of the inhibitory system is delayed; and the number of NMDA receptors that respond to glutamate is increased (Fox et al, 1996; Fitzgerald & Jennings, 1999; Holmes & Ben-Ari, 2001). Seizure activity in these infants is more likely to be generated in areas of the brain that are maturer, such as the temporal lobe and subcortical structures, especially in the limbic area. The limbic area, located in the gyrus area above the corpus callosum, is one of the oldest parts of the brain in terms of embryologic development. This area is involved with behaviors such as sucking, drooling, chewing, swallowing, oculomotor deviations, and apneic episodes, behaviors typical of those seen with subtle seizures in the neonate (Volpe, 2001b).

Risk Factors. Seizures are a clinical manifestation associated with various underlying pathologic processes (Table 31-5). The two events that most often place the neonate at risk for seizures are perinatal asphyxia and metabolic disturbances, such as hypoglycemia and hypocalcemia (Scher, 1997). Other problems that increase the risk of seizures in the neonate include intracranial hemorrhage, infection (meningitis, congenital viral infections, viral encephalopathy), congenital anom-

(6) lactate/H$^+$-stimulated local vasodilation, which increases local blood flow and substrate availability (Volpe, 2001a). The rise in blood pressure associated with seizures also increases cerebral blood flow and substrate availability. Seizures result in a marked decrease in brain glucose concentrations because the cells to replenish ATP supplies use much of the available glucose.

Repetitive seizures in the neonate eventually alter brain lipid and protein metabolism and energy metabolism, resulting in a reduction in total brain DNA, RNA, protein, and cholesterol. In animal models these deficiencies lead to impairment of cellular proliferation, differentiation, and myelinization (Volpe, 2001a, b). The effects in the human neonate are unclear but of concern. Brain damage caused by seizure activity could be the result of alterations in protein metabolism or the energy supply, or it could be the result of damage from asphyxia or edema.

Seizures in Neonates Compared with Those in Older Children and Adults. Seizures are more common and expressed differently in the neonate than in older individuals because of

| TABLE **31-5** | Major Causes of Neonatal Seizures |

Cause and Frequency (% of Total)	Usual Age at Onset (Days)	Predominant Type of Seizure	RELATIVE FREQUENCY	
			Partial Tremor	Focal Tremor
Perinatal asphyxia (30% to 65%)	After 1 (often 6 to 18 hours after birth); 90% in first 72 hours'	Subtle (all), generalized tonic, multifocal clonic	++++	+++
Intracranial hemorrhage				
IVH	1 to 4	Subtle progressing to tonic	+++	—
SAH	2 to 3	Any type	++	+
SDH	1 to 2	May be focal	+/−	+
Hypocalcemia (15%)				
Early	1 to 3	Usually focal or multifocal	+++	+/−
Late	4 to 7	Usually focal or multifocal	++	+
Hypoglycemia (10%)	1 to 2	Usually focal or multifocal	++	+/−
Infections (10% to 15%)				
Bacterial meningitis	4 to 7	Any type; may be tonic	++	+
Viral encephalopathy	2 to 15	Any type	+	+
Congenital viral infection	3 to 7	Tonic, myoclonic	+/−	+/−
CNS malformations (fewer than 10%)	2 to 10 (often not until several months of age)	Tonic, myoclonic	+	+/−
Drug withdrawal (rare)	3 to 34	Tonic or myoclonic	+/−	+/−
Local anesthetic intoxication* (uncommon)	Before 1 (1 to 6 hours after birth)	Tonic	+/−	+/−

Modified from Brown JK, Minns RA (1988). Seizure disorders. In Levene MI et al, editors. Fetal and neonatal neurology and neurosurgery. Churchill Livingstone: Edinburgh; Clancy RR (1989). Neonatal seizures. In Stevenson DK, Sunshine P, editors. Fetal and neonatal brain injury. BC Decker: Toronto; Torrence C (1985). Neonatal seizures. I. A developmental and clinical understanding. Neonatal Network 4:9-16; Scher M (2001). Brain disorders of the fetus and neonate. In Klaus MH, Fanaroff AA, editors. Care of the high-risk neonate, ed 5. WB Saunders: Philadelphia; Torrence C (1985). Neonatal seizures. II. Recognition, treatment, and prognosis. Neonatal Network 4:21-22; and Volpe JJ (2001). Neurology of the newborn, ed 4. WB Saunders: Philadelphia.

Caused by accidental injection of local anesthetic into the scalp during placement of paracervical, pudendal, or epidural blocks or during injection of local anesthetics at delivery.

++++, Most common; +, least common; —, not seen; +/−, may or may not be seen; IVH, intraventricular hemorrhage; SAH, subarachnoid hemorrhage; SDH, subdural hemorrhage; CNS, central nervous system.

alies of the CNS, and other metabolic disturbances, such as alkalosis, hypomagnesemia, hypernatremia, and hyponatremia. Less common causes of seizures are drug withdrawal from opiates or barbiturates, genetic disorders of amino and organic acid metabolism, kernicterus, hyperviscosity, and local anesthetic intoxication.

Differential Diagnosis.   Seizures can be difficult to recognize in neonates because the clinical manifestations often are subtle and can be associated with other disorders or can involve individual behaviors such as grimacing, startle, sucking, and twitching. Seizures also can occur with minimal or no outward signs. In addition, the individual behaviors just mentioned are normally seen during active sleep and thus can also be benign.

Seizure and jitteriness may be confused in the neonate, although the predominant type of movement is different. With jitteriness, the predominant movements are tremors characterized by alternating rhythmic movements of equal rate and magnitude. Seizures that may be confused with jitteriness involve primarily clonic movements that have characteristic fast and slow components (Scher, 1997; Volpe, 2001b). Jitteriness sometimes occurs along with seizures in such disorders as hypoglycemia and hypocalcemia and after perinatal asphyxia. Tonic seizures sometimes are confused with decorticate posturing and

opisthotonos. (See Table 31-2 for a summary of the characteristics of each of these signs.)

Clinical Manifestations.   Recognition of seizures in the neonatal period requires careful, continuous assessment by the nurse of all infants at risk. As mentioned before, clinical manifestations of seizures in the neonate differ from those seen in older children and adults because of the immaturity of the CNS. Consequently, seizure manifestations tend to be subtler. Clinical manifestations may include abnormal movements or alterations in tone of the trunk or extremities; abnormal facial, oral, tongue, or ocular movements; and respiratory problems (Mizrahi, 2001). Specific examples of each of these are listed in Table 31-6.

Types of Seizures.   The types of seizures seen in the neonate are, in order of decreasing frequency, subtle, tonic, clonic (multifocal and focal), and myoclonic (Scher, 1997; Mizrahi, 2001; Volpe, 2001b).

Subtle Seizures.   Subtle seizures are the most common type of seizure seen in neonates, particularly among preterm infants. This type of seizure often is missed because the clinical manifestations may be difficult to recognize and distinguish from other events. The behaviors most commonly seen with subtle seizures are (1) tonic, horizontal deviations of the eyes

TABLE 31-6	Clinical Manifestations of Seizures in the Neonate
Type of Manifestation	**Specific Alterations**
Abnormal movement or alterations of tone in the trunk and extremities	Clonic (generalized or multi-focal, migratory)
	Altering hemiclonic tonic (single extremity), extension of arms and legs ("decerebrate-like"), extension of legs and flexion of arms ("decorticate-like"), or generalized
	Myoclonic (isolated or general)
	Bicycling movements of legs
	Swimming or rowing arm movements
	Loss of tone with general flaccidity
Facial, oral, and tongue movements	Sucking
	Grimacing
	Twitching
	Chewing, swallowing, yawning
Ocular movements	Tonic horizontal eye deviation
	Staring, blinking
	Nystagmoid jerks
Respiratory manifestations	Apnea (usually preceded or accompanied by one or more subtle manifestations)
	Hyperpneic or stertorous breathing

Modified from Clancy RR (1983). Neonatal seizures. In Polin RA, Berg F, editors. Workbook in practical neonatology. WB Saunders: Philadelphia; Gale E (1981). Neonatal seizures. In Perez R, editor. Protocols for perinatal nursing practice. Mosby: St Louis; and Mizrahi EM (2001). Neonatal seizures and neonatal epileptic syndromes. Neurology clinics 19:427-463.

with or without nystagmoid jerking; (2) repetitive blinking or fluttering of the eyelids; (3) drooling, sucking, and/or tongue thrusting; and (4) swimming or rowing movements of the arms with occasional bicycling movements of the legs (Goddard-Finegold et al, 1998; Volpe, 2001b). Apnea may occur but usually is the result of the underlying cause of the seizure rather than of the seizure per se and rarely occurs as an isolated seizure event (Bernes & Kaplan, 1994).

Tonic Seizures. The most common form of tonic seizure is the generalized tonic seizure, which usually involves tonic extension of all the extremities but sometimes is limited to one extremity or is manifested by tonic flexion of all limbs. Generalized tonic seizures can be confused with decorticate or decerebrate posturing (Table 31-2). Other signs may include eye deviations, apnea, and occasional clonic movements. This type of seizure is the one seen most frequently in preterm infants, especially those with intraventricular hemorrhage and hypoxic-ischemic insults. Generalized tonic seizures often are accompanied by apnea or decerebrate-type postures or both. Occasionally, focal tonic seizures may occur, which are char-

acterized by sustained asymmetric posturing of the limbs, trunk, and/or neck. Focal tonic seizure activity may be difficult to differentiate from voluntary movement (Scher, 1997; Volpe, 2001b).

Clonic Seizures. Clonic seizures may be multifocal or focal. Because multifocal clonic (migratory) seizures involve the cortex, they are more characteristic of term infants but occasionally may be seen in older preterm infants. This type of seizure involves rhythmic, jerky clonic movements of one or more limbs that migrate to other parts of the body in a random fashion. Multifocal clonic seizures can be confused with jitteriness. These seizures are associated with diffuse hyperexcitability of the cortex, such as occurs with metabolic derangements (Mizrahi, 2001). Focal clonic seizures are also seen more frequently in term than in preterm infants. This relatively uncommon form of seizure is characterized by localized clonic jerking that usually is confined to one limb or the face. Focal clonic seizures may be associated with focal traumatic CNS injuries, such as cerebral contusions and infarcts, or they may be a response to a severe metabolic disturbance or asphyxia. These seizures often are seen in combination with other seizure types (Mizrahi, 2001).

Myoclonic Seizures. Myoclonic seizures are uncommon in term infants and are rarely seen in preterm infants. These seizures are characterized by single or multiple sudden jerks with flexion of the upper (most common) or lower extremities and occasionally the trunk and neck. Myoclonic seizures are most often seen with inborn errors of metabolism or other metabolic problems.

Prognosis. The mortality rate for infants with seizures has declined in recent years, from approximately 40% before 1969 to less than 15% currently. Benign seizures in otherwise healthy infants during the first week have a good prognosis (Mizrahi, 2001). Among infants who have repeated seizures, the percentage that show later developmental problems is 25% to 35% or higher (Mizrahi & Clancy, 2000; Holmes & Ben-Ari, 2001; Volpe, 2001b). Preterm infants tend to recover more rapidly from a seizure than do term infants; however, mortality and later morbidity are higher in preterm infants. The prognosis for infants who have seizures during the neonatal period is influenced by (1) the time of onset, (2) the cause of the seizure, (3) the interictal EEG results, and (4) the frequency and duration of the seizures (Mizrahi, 2001; Scher, 2001). Seizure onset less than 48 hours after birth has a poor prognosis, whereas onset after 4 days generally has a good prognosis. Clonic seizures have a better prognosis than the other types (Mizrahi, 2001). The EEG results are a better prognostic sign in term than in preterm infants. The prognosis should not be based on a single EEG; fewer than 10% of infants with normal interictal EEG results have neurologic sequelae (Scher, 1997). Among neonates who have had documented seizures, 20% to 25% are at risk of developing epilepsy in childhood (Scher, 1997).

Seizures are actually relatively difficult to produce and maintain in most newborn animals, including human infants, because of CNS immaturity. Therefore the increased frequency of seizures during the neonatal period is thought to be due to the many severe pathologic events to which the neonate is exposed that have the potential to cause seizures. The poorest prognosis is seen with seizures associated with severe birth asphyxia, grade III or grade IV intraventricular hemorrhage, herpes infection, some bacterial meningitis, and CNS malformations. The best prognosis is seen in infants with seizures that occur secondary to late hypocalcemia, hyponatremia, and uncomplicated subarachnoid hemorrhage. Other causes have a mixed prognosis (Volpe, 2001b).

The seizure itself, unless prolonged or repeated, probably causes little damage. CNS damage associated with neonatal seizures usually occurs secondary to underlying pathologic processes that are severe enough to cause a seizure. Repeated or prolonged seizures can lead to brain injury by altering cerebral blood flow and delivery of oxygen and nutrients, by depleting brain glucose and energy stores, and by interfering with ventilation (Volpe, 2001b). The interaction of these events is summarized in Figure 31-7.

Collaborative Management.   Management of neonatal seizures has two goals: (1) to determine and treat the underlying cause of the seizures and (2) to protect the infant from injury during and after the seizure. Determining the cause involves assessment of the perinatal and neonatal history, a physical examination, laboratory evaluation, and other diagnostic studies. Previous events that may indicate the underlying cause include the delivery history, bleeding, birth trauma, perinatal asphyxia, exposure to infectious agents and other teratogens, maternal substance abuse, and postbirth illnesses.

The physical examination includes evaluation of the infant's general health and neurologic status. Routine laboratory studies include electrolyte levels; glucose, calcium, magnesium, and blood urea nitrogen levels; hematocrit value, blood gases, and pH. A blood culture and lumbar puncture also are often performed. A lumbar puncture helps to rule out both infection and

CNS bleeding. Other laboratory and diagnostic studies may include CT, ultrasonography, MRI, skull radiography, TORCH screening, amino acid screening (for inborn errors of metabolism), or EEG. The results of an interictal EEG can provide information for the prognosis, more so in a term than a preterm infant. The timing of seizure onset and the type of seizure also can aid in the determination of the cause (Table 31-5).

Treatment of the underlying cause of the seizure is a priority for preventing more seizures and neurologic damage. Management of intracranial hemorrhage and CNS anomalies is discussed later in this chapter. Management of other conditions, such as perinatal asphyxia, metabolic and electrolyte disorders, infections, and drug withdrawal, are discussed in detail in other chapters.

Continual monitoring of blood gases, acid-base status, serum glucose, and fluid and electrolyte status is important for any infant with seizures. Infants who have seizures, regardless of the cause, require intravenous administration of glucose because seizure activity depletes brain glucose and energy supplies (Scher, 1997). Alterations in oxygenation and acid-base status can occur as a complication of the apnea associated with a seizure or the physiologic consequences of seizure activity. Fluid and electrolyte management should be appropriate to the underlying cause of the seizures. For example, fluids are restricted initially in infants with cerebral edema and perinatal asphyxia.

The issues of when to treat with anticonvulsant drugs and for how long are controversial. Some clinicians favor early, aggressive therapy, whereas others do not because neonatal

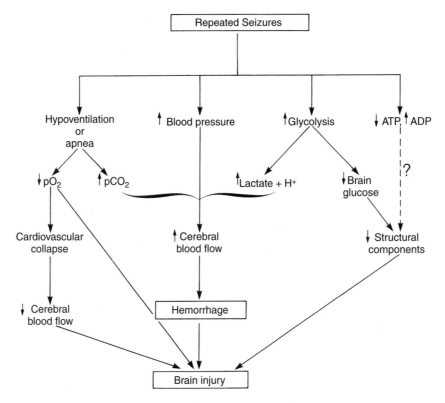

FIGURE **31-7**
Mechanisms of brain injury with repeated seizures. *ATP,* Adenosine triphosphate; *ADP,* adenosine diphosphate; *PO₂,* partial pressure of oxygen; *PCO₂,* partial pressure of carbon dioxide; *H⁺,* hydrogen ion. Modified from Volpe JJ (1987). *Neurology of the newborn,* ed 2. WB Saunders: Philadelphia.

seizures often abate spontaneously. Recurrent or prolonged seizures require treatment with anticonvulsants to reduce the risk of brain injury. The anticonvulsants most often used in the neonate are phenobarbital (usually the first-line drug) and phenytoin (Dilantin), followed by benzodiazepines such as diazepam and lorazepam (Mizrahi, 2001). Blood levels of these drugs must be monitored carefully to ensure therapeutic levels and prevent toxicity. Cardiovascular status and respiratory function must also be monitored. Refractory seizure may require alternative agents such as clonesepam, lidocaine, carbomazepam, midazolam, or primidone (Goodard-Finegold et al, Mizrahi, 2001). Administration of anticonvulsants should be discontinued before discharge whenever possible. Volpe (2001b) indicates that anticonvulsant therapy can be discontinued if the infant has a normal neurologic examination and EEG result and if no brain lesions are seen on cranial imaging.

Nursing Management.   The nurse is the individual most likely to observe seizure activity in the nursery. Nursing management, therefore, focuses on recognizing and documenting seizure activity and protecting and supporting the infant during and after the seizure. Observing and documenting seizure activity involves noting and recording (1) the time the seizure begins and ends; (2) the body parts involved (e.g., extremities, eyes, head); (3) a description of motor movement, eye deviations, and pupillary reactions; and (4) the infant's respiratory status, color, state, level of consciousness, and postictal status.

Nursing interventions during a seizure vary with the severity, duration, and type of seizure. During the seizure, the nurse must ensure that the infant's airway is maintained, monitor vital signs, and assess for adequacy of respiration and heart rate to maintain ventilation and perfusion. To protect the infant from injury during the seizure, the nurse should not force anything into the infant's mouth or try to restrain the infant's extremities. The nurse should try to turn the infant's head to the side, if possible. After the seizure, the infant's condition should be monitored, and supportive care should be provided so that ventilation, oxygenation, adequate fluids, glucose, and warmth are maintained. The nurse also should assess the infant for signs related to the events that can cause seizure activity in the neonate to help determine the cause of the seizure and prevent additional seizures.

Nursing management also involves administering and monitoring anticonvulsants and performing interventions aimed at treating the underlying cause of the seizures. Because anticonvulsants can be respiratory, myocardial, and CNS depressants or can compete with bilirubin for albumin binding, the infant's cardiorespiratory status, color, and neurologic status are monitored in addition to drug effectiveness. Parent teaching includes helping the family to understand the cause and significance of the seizure or seizures and any diagnostic tests that are planned. Discharge teaching of parents includes recognition of seizure manifestations, care of the infant during and after a seizure, and administration of anticonvulsants (dosage and side effects) if administration of these drugs is to be continued after discharge.

Periventricular/Intraventricular Hemorrhage

Periventricular/intraventricular hemorrhage (P/IVH) is the most common type of intracranial hemorrhage seen in the neonatal period. P/IVH is seen almost exclusively in preterm infants, particularly those born at less than 32 weeks' gestation

or weighing less than 1500 g, or both. The incidence in this group of infants has declined and currently ranges from 15% to 20% (Bulas & Vezina, 1999; Volpe, 2001b). The incidence in infants of less than 26 weeks' gestation may approach 60% (Tortorolo et al, 1999; Scher, 2001). The risk of P/IVH increases with decreasing gestational age. P/IVH occurs but is rare after 35 to 36 weeks' gestation because of the involution of the subependymal germinal matrix and alterations in cerebral blood flow patterns that occur after this time (Levene, 1995b).

Pathophysiology.   The neuropathophysiology of P/IVH involves a complex interaction of intravascular, vascular, and extravascular factors. In infants of less than 28 to 32 weeks' gestation, the hemorrhage generally arises from the subependymal germinal matrix at the head of the caudate nucleus near the foramen of Monro. On those rare occasions when P/IVH occurs in term infants, bleeding usually arises from the choroid plexus rather than from the germinal matrix (Volpe, 1998b; Tortorolo et al, 1999).

The germinal matrix includes the tissue underlying the ependymal wall of the lateral ventricles. In many preterm infants, the hemorrhage begins as a microvascular event in the germinal matrix and is confined to the subependymal area. In the rest, the original hemorrhage ruptures into the lateral ventricles and then into the third and fourth ventricles. The blood eventually collects in the subarachnoid space of the posterior fossa, often extending into the basal cistern (Figure 31-1) (Levene & de Vries, 1995). Rupture of the hemorrhage from the germinal matrix into the ventricles may serve a protective function by decompressing the hemorrhagic area and reducing further tissue destruction. Progressive ventricular dilation may occur as the result of obstruction of CSF flow by an obliterative arachnoiditis or as the result of blood clots at the level of the aqueduct of Sylvius or the foramen of Monro (Scher, 2001). With severe hemorrhages, blood may also be found in the periventricular white matter. This usually is not due to extravasation of blood from the ventricles but to an associated insult in the white matter (Goddard-Finegold et al, 1998).

The neuropathologic consequences of P/IVH include (1) destruction of the germinal matrix and its glial precursor cells, (2) infarction and necrosis of periventricular white matter, and (3) posthemorrhagic hydrocephalus (Volpe, 2001b). As the IVH moves from the germinal matrix area into the surrounding white matter, periventricular hemorrhagic infarction associated with intraparenchymal echodensities develops. The appearance of this parenchymal lesion is associated with increased mortality and neurodevelopmental sequelae (Volpe, 2001b). Infants with P/IVH may also have periventricular leukomalacia (PVL). However, PVL is thought to arise as a consequence of hypoxic-ischemic injury and is not caused by the P/IVH per se (Goddard-Finegold et al, 1998; Volpe, 2001b).

Pathogenic Factors

Intravascular Factors.   Intravascular hemodynamic factors play a prominent role in the pathogenesis of P/IVH. These factors include distribution of blood to the periventricular region, pressure-passive cerebral blood flow, and venous hemodynamics. The stages of CNS development characteristic of preterm infants born at less than 32 to 33 weeks' gestation increase the risk of hemorrhage in the periventricular area.

Periventricular Blood Flow.   The subependymal germinal matrix is a transient structure that begins to thin after 14 weeks and has almost completely involuted by 36 weeks' gestation (Tortorolo et al, 1999). This is the site where neuroectodermal cells that serve as precursors for neurons (before about 24 weeks' gestation) and glial cells develop. These cells subsequently migrate to their eventual locus in the cerebral cortex. Processes involved in the proliferation, differentiation, and migration of these cells result in an area that is highly vascularized and metabolically active. Before 32 weeks' gestation, a significant portion of the total cerebral blood flow goes to the periventricular germinal matrix, primarily to support neuroblast and glioblast mitotic activity and migration. Any factor that increases cerebral blood flow can result in overperfusion of the periventricular region. After 32 to 34 weeks' gestation, cell proliferation and migration decline. The germinal matrix becomes less prominent and receives a smaller proportion of the cerebral blood supply. At this point, the greater proportion of blood flow is to the rapidly differentiating cerebral cortex (Volpe, 2001b; Papile, 2002).

Cerebral Autoregulation.   The blood vessels of the brain normally are protected from marked alterations in flow by autoregulatory processes. If cerebral autoregulation is intact, the arterioles constrict or dilate to maintain a constant cerebral blood flow despite fluctuations in systemic blood pressure. Asphyxia or hypoxemia in the neonate alters cerebral autoregulation. This alteration can lead to a pressure-passive system in which cerebral blood flow varies directly with arterial pressure. Subsequent alterations in systemic blood pressure or cerebral blood flow, or both, are transmitted directly to the brain and, in particular, to the area receiving the greatest proportion of cerebral blood flow; that is, the fragile, thin-walled vessels of the germinal matrix. Thus rapid fluctuations in systemic blood pressure or cerebral blood flow (i.e., moving from increased to decreased flow and vice versa) also increase the risk of vessel rupture (Levene & de Vries, 1995; Hardy et al, 1997; Bulas & Vezina, 1999; Tortorolo et al, 1999; Volpe, 2001b). Altered hemodynamics with fluctuations in blood flow can occur with positive pressure ventilation, rapid volume expansion, hypercapnia, and possibly reduced hematocrit and blood glucose values. Increased systemic blood pressure and, potentially, cerebral blood flow also can occur with caregiving events, handling, suctioning, and chest physical therapy (Tortorolo et al, 1999; Volpe, 2001b). Even without altered cerebral autoregulation, hypoxia, acidosis, and hypercarbia silate, the cerebral blood vessels, increasing the risk of damage to the vessel epithelium and of P/IVH after reperfusion (Tortorolo et al, 1999).

Venous Hemodynamics.   Increased venous pressure, arising from events such as myocardial failure or positive-pressure ventilation, can also be transmitted directly to the capillaries of the germinal matrix. These events can impede cerebral venous return, leading to stasis and venous congestion, which then lead to increased venous pressure and vessel rupture. The point of vulnerability in the venous drainage system of the brain is at the level of the foramen of Monro and the caudate nucleus (the usual site of P/IVH). At this location there is a U-shaped turn in the venous drainage system where the confluence of the thalamostriate, terminal, and choroidal veins forms the internal cerebral vein, which empties into the great vein of Galen. This results in a sharp change in the direction of blood flow and predisposes to turbulent venous flow with stasis and thrombi formation and an area vulnerable to increased intravascular pressure (Tortorolo et al, 1999; Volpe, 2001b). In addition, the pliable skull of the preterm infant can easily be deformed, obstructing the major venous sinuses and increasing venous pressure.

Vascular Factors.   The capillary bed of the germinal matrix is immature and has large, irregular, thin-walled vessels, a feature that increases its vulnerability to rupture. The capillary walls thicken with increasing gestational age. The fragility of these vessels is due partly to the lack of thickness and strength of the basement membrane and the lack of collagen and smooth muscle. With migration of the neuronal and glial cells and their derivatives, the germinal matrix undergoes involution. The immature capillary bed is remodeled into the definitive, mature capillary bed (Goodard-Finegold et al, 1998; Tortorolo et al, 1999; Volpe, 2001b). The epithelial cells of these capillaries are dependent on oxidative metabolism and thus are easily injured by hypoxic events. This characteristic increases the likelihood of leakage or rupture if transmural pressure increases. Because these vessels require an adequate supply of oxygen to maintain their functional integrity, decreased cerebral blood flow can lead to hypoxic-ischemic injury. These vessels are also susceptible to ischemia because they tend to lie in the vascular border zone, or "watershed" area (see the section on Hypoxic-Ischemic Encephalopathy). Both increased and decreased cerebral blood flow, therefore, can be involved in the pathogenesis of P/IVH.

Extravascular Factors.   The capillary bed of the highly vascularized germinal matrix is embedded in gelatinous material that is deficient in supportive mesenchymal elements, thus providing poor support for the fragile blood vessels. In addition, excessive fibrinolytic activity occurs in the periventricular area. As a result, a small initial bleed may not clot off and be localized, but rather may continue to enlarge and rupture into the ventricles, or the cerebral parenchyma, or both (Volpe, 2001b).

Risk Factors.   The overall major risk factors for P/IVH in the neonate are prematurity and hypoxic events interrelated with the anatomic and physiologic processes that make the periventricular site particularly vulnerable. From a clinical perspective, any perinatal or neonatal event that results in hypoxia or alters cerebral blood flow or intravascular pressure increases the risk of P/IVH. Perinatal events that can lead to fetal and neonatal hypoxia include maternal bleeding, fetal distress, perinatal asphyxia, prolonged labor, preterm labor, and abnormal presentation. Neonatal hypoxic events, such as respiratory distress, apnea, and hypotension, further increase the risk of intraventricular hemorrhage. The most consistent risk factors for P/IVH in the preterm infant are respiratory distress syndrome with severe hypoxia and mechanical ventilation (Levene & de Vries, 1995; Tortorolo et al, 1999). An increased risk of P/IVH has been reported with use of maternal sympathomimetic tocolytic therapy. The effects of high-frequency ventilation and surfactant administration vary (Roland & Hill, 1997). Alterations in the coagulation system increase the risk both of an initial hemorrhage and of extension of that hemorrhage or subsequent hemorrhages.

Events associated with impeded venous return, increased venous pressure, or both, include assisted ventilation, high positive inspiratory pressure, prolonged inspiratory duration, continuous positive airway pressure, and air leak. Venous pressure can also be increased by compression of the infant's skull during vaginal delivery, application of forceps, and use of constricting head bands. Rapid administration of hypertonic solutions (e.g., sodium bicarbonate and glucose), rapid volume expansion, hypernatremia, hypercarbia, caregiving interventions, and environmental stress can increase cerebral blood flow. Hypercarbia causes cerebral vasodilation, thus increasing blood flow. Hypertonic solutions given rapidly or in a large bolus alter osmotic gradients between the brain and the blood. Repeated or prolonged seizures raise the blood pressure and can lead to hypoxia (Goddard-Finegold et al, 1998; Tortorolo et al, 1999; Volpe, 2001b).

Differential Diagnosis. P/IVH usually occurs in preterm infants who have sustained some form of hypoxic insult. Many of these infants are ill with other problems. The clinical manifestations of this disorder often are nonspecific and are not well correlated with later sonographic evidence of bleeding. Therefore a high index of suspicion, along with careful monitoring, is important for infants at risk.

The diagnosis usually is made by cranial ultrasonography. Ultrasonography is the preferred method because it can be performed at the patient's bedside and does not expose the infant to ionizing radiation. Cranial ultrasonography can be used to determine the presence and severity of P/IVH and the progression of the hemorrhage, as well as to monitor later complications such as PVL and progressive ventricular dilation. However, ultrasonography is limited in its ability to identify small amounts of blood in normal size ventricles (Papile, 2002).

Clinical Manifestations. More than 90% of infants with P/IVH bleed within the first 72 hours after birth; 50% of the bleeding occurs in the first 24 hours after birth (Tortorolo et al, 1999; Volpe, 2001b). Approximately 10% to 20% of infants observed serially with cranial ultrasonography after bleeding demonstrate progressive increases in the size of the hemorrhage over a 24- to 48-hour period (Levene & de Vries, 1995). Late hemorrhages are seen after a few days or weeks in about 10% of infants. Late hemorrhages are seen primarily in preterm infants with severe, prolonged respiratory problems. A new hemorrhage or an extension of a previous one may develop in these infants. A P/IVH may also develop before birth in some infants.

The signs and symptoms of P/IVH are often nonspecific and subtle. The clinical signs that correlate most closely with CT evidence of hemorrhage are (1) a decreasing hematocrit value or failure of the hematocrit value to increase after a transfusion; (2) a full anterior fontanel; (3) changes in activity level; and (4) decreased tone (Volpe, 2001b). Other clinical signs associated with P/IVH are impaired visual tracking, increased tone of the lower limbs, neck flexor hypotonia, and brisk tendon reflexes (Levene & de Vries, 1995; Tortorolo et al, 1999).

P/IVH is classified into grades I to IV, depending on the location and severity of the hemorrhage (Table 31-7). Besides a declining hematocrit value, laboratory evidence suggestive of P/IVH involves CSF findings indicative of hemorrhage: increased red blood cell levels, increased protein levels, decreased glucose levels, and xanthochromia (often a later finding and caused by increased protein). Extremely low CSF glucose levels, or hypoglycorrhachia, can be found several days to a week (usually 5 to 15 days) after the hemorrhage in some infants. The CSF glucose level remains depressed for up to 2 to 3 months. The etiology for this finding is unclear, but it may be caused by inhibition or alteration in glucose transport between the CNS and the CSF (Tortorolo et al, 1999).

The patterns of clinical manifestations seen in individual infants vary widely and range from silent or subtle to catastrophic. At one end of the continuum are most infants; these babies have only silent, subependymal bleeding with no or minimal clinical signs. The hemorrhage is discovered during routine ultrasonographic screening. Other infants may show

TABLE 31-7	Grading System for Periventricular/ Intraventricular Hemorrhage	
Grade	**Degree of Hemorrhage**	**Characteristics**
I	Slight	Isolated germinal matrix hemorrhage
II	Slight	Intraventricular hemorrhage with normal ventricular size
III	Moderate	Intraventricular hemorrhage with acute ventricular dilation
IV	Severe	Intraventricular hemorrhage with parenchymal hemorrhage

From Papile L (2002). Intracranial hemorrhage. In Fanaroff AA, Martin RJ, editors. Neonatal-perinatal medicine: diseases of the fetus and infant, ed 7. Mosby: St Louis.

an unexplained fall in hematocrit (by 10% or more) or failure of the hematocrit to rise after a transfusion (Volpe, 2001b). Other clinical manifestations, if present, include alterations in level of consciousness or stupor, hypotonia, abnormal eye movements or positions, and altered mobility. These infants generally survive. Later developmental outcome varies, depending on the severity of the hemorrhage.

Catastrophic deterioration usually involves major hemorrhages that evolve rapidly over several minutes or hours. Clinical findings include stupor progressing to coma, respiratory distress progressing to apnea, generalized tonic seizures, decerebrate posturing, fixation of pupils to light, and flaccid quadriparesis. This clinical presentation is associated with a declining hematocrit value, bulging fontanel, hypotension, bradycardia, temperature alterations, hypoglycemia, and syndrome of inappropriate antidiuretic hormone. Infants with catastrophic hemorrhages have a high mortality rate and, if they survive, a poor prognosis for later development.

Prognosis. The severity and extent of the hemorrhage and the presence of associated problems (e.g., respiratory distress syndrome, perinatal asphyxia, and sepsis) influence mortality and morbidity. Infants with a history of P/IVH are also at risk for developing posthemorrhagic ventricular dilation, which may be normopressive or associated with increased ICP. Infants with small or mild hemorrhages survive and generally have a good outcome, with a low incidence of major neurologic sequelae and posthemorrhagic ventricular dilation. Infants with moderate hemorrhage have a 5% to 20% mortality rate, and ventricular dilation develops in 15% to 25% of survivors. Mortality in infants with severe hemorrhage averages 50%, with development of progressive ventricular dilation in 55% to 80%. Although infants with severe hemorrhages tend to have significant motor and cognitive deficits, some seem to escape significant long-term sequelae. The incidence of neurologic sequelae ranges from 15% in infants with moderate hemorrhage to 35% to 90% in infants with severe hemorrhages. Sequelae include cerebral palsy (CP), developmental retardation, sensory and attention problems, learning disorders, and hydrocephalus (Levene & de Vries, 1995; Wildrick, 1997; Bulas & Vezina, 1999; Volpe, 2001b).

Collaborative Management. Routine ultrasonographic screening of infants at risk for P/IVH can identify infants with silent bleeding or bleeding associated with nonspecific, subtle symptoms. By identifying these vulnerable infants, interventions can be instituted to prevent new bleeding or extensions of existing hemorrhage. Management of P/IVH involves prevention of hemorrhage in infants at risk, acute care of infants with current bleeding, pharmacologic therapies, and management of posthemorrhagic ventricular dilation.

Prevention begins in the perinatal period, with the prevention of preterm birth, perinatal asphyxia, and birth trauma. Continual assessment of fetal and neonatal oxygenation and perfusion is important so that subtle alterations can be recognized and clinicians can intervene early to prevent cerebral hyperperfusion and stabilize cerebral blood flow and pressures. Prompt resuscitation at birth minimizes hypoxemia and hypercarbia, which can alter cerebral autoregulation. Hypertonic solutions and volume expanders are administered slowly, with careful monitoring of vital signs and color. This may be particularly important during delivery resuscitation and early stabilization efforts. Activities that can increase ICP or cause wide swings in arterial or venous pressure are avoided or minimized when possible, especially during the first 72 hours of life. Because seizures can alter cerebral blood flow and ICP, they must be recognized promptly and treated. Acute care of infants with bleeding focuses on monitoring, maintenance of oxygenation and perfusion to prevent further damage or extension of the bleeding, minimal handling, and stress reduction interventions. A single course of antenatal corticosteroids (betamethasone) has been associated with a decrease in P/IVH (Perlman, 1998; Whitelaw & Thoresen, 2000).

Pharmacologic therapies, including administration of phenobarbital, indomethacin, vitamin E, and fibrinolytic agents, have been tried prophylactically to reduce the incidence of hemorrhage or to prevent more severe bleeding or neurologic damage, or both. Ethamsylate, an agent currently under investigation, appears to offer hope of promoting platelet aggregation (Papile, 2002). Research findings have been inconsistent for all of these therapies (du Plessis, 1998; Goddard-Finegold et al, 1998; Hill, 1998; Haines & Lapointe, 1999; Tortorolo et al, 1999). Additional research is needed and is under way.

Management of Progressive Ventricular Dilation.   Because progressive posthemorrhagic ventricular dilation is a common complication of P/IVH, all infants with a history of P/IVH should have serial cranial ultrasonography. In most infants, ventricular dilation occurs slowly, without increased ICP (normopressive hydrocephalus). Ventricular growth spontaneously arrests in approximately half of these infants within about 30 days. The remaining infants continue to demonstrate ventricular dilation and increased ICP (Volpe, 2001a).

The initial treatment for normopressive hydrocephalus is observation, because in many of these infants, ventricular growth arrests spontaneously without therapy. Clinicians may use serial lumbar punctures to remove CSF and reduce ventricle size. Progressive ventricular dilation with increasing ICP is managed with a ventriculoperitoneal shunt or, if the infant is too ill or too small for surgery, with temporary ventricular drainage. An external ventricular drain or a tunneled catheter attached to a subcutaneous reservoir can accomplish ventricular drainage (Volpe, 2001). The long-term outcome generally has not been improved by the use of serial lumbar puncture and administration of drugs to reduce CSF production (e.g., furosemide and acetazolamide) or use of fibrinolytic agents to dissolve clots (Tortorolo et al, 1999; Whitelaw, 2000a, 2000b).

Nursing Management.   Nursing management involves recognition of factors that increase the risk of P/IVH, interventions to reduce the risk of bleeding, and supportive care of infants with acute bleeding or posthemorrhagic ventricular dilation. Prevention or risk reduction begins in the perinatal period and is especially critical during the intrapartum period and the first 3 to 4 days after birth, the period of greatest vulnerability. Interventions are directed at reducing stress and inappropriate stimulation. Prevention and risk-reduction activities include interventions to prevent or reduce hypoxic or asphyxial events; to prevent rapid changes in cerebral blood flow, fluctuations in systemic blood pressure, and hyperosmolarity; and to prevent or minimize fluctuations in ICP. Specific nursing interventions to accomplish these goals are listed in Table 31-8. Developmental interventions, such as containment or swaddling during aversive procedures such as endotracheal suctioning, may promote greater physiologic stability during these procedures and a more rapid return to baseline.

Acute treatment of infants with P/IVH involves providing physiologic support by maintaining oxygenation, perfusion, normothermia, and normoglycemia. Physical manipulations and handling are minimized, as are environmental stressors, to reduce the risk of hypoxia and of fluctuations in arterial blood pressure and cerebral blood flow. The infant's position is also important. The infant can be placed prone or side lying. The head is positioned in the midline or to the side, but without flexing the neck. The head of the bed can be elevated slightly. The Trendelenburg position is avoided. Vital signs, blood pressure, tone, activity, and level of consciousness are monitored frequently. The care of infants with progressive ventricular dilation is discussed in the section on hydrocephalus.

Parent care involves recognition and discussion of parental concerns about their infant's immediate and long-term prognosis and teaching regarding P/IVH, its implications and management. The parents need to be shown how to interact with and care for the infant at risk for P/IVH in a developmentally appropriate manner, with the goal of promoting opportunities for interaction while minimizing stressful events. The nurse can model this type of care for parents and provide anticipatory guidance in the ways in which the infant's needs and care will change as the baby matures. Parents can also be involved in devising and implementing a developmental plan of care for their infant to reduce environmental stressors.

Other Types of Intracranial Hemorrhage

In addition to P/IVH, several other clinically important types of intracranial bleeding can occur in the neonate, including primary subarachnoid hemorrhage, subdural hemorrhage, and intracerebellar hemorrhage. These types of hemorrhage arise from trauma or hypoxia during the perinatal period.

Primary Subarachnoid Hemorrhage.   Primary subarachnoid hemorrhage (SAH) is the most prevalent form of intracranial hemorrhage in neonates and the least clinically significant for most infants. SAH occurs in both preterm and term infants but is more common in preterm infants. SAH may occur alone (primary SAH) or as a secondary event with other forms of intracranial hemorrhage. For example, with P/IVH, blood moves into the subarachnoid space via the fourth ventricle.

Pathophysiology and Risk Factors.   Primary SAH consists of bleeding into the subarachnoid space that is not secondary

TABLE 31-8	Nursing Care to Reduce the Risk of Periventricular/Intraventricular Hemorrhage*	

Intervention	Rationale
1. Position the infant with the head in the midline and the head of the bed slightly elevated.	Intracranial pressure (ICP) is lowest with the head in the midline and the head of the bed elevated 30 degrees. Turning the head sharply to the side causes obstruction of the ipsilateral jugular vein and can increase ICP.
2. Avoid tight, encircling phototherapy masks.	Pressure on the occiput can increase ICP by impeding venous drainage.
3. Avoid rapid fluid infusions for volume expansion. • Know the normal blood pressure (BP) for the infant's weight and age. • If the infant is not hypovolemic, suggest dopamine therapy to maintain BP.	Rapid increases in intravascular volume can rupture the capillaries in the germinal matrix, and this risk may be even greater if the infant has a history of hypoxia and hypotension. Even modest, abrupt increases in BP may cause periventricular/intraventricular hemorrhage (P/IVH).
4. If sodium bicarbonate ($NaHCO_3$) therapy is necessary to correct a documented metabolic acidosis, give a dilute solution slowly.	The role of $NaHCO_3$ is unclear, but rapid infusions may cause elevations in carbon dioxide, possibly dilating cerebral vessels and contributing to a pressure-passive cerebral circulation.
5. Monitor BP diligently. Inform physician if a fluctuating pattern in the arterial pressure tracing is noted in high-risk infants receiving ventilation.	The blood flow velocity in the anterior cerebral artery is reflected by the pattern of the simultaneously recorded arterial BP. A fluctuating pattern, which is associated with the development of P/IVH, can be stabilized by administration of pancuronium bromide.
6. Monitor closely for signs of pneumothorax, including: (a) Increase in mean BP, especially increases in diastolic BP (early) (b) Increased heart rate (c) Changes in breath sounds, which may or may not be appreciated (d) Diminished arterial oxygen pressure (PaO_2) (e) Increased arterial carbon dioxide pressure ($PaCO_2$) (f) Shift in cardiac point of maximum impulse (g) Hypotension and bradycardia (late)	Pneumothorax frequently precedes P/IVH. The sum of hemodynamic changes caused by pneumothorax is flow under increased pressure in the germinal matrix capillaries. Changes in vital signs can be early indicators of pneumothorax.
7. Maintain temperature in neutral thermal range.	Hypothermia has been associated with P/IVH.
8. Suction only as needed.	Even brief suctioning episodes (20 seconds) can increase cerebral blood flow velocity, BP, and ICP and reduce oxygenation.
9. Avoid interventions that cause crying. • Consider long-term methods of achieving venous access to avoid frequent venipunctures. • Critically evaluate all manipulations and handling. • Use analgesics for stressful procedures.	Crying can impede venous return, increase cerebral blood volume, and compromise cerebral oxygenation in sick infants.
10. Maintain blood gas values within a normal range. • Use continuous noninvasive monitoring of oxygenation. • Adjust the fractional concentration of oxygen in inspired gas (FiO_2) as needed to maintain the transcutaneous oxygen pressure ($TcPO_2$) or pulse oximeter values within desired range. • Avoid interventions that cause hypoxia.	Hypoxia and hypercapnia are associated with the development of P/IVH. These events increase cerebral blood flow and may impair the neonate's already limited ability to autoregulate the cerebral blood flow. Hypoxia can injure the germinal matrix capillary endothelium.

From Kling P (1989). Nursing interventions to decrease the risk of periventricular-intraventricular hemorrhage. Journal of obstetric, gynecologic, and neonatal nursing 18:462.

*Premature neonates are most vulnerable to P/IVH during the first 4 days of life; approximately 50% of hemorrhages occur in the first 24 hours. Attempts to minimize the risk of P/IVH should begin immediately after birth, even before the infant has reached the special care nursery.

to subdural or intraventricular bleeding. In neonates, the source of the bleeding is venous blood; in older children and adults, SAH usually involves arterial blood. With primary SAH, blood leaks from the leptomeningeal plexus, bridging veins, or ruptured vessels in the subarachnoid space (Levene & de Vries,

1995). This type of hemorrhage is associated with trauma or asphyxia. Trauma that causes increased intravascular pressure and capillary rupture is the underlying causal event in most term infants with SAH. In preterm infants, SAH usually is the result of asphyxial events. Factors that place an infant at risk for SAH include birth trauma, prolonged labor, difficult delivery, fetal distress, and perinatal asphyxia.

Differential Diagnosis. Subarachnoid hemorrhage must be distinguished from other forms of intracranial hemorrhage and other neurologic problems. Differentiation often can be accomplished by evaluating the infant's history and presentation and, if the infant is having seizure activity, by eliminating other causes of seizures. Blood in the CSF on lumbar puncture indicates the possibility of SAH, but true hemorrhage must be distinguished from a bloody tap. Ultrasonography and CT also can help confirm the diagnosis; CT may be more useful than ultrasonography (Levene & de Vries, 1995).

Clinical Manifestations. Three clinical presentations have been described for infants with SAH (Volpe, 2001b). The most common is a preterm infant with a minor SAH. These infants are asymptomatic. The hemorrhage is discovered accidentally, for example, during a lumbar puncture as part of a sepsis workup. With the second type of clinical presentation, term or preterm infants may show isolated seizure activity at 2 to 3 days of age (Table 31-5) or preterm infants occasionally may present with apnea. Between seizures, the infant appears and acts healthy ("well baby with seizures"). Infants in both of these groups survive and usually do well developmentally. The third type of clinical presentation involves infants with a massive SAH that has a rapid and fatal course. This presentation is rare and often is associated with both a severe asphyxial event and birth trauma.

Prognosis. Generally, infants with SAH survive, and asymptomatic infants do well. Up to half of symptomatic infants with severe, sustained traumatic or hypoxic injury with further damage to the CNS have neurologic sequelae (Volpe, 2001b). Hydrocephalus occasionally develops in infants with a history of SAH as a result of obstruction of CSF flow by adhesions. These infants should undergo repeat ultrasonographic examinations to monitor ventricular dilation.

Collaborative and Nursing Management. Collaborative and nursing management of these infants begins with efforts to prevent or reduce the risk of trauma and hypoxia during the perinatal period, so as to reduce the risk of development of SAH. Infants with SAH are observed for seizures and other neurologic signs during the early neonatal period. Nursing care is primarily supportive and includes maintenance of oxygenation and perfusion and provision of warmth, fluids, and nutrients. Nursing management also involves helping the parents to understand the basis for and cause and prognosis of SAH, as well as the care of their infant. Occasionally, infants with massive, acute SAH may require a craniotomy.

Subdural Hemorrhage. Subdural hemorrhage (SDH) is more common in term than preterm infants. The incidence of SDH has declined markedly as a result of improvements in obstetrical care. This decrease has been particularly notable in term infants. SDH may account for 4% to 11% of cases of intracranial hemorrhage in preterm infants (Levene & de Vries, 1995). Early recognition of SDH is critical for infants with severe bleeding who require surgical intervention.

Pathophysiology. SDH in newborns is almost always caused by trauma during the perinatal period. Bleeding occurs between the dura and the arachnoid and may be unilateral or bilateral. The bleeding occurs over the cerebral hemispheres or posterior fossa with or without tentorium or falx cerebri lacerations (Figure 31-1). The cerebral hemispheres are the most common site for SDH. Bleeding usually occurs over the temporal convexity, with rupture of superficial cerebral veins or of "bridging" veins between the superomedial aspect of the cerebrum and the superior sagittal sinus. Because the superficial veins over the cerebrum are poorly developed in the preterm infant, this type of hemorrhage is seen less often in these infants. Bleeding over the posterior fossa involves bleeding below the tentorium and compression of the brainstem. Dural tears at the junction of the falx and tentorium near the attachment of the great vein of Galen are also associated with compression of the brainstem and midbrain (Levene & de Vries, 1995; Volpe, 2001b).

Risk Factors. Risk factors include precipitous, prolonged, or difficult delivery, use of midforceps or high forceps, prematurity, cerebropelvic disproportion, and LGA infants. SDH is seen more often in infants born to primiparas, possibly because of the more rigid birth canal. Infants with abnormal presentations (e.g., breech, foot, brow, or face) are also at higher risk for SDH.

Differential Diagnosis. SDH must be distinguished from other types of intracranial hemorrhage and neurologic problems. This differentiation often can be accomplished by evaluating the infant's history and presentation and, if the infant is having seizure activity, by ruling out other causes of seizures. SDH over the cerebral hemispheres often is associated with SAH. SDH also occurs with extracranial hemorrhages, such as cephalohematoma and subgaleal, subconjunctival, and retinal hemorrhages; skull fractures; and brachial plexus or facial palsies (Levene & deVries, 1995; Volpe 2001b). MRI or CT can assist in confirming the diagnosis; HUS is less reliable (Barnes & Taylor, 1998).

Clinical Manifestations. Clinical signs of SDH relate to the site of the bleeding and the severity of the hemorrhage. Three patterns are seen in infants with bleeding over the cerebral hemispheres (Volpe, 2001b). The first pattern is seen in most neonates with SDH; these infants have a minor hemorrhage and are asymptomatic or have signs such as irritability and hyperalertness. With the second pattern, seizures develop during the first 2 to 3 days of life and usually are focal. Other neurologic signs, which may be absent or present, include hemiparesis; pupils that are unequal and respond sluggishly to light; full or tense fontanel; bradycardia; and irregular respirations. The third pattern is seen in a few infants who have no or nonspecific signs in the neonatal period but in whom signs appear at 4 weeks to 6 months of age. These infants generally show increasing head size as a result of continued hematoma formation, poor feeding, failure to thrive, altered level of consciousness and, occasionally, seizures caused by the chronic subdural effusion.

Infants with abnormal neurologic signs from birth often have had bleeding over the posterior fossa with tentorial lacerations. Signs include stupor or coma, eye deviation, asymmetric pupil size, altered pupillary response to light, tachypnea, bradycardia, and opisthotonos. As the clot enlarges, these infants rapidly deteriorate, with signs of shock appearing over minutes to hours. The infant becomes comatose and has fixed, dilated pupils and altered respirations and heart rate, which culminate in respiratory arrest. Infants with small tears in the posterior fossa may have no clinical manifestations for the first 3 to 4 days of life. During this time, the clot gradually enlarges until signs of increased ICP appear. As the brainstem becomes compressed, the infant's condition deteriorates, and oculomotor abnormalities, altered respiration, bradycardia, and seizures occur (Volpe, 2001b).

Prognosis.   The prognosis varies with the location and severity of the hemorrhage. Infants with bleeding over the cerebral hemispheres who are asymptomatic do well, as do most infants who have transient seizures in the neonatal period if no associated cerebral injury is present. In recent years, early diagnosis with CT or MRI has improved the outcome for infants with posterior fossa hemorrhage (Volpe, 2001b). Most infants with bleeding over the tentorium or falx cerebri die. Severe hydrocephalus and neurologic sequelae usually develop in those that survive.

Collaborative and Nursing Management.   SDH often can be prevented or its severity diminished by reducing trauma during the perinatal period. Treatment of infants who have bleeding over the cerebral hemispheres is supportive. Infants with a history of perinatal trauma or other risk factors are observed for seizures and other neurologic signs. Care is primarily supportive and includes maintenance of oxygenation and perfusion and provision of warmth, fluids, and nutrients. Nursing management also involves helping the parents to understand the basis for and the cause and prognosis of this type of hemorrhage, as well as the care of their infant.

Symptomatic infants with bleeding over the temporal convexity and increased ICP may require surgical evacuation if the infant's condition cannot be stabilized neurologically. Massive posterior fossa hemorrhage requires craniotomy and surgical aspiration of the clot (Levene & de Vries, 1995). Infants at risk for SDH should be monitored carefully over the first 4 to 6 months after birth for late signs of bleeding and hematoma formation. Monitoring of these infants includes observation of head size, growth, feeding, activity, and level of consciousness, as well as monitoring for seizure activity.

Intracerebellar Hemorrhage.   Intracerebellar hemorrhage is rare and is thought to be the result of hypoxia. These hemorrhages occur in both term and preterm infants but are more common in preterm infants. Intracerebellar hemorrhage is seen during autopsy in infants with a history of perinatal asphyxia or severe respiratory distress syndrome (or both) and P/IVH. Intracerebellar hemorrhage also occurs secondary to trauma, especially in very-low-birth-weight (VLBW) infants. Mechanical deformation of the occiput during forceps or breech delivery and compression of the compliant skull during fixation of the head for caregiving procedures or with use of constrictive head bands may also be predisposing factors (Volpe, 2001b).

Two presentations have been described. Many infants are critically ill from birth, with rapidly progressive apnea, a declining hematocrit value, and death within 24 to 36 hours. Other infants are less ill initially, and symptoms develop up to 2 to 3 weeks of age. Clinical manifestations include apnea, bradycardia, hoarse or high-pitched cry, eye deviations, opisthotonos, seizures, vomiting, hypotonia, and diminished or absent Moro reflex. Hydrocephalus often develops in these infants as early as

the end of the first week after birth. The prognosis is poor in survivors, especially those born prematurely.

Hypoxic-Ischemic Encephalopathy

Hypoxic-ischemic encephalopathy (HIE) occurs as a result of injury to the brain from a combination of systemic hypoxemia and diminished cerebral perfusion that leads to ischemia. The hypoxemia and ischemia may occur simultaneously or sequentially. Hypoxic-ischemic damage to the brain occurs in both preterm and term infants. The site of injury varies with maturational changes in the vascular anatomy and metabolic activity of the brain. In the preterm infant younger than 32 to 34 weeks' gestation, hypoxic-ischemic damage usually is associated with P/IVH. The incidence of severe forms of HIE has declined markedly as a result of advances in perinatal care. The incidence of HIE is 2% to 6% per 1000 births (Saugstad, 2001).

Pathophysiology.   After 33 to 34 weeks' gestation, blood flow and brain metabolic activity become less prominent in the germinal matrix and periventricular area and shift to the cortical area. Hypoxia and ischemia in older preterm and term infants, therefore, are more likely to damage areas of the peripheral and dorsal cerebral cortex. Five types of lesions have been identified in infants with HIE: (1) selective neuronal necrosis; (2) status marmoratus of the neurons of the basal ganglia and thalamus, with loss of neurons in these areas; (3) parasagittal cerebral injury; (4) PVL (primarily in preterm infants); and (5) focal or multifocal ischemic brain necrosis (Volpe, 2001b).

The primary lesion for the hypoxic injury is necrosis of neurons in the cortices of the cerebrum and cerebellum, with damage to the gray matter at the depths of the sulci. Neurons of the brainstem may also be injured. Areas of necrosis may extend into the white matter and into the gray matter of the basal ganglia (Berger & Garnier, 2000). The primary ischemic injury occurs in the posterior portion of the parasagittal region secondary to watershed or border zone infarcts. The border zone is at the junctions of the anterior, middle, and posterior cerebral arteries and the superior and inferior cerebellar arteries. This area is farthest from the original source of the brain blood supply of the major cerebral vessels. Thus, with localized ischemia, such as occurs when the infant has systemic hypotension or hypoperfusion as a consequence of perinatal asphyxia, this area receives the least amount of blood.

With asphyxia and systemic hypotension, cerebral perfusion is maintained at first by cerebral vasodilation and redistribution of blood flow to the brain from other organs. If the asphyxia continues, brain water balance and cerebral blood flow are altered; energy is depleted; ischemia and edema develop; and neurophysiologic activity is disrupted.

At the cellular level, neurologic injury is caused by energy depletion, accumulation of extracellular glutamate, and activation of glutamate NMDA receptors (Volpe, 2001b). This process occurs in two phases. The initial insult and effects of hypoxia lead to hyperpolarization with an influx of sodium, potassium, and water into the cell. This interferes with the cell's ability to produce an action potential, with failure of the sodium-potassium pump and cell edema. Calcium moves into the cell via voltage-dependent ion channels opened by the changes in the sodium-potassium pump. This reduces calcium currents and release of neurotransmitters. These events may be protective mechanisms to reduce neuronal excitability and conserve oxygen.* If hypoxia and ischemia persist, NMDA receptors are activated, which further increases intracellular calcium (entering the cell via glutamate-controlled ion channels). More glutamate (a major excitatory neurotransmitter) is released and accumulates to toxic levels. Nitric oxide (NO) is also released and accumulates. NO, which at normal levels promotes vasodilation and increased blood flow, reaches toxic levels, leading to production of excess free oxygen radicals and further activation of NMDA receptors. NO combines with superoxide free radicals to produce the toxic peroxynitrate, causing further cell damage.* The late reperfusion phase (8 to 48 hours after the initial insult) is characterized by hyperexcitability and cytotoxic edema and damage caused by the release of free oxygen radicals and NO, inflammatory changes, and imbalances in inhibitory and excitatory neurotransmitters (Berger & Garnier, 2000; Saugstad, 2001) After a hypoxic-ischemic insult, the entire cortex initially may be edematous, and further ischemic damage may occur as a result of compression of the cortex against the skull.

Risk Factors. HIE may occur secondary to prenatal, intrapartal, or postnatal insults. Prenatal-intrapartal risk factors include fetal distress, perinatal asphyxia, abruptio placentae, placenta previa, maternal hypertension, prematurity, postmaturity, intrauterine growth retardation, prolapsed or nuchal cord, dystocia, and precipitate or prolonged labor. Injury during the postbirth period generally occurs in infants with a history of severe respiratory distress, persistent pulmonary hypertension, recurrent apnea, hypotension, or septic shock (Goddard-Finegold et al, 1998; Vannucci, 2000).

Differential Diagnosis. HIE must be differentiated from other neurologic dysfunctions caused by trauma, infection, or CNS anomalies. An extensive workup to define the type, extent, and location of the injury may include cranial ultrasonography, brainstem auditory evoked potentials, MRI, EEG, and measurements of cerebral blood flow, ICP, and the creatinine kinase level.

Clinical Manifestations. HIE in term or older preterm infants usually is found in infants with perinatal asphyxia. Nonneurologic signs and symptoms related to the underlying perinatal asphyxia are discussed elsewhere. Most term infants with HIE demonstrate a characteristic pattern of neurologic findings over the first 72 hours of life, including seizures, altered level of consciousness, altered tone, altered activity, irregular respirations, apnea, poor or absent Moro reflex, abnormal cry, poor suck, and altered pupillary responses and eye movements.

Clinical signs can be graded, ranging from mild to severe. Mild HIE is characterized by mild depression or hyperalertness and sympathetic nervous system excitation. These infants have a good Moro reflex and deep tendon reflexes and generally are symptomatic for less than 24 hours. Infants with moderate to severe insults have varying levels of consciousness initially but then become stuporous or comatose. These infants have depressed deep tendon and Moro reflexes, hypotonia, and seizures. Symptoms last longer than 24 hours (Rivkin, 1997).

The neurologic findings of most concern in terms of severity of injury and outcome are seizures, altered level of consciousness, and abnormal tone. Seizures occur in 30% to 60% of these infants, and the usual onset is 12 to 14 hours of age. The types of seizures most often seen are multifocal clonic seizures in term infants. Subtle seizures may occur as early as 2 to 6 hours after birth.

Prognosis. The prognosis, which varies with the extent and severity of the insult and the resulting brain injury, ranges from death before or shortly after birth to severe neurologic impairment to minimal or no sequelae. Specific sequelae may not be apparent for several months or longer. Some infants make a significant recovery, although the rate and degree of recovery vary. MRI or CT can be used to assess the location, degree, and extent of the injury (Rivkin, 1997).

Sequelae of HIE in term infants are related to the site of injury (e.g., the cortex); they include mental retardation, microcephaly, cortical blindness, hearing deficits, and epilepsy. CP is more common in preterm infants than in term infants but does occur in term infants with HIE. Term infants are likely to have involvement of the upper extremities and speech in addition to involvement of the lower extremities; most preterm infants primarily have involvement of the lower extremities. Generally, infants with mild HIE do well, as do most infants with moderate HIE of less than 5 days' duration. Infants with moderate HIE of longer duration or severe HIE have a higher mortality rate, and later cognitive and motor problems are seen in more than 50% (Rivkin, 1997).

Collaborative Management. According to Rivkin (1997), "Currently the most effective intervention against hypoxic-ischemic brain injury is prevention." Infants with HIE have multiorgan and multisystem problems that arise from the original hypoxic-ischemic insult. As a result, management of these infants is complex and requires a coordinated team effort. Acute management of infants with HIE focuses on delivery room resuscitation and stabilization and management of the primary problem (usually perinatal asphyxia) and related alterations in the cardiovascular, pulmonary, gastrointestinal, and renal systems. Management of these systems is discussed elsewhere. Prompt identification and treatment of seizures is needed to prevent further alterations in ICP and cerebral blood flow. Management of these infants in relation to neurologic problems focuses on elimination of the original hypoxia, alleviation of tissue hypoxia, and promotion of adequate cerebral perfusion and brain oxygenation (Rivkin, 1997; Volpe, 2001b). Interventions are directed toward establishing ventilation and adequate perfusion and preventing or minimizing hypotension, hypoxia, acidosis, and severe apneic and bradycardic episodes.

Hyperoxia is also avoided because this state can result in cerebral vasoconstriction and diminished perfusion. Fluid management is critical not only for treating the cerebral edema but also for managing the alterations in renal function and problems such as acute tubular necrosis that frequently accompany moderate to severe forms of HIE.

The infant's neurologic status is continually monitored and documented, as are oxygenation, temperature, and blood pressure. Other parameters that are monitored are the serum and urinary electrolyte levels and osmolality; blood urea nitrogen, serum creatinine, and glucose levels; and fluid and electrolyte balance. These infants are at risk for hypocalcemia secondary to release of excessive phosphorus from the breakdown of ATP

---

*Goddard-Finegold et al, 1998a; Amato & Donati, 2000; Berger & Garnier, 2000; Guzzetta et al, 2000; and Inder & Volpe, 2000; Saugstad, 2001.

that occurred to produce energy; the need for energy arises in response to the stress induced by perinatal asphyxia. The excess phosphorus is also related to use of bicarbonate to correct acidosis induced by asphyxia.

The blood glucose level should be monitored closely in infants with HIE, and any deviations should be treated promptly to maintain blood glucose levels between 75 and 100 mg/dl. After perinatal asphyxia, an infant is at risk for hypoglycemia as a result of depletion of stores from high energy demands. Use of high levels of glucose in the management of HIE is controversial, and conflicting evidence exists as to whether this is an effective or a dangerous therapy (Vannucci & Perlman, 1997). Glucose administration may be therapeutic because glucose is the major substrate for brain metabolism. Concerns have been raised, however, that under anaerobic conditions, such as occur in infants with perinatal asphyxia, glucose is converted to lactate, which may cause a localized metabolic acidosis and aggravate existing problems (Levene, 1995a, 1995b; Vannucci & Perlman, 1997).

Acute intracranial hypertension may be managed with osmotically active agents such as furosemide, barbiturates, and corticosteroids, as well as with fluid restriction. Use of agents to reduce cerebral edema is controversial, and few data are available. Management is directed toward reducing localized increases in pressure with fluid restriction and reducing energy requirements. Barbiturates have also been proposed as a therapeutic measure to reduce the cerebral metabolic rate, cerebral blood flow, and cerebral edema and to promote consumption of oxygen free radicals and modification of cell physiology. Barbiturates seem to be most effective when used before the hypoxic-ischemic event or within 1 to 6 hours after birth (Vannucci & Perlman, 1997; Vannucci & Vannucci, 2000). Corticosteroids may also have a protective benefit, although additional research is needed to clarify their effect (Vannucci & Perlman, 1997). Research continues into newer therapeutic strategies, including head cooling, calcium channel blockers, antioxidants, xanthine oxidase inhibitors, free radical scavengers, and nitric oxidase synthetase inhibitors (Berger & Garnier, 2000; Marret et al, 2001; Peeters & Van Bel, 2001; Saugstad, 2001).

Nursing Management.   Nursing management involves recognition of factors that increase the risk of further hypoxia, interventions to restore oxygenation, and supportive care of infants and their families. Nursing care activities include interventions to prevent or reduce hypoxic or asphyxial events; to prevent rapid alterations in cerebral blood flow and fluctuations in systemic blood pressure and hyperosmolarity; and to prevent or minimize fluctuations in ICP. The interventions listed in Table 31-8 to alter ICP and promote oxygenation in infants at risk for P/IVH can also be used for infants with HIE.

Nursing management involves promotion of oxygenation, perfusion, normothermia, and normoglycemia. Fluid status and intake and output are monitored to prevent fluid overload. The infant is monitored for hypoglycemia, hypocalcemia, and electrolyte disturbances. Fluctuations in systemic blood pressure with increased ICP and altered cerebral hemodynamics can occur as a result of caregiving or environmental stress, therefore developmentally supportive care of these infants to reduce stress is essential. As the infant recovers, opportunities for sensory experiences are an important part of care. These experiences can be introduced slowly, as the infant can tolerate them without becoming stressed and overloaded. Physiologic and

neurologic status is monitored and documented at regular intervals. The infant is observed for changes in level of consciousness, tone, and activity and for evidence of seizures. Seizures are recognized and treated promptly to prevent further injury. Positioning and skin care are important, especially for hypoactive, obtunded, or comatose infants.

Parents need initial and continuing support in dealing with their infant's critical illness; the lack of infant responsiveness if the infant is hypoactive, stuporous, or comatose; the possibility of death; and the implications for later neurologic deficits. Parent teaching focuses on promoting an understanding of the infant's health status and care and providing anticipatory guidance regarding changes in the infant's state, as well as the outcome. The parents need to be shown how to interact with and care for their infant in a developmentally appropriate manner, with the goal of promoting opportunities for interaction while minimizing stressful events. The nurse can model this type of care for the parents and provide anticipatory guidance in the ways the infant's needs and care will change as the baby matures. Parents can also be involved in devising and implementing a developmental plan of care for their infant.

Periventricular Leukomalacia

Two forms of white matter hypoxic-ischemic injury are seen in preterm infants, periventicular leukomalacia and ipsilateral hemorrhage into the white matter (periventricular hemorrhagic infarction) associated with P/IVH (Perlman, 1998). PVL is the ischemic brain lesion most commonly seen in preterm infants. Leukomalacia refers to change in the brain's white matter reflective of softening. PVL often is associated with P/IVH, but it is a separate lesion that may also occur in the absence of P/IVH. PVL is a symmetric, nonhemorrhagic, usually bilateral lesion caused by ischemia from alterations in arterial circulation. PVL is characterized by focal periventricular necrosis and diffuse cerebral white matter injury (Volpe, 1997; Perlman, 1998). Periventricular hemorrhagic infarction that develops with P/IVH is associated with the development of intraparenchymal echodensities. Periventricular hemorrhagic infarction differs from PVL in that it is an asymmetric, hemorrhagic lesion that primarily arises from alterations in the venous circulation (Volpe, 2001b).

Pathophysiology.   PVL begins with ischemic necrosis of the white matter dorsal and lateral to the external angles of the lateral ventricles, especially in the border zone area. The border zone is the area farthest from the original source of the cerebral blood supply and thus is most susceptible to ischemic damage from diminished cerebral blood flow. PVL often extends into the cortical white matter (Volpe, 2001b). Pathologic changes begin with patchy areas of focal ischemic coagulation that may occur as early as 5 to 8 hours after the initial hypoxic-ischemic insult. This is followed within a few days by proliferation of macrophages and astrocytes, along with endothelial and glial infiltration. Later changes include thinning of the white matter and liquefaction in the central portion of the necrotic area, as well as cavitation, cystic changes, and decreased myelinization (de Vries, 1995). Cerebral atrophy leads to expansion of the lateral ventricles and hydrocephalus.

The two main pathogenic events seen with PVL are (1) reduction of oxygen delivery to vulnerable areas of the brain, resulting in hypoxic-ischemic injury, and (2) damage to the myelin-producing oligodendroglia by the subsequent release of cytokines (indicating an inflammatory process), glutamate, and free radicals (Jacobson & Dutton, 2000). Oligodendrocyte development and survival are impaired, and myelinization is altered. Axonal damage and disruption also occur, although it is unclear which is the primary event (Kinney & Back, 1998; Dammann et al, 2001). Perinatal infection and an immune-mediated inflammatory response with release of proinflammatory cytokines are increasingly thought to play a prominent role in PVL pathogenesis (Kadhim et al, 2001).

Risk Factors. PVL occurs in both term and preterm infants. However, approximately 75% of infants with PVL are preterm. Risk factors include any event during the prenatal, intrapartal, or postbirth periods that results in cerebral ischemia; this includes perinatal asphyxia, P/IVH, hypoxia, hypercarbia, hypotension, cardiac arrest, and infection (in which blood flow is diminished by the action of endotoxins). The major risk factors are P/IVH, perinatal asphyxia, and infection.

Differential Diagnosis and Clinical Manifestations. PVL is a compilation of prenatal or postnatal insults or both. Often no clinical findings are specific to PVL during the first weeks of life unless the damage is severe. Cranial ultrasonography can identify infants at risk for or who have early signs of PVL, although HUS is not as sensitive in the diagnosis of PVL as it is with P/IVH; MRI can identify changes as soon as 3 days of age (Bulas & Vezina, 1999). Infants at risk for PVL should undergo serial cranial ultrasonographic examinations and again at discharge and with later follow-up. With severe damage, neuromotor abnormalities and signs of ventricular enlargement develop. As the infant matures, neurologic and motor deficits become apparent.

Prognosis. Infants with PVL may die in the neonatal period, usually from the original hypoxic, hemorrhagic, or infectious insult rather than from PVL per se. Infants with PVL are at higher risk for later developmental problems that affect motor, cognitive, and visual function (Perlman, 1998). The later outcome is related to the progression of the PVL abnormalities.

The most prominent sequelae in survivors, especially those who progress to cystic lesions, is spastic diplegia with or without hydrocephalus. In infants with spastic diplegia, 72% to 90% have PVL (Jacobson & Dutton, 2000), descending fibers from the motor cortex cross the affected area around the ventricles. Because the leg motor fibers are closest to the ventricles, spastic diplegia of the leg is the most common sequela. With extension of the damage, arm involvement, with spastic quadriplegia, may occur. Damage to the optic radiations in this area leads to visual deficits. Extensive cystic changes are predictive of cerebral visual impairment (Jacobson & Dutton, 2000).

Collaborative Management. Initial management focuses on treating the primary insult and its attendant complications and preventing further hypoxic-ischemic damage. This involves preventing or minimizing hypotension, hypoxia, acidosis, and severe apneic and bradycardic episodes. HUS and MRI are used serially to diagnose PVL and to follow its progression in infants at risk. Later management involves care related to residual problems, such as spastic diplegia and hydrocephalus.

Nursing Management. Nursing interventions focus on acute management of the primary problem and supportive care for the infant and parents. Nurses have a major role in identifying signs of hypoxia and asphyxia and instituting interventions to prevent further ischemic damage. These interventions are similar to those described earlier and in Table 31-8. Environmental stressors may increase the risk for development of P/IVH and subsequent PVL or may cause associated developmental problems. Developmental and environmental interventions, therefore, are important aspects of nursing care.

Parents need initial and continuing support in dealing with their infant's illness and the risk of later neurologic problems. Parent teaching should focus on promoting an understanding of the infant's health status and care and providing anticipatory guidance and follow-up care. The parents can be shown how to interact with and care for their infant in a developmentally appropriate manner to foster parent-infant interaction and to promote infant organization and development. The nurse can model this type of care for the parents and can provide anticipatory guidance as the infant's needs and care change.

Birth Injuries

Traumatic injury to the central or peripheral nervous system can occur during the perinatal or postnatal period. Most of these injuries happen during the intrapartum period and may occur with perinatal asphyxia. The incidence of birth trauma in the United States is 6 to 8 per 1000 live births (Goddard-Finegold, 1998). Perinatal events most frequently associated with birth injury include midforceps delivery, shoulder dystocia, low forceps delivery, birth weight exceeding 3500 g, and second stage of labor lasting longer than 60 minutes (Medlock & Hanigan, 1997). The incidence of injury has declined markedly in recent years as a result of improvement in obstetrical care and increased use of cesarean sections for abnormal presentations. However, birth injuries can also arise from trauma during a cesarean section or resuscitation.

Injuries that occur before the intrapartum period usually are caused by compression or pressure injuries from an unusual fetal position. The risk of injury to the central or peripheral nervous system is greater with malpresentation (especially breech), malposition, prolonged or precipitate labor, prematurity, multiple gestation, shoulder dystocia, macrosomia, and instrumental delivery. The most prevalent types of injury to the nervous system are extracranial hemorrhage, intracranial hemorrhage (described previously), skull fractures, spinal cord injury, and peripheral nerve injury.

Extracranial Hemorrhage. Caput succedaneum and cephalohematoma are the most common types of birth injury, as well as the most benign. Caput succedaneum is characterized by soft, pitting, superficial edema that is several millimeters thick and overlies the presenting part in a vertex delivery. This edematous area lies above the periosteum and thus crosses suture lines. The edema consists of serum or blood, or both. Infants with caput succedaneum may also have ecchymosis, petechiae, or purpura over the presenting part. Caput succedaneum occurs in infants after a spontaneous vertex delivery or after the use of a vacuum extractor. This type of extracranial hemorrhage requires no care other than parent teaching regarding its cause and significance. It resolves within a few days after birth with no sequelae.

Cephalohematoma occurs in 0.2% to 2.5% of newborns (Steinbach, 1999). It involves subperiosteal bleeding, usually over the parietal bone but possibly over other cranial bones. Cephalohematoma usually is unilateral but can be bilateral.

This type of hemorrhage is seen most often in males, after the use of forceps, after a prolonged, difficult delivery, and in infants born to primiparas. The characteristic finding is a firm, fluctuant mass that does not cross the suture lines. The mass often enlarges slightly by 2 to 3 days of age. Approximately 10% to 25% of cases have a linear skull fracture underlying the mass (Moe & Paige, 1998). In rare cases an infant may have a subdural or subarachnoid hemorrhage.

A cephalohematoma is limited to the periosteal area and does not cross suture lines; it can take weeks to months to resolve completely. Conversely, caput succedaneum crosses suture lines, may be accompanied by ecchymosis, and resolves within a few days after birth. Caput succedaneum and cephalohematoma over the occipital bone must be differentiated from encephalocele. In contrast to extracranial hemorrhage, an encephalocele is characterized by pulsations, increased pressure (tenseness) with crying, and the appearance of a bony defect on radiographic studies.

Infants with a cephalohematoma generally have no symptoms. Management includes parent teaching and monitoring for the development of hyperbilirubinemia. Occasionally an infant with a large cephalohematoma becomes anemic. These infants should also be monitored for symptoms of intracranial hemorrhage or skull fracture. Generally, cephalohematomas resolve between 2 weeks and 6 months of age, and most resolve by 6 weeks. Calcium deposits occasionally develop, and the swelling may remain for the first year.

Skull Fracture.   Two types of skull fractures, linear and depressed, are seen in newborns.

Pathophysiology and Risk Factors.   Skull fractures occur in utero, during labor, with forceps delivery, or during a prolonged, difficult labor with compression and battering of the fetal skull against the maternal ischial spines, sacral promontory, or symphysis pubis (Goddard-Finegold, 1998). The fetal skull often is able to tolerate mechanical stressors relatively well, because it is flexible, malleable, poorly ossified, and less mineralized than the adult skull. Depressed fractures occur after forceps delivery but occasionally are seen after a vaginal or cesarean birth. Compression of the skull causes buckling of the inner table without a break in the continuity of the skull.

Differential Diagnosis and Clinical Manifestations.   Linear fractures usually occur over the frontal or parietal bones. These fractures often are associated with extracranial hemorrhage and may underlie a cephalohematoma; they usually are asymptomatic. Skull radiographs are required for the diagnosis. Intracranial hemorrhage rarely complicates linear fractures. Some infants may have underlying cerebral injury or may have a "growing fracture," which is a rare complication in which a dural tear allows the leptomeninges to extrude into the fracture site. A leptomeningeal cyst may develop in these infants. Enlargement of the cyst results in growth of the fracture and failure to fuse (Moe & Paige, 1998).

A depressed skull fracture manifests as a visible, palpable depression or dent in the skull, usually over the parietal area. These fractures often are described as resembling a Ping-Pong ball because the depression does not involve any loss of bone continuity. Unless underlying cerebral contusion or hemorrhage is present, no other signs or symptoms are seen.

Prognosis.   Linear fractures heal spontaneously with no sequelae unless underlying cerebral damage or a growing fracture

is present. Basal fractures are associated with high mortality and poor developmental outcome. Infants with depressed fractures that are small or treated early (or both) have a good prognosis. Infants with large fractures, especially if treatment is delayed, have a greater risk of sequelae. Unless a depressed fracture has lacerated the dura (a rare occurrence), neurologic deficits in these infants usually are caused by cerebral injury from the original trauma or a hypoxic event, or both, rather than by the fracture per se (Moe & Paige, 1998). Infants with skull fractures should undergo regular evaluation of growth and developmental during infancy and early childhood.

Collaborative and Nursing Management.   The diagnosis is confirmed with skull radiographs or CT scans. CT is performed to identify cerebral contusions or hemorrhage. Nursing assessment includes monitoring these infants for signs of neurologic dysfunction, intracranial hemorrhage, meningitis, and seizures, although these findings are rare. Parents usually are concerned about their infant's appearance (with a depressed fracture) and the possibility of brain damage. They need support and teaching. Infants with uncomplicated linear fractures require no special management. Follow-up monitoring usually is recommended so that a growing fracture and development of a leptomeningeal cyst can be ruled out. Infants with basal fractures are treated for shock and hemorrhage. If the infant has leakage of CSF, antibiotics usually are given prophylactically to prevent meningitis.

In some infants with a depressed fracture, the fracture elevates spontaneously within the first week. Most clinicians recommend manually elevating an uncomplicated depressed fracture that does not elevate spontaneously within a few days (Moe & Paige, 1998). After this time, manual elevation is more difficult or impossible. Several techniques have been used for manual elevation, including gentle pressure and use of a breast pump or vacuum extractor, with varying results (Moe & Paige, 1998). Surgical intervention usually is necessary if manual elevation fails; if the fracture is more severe and bone fragments are in the cerebrum; if neurologic deficits exist, or if ICP is increased.

Spinal Cord Injury.   Spinal cord injuries usually occur in the midcervical to lower cervical and upper thoracic areas. Injury can occur at any point along the cord. Lower cervical to midthoracic injuries are usually seen in association with breech deliveries, midcervical to high cervical injuries, and vertex deliveries.

Pathophysiology.   Spinal cord injuries are caused by excessive traction, rotation, and torsion of the vertebral column and neck. Injury usually does not result from compression, but rather from stretching of the spinal cord, which is less flexible than the bony vertebral column. Damage to the spinal cord ranges from complete transection to laceration, edema, hemorrhage, and hematoma formation. Hemorrhage into the lining of the arteries may result in thrombosis, infarction, and ischemic cord damage.

Risk Factors.   Risk factors are breech delivery (major factor), dystocia, macrosomia, and cephalopelvic disproportion.

Spinal cord injuries occur most often in breech deliveries in which hyperextension of the head or version and extraction occur. This type of injury can also occur in infants with shoulder dystocia, with cord traction via the brachial plexus, or in a vertex secondary to torsional forces and rotation of the head (Levene, 1995c).

Differential Diagnosis. Infants with severe injuries initially may appear similar to those who have experienced severe birth asphyxia. Other problems that can have similar presentations include spina bifida occulta, neuromuscular disorders, tumors of the spinal cord, and bilateral brachial plexus injury.

Clinical Manifestations. Infants with partial spinal cord injury have subtle neurologic signs and variable degrees of spasticity. Infants with high cervical or brainstem injuries are stillborn or die shortly after birth from respiratory depression, shock, and hypothermia. Infants with midcervical or upper cervical injury may be stillborn, born with marked respiratory depression, or have respiratory depression, with the neurologic injury going unrecognized until flaccidity, immobility of the legs, urine retention, or all three are noted. If born alive, these infants usually die within the first week, after development of progressive central respiratory depression that often is complicated by pneumonia. Other clinical findings in this group of infants include relaxation of the abdominal wall, absent sensation in the lower half of the body, absent deep tendon and spontaneous reflexes, brachial plexus injury (20%), and constipation. This group also includes infants with injuries at the C8 to T1 level. These infants usually survive. Infants with this type of injury may have a transient paraplegic paralysis at birth. Infants with mild injury may recover most or all of their function. Infants with moderate to severe damage are paraplegic or quadriplegic and have permanent neurologic damage (Miller, 1997).

Initially, the clinical manifestations are those of spinal cord shock, with hypotonia, weakness, flaccid extremities, sensory deficits, relaxed abdominal muscles, diaphragmatic breathing, Horner syndrome (ipsilateral ptosis, anhidrosis, and miosis), and a distended bladder. Infants with low cervical lesions have shallow, paradoxical respirations; these infants do not sweat. The skin over the affected area is dry and warm. Pinprick and deep tendon reflexes are absent. Areflexia may be noted over the upper and lower extremities in some infants. The degree of neurologic insult often cannot be accurately evaluated until the infant has recovered from the initial period of spinal shock and any edema or hemorrhage has been reabsorbed (Moe & Paige, 1998). After several weeks or months, a paraplegic autonomic hyperreflexia develops that is characterized by periodic mass reflex response. This results in tonic spasms of extremities, spontaneous micturition, and profuse sweating over the paralyzed area.

Prognosis. The prognosis depends on the level and severity of the injury, but it generally is poor. Many infants with spinal cord injury are stillborn or die shortly after birth, particularly those with midcervical to high cervical or brainstem injuries. Those that survive have varying degrees of residual paralysis, respiratory problems, and bowel and bladder dysfunction, depending on the level of the injury. Most surviving infants have a spastic quadriplegia. Infants with involvement of the intercostal muscles and diaphragm often are ventilator dependent.

Collaborative Management. At birth the infant may be in shock and require delivery room resuscitation. Initial management focuses on stabilization, treatment of associated problems (e.g., perinatal asphyxia and hemorrhage), and management of respiratory depression. Infants with midcervical to upper cervical or brainstem lesions require assisted ventilation. Parents are in shock initially and need time to grieve. They need continu-

ing support and teaching regarding the care of the infant. Ongoing management of these infants and their families requires a multidisciplinary team that includes the disciplines of nursing, medicine, neurology, neurosurgery, physical therapy, orthopedics, urology, social work, and psychology. Ultrasonography, CT, or MRI may be performed to determine the level and the extent of injury.

Nursing Management. Nursing management focuses on caring for the infant and providing support to the shocked, grieving parents. Care of the infant in the delivery room and neonatal intensive care unit involves initial stabilization, management related to accompanying perinatal asphyxia or hemorrhage, and promotion of ventilation. Management of these infants presents a major challenge to the nurse to support the infant and to prevent further complications.

Skin integrity over the paralyzed area must be maintained to prevent pressure areas and skin breakdown. Thermoregulation may be a problem, because evaporative loss through the skin is reduced over the affected body parts in the initial period of the recovery process. The infant is positioned and repositioned regularly to promote normal alignment of body parts and prevent development of contractures and decubiti. Infants can be placed on soft foam, sheepskin, lambskin, or similar material or on a waterbed, and their position should be changed every 2 to 3 hours. The affected areas should be kept clean and dry and massaged with gentle, passive range-of-motion exercises. These infants need meticulous bowel and bladder care to prevent urinary tract infection and skin excoriation. Glycerin suppositories at regular intervals can help normalize bowel function. Infants are also monitored for signs of respiratory infection and pneumonia. Parental teaching before discharge focuses on normal baby care issues and concerns, as well as the special needs of a paralyzed infant.

Peripheral Nerve Injuries. Peripheral nerve injuries result from stretching, compression, twisting, hyperextension, or separation of nerve tissue (Moe & Paige, 1998). Injury can occur before, during, or after birth. Damage can range from swelling of the nerve to complete peripheral degeneration (with later total recovery) to complete division of all structures. The more common sites affected are the brachial plexus and the facial, phrenic, radial, median, and sciatic nerves. This type of injury is seen predominantly in term or LGA infants.

Injury to the radial nerve usually results from compression of the nerve caused by fracture of the humerus during a breech delivery or by intrauterine compression of the arm. The infant has wrist drop with a normal grasp reflex. Recovery usually occurs over the first few weeks to months. Median and sciatic nerve injuries are generally postnatal iatrogenic events. Median nerve injury can be a complication of brachial or radial arterial punctures. These infants have diminished pincer grasp and thumb strength and a flexed fourth finger. Recovery is variable. Sciatic nerve injuries are often permanent. They arise from trauma from a misplaced intramuscular injection or from ischemia from an injection of hypertonic solutions into the gluteal muscle. Infants with this type of injury have diminished abduction and distal joint movement. Hip adduction, rotation, and flexion are unaffected (Moe & Paige, 1998).

Facial Nerve Palsy. Facial nerve palsy is one of the more common types of peripheral nerve injury. The incidence is 0.23%.

Pathophysiology and Risk Factors.   Injury to the peripheral nerve is caused by trauma from oblique application of forceps, prolonged pressure on the nerve during labor from the maternal sacral promontory, or pressure from an abnormal fetal posture. Although some investigators have not found any differences in incidence between forceps and spontaneous vaginal deliveries, others have noted a correlation between the type of forceps and the incidence of injury. The facial nerve of the newborn is superficial after it emerges from the stylomastoid foramen. As a result, the nerve is vulnerable to compression injury at this site or as it traverses the ramus of the mandible. The temporofacial and cervicofacial nerve branches are most often involved. The injury is most common on the left. Because the prognosis is favorable, the injury appears to be caused by hemorrhage or edema into the nerve sheath rather than by disruption of the nerve fibers (Volpe, 2001b).

Differential Diagnosis.   Facial nerve paralysis must be distinguished from asymmetric crying facies and nuclear agenesis. Asymmetric crying facies results from absence of the depressor muscle of the angle of the mouth. These infants close their eyes normally when crying, but the mouth does not move down and out. They suck without dribbling. This disorder generally is benign. Nuclear agenesis (Mobius syndrome) is a more severe disorder characterized by congenital paralysis of the facial muscles.

Clinical Manifestations.   Clinical manifestations vary, depending on whether the injury is to the central nerve, the peripheral nerve, or the peripheral nerve branch. The complete peripheral nerve injury results in a unilateral inability to close the eye or open the mouth. The lower lip on the affected side does not depress during crying, nor does the forehead wrinkle. The affected side appears full and smooth, with obliteration of the nasolabial fold. These infants dribble milk while feeding. The infant may be unable to close the eye on the affected side. Central injury usually results in a spastic paralysis of the lower portion of the face contralateral to the side of CNS injury without involvement of the eyes or forehead. Peripheral nerve branch injury results in varying degrees of paralysis of the forehead, eye, or lower face, depending on the branch involved. The paralysis is apparent at birth or within 1 to 2 days after birth.

Prognosis.   Almost all infants recover completely. Improvement usually is apparent by 1 to 4 weeks, and complete recovery occurs after several months in most infants. Infants with severe nerve regeneration have a longer recovery period and may occasionally require later cosmetic surgery.

Collaborative and Nursing Management.   Nursing management involves parent counseling and teaching and prevention of complications. The eye on the affected side is patched, and 1% methylcellulose eye drops are instilled every 3 to 4 hours to prevent corneal damage. Dribbling with sucking can be a transient problem. If no improvement is noted by 7 to 10 days or if further loss of function occurs, a neurosurgical consultation usually is recommended. With partial degeneration, physical therapy, massage, or electrical stimulation may be used, although the efficacy of these therapies is controversial and not well documented. Electromyography, nerve excitability, or nerve conduction latency examinations may be performed to evaluate the extent of the damage.

Brachial Plexus Injury.   Brachial plexus palsy involves injury of the C5 to T1 nerve roots and is seen almost exclusively in term infants. The incidence ranges from 0.5% (in infants weighing less than 4000 g at birth) to 2.6% (in infants weighing more than 4500 g) (Rouse et al, 1996).

Pathophysiology and Risk Factors.   Injury to the brachial plexus results from excessive lateral flexion, rotation, or traction on the neck (Dodds & Wolfe, 2000). The degree of injury varies, ranging from edema and hemorrhage of the nerve sheath to avulsion of the nerve root from the spinal cord. With mild to moderate injury the axons are shattered, but the nerve sheaths remain intact. This degree of intactness of the nerve sheaths promotes regeneration of the nerve by 3 to 4 months, with full recovery. Severe injuries result in radicular rupture or intraspinal tearing of the nerve and division of the nerve into radicles. If radicular rupture occurs, the root loses contact with the spinal cord. These injuries do not recover spontaneously (Levene, 1995c; Dodds & Wolfe, 2000).

Brachial plexus injuries usually are unilateral and on the left side. Fracture of the clavicle may occur in conjunction with this type of injury. Brachial plexus injury can be seen in uncomplicated deliveries and after cesarean birth but is usually associated with vaginal delivery of LGA infants, shoulder dystocia, breech and other abnormal presentations, and prolonged labor or difficult delivery. Spontaneous injuries may occur from compression of the shoulder as it passes over the sacral prominence (Gherman et al, 1999).

Differential Diagnosis.   Cerebral and spinal cord injuries can manifest with similar initial findings. Other disorders that should be considered include injury to the clavicle or humerus and to the soft tissues of the shoulder and upper arm.

Clinical Manifestations.   Clinical manifestations vary with the location and severity of the injury. Signs of injury usually are apparent from birth but may be delayed for several days to a few weeks in some infants. The three major types of injury and their relative incidences are (1) Erb palsy, or upper plexus injury (73% to 86%), (2) Klumpke palsy, or lower plexus injury (less than 1%), and (3) Erb-Klumpke palsy, or both upper and lower plexus injury (20%) (Dodds & Wolfe, 2000).

Erb palsy results from injury to the C5 and C6 nerve roots. The shoulder and upper arm are involved, and denervation of the deltoid, supraspinous, biceps, and brachioradialis muscles occurs. The arm lies passively at the infant's side, abducted and internally rotated, and the forearm is pronated. The wrist and fingers are flexed. This posture is referred to as the "waiter's tip" position. The Moro reflex is absent, and the biceps and radial reflexes are diminished or absent on the affected side; the grasp reflex is normal. Klumpke palsy, seen primarily in breech infants whose arm has been hyperabducted and delivered with the head, involves the C8 to T1 roots, affecting the flexors of the wrist and hand. Cervical sympathetic fibers may also be affected; sweating and sensation are absent in the affected hand and arm. The infant holds the affected arm at the side of the thorax with the hand in a claw hand posture. The Moro and grasp reflexes are absent, and the triceps reflex is diminished or absent on the affected side; biceps and radial reflexes are present. If the T1 root is affected, the infant manifests Horner syndrome (ipsilateral ptosis, anhidrosis, and miosis) (Levene, 1995c; Dodds & Wolfe, 2000).

Total (Erb-Klumpke) palsy has the worst prognosis. The entire arm and hand are involved as a result of injury to the nerve roots of the brachial plexus from C5 to T1. Complete paralysis of the upper and lower arm and hand, flaccidity, and accompanying sensory, trophic, and circulatory changes are noted. Deep tendon and Moro reflexes are absent. If the C4 roots are also affected, an associated phrenic nerve (diaphragmatic) paralysis occurs. Involvement of the T1 root leads to Horner syndrome in about one third of these infants (Dodds & Wolfe, 2000).

Prognosis. The prognosis depends on the level and severity of the injury. Approximately 65% to 95% of infants have full recovery with supportive care (Noetzel & Wolpaw, 2000). Most (75%) have complete recovery by 3 to 4 months of age. Lack of significant recovery by this time is associated with a high risk of residual deficit. Erb palsy, the most common type of injury, has the best prognosis for full recovery. Infants with total paralysis are most likely to have residual paralysis. Residual functional deficits include alteration in abduction and external rotation of the shoulder; restricted movement of the elbow, forearm, and hand; and hand weakness (Noetzel & Wolpaw, 2000). These functional impairments can lead to abnormal muscle development and arm growth.

Collaborative Management. Initial management focuses on protecting the arm until localized edema and pain have subsided. MRI or CT are used to visualize the degree of injury. The affected arm is immobilized with shoulder and elbow splints to prevent contractures and further stretching of the plexus. After edema subsides, at about 7 to 10 days, physical therapy gradually is instituted as the infant can tolerate it. Initially the regimen may involve gentle, passive range-of-motion exercises. These infants have continued physical therapy consisting of massage and exercise over the first months until total or partial recovery occurs. Infants with a brachial plexus injury should be evaluated for associated problems, including fractures and respiratory difficulty secondary to phrenic nerve paralysis.

If improvement is not noted within the first few months, electromyography and nerve conduction studies are performed to determine the extent of the damage, to follow recovery, and to determine if surgical intervention is needed (Dodds & Wolfe, 2000). Radicular ruptures can be repaired with microsurgical reconstruction, tendon transfers, and nerve grafts. Surgery usually is done at 3 to 6 months. Muscle contractions of the shoulder and elbow may develop and require surgical release (Dodds & Wolfe, 2000).

Nursing Management. Infants with brachial plexus injuries often experience considerable pain during movement of the affected arm in the first few weeks after birth. Nursing management is directed at reducing passive and active movement of the arm and providing comfort measures to reduce pain. Splints are removed intermittently to reduce the risk of abduction contractures. The paralyzed arm is supported in a position of relaxation. Parent teaching regarding positioning, prevention of contractures, and exercise is essential.

Phrenic Nerve Palsy

Pathophysiology and Risk Factors. Phrenic nerve palsy is caused by injury of the cervical nerve roots at C3 to C5. The injury results from tearing of the nerve sheath, which is accompanied by edema and hemorrhage. Phrenic nerve palsy is frequently associated with Erb-Klumpke paralysis. Risk factors, especially breech delivery, are similar to those for brachial plexus injury. Paralysis of the diaphragm is a result of damage to the phrenic nerve. The injury usually is unilateral and on the right side.

Differential Diagnosis. Because the diaphragm is paralyzed, infants with phrenic nerve injury have respiratory difficulty. This phenomenon must be differentiated from CNS, cardiac, and pulmonary problems. The differential diagnosis also includes neuromuscular disorders, such as myogenic dystonia.

A radiographic finding of an elevated hemidiaphragm and paradoxical diaphragmatic movements on fluoroscopy confirm the diagnosis (Moe & Paige, 1998). Real time ultrasonography also is useful. Up to 90% of these infants also have plexus injuries (Moe & Paige, 1998).

Clinical Manifestations. Infants with mild to moderate phrenic nerve injury may have early respiratory difficulty, suggestive of hypoventilation, that stabilizes or improves. The infant may have recurrent episodes of cyanosis and dyspnea. The breathing pattern is altered. In these infants, breathing involves primarily thoracic movement with minimal or no abdominal excursions. Infants with complete avulsion or bilateral injuries have severe respiratory distress from birth, with tachypnea, apnea, and a weak cry (Miller, 1997).

Prognosis. A mortality rate of 10% to 20% has been reported with unilateral injury and up to 50% with bilateral injury (Moe & Paige, 1998). Most infants recover by 6 to 12 months of age. Other infants recover clinically but have residual abnormalities of diaphragmatic movement on radiography.

Collaborative Management. Management focuses on promoting ventilation and oxygenation. Infants may be placed on nothing by mouth status (NPO) initially, and feeding may be instituted as the infant's respiratory status improves. Infants with severe distress require positive pressure ventilation or constant positive airway pressure for support until recovery occurs. Electrical pacing of the diaphragm, constant positive airway pressure, and rocking beds have also been used (Moe & Paige, 1998). Surgical plication of the diaphragm is performed if no improvement is noted or if the infant is still ventilator dependent at 4 to 6 weeks of age.

Nursing Management. The infant is positioned on the affected side. If the infant cannot be fed, adequate fluid and calories must be provided. Feeding is instituted gradually. Initially, the infant may need to be gavage fed. When oral feeding is started, the infant is fed slowly and is given ample opportunity for rest and monitoring of respiratory status. Because recovery takes several months, parents must be taught feeding, positioning, and comfort techniques. Nursing management of infants with respiratory problems is similar to that for any infant with respiratory distress. The developmental needs of infants requiring prolonged hospitalization must be met; sensory input and play activities appropriate to their maturity and health status must be provided.

Neurologic Structural Dysfunction

Neurologic structural dysfunctions are primary disorders caused either by alterations in developmental processes in the embryo or fetus or, in the case of some forms of hydrocephalus, by postnatal problems such as intracranial hemorrhage or infection. This section focuses on the management of the two most common forms of neurologic structural abnormalities, NTDs and hydrocephalus.

Neural Tube Defects. The prevalence of CNS defects is declining as a result of prenatal diagnosis and folic acid supplementation (Marks & Khoshnood, 1998). Of these defects, 80% result from failure of neural tube closure at either the cranial or the caudal end (Moore & Persaud, 1998). NTDs include anencephaly, encephalocele, and spina bifida. Management of anencephaly, encephalocele, and spina bifida occulta are described in the section on embryologic development of the CNS. This section focuses on assessment and management of spina bifida cystica, especially myelomeningocele.

Pathophysiology. NTDs are caused by alterations in closure of the neural tube and in formation of the vertebrae. These processes and their alterations were described earlier. The three main forms of spina bifida cystica are meningocele, myelomeningocele, and myeloschisis. Spina bifida cystica can occur anywhere along the spinal column but is seen most often in the lumbar or lumbosacral area. A meningocele involves a sac that contains meninges and CSF; the spinal cord and nerve roots are in their normal position. With myelomeningocele, the most common form of spina bifida cystica, the sac contains spinal cord or nerve roots, or both, in addition to meninges and CSF. Myeloschisis is a severe defect in which no cystic covering exists, and the spinal cord is left open and exposed. The entire length of the spinal cord may be involved, and the infant may also be anencephalic (Moore & Persaud, 1998).

With myelomeningocele or myeloschisis, the spinal cord or nerve roots, or both, are displaced dorsally; defects of the muscle and bony structures exist lateral to the defect. The lesions are covered with skin or meninges or both. If the sac is covered with meninges, there is a risk of rupture during delivery, along with leakage of CSF and the risk of infection and dehydration. Many infants also have an associated Arnold-Chiari malformation, with secondary aqueductal stenosis in 40% to 75% that results in a noncommunicating form of hydrocephalus.

The Arnold-Chiari malformation is also a defect in neural tube closure. This malformation involves a group of anomalies, including displacement of the medulla, fourth ventricle, and lower cerebellum into the cervical canal; bony defects of the occiput, foramen magnum, and cervical vertebrae; and obstruction of the foramen magnum, leading to hydrocephalus (Hirose et al, 2001). Infants with NTDs may also have cardiac, intestinal, orthopedic, and other neurologic anomalies. Common associated orthopedic anomalies are congenital dislocated hips and talipes equinovarus.

Risk Factors. NTDs arise from genetic and environmental influences. They have a familial incidence and an increased genetic susceptibility. With one affected family member, the overall risk for defects in subsequent offspring in the United States is 2% to 3%, which doubles with two or more affected family members; the risk is greater if the previously affected offspring had a lesion at T11 or higher (Volpe, 2001b). NTDs are seen slightly more often in females than in males. The incidence is also higher with younger and older mothers, maternal diabetes, a history of miscarriages, maternal folate deficiency, and maternal exposure to drugs such as valproic acid and aminopterin. Geographic and seasonal patterns are seen, and seasonal outbreaks have been reported (Marks & Khoshnood, 1998).

Antenatal screening for NTDs involves analysis of maternal serum alpha-fetoprotein (AFP), which is done as part of the multiple marker test, along with estriol and human chorionic gonadotropin, at 16 to 18 weeks' gestation. Elevated AFP levels (greater than 2.5 multiples of the median) are followed up with an ultrasonographic examination and, if that is not definitive, by analysis of amniotic fluid AFP levels (Marks & Khoshnood, 1998). AFP is a major fetal glycoprotein, similar to the albumin produced in the fetal liver from 6 weeks' gestation. Concentrations of AFP peak at 13 to 15 weeks' gestation. AFP is found in fetal serum, CSF, and amniotic fluid. Normally the AFP concentration of the cerebrospinal fluid is significantly higher than that of the amniotic fluid, therefore when CSF leaks into the amniotic fluid, as occurs with an open neural tube defect, the AFP level of the amniotic fluid is elevated.

Differential Diagnosis and Clinical Manifestations. The defect may vary greatly in size but is apparent on examination of the infant. The protruding sac usually is in the lumbosacral area and is covered with skin or meninges. Fluid may be leaking from a partly or completely ruptured sac. Infants with this defect have altered tone and activity of the lower extremities and may assume a froglike posture. With bowel and bladder involvement, dribbling of urine and feces may be noted. The neurologic deficit varies with the level of the defect. The sensory level generally tends to approximate the motor level but may be several segments lower because of differences in the pattern of innervation between sensory and motor fibers. The sensory level can be useful for reaching a prognosis (McComb, 1997).

Infants with NTDs may have evidence of hydrocephalus at birth. Ultrasonography, CT, or MRI can be used to determine the size of the ventricular system, to rule out aqueductal stenosis or Arnold-Chiari malformation (or both), and to monitor ventricular status and the development of hydrocephalus. Renal dysfunction may develop as a result of recurring urinary tract infections. Hydronephrosis may be present at birth. An intravenous pyelogram may be obtained to evaluate renal status and to determine whether hydronephrosis is a factor (Miller, 1997).

Prognosis. The prognosis varies with the level and severity of the defect. Most infants with lesions lower than S1 will walk unaided; those with lesions higher than L2 generally will have some wheelchair dependency; bowel and bladder function are controlled at the level of S2-S4 (Hirose et al, 2001; Volpe, 2001b). However, these limitations are changing as a result of improved perinatal management and new technologies and aids, and more children are ambulatory now than previously. In some but not all studies, diagnosis before birth and delivery by elective cesarean section have been associated with prevention of sac rupture and improved motor function for the level of the lesion (Wilkins-Haug, 1999). Infants with a myelomeningocele involving a small lumbosacral lesion, without accompanying hydrocephalus or other anomalies, have some degree of neurologic deficit. These infants may be paraplegic but have a good prognosis for eventual independent function. Infants with myeloschisis have a poor prognosis. Many of these infants die of sepsis in the neonatal period. Those that survive have severe neurologic impairments. The prognosis has also improved with the current early and aggressive treatment of infants without major cerebral lesions, hemorrhage, infection, high spinal cord lesions, or advanced hydrocephalus (Volpe, 2001b).

Collaborative Management. Management begins with prevention, which is accomplished through folic acid supplementation for childbearing women to reduce the risk of NTDs and prevent recurrence (Marks & Khoshnood, 1998; AAP, 1999; Kadir et al, 1999; Ali & Economides, 2000; Northrup & Volcik, 2000). For many infants with NTDs, immediate closure and aggressive care constitute the appropriate management. Unless the defect is severe or is associated with multiple life-threatening anomalies, more than 90% of infants with myelomeningocele survive the neonatal period. If the defect goes untreated, 15% to 30% survive and are left with increased deficit. Immediate closure, therefore, is the treatment of choice for most infants.

Immediate closure reduces the risk of infection and improves the prognosis by reducing further deterioration of the spinal cord and nerve tracts. Early closure also facilitates caregiving. Surgical closure is performed within the first 24 to 48 hours, often in the first few hours after birth. A large defect may require several surgical procedures for complete closure. If the defect is completely covered by epithelium, surgery may be delayed for a short period so that function can be evaluated further. All infants with NTDs are evaluated and monitored for hydrocephalus. Urologic function and renal function also are assessed continually. All infants with involvement of the spinal cord or nerve roots, or both, require multidisciplinary follow-up and continuing care to deal with neurologic, urologic, orthopedic, and psychologic problems.

In utero repair of neural tube defects at 22 to 30 weeks' gestation, in an attempt to reduce postnatal complications such as hindbrain herniation and hydrocephalus, has been reported. However, an increase in obstetrical complications, such as preterm labor, oligohydramnios, and premature rupture of the membranes, has been reported. This procedure is controversial and still experimental, and the long-term outcomes are unclear (Olutoye & Adzick, 1999; Bannister, 2000; Hirose et al, 2001).

Nursing Management. Immediate nursing management of an infant with an NTD includes stabilization and prevention of trauma to or infection of the sac and its contents. The infant is monitored for signs of infection, including signs of sepsis or meningitis and localized infection, including redness or discharge from the sac. Warmth and hydration are provided, and fluid and electrolyte status is monitored. These infants are at greater risk of hypothermia and dehydration because of the open lesion, which lacks the normal protective skin covering.

The infant is positioned prone or on the side to reduce tension on the sac. A roll between the legs at hip level assists in maintaining abduction of the legs; a foot roll is used to maintain the feet in a neutral position. Change of position from prone to side lying or side to side, as well as range-of-motion exercises, helps prevent skin breakdown and contractures. Low Trendelenburg position may be used to reduce CSF pressure on the sac. If the infant must be temporarily placed in a supine position for a procedure, a donut roll can be used to prevent pressure on the sac. Postoperative positioning also involves use of the prone or side-lying position, maintenance of body alignment, prevention of hip abduction, and prevention of pressure on the operative site with holding.

The sac must be kept free of fecal or urine contamination. Meticulous skin care, consisting of keeping the skin clean and dry and removing urine and stool, helps prevent skin breakdown and infection. The timing and characteristics of urination and stool excretion are observed to help determine the degree of deficit.

Tone, spontaneous movement, range-of-motion, and reflex activity are assessed. Head circumference is monitored serially, and signs of increasing ICP are noted. These infants have an intravenous drip and are placed on NPO status initially because surgery usually is performed within the first hours after birth. After surgery, the infants are also placed in a prone position initially until the surgical site heals. Skin care to prevent excoriation and contamination of the excision site continues to be critical during this period, as does prevention of contractures.

Families of infants with NTDs need initial and continuing support and counseling. Initial parental care involves assisting parents with the shock of the defect and its appearance and with their grief over having an infant with an anomaly. Nursing care also involves enhancing parent-infant interaction and involving the parents in the infant's care when they are ready. Teaching before discharge includes skin care, positioning, exercises, handling and feeding techniques, and provision of activities to promote development. Many areas have spina bifida associations and parent to parent support programs to which parents can be referred for peer support.

Care of untreated infants is supportive, consisting of provision of warmth, hydration, and comfort. Decisions not to treat these types of infants, however, are controversial. A case of an infant with an NTD was the basis for Baby Doe regulations. In any case, the birth of an infant with an NTD is a difficult situation for the family and for nurses and other staff members, one that requires mutual understanding, support, and discussion of feelings.

Hydrocephalus. Hydrocephalus is the most common cause of head enlargement in the neonate. It may be congenital or acquired. The incidence of congenital hydrocephalus is 0.48 to 0.81 per 1000 live births (McAllister & Chovan, 1998). The disorder is caused by an abnormal accumulation of CSF in the ventricles and subarachnoid space. Hydrocephalus arises from alterations in circulation or production of CSF caused by a congenital defect or postbirth problems, such as infection or hemorrhage.

Pathophysiology. CSF is produced in the choroid plexus. It circulates from the lateral ventricles through the foramen of Monro to the third ventricle and, via the aqueduct of Sylvius, to the fourth ventricle. From there, CSF flows through the foramina of Luschka and Magendie, along the base of the brain, and around the hemispheres. CSF is absorbed by bulk flow through valves along the sagittal sinus. Although hydrocephalus can arise from overproduction of CSF by the choroid plexus, this cause is rare. Hydrocephalus almost always arises from an obstruction in the ventricular system or external to the ventricles. The primary mechanism of injury with hydrocephalus is compression and stretching of the brain parenchyma, ischemia, anoxia, cerebral edema, and dysfunction of the blood-brain barrier (McAllister & Chovan, 1998).

Congenital hydrocephalus usually is associated with malformations in the ventricular system proximal to the subarachnoid space. This is a noncommunicating form of hydrocephalus, meaning that no free communication exists between the ventricles and the subarachnoid space. The common malformations are stenosis of the aqueduct of Sylvius, Dandy-Walker syndrome, and Arnold-Chiari malformation. Aqueductal stenosis is the most common malformation associated with congenital hydrocephalus. The aqueduct is divided into many small channels that have varying amounts of occlusion. This abnormality is thought to arise at 15 to 17 weeks' gestation as the result of an alteration in the normal constriction of the aqueduct that occurs during this period (Whitelaw, 1995). Dandy-Walker syndrome is often associated with other CNS malformations. Infants with this defect have a cystic enlargement of the fourth ventricle, atresia of the foramina of Luschka and Magendie, and abnormal cerebellar development. Arnold-Chiari malformation varies in severity and often is associated with NTDs.

Acquired hydrocephalus involves arachnoiditis with arachnoidal adhesions that arise after intracranial hemorrhage or postinfection inflammation in the fetal or neonatal periods. In this type of hydrocephalus, some degree of communication usually exists between the ventricles and the subarachnoid space. The most common cause of posthemorrhagic hydrocephalus in the newborn is P/IVH. This P/IVH results in an obliterative arachnoiditis in the posterior fossa, which impedes CSF flow from the fourth ventricle or through the subarachnoid space or cisterns. Hydrocephalus also occurs after meningitis as a result of impediment of CSF flow by fibrotic areas and adhesions at the exit of the fourth ventricle or in the subarachnoid space (Madsen & Frim, 1999).

Hydrocephalus can involve static or progressive increase in ventricular volume with enlargement of the ventricles and compression of the cortex. Compression of the cortex may occur before clinical signs are apparent, such as changes in head size and separation of the sutures. In the newborn, progressive ventricular dilation results in diffuse atrophy of the white matter and destruction of glial cells and axons, spongy edema of the periventricular area, and fibrosis of the choroid plexus. Neurons tend to be selectively spared (Whitelaw, 1995; McAllister & Chovan, 1998).

Risk Factors.   Risk factors vary with the type of hydrocephalus. Congenital hydrocephalus arises from genetic influences or environmental influences, or both, during the period of embryonic or fetal development. Risk factors for hydrocephalus that develops after birth include intraventricular hemorrhage and other forms of intracranial hemorrhage, meningitis, and any factor that predisposes the infant to intracranial bleeding or sepsis.

Differential Diagnosis.   Hydrocephalus must be differentiated from other problems associated with increased or increasing head size. These include subdural hemorrhage, hydranencephaly (congenital absence of the brain but with normal dura, scalp, and skull), porencephaly (cystic cavitation of the brain that usually communicates with the ventricles or subarachnoid space), arachnoid cysts, achondroplasia, and macrencephaly with disorders such as Tay-Sachs disease. Hydrocephalus in LBW infants must be differentiated from normal head growth, catch-up growth, or the large head to body size of small-for-gestational-age (SGA) infants. Hydrocephalus can be differentiated from these disorders by cranial ultrasonography (most often used), MRI, or CT.

Clinical Manifestations.   Often, few signs and symptoms of hydrocephalus are present in the neonate. Enlargement of the head may be noted at birth in infants with congenital hydrocephalus, or it may develop gradually. Posthemorrhagic and infection hydrocephalus develop after birth at varying times after the initial insult. Head size can increase without increases in ICP (normopressive hydrocephalus) because of the neonate's soft, malleable skull and open sutures and fontanels (Madsen & Frim, 1999). A tense fontanel may be noted when the infant is placed in an upright position. Progressive ventricular dilation initially may cause compression and damage to the cortex without causing any change in head size. The developing hydrocephalus may be apparent only on a sonogram. Signs of increased ICP (e.g., bulging anterior fontanel, setting sun sign, dilated scalp veins, and widely separated sutures) tend to be later findings. In normal infants, sutures should be separated only by a few millimeters in the first few days after birth because of overriding of the bones. Separation of the squamosal

suture above the ear between the temporal and parietal bones is a good indicator of markedly increased ICP.

Prognosis.   The prognosis depends on the cause of the hydrocephalus and the presence and severity of associated problems. The prognosis tends to be better for infants with neonatal onset than for those with fetal onset. Infants with congenital hydrocephalus associated with NTDs or Dandy-Walker syndrome tend to have a high incidence of later neurologic problems, as do infants who have hydrocephalus after grade III or grade IV P/IVH (see section on P/IVH) or meningitis. On the other hand, infants with aqueductal stenosis as an isolated defect have a good prognosis.

Collaborative Management.   Serial head circumference measurements are plotted on all infants at risk for progressive ventricular enlargement and hydrocephalus. Management can involve either surgical or medical therapy.

Surgical management involves placement of a shunt to drain excess CSF. Other, less common, surgical procedures include removal of arachnoidal cysts or tumors or fenestration procedures for infants with Dandy-Walker syndrome. In infants with congenital hydrocephalus (who usually are term infants), a shunt may be inserted within a few days of birth, depending on the infant's health status and size (Madsen & Frim, 1999). A ventriculoperitoneal shunt is the shunt of choice in infants and children because this type is easier to insert, revise, and lengthen and has a lower risk of infection than a ventriculoatrial shunt. One end of a radiopaque catheter is placed in the lateral ventricle, usually on the right side, and the other end is placed in the peritoneal cavity. The catheter contains a one-way valve that is palpable on the side of the head near the ear. The shunt needs multiple revisions during childhood for growth and for malfunctioning. Major complications of ventriculoperitoneal shunts are infection and obstruction. Too rapid drainage of CSF immediately after insertion of the shunt can lead to herniation of the brain or subdural hematoma.

Infants with uncomplicated hydrocephalus may not need shunting if the hydrocephalus arrests, as it does spontaneously in about 50% of infants. These infants are managed by close follow-up and monitoring of ventricular size and cortical mantle thickness with serial cranial ultrasonography. Medical therapy is used primarily with acquired hydrocephalus. Serial lumbar punctures, intermittent CSF drainage with a ventricular access device, and administration of pharmacologic agents such as acetazolamide to reduce CSF may be used while these infants are monitored for cessation of progressive ventricular dilation. As noted in the section on P/IVH, serial lumbar punctures and most pharmacologic agents do not appear to significantly improve the long-term outcome (Tortorolo et al, 1999; Whitelaw, 2000a, 2000b). Medical therapies may also be used in infants who are too ill to tolerate surgery and shunt placement (Madsen & Frim, 1999).

Nursing Management.   Head circumference is monitored serially on all infants with or at risk for hydrocephalus. These infants are also monitored for signs of progressive ventricular enlargement and increased ICP. Skin care; use of soft foam, sheepskin, lambskin, or other materials that minimize pressure and excoriation; and regular position changes help prevent skin breakdown from pressure. The head of the hydrocephalic

---

BOX 31-1

Nursing Management of an Infant with a Ventriculoperitoneal Shunt

1. Ensure proper positioning:
   - Place infant on unaffected side (may position on shunt side with "donut" over operative site once incision has healed). Keep head of bed flat to 15 to 30 degrees to prevent too rapid fluid loss.
   - Support head carefully when moving infant.
   - Turn every 2 hours from unaffected side of head to back.
2. Provide care for shunt site:
   - Use strict aseptic technique when changing dressing.
   - Pump shunt if and only as directed by neurosurgeon.
   - Observe for fluid leakage around pump.
3. Observe and document all intake and output. Watch for symptoms of excessive drainage of CSF:
   - Sunken fontanel
   - Increased urine output
   - Increased sodium loss
4. Observe, document, and report any seizure activity or paresis.
5. Observe for signs of ileus:
   - Abdominal distention (serially measure abdominal girth)
   - Absence of bowel sounds
   - Loss of gastric content by emesis or through orogastric tube
6. Perform range-of-motion exercises to all extremities.
7. Observe and assess for symptoms of increased intracranial pressure (shunt failure):
   - Increasing head circumference (measure head daily)
   - Full and/or tense fontanel
   - Sutures palpable, more separated
   - High-pitched, shrill cry
   - Irritability or sleeplessness
   - Vomiting
   - Poor feeding
   - Nystagmus
   - Sunset sign of eyes
   - Shiny scalp with distended vessels
   - Hypotonia or hypertonia
8. Observe and assess for signs of infection:
   - Redness or drainage at shunt site
   - Hypothermia or hyperthermia
   - Lethargy or irritability
   - Poor feeding or weight gain
   - Pallor
9. Provide parent teaching:
   - Teach parents the signs and symptoms of increased intracranial pressure, infection, and dehydration; given them a written copy of these signs and symptoms.
   - Emphasize the importance of notifying the physician if any signs or symptoms are noted.
   - Demonstrate and receive return demonstration of proper head positioning (at rest, lifting, and carrying).
   - Demonstrate and receive return demonstration of drug administration. Teach parents the side effects of medications.
   - Emphasize the importance of follow-up medical care for assessment and medication adjustment.

Adapted from Moe P, Paige PL (1998). Neurologic disorders. In Merenstein G, Gardner S, editors. Handbook of neonatal intensive care, ed 4. Mosby: St Louis.

---

infant requires additional support, consisting of repositioning and holding. The infant may feed poorly and require small, frequent feedings. Reduction of environmental stressors and institution of comforting measures can reduce irritability.

After surgery, these infants are positioned on the side opposite the shunt, with the head of the bed flat or slightly elevated to prevent rapid loss of CSF and decompression. The valve should not be pumped unless this action is specifically ordered. The position can be rotated to supine every few hours to prevent skin breakdown. The skin should be kept clean and dry. The infant can also be placed on sheepskin or lambskin to prevent skin breakdown.

Infants with a shunt are observed for signs of localized or systemic infection, ileus, and shunt obstruction. Obstruction of the shunt leads to accumulation of CSF, enlargement of the head, and signs of increased ICP. Infection of the shunt may appear as localized redness or drainage around the incision, temperature instability, altered activity, or poor feeding. Fluid status and intake and output are monitored, and the infant is observed for signs of dehydration from too rapid loss of CSF. Signs of too rapid decompression include a sunken fontanel, agitation or restlessness, increased urine output, and electrolyte abnormalities. The postoperative management of infants with a ventriculoperitoneal shunt is summarized in Box 31-1.

Parent teaching before discharge includes care of the infant and shunt, including positioning and skin care. Parents must be comfortable in handling and caring for their infant before discharge. They should know the signs of shunt malfunction, increased ICP, infection, and dehydration. Continuing follow-up care of the infant and parental support are important. Parents may be referred to parent groups for peer support.

SUMMARY

Infants with neurologic dysfunction present a significant challenge to the neonatal nurse. The nurse must respond to infants with life-threatening conditions, such as perinatal asphyxia and intracranial hemorrhage; to those with transient problems, such as an isolated seizure; and to those with chronic problems, such as NTDs. Nurses must also deal with their own responses and those of the families of infants who may die during the neonatal or early infancy periods or whose short-term and long-term outcome may be altered by the extent of neurologic insult. To optimally care for these infants and their families, nurses must understand the basis for and the implications of specific types of neurologic dysfunction; they must recognize the clinical manifestations of these types of dysfunction; and they must respond appropriately in concert with other health care professionals.

The nursing care of infants who have or who are at risk for neurologic dysfunction involves assessment and monitoring of the infant's neurologic status and responses to the extrauterine environment, as well as of subtle signs that may indicate a change in status. Nursing management of the infant involves activities to address alteration in level of consciousness, potential for injury related to trauma or infection, impairment of skin integrity, alterations in comfort, impaired mobility, alterations in thermoregulation, alterations in nutrition and fluid and electrolyte status, and promotion of neurobehavioral organization and development. The nurse must also assess family coping, interactive processes, knowledge, and grieving to assist the family in coping with the birth of an ill infant and, for many families, with the uncertainty or certainty of long-term neurologic deficits in their infant.

REFERENCES

Ali SA, Economides DL (2000). Folic acid supplementation. *Current opinion in obstetrics and gynecology* 12:507-512.

Amato M, Donati F (2000). Update on perinatal hypoxic insult: mechanism, diagnosis, and interventions. *European journal of paediatric neurology* 4:203-209.

American Academy of Pediatrics, Committee on Genetics (1999). Folic acid for the prevention of neural tube defects. *Pediatrics* 104:325.

Amiel-Tison C (1995). Clinical assessment of the nervous system. In Levene MI, Lilford RJ, editors. *Fetal and neonatal neurology and neurosurgery*, ed 2. Churchill Livingstone: Edinburgh.

Bannister CM (2000). The case for and against intrauterine surgery for myelomeningoceles. *European journal of obstetrics, gynecology and reproductive biology* 92:109-113.

Barnes PD, Taylor GA (1998). Imaging of the neonatal central nervous system. *Neurosurgery clinics of North America* 9:17-47.

Berger R, Garnier Y (2000). Perinatal brain injury. *Journal of perinatal medicine* 28:261-285.

Bernes SM, Kaplan AM (1994). Evolution of neonatal seizures. *Pediatric clinics of North America* 45:1069-1104.

Bulas DI, Vezina GL (1999). Preterm anoxic injury: radiologic evaluation. *Radiology clinics of North America* 37:1147-1161.

Dammann O et al (2001). Is periventricular leukomalacia an axonopathy as well as an oligopathy? *Pediatric research* 49:453-457.

de Vries LS (1995). Cerebral ischemic lesions. In Levene MI, Lilford RJ, editors. *Fetal and neonatal neurology and neurosurgery*, ed 2. Churchill Livingstone: Edinburgh.

Dodds SD, Wolfe SW (2000). Perinatal brachial plexus palsy. *Current opinion in pediatrics* 12:40-47.

du Plessis AJ (1998). Posthemorrhagic hydrocephalus and brain injury in the preterm infant: dilemmas in diagnosis and management. *Seminars in pediatric neurology* 5:161-179.

Fieggen PG (1999). Congenital malformations of the brain: a neurosurgical perspective at the close of the twentieth century. *Child's nervous system* 15:635-645.

Fitzgerald M, Jennings E (1999). The postnatal development of spinal sensory processing. *Proceedings of the National Academy of Science USA* 96:7719-7722.

Fox K et al (1996). Glutamate receptor blockage at cortical synapses disrupts development of thalamocortical and columnar organization in somatosensory cortex. *Proceedings of the National Academy of Science USA* 93:5584-5589.

Gherman RB et al (1999). Brachial plexus palsy: an in utero injury? *American journal of obstetrics and gynecology* 180:1303-1307.

Goddard-Finegold J (1998). The intrauterine nervous system. In Taeusch HW, Ballard RA, editors. *Avery's diseases of the newborn*, ed 7. WB Saunders: Philadelphia.

Goddard-Finegold J et al (1998). The newborn nervous system. In Taeusch HW, Ballard RA, editors. *Avery's diseases of the newborn*, ed 7. WB Saunders: Philadelphia.

Guzzetta F et al (2000). Brain ischemic lesions of the newborn. *Child's nervous system* 16:633-637.

Haines SJ, Lapointe M (1999). Fibrinolytic agents in the management of posthemorrhagic hydrocephalus in preterm infants: the evidence. *Child's nervous system* 15:226-234.

Hardy P et al (1997). Control of cerebral and ocular blood flow autoregulation in neonates. *Pediatric clinics of North America* 44:137-152.

Hill A (1998). Intraventricular hemorrhage: emphasis on prevention. *Seminars in pediatric neurology* 5:152-160.

Hirose S et al (2001). Fetal surgery for myelomeningocele. *Current opinion in obstetrics and gynecology* 13:215-222.

Holmes GL, Ben-Ari Y (2001). The neurobiology and consequences of epilepsy in the developing brain. *Pediatric research* 49:320-325.

Ikonomidou C et al (2001). Neurotransmitters and apoptosis in the developing brain. *Biochemistry and pharmacology* 62:401-405.

Inder TE, Volpe JJ (2000). Mechanisms of perinatal brain injury. *Seminars in neonatology* 5:3-16.

Jacobson LK, Dutton GN (2000). Periventricular leukomalacia: an important cause of visual and ocular motility dysfunction in children. *Survey of ophthalmology* 45:1-13.

Kadhim H et al (2001). Inflammatory cytokines in the pathogenesis of periventricular leukomalacia. *Neurology* 56:1278-1284.

Kadir RA et al (1999). Neural tube defects and periconceptional folic acid in England and Wales: retrospective study. *British medical journal* 319:92-93.

Kinney HC, Back SA (1998). Human oligodendroglial development: relationship to periventricular leukomalacia. *Seminars in pediatric neurology* 5:180-189.

Levene MI (1995a). Management and outcome of birth asphyxia. In Levene MI, Lilford RJ, editors. *Fetal and neonatal neurology and neurosurgery*, ed 2. Churchill Livingstone: Edinburgh.

Levene MI (1995b). The asphyxiated newborn infant. In Levene MI, Lilford RJ, editors. *Fetal and neonatal neurology and neurosurgery*, ed 2. Churchill Livingstone: Edinburgh.

Levene MI (1995c). Disorders of the spinal cord and cranial and peripheral nerves. In Levene MI, Lilford RJ, editors. *Fetal and neonatal neurology and neurosurgery*, ed 2. Churchill Livingstone: Edinburgh.

Levene MI, de Vries (1995). Neonatal intracranial hemorrhage. In Levene MI, Lilford RJ, editors. *Fetal and neonatal neurology and neurosurgery*, ed 2. Churchill Livingstone: Edinburgh.

Madsen JR, Frim DM (1999). Neurosurgery of the newborn. In Avery GB et al, editors. *Neonatology: pathophysiology and management of the newborn*, ed 5. Lippincott, Williams & Wilkins: Philadelphia.

Marks JD, Khoshnood B (1998). Epidemiology of common neurosurgical diseases in the neonate. *Neurosurgery clinics of North America* 9:63-72.

Marret S et al (2001). Fetal and neonatal cerebral infarcts. *Biology of the neonate* 79:236-240.

McAllister JP, Chovan P (1998). Neonatal hydrocephalus: mechanisms and consequences. *Neurosurgery clinics of North America* 9:73-93.

McComb JG (1997). Spinal and cranial neural tube defects. *Seminars in pediatric neurology* 4:156-166.

Medlock MD, Hanigan WC (1997). Neurologic birth trauma: intracranial, spinal cord, and brachial plexus injury. *Clinics in perinatology* 4:845-853.

Miller G (1997). Hypotonia and neuromuscular disease. In Fanaroff AA, Martin RJ, editors. *Neonatal-perinatal medicine*, ed 6. Mosby: St Louis.

Mizrahi EM (2001). Neonatal seizures and neonatal epileptic syndromes. *Neurology clinics* 19:427-463.

Mizrahi EM, Clancy RR (2000). Neonatal seizures: early onset seizure syndromes and their consequences for development. *Mental retardation and developmental disabilities research review* 6:229.

Moe P, Paige PL (1998). Neurologic disorders. In Merenstein G, Gardner S, editors. *Handbook of neonatal intensive care*, ed 4. Mosby: St Louis.

Moore KL, Persaud TVN (1998). *The developing human: clinically oriented embryology*, ed 6. WB Saunders: Philadelphia.

Noetzel M, Wolpaw JR (2000). Emerging concepts in the pathophysiology of recovery from neonatal brachial plexus injury. *Neurology* 55:5-6.

Northrup H, Volcik KA (2000). Spina bifida and other neural tube defects. *Current problems in pediatrics* 10:313-332.

Olutoye OO, Adzick NS (1999). Fetal surgery for myelomeningocele. *Seminars in perinatology* 23:462-473.

Papile L (2002). Intracranial hemorrhage. In Fanaroff AA, Martin RJ. editors. *Neonatal-perinatal medicine*, ed 7. Mosby: St Louis.

Peeters C, Van Bel F (2001). Pharmacotherapeutical reduction of posthypoxic-ischemic brain injury in the newborn. *Biology of the neonate* 79:274-280.

Perlman JM (1998). White matter injury in the preterm infant: an important determination of abnormal neurodevelopment outcome. *Early human development* 53:99-120.

Rivkin MJ (1997). Hypoxic-ischemic brain injury in term newborn: neuropathology, clinical aspects, and neuroimaging. *Clinics in perinatology* 3:607-625.

Roland EH, Hill A (1997). Intraventricular hemorrhage and post-hemorrhagic hydrocephalus: current and potential future interventions. *Clinics in perinatology* 24:589-605.

Rouse DJ et al (1996). The effectiveness and costs of elective cesarean delivery for fetal macrosomia diagnosed by ultrasound. *Journal of the American Medical Association* 276:1480-1488.

Sanchez RM, Jensen FE (2001). Maturational aspects of epilepsy mechanisms and consequences for the immature brain. *Epilepsia* 42:577.

Saugstad OD (2001). Resuscitation of the asphyxic newborn infant: new insight leads to new therapeutic possibilities. *Biology of the neonate* 79:258-260.

Scher MS (1997). Seizures in the newborn infant: diagnosis, treatment, and outcome. *Clinics in perinatology* 24:735-772.

Scher MS (2001). Brain disorders of the fetus and neonate. In Klaus MH, Fanaroff AA, editors. *Care of the high-risk neonate,* ed 5. WB Saunders: Philadelphia.

Steinbach MT (1999). Traumatic birth injury: intracranial injury. *Mother baby journal* 4:513-519.

Tortorolo G et al (1999). Intraventricular hemorrhage: past, present, and future, focusing on classification, pathogenesis, and prevention. *Child's nervous system* 11-12:652-661.

Vannucci RC (2000). Hypoxic-ischemic encephalopathy. *American journal of perinatology* 17:113-120.

Vannucci RC, Perlman JM (1997). Interventions for perinatal hypoxic-ischemic encephalopathy. *Pediatrics* 100:1004-1014.

Vannucci RC, Vannucci SJ (2000). Glucose metabolism in the developing brain. *Seminars in Perinatology* 24:107-115.

Volpe JJ (1997). Brain injury in the premature infant: neuropathology, clinical aspects, pathogenesis, and prevention. *Clinics in perinatology* 24:567-587.

Volpe JJ (1998a). Neonatal neurologic evaluation by the neurosurgeon. *Neurosurgery clinics of North America* 9:1-16.

Volpe JJ (1998b). Brain injury in the premature infant: overview of clinical aspects, neuropathology, and pathogenesis. *Seminars in pediatric neurology* 5:135-151.

Volpe JJ (2001a). Perinatal brain injury: from pathogenesis to neuroprotection. *Mental retardation and developmental disabilities research review* 7:56-64.

Volpe JJ (2001b). *Neurology of the newborn,* ed 4. WB Saunders: Philadelphia.

Whitelaw A (1995). Neonatal hydrocephalus and clinical assessment and nonsurgical treatment. In Levene MI, Lilford RJ, editors. *Fetal and neonatal neurology and neurosurgery,* ed 2. Churchill Livingstone: Edinburgh.

Whitelaw A (2000a). Postnatal phenobarbitone for the prevention of intraventricular hemorrhage in preterm infants. *Cochrane database systemic reviews* 2:CD001691.

Whitelaw A (2000b). Repeated lumbar or ventricular punctures for preventing disability or shunt dependence in newborn infants with intraventricular hemorrhage. *Cochrane database systemic reviews* 2: CD000216.

Whitelaw A, Thoresen M (2000). Antenatal steroids and the developing brain. *Archives of diseases of childhood (fetal & neonatal)* 83:F154-F157.

Wildrick D (1997). Intraventricular hemorrhage and long-term outcome in the premature infant. *Journal of neuroscience nursing* 29: 281-289.

Wilkins-Haug L (1999). Considerations for delivery of infants with congenital abnormalities. *Obstetrics and gynecology clinics* 26:399-412.

CHAPTER 32

ASSESSMENT AND MANAGEMENT OF THE MUSCULOSKELETAL SYSTEM

JOYCE M. BUTLER

INTRODUCTION

Abnormalities of the neonatal musculoskeletal system range from a subtle brachydactyly to a fatalistic form of osteogenesis imperfecta congenita. Causes range from uterine malpositioning of the fetus to autosomal dominant disorders. Regardless of the clinical significance, an overt structural defect can become the focus of parental attention. Assessment of the musculoskeletal system—which can have multiple normal variants—and knowledge of pathogenesis, sequelae, treatment, and prognoses for deformities of this system is imperative to the clinician. Delay in diagnosis and treatment may be implicated as a cause of a less than favorable outcome of the musculoskeletal deformity. Appropriate education of the family by the health care professional is often paramount to a beneficial outcome because many musculoskeletal disorders require compliance with long-term therapy.

The following are common terms that are used when discussing the musculoskeletal system:
- Valgus refers to a deformity in which a body part is bent outward and away from the midline of the body; it is a part that is in abduction.
- Varus implies a body part positioned inward, toward the midline of the body; it is a part that is in adduction.
- Talipes refers to any one of various foot deformities.
- Reduction is restoration to a normal position.
- Avulsion is the tearing away of a part or segment.
- Plagiocephaly describes a misshapen skull/head.

Deformities of the musculoskeletal system create not only functional problems but, in some cases, visible defects as well. The type of dysfunction may greatly affect how the parent views the neonate and the infant's potential for positive growth and development.

This chapter outlines the common musculoskeletal dysfunctions seen during the neonatal period. In addition, it describes the collaborative management as well as the long-term implications of the functional and aesthetic problems encountered with musculoskeletal dysfunction.

EMBRYOLOGY

The embryonic period is characterized by maximal organogenesis and lasts from the end of the first week until the eighth week of gestation. The embryo originates from three cell layers—termed the ectoderm, endoderm, and mesoderm. The embryonic mesoderm gives rise to the articular, muscular, and skeletal systems.

The articular system, or joints, can be classified into three types: fibrous, cartilaginous, and synovial. Fibrous joints are those in which two bones are separated only by dense fibrous connective tissue, as seen in cranial sutures. Cartilaginous joints (such as the symphysis pubis) have hyaline cartilage or fibrocartilage between the two bony surfaces. The elbow and knee are examples of synovial joints. In these joints, the adjoining bone ends are covered with a thin cartilaginous layer and joined by a ligament lined with a synovial membrane. This synovial membrane secretes a lubricant referred to as synovial fluid, a source of nutrition for the articular cartilage. The articular system begins to develop during the sixth week of gestation, with functional joints being present by the end of the eighth week.

Groups of myotubes, the primordia of skeletal or striated muscle, are apparent by the end of the eighth week of gestation. As the myotubes enlarge, the appearance of myofilaments is evident in interior regions. Growth of myofilaments leads to mature muscle fibers. Postnatal development of muscle fibers continues both in number and in size. Muscle development depends on proper innervation, evident at 8 to 10 weeks of gestation. Without this innervation, the muscles atrophy. The mother can detect intrauterine fetal movements at 16 weeks of gestation. The upper and lower limb buds first appear by the end of the fourth week of gestation. Sequential development progresses from limb buds, to hand and foot plates with digital rays, to hand and foot with separate digits at 8 weeks' gestation. The upper limbs develop more quickly than the lower limbs, and several days elapse between the development of the upper limbs and that of the lower limbs.

The skeleton develops by intramembranous bone formation and endochondral ossification. The vertebral column is initially of a cartilaginous form, with ossification beginning during the embryonic period and reaching completion in early adulthood. Ossification is evident in all long bones by 12 weeks' gestation.

Rapid cell division during organogenesis renders an organ vulnerable to any disturbance that might result in aberrant development. The most sensitive period for the development of major morphologic deformation of the limbs is from the beginning of the fourth until just shortly after the sixth week of gestation. Functional and minor morphologic abnormalities may occur any time during gestation. The skeletal system, because of rapid growth through puberty, has a prolonged period of sensitivity.

ASSESSMENT

Astute systematic observation is the key tool for assessing the neonatal musculoskeletal system. Visual inspection should begin in one body region—that is, cephalic or caudal—and progress along the body in an organized fashion. For the initial examination, place the infant in a quiet resting state to assess posture, positioning, and identification of any overt anomalies. Active movement by the infant allows the clinician to view muscle tone and active ranges of motion. Manipulation is used to assess passive range of motion, including joint mobility. Radiologic studies as well as simple body measurements aid the clinician in the collection of evidence of covert musculoskeletal deformities.

Maternal history is reviewed for uterine anomalies such as the bifid uterus, thereby dividing the uterine cavity into two segments. Additional maternal and family history that are important include previous family members, especially siblings, with musculoskeletal anomalies; presence of oligohydramnios; fetal movement during gestation, and the birthing process.

In developing a differential diagnosis, the clinician must be aware that a combination of deformities present in a neonate may be a small part of a larger syndrome. Conversely, congenital anomalies that present in combination may be a coincidental finding (Box 32-1).

TYPES OF MUSCULOSKELETAL DYSFUNCTION

Osteogenesis Imperfecta

Osteogenesis imperfecta (OI) is a connective tissue disorder with genetic origins. The primary pathophysiologic defect involves the collagen structure. A genetic mutuation occurs either in the COL1A1 or COL1A2 gene response for collagen formation (Lashley, 1998). Many mutations occur, most of

---

BOX **32-1**

Common Musculoskeletal Conditions

Skeletal Dysplasias
Osteogenesis imperfecta
Achondroplasia
Arthrogryposis
Congenital hip dislocation

Limb Defects
Clubfoot
Syndactyly
Polydactyly
Amniotic band syndrome
Miscellaneous
Birth trauma
Torticollis

---

which substitute glycerin with another substance. Collagen (the major extracellular protein) formation fails to progress beyond the reticulin fiber stage. Further significant disruption in the collagen formation in OI includes a defect in cross-linking that results in decreased collagen stability. Although osteoblastic activity appears normal, typically no collagen is produced. Any tissue containing collagen, such as sclerae, bones, ligaments, and teeth, may be affected. Through various clinical, genetic, and biochemical studies OI has been determined to be heterogenous; it may result from autosomal recessive or autosomal dominant disorders as well as from spontaneous mutations (Spitz, 1996). Clinical presentations of OI range from mild affectations to individuals with fatalistic prognoses. The overall incidence in Western countries is reported as 1:20,000 live births (Lashley, 1998).

Numerous attempts have been made to develop a taxonomy for OI. Because of limited knowledge as to the exact pathomechanics of the disease, however, a precise classification system remains elusive. Sillence and Danks (1978) developed the most widely used classification system in the late 1970s. This system is a numerical classification based on clinical and genetic factors. There are four major groups; two are autosomal recessive, and two are autosomal dominant. Two of the groups (OI types I and IV) are subdivided according to the absence or presence of dentin abnormalities (dentinogenesis imperfecta). Dentinogenesis imperfecta occurs when the dentin layer is affected concomitant with constriction of the pulp space. The clinical appearance of dentinogenesis imperfecta involves teeth that are grayish blue to brown in color. The teeth are typically worn down because of decreased resistance to pressure. The deciduous teeth are more often affected than the permanent teeth. It is important to explain to the parents that the aesthetic appearance of the child may improve with the emergence of permanent teeth.

Osteogenesis Imperfecta Type I.   OI type I is an autosomal dominant disorder. As with many other dominant disorders, penetrance varies. This means that the clinical appearance of affected individuals in the same family may range from mild to severe. Severe forms of OI present with early-onset fractures, and the frequency of fractures is increased. Other clinical features include severe hearing impairment, with an incidence of 40:1, and a preponderance for bruising (75:1). The sclera is often bluish as well.

OI type I is subdivided into types IA and IB. Type IA occurs without dentinogenesis imperfecta, whereas evidence of dentin abnormalities is seen in type IB.

The clinical presentation of this disorder is evident in the neonatal period in 10% of affected individuals. Fractures are the primary sign in neonates. Affected neonates typically have normal height and weight for their gestational age. Because of the progressive nature of kyphoscoliosis (a component of OI disorders), however, short stature develops in most affected persons.

Prenatal diagnosis of type I is difficult, as most cases do not exhibit fractures *in utero* as do the more severe forms of OI, which exhibit repeated fractures and bowing of the fetal extremities. In one recent study, the percentage of OI type I diagnosed prenatally was 3.4 versus 49% of OI type II diagnosed in the prenatal period (Cubert et al, 2001).

Osteogenesis Imperfecta Type II.   OI type II is an autosomal recessive disorder. This extremely severe OI disorder results in death either in the prenatal or neonatal period. Prenatal diagnosis is possible with this condition. Death occurs through damage to vital organs—brain, liver, and lungs—not protected by the fragile bony structures.

Neonates affected with this disorder are typically small-for-gestational-age and appear dwarf-like. The extremities are deformed and short as a result of multiple fractures and crumbling of the long bones. Chest radiographs exhibit beaded ribs with numerous fractures, both old and new. Blue sclera are characteristic features in both OI type I and OI type II. Blue sclera can be a normal neonatal finding and cannot serve as a diagnostic criterion for this age group.

Trauma of birth exacts a further toll on the appearance of these infants and contributes to the maceration of the head and limbs. This form of OI is also referred to as the perinatal lethal form.

Osteogenesis Imperfecta Type III.

OI type III is a rare, severe disorder with autosomal recessive inheritance patterns. Fractures may be present at birth, and the clinical course may simulate OI type II. Variations between types II and III are identified on physical examination. Neonates affected with OI type III have normal height and weight for gestational age at birth. Although multiple rib fractures may appear on chest radiograph, the beaded rib appearance is absent. The long bones in OI type II are crumbled, whereas the bones have multiple fractures and calcifications in OI type III. The extremities do not usually appear deformed as in OI type II; however, individuals affected with OI type III have the shortest stature for all OI disorders. Mortality rates for children with OI type III are high because of the development of severe kyphoscoliosis.

Osteogenesis Imperfecta Type IV.

OI type IV is similar to type I in that it is an autosomal dominant disorder with variable penetrance. OI type IV is subdivided into types IVA and IVB, depending on the absence or presence of dentinogenesis imperfecta. OI type IV resembles types I and III in clinical presentation and course. Incidence rates for OI types III and IV have not yet been established.

Glorieux et al (2000) have proposed a new form of OI—an autosomal dominant form that does not appear to be associated with type I mutations. This form has been classified OI type V.

Clinical presentation of this form of OI has included: ligamental laxity similar to type IV, moderate to severe increased fragility of long bones and vertebral bodies, and limitations in the range of pronation/supination in one or both forearms. Incidence rates and genetic etiology have not been determined.

Diagnosis.

Accurate diagnosis of OI disorders is of primary concern for the affected individual and family. Recurrence rates and inheritance patterns vary among the recessive and dominant forms. Instances of OI have resulted from spontaneous mutations.

Any of the forms of OI can be present at birth, although severity varies among the different types. In the milder cases, fractures in the neonatal period may result from birth trauma. Fractures are most abundant in the arms, legs, clavicles, and ribs. As the infant ages, the lower extremities more often are affected as a result of increased weight-bearing trauma.

Calcification is rapid in neonates; callus formation usually occurs within 10 days. No deficiency seems to exist in callus formation in OI disorders; however, the callus is weaker than in normal individuals and predisposes the bone to further fractures in that area.

Multiple rib fractures in a neonate may prompt respiratory compromise, because the pain from the fracture thwarts the infant's breathing attempts. OI may be suspected when it is difficult to wean an infant from ventilatory support and other pathologic causes have been ruled out. In such cases, chest radiographs should be closely inspected for rib fractures and callus formation.

Case reports have identified newborns who sustain fractures of the femurs during routine examination of the hip for dysplasia. Some cases of OI are not recognized until either one or both femurs sustained fractures during hip examination. Some of the infants exhibit significant distress, immediately followed by prolonged crying, decreased movement of the extremity, or both. Whether increased incidence of birth trauma occurs with the delivery methods for infants with OI has been of concern. Cubert and colleagues (2001) evaluated 167 pregnancies affected with neonatal OI, the majority of which were diagnosed postnatally, and concluded that cesarean section delivery did not decrease fracture rates at birth in infants with nonlethal forms of OI. Cesarean delivery also did not prolong survival for those infants with the perinatal lethal form of OI.

Treatment.

No treatment for the underlying pathologic cause of OI disorders exists. Therefore management of OI centers around support and promotion of independence in terms of mobility, function, and social integration. Rehabilitation techniques include active range of motion, strengthening exercises, stretching, and coordination exercises. Water activities are well tolerated, even in patients with severe affectations. Outcome appears to be enhanced when physical and occupational therapies are instituted promptly after birth, condition allowing. Independent living is improved in this population when the affected individual is mobile. One study evaluated the ability of children with OI to walk and reported that the type of OI was the most important clinical indicator for the ability to walk (Engelbert et al, 2000). Children with type III and IV had a lower chance of walking than those with type I. Positive clinical signs associated with the development of the ability to walk included rolling over before 8 months, unsupported sitting before 9 months, sitting without support by 12 months, and pulling to a standing position without support before 12 months. (Engelbert et al, 2000).

Collaborative Management.

In the neonatal period, infants with OI are managed according to clinical presentation and protocol for that particular gestational age. Health care professionals and the patient's family must handle the infant carefully. Padded splints for the extremities may help reduce the incidence of accidental fractures, and signs should be posted on the infant's bed to warn all individuals of the consequences of improper handling. As the infant grows, padded orthotic devices support the trunk and extremities to reduce the incidence of skeletal deformities such as kyphoscoliosis.

Vascular checks of the casted or splinted extremity are required. A pink color of the capillary bed indicates adequate arterial flow; white (or pallor) symbolizes decreased or poor arterial flow; and cyanosis of the extremity indicates venous stasis. Although pulse checks may be helpful, the care giver should realize that, by the time a pulse is absent, irreparable harm has probably occurred. For this reason, parents should be taught how to assess color and capillary refill rather than pulse palpation.

An infant with OI necessitates skin care in terms of positioning. Bedding should be such that discourages decubitus formation, because the infant may have minimal spontaneous movement secondary to pain from the fractures. It is wise for the caregiver to ask a colleague for assistance when repositioning these infants. Splints (e.g., rolled blankets or sandbags) placed beside the infant's chest stabilize the thoracic wall and potentiate effective ventilation. These splints are most effective in cases of multiple rib fractures.

Pain relief through medication and supportive measures should be considered for the infant. The infant may react to pain caused by multiple fractures through facial grimacing and crying upon movement. Alterations in vital signs (e.g., tachycardia, tachypnea, hypertension), irritability, and restlessness have also been attributed to pain in the neonate (Chapter 42).

Family education and support are integral components in the management of the neonate's care. Parents and other family members may be reluctant to hold and cuddle the infant for fear of causing additional fractures. The clinician should educate the family on proper handling of the infant. It should be stressed to the family that fractures are inevitable in the infant with OI.

SKELETAL DYSPLASIA

Skeletal dysplasia identifies a group of clinical disorders that involve abnormal endochondral ossification. It includes achondroplasia, hypochondroplasia and thanatophoric dysplasia, all of which present with a short-limbed skeletal dysplasia at varying times of presentation.

Achondroplasia

Although the word achondroplasia was once used to describe any form of dwarfism, it is now recognized as one distinct type of dwarfism having characteristic features. Achondroplasia has an autosomal dominant pattern of inheritance and is the most common nonlethal skeletal dysplasia. Most cases occur by spontaneous mutation. The incidence of achondroplasia has varied in the past as a result of multiple forms of skeletal dysplasia diagnosed as achondroplasia. The incidence is 2.5 per 100,000 live births.

One risk factor for spontaneous mutation that involves achondroplasia appears to be advanced paternal age. Achondroplastic infants can be identified at birth with a rhizomelic shortening of the extremities meaning the proximal portion of the arm/leg is shorter in length than the distal portion. The infant who is affected with achondroplasia also presents with a disproportionately large head with frontal bossing and depressed nasal bridge. The hands are small with a trident configuration that describes the appearance of the fingers and an increased spacing between the long and ring fingers. Identification of mild hypotonia and limitation of elbow extension with laxity in most other joints is also noted in the achondroplastic child. These neuromuscular and skeletal anomalies—including the mild hypotonia, rhizomelia, joint laxity and reduced elbow extension—can produce a delay in gross motor milestones but generally improves to normal over the first few years of life. Central intelligence is normal in most cases.

Hypochondroplasia

Hypochondroplasia is rarely noted at birth, as the length of the infant is often normal. The short stature becomes clinically apparent around 24 months of age. This condition is rarely diagnosed in the neonatal period but may present with macro-cephaly. Hypochondroplastic children and adults experience the some of the similar orthopedic complications as the achondroplastic individual. Some of these include joint and lower back pain.

Thanatophoric Dysplasia

Thanatophoric dysplasia is the third in this series of skeletal dysplasias. It is a lethal defect and is often compared to osteogenesis type II in terms of its clinical scenario after birth with death usually in several hours or days. Death occurs secondary to lung hypoplasia.

The clinical presentation of thanatophoric dysplasia describes a fetal environment of reduced fetal movements and polyhydramnios. Hypotonia in the neonate with macrocephaly often presenting as a clover leaf-shaped skull. This is believed secondary to the fusion of the coronal and lambdoidal sutures. The limbs are short and bowed with severe brachydactyly or short digits. The thorax is very narrow and short, thus reminding the clinician of the abnormal pulmonary development and severe pulmonary hypoplasia. The abdomen has a protuberant appearance. Almost all cases of thanatophoric dysplasia result from a new genetic mutation.

Differential Diagnosis. The differential diagnosis of a neonate with dwarfism includes achondroplasia, OI type II, thanatophoric dwarfism, asphyxiating thoracic dysplasia, lethal short limb-polydactyly syndromes, and achondrogenesis. In achondroplasia, the patient has markedly shortened limbs and often bowing of the lower limbs, but radiographic studies do not show evidence of multiple fractures and long-bone crumbling as is seen in OI type II. Thanatophoric dwarfism and achondrogenesis, both typically fatal in the neonatal period, are characterized by an extremely narrow chest and marked defective ossification, respectively.

Collaborative Management. Respiratory or ventilatory management of the severely affected achondroplastic dwarf is the primary concern. Supporting positive pulmonary function in the face of reduced lung volume capacity within the narrow thorax can be challenging. Mildly affected infants may compensate for decreased lung volume with a mild to moderate increase in the work of breathing. As the infant grows, this compensation becomes more difficult.

Compensatory mechanisms, such as increased work of breathing in the mildly affected achondroplastic dwarf, require that meticulous attention be paid to nutritional support for the increased energy needs. An infant who exhibits tachypnea or retractions must have increased caloric intake for positive growth to occur. If growth proceeds too rapidly, however, the infant's body mass may exceed the pulmonary capacity and decompensation may occur. Nutritionists may provide insights into the daily management of providing calories but not adding to the work of the infant.

Parental and family needs may be satisfied through education and collaboration with social services. Support groups specifically for parents of dwarfed infants are organized in many cities. From these groups, parents can gain a better perspective of the long-term development of their infant.

Long-Term Consequences of Achondroplasia. Complications of achondroplasia are primarily neurologic and involve the spinal nerves. Anatomic configuration of the intraspinal canal results in pressure on the cord and spinal nerves. This pressure produces chronic backache and, in the most severe scenario, paraplegia. Referrals to physical and occupational therapists; along with long-term orthopedic follow-up, can reduce some of the complications. If these changes in the spinal column do occur, the child is at greater risk for development of increased respiratory difficulties, mobility problems, self-concept and self-esteem concerns, physical pain, and central or peripheral nervous system neuropathies.

Sisk and colleagues (1999) described a 38% incidence of obstructive sleep apnea in children with achondroplasia. Apnea usually presented in early childhood. Adenotonsillectomy was more successful than adenoidectomy; follow-up surgery in the two groups were reported as 18% and 90%, respectively.

Because children with achondroplasia have a different appearance than their peers, any exaggeration of the condition can add to a faulty self-concept. As the child grows, continual assessment by both health professionals and parents of the mental personal image that the child is forming. Positive support of parents during the neonatal period through comments about what the infant is doing and how the infant looks may provide a role model of positive behavior that the parents can emulate with the child.

ARTHROGRYPOSIS

Historically, the term arthrogryposis (curved, hooked joint) has been used not only to provide a description of a clinical appearance but also as a diagnosis for various conditions. The one common denominator for conditions termed arthrogryposis is the presence of multiple congenital joint contractures. More than 150 known conditions feature multiple congenital contractures as the dominant feature; many of these conditions are syndromes unrelated to a chromosomal or genetic problem. The most common forms are autosomal dominant distal arthrogryposis, amyoplasia, multiple pterygium syndrome, and cerebro-oculo-facio-skeletal syndrome. A less common form that geneticists currently are examining is Pena-Shokeir syndrome. Consequently, the name arthrogryposis multiplex congenita is often used to incorporate these many uses of the word.

An infant born with multiple congenital contractures may have either a specific syndrome or a chromosomal anomaly. Achieving a precise diagnosis of the infant with multiple congenital contractures is important because recurrence risks vary among the different entities and because genetic counseling depends on knowledge of recurrences.

Arthrogryposis involves congenital, nonprogressive limitation of movement in two or more joints in different body areas. The deformity primarily results from fibrous and fatty changes in muscles secondary to decreased fetal movement. Although muscles undergo normal embryologic development, they are replaced by fibrous and fatty tissue after a reduction of normal fetal movement. The physiologic muscle changes subsequently produce contracted joints. Animal studies have produced congenital joint contractures by decreasing fetal movement through various processes. Ultimately, any process that result in limited intrauterine movement by the fetus can lead to multiple congenital contractures. The severity of such contractures increases with a longer duration of limited movement. The earlier in fetal development that the limitation is imposed, the greater the severity of contractures. The causes of decreased fetal movement can be classified into three categories, which are listed in Table 32-1.

TABLE 32-1	Etiology of Decreased Fetal Movement
Category	**Examples**
Myopathic Abnormal muscle function secondary to failure of muscle formation or degeneration	Congenital muscular dystrophy Absence of muscles
Neuropathic Abnormal nerve function or innervation that involves either CNS or peripheral nervous system	Drugs or toxins CNS malformations: decreased number of anterior horn cells
Abnormal connective tissue	Abnormal formation of bone, cartilage, tendons, or connective tissue
Mechanical Limitation Produces compression within the uterus	Twins Amniotic rupture Oligohydramnios Uterine myomas

Incidence and Inheritance Patterns

The incidence of multiple congenital contractures is 1 in 3,000 live births. Hall (1981) examined 350 infants and divided them into three categories based on the body areas affected by the contractures. This classification system, which is still in use, can provide a prognostic indicator for the clinician.

The first category primarily involves the limbs. Most affected infants are in this category, and otherwise they are normal. The second category primarily involves contractures in the limbs but also involves other organ systems, predominantly the visceral organs. The third category involves multiple congenital contractures concurrent with central nervous system (CNS) dysfunction.

The first category can be subdivided into amyoplasia and distal arthrogryposis. Amyoplasia, a sporadic condition, is considered to be classic arthrogryposis. The sporadic nature of this condition reflects the lack of an identifiable inheritance pattern when a family history is examined. Thus families with an affected member are not at increased risk for recurrence. Distal arthrogryposis is inherited by an autosomal dominant pattern. Parents with an infant with distal arthrogryposis can have a risk calculation done by a genetics counselor to give them an idea of their potential for having another child with this same condition.

Two other types of arthrogryposis have an autosomal recessive inheritance pattern. The first is multiple pterygium syndrome, which consists of webbed, contracted fingers with later development of camptodactyly; micrognathia; low-set rotated ears; palpebral fissures that appear to have a downward slant; ptosis; rocker-bottom feet, much like those of an infant with trisomy 13 or 18; possibly neck webbing; and possibly cleft palate. The second syndrome is cerebro-oculo-facio-skeletal syndrome. It is associated with postnatal failure to thrive, microcephaly, intracranial calcifications, shortened palpebral fissures, and congenital cataracts. These children usually die by school age.

Another form of arthrogryposis, which is very rare, is Pena-Shokeir syndrome. An infant with this syndrome has a short umbilical cord, pulmonary hypoplasia, intrauterine growth retardation, ankyloses, and camptodactyly. The maternal history includes oligohydramnios and fetal akinesia, or decreased fetal movement. This condition may have an autosomal recessive inheritance pattern, but this idea has not been confirmed. This condition is the second most common condition that involves multiple congenital contractures of the limbs. Distal arthrogryposis is an autosomal dominant disorder with variable penetrance.

Clinical Manifestations. On physical examination, amyoplasia has a typical appearance, with symmetric joint involvement, usually of all four limbs, and decreased muscle mass. Frequency of joint involvement increases from proximal to distal joints. Therefore severe equinovarus deformity is almost universal, and the wrists are typically flexed. The elbows and knees can be in a flexed or extended position; however, in most cases, both upper and lower extremities are in extension. Dimpling may be notable at the elbows and knees. Shoulders are internally rotated, and hips are frequently dislocated. Normal skin creases overlying the joints are absent, and the skin is tense and glossy.

The faces of an infant with amyoplasia are characterized by mild micrognathia. A midline hemangioma of the eyes, nasal bridge, and forehead may be present and usually fades with time.

Newborn infants affected with amyoplasia are usually active but with decreased limb movement. They feed well, although positioning of the infant during feeding and routine baby care presents a challenge. Distal arthrogryposis primarily involves the hands and feet. On physical examination, the hands of the newborn with distal arthrogryposis have a typical appearance and thus are easily recognized. Hands are clenched, with the thumb flexed into the palm. Fingers cross over the thumb and palm, usually overlapping each other. This hand position resembles that of an infant with trisomy 18.

Collaborative Management. Excluding infants with concurrent CNS dysfunction, infants with multiple congenital contractures have excellent prognoses. The goal of collaborative management is to achieve and maintain an acceptable range of motion in the affected joints. With appropriate management, independent living is attainable for many individuals.

Physical therapy should be initiated early in the neonatal period. Collaboration with physical and occupational therapists should begin in the neonatal intensive care unit. In the past, infants with multiple congenital contractures were casted; however, this therapy was found to produce additional muscle atrophy secondary to the immobilization. Currently, physical therapy is used in conjunction with splinting when necessary.

Physical therapy is a lifetime process, and parents are taught the techniques to use with their children. Parental or family involvement is a key factor in the success of the physical therapy for these infants. Creativity on the part of the health care professional as well as on the part of the parents complements efforts to manipulate the rather rigid infant during feedings, sleeping, holding, and daily care activities. Parents may need referrals to agencies that can provide respite care or assistance from volunteers to carry out these physical therapies on a daily basis. The nurse may collaborate with social workers and financial counselors on behalf of the families for help with services and financing.

Research Findings. Because of the theory that multiple congenital contractures are a direct result of decreased fetal movement, researchers continue to examine ways to stimulate fetal movement for fetuses considered to be at high risk for the development of multiple congenital contractures. High-risk attributes include positive family history of arthrogryposis; maternal complaints of decreased fetal movement; oligohydramnios; and known or family history of muscle, nerve, CNS, or connective tissue abnormalities that might lead to decreased ability to move fetal body parts during development.

If in utero contractures occur because of fetal akinesia, any stimulation of movement during development has the potential for preventing contracted joints. Stimulation could be in the form of intrauterine physical therapy and drugs such as caffeine to stimulate fetal activity.

Prognosis. The long-term prognosis for multiple congenital contractures depends on the extent of involvement. Mortality rates have been reported from 1% to 7% when the primary problem is limb involvement. When the CNS is compromised, the rate rises to almost 50%. Maternal/neonatal characteristics that place the fetus in a high-risk category for contractures included history of decreased fetal movements, hydramnios, contractures, micrognathia, and, on radiologic examination, thin ribs.

DEVELOPMENTAL DYSPLASIA OF THE HIP (DDH)

Developmental dysplasia of the hip (DDH) refers to any manifestation of hip instability, ranging from subluxation to complete dislocation. DDH remains a common problem despite almost universal neonatal screening. Reports indicate success rates as high as 100% for the diagnosis of DDH in the neonatal period, yet these same reports also suggest that neonatal screening programs are ineffective. Although controversy surrounds the usefulness of neonatal screening programs for the diagnosis of DDH, these programs have led to earlier diagnosis and treatment for many infants. Because some infants possess normal hip movement, some examinations may initially be normal, yet later exhibit abnormal hip development. Dysplastic hip screenings should be performed at routine health visits at 2 weeks and at 2, 4, 6, 9, and 12 months of age.

Incidence Rates and Risk Factors
Reports of the incidence of DDH vary. The incidence of DDH in the United States is approximately 10 in 1,000 live births. Differences in DHH incidence rates across ethnic groups can be attributed to genetic, ethnic, and environmental influences. Other influential factors include the age of the infant at the time of examination, the expertise of the examiner, and the definition used by the examiner for the diagnosis of DDH.

Incidence of DDH is increased in first-born children. This increase may be due to the unstretched uterine and abdominal muscles, oligohydramnios, and the high association of fetal breech positioning in primigravidas. A definite preponderance toward DDH occurs in female children. The ratio of occurrence of DDH in girls to boys is 6:1. Females account for 80% of all cases of DDH. Factors that may contribute to this finding include the fact that twice as many females as males present in the breech position, and females appear to have heightened laxity in response to maternal relaxin hormones.

The breech position remains a major contributory factor to the development of DDH. Authors have reported that anywhere from 16% to 25% of affected infants are born in the breech presentation. Specific incidences of DDH in relationship to positioning are 0.7% for cephalic, 2% for footling, and 20% for single breech. The incidence of DDH for infants in the breech presentation is not altered by delivery methods. Breech-positioned infants delivered by cesarean section have the same predisposition to hip dislocation as those delivered vaginally. The left hip is involved three times more often than the right hip. Approximately 60% of DDH is on the left side, 20% on the right side, and 20% bilateral. This finding is attributed to the tendency of the fetus to lie with its left thigh against the maternal sacrum. This position forces the left hip into a posture of flexion and adduction. Thus the femoral head is covered more by the joint capsule than by the acetabulum.

For infants born with other musculoskeletal and congenital renal abnormalities, such as torticollis and Potter's association, the incidence of DDH is increased. Congenital renal abnormalities can result in fetal oliguria, thus subsequently producing oligohydramnios (Chapter 33). Oligohydramnios can cause postural deformities because of the mechanical pressure on the fetus. Torticollis, arthrogryposis, and metatarsus adductus are thought to result from intrauterine compression, as does DDH.

After 40 weeks' gestation, the femoral head in the normal infant is firmly seated in the acetabulum and remains positioned there by the surface tension of the synovial fluid. The hips of a normal infant are difficult to dislocate. Conversely, the infant with a dysplastic hip has a loosely fitting femoral head and acetabulum. Because of this pathophysiologic phenomenon, the femoral head can assume several abnormal positions in an infant with DDH. One such position is termed subluxation. Subluxation occurs when the femoral head can be moved to the edge of the acetabulum but not completely out of it. Another position is termed a dislocatable hip. A dislocatable hip exists when the femoral head can be displaced from the acetabulum by manipulation but returns to the acetabulum afterward. The femoral head can also be found in a completely dislocated position at birth. Dislocated hips may or may not be reduced by manipulation.

DDH is a dynamic disorder that may improve or deteriorate with or without treatment. Thus the joint may spontaneously dislocate and reduce (return to normal position) with normal neonatal movement. At the initial phase of the disorder, seen during the neonatal period, no other significant pathologic concern exists. With time, this simple mechanism progresses in complexity secondary to adaptive changes. DDH can eventually progress either to permanent reduction, complete dislocation, or dysplasia (abnormal development). More than 60% of infants with hip instability stabilize within the first week of life, and 88% stabilize postnatally within the second month. Only 12% of infants with initial hip instability are considered to have DDH with potential for progression.

When complete dislocation occurs, pathologic changes occur to the femoral head, acetabulum, and ilium. This complete dislocation is due to the adaptive changes that occur in the adjacent tissue and bone. The long-term complication of dislocation, when adequate treatment has not occurred, is degenerative changes of both the femoral head and the acetabulum. Once adaptive changes occur, risk for progressive degeneration despite treatment increases. The subluxated hip, when not diagnosed in the neonatal period, is generally diagnosed at adolescence, when the strain of puberty and rapid growth spurts occur. With subluxation, the femoral head is laterally displaced and pushed upward into the joint; it is not completely out of the acetabulum.

As the child grows and increased weight bearing occurs, the femoral head slides around and moves to the joint's edge. Degenerative changes result from this continual sliding. Sclerosis of the underlying bone, loss of cartilage, and formation of degenerative cysts are the most common degenerative changes (Cooperman & Thompson, 2002).

Diagnosis and Clinical Manifestations

In the neonatal period, the Ortolani and Barlow maneuvers are useful in making the diagnosis of DDH. The Ortolani test is used to determine dislocation in the hip of a newborn, and the Barlow test is used to determine whether the hip is dislocatable (Barlow, 1962; Ortolani, 1976). In practice, both procedures are done in sequence. For examination, the infant is placed on a firm surface in the supine position.

The infant should be relaxed and quiet. Only one hip should be examined at a time. To perform the Ortolani test, the clinician stabilizes the infant's pelvis with one hand and with the other hand grasps the infant's thigh on the side to be tested. The examiner's middle finger is located over the greater trochanter (lateral aspect of the upper thigh), and the thumb is across the knee. The hip is flexed to 90 degrees while bending the infant's knee. The infant's leg is then gently abducted with an anterior lift. In a positive Ortolani test, a "clunk" is heard with abduction. This clunk occurs as the dislocated femoral head slides over the posterior rim of the acetabulum and into the hip socket. Next, the hip is adducted, and, for the infant with DDH, a second clunk can be heard as the femoral head is displaced out of the acetabulum.

False-positive diagnoses of DDH have occurred when the examiner misinterprets a normal "click" (high-pitched sound) for a clunk. A click is not a sign of DDH. Clicks may be heard as a result of snapping of ligaments or tendons, and the majority are normal.

Barlow's test determines instability of the hip and identifies those hips that can be dislocated upon manipulation. Both hips and knees are flexed, with the hip to be tested in slight adduction. The examiner's middle finger remains positioned as for the Ortolani test, over the greater trochanter. However, the thumb is located over the medial aspect of the infant's lower thigh. Gentle pressure is exerted by the thumb posteriorly and laterally (down and out). For the infant with DDH, the femoral head can be felt to move out of the acetabulum with the typical clunk. The hip can then be reduced by the Ortolani maneuver or simply by releasing thumb pressure and abducting and flexing the hips.

When the femoral head is subluxated, the examiner may observe a sliding motion in the hip joint during physical examination. This sliding motion can be characteristic of an unstable hip joint. Most cases of unstable hips spontaneously resolve without treatment. Because no way to determine which hips will reduce and stabilize without treatment exists, treating all unstable hips is the best approach. The use of sonography is valuable for DDH detection, but, because of the cartilaginous composition of the neonatal pelvis, radiographic examination is not.

The American Academy of Pediatrics (AAP) committee on quality improvement has issued guidelines to assist in the diagnosis and management of the infant with DDH. All newborn should receive a screening exam. The Barlow and Ortolani maneuvers are not useful after 8 to 12 weeks of age. Ultrasonography is not recommended as a screening tool. If the physical exam of the neonate is equivocal, a repeat exam should be performed at 2 weeks of age. Certain physical signs that would result in an equivocal hip exam for DDH would include a persistent soft click and mild asymmetry of the gluteal folds. If the Ortolani/Barlow exam is positive with a hip clunk at 2 weeks of age, a referral to an orthopedic specialist is required. This is not an emergency but should be completed in a timely matter over the next few weeks. The infant presenting at 2 weeks with a persistent soft click should receive ultrasonography of the hip within the next 3 to 4 weeks or referral to an orthopedic specialist at this time. For the infant who exhibits a normal hip exam with resolution of the soft hip click, routine screening with well baby checks during the first year of life is the recommendation. It is important to note that, according to the AAP recommendations, a newborn who is discharged before 48 hours of age should receive repeat hip exam at 2 to 4 days after discharge.

If the family has a history of DDH, the incidence increased 9.4/1,000 in males and 44/1,000 in females. Because of this increased risk, even with a negative hip exam, an ultrasound at 6 weeks should be considered, or an x-ray of the hips at 4 months can be an alternative (Morey, 2001).

Collaborative Management. The goal of collaborative management is to achieve and maintain reduction of the unstable hip. The sooner treatment is implemented, the greater the chance for successful outcome. Various splinting devices are used to treat DDH in infants. Examples of splints include the Pavlik harness, von Rosen splint, Denis Browne hip adduction splint, and Frejka pillow splint. The most commonly used splint for neonates is the Pavlik harness.

The Pavlik harness allows for spontaneous hip and lower extremity movement while maintaining reduction of the hip joint. It can be worn comfortably during all aspects of normal newborn care, including diaper changes. The Pavlik harness can be adjusted for growth. It is indicated for use in newborns and infants up to 6 months of age. Use of the Pavlik harness is contraindicated for infants able to stand and for those infants in whom the hip joint is not reducible by manipulation, specifically the Ortolani procedure, because the infant may attempt to bear weight while wearing the harness, thus potentially pushing the hip out of alignment. This movement counteracts reduction of the hip joint. The greatest danger is that the child will become entangled in the parachute-like straps while attempting to push up to a standing position. Children could hang themselves in the straps. A major factor influencing the success of the Pavlik harness is parental compliance with the treatment. With this condition extensive parental education is imperative.

Parent and Family Education and Support. In addition to providing information regarding the pathology and treatment goals of DDH, the nurse should provide the parents with an opportunity to remove and reapply the harness while under supervision. Parental support groups can help parents adjust to the infant's temporary awkward condition. Parents should also be educated in the procedure used to reduce the dislocated hip because complete reduction must be achieved before the harness is applied.

Long-Term Consequences and Complications. As with most therapeutic treatments, the potential for iatrogenic complications exists. Complications observed following DDH treatment include avascular necrosis, redislocation, and acetabular dysplasia. Complications can result from either inadequate or overly aggressive treatment.

An additional complication that has been reported with the use of the Pavlik harness is the development of brachial plexus palsy (Mostert et al, 2000). The tension of the shoulder harness appears related to this complication. The harness may be applied too tightly or may not be modified with the infant's growth, thus causing downward pressure on the brachial plexus nerves and subsequent neuropathy.

Such alternatives include closed reduction with traction or open reduction with casting. A hip spica cast is most often used with these infants. Care then includes observance for poor pedal pulses, decreased peripheral circulation, pain, skin excoriation or abrasions, and possible development of respiratory infections resulting from decreased mobility. Parents should learn cast care, because the child is discharged with the cast in place.

CLUBFOOT

The classic clubfoot, talipes equinovarus, refers to a dysmorphic-appearing foot with hindfoot equinus, forefoot adduction, and midfoot supination. The term clubfoot may also be used to describe milder talipes conditions, including talipes calcaneus and talipes varus.

Foot deformities are among the most common birth defects. Clubfoot has an incidence of 1 in 1,000 live births. Males are affected nearly twice as often as females, and, in infants with unilateral presentation, the majority appear on the right.

Mechanism of Development

The precise mechanism of development of clubfoot has not been irrefutably established. Some researchers allude to the theory of intrauterine malposition, whereas others, noting a higher incidence of clubfoot in families with a positive history of the disorder, ascribe it to a genetic cause.

Gaining popularity is the theory that clubfoot is a multifactorial disorder involving a genetic predisposition coupled with environmental forces such as oligohydramnios, primiparity, macrosomia, and multiple fetuses.

Clinical Manifestations. Clubfoot deformities are apparent at birth. The skin overlying the lateral aspect of the foot may be taut, whereas the medial aspect may have increased skin folds. The affected foot may be smaller in size than a normal foot. In older children, the calf muscle may be noticeably decreased in size. Milder talipes conditions may be returned to the neutral position by manipulation.

Collaborative Management. Early diagnosis and treatment of clubfoot are essential. In the early newborn period, joints, muscles, and ligaments may be more compliant to corrective manipulation without surgical intervention. This may involve serial casting as frequently as 2- to 4-day intervals. As many as 50% of clubfoot deformities may require surgery. Difficulty with skin closure has been reported as a complication following correction of severe clubfoot. This is especially true if the affected foot has received prior surgery. Special shoe splints or braces may be used toward the end of any successful treatment.

Parental education includes implementation of routine newborn care for an infant wearing either splints or bilateral casts. Problems and solutions associated with clothing, sleeping, feeding, and bathing should be addressed. Compliance by parents in using splints may vary. Because consistent treatment is necessary for a favorable outcome, health care professionals must explore parental feelings and actions while providing anticipatory guidance.

SYNDACTYLY

Fusion, or webbing, between two digits is referred to as syndactyly. This condition is the most common anomaly of the hand, with an incidence of 1 in 2,250 live births. Males are affected slightly more than females. Half of the time, both hands are involved in a symmetric presentation. Syndactyly of the fingers may be accompanied by syndactyly of the toes.

Mechanism of Development

Although most occurrences of syndactyly appear to be through spontaneous mutation, familial predisposition has been reported, thus indicating an autosomal dominant pattern. Syndactyly may also be associated with a specific syndrome such as Apert's syndrome.

There are four classifications of syndactyly. Complete syndactyly occurs when the fusion is from the base to the tip of the digit. Fusion that does not extend to the tip of the digit is termed incomplete. Simple syndactyly refers to digits connected by skin and soft tissue. Fused digits involving an osseous connection is considered complex. Abnormal nerve and vessel configurations may accompany complex syndactyly.

Treatment.   The type and timing of treatment of syndactyly depends on its classification. Surgery is directed toward promoting normal function and appearance. Fingers of unequal length should be separated within 6 to 12 months of age to prevent curvature of the longer finger from deviating toward the shorter finger. If more than two adjacent digits are involved, surgery should be performed in stages to prevent vascular compromise of the middle digits.

Prognosis.   Prognosis is favorable for normal function and appearance, except in cases of complex syndactyly involving not only bone but also vascular and nervous tissue. These cases may be associated with some postoperative loss of function.

Collaborative Management.   Parents of infants with syndactyly are instructed in physical therapy, specifically in massage of the interconnecting skin. Massage the webbed area to be stretched, which allows for easier repair, is indicated.

POLYDACTYLY

Polydactyly is any duplication of digits beyond the normal five. It is the second most common hand anomaly. Polydactyly is believed to be caused by duplication of a single embryonic bud. African Americans are affected 10 times more often than Caucasians. African Americans more often have postaxial polydactyly (duplication of the little finger), whereas preaxial polydactyly (duplication of the thumb) occurs primarily in Caucasians. In African Americans, postaxial polydactyly is typically an isolated incidence, whereas in Caucasians it is associated with syndromes and chromosomal anomalies. Central axial polydactyly is the duplication of the ring, long, or index finger. Central axial polydactyly is often associated with complex syndactyly. Polydactyly may be further classified into three types. Type I is merely a rudimentary soft tissue mass connected by a pedicle. Treatment of this type involves simple excision, which is often done in the newborn nursery before discharge. Type II is a partial duplication with involvement of the phalanges.

Type III, a rare occurrence, involves complete duplication of the metacarpal and phalanges.

Collaborative Management

Treatment of polydactyly types II and III, centers around functional capacity first and appearance second. The infant is observed for which duplication is dominant and most functional, and efforts are made to remove the least functional counterpart. If both duplicated digits appear to be equally functional, surgery should then be used to promote aesthetic appearance. Reparative surgery should be completed by 3 years of age.

AMNIOTIC BAND SYNDROME

Amniotic band syndrome, with an incidence ranging from 1 in 1,250 to 1 in 15,000 live births, is characterized by uncommon, asymmetric fetal deformities. Deformities that have been attributed to the amniotic band syndrome include congenital limb amputation, syndactyly, constriction bands, clubfoot, craniofacial defects such as cleft lip and palate, and visceral defects such as gastroschisis and omphalocele (Baraitser & Winter, 1996).

Mechanism of Development

Etiologic factors in the amniotic band syndrome are unclear. Part of the difficulty is that some of the same deformities that occur with this syndrome can also occur for other reasons. Thus the exact cause of the deformities is not always identified. This area needs further research.

Diagnosis.   Many clinicians believe that amniotic bands must be present for the diagnosis of amniotic band syndrome to be made. However, others believe that the presence of fetal deformities in a nonanatomic pattern, without obvious bands, is sufficient to establish the diagnosis of the syndrome. Congenital deformations, such as the visceral and craniofacial types, in the absence of amniotic bands may go undiagnosed as amniotic band syndrome because they could represent a faulty midline developmental pattern during the first trimester of pregnancy instead of the production of amniotic bands that constricted or restricted growth. Therefore the true incidence of this syndrome may be much higher than it generally appears—not only because of the difficulty establishing a diagnosis but also because of the high mortality rate that exists during gestation.

Amniotic band syndrome has been implicated in fetal deaths secondary to cord compression by the constricting bands. Strauss and colleagues provide a clinical report of fetal demise involving a normal karyotype male secondary to torsion and strangulation of the umbilical cord by an amniotic band. The only significant history in the gestation was an early second trimester amniocentesis. It has been speculated that amniotic rupture may follow amniocentesis and fetal blood sampling. Strangulation furrows, limb reduction defects, and cleft lip or palate can be late sequelae of invasive prenatal procedures in animal models.

Pathophysiology.   Two theories—endogenous and exogenous—explain the cause of amniotic band syndrome. The endogenous theory postulates that the deformities are caused by an innate derangement of the primary embryonic cell layers from which the tissues and organs develop. The presence of amniotic bands, according to the endogenous theory, is a late development with no clinical significance.

The exogenous—and seemingly more popular—theory contends that early amniotic rupture allows the fetus to move into close approximation to the chorion by entering the chorionic cavity. The ruptured amnion then forms fibrous strings or bands. These bands can adhere to the skin, thus altering normal morphogenesis (e.g., cleft lip or palate, omphalocele) or disrupt the vascular integrity, resulting in gastroschisis. Amniotic bands have been found encircling normally developed structures, thus resulting in congenital amputations, constriction rings with lymphedema distal to the ring, and facial clefts in nonanatomic distribution. Postural deformities such as clubfoot are believed to be caused by the fetus' close approximation to the chorion (Chapter 11.)

Collaborative Management. Notwithstanding the inherent problems associated with omphaloceles, gastroschisis, encephaloceles, clubfoot, syndactyly, and facial clefts, the clinician must be attuned to the unique complications of constricting bands. Constricting bands are usually associated with edema distal to the band. The resulting edema and vascular compromise contribute to complications such as skin breakdown, necrosis, thromboemboli formation that results from venostasis, and infection. Care should include frequent vascular checks to assess perfusion. Trauma and tissue breakdown are discouraged through positioning and skin care. Observation for localized areas of necrosis is stressed.

As with other aesthetically disappointing musculoskeletal disorders, the family requires emotional and psychological support as adjustment to and acceptance of the infant are allowed to occur. Parents may be fearful that an extremity will be lost because of necrotic tissue formation or infection. These fears may be justified, and the parents should be prepared for such a possibility. Complete surgical repair may not be possible during the infant's initial hospitalization, thus necessitating frequent hospitalizations during the early developing years. The delay in repair may necessitate that parents be taught to observe for vascular perfusion of an extremity, to recognize signs of infection, and to change dressings over open or healing areas. Preparation for discharge requires a multidisciplinary approach. The family may need surgical supplies, follow-up visitations by a home-visiting nurse, orthopedic or surgical consultations, pediatrician visits for general well-child care, and support of social or financial services to meet the long-term responsibilities of caring for their infants.

In addition, the nurse, working with the perinatal social worker, must attempt to provide opportunities for parent-infant bonding if the parents are to feel somewhat prepared for discharge. While the infant is still in the hospital, the parents must be encouraged to touch and talk to the infant and to participate in the infant's care. They must also be encouraged to verbalize their own feelings about their infant's condition. Every attempt should be made to attend to their fears, concerns, or misconceptions about the cause of their infant's problem. Only then will positive transition to home be possible.

BIRTH TRAUMA

Birth trauma encompasses both mechanical and asphyxial events occurring during delivery. This trauma may be due to pressure and distortion. Trauma can occur despite exemplary obstetrical care. Birth trauma occurs in approximately 2 to 7 in 1,000 live births. A positive association exists between birth trauma and macrosomia, prematurity, breech presentation, dystocia, and cephalopelvic disproportion.

Clinical Manifestations

Birth trauma includes abrasions, ecchymoses, erythema, cephalhematomas, caput succedaneum, fractures (especially of the clavicle), brachial plexus damage, and nerve palsies. Clavicular fractures are the most common fractures diagnosed as birth trauma. Clavicles are at an increased risk for fractures during shoulder dystocias in a vertex presentation or with arms extended during a breech delivery (Cooperman & Thompson, 2002).

Physical examination findings related to birth trauma may appear only as bruising, abrasions, and petechiae that overlie the affected part. Further diagnostic methods should be used when the infant exhibits pain on movement, limited motion, and abnormal passive positioning of an extremity or head movement.

Skull fractures may present as cephalhematomas. Skull fractures are most often linear and typically involve the parietal bones. Symptomatic evidence of a nondepressed skull fracture may resemble signs of increased intracranial pressure secondary to epidural hemorrhage. Clinical presentation may include changes in tone, hypertonicity or hypotonicity, arching of the back with the head in hyperextension, and respiratory compromise. Usually, no treatment is indicated for asymptomatic skull fractures. Depressed skull fractures, however, may require elevation of the depressed area.

Vertebral fractures are incurred in difficult breech deliveries in which longitudinal traction in combination with a twisting motion may occur. These features commonly involve the seventh cervical and first thoracic vertebrae. Treatment depends on the extent of resultant nerve damage but often requires traction.

The most common nerve injury attributed to birth trauma is brachial plexus damage and resulting nerve palsy. This injury involves damage to the network of nerve fibers in the neck and shoulders referred to as the brachial plexus. Involvement may occur in the upper portion (Erb-Duchenne palsy), lower portion (Klumpke's paralysis), or both portions (complete brachial plexus palsy).

Erb-Duchenne paralysis is the most common form. The affected arm is limp and in a position of elbow extension and internal rotation. The Moro reflex is diminished and the grasp reflex intact. Klumpke's paralysis involves paralysis of the hand and wrist. Complete brachial plexus paralysis results in paralysis of the entire arm.

Diagnosis

Diagnosis of birth trauma is based on physical assessment findings. These are usually fairly visible at birth or in the immediate postnatal period. Physical findings should be confirmed, when necessary, by radiologic evaluation to establish whether a fracture is present. For large cephalhematomas, evaluation of the skull by x-ray is prudent.

Collaborative Management. Treatment of birth trauma depends on the type and severity of the trauma. Often, supportive measures may be the only intervention required. For instance, brachial plexus injuries require immobilization in a neutral position using braces or splints. Passive range-of-motion exercises should be instituted at 7 to 10 days.

Clavicular fractures also respond to supportive management. Typically, the arm is held flexed, and the elbow is held against the chest. This position limits movement, thereby decreasing pain and possible trauma to the site. Callus formation stabilizes the fracture by 10 days of age. A hard, palpable knot can often be felt with this callus formation.

Parent Education and Support.   Diagnosing a disorder resulting from birth trauma can evoke anxiety in a parent. Birth trauma may connote thoughts of violence. The manner in which such information is taken from and conveyed to the family is important. Nonjudgmental, supportive care by health professionals along with consistent primary care by one individual may diminish some anxiety and allow the parents to establish trust. The mother may especially feel that she is to blame for the neonatal problem. Calm reassurance about the nature of the trauma is important. It also helps to allay fears that something was done incorrectly during the delivery process if parents understand that many of these injuries cannot be avoided or anticipated. Parental education is prerequisite if the parents are to understand the need for continued, long-term treatment, which many of these infants require. Many birth trauma injuries require long-term follow-up care by orthopedists, neurologists, or physical and occupational specialists (Chapter 31).

CONGENITAL MUSCULAR TORTICOLLIS

Congenital muscular torticollis, with an incidence of 0.4% of all live births, is another musculoskeletal deformity with unknown pathogenesis. It is known to be primarily a disorder of the sternocleidomastoid muscle.

Pathophysiology
Several theories exist as to the cause of congenital torticollis, including genetics, abnormal uterine positioning, neurogenic disorders, and ischemic injury to the sternocleidomastoid muscle. Whatever the cause, this pathologic disorder consists of a fibrous contraction of the sternocleidomastoid muscle. Typically, the ipsilateral trapezius muscle is atrophic.

Diagnosis
Congenital torticollis can present within the neonatal period. Presentation may include a 1- to 3-cm hard palpable mass in the neck on the affected side accompanied by an abnormal positioning of the head. Infants with congenital torticollis tilt the head to the affected side, and the chin is pointed upward in the opposite direction. Facial asymmetry may be a later sign. The face and skull on the affected side appear smaller.

In children with untreated congenital torticollis or in cases with torticollis unresponsive to therapy, the shoulder on the affected side is raised to compensate for the abnormal head positioning. This form of compensation may lead to cervical and lumbar scoliosis as well as chronic back pain.

Collaborative Management.   Traditionally, physical therapy for congenital torticollis is instituted immediately. Because congenital torticollis may resolve naturally within the first year of life, surgery is typically delayed until after 1 year of age. Persistent congenital torticollis past 1 year of age should be surgically treated to prevent the compensatory complications described.

Physical therapists and orthopedic surgeons should be consulted to assist in the management and subsequent follow-up of these infants. Family members should be taught home physical therapy, which should be performed at least twice daily. Parents should be counseled regarding the possibility of a neck brace to be postoperatively worn by the infant. It is usually the nurse's responsibility to coordinate consultations and to prepare the family with discharge instructions. In addition, the nurse must determine whether the family lives in an area accessible to follow-up care. If not, a referral to social services or financial counseling may be needed so the family can participate in follow-up.

CRANIOSYNOSTOSIS

The bones that constitute the skull are joined with fibrous joints. As previously mentioned, these joints are lined with a thin layer of fibrous tissue. Separation of these joints allows for remodeling of the skull at the time of delivery and for rapid growth of the head during the early developmental years. The skull consists of five main sutures. The coronal, lambdoidal, and squamosal are each paired with an opposing suture. The sagittal and metopic sutures are present in solo along the calvaria (skull). The signal for normal closure of these sutures is not very clear but is believed secondary to multiple factors—including vascular, hormonal, genetic, mechanical, and local factors. Complete sutural fusion is anticipated in the second or third decade of life.

Premature closure of any suture in the skull results in a clinical condition called craniostenosis, also commonly referred to as craniosynostosis. The early closure of a cranial suture typically starts at one point and progresses along the suture line. Premature closure may occur prenatally or postnatally. Simple craniosynostosis defines the premature fusion of one suture; complex craniosynostosis indicates that two or more sutures are fused. Primary craniosynostosis is the most common type of premature suture fusion. It is not associated with a known disorder. Secondary craniosynostosis is associated with an underlying disorder, such as hyperthyroidism, thalassemia, Apert syndrome, Crouzon syndrome and Cole-Carpenter syndrome.

Clinical characteristics depend on which suture is affected. The closure of one suture does not allow growth in that area but generally increases growth in the other areas of the skull. When the sagittal suture is involved, the head presents as dolichocephalic, with increased length from front to back and a long and narrow skull on exam. A bossing of the skull also occurs, both in the frontal and occipital regions. The coronal suture is the second most common for premature closure, behind the incidence rates of the sagittal suture. The clinical appearance involves a skull that is wide from side to side and short from front to back, also termed brachydactyly. Bilateral lambdoidal craniosynostosis could be identified with a flattened occipital region, whereas unilateral lambdoidal craniosynostosis has a flattened area on one side of the back of the head and is asymmetric when compared to the other. Long term supine positioning of the infant can produce this same appearance. Positional asymmetric skull appearance, not related to abnormal suture closure, is generally seen in those infants with a neuromusculoskeletal defect that will not allow the child to move its head from side to side spontaneously. Congenital torticollis can result in an asymmetrical flat occipital region as the infant tilts the head toward the contracted and fibrous sternocleidomastoid muscle.

Isolated metopic craniosynostosis will produce a deformity with a narrow, protruding forehead. Facial development of the skull is also affected, and orbital hypotelorism is also associated with this defect.

Diagnosis is usually confirmed with CT scan of the skull. Suspicion of the defect occurs with persistent and/or progressive abnormal skull growth—often with the head circumference intact for age.

Developmental anomalies may include mental dysfunction secondary to intracranial pressure, abnormal brain growth, or a primary CNS abnormality. The incidence of mental dysfunction is increased beyond simple craniosynostosis when more than one suture is involved.

Surgical therapy is required for treatment of this disorder. The complexity of the procedure increases with the number of sutures involved and the cranial remodeling at the time of surgery. Often serial craniotomies are required for full correction. The fused suture is removed, and to prevent repeat early closure and reduce osteoblastic activity, a material is used to line the sutures. Often a helmet is required for the child to wear for a period of time to improve cranial remodeling.

TAR SYNDROME: THROMBOCYTOPENIA ABSENT RADIUS

Thrombocytopenia absent radius syndrome is classified by the bilateral absence of radii and hypomegakaryocytic thrombocytopenia, less than 150,000 mm^3. This anomaly is associated with some degree of ulnar hypoplasia 100% of the time. The ulna may be either hypoplastic or absent.

In addition to the forearm anomalies, multiple other defects may be present—including congenital heart disease (33%) and mental deficiency (7%). Cognitive delay is usually associated with intracranial hemorrhage during the first year of life.

Prenatal diagnosis has been documented with ultrasound and cordocentesis. Management for the type of delivery can be a concern for the obstetrician secondary to the increased risk of bleeding in this population. One author describes the vaginal delivery of a fetus diagnosed with TAR syndrome without clinical complications. It might be assumed that the level of platelets in the fetus at the time of delivery could be prognostic for a safe vaginal delivery; however, further research is required.

Complications of this syndrome, assuming no other anomalies other than thrombocytopenia and absent radii, can be segregated by age. In the neonatal period and during the first year of life, the incidence of life-threatening hemorrhage is at its highest. Dramatic decline in platelet count and function is associated with viral illnesses. Infants who develop viral infections, especially gastrointestinal, have an increased risk of hemorrhagic death. The incidence has been reported at 40% (Jones, 1997).

Hematologic complications improve with age—thus the reduced mortality and morbidity associated with this disorder after the first year of life. The complication encountered as the child matures is the gross motor developmental delay experienced by the abnormal hands/arms. Most children who are affected with this disorder require some type of adaptive device but rarely perform well with extremity prostheses, as they learn to compensate with their existing limbs (McLaurin, 1999).

Platelet transfusions are required with hemorrhagic events. Reports of isolated therapies with improvement in platelet count and function have been reported, but large population studies are required for significance.

SUMMARY

Although the majority of musculoskeletal defects in the newborn are nonlethal and often not functional problems, they may become the focus of the parents' attention. This can be attributed to the perception that the infant does not meet their preconceived idea of the "perfect child." An understanding of the development of the musculoskeletal system and pathology for various defects can assist the clinician in teaching and supporting the family and infant. In addition, recognizing the subtle abnormalities can prompt the clinician to evaluate for additional, often subtle, associated defects that could have serious genetic implications.

When a clinician recounts a case involving a musculoskeletal defect, it is often one of the more rare, yet clinically impressive, defects such as thanatophoric dwarfism and osteogenesis imperfecta. This chapter helps to identify the epidemiological and clinical aspects of the rare and the common defects in an effort to improve the understanding of the defect as well as to provide guidelines for management based on the pathology, complications, and prognosis of the defect.

REFERENCES

Baraitser M, Winter RM (1996). *Color atlas of congenital malformation syndromes*. St Louis: Mosby.

Barlow TG (1962). Early diagnosis and treatment of congenital dislocation of the hip. *Journal of bone and joint surgery*, 44B, 292-301.

Cooperman DR, Thompson GH (2002). Neonatal orthopedics. In Fanaroff AA, Martin RJ (Eds.), *Neonatal-perinatal medicine: diseases of the fetus and infant*, ed 7, St Louis: Mosby.

Cubert RR et al (2001). Osteogenesis imperfecta: mode of delivery. *Obstetrics & gynecology*, 97, 66-69.

Engelbert RH et al (2000). Osteogenesis imperfecta in childhood: prognosis for walking. *Journal of pediatrics*, 137, 397-402.

Glorieux FH et al (2000). Type V Osteogenesis imperfecta: a new form of brittle bone disease. *Journal of bone and mineral research*, 15(9), 1650-1658.

Hall IG (1981). An approach to congenital contractures (arthrogryposis) [review]. *Pediatric annals*, 10(7), 15-26.

Jones KL (1997). *Smith's recognizable patterns of human malformation*, ed 5, Philadelphia: WB Saunders.

Lashley FC (1998). *Clinigenetics in nursing practice*, ed 2, New York: Springer Publishing Company.

McLaurin TM et al (1999). Management of thrombocytopenia-absent radius (TAR) syndrome. *Journal of pediatric orthopedics*, 19, 289-296.

Morey SS (2001). The American Academy of Pediatrics: AAP develops guidelines for early detection of dislocated hips. *American family physician*, 63, 565-566.

Mostert AK et al (2000). Results of Pavlik harness treatment for neonatal hip dislocation to Graf's sonographic classification. *Journal of pediatric orthopedics*, 20, 306-310.

Ortolani M (1976). Congenital hip dysplasia in the light of early and very early diagnosis. *Clinical orthopedics and related research*, 119, 6-10.

Sillence D, Danks D (1978). The differentiation of genetically distinct varieties of osteogenesis imperfecta in the newborn period. *Clinical research*, 26, 178A.

Sisk EA et al (1999). Obstructive sleep apnea in children with achondroplasia: surgical and anesthetic considerations. *Otolaryngology-head and neck surgery*, 120, 248-254.

Spitz JL (1996). *Genodermatosis: a full-color clinical guide to genetic skin disorders*, Baltimore, Williams & Wilkins.

CHAPTER 33

ASSESSMENT AND MANAGEMENT OF THE GENITOURINARY SYSTEM

KAREN SWEETWYNE THOMAS

INTRODUCTION

Comprehensive nursing care of infants with renal or genital disorders requires thorough understanding of normal anatomy and physiology of the complete system. Because the development of the renal and genital systems arises from shared structures, aberrations in one can affect the development of the other. Genital conditions that present in the neonatal period are seldom life-threatening. However, many times parents have difficulty with their own sexuality, and having a child with a genital abnormality may be very upsetting. In addition to providing physical are to the infant, many times the neonatal nurse is the first person to identify parental concerns.

Unlike genital abnormalities, renal disease can cause life-threatening events in the neonatal period. The kidneys function to maintain fluid and electrolyte balance and acid-base balance as well as to rid the body of nitrogenous waste. In utero, the placenta functions as the excretory organ. Many times serious and sometimes fatal pathology may not be evident until the time of birth. In some instances, intact kidneys are damaged due to perinatal events. Trauma surrounding births, medical management for common neonatal conditions, and fluid overhydration or underhydration are only a few of many factors that place the newborn at risk for renal compromise. Timely, accurate nursing assessment and intervention is of utmost priority to ensure optimal outcome for the infant and their families.

This chapter outlines embryonic development and anatomy and physiology of the genitourinary system. It also describes various abnormalities and disease processes commonly identified in the neonatal period—including risk factors, medical and nursing management, and prognosis.

EMBRYOLOGIC DEVELOPMENT OF THE UROGENITAL SYSTEM

During the first weeks of gestation, the mesoderm is divided into three segments: the lateral, intermediate, and paraxial. The intermediate mesoderm separates from the paraxial mesoderm and migrates ventrally as the nephrogenic cords located on either side of the primitive aorta. Cells on the dorsal end of the nephrogenic cords join to form the urogenital ridges from which components of both the urinary and genital structures are developed.

THE URINARY SYSTEM

The urinary system consists of the kidneys, ureters, urinary bladder and the urethra (Figure 33-1). Development of the primary excretory organ begins around the fourth week of gestation with the production of fetal urine by week 10. At approximately 36 weeks, renal anatomic development is completed. Functional maturity increases after birth and continues until approximately 2 years of age.

Development of the kidneys occurs with the progressive formation of three nephric structures within the nephrogenic cord: the pronephros, the mesonephros, and the metanephros. The pronephros or primitive kidney develops during the first month of gestation, then gradually degenerates, thus contributing the duct system for the next developmental stage. The pronephros has no excretory function.

The second excretory organ to develop is the mesonephros. The mesonephric development begins at the caudal end of the pronephros during the fourth to sixth week of gestation. The mesonephros contains thin-walled glomeruli and tubules that are functional. Ultra urine is produced by these mesonephric nephrons at 8 to 10 weeks. Mesonephric nephrons that are located more cranially along the nephrogenic cord begin to degenerate as those located more caudally are still developing. During this time—approximately the 4th week—the gonadal blastema begins to form in the genital ridge located on the medial aspect of each mesonephros, thus creating a urogenital ridge between the developing kidney and the genitals. As the mesonephric structure begins to degenerate in a caudal direction, it leaves a duct system for the following stage. In addition, the mesonephric duct eventually matures into the epididymis, vas deferens, and ejaculatory duct in the male or the vestigial Garner in the female. Thus failure of the mesonephric duct to develop may result in anomalies in both the urinary and genital systems (Maizels, 1998).

The third and final stage of kidney development, which begins in the fifth week of gestation, is the formation of the metanephros or definitive kidney. The metanephros develops from the induction of the metanephrogenic blastema (metanephric mesoderm) by the ureteric bud. The ureteric bud, also called the metanephric diverticulum, is an outgrowth of the mesonephric duct, and the metanephrogenic blastema originates from the lower segment of the nephrogenic cord

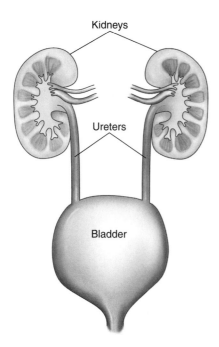

FIGURE **33-1**
The renal system.

(Figure 33-2). As this stage progresses, the stalk of ureteric bud becomes the ureter. Continued elongating and branching of the cranial end of the ureteric bud results in the development of the renal pelvis, major and minor calices, and finally the collecting tubules. At the ends of the collecting tubules, the cells of the metanephric blastema clump and stimulate the formation of the glomerulus, proximal tubule, loop of Henle, and distal tubule, which eventually empties into the collecting duct. Thus a nephron is formed.

To complete the formation of the urinary system, a bladder and urethra are produced. The epithelium of the bladder and most of the urethra derive from the embryologic hindgut. The expanded terminal end of the hindgut is the cloaca. The allantois, an outgrowth of the yolk sac, is attached to the ventral side of the cloaca. The urorectal septum creates a compartmentalized cloaca that consists of the anorectal canal and the urogenital sinus. With the exception of the bladder trigone—the area between the urethra and ureters—the bladder arises from this urogenital sinus. The primitive structures regress, fibrose, or become a part of the newly formed structures. The point of origin of ureteric bud marks the point of insertion for the ureters. The ureters, formerly the metanephric ducts, then open bilaterally into the urinary bladder as the developing bladder reabsorbs the distal portions of the mesonephric ducts into its dorsal wall (trigone).

The allantois narrows into a fibrous band called the urachus that runs from the apex of the bladder to the umbilicus. Abnormalities of the urachus occur when it either remains patent or forms an urachal sinus. A patent urachus may occur in association with another anomalous condition and may allow development of a functional kidney by alleviating the effects of urinary obstruction. An urachal sinus is usually an isolated anomaly and causes a leakage of urine from the umbilical stump (Brion et al, 1997).

Urethral development in the male and female begins in the same manner. The urogenital sinus is visible at 6 weeks and

consists of a narrow portion near the bladder, the pelvic urethra, and an expanded portion near the urogenital membrane (cloacal membrane), called the phallic urethra. Through several processes and stages, the phallic end of the urogenital sinus eventually becomes the bulbar and the penile urethra, and the pelvic urethra develops into the permanent urethra and vagina. Differentiation of the urethra in the male and female fetus can be detected by 12 to 14 weeks' gestation (Maizels, 1998).

Initially, the kidneys are located within the pelvic region. They make a gradual ascent into to their final location in the flank position or lumbothoracic area. Normal renal ascent is achieved as the result of caudal growth of the fetal spine, lengthening of the ureter, molding of the renal parenchyma, and fixation of the kidney to the retroperitoneum (Maizels, 1998). Failure of normal ascent of the kidneys results in abnormalities such as horseshoe kidneys or pelvic kidneys. Blood supply to the ascending kidneys changes from lower arteries that gradually regress to arteries that arise from the aorta.

In utero, the placenta functions as the excretory organ for the fetus. Functional kidneys are therefore not necessary for fetal homeostasis. Consequently, pathological problems such as aplastic, hypoplastic, and otherwise nonfunctioning kidneys may not be detected until the neonatal period. Fetal urination, swallowing, and breathing impact amniotic fluid volume. Excretion of fetal urine contributes significantly to amniotic fluid volume, especially during the third trimester. A reduction in fetal urine excretion results in oligohydramnios. Failure of the fetus to swallow amniotic fluid because of gastrointestinal obstruction or central nervous system anomaly results in overaccumulation of amniotic fluid or polyhydramnios. Abnormalities in amniotic fluid volume can therefore signal pathology in various fetal organ systems.

A balance between genetic influences, cellular mediators, and the interaction of various molecular mechanisms is necessary for the initiation and development of the kidney. Depending on the timing of development, insult or failure of the primitive structures to grow or to branch appropriately may result in a variety of uropathies—including dysplasia and renal agenesis (Gomez & Norwood, 1999; Maizels, 1998).

PHYSIOLOGY OF KIDNEY FUNCTION

The structure of the kidney includes the cortex, the major and minor calices, and the renal pelvis (Figure 33-3). The kidneys function to regulate fluid and electrolyte balance, arterial blood pressure, and toxin levels in the body. These regulatory mechanisms are all intimately tied to the formation of urine. Three basic processes are involved in the formation of urine: ultrafiltration of plasma by the glomerulus, reabsorption of water and solutes from the ultrafiltrate, and secretion of certain solutes into the tubular fluid (Koeppen & Stanton, 1997). Urine formation begins with renal blood flow.

The nephron, which is the site of urine formation, is the functional unit of the kidney. It consists of a glomerulus (Bowman's capsule and glomerular capillaries), proximal tubule, loop of Henle, and distal tubule (Figure 33-4). The process of nephron formation—nephrogenesis—begins during the second month of gestation and is anatomically complete by approximately the 35 weeks' gestation. Renal development will progress at the same rate regardless of gestation at birth. At the completion of nephrogenesis, each kidney contains approximately 1 million nephrons.

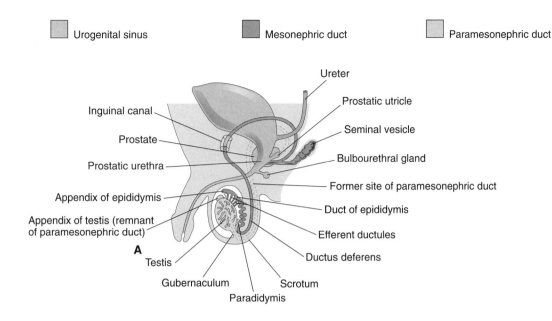

Urogenital sinus   Mesonephric duct   Paramesonephric duct

A

Ureter
Prostatic utricle
Seminal vesicle
Bulbourethral gland
Former site of paramesonephric duct
Duct of epididymis
Efferent ductules
Ductus deferens

Inguinal canal
Prostate
Prostatic urethra
Appendix of epididymis
Appendix of testis (remnant of paramesonephric duct)
Testis
Gubernaculum
Paradidymis
Scrotum

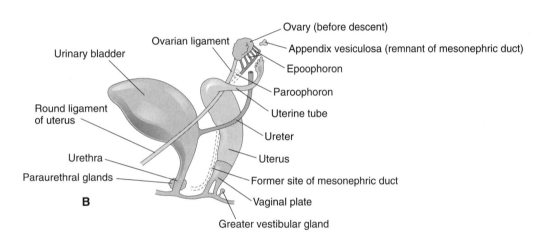

B

Ovary (before descent)
Appendix vesiculosa (remnant of mesonephric duct)
Epoophoron
Paroophoron
Uterine tube
Ureter
Uterus
Former site of mesonephric duct
Vaginal plate
Greater vestibular gland

Ovarian ligament
Urinary bladder
Round ligament of uterus
Urethra
Paraurethral glands

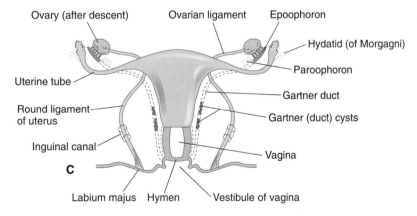

C

Ovary (after descent)
Ovarian ligament
Epoophoron
Hydatid (of Morgagni)
Paroophoron
Gartner duct
Gartner (duct) cysts
Vagina

Uterine tube
Round ligament of uterus
Inguinal canal
Labium majus
Hymen
Vestibule of vagina

FIGURE 33-2

Genitourinary embryonic structures. From Moore K, Persaud T (1998): *The developing human: clinically oriented embryology,* ed 6, Philadelphia: WB Saunders.

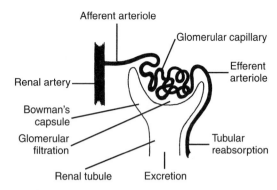

FIGURE 33-3
Glomerular apparatus.

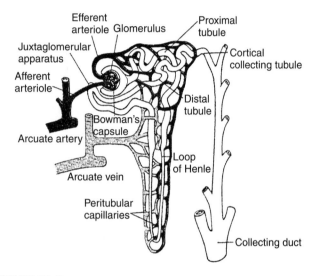

FIGURE 33-4
The nephron. From Guyton AC, Hall JE (1997): *Human physiology and mechanisms of disease*, ed 6, Philadelphia: WB Saunders.

Nephrogenesis begins deep within the renal cortex near the medulla in the juxtamedullary region and continues outwardly (Koeppen & Stanton, 1997). The juxtamedullary nephrons differ from the superficial cortical nephrons in that their glomeruli are larger; the loop of Henle is longer; and the efferent arteriole forms a more complex vascular system. The less mature superficial cortical nephrons make up the majority of nephrons; the more mature juxtamedullary nephrons account for a very small percentage of the total number (Brion et al, 1997). Altered renal function in the premature infant may therefore be caused by anatomic as well as physiologic immaturity.

The nephron's tubules are formed as the proximal tubule coils several times and as it then straightens and descends toward the medulla. The next segment is the loop of Henle, which consists of the straight portion of the proximal tubule, a descending thin limb, an ascending thin limb if the nephron contains long loops of Henle, and a thick ascending limb. A small portion of the thick ascending limb passes between the afferent and efferent arteries of the same nephron. This area is called the macula densa. Just beyond the macula densa, the distal tubule begins. The distal tubule extends into the cortex, where two or more nephrons join to form a cortical collecting duct. The duct then enters the medulla and becomes the outer and inner medullary, collecting duct (Koeppen & Stanton, 1997).

Renal Blood Flow and Glomerular Filtration

Urine formation begins with blood flow. Hydrostatic pressure within the renal capillaries depends on blood flow. The pressure-driven process of ultrafiltration depends on optimal arterial pressure and is regulated by the dilatation and constriction of afferent and efferent arterioles (Koeppen & Stratton, 1997). Adequate renal blood flow is therefore essential to kidney function. Although the kidneys account for only 0.5% of total body weight, approximately 25% of cardiac output is directed toward the kidneys (Koeppen & Stanton, 1997). Renal blood flow not only provides oxygen and nutrients to the kidneys but also affects the rate of solute and water reabsorption by the proximal tubule, participates in the concentration and dilution of the urine, and delivers substrates for excretion in the urine.

The renal arteries arise from the aorta. They enter the kidneys after dividing and branching several times to eventually give rise to the afferent arterioles that then lead to the glomerular capillaries. The distal ends of the glomerular capillaries merge to form the efferent arterioles, from which the peritubular capillaries emerge. The juxtamedullary efferent arterioles give rise to the vasa recta capillaries. The peritubular capillary bed surrounds the renal tubules and is considered a low-pressure bed that facilitates rapid fluid reabsorption. The peritubular capillaries empty into the venous system and eventually leave the kidneys in the form of the renal vein. The glomerular capillary bed is considered a high-pressure bed that facilitates rapid filtration of fluid from the glomerulus to Bowman's capsule.

As blood flows into the kidney via the renal artery, it is directed into the afferent arteriole that carries it into the glomerulus, which consists of the glomerular capillaries and Bowman's capsule. Plasma that is driven through the glomerular capillaries is filtered through the filtration barrier, and the protein-free plasma, or ultrafiltrate, is forced into Bowman's capsule or leaves via the efferent arteriole and enters into the renal vein. To produce this ultrafiltrate, the glomerulus functions as a filtering site. Glomerular capillaries are lined with epithelial cells that are called podocytes. These podocytes form one of the layers of Bowman's capsule (Figure 33-4). The endothelial cells of the glomerular capillaries are covered by a basement membrane that is also surrounded by podocytes. The basement membrane, podocytes, and the endothelial cell of the glomerular capillaries form the filtration barrier. The epithelial cells of this filtration barrier express negatively charged glycoproteins and contain many very small openings that are called fenestrations. The size of the fenestrations inhibits passage of large proteins but is highly permeable to passage of water, small solutes, urea, and glucose. In addition, positively charged large proteins are repelled by the cationic cell membrane. Albumin is an exception to the filtration rule because it possesses a large molecular structure, passes through the filtration system, and finds its way in small quantities into the urine (Koeppen & Stanton, 1997).

The glomerular filtration rate (GFR) is the rate at which fluid is filtered through the glomerulus. Because it is equal to the sum of all filtration rates of all nephrons in both kidneys, the GFR reflects kidney function, with a decrease in GFR signaling renal disease. Oncotic and hydrostatic pressures (Starling forces) drive the ultraflitration process. Oncotic pressure is osmotic pressure generated by large proteins or colloids. Hydrostatic pressure, on the other hand, is pressure exerted by fluids in equilibrium and depends on arterial pressure and vascular resistance (Koeppen & Stanton, 1997; Baylis & Lemley, 1997). Oncotic pressure in Bowman's space is very near zero because ultrafiltrate is nearly protein-free. Filtration at this level is therefore driven by hydrostatic pressure across the glomerular capillaries. Hydrostatic pressure within Bowman's space and glomerular oncotic pressure oppose glomerular hydrostatic pressure in the capillaries. The GFR is proportional to the sum of hydrostatic and oncotic pressures that exist along the renal capillaries multiplied by the ultrafiltration coefficient. The difference between the permeability of the glomerular capillary and the glomerular surface area available for filtration is the ultrafiltration coefficient (Koeppen & Stanton, 1997). GFR is therefore affected by changes in arterial blood pressure, vascular resistance, concentration of plasma proteins, and glomerular capillary permeability. Alteration in the permeability of the glomerular capillaries may result from inherent damage to the capillary, thus altering the pore size or changing the electrical charge within the membrane. GFR is also affected by urinary system obstruction.

GFR in the fetus is relatively low because of increased renal vascular resistance and decreased renal blood flow. The filtration rate increases with increasing gestational age and continues after birth, even in the premature infant. When corrected for body surface area, GFR is reportedly 10-ml/min/1.73 m^2 at 28 weeks' gestation and rises to 30-ml/min/1.73 m^2 at term. The rise in GFR is not caused by an increase in nephrons; rather it is believed to reflect a decrease in vascular resistance and an increase in glomerular surface area (Brion et al, 1997). Various medications given to control various maternal conditions have had detrimental effects on fetal GFR and subsequent neonatal renal function. Examples of these drugs have included beta-adrenergic antagonists (ritodrine hydrochloride), prostaglandin inhibitors (indomethacin), and angiotensin-converting enzyme inhibitor (captopril) (Chevalier, 1999; Brook et al, 1998).

Assessment of GFR is important in evaluating renal function. One method of assessing GFR is measurement of the renal clearance of a substance. Renal clearance represents a volume of plasma completely cleared of a substance by the kidneys over a specified period of time (Baylis & Lemley, 1997; Koeppen & Stratton, 1997). Various substances are used as markers for measuring GFR. Marker substances must do the following: (1) freely filter across the glomerulus into Bowman's space; (2) not be reabsorbed or secreted by the nephron; (3) not be metabolized or produced by the kidney; and 4) not alter GFR (Koeppen & Stratton, 1997). Para-aminohippurate (PAH) is a substance that the body does not produce, that is secreted by the proximal tubules, and that meets the marker criteria. PAH, which is nearly completely cleared, moves through the renal tubules so that it is effectively cleared via plasma movement within the kidney. Therefore measurement of the renal clearance of PAH can determine the effective renal plasma flow. This is significant because measurement of the effective renal plasma flow is a direct way of determining the renal functioning. However, this measurement is only accurate at low plasma concentrations of PAH. PAH is not produced by the body; therefore, it must be administered by infusion. Insulin also may be used as a tag substance for testing the intactness of the kidney's filtering system and glomerular filtration rate (Koeppen & Stratton, 1997). However, it too must be administered via infusion.

Creatinine, a by-product of muscle metabolism, also meets the marker criteria. Urine creatinine clearance is usually calculated on a 24-hour urine specimen. An accurate specimen of this type is difficult to obtain in a neonate. Measurement of serum creatinine levels is clinically the most useful method

of estimating renal function in neonates. Because creatinine readily crosses the placenta, levels obtained during the first week may reflect maternal levels. After birth, the GFR in term infants increases as renal blood flow increases and vascular resistance decreases. This increase in function usually occurs over the first week of life and results in a drop in creatinine levels to nearly 0.4 mg/dl, depending on hydration and clinical status. GFR typically does not increase until the completion of nephrogenesis. Therefore premature infants do not demonstrate the same decline in serum creatinine levels as infants born after 36 weeks' gestation. In addition, small increments of increase in serum creatinine levels may indicate a significant decrease in GFR. Monitoring trends in serial creatinine levels renders a more accurate evaluation of renal function.

Regulation of renal blood flow—and consequently GFR—is achieved by hormonal and sympathetic nervous system (SNS) influences. The renal vessels, including the afferent and efferent arterioles, are highly innervated by sympathetic nerve fibers. Mild stimulation of the SNS does not cause a change in renal vascular tone. However, under severe physiologic stress such as that caused by significant fluid loss, activation of the renal sympathetic nerve fibers causes vasoconstriction of the renal arteries, which in turn decreases GFR.

Hormonal control is exerted mainly via activation of the renin-angiotensin-aldosterone system (RAS). The RAS plays a significant role in blood pressure regulation and sodium homeostasis. Renin is found in high levels in the plasma. Renal renin is produced and stored in the specialized cells of the juxtaglomerular apparatus. It is also found in the fetus, beginning at about 3 months' gestation. Newborns have a significantly higher renin level than their adults do. This high level may be related to the neonate's altered glomerular filtration rate, vascular resistance, and renal blood flow. When renal blood flow is diminished as the result of a decrease in arterial pressure, the sympathetic nervous system responds to maintain homeostasis at the level of the kidney. As the result of the decrease in GFR, the concentration of sodium and chloride ions decreases, and renin secretion is stimulated. Renin then leads to the production of angiotensin I, which is then converted to angiotensin II in the lungs. Angiotensin II then stimulates secretion of aldosterone by the adrenal cortex. Aldosterone in turn triggers the reabsorption of sodium and water, thereby increasing extracellular fluid volume and renal perfusion (Figure 33-5). The ultimate goal of the rennin-angiotensin cycle is to maintain adequate systemic blood flow to supply the body's vital organs.

Renal prostaglandins are very potent vasoactive hormones. They are manufactured in the renal medulla and act to balance the RAS via vasodilatation, natriuresis, and diuresis. This action opposes the hormone angiotensin II, which acts as a vasoconstrictor and stops or reduces renin secretion.

Similar to other organs, the renal blood flow and GFR are maintained fairly constantly over a range of arterial blood pressures, mainly via autoregulation. Renal autoregulation is accomplished by at least two mechanisms: the pressure sensitive myogenic mechanism and the flow-dependent tubuloglomerular feedback mechanism. When smooth vascular muscles are stretched, they tend to contract. When arterial pressure increases, the renal afferent arteriole stretches, thus causing the smooth muscle to contract. The increase in resistance within the arteriole offsets the increase in pressure, and thus this myogenic mechanism maintains renal blood flow and GFR at a relatively constant state. Although the myogenic mechanism may be intrinsic to all organ systems, the tubuloglomerular feedback mechanism is unique to the renal system. The tubu-

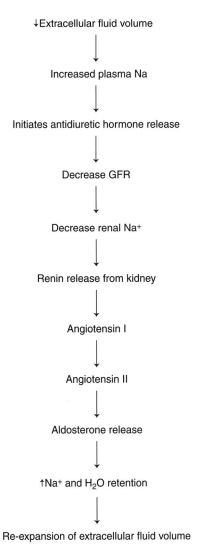

↓Extracellular fluid volume

↓

Increased plasma Na

↓

Initiates antidiuretic hormone release

↓

Decrease GFR

↓

Decrease renal Na⁺

↓

Renin release from kidney

↓

Angiotensin I

↓

Angiotensin II

↓

Aldosterone release

↓

↑Na⁺ and H₂O retention

↓

Re-expansion of extracellular fluid volume

FIGURE **33-5**
The Renin-Angiotensin-Aldosterone regulation of extracellular fluid.

loglomerular feedback mechanism causes an increase or decrease in GFR and renal blood flow in response to the flow of tubular fluid within the nephrons. A key component of the tubuloglomerular feedback mechanism is the juxtaglomerular apparatus (JGA). The JGA consists of the macula densa, the extraglomerular mesangial cells, and the granular cells of the afferent and efferent arterioles that produce renin (Koeppen & Stratton, 1997). A change in the flow of tubular fluid is sensed by the macula densa, which in turn triggers a signal that causes a change in afferent artery resistance. The change in resistance in the afferent arteriole then either increases or decreases GFR and renal blood flow. It is unclear as to what is sensed at the macula densa and what mediator actually effects the change in afferent arteriole resistance. Some researchers postulate that changes in flow-dependent sodium chloride reabsorption is sensed at the macula densa. Likewise, what actually causes the change in resistance at the afferent arteriole is in question. A mediator such as adenosine, which acts as a vasoconstrictor specifically on the afferent arteriole, could be present. Afferent arteriole vasoconstriction increases resistance and subsequently reduces GFR and renal blood flow (Baylis & Lemley, 1997; Koeppen & Stanton, 1997).

Secretion and Absorption

The kidneys control fluid and electrolyte balance by reabsorption and secretion of sodium and water. The four segments of the nephron—the proximal tubule, loop of Henle, distal tubule, and the collecting duct—determine the composition and volume of urine. In the neonate, the thin ascending portion, which controls reabsorption, is not fully formed, because nephron formation starts in the medullary area. By birth, it has extended from the medullary to the juxtamedullary area. The descending portion of the tubular system, which controls urine secretion, thus is more fully developed than the ascending segment at birth. The ability to concentrate urine is decreased in the newborn because although urine secretion occurs readily, reabsorption is limited.

Tubular reabsorption, secretion, and excretion are tied closely together. These processes are concerned with the maintenance of the internal homeostasis. This maintenance depends on a flexible and dynamic reabsorption pattern that responds to other body systems.

Tubular reabsorption occurs via transport and diffusion of substances across a semipermeable membrane in the direction of the lumen into the epithelial lining of the tubule to the efferent arteriole. Many of the body's nutrients, electrolytes, and water are reabsorbed, thus achieving a balance for continued growth and normal physiologic function. Simple diffusion or passive transport involves movement of substances down a gradient—from an area of higher to an area of lower concentration—or, according to polarization of the molecules, migration of anions toward cations. Active transport requires energy derived directly from adenosine triphosphate because the net movement of substances is against a gradient. Molecular structures may link together to piggyback—or carry one another—across the membrane. Sodium first undergoes simple diffusion across the tubular membrane and then is transported via this mechanism of active transport by the sodium pump into the interstitial fluid. Sodium filtration depends on the glomerular filtration rate. Thus a higher glomerular filtration rate results in an increase in sodium reabsorption into the vascular space. If the extracellular fluid volume increases, sodium reabsorption is decreased. Thus the regulation of fluids and electrolytes is highly complex because sodium, in turn, influences other substances to move against their gradients.

Water follows the sodium ion across the membrane and into the capillary bed. This type of transport of a second substance is often referred to as secondary active transport. Simple facilitated diffusion is similar to active transport in that a carrier substance is used but the net movement is not against a gradient. Glucose is one secondary substance that secondary active transport carries along with sodium across the membrane. Glucose is reabsorbed by the proximal tubules, thus appearing in the urine only when the renal threshold or the maximal tubular transport capacity has been exceeded or when the permeability of the filtering capillaries has been altered. Amino acids, water-soluble vitamins, albumin, and lactate are also transported in this fashion. Therefore errors of metabolism, for example, may alter tubular reabsorption of amino acids. Tubular secretion moves substances from the epithelial lining of the tubules' capillaries into the interstitial fluid and finally into the lumen. Thus the substances are secreted into the tubular lumen. Potassium and hydrogen undergo tubular secretion. Tubular excretion—the process by which substances enter into the filtrate that will eventually exit the body as urine—is linked with the secretion just described. Ions such as potassium, which are secreted in the distal tubule (a portion is also reabsorbed in the proximal tubule), find their way into the urine when the body has no need for higher concentration levels. The movement of hydrogen ions influences the excretion of potassium; thus metabolic acidosis and alkalosis affect potassium levels. Hormones and drugs, especially diuretics, affect potassium movement. In the presence of aldosterone, potassium is secreted; thiazides, in contrast, result in potassium excretion. Other filtrates that show up in the urine are urea, creatinine, and other ions that are not needed by the body.

The regulation of fluids and electrolytes is an important function of the processes of tubular secretion, reabsorption, and excretion. Excretion of toxins, drugs, and other by-products of metabolism is also important and has been previously mentioned.

PHYSIOLOGIC DEVELOPMENT OF THE GENITALIA

Although sexuality is determined at the time of fertilization, external characteristics are not present until the end of the second month of gestation. Development and maturation of the fetal genital system represent the first steps in gender identification. Gonadal development begins in the fifth week of gestation, when thickened areas of epithelium form ridges along the mesonephros. These epithelial ridges continue to grow along with the underlying mesenchyme. These thickened areas or ridges are known as gonadal or genital ridges. Soon fibrinous projections—called primary or primitive sex cords—appear and extend into the mesenchymal tissue. The gonad now has an outer portion called the cortex and an inner portion called the medulla. Before the seventh week, the gonads of both sexes are identical and are called indifferent or undifferentiated relative to sex. At 7 weeks' gestation, sexual differentiation begins. If the Y chromosome is present, the gonad will differentiate into a testis or into an ovary if the Y chromosome is absent. Control mechanisms that affect sex differentiation involve steps in male differentiation. Male differentiation requires all steps must be present. If any of the necessary steps fail to occur, the gonad will follow female lines of development.

Each gonad contains mesonephric and paramesonephric ducts. The mesonephric duct evolves from the urogenital ridge. The upper portion communicates with the peritoneal cavity. At midline, the mesonephric and paramesonephric ducts join to form the uterovaginal canal. Invagination of the urogenital sinus ends in a protrusion called the müllerian (paramesonephric) tubercle. During the sixth week of fetal development, primordial germ cells appear near the allantois along the wall of the yolk sac and begin their migration from the hindgut to the genital ridges. These germ cells influence the development of the male and female gonads.

If an XX chromosome pair is present, the outer portion of the gonad—or the cortex—becomes an ovary, and the medullary portion degenerates. Development of the ovary is slow and occurs in at 10 to 12 weeks' gestation. A primitive ovary initially forms and is called rete ovarii. This structure eventually regresses, thus giving way to the permanent ovary. In the female, mitosis of the primordial follicles (groups of cells that form from the cortical cords and the germ cells) begins and is completed during fetal life. Development of oogonia, or female eggs, occurs only in utero. No new oogonia are produced postnatally.

If an XY chromosome pair is present, the opposite phenomenon occurs. The medullary portion becomes a testis cord and later forms the rete testis, which is grounded in epithelial tissue. As this cord grows, it separates from the epithelium and leaves a fibrinous, thick band of connective tissue known as the tunica albuginea. The primary sex cords become seminiferous cords and—at puberty—become patent tubules composed of sustentacular cells of Sertoli and spermatogonia. These seminiferous cords subdivide into branches called the ductuli efferentes testis. During the second trimester, mesenchymal cells—called interstitial cells of Leydig—appear. By the sixth month of gestation, the testis is mature enough to influence development of the external genitalia. In the male, a primitive connection between the mesonephros and the rete testis remains. It is called the mesonephric duct, or the ductus deferens.

DIFFERENTIATION OF THE GENITALIA AND THE DUCT SYSTEM

Differentiation of the genitalia continues as the duct system and the external genitals flourish under hormonal influence. In the female, genital development is influenced by estrogen production coupled with the absence of androgens, in stimulating the formation of the clitoris from the phallus, the labia minora from the opened urogenital ridges, and the labia majora from the labioscrotal folds. A uterine tube or canal is evolved as the ovary descends slightly to just above the true pelvis. The posterior portion of the paramesonephric duct is stimulated by estrogen to develop into the uterine canal. The caudal portion of the paramesonephric ducts in a fused state creates two major structures, the uterus and the cervix. The caudal portion further fuses with endodermal cells and develops into a müllerian (paramesonephric) tubercle, thus forming the uterine tube. This tubercle stimulates the formation and canalization of the vagina by 18 to 20 weeks' gestation. Enfolding of the peritoneal tissue occurs, creating the uterus's broad ligament, which subdivides the pelvic cavity into the uterorectal and the uterovesical pouches. The hymen acts as a partition between the vaginal opening and the urogenital sinus.

In the male, or mesonephros, gradually diminishes, leaving a few rudimentary tubules under the influences of androgens and müllerian inhibiting substance that form the efferent testicular ducts. These ducts are in communication with the epididymal ducts. The ductus deferens forms from the tortuous epididymal ducts. This duct system is composed of smooth muscle that leads to an outgrowth or appendage, called the seminal vesicle, and finally into the most distal portion, called the ejaculatory duct. The male's external genitalia develop, as the phallic projection, which in the female creates the clitoris, continues to grow and form the penile organ. On the penis's ventral surface, the male urethral opening develops. Its formation is complete by 16 weeks' gestation. The patency and positioning of the urethral opening depend on the posterior-to-anterior progressive joining of the urogenital folds. The normal urethral position is midline on the ventral surface of the glans penis. With the development of the male urethra comes Cowper's or bulbourethral glands, which form just below the prostatic portion of the urethra. This portion of the urethra swells and engulfs a portion of the mesenchymal tissue, thus forming the prostatic gland. The scrotum begins to form as outpouches of tissue (scrotal swelling) first found in the inguinal area and later located on either side of the urogenital folds anterior to the anal and peritoneal tissue.

The final stage of the development in the male is the descent of the testes. This process involves two simultaneous-actions. First is the development of the gubernaculum testis. This occurs as the mesonephros degenerates and leaves a band rudimentary band of mesentery called the urogenital mesentery. The fibrosed urogenital mesentery gradually becomes the caudal genital ligament. A portion of the ligament communicates with the developing scrotal swellings. This area is known as the inguinal region. The product of these transformations is the gubernaculum testis. Once this communication is no longer open, the testes begin to descend through the inguinal canals and move from within the peritoneal cavity to reach their final position in the scrotal sac at around 32 to 34 weeks' gestation. The female vaginal process occurs at the same stage in development. This process involves the differentiation of the inguinal region into the inguinal canal and the partitioning of the peritoneal cavity and the tunica vaginalis. The complete obliteration of the communication between the scrotal portion of the peritoneal cavity and the vaginal process occurs several months after birth.

ASSESSMENT OF THE GENITOURINARY SYSTEM

History

Having a thorough familial history on record for neonates suspected of having urogenital abnormalities is imperative. Many urogenital problems have an inheritance pattern, which suggests genetic predisposition. The history should focus on any family members who have renal transplants or undergone dialysis, those with a history of renal failure, and those with cystic kidney disease or anomalies of the GU system. Investigate family history for members who may have the fragile X syndrome or Turner's syndrome. Are there any abnormalities of the external genitalia, like hypospadias, ambiguous genitalia, or undescended testicles? Do any members have low-set ears, or were they born with a single umbilical artery? Prenatal histories should be reviewed for antepartal factors that may predispose the infant to renal problems. Were polyhydramnios or oligohydramnios or an increased fetal abdominal area present on ultrasonography?

Neonatal history should include the following questions:

1. Has micturition taken place? If so, at what age? (The first voiding may occur in the delivery room or by 24 hours of life.)
2. Has the infant undergone any hypoxic episodes that may result in delayed voiding?
3. Is the infant receiving enteral or parenteral nutrition? If so, is the fluid intake sufficient relative to clinical status, gestational age, and immediate environment (radiant warmer or humidified isolette)? The radiant warmer increases insensible water loss.
4. Is the infant under treatment for jaundice? (Phototherapy increases fluid losses.)
5. Is the infant experiencing any frank blood loss or increased GI losses such as are caused by nasogastric suctioning, vomiting, diarrhea, or increased ostomy losses?
6. What is the specific gravity of urine? (Normal range is 1.003 to 1.015.)
7. How old is the infant?

Physical Assessment

Physical examination should include inspection, palpation, and percussion. Auscultation is not generally useful for the renal system.

Inspection. Observation of the abdominal region is an important place to start. Is distention present? If so, is it unilateral or generalized? Mild abdominal protuberance in the neonate may be a normal finding because the abdominal musculature is relatively weak at birth in comparison to the eventual state of the musculature several months after birth. Absence of muscle tone is a characteristic finding in prune-belly syndrome. Abdominal asymmetry is an abnormal finding. Is drainage coming from the umbilicus? Does the bladder appear distended?

Next, the genital area is inspected. Peritoneal tissue that leads to the anal opening should be intact and smooth in appearance. Any abnormal openings, depressions, or swellings should be noted. The anus is normally located midline and should be tested for patency by gentle insertion of a gloved, well-lubricated small finger. Gentle stroking of the anal tissue and observation for anal sphincter constriction may test the anal wink, which indicates muscle tone. Inspection is also made for meconium or stool.

Male. Inspect the skin over the scrotum for color, rugae, edema or ecchymosis. If the infant is a full-term male, the scrotal sac should be full, and rugae should be present. The premature male exhibits a generally flaccid, smooth scrotal sac. The scrotum is generally darkly pigmented, without bluish discoloration. A blue color may denote disruption of circulation to the area, and when coupled with dimpling, torsion of the testicles must be suspected. The scrotum that is enlarged or very edematous may accompany a hydrocele (a trapping of fluid in the tunica vaginalis), or it may result from pressure on this tissue during the birth process, which is especially true in a breech birth. If a hydrocele is suspected, transillumination of the scrotum with a good light source, such as a transilluminator and a flashlight, helps determine the presence of fluid. On transillumination, fluid allows light to pass through it and shows as a highly lightened area.

Penile size, resting position, and position of the urinary meatus should be assessed. If the penile structure is abnormally large or small in proportion to the gestational age and the rest of the body parts, a renal problem may be present. Micropenis— penile hypoplasia with an otherwise normal appearance—is associated with a number of clinical syndromes or chromosomal aberrations (Fletcher, 1998). The penis is generally straight. Downward incurvation, bowing, or chordee is most often associated with hypospadias. Priapism, or a constantly erect penis, is also an abnormal finding. The urinary meatus is usually located midline on the ventral portion of the glans penis. Alterations of position result in dorsal or ventral placement anywhere along the shaft of the penis. This condition is known as epispadias if the urinary meatus is on the dorsum of the penis or as hypospadias if the opening is displaced along the ventral penile surface. The foreskin of the uncircumcised male is gently retracted for accurate observation and then should be returned to its unretracted state after inspection; otherwise, swelling with associated decreased circulation to the glans penis may occur.

Female. Inspect the female infant's labia, clitoris, urinary meatus, and external vaginal orifice. In the full-term female, inspect for presence of labia majora. The labia minora in the term infant should be well-formed. The labia majora should be present and should extend beyond the labia minora. The labia minora in the premature female infant may be larger than the labia majora. The less mature the female infant, the smaller the labia majora. The labia may have a dark pigmentation. This is of no clinical significance. Clitoral tissue should be present.

The clitoris may be enlarged in both fullterm and preterm infants. Because the labia may not be fully developed, the clitoris of preterm infants may be quite prominent. The urinary meatus should be patent and anterior to the vaginal orifice. The vagina should be inspected for patency, and any vaginal secretions should be noted. A white milky vaginal secretion in the first few days of life followed by pseudomenses or slight vaginal bleeding is a normal finding. A hymenal tag may be present. The hymenal tag usually disappears within a few weeks and is a normal finding with no clinical significance.

Both Sexes.   Bruising and related swelling of the genitalia following breech delivery should be appropriately documented. Ecchymosis and sometimes hematomas may also be observed after traumatic delivery. These birth-related findings are transient and should resolve within several days. Although inguinal hernias may be found in either sex, they occur less often in females. The urinary stream should be continuous and straight. The genital and peritoneal regions must be observed to ensure that a clear differentiation of the sexes is possible. If it is not, a genetics consult must be made.

Palpation.   This portion of the physical examination may be upsetting to the neonate and thus is best left until last. Place the infant in the supine position with the knees and hips flexed and provide a means of nonnutritive sucking for the infant. This position usually puts the infant at ease and facilitates relaxation of the abdominal muscles. The abdomen is gently palpated with a gradual downward movement, anteriorly to posteriorly. The kidneys may be felt on deep palpation. Another technique that is sometimes successful is placing the infant again in the supine position and then placing the fingers of one hand along the flank with the thumb while palpating the abdomen. This technique allows the examiner to possibly trap the kidney's pole between the fingers and the thumb (ballottement).

On palpation, the kidneys should be bilaterally equal in size. The right kidney may be slightly lower than the left kidney because of the position of other abdominal organs. No masses should be felt during abdominal palpation. However, if one is encountered, its position, mobility on palpation, and contour (either flat, lumpy, or depressed) must be accurately described. Bladder distention or ureterocele may present as a mobile mass. If Wilms' tumor is suspected, palpation should not be performed. Palpation in this instance may break the tumor into small fragments, thus leading to tumor seeding.

Male.   Palpate scrotal sac for each testis and cord. If the testis is absent, palpate along the canal to assess location. The scrotal sac may be palpated by gentle pressing of the tissue between two fingers—one on the anterior surface and the other on the posterior surface. Gentle movement of the fingers upward over the scrotum until the testes are detected bilaterally indicates whether one or both testes are descended and their location in relationship to the internal ring in the inguinal canal. Up until 28 weeks' gestation, the testes are abdominal organs. Between 28 to 30 weeks, they begin to descend into the inguinal canal. The cremasteric reflex, recoil of the testes toward the inguinal canal, may be elicited by gentle stroking of the upper thigh or scrotal sac.

Percussion.   If bladder distention is palpated or observed, percussion should be performed. This technique is useful in

determining whether fluid is filling the bladder, a situation denoted by a somewhat tympanic sound; if a solid mass is present, dullness is noted. Percussion may also be used over the entire abdominal region. Examination of the abdomen and intestinal area is discussed in depth in the Chapter 26.

Related Findings
Neonates should be inspected for general characteristics that strongly suggest renal abnormalities. Potter's facies (flattened, beak-like nose, wide-set eyes, micrognathia, and disproportionately large ears, short neck) accompanied by abnormal positioning of the hands and feet and pulmonary hypoplasia are all associated with oligohydramnios. These characteristics often accompany syndromes in which renal disorders are a component. Presence of a single umbilical artery is also a common finding when renal problems are present.

Meningomyelocele and other neural tube defects may result in decreased or absent innervation to the bladder. The result may be a neurogenic bladder characterized by bladder distention. If untreated, the urinary stasis ultimately leads to urinary and cystic infection.

Various syndromes that have associated renal and genital problems are listed in Table 33-1.

RISK FACTORS

Table 33-2 lists maternal, neonatal, and other risks associated with urogenital disorders. Specific risk factors for each of the urogenital dysfunctions are addressed in the appropriate sections.

DIAGNOSTIC WORK-UP

The diagnostic work-up for potential renal problems includes several diagnostic screening tests.

Urine Collection
Urine collection is a relatively simple procedure in the neonate. Several adhesive-backed collection bags are available. Care should be taken not to include the rectum or scrotum within the opening of the bag. The penis should not be left in urine, because infection and skin irritation may occur. Skin irritation with the use of these bags is possible; therefore care should be taken to maintain skin integrity. Alternative collection systems can be used if sterile specimens are not required and accurate measurement of output is not needed. Cotton balls can be placed inside diapers to catch a small specimen for dipstick analysis or for measurement of specific gravity. Many institutions now use super-absorbency disposable diapers. The super-absorbent material can potentially alter the results of the urine test. Further nursing research is needed to evaluate accuracy of laboratory values in these newer products. In male infants, test tubes or syringe barrels may be secured to the penis to collect small specimens.

When sterile urine specimens are required for blood culture, a suprapubic bladder tap or urethreal catheterization may be performed. The performance of the suprapubic tap requires minimal equipment and time. The lower abdomen is prepared with an antimicrobial solution and allowed to dry. Palpation of the bladder is attempted, although it may not be felt in the neonate. If the infant has voided within the previous hour, the attempt should be delayed until the infant has a full bladder. If severe dehydration, abdominal congenital

ABLE **33-1**	Syndromes Associated with the Development of Urogenital Disorders	
Syndromes	**Renal Component**	**Genital Component**
Potter's association	Renal agenesis	Absence of vas deferens, seminal vesical, upper vagina, uterus
Meckel's syndrome	Polycystic kidneys	Ambiguous genitalia Hypoplastic phallus Cryptorchidism
Trisomy 21	Cystic kidneys and other renal anomalies	Hypoplastic penis and scrotum Cryptorchidism
Trisomy 18	Dysplastic renal system	Hypoplastic clitoris and labia minora Cryptorchidism
Turner's syndrome	Horseshoe kidney Duplications of the collecting system	Infantile genitalia
Prune-belly syndrome	Urinary tract dysplasia Bladder and ureter dilation Patent urachus	Cryptorchidism
Errors of metabolism Galactosemia Tyrosinemia Glycogen storage (Gierke's) disease	Renal tubular dysfunction	
Adrenogenital the syndrome		Masculinization of female Incomplete mas- culinization of the male Clitoral hypertrophy
Hypospadias Hypoplastic penis Cryptorchidism		

ABLE **33-2**	Risk Factors Associated with Genitourinary Dysfunction	
Risk Factor	**Urogenital Defect**	
Maternal		
Fetal alcohol syndrome	Hydronephrosis Hypospadias Small, rotated kidneys	
Maternal cocaine use	Genitourinary anomalies	
Rubella	Renal artery stenosis	
Maternal diabetes	Maternal hypertension	
Oligohydramnios	Renal agenesis	
Positive familial history: Polycystic kidneys Renal transplants Medullary cystic disease Nephritis Tubular acidosis Renal tubular necrosis Renal tubular necrosis	Other similar renal anomalies	
Neonatal		
Asphyxia	Renal tubular necrosis	
Resuscitation	Renal tubular necrosis	
Vascular catheterization	Renal vessel thrombosis	
Birth and other trauma	Renal tubular necrosis Physical renal damage Renal hemorrhage Peritoneal lacerations	
Polycythemia; dehydration	Renal vessel thrombosis Renal necrosis	
Nephrotoxic drugs Gentamicin Hyperosmotic fluids Metabolic buffers Disseminated intra- vascular coagulation		
Other Defects		
Spina bifida	Urinary stasis	
Meningomyelocele	Urinary stasis, infection	
Compression of aorta	Acute renal failure	
Abdominal wall defects	Multiple urogenital deformities	

anomalies, or distention are present, a suprapubic tap may not be warranted. The procedure is usually performed with a 3-ml syringe with a 23- to 25-gauge straight needle. The needle is placed midline, 1 to 1.5 cm above the symphysis pubis and is inserted perpendicularly or at a slight angle, pointing toward the head. Entry into the bladder is determined when resistance decreases as the needle is inserted. A slight traction on the plunger facilitates aspiration of urine into the syringe. If no urine is obtained on the first attempt, a second attempt should be delayed until sufficient urine build-up has occurred. At the completion of the procedure, pressure should be applied over the puncture site until all evidence of bleeding has ceased.

This procedure may have complications. Uterine and bowel perforations, trauma to other portions of the renal system, and infection are known complications. The procedure is not rec-

ommended for any neonate with clotting disorders or known disseminated intravascular coagulation. Uretheral catheterization may also be performed to obtain sterile urine specimens. Bladder catheterization may be performed with a 3.5 or 5 Fr catheter. Catheterization and suprapubic bladder taps have a lower contamination risk than that associated with bagged specimens.

Urinalysis

One of the first steps in a urogenital work-up is urinalysis. Variables normally assessed in urinalysis include color, odor, pH, specific gravity, cells, blood, and protein. It includes gross assessment as well as dipstick and microscopic evaluation. The urine is most often straw-colored, but this may be altered by the type and amount of solutes. Dipstick testing of urine can provide a wide range of information. This test requires that only one to two drops of urine be placed on the dipstick, or the stick may be dipped into a specimen of urine. The results are obtained within 30 seconds to 1 minute after the stick is wet with urine. The exact timing for the most accurate reading is found on the bottles of the dipstick materials, based on the manufacturer's suggested clinical timing cycle. In addition to pH, specific gravity, protein, and blood the dipstick test may also assess the presence of blood, nitrites, glucose, bilirubin, and ketones in the urine.

Renal regulation of acid base balance has previously been discussed. Urinary pH values range from 4.5 to 8 and reflect the kidney's attempt to maintain acid base balance. The newborn initially excretes alkalotic urine with a pH of 6. Urine pH values in the newborn should be evaluated in relation to the serum bicarbonate values. Production of alkaline urine with documented metabolic acidosis may indicate renal pathology.

Specific gravity indicates the kidney's ability to concentrate and dilute urine. Specific gravity measurement in the newborn can be misleading in its interpretation. Normal levels often range from 1.001 to 1.020. A low specific gravity may appear normal yet may not be an accurate reflection of renal functioning because the infant has a decreased ability to concentrate urine. High specific gravities often reflect dehydration versus high solute excretion. Excretion of glucose and protein in the urine may artificially increase the specific gravity in the newborn. Urine osmolality is a more accurate measure of the kidney's urine concentrating ability.

Small amounts of protein are normally found in urine. Glomerular filtrate is nearly protein-free, and the majority of the protein that is filtered is reabsorbed along the nephron's tubular system. Glomerular and tubular damage can result in excessive proteinuria. Extra-renal pathology may also result in proteinuria. The source of persistent, large quantities of proteinuria must therefore be evaluated (Brion et al, 1997).

Sources of hematuria include infection, urinary obstruction, renal necrosis, renal thrombosis, trauma, or administration of hyperosmotic or nephrotoxic drugs. Because of the various sources of red cells in urine, the source should be quickly determined. Blood is a protein; therefore if blood is present, a positive protein test result should also be expected.

Trace amounts of glucose may be detected in the fullterm infant's urine but is found more often in the premature infant's urine. Glucosuria occurs in when the renal tubules have reached their threshold for reabsorption of glucose, thus resulting in excretion. Glucosuria also occurs with increased glucose loads that are sometimes given via parenteral nutrition. This increased glucose load and can lead to osmotic diuresis.

Renal Clearance Tests

Renal clearance tests are of little value in the newborn. Although inulin clearance tests may be performed, other measurements may be more diagnostic in the newborn period.

Urine Chemistries

Urine chemistries are helpful in determining fluid and electrolyte balance when evaluated in comparison to serum electrolyte levels.

Sodium excretion is very high in the fetus and premature infant but decreases with increasing gestational age. The fullterm infant conserves renal sodium, and renal sodium loss is small. Increasing GFR, combined with impaired reabsorption of sodium in the renal tubules, is thought to cause the high level of excretion in the premature neonate. In addition, kidneys of premature infants display a relative unresponsiveness to aldosterone. Sodium is regulated by extracellular fluid volume and hormonal influences.

Potassium is freely filtered by the glomerulus. Urinary potassium levels are low, however, because the majority of filtered potassium is reabsorbed by the proximal tubule and, to a lesser extent, the loop of Henle. Urinary potassium levels reflect the amount secreted by the collecting tubule. As a result, increased potassium load can significantly increase serum potassium levels. Urinary potassium loss is the result of increased mineralocorticoid concentrations and increased delivery of sodium to the collecting tubule where it is secreted.

Osmolality is a more accurate measure of concentration or dilution of urine. It is the measure of the number of solute particles dissolved in a given volume of solution.

Serum Chemistries

The measurement of serum chemistries plays a large role in assessing renal functioning. In the premature or compromised infant, serum electrolyte levels may indicate a wider range of problems than occurs in the healthy newborn. Dehydration, fluid overload, metabolic disorders, fluid-losing and electrolyte-losing disorders, and respiratory compromise all lead to alterations in serum electrolyte levels. High serum sodium levels may reflect dehydration, excessive fluid loss, or administration of high-solute loads. Low sodium levels can occur with overhydration or possibly with inappropriate antidiuretic hormone secretion. Potassium losses are apparent with diuretic use and with episodes of diarrhea.

Blood Urea Nitrogen and Creatinine.   Another indication of renal functioning is the determination of blood urea nitrogen (BUN) and creatinine levels. Although these indices are not absolute indicators of long-term renal problems, these values can be used to identify and treat acute problems. During the first few days of life, BUN levels may not be greater than 20 mg/dl. Until this point, placental function has maintained normal serum fetal levels, which remain stable in the early newborn period. In many cases, dehydration can cause dramatic increases in serum levels to levels higher than adult norms. Ingestion of high protein loads may affect levels in infants with normal renal function. Creatinine levels at birth often reflect maternal levels. Creatinine levels should begin to decrease gradually over the first 10 days as GFR increases. Serial levels should be obtained to better evaluate renal function. Table 33-3 provides a summary of urine chemistries in term and preterm infants.

Urine Culture

Urine culture in the newborn is used as an assessment for neonatal sepsis. Although urine infections are rare in the newborn, they can occur when urinary tract deformities are present or when organisms have been introduced via invasive procedures. In many cases, clean-catch specimens are obtained by use of either sterile or clean infant specimen collectors. When organisms appear on a culture report, a repeat culture is usually performed. The presence of leukocytes may not be an indication of infection, especially in the female, because of vaginal secretions.

Adrenocorticosteroid Levels

In the infant with adrenogenital syndrome, adrenocorticosteroid levels help to determine the specific disorder and treat-

TABLE **33-3**	Differences in Renal Function Between Fullterm and Preterm Infants	
	Preterm	**Fullterm**
Creatinine clearance 1 week after birth (ml/min/ 1.73m²)	11 ± 5 (GA 25 to 28 wk) 15 ± 6 (GA 29 to 34 wk)	46 ± 15
Plasma creatinine 1 wk after birth (mg/dL)	1.4 ± 0.8 (GA 25 to 28 wk)	0.5 ± 0.1
Maximum urine osmolality (mOsm/kg H₂O)	400 to 700	600 to 900
Proteinuria (mg/m²/d)	88 to 377	68 to 309
Plasma bicarbonate (mEq/L)	19.5 ± 2.9	21.0 ± 1.8
Mean fractional excretion of sodium (%)	4 (GA <30 wk)	<2

GA, gestational age.
From Springate JE et al (1987). Assessment of renal function in newborn infants. Pediatrics in review, 9(2), 56. Reprinted with permission from Pediatrics in review.

ment. The most common form is 21-hydroxylase deficiency. In addition to physical evidence of deficiency on external genitalia examination, urine or plasma levels of 17-ketosteroids, pregnanediol, and 17α-hydroxyprogesterone are deficient. The development of the adrenals is addressed in Chapter 28.

Radiologic Examination

Radiologic examination includes a range of tests available for determining anatomic and physiologic function. The injection of contrast material can be used to visualize kidney mass as well as ureter and bladder outline and to help determine the amount of functioning kidney. In the premature infant, contrast material should be used selectively because the solution is hyperosmolar and may lead to further renal compromise. In instances in which an intravenous pyelogram is ineffective in determining structural outlines, retrograde instillation of dye may be used.

Radionuclide Evaluation. Radionuclide evaluation may be necessary if pyelographic studies do not indicate accurate renal mass. The amount of uptake and the timing of excretion both may indicate renal deficiencies. Excretion of the dye via the urinary tract should be handled according to institutional policy regarding radioactive waste.

Another radionuclide test is diuretic renography, which is used most often if hydronephrosis is suspected. A radioisotope injection is given, followed 15 to 30 minutes later by a diuretic injection. The diuretic facilitates the movement of the radioisotope through the renal system. A gamma computer tracks the isotope's movement. If a urinary obstruction is present, the isotope's progress is slowed or impeded, thus showing retention

of the radioactive substance. If dilation exists along the renal system, urine is retained at the uteropelvic junction until overflow occurs with diuretic action. The stretching of the muscle fibers at this point causes strong contractions to begin. Soon, the urine is released, thus rapidly moving the isotope along (about 10 to 15 minutes) and showing a sharp, immediate decline in isotope concentration. In a normal kidney, the isotope takes about 25 minutes to clear the system, and the isotope concentration gradually declines. Institutional variations in the selection of the diuretic and isotope exist. Because of the uniqueness of performing this type of study in newborns, a standardized method of performing diuretic renograms in infants has been developed and is used widely.

Renal Ultrasonography. The safest and one of the most useful tests to determine renal anomalies is ultrasonography. The two dimensional mode and Doppler imaging are the usual techniques. The two-dimensional mode may be used to illustrate kidney structure, and Doppler imaging provides information relative to flow in the renal arteries and veins. Analysis can often determine differences in normal versus cystic tissue. Solid tumors and masses may be readily apparent. In most institutions, ultrasound examinations are performed before invasive studies. In many cases, accurate and specific diagnosis may be determined from ultrasonography alone. Ultrasonography is useful in identifying renal obstruction, presence of calculi, and in some cases, advanced parenchymal disease.

Computed Tomography. Computed tomography can be helpful in locating major structures. Its use is limited in providing specific diagnoses, and the cost may be prohibitive in relation to other available testing methods.

Genetic Consultation

Genetic consultation is an important part of the care for the infant with genital abnormalities. Chromosome banding and karyotyping should be performed if the infant has a positive family history of GU anomalies or if a visible neonatal GU malformation is present. Chromosomal analysis may take several weeks before final reports are completed. Fetal chromosomal studies can be performed if a defect is suspected.

COLLABORATIVE AND NURSING MANAGEMENT

Fluid, Electrolytes, and Nutrition

When urine output decreases, serum electrolytes, phosphorous, and calcium levels should be monitored serially to prevent overload. Urine and serum chemistries should be monitored as frequently as clinically indicated. Fluids should be carefully managed relative to clinical presentation and response to therapy.

Hyperkalemia is a consequence of renal failure. Maintenance of appropriate potassium levels is most important in the management of renal failure. Careful cardiac monitoring is extremely important to detect any abnormal rhythms or patterns that result from alterations in potassium levels. Potassium should not be added to parenteral fluids until an appropriate urine output has been established. The goals of hyperkalemia management are to decrease myocardial excitability, enhance cellular potassium uptake, and facilitate potassium excretion. Administration of intravenous calcium gluconate aids in decreasing myocardial excitability. Cellular uptake of potassium can often be achieved through combined administration of glucose and insulin, administration of sodium bicarbonate

(1 Meq/kg), and exchange transfusion. Dialysis can be used to return the body to normal potassium levels, but the use of long-term dialysis in the neonate is limited (Brion et al, 1997).

Furosemide (Lasix) is used to treat congestive heart failure as well as fluid balance problems caused by genitourinary problems. Hypokalemia may result from the use of potassium-wasting diuretics such as furosemide. One experimental therapy aimed at decreasing the incidence of electrolyte imbalance is nebulized furosemide. A single dose of 1 mg/kg of inhaled furosemide is thought to be more effective than the intravenous route and has fewer side effects. Although this therapy is experimental, it certainly merits further investigation if side effects such as hypokalemia can be diminished.

Optimal nutritional status should always be an intergral part of management. Adequate nutritional status positively impacts the outcome of infants who experience renal compromise. Nursing management involves the ongoing assessment and reporting of aberrant signs and symptoms. Daily or twice-daily weights may be required for a baseline determination of excessive fluid retention or loss. Accurate intake and output must be measured. Urine-specific gravity should be frequently monitored. Sodium and phosphorus restrictions may also be imposed, although if the infant is asymptomatic, such electrolyte restrictions may not be necessary. Protein intake should be determined by evaluation of overall caloric intake and by BUN levels.

Renal disease may also lead to elevated phosphorus levels. Use of aluminum hydroxide to bind phosphorus in the intestines may be helpful if management is warranted. A formula that is low in phosphorus may be given in the form of Similac PM 60/40 or SMA. Calcium levels often stabilize without intervention. Calcium supplements can be used after the phosphorus level has been normalized. However, calcium supplementation may also be needed because the phosphorus level affects the calcium level. These levels are inversely proportional; as one increases, the other decreases. Caution should be practiced during intravenous administration. Rapid administration of calcium can precipitate a cardiac arrest; thus administration of this agent requires close nursing observation.

Dihydrotachysterol or vitamin D supplementation is also a useful adjunct for the correction of calcium levels because it facilitates the movement of calcium from the bones so that it is freed for absorption by the body.

In addition to these concerns, positive growth and nutrition may be compromised. If a fluid restriction has been imposed, the caloric consumption must be increased without increasing fluid volume. Hyperalimentation may be initiated in infants who are not capable of receiving enteral feedings once electrolyte and mineral balance has been achieved (Chapter 25). The overall goal of nutritional therapy is the preservation of a positive nitrogen balance and the avoidance of increases in nitrogenous waste products that can lead to further increases in urea nitrogen levels and uremia.

In addition, fluid shifts may occur secondarily to fluid overload or to a change in electrolyte balance, thus resulting in edema. Assessment for the presence of edema includes observation of periorbital area and observation of dependent surfaces, including examination of the hands, feet, labia and scrotum. Pitting should be determined by gentle depression of a fingertip into the suspected edematous site. Caution should be taken around the ocular area because direct pressure on the eyeball may precipitate bradycardia. A late manifestation of renal disease is ascites.

Skin Management

Skin integrity is a concern, especially when pitting edema is present. The infant's position should be changed every 2 hours to decrease effects of dependent edema. Skin around any operative site should be inspected with every dressing change for any signs of irritation or infection. The skin must be kept dry and clean to prevent skin breakdown and infection.

Respiratory Management

Respiratory compromise is common in the infant who is experiencing alterations in urinary elimination. During fetal life, insufficient amniotic fluid is linked to decreased development of the respiratory tree (see discussion on Potter's association). Varying degrees of lung hypoplasia may exist. As a result, the chest may be small in comparison with the rest of the body and concave.

The ability to use accessory muscles that help achieve effective respiration may be lacking. This situation can lead to an increase in respiratory effort. Before extensive therapy is initiated for the treatment of renal anomalies, careful evaluation of respiratory status should be performed (Chapter 21). Measures to improve renal function should not be undertaken if respiratory capacity is insufficient to support life.

General Preoperative Management

If surgical intervention is indicated, preoperative care is directed toward achieving and maintaining the stability of the fluid and electrolyte balance and the hemodynamic status of the infant. Assessment for any signs of urinary tract infection—such as poor feeding, temperature instability, cyanosis, and any other detectable subtle change from the infant's baseline norm—should be ongoing.

General Postoperative Management

Postoperatively, nursing management is again focused on careful assessment and monitoring of the fluid and electrolyte status as well as the hemodynamic system—including blood pressure, pulse, and respiration of the infant. Accurate measurement of fluid intake and output is critical. If poor renal function develops in one of the infant's kidneys, surgical placement of a nephrostomy tube may be indicated. This tube's insertion site is covered with a sterile dressing.

Because the renal system is a highly vascular system, the chance for bleeding or infection is great. After the insertion of a nephrostomy tube or tubes, pink-tinged urine or even urine with visible bloody streaks is common. Because they are located within the renal pelvis, these tubes should not be irrigated (see Figure 33-3). The tubes should be connected to a closed drainage system to maintain sterility. A clean dressing surrounding the tube should be used to maintain the position and protect the underlying skin. On removal of such tubes, urine leakage for as long as 48 hours is not unusual.

Maintenance of an aseptic suture line is important. Any dressings, especially over a nephrostomy site, should be closely observed for bleeding or drainage. An infant with a nephrostomy tube or who has undergone other renal surgery is at risk for infection. Broad-spectrum antibiotics, such as ampicillin and gentamicin, are useful. Use of trimethoprim-sulfamethoxazole (Bactrim) is appropriate in the infant older than 2 months of age who does not have severe renal impairment. This drug is specific to the bacteria that most often cause urinary tract infections.

A urinary stent may also be placed in the ureter to splint the site of the anastomosis that has been performed. Although no drainage is expected through the stent, a closed drainage system is necessary to protect the neonate from infection. The infant may have a Foley catheter as well. Eventually, the neonate may require an ureterostomy followed by a nephrectomy if kidney function cannot be restored.

When urinary stents or suprapubic or nephrostomy tubes are used, maintaining the infant's position by placement in traction may be necessary.

Parental Support

The parents' response to their infants' conditions will vary and must be addressed individually. Consenting to a major surgical procedure on their infant so early in life may be very difficult. The parents must be given accurate information as to the prognosis for their infant and should be encouraged to express their concerns. Use of the interdisciplinary team is essential. Collaboration among the neonatologist, pediatric urologist, nurse, clergy, and social worker helps the parents adjust to this frightening situation. If the infant's clinical status is terminal, early identification and involvement of their support network—other parents, family, or friends—or the clergy can assist the parents in coping with the reality that their child may not survive. When the bedside nurse anticipates this need responds early, the optimal possible outcome is ensured.

Nursing Considerations for the Protection of Health Professionals

The child who is born with cytomegalic inclusion disease sheds the virus in the urine for an unknown period of time, often years. The implications for nurses are twofold. When contracted by pregnant women, cytomegalovirus may result in damage to the central nervous system of the developing fetus. In the first trimester, exposure to cytomegalovirus sometimes results in miscarriage. Nurses who are of childbearing age must be cautious and use meticulous hand-washing when caring for these infants. Gloves should be worn when diapers of any infant believed to be at risk for cytomegalovirus are changed. Good hand-washing is essential after diaper changes and any type of urine-testing.

Compromised newborns must also be protected against exposure to the virus because their immune system is not adequate to fight such an infection and it could result in death. Thus cross-contamination is a vital consideration. Excretion-secretion precautions should be used in caring for neonates who are known to be cytomegalovirus-positive to ensure protection against accidental passage of the virus. Diapers should be discarded in a bedside receptacle rather than in a receptacle across the nursery.

In addition, an infant with acquired immunodeficiency syndrome may be asymptomatic in the nursery; however, universal precautions should be used any time an infant is suspected to be at high risk for acquired immunodeficiency syndrome (Chapter 29).

The general principles of nursing management have been outlined. The remainder of the chapter addresses the most common GU neonatal problems.

URINARY TRACT INFECTION

Pathophysiology

Full-term neonates are at risk for developing any type of infection because of their immature immune status. In the newborn, the specific and the nonspecific immunity as well as the complement system are diminished, thus predisposing the infant to difficulty in locating the source or the site of an infection and in mounting an effective response to invasion (Chapter 29).

Urinary tract infections (UTI) in neonates are not particularly common. Such neonatal infections are iatrogenic or result from urinary malformation or obstructions. Many iatrogenic factors can be eliminated with strict adherence to aseptic technique. Urinary obstruction along the renal or urinary pathways typically causes urinary flow to be slowed or stopped. As a result, urinary stasis occurs and thus predisposes the neonate to bacterial colonization and ultimately bladder or UTI. A neurogenic bladder—that is, one that lacks innervation—often accompanies spinal or neural tube deformities such as spina bifida or meningomyelocele. It also predisposes the infant to the effects of urinary stasis. Vesicoureteral reflux, retrograde flow of urine from the bladder toward the kidney, is another risk factor for development of UTI. If retrograde flow of infected urine reaches the upper urinary tract, pyelonephritis can occur.

UTIs are more frequently found in males than females. Evidence also suggests that uncircumcised males have a higher rate of UTI than circumcised males do (Schoen et al, 2000). Others, however, note that UTI is influenced by numerous factors and not definitively increased in the uncircumcised male neonate.

E. coli is the most commonly found causative agent in UTI. However, Klebsiella, Pseudomonas, Proteus, Enterococcus, and Staphylococcus have been identified as causative agents in infants as well.

Fungal infections are becoming more common in neonates with long-term health problems who have required invasive procedures and prolonged antibiotic therapy. Percutaneous nephrostomy tubes have been found to provide an effective method of diagnosing the exact fungal agent and of administering amphotericin B in conjunction with intravenous systemic amphotericin B and 5-fluorocytosine to combat *Candida albicans* and *Torulopsis glabrata* infections.

Clinical Manifestations

Because neonates have immature nonspecific and specific immune systems, localization of infection is not usually possible. The clinical manifestations of a UTI are often subtle. The affected infant is often asymptomatic. General signs and symptoms of infection are commonly present. Characteristics, if demonstrated, are temperature instability, poor feeding, cyanosis, abdominal distention, poor weight gain, hepatomegaly, jaundice, thrombocytopenia purpura, and fever; the infant may or may not have proteinuria. These characteristics result from the immune system's response to infection. The nurse should report these signs to the medical team for further diagnostic work-up. Nurses must perform an ongoing assessment of all newborns who are suspected of having any type of infection, including UTIs.

Differential Diagnosis

In any neonate suspected of having a urinary tract infection, a blood culture should accompany the urine culture. The UTI may be the first sign of systemic infection. Other physical and internal anomalies must be considered whenever a urinary tract infection is suspected. Positive diagnosis of a urinary tract infection is made when a urine culture grows the causative agent.

Prognosis

The prognosis is generally good for an isolated urinary tract infection. However, the potential for serious complications, including severe damage to the renal system, exists. Septicemia may be life-threatening. The prognosis is directly dependent on the cause of such an infection. Therefore the exact cause of the infection must be determined as early as possible if complications are to be prevented.

Collaborative Management

A sepsis work-up should be performed on any infant who is suspected of having a UTI. Intravenous broad spectrum antibiotic therapy is then initiated based on clinical presentation. Antibiotic therapy may be adjusted once the causative organism is identified and sensitivities are obtained. The physician or practitioner should be notified immediately if urinary output is diminished. At the completion of antibiotic therapy—and once repeat cultures are negative—evaluation for presence of residual renal damage should be done. Voiding cystourethrogram (VCUG) and renal ultrasound are the studies most often used. These tests are performed to ensure that no damage to the urinary tract exists. If the infection results from a suspected urinary or renal obstruction, further diagnostic studies should be performed. After an initial UTI in the male infant, a renal ultrasound and VCUG can be used for a further diagnostic workup. It is recommended the dimercaptosuccinic acid (DSMA) scan be used as an adjunct assessment tool when ultrasound and VCUG illustrate abnormal findings.

Collaborative and Nursing Management

An ongoing holistic assessment of the infant should be conducted. A review of the maternal and newborn history is essential. Any positive familial history of pyelonephritis or nephritis should be considered. Maternal infections, especially of the genital tract, should be noted. Neonatal procedures such as suprapubic bladder taps should be noted along with the dates the procedures were performed. These dates estimate the incubation time for possible pathogens.

A neonate with hepatomegaly, jaundice, or thrombocytopenia purpura may actually exhibit associated symptoms of UTIs. Such an infant should be monitored closely for any baseline deviations and considered at risk for development of a urinary tract infection. Familial pyelonephritis is a risk factor for the development of neonatal renal dysfunction. However, pyelonephritis is not a common finding in the newborn period.

Careful assessment of the infant includes observation for general signs of neonatal infection as well as of fluctuations in temperature or the presence of fever. An elevated temperature may be the only indication of onset of a UTI. If wide temperature fluctuations are present or if a persistent temperature of greater than 37.5° C exists rectally, temperature checks should be made every 1 to 2 hours. If fever is present, tachycardia of greater than 160 beats per minute or tachypnea of greater than 60 breaths per minute may also occur. Each infant's baseline norm should be used for each individual infant. If the temperature is consistently greater than previous temperatures, a fever should be suspected.

If the infant has an indwelling urinary catheter, urine clarity and presence of hematuria should be noted. A urine culture should be sent any time a urinary tract infection is suspected. It should be noted in the patient's chart that hematuria may be present as the result of a traumatic catheterization or postsurgical trauma, especially if incurred during placement of nephrostomy tubes. Hematuria alone is therefore not a good indicator of UTI. A urine dipstick assessment may or may not be helpful. Although proteinuria can indicate the presence of urinary bacteria, dipstick protein levels may be exaggerated in the presence of blood because it is a protein. However, if hematuria is present, this finding is essentially useless because blood is a protein.

Observation of the infant's weight and ability to take feedings is important. Especially worrisome is a neonate who begins to progressively lose weight or does not feed as well as he or she did in the past. A good baseline of the typical feeding pattern and weight and thorough documentation of feeding and weight changes are imperative. An infant's well-being should be measured against a documented baseline.

CIRCUMCISION

Historically, the practice of male circumcision has been based on the premise that this surgical procedure helped promote positive hygiene and prevent UTIs. It was also believed that the circumcised male was less likely than an uncircumcised male to transmit sexually transmitted diseases to partners. Since the early 1990s the American Academy of Pediatrics has not advocated circumcision on a routine basis. The actual decision to circumcise is usually based on parental cultural values and beliefs.

Circumcision makes cleansing the penis and removing smegma (the whitish secretions generally found lying underneath the foreskin) easier. Several research teams have found an increase in the incidence of UTIs as the number of circumcisions declined (Schoen et al, 2000; see section on neonatal UTI). Circumcision requires surgical intervention and causes discomfort. Neonatal local anesthesia should be used to reduce the discomfort. Parents should be taught to observe the penis for any drainage or bleeding. They should receive an explanation about the Plastibell clamp, if it is left in place, including how long it will be on the penis and the fact that it will fall off. They need to be shown how to cleanse the penis without introducing bacteria.

ACUTE RENAL FAILURE

Pathophysiology

Acute renal failure is defined as an abrupt severe decrease or complete halt of kidney function. Neonatal renal failure is suspected when urinary output falls below 1 ml/kg/hr and is accompanied by serum creatinine levels greater than 1.5 mg/dl and BUN greater than 20 mg/dl. Because the placenta functioned as the major excretory organ in utero, symptoms of renal in the newborn may take several days to manifest. Therefore manifestation of renal failure in the newborn may have occurred in utero because of congenital renal abnormality or adverse birth events in normal kidneys. Any condition that interferes with kidney function can lead to acute renal failure (Table 33-4). Acute renal failure has been estimated to affect as many as 23% of all neonates admitted to an intensive care unit (Brion et al, 1997).

Acute renal failure occurs in three forms: prerenal, intrarenal (intrinsic), and postrenal. Prerenal failure results from inadequate systemic and/or renal blood flow that in turn leads to renal hypoperfusion. Hypoxia plays a large role in the development of the acute prerenal type of renal failure. Persistence of hypoxia leads to shunting of blood away from the kidneys.

TABLE 33-4	Major Causes of Acute Renal Failure in the Newborn	
Prerenal Failure	**Intrinsic Renal Failure**	**Postrenal Failure**
Systemic hypovolemia	Acute tubular necrosis	Congenital malformations
Fetal/neonatal hemorrhage	Congenital malformations	Imperforate anus
Septic shock	Bilateral agenesis	Urethral stricture
Necrotizing enterocolitis	Renal dysplasia	Posterior urethral valves
Dehydration	Polycystic kidney disease	Urethral diverticulum
Renal hypo-perfusion	Glomerular immaturity	Primary vesi-coureteral
Perinatal asphyxia	Infection	Reflux
Congestive heart failure	Congenital syphilis	Ureterocele
Cardiac surgery	Toxoplasmosis	Megacystis
Respiratory distress syndrome	Pyelonephritis	megaureter
	Renal vascular	Eagle-Barrett
Pharmacologic	Renal artery thrombosis	syndrome
Tolazoline	Renal venous thrombosis	(Prune-belly syndrome)
Captopril	Disseminated intravascular coagulation	Ureteropelvic junction obstruction
Indomethacin	Nephrotoxins	Extrinsic compression
	Aminoglycosides	Sacrococcygeal teratoma
	Indomethacin	Hematocolpos
	Amphotericin B	Intrinsic
	Contrast media	obstruction
	Intrarenal obstruction	Renal calculi
	Uric acid nephropathy	Fungus balls
	Myoglobinuria	Neurogenic bladder
	Hemoglobinuria	

Vogt BA, Avner ED (2002). *The kidney and urinary tract.* In Fanaroff AA, Martin RJ (Eds.), Neonatal-perinatal medicine: diseases of the fetus and infant, *ed 7, St Louis: Mosby.*

Renal hypoperfusion occurs. When blood pressure decreases, GFR and subsequently urine output decrease. Prerenal failure is the most common type of neonatal renal failure and responds positively to treatment with early identification. Reversing the effects of hypovolemia and hypotension may prevent the occurrence of renal damage and resultant intrinsic renal failure. Intrinsic renal failure results from parenchymal injury. It can result from progression of prerenal and postrenal failure. Other causes include infection, nephrotoxicity, renal vein thrombosis, or acute tubular necrosis. Intrinsic renal failure occurs in three phases: initiation, maintenance, and recovery. During the initiation phase, an insult occurs that leads to tubular cell injury. Sustained decreased GFR, and azotemia occur in the maintenance phase. How long the maintenance phase will last depends on the severity and duration of the initial insult. A gradual return to normal GFR and tubular function occurs during the recovery phase. The pathophysiol-ogy of intrinsic renal failure is often related to impairment in glomerular capillary filtration, tubular obstruction, and back-leak of glomerular filtrate. Glomerular capillary filtration is thought to be impaired by a change in glomerular permeability. Glomerular permeability can be affected because of a reduction in size and number of endothelial fenestrations and fusion of podocytes. Severely damaged cells separate from the basement membrane and slough into the tubular lumen. This leads to obstruction that then results in increased tubular pressure that eventually culminates in a reduction in GFR. Back leakage of filtrate results in nitrogenous waste and creatinine returning to circulation.

Postrenal failure is usually caused by congenital anomalies that obstruct the flow of urine. These anomalies include ureteropelvic junction and urethrovesical obstruction, prune-belly syndrome, and neurogenic bladder. A back-up of urine into the kidney pelvis inhibits the ability of the kidneys to function. If this condition persists, fluid permanently fills the tissue spaces with resultant hydronephrosis. Damage can occur as early as the sixteenth to eighteenth weeks of gestation. Hydronephrosis may be nonreversible, thus leading to renal failure in one or both kidneys. Obstructive uropathies can most often be diagnosed with antenatal testing and thereby treated before significant renal damage occurs (Roth et al, 2001; Saphier et al, 2000). Oliguria of the fetus leads to oligohydramnios, which may be detected on maternal physical examination. Familial tendency for some renal disorders may suggest that antenatal testing for fetal renal disease be performed in identified groups. Table 33-5 provides a list of diagnostic indices for neonatal acute renal failure.

Risk Factors
Treatments such as mechanical ventilation and umbilical and femoral vessel catheterization may predispose the infant to renal failure because of renal vein and artery thrombosis. Birth injury, hypovolemia, and hypoxemia may compromise renal blood flow. Congenital causes of intrinsic renal failure include aplastic kidney, polycystic renal disease, necrosis, and maternal ingestion of nephrotoxic agents. Other infants at risk for renal disease include premature infants and infants with respiratory distress syndrome or trisomy defects and other genetic disorders. Prenatal exposure to various drugs has been linked with renal insufficiency and acute renal failure in the first few days of postnatal life of the premature infant (Brock et al, 1998). Maternal use of certain drugs has also been implicated in the development of neonatal renal failure. Excessive prenatal use of acetaminophen can lead to nephrotoxic effects in the fetus.

Differential Diagnosis
Acute renal failure is a manifestation of many other problems. The diagnosis is aimed at identifying the causative agent and is not simply limited to determining the presence of acute renal failure. The specific diagnostic tests are determined by the contributing process suspected by the practitioner. This hypothesis requires a thorough nursing assessment in conjunction with an aggressive medical work-up.

Clinical Manifestations
Decreased urine output, edema, and lethargy are clinical signs that may point to acute renal failure. Oliguria is the most significant sign of acute renal failure, but a high output failure also occurs. Edema is usually caused by fluid overload rather than by

TABLE **33-5**	Diagnostic Indices in Neonatal Acute Renal Failure	
	Prerenal Oliguria without Renal Failure	**Prerenal and Intrinsic Renal Failure**
Serum Findings		
Na	Normal or elevated	Low normal or elevated
K	Normal or elevated	Normal or elevated
BUN	Normal or elevated	Elevated
Creatinine	Normal or elevated	Elevated
Ca	Normal	Low
P	Normal	Normal or elevated
Urine Findings		
RBC, protein, casts, and tubular cell casts	Usually absent	Present
Specific gravity	Increased	Low
Urine volume	Low	Low in 60% to 80% (1 ml/kg/hr), normal or high in 40% (>2.4 ml/kg/hr)
Urine osmolarity (mOsm/kg water)	Increased >300 to 400	Decreased <300
Urine Na (mEq/L)	<30 mEq/L (preterm infant) <20 mEq/L	>30 mEq/L
Creatinine clearance	Normal or decreased	Decreased
U/P creatinine	>20:1	<10:1
U/P urea	>20:1	<10:1
U/P osmolarity	<1.5:1	>1.5:1
FE_{Na}%	<1% (term infant) <3% (preterm infant)	>2% (term infant) >3% (preterm infant)
RFI	<3%	>3%

U/P, urine:plasma ratio; RFI, renal failure index; BUN, blood urea nitrogen
Modified from John EG, Yeh TF (1985). Renal failure. In Yeh TF (Ed.), Drug therapy in the neonate and small infant, Chicago: Year Book Medical Publishers. Reprinted with permission.

the condition itself. Hematuria and proteinuria are common signs of failure. Some neonates also present with abdominal distention or a flank mass. Because hypoperfusion of the kidneys may be common in the neonate, efforts should be made to determine the cause of the oliguria. In true renal failure, hematuria and hemoglobinuria may occur. Urine-to-plasma osmolality ratio of 1:1 or less may indicate renal failure. Renal compromise can be detected even in utero through evaluation of fetal urine samples. The maximum fetal urine electrolyte levels considered within normal limits are sodium, 100 mEq/L; chloride, 90 mEq/L; and osmolality, 210 mOsm/kg. Levels greater than these values are indicative of renal failure and poor prognosis. BUN and serum creatinine levels increase.

Urine output should be at least 1 ml/kg/hour. Urine output, at least initially, may be within normal limits. The use of diuretics may alter the results of urine tests, thus causing decreased specific gravity (dilute urine) and changes in urine electrolytes (increased loss of potassium with loop or thiazide diuretics and increased loss of chloride ions). Diuretic use should be documented when renal function studies are performed. Shock and volume depletion should always be evaluated when oliguria results. In the presence of open or draining congenital anomalies, hidden fluid losses may occur. Surgery to repair defects can lead to third spacing of fluids, leaving the infant further fluid-compromised.

Complications of renal failure include hyperkalemia, volume overload, hyponatremia, hypertension, acidosis, hypocalcemia, hyperphosphatemia, sepsis, anemia, azotemia (increased level of nitrogenous waste products in the blood), and nutritional compromise.

The blood pressure may at first decrease and then rebound to an above-normal level. Hypertension, or a blood pressure of greater than 90/65 mm/Hg in fullterm infants, is often the result of fluid overload or increased secretion of renin and aldosterone. Less common signs of renal failure are usually due to hypoxemia. Seizures, for example, may follow, as may intraventricular hemorrhage or cerebral edema.

Prognosis
The prognosis of acute renal failure depends solely on the ability to treat the underlying problem. Early detection—sometimes even in utero—and treatment of acute renal failure guide the treatment course, possibly preventing life-threatening complications.

Collaborative Management
The treatment aims to prevent the long-term complications of acute renal failure. Symptomatic treatment is administered until a definitive cause is determined and treated. Once absence of a urinary obstruction is established, a fluid challenge to intravenous isotonic solution, 10 to 20 ml/kg given over 1 hour, may be helpful in differentiating prerenal from intrinsic failure. If urine output is at least 1 ml/kg/hr within two hours of the fluid infusion, the cause of the renal failure is probably related to hypoperfusion. Use of a diuretic after the fluid challenge may be necessary if urine output does not increase immediately after the fluid challenge. To treat prerenal renal failure, low-dose dopamine may also be tried in an attempt to increase renal perfusion.

Fluid replacement depends on the type of renal failure the infant exhibits. If intrinsic failure exists, fluid replacement is limited to insensible loss and replacement of renal output. If the infant is acidotic, sodium acetate may be used instead of sodium chloride in intravenous solutions. Sodium bicarbonate should be used with caution because it is hypertonic and has been found to increase intracranial pressure and resultant intraventricular hemorrhage and may also cause a transient hypercarbia.

Peritoneal dialysis or hemodialysis should be used only in infants with severe congestive heart failure, fluid overload, or uremia. Peritoneal dialysis seems to be the method of choice in neonatal care. Either method can be used within the neonatal intensive care unit; however, expert professionals must be in charge of this procedure because close monitoring of the infant's status is needed. The cycle of dialysis infusion, dwell time, and release—as well as the accurate measurement of fluid intake and output and serum electrolyte levels—is critical. Exact parameters of dialysis are beyond the scope of this text.

Drugs with high sodium levels—such as carbenicillin, penicillin G, ampicillin, and cephalothin—or drugs diluted in sodium chloride should be used with caution in patients with renal failure because they may add to the problem of maintaining fluid and electrolyte balance.

Nursing assessment is critical in prompt identification of renal failure. Accurate calculation of fluid intake and output is vital in guarding against fluid overload and resultant hypertension and edema. Nurses should also remember that potassium affects cardiac conduction. Therefore, because these neonates may experience hyperkalemia, all intake of potassium must be eliminated. This measure includes the use of only fresh blood for transfusions because the older the blood, the more likely the cells are to have broken down and release potassium. Calcium gluconate (10%) or calcium carbonate helps decrease the effect of potassium on the heart. Acidosis is inevitable, and its management is complicated by the need to restrict sodium.

Increased serum phosphorus and decreased calcium levels are treated by protein restriction. Calcium supplementation and phosphorus-binding substances may be needed. Anemia is a potential consequence of renal failure. The infant's hematocrit value and/or hemoglobin level must be serially measured at least daily. Changes in the vital signs or color should be assessed so that subtle changes that indicate anemia may be detected.

Hypertension secondary to fluid overload may be treated by sodium and fluid restriction. Antihypertensive agents may also be effective in management. These infants are prone to infections. The infant should be monitored for signs of infection and any abnormality reported so that treatment is begun immediately.

Because the kidney is the clearinghouse for many drugs, the metabolism of drugs is altered when renal failure occurs. Aminoglycosides, penicillins, cephalosporins, theophylline, indomethacin, tolazoline, and magnesium should all be used with caution.

Nutritional needs for the infant are 1 to 1.5 g/kg/day of protein with 30 to 50 cal/kg/day. Vitamin D, vitamin B complex, and folic acid supplements may be needed. If the infant is taking enteral nutrition some institutions recommend feedings, breast milk, Similac PM 60/40, and SMA because of their decreased sodium, potassium, and phosphorus loads.

Nursing Management

If the infant's condition continues to deteriorate and high BUN levels coupled with increasing ammonia levels are present, dialysis may be necessary. This procedure may be performed in the NICU and necessitates one-on-one nursing care. The dialyzing cycle depends on the medical treatment and the severity of the condition. Nursing responsibility includes monitoring the equipment, monitoring the cycles if performed manually, performing clotting studies, and administering heparin and other drugs via the dialysis setup. Either hemodialysis or peritoneal dialysis may be performed. Catheter care includes maintenance of aseptic technique, prevention of hemorrhage and clotting, and observation of the insertion site for signs of infection or dislodgment. The nurse should observe for signs and symptoms of chemical imbalances during the entire dialysis procedure. Fluid shifts affecting blood pressure and electrolyte balance can occur rapidly and cause cardiac arrhythmias, muscle spasms, seizures, and shock.

POTTER'S ASSOCIATION (POTTER'S SYNDROME)

Pathophysiology

Potter's syndrome is an association of defects and begins with bilateral renal agenesis. For this reason, the word *association* is generally replacing the term *syndrome*. It occurs when the ureteric bud fails to divide and develop, culminating the complete absence of the kidney. Because fetal urine is a major component of amniotic fluid, especially in the third trimester, oligohydramnios is present. In the severest form, no amniotic fluid may be present. The developing fetal structures are compressed as a result of this lack of fluid, thus leading to the characteristic Potter facies (Potter, 1965).

Clinical Manifestations

A typical appearance of the facies includes low set, malformed ears and micrognathia, "senile" appearance, wrinkled skin, parrot-beak nose, and eyes that are wide-set with obvious epicanthal folds (Potter, 1965). Other associated defects include abnormal genital development, leg deformities, GI defects, and arthrogryposis, a condition associated with contractures of the extremities (Chapter 32).

Infants may be premature or stillborn. The infant is usually born in the breech position and is small-for-gestational-age. In the absence of severe respiratory compromise, oliguria or anuria may be the only presenting symptoms.

Risk Factors

The incidence of Potter's association is approximately 1 in 10,000 births, predominantly in males. Although no strong genetic predisposition exists, a multifactorial inheritance pattern has been suggested. Evidence that siblings of infants with Potter's association have a higher-than-average incidence of neural tube defects does exist

Differential Diagnosis

Potter's association is usually readily identifiable on direct observation because of its characteristic facies. Most often, no other diagnosis is even considered. Potter's association is also a part of the XYY syndrome.

Prognosis

The infant may die within the first several days of life because of lack of kidney tissue to support life. Because of the association of renal agenesis with lung hypoplasia, death often occurs as the result of respiratory insufficiency. The exact reason the lungs do not fully develop in the presence of renal agenesis has eluded researchers. Researchers have hypothesized that pulmonary development depends on adequate levels of amniotic fluid. This principle has been demonstrated in fetuses with esophageal atresia or other defects that interfered with fetal swallowing. Although the circulation of the amniotic fluid was disrupted, the amount of fluid was normal; therefore, lung development followed the usual course. If the fluid was diminished or scanty, as with Potter's association, the pulmonary development was disrupted.

It is hypothesized that a mechanical element that stops or slows alveolar development may be involved. The fetal kidney may secrete a substance that assists lung development. Researchers have demonstrated that when damage to the metanephros of the kidney occurs, the substance arginase is not produced. Arginase is necessary for the conversion of ornithine to proline; the latter substance is required for mesenchymal development and thus the development of the bronchial and alveolar tree. Because of irreversible pulmonary hypoplasia, current treatment of neonates with Potter's association does not include renal transplantation or long-term dialysis.

Collaborative and Nursing Management

Focus on the parents is the most important aspect of nursing care. Denial and feelings of guilt are usual and are often a necessary defense mechanism in the first few days. The nurse should encourage parents to visit and hold their children. If one or both parents choose not be involved with the infant, they should be supported in their choice. Grandparents need support as well because they often feel guilt because they could not shield their children from this "hurt" (Chapter 8).

RENAL APLASIA

Pathophysiology

When the ureteric bud fails to form in utero, aplasia or absence of the kidney occurs. One kidney develops, but the other kidney does not. This is also called unilateral renal agenesis.

Risk Factors

The rate of occurrence may be as high as 1 in 500 births. It is most often associated with other structural defects, such as spinal deviations—especially scoliosis, imperforate anus, and, in the female, uterine and vaginal agenesis (Kaplan, 1994). No specific inheritance pattern is noted.

Clinical Manifestations

The infant may be asymptomatic if no renal disease is present in the unaffected kidney. Renal function of a single kidney is sufficient to support life. However, if the remaining kidney is dysfunctional, the infant may exhibit signs of renal problems. The exact symptoms exhibited are directly associated with the infant's particular renal problem.

Differential Diagnosis

The differential diagnosis centers on the confirmation of the presence of a single kidney. This determination is best made by renal ultrasonography.

Prognosis

The prognosis for survival with a single kidney is excellent if the remaining kidney is disease-free.

Collaborative and Nursing Management

The major focus of care is preparation of the infant and family for preliminary testing. If kidney function is not compromised, no nursing care beyond normal newborn care may be necessary. The sections on the specific disorders contain more information on nursing management to be implemented if kidney disease is found. This condition often goes undetected in the newborn period because no symptoms may be exhibited.

CYSTIC KIDNEY DISEASE

Pathophysiology

Cystic disease of the kidney involves replacement of normal kidney mass with cysts. The amount of cystic formation within each or both kidneys determines the severity of the disease. If the kidney is severely affected, ureteral agenesis may also exist. Cystic disease includes a variety of disorders, such as polycystic disease and multicystic disease.

Infantile polycystic disease is a genetic autosomal recessive disease. The cystic lesions occur in the collecting and result in the inability to concentrate urine. Cystic lesions may also occur in the liver, bile duct, and pancreas. Infantile polycystic disease generally involves both kidneys and has a poor prognosis related to pulmonary hypoplasia and respiratory failure. If these infants survive beyond the neonatal period, renal failure becomes a less common finding. Congenital hepatic fibrosis and bilateral dysgenesis is also usually present in these infants. Adult-type polycystic disease is an autosomal dominant disease that leads to serious renal compromise and death. It is rarely seen in infants.

Multicystic kidney disease is a noninherited disorder. It usually follows an obstructive uropathy in utero and is most often unilateral. Back-up of urine causes the fluid-filled kidney mass to develop into cystic lesions.

Risk Factors

No specific risk factors exist for the development of this complex of dysfunctions. Either of these types of family inheritance patterns should be considered a risk for the development of cystic kidney disease.

Clinical Manifestations

In the newborn, the abdomen may be enlarged and have an apparent palpable mass. The mass may not be perceived as a kidney, because the cystic lesions distort its normal shape. In single-kidney cystic disease, normal urine output is maintained. The affected kidney has a high potential for infection, owing to urinary stasis. Albuminuria occurs in polycystic kidney disease.

Differential Diagnosis

Cystic kidney disease must be differentiated from hydronephrosis, Wilms' tumor, and anatomic deformities. Palpation alone cannot lead to an accurate diagnosis. Ultrasonography and pyelography are necessary to differentiate between normal renal mass and cystic lesions. These tests should be delayed until the infant is 48 hours old to allow the neonate to become hydrated and to restore the fluid balance after birth. This delay helps in the detection of possible hydronephrosis or cystic kidney disease. Voiding cystography should be performed in infants highly suspected of having cystic disease. A renal scan helps differentiate between ureteropelvic junction obstruction and multicystic kidney disease. In multicystic kidney disease, the radioactive isotope is concentrated in a mass, whereas in ureteropelvic junction obstruction, the isotope continues on into the renal pelvis.

Prognosis

The prognosis is poor for infantile polycystic disease. The prognosis for multicystic disease directly depends on the severity of kidney damage. In addition, infants with multicystic disease are at greater risk for later development of Wilms' tumor, a malignancy with a relatively poor prognosis. More research is needed in tracking this possible relationship.

Tissue hypertrophy in the contralateral, normal kidney begins at birth. This increase in renal tissue increases the functional ability of the kidney. Thus the body compensates for the loss of one kidney.

Collaborative Management

Treatment entails complete or partial nephrectomy of the affected kidney. The treatment for single-kidney cystic disease is complete nephrectomy because the diseased kidney may continue to harbor infection. This infection may spread to the unaffected kidney. A partial nephrectomy may be performed if sufficient unaffected renal mass is found. If the cystic disease results from ureteropelvic junction obstruction, pyeloplasty has been successful. In either case, careful medical and nursing management follows the surgical intervention.

Nursing Management

The health professional must thoroughly assess the infant for the presence of a mass, which is usually in the flank area. If Wilms' tumor is suspected, no palpation should be performed. Manipulation can cause the tumor to break up and spread. If urine output is normal, careful consideration of the fluid intake and output may not be necessary; if renal function is compromised, strict attention must be paid to fluid balance. Electrolyte status should be monitored at least daily. Urine should be checked for the presence of albumin. Because hydronephrosis may be present, hematuria is also a consideration. Before surgery, a complete blood count with differential and a urine culture should be obtained to rule out presence of urinary tract infection.

Hypertension has been documented in this condition. It is believed that the blood pressure change is related to decreased arterial renal perfusion and to concomitant elevations in renin levels. A nephrectomy reverses this trend.

If the infant undergoes a complete nephrectomy, strict adherence to aseptic technique must be followed. Because the infant is prone to infection, vital signs should be monitored at least every 2 to 4 hours after the immediate postoperative period. Any dressings should be inspected for the presence of bloody drainage or secretions. Initially, a small amount of bleeding at the site is common, but it should be short-lived. No urine drainage should be noted on the dressing because the entire kidney has been removed. Abdominal decompression is often necessary to prevent distention that could cause pressure and pull the suture line apart. If a nasogastric tube is in place, it should be irrigated with 2 ml of saline or air every 2 to 4 hours to maintain patency. Feedings may be resumed once bowel sounds can be auscultated and the nasogastric tube has been removed. Feedings are usually tolerated 2 to 3 days after surgery.

PRUNE-BELLY SYNDROME (EAGLE-BARRETT SYNDROME)

Pathophysiology

An infant born with prune-belly syndrome has a congenital lack of appropriate abdominal musculature, undescended testicles, and urinary tract malformations (Brion et al, 1997). The abdominal muscles may be so weakened that the abdominal region actually appears wrinkled, much like a prune's surface. It typically affects males; in females, the true syndrome does not exist. Pseudohermaphroditism may be associated with prune-belly syndrome, or it may even be the diagnosis of record in the female. The incidence rate is approximately 1 in every 50,000 births. The associated urinary problems include an enlarged bladder and dilated, curved ureters. Dilation of the ureter is referred to as megaureter (primary reflux megaureter). This condition can be diagnosed before birth via ultrasonography. It is not always associated only with prune-belly syndrome but can be due to infection or other accompanying renal anomalies. Kidney development may have been diminished, thus

resulting in hypoplastic kidneys. A patent urachus may also be associated with this anomaly. Other associated problems include hip and feet deformities, respiratory insufficiency, imperforate anus, and cardiac anomalies. Spinal deformities may result from imbalance of muscle pull.

No clear cause for prune-belly syndrome is known, but the defect may occur between the 23rd day and the 10th week of fetal development. During this time period, the bladder is taking shape and being separated from the allantois, and the abdominal wall is forming. The question arises as to whether the obstruction of the urethra causes back-up of urine and thus causes bladder distention and ultimately muscle deformity or whether musculature defects lead to the obstructive uropathies.

Risk Factors

No clear-cut genetic predisposition for this syndrome exists. The presence of oligohydramnios suggests a renal problem. Ultrasound examination may reveal bladder distention and dilated ureters, again leading only to a highly suspicious status of the renal system. No other clear risk factors are known to precipitate this syndrome. Maternal use of cocaine, however, has been documented as a known teratogen that results in prune-belly syndrome, among other GU anomalies.

Clinical Manifestations

The musculature defect may be small or may cover the entire surface of the abdomen. Although all layers of musculature are present, the degree of development of these muscle layers varies. A thin layer of subcutaneous tissue, coupled with distention, gives the abdomen a wrinkled appearance. Cryptorchidism (undescended testes), prostatic urethral dilation, bladder distention, patent urachus, abdominal distention or protuberance, malrotation of the intestines, cardiac defects, congenital hip dysplasia and associated "click," and clubfoot (talipes equinovarus) are some of the other associated clinical findings. Not all of these disorders are present in all infants, but they should be considered as potential problems.

Differential Diagnosis

Prune-belly syndrome may be obvious on observation. However, other conditions can result in abdominal distention and apparent weakened abdominal musculature. Any infant with severe uropathy and urethral obstruction may also demonstrate these signs. Differentiation should be made by palpation of bladder distention, as opposed to the finding of distended bowel loops. The latter would indicate an intestinal rather than a renal problem. Underlying renal disease must be distinguished from abdominal muscle defects with accompanying renal dysfunction. The exact nature of the renal problem, the degree to which renal function is compromised, and the other deformities that might also be present must be determined. The exact diagnosis can be made only when a demonstrable lack of abdominal musculature is present.

Prognosis

The prognosis is directly related to the degree of severity of the underlying renal dysfunction. Half of infants with prune-belly syndrome will die in the first two years of life if severe renal dysfunction or chronic renal failure is present.

Collaborative Management

This triadic anomaly leads to severe urinary tract complications. The condition of the kidney can range from normal kidney mass to complete atresia. In many cases, dilation of the ureter, bladder, and urethra occurs and may be caused by a lack of muscle fiber in the lining of the structures. The lack of muscle in the ureters leads to their elongation and distention. If obstruction occurs as a result of the tortuous nature of the ureters, surgical intervention may be necessary. Reimplantation or diversion may be necessary to prevent urine stasis and renal failure.

Obstruction of the urethra may be caused by angulation that results from a lack of musculature in the urethra or by an obstructive action that results from a distention of the enlarged prostatic urethra. Surgical correction may not achieve bladder functioning, because bladder atonia persists.

Undescended testes accompany this syndrome. Orchiopexy may be performed, but it has not been found to improve fertility in the adult who has survived with prune-belly syndrome. Testosterone levels have been found to be adequate in two thirds of men studied.

Bladder decompression is necessary for the prevention of stasis. A skilled practitioner should perform catheterization to prevent trauma to the distorted urethra and bladder. Any severe abdominal distention and insufficient urinary output in the first day of life observed by the nurse should be evaluated by other members of the health care team to rule out the possibility of this syndrome. A large amount of urine may have accumulated in the fetal period and may result in a greatly distended bladder. Renal dysplasia, an abnormal development of the kidney or its associated structures, is common in more than half of the infants born with prune-belly syndrome. It is most commonly seen as aplastic kidneys and multicystic disease.

A nephrostomy or ureterostomy diversion should be considered if urine drainage is compromised. Because peristalsis may be absent or deficient, a vesicostomy may allow temporary drainage until the infant can tolerate extensive surgical intervention. Long-term use of antimicrobial therapy may be necessary to prevent sepsis. In the presence of a patent urachus (fetal communication between the bladder and umbilicus), closure may not be necessary in the neonatal period if adequate drainage and prevention of infection can be maintained. If the bladder is distended, reduction cystoplasty is performed to relieve the tension on the bladder and to promote emptying.

Long-term therapy includes exercise, use of abdominal binders, and reconstructive surgery. Although not curative, these methods provide some palliative benefit to the appearance and function of the distended and sagging abdomen.

The effects of renal damage that occur in the early stages of life require careful attention to fluid and electrolyte balance, removal of wastes, and adequate nutrition for growth and development. Growing children should be monitored for adequate growth and calcification of bones because both depend on good renal functioning. Frequent hospitalizations may be necessary during childhood. Parents need to be prepared for this and need to be assisted with financial as well as psychosocial support.

Nursing Management

The focus of nursing management is assessment and maintenance of renal functioning. Fluid intake and output should be strictly measured and recorded. If an appliance is used, skin surfaces must be kept clean and dry. The use of adhesives may be necessary to prevent leakage that results from skin folds and wrinkling around the stoma. Turning and repositioning every 2 hours also helps decrease skin breakdown. Bladder decompression may be accomplished by intermittent catheterization or the Crede© method. The Crede© method may be sufficient to empty the bladder. This method involves the practitioner's

placing both hands under the infant's flank area and bringing the thumbs together at the umbilicus. Pressure is gently applied, and the thumbs are rolled downward from the umbilicus to the symphysis pubis.

If bladder distention and urinary retention continue to occur until the infant is discharged, parents must be taught a method of emptying the bladder. This may involve the Crede© method or intermittent catheterization. Parents must be taught the signs and symptoms of a UTI—including increased irritability with urination, temperature instability, increase or decrease in urine output, and cloudy or foul-smelling urine. They must understand the importance of early detection and intervention to prevent long-term renal compromise. The vesicostomy has been found to be an effective treatment to prevent urinary stasis and infection before reconstruction of this and other cloacal anomalies. If a vesicostomy or other urinary diversion has been performed, specific instructions are necessary to prevent bladder contamination. Stoma care is another aspect of parent education and discharge planning.

Lack of abdominal musculature also can lead to constipation, even in the newborn period. Long-term suppository use and bowel training may be necessary. Feedings should not promote distention and respiratory compromise. Parents should be well-informed of dietary approaches to help promote appropriate GI functioning. Consideration for parental feelings must also center on the physical appearance of their baby. Because the American culture places great value on appearance, it may be difficult for parents to accept the loss of their "perfect" dream baby. Parental support is a must. A good strategy for increasing the parent-infant interaction is to include them as much as possible in the daily care of their infants.

EXSTROPHY OF THE BLADDER

Pathophysiology

In exstrophy of the bladder, the anterior abdominal wall fails to close at the point of the bladder. During the first 4 weeks of gestation, the abdominal wall begins to fuse. When the mesenchymal cells fail to migrate over the abdomen, exstrophy results. A thin membrane forms over the abdominal contents, which may later rupture and leave the bladder exposed.

Risk Factors

The incidence of this defect is 1 in 24,000 to 40,000 live births, with males being affected more than females. Exact risk factors are not known, because exstrophy of the bladder is just one of many exstrophies of the cloacal membrane.

Clinical Manifestations

This condition is obvious on visual inspection. The bladder region appears open or uncovered. Because of the failure of the abdominal and anterior bladder wall to close, the posterior wall of the bladder is exposed. The implantation of the ureters may be visible as urine continues to pass from the orifices. A concomitant defect exists in the genitalia. In the male, the penis may be short, flat, and angulated. Epispadias may occur to the extent that proper sex identification may be difficult. In the female, the labia do not meet in the midline, and a divided clitoris exists. Prolapse of the rectum may also be evident with this condition and may occur through the abdominal wall defect, thus requiring an intestinal diversion. The failure of the pubic bones to meet anteriorly may lead to hip and leg deformities. Neurospinal defects, omphalocele, and other chromosomal abnormalities may also occur with this defect.

Differential Diagnosis

The diagnosis of exstrophy of the bladder may be determined on visual inspection. However, the concomitantly occurring deformities, as mentioned previously, must be assessed.

Prognosis

The exact prognosis is directly related to the presence of other deformities. In and of itself, exstrophy of the bladder has a good prognosis for survival. However, the infant may have chronic problems. If this condition has been associated with intestinal problems that led to an ileostomy, it may or may not be permanent, depending on the degree of severe intestinal malformation. As for the renal system, the infant may have permanent incontinence. An ileal conduit may be permanent. Neurologic or orthopedic deformities require consultation from health care professionals in these specialties and again may result in chronic problems.

Collaborative Management

If the infant with exstrophy of the bladder must be transported to a tertiary center for treatment, the exstrophy is covered with plastic wrap or a similar material to protect the open area. Before surgical correction, the defect is covered with a petroleum dressing and sufficient gauze to absorb urine flow. Dressing should be changed as needed to prevent skin irritation occurs. Extreme dryness of the skin should be prevented as it promotes skin breakdown. Incubator humidification helps to prevent excess drying. Diapers should be kept folded well below the defect if wound infections are to be avoided.

Because bladder extrophy exposes the urinary tract to the environment, care attention should be given to prevention of infection in these infants before and after surgical correction of the defect. Some infants may not have the defect closed during initial hospitalization and require that dressings continue to be used at home. Parents must be taught the principles of skin management and the importance of the regularity of the changes as a method of preventing infection.

Primary closure of the defect is usually performed in the neonatal period. Some institutions perform a staged approach to closure and correction of genital defects. Closure in some cases may be delayed for a year or longer without serious complications. Before surgery is performed, broad-spectrum antibiotic therapy (ampicillin and gentamicin) is initiated to give protection against infections. This therapy is continued for at least 7 days after surgery because 42% of wound dehiscence is caused by infections. Strict observation of aseptic technique is essential. If infection is suspected, aggressive treatment should be started.

Surgical correction of the defect does not guarantee continence. In some cases, urinary diversion or use of ileal conduits may be necessary. In the infant with concomitant neurospinal defects, continence might never be achieved. The nurse may need to coordinate follow-up by surgical, medical, and neurosurgical teams. Long-term follow-up may include the use of social services and financial counseling.

Nursing Management

Care of the infant with an exposed bladder includes protection as well as output measurement. Petroleum jelly-impregnated gauze should be used to protect the moist surface from trauma or drying. Preweighed gauze dressings can be used to collect and measure urine output. If accurate output measurement is not necessary, diapers may be used to collect urine drainage. If rectal prolapse has occurred through the abdominal defect, separate dressings should be maintained, if possible.

Parents should be told what to expect after surgery. Although closure of the abdominal defect may be accomplished in one stage, repair of the epispadias is performed when the child is older. If closure is delayed for a period of time, parents must be taught how to dress and care for the defect.

HYDRONEPHROSIS

Pathophysiology

Hydronephrosis is the accumulation of urine within the renal pelvis and calices to the point of overdistention. Hydronephrosis often follows obstruction of urine flow at the junction of the ureteropelvis, the ureterovesical valve, or the urethrovesical valve. Nonobstructive lesions such as vesicourethral reflux, multicystic kidneys, and abnormalities of the ureteropelvic and ureterovesical junction can cause hydronephrosis. The buildup of fluid that then accumulates in the kidney leads to distention of the renal pelvis and damage of the kidney mass. If only one ureter is affected, then damage occurs to that kidney only and leaves the other capable of supporting life. Removing the source of the urinary obstruction before permanent renal damage has occurred has been beneficial in treating hydronephrosis.

Prenatal prevention of hydronephrosis is possible in some circumstances. Fetal surgery is possible; this practice can relieve the obstruction in utero by placing a catheter into the bladder to drain the urine, thus preventing the infant from being born with permanently damaged kidneys (Figure 33-6). After birth, definitive surgery is performed to correct the obstructive defect or to provide a diversion of urine flow. Early detection is necessary because damage to the kidneys may occur as early as the fourth month of gestation (Chapter 13).

Risk Factors

The presence of a urinary tract infection may result in an inflammatory response so severe that urinary obstruction and ultimately hydronephrosis occur. Renal or GU tumors or masses may precipitate this condition. Maternal oligohydramnios suggests renal obstruction and may accompany hydronephrosis. Any factor or condition that potentially obstructs renal or urinary flow may contribute to the development of hydronephrosis.

Clinical Manifestations

Antenatal ultrasound after 16 weeks assists in the early detection of fetal renal anomaly by providing an anatomic view of the system as well as by detecting abnormalities in amniotic fluid volume (Saphier et al, 2000). In the newborn, hydronephrosis may be detected as a large, solid, palpable smooth mass at the region of the kidney. Urine output may be decreased or normal, depending on the amount of functioning kidney mass. If only one kidney is involved, urine output may be normal because a single kidney is sufficient for adequate removal of water and waste. UTI often accompanies hydronephrosis and makes fever and discomfort observable signs. Gross hematuria may be present and must be differentiated from the hematuria associated with Wilms' tumor and renal vein thrombosis.

Differential Diagnosis

Clinical diagnostic studies include pyelography, ultrasonography, and computed tomography. Intravenous pyelograms may

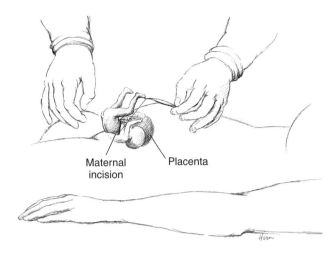

Maternal incision   Placenta

FIGURE **33-6**
Fetal surgery to prevent hydronephrosis.

not be definitive in that interpretation of the results could indicate nonexistence of the kidney because the fluid-filled mass does not readily pick up the dye. The kidney outline can be determined with retrograde pyelography. Before drastic reparative procedures are attempted, respiratory status must be assessed. During fetal life, oligohydramnios and distention of the abdomen can precipitate a cessation of growth of the respiratory tree.

Because many different forms of abdominal masses may occur, determination of the origin of the mass is essential. This condition must be differentiated from cystic kidney disease, urogenital tumors, and renal vein thrombosis (Saphier et al, 2000).

Prognosis

The prognosis for this condition depends on the underlying causative factor and on the degree of severity of the permanent renal damage. If severe renal damage is present, the prognosis is grave. The more kidney damage present, the less likely the infant will survive. However, if only one ureter or kidney is affected, the other kidney should be able to support life.

Collaborative Management

Hydronephrosis is managed according to its cause. In the case of repairable obstructive uropathies, surgical treatment of the cause removes the source of the process, which may reverse itself in time. This correction is usually performed via pyeloplasty and nephrostomy tube insertion for drainage. If surgery is not required, nutritional support may be the only treatment necessary. The nurse should work with the nutritional support team to plan the course of care.

If irreversible damage has occurred to the entire kidney, nephrectomy may be necessary. The hydronephrotic kidney is a source for frequent UTIs. Nephrectomy may be performed in the neonatal period to prevent the occurrence of infection, or it may be delayed until infection becomes a serious problem.

Nursing Management

Careful assessment is necessary for the infant who is thought to have hydronephrosis. First of all, the infant's respiratory status must be determined. The presence of cyanosis, grunting, nasal flaring, and retractions is important because the lungs may not have fully developed. The chest should be observed for any alterations in the anteroposterior diameter or asymmetry. Vital signs, including blood pressure, must be monitored at least every 4 hours—more frequently if they are unstable. The blood pressure is especially important because hypertension is common in the infant with hydronephrosis. If hypertension is severe, antihypertensives may be given. Some institutions use intravenous hydralazine, intravenous diazoxide, or methyldopa. Use of any of these drugs requires extremely close monitoring of the cardiorespiratory system. Fluid and electrolyte status also must be carefully watched. Fluid intake and output should be recorded at least every 2 to 4 hours. Specific gravity may be checked every 4 to 8 hours. A urine dipstick assessment may be useful for determining the presence of protein or blood in the urine. Assessment of hydration status is important. The fontanelles should be observed to determine whether they are sunken or bulging. Skin turgor should demonstrate instant recoil.

Assessment for the presence of any dependent or pitting edema should be performed and recorded. The nurse often detects the early cues that an infant has hydronephrosis. If hydronephrosis is even suspected, the medical team must be notified so that early intervention and prevention of long-term complications can occur. Palpation of the abdomen is also helpful to determine whether a mass is present.

After surgery, a nephrostomy or a urinary stent may be placed and connected to a closed drainage system.

URETERAL OBSTRUCTION

Pathophysiology

Ureteral obstruction occurs when the developing ureter fails to form a tube or the junction of the kidney pelvis or bladder is constricted. Most commonly, the obstruction occurs at the ureteral junction of the kidney pelvis; the second most common site is the junction of the bladder. Unilateral or bilateral obstructions may occur. The result is a back-up of urine into the affected kidney and thus a fluid-filled kidney. In some instances, complete obstruction does not occur, and minimal functioning persists until the child is older and symptomatology increases. Recurrent infection of the urinary tract should be investigated in the young child. The presence of static fluid in the kidney leads to permanent damage of renal tissue. The fluid may be contained in a sac or a cyst-like lesion on the ureter.

Risk Factors

The risk factors for the development of ureteral obstruction are actually the underlying causes of such an impingement. Cystic kidney disease, polycystic kidney disease, ureteropelvic junction obstruction, and urethral atresia are among the most common causes of this entity. Any one of these problems is considered to precipitate urethral obstruction.

Clinical Manifestations

An infant may be asymptomatic unless complete obstruction is present. Delayed voiding or failure to void may be the initial signs of pathology. Hematuria may or may not be present. Because the presence of a blocked ureter may lead to hydronephrosis, an enlarged, palpable kidney may be the first indication of a problem.

Differential Diagnosis

The following determinations must be made: (1) whether urethral obstruction is occurring by itself as urethral atresia; (2) whether hydronephrosis or cystic or polycystic kidney disease is present; and (3) whether a ureteropelvic junction obstruction exists. A radiologic examination after renal scanning or ultrasonography helps definitely differentiate among these entities.

Prognosis

The prognosis depends directly on the severity of kidney damage. The less the damage, the greater the chances for survival if no other lethal conditions are present.

Collaborative Management

Correction or repair of the blocked ureter may lead to reversal of hydronephrosis. If permanent damage has occurred, nephrectomy may be performed. Once surgical correction is completed, long-term medical care is essential for the early detection of chronic renal problems. The nurse should educate parents about the need for follow-up care.

Nursing Management

The nurse must observe for signs of decreasing urine output. The infant may be edematous, thus making good skin care a high priority. Infection may be present and should be treated before any surgical intervention.

HYDROCELE

Pathophysiology

Hydrocele, the collection of fluid in the scrotal sac, is a common finding in the neonate. Hydrocele occurs as the result of the failure of the processus vaginalis to close. At birth, this area is still open; however, during the first few months of postnatal life, this communicating space gradually closes. If small cysts develop along this closure, fluid may be secreted from them. This secretory process leads to the accumulation of fluid between the layers of the tunica vaginalis within the scrotal sac.

Risk Factors

The premature infant and the infant who experiences increased abdominal pressure secondary to manual resuscitation and high ventilatory pressures are at risk for hydrocele. It occurs as fluid accumulation in the scrotal sac through failure of the processus vaginalis to close.

Clinical Manifestations

Fluid accumulation in the scrotum readily transilluminates with the use of a good light source. Palpation reveals no masses. Some infants may have a mass in the groin that fades when abdominal pressure is decreased, such as after an infant stops crying. This mass is most often associated with a hernia, but a hydrocele may exist also. If the defect is large enough, fluid may continue to shift from the abdomen into the scrotal sac and back into the abdomen. As abdominal pressure increases, the shift of fluid becomes unidirectional into the scrotal sac. If the defect is large enough, intestines may also pass into the scrotal sac, thus leading the formation of an inguinal hernia. In rare instances, female infants may have fluid accumulation in the labia that causes edema. They may also experience herniation into the patent passageway, which is called the processus vaginalis.

Differential Diagnosis

Because the hydrocele may be asymptomatic, if it does not occur in conjunction with an inguinal hernia and is not large enough to create observable scrotal swelling, it may be difficult to detect. The "silk glove" test is useful in an older infant but is generally not useful in the neonatal period. In this test, the examiner places pressure on the peritoneal surfaces by rubbing gently on the scrotal tissue that follows the inguinal canal. If a hydrocele is present, the two distinct open layers of tissue should be felt sliding over each other. If the hydrocele is palpable, it feels smooth and is painless. In the neonate, direct observation and transillumination with a strong light source should reveal a lightened area of scrotum where the fluid has accumulated. Observation of the infant during a crying episode, in which the intra-abdominal pressure is the greatest, may also demonstrate a hydrocele or scrotal swelling. If scrotal swelling is detected, the nurse should report this finding immediately to the medical team.

The most important element of the differential diagnosis is distinguishing a hydrocele from an incarcerated inguinal hernia. This distinction can best be made by rectal examination and simultaneous palpation of the inguinal canal. If the examiner encounters loops of intestine near the vas deferens or the ductus deferens within the scrotal sac, an inguinal hernia is present.

Prognosis

The prognosis for infants with hydrocele is excellent.

Collaborative Management

The treatment for hydrocele involves removal of the fluid by the physician. The fluid may be aspirated, or actual tissue removal may be necessary to close the freely communicating space. Treatment is often not attempted until the infant is 1 year of age. Until the hydrocele is corrected, the infant should be closely assessed for signs of herniation. If any herniation is suspected or if the bowel is possibly incarcerated, immediate surgical intervention is indicated.

Nursing Management

Hydrocele repair is usually not performed in the newborn stage because resolution often occurs spontaneously. Parents must be taught the signs of herniation and incarceration before discharge. These signs are the presence of a lump found in the groin (this lump is especially noticeable when the infant is crying) and increased irritability on the part of the infant. They must understand the need to seek immediate medical attention if either of these symptoms appears. Careful attention must be paid to skin care of the edematous scrotum.

If surgery is postoperatively indicated, the infant may experience abdominal distention that could place pressure on the suture line and pull it apart. Therefore the use of a nasogastric tube attached to low intermittent suction may be necessary. The infant should be placed in the side-lying or supine position with the head turned to the side to prevent rubbing or pressure on the suture line. The bed should be flat. Maintenance of a dry sterile or waterproof occlusive dressing over the operative site is essential to prevent infection and skin breakdown. The perineum should be carefully cleaned after every void and stool.

INGUINAL HERNIA

Pathophysiology
Inguinal hernia is one of the most common surgical problems in the infant. It occurs more often in the premature infant. Inguinal hernia occurs when the small intestine and gonads pass through the open processus vaginalis. In the female, the herniation may occur into soft tissue of the labia. Small hernias without complications may be allowed to close on their own. Often, hernia repair is deferred until the infant is older and can tolerate anesthesia. The matured premature infant must be closely observed for respiratory and cardiac compromise in the postoperative period because he or she is prone to apnea and bradycardia. When the intestines are caught within the processus, incarceration can occur. Vomiting and abdominal distention may indicate obstruction of the herniated intestine. Strangulation of the bowel and gonads occurs when the circulation becomes compromised. Necrosis may follow a few hours later.

Risk Factors
Right-sided hernias occur more often than left-sided ones, and bilateral hernias make up only a small percentage of occurrences. Males are commonly affected more than females, and a high incidence exists in the premature population. A rare genetic syndrome called deficiency of müllerian inhibition substance results in a phenotypic male; however, a uterus and fallopian tube can be found in the scrotal sac.

Clinical Manifestations
The inguinal hernia can be felt as a mass in the groin. In many cases, crying or increased abdominal pressure can exaggerate the hernia. In reducible hernias, the intestine can be gently manipulated back into the abdomen. Transillumination may not be helpful in diagnosis, because bowel air may be difficult to differentiate from a hydrocele.

Differential Diagnosis
In the differential diagnosis, an inguinal hernia that occurs in isolation should be distinguished from one accompanying a hydrocele. Some experts do not believe that such a distinction is possible. A distinction should be made between a hydrocele and undescended testicles by scrotal examination for the presence of testes. A hydrocele may or may not be palpated, but a hernia appears as a lump or swelling within the groin. Another

concern is whether the hernia is incarcerated. Performing a rectal examination and palpating the scrotum simultaneously is necessary to reveal whether an intestinal loop is present in the scrotal sac versus a fluid-filled hydrocele.

A reducible hernia may be easily popped back into place, whereas an incarcerated hernia is thick and nonreducible.

Prognosis
The prognosis for survival is excellent in inguinal hernias.

Collaborative Management
Surgery is indicated in all inguinal hernias that do not resolve spontaneously. Surgical intervention is also required if strangulation or incarceration occurs. It involves repair of the hernia and separation of the hernia from the inguinal canal. The nurse must instruct the parents to recognize symptoms of intestinal obstruction or protrusion of bowel loops through the hernia that do not reduce easily or become discolored. These symptoms indicate the need for immediate surgery.

Nursing Management
The focus of preoperative nursing care is on keeping the infant quiet and comfortable. If vomiting has occurred, the infant should be assessed for dehydration, and the fluid and electrolyte status should be monitored closely. After surgery, the aim is adherence to aseptic technique with regard to suture line maintenance. The infant should be placed in a side-lying or supine position with the head turned to the side to prevent disruption of the suture line. If abdominal distention is present, a nasogastric tube for decompression may be necessary. Operative dressings should be observed for any drainage and bleeding. They should be kept dry, and the underlying skin should be inspected for irritation or breakdown.

TORSION OF THE TESTICLE

Pathophysiology
Torsion of the testicle occurs when the testis or sperm cord twists, thus restricting circulation to the testicle. If circulation is allowed to remain compromised, permanent damage to the testicle results. In the newborn, permanent damage may have resulted in utero, with consequent necrosis of the testicle. In the female, torsion of the fallopian tube may result in compromised circulation to the ovary.

Neonatal torsion occurs as the result of twisting of the tunical vaginalic testis during testicular descent into the scrotal sac. This problem can be unilateral or bilateral.

Risk Factors
No specific risk factors are known. Torsion of the testicle is a common finding in the newborn period.

Clinical Manifestations
Common to many scrotal problems are enlargement and edema. In torsion, the scrotum is firm to the touch, is very tender, and is often discolored. The surrounding abdomen may also show significant discoloration and be either plethoric or cyanotic. The mass itself does not transilluminate.

Differential Diagnosis
Because of its similarities with other benign scrotal problems, torsion must always be considered in the diagnosis. The diag-

nosis is usually made on the basis of the presence of the discoloration of the scrotum and the nontransilluminating consistency of the scrotal sac.

Prognosis

The prognosis for survival is very good; however, maintenance of testicular function may not be possible.

Collaborative Management

The treatment is aimed at surgical relief of the twisting of the testicle. Correction can be performed either transscrotally or inguinally. In certain instances, the twisted testis has been left in place to atrophy and necrose, in an attempt to preserve the function of the Leydig cells so as to avoid testosterone therapy. However, infertility is a potential long-term complication of neonatal torsion. This is an area for future research.

Nursing Management

The focus of nursing care is on keeping the infant comfortable and as quiet as possible. The abdominal girth should be measured every 4 hours for any signs of distention. The scrotum must be inspected for edema, discoloration, and skin temperature. If the infant is experiencing vomiting because of abdominal distention, the use of a nasogastric tube attached to intermittent low suction may be necessary. The tube should be irrigated every 2 to 4 hours with 2 ml of saline or air to maintain patency. Positioning of the infant should be only on the back with head turned to the side or in a side-lying position so as to avoid too much pressure being placed on the abdominal and scrotal areas.

After surgery, the nursing care is centered on stability of the vital signs and prevention of infection. The respiratory status must be carefully assessed because abdominal distention may compromise the respiratory function. Nasopharyngeal suctioning may be necessary. The suture line is generally small but still requires aseptic technique. The site should be assessed for the presence of edema, drainage, or discoloration. A urinary drainage bag may be necessary to protect the skin and to prevent infection if excessive drainage is present.

NEPHROBLASTOMA

Pathophysiology

The occurrence of malignant tumor in the neonate is rare, but Wilms' tumor occurs in the young infant. Associated with Wilms' tumor are aniridia, GU tract defects, and hemihypertrophy. The presence of these signs in the neonate should alert the health care professional to the potential development of Wilms' tumor beyond the neonatal period.

Risk Factors

When hemihypertrophy is present, the infant may be at risk for nephroblastoma.

Clinical Manifestations

The usual finding is a smooth, solid abdominal or flank mass that is actually a renal mass. It may be accompanied by hypertension because of the possibility of renal artery stenosis. Fever is another common symptom of Wilms' tumor.

Differential Diagnosis

The diagnosis may be made on the basis of an intravenous pyelogram that shows distorted renal calices, and on an abdominal radiograph, the mass will appear coarse. A chest radiograph should be taken to determine the presence of any lung metastatic lesions. This condition must be differentiated from other abdominal masses.

Prognosis

Although the prognosis is generally good, this may be because mesoblastic nephroma, a benign tumor, was mislabeled as Wilms' tumor. In the newborn period, metastasis may occur and may make treatment difficult.

Nursing Management

The mass must not be palpated, because palpation may seed the tumor to other areas of the body. The major focus of nursing management—at least initially—is support of the parents. They may fear attachment to the infant. Otherwise, the neonatal nurse may not see an infant with Wilms' tumor because it is often not diagnosed in the newborn period.

AMBIGUOUS GENITALIA

The most common cause of ambiguous genitalia is an adrenal problem. This neonatal problem is discussed in Chapter 28.

SUMMARY

The infant who presents with genitourinary abnormality presents unique challenges to the neonatal care team. Although aberrations in the genital system are not life-threatening, their appearance can very traumatic for the parents. Urinary tract pathology, on the other hand, can result in emergent life-threatening events at any age. Renal abnormality and disease that manifest in the neonatal period can have lifelong consequences. The neonatal nurse must be able to accurately assess and respond to alterations in renal function. Astute nursing care of the infant and parents is paramount to optimal management and outcome. The neonatal nurse is in the position to be the first member of the health care team to detect the minor changes in neonatal physiologic functions that could signal onset of significant compromise. To do this, the neonatal nurse must have knowledge of normal renal physiology.

Parental support is another aspect of nursing care that is of major importance when caring for the infant with GU conditions. Timely assessment of parental coping mechanisms, alterations in parent-infant attachment, and evaluation of the parents' response to teaching provides vital information that will ultimately affect the infant's overall well-being.

REFERENCES

Baylis C, Lemley K (1997). Glomerular filtration. In Jamison R, Wilkinson R (Eds.) Nephrology, London: Chapman & Hall.

Brion LP et al (1997). The kidney and the urinary tract. In Fanaroff A, Martin R (Ed.), Neonatal-perinatal medicine: diseases of the fetus and infant, ed 6, Philadelphia: WB Saunders.

Brook J et al (1998). Role of the renin-angiotensin system in disorders of the urinary tract. The journal of urology, 160(5), 1812-1819.

Chevalier R (1999). Prenatal and perinatal nephrology: compensatory renal growth. In Gonzales E, Bauer S (Eds), Pediatric urology practice, Philadelphia: Lippincott, Williams & Wilkins.

Fletcher MA (1998). Physical diagnosis in neonatology, Philadelphia: Lippincott-Raven.

Gomez R, Norwood V (1999). Recent advances in renal development. *Current opinion in pediatrics,* 11(2), 135.

Kaplan GW (1994). Structural abnormalities of the genitourinary system. In Avery GB et al (Eds.), *Neonatology: pathophysiology and management of the newborn,* ed 4, Philadelphia: WB Saunders.

Koeppen B, Stanton B (1997). *Renal physiology,* ed 2, St Louis: Mosby.

Maizels M (1998). Normal and anomalous development of the urinary tract. In Walsh P et al (Eds.), *Campbell's urology,* ed 7, Philadelphia: WB Saunders.

Potter E (1965). Bilateral absence of ureters and kidneys: a report of 50 cases. *Obstetrics & gynecology,* 25(1), 3-12.

Roth K et al (2001). Obstructive nephropathy in children: long-term progression after relief of posterior urethral valve. *Pediatrics,* 107(5), 1004-1010.

Saphier C et al (2000). Prenatal diagnosis and management of abnormalities in the urologic system. *Clinics in perinatology,* 27(4), 921-945.

Schoen E et al (2000). Newborn circumcision decreases incidence and costs of urinary tract infections during the first year of life. *Pediatrics,* 105(4), 789-793.

ASSESSMENT AND MANAGEMENT OF THE INTEGUMENTARY SYSTEM

CAROLYN HOUSKA LUND, JOANNE MCMANUS KULLER

INTRODUCTION

In neonatology, skin phenomena, along with other examination findings, are used to assess maturity, duration of pregnancy, and neonatal vitality. The skin is a major organ of the premature infant; it makes up 13% of the body weight, compared with 3% in adults. This large organ provides a barrier against infection, protects internal organs, contributes to temperature regulation and insensible water loss, stores fats, excretes electrolytes and water, and provides tactile sensory input. The sensations of touch, pressure, temperature, pain, and itch are received by millions of microscopic dermal nerve endings. As a means of communication, the skin is instrumental in early establishment of the mother-infant relationship and in that the quality of touch and stimulation that an infant receives is responsible for the infant's later responses to other people and to the environment. In this sense, it fulfills a task of vital importance, particularly in the area of maternal-child nursing.

Nursing care practices that affect the fragile, underdeveloped skin of the premature infant, present major concerns as well as dilemmas for care providers. Life support and monitoring equipment must be securely attached and frequently removed or replaced; this practice can cause trauma to the skin. Numerous invasive procedures, such as vascular access, blood sampling, and chest tube insertion, are necessary but invade the skin's barrier. Because the skin of the premature infant makes up such a large percentage of body weight, trauma to skin can result in the diversion of an excessive proportion of caloric intake to tissue repair. Other concerns about the effects of trauma to premature skin include the energy demands of electrolyte imbalances and increased evaporative heat loss through damaged or immature skin and the risk of toxicity when substances are applied to the skin surface.

Another major concern is infection. Because of trauma to the skin, large areas of the skin are portals to bacteria and fungus in an already immune compromised host. Even common skin flora—such as coagulase-negative staphylococci and *Candida* species—can have serious pathogenic capabilities in these hosts and often enter the system through mucocutaneous inoculation (Rowen et al, 1995). Thus significant morbidity and mortality can be attributed to practices that cause either trauma to skin or alterations in normal skin function.

Iatrogenically caused skin problems—including burns and caustic lesions from isopropyl alcohol and erythema and skin craters from transcutaneous oxygen monitoring—have been reported. Increased skin permeability of preterm infants and percutaneous toxicity from drugs and chemicals have also been documented.

This chapter covers the development and structure of skin, the normal physiologic variations in newborn skin, and dermatologic diseases. This information is then incorporated into the nursing management of the neonatal skin.

SKIN STRUCTURE AND FUNCTION

All skin consists of three anatomically distinct layers: the epidermis, the dermis, and the subcutaneous tissue. The principal functional compartment of the epidermis is the stratum corneum epidermidis, the horny outer layer of the epidermis. It is primarily composed of closely packed dead cells that are being continually brushed off by clothing and washing. These exfoliated cells form part of the vernix caseosa, the cheese-like substance that covers and protects fetal skin. The bottom, living basal layer constantly replaces these cells. It takes approximately 26 days for cells from this layer to migrate up to the stratum corneum. Approximately 20% of an adult's protein requirement is needed for this purpose. Keratin-forming cells—which cornify the outer layer of the epidermis—and melanocytes are contained in the lower levels of the epidermis. Melanocytes begin producing melanin, or pigment, before birth and distribute it to the epidermal cells. Active pigmentary activity can be observed before birth in the epidermis of infants of dark-skinned races, but little evidence of such activity exists in white fetuses (Moore & Persaud, 1998).

The dermis lies directly under the epidermis and is 2 to 4 mm thick at birth. It is a closely woven layer of collagen, which is a fibrous protein, and elastin fibers. This fibrous complex provides mechanical strength as well as elasticity and allows the skin to withstand frictional stress while extending easily over joints. At term, the dermis is thick and well organized but is thinner and has a higher water content compared to the adult dermis (Loomis & Birge, 2001). Many nerves and a rich supply of blood vessels are contained there. They nourish the skin cells and act as carriers of the sensations of heat, touch, pressure, and pain from the skin to the brain.

Hair originates from deep in the dermis. Down-growths, called epidermal ridges, which extend into the developing dermis, result from a proliferation of cells in the basal layer. These ridges are permanently established by 17 weeks' gestation and produce ridges and grooves on the surface of the palms—including the fingers—and on the soles of the feet—including the toes. Determined genetically; this type of pattern constitutes the basis for the use of fingerprints in criminal investigations and medical genetics. Dermatoglyphics is the study of the pattern of these epidermal ridges. The presence of abnormal chromosome complements affects the development of the ridge patterns. For example, infants with Down syndrome exhibit distinctive hand and feet patterns that are of diagnostic value (Moore & Persaud, 1998).

The major component of the subcutaneous layer is fatty connective tissue. The subcutaneous fat functions as a heat insulator, a shock absorber, and a calorie reserve area. Fat accumulation occurs predominantly in the last trimester.

Sebaceous glands are found in both the dermis and the subcutaneous layer. Well developed and potentially functional at birth, these glands have only minimal function until puberty. Sweat glands are also found in the dermis and the subcutaneous layer and are affected directly by external environmental temperature. In premature infants, sweat gland maturation occurs between 21 and 33 days of age. In term infants, this maturation occurs at about 5 days of age. Poor sweat production in the premature infant is caused by sweat gland immaturity. However, adult function is not achieved until the second or third year of life.

Normal term infant skin is soft, wrinkled, velvety, and covered with vernix caseosa. Transformation of the fetal circulation is evident soon after the cord is cut, as the skin develops the intense red coloration that is characteristic of the newborn. This color may remain for hours. A blue, blotchy appearance may occur if the infant is exposed to a cool environment.

The insulating layer of vernix is usually lost during the first few days of life through traditional newborn skin care. This results in a loss of insulation for the stratum corneum, which then peels off, thus resulting in skin with a grayish-white or yellowish hue. Visible desquamation of newborn skin comes to an end after about 7 days. Vernix may provide bactericidal protestion and may contribute to the development of epidermal barrier function and regulate postnatal surface adhesion properties, heat flux, and surface adhesion properties (Hoath et al, 2001; Okah et al, 1994).

In comparison with that of the term infant, the premature infant's skin at birth is more transparent and gelatinous and tends to be free of wrinkles. Lanugo, which has been lost in the fullterm infant, may be present in varying degrees and is one criterion used to estimate gestational age. Additionally, subcutaneous edema may be present and is clinical evidence of a cutaneous excess of water and sodium. This edema decreases within the first few days of life, and the skin then lies loosely over the infant's entire body. The immaturity of the infant's skin is linked to the premature newborn's difficulty maintaining body temperature. A poorly developed fat supply and a large body surface area in relation to body weight add to this difficulty.

The skin of the fullterm infant has a well developed epidermis; the stratum corneum is structured to perform efficiently to control transepidermal water loss (TEWL) and prevent absorption of toxic substances, similar to the function of the adult epidermis. The stratum corneum, the nonliving layer of the epidermis, contains 10 to 20 layers in adults and term infants. The stratum corneum of term newborns has been shown to have lower TEWL and stratum corneum hydration (SCH) than adults, with the lowest levels seen on the first day of life. This suggests that the barrier is relatively impermeable to water to protect from maceration in utero and that a gradual drying process occurs over the first few days of life. In addition, the TEWL in different areas—such as the forehead, palms, and soles—is lower in newborns, whereas levels are higher on the forearm region (Yosipovitch et al, 2000).

The premature infant, in contrast, has been shown to have a less well developed stratum corneum; at less than 30 weeks' gestation there may be only 2 to 3 layers of stratum corneum (Figure 34-1). This immaturity results in the premature infant's decreased capacity to resist particles, viruses, parasites, and bacteria in the external environment, thus leaving the infant readily susceptible to infection and irritation of the skin.

Transferring from the intrauterine aquatic environment to the external atmospheric environment stimulates and accelerates maturation of skin function. Harpin and Rutter (1983) reported that by 10 days' postnatal age or with increasing gestational age, the integrity of the premature infant's skin improves and approaches that of the term infant or adult. However,

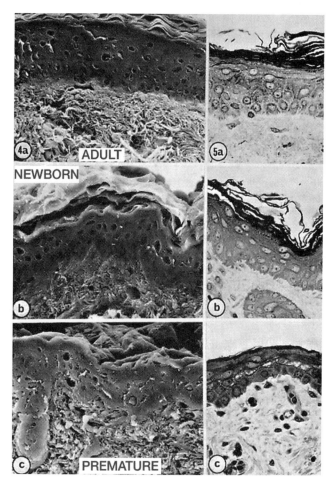

FIGURE **34-1**

Photomicrograph of stratum corneum in an adult, in a full-term newborn, and in a premature infant of 28 weeks' gestation. From Holbrook KA (1982). A histological comparison of infant and adult skin. In Maibach HI, Boisits EK (Eds.), *Neonatal skin: structure and function,* New York, Marcel Dekker. Reprinted with permission.

other authors cite a slower process in premature infants less than 27 weeks' gestation, with rates of TEWL nearly double adult levels even at 28 days of life (Agren et al, 1998). In infants of 23 to 25 weeks' gestation, skin barrier function has been shown reach mature levels at a much slower rate, with mature levels seen at 30 to 32 weeks' postconceptional age (Kalia et al, 1998).

Embryologic Development of Skin

The skin consists of two morphologically different layers, which are derived from two different germ layers. The epithelial structures (epidermis, pilosebaceous-apocrine unit, eccrine unit, and nails) are ectodermal derivatives. The ectoderm also gives rise to the hair, the teeth, and the sense organs of smell, taste, hearing, vision, and touch—everything involved with events that occur outside the organism. Mesenchymal structures (collagen, reticular, and elastic fibers; blood vessels; muscles; and fat) originate from mesoderm. These developments are outlined in Table 34-1.

The epidermis, which develops from the surface ectoderm, consists of one layer of undifferentiated cells in a 3-week-old embryo. By 4 weeks' gestational age, it has an inner germinative layer of cuboidal cells with dark, compact nuclei and an outer layer of slightly flatter cells covered by microvilli. About the middle of the second month of gestation, some of the cells begin to be crowded to the surface and form a thin, protective layer of flattened cells known as the periderm. The cells of this layer continually undergo keratinization and desquamation and are replaced by cells arising from the basal layer. The periderm is often called the epitrichial ("upon the hair") layer of the epidermis because the hairs that later grow up from the deeper layers are said not to penetrate this thin surface layer but to push it up on their growing tips, thus causing it to be cast off if it has not already disappeared. These exfoliated cells form part of the vernix caseosa.

During the later part of the second month, the epithelium tends to become thicker. This occurs (at first) by a staggering of the nuclei and the beginning of cell rearrangement, which leads rapidly to the formation of an intermediate layer between the flattened cells of the epitrichial layer and the basal layer adjacent to the underlying dermis. The cells of this intermediate layer tend to become enlarged and show a high degree of vacuolation. The basal layer of the epidermis is later called the stratum germinativum (Moore & Persaud, 1998).

At the end of the second month of gestation, the cutaneous nerves, which are detectable in embryonic dermis about the fifth week of gestation, appear to be functional, although the skin is primitive by comparison with that of an adult.

At about 10 weeks' gestation, fingernail development begins at the tips of the digits. A thickened area of epithelium on the dorsum of each digit is the first sign of nail formation. Our nails are adaptations of the epidermis, homologous to the claws and hoofs of lower mammals, and are formed by a modified process of keratinization. Development of the fingernails is begun and completed (30 to 34 weeks) before that of the toenails (35 to 38 weeks).

By about 11 weeks' gestation, collagen, and elastic connective tissue fibers begin to develop in the dermis. The epidermal-dermal junction, which has been smooth up to this time, now becomes wavy as epidermal thickenings grow down into the dermis of the palm and the soles of the feet. Dermal papillae develop in these dermal projections. Capillary loops develop in some dermal papillae, and Meissner's corpuscles, which

TABLE 34-1	Embryonic and Fetal Development of Skin

Embryonic period: undoubtedly the most important period of human development because the beginnings of all major external and internal structures develop.

Fetal period (9th week to birth): primarily concerned with growth and differentiation of tissue and organs that started to develop during the embryonic period.

Weeks of Gestation

3	Epidermis, which develops from surface ectoderm, consists of one layer of cells.
5	Cutaneous nerves are detectable in embryonic dermis.
6-7	Periderm, a thin protective layer of flattened cells, is formed.
11	Collagen and elastic fibers are developing in the dermis.
	Epidermal ridges (fingerprints) are forming.
	Nails begin to develop at the tips of the digits.
13-16	Scalp hair patterning is determined.
17-20	Melanocytes migrate to the epidermal-dermal junction and begin to produce melanin.
	Skin is covered with vernix caseosa and lanugo.
	Keratin is accumulating in the epidermis.
21-25	Skin is wrinkled, translucent, and pink to red because blood in the capillaries has become visible.
26-29	Subcutaneous fat begins to be deposited and starts to smooth out the many wrinkles in the skin.
	Eccrine sweat glands are anatomically developed and found over the entire body; their function, however, is somewhat immature in the perinatal period.
30-34	Skin is pink and smooth.
	Fingernails reach fingertips.
	Lanugo begins to shed.
35-38	Fetuses are usually plump.
	Skin is usually white or bluish-pink.
	Toenails reach toe tips.

Data from Ackerman A. (1985). Structure and function of the skin. In Moschella S, Hurley H (Eds.), Dermatology (Vol. II, 2nd ed.), Philadelphia, WB Saunders.

are the sensory nerve endings of touch, form in others (Moore & Persaud, 1998). These epidermal ridges produce ridges and grooves in a genetically determined pattern and are the basis for fingerprinting and footprinting. The development of these ridges can be distinctly affected by the presence of abnormal chromosome complements (e.g., as occurs in Down syndrome). These ridges are permanently established by about 17 weeks' gestation.

During the third to fourth month of gestation, the stratum germinativum differentiates from the rest of the epithelium. These cells are termed the germinative layer because they undergo the repeated cell divisions that are responsible for the growth of the epidermis.

During the fourth month of gestation, the epithelium starts to become many cells thick, and keratin begins to accumulate in the cells above the stratum germinativum layer. Daughter cells from the basal layer are crowded upward and undergo progressive changes in each layer and finalize in cornification. The thin stratum granulosum epidermidis, which contains keratohyalin granules, is the layer directly above the stratum germinativum. The next higher layer is the thin and clear stratum lucidum epidermidis, the content of which is a fluid—eleidin—that replaces the granules. Above that is the keratinized multilayered stratum corneum epidermidis (Moore & Persaud, 1998). As the keratin accumulates in these cells, they become more and more sluggish and finally die, so that the surface layer of the epidermis is made up of tough, scale-like, dead cells that form a relatively impermeable membrane.

In areas such as the soles of the feet and the palms of the hands, where the skin is subjected to more than ordinary wear, the keratinization of the outer layer is much heavier than in the general body surface. Of interest, however, is that the greater thickness of palmar and plantar epidermis becomes evident in the embryo long before it is possible for these areas to have been subjected to any more wear than other parts of the skin. When the aforementioned layers are all completely differentiated, the structure of fetal epidermis resembles that of adult epidermis.

During the early fetal period, neural crest cells migrate into the dermis and differentiate into melanoblasts. At about 17 to 20 weeks of gestation, these melanoblasts differentiate into melanocytes, migrate to the epidermal-dermal border, and begin to produce melanin. Fetal melanocytes in white races contain little or no pigment, whereas in dark-skinned races, they produce melanin granules. The skin of black newborns is only a little darker than that of white newborns. The skin at the bases of the fingernails and toenails is often noticeably darker, however.

The skin of black infants continues to darken after birth, as increased melanin production occurs in response to light. When melanocytes remain behind in the dermis, they appear bluish through the overlying cutaneous tissue and are called mongolian spots. Some believe that it is not the number of melanocytes present that is important but rather their activity level. The hormone secreted by the pituitary gland that controls the clumping or dispersion of the melanin granules is melanocytestimulating hormone.

Around 20 weeks of gestation, the eyebrows, upper lip, and chin hair are first recognizable. On the general body surface, the hair makes its appearance about a month later. These fine hairs are called lanugo. As stated earlier, the emergence of this hair breaks off the periderm, and the periderm becomes one component of the vernix caseosa. The other components of vernix are sebum from the sebaceous glands, fetal hair, and desquamated cells from the amnion (Moore & Persaud, 1998). Vernix protects the epidermis against a macerating influence that would be exerted by the amniotic fluid and acts as a lubricant to prevent chafing injuries from the amnion as the growing fetus becomes progressively confined in its fluid-filled sac.

Between 21 and 24 weeks' gestation, the fetus's skin is wrinkled, translucent, and pinkish-red because blood in the capillaries has become visible. Head and lanugo hair are well developed in a 26- to 29-week fetus. At this same time, eccrine sweat glands are anatomically developed and are found over the entire body. Their function, however, is somewhat immature in the perinatal period.

Brown adipose tissue cells begin to differentiate in the seventh month of gestation, and the accumulation of subcuta-neous fat begins to smooth out the many skin wrinkles. Between the 30th and 34th week of gestation, the skin is pink and smooth, and the lanugo is beginning to shed. The fingernails reach the fingertips, but the distal part of the nail is still thin and soft (Moore & Persaud, 1998). During the last trimester of pregnancy, subcutaneous fat accumulates, and the fetus acquires a plump appearance. The composition of amniotic fluid tested at this time reflects skin function. The number of anucleated cells and keratinized lipid-containing skin flakes increases.

Developmental Variations

Several factors are responsible for the functional differences between premature and term infants' skin. These differences subside with increasing gestational and postnatal age (Table 34-2).

Thickness of the Stratum Corneum and Permeability.   The barrier function of the skin resides in the outermost layer of the epidermis, the stratum corneum. This barrier is composed of keratinocytes coated by intercellular lipids. The stratum corneum begins to develop in the fetus after 21 weeks' estimated gestational age (EGA). The stratum corneum in infants of 28 weeks' gestation consists of only a few cell layers and is markedly thinner than that of term infants (Figure 34-1). These findings correlate with the immaturity of barrier function of the stratum corneum; this immaturity is characterized by increased permeability and increased TEWL.

By 32 to 34 weeks' EGA, the stratum corneum has developed sufficiently to offer some protection. The fullterm infant has a fully functional stratum corneum.

After birth, rapid postnatal maturation occurs with thickening of the epidermis and development of the stratum corneum. As noted previously, the stratum corneum of premature infants is thought to rapidly mature and reach adult barrier function in approximately 2 weeks after birth. A slower process in premature infants less than 27 weeks' gestation is noted; rates of TEWL are nearly double adult levels even at 28 days of life. In infants of 23 to 25 weeks' gestation, skin barrier function reaches mature levels much more slowly (Agren et al, 1998), as long as 8 weeks after birth in a 23-week gestation infant (Kalia et al, 1998).

The undeveloped stratum corneum of the premature infant's skin also produces increased transepidermal water loss and evaporative heat loss and contributes to the difficulty the premature newborn experiences in maintaining fluid balance and body temperature.

Neonatal skin is 40% to 60% thinner than adult skin, and their body surface/weight ratio is nearly five times greater. Thus the newborn is at risk for toxicity from topically applied substances (Siegfried, 2001). Due to their deficient stratum corneum, the skin of a premature infant is remarkably permeable; permeability correlates inversely with gestational age.

Toxicity due to topically applied substances secondary to the increased permeability of both preterm and term infants' skin has been reported in numerous cases (Siegfried, 2001).

Based on this information, all solutions topically applied to the infant's skin, especially to the premature infant's skin, during the first 2 to 3 weeks of life should be carefully evaluated as to their necessity and should be applied appropriately and sparingly if they are deemed beneficial to the infant's care.

Dermal Instability.   Collagen in the dermis increases with gestational age as the tendency toward water fixation and edema decreases. The other component of the dermis, the

TABLE 34-2	Structural Differences Between Infant and Adult Skin		
	Premature	**Full-Term**	**Adult**
Epidermis	Thinner cells compressed Fewer desmosomes Fewer layers of stratum corneum Melanin production low	Stratum corneum appears as adherent cell layers Melanin production low	Good resistance to penetration
Dermoepidermal junction	Fewer hemidesmosomes Less cohesion between layers		
Dermis	Fewer elastin fibers Thinner than in the adult	Fewer elastin fibers Thinner than in the adult	Full complement of elastin fibers
Eccrine glands	May be more typical of fetus than adult Ducts patent Secretory cells undifferentiated	Equivalent in structure to adult Denser distribution	Distribution less dense than in infant
Hair	Lanugo hair may be present Hair growth synchronous	Vellus hair characteristic Hair growth synchronous	Both vellus and terminal hairs Hair growth dyssynchronous
Sebaceous glands	Large and active	Large and active but diminishing rapidly in both size and activity for several weeks after birth	Large and active
Nerve and vascular system	Not fully organized Most nerves are small in diameter, unmyelinated, sensory, and autonomic Unmyelinated nerves are typically fetal in structure Meissner's touch receptors not fully formed	Vascular system not fully organized until 3 months Cutaneous nerve network not fully developed, may continue to develop until puberty Most nerves are small in diameter, unmyelinated, sensory, and autonomic Meissner's touch receptors not fully formed	Adult pattern
Permeability	Highly permeable Higher penetrability of fat-soluble substances Greater absorption because of higher skin surface: body weight ratio	Good resistance to penetration Higher penetrability of fat-soluble substances Greater absorption because of higher skin surface: body weight ratio	Good resistance to penetration
Eccrine sweating	Reduced sweating capability, especially for first 13-24 days	Reduced sweating capability, especially for first 2-5 days	Full sweating capability
Photosensitivity	Melanin production low; will sunburn readily	Melanin production low; will sunburn readily	Sensitivity to sun depends on skin type
Related conditions	Reduced ability to ward off infection because of deficient immune system Low reactivity to allergens	Reduced ability to ward off infection Low reactivity to allergens	Readily sensitized to allergens

From Shalita A (1981). Principles of infant skin care, Skillman NJ, Johnson & Johnson Baby Products.

elastin fibers, is formed mostly after birth and may not become fully mature until 3 years of age. Protection from pressure and ischemic injury includes routine turning and repositioning and surfaces such as gelled pads or water mattresses (Lund, 1999).

Diminished Cohesion. Another variation in the premature infant's skin structure and function is the diminished cohesion between the dermis and the epidermis. The junction of the epidermis and the dermis, which is normally connected by numerous fibrils, has fewer and more widely spaced fibrils in the premature infant than in term infants or adults (Figure 34-2). These fibrils become stronger with increasing gestational and postnatal age. Because the premature infant in the neonatal intensive care unit (NICU) is usually covered with some

type of adhesive to secure intravenous lines, cardiorespiratory electrodes, endotracheal tubes, and umbilical artery catheters, the premature infant is at higher risk for blistering and stripping of the epidermis when adhesives are removed. The cohesion between many of the currently used adhesives and the stratum corneum may be stronger than the bond between the dermis and the epidermis.

Skin pH. Another developmental variation of infant skin resides in the functional capacity of the skin to form a surface pH of less than 5.0, which is the acid mantle. A skin surface pH of less than 5 is ordinarily seen in both children and adults.

In the large number of term newborns studied, the skin was found to have a mean pH of 6.34 immediately after birth.

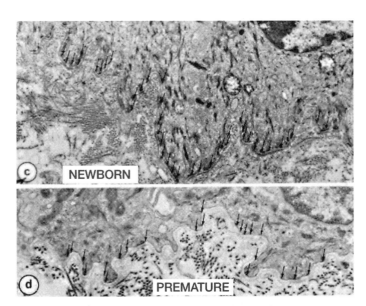

FIGURE **34-2**
Arrows indicate anchoring fibrils at dermoepidermal junction in a full-term and a premature infant. From Holbrook KA (1982). A histological comparison of infant and adult skin. In Maibach HI, Boisits EK (Eds.), *Neonatal skin: structure and function*, New York, Marcel Dekker. Reprinted with permission.

Within 4 days, the pH decreased to a mean of 4.95, and between 7 and 30 days it further decreased to 4.7. In a later study of 127 low-birth-weight infants, these authors documented that the mean pH decreased from 6.7 (day 1) to 5.04 (day 9). However, a different technique for measuring pH was used than in the previous study; thus the absolute values for pH may not be comparable. They concluded that acidification of the skin is independent of gestational age (Fox et al, 1998).

An acidic skin surface is credited with having bactericidal qualities against some pathogens and serves in the defense against microorganisms. Microbial colonization also begins immediately after birth. An increased skin pH, from acidic to neutral, can increase the total numbers of bacteria and TEWL and shift the species present.

Melanin Production. One of the primary functions of melanin is to screen the skin from the sun's harmful rays by absorbing their radiant energy. Although melanin production—and therefore pigmentation—are lower during the neonatal period than later in life, certain areas—such as the linea alba, the areola, and the scrotum—are often deeply pigmented as a result of high circulating levels of maternal and placental hormones. Melanin production in premature infants is even less than in term infants, thus placing them at greater risk for damage from sunlight and ultraviolet light (Williams, 2001).

ASSESSMENT AND PHYSIOLOGIC VARIATIONS

Acrocyanosis, or peripheral cyanosis involving the hands, feet, and circumoral area, is a common finding in the newborn. It occurs because of sluggish blood flow in the feet and hands that results from limited development of the peripheral capillary circulation. Acrocyanosis usually resolves within the first few days of life but may reappear with cold stress.

Pallor is most commonly a sign of anemia, hypoxia, or poor peripheral perfusion that results from hypotension or infection. Meconium staining is caused by the passage of meconium in utero and usually requires at least 6 hours of meconium contact to stain the skin.

Jaundice, which occurs in 50% to 70% of newborns, is a yellowing of the skin and develops because of the presence of indirect bilirubin in the blood. Bilirubin is normally processed by the liver and is eliminated in the urine and feces. In newborns, the body cannot eliminate bilirubin as fast as it is produced.

For visible staining of the skin and sclera, a bilirubin level of at least 5 mg/100 ml is required. The head-to-toe progression of jaundice over the body gives a crude estimate of the level of bilirubin.

Linea nigra is a line of increased pigmentation from the umbilicus to the genitals. This area of benign pigmentation may become less noticeable as the infant's skin darkens.

Mongolian spots are collections of melanocytes located in the dermis that are most frequently seen at birth. They are slate blue, gray, or black, shaped as irregular, bruise-like spots that are seen primarily over the sacrum and the buttocks but may extend over the back and shoulders. Most commonly seen in newborns with darkly pigmented skin, they are found in 96% of African American, 86% of Asian, and 13% of Caucasian infants (Lucky 2001). Although they look like bruises, they are harmless and resolve over several years.

Lanugo is the fine downy hair that is most commonly seen over the back, shoulders, and facial areas of a premature newborn. It is shed at the seventh to eighth month of gestation and is one criterion used to estimate gestational age.

Milia are common papules that occur primarily on the face but may also occur in other locations. They are seen as small, white, pinhead-sized bumps that are scattered over the chin, cheeks, noses, and forehead of 25% to 40% of fullterm babies (Margileth, 1999). They spontaneously resolve within the first month of life. Mothers should be instructed not to squeeze or prick these pimple-like spots. Milia can develop on the foreskin of infant boys; these are called epidermal inclusion cysts; when they occur on the palate, they are called Epstein's pearls.

Miliaria is a general term for describing obstructions of the eccrine duct. The cause is retention of sweat as a result of edema of the stratum corneum; this edema blocks eccrine pores, thus resulting in four types of miliaria: rubra (prickly heat), crystallina, pustulosa, and profunda.

Miliaria pustulosa and miliaria profunda are rarely seen in temperate climates. Miliaria rubra is commonly observed in infants exposed to excessive environmental temperatures with humidity. It appears as pink or white pimples with a little redness around them. They resolve when the infant is moved to cooler temperatures. Miliaria crystallina presents as clear, 1- to 2-mm superficial water blisters without inflammation (Margileth, 1999). The distribution and grouping of vesicles that contains no eosinophils help to differentiate them from erythema toxicum neonatorum.

Harlequin color change is a dramatic but benign phenomenon in which the color on the dependent half of an infant in a side-lying position turns deep red while the upper half is pale. The color reverses when the infant is turned. Attributed to a temporary imbalance in the autonomic regulatory mechanism of the cutaneous vessels, this phenomenon is more common in low-birth-weight infants—whether well or sick.

Vernix caseosa is a grayish-white cheesy substance that is protective to the fetal skin while the fetus is in utero and helps the infant slide through the birth canal. The vernix covering diminishes as the fetus reaches term and is one determinant of gestational age.

Cutis marmorata, or mottling, is a normal physiologic vascular response to cool air. This generalized mottling reflects the infant's vasomotor instability. The marbling disappears with rewarming and is uncommon after several months of age. Mottling is often prominent in infants with Cornelia de Lange's syndrome and Down syndrome.

Erythema toxicum neonatorum, the most common rash of newborns, usually occurs within 5 days of birth and affects approximately half of term infants, although it is almost never seen in premature infants or those less than 2500 grams. It appears as small, firm, white, or pale yellow pustules with an erythematous margin. Lesions may first appear on the face and spread to the trunk and extremities but may appear anywhere on the body except the soles and palms (Lucky, 2001).

A smear and Wright's stain of the pustules reveal numerous infiltrates of eosinophils that are devoid of bacteria. The differential diagnosis includes transient neonatal pustular melanosis, candidiasis, staphylococcal pyoderma, and miliaria. No treatment is necessary.

Neonatal and infantile acne are two distinct conditions distinguished by the time of onset and clinical features. Neonatal acne involves inflammatory, erythematous papules and pustules located primarily on the cheeks, often scattered over the face and extending into the scalp. Recently, a hypothesis that neonatal acne may be an inflammatory response to malssezia species of fungus has been proposed (Niamba et al, 1998; Rapelanoro et al, 1996). A later form of acne has been termed infantile acne.

Infantile acne is considered an androgen-driven condition with hyperplasia of sebaceous activity. It is found primarily on the face. Neonatal acne generally resolves without treatment. Infantile acne may be more persistent and even cause scarring. Treatment for infantile acne may benefit from treatment with topical benzyl alcohol peroxide or erythromicin (Lucky, 2001).

Transient neonatal pustular melanosis is a lesion that is similar to miliaria but is present at birth, usually causing the infant to be unnecessarily isolated. It occurs most commonly on the face, the palms of the hands, and the soles of the feet. It is most commonly seen in black infants. The differential diagnosis includes erythema toxicum neonatorum, staphylcoccal impetigo, neonatal candidiasis, miliaria crystallina or rubra, and acropustulosis of infancy. If the lesions are ruptured, smeared on a slide, and stained, the contents are found to be amorphous debris. The lesion is neither infectious nor contagious. It is self-limiting and requires no treatment.

Sucking blisters that contain sterile, serous fluid may be seen on the thumb, index finger, or lip. Presumably, they are the result of vigorous sucking in utero and resolve without treatment.

Pigmentary Lesions

Hyperpigmented lesions may be present at birth or during the first weeks of life. Some pigmentary problems are benign, such as mongolian spots, whereas others can be signs or systemic or genetic disorder. Some of the more common are included in this section.

Café au lait spots are irregularly shaped, oval lesions. Their color resembles coffee to which milk has been added. They should be noted on the newborn's initial physical examination, and if they are larger than 4 to 6 cm or if more than six are present, a diagnosis of neurofibromatosis should be considered (Landau & Krafchik, 1999).

Hyperpigmentation that presents in a diffuse pattern is unusual in the newborn. When present, it may be caused by congenital Addison's disease, hepatic or biliary atresia, metabolic disease (Hartnup's disease, porphyria), nutritional disorders (pellagra, sprue), hereditary disorders (lentiginosis, melanism), or unknown causes (the bronze discoloration seen in Niemann-Pick disease). Hyperpigmentation of the labial folds with clitoral hypertrophy may result from the transplacental passage of androgens (Margileth, 1999).

Hypopigmentation that presents as a diffuse or localized loss of pigment in the neonate may stem from metabolic (phenylketonuria), endocrine (Addison's), genetic (vitiligo, piebaldism, tuberous sclerosis, albinism), traumatic, or postinflammatory causes (Margileth, 1999).

Piebaldism, or partial albinism, an autosomal dominant disorder that is present at birth, is easily detected in the dark-skinned infant. Off-white macules are seen on the scalp, widow's peakand forehead and extend to the base of the nose, trunk, and extremities. Differential diagnoses are Klein-Waardenburg syndrome, vitiligo, nevus anemicus, Addison's disease, and white macules of tuberous sclerosis. When illuminated with a Wood light, the amelanotic areas of piebaldism exhibit a brilliant whiteness (Margileth, 1999).

Albinism refers to a group of genetic disorders involving abnormal melanin synthesis. It may occur in any race, with the incidence approximately 1 in 20,000, with a slightly higher rate in African Americans (Sethi et al, 1996). An autosomal recessive gene usually causes it, but rare cases of autosomal dominant inheritance have occurred (Margileth, 1999).

White leaf macules are the earliest cutaneous manifestations of tuberous sclerosis, an autosomal dominant neurocutaneous syndrome. They vary in size and shape but most often resemble a mountain ash leaflet. They may be difficult to see in a newborn infant and may be more readily observed by examination with a Wood lamp, which heightens the contrast between the macule and normal skin. Normal infants occasionally have a single lesion, but the presence of one or more of these macules in an infant with neurologic problems strongly suggests the diagnosis of tuberous sclerosis. Skin biopsy is nondiagnostic. A careful family history, physical examination, and, when appropriate, additional diagnostic studies are indicated in infants with these lesions.

Lesions Related to the Birth Process

Caput succedaneum is a diffuse, generalized edema of the scalp that is caused by local pressure and trauma during labor. The borders are not well defined, and the swelling crosses suture lines.

Cephalhematoma is a subperiosteal hemorrhage caused by the trauma of labor and delivery. The margins of the suture lines are clearly demarcated, and the swelling never crosses suture lines. Sclerema neonatorum may have the same cause and adipose tissue abnormality in the subcutaneous tissues as those noted in fat necrosis. However, sclerema more commonly affects the premature or debilitated infant. It is a diffuse hardening of the subcutaneous tissue that results in cold, nonpitting skin. Low environmental temperature alone can produce this injury. The extremities may be involved at first, but generalized involvement occurs within 3 to 4 days.

Infants with this disorder are usually critically ill, but if they survive, the sclerematous changes rarely last beyond 2 weeks. Treatment is based on therapy for the underlying systemic disease, restoration of body temperature, and adequate nutrition.

Forceps marks are identified by their rounded contours and position. The bruised area should be checked for underlying tissue and nerve damage.

Scalp lacerations can occur in many ways. A laceration can be caused by the placement of an inrnal monitoring lead or by the artificial rupture of membranes. A circular red or ecchymotic area may be caused by the use of a vacuum extractor. Any abraded area may serve as a portal of entry for infection; therefore a scalp laceration should be carefully and continuously assessed for the presence of infection. Lacerations can also occur to other body surfaces from scalpel injuries during cesarean birth; an incidence of 1.9% was noted in a series of 896 cesarean section deliveries (Smith et al, 1997).

Subcutaneous fat necrosis is an uncommon disorder that occurs primarily in fullterm infants. It has been associated with birth trauma, shock, asphyxia, hypothermia, seizures, preeclampsia, meconium aspiration, and intrapartum medications (Scales et al, 1998). One or several indurated, violet or red plaques or sharply defined subcutaneous nodules on the buttocks, thighs, trunk, face, or arms may appear (Cohen, 2001). Most areas of subcutaneous fat necrosis gradually reabsorb over weeks to months if it is left alone. Residual atrophy or scarring is unusual.

Internal fetal monitoring sites are at risk for infection, owing to the introduction of the maternal vaginal flora directly into the subcutaneous tissue of the fetus. Scalp abscesses caused by implantation of a fetal electrode are generally benign, self-limited occurrences. Rare instances have been reported of major complications, however—including significant areas of cellulitis, osteomyelitis, and sepsis.

DERMATOLOGIC DISEASES

Diseases of the skin in newborns often present patterns that are different from the presentation of the same disease in adults. Therefore a careful physical examination of the skin is necessary for an accurate dermatologic diagnosis to be made. All lesions should be described and their location and pattern noted.

Lesions can be classified as either primary or secondary. Primary lesions are described as the initial or principal lesion that is identified when the disease begins. Primary lesions are classified as macule, patch, papule, plaque, nodule, tumor, vesicle, bulla, wheal, pustule, or abscess. Secondary lesions are brought about the modification of a primary lesion. The secondary lesion may be called a crust, scale, erosion, ulcer, fissure, lichenification, atrophy, or scar.

Terminology
Ecchymoses appear as black and blue bruises of varying sizes anywhere over the body. Primarily seen over the presenting part in a difficult vertex delivery or a vaginal breech delivery, ecchymosis is most frequently due to trauma associated with labor and delivery. It occurs more commonly in the fragile premature infant. This bruising, however, can be indicative of serious infection or bleeding disorders.

Petechiae are pinpoint hemorrhagic areas, less than 1 mm, scattered over the upper trunk and face as a result of pressure during the descent and rotation of birth. Their incidence is increased when the umbilical cord has been around the neck or when the cervix clamps down after delivery of the head. They usually fade within 24 to 48 hours. If they continue to develop or are unusually numerous, a complete work-up for infection or bleeding disorders should be performed.

Intracutaneous hemorrhage may be caused by thrombocytopenia, inherited disorders of coagulation, transient deficiency of vitamin K, disseminated intravascular coagulation, and trauma.

Disseminated intravascular coagulation should be suspected in an acutely ill infant who has an intracutaneous hemorrhage. Thrombocytopenia and disorders of coagulation generally occur in infants who seem well otherwise. Thrombocytopenia should be suspected when the infant presents with general cutaneous petechiae. It frequently accompanies neonatal infections and is most commonly associated with the TORCH diseases (toxoplasmosis, rubella, cytomegalovirus, and herpes simplex).

Ecchymoses and petechiae are purple discolorations caused by hemorrhage into the superficial skin layers. They do not disappear with blanching, because the blood is contained in the tissues. Macules are nonpalpable, nonraised lesions less than 1 cm in diameter that are identified only by color change. They are seen in measles, rubella, scarlet fever, roseola, typhoid fever, and drug reactions.

Papules are superficial elevated solid lesions less than 1 cm in diameter. They are firm and not fluid-filled. They may follow the macular stage in many eruptive diseases.

Vesicles are skin elevations that contain serous fluid (blisters). They are commonly seen with herpes simplex, insect bites, and poison ivy.

Pustules are localized accumulations of pus in or just beneath the epidermis. They are often centered around appendageal structures (e.g., hair follicles) and are usually caused by bacterial infections or skin abscesses. When a pustule breaks, the degree of crusting is more marked than occurs with the rupture of a vesicle.

Nodules are deep solid lesions larger than 1 cm in diameter. Nodules are similar to papules but are larger. Because of their size, they are more likely to have a dermal component than are papules.

Developmental Vascular Abnormalities
The following two major groups of vascular birthmarks are seen:
- Vascular malformations composed of dysplastic vessels
- Vascular tumors that demonstrate cellular hyperplasia

Vascular malformations have various subcategories determined by the anomalous vessels involved—including capillary, venous, arteriovenous, or lymphatic. Hemangiomas or vascular nevi are the most common cutaneous congenital malformations seen during early infancy. They may be either involuting or noninvoluting vascular lesions, as well as flat (telangiectatic) or raised (hemangiomatous). The common involuting types include salmon patch, spider nevi (telangiectases), and strawberry and cavernous hemangiomas. Noninvoluting lesions, which are seen less commonly in newborns, are the port-wine stain and, rarely, the pyogenic granuloma (Enjolras & Garzon, 2001).

Pigmented Nevus. Pigmented nevi are benign tumors of the skin that contain nevus cells. Nevus cells can produce melanin and are closely related to melanocytes. In contrast to melanocytes, they tend to lie in groups or nests. Congenital pigmented nevi are different from pigmented nevi that arise later in that they are usually larger and more extensive. As the infant grows, the area becomes thicker and darker (Margileth, 1999).

Flat, junctional nevi are seen in about 1% of newborns. They are brown or black, and their size varies from one to sev-

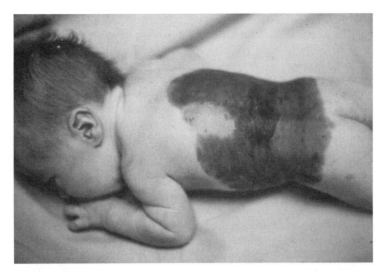

FIGURE **34-3**
The giant pigmented hairy nevus of this infant involves the thorax, abdomen, and back and is commonly called a "bathing trunk" nevus. It is raised with fleshy elements and has a somewhat leathery texture. From Clark D, Thompson J (1986). Dermatology of the newborn. Parts 1 and 2. In *Pathology of the neonate slide series* (Vol. III, No. 4). Philadelphia: Wyeth-Ayerst Laboratories. Copyright© Wyeth; used with permission.

eral centimeters. When they are present at birth, they may be associated with neurofibromatosis, tuberous sclerosis, or bathing trunk nevi. Therapy is rarely needed, but lesions larger than 3 cm should be removed.

Giant Hairy Nevus. A giant hairy nevus is characterized by a pigmented, hairy, and softly infiltrated area. The color varies from pale brown to black. When the nevi are large, they tend to have a dermatomic distribution, and their location and size give them their name (e.g., bathing trunk nevus, vest nevus, shoulder stole nevus) (Figure 34-3). On histologic examination of a biopsy specimen, the nevus cells are seen penetrating deeply into the dermis and subcutaneous tissue.

When a giant nevus is situated on the head or neck, it may be associated with mental retardation, epilepsy, or hydrocephalus. Spina bifida or meningocele may occur when this nevus is present over the spine (Margileth, 1999). Other abnormalities that are sometimes associated with a giant pigmented nevus are clubfoot, hypertrophy or hypotrophy of the affected limb, and von Recklinghausen's disease (neurofibromatosis).

Besides being a cosmetic problem, the giant nevus is associated with a higher incidence of malignancy. Malignant melanomas develop in as many as 15% of these patients.

Collaborative Management. Management involves surgical excision of the entire lesion at or near puberty to prevent the development of skin cancer in the lesion. Plastic surgical reconstruction may be needed if the excision is extensive.

Hemangiomas. Hemangioma of infancy is an angiomatous disorder characterized by the proliferation of capillary endothelium and multilamination of the basement membrane and accumulation of mast cells, fibroblasts, and macrophages. Hemangiomas appear on 1% to 3% of infants at birth and develop on another 10%, usually within the first 3 to 4 weeks of life. The incidence is 22% in preterm babies who weigh less than 1000 grams and 15% in infants with birth weights of 1000 to

1500 grams. When examined microscopically, hemangiomas are one of two kinds: capillary or cavernous. They most often appear in the skin as a single tumor, but multiple cutaneous lesions also occur, often with involvement of other organ systems.

The natural history of the hemangioma is characterized by their appearance during the first few weeks of life, rapid postnatal growth for 8 to 18 months (proliferative phase), which is followed by very slow but inevitable regression for the next 5 to 8 years (involutive phase). Hemangiomas completely resolve in more than 50% of children by the age of 5 years of age and in more than 70% by 7 years of age, and continued improvement occurs in the remaining children until 10 to 12 years of age. The rate of regression does not seem to be related to the sex or age of the infant or to the site, size, or appearance of the hemangioma or the duration of the proliferative phase.

Strawberry hemangiomas consist of a dilated mass of capillaries in the dermal and subdermal layers that protrude above the skin surface. They are bright red, soft, compressible tumors that can appear anywhere on the body (Figure 34-4). These marks require no treatment, and no permanent scars occur if the marks are left alone. However, when these lesions interfere with vital functions such as vision, feeding, and respiration, intervention is required.

Cavernous hemangiomas are more deeply situated in the skin than strawberry hemangiomas are. They are bluish-red and feel spongy when touched. Most hemangiomas are small, harmless birthmarks that involute to leave either normal or slightly blemished skin. However, even a small hemangioma can obstruct the airway or impair vision. A large hemangioma in the liver or an extensive cutaneous hemangioma can divert a considerable volume of blood through its extensive labyrinth of capillaries and produce high-output heart failure. The increased capillary endothelial surface that characterizes a giant hemangioma can also trap platelets and may cause thrombocytopenic coagulopathy (Kasabach-Merritt syndrome).

A few hemangiomas grow to an alarming size or proliferate simultaneously in several organs and cause life-endangering

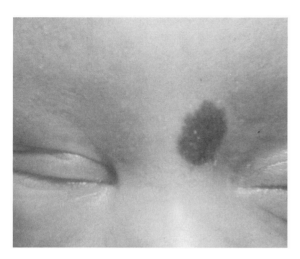

FIGURE **34-4**
This photograph shows the early hemangioma in a 28-weeks'-gestation premature infant. Approximately 5 weeks after birth the first area of discoloration appeared. The irregular surface with sharp demarcation is typical of strawberry hemangioma, which eventually enlarges to twice the size as it appears in this photograph before involution. From Clark D, Thompson J (1986). Dermatology of the newborn: parts 1 and 2. In *Pathology of the neonate slide series* (Vol. III, No. 3). Philadelphia, Wyeth-Ayerst Laboratories. Copyright© Wyeth and used with permission.

conditions, such as soft tissue destruction, deformation or obstruction of vital structures, serious bleeding, congestive heart failure, and sepsis. Large lesions can expand the skin, and even after they regress, they can result in excess slack skin, pigment changes, and a fibro-fatty residuum.

Visceral hemangiomas may arise in many organs, most commonly in the liver and larynx, with or without cutaneous involvement; a singe lesion or multiple hemangiomas may occur (Boon et al, 1996). Flow through extensive hemangiomas increases the total blood volume, causes hemodeviation, and disturbs the hemodynamic equilibrium. The hyperdynamic cardiovascular state of the hemangiomas decreases or shunts blood away from other tissues, thus resulting in hypoperfusion of other tissues. This hypoperfusion may cause brain hypoxia and acidosis and predispose to the seizures, as seen in some cases. Close surveillance of the cardiovascular system is necessary to determine the proper time to begin digitalization.

Collaborative Management.   Management of both strawberry and cavernous hemangiomas consists of a detailed history; close scrutiny of the lesion or lesions—including three-dimensional measurements—and evaluation of the growth pattern of the hemangioma. As involution progresses, the color gradually changes from grayish-pink to white or pink, and the tension of the lesion decreases. Ulcerated hemangiomas should be treated with topical antibiotics to prevent infection.

While the cutaneous lesions are being monitored, the infant's clinical course and physical development must be closely observed for poor growth, altered cry, stridor, dyspnea, cyanosis, feeding difficulties, or swallowing impairment. If any abnormal sign or symptoms—such as tachycardia, heart murmur, hepatomegaly, and bruit heard over the liver—appear, the infant should be examined for evidence of heart failure. Ultrasonography, echocardiography, and computed tomography may be needed.

In general, management consists of planned neglect, which is essential in avoiding disfiguring scars. Complications of therapy may be significant, but residual scarring after complete involution is uncommon. Hemangiomas located in exposed areas often cause great parental anxiety, which increases as the hemangioma grows. This anxiety often puts pressure on the physician to do something. However, the hemangioma should be left to regress spontaneously, and preconceived notions about birthmarks should be discussed with the family.

Treatment of hemangiomas may be needed. The following indications for treatment have been proposed: life-threatening or function-threatening hemangiomas, including those that cause impairment of vision, respiratory compromise, or congestive heart failure; hemangiomoas in certain anatomic locations such as the nose, lip, glabellar areas and ear and may cause permanent deformity or scars; large facial hemangimoas, especially those with a large dermal component; and ulcerated hemangiomas (Enjolras & Garzon, 2001).

Alarming hemangiomas is a term used to categorize lesions that impair vital functions or cause life-threatening complications. A vascular mark was present at birth in 68% of these infants. Visceral hemangiomas are associated with cervicocephalic hemangiomas or with small hemangiomas scattered over the body. About a third of these life-threatening hemangiomas respond to treatment with corticosteroids, but for the others, no safe and effective treatment exists. The mortality rate can be as high as 54% for life-threatening visceral or hepatic hemangiomas and may be up to 30% to 40% with platelet consumptive coagulopathy, despite the administration of steroids.

High-dose corticosteroid therapy is the primary means of controlling hemangiomas pharmacologically. These agents inhibit the activators of fibrinolysis in vessel walls, decrease plasminogen activator content of endothelium, and increase sensitivity to vasoactive amines, thus causing constriction of arterioles. When steroids fail, less conventional modalities, such as embolization, operative excision, and radiotherapy, are used.

Subcutaneous interferon alfa-2a (2 million units per square meter of body surface area) has been used with life-threatening or vison-threatening hemangiomas that failed to respond to corticosteriod therapy. Their mechanisms of action includes inhibition of motility and proliferation of endothelial cells and interference with new capillary vessel formation, thereby preventing platelet trapping. These daily injections seemed to reduce the local and systemic complications and appeared to shorten the length of time to involution in some infants. Sustained therapy for 9 to 14 months appeared to be desirable because earlier withdrawal was followed by regrowth of the lesion that was halted and reversed by reintroduction of the drug. Interferon alfa therapy was not found to have toxic effects.

Transexamic acid has been used in the treatment of giant hemangiomas. It is a fibrinolytic inhibitor that exerts its effect through inhibition of plasminogen activator and plasmin and through inhibition of tumor vessel proliferation. One of the infants had a measurable response in the size of the hemangioma and the extent of the coagulopathy. The other two had progression of their lesions. It appears that tranexamic acid is an additional agent for treatment of giant hemangiomas, but its efficacy is limited. Further study of this treatment is needed to determine which patients may respond best. Surgical therapy involving laser removal or surgical excision are also treatment options. Excision is usually done once the hemangioma has involuted, so as to remove residual tissue and redundant skin. Early excision is generally not recommended.

Port-wine Stain. Port-wine stain is a capillary angioma consisting of dilated and congested capillaries lying directly beneath the epidermis. It appears in approximately 3 of 1000 newborns. This birthmark appears pink at birth but gradually darkens to purple. Most commonly found on the face and neck, it is a permanent developmental defect. Although a port-wine stain is primarily a cosmetic problem, it is occasionally an indicator of a multisystem disorder, such as the Sturge-Weber syndrome or the Klippel-Trenaunay-Weber syndrome. The presence of convulsions, mental retardation, hemiplegia, or intracortical calcification suggests the presence of Sturge-Weber syndrome. An ophthalmologic examination is extremely important in these infants. Gradual thickening and nodule formation can occur with port-wine stain and thus support the need for early treatment in infancy and childhood. Recent advances in laser therapy techniques are shown to be more effective in previously resistant lesions. Although the timing of intervention is somewhat controversial, many dermatologists now advise laser treatment as early as possible in infancy to decrease the stigma associated with this lesion and to prevent skin thickening (Enjolras & Garzon, 2001).

Blistering Diseases

Epidermolysis Bullosa. Epidermolysis bullosa (EB) is a group of rare congenital blistering disorders, all of which are inherited. They are considered mechanobullous diseases, meaning that trauma to or friction on the skin induces blister formation. EB is caused by defects in the complex meshwork of proteins in the epidermis, dermis, and dermoepidermal junction that allow the skin to adhere in the presence of frictional stress. The underlying defect appears to be a lack of cellular glue in squamous epithelium, which is responsible for the maintenance of cellular integrity. Diagnostic studies should include a skin biopsy for light and electron microscopy.

EB is classified by the clinical extent and ultrastructural level of blistering, by inheritance pattern, and by specific molecular defect (Fine et al, 2000; Fine et al, 1999; Marinkovich, 1999). Although some subtypes of EB are severe in the neonatal period and milder later, others can be fatal in the first weeks as a result of severe generalized blistering and complications that arise from this. EB can be nonscarring or scarring. Inheritance may be either autosomal dominant or autosomal recessive.

Epidermolysis bullosa simplex is the mildest form of EB. Most cases are autosomal dominant. The lesions occur at the basal layer of epidermis and do not lead to scarring and hyperkeratosis. Usually present at birth, the vesicles and bullae appear over the joints and the bony protuberances and at sites subjected to repeated trauma. The differential diagnosis may be aided by the absence of milia, which are commonly seen in the dystrophic types of epidermolysis bullosa. Little or no scarring is seen with EB simplex.

Junctional epidermolysis bullosa is the least common type of EB with autosomal recessive inheritance. In junctional EB, severe generalized blistering is present at birth, with subsequent extensive denudation. Marked mucosal blistering occurs, and erosions of the larynx, respiratory, gastrointestinal, and urinary tract may also be present. It may be fatal in a few days to a few months because of fluid loss or sepsis. Histopathologically, a separation occurs between the plasma membrane of the basal cells and the basal lamina. In junctional EB, healing is poor, and scarring is extensive.

Dystrophic epidermolysis bullosa results in blistering that occurs below the dermoepidermal junction and has either dominant or recessive inheritance. In the recessive form, blistering is severe, begins at birth, and can lead to marked scarring and joint contractures.

The dominant form of dystrophic EB is milder, with moderately severe blisters seen on the distal extremities and bony protuberances (Figure 34-5). Some scar formation occurs, and the nails may be mildly dystrophic. Atrophy may occur with healing. The external skin layer can be easily rubbed off by slight friction or injury. Milia, due to a functional disorder of the sweat glands, are found on the rims of the ears, the dorsa of the hands, and the extensor surfaces of the arms and legs. The oral, anal, and esophageal mucosa are frequently involved. Complications include infections and hemolytic, nutritional, orthopedic, gastrointestinal, and psychiatric sequelae. These vary according to the severity of the disease.

Collaborative Management. EB can be a great challenge in the newborn period, particularly with the more severe forms. Nursing care centers around three main issues: (1) skin breakdown; (2) prevention of infection; and (3) dysphagia. Many of the techniques used to protect the skin of very premature infants are useful with EB patients. Avoiding the use of tape and preventing traumatic injuries is important. Clean, soft dressings may be helpful over bony pressure points. Wound care involves providing a moist healing environment by covering open lesions with a thick coating of petrolatum-based emollients combined with topical antibiotic ointments and covered with nonstick dressings.

Many dermatologists will rotate topical antibiotics every few months to prevent resistance, and may use wound cultures to guide selection of agents (Lin, 1996). Nonstick dressings include petrolatum gauze, Exu-dry or silicone based products such as Mepitel (Direct Medical Inc., Houston, TX). After this layer, the wound is further protected by wrapping with nonad-

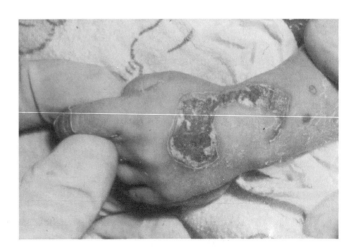

FIGURE **34-5**

This photograph of epidermolysis bullosa shows the scaling broken bullae with underlying erythroderma. From Clark D & Thompson J (1986). Dermatology of the newborn: parts 1 and 2. In *Pathology of the neonate slide series* (Vol. III, No. 4). Philadelphia, Wyeth-Ayerst Laboratories. Copyright© Wyeth; used with permission.

hesive cotton gauze; some practitioners prefer cotton mesh, and others use Coban (3M, Indianapolis), a wrap that adheres to itself without adhesives. When blisters are tense and fluid filled, they should be "unroofed" to prevent extension. This procedure is done with sharp, clean scissors, leaving the blister roof in place. Dressings are changed daily and removed gently; some prefer to remove dressings during immersion bathing (Frieden & Howard, 2001).

From birth to 6 months of age, the environment is easy to control through the use of sheepskin, loose-fitting clothes, and mittens for the infant's hands and feet. Cloth diapers softened with fabric softener are preferred over rougher, disposable diapers. Any person handling the infant should avoid wearing jewelry. Protection of the infant becomes more difficult once the infant is mobile.

The infant should always wear long pants, and foam rubber pads sewn into the knees help avoid trauma during crawling. Contractures may form quickly as scarring begins to occur. The pathologic increase in elastic skin fiber adds to this process. Gentle range-of-motion exercises lessen contracture formation.

Dysphagia can occur from facial and pharyngeal scarring, which is secondary to erosions on the buccal mucosa, tongue, palate, esophagus, and pharynx. Feedings should be performed slowly and carefully to avoid aspiration and to maintain adequate nutrition. The metabolic needs of these infants are high because of the continuous sloughing of epithelium, which results in large protein, fluid, and electrolyte losses. Adding additional puncture holes to a nipple may help prevent oral mucosal trauma. If oral ulcerations do occur, several weeks of hyperalimentation and high-dose steroid therapy are instituted. Gavage feedings are discouraged because of the possibility of trauma. It is essential that the family receive genetic counseling regarding the inheritance pattern associated with epidermolysis bullosa; a negative family history does not exclude its occurrence.

Infections of the Skin

Normal skin flora includes 13 species of coagulase-negative staphylococci (CONS) (Darmstadt & Dinulos, 2001). CONS colonize the skin of newborns within 2 to 4 days after birth. Skin infections and skin manifestations of systemic infection can be of bacterial, viral, or fungal origin. In this section, the various skin infections from each type of microorganism are discussed, along with implications for nursing care.

Bacterial

Staphylococcus Aureus.   Infections resulting from *Staphylococcus aureus* are seen in newborns and can result in two types of skin lesions. Nonbullous impetigo is a superficial infection localized to the epidermis and is characterized by erythematous, honey-colored crusted plaques. Bullous impetigo of the newborn involves blisters that originate in the subcorneal portion of the epidermis and are filled with clear or straw-colored fluid. Bullous impetigo often presents during the first two weeks of life. Few or many blisters may be dispersed widely over all areas of the body and may rupture easily, thus leaving denuded areas of skin. *S. aureus* is most commonly cultured, but other bacteria, such as group A streptococci and beta-hemolytic streptococci, are sometimes seen.

Collaborative Management.   Medical and nursing management is focused on treatment of the affected infant and on prevention of the spread of infection to other infants, because this condition is highly contagious. Systemic antibiotics are administered parenterally initially and may be followed by oral treatment once the infection begins to subside. Antibiotics include oxacillin, nafcillin, or methicillin; vancomycin is used if the culture indicated methicillin-resistant *S. aureus*. Topical antibiotics are not indicated for treatment of bullous impetigo (Darmstadt & Dinulos, 2001). Fluid and electrolyte monitoring is necessary if the denuded areas cover a large surface or if the infant is of low birth weight. Isolation of the affected infant is necessary to prevent the spread of the infection throughout the nursery.

Scalded Skin Syndrome.   *S. aureus* can also result in a severe bullous eruption called scalded skin syndrome. Initially, the infant's skin is bright red and resembles a scald. This finding is followed by the formation of large flaccid blisters that quickly progress to large sheets of shed skin (Figure 34-6). The entire epidermis is often shed during the course of this disease. The mechanism for this severe injury involves the production of an endotoxin, called exfoliatin, that causes the skin manifestations. Usually, the skin lesions do not culture positive for the responsible organism; thus culturing the nasopharynx, blood, conjunctiva, and normal skin is recommended to recover the organism for appropriate sensitivity assessment (Drolet & Esterly, 2002).

Collaborative Management.   Medical and nursing management also involves administration of the appropriate antibiotic regimen and supportive measures in terms of fluid and electrolytic replacement, prevention of secondary infection through the damaged epidermis, and comfort. Applying local antibiotic solutions or ointments is not recommended; cleansing open skin areas with gentle irrigation using half normal saline promotes healing and prevents secondary infection. The infant may be more comfortable in an incubator rather than in a radiant warmer because the incubator is a convective heat source that does not have a direct cutaneous effect, whereas

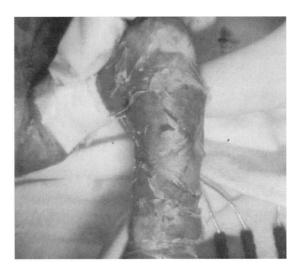

FIGURE **34-6**
The peeling, scaling skin of this premature infant had an acute onset at approximately 2 weeks of age. This is the scalded skin syndrome that results from *Staphylococcus aureus*. From Clark D & Thompson J (1986). Dermatology of the newborn: parts 1 and 2. In *Pathology of the neonate slide series* (Vol. III, No. 4). Philadelphia, Wyeth-Ayerst Laboratories. Copyright© Wyeth; used with permission.

the radiant heat source heats directly through the skin. In addition, the radiant heat source may further increase the degree of insensible water loss through the damaged epidermis. Usually, a flaking process is observed on the skin during the healing process. Emollients may be helpful in treating dry skin at this point.

Listeria Monocytogenes.   Another bacterial skin disease is listeriosis, caused by *L. monocytogenes*. This organism, which can cause severe systemic disease, can also result in a disseminated miliary granulomatosis in neonates (Drolet & Esterly, 2002). In some cases, miliary abscesses can occur; occasionally, more generalized erythema or petechiae may be present. Systemic listeriosis is a very severe infection that causes blood hemolysis and a high mortality rate. Prompt recognition and treatment with intravenous penicillin or ampicillin are indicated for the best prognosis. No direct skin therapy has been described as being necessary in this disease.

Syphilis.   Congenital syphilis is another bacterial infection that has skin manifestations. If the infant with congenital syphilis is not treated after birth, a maculopapular or bullous skin eruption develops between 2 and 6 weeks of age (Margileth, 1999). Sometimes the bullous lesions may be observed at birth on the palms or the soles, thus signifying the presence of more severe disease. Fluid contained in the blisters contains spirochetes.

The lesions most commonly seen in congenital syphilis are copper-colored and maculopapular and are located on the soles and palms. In addition, open lesions may be present around the mouth, anus, or genitals, and a highly contagious nasal discharge is occasionally seen. If the syphilis remains untreated, the lesions regress in 1 to 3 months, leaving areas on the skin with either hyperpigmentation or hypopigmentation.

Collaborative Management.   Medical and nursing management for the infant with congenital syphilis involves prompt, consistent administration of penicillin—usually a 10-day course. Titers are obtained over the next year at 3-month intervals, and a negative serologic finding is expected at 1 year. Care of the skin lesions is primarily directed toward preventing the spread of infection during the active phase of the illness, especially when bullous lesions or open areas are apparent. No direct topical therapies have been advocated in the literature.

Viral.   Viral infections can display a broad range of cutaneous manifestations in the neonate and can occur in utero, perinatally, or postnatally. Skin manifestations can be a direct result of skin infection or be a consequence of viral infection in other tissues. Viral infections that have skin symptoms include several of the herpes conditions, cytomegalovirus, and rubella. Toxoplasmosis, which has cutaneous manifestations and is caused by a parasite, is also discussed in this section.

Herpes Simplex.   Herpes simplex virus types 1 and 2 are serious pathogens in newborns. The majority of newborns acquire infections from infectious vaginal secretions at the time of delivery. Infections range from systemic, disseminated infections, CNS infection, and infection involving the skin, eye or mouth. Vesicles that occur on the skin with this disease vary; a few faint scars may be present, or actual vesicle formations may be present with either one large swelling or discrete groups of vesicles. Vesicles may recede and then recur over months.

Collaborative Management.   Medical and nursing management is centered primarily on early recognition and treatment with the antiviral medication, acyclovir. The prognosis of systemic herpes simplex is extremely poor if encephalitis develops, with either a high risk of death or severe mental retardation. An important consideration in the care of infants with known or suspected herpes simplex infection is isolation from other patients to prevent transmission.

Varicella.   Another viral infection with manifestation in the skin is varicella. Varicella infection is rare, but when it occurs in the first 10 days of life, it is generally thought to have been acquired in utero. The vesicular eruptions are the same as those in chickenpox acquired at any age. A mortality rate of 20% is associated with varicella infection in newborns, and certainly this infection poses a significant risk for the immunocompromised infants in premature and intensive care nurseries. No systemic medication or topical treatment is required for these lesions. Occasionally scarring can occur. Strict isolation is absolutely necessary to protect other infants from exposure because this virus is airborne. Passive immunization of infants exposed to the affected infant may also be necessary.

Toxoplasmosis.   Toxoplasmosis, which is caused by an intracellular parasite (*Toxoplasma gondii*), can be transmitted transplacentally and can result in systemic infection. Some infants may have a generalized maculopapular rash as well as hepatosplenomegaly, jaundice, fever, and anemia. The rash may progress to desquamation and hypopigmentation in very severe cases. Direct topical therapy is not reported to be necessary or efficacious; systemic therapy may be considered.

Cytomegalovirus and Rubella.   Both cytomegalovirus and rubella have symptoms that are manifested in the skin. Petechial lesions can occur with both infections. These are the result of thrombocytopenia and usually disappear in 2 to 6 weeks. In severe rubella infection, and very rarely in cytomegalovirus, bluish-red papules that are 2 to 8 mm in diameter can occur on the head, trunk, and extremities (Figure 34-7).

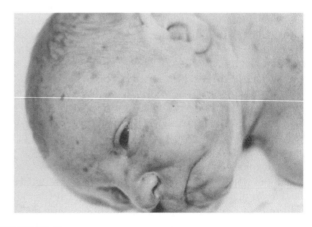

FIGURE **34-7**
This is an example of the "blueberry muffin" syndrome, seen in an infant with congenital cytomegalovirus infection. The infant has multiple petechiae and purpura from thrombocytopenia in this systemic infection. From Clark D & Thompson J (1986). Dermatology of the newborn: parts 1 and 2. In *Pathology of the neonate slide series* (Vol. III, No. 4). Philadelphia, Wyeth-Ayerst Laboratories. Copyright © Wyeth; used with permission.

This so-called blueberry muffin syndrome is the result of erythropoiesis in the dermis and usually subsides in 2 to 3 weeks. Neither of these lesions requires topical therapy (for a complete discussion of infections, see Chapter 29).

Fungal. *Candida albicans* infection is the primary fungal infection with cutaneous manifestations, although other species—such as *C. parapsilosis, C. tropicalis, C. lusitaniae, C. glabrata,* and *Malassezia furfur*—can also potentially colonize the skin of term and preterm newborns, particularly those who are hospitalized in an intensive care nursery. Manifestations of infection with *Candida* species can range from diaper dermatitis or other localized skin or mucous membrane eruptions to disseminated candidiasis, thus resulting in significant morbidity and mortality. *Candida* is not normally found in the skin flora of the newborn. The gastrointestinal system is the primary reservoir, but the skin may also be colonized during passage through a colonized vaginal canal. The incidence of *Candida* colonization is also increased with the frequent use of broad-spectrum antibiotics that alter normal skin flora in infants after delivery.

Infants with systemic candidiasis may demonstrate cutaneous involvement. This cutaneous pattern may be a diffuse burn-like dermatitis that affects large areas on the lower back, buttocks, chest, and abdomen. In a few infants, the axilla and groin are affected. Scaling followed the erythematous macular patches, and severe cases desquamation develops in a manner similar to that seen in staphylococcal scalded skin syndrome. These infants do not always have the satellite papules and pustules normally seen with *Candida* diaper dermatitis. The onset of the generalized rash often occurs within the first 3 days of life, but it can appear later.

A monilial diaper rash was the other dermatologic condition exhibited by some infants. This rash consisted of a red, scaling dermatitis in the groin, and the rash spread to other body parts.

Erosive crusting lesions in a cohort of extremely premature infants as an invasive fungal dermatitis, leading also to systemic disease, was reported (Rowen et al, 1995). Primarily due to candida albicans or other candida species, other fungal species were also seen and included Aspergillus, Trichosporum beigelii, and Curvularia. Skin biopsies performed on patients with this condition revealed fungal invasion that extended beyond the epidermis into the dermis. The onset is several days after birth, and associated factors included maternal colonization with vaginal birth, steroid administration, hyperglycemia and skin trauma from adhesive removal.

Collaborative Management. Medical and nursing management of infants with systemic or local *Candida* infection involves therapy with systemic antifungal medications and antifungal ointments and creams. Cutaneous candida in the extremely premature infant less than a week of age requires aggressive monitoring for systemic infection and may warrant parenteral antifungal agents to prevent dissemination of the fungal infection. Yeast is sometimes difficult to culture; techniques include obtaining urine to look for hyphae or budding yeast, blood cultures, and skin scrapings prepared with potassium hydroxide (KOH) obtained from the margins of the affected areas since this is the area of active growth, and examined for pseudohyphae (Cunningham & Wagner, 2001). Nursing observation in low-birth-weight infants for evidence of the diffuse burnlike dermatitis or a spreading monilial diaper rash is essential and may expedite the initiation of parenteral antifungal therapy with amphotericin B for systemic candidiasis.

Scaling Disorders

A scaly appearance in the skin of a newborn can have a range of causes, from relatively benign to long-term and potentially life-threatening. In this section, scaly skin due to postmaturity, essential fatty acid deficiency, congenital ichthyosis, and eczema is discussed, and areas of nursing management are determined.

Postmaturity. Many term infants born between 40 and 42 weeks' gestation experience a period of shedding or desquamation that is considered to be a normal physiologic process. Postmature infants born after 42 weeks' gestation may also have this appearance, but other characteristics are different. The postmature infant may have a lean appearance, with little subcutaneous fat; the weight is low in relationship to length. The skin resembles parchment paper and may literally peel off in sheets. Fingernails may be stained with meconium and may be long. Long hair may also be present.

Skin care is not the major problem, nor is it the focus of medical or nursing management. Eventually, the skin underneath the peeling layers predominates; even during the period of desquamation, the skin functions well as a barrier because these infants have all the layers of stratum corneum of a term infant or adult. Aside from bathing with a mild soap initially, a moisturizing with a petrolatum-based ointment may be used. More careful attention is paid to the more compelling problems associated with postmaturity, such as hypoglycemia and meconium aspiration.

Essential Fatty Acid Deficiency. In some newborns who are unable to receive an adequate diet because of other illnesses or surgical condition, scaly dry skin may signify the development of essential fatty acid deficiency syndrome. Infants may be more prone to the development of this syndrome, especially if they are premature or postmature because of the decreased fat stores available. It may also occur in infants with severe fat malabsorption, such as those with cystic fibrosis.

The skin appearance in essential fatty acid deficiency includes a superficial scaling and, in some cases, desquamation. Later presentation may involve oozing and irritation in the neck, groin, or perianal region.

This syndrome is sometimes confused with other conditions that cause scaling or other skin disruptions, including ichthyosis, acrodermatitis enteropathica, and candidal infection. Laboratory findings that confirm this diagnosis are decreased serum essential fatty acid levels, possibly in conjunction with thrombocytopenia and impaired platelet aggregation, because essential fatty acids are necessary to ensure platelet function.

Collaborative Management. Medical and nursing management consists of replacement of essential fatty acids through the administration of intravenous lipid solutions or diet. Human breast milk and most infant formulas contain more than adequate amounts of essential fatty acids. However, if the gastrointestinal system is not functioning well in the digestion and absorption of nutrients, intravenous therapy is required.

Once skin symptoms are present, administration of intravenous lipid solution can reverse the process in 1 to 2 weeks. Dietary replacement takes longer and is effective only in the presence of healthy gastrointestinal function.

Prevention of essential fatty acid deficiency is possible and should be the goal. Early administration of intravenous lipid solutions in the first weeks of life in a dose as low as 0.5 g/kg/day can prevent the development of essential fatty acid deficiency.

Ichthyosis. The most serious cause of scaly skin in the newborn is ichthyosis dermatosis. Four major types of ichthyosis exist: (1) X-linked ichthyosis; (2) lamellar ichthyosis; (3) bullous congenital ichthyosiform erythroderma, which is present at birth; and (4) ichthyosis vulgaris, which usually appears after the third month of life. Terms commonly used to describe infants with ichthyosis may include harlequin fetus and collodion baby, but these terms do not define which form of ichthyosis is present.

In the X-linked type of ichthyosis, males are affected. Some female heterozygotes may exhibit mild scaling of the arms and lower extremities. Affected male newborns have large yellow or brown plaques that cover the whole body except the palms, soles, and midface and over joints. At birth, some affected males may appear scaly, whereas others are often called collodion babies.

Lamellar ichthyosis, formerly called nonbullous congenital ichthyosiform erythroderma, is an autosomal recessive disorder. Initially, affected newborns may have a bright red appearance that rapidly progresses to desquamation; rarely is a collodion-baby appearance present at birth. Later, scales develop that are yellow to brown and that may eventually become thick, horny plates. Although the prognosis is usually good, infants who are severely affected—the so-called harlequin fetuses—may die of sepsis or require extensive plastic surgery (Figure 34-8).

In bullous congenital ichthyosiform erythroderma, autosomal dominance is the mode of heredity; thus several family members may be affected. Large bullae are initially seen, as are erythema and dry scaly skin; the blistering that recurs throughout childhood differentiates this form from the lamellar type. Extensive denuded areas of the skin can present a problem in

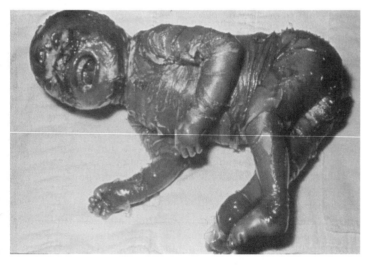

FIGURE 34-8
This harlequin infant is an example of the most severely affected ichthyotic infant. The skin is hard and thick, with deep crevices. The lack of elasticity of the skin results in fleshy deformities of joints and limbs. From Clark D & Thompson J (1986). Dermatology of the newborn: parts 1 and 2. In *Pathology of the neonate slide series* (Vol. III, No. 4). Philadelphia, Wyeth-Ayerst Laboratories. Copyright© Wyeth; used with permission.

the newborn as the blisters burst because secondary infections with *Streptococcus* or *Staphylococcus* can occur and are life-threatening.

Collaborative Management. Medical and nursing management of all forms of ichthyosis involves the continual use of topical therapies and prescription bathing techniques and the prevention of infection. Bathing is performed with a water-dispersible bath oil, and soaps that are excessively drying or irritating should be avoided. Colloidion babies should be placed in a high humidity incubator to increase hydration. Emollients that preserve moisturization, such as Aquaphor ointment (Beiersdorf, Inc., Wilton, CT), are applied several times daily.

Infants with severe skin involvement from ichthyosis may require protective isolation if they receive care in an intensive care nursery because of the higher risk of contact with nosocomial infections. Incubators provide a barrier to infection. Use of sterile linen and sterile gloves and other measures are needed if larger areas of denuded skin are present.

Comfort is another key nursing concern in the care of the infant who is significantly affected with ichthyosis. Fussy, irritable agitation may be seen and is related to pruritus or inflammation. Some form of analgesia may help, although the topical therapies prescribed have the most direct effect. Some authors describe the use of diphenhydramine (Benadryl) if severe pruritus exists, but this would be very hard to determine in a neonate, who lacks verbal or fine motor skills to communicate this symptom. A trial of this medication with careful observation might be helpful in the case of a very frantic or irritable infant when other measures (e.g., topical treatment, pacifiers, feeding) are unsuccessful.

Working with the parents of an infant with ichthyosis has many facets. The appearance of the infant, especially if he or she is severely affected, could be shocking and traumatic to the parents and could require careful interventions. As with parents of infants with other congenital abnormalities, a period of shock, denial, and grief occurs over the loss of a perfect baby. In addition, the genetic nature of this disorder and the implications for future children must be comprehended. Parents of these infants need genetic counseling, support, and education as they come to terms with this disease.

Eczema. Eczema, which is a skin disorder that causes several degrees of skin irritation and has multiple causes, is rarely seen in the newborn period. It is more commonly seen after 2 months of age and involves an eruption that proceeds to the development of microvesicles and oozing, which later turns into scaling of the epidermis, as this layer tries to regenerate rapidly. Lichenification, or thickening of the skin, which occurs in adult skin with eczema, is not seen in infants. Primary irritants—such as saliva, feces, and some soaps or skin preparations—rather than allergies are the usual causes of eczema in infants. It is important to have a good history of all products that have been applied to the skin to sort out the causes. If external agents have been ruled out, other diagnoses are considered, such as seborrheic dermatitis and Leiner's disease, which involves a total exfoliation of the entire body.

Collaborative Management. Medical and nursing treatment of eczema involves prevention by avoiding the primary irritant source, if it has been identified, or protection, as in the use of zinc oxide paste to the perianal area to prevent contact with feces. For more generalized eruptions, short-term therapy with topical steroids may be used. Bathing should be carried out in tepid water with water-dispersible oil; use of irritating or drying soaps should be avoided. If large areas of skin are involved, thermoregulation may be a concern, especially in dry climates. Humidification may be desirable in some climates, especially during the summer months. Air conditioning may also be necessary during the summer months.

Discomfort is also a significant concern because infants with eczema may experience considerable pruritus. Topical therapy is generally the first consideration, followed by the judicious use of diphenhydramine in severe cases.

SKIN CARE PRACTICES

The most basic aspects of skin care for newborns include daily bath; moisturizing with emollients; skin preparation with disinfectant solutions; and use of adhesives for life support devices, monitoring of vital signs, and oxygenation, if the newborns are hospitalized. During all these practices, the skin of the newborn has the potential for trauma or alterations in normal barrier function and pH. The literature is reviewed to determine what is currently known about these and other common nursing practices and the impact on the skin of newborns.

Bathing

The purposes of bathing newborns includes providing overall hygiene, aesthetics, and protection of health care workers by removing blood and body fluids. However, bathing is not an innocuous procedure and during the immediate postbirth period can result in hypothermia, increased oxygen consumption, and respiratory distress. The first bath should be delayed until the infant's temperature has been stabilized in the normal range for 1 to 4 hours (Penny-MacGillivay 1996; Varda & Behnke, 2000) Bathing has also been shown to destabilize vital signs and temperature in premature infants (Peters, 1998).

Bathing with antiseptic soaps and cleansers is still practiced in some nurseries. Studies have shown that although hexachlorophene reduced the number of *Staphylococcus aureus* strains, toxicity was reported, especially in premature infants and was associated with absorption through the skin; thus it should not be used (American Academy of Pediatrics, 1997). Both povidone-iodine and chlorhexidine are sometimes used for the initial bath in newborn nurseries, although the effect on bacterial colonization is transient. Chlorhexidine has proven effective in reducing colonization for up to 4 hours but can also be absorbed. Although toxicity from chlorhexidine has not been identified, many nurseries do not use chlorhexidine for routine bathing because of the potential risk. No guidelines from the Centers for Disease Control or the American Academy of Pediatrics recommend that antimicrobial cleansers be used for the newborn's first or subsequent baths (American Academy of Pediatrics, 1997).

Products used in bathing include soaps made with lye and animal fats which are alkaline (pH >7.0) and cleansing bars and liquids made with synthetic detergents that are formulated to a more neutral pH of 5.5 to 7.0. All soaps and cleansers are at least mildly irritating and drying to skin surfaces. Study of bathing with soap, cleansing liquid, or cleansing bar in infants ages 2 weeks to 16 months showed alterations in fat content, hydration, and skin surface pH—most significantly with alkaline soap (Gfatter et al, 1997). In addition, the degree to which the skin is irritated also depends on the length of contact and the frequency of bathing.

Selecting cleansers that have a neutral pH and minimal dyes and perfumes to reduce risk of future sensitization to these products and bathing only 2 to 3 times per week is the best course to follow. Reducing the frequency of bathing even to four-day intervals did not increase colonization with pathogens or result in infections in a study of healthy premature infants (Franck et al, 2000). For extremely premature infants, skin surfaces should be cleaned with warm water for the first week, with soft materials such as cotton balls or cloth. A rinsing technique is best during cleansing because rubbing is irritating to immature skin and potentially is uncomfortable. If areas of skin breakdown are evident, use warm sterile water.

Immersion bathing may be beneficial, when clinically possible, from a developmental perspective (Anderson et al, 1995). Immersion bathing places the infant's entire body, except the head and neck, into warm water (100.4° F), deep enough to cover the shoulders. Stable premature infants (after umbilical catheters are removed) and term infants with umbilical clamp in place can safely be bathed in this way (AWHONN/NANN Guideline, 2001). Bathing is also an excellent time to educate parents about how to physically care for their babies and may also integrate information about their children's neurobehavioral status and social characteristics (Karl, 1999).

Emollients

The skin surface of term newborns is drier than that of adults but becomes gradually better hydrated as the eccrine sweat glands mature during the first year of life. Maintaining the hydration of the stratum corneum is necessary for an intact skin surface and normal barrier function. Skin that is dry, scaly, or cracking is not only uncomfortable but also can also be a portal of entry for microorganisms. Products used to counteract dryness are called moisturizers, emollients, or lubricants. Common emollients include mineral oils, petrolatum, and lanolin and its derivatives. Emollients are divided into oil-in-water or water-in-oil emulsions (Hoath & Narendran, 2000).

Emollient use to prevent dermatitis and improve skin integrity in premature infants has been studied recently. Premature infants of 29 to 36 weeks' gestation treated daily with Eucerin cream (Beiersdorf, Inc., Wilton, CT) had less visible dermatitis but no differences in direct measurements of TEWL with an evaporimeter.

In a later study, premature infants of both younger gestation and postnatal age were treated with Aquaphor ointment (Beiersdorf, Inc., Wilton, CT), a water miscible oil-in-water preparation that contains neither dyes nor perfumes. In this study, both TEWL and visual scale dermatitis improved.

No increase in skin surface temperatures or thermal burns were seen, even when the emollient was applied to infants under radiant heaters or phototherapy lights. In addition, cutaneous cultures revealed no increase in bacterial or fungal colonization on skin treated with emollients, and fewer treated infants had positive blood or cerebrospinal fluid cultures compared with controls (Nopper et al, 1996).

A large, randomized controlled trial of 1191 infants with birth weights of 501 to 1000 grams was conducted to determine whether a twice-daily application of Aquaphor ointment would reduce combined outcome measures of mortality and sepsis. Although skin integrity appeared improved with routine emollient use, no effect on the outcomes of sepsis plus mortality was seen. Of note, an increase in coagulase-negative staphylococcus epidermidis bloodstream infections was seen in infants with birth weights <750 grams, although the mechanism and relationship to emollient use are not clearly understood (Edwards et al, 2000). Although a small case-control study had previously associated petrolatum-based emollients to a higher incidence of fungal infections, this was not seen in the larger study. The effects of emollients on TEWL or fluid balance were not studied in this trial (Edwards et al, 2000).

The benefits of emollient use must be carefully weighed against the risk of infection. In general, emollients can be safely used to treat skin with excessive drying, skin cracking, and fissures. They may also be beneficial in reducing TEWL and evaporative heat loss, although other methods, such as using a high humidity environment or transparent adhesive dressings, are also available for this purpose (AWHONN/NANN Guideline, 2001). Avoiding products with perfumes or dyes is prudent because these can be absorbed and are potential contact irritants. Small tubes or jars for single patient use are recommended to prevent contamination with microorganisms.

Disinfectants

Disinfection of the skin before invasive procedures such as venipuncture and placement of umbilical catheters and chest tubes is common practice in neonatal intensive care nurseries. Anecdotal reports of skin injury include blistering, burns, and sloughing from both isopropyl alcohol and povidone-iodine use in premature infants. High iodine levels, iodine goiter, and hypothyroidism associated with povidone-iodine use in premature infants have also been reported. Several prospective studies of routine povidone-iodine use in intensive care nurseries (Linder et al, 1997; Parravicini et al, 1996) and one study of presurgical skin preparation of infants under 3 months of age found alterations in iodine levels and potential thyroid effects from povidone-iodine exposure due to absorption through the skin. Although one study did not find thyroid effects from iodine absorption in neonates (Gordon et al, 1995), the study period (10 days) may be too short a period of time to see the effect.

Another important aspect of skin disinfection is the efficacy of the solutions. During skin preparation before blood culture sampling in children and adults, lower rates of microbial colonization were seen with povidone-iodine compared to isopropyl alcohol. A larger study of blood culture sampling in adults found fewer contaminated cultures with chlorhexidine compared to povidone-iodine (Mimoz et al, 1999). Two studies in premature infants compared skin and peripheral intravenous catheter colonization with bacteria after skin preparation with either chlorhexidine or povidone-iodine. Malathi et al (1993) found the rate of colonization was no different between disinfectants but that the technique of application was important; the authors recommended longer periods of cleansing (>30 seconds) or two consecutive cleansings for maximum reductions of colonization. Garland et al (1995) reported that chlorhexidine reduced the rate of catheter colonization in premature infants: 4.3% with chlorhexine, in comparison to 9.3% with povidone-iodine.

A comparison of isopropyl alcohol, povidone-iodine, and 2% chlorhexidine aqueous solution for disinfection of 668 central venous catheters in adults during insertion and routine dressing changes showed chlorhexidine to be significantly more effective in reducing catheter related infections.

Skin disinfectants used for newborns include both chlorhexidine or povidone-iodine solutions and, less frequently, 70% isopropyl alcohol. Chlorhexidine is available as a tincture (0.5% in isopropyl alcohol) or as a surgical scrub (2% or 4% in an aqueous solution). A single-use applicator of 2% chlorhexidine in isopropyl alcohol has recently been approved for preoperative skin preparation in adults. Other chlorhexidine products must be poured from bottles or packages onto sterile gauze for application. Chlorhexidine should not be used as preoperative skin disinfection on the face or head, because misuse has been reported to result in injury if it remains in contact with either the eye or ear during surgical procedures. However, careful use before scalp intravenous or central line insertion is acceptable, providing that splashing or using excessive amounts of chlorhexidine is avoided. Chlorhexidine is applied in two consecutive wipings or for a 30-second scrubbing period and is removed with sterile water or saline when the procedure is completed.

Povidone-iodine is available in a 10% aqueous solution in a variety of single use applications. It is also applied in two consecutive wipings or for a 30 second scrubbing period and then allowed to dry for at least 30 seconds before the procedure. Any solution should then be completely removed with sterile water or saline to prevent any further absorption. Disinfection with isopropyl alcohol is questionable in the neonatal intensive care nursery because it is less efficacious than either povidone-iodine or chlorhexidine and can be irritating and drying to skin surfaces.

Use of disinfectants for umbilical cord care is debatable. The use of antibiotic ointments and antiseptics can prolong the time to cord separation and seems to have no beneficial effect on the frequency of infection (Zupan & Gardner, 2000).

A study of 1811 newborns randomized to receive either routine isopropyl alcohol with each diaper change or natural drying found no umbilical infections in either group, and time to cord separation was reduced from 9.8 days in the alcohol-treated group to 8.16 days in the natural drying group (Dore et al, 1998). Therefore routine use of alcohol for cord care is not helpful in facilitating cord separation or reducing risk of infection (AWHONN/NANN Guideline, 2001).

Adhesives

One of the most common practices in the neonatal intensive care nursery is the application and removal of adhesives that secure endotracheal tubes, IV devices, and monitoring probes and electrodes. A research utilization project that involved 2820 premature and term newborns found that adhesives were the primary cause of skin breakdown among NICU patients (Lund et al, 2001).

Changes in TEWL and skin barrier function are seen in adults after 10 consecutive removals of adhesive tape and after one removal of adhesive tape in a premature infant. Types of damage from adhesive removal include epidermal stripping, tearing, maceration, tension blisters, chemical irritation, sensitization, and folliculitis (Hoath & Narendran, 2000).

Solvents are sometimes used to prevent discomfort and skin disruption from adhesive removal. They contain hydrocarbon derivatives or petroleum distillates that have potential or proven toxicities. Toxicity is a major concern, especially in premature infants with their underdeveloped stratum corneum, increased skin permeability, larger surface area to body weight, and immature hepatic and renal function. A case report of toxic epidermal necrosis in a premature infant resulted from the use of a solvent. Mineral oil or petrolatum products may be helpful in removing adhesives but cannot be used if the site must be used again for reapplication of adhesives, such as with the retaping of an endotracheal tube.

Skin bonding agents promote adherence. Unfortunately, they may create a stronger bond between adhesive and epidermis than the fragile cohesion of the epidermis to the dermis; when removed, epidermal stripping may result. Plastic polymers have been studied and are reported to reduce skin trauma. An alcohol-free skin protectant that is less irritating to skin surfaces in adults than comparable products that contain alcohol is available. This product has been approved for infants over 30 days of age to treat mild diaper dermatitis and to prevent skin injury from adhesive removal (3M Health Care, 2000). Although a single study from England reports positive effects when using this skin protectant to tape intravenous lines in newborns (Irving, 2001), it has not yet been approved for use in premature infants or term newborns in the United States.

Skin barriers such as karaya rings and pectin products have been used to protect the peristomal skin in adult ostomy patients. A comparison of regular adhesive electrodes and karaya electrodes found less skin disruption, as measured by TEWL, from the karaya electrodes in premature infants. However, some premature infants developed skin irritation from the karaya electrodes, and they are no longer available. Pectin barriers (Hollihesive, Hollister, Libertyville, IL; Duoderm, Conbatec, Gillman, NJ; Comfeel, Coloplast North America, Marietta, GA) have been used beneath adhesives in premature infants and are reported as leaving less visible skin trauma when removed (Dollison & Beckstrand, 1995). Following these reports, a controlled trial of pectin barrier (Hollihesive), plastic tape (Transpore, 3M), and hydrophilic gelled adhesive was done and found significant skin disruption, as measured by TEWL and visual inspection, occurred after removal of both the pectin barrier and plastic tape. Because the adhesives were left in place 24 hours before removal in this study, a time effect of peak adhesive aggressiveness may have been reached. It is interesting to note that significant changes were identified after a single adhesive removal in all three weight groups that were studied (<1000 g, 1001 to 1500 g, >1501 g), thus indicating that even larger premature infants are at risk for skin injury from tape removal.

Prevention of skin trauma from adhesive removal includes minimizing tape use when possible by using smaller pieces, backing the adhesive with cotton, and delaying tape removal until adherence is reduced. Pectin barriers and hydrocolloid adhesives may prove helpful because they mold and adhere well to body contours and often attach better in moist conditions. As with tape, removal of pectin barriers and hydrocolloid should be delayed, if possible, until the adherence lessens. Soft gauze wraps to secure probes and the use of hydrogel ECG electrodes and hydrogel tapes are helpful. Adhesives should be removed with warm water and cotton balls slowly and carefully. Mineral oil or an emollient may facilitate adhesive removal if reapplication of adhesives at the site of removal is not necessary.

Transepidermal Water Loss

Because of the poorly keratinized stratum corneum, which provides minimal resistance to the diffusion of water, the preterm infant is subjected to transepidermal water loss (TEWL) and heat loss via evaporation that results in low body temperatures during the first few days after birth. Characteristic skin factors that predispose infants to water loss include larger surface area in relation to body weight, thinner epidermis, increased water content, increased permeability, and increased blood supply that is closer to the skin surface.

TEWL is directly correlated to gestational age and degree of maturation of the epidermal stratum corneum. Mature keratin, which is a major component of the tough, nonliving outer layer of the epidermis, is relatively water impermeable. Because keratin formation is directly related to gestational age, the ex-

tremely premature infant is at increased risk for increased evaporative losses. Water easily diffuses across the permeable skin barrier and evaporates. TEWL is influenced by many factors: ambient humidity, gestational age at birth, postnatal age, ambient temperature, weight, activity, and body temperature. Term infants have been shown to have lower TEWL levels compared to adults, with the exception of the antecubital region (Yosipovitch et al, 2000). Infants who are small-for-gestational-age have a lower TEWL in the first day after birth than that of infants of the same gestational age whose weight is appropriate for gestational age.

The highest TEWL levels are seen in extremely premature infants. Water losses of 130 to 160 cc/kg/day have been measured in infants of 23 to 25 weeks' gestation (Agren et al, 1998). Mature barrier function—thought at one time thought to advance rapidly over a two week period in premature infants less than 30 weeks' gestation—has been shown to take longer in extremely premature infants of 23 to 24 weeks' gestation and occurs when the infant reaches approximately 30 to 31 weeks' postconceptional age (Kalia et al, 1998).

Several techniques that have been shown to reduce evaporative heat and transepidermal water loss (TEWL) in very-lowbirth-weight infants and include the use of double-walled incubators, increased ambient humidity, transparent adhesive dressings, and coating the skin with petrolatum-based emolients.

For the past two decades it has been known that insensible water loss is greater under radiant warmers than incubators without shields. The addition of the heat shield reduced insensible water loss in the incubator but not under the radiant warmer. A plastic blanket under a radiant warmer reduces oxygen consumption, insensible water loss, and radiant warmer demands.

In 1995, Kjartansson et al measured the rate of evaporation from the skin of 12 fullterm and 16 preterm infants (gestational age of 25 to 34 weeks), both during incubator care and in care under a radiant warmer. They concluded that the evaporative water loss from the skin depends on the ambient water vapor pressure, irrespective of whether the infant is nursed under a radiant warmer or in an incubator. The higher rate of evaporation during care under a radiant warmer is due to the lower ambient water vapor pressure and not to any direct effect of the nonionizing radiation on the skin. Thus the effect of each heating device on the immediate "microclimate" surrounding the infant needs to be assessed not only in terms of temperature but also the relative humidity (RH). A RH below 40% is drying to the skin and leads to excessive TEWL in the extremely premature infant.

Plastic wraps and transparent adhesive dressings have also been shown to reduce TEWL and evaporative heat loss. Immediately after delivery, infants <28 weeks' gestation wrapped with occlusive polyethylene bags covering their torso and extremities had significantly better temperatures than infants who received drying and radiant heat in the delivery room due to significantly reduced evaporative heat and water loss; the wrapping was removed upon admission to the NICU. Mortality also significantly decreased in the infants who were wrapped (Vohra et al, 1999).

Transparent adhesive dressings such as Tegaderm (3M Healthcare, St. Paul), OpSite (Smith-Nephew, Inc., Largo, FL), or Biocclusive (3M) applied to large areas of skin surfaces reduce TEWL. Mancini et al (1994) studied the effect of a nonadhesive semipermeable dressing on the epidermal barrier of 15 premature infants by measuring TEWL on control and on

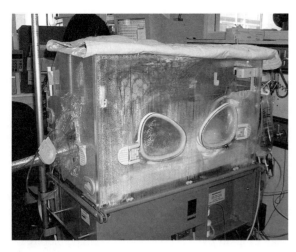

FIGURE **34-9**
Incubator with >70% relative humidity; humidity is generated by heating system that is separate from circulating convective heat to prevent contamination with microorganisms.

BOX **34-1**

Neonatal Skin Condition Score

Dryness
1=normal, no sign of dry skin
2=dry skin, visible scaling
3=very dry skin, cracking/fissures

Erythema
1=no evidence erythema
2=visible erythema <50% of body surface
3=visible erythema >50% of body surface

Breakdown/excoriation
1=none evident
2=small localized areas
3=extensive

Perfect score=3; worst score=9

From the Association of Women's Health, Obstetric, and Neonatal Nurses (AWHONN) and the National Association of Neonatal Nurses, Skin Care Utilization Project. Copyright 2001, AWHONN.

treated skin. Treated skin showed a significantly decreased TEWL on the treated site; TEWL was measured after temporary dressing removal on days 1, 2, 4, and 7. Increased cellular proliferation was documented; this phenomenon is associated with improved epidermal barrier function. High humidity (>70% RH) added to the incubator has been shown to effectively reduce evaporative heat loss and TEWL; using incubators that actively heat and evaporate water separately from circulating heat prevents contamination with microorganisms (Figure 34-9) (Drucker & Marshall 1995; Marshall 1997). Application of petrolatum-based emollients, such as Aquaphor ointment (Beirsdore) every 6 to 12 hours also reduces TEWL and can be used on infants on radiant warmers or under phototherapy without temperature increases or burns (Nopper et al, 1996). Although each of three techniques has been shown to be effective, none have been compared; thus it is not clear which is most effective with the fewest side effects. However, addressing the important area of reducing excessive heat loss and TEWL is necessary in the care of the small premature with lung disease to maintain adequate hydration without excessive fluid intake. The goal of maintaining hydration and normal serum sodium levels on an intake of less than 150 cc/kg/day is optimal and achievable using of these preventive strategies.

MANAGEMENT OF SKIN CARE PROBLEMS

The stratum corneum can be traumatized by a variety of insults, including epidermal stripping from removal of adhesives; burns from transcutaneous oxygen electrodes; pressure sores; infection; nutritional inadequacies, such as zinc and essential fatty acid deficiency; extravasation of intravenous fluids; and diaper dermatitis. The goal of all skin care for neonates should be the maintenance of skin integrity; however, even with meticulous care, skin breakdown can occur.

Skin Assessment
A thorough examination of all skin surfaces on a daily basis will reveal the state of skin integrity in critically ill or extremely premature infants in the NICU. Early signs of skin abrasions or small excoriations may call for either diagnostic or treatment procedures. A skin assessment tool such as the

Neonatal Skin Condition Score (NSCS) (Box 34-1, Figure 34-10) used in the AWHONN/NANN research-based practice project may be beneficial when assessing skin conditions (Lund et al, 2001). Identifying risk factors for skin injury in individual patients may include gestational age <32 weeks, use of paralytic medications and vasopressors, multiple tubes and lines, numerous monitors and probes, surgical wounds, ostomies, and technologies that limit patient movement such as high frequency ventilation and extracorporeal membrane oxygenation (ECMO).

Skin Excoriations
When a skin excoriation is noted, the first step is to identify the cause of the injury before determining a treatment strategy. In cases in which no trauma has been known to occur, ruling out infectious causes—such as staphylococcal scalded skin syndrome and cutaneous candidiasis—is especially important because these conditions may require culturing and either systemic or topical treatment.

Ointments are sometimes used because of their antibacterial or antifungal properties and also because covering the wound with a semiocclusive layer promotes healing by facilitating the migration of epithelial cells across the surface. Petrolatum-based emollients and ointments are used to cover wounds and provide a semiocclusive layer that facilitates the migrations of epithelial cells across the surface and may actually become part of the stratum corneum layer during the healing process. Antibacterial ointments such as Polysporin, Bacitracin, or Bactroban ointment is useful to treat gram-positive colonized surfaces but can actually promote the growth of gram-negative organisms (Smack et al, 1996). Many dermatologists recommend against the use of Neosporin because of the potential for developing later sensitization to this ointment, although sensitization to Bacitracin is being reported with increasing frequency (Marks et al, 1995). If fungal infection is suspected, Nystatin ointment is used and can also be applied to surrounding intact skin to prevent extension of the infection. In general, ointments are preferable to creams in

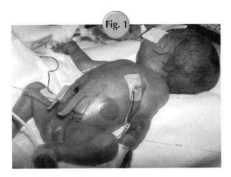

Dryness: 1 = normal, no
              sign of dry skin
Eythema: 2 = visible
              erythema <50%
              body surface
Breakdown: 3 = extensive

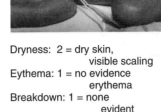

Dryness: 2 = dry skin,
              visible scaling
Eythema: 1 = no evidence
              erythema
Breakdown: 1 = none
              evident

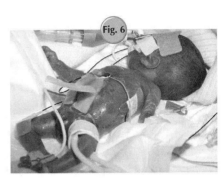

Dryness: 2 = dry skin,
              visible scaling
Eythema: 3 = visible erythema
              >50% body surface
Breakdown: 3 = extensive

FIGURE **34-10**
Examples of skin assessments in three infants using the Neonatal Skin Condition Score (NSCS).

this application because of better adherence and healing properties.

Transparent adhesive dressings are made from a polyurethane film backed with adhesive that is impermeable to water and bacteria but allows airflow. There must be a rim of intact skin around the wound to attach the dressing. Uses include wound care, dressings for IV devices—including central venous lines and percutaneous silicone catheters—and prevention of friction injuries to areas such as the knees or sacrum. When used for wound care, transparent adhesive dressing promotes "moist healing" that allows the rapid migration of epithelial cells across the site. These dressings should only be used on "clean wounds" (uninfected) because bacteria and fungus can proliferate under the dressing. When placed over a clean wound, a serous or milky exudate often forms and is composed of leukocytes that actually aid in the prevention of infection. The dressings can be left in place for days at a time or until they become loose. Removing and reattaching the dressings on a daily basis is not recommended because the adhesive can injure the intact skin around the wound and further impede healing.

Some of the skin excoriations seen in the patient in the NICU cannot be easily covered with transparent adhesive dressings if no rim of intact skin exists around the site or if it is located in close proximity to other skin that cannot be separated or folds over the excoriation, such as the neck folds and the groin. Treatment of excoriations includes irrigating with sterile normal or half-normal saline every 4 to 6 hours and then leaving the area exposed to air. This simple, basic procedure is effective in keeping the excoriation clean, and it promotes healing with little risk of sensitization or infection. Other types of dressings used in wound management include hydrogel dressings (Vigilon) and hydrocolloid and pectin dressings (Duoderm), both of which promote moist healing. Hydrogel dressings can be used after irrigation of the wound and in conjunction with either antibacterial or antifungal ointment if the wound is infected. These dressings must be changed every 8 to 12 hours because they can dry out. No adhesive can attach these dressings. It is best to avoid placing hydrogel dressings on intact skin surfaces because they can macerate the skin and actually reduce barrier function. Hydrocolloid dressings are used over uninfected wounds and can be left in place for 5 to 7 days while healing takes place (Lund, 1999). Surgical wounds that

open or dehisce are infrequent but require expert wound management. Nutrition is often a part of the process in getting these wounds to heal, as is the prevention of infection. Often the surgeon or enterostomal therapist will design the appropriate wound management program for these situations.

Nutritional Deficiencies

Zinc is an essential trace element—essential because it is crucial for growth and development and a trace element because it is present in humans in quantities equal to or less than the quantities in which iron is present. Zinc is a cofactor in the reaction of more than 15 enzymes in many areas of metabolism. It is essential for lymphocyte transformation and is important for the metabolism of proteins, nucleic acids, and mucopolysaccharides of the skin and subcutaneous tissues. It is also an essential part of the enzyme structure of alkaline phosphatase (Prasad, 1995). In addition, zinc is required for normal taste, smell, and wound healing.

Zinc deficiency can result from inadequate intake, malabsorption, excessive loss, or a combination of factors (Stevens & Lubitz, 1998). Absorption and excretion of zinc occur primarily through the gastrointestinal tract. Deficiencies are related to abnormal losses of zinc in stool or urine, poor stores, or increased demands, as occur during rapid growth phases or stress. Total body zinc doubles between 32 and 40 weeks' gestation, with two thirds of the maternal-fetal transport occurring during the last 10 weeks of gestation. Premature infants are at special risk for developing a zinc deficiency. Because they have trouble absorbing zinc and have not received adequate stores before birth, they may be in negative zinc balance for several weeks after birth. Other infants at risk for zinc deficiency include those with gastrointestinal pathology, chronic diarrhea, short-gut or short-bowel syndrome with jejunoileal bypass, necrotizing enterocolitis, or an ileostomy.

The clinical manifestations of zinc deficiency include lethargy, growth retardation, skin lesions, alopecia, and diarrhea; the striking sign of zinc deficiency, however, is some form of skin lesions. Common sites of involvement are the groin and perianal area, the neck folds, and the face, particularly the angles of the mouth and the cheeks. Lesions have also been noted at sites of trauma, such as endotracheal and cardiac monitor tape sites. The skin lesions are reddened, scaly, and moist. The skin eruption of zinc deficiency strongly resembles acrodermatitis enteropathica, a rare autosomal recessive disorder of zinc malabsorption and deficiency, in its morphologic features and distribution.

Zinc deficiency can result from inadequate intake of zinc. The routine supplementation of trace minerals in parenteral nutrition solutions has eliminated much of the zinc deficiency seen in the past. It is still seen in some premature infants who are exclusively breastfed. For infants receiving total parenteral nutrition, zinc supplementation is 250 mcg/kg/day for term infants under three months of age and 400 mcg/kg/day for premature infants (Zenk, 1999). Oral supplementation for with zinc sulfate ranges from 1 to 3 mg/kg/day. Recovery from zinc deficiency is dramatic once adequate zinc supplementation has begun. In general, skin conditions caused by nutritional deficiencies are often confused with infections and other irritants but do not respond until the deficiency state itself is treated.

Intravenous Extravasations

The extravasation of intravenous fluids and medications can result in skin injury and, in some cases, deep tissue injury to muscle and nerves (Figure 34-11). The most serious extravasation injuries are iatrogenic complications that can lead to pain, prolonged hospitalization, and increased morbidity, such as infection. Extravasation injuries can also result in increased hospital costs and the potential for legal action. Despite vigilant nursing assessment, intravenous extravasations do occur in about 11% of patients in the NICU. Tissue sloughing occurs in as many as 43.6% of these infants. Therefore nursing actions such as the monitoring of intravenous sites and other preventive strategies as well as immediate interventions that can reduce the extent of tissue injury are important considerations for all nurseries that care for newborns with intravenous devices for fluid administration and medications.

Some of the factors known to increase the risk of tissue injury include the following:

1. The length of exposure after extravasation occurs, especially when the patients are unable to verbalize the discomfort of pain or pressure.
2. The nature of the drug or solution; hypertonic solutions with high concentrations of calcium, potassium, glucose, or amino acids,

and medications such as nafcillin have been identified as high-risk for causing injury.
3. The mechanical compression caused by electronic infusion pumps.

Another risk factor is compromised perfusion to the skin, as evidenced by the poor capillary refill exhibited by the most critically ill neonates or by the obstructed venous circulations seen with taping methods that constrict the extremities in which the intravenous device is placed.

Prevention of skin injury after infiltration is the first important consideration. Strategies include ensuring that the insertion site is clearly visible by using transparent adhesive dressing or clear tape to secure the device and observing the site with appropriate documentation every hour. In addition, the tape should be carefully placed on the extremity to avoid obstruction of venous return. Tape placed loosely over a bony prominence, such as the knee or elbow, permits extravasated fluids and medications to disperse over a larger surface area and thus reduce the risk of injury, compared with extravasation that is limited to a small surface area. Avoiding extremities with poor perfusion in favor of better-perfused scalp veins (except, of course, those on the forehead) may also be prudent; in some cases, the wiser choice may be the placement of central venous lines for access. Nursery policies that limit the glucose (<12.5%), amino acid (<2%), and calcium (10%) concentrations are also strategies to reduce the risk of tissue injury from the extravasation of intravenous fluids and medications.

Once an intravenous extravasation has been identified, immediate measures to reduce injury are instituted. The device should be carefully removed, and the extremity should be elevated (if it is an arm or leg). Treatment with heat or moisture is not recommended, because the delicate tissue could be further injured by a burn or the effects of maceration. If tissue damage is visible, the use of a topical antimicrobial ointment and petrolatum-impregnated gauze to facilitate healing is instituted. In the most severe cases of deep tissue necrosis after extravasation injury, a surgical or plastic surgical consultation is necessary, and skin grafts may be needed (Figure 34-12). In all cases of tissue injury, the open wound should be considered to be a potential portal for infection, and topical or systemic treatment may be required.

Wydase has been taken off the market in the United States and will not be manufactured any longer. An alternative to

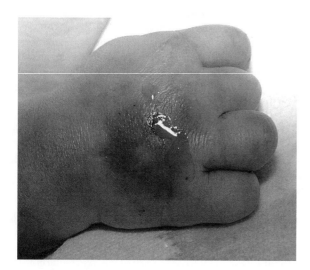

FIGURE 34-11
IV extravasation injury with swelling, discoloration, and leaking of fluid.

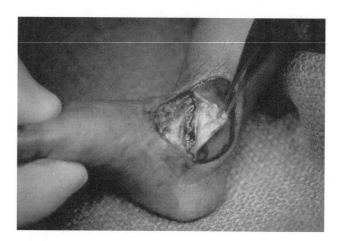

FIGURE 34-12
This IV extravasation injury will require plastic surgery.

this intervention includes making multiple puncture holes over the area of greatest swelling and squeezing or allowing the fluid to leak out of the tissue to release the infiltrated fluid and potentially prevent skin injury.

Diaper Dermatitis

A common skin disruption that occurs in neonates and infants is diaper dermatitis. This term encompasses a range of processes that affect the perineum, groin, thighs, buttocks, and anal area of infants who are incontinent and wear some covering to collect urine and feces. Diaper dermatitis can be caused by many different mechanisms, but the condition of the skin has a direct role in the progression of skin injury.

The pathogenesis of diaper dermatitis is partly related to the degree of wetness of the skin. Skin that is moist and macerated becomes more permeable and susceptible to injury because wetness increases friction. In addition, moisture-laden skin is more likely to contain microorganisms than dry skin is.

Another component in the process of skin injury from diaper dermatitis is the effect of an alkaline pH. The normal skin pH is acidic—ranging between 4.0 and 5.5—but can become alkaline when it is exposed to urine, which generally has a higher pH. It is the resulting increased pH of the skin—not the effect of ammonia in urine, as previously thought—that increases its vulnerability to injury and penetration by microorganisms. Another problem associated with increased pH of the skin is that it stimulates fecal enzyme activity. Specifically, both protease and lipase, which are found in stool, can injure the skin, that is made up of protein and fat components. These enzymes can cause significant injury to the epidermis fairly quickly and are responsible for the contact irritant diaper dermatitis that is commonly seen.

Once the epidermis has been impaired or becomes a less efficient barrier because of one of the aforementioned mechanisms, invasion by bacteria or fungus can occur. Thus a contact irritant diaper dermatitis can turn into a staphylococcal or fungal rash if this progression occurs. *S. aureus* can be found in large numbers on the skin surface, especially if it is inflamed or impaired, and can result in secondary infection. The classic presentation for *S. aureus* is pustule formation at the site of hair follicles, although the overall incidence of *S. aureus* complicated diaper dermatitis is quite low.

Fungal rashes, primarily those caused by *C. albicans*, may have different mechanisms of invasion. Many researchers have identified *C. albicans* as a secondary invader of skin that has been injured by other mechanisms, whereas others suggest that *C. albicans* is a primary causative factor in diaper dermatitis. This theory is based on the ability of *C. albicans* to penetrate the stratum corneum, especially in a warm and moist environment, such as that found under an occlusive diaper. The resulting intense inflammation is significant and appears as brightly erythematous, sharply marginated dermatitis that involves the inguinal folds as well as the buttocks, thighs, abdomen, and genitalia, characteristically with satellite lesions that may extend the rash over the trunk (Figure 34-13). The gastrointestinal tract is often the reservoir for *C. albicans*, and it can frequently be recovered in stool. Thus oral therapy may be indicated, especially if evidence of oral infection, such as thrush, is apparent.

Some diaper dermatitis can be the result of a primary dermatologic condition, such as psoriasis, eczema, and seborrheic dermatitis. Significant family history of these skin conditions may identify infants who are especially vulnerable to developing severe reactions to inflammation in the diaper area.

Collaborative Management. Prevention is the first goal of intervention and is paramount in breaking the cycle of diaper dermatitis. Frequent diaper changes result in skin that is drier with a more normal pH and thus maintain the functional barrier of the skin. Strategies to keep the skin dry also include the use of highly absorbent gelled diapers that act to "wick" moisture away from the skin. Use of talcum powders has been discouraged because of the risk of inhalation of silicone particles into the respiratory tract.

Once diaper dermatitis occurs—and it is not completely avoidable in most infants—protection of injured skin during healing is the primary goal. Use of a generous layer of protective skin barriers that contain zinc oxide prevents further trauma and allows impaired skin to heal (Figure 34-14).

Opening the skin to light and air is not effective if the fecal contents are allowed to have direct contact with already injured areas. Because protective skin barriers tend to adhere well to the skin, it is neither necessary nor desirable to completely remove them during diaper changes before more cream is applied. It is best to generously apply more cream to the site to protect the area from further injury.

Multiple products are used in the care of diaper dermatitis—including topical emollients, diaper rash balms, and wipes—

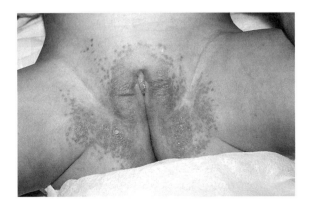

FIGURE **34-13**
Candida diaper dermatitis involving labia and inguinal folds with characteristic satellite lesions.

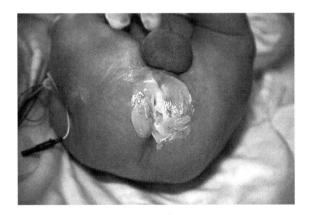

FIGURE **34-14**
Use of thick layer of a skin barrier such as zinc oxide or pectin paste will prevent reinjury of skin damage in diaper dermatitis.

but product selection is often affected by myth and tradition, rather than science. A damp diaper covered with a plastic coating enhances the risk of irritation and percutaneous absorption. The risk of absorption is even greater in newborns and premature infants due to their large surface area to body weight ratio and immature. The various compounds and numerous chemicals used have been described extensively (Siegfried & Shah, 1999; Siegfried, 2001), with concerns raised about potential toxicity, irritancy, and later sensitization. Simple, inexpensive products such as zinc oxide ointment are recommended over more complex compounds.

Treatment of diaper dermatitis that is solely due to invasion with C. albicans requires the use of antifungal creams or ointments. Some of the antifungal preparations include nystatin, miconazole, and clotrimazole. If the diaper dermatitis involves both fungus and a contact irritant component, alternating applications of the topical creams or ointments is effective.

Severe diaper dermatitis with deep excoriations can be seen in infants with severe malabsorption syndrome secondary to intestinal resection or mucosal injury. Other infants at risk for severe diaper dermatitis include those with symptomatic opiate withdrawl, spina bifida, and exstrophy of the bladder with loss of anal sphincter tone. In these cases, the stool is extremely caustic and contains a higher level of enzyme activity, a lower pH as the result of rapid transit through the intestine, and significant amounts of undigested carbohydrates. Stool frequency is often greatly increased. In cases of loss of sphincter tone, fecal material constantly dribbles to the perianal area.

Although skin disruption frequently becomes the focus of nursing interventions, this symptom may be a significant indication of more serious physiologic concerns. These infants' stools should be carefully monitored by documentation of number, volume, pH, and carbohydrate testing. The infants must be observed for the dehydration caused by extensive water losses in diarrhea. Once dietary manipulations and hydration have stabilized the general physiologic status, a program of skin protection is imperative because some level of chronic diarrhea may be ongoing for many weeks or months. Products such as pectin-based powders or pectin-containing pastes without alcohol may be better barriers to the caustic, constant fecal irritation if traditional zinc oxide creams do not work adequately. If yeast is present, antifungal creams may be applied in conjunction with protective barriers.

EVIDENCE-BASED SKIN CARE GUIDELINE

Many intensive care and newborn nurseries have written protocols for various aspects of neonatal skin care. Recently, two national nursing organizations, the Association of Women's Health, Obstetrics and Neonatal Nurses (AWHONN) and the National Association of Neonatal Nurses (NANN), collaborated in the development of a comprehensive evidence-based neonatal skin care guideline. An extensive review of the scientific basis for neonatal skin care was undertaken by a team including advanced practice nurses and a pediatric dermatologist (Lund et al, 1999), and a neonatal skin guideline was written to address 11 aspects of skin care (Box 34-2). Following this report, 50 nurseries agreed to participate in a research-based practice project to implement and evaluate this guideline for their patients. The project involved identifying site coordinators at each site who were willing to collect baseline information about the skin condition of infants in their units, implement the practice guideline in their respective units, and then

---

BOX 34-2

Elements of the AWHONN/NANN Evidence-Based Practice Guideline: Neonatal Skin Care

1. Newborn skin assessment
2. Bathing, including first bath, routine, and immersion bathing
3. Cord care
4. Circumcision care
5. Disinfectants
6. Diaper dermaitis
7. Adhesives
8. Transepidermal water loss (TEWL)
9. Skin breakdown
10. IV infiltration
11. Skin nutrition

From the Association of Women's Health, Obstetric, and Neonatal Nurses (AWHONN) and the National Association of Neonatal Nurses Skin Care Utilitation Project. Copyright 2001, AWHONN.

collect skin condition information again once the guideline had been introduced. Issues of safety and feasibility were important, as was the evaluation of the impact of evidence-based practice on skin condition.

Over 11,000 skin observations using the Neonatal Skin Condition Score (NSCS) were performed on 2820 newborns of varying gestational ages and weights. An improvement in skin condition was observed after implementation of the guideline, as evidenced by overall lower scores on the NSCS during the observation period. Initial scores were similar in both the preguideline and postguideline groups but improved more rapidly after the guideline had been implemented. The results were more dramatic in the low-birth-weight infants, but improvement was seen in the "well-baby" sample as well. Reduction in the frequency of bathing and fewer baths given with cleansers were noted, thus showing compliance with the guideline. An increase in the use of emollients was also documented.

Positive blood cultures did not increase after the guideline had been implemented (Lund et al, 2001).

AWHONN and NANN both offer the neonatal skin care evidence-based clinical practice guideline as well as educational materials for both members and non-members (AWHONN/NANN Guideline 2001).

SUMMARY

Neonatal skin management is a complex problem that requires a collaborative approach. Some research has been conducted in this area, but a lot remains to be done regarding the use of routine NICU equipment and its impact on neonatal skin, the use of skin barriers for protection, and the effect of a consistent approach to skin care on the integrity of neonatal skin. This chapter has outlined the development and structure of the skin. It has addressed differences in the skin based on gestational age variations. Normal physiologic as well as common dermatologic abnormalities have been presented. Evidence-based neonatal skin care is recommended and has proven to be feasible and safe and results in improvement in skin condition for newborns.

REFERENCES

3M Health Care (2000). *3M Cavilon No Sting Skin Barrier Film* (Brochure), St. Paul, MN.

Agren J et al (1998). Transepidermal water loss in infants born at 24 and 25 weeks of gestation. *Acta paediatrica*, 87, 1185-1190.

American Academy of Pediatrics (1997). *Red book: report of the committee on infectious diseases*, ed 24, Elk Grove Village, IL.

Anderson GC et al (1995). Axillary temperature in transitional newborn infants before and after tub bath. *Applied nursing research*, 8, 123-128.

Association of Women's Health, Obstetric, and Neonatal Nurses (AWHONN) and National Association of Neonatal Nurses (NANN) (2001). *Evidence-based clinical practice guideline: neonatal Skin Care*, Washington, DC, AWHONN.

Boon LM et al (1996). Hepatic vascular anomalies in infancy: a twenty-seven year experience. *Journal of pediatrics*, 129, 346-354.

Cohen BA (2001). Disorders of the subcutaneous tissue. In Eichenfield LA et al: *Textbook of neonatal dermatology*, Philadelphia, WB Saunders.

Cunningham BB, Wagner AM (2001). Diagnostic and therapeutic procedures. In Eichenfield LA et al: *Textbook of neonatal dermatology*, Philadelphia, WB Saunders.

Darmstadt GL, Dinulos JG (2001). Bacterial infections. In Eichenfield LA et al: *Textbook of neonatal dermatology*, Philadelphia, WB Saunders.

Dollison E, Beckstrand J (1995). Adhesive tape vs. pectin-based barrier use in preterm infants, *Neonatal network*, 14, 35-39.

Dore S et al (1998). Alcohol versus natural drying for newborn cord care. *Journal of obstetrics, gynecology, and neonatal nursing*, 27, 621-627.

Drolet BA, Esterly NB (2002). The skin. In Fanaroff AA, Martin RJ (Eds.), *Neonatal-perinatal medicine: diseases of the fetus and infant*, ed 7, St Louis, Mosby.

Drucker D, Marshall N (1995). Humidification without risk of infection in the Drager incubator 8000. *Neonatal intensive care*, 8, 44-46.

Edwards W et al (2000, December). The effect of Aquaphor emollient ointment on nosocomial sepsis rates and skin integrity in infants of birthweights 501-1000 grams. Paper presented at the Hot Topics Neonatology Conference, Washington, DC.

Enjolras O, Garzon MC (2001). Vascular stains, malformations, and tumors. In Eichenfield LA et al: *Textbook of neonatal dermatology*, Philadelphia, WB Saunders.

Fine JD et al (1999). *Epidermolysis bullosa: clinical, epidemiologic, and laboratory advances and the findings of the National Epidermolysis Bullosa Registry*. Baltimore, Johns Hopkins University Press.

Fine JD et al (2000). Revised classification system for inherited epidermolysis bullosa: report of the Second International Consensus Meeting on diagnosis and classification of epidermolysis bullosa. *Journal of the American academy of dermatology*, 42, 700-702.

Fox C et al (1998). The timing of skin acidification in very low birth weight infants. *Journal of perinatology*, 18, 272-275.

Franck L et al (2000). Effect of less frequent bathing of preterm infants on skin flora and pathogen colonization. *Journal of obstetrics, gynecology, and neonatal nursing*, 29, 584-589.

Frieden IJ, Howard R (2001). Vesicles, pustules, bullae, erosions, and ulcerations. In Eichenfield LA et al: *Textbook of neonatal dermatology*, Philadelphia, WB Saunders.

Garland J et al (1995). Comparison of 10% povidone-iodine and 0.5% chlorhexidine gluconate for the prevention of peripheral intravenous catheter colonization in neonates: a prospective trial. *Pediatric infectious disease journal*, 14, 510-516.

Gfatter R et al (1997). Effects of soap and detergents on skin surface pH, stratum corneum hydration and fat content in infants. *Dermatology*, 195, 258-262.

Gordon C et al (1995). Topical iodine and neonatal hypothyroidism. *Archives of pediatric and adolescent medicine*, 149, 1336-1339.

Harpin VA, Rutter N (1983). Barrier properties of the newborn infant's skin. *Journal of pediatrics*, 102(3), 419-425.

Hoath S, Narendran V (2000). Adhesives and emollients in the preterm infant. *Seminars in neonatology*, 5, 112-119.

Hoath S et al (2001). The biology and role of vernix. *Newborn and infant nursing reviews*, 1, 53-58.

Irving V (2001). Reducing the risk of epidermal stripping in the neonatal population: an evaluation of an alcohol free barrier film. *Journal of neonatal nursing*, 7, 5-8.

Kalia YN et al (1998). Development of the skin barrier function in premature infants. *Journal of investigative dermatology*, 111, 320-326.

Karl D (1999). The interactive newborn bath: using infant behavior to connect parents and newborns. *MCN*, 24, 280-286.

Kjartansson S et al (1995). Water loss from the skin of term and preterm infants nursed under a radiant heater. *Pediatric research*, 37(2), 233-238.

Landau M, Krafchik B (1999). The diagnostic values of café au lait macules. *Journal of the American academy of dermatology*, 40, 877-890.

Lin AN (1996). Management of patients with epidermolysis bullosa. *Dermatology clinics*, 14, 381-387.

Linder N et al (1997). Topical iodine-containing antiseptics and subclinical hypothyroidism in preterm infants. *Journal of pediatrics*, 131, 434-439.

Loomis CA, Birge MB (2001). Fetal skin development. In Eichenfield LA et al: *Textbook of neonatal dermatology*, Philadelphia, WB Saunders.

Lucky AW (2001). Transient benign cutaneous lesions in the newborn. In Eichenfield LA et al: *Textbook of neonatal dermatology*, Philadelphia, WB Saunders.

Lund C (1999). Prevention and management of infant skin breakdown. *Nursing clinics of North America*, 34, 907-920.

Lund C et al (1999). Neonatal skin care: the scientific basis for practice. *Journal of obstetrics, gynecology, and neonatal nursing*, 28, 241-254.

Lund C et al (2001). Neonatal skin care: clinical outcomes of the AWHONN/NANN evidence-based clinical practice guideline. *Journal of obstetrics, gynecology, and neonatal nursing*, 30, 41-51.

Lund C et al (2001). Neonatal skin care: evaluation of the AWHONN/NANN research-based practice project on knowledge and skin care practices. *Journal of obstetrics, gynecology, and neonatal nursing*, 30, 30-40.

Malathi I et al (1993). Skin disinfection in preterm infants. *Archives of disease in children*, 69, 312-316.

Mancini A et al (1994). Semipermeable dressings improve epidermal barrier function in premature infants. *Pediatric research*, 36, 306-314.

Margileth AM (1999). Dermatologic conditions. In Avery G et al (Eds.), *Neonatology: pathophysiology and management of the newborn*, ed 5, Philadelphia, JB Lippincott.

Marinkovich MP (1999). Update on inherited bullous dermatoses. *Dermatology clinics*, 17(3), 473-485.

Marks J et al (1995). North American Contact Dermatitis Group standard tray patch test results. *American journal of contact dermatitis*, 6, 160-165.

Marshall A (1997). Humidifying the environment for the premature neonate: maintenance of a thermoneutral environment. *Journal of neonatal nursing*, 3, 32-36.

Mimoz O et al (1999). Chlorhexidine compared with povidone-iodine as skin preparation before blood culture. *Annals of internal medicine*, 131, 834-837.

Moore KL, Persaud TVN (1998). *The developing human: clinically oriented embryology*, ed 6, Philadelphia, WB Saunders.

Niamba P et al (1998). Is common neonatal cephalic pustulosis (neonatal acne) triggered by Malassezia furfur? *Archives of dermatology*, 134, 995.

Nopper A et al (1996). Topical ointment therapy benefits premature infants. *Journal of pediatrics*, 128, 660-669.

Okah FA et al (1994). Human newborn skin: the effect of isopropanol on the skin surface hydrophobicity. *Pediatric research*, 35, 443-446.

Parravicini E et al (1996). Iodine, thyroid function, and very low birth weight infants. *Pediatrics*, 98, 730-734.

Penny-MacGillivray T (1996). A newborn's first bath: when? *Journal of obstetrics, gynecology, and neonatal nursing*, 25, 481-487.

Peters K (1998). Bathing premature infants: physiological and behavioral consequences. *American journal of critical care*, 7, 90-100.

Prasad AS (1995). Zinc: an overview. *Nutrition*, 11, 93-99.

Rapelanoro R et al (1996). Neonatal *Malassezia furfur* pustulosis. *Archives of dermatology*, 132, 190-193.

Rowen JL et al (1995). Invasive fungal dermatitis in the <1000 gram neonate. *Pediatrics*, 95, 682-687.

Scales JW et al (1998). An infant with firm fixed plaques. *Archives in dermatology*, 134, 425-426.

Sethi R et al (1996). Oculocutaneous albinism. *Cutis*, 57, 397-400.

Siegfried EG (2001). Neonatal skin care and toxicology. In Eichenfield LA et al: *Textbook of neonatal dermatology*, Philadelphia: WB Saunders.

Siegfried EC, Shah PY (1999). Skin care practices in the neonatal nursery: a clinical survey. *Journal of perinatology*, 19, 31-39.

Smack DP et al (1996). Infection and allergy incidence in ambulatory surgery patients using white petrolatum vs. bacitracin ointment: a randomized controlled trial. *Journal of the American Medical Association*, 276, 972-977.

Smith JF et al (1997). Fetal laceration injury at cesarean delivery. *Obstetrics gynecology*, 90, 344-346.

Stevens J et al (1998). Symptomatic zinc deficiency in breastfed term and premature infants. *Journal of paediatric child health*, 34, 97-100.

Varda K, Behnke R (2000). The effect of timing of initial bath on newborn's temperature. *Journal of obstetrics, gynecology, and neonatal nursing*, 29, 27-32.

Vohra S et al (1999). Effect of polyethylene occlusive skin wrapping on heat loss in very low birth weight infants at delivery: a randomized trial. *Journal of pediatrics*, 134, 547-551.

Williams ML (2001). Skin of the premature infant. In Eichenfield LA et al: *Textbook of neonatal dermatology*, Philadelphia: WB Saunders.

Yosipovitch G et al (2000). Skin barrier properties in different body areas in neonates. *Pediatrics*, 106, 105-108.

Zenk K (1999). *Neonatal medications and nutrition: a comprehensive guide*. Santa Rosa, CA, NICU Ink.

Zupan J, Gardner P (2000). Topical umbilical cord care at birth. *The Cochrane database of systematic reviews*, 3, 34-82.

CHAPTER 35

ASSESSMENT AND MANAGEMENT OF THE AUDITORY SYSTEM

KATHLEEN HAUBRICH

Hearing is a prerequisite to cognitive, social, and emotional development. Any impairment of hearing from birth to 18 months can have a profound effect on the auditory stimulation necessary for language development. The importance of early identification of hearing impairment in the neonate has been well documented in the literature (Kennedy et al, 2000). Sensory deprivation affects the acquisition of communication skills, even though the hearing loss may be corrected.

A study of childhood language development and academic achievement found that hearing impairment has a significant impact on the development of a child (Gallaudet and University Center for Assessment and Demographic Study, 1998). This investigation further substantiated earlier findings that children with a hearing impairment demonstrate limited speech-production skills. Karchmer and Allen (1999) looked at another aspect of childhood development, receptive and expressive language skills, and found that children with a hearing impairment demonstrated a significant delay in the development of these skills. These researchers also studied the outcomes and vocational opportunities of children, and their report further supported earlier findings that hearing-impaired children show lower academic achievement.

To prevent or minimize its detrimental effects on social, cognitive, and educational development, hearing impairment must be identified as early as possible. Reliable data on the incidence of hearing loss in infants and young children are difficult to obtain. However, national statistics indicate that the incidence of significant bilateral hearing loss is about 1 to 3 per 1000 newborn infants in a well baby nursery and about 2 to 4 per 100 infants in the neonatal intensive care unit (White et al., 2000). Moderate to profound hearing impairment is reported in fewer than 2% of infants at risk, and approximately 1 in 100 infants is born deaf.

Despite the sequelae of auditory impairment in infants and young children, the average age at which hearing impairment is identified is beyond age 1½ years, the critical stage for speech and language development.

The American Academy of Pediatrics (AAP) Task Force on Newborn and Infant Hearing (1999), reporting on early identification of hearing impairment in infants and young children, concluded that all infants should be screened for hearing impairment. The task force based its conclusion on two premises: first, advances in technology have led to better screening methods, and second, current criteria fail to identify 50% to 70% of children born with impairment. Nevertheless, current practice indicates that not all states require universal newborn hearing screening.

The assessment and management of auditory dysfunction present a challenge to nurses committed to the welfare of the neonate and infant. This chapter describes a comprehensive nursing approach that identifies current practice and future trends, as well as management of infants at risk for hearing impairment.

AUDITORY DEVELOPMENT AND MECHANISM OF FUNCTION

A basic understanding of the embryologic development of the ear is essential to early identification and management of hearing loss. By understanding the developmental timetable of the various structures and the relationship of the processes to the final structure, the nurse can apply estimates of developmental deviations and of the association of hearing loss with other disorders that may cluster with an auditory abnormality. For example, if malformation of a pinna is assessed during physical examination of the newborn, then malformation of the ossicles in the middle ear may be suspected because these two structures develop simultaneously. Table 35-1 presents a timetable of the important events in the development of the ear.

Embryology

The ear is a singular organ that functions in both hearing and equilibrium. In the embryo, the ear develops from three different parts.

Internal Ear.   The internal ear is the first area of the ear to develop in the embryo. As early as the fourth week of gestation, a thickening of the surface ectoderm on the sides of the rhombencephalon appears as the otic placodes. Each otic placode invaginates to the underlying mesenchyma of the surface ectoderm, eventually forming an otic pit. The periphery of the otic pit fuses to form the otic vesicle, which is the rudimentary membranous labyrinth.

As the otic vesicle loses its connection with the surface ectoderm, a diverticulum develops from the otic vesicle and lengthens to form the endolymphatic duct. The dorsal portion

TABLE 35-1	Important Events in the Embryologic Development of the Ear		
Fetal Week	**Inner Ear**	**Middle Ear**	**External Ear**
Third	Auditory placode, auditory pit begin to develop.	Tubotympanic recess begins to develop.	
Fourth	Auditory vesicle (otocyst), vestibular-cochlear division begin to develop.		Tissue thickenings begin to form.
Fifth			Primary auditory meatus begins to develop.
Sixth	Utricle and saccule are present; semicircular canals begin to develop.		Six hillocks are evident; cartilage begins to form.
Seventh	One cochlear coil is present; sensory cells in utricle and saccule are present.		Auricles move dorsolaterally.
Eighth	Ductus reuniens is present; sensory cells in semicircular canals begin to develop.	Incus and malleus are present in cartilage; lower half of tympanic cavity is formed.	Outer cartilaginous third of external canal is formed.
Ninth		Three tissue layers at tympanic membrane are present.	
Eleventh	Two and one half cochlear coils are present; nerve VIII attaches to cochlear duct.		
Twelfth	Sensory cells in cochlea begin to develop; membranous labyrinth is complete; otic capsule begins to ossify.		
Fifteenth		Cartilaginous stapes is formed.	
Sixteenth		Ossification of malleus and incus begins.	
Eighteenth		Stapes begins to ossify.	
Twentieth	Inner ear matures and reaches adult size.		Auricle assumes adult shape but continues to grow until age 9.
Twenty-first		Meatal plug disintegrates, exposing tympanic membrane.	
Thirtieth		Tympanum is pneumatized.	External auditory canal continues to mature until age 7.
Thirty-second		Ossification of malleus and incus is complete.	
Thirty-fourth		Mastoid air cells develop.	
Thirty-fifth		Antrum is pneumatized.	
Thirty-seventh		Epitympanum is pneumatized; stapes continues to develop until adulthood; tympanic membrane changes relative position during first 2 years of life.	

From Northern J, Downs M (1984). Hearing in children. Williams & Wilkins: Baltimore.

of the otic vesicle gives rise to the semicircular canals of the utricle and the endolymphatic duct. A ventral component gives rise to the saccule and the cochlear duct.

Diverticula extend from the utricular portion of the membranous labyrinth. Central portions eventually fuse and disappear. Peripheral portions of the diverticula eventually become the semicircular canals.

Ampullae develop at the end of each semicircular duct, with the sensory nerve ending differentiating in the specific regions. Cells of the ampulla form a crest; the crista ampullaris contains cells for maintaining equilibrium. Sensory areas of the utricle and the saccule, known as maculae acousticae, develop similarly. Impulses generated from these areas are transmitted to the brain by the eighth cranial nerve.

By the sixth week of gestation, the ventral saccule of the otic vesicle forms an outpouching at its lower end known as the cochlear duct, which grows in a spiral fashion to form the cochlea. A narrow pathway, the ductus reuniens, remains between the saccule and the cochlea.

Mesenchyma surrounding the cochlear duct differentiates into a cartilaginous shell that gives rise to the formation of vacuoles and two perilymphatic spaces, the scala vestibuli and the scala tympani. Further differentiation in the cochlear duct is accomplished through separation of the scala vestibuli by the vestibular membrane and of the scala tympani by the basilar membrane. The lateral walls of the cochlear duct remain attached to the surrounding cartilage by the spiral ligament.

Epithelial cells of the cochlear duct further develop to form an inner ridge and an outer ridge. The outer ridge forms hair cells, which are the sensory cells of the auditory system. The tectorial membranes cover the hair cells. The sensory cells and tectorial membrane are called the spiral organ of Corti. Impulses are transmitted by the organ of Corti to the spiral ganglion and then to the nervous system by the auditory fibers of the eighth cranial nerve. The internal ear reaches its adult size and shape by 20 to 22 weeks' gestation.

Middle Ear.   The tympanic cavity is derived from the first pharyngeal pouch. The distal portion of the pouch, the tubotympanic recess, widens to become the primitive tympanic cavity, and the proximal end narrows to form the auditory, or eustachian, tube.

The malleus and the incus develop from the cartilage of the first pharyngeal arch, and the stapes develops from the second arch. During the first half of fetal life, the ossicles are embedded in mesenchyma until the tissue dissolves. The endodermal lining of the tympanic cavity extends into the new developing space. The ossicles are free of the surrounding mesenchyma, and the endodermal epithelium connects them to the wall of the cavity. Ligaments that support these ossicles are developed from mesenteries.

The tympanic cavity expands dorsally to form the mastoid antrum through the formation of vacuoles. The mastoid antrum is well developed in the newborn, although no mastoid cells are present. Mastoid cells, which are well developed by 2 years of age, produce projections called mastoid processes.

External Ear.   The external ear develops around the first branchial groove. The meatal plug is derived as the ectodermal cells form a funnel-shaped tube. Central cells of the meatal plug degenerate to form a cavity known as the external auditory meatus.

The tympanic membrane is derived from the first branchial membrane. As embryonic development continues, the mesenchyma separates two parts of the branchial membrane that later develop into two layers of fiber in the tympanic membrane. The external covering of the tympanic membrane is derived from the surface ectoderm, and the internal lining is derived from the endoderm of the tympanic recess.

The auricle, or pinna, is derived from six mesenchymal swellings, known as auricular hillocks, around the first branchial groove. Mesenchyma in the hillock is derived from mesoderm in the first and second branchial arches. The lobule of the auricle is the last part to develop.

STRUCTURE OF THE EAR

The ear is the anatomic unit involved in hearing and equilibrium. It consists of three parts: the external ear, the middle ear, and the inner ear. The external ear is composed of the auricle (pinna) and the external ear canal (Figure 35-1). A complex cartilage framework gives structure to the auricle. Because of this anatomic position, the auricle is susceptible to trauma from external forces. The external ear canal is curved posterosuperiorly and anteromedially. The canal is oval in shape, and the long axis is positioned superoinferiorly. Normally, the outer portion of the canal is cartilaginous, and the medial por-

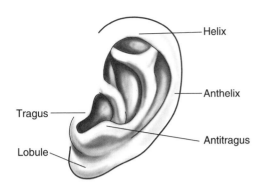

FIGURE **35-1**
Anatomy of the external ear.

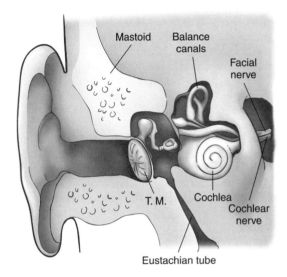

FIGURE **35-2**
General framework of the outer, middle, and inner ear. *T.M.*, Tympanic membrane. Redrawn from Pappas D (1985). *Diagnosis and treatment of hearing impairment in children.* College-Hill Press: San Diego.

tion is bony. Before 34 weeks' gestation, the pinna is a slightly formed, cartilage-free double thickness of skin. In the newborn, however, most of the canal is cartilaginous and collapsed. But as ear development ensues, the cartilage becomes firmer, making the outer two thirds of the canal more patent. Cerumen glands and tiny hairs are present in the outer portion of the cartilaginous canal. The medial two thirds of the canal lies immediately over a bony area and is referred to as the osseous region. The auditory meatus assumes an irregular path from the concha to the tympanic membrane.

At the termination of the external canal is the eardrum, or tympanic membrane, which forms the boundary between the outer and the middle ear (Figure 35-2). This membrane, which has a complicated shape that loosely resembles a flat cone, moves with changes in air pressure. Because the tympanic membrane is oval and translucent, the middle ear structure often can be visualized through it. The short and long processes of the malleus are attached to the fibrous layer of the tympanic membrane and are visible on the lateral surface. The middle ear cavity is an air-filled space connected by an air cell system posterior to the mastoid and by the eustachian tube anterior to the nasopharynx. Neither of these communications is in a dependent position for drainage of fluids. Ciliated columnar cells cover the walls of the tympanic cavity and mastoid air cells. Secretory cells are distributed throughout the middle ear, with the greatest number in the eustachian tube. In the middle ear, the malleus, incus, and stapes occupy the region between the tympanic membrane and the oval window of the middle ear. During otoscopic examination, the long process of the incus often can be seen through the tympanic membrane.

The stapedius and the tensor muscles of the tympanic membrane attach in the middle ear to the malleus and the stapes by tendons. The chorda tympani nerve passes across the posterior surface. The medial wall of the middle ear cavity contains the oval and round windows. Between these two windows, the lower portion of the cochlea forms a prominence known as the promontorium tympani on the medial wall of the middle ear.

The inner ear consists of a bony labyrinth composed of three parts: the semicircular canals, the vestibule, and the cochlea. A dense, bony capsule in the petrous protein of the temporal bone surrounds these hollow spaces; this capsule contains perilymph and endolymph. Each of the semicircular canals has a dilated portion at the end, referred to as ampullae, which contain the crista ampullaris, a vestibular sense organ. In the vestibule, the utricle and saccules are formed; these structures saccules contain sensory endings important for maintaining equilibrium.

The cochlea is a tubular structure with 212 spirals; it closely resembles a snail shell, having a base and an apex. The cochlea is divided into the scala vestibuli and the scala tympani. The two tracts connect at the apex. The scala vestibuli begins at the oval window, and the scala tympani terminates at the round window. The basilar membrane side of the duct gives rise to the organ of Corti, the organ of hearing. The organ of Corti includes hair cells and supporting cells; attached to the hair cells is a gelatinous membrane called the tectorial membrane.

The membranous labyrinth of the inner ear is composed of connective tissue filled with endolymph that forms in the bony labyrinth. Hair cells of the cochlea and the vestibular labyrinth are attached by afferent nerve fibers to the neurons of the auditory system, the spiral ganglion, and the Scarpa ganglion in the temporal bone. Efferent nerve fibers from ganglia form the auditory and vestibular division of the eighth cranial nerve and exit the temporal bone on its posterior surface to enter the brainstem.

PHYSIOLOGY OF AUDIOLOGIC FUNCTION

External Ear

The external ear consists of the auricle (pinna) and the external auditory meatus (external canal). The primary function of the external ear is to funnel sound to the tympanic membrane. Absence of the auricle contributes to difficulty in sound localization.

Middle Ear

Advancing sound entering the auditory canal directly strikes the tympanic membrane. This membrane and the ossicles serve as transmitters from the outer ear to the inner ear. The malleus, which is continuous with the tympanic membrane and is connected with the incus and stapes, moves the ossicles. Ossicles transfer sound energy into the inner ear through the oval window, which holds the stapes by means of an angular ligament.

The middle ear is lined with respiratory mucosa composed of ciliated columnar epithelial cells, supporting cells, and secretory cells. Secretory cells secrete mucus that forms a complex mucous layer. The cilia of the middle ear interact with the mucus by transporting mastoid and middle ear secretions through the eustachian tube to the nasopharynx, where they are swallowed. This mechanism is known as the mucociliary transport system. Glycoproteins in the mucus determine the viscosity and elasticity of the middle ear mucus. Mucus that is too thick or too thin impedes effective transport of bacteria and cellular debris from the mastoid and middle ear cleft: this transport has a protective effect against ear infections. In addition to serving as an exit for secretions into the nasopharynx, the eustachian tube equalizes the pressure between the middle ear and the ambient atmosphere.

Inner Ear

Before this point in the hearing mechanism, all of the sound energy is contained in the air-filled spaces of the external and middle ear. From the stapes onward, the pathway for sound moves through fluid-filled spaces. When sound is transferred from the tympanic membrane to the inner ear, the stapes creates a fluid wave that is transmitted to the round window. This transmission creates fluid waves that travel from the basal aspect of the cochlea to the apex. As the fluid wave moves, it displaces the basilar membrane. Maximum movement of the basilar membrane occurs at the point specific to the frequency of sound entering the ear; that is, high-frequency sounds cause minimal disturbance at the basal end of the cochlea, and low-frequency sounds cause minimal disturbance at the apex.

Vibrations in the basilar membrane cause movement of the organ of Corti. This organ contains receptor hair cells that are on the basilar membrane. Vibrations of the hair on the hair cells cause either polarization or depolarization, depending on the direction of the bend. When sufficient depolarization occurs, action potentials are produced that are propagated along the auditory pathway to the auditory cortex. The cochlea provides input by coding information about loudness and frequency in the action potentials sent to the cortex, giving meaning to the sound. Hair cells of the spiral organ of Corti are stimulated as they touch the tectorial membrane. Hair cells act as transducers that convert mechanical energy into electrical impulses; this action occurs in the fibers of the spiral ganglion. Axons of these cells become the auditory nerve (vestibulocochlear nerve). Nerve fibers pass to the medulla, the pons, and the midbrain, and finally to the temporal lobes of the cortex, where the impulses are interpreted as sound.

The vestibular system is similar to the auditory system. Fluid moves within the vestibular labyrinth when the head moves. The semicircular canals respond to angular acceleration (rotation), and the utricle and saccule respond to linear acceleration (position). Movement of endolymph exerts force on the hairs of the sensory cells of the cristae and the maculae. Depolarization of the sensory cells produces action potentials, which are transmitted to the vestibular cortex. The vestibular apparatus functions in conjunction with proprioception and visual orientation to maintain balance.

PERINATAL AUDITORY DEVELOPMENT

Evidence is growing that the fetus can perceive auditory stimulation and can act on it at an early age. Womb music (music placed on the mother's abdomen and transmitted to the womb) and tapes used by parents to stimulate the fetus are popular in the lay press. External stimuli are shaped by the tissues and fluid of the uterus with background noise associated with the maternal respiratory, cardiovascular, and intestinal activity as the backdrop and voicing information from male and female talkers reserved in the uterus. Auditory, brainstem, middle latency, and cortical responses emerge around 25 weeks' gestation. Maturation of the nerve fibers continues well into the first year of life.

During the remainder of the pregnancy, exogenous sounds affect fetal behavior, the fetal pulse rate, and fetal activity or inactivity (Hepper & Shahidullah, 1994). Vibroacustic stimulation is now used as an indicator of fetal well-being.

Overt reactions to auditory stimuli include arousal, gross body movements, orienting behavior, turning of the head, wide-eyed appearance, papillary dilation, motor reflexes, facial grimaces, displacement of a single digit, crying or cessation of crying, and acceleration or deceleration of the heart rate (Kaminski & Hall, 1996). Preterm infants also show changes in heart rate and various types of body movements in response to sound (Graven, 1996, 2000).

It is important that the auditory centers be highly stimulated and that early vocalization attempts be rewarded in the prelinguistic period. The babbling response in both deaf and hearing infants appears to represent an innate, preprogrammed linguistic process unique to the human infant. During certain critical periods in development, the neonate is programmed to receive and use particular types of stimuli for important prelinguistic activities, but once the period has passed, effective use of these stimuli diminishes. Environmental sounds have their greatest impact in shaping auditory ability from the time the inner ear and the eighth cranial nerve become functional to the time of central nervous system (CNS) maturation; that is, from approximately 5 months' gestation to between 18 and 28 months of age. A long period of receiving complex adult auditory language symbols exists, before which speech and language manifest as a culmination of coding and organizing grammatic structure into the child's language structure.

Early identification and intervention are imperative to achieve the optimum outcome. Auditory development is an area in which neonatal nurses assume important roles in parental teaching, role modeling, and evaluation of the child. Additional research studies are needed in all areas of in utero and early neonatal auditory stimulation. Protocols for supporting parents' early verbal encounters with their infants must continue to be developed and tested to ensure positive outcomes. This area of perinatal auditory behavior holds great potential as another surveillance tool for identification of hearing loss. The emphasis on neonatal hearing screening is an indication of the importance of early identification and intervention for hearing problems if long-term complications are to be diminished. Evidence is needed to support screening protocols for early identification of problems and of their long-term consequences for speech, hearing, and language acquisition. Also, parents' concerns about screening and its implications must be addressed (Weichbold & Welzl-Mueller, 2001).

HEARING IMPAIRMENT

The American Speech-Language-Hearing Association (ASHA) defines hearing impairment as "a loss of auditory sensitivity that can be measured at birth and for which intervention strategies are known and available." Hearing impairment represents a spectrum of hearing loss classified as mild, moderate, severe, or prolonged (Spivak, 1998). The criterion for measuring bilateral conductive and sensorineural hearing deficit in children is 1000 to 4000 Hz, the frequency range that is important for speech recognition.

Types of Hearing Impairment

The types of hearing impairment have been classified according to the location of the problem. An impairment may be one of three types: conductive, sensorineural, or a combination of these. Conductive losses arise from conditions that affect the outer and middle ear; sensorineural loss results from inner ear disorders; and combination losses result from disruptions in both areas of the ear.

A conductive hearing loss exists when dysfunction in the outer or middle ear disrupts the normal sequence of sound localization and vibration. Frequently the external auditory meatus becomes occluded by cerumen (wax), which impedes the transmission of sound. Otitis media, an infection of the middle ear, is the most common cause of conductive hearing loss. In this instance, fluid accumulates in the middle ear, preventing the tympanic membrane and ossicular chain from vibrating normally. The infection also can occur secondary to newborn diseases such as bronchopulmonary dysplasia (Gray et al, 2001). Congenital syndromes, such as CHARGE (posterior coloboma, hearing defect, choanal atresia, retardation, and genital and ear anomalies), often are related to hearing loss (Acham & Walch, 2001).

Congenital deformities of the outer ear also can affect the neonate's ability to hear. Because the function of the external ear is to funnel sound, variations in the structure and protrusion of the pinna may contribute to conductive hearing loss.

A missing or deformed pinna can result from a malformation of the auricular folds. Atresia of the auditory meatus or abnormal development of the ossicular chain may arise from defective development of the branchial chain.

Auditory pure-tone testing can reveal disorders of conduction. Individuals with conductive hearing loss have difficulty hearing low-frequency sounds (i.e., those in the 125- to 500-Hz range). Collaborative management of the neonate with conductive hearing loss is directed toward early observation, detection, and intervention to eliminate the source of infection, to remove the blockage, and to provide amplification, resulting in the restoration of normal hearing.

Sensorineural hearing impairment results from damage to the sensory nerve endings of the cochlea or dysfunction of the auditory nerve (eighth cranial nerve). A typical characteristic of inner ear dysfunction is the inability of the inner ear to interpret fluid changes in the cochlea. With sensorineural loss, hearing is normal at low frequencies; sound deficits are evident at frequencies above 1000 Hz.

Sensorineural hearing loss may manifest as a congenital inner ear abnormality, resulting in congenital deafness. Other conditions that may cause sensorineural hearing loss are trauma to the inner ear, the effects of certain drugs, prolonged exposure to loud noise, infections, infectious conditions such as measles, and the effects of aging.

Collaborative Management

Collaborative management of the neonate with hearing loss is directed toward early identification, detection, and restoration with amplification of sound, if indicated. For some neonates, the hearing deficit may cause a severe distortion of sound, and amplification for correction is indicated. However, for other neonates with severe sound distortion, amplification might not be an appropriate treatment; rather, in these cases early intervention with visual cues offers the greatest potential for the child's growth and development.

IDENTIFICATION OF THE HEARING-IMPAIRED INFANT

Physical Examination

The physical examination of the infant should be performed in a quiet, warm, draft-free area appropriate for observation and inspection of auditory structures and function. Observing the infant's behavior before examining the ear yields valuable baseline assessments. The alert, normal newborn reacts by turning toward the sound of human speech or a ringing bell; this infant also startles at the stimulus of a loud noise. Observation of the preterm infant (34 to 38 weeks' gestation) is deferred to a later time, when behavioral response has matured. Observation provides a crude estimate of neonatal hearing ability. If the neonate does not respond as expected, the examiner should suspect audiologic dysfunction.

Inspection of the ear begins with the medial and lateral surfaces of the pinna and the surface of the scalp, face, and neck. Development of the pinna correlates with the infant's gestational age. At term, the pinna of the newborn is well shaped and has sufficient cartilage to maintain normal shape and resistance (Figure 35-3). Before 34 weeks' gestation, the pinna is a slightly formed double thickness of skin.

The pinna of the term infant, when folded, demonstrates instant recoil and remains erect from the head. In contrast, the pinna of the premature infant is flat and shapeless and remains folded. As gestation continues, the pinna develops more cartilage, resulting in better form.

The pinna should be inspected for location and for its relationship to other facial structures. Normal attachment is to the side, level with the middle third of the face, and fixed in position to the lateral aspect of the external auditory canal. The major convolutions of the pinna are the helix, anthelix, tragus, antitragus, and lobule. The lobule of the external ear has no cartilage. The angle of placement of the pinna is almost vertical, and if the angle is more than 10 degrees off normal, it is considered abnormal. The superior helix is located at the outer canthus of the eye, and the tragus is roughly level with the infraorbital rim.

Low-set auricles frequently are associated with other abnormalities of the first and second branchial cleft and with abnormalities of the urinary system. Other abnormalities that may be noted are skin tags, sinuses, or pits, which often are associated with other auditory or renal malformations. The pinna often may be observed to have bruising from a forceps delivery. Depending on the degree of bruising, the discoloration should subside within the first week of life.

The external auditory meatus should then be observed for patency. Atresia or stenosis of the external meatus may be seen. This abnormality results in a conductive hearing loss because sound transmissions are blocked; the condition should be noted as part of the physical findings.

The next phase of the examination is directed toward inspection of the middle ear and the tympanic membrane. The depths of the external meatus can be examined with a brightly illuminated pneumatic otoscope. Vernix caseosa frequently is encountered in the ear canal of the neonate. The otoscope is introduced into the ear canal by exerting gentle traction posterosuperiorly on the auricle. In the neonate, the tympanic membrane lies in a nearly horizontal plane. The tympanic membrane is visualized through the collapsed neonatal ear by gently dilating the ear canal with the speculum as the cartilaginous canal is traversed. The tympanic membrane should be examined for thickness, vascularity, and contour. All areas, including the area above the short process of the malleus (pars flaccida), should be visualized for completeness. Normally the tympanic membrane appears translucent. White shadows of the ossicles usually can be seen through the membrane. The mobility of the tympanic membrane can be assessed by applying intermittent pressure through a bulb or by blowing through a polyethylene tube connected to an otoscope.

Otitis media can occur in the first days of life and can be di-

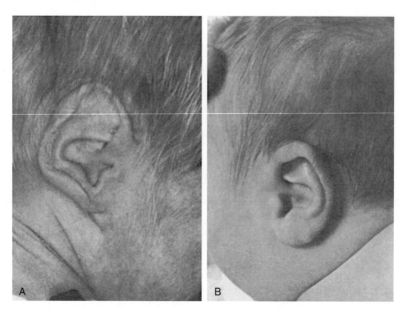

FIGURE **35-3**
Premature (**A**) and full-term (**B**) ear. From Schreiner RL, Bradburn NC (1987). *Care of the newborn*, ed 2. Raven Press: New York.

agnosed by otoscopic examination. Otitis media often manifests as a poorly mobile, bulging, yellow, opacified tympanic membrane. Complications of otitis media are common. Otitis media with middle ear effusion may cause hearing loss, perforation of the tympanic membrane, and possibly intracranial complications, including meningitis, encephalitis, and brain abscess (Vartiainen, 2000). Middle ear effusion occurs in both outpatient and inpatient groups of neonates.

History.   The importance of a comprehensive history for identifying the infant at risk cannot be overemphasized. The newborn carries a history extending back to the time of conception and is influenced by both perinatal events and parental genetic composition. Gathering of data on the infant's history is the first step in identifying infants at risk for hearing impairment. Early identification of hearing-impaired infants aids in minimizing the detrimental effects of reduced auditory input.

In 1974 the Joint Committee on Newborn Hearing developed a high-risk register, a list of categories that would identify a satisfactory number of infants at risk. Expansion and revision of the guidelines resulted in a new list in 1994 and in 2000. The 1994 and 2000 lists of risk factors offer a format for screening elements in the perinatal or genetic history that place the neonate at risk for hearing impairment. An abundance of information is available from studies on various aspects of the high-risk register.

Factors are presented to facilitate identification of infants at risk for hearing impairment (American Speech-Language-Hearing Association Joint Committee on Hearing, 1994, 2000). In the absence of universal screening of all newborns, institutions are advised to use the ASHA Joint Committee's high-risk neonatal indicators associated with sensorineural and/or conductive hearing loss (Box 35-1) as a guide to identifying infants in need of hearing screening. These factors are also used to determine which infants need follow-up despite a normal screening result.

Asphyxia.   Asphyxia, or anoxia, a condition involving a lack of oxygen with an increase in the carbon dioxide level in

---

BOX 35-1

Risk Identification Criteria: Neonates (Birth to 28 Days)

The risk factors that identify those neonates at risk for sensorineural hearing impairment include:
1. An illness or condition requiring admission of $\leq$ 48 hours to a NICU.
2. Stigmata or other findings associated with a syndrome known to include a sensorineural and/or conductive hearing loss.
3. Family history of permanent childhood sensorineural hearing loss.
4. Craniofacial anomalies, including those with morphological abnormalities of the pinna and ear canal.
5. In-utero infection such as cytomegalovirus, herpes, toxoplasmosis, or rubella.

From Joint Committee on Infant Hearing (2000). Year 2000 position statement: Principles and guidelines for early hearing detection and intervention program. *American journal of audiology, 9,* 9-29.

---

the tissue, is particularly damaging to the CNS. The incidence of asphyxia is indirectly related to gestational age and birth weight, with the preterm infant at greater risk for anoxic episodes than the full-term infant. A postulated cause of asphyxia is hypoxic-ischemic injury to the brainstem. It is essential that an adequate supply of oxygen be available for adequate functioning of the organ of Corti. The incidence of sensorineural hearing loss in children with severe perinatal asphyxia has been reported to be approximately 4% (Eichwald & Mahoney, 1993).

The clinical definition of asphyxia remains a matter of debate among authors and clinicians. Use of multiple measures to determine clinically significant asphyxia has been suggested. The hearing loss evident in cases of asphyxia is the sensorineural type, with a steep slope noted, especially in the high-frequency range. Because this type of hearing impairment is not progressive, screening can be done early in the neonatal period.

Bacterial Meningitis.   Bacterial meningitis is a common infection and a sequela of bacterial infection in the neonate. Meningitis, which is a disease of the CNS, manifests as an inflammation of the meninges and the cerebrospinal fluid (CSF) that may extend to adjacent organs, such as the brain and the ear. Meningitis is seen in approximately 1 in 2500 live births. In the neonate, meningitis may be acquired from a maternal infection transmitted transplacentally or at the time of delivery. The mode of transmission may also be infant to infant via nursery personnel or contaminated equipment. In most cases meningitis is acquired after birth; it is the most common cause of hearing loss in infants (Hristeva et al, 1999). It has been proposed that the infection passes from the meninges to the inner ear via the cochlear aqueduct and along vessels and nerves from the internal and auditory meatus. Because clinical manifestations of neonatal meningitis often are subtle and deceptive, clinical vigilance and verification by laboratory studies are the only means of diagnosis in the newborn. Factors implicated in neurologic damage include host differences, bacterial virulence, the infant's age, the time between exposure to the disease and the onset of treatment, the intensity of treatment, and the duration of the disease.

Meningitis may be viral in origin, but bacteria cause most cases that result in neurologic deficits. Two organisms, group B *Streptococcus* and *Escherichia coli,* have been identified as the responsible agent in 89% of cases. Of these two, group B *Streptococcus* is the more commonly seen.

The treatment for infants with meningitis is supportive, and antibiotic therapy is an important aspect of the regimen. Antibiotics, such as gentamicin and kanamycin, which are widely used in treatment, often are potentially ototoxic. Careful monitoring of drug levels is imperative to reduce the risk of hearing loss.

Sensorineural hearing loss has been reported after bacterial meningitis. The hearing loss generally is bilateral and ranges from severe to profound. Reports of mild to moderate hearing loss have also been documented. Meningitic hearing loss may be recovered to some degree.

Congenital Perinatal Infection.   The occurrence of certain infections during the perinatal period places the fetus at risk for various congenital malformations that affect auditory function. The most common and best-referenced infections are represented by the acronym TORCH (i.e., toxoplasmosis, other infections, rubella, cytomegalovirus [CMV], and herpes simplex). Although "other infections" does not include syphilis, that infection is discussed here because of its potential impact on hearing. Exposure to these infectious agents early in development often results in a pregnancy loss. With late gestation exposure, the degree of involvement may range from subclinical to severe multisystem disease.

Lack of symptomatology, which often is associated with the TORCH infections, makes identification difficult in the prenatal period. In general, infants exposed to congenital perinatal infections experience varying degrees of ocular, cardiovascular, and psychoneurologic problems, among which is hearing impairment.

Toxoplasmosis. Toxoplasmosis is caused by the parasite *Toxoplasma gondii*. The route of transmission is transplacental, and infection occurs through maternal contact with the organism in uncooked meat or in cat feces. The most severe impact on the fetus results from exposure during the first and second trimesters. Congenital toxoplasmosis is manifested by chorioretinitis, cerebral calcification, psychomotor retardation, hydrocephalus or microcephaly, and convulsions.

Although research directly relating toxoplasmosis to hearing disorders is sparse, the disease is similar to CMV infection and therefore may have a similar impact on hearing. Pathologic studies have demonstrated changes in the soft tissue mesenchyma and mucoperiosteum and calcium deposits in the spiral ligament of the inner ear.

More than 70% of infants with toxoplasmosis do not show clinical signs in the neonatal period. Infants who do demonstrate generalized disease are likely to have low birth weight, hepatosplenomegaly, icterus, and anemia in the first weeks of life. Findings indicating neurologic disease are convulsions, intracranial calcification, and hydrocephalus or microcephaly; however, these are not seen until 1 month of age in most infants. In follow-up studies of infants with newborn toxoplasmosis who showed infectious symptoms, fewer than 25% demonstrated hearing loss. Yet when asymptomatic infants were examined, the proportion with neurologic sequelae was closer to 75%. These observations indicate the need for follow-up of infants at risk because of the maternal and neonatal histories until 1 year of age. Collaborative studies with larger sample sizes need to be conducted to replicate reports currently in the literature.

Syphilis. Now thought to be on the increase, syphilis poses a threat to the mother and fetus. The disease is caused by the spirochete *Treponema pallidum*, which is transmitted in utero to the fetus from an infected mother. It previously was thought that before the eighteenth week of gestation, the Langhans layer of the chorion acted as a barrier, preventing transmission of the spirochete to the fetus. However, infection occurs before the eighteenth week, although pathologic changes do not develop until the fifth month of gestation, when the fetus becomes immunocompetent and inflammatory cells can be found. Treatment of the disease before 18 weeks' gestation almost always prevents signs of infection in the fetus. Transmission of the spirochete to the fetus occurs in 70% to 100% of pregnancies with untreated primary syphilis and in approximately 30% of pregnancies with latent syphilis.

Early symptoms of congenital syphilis in the neonate include nasal discharge (snuffles), rash, anemia, jaundice, and osteochondritis. Late symptoms include saddle nose, saber skin, and dental abnormalities. Congenital syphilis has a profound effect on the inner ear. Pathologic changes include osteitis of all three layers of the otic capsule, with inflammatory infiltration of the membranes of the cochlea and the vestibular labyrinth. Hear-

ing impairment may be profound as a result of severe degeneration of the organ of Corti, spiral ganglion, and nerve cells, along with destruction of the membranous labyrinth. Spirochetes remain visible in the perilymph of the ear despite massive therapy because penicillin does not readily cross the perilymph barrier to enter the endolymphatic fluid of the inner ear.

Congenital syphilis affects hearing in approximately 35% of children, and the hearing deficit associated with this disease presents a challenge to health care providers. Some of the complex issues surrounding these cases include the following:

1. Congenital syphilis may be asymptomatic in as many as 50% of neonatal cases.
2. Routine hospital screening for syphilis done through the Venereal Disease Research Laboratory (VDRL) test has high false-positive and false-negative rates and may show a positive reaction when other diseases are present, such as malaria, infectious hepatitis, infectious mononucleosis, and disseminated lupus erythematosus. The fluorescent treponemal antibody absorption test is more sensitive but also more expensive.
3. The progressive pattern of hearing impairment demonstrates variations as to the time of onset and the rapidity of progression.
4. The onset of infantile congenital syphilis usually is between 8 and 20 years of age. Hearing loss is sudden, bilateral, symmetric, and profound and has no accompanying symptoms.
5. Hearing loss caused by congenital syphilis manifests as poor function and limited use of hearing aid devices as a result of neural atrophy with poor discrimination.
6. Penicillin therapy does not prevent or retard the progressive hearing loss.

Treatment includes early identification of infants suspected of having a syphilitic infection and prompt treatment with large doses of penicillin. Steroids are the drugs of choice for treating hearing loss that occurs secondary to congenital syphilis. However, not all patients improve with steroid therapy.

Because syphilitic hearing impairments pose a grave threat to developmental milestones, early identification and testing, as well as lengthy follow-up, are imperative.

Rubella. Congenital rubella infection is a major threat to the fetus and newborn. Before immunization became widespread, rubella was the leading cause of deafness in children attending schools for the hearing impaired in the United States.

Acquired rubella is a mild disease of children and adults that is transmitted by droplet contact with the virus. The fetus acquires the virus congenitally through placental transfer. The critical factor in determining the pregnancy outcome is the gestational age of the fetus at the time of exposure. A 50% prevalence of congenital rubella defects has been noted in infants exposed during the first month of pregnancy. The prevalence declines to 22% in infants exposed during the second month of pregnancy and drops to 6% to 10% in those exposed during the third, fourth, and fifth months. Clinically, the infant with congenital rubella may show a wide range of effects. Many appear to be normal newborns, whereas others have cardiac lesions, low birth weight, eye defects, growth retardation, thrombocytopenia purpura, hepatosplenomegaly, hepatitis, and CNS defects, such as psychomotor retardation. Hearing defects are the most common result of the viral insult. Congenital rubella is manifested as a chronic infection in fetal tissues that inhibits fetal cell multiplication; therefore it is not a static disease. The severity of the pathologic effect caused by the arrest of development varies and reflects the clinical variations demonstrated in hearing loss. Histopathologic studies after rubella infection have revealed degeneration of the organ of Corti and anomalies of the middle ear, such as a fixed stapedial footplate.

The hearing deficit associated with congenital rubella syndrome is severe to profound bilateral sensorineural loss, with an audiometric configuration that depicts the greatest degree of loss in the midrange, from 500 to 2000 Hz. Although the incidence of congenital rubella defects is related to the time of onset, no special relationship appears to exist between the degree of loss and the time of the infection.

Rubella exposure during pregnancy is difficult to verify because the disorder often passes a mild, unrecognized disease. Because of the possible late onset and the progressive nature of congenital rubella syndrome, infants with a history of rubella or of rubella exposure should be observed with serial audiograms until they are 18 to 24 months of age.

Cytomegalovirus.   CMV, a member of the herpes family, is the most common cause of congenital viral infection in human beings. An estimated 20% of pregnant women carry CMV; 2.5% of the infants are infected at birth, and 10% to 20% of these infants are at risk for later sequelae.

The virus can be transmitted to the fetus transplacentally or at the time of delivery via the cervix. CMV can also be transmitted after birth through infected urine, saliva, breast milk, tears, feces, and blood transfusions. Nearly all congenital infections occur in infants whose mothers had the antibody to the virus before conception; the congenital infection represents reactivation of a latent infection. During pregnancy, cervical reactivation of the CMV infection is common, and there is a high probability that the infant will be infected. The risk to the fetus may be related both to the time of infection in utero and to the mother's immune status.

The effects of CMV infection range from severe CNS involvement to asymptomatic carrying of the virus. Asymptomatic infants are at risk for late sequelae, manifested as bilateral sensorineural hearing loss that may be mild to profound. About 25% of these infants show severe hearing loss by the end of the first year of life.

Symptomatic congenital infection, also known as cytomegalic inclusion disease (CID), occurs in only 5% to 10% of infected infants and is nearly always associated with maternal infection around the time of conception. Manifestations of CID include enlargement of the liver and spleen, jaundice, petechial rash, chorioretinitis, cerebral calcifications, and microcephaly.

CMV infections of the inner ear cause either partial or total cochlear and labyrinthine end-organ destruction. The damaged cell reaction is clearly manifested among the cells of the organ of Corti and the neurons of the spiral ganglion. In a follow-up study of symptomatic infants with CID, 30% were found to have severe to profound bilateral sensorineural hearing loss.

The following basic tenets should be considered in the care of a neonate identified as being at risk for CMV infection (Downs, 1994):

1. Excretion of the virus may continue for several years after birth, contributing to degenerative hearing loss. Follow-up testing, therefore, should be done at shorter intervals than for nonprogressive diseases. Audiologic evaluation every 3 months is recommended.
2. With CID, any pattern and degree of hearing loss can occur. These infants should be screened with electrophysiologic testing, because detection of mild to moderate hearing loss is greater with this technique.
3. With asymptomatic viral infection, hearing loss may occur at a later date. This knowledge may help determine the cause of childhood-onset hearing loss.

Herpes Simplex Virus.   The herpes simplex virus (HSV) is a member of a group of DNA viruses that cause latent infection characterized by periodic recurrences. HSV poses a threat to the health of both the mother and the neonate. Infection with HSV type 1 (HSV-1) generally occurs in the oral cavity or above the waist and is most prevalent among children and young adults. Transmission usually occurs via the respiratory route through contact with asymptomatic family members. The oral lesions recur in 20% to 45% of those with the disease.

HSV type 2 (HSV-2) infection generally occurs in the genital region and is transmitted by sexual contact. The virus can be isolated in sexually active individuals. Most genital infections are asymptomatic. Patients who are symptomatic report local tenderness and burning involving the labia and vaginal mucosa. Both symptomatic and asymptomatic individuals may transmit the infection.

Many women are infected before pregnancy, but the infection blooms during the pregnancy. If the mother is actively infected, the most common means by which HSV is transmitted to the fetus is vaginal birth. The risk to the infant of genital herpes infection during vaginal delivery has not been clearly defined but may be as high as 50%. Fewer than 10% of infants are infected after birth through airborne infection or through direct contact with the virus from labial sores on the mother or open lesions on the face, lips, or hands of the father or nursery personnel. An ascending mechanism of infection has also been reported as a mode of transmission, despite the presence of intact membranes. Transplacental transmission of the virus, although rare, may occur during maternal viremia.

Although HSV infections often are asymptomatic in adults, they rarely are so in neonates. Vaginally contracted HSV in the neonate does not manifest initially; an incubation period of 6 to 12 days elapses before clinical symptoms appear. Neonatal infections are classified as disseminated with or without CNS involvement, or localized. Disseminated infections may involve virtually every organ system. Most cases with CNS involvement result in death; of the survivors, only 4% are free of sequelae. Of infants in whom there is no CNS involvement, 12% survive without sequelae. About 40% of infants with localized infection suffer from progressive neurologic damage resulting in death, and about 40% of those who survive have severe neurologic sequelae.

Histopathologic studies have demonstrated that HSV infects the sensory cells of the labyrinth. In light of the similarities of all the perinatal viral infections, nurses should ensure careful follow-up of this at-risk group.

Collaborative research studies need to be conducted in many different areas. The incidence of HSV infection during various stages of pregnancy and at the time of delivery must be documented. Longitudinal studies of neonates exposed to HSV must be done to ascertain if the virus contributes to progressive hearing loss.

DEFECTS OF THE HEAD AND NECK

The anatomy of the head and neck should be assessed for deficits as part of the screening process for all neonates. Ear anomalies associated with head and neck anomalies may occur as a result of a primary regional defect; secondary to a primary defect in an area contiguous to the temporal bone; as part of an inherited defect involving the skeletal system; or as part of a chromosomal disorder. Malformations of the head and neck may be relatively simple or complex. Any neonate with a defect, even a minor one, should be closely examined for hidden major malformations.

Ear

The relationship of the pinna to the other structures of the head and face is important in the initial assessment. With normal placement, the helix is located at the level of the outer canthus and the tragus is roughly level with the intraorbital rim. Low-set auricles frequently are associated with abnormalities of the urinary system. Unilateral conductive hearing loss may be present in children with normal-size pinnae and unilateral absence of the superior crus or in patients with a fused anthelix-helix; thickened, hypertrophied ear lobes; a "cup" ear; and a protruding pinna. The pinna may be abnormally small (microtia) or absent (anotia). Atresia (closure of the external auditory canal) may be observed. The condition is classified as mild, indicating a small ear canal; medium, indicating that a bony atretic plate has replaced the canal with ossicular malformation; or severe, indicating a small or absent ear canal and middle ear space.

Several combinations of atresia and microtia may be seen, therefore all children with these abnormalities should be suspected of having middle ear abnormalities. These infants may also have sensorineural hearing loss. Atresia often is observed with cranial, facial, mandibular, or acrofacial dysostoses. Abnormalities of the skeletal system or chromosomal aberration may also be accompanied by atresia. Aural atresia may be associated with facial, labial, or palatal clefts. Infants with atresia often have conductive hearing loss related to the inability of the ear canal to transmit sound.

Preauricular abnormalities, including pits or tags (Figure 35-4) and branchial fistulas, often are accompanied by external or middle ear malformations. These appendages may be present with an otherwise normal-appearing pinna. Preauricular tags or pits usually require only cosmetic surgery or excision if they are draining.

Nose

Examination of the nose should be directed toward identification of suspicious defects, such as unusual broadness with a flat base and a short length (saddle nose), small nostrils, and notched alae. Deformities of the nose often appear with other craniofacial abnormalities.

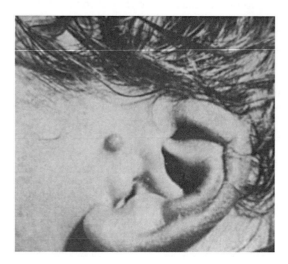

FIGURE **35-4**
Preauricular tag. From Schreiner RL, Bradburn NC (1987). *Care of the newborn*, ed 2. Raven Press: New York.

Mouth

Defects in the oral cavity are the most common defect associated with hearing impairment. A child with cleft lip or palate has a deficiency in the palate musculature that is primarily related to the inability of the tensor muscle of the velum palatinum to dilate the eustachian tube actively during swallowing. Hearing problems may be observed in patients with cleft palate, depending on the patient's age on examination and the means of the exploration.

Cleft palate or palate leaves the child vulnerable to the effusion of fluid and, as a result, to varying degrees of hearing loss. The consequences of effusion of fluid raise the rate of otitis media, for which 50% to 90% incidences have been reported. The hearing loss associated with cleft lip or palate generally is conductive; however, sensorineural and combination losses have been reported. Infants younger than 12 months of age who had cleft palate that was surgically repaired often have a detectable degree of hearing loss. The degree of loss is directly related to the severity of the palatal defect.

Eyes

Deformities of the eyelids are the most common abnormality involving the eyes. A variation in eyelid configuration has been noted in which the upper eyelid forms an almost vertical curve at the level of the medial limit of the cornea and fuses with the lower eyelid. The distance of the two medial angles is increased. These findings typically are noted in Waardenburg syndrome, an autosomal dominant disorder that results in mild to severe sensorineural hearing loss in 50% of patients. The hearing loss may be unilateral or bilateral and progressive.

Epicanthal folds, which are true vertical folds extending from the nasal fold into the upper eyelid, are commonly noted in infants with Down syndrome, or trisomy 21. Other physical features seen in Down syndrome are low-set ears, small pinnae, and a narrow external ear canal. Infants with this syndrome tend to have recurrent otitis media and anomalies of the middle ear ossicles. The incidence of hearing loss is high, and the condition may be the sensorineural, conductive, or combination type.

Hair

An unusual hair texture or hairline should raise suspicion in the assessment for abnormalities associated with hearing loss. Twisted hair (pili torti) has been associated with sensorineural hearing loss. The hair may be twisted, dry, brittle, or easily broken. Aberrant scalp hair patterns may also be significant.

Neck

Defects of the neck that may be associated with hearing impairment are branchial cleft fistulas and mildly webbed or shortened neck. Not all infants with defects of the head or neck also have hearing impairments; many variations may be observed in the normal neonate (Jones, 1988). The presence of such defects does increase the risk of hearing impairment, however, and should be followed up in the long-term interest of the child.

Elevated Bilirubin Level

Hyperbilirubinemia, also referred to as neonatal jaundice, occurs when an excess of bilirubin is present in the blood. The condition can be neurotoxic to the infant at high concentrations. Jaundice is observed in approximately 60% of term infants and in 80% of preterm infants. Any number of factors that interfere with the transport of bilirubin to the liver or that reduce or prevent the metabolization of bilirubin in the liver can lead to toxic levels of the unconjugated bilirubin. Unconjugated bilirubin can cross the blood-brain barrier. Kernicterus, a neurologic syndrome, results from the deposit of unconjugated bilirubin in the basal ganglia of the brain, causing motor and sensory deficits, mental deficits, or death. Exchange transfusions are performed to lower the bilirubin level in infants at risk of developing kernicterus. For neonatal problems, hyperbilirubinemia is the most common sequela that results in deafness.

The AAP Joint Committee on Infant Hearing (2000) has suggested that infants with a bilirubin level that exceeds the indications for an exchange transfusion are at risk for hearing impairment. The committee has suggested that certain birth weights and bilirubin levels be used as guidelines for deciding whether an infant should be placed on the high-risk register (Table 35-2).

Family History

More than 50 types of hereditary hearing loss have been described. A significant number of hearing impairments may be classified as genetically based. Hereditary hearing loss must be identified on the basis of a thorough medical and family history, which should include the following components:

1. Determination of the cause and circumstances under which the hearing impairment was first noticed: Many different circumstances surrounding the onset of the hearing loss may cause it to be labeled as congenital or hereditary or both. An example of hearing loss that is hereditary and not congenital is Alport syndrome, an autosomal dominant trait resulting in deafness that appears at 8 years of age.
2. A complete family history: This should include a history of previous and current pregnancies.
3. An extended family history of data relating to hearing impairments of both immediate and extended family members.
4. A thorough physical examination: The head and neck region, particularly, should be examined for abnormalities.
5. Selective testing procedures for assessing possible causes of sensorineural hearing loss.

Figure 35-5 shows a form that can be used to obtain information from the mother. Although the questions easily may be asked orally, the form provides a structure that can

TABLE 35-2	Birth Weight and Bilirubin Levels Indicating a High Risk of Sensorineural Hearing Impairment	
Birth Weight (g)	**Bilirubin Level (mg)**
Under 1000	10
1001 to 1250	10
1251 to 1500	13
1501 to 2000	15
2001 to 2500	17
Over 2500	18

MOTHER'S NAME:_____

ROOM NO.:_____

1. Do you know any of the baby's relatives who now have a hearing loss which started before the age of five? Think hard about all of your family and the baby's father's family . . . .
   Yes_____ No_____
   A. In no, proceed to question No. 2.
   B. If yes, ask the following:
      (1) Who were they? (relationship to baby)
          (A)_____ (B)_____ (C)_____
      (2) Do you know what caused the loss? . . . .
          Yes_____ No_____
          (A)_____ (B)_____ (C)_____
      (3) What makes you think the onset of the hearing loss was before age five?
          (A)_____ (B)_____ (C)_____
      (4) Did he/she wear a hearing aid before age five? . . (A)_____ (B)_____ (C)_____
          Does he/she still wear an aid? . . . .(A)_____ (B)_____ (C)_____
      (5) Did he/she attend a special school for the deaf? . (A)_____ (B)_____ (C)_____
          Did the person attend public school? . . . .(A)_____ (B)_____ (C)_____
      (6) Did he/she have a speech problem? . . . .(A)_____ (B)_____ (C)_____
2. During your pregnancy, did you have 3-day measles, German measles, rubella, or a rash with a fever? . . . . Yes_____ No_____
   WHEN: 1st 3 mo._____ Middle 3 mo._____ Last 3 mo._____
3. During your pregnancy, were you around anyone who had 3-day measles, German measles, rubella, or a rash with fever? . . . . Yes_____ No_____
   WHEN: 1st 3 mo._____ Middle 3 mo._____ Last 3 mo._____
4. Do you have any reason to be concerned about your baby's hearing? . . . .
   Yes_____ No_____
   If yes, why?_____
5. What pediatrician or clinic will be caring for your baby when he/she leaves the hospital? _____

   Approximate location_____
6. Nearest relative or friend: Name:_____
                                 Address:_____
                                 Phone:_____

FIGURE 35-5
Mother's interview. From Northern J, Downs M (1984). *Hearing in children*. Williams & Wilkins: Baltimore.

help ensure consistency during the interview. The questionnaire should be given to all new mothers and should be completed before discharge. This tool provides an excellent opportunity for educating the mother on normal speech and language development.

HEREDITARY HEARING LOSS

Autosomal Dominant Inheritance

Autosomal dominant inheritance accounts for 10% to 25% of cases of hereditary hearing impairment. The hearing loss may be unilateral or bilateral, and males and females are affected equally. Autosomal dominant hearing disorders vary in severity ("variable expressivity") and in progression of hearing loss. A typical example of an autosomal dominant hearing disorder occurs in Waardenburg syndrome, which is characterized by hypertelorism, a high nasal bridge, synophrys, and hypoplastic alae nasi. Pigmentation abnormalities include a white forelock, partial albinism, hypopigmentation of the fundi, blue irises, and premature graying. In this syndrome, severe to profound bilateral sensorineural hearing loss is present with integumentary system involvement. The histopathologic characteristics are absence of the organ of Corti and atrophy of the spiral ganglion.

Another example of an autosomal dominant hearing loss with incomplete penetrance and variable expression occurs in Treacher Collins syndrome. Major features of the syndrome include facial anomalies; small, displaced, or absent external ears; external auditory canal atresia; and poorly developed or malformed tympanic ossicles. Deafness generally is complete and conductive.

Klippel-Feil syndrome, if familial, is another example of autosomal dominance with variable expression. The characteristics of this syndrome are craniofacial disorders, fusion of some or all of the cervical vertebrae, cleft palate (occasionally), and severe sensorineural hearing loss. Crouzon disease is another disorder in which hearing loss is attributed to autosomal dominance with variable expression. An abnormally shaped head, a beaked nose, and marked bilateral exophthalmos caused by premature closure of the cranial sutures characterize this disease. Hearing loss may be conductive or sensorineural because of middle ear deformities.

Autosomal Recessive Inheritance

Autosomal recessive inheritance accounts for about 40% of childhood deafness. An estimated 1 in 8 individuals is a carrier for a recessive form of hearing impairment. The incidence of recessive inheritance is higher in marriages of recent common ancestry. This type of union increases the possibility that each parent will be the carrier of an identical defective gene that may express itself as an abnormal trait. Hearing loss in people with an autosomal recessive gene tends to be more severe than in those with autosomal dominant inheritance, because most cases of recessive hearing loss are associated with the Scheibe deformity of the cochlea. With Scheibe dysplasia, the entire organ of Corti is rudimentary; hair cells are missing, and the supporting cells are distorted or collapsed. The vestibular membrane usually is collapsed. Pendred syndrome, a condition marked by hearing loss and goiter detected in the first 2 years of life, is an example of an autosomal recessive disorder.

X-Linked Disorders. Approximately 3% of hereditary deafness is due to the X-linked mode of transmission (Northern & Downs, 1984). The mutant gene is on the X chromosome, and males transmit only Y chromosomes to their male offspring; therefore only males are affected. The female is the carrier and has the chance to transmit the gene to 50% of her sons, who manifest the disease, and 50% of her daughters, who carry the abnormality. The hearing loss characteristically is not present at birth but develops in infancy to varying degrees. X-linked hearing losses, with exceptions, are sensorineural, and some retention of hearing in all frequencies often occurs. Recessive, or X-linked, Duchenne muscular dystrophy is an example of this type of disorder. Characterized by muscle wasting, the severe infantile form of muscular dystrophy also is associated with mild to moderate sensorineural hearing loss. (See Chapter 10 for a complete discussion of genetic inheritance patterns.)

Cytogenetic Disorders. Cytogenetic disorders are caused by structural changes in one or more of the chromosomes or by errors in the distribution of the chromosomes. Down syndrome, which is caused by an extra chromosome 21, is the most common chromosomal aberration syndrome, with an incidence of 1 in 600 to 800 births. Approximately 5% of cases of Down syndrome are due to translocation and fusion of part of chromosome 21 to chromosome 14. Children with trisomy 21 have a high incidence of hearing loss.

Characteristic otologic findings that have an impact on the hearing performance of these children during the early years are (1) a high incidence of stenosis of the external auditory canal, (2) a high incidence of serous otitis media, and (3) a high incidence of cholesteatoma-persistent growth of squamous epithelium from the ear canal into the middle ear or mastoid through a tear in the tympanic membrane.

The narrowed segment is located at the junction of the cartilaginous and bony portions of the canal. With increasing age, the canal has been noted to assume a more typical appearance as the thickened tissue recedes.

The degree of hearing loss in these infants varies but is rarely ever profound. On examination of the aperture, some of these children are found to have congenital ossicular malformations and destruction caused by inflammations arising from chronic infection.

Mental retardation is a clinical condition frequently seen with Down syndrome. The impact of the otologic handicap on the developmental potential of these children is uncertain. Because of the high incidence of hearing loss in this group, early and frequent monitoring is imperative. Collaborative research studies must be done to identify factors affecting the otologic problems of infants with Down syndrome and to devise early strategies to optimize these infants' potential.

Low Birth Weight

Low birth weight (under 1500 g), especially when associated with such complications as hyperbilirubinemia and perinatal asphyxia, is widely accepted as a risk factor for congenitally acquired hearing impairment. Reports of hearing loss in low-birth-weight (LBW) infants put the incidence in the range of 4% to 16%. Other conditions that have been reported to enhance the risk of neurologic sequelae, including hearing impairment, are acidosis, sepsis, ototoxic drug therapy, sound trauma, and hypoglycemia. Determining the exact cause of hearing loss in neonates with multiple risk factors remains difficult. Any of these factors alone may cause hearing impairment, but when they are associated with immature physiologic status, the risk of hearing impairment increases. The hearing loss most often demonstrated in LBW infants is the sensorineural type, particularly in the high-frequency range. Prolonged intubation and otitis media have been correlated with hearing loss in LBW infants.

The higher incidence of hearing loss in LBW infants has been attributed to several factors, including (1) the infant's premature physiologic status; (2) perinatal complications (e.g., hyperbilirubinemia, hypoxia, acidosis, and apneic spells), which are likely to cause brain damage in LBW infants; (3) the constraints of intensive care; and (4) the combined effects of the preceding factors.

The "constraints of intensive care" refers to the iatrogenic factors common in the care of newborns admitted to the neonatal intensive care unit (NICU) that have an impact on the incidence of hearing impairment. These factors include ambient noise and exposure to ototoxic drugs.

Galambos and colleagues (1994) presented a retrospective study of hearing loss in level two (n = 1527) and level three (n = 4374) graduates. Their findings indicated that 1.4% of level two and 2.1% of level three infants failed two rounds of auditory brainstem response (ABR) testing and subsequently required hearing aid devices within the first year of life.

Ototoxic Drugs

The effects of ototoxic drugs commonly used in the care of LBW infants, which potentiate damage to the cochlea or to the vestibular portion of the inner ear, have been well documented. Drugs that have been reported to be potentially ototoxic include antibiotics, diuretics, and antimalarial pharmaceuticals. There appears to be considerable individual susceptibility to these ototoxic drugs, which usually cause bilateral symmetric hearing loss of varying degrees. Numerous factors may enhance the risk of ototoxicity, including elevated serum drug levels; decreased renal function; use of more than one ototoxic drug simultaneously or in increased doses or for an extended period; the infant's age, health, and heredity; and concurrent noise.

Specific aminoglycosides reported for more than a decade to have ototoxic potential include amikacin, clindamycin, gentamicin, kanamycin, tobramycin, and vancomycin. The American Speech-Language-Hearing Association (1994) guidelines suggested that aminoglycoside therapy administered for longer than 5 days in combination with loop diuretics be added to the risk criteria for potential sensorineural hearing loss.

Neonatal nurses are urged to monitor peak and trough serum concentrations of antibiotics, as well as creatinine clearance, to avoid high systemic levels in infants with impaired renal function.

Sound Trauma

The potential for noise-induced hearing loss in the neonate has been the subject of numerous reports in the literature. In the NICU, numerous sources constantly generate background and alarm noise.

The noise level in the NICU has been reported to be 20 dB higher than that in the well-baby nursery. The noise level of incubators per se does not cause sensorineural hearing loss in otherwise healthy preterm infants. Sudden noises in the NICU have been reported to cause hypoxemia in preterm infants, which leads to a decrease in transcutaneous oxygen tension and an increase in intracranial pressure, heart rate, and respiratory rate.

Nearly all the reported sound pressure levels of incubators (60 to 80 dB) are consistently lower than the risk level for adults. However, the damage risk level for adults, 90 dB, is based on intermittent exposure to noise; neonates are subject to continuous exposure for weeks and months at a time.

In recent years more research has focused on sound levels in the NICU and ways to reduce them (Walsh-Sukys et al, 2001). Graven (2000) performed a systematic review of NICU noise levels to determine the adverse reactions that were found, such as hearing loss. Philbin and associates (1999) recommended that the overall continuous sound level in any bed space or patient care area not exceed 55 dB. When background noise exceeds 50 dB, sleep is disturbed (Robertson & Philbin, 1996). Operating an NICU at sound levels below 50 dB requires careful attention to design and the cooperation of all those working on the unit.

Newborns at risk for hearing impairment may be exposed to hazardous sound levels during transport. For example, in a helicopter the noise level can reach 90 to 110 dB. Use of ear protectors during air transport has been suggested. These earmuffs also are used worldwide in many units to reduce noise for infants transported by ground or air.

Adding recorded voice and music to the environment of the preterm infant is a practice widely used to enhance the auditory environment. Sound sources should be kept a reasonable distance from infants' ears, and the sound level should be kept below 55dB (Philbin & Klass, 2000). White and associates (2000) have developed NICU design standards that include recommendations both for safe lighting and for sound levels.

SCREENING METHODS FOR IDENTIFICATION OF HEARING LOSS

Hearing screening is a method of detecting hearing impairment before the deficit becomes obvious in the infant. In the past 15 years, programs and procedures for screening newborns have been developed, modified, and improved.

The goal of any screening program is to accomplish the task rapidly, accurately, and economically. None of the current diagnostic screening methods fully meet all those criteria.

The AAP Task Force on Newborn and Infant Hearing (1999) has endorsed universal screening of all newborns. Audiologic follow-up is required for infants whose history indicates that degenerative disease or intrauterine infection may cause progressive, fluctuating, or late-onset hearing loss. In all cases, before discharge the neonatal nurse should teach the parents about the speech and hearing milestones and should provide them with information about community agencies available for long-term follow-up if needed. Because the intent of all screening programs is to identify hearing impairment before 3 months of age and to habilitate hearing-impaired children no later than 6 months of age, program development is essential (Joint Committee on Infant Hearing, 2000). If only infants who are identified as having one or more high-risk factors are screened, 50% to 70% of children with impairment remain unidentified.

Infant screening is a collaborative effort involving nurses, physicians, audiologists, and public health agency members. Each of these individuals plays a vital role in the program's success.

Behavioral Measurements of Hearing Function

Early attempts at infant behavioral screening focused on observational assessments of the neonatal behavioral response to sound, using noisemakers to obtain orienting responses. A squeeze toy, bell, or rattle was used to test for a behavioral response based on the maturational level of the subject (Figure

35-6). The expected response at 0 to 4 months included eye widening, eye blink, and arousal from sleep. However, with this method, the false-positive and false-negative results were found to be unacceptably high. Having more than one observer can minimize errors. The response to auditory stimulation should be eye movement and movement of at least one limb; both reactions should occur within 2½ seconds of the signal, and both must be observed by two independent observers or by one observer subjected to auditory masking. The validity of the test depends partly on identification of the infant's state and control of environmental noise. For testing purposes, a light sleep state is best. Because of this method's lack of specificity, the Joint Committee on Infant Hearing

(2000) excludes behavioral screening for use with infants under 6 months of age.

Automated Screening Devices

Disappointing results from observational screening methods prompted the development of automated methods of detecting hearing loss.

Crib-O-Gram

The Crib-O-Gram was an ingenious automated system aimed at monitoring behavioral and physiologic responses to auditory stimuli. For the test, a motion-sensitive transducer is placed under the crib mattress. The infant's state is monitored auto-

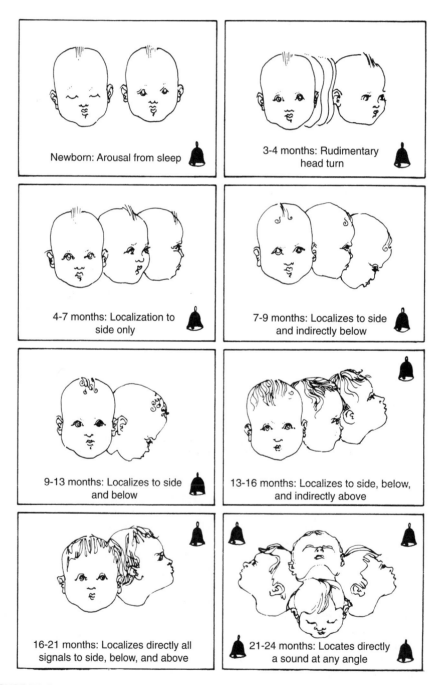

FIGURE **35-6**

Maturation of auditory response. From Northern J, Downs M (1984). *Hearing in children.* Williams & Wilkins: Baltimore.

matically by measurement of crib movement before and after each sound presentation. An earphone placed in the bassinet presents the test sound, 92 dB. Responses are recorded from 10 seconds before until 3½ seconds after the stimulus. This pattern of testing is continued until a microprocessing unit makes a statistically valid determination.

Auditory Response Cradle

Like the Crib-O-Gram, the auditory response cradle (ARC) monitors behavioral and physiologic responses to auditory stimuli by an automatic, microprocessor-controlled device. The system, which was designed by Bennett and Lawrence in 1980, is composed of a cradle that houses the electronic components of the device, including the microprocessor. Four types of response are monitored during the test: (1) head and trunk movements are monitored by a pressure-sensitive mattress; (2) startle responses are detected by the microprocessor and transducer; (3) body movements are detected by pressure transducers beneath the mattress; and (4) respiratory movements of the chest are monitored by a transducer inside a band fixed around the infant's chest or abdomen. Noise stimulus is presented through earphones at 85 dB, and the analysis procedure takes into account the number of responses that occur with sound and control trials. The device assesses infant activity in the prestimulus period and defers testing if the subject is restless.

Peripheral Measurements of Hearing Function

Assessment of hearing function in the neonate has focused on a two-tiered approach in which the evoked otoacoustic emissions (EOAE) test is used initially, and the automated ABR test is used as follow-up for infants who show hearing impairment on the initial screening. Otoacoustic emissions are low-intensity sounds that can be measured by placing a sensitive microphone in the ear canal. Hearing screening using otoacoustic emissions is quick, inexpensive, and relatively accurate.

If hearing impairment is detected on the EOAE test, the ABR test can confirm the validity of that result. The ABR test records the electrical potentials that arise from the auditory nerve system. During this test, disk electrodes are attached to the vertex and mastoid areas, and repetitive sounds are presented to the ear in the form of clicks caused by a direct current pulse. The recorded response is a sequence of waves that represents the action potential of the auditory nerve. The wave latencies in infants at risk tend to show smaller and more prolonged responses. The absolute latency of the ABR waves depends on the intensity of the click stimulus. Reducing the click stimuli from 60 dB to 30 to 40 dB identifies thresholds of hearing. Absence of all waves indicates the presence of a peripheral lesion.

An abnormal ABR result may be defined as one that shows an absence of response at 40 dB or a wave V latency that exceeds the norm by two standard deviations. Wave V responses are used to determine abnormality because they are highly repeatable in infants and show little variability in normal-hearing subjects. The ABR test appears to be a sensitive method in that no false-negative results have been reported. Considering that any screening method should be quick, inexpensive, and easily administered and should allow easy interpretation of a large number of infants, the drawback to the ABR test is that it is more costly than the EOAE test. Nevertheless, the ABR test can be justified as the initial neonatal hearing test, especially in preterm or high-risk infants. The Joint Committee

on Infant Hearing (1994, 2000) specifies that an audiologist should supervise the infant hearing screening program.

In some infants whose initial ABR test results meet risk criteria, continuing audiologic follow-up and management may be appropriate. These infants include those with risk factors associated with possible progressive or fluctuant loss, such as a family history of progressive hearing loss, CMV infection, and persistent fetal circulation.

Infants who do not demonstrate a repeatable ABR wave V to the signal presented at 40 dB in at least one ear should have a comprehensive hearing evaluation at no later than 6 months of age. This follow-up includes a general physical examination, including examination of the head and neck; otoscopy and otomicroscopy; identification of relevant physical abnormalities; and laboratory tests for perinatal infections. A comprehensive audiologic evaluation may include additional evoked potential evaluation and acoustic emittance measurements. Although precise data on hearing sensitivity cannot be obtained until the infant can respond to operant conditioning test procedures at approximately 6 months of age, habilitation should not be delayed. The treatment protocols can be modified as additional hearing evaluation data become available. Many institutions are now using the ABR and EOAE tests as early as 24 hours of age. The rationale is that the earlier a problem is identified, the sooner treatment can be started (Ronge, 1997).

Infants can be fitted with hearing aids before 3 months of age. Attention to early identification, amplification, and education does not necessarily ensure speech and language acquisition but certainly facilitates it, even in the most profoundly hearing-impaired child.

MANAGEMENT OF THE HEARING-IMPAIRED NEONATE

Two of the recommendations of the Joint Committee on Infant Hearing (1994, 2000) are that hearing screening of all infants be completed before discharge or no later than 3 months of age, and that whenever possible, the diagnostic process be completed and habilitation begun by 6 months of age. An infant with a positive hearing test result should be retested within 6 weeks of the initial screening procedure. Infants whose history indicates that they are at risk for late-onset hearing loss should be observed by periodic audiologic testing.

For the infant with a confirmed hearing loss, efforts are directed at treatment. In accordance with Public Law 99, early intervention services are (1) evaluation and assessment and (2) development of an individualized family service plan. The full evaluation plan is to be completed within 45 days of referral. This plan may include various methods directed at treatment of serous otitis media, which is a major cause of temporary conductive hearing loss. For the infant with a permanent conductive hearing loss, amplification with a hearing aid may facilitate stimulation in the early critical period. Infants can be fitted with a hearing aid device as soon as the impairment is diagnosed. In addition to amplification, the family should be taught total communication skills that will enhance interaction between the sender and the receiver. The basic premise is to use every means to communicate, such as gesturing, touching, and attending to stimuli.

Hearing screening is a task for a team of professionals that includes pediatricians, otolaryngologists, audiologists, and nurses. Local public health agencies may provide services such as data collection and referral. Many large metropolitan medical centers have speech and hearing centers as part of a broad base of services ranging from diagnosis to rehabilitation. At the national level, the following organizations provide health professionals and consumers with information on the diagnosis and treatment of hearing impairments:

American Speech-Language-Hearing Association (ASHA)
10801 Rockville Pike
Rockville, MD 20852
www.professional.asha.org

National Institute on Deafness and other
Communication Disorders
Wise Ears
www.nih.gov/nidcd/health/wise

The overall goal of any treatment program for the hearing impaired is to optimize the infant's potential communication skills and abilities. To achieve this goal, a comprehensive evaluation, follow-up, and management system must be implemented. The multidisciplinary, multiservices approach should be instituted only when all components are available to the infant and the family (American Speech-Language-Hearing Association, 1994).

In addition to qualified professionals and services, other factors influence the management and habilitation of the hearing-impaired infant. These factors can facilitate or hamper entry into the system and compliance with the treatment regimen (Box 35-2).

Outcome measures of the treatment program are early identification and implementation of a comprehensive habilitation plan to maximize communication potential and parental acceptance of the infant's disability.

The infant with severe to profound hearing impairment who is not at risk for recurrent otitis media and who does not get satisfactory results with a hearing aid is a candidate for cochlear implants (discussed below).

For the hearing-impaired infant, multiple referral sources exist in which a multidisciplinary approach optimizes the infant's potential for growth and development.

Cochlear Implants

Cochlear implants are not new, but they increasingly are being used to treat infants with sensorineural hearing loss. The implants are electronic devices that are more sensitive to sound than traditional hearing aids. The external part of the device is surgically placed in the skin behind the ear, and the internal electrodes are placed in the inner ear at the cochlea. Rather than amplifying sound, the implant replaces the nonfunctional transmission of sound in the inner ear; it allows the brain to understand sound signals. In the United States about 7000 children have received cochlear implants (www.nidcd.nih.gov, 2001). Implants work only if some spiral ganglion cells are present to transmit the auditory signal. The implants take sound signals and convert them to electrical stimuli. The sound is conveyed by electrodes, which can be placed in several arrangements, and then transmitted to an external processor. A single-channel or multiple-channel (as many as 22) unit can be used to process the sound.

An issue for patients of any age with any type of cochlear implant is the comfortable level of sound (Donaldson et al, 2001). This sometimes is difficult to determine in infants, who are easily stimulated. The impact of implants on speech and language development is also an area of research (Sarant et al, 2001). The implant consists of a microphone, speech processor, transmitter, receiver, and electrodes. More studies are needed to determine if implants have a positive effect on language acquisition and speech perception and at what age should they be done? To date the outcome has been promising; children who received implants before language acquisition are in some cases developing close to the normal range. The later the child receives the implants, the more likely it is that speech patterns will remain disturbed. (More information on cochlear implants is available online at http://www.nidcd.nih.gov/health/pubs_hb/coch.htm).

Parental Support

Support for the parents of a hearing-impaired child is based on the foundation of trust and acceptance between the nurse and the family. Notification of a hearing impairment is an extremely traumatic and deeply disturbing situation for the parents, one that often provokes denial. Often, identification of the problem is delayed because the parents cannot admit that something is wrong. Some practices in the diagnostic workup for hearing impairment seem to favor separation of the parents from the diagnostic process. EOAE and ABR testing may foster denial because the findings are abstract, and parents need to have visible, tangible evidence of the impairment. The nurse plays a major role in reiterating, interpreting, and reinforcing the information conveyed by the audiologist. Sensitivity to the parents' need to grieve the loss of the "perfect child" is important. Acceptance of the handicap can be aided by enlisting the parents as codiagnosticians. Asking the parents what they think the problem is and making them part of the decision-making process objectifies the diagnoses and aids future compliance with the habilitative regimen. By listening to the parents' feelings of inadequacy and by indirect teaching, nurses can help the parents acquire more fruitful coping strategies.

The mother-infant relationship is potentially damaged when the infant is hearing impaired. Reciprocal communication that normally occurs between the mother and the infant on an affective and a verbal level has been reported to be diminished with infants who are hearing impaired. The handicapped infant may miss intended signals from parents and may emit signals that are not understood. The parents must capture their infant's visual attention so that their efforts are effectively stimulating. An asynchrony may develop that can retard the infant's ability to acquire language even beyond the limits of the hearing loss itself. The family can be taught total communication skills (gesturing, touching, and attending) to support interaction with the infant.

BOX 35-2

Factors Influencing the Management and Habilitation of the Hearing-Impaired Infant

Factors that Facilitate Management
Parental involvement
Expeditious arrangements for referral

Factors that Hamper Management
Long waiting list
Poor communication between speech and hearing departments

SUMMARY

This chapter supports the following concepts: (1) significant hearing loss is one of the common major abnormalities present at birth; (2) if undetected and unremediated, hearing loss impedes speech, language, and cognitive development and later academic achievement; (3) use of the high-risk registry is not an effective screening tool for identifying infants at risk for a hearing impairment, especially in the well baby nursery group; (4) screening of all infants for hearing loss in the neonatal period is critical for early identification, comprehensive evaluation, and timely referral.

REFERENCES

Acham A, Walch C (2001). Mondini dysplasia without functional impairment in the framework of a CHARGE association. *Laryngorhinootologie*, 80(7), 381-384.

American Academy of Pediatrics (AAP). Joint Committee on Infant Hearing 1994 position statement. *Pediatrics*, 95, 152-156.

Donaldson GS et al (2001). Effects of the clarion electrode positioning system on auditory thresholds and comfortable loudness levels in pediatric patients with cochlear implants. *Archives of otolaryngology, head neck surgery*, 127(8), 956-960.

Downs MP (1994). The case for detection and intervention at birth. *Seminars in hearing*, 15, 76-83.

Eichwald J, Mahoney T (1993). Apgar scores in the identification of sensorineural hearing loss. *Journal of the American Medical Association*, 3, 133-138.

Galambos R et al (1994). Identifying hearing loss in the intensive care nursery: a 20-year summary. *Journal of the American Academy of Audiology*, 5(3), 151-162.

Gallaudet University, Center for Assessment and Demographic Study (1998). Thirty years of the annual survey of deaf and hard of hearing children and youth: a glance over the decades. *American annals of the deaf*, 142(2), 72-76.

Graven SN (1996). Concepts of fetal sensory development. Paper presented at the conference on the Physical and Developmental Environment of the High Risk Neonate, January 31, 1996. University of South Florida College of Medicine: Clearwater Beach.

Graven SN (2000). Sound and the developing infant in the NICU: conclusions and recommendations for care. *Journal of perinatology*, 20(8 part 2), S88-S93.

Gray PH et al (2001). Conductive hearing loss in preterm infants with bronchopulmonary dysplasia. *Journal of paediatric child health*, 37(3), 278-282.

Hepper PG, Shahidullah SB (1994). The development of fetal hearing. *Fetal maternal medical review*, 6, 167-179.

Hristeva L et al (1999). Prospective surveillance of neonatal meningitis. *Archives of disease in childhood*, 69, 14-18.

Joint Committee on Infant Hearing (1994). Joint Committee on Infant Hearing Year 1994 position statement. Available online at http://professional/asha.org/resources/legislative/joint_statement.cfm.

Joint Committee on Infant Hearing (2000). Joint Committee on Infant Hearing year 2000 position statement: principles and guidelines for early hearing detection and intervention programs. Available online at http://www.infanthearing.org/jcih/.

Jones KL, editor (1988). *Smith's recognizable patterns of human malformation*, ed 4. WB Saunders: Philadelphia.

Kaminski J, Hall W (1996). The effect of soothing music on neonatal behavioral states in the hospital newborn nursery. *Neonatal nursing*, 15(1), 45-54.

Karchmer MA, Allen TE (1999). The functional assessment of deaf and hard of hearing students. *American annals of the deaf*, 144(2), 68-77.

Kennedy CR et al (2000). Current topic: neonatal screening for hearing impairment. *Archives of disease in childhood*, 83, 377-383.

Northern JL, Downs MP (1984). *Hearing in children*. Williams & Wilkins: Baltimore.

Nyhan WL (1983). Cytogenetic diseases. *Clinical symposia*, 35(1), 1-32.

Philbin MK, Klass P (2000). Behavior effects of auditory experience on the term newborn. *Journal of perinatology*, 20(8), 68-76.

Philbin MK et al (1999). Recommended permissible noise criteria for occupied, newly constructed, or renovated hospital nurseries. *Journal of perinatology*, 19(8 part 1), 559-563.

Robertson A, Philbin MK (1996). Studies of sound and auditory development. Paper presented at the conference on the Physical and Developmental Environment of the High Risk Neonate, January 31, 1996. University of South Florida College of Medicine: Clearwater Beach.

Ronge LJ (1997). Making a sound decision. *AAP news*, 13(4), 10-11.

Sarant JZ et al (2001). Variation in speech perception scores among children with cochlear implants. *Early hearing*, 1, 18-28.

Spivak LG, editor (1998). *Universal newborn hearing screening*. Thieme: New York.

Task Force on Newborn and Infant Hearing (1999). Early identification of hearing impairment in infants and young children. American Academy of Pediatrics: Elk Grove Village, IL.

Vartiainen E (2000). Otitis media with effusion in children with congenital or early onset hearing impairment. *Journal of otolaryngology*, 29(4), 221-223.

Walsh-Sukys M et al (2001). Reducing light and sound in the neonatal intensive care unit: an evaluation of patient safety, staff satisfaction, and costs. *Journal of perinatology*, 21(4), 230-235.

Weichbold V, Welzl-Mueller K (2001). Maternal concern about positive test results in universal newborn hearing screening. *Pediatrics*, 108(5), 1111-1116.

White R et al (2000). Neonatal intensive care unit structure and design: recommended standards. University of South Florida: Tampa.

ASSESSMENT AND MANAGEMENT OF THE OPHTHALMIC SYSTEM

FRANCES STRODTBECK

The eye begins to develop early in gestation, making this body system vulnerable to insults during the growth process. Neonatal visual problems occur as a result of transplacental, congenital, or neonatal infections; congenital or genetic malformation; exposure to drugs; or abnormal adaptation of the developing eye and its vascularity to stimuli such as oxygen. Visual disturbances in the newborn can range from minor refractory problems to complete blindness. Early detection and treatment are essential if the best possible outcome is to be achieved.

This chapter briefly outlines the embryologic development of the eye, reviews the key points of assessment of the newborn's eyes, and describes specific ophthalmic dysfunctions. Collaborative management and appropriate nursing care are also discussed.

EMBRYOLOGY

Our understanding of the forces that control and govern the development of the eye is growing but limited. About 2 weeks after fertilization, the embryonic plate elongates, and the primitive streak develops along the dorsal surface. The brain and eye develop from the neuroectoderm anterior to the primitive streak. The optic pits (optic sulci) are formed by the indentation of neuroectoderm. Closing of the neural tube leads to movement of the optic pits laterally and outward, toward the surface ectoderm. This movement results in the formation of the optic vesicles (Moore et al, 2001).

As the optic vesicle approaches the outer wall of the embryo, it stimulates a focal thickening of cells called the lens placode. At the fourth week of gestation, this tissue invaginates, forming the optic cup. The inferior portion of the cup is the last to close. The two layers of the optic cup oppose one another to form the retina. At the same time, the lens placode sinks beneath the ectoderm and later becomes the crystalline lens. Mesoderm surrounding the optic cup differentiates to form the sclera, choroid, and part of the cornea (Moore et al, 2001).

Mesoderm anterior to the lens develops into the pupillary membrane; the periphery of the pupillary membrane becomes the iris. The center degenerates to form the pupil. Ectoderm that covers the mesodermal folds appears above and below the lens placode to form the eyelids. The eyelids are fused until

about 26 weeks' gestation. The lacrimal gland, the lacrimal drainage system, and the eyelashes form from the ectoderm that covers these folds. Tear production does not begin until 2 to 4 months after birth, when the lacrimal system process is complete (Moore et al, 2001).

ASSESSMENT OF THE EYES

History

A thorough history is imperative to determine whether risk factors for eye problems are present. A complete family, medical, pregnancy, and psychosocial history, along with a maternal review of systems, should be obtained. The interviewer should ask questions related to the family history of vision problems (e.g., strabismus, glaucoma, retinoblastoma) and refractive errors (e.g., myopia). The maternal history should include questions about exposure to infectious diseases such as gonorrhea, chlamydiosis, rubella, and cytomegalovirus (CMV) infection, which are known to cause significant eye problems in newborns. The perinatal history should include questions about any difficulties that might have resulted in hypoxia or anoxia, conditions associated with adverse optical changes. Previous pregnancies that resulted in preterm births can provide important information about prior experience with retinopathy of prematurity (ROP).

Examination

Examining the eyes of a newborn can be a challenge. Care must be taken during the examination process to protect the newborn from injury and cold stress. The infant's state is also important for a successful examination. Newborns in the quiet alert state are more responsive to visual stimuli.

Most important information about the eyes of the newborn can be obtained from inspection and observation. An examination with an ophthalmoscope usually is not indicated, except when the inspection and observation findings suggest serious problems, such as cataracts or glaucoma.

It is easier to examine the newborn's eyes when they are spontaneously open. Dimming the lights, talking to the infant, and holding the baby upright may facilitate natural opening of the eyes. Newborn eyes should be assessed for their shape, symmetry, and size and for the presence of obvious features, such as eyebrows and eyelashes. The eyes should appear clear, unswollen, and without discharge. Occasionally, irritation may result from the prophylactic drops or ointment used to prevent ophthalmia neonatorum. The eyelids should be evaluated for redness or swelling and for evidence of colobomas and abnormal tumor masses. Inability to elevate the eyelids or ptosis (drooping) of one or both eyelids may lead to amblyopia or poor visual development. The presence of unusual folds and the slant of the eye should be noted. The pupils should be checked for size, equality, reaction to light, and accommodation. The color and clarity of the red reflex should be checked. In African-American infants, the reflex may be pale orange rather than red (Fletcher, 1998).

The cornea should be evaluated for clarity and size. A cloudy cornea may be caused by congenital glaucoma, errors of metabolism, or congenital corneal dystrophy. Trauma at birth can result in injury to the cornea, giving the cornea a hazy appearance.

Directly behind the iris is the lens. Cloudiness or opacity in the lens is by definition a cataract. An ophthalmologist should evaluate any cataract found in a newborn as soon as possible to determine if it is visually significant. Surgery should be performed to remove vision-threatening cataracts as soon as the infant is able to tolerate the procedure. Early surgery is critical to the prevention of amblyopia (lazy eye), which develops in these eyes when the condition is ignored for a few months.

Leukocoria is the descriptive term for a whitish-appearing pupil. This condition is almost always indicative of a serious eye problem. The differential diagnosis of leukocoria includes cataract, retinoblastoma, persistent hyperplastic primary vitreous, retrolental fibroplasia, toxocariasis, and Coats' disease.

Because infants with fetal alcohol syndrome can have coloboma, cataract, and microphthalmos, the presence of these findings should alert the examiner to look for other features of the syndrome (Hug et al, 2000). The maternal history should also be re-evaluated for alcohol use during the pregnancy.

The posterior pole of the eye (optic nerve, macula, and blood vessels) is examined with a direct ophthalmoscope with the pupil dilated. Because a newborn often squirms and moves the head to avoid the light of the ophthalmoscope, an assistant should stabilize the infant's head and body. Giving the infant a bottle or pacifier as a calming measure often is helpful. A topical anesthetic, such as 0.5% proparacaine, may be instilled to dull the corneal and conjunctival sensitivity. The assistant may separate the eyelids, or a small pediatric eyelid speculum can be used. Care should be taken to avoid causing a corneal abrasion while the speculum is inserted. Normal saline should be used to prevent corneal drying, especially under the heat of a radiant warmer.

About 34% of newborns show retinal hemorrhage, most often in the posterior pole. The risk of retinal hemorrhage is greater with vacuum-assisted delivery and diminished with delivery by cesarean section. More than 90% of the hemorrhages resolve within 2 weeks; however, resolution of retinal hemorrhage in the newborns of women who have had induced labor may take up to 5 weeks.

The infant's ability to see can be assessed by getting the newborn to fix on and follow brightly colored objects. The examiner should hold the object steady about 7 to 9 inches from the infant's eye until the newborn fixes on it (the examiner notes the reflection of the object in the middle of the newborn's pupil). Newborns should be able to follow an object about 90 inches either left or right from a midline or central position. Care should be taken to eliminate distractions and to avoid talking because infants respond best to the presentation of one stimulus at a time.

Several important measurements should be obtained. The interpupillary distance and the width of the palpebral fissure should be determined; abnormal values may indicate an underlying syndrome, such as fetal alcohol syndrome. The interpupillary distance (the distance from midpupil to midpupil when the eyes are looking forward) determines whether the eyes are spaced appropriately. Abnormal findings are hypotelorism (eyes too close together) or hypertelorism (eyes too far apart). The width of the palpebral fissure is the distance from the medial canthus to the lateral canthus of each eye; this measurement determines the appropriateness of the opening for the eye. The measurements obtained should be compared with published norms to determine if the value is normal or abnormal. Infants of diabetic mothers (except those born to women with gestational diabetes) should be carefully examined for displaced inner canthi, lens opacity, microphthalmos, tear duct obstruction, and ocular lipoma.

Determining visual acuity in a newborn is difficult. Several methods can be used, including visual preference charts and visual evoked potentials. At term, newborn visual acuity ranges from 20/100 to 20/400, depending on the testing method used. This improves to 20/80 to 20/200 by 4 months of age, 20/40 to 20/80 by 12 months of age, and 20/20 by 2 years of age. Attention should also be given to an eye motility examination. In the neonate, the position of the eyes varies greatly. Most infants display intermittent outward deviation (exotropia), which usually disappears within the first few months of life. Any constant inward (esotropia) or outward deviation should be evaluated for a possible nerve or muscle palsy. Intermittent nystagmus (rapid movements of the eye) is a common finding in the newborn. Persistent nystagmus is abnormal; patients with this disorder should be referred for further evaluation (Fletcher, 1998).

Eye Drops

Great care must be taken in the selection of dilating drops for use in newborns. Systemic absorption of the eye drops, although unavoidable to some extent, can cause severe reactions, including death. Cardiovascular consequences, including arterial hypertension, a predisposing factor for intracranial hemorrhage, have been reported in premature infants. Necrotizing enterocolitis (NEC) has also been reported in premature infants after eye examinations.

Excess medication that flows out of the eyelids is easily absorbed through the porous skin of the newborn and should be wiped off to prevent systemic absorption. Medication can also be absorbed from the nasolacrimal system; this can be minimized by applying pressure with a fingertip over the nasolacrimal duct for approximately 1 minute after instillation of the drops.

The mydriatics most often used are cyclopentolate, phenylephrine, and tropicamide. For maximum dilation and minimum risk of side effects, a combination of drugs routinely is used in most clinical settings. According to Bolt and colleagues (1992), the combination of phenylephrine 2.5% and tropicamide 0.5% (one drop of each, then a second drop of tropicamide 20 minutes later) produced better mydriasis with no systemic side effects than the combination of cyclopentolate and tropicamide. Table 36-1 presents a complete list of ophthalmic medications commonly used in the newborn.

TABLE **36-1** Commonly Used Eye Medications	
Generic Name	**Brand Name**
Topical Anesthetics	
Proparacaine hydrochloride	Alcaine, Ophthaine, Ophthetic
Tetracaine hydrochloride	Anacel, Pontocaine
Mydriatics (Dilating Drops)	
Atropine sulfate	Atropisol, BufOpto Atropine, Isopto-Atropine
Cyclopentolate hydrochloride	Cyclogyl
Homatropine hydrobromide	Isopto Homatropine
Scopolamine hydrobromide	Isopto Hyoscine
Tropicamide	Mydriacyl
Phenylephrine hydrochloride	Mydfrin, Neo-Synephrine
Antiinflammatory Agents	
Dexamethasone	Maxidex Ophthalmic Suspension
Dexamethasone sodium phosphate	Decadron Phosphate
Fluorometholone	FML Liquifilm Ophthalmic
Prednisolone acetate	Econopred, Pred Forte, Pred Mild
Prednisolone sodium phosphate	AK-Pred, Inflamase Forte, Inflamase, Metreton
Antiinfectives	
Antibacterials	
Bacitracin	
Chloramphenicol	Chloromycetin, Chloroptic, Econochlor
Erythromycin	Ilotycin
Gentamicin sulfate	Garamycin
Polymyxin B sulfate	
Silver nitrate 1%	
Sulfacetamide sodium	Bleph-10, Cetamide, Sodium Sulamyd
Tetracycline hydrochloride	Achromycin
Tobramycin	Tobrex
Antivirals	
Idoxuridine	IDU
Trifluridine	Viroptic
Vidarabine	Vira-A
Miscellaneous	
Timolol maleate	Timoptic (antiglaucoma medication)
Fluorescein sodium	Diagnostic drops for corneal abnormalities

After the examination, the infant's eyes should be shielded from light until the pupils have returned to normal size. The eyes can be covered with occlusive eye shields, such as phototherapy shields, or a cover can be placed over the baby's incubator. Unshielded, dilated eyes are very sensitive to light. Excessive light entering a dilated pupil can cause intense pain in an infant. In premature infants or those with underlying health problems, the reaction to the pain may involve systemic responses, such as apnea, bradycardia, cyanosis, and agitation.

DIAGNOSTIC TESTS

Several relatively new diagnostic tests can be used to further evaluate the newborn for eye abnormalities. These tests are not routinely performed and require the expertise of specially trained ophthalmologists.

Electroretinography

An electroretinogram (ERG) may be obtained when retinal disease is suspected. The ERG provides information about retinal and photoreceptor function. Before an ERG is done, the infant should be sedated and the pupils pharmacologically dilated. Black, opaque patches are placed over each eye for a minimum of 30 minutes before testing, which is done in a special darkroom. The examiner wears a red light similar to that used in photographic darkrooms; this allows the examiner to operate the equipment and visualize the patient. For the test, the examiner removes one patch, instills another drop of dilating drug, and places a special contact lens electrode on the eye's surface. A photic stimulator then generates white flashes of varying intensities. The eye's response to these stimuli is recorded continuously in a manner similar to that used to obtain an electroencephalogram (EEG).

Visual Evoked Potentials

Visual evoked potentials (VEPs) provide information about the functioning of the visual system by measuring activity evoked by neurons in different afferent pathways. Unlike ERGs, VEP testing does not require any medication. The testing is done in a darkened room with the infant held on an assistant's lap. EEG electrodes are placed on the infant's head, and a light flash stimulating lamp is directed toward the baby's eyes. Responses to light stimuli, called flash evoked responses, are then recorded. VEP testing can be used to estimate function and maturation of the primary cortex and the geniculocortical visual system. This may provide useful information in the management of infants with delayed visual maturation and other neurologic problems, including hydrocephalus and intraventricular hemorrhage (Kraemer et al, 1999).

Digital Image Analysis

Digital image analysis (DIA) is used in conjunction with optic fundal photographs to evaluate the morphology of the optic nerve. Because the retina develops from the brain, studying the eye can provide clues to central nervous system (CNS) problems. With DIA, a computer-assisted digital mapping system is used to analyze photographs of the fundus. This technology may provide information helpful to an understanding of the relationship between pathologic conditions of the CNS and retinal problems (Hellström, 1999).

NEONATAL CONJUNCTIVITIS

Any conjunctivitis that occurs in the first 28 days of life is classified as neonatal conjunctivitis, according to the World Health Organization (WHO). Neonatal conjunctivitis can be classified as aseptic or septic. Aseptic conjunctivitis is often a chemical reaction to prophylactic medication administered shortly after birth to prevent gonorrheal disease of the newborn's eyes.

Septic conjunctivitis in the newborn is an infection of the conjunctiva (the thin, translucent mucous membrane covering the cornea) caused by a variety of bacteria, viruses, and other organisms. The incidence of septic neonatal conjunctivitis in the United States is 1% to 2%. Chlamydial infection has replaced gonorrhea as the most common cause of septic eye infection (Nelson, 1998). Septic neonatal conjunctivitis usually manifests with a discharge that develops shortly after birth. Because the origins of newborn conjunctivitis can vary, laboratory investigations are important in determining the exact cause. In some cases of conjunctivitis, rapid treatment is important to prevent vision loss.

The presentation of neonatal conjunctivitis varies with the cause of the inflammation or infection. Some findings, such as purulent eye discharge and erythema and edema of the eyelids and conjunctivae, are present in most cases. Transient tearing or watery discharge may be noticed early in the infection process.

Aseptic Neonatal Conjunctivitis

Most states in the United States require prophylaxis against neonatal gonorrheal conjunctivitis. According to the American Academy of Pediatrics (AAP), topical 1% silver nitrate solution, 0.5% erythromycin ointment, and 1% tetracycline ointment are equally effective (AAP, 2000). Although not available commercially as single-dose vials or tubes, 2.5% povidone-iodine solution is gaining recognition as another treatment option.

Although silver nitrate has largely been replaced by erythromycin as the drug of choice for neonatal ocular prophylaxis, it still is used in some units. Silver nitrate drops typically cause an irritant reaction that leads to conjunctival edema, redness, and watery discharge. The reaction starts within a few hours of instillation of the drops, usually resolves within 48 hours, and is self-limiting. Laboratory cultures and smears should be obtained to rule out an infectious cause for the conjunctivitis. Parents should be informed of the benign nature of the inflammation once the proper diagnosis has been made. The eyes should be cleansed frequently of any secretions to prevent skin irritation.

Silver nitrate is effective against Neisseria gonorrhoeae and most bacteria; however, it is not effective against Chlamydia organisms. For this reason, some states substitute tetracycline ointment or erythromycin ointment for routine prophylaxis. In areas with a high incidence of penicillinase-producing N. gonorrhoeae, silver nitrate is the drug of choice (Zhao & Enzenauer, 2001).

Erythromycin and tetracycline ointments are effective against a variety of microorganisms, including chlamydia. These ointments rarely cause irritation to the newborn's eyes. Because erythromycin is only about 80% effective, a second dose may be needed.

Chlamydial Conjunctivitis (Inclusion Conjunctivitis)

In recent years Chlamydia trachomatis has been recognized as the most common cause of conjunctivitis in the newborn. The bacteria are transmitted from the infected mother to the infant at birth, and conjunctivitis usually appears 4 to 14 days later. The condition may be mild or moderate, and with proper treatment it resolves within 6 weeks. Clinical symptoms include swelling of one or both eyelids and mucopurulent discharge. Chronic infection can lead to more serious consequences, such as conjunctival scarring, adhesions of the eyelid, and deposits of connective tissue under the cornea.

The diagnosis is made from laboratory tests. The conjunctiva is scraped with a spatula, and a smear is made for Giemsa staining; classically this reveals a dark-staining cytoplasmic inclusion body. Direct immunofluorescent antibody staining or enzyme immunoassay should be done to confirm the diagnosis.

Topical eye treatment should consist of application of sulfacetamide or tetracycline drops or ointment for 3 weeks. Although the eye infection generally is not serious, a chlamydial pneumonitis develops in 11% to 20% of infected neonates. Systemic therapy with oral erythromycin estolate or erythromycin ethylsuccinate for 3 weeks often is necessary to eradicate the organism from the respiratory tract.

Gonorrheal Conjunctivitis

Routine prophylaxis of neonates has greatly reduced the incidence of gonorrheal conjunctivitis. Because of the potential for blindness from this infection, early detection and prompt treatment are critical. Gonorrheal conjunctivitis typically manifests as an acute, purulent, bilateral conjunctivitis with eyelid edema. If not treated appropriately, the infection may progress rapidly to corneal ulceration and endophthalmitis. Gram stains and cultures should be performed routinely in all cases of neonatal conjunctivitis. The presence of N. gonorrhoeae confirms the diagnosis. Treatment consists of administration of intravenous or intramuscular antibiotics and application of topical ointment to the eye. Irrigation of the eye with sterile saline may be necessary to remove drainage.

Staphylococcal Conjunctivitis

Staphylococcal conjunctivitis is a bacterial infection usually acquired during vaginal delivery or by contact with an infected mother or nursery personnel. Symptoms normally appear 2 to 4 weeks after birth. In most cases the conjunctivitis is mild and produces a purulent discharge. It may progress to corneal ulceration, endophthalmitis, or generalized skin infection. The diagnosis is made with cultures and Gram stain. Because staphylococci can be found in the conjunctivae of healthy neonates, laboratory results should be interpreted cautiously. Treatment includes application of topical bacitracin or erythromycin ointment and cleansing of exudate from the eyelids.

Herpes Simplex Conjunctivitis

Herpes simplex infection at birth may be a feature of either localized or systemic disease. The neonate usually is infected during passage through the birth canal. The conjunctivitis manifests with eyelid swelling, conjunctival inflammation, corneal opacity, and epithelial dendrites. The dendrites can best be seen if the cornea is stained with a fluorescein dye and then examined under the blue light of a portable slitlamp. The onset of the conjunctivitis usually is 2 to 14 days after birth. The disseminated form of the disease may also lead to cataracts and optic neuritis.

Diagnosis through laboratory findings is based on conjunctival epithelia scrapings for Giemsa staining and tissue cultures. The Giemsa stain should reveal multinucleated giant cells and intranuclear inclusion. Fluorescent antibody techniques are also helpful for making the diagnosis. This disease should always be kept in mind when the mother or father has a history of genital herpes. Treatment should be instituted with application of the topical antiviral trifluridine. Systemic treatment may be helpful in disseminated cases.

Infectious Conjunctivitis Caused by Other Microorganisms

Case reports describing neonatal infectious conjunctivitis caused by unusual microorganisms are increasing in the professional literature. Although most of the case reports describe infections in hospitalized premature infants, two reports concerned full-term infants who were readmitted with conjunctivitis caused by *Neisseria meningitidis* (Dinakaran & Desai, 1999; Lehman, 1999). Both infants required local and systemic treatment and were discharged home. Because *N. meningitidis* can cause a serious infection resulting in significant morbidity and mortality, it is important to differentiate this organism from other gram-negative diploccoci, such as *N. gonorrhoeae* (Lehman, 1999). Individuals exposed to *N. meningitidis* are considered high-risk contacts and should be treated with chemoprophylaxis (Lehman, 1999).

Two cases of serious eye infection in preterm infants caused by *Pseudomonas aeruginosa* have been reported (Shah et al, 1999; Wasserman et al, 1999). A 910-g boy born at 27 weeks' gestation developed meningitis and multiple brain abscesses subsequent to the conjunctivitis. This infant was discharged at 2 months of age with no apparent visual impairment. The other infant, a 736-g boy born at 24 weeks' gestation, was found to have *P. aeruginosa* sepsis. Several days later a purulent discharge from the eyes was noted. Examination of the eyes revealed bilateral endophthalmitis, perforated cornea, and possible total retinal detachment in one eye. A detailed eye examination was not possible because of the infant's unstable condition. The baby subsequently died of overwhelming sepsis, and no autopsy was performed (Wasserman et al, 1999).

Premature infants in the neonatal intensive care unit (NICU) frequently are colonized with a variety of *Candida* species. Despite the increased incidence of *Candida* sepsis in premature infants, ocular involvement usually is limited to a retinochoroiditis that resolves with systemic antifungal therapy. Three reports have been published describing severe candidal eye disease that required surgical intervention (Shah et al, 2000; Todd Johnston & Cogen, 2000). Two of the reports described the development of a cataract, one in an infant born at 29 weeks' gestation and the other in an infant born at 32 weeks' gestation. Both infants required a lensectomy and vitrectomy (Shah et al, 2000; Todd Johnston & Cogen, 2000). The third report concerned an infant born at 24 weeks' gestation who developed recurrent candidal endophthalmitis, which required vitrectomy for treatment.

Lacrimal Dysfunction

Obstructed Nasolacrimal Duct. Blockage of the nasolacrimal duct occurs when the duct fails to canalize at the entrance to the nose. This blockage occurs in 2% of all newborns and is the most common cause of chronic conjunctivitis in infants. After 1 month of age, the infant shows excessive tearing and pooling in the medial canthal region and signs of infection. Pressure on the lacrimal sac area usually causes pus or mucus to exude from the puncta. Because the problem resolves spontaneously in 50% of affected neonates by 6 months of age, conservative treatment involving lacrimal massage and application of topical antibiotics is recommended. Obstruction that lasts beyond this point may require lacrimal probing. Nasolacrimal duct blockage must be differentiated from congenital glaucoma, a foreign body on the eye, or corneal injury or inflammation.

Mucocele

Mucoceles occur because of the one-way valve effect at the end of the nasolacrimal duct. Mucus accumulates or amniotic fluid is trapped in the nasolacrimal sac, and the infant develops a bluish mass in the inferomedial region of the eyelid. This swelling most often is confused with a hemangioma. If simple massage does not decompress the mucocele, probing of the nasolacrimal duct may be necessary.

RETINOPATHY OF PREMATURITY

Retinopathy of prematurity (ROP), a disease arising from proliferation of abnormal blood vessels in the newborn retina, was first reported by Terry in 1942. His description of a fibrous growth behind the lens and retinal detachment in premature infants gave birth to the name retrolental fibroplasia (RLF). The name was changed to retinopathy of prematurity in 1984 by an international committee charged with providing a uniform classification system for the disease (Figure 36-1). The classification system uses a standard description of the location of retinopathy (using zones and clock hours), the severity of the disease (stage), the presence of special risk factors (plus disease), and the features of regression (International Committee on Retinopathy of Prematurity, 1984).

ROP was responsible for an epidemic of blindness in young children in the 1940s and early 1950s until the link to supplemental oxygen therapy was made in 1952. Subsequently, the practice of limiting oxygen administration in the care of premature infants led to the near disappearance of the disorder. Improvements in neonatal health care in the past 30 years have increased the survival of preterm infants, yet ROP remains the leading cause of blindness in premature infants. According to data from a multicenter cryotherapy trial of more than 4000 infants, the two groups with the greatest risk are premature infants weighing less than 750 g at birth (90%) and those whose birth weight is 751 to 1000 g (78%) (Phelps, 1992). The overall incidence of ROP is increasing and currently is estimated to be 25% annually (Hunter & Mukai, 1994). Although most of these cases regress, the incidence of severe disease has reached a plateau of 5% to 10%, with more than 500 new cases of blind infants reported annually in the United States (Hunter & Mukai, 1994; Vander, 1994). This percentage holds fairly steady even today.

Pathophysiology

ROP is a disease caused by an abnormal adaptation of normal maturational processes in the face of physiologic stress. The disease develops gradually and is divided into five stages of increasing severity (Table 36-2). The key factor in the development of ROP, especially in premature infants, is the developing retinal blood vessels. Mature retinal vasculature is not susceptible to the adverse effects of severe stress. Retinal vascularization begins at the optic nerve at about 16 weeks' gestation. Retinal vascular development proceeds slowly and reaches the retinal periphery (ora serrata retinae) during the ninth month of gestation (Vander, 1994). If undifferentiated mesenchymal cells, which are critical to the process of capillary development, are exposed to severe physiologic stress during this migration, the cells may die or lose their orientation. The newly developing capillaries are obliterated, resulting in retinal ischemia.

The ischemia becomes a potent inducer of new vessel growth (neovascularization). As the new blood vessels proliferate, they tend to grow into the vitreous and can cause bleeding and the formation of fibrous tissue. Mild degrees of ROP are often transient and regress once the abnormal stimuli are removed or corrected. Moderate retinopathy can lead to excessive fibrous tissue formation or scarring in the peripheral retina, which may lead to traction on the macula and reduced

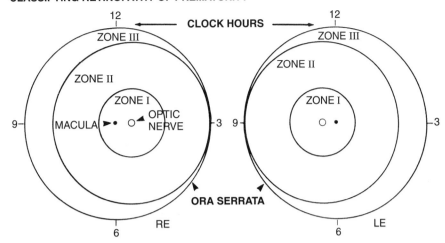

FIGURE 36-1
International classification of retinopathy of prematurity. Zones and clock hours are used to describe the location and extent of ROP in the retinas of the right eye *(RE)* and the left eye *(LE)*. From Martin RJ et al (2001). Respiratory problems. In Klaus MH, Fanaroff AA, editors. *Care of the high-risk neonate,* ed 5. WB Saunders: Philadelphia.

TABLE 36-2	Stages of Retinopathy of Prematurity
Stage	**Finding**
1	Demarcation line at avascular retina
2	Ridge with height and width
3	Ridge with fibrosis extending into vitreous
4	Partial retinal detachment with or without fovea
5	Complete retinal detachment

From George DS et al (1988). The latest on retinopathy of prematurity. MCN, American journal of maternal child nursing, *13(4), 256.*

vision. In severe cases of ROP, fibrous tissue development may lead to retinal detachment and blindness (Hunter & Mukai, 1994). Severely affected neonates may also have leukocoria or glaucoma, or both.

Risk Factors

ROP is a multifactorial disease related to conceptual age that occurs primarily in premature infants. Although many risk factors have been identified, prematurity is the single most important factor leading to the development of ROP (Phelps, 1992; Hunter & Mukai, 1994). Other risk factors include use of supplemental oxygen, low birth weight, intraventricular hemorrhage, sepsis, multiple births, acidosis, and blood transfusions (Fielder & Levene, 1992; Phelps, 1992; Todd et al, 1994).

For some variables linked to the development of ROP, the evidence is less conclusive, and no direct link to the treatment or management of medically unstable premature infants has been established. Often these factors are interlinked; they include antioxidant deficiencies; administration of beta-adrenergic blockers late in pregnancy for preterm labor; maternal bleeding; apnea of prematurity; use of xanthines, such as caffeine and theophylline; abnormal blood gas findings; the number of days on mechanical ventilation; early intubation; ambient lighting; hypotension; NEC; and patent ductus arte-

riosus treated with indomethacin (Phelps, 1992; Arroe & Peitersen, 1994; Todd et al, 1994). An association between ROP and glucocorticoid steroid use has not been substantiated (Wright & Wright, 1994), although the use of steroids may increase the chance of surgical intervention for ROP (Todd et al, 1994). The impact of surfactant therapy on ROP is a major concern. Preliminary reports suggest that the incidence and severity of ROP are not altered by surfactant therapy (Holmes et al, 1994).

Although most ROP occurs in premature infants, rare cases of the disease have been reported in full-term infants, stillborn infants, infants with hypoxia, and infants who were not given supplemental oxygen. These reports, along with the striking similarity of disease presentation from infant to infant, have led some to conclude that ROP may have a genetic component. Further research is needed to further our understanding of the cause and the pathophysiology of this disease.

Treatment

Treatment of ROP can be divided into three categories: preventive, interdictive, and corrective. Until premature birth can be abolished, the major focus of ROP treatment is early detection and appropriate follow-up of significant disease. Javitt and colleagues (1993) estimated that properly timed screening and treatment for ROP is not only cost saving but also may save approximately 320 infants per year from a lifetime of blindness. Despite the international effort to standardize ROP and the efforts of the multicenter, randomized clinical trial known as the Cryotherapy for Retinopathy of Prematurity Study (1988), no universally accepted guidelines exist for the screening of premature infants for ROP. Screening protocols vary from institution to institution. Several widely used, published guidelines are summarized in Table 36-3.

Preventive Treatment.   Other preventive strategies that have been used or are under consideration are antioxidant therapy, oxygen monitoring, and modification of environmental light. High doses of vitamin E, an antioxidant, gained popularity in the 1980s as a prophylactic therapy for ROP; how-

TABLE **36-3**	Guidelines for Retinopathy of Prematurity Screening Examinations	
Recommending Group	**Infant Criteria**	**Examination Protocol**
Cryotherapy for Retinopathy of Prematurity Cooperative Group (1988)	Birth weight under 1251 g	First examination, 4 to 6 weeks after birth; continue every 2 weeks. Increase to weekly examinations if prethreshold disease develops.
American Academy of Pediatrics, *Guidelines for Perinatal Care* (1988)	Birth weight under 1800 g *or* infants of less than 35 weeks' gestational age who require oxygen Birth weight under 1300 g *or* gestational age less than 30 weeks	Examine 5 to 7 weeks after birth or before discharge to home (whichever comes first).
British College of Ophthalmologists and British Association of Perinatal Medicine (Fielder & Levene, 1992)	Birth weight under 1500 g *or* gestational age less than 31 weeks	*Infants of less than 25 weeks' gestation:* first examination, 6 to 7 weeks after birth; continue every 2 weeks. *Infants of 26 to 31 weeks' gestation:* first examination, 6 to 7 weeks after birth; continue every 2 weeks.

ever, most clinical studies failed to document a protective effect (Muller, 1992). Significant side effects, such as sepsis, NEC, intraventricular hemorrhage, and death, were noted in numerous studies, prompting most nurseries to avoid the use of high-dose vitamin E (Pierce & Mukai, 1994). Preliminary evidence suggests that penicillamine, an antioxidant used in the treatment of hyperbilirubinemia in Hungary, may lower the incidence of ROP; however, the substance has not been tested for this purpose outside of Hungary. Inositol, an antioxidant found in breast milk and other dietary sources, is being investigated for a possible role in reducing the incidence of chronic lung disease. Preliminary data reveal an unexpected reduction in the incidence of ROP in treated infants (Phelps, 1992). Other investigators are exploring whether bilirubin is protective against ROP. Multicenter, randomized, controlled studies are needed to determine the true value of these antioxidants.

Oxygen monitoring has been the major emphasis in the prevention of ROP. Elaborate policies and practices for continuous monitoring of oxygenation have evolved over the years, including invasive methods (fiberoptic umbilical catheters) and noninvasive techniques (transcutaneous oxygen monitoring, pulse oximetry). Despite these efforts, few data indicate a safe level of oxygenation in infants at risk for ROP. Early efforts at restricting oxygen delivery in the 1950s and 1960s traded visual problems for neurologic sequelae. The current practice of minimizing oxygen exposure while preserving optimum functioning of vital organs must continue until research determines the appropriate strategies.

Environmental lighting in nurseries has been implicated as a contributing factor in the development of ROP. Although the clinical studies that claim to show this relationship have many limitations, some authorities believe the data are sufficient to warrant concern (Phelps, 1992). It is hoped that multicenter clinical trials will shed some light on the subject (Seiberth et al, 1994). Many nurseries have already instituted reduced environmental lighting and shielding of incubators as part of a developmental approach to care (Blackburn, 1996).

Interdictive Treatment. The second strategy for treating ROP focuses on therapies aimed at minimizing or preventing blindness once the disease has developed. Interdictive therapies include cryotherapy and laser photocoagulation.

Cryotherapy, the most widely used technique, was developed in the 1970s in Japan. It gained popularity in the United States in the 1980s after the release of data from the Cryotherapy for Retinopathy of Prematurity Study. The study was terminated early, when preliminary analysis revealed a significant benefit in eyes treated with cryotherapy (Phelps, 1992). The improvements noted in study subjects persisted in follow-up studies (Cryotherapy for Retinopathy of Prematurity Cooperative Group [CRPCG], 1988).

Cryotherapy is a surgical procedure involving insertion of a probe cooled with liquid nitrogen on the medial aspect of the eye. Confluent spots on the avascular retina are ablated (destroyed by freezing), reducing the release of an angiogenic factor that appears to induce retinal vasoproliferation. Although the exact way in which cryotherapy works remains unknown, substantial evidence indicates that the therapy works and improves the outcome of ROP (CRPCG, 1988; Trese, 1994).

Despite its proven benefits, cryotherapy is not a benign procedure. Ocular and other complications can occur. Ocular complications include edema of one or both eyelids, laceration of the conjunctiva, intraocular hemorrhage, and late retinal detachment (Vander, 1994). Other complications reported include apnea, bradycardia, arrhythmias, increased oxygen requirement, seizures and, in rare cases, cardiorespiratory arrest.

Neonatal nurses and other health care professionals should work closely with the ophthalmologist performing the cryotherapy. Infants undergoing the procedure must have their pupils dilated because of the need for indirect ophthalmoscopy. Although the procedure usually is performed using local or general anesthesia, it can severely stress the infant. The oculocardiac reflex, a vagal nerve-mediated reflex, may be set off during the procedure, causing bradycardia. Triggering of this reflex can be prevented by preoperative administration of atropine. It is imperative that the infant's cardiorespiratory status be closely monitored throughout the procedure and the immediate postoperative period. Analgesia during and after the procedure also is recommended. Premature infants, especially those with bronchopulmonary dysplasia, often have increased oxygen requirements and apnea episodes after cryotherapy. Nasal stuffiness, another common side effect of cryotherapy, may be partly responsible for the increase in apnea or oxygen requirements or both (Phelps, 1992).

Laser photocoagulation, a recent technique used in the treatment of ROP, is showing promise and eventually may replace cryotherapy. Argon and infrared diode lasers have been used successfully to ablate the avascular retina in a manner similar to that used in cryotherapy. The rationale for this ablation is that the peripheral avascular retina is believed to produce angiogenic factors, such as vascular-endothelial growth factor (VEGF), that act on the vascular system of the eye (Gupta et al, 2002). The result is abnormal growth which, if allowed to continue, further impairs vision. Evidence to date suggests that laser therapy is as effective as cryotherapy, although no conclusive evidence indicates that it is better than cryotherapy (Pierce & Mukai, 1994). The described advantages of laser photocoagulation therapy have included technical ease of performance; usefulness in posterior ROP, which is difficult to treat with cryotherapy; less stress to the infant; fewer side effects; and fewer delayed consequences of myopia and retinal detachment. However, some evidence indicates that laser therapy may increase the risk of cataracts.

Corrective Treatment.   The focus of corrective treatment is surgery for the repair of detached retinas. Scleral buckling or vitrectomy, or both, with or without lensectomy are the techniques currently available (Trese, 1994). Scleral buckling involves the placement of a silicone or plastic band around the globe of the eye. The band is constricted, which brings the sclera closer to the retina, facilitating retinal reattachment. This procedure often is performed in conjunction with cryotherapy or laser therapy to salvage any remaining vision (Gupta et al, 2002).

When retinal detachment progresses beyond the point of scleral buckling, the ophthalmologist must consider anatomic reattachment of the retina. Vitrectomy involves surgically opening the eye, removing the lens, and gently excising the proliferative scar tissue; this allows the retina to lie against the pigmented epithelium and reattach (Trese, 1994). Despite the skill required for these procedures, most infants who undergo corrective therapy do not have significant improvement in their vision. Functional success rates range from 3% to 43%.

Nursing Care

Parents often express concern about the development of ROP in their premature infant. Open communication between the neonatal health care team and the parents is crucial for helping the parents to cope successfully with the stress of having a hospitalized premature infant. It is important to determine the amount of information a parent can handle. At first, general information about the relationship of ROP and prematurity can be shared with the parents. After the first eye examination has been performed, the information can be specific to their baby. The neonatal health care team must work closely with the ophthalmologist to provide a consistent message to the family. Information shared should take into account known cultural differences, such as that the occurrence of severe ROP is higher in white infants than in those of other racial groups (Gupta et al, 2002). Parent teaching should focus on providing a basic understanding of ROP, the purpose of the screening examinations, and the importance of regular vision testing for their infant after discharge (Box 36-1). Explanations of eye examination results may need reinforcing as parents try to assimilate an overwhelming amount of information. Misconceptions about the disease and the use of oxygen need to be corrected.

BOX **36-1**

Schedule for First Indirect Ophthalmoscopy in Premature Infants

Who
- All infants of less than 29 weeks' gestation or weighing less than 1500 g at birth
- Infants born at 29 to 34 weeks' gestation who have a medically unstable course

When
- By the latter of 32 weeks' postmenstrual age* or 4 weeks after birth
- Recommended before discharge from the hospital

*Postmenstrual age in weeks is equal to the gestational age at birth plus the chronologic age in weeks after birth.
From Gupta BK et al (2002). The eye. In Fanaroff AA, Martin RJ, editors. Neonatal-perinatal medicine: diseases of the fetus and infant, ed 7. Mosby: St Louis.

Once ROP has been diagnosed in an infant, parents may need more support than usual. Some parents may exhibit denial because they cannot see any physical evidence of a problem. Families of infants who need surgical intervention may feel greater stress from their concern for their infant's vision and the added communication with an ophthalmologist or retinal surgeon. Nursery staff members can help parents cope by providing support during decision-making sessions with the eye specialists, by asking questions to clarify information, and by reinforcing information provided.

Information given to the parents about the prognosis of ROP in their infant must be included in any discharge planning. Parents need to understand that eye problems are more common in premature infants and may develop in infants with regressed ROP. Myopia (nearsightedness), strabismus (crossed eye), astigmatism, and amblyopia (lazy eye) are common sequelae. Glaucoma and late retinal detachment are common sequelae in infants with severe ROP.

Outcome studies suggest that the incidence of long-term problems has been underestimated. McGinnity & Bryars (1992) compared 200 low-birth-weight (LBW) infants with a matched group of full-term infants at 9 years of age. They found significantly more visual problems, such as strabismus, refractive errors, cicatricial ROP, and optic atrophy, in the LBW group. They also found that 70% of children with poor vision needed special resources to succeed in school. Clearly, early detection and referral to programs for visual impairment are essential. Parents need to understand the importance of regular eye examinations by a pediatric ophthalmologist or by an ophthalmologist knowledgeable about ROP and its complications (Blackburn, 1995). Many families may benefit from referral to community resources, support groups, and special programs for children with visual problems.

CONGENITAL DEFECTS

Aniridia

Aniridia is a severe ocular abnormality that manifests as a bilateral absence of the iris. Cataracts, corneal pannus, macular dysfunction, and glaucoma usually accompany the defect. Most of these infants have significantly diminished visual acuity, to a level of 20/200 or worse. About 20% to 30% of children with the noninherited form of aniridia eventually develop Wilms' tumor of the kidney.

Persistent Hyperplastic Primary Vitreous

Persistent hyperplastic primary vitreous is a unilateral disorder that affects both genders equally. It results from persistence of the hyoid vessels that connect the optic nerve and the posterior surface of the lens. It should be considered in the differential diagnosis of leukocoria. The involved eye invariably is small, and a mature cataract often is present. Surgery may improve the integrity of the eye, but useful vision usually is not restored.

Capillary Hemangioma of the Eyelid

Capillary hemangioma of the eyelid, a blood vessel tumor, usually appears before 6 months of age. It tends to enlarge, stabilize, and then regress by the time the child is 5 years old. The tumor usually is elevated and reddish purple. Capillary hemangiomas often are referred to as strawberry nevi because of their appearance.

Superficial tumors of the eyelid cause cosmetic and visual problems. Pressure on the globe from the tumor may result in significant astigmatism and subsequently amblyopia. If the tumor is large, it may cover the pupil and prevent normal visual development. Deep tumors in the orbit may manifest with proptosis. These tumors may be treated with surgical removal, radiation, or steroid injection. Tumors that are exclusively cosmetic should be allowed to regress without intervention.

Ptosis

Ptosis is a drooping of one or both eyelids as a result of neurologic, muscular, or mechanical factors. If the ptosis is significant enough to cover the pupil, a dense amblyopia may result. If bilateral ptosis is present, the infant may have slowed motor development and delayed ambulation later in life. These problems are caused by the awkward, chin-up position the child must maintain in order to see. Mild ptosis that causes a problem with appearance generally is not repaired until the child is 4 or 5 years old because the results usually are better at this age.

A thorough family history should be obtained. Several familial syndromes are associated with ptosis, including blepharophimosis syndrome and double-elevator palsy. Significant birth trauma may result in damage to the cervical ganglion and in an infantile Horner syndrome, in which the infant has different-colored pupils, miosis, anhidrosis (lack of sweating), and mild ptosis. Direct trauma to the eyelid or a tumor in the eyelid may also cause ptosis. Surgical repair corrects this defect easily.

Congenital Glaucoma

Congenital glaucoma occurs in approximately 1 in 25,000 births. Glaucoma is a disease in which the intraocular pressure is elevated to a level sufficient to damage the optic nerve. Because of the blinding potential of this disease, it must be detected early in the infant's life and treated properly. The affected neonate shows tearing, light sensitivity, eyelid spasm, and a large, cloudy cornea. The disease is slightly more common in males than in females. The diagnosis often is missed until the child is about 2 to 3 months of age. Conditions associated with glaucoma include trisomy 21, congenital rubella, Marfan syndrome, neurofibromatosis, oculodentodigital syndrome, Rieger

syndrome, Sturge-Weber syndrome, Rubinstein-Taybi syndrome, and Weill-Marchesani syndrome (Gupta et al, 2002).

It is critical that congenital glaucoma be differentiated from other diseases that have similar symptoms. Nasolacrimal duct obstruction involves tearing but does not cause light sensitivity or a cloudy cornea. Difficult labor or forceps injury may damage the cornea and cause temporary clouding, but the intraocular pressure is not elevated, a hallmark feature of glaucoma. The large eyes of the infant with congenital glaucoma may appear beautiful to the parents, but health professionals should be alert to the possibility of this disease.

The abnormality in congenital glaucoma is a deformity of the filtering system that controls the level of intraocular pressure in the eye. Congenital glaucoma is treated surgically. The results usually are good, but parents must be educated about the need for continued monitoring of this condition throughout the child's life.

Congenital Cataracts

The causes of significant lens opacity in the newborn are numerous. Cataracts are an important cause of blindness because they may interfere with the process of visual development early in the infant's life. For this reason, visually significant cataracts must be detected and treated before they cause amblyopia, which may be unresponsive to the most persistent treatment.

Heredity is an important cause of congenital cataracts. A thorough family history is critical in determining the cause of the lens opacity. The inheritance pattern may be autosomal dominant, autosomal recessive, or sex linked. A maternal history of diabetes, x-ray exposure, or malnutrition may be an important factor in cataract formation. In premature infants, transient cataracts or insignificant opacities are commonly seen as a result of remnants of developmental tissues. ROP can also lead to cataracts in premature infants. Several inborn errors of metabolism cause cataracts, including galactosemia, Alport syndrome, Fabry disease, and Lowe syndrome. Intrauterine rubella infection is also associated with cataracts in the neonate.

Cataract surgery early in life is critical to the infant's visual rehabilitation. Useful vision is especially difficult to achieve in eyes with monocular cataracts. It is important for nurses to work closely with the infant's parents. The parents' persistence in handling contact lenses and in amblyopia therapy often determines the outcome for their child's vision.

Retinoblastoma

Retinoblastoma is the most common intraocular neoplasm in childhood. The tumor occurs in approximately 1 in 20,000 live births. Most cases appear sporadically and occur in infants with no family history of the disease. An autosomal dominant pattern usually is responsible for the 5% to 10% of inherited retinoblastomas, most of which are bilateral. Autosomal dominant transmission occurs with an estimated 85% penetrance (Brantley & Harbour, 2001). A somatic mutation accounts for 80% of unilateral tumors.

The most common presenting symptom is leukocoria. Most of the tumors are not detected in the neonatal period, except in infants with a positive family history. The tumor is highly malignant and may spread to the bone marrow, CNS, or other organs. Untreated patients rarely survive. The standard treatment for advanced cases of retinoblastoma is enucleation. Less severe cases are treated with radiation, laser photocoagulation, or cryotherapy. Children with this tumor require close follow-up for possible recurrence after treatment. Parents must be educated about the disease so that they are aware of the need for constant monitoring of their child.

CONGENITAL INFECTIONS

Cytomegalovirus Infection

Congenital cytomegalovirus (CMV) infection occurs in most infants with symptomatic disease and infrequently in asymptomatic infants. Ocular lesions include chorioretinitis, optic nerve atrophy, strabismus, cataract, macular scarring, and visual impairment. In a recent report from the Congenital CMV Longitudinal Study Group, 22% of the infants with symptomatic CMV disease had moderate to severe vision impairment, compared with 1% of the asymptomatic infants with CMV disease (Coats et al, 2000). The two common causes of severe visual impairment were optic atrophy and cortical visual impairment. Strabismus was also present in many of the symptomatic infants (Coats et al, 2000). Because of the risk for later development of strabismus and amblyopia, the authors recommend lifelong eye examinations for symptomatic infants (Coats et al, 2000).

Like many of the herpes family viruses, CMV can become active after periods of dormancy. Parents should be advised of this so that they can seek appropriate eye care if their child develops vision problems later in life.

Rubella

Congenital rubella is responsible for a wide variety of ocular complications, including pigmentary retinopathy, glaucoma, cataract, and microphthalmos. Although the clinical presentations range across a wide spectrum, newborns classically have hearing, eye, and cardiac defects.

Currently the incidence of congenital rubella syndrome is low; however, new information from long-term follow-up studies suggests that the prevalence of ocular problems is nearly twice the previously thought rate (78% instead of 43%). Several trends have also been noted, including an increase in cases of delayed disease and new associations of combination problems. Microphthalmia, cataracts, and glaucoma are more likely to occur in combination than independently. Pigmentary retinopathy produces a characteristic salt and pepper appearance and can result in sudden vision loss during adulthood. Poor visual acuity and diabetic retinopathy are also of concern in individuals with congenital rubella syndrome. The parents of an infant with congenital rubella need to understand that vision problems may occur at any time and that they must have their child screened regularly.

Herpes Simplex Virus

Herpes simplex virus causes a wide variety of eye disorders in newborns. Corey and Flynn (2000) recently reported a case of congenital herpes simplex infection that resulted in bilateral persistent fetal vasculature of the eye. Persistent fetal vasculature occurs when intraocular vessels fail to involute in utero. This involution is a normal part of eye development.

Varicella

Although rare, congenital infection caused by varicella, commonly known as chickenpox, produces eye anomalies in more than 50% of affected infants. These defects include microphthalmia, chorioretinitis, enophthalmia, cataract, optic nerve atrophy, nystagmus, and anisocoria (Choong et al, 2000).

Toxoplasmosis

Toxoplasma gondii is a parasitic organism with an affinity for brain and eye tissue. As with many other congenital infections, ocular anomalies vary depending on fetal age at the time of infection. The most common clinical presentation is a focal necrotizing retinochoroiditis. Other ocular manifestations include microphthalmia, traction retinal detachment, nystagmus, strabismus, cataracts, disruption of the retinal pigment epithelium, retinal dysplasia, and vitreitis (Berk et al, 2000; Roberts et al, 2001). A recent study of congenital toxoplasmosis suggests that the inflammatory response mounted by the fetus and newborn contributes to irreversible retinal damage (Roberts et al, 2001).

Lymphocytic Choriomeningitis Virus

A new congenital viral infection, lymphocytic choriomeningitis virus (LCV), must be added to the list of viruses that cause ocular defects. Congenital LCV infection was first reported in the United States in 1993. The number of cases reported in the world literature currently stands at 32. LCV is a single-strand RNA virus found in rodents, including house mice and hamsters. Outbreaks of LCV infection associated with mice tend to occur in trailer parks, inner city dwellings, and substandard housing. Laboratory mice and hamsters can also cause outbreaks among laboratory personnel. The virus probably is transmitted by airborne droplets and by food contaminated by rodent urine or feces. It also may be transmitted by the bite of an infected animal (Mets et al, 2000).

Neonates with congenital infection usually have microcephaly, hydrocephaly, and chorioretinitis. In a recent report, a 3-day-old boy who had microcephaly at birth was found to have chorioretinitis, conjunctivitis, congenital glaucoma, and a serious cardiac defect (single ventricle and pulmonary atresia). Further testing revealed positive antibody titers for LCV (Mets et al, 2000). Mets and colleagues concluded that "congenital lymphocytic choriomeningitis virus infection may be more common than previously appreciated" and that "serologic testing . . . should be part of the standard workup for congenital chorioretinitis" (Mets et al, 2000). It also might be prudent to counsel women to avoid handling pet mice and hamsters during pregnancy.

OTHER DISORDERS THAT AFFECT THE EYES

Fetal Alcohol Syndrome

Ocular abnormalities often are overlooked in infants with fetal alcohol syndrome (FAS) because of the CNS damage, facial dysmorphia, and severe intrauterine growth retardation present in these infants. Abnormalities of the eyes common in infants with FAS include microphthalmos, coloboma, nystagmus, cataracts, glaucoma, microcornea, amblyopia, phthisis, persistent hyperplastic primary vitreous, and refractive errors. Most affected infants have diminished visual acuity. A recent study found ocular evidence of FAS in previously undiagnosed children evaluated for developmental delay or hyperactivity disorders or both (Hug et al., 2000). This study suggests that FAS should be included in the differential diagnosis of infants undergoing eye examination for developmental delay or hyperactivity disorders.

Maternal Diabetes

Although maternal diabetes is recognized for its teratogenic effects, craniofacial anomalies are rarely reported. A recent study documents the presence of oculoauriculovertebral (OAV) complex in 14 infants of diabetic mothers who were insulin dependent or who were treated with oral hyperglycemic medications throughout their pregnancies. Women with gestational diabetes were excluded from the study. The specific ocular anomalies noted in these infants were lens opacity, microphthalmia, optic nerve hypoplasia, laterally displaced inner canthi, tear duct obstruction, and ocular lipomas.

Periventricular Leukomalacia

Periventricular leukomalacia (PVL) has replaced ROP as the major cause of visual impairment in premature infants (Jacobson et al, 1998). Impairments found in infants with PVL included diminished visual acuity, eye movement disorders, and visual field restriction. Other eye problems included optic disc anomalies, nystagmus, strabismus, delayed visual maturation, and visual perceptual-cognitive problems (Jacobson & Dutton, 2000). These visual problems persist into childhood, according to a recent report from France (Porton-Deterne et al, 2000).

Intraventricular Hemorrhage

Intraventricular hemorrhage (IVH) without PVL is also associated with ocular morbidity (O'Keefe et al, 2001). Strabismus was present in 47% of infants with grade I and grade II IVH and in 42% of infants with grade III and grade IV IVH. Optical atrophy was present in 25% of infants with IVH. The incidence of ROP was also higher in this population of infants; no significant relationship to the grade of IVH was noted. Visual impairments were also common in infants with IVH, including smaller than average visual field, poor grating acuity, and poor recognition acuity (O'Keefe et al, 2001).

SUMMARY

Visual disturbances, although sometimes difficult to detect, have a dramatic impact on a newborn's behavioral and psychosocial development. PVL has replaced ROP as the most common cause of serious eye disease in premature infants. Despite significant advances in the diagnosis, treatment, and follow-up of infants with very low birth weight and prematurity, visual morbidity continues to be a concern as smaller neonates survive neonatal intensive care.

Treatment of vision problems requires collaborative efforts among the neonatal health care team, the ophthalmologist, and the families of affected children. Clear, consistent communication between health care providers and parents, parental education, and good follow-up are important to the quality of care.

REFERENCES

American Academy of Pediatrics Committee on Infectious Disease (2000). Red book 2000. APA: Elk Grove Village, IL.

Arroe M, Peitersen B (1994). Retinopathy of prematurity: review of a seven-year period in a Danish neonatal intensive care unit. Acta paediatrica, 83(5), 501-505.

Berk TA et al (2000). Underlying pathologies in secondary strabismus. Strabismus, 8(2), 69-75.

Blackburn S (1995). Problems of premature infants after discharge. Journal of gynecologic and neonatal nursing, 24(1), 43-49.

Blackburn S (1996). Studies of light and its application to clinical practice. Paper presented at the Physical and Developmental Environment of the High-Risk Neonate, January 31, 1996. University of South Florida College of Medicine: Clearwater Beach.

Bolt B et al (1992). A mydriatic eye drop combination without systemic effects for premature infants: a prospective double-blind study. Journal of pediatric ophthalmology and strabismus, 29(3), 157-162.

Brantley MA Jr, Harbour JW (2001). The molecular biology of retinoblastoma. Ocular immunology inflammation, 9(1), 1-8 (review).

Choong CS et al (2000). Congenital varicella syndrome in the absence of cutaneous lesions. Journal of paediatrics and child health, 36(2), 184-185.

Coats DK et al (2000). Ophthalmologic findings in children with congenital cytomegalovirus infection. JAAPOS, 4(2), 110-116.

Corey RP, Flynn JT (2000). Maternal intrauterine herpes simplex virus infection leading to persistent fetal vasculature. Archives of ophthalmology, 18(6), 837-840.

Cryotherapy for Retinopathy of Prematurity Cooperative Group (CRPCG) (1988). Multicenter trial of cryotherapy for retinopathy of prematurity: preliminary results. Archives of ophthalmology, 106(4), 471-499.

Dinakaran S, Desai SP (1999). Central serous retinopathy associated with Weber-Christian disease. European journal of ophthalmology, 9(2), 139-141.

Fielder AR, Levene MI (1992). Screening for retinopathy of prematurity. Archives of disease in childhood, 67(7), 860-867 (review).

Fletcher MA (1998). Physical diagnosis in neonatology. Lippincott, Williams & Wilkins: Baltimore.

Gupta BK et al (2002). The eye. In Fanaroff AA, Martin RJ, editors. Neonatal-perinatal medicine: diseases of the fetus and newborn, ed 7. Mosby: St Louis.

Hellström A (1999). Optic nerve morphology may reveal adverse events during prenatal and perinatal life: digital image analysis. Survey of ophthalmology, 44(suppl 1), S63-S73.

Holmes JM et al (1994). Randomized clinical trial of surfactant prophylaxis in retinopathy of prematurity. Journal of pediatric ophthalmology and strabismus, 31(3), 189-191.

Hug TE et al (2000). Clinical and electroretinographic findings in fetal alcohol syndrome. JAAPOS, 4(4), 200-204.

Hunter DG, Mukai S (1994). Retinopathy of prematurity: pathogenesis, diagnosis, and treatment. International ophthalmology clinics, 34(3), 163-184.

International Committee on Retinopathy of Prematurity (ICROP) (1984). An international classification of retinopathy of prematurity. Pediatrics, 74(1), 127-133.

Jacobson LK, Dutton GN (2000). Periventricular leukomalacia: an important cause of visual and ocular motility dysfunction in children. Survey of ophthalmology, 45(1), 1-13 (review).

Jacobson L et al (1998). Periventricular leukomalacia causes visual impairment in preterm children: a study on the aetiologies of visual impairment in a population-based group of preterm children born 1989-95 in the county of Varmland, Sweden. Acta ophthalmologica Scandinavica, 76(5), 593-598.

Javitt J et al (1993). Cost-effectiveness of screening and cryotherapy for threshold retinopathy of prematurity. Pediatrics, 91(5), 859-866.

Kraemer M et al (1999). The neonatal development of the light flash visual evoked potential. Documenta ophthalmologica, 99(1), 21-39.

Lehman SS (1999). An uncommon cause of ophthalmia neonatorum: Neisseria meningitidis. JAAPOS, 3(5), 316.

Moore K et al (2001). The developing human: clinically oriented embryology. WB Saunders: Philadelphia.

Muller DP (1992). Vitamin E therapy in retinopathy of prematurity. Eye, 6(part 2), 221-225 (review).

Nelson LB (1998). Disorders of the conjunctiva. In Nelson LB, Harley RD, editors. Harley's pediatric ophthalmology, ed 4. WB Saunders: Philadelphia.

Palmer EA (2001). Ocular significance of intraventricular haemorrhage in premature infants. British journal of ophthalmology, 85(3), 357-359.

Phelps DL (1992). Retinopathy of prematurity. Current problems in pediatrics, 22(8), 349-371.

Pierce EA, Mukai S (1994). Controversies in the management of retinopathy of prematurity. *International ophthalmology clinics*, 34(3), 121-148.

Porton-Deterne IF et al (2000). Ocular motility and visuo-spatial attention in children with periventricular leukomalacia. *Brain and cognition*, 43(1-3), 362-364.

Seiberth V et al (1994). A controlled clinical trial of light and retinopathy of prematurity. *American journal of ophthalmology*, 118(4), 492-495.

Shah GK et al (2000). Intralenticular *Candida* species abscess in a premature infant. *American journal of ophthalmology*, 129(3), 390-391.

Todd DA et al (1994). Retinopathy of prematurity in infants less than 29 weeks' gestation at birth. *Australian and New Zealand journal of ophthalmology*, 22(1), 19-23.

Todd Johnston W, Cogen MS (2000). Systemic candidiasis with cataract formation in a premature infant. *JAAPOS*, 4(6), 386-388.

Trese MT (1994). Surgery for retinopathy of prematurity. *International ophthalmology clinics*, 34(3), 105-111.

Vander JF (1994). Retinopathy of prematurity: diagnosis and management. *Journal of ophthalmic nursing and technology*, 13(5), 207-212.

Wasserman BN et al (1999). *Pseudomonas*-induced bilateral endophthalmitis with corneal perforation in a neonate. *JAAPOS*, 3(3), 183-184.

Wright K, Wright P (1994). Lack of association of glucocorticoid therapy and retinopathy of prematurity. *Archives of pediatric and adolescent medicine*, 148(8), 848-852.

Zhao F, Enzenauer RW (2001): Neonatal conjunctivitis. *Emedicine journal*, 2(1). Downloaded November 15, 2001, from www.emedicine.com/oph/topic325.htm.

ASSESSMENT AND MANAGEMENT OF THE SURGICAL NEWBORN AND INFANT

JUDITH POLAK

Care of the surgical neonate is an exciting challenge. Providing for the needs of the surgical neonate requires a knowledge of pathophysiology and current neonatal care practices, the training to recognize and respond to complications, and the ability to extend supportive care to the family. Providing complete care and achieving optimum survival require the skills of a multidisciplinary team. This team must include neonatal nurses, neonatologists, pediatric surgeons, radiologists, anesthesiologists, respiratory therapists, and parents. The members of this team must work together, guided by the knowledge that all of principles of neonatal care, as well as additional considerations related to surgical care, apply in each case.

This chapter discusses the challenges faced by the surgical neonate in the preoperative, intraoperative, and postoperative periods. Neonates, especially those whose condition is complicated by prematurity, poorly tolerate stressors such as hypoxia, acidosis, hypothermia, and fluid and electrolyte imbalances. However, when these stressors are prevented or minimized, surgical stress is tolerated remarkably well. In addition, parenting the surgical neonate is unlike parenting a well newborn. Different approaches to supporting these parents are discussed. This chapter is an overview of the concerns surrounding any neonate facing surgery. The specific care regimens of the surgical problems are discussed in detail in the respective assessment and management chapters of the text.

PREOPERATIVE PERIOD

Stabilization of the neonate's condition in the preoperative period determines the infant's ability to survive the trauma of surgical intervention. The major factors to be considered for effective stabilization are oxygenation and ventilation, acid-base balance, thermoregulation, fluid and electrolyte balance, and pharmacologic support.

Oxygenation and Ventilation

Assessment of the surgical neonate immediately after birth includes observing the infant's ability to complete the transition from intrauterine to extrauterine life. Adequate tissue oxygenation is necessary to prevent irreversible organ damage resulting from hypoxia. Establishing effective ventilation is a primary concern in providing optimum air exchange and oxygenation.

Ventilatory insufficiency can occur with various surgical problems. For example, airway obstruction occurs with choanal atresia, whereas an ineffective airway clearance mechanism is seen with a tracheoesophageal fistula with esophageal atresia. Hypoventilation is encountered with a diaphragmatic hernia and with defects that cause increased abdominal pressure on the diaphragm and lungs. Defects that manifest this type of problem include omphalocele or gastroschisis, necrotizing enterocolitis, and bowel obstructions.

It is imperative that the numerous causes of altered neonatal ventilation be considered and properly treated. A surgical neonate is not immune to problems such as prematurity, respiratory distress syndrome, persistent pulmonary hypertension, atelectasis, aspiration pneumonia, and bronchopulmonary dysplasia.

Neonates are obligate nose breathers. With choanal atresia, an oral airway is required to establish adequate ventilation. Intubation, if required, is performed by the orotracheal route. Diaphragmatic breathing is also characteristic of neonates. Any intraabdominal pressure change can lead to respiratory compromise. To minimize this problem, care must be taken to position the infant so as to avoid abdominal pressure from an abdominal wall defect. Placing these infants in the side-lying or semi-side-lying position may relieve diaphragmatic pressure from the defect and enhance ventilator assistance and pulmonary function.

Omphalocele or gastroschisis, necrotizing enterocolitis, and bowel obstruction all cause increased abdominal distention. Gastric decompression is necessary to reduce this source of pressure on the diaphragm and increasing difficulty in lung expansion. Decompression is achieved by use of an orogastric or nasogastric tube attached to a gravity drain or low intermittent suction. The patency of this tube must be maintained to allow for adequate gastrointestinal decompression. Continued abdominal distention may further compromise respiratory effort. Increased oxygenation or ventilation needs may reflect unresolved abdominal distention and worsening of the disease process. In addition, the ascites encountered in renal defects, such as ureteropelvic junction obstructions, can cause respiratory difficulty. Mechanical ventilation may be required until surgical intervention relieves the abdominal pressure.

A neonate with a diaphragmatic hernia has special respiratory needs. Mask ventilation must be avoided. This method of oxygenation is contraindicated because air is forced into the gastrointestinal tract, causing an increase in the volume in the chest and thereby increasing respiratory compromise in an infant with already limited lung function. Ventilation strategies that minimize airway pressure and reduce barotrauma to severely hypoplastic lungs improve survival. Prevention of persistent pulmonary hypertension must also be a primary concern. To accomplish this, adequate ventilation must be established to avoid hypoxia, hypercarbia, and acidosis, which are known factors in the pathophysiology of pulmonary hypertension.

Mask ventilation is also contraindicated when a tracheoesophageal fistula with esophageal atresia is present. Rupture of the esophageal pouch and overdistention of the stomach may occur. As a result, stomach contents can reflux through the fistula into the trachea, causing pneumonia. Proper positioning of the endotracheal tube, if needed, and the use of minimum ventilator pressure minimize these complications.

Prevention of aspiration pneumonia is a major concern with a tracheoesophageal fistula with esophageal atresia. If the blind esophageal pouch fills with saliva, overflow into the lungs occurs, causing pneumonia. Maintaining the patency of a double-lumen suction tube to drain the esophageal pouch prevents this complication. If diagnostic testing is necessary to evaluate the esophageal pouch, the contrast fluid must be kept from spilling out of the pouch because this, too, can cause aspiration pneumonia. This danger can be avoided by using a plain anteroposterior chest and abdomen radiograph taken with a radiopaque tube placed in the esophageal pouch. The esophageal pouch is clearly outlined, and visualization of air in the stomach confirms the presence of a tracheoesophageal fistula. Elevating the head of the infant's bed or placing the infant in the prone position minimizes possible reflux of gastric secretions through the tracheoesophageal fistula, preventing aspiration pneumonia.

Maintenance of a patent airway can be a concern with various defects. In some circumstances, intubation may be avoided if proper positioning is used. Extension of the neck may be necessary when a large, obstructing cystic hygroma is present. Hydrocephalus of severe proportions may also require slight extension of the neck and turning of the head to either side.

Regardless of the type of defect, nursing priorities with regard to oxygenation status include respiratory assessment for the quantity and quality of respiratory effort. Significant changes in the respiratory rate should be investigated. Adequate ventilation can be demonstrated by ease of respirations, absence of retractions or nasal flaring, and appropriate pink color of lips, mucous membranes, or nail beds.

Acid-Base Balance

A variety of factors can alter the acid-base balance in the surgical neonate. Major conditions that can result in acidosis include inadequate respiratory support and fluid or electrolyte imbalances. The effects of sepsis and tissue necrosis are also significant causes of acidosis. Acidosis in the surgical neonate can be the respiratory, metabolic, or mixed type.

Respiratory acidosis could occur with decreased ventilation, resulting in an increased partial pressure of carbon dioxide (PCO_2) and a decreased pH. An overproduction of acids may occur with any condition that causes a decrease in oxygenation or perfusion. Impaired kidney function, such as that which occurs in acute renal failure or renal tubular necrosis, reduces elimination of hydrogen ions, contributing to the development of metabolic acidosis. Bicarbonate losses are increased with severe diarrhea, intestinal fistulas, vomiting, and gastric drainage, resulting in metabolic acidosis.

The neonate with a diaphragmatic hernia is at great risk for the development of respiratory acidosis or metabolic acidosis, or both. Such an infant requires aggressive ventilation and administration of a buffering agent (e.g., sodium bicarbonate, tromethamine [Tham]) to prevent acidosis, which could contribute to the development of persistent pulmonary hypertension.

Poor tissue perfusion causes acidosis, as is seen with multiple gastrointestinal anomalies that are accompanied by large fluid losses. These anomalies include tracheoesophageal fistula with esophageal atresia, ruptured omphalocele and gastroschisis, bowel obstruction, and necrotizing enterocolitis. Adequately replenishing fluid or blood volume usually corrects this metabolic acidosis. When necrosis or perforation occurs, however, the acidosis may not be correctable until the necrotic bowel has been removed and any resulting sepsis treated.

Thermoregulation

Neonates are uniquely vulnerable to cold stress and overheating. The consequences of either can be devastating if the problem is not recognized early and corrected. Ultimately, prevention is the key.

Neonates may have poorly developed mechanisms for thermoregulation. The neonate's large body surface area coupled with the lack of insulating subcutaneous fat enhances heat loss. Also, oxygen consumption is not reduced with prolonged cooling of a neonate; rather, oxygen consumption increases as the metabolic rate increases to maintain body temperature. This increased metabolic work results in acidosis and tissue hypoxia.

Prevention of hypothermia in the surgical neonate is imperative in the preoperative period. Maintaining a neutral thermal environment is a constant challenge. In a neutral thermal environment, metabolic activity is minimal because body temperature is kept stable. Oxygen consumption is reduced, and acidosis is prevented. Any prolonged deviations from the neutral thermal environment further stress the infant's already limited thermoregulatory abilities.

Heat loss occurs through evaporation, conduction, convection, and radiation. Evaporative heat loss occurs with exposure of the intestinal contents of a ruptured omphalocele or gastroschisis. In the case of an encephalocele or a myelomeningocele, the unprotected spinal cord may allow heat loss. The exposed bladder mucosa in exstrophy of the bladder also contributes to heat loss. This type of heat loss can be prevented by applying warm dressings to the defects and then covering these areas with plastic.

Conductive heat loss occurs with direct skin contact with a cold surface, such as cold or wet linens, a weight scale, an examining table, x-ray plates, or an unwarmed bed. To prevent this type of heat loss, linens should be prewarmed as the bed or incubator is warmed. Examining or x-ray tables can be warmed with heat lamps before and during procedures. Linens that become wet should be replaced with dry, warmed linens; x-ray plates and scales should be covered with warmed linens before the infant is placed on them.

Heat loss by convection occurs when air blows over the infant. Use of warmed oxygen in head hoods and ventilators can reduce this type of heat loss. Also, it is essential that the incubator door not be open for prolonged periods. Insertion of nasogastric tubes, placement of intravenous lines, x-ray studies, physical examinations, and phlebotomy procedures should be performed through the incubator portholes to reduce heat loss. An additional heat source may be placed over the incubator when the door must be open.

Heat loss by radiation is the most difficult to control. This type of heat loss occurs during transportation of the neonate in cold hallways, in cold examining rooms, or in the cold operating room. To prevent this cold stress, the infant should be covered with warmed linens during transport. Examining rooms and operating rooms should be prewarmed to well above the "comfortable" temperature.

Nursing care that focuses on the thermoregulatory process of the neonate is vital to the prevention of complications related to poor temperature control. Maintaining a constant temperature, whether inside an incubator or in a radiant warmer bed, is a top priority. It is also beneficial to use warmed solutions for suctioning and dressing changes. Frequent monitoring of the infant's temperature is extremely important. Consistency in the method of measuring temperature and appropriate documentation are also essential. Prevention of cold stress reduces the chance of surgical complications, resulting in more neonatal surgeries (e.g., patent ductus arteriosus ligations) to be performed in the neonatal intensive care unit (NICU). Because no transport to the operating room suite is required, the infant is not subjected to environmental temperature changes during the move to and from the operating room and in the operating room itself. Some newer NICUs include a room that serves as a surgical unit so that no transport is needed. This design feature is intended to reduce the incidence of problems with thermoregulation.

Fluid and Electrolyte Balance

Fluid Losses.   Adequate fluid volume is required to ensure adequate perfusion of all organ systems. An inadequate vascular volume interferes with the oxygen supply to peripheral tissues, resulting in cellular damage and acidosis.

A neonate with a normally functioning cardiovascular system can tolerate the administration of intravenous fluids and blood products as long as the delivery of these fluids is precise and appropriate. Precision in fluid management is essential; there is little margin for error.

All fluid losses must be measured accurately to ensure adequate replacement. Estimation of insensible fluid losses is essential, including those caused by humidification through ventilation, radiant heating, and phototherapy. Unexpected fluid losses and inadequate fluid replacement delay preoperative stabilization of the neonate's condition.

With an esophageal atresia, continuous losses of saliva suctioned from the esophageal pouch must be measured and replaced. The large exposed intestinal area seen with a ruptured omphalocele or gastroschisis results in tremendous amounts of fluid losses. Replacement of these losses may involve up to twice the normal maintenance fluids of a neonate. If a membranous sac protects an omphalocele, the fluid requirement is less.

Gastrointestinal obstructions cause fluid losses from vomiting and from the suctioning required for gastric decompression. Peritonitis, such as occurs with perforations in necrotizing enterocolitis, midgut volvulus, or ruptured meconium ileus, causes third spacing of fluid (capillary leak syndrome) or fluid shifts into the bowel, necessitating increased fluid replacement.

Infants with open neural tube defects also have increased fluid losses. A leaking myelomeningocele requires increased fluid administration to keep up with the loss of cerebrospinal fluid.

Third spacing of fluids, or capillary leak syndrome, is the result of trauma to the gastrointestinal system. The capillary membrane's permeability is changed. This phenomenon may be due to secretion of natural fibronectin, a glycoprotein secreted by epithelial cells in the pulmonary and gastrointestinal trees. It is secreted in response to stimulation of the immune system to heal a wound. Fibronectin alters capillary permeability, shifting fluid and resulting in a "leaky capillary" and the third spacing of fluid. The body's compensatory response to any gastrointestinal trauma, then, can result in a movement of fluid across this "leaky" membrane. Fluid moves out of the vascular compartment and into the tissues, and the infant develops generalized edema. Abdominal swelling exerts pressure on the thoracic cavity, increasing the work of breathing. Gas exchange and ventilation are compromised as a result of (1) the pressure, (2) the decreased circulation, (3) the increased workload of the heart, which delivers oxygen to the tissues, and (4) the increasing loss of the buffer system through the mechanisms of diminished kidney perfusion and gastric losses.

The immediate reaction of inexperienced health professionals is to restrict fluids in this edematous infant, even though the vascular compartment is severely depleted of fluids. The infant is hypotensive, which increases cardiopulmonary compromise. Liberalization of fluids, therefore, is necessary to avoid total vascular collapse.

Diagnostic enemas with hyperosmolar solutions can have catastrophic results in a neonate who is not properly hydrated. Adequate intravenous access and good hydration are essential. Vascular collapse and even shock can occur rapidly if the fluid is shifted from the vascular bed to the bowel and is extracted with the enema and not appropriately replaced.

Glucose Level.   Fluctuation in the glucose level is a major indication of stress and infection. Preoperative hyperglycemia can result from sepsis or excessive intravenous administration of glucose. Hypoglycemia may result from a multitude of problems. For example, reduced glycogen stores are seen in premature infants and in infants with intrauterine growth retardation. Excessive insulin production occurs in the infant of a diabetic mother and with sudden or prolonged cessation of glucose infusions, as may occur with difficult or delayed insertion of intravenous lines. Abnormalities in glucose metabolism are evident with sepsis, shock, and asphyxia, as well as with various central nervous system (CNS) abnormalities. Glucose infusions must be carefully titrated to provide adequate hydration while the serum glucose is slowly restored to an acceptable concentration, avoiding extremes in the serum glucose level.

Electrolyte Imbalances.   The numerous conditions that affect the surgical neonate may result in imbalances of serum electrolytes, especially sodium and potassium. Fluid losses and inadequate intake result in hypokalemia and hyponatremia.

Hyperkalemia occurs with acidosis, excessive potassium intake, and renal failure. Renal failure may result from genitourinary obstructions or from sepsis and poor perfusion, as is seen with necrotizing enterocolitis with perforation or peritonitis.

The causes of hypernatremia generally are iatrogenic. An excessive intake of sodium occurs with administration of hypertonic solutions, intravenous flushes with normal saline or heparinized normal saline, or sodium bicarbonate for treatment of acidosis. Therapy with antibiotics such as ampicillin enhances the risk of hypernatremia.

Return to proper fluid and electrolyte balance is needed to improve the neonate's ability to tolerate any necessary operative procedure and to reduce the likelihood of complications.

Pharmacologic Support

Calculation of medication doses must be carefully individualized to the neonate. The infant's weight is only one factor to be considered in these calculations. An immature renal and hepatic system may result in a decreased ability to metabolize and excrete drugs. Serum levels of medications should be closely monitored to prevent toxicity (Chapter 43).

Preoperative antibiotic therapy may be required to treat sepsis. Untreated sepsis may progress, causing deterioration of the respiratory and cardiovascular systems. Respiratory distress requires increased ventilation. Inotropic drugs may be needed to support the cardiovascular system. In many NICUs, sepsis is treated with the antibiotic gentamicin sulfate combined with aminoglycoside therapy. Gentamicin sulfate increases sodium intake, which must be considered in monitoring electrolyte balance. Clindamycin is an effective agent for the treatment of anaerobic organisms, which generally are found in gastrointestinal infections.

Surgical problems in the neonate require antibiotic therapy. With suspected gastrointestinal obstructions, antibiotics may be needed to treat peritonitis or enterocolitis. The progression of necrotizing enterocolitis may be slowed with vigorous antibiotic therapy. Treatment of omphalocele and gastroschisis should include antibiotics to protect the exposed gastrointestinal contents and to help prevent ischemic injury to the abdominal contents. If pneumonia accompanies an esophageal atresia with tracheoesophageal fistula, aggressive antibiotic therapy should be instituted to clear the pneumonia and promote optimum surgical repair of the defect. The infant with a myelomeningocele requires antibiotic treatment to prevent meningitis.

Inotropic agents may be necessary to improve cardiac function and thus improve organ perfusion impaired by sepsis and stress. The most frequently used agents are dobutamine and dopamine. Dobutamine achieves organ perfusion by increasing cardiac output. Dopamine, used in low to moderate doses, causes vasodilation with resultant improvement in cardiac, renal, gastrointestinal, and cerebral blood flow. Use of dopamine at high doses, however, causes vasoconstriction of renal and gastrointestinal vessels. This vasoconstriction could worsen the condition of a renal system affected by obstruction or poor flow status, as well as the gastrointestinal system already compromised by necrotizing enterocolitis, omphalocele, gastroschisis, or obstruction. Dobutamine and dopamine doses, therefore, must be carefully calculated and continually titrated to achieve the desired effect. Furthermore, these medications are incompatible with many other drugs. For example, alkaline solutions (e.g., sodium bicarbonate, ampicillin, gentamicin, and furosemide) can inactivate dobutamine and dopamine. These inotropic agents are also irritating to vessels, and close monitoring of intravenous sites for infiltration is essential.

A buffering agent may be required to treat the acidosis that may accompany a diaphragmatic hernia, necrotizing enterocolitis, omphalocele, gastroschisis, or obstruction with resulting ischemic injury. Adequate ventilation and tissue perfusion must be established and maintained before medication is used to treat acidotic conditions.

Family

Through routine prenatal screening, many congenital surgical defects are diagnosed in utero, meaning that the cascade of events leading to successful neonatal surgery begins prenatally. For the family, this provides time for education and emotional support. If possible, a tour of the NICU should be arranged before delivery. Also, the parents should meet with members of the surgical and neonatal teams to discuss the findings and probable prognosis for their infant. Information given to the family should include the natural history of the abnormality, timing of surgery, anticipated surgical outcomes, possible long-term sequelae, and any other possible problems that may be involved with the neonate's course.

Decisions on the management and treatment of the infant require a team approach that includes the parents, nurses, obstetricians, pediatric surgeons, neonatologists, nurse practitioners, and radiologists. Supportive services should be provided to the family as indicated.

OPERATIVE PERIOD

Timing of the Operation

Proper timing of a surgical procedure is an important factor in minimizing stress for the surgical neonate. If the infant is hemodynamically stable, major intervention may be tolerated with surprisingly few complications. However, the infant with untreated sepsis or acidosis may not even survive the induction of anesthesia without severe problems.

A surgical neonate may suffer from a multitude of medical and surgical problems. A complete evaluation is needed, as long as the infant can tolerate this delay. A metabolically stable, growing infant is a much better surgical risk than an acidotic, premature baby whose condition is unstable.

The emergent nature of any surgical problem takes precedence over minor defects. For example, resection of a perforated bowel requires intervention before the repair of a mild congenital heart defect; however, severe congenital heart disease may be repaired before an uncomplicated intestinal atresia is corrected.

Perforation of the stomach or intestines is one of the few reasons an emergency surgical repair is performed. If such a case goes untreated, hypovolemia, acidosis, and shock occur. Delay in treating necrotizing enterocolitis with perforation or midgut volvulus results in further infarction of an already compromised bowel, leading to further shock and then death. The physiologic response to perforation is not correctable until the diseased bowel is resected. Even in these emergent situations, hypovolemia must be aggressively treated to attain an optimum surgical outcome.

Treatment of a congenital diaphragmatic hernia is directed toward aggressive stabilization of the infant's respiratory status. In the past, neonates with this defect were rushed to the operating room immediately after birth. The change in practice, to delay surgery until the respiratory problems have been stabilized, reflects the current belief that surgery cannot correct the respiratory insufficiency. Neonates now are managed medically until their respiratory status and cardiovascular status are stable (Clark et al, 1998).

For an infant with a tracheoesophageal fistula with esophageal atresia, a gastrostomy tube may be inserted as soon as possible to prevent reflux of gastric contents into the lungs through the fistula. Repair of the atresia and fistula can be delayed until the infant's condition is stable and a complete evaluation has been performed for other anomalies. The fistula may be ligated and esophageal anastomosis delayed to allow for better growth and an optimum surgical outcome. Pneumonia must be treated before any surgical procedure is undertaken.

If a neonate is not stable enough for primary closure of an omphalocele or gastroschisis or if the defect is too large, a Silastic pouch, or "silo," may be created. This pouch helps to prevent infection, alleviate the restriction of venous return to the extremities, and reduce renal compromise. This procedure relieves abdominal pressure, which may cause respiratory compromise by suspending the defect above the abdomen. Slow, daily reduction of this "silo" over 7 to 10 days allows closure with minimum complications.

A myelomeningocele can be protected with dressings soaked in sterile normal saline to allow for full evaluation of the infant's neurologic status before the defect is repaired. A sonogram of the head helps determine whether placement of a ventriculoperitoneal shunt is needed. Evaluation by an orthopedist to determine if intervention is needed for the lower extremities can be delayed until the back repair is done and is healing.

If the infant with an encephalocele is in stable condition, a full evaluation should be performed to determine the type of tissue and vascular access involved in the defect. This information is useful to the surgeon who removes the encephalocele and allows for preparation of the family for the infant's postoperative prognosis.

The timing factor is important when a sacrococcygeal teratoma is present. Evaluation of the defect preoperatively is essential to determine the surgical technique and the postoperative outcome. Relevant questions include the following:

- Is the spinal cord involved?
- Is the defect extremely vascular?
- What will be the result if the defect is excised?

A great loss of blood can occur and should be anticipated. Preoperative stabilization of the infant's hematologic status is imperative to optimize the surgical outcome.

An infant with an imperforate anus requires radiologic evaluation to identify the location of the rectum. This evaluation determines whether an anoplasty or a colostomy is required.

The timing of the operation can also be extremely important to the family. For an infant in stable condition, thorough evaluation of a surgical defect is essential. This information, as complete and accurate as time allows, enables the family to give truly informed consent.

Intraoperative Care

The stressors encountered by the surgical neonate during the preoperative period continue to present a challenge for patient management during the intraoperative period. Although stabilization of the infant's condition remains a major consideration, the effects of anesthesia during the surgical procedure present additional problems. Vascular access must be established so that drugs, fluids, and blood products can be administered rapidly. Arterial lines may be needed for monitoring blood gases and arterial pressures. Critical assessments of vital signs and exact fluid management directly affect the positive or negative outcome of surgical intervention.

Oxygenation and Ventilation.   A number of factors can limit gas exchange during induction of anesthesia in the neonate. The infant's gestational age and birth weight dictate the size of the endotracheal tube used for intubation. Smaller gauge tubes create increased airway resistance and thus increased difficulty with ventilation. Specific defects, such as a diaphragmatic hernia, an omphalocele, and gastroschisis, create additional considerations. When the abdominal contents of the defects are replaced in the abdominal cavity, pressure on the diaphragm is increased and ventilation must be adjusted to compensate for this change. Stress and fatigue in the infant also diminish respiratory effort and necessitate prolonged manual or mechanical ventilation.

Anesthetic agents can cause respiratory depression, as can narcotic and sedative medications. The neonate has a limited capacity to tolerate prolonged anesthesia. Residual effects of anesthesia can delay recovery from the surgical procedure, as is seen by the infant's diminished respiratory effort or apnea. Oxygenation of the neonate should be directed toward maintaining a partial pressure of oxygen (PO_2) in the range of 60 to 80 mm Hg or an O_2 saturation range of 90% to 95%. Oxygenation levels are higher for infants at risk for or who have documented persistent pulmonary hypertension.

Acid-Base Balance.   Acidosis during surgery remains a challenge for management. As previously discussed, the effects of sepsis and tissue necrosis, as well as poor tissue perfusion, add to the potential for an acidotic state. Acid-base balance may also continue to be altered as a result of impaired renal function or prolonged fluid imbalances. Monitoring of blood gases and administration of buffering agents are important aspects of patient care throughout the surgical procedure, as discussed for the preoperative period.

Thermoregulation.   Concerns regarding temperature regulation continue during the intraoperative period. Although achieving a normal core temperature in the infant before surgery is always helpful, it is not always possible. Body temperature should be monitored throughout the procedure using either a skin or a rectal probe. A radiant warmer should be used during line placement, preparation, draping, and induction of anesthesia. A warming blanket can also be used to achieve constant temperature control. In addition, the room temperature should be increased to help compensate for the neonate's inability to stabilize temperature. Another mechanism for improving temperature control is humidification and warming of anesthetic gases. Slightly warming blood products, irrigation fluids, and intravenous fluids also assists in temperature maintenance. Surgical drapes should be replaced, if possible, when they become wet.

Another challenge in temperature maintenance is encountered during transport of the neonate to and from the operating room. To ensure temperature stability, the infant should be covered with warmed linen during transport. During the operative procedure, the bed should be warmed to allow for some warmth during transport postoperatively.

Fluid and Electrolyte Balance.   The goal of intraoperative fluid management is to replace the fasting fluid deficit, maintenance and third space fluid losses, and blood loss to maintain homeostasis (Aker & O'Sullivan, 1998). Constant monitoring of fluid balance should continue throughout the surgical procedure. During the operative procedure, the fluid choice reflects the most dominant fluid loss. Early treatment of hypovolemia is essential. Intravenous fluid administration rates must be monitored to prevent fluid boluses, which could compromise fluid and electrolyte balance. Fluid loss from the surgical defect and blood loss during the operative procedure must be monitored and replaced. The metabolic response to surgery may also alter the infant's fluid and electrolyte balance. Hyperglycemia is a common response to surgical stress. Cold stress adds to this metabolic response and consequent fluid needs.

Glucose stability is an additional consideration during surgery. Glucose metabolism is not stable in the neonate, and prematurity magnifies this problem. The glucose level should be monitored frequently to maintain a narrow range of normal. As discussed, the infusions of intravenous fluids should be monitored closely to prevent inaccurate rates of administration, resulting in hypoglycemia or hyperglycemia.

Pharmacologic Support.   Use of medications during the intraoperative period can be affected by many variables. Irregular patterns of metabolism, immature or compromised renal function, and variations in hepatic blood flow can influence the action and effectiveness of medications. Bradycardia can result from narcotics such as fentanyl and morphine, inhalation anesthetics, and muscle relaxants. The resultant hypoxia must be considered a major problem and must be resolved quickly to ensure a successful surgical outcome.

When use of muscle relaxants is considered, it must be remembered that neonates are particularly sensitive to succinylcholine. Bradycardia can be associated with this drug, and a predose of atropine may be given to prevent this complication. Intermediate and long-acting muscle relaxants, such as pancuronium or vecuronium, are commonly preferred for their ability to achieve or maintain a hemostatic state by increasing the heart rate and blood pressure.

Inhalation anesthetics and intravenous anesthetics can depress the ventilatory response to hypoxemia and hypercarbia. An increased pulmonary uptake of some agents causes high tissue levels and eventual cardiac compromise. Successful use of inhalation anesthetics in combination with narcotics has been achieved in neonates (Watcha, 1997). However, careful monitoring of fluid status and of cardiovascular and renal function is essential throughout the surgical procedure.

Latex Allergy.   A significant issue that affects perioperative care in this era is latex allergy. A correlation between children with spina bifida or genitourinary anomalies and latex allergies has been made. Latex allergy increases in populations that have frequent exposure to latex, such as bladder catheterizations, operative procedures, and universal precautions. The allergic reaction occurs when the patient is exposed to an allergen to which he or she is sensitized (Young & Meyers, 1997).

Because the correlation has been made between latex and direct patient exposure, many institutions now have policies to protect patients from latex exposure. Some interventions include a latex-free cart and a frequently updated listing of institutionally used products and their latex content. Other institutions are developing a latex-free environment to reduce exposure for patients and health care workers.

Family.   Parents want comprehensive information, especially during the waiting periods. Parental coping may be greatly enhanced by timely updates from the operating room while the parents are waiting for their infant in surgery. It is also important for the surgeon to speak with the parents immediately after surgery to discuss findings and the infant's condition.

POSTOPERATIVE PERIOD

The initial postoperative period is a critical time in the recovery of the surgical neonate. Neonatal surgery is done only when absolutely necessary, therefore the infant is already in a compromised condition before the procedure. Skillful assessment and management of the neonate is required to achieve a positive surgical outcome. This requires experience and collaborative care before, during, and after surgery. At times, no matter how careful and diligent the care before surgery, the outcome in terms of morbidity and mortality is not good.

Close monitoring of the neonate includes frequent assessment of core temperature, surface temperature, heart and respiratory rate, blood pressure, perfusion, and oxygen saturation. Ventilatory assistance must also be evaluated frequently for rate, pressure, and oxygen administration. The rate of intravenous infusions should also be assessed to ensure an adequate urine output of at least 1 to 2 ml/kg/hour (Aker & O'Sullivan, 1998). Serum glucose levels should be monitored and adjusted appropriately.

Oxygenation and Ventilation

Respiratory care in the postoperative period can present a great challenge to the caregiver. Intubation, anesthetic gases, and the stress of the procedure can traumatize the infant's respiratory tract. Depression of respiratory drive may be seen as a residual effect of anesthesia, and airway clearance may be difficult to maintain. These alterations in respiratory mechanics may lead to respiratory insufficiency and the need for prolonged mechanical support. Although specific respiratory needs may vary depending on the surgical procedure, a conservative approach to respiratory care is essential to maintain optimum oxygenation. An aggressive plan of weaning may cause recurring acidosis, hypoxia, or damage to the surgical repair.

In the postoperative neonate with a diaphragmatic hernia, care should focus on prevention of persistent pulmonary hypertension, which is caused by pulmonary vasoconstriction, and prevention of damage to the "good lung" resulting from excessive ventilator pressures. Paralysis with pancuronium or vecuronium can be beneficial in the postoperative period to assist in adequate ventilation and oxygenation. Such an infant should be weaned cautiously.

Respiratory support for the postoperative infant with a tracheoesophageal fistula may range from humidified mist to endotracheal intubation, depending on the type of repair and the complications encountered in surgery. The infant should be suctioned frequently to minimize both endotracheal and oropharyngeal secretions. A measured catheter should be used to avoid damage to the surgical sites. A thoracotomy may also be done to prevent atelectasis or pneumothorax and to promote expansion of the lung.

Respiratory compromise is a common complication after primary closure of an omphalocele or gastroschisis. Excessive pressure on the diaphragm and poor peripheral perfusion related to pressure on the inferior vena cava may require ventilatory support to improve lung expansion and oxygenation status. Paralysis with pancuronium may aid ventilation efforts and help prevent rupture of incisions.

Postoperative care of the neonate with necrotizing enterocolitis includes aggressive ventilation. Many of these infants are small, premature, or of low birth weight and have already compromised lung function. The stress of severe infection and the surgical procedure itself, as well as the prematurity of the lungs, may necessitate prolonged ventilation with a slow weaning process.

Acid-Base Balance

As in the preoperative and intraoperative periods, acid-base balance presents a challenge postoperatively. Although the neonate's initial reaction to the stress of surgery influences this balance, the concern over acidosis continues for a significant period. Monitoring of blood gases, attention to fluid balance, and delivery of appropriate respiratory support are important aspects of postoperative care. As sepsis resolves, fluid status stabilizes, and urine output is optimized, the acid-base balance also stabilizes.

Thermoregulation

Temperature regulation in the neonate may remain a problem in the immediate postoperative period. Use of radiant warmers is the method of choice for maintaining both core and surface temperatures. The premature infant may require enclosure in an incubator to maintain consistent temperature control.

The principles of thermoregulation used in the preoperative and intraoperative periods are also useful in the postoperative plan of care for the surgical neonate. The use of warmed linens immediately after transport of the infant may help in maintaining temperature stability. Removal of wet dressings and warming of irrigation fluids also help alleviate variations in body temperature.

Fluid and Electrolyte Balance

The goal of postoperative care is to provide fluid and electrolyte balance without overhydration. Hypovolemia is a major cause of hypotension and must be resolved quickly to ensure adequate perfusion to all organ systems and to combat acidosis. However, extreme care must be taken in administering fluids because premature infants are susceptible to third spacing and edema. Neonates are also very easily overloaded with excessive fluids.

Vital signs should be monitored frequently, initially every 15 to 30 minutes. Drastic changes in heart rate or blood pressure could indicate shock or undetected fluid loss for which the body is trying to compensate. Assessment of temperature continues to be an important factor and must be considered when evaluating fluid needs.

The serum electrolyte and glucose levels should be evaluated immediately postoperatively and then intermittently until the infant's condition is stable. The frequency of laboratory evaluation should be individualized to the neonate's condition. Sodium losses may continue through wound drainage as well as through gastric decompression. Thus re-evaluation of intravenous fluids, both maintenance and replacement, is required to achieve and maintain electrolyte balance. Glucose metabolism may be altered as a response to surgery. Serum glucose levels should be monitored every 1 to 2 hours after surgery.

Replacement fluid therapy is designed to make up for abnormal fluid and electrolyte losses during therapy to reduce vomiting and for losses incurred through diarrhea, nasogastric tube drainage, stoma output, wound drainage, pleural fluid, and fistula losses. Because the constituents of these losses frequently are quite different from the composition of maintenance fluids, it may be hazardous to simply increase the volume of maintenance fluids in an attempt to compensate for these losses. In some cases, it is preferable to actually measure and analyze the electrolyte content of these losses and replace them milliequivalent for milliequivalent and milliliter for milliliter. Samples may be sent to the laboratory as needed for exact determination of the electrolyte content of theses different body fluids.

The rate at which abnormal losses are replaced depends on the rate at which the fluid is lost and the patient's size. In small infants, even modest abnormal losses should be replaced every 2 to 4 hours.

Overzealous attempts to correct glucose or electrolyte problems can produce a rebound effect. The neonate may change from being hyperglycemic to being hypoglycemic without intervention over a period of minutes or hours. The neonate moves from a catabolic to an anabolic state fairly rapidly compared with an older child or adult. These phases may occur over a few days or weeks in the infant instead of over months as in the adult. Therefore it is best to obtain baseline serum electrolyte and glucose levels. These values should be obtained every 1 to 4 hours, depending on how extreme the levels are. When intervention is needed, the sodium, potassium, or other electrolyte should be increased or decreased slowly and in small increments. These incremental changes should be followed by repeated measurement of serum levels, which must be closely monitored.

Third spacing of fluids that causes edema in the first few postoperative days is an additional consideration. The infant's weight, renal function, and nutritional needs must continue to be evaluated, and nursing care must include measures to maintain skin integrity during this period of edema and fluid mobilization.

Nutritional Needs

For some surgical neonates, concern during the convalescent period goes beyond fluid and electrolyte balance. The nutritional needs of infants with altered function of the gastrointestinal tract present unique problems. A small stomach size with altered emptying ability, as is sometimes seen with a diaphragmatic hernia, gastroschisis, omphalocele, and bowel resection, may present paramount problems in providing proper nutrition when feedings are started. Use of continuous feedings may help with these problems.

Gastroesophageal reflux (GER) may present challenges in feeding. Assessments of vomiting and large gastric aspirates must be made. Treatment of reflux may include positioning the infant prone or in an upright position after feedings and thickening the feeding. Pharmacologic treatment may be initiated in the immediate postoperative period in anticipation of GER, or it may be started once symptoms appear.

The neonate who has had a bowel resection after perforation (as in necrotizing enterocolitis) can present a significant challenge. Concerns should center on vomiting, diarrhea, distention, or the presence of glucose or blood in the stool. The infant may not tolerate standard formulas, and an alternative formula, such as Pregestimil, may be required (Chapter 25).

Pharmacologic Support

Antibiotic therapy remains aggressive during the postoperative period. Ampicillin sodium plus gentamicin sulfate is the most commonly used combination of drugs. Penicillin G, clindamycin, cefotaxime sodium, and ceftriaxone sodium are also frequently used.

Inotropic agents, dopamine and dobutamine, may be needed postoperatively to maintain organ perfusion and renal function. As fluid balance is achieved and cardiac compromise resolves, monitoring and titration of these drugs remains essential.

Management of pain in the surgical neonate is important in the postoperative period (Hummel & Puchalski, 2001). Pain must be anticipated, recognized, and treated (see Chapter 42 for a more complete discussion of neonatal pain and its treatment).

Wound Care

Surgical neonates are vulnerable to infection throughout their hospital course. To prevent infection, the nurse must provide careful wound care. Wound infections can occur during or after the surgical procedure and can be a complicating factor. Infection occurs more often after "contaminated" surgeries, such as an intestinal perforation, compared with "clean" surgeries, such as ductal ligation (Jankelelvich, 1998). These wound infections often require treatment with antibiotics.

The surgery team typically performs the first dressing change. Gentle restraints or analgesia may be required if the dressing change is painful or if the infant is vigorous. Nursing assessment of the site must be continual, because these observations may provide the first indication of poor healing or wound infection. The neonatal or surgery team (or both) should be made aware of any changes. If any suspicion of infection exists, blood cultures should be drawn before treatment is started with broad-spectrum antibiotics that target anaerobes and aerobes, gram-positive and gram-negative organisms.

Family

Once the infant is back from the operating room, the parents should be allowed to visit in a timely manner to reduce anticipatory stress. The nurse should discuss the infant's current condition, the equipment used, and anticipatory care in the short term.

In the postoperative period, parents need to be able to negotiate their parental role with the staff members caring for their infant and should be supported in their attempts to advocate for their infant. Parents should also be encouraged to participate in their child's care to the extent that is comfortable for them. This means that parents must be provided with adequate information, guidance regarding their role, coping instructions, and support.

SUMMARY

Care of the surgical neonate is a multidimensional challenge. These infants have much strength, which assists them in tolerating the surgical procedure and promotes recovery. Rebound from surgery can occur rapidly if the case is properly managed and complications are anticipated. Nursing care requires continual assessment and timely intervention to produce optimum outcomes in the surgical neonate.

Some neonates present many challenges for medical and surgical management that requires immediate intervention. The infant's condition must be stabilized before surgery to optimize the neonate's ability to tolerate anesthesia and the surgical procedure with minimum complications. These infants are at risk for problems with ventilation and oxygenation, thermoregulation, fluid and electrolyte abnormalities, pain, inadequate nutrition, and infection.

Family support from the time of diagnosis to discharge is the responsibility of all health care providers. Parental participation in care and decision making builds confidence and familiarity with the skills parents need to care for their infant. Achieving the best possible outcome for these infants requires the expertise of a multidisciplinary team that is well trained in the principles of management during the preoperative, intraoperative, and postoperative phases.

REFERENCES

Aker J, O'Sullivan C (1998). The selection and administration of perioperative intravenous fluids for the pediatric patient. *Journal of perianesthesia nursing*, 13(3), 172-181.

Clark RH et al (1998). Current surgical management of congenital diaphragmatic hernia: a report from the congenital diaphragmatic hernia study group. *Journal of pediatric surgery*, 33, 1004-1009.

Jankelelvich J (1998). Wounds, abscesses, and other infections caused by anaerobic bacteria. In Katz S et al, editors. *Krugman's infectious diseases of children*. Mosby: St Louis.

Hummel MA, Puchalski M (2001). Assessment and management of pain in infancy. *Newborn and infant nursing reviews*, 1(2), 114-121.

Watcha MF (1997). Anesthesia. In Levin DL, Morris FC, editors. *Essentials of pediatric intensive care*. Churchill Livingstone: New York.

Young MA, Meyers M (1997). Latex allergy: considerations for the care of pediatric patients and employee safety. *Nursing clinics of North America*, 32(1), 169-182.

CHAPTER 38

ASSESSMENT AND MANAGEMENT OF THE NEWBORN AND INFANT UNDERGOING TRANSPLANTATION

CAROLE KENNER

Transplantation in newborns and infants is on the rise. For the past few decades, most of the transplants in this age group have centered on livers. Currently the growing trends are toward stem cell and whole organ transplants. Through the use of high level ultrasonographic and endoscopic techniques, transplantation has become technically possible. However, just because we can perform a procedure does not mean we always should.

This chapter outlines the common types of newborn and infant transplantations. It is meant to serve only as an overview and to describe the state of science in this area of newborn care.

HEPATIC TRANSPLANTATION IN INFANTS AND CHILDREN

Transplantation of the liver in infants and children has been recognized for many years as a possible solution to numerous inherited metabolic diseases and primary abnormalities of liver function. The first attempts at clinical transplantation failed, but in 1967 the prolonged survival of a child who received a transplant after hepatoma resection was reported. With improving survival rates, the indications for transplantation have broadened, and the number of transplantations performed has risen. For example, after the introduction of cyclosporine in 1980, the number of liver transplants greatly increased because the drug improved the survival rate among recipients. Currently, liver transplantation is offered to all children with progressive liver failure, regardless of age or weight.

Etiology

Liver transplantion most often is performed because of biliary atresia, errors of metabolism, or liver failure.

Biliary Atresia. Within the first 60 days of life, most infants with biliary atresia show signs of progressive jaundice and acholic stools. A percutaneous liver biopsy demonstrates bile duct obliteration, and ultrasonographic examination does not visualize a gallbladder. The primary use of hepatic portoenterostomy (Kasai procedure) is indicated in patients diagnosed in infancy. Long-term correction of liver function is achieved in approximately one third of all cases, and although these patients require careful follow-up, transplantation may not be

necessary. In the remaining children, progressive cirrhosis, portal hypertension, and nutritional failure develop, requiring liver transplantation. Vigorous institution of nutritional support is essential to maintain growth and development while sufficient hepatic function exists. Transplantation should be undertaken when growth failure develops; portal hypertensive complications occur; or the synthetic function of the liver deteriorates. Transplantation in these infants is more difficult because of their small size, because intra-abdominal adhesions often have developed as a result of previous operations, and because associated anomalies of the portal vein, hepatic artery, and inferior vena cava frequently are present. In addition, malrotation or abdominal situs inversus can complicate organ placement (Chapter 26).

Errors of Metabolism. Many errors of metabolism have been addressed by liver transplantation. Although these errors are often diagnosed in infancy, the need for transplantation during this period is rare. Alpha$_1$-antitrypsin deficiency, Wilson's disease, tyrosinemia, glycogen storage disease, and familial hypercholesterolemia have all been significantly improved or cured by liver replacement (Chapter 27). Appropriate genetic counseling is indicated when the diagnosis is made. The prognosis for these patients is good, owing to the predictability of transplantation and the patients' larger size. Inherited urea cycle abnormalities, such as ornithine transcarbamylase deficiency, can also be cured by liver transplantation. However, careful dietary intervention to prevent irreversible central nervous system injury secondary to hyperammonemia is required in infancy (Chapter 28).

Acute Hepatic Failure. Liver replacement for acute fulminant liver failure is performed more frequently in children than in infants. The primary cause may range from viral hepatitis to unrecognized metabolic disturbances. The prognosis is directly related to the primary disease and the severity of the neurologic impairment at the time of transplantation. The rapidity of hepatic failure in these patients makes pretransplant diagnosis uncommon, and the prognosis is impaired by the rapidity of disease progression and the common neurologic abnormalities.

Other Diagnoses. Familial cholestasis, chronic active hepatitis, biliary hypoplasia, cryptogenic cirrhosis, and hepatic tumors are other indications for hepatic replacement in selected infants and children.

Pretransplant Management

The pretransplant management of infants and children with progressive end-stage liver disease is paramount in achieving later success with liver transplantation.

Selection of Candidates for Transplantation

In general, indications for transplantation in children include (1) progressive end-stage liver disease, (2) stable liver disease with a known lethality, (3) fatal hepatic-based metabolic disease, (4) metabolic disease correctable by liver cell replacement, and (5) social invalidism, or inability to participate in any social or extracurricular activities. Although specific size and age limitations do not exist, complications and technical difficulties with transplantation increase greatly in small donors and recipients. Currently transplantation is limited to infants of term gestation without other life-threatening abnormalities.

The selection of candidates for transplantation and the most appropriate allocation of available organs have been difficult issues in pediatric transplantation. Standard liver function tests do not quantitate hepatic reserve or disease progression. Several attempts at quantitating and stratifying infants and children have been undertaken. Through a retrospective review of 70 variables, 23 of which had prognostic significance, Malatack and associates (1987) developed a scoring system. Patients were stratified into one of three risk groups—high, medium, or low—according to their overall score. This score was complex and, although helpful, assessed the severity of hepatic disease and its complications rather than the degree of potential hepatic reserve. Further attempts to quantitate hepatic functional reserve and to predict patient deterioration using a quantitative assessment of lidocaine metabolism have been undertaken in pediatric candidates. The formation of monoethylglycinexylidide (MEGX), a product of lidocaine metabolism in the liver, is decreased in proportion to the severity of the liver disease. MEGX has been shown to be predictive of hepatic function, not only in potential recipients but also in transplant donors (Colombani & McDonald, 2001). This test is simpler to administer and correlates well with the more complex Malatack score. Quantitative stratification of the severity of liver disease in the potential recipient should allow earlier referral of patients with deteriorating hepatic status before they reach the point at which transplantation is not practical and survival is not possible. Although each of these tests is helpful in the assessment of potential recipients, no single test reliably predicts hepatic reserve or impending failure.

Interventional radiology has been helpful in the selection not only of potential candidates for liver transplants but also of potential donors. This technology uses three-dimensional ultrasound (3D US).

Nutritional Support.

Attention to nutritional assessment and support is particularly important. The initial assessment, height, weight, anthropometric data, and growth velocity properly establish a nutritional database. Growth failure is considered a concern among chronically ill children but especially those awaiting a transplant (UNOS, 2001). Growth failure and malnutrition lead to increased morbidity and mortality after the transplantation procedure. It is important, therefore, to anticipate and to try to prevent these problems both before and after transplantation.

Chronic intake and oxygen consumption measurement allows nutritional goals to be set. The goal of nutritional management should be a positive nitrogen balance and progressive weight gain. Management of complications of liver failure, such as ascites, coagulopathy, and increased risk of infection, requires meticulous coordination of fluid and dietary intake. Fat-soluble vitamins (A, D, E, and K) are administered. Early institution of nocturnal supplemental nasogastric or nasojejunal feedings is often necessary to achieve an adequate caloric intake. Periodic reassessment is essential to ensure timely adjustment of the feeding schedule.

Portal Hypertension.

Regardless of the primary diagnosis, the common complications of portal hypertension develop in most patients with progressive cirrhosis. These include esophageal varices, gastrointestinal hemorrhage, and hypersplenism. Esophageal varices complicated by hemorrhage are the most common manifestation of this process. Endoscopic assessment with sclerotherapy of the varices is used to treat both acute and chronic bleeding. Sequential reevaluation and repeat sclerotherapy can prevent recurrent hemorrhage while attempts at donor organ acquisition occur. Pharmacologic management of acute hemorrhage includes administration of vasopressin and octreotide (somatostatin). Use of a Sengstaken-Blakemore tube to achieve direct balloon tamponade of bleeding varices or transthoracic ligation of the bleeding varices is rarely necessary. Portal azygos venous disconnection (Segura procedure) is an accepted long-term alternative when transplantation is not immediately required. Portacaval shunting should be avoided when possible in transplant candidates.

Other complications of portal hypertension also can occur, such as hypersplenism and ascites. Splenic sequestration of blood components can be recognized by the development of leukopenia, thrombocytopenia, or anemia. Most instances resolve with transplantation and resolution of the portal hypertension. When severe leukopenia (white blood cell count less than 3000) or thrombocytopenia (platelet count less than 50,000) occurs, splenectomy may be necessary at the time of transplantation. This splenectomy is rarely, if ever, necessary in infants and small children because there is an increased risk of sepsis and a likelihood of resolution after transplantation. Dietary salt restriction, caloric support, and occasional albumin supplementation in association with diuretics are used to control ascites.

Infection.

Patients with end-stage liver disease are especially prone both to infections normally seen in infants and children (e.g., meningitis, otitis media, pneumonia) and to infections from unique sources. Any fever or physical examination suggestive of infection requires vigorous investigation. Identification of specific organisms by blood, urine, sputum, nasal wash, or spinal fluid cultures allows directed antibiotic treatment. Paracentesis to exclude peritonitis is essential in patients with increased or newly recognized ascites and in those with chronic ascites. Cholangitis is particularly common in patients with biliary tract abnormalities or biliary atresia. Direct bile cultures are rarely available, but percutaneous liver biopsy cultures often reveal the specific organisms in refractory cases.

Antibiotic treatment should be instituted empirically and modified according to culture and sensitivity results. The potential for rapid clinical progression in these patients necessitates hospital admission for the initiation of treatment in most cases. Antibiotic coverage to include *Staphylococcus epidermidis*, enterococci, and gram-negative enteric organisms should be administered until culture evidence is available. Use of long-term prophylactic antibiotics promotes the development of resistant organisms and is not recommended. Prophylactic administration of hepatitis B vaccine should be undertaken. Older infants and children should receive all scheduled immunizations and polio vaccine before transplant evaluation when possible. Influenza immunizations are administered to older children but not to neonates or infants.

Education and Psychosocial Concerns.
The family of an infant or child facing liver transplantation must acquire a significant amount of knowledge related to the disease and the transplant process and must become integrated into a complex health care system. This acquisition of knowledge is most appropriately facilitated by the efforts of an interdisciplinary transplant team composed of medical, surgical, nursing, social service, nutritional, and hospital administrative services. Preparation of the patient and the family for transplantation optimally begins at the time of initial diagnosis and progresses throughout the transplant process. A variety of media can be used for family and age-appropriate patient education, including written materials, play therapy, and frequent, direct communication with members of the interdisciplinary transplant team. Liver transplantation disrupts the family's lifestyle and expectations and has profound financial ramifications. For these reasons, anticipatory emotional, spiritual, and financial assessments of the family unit are critical and continue throughout the transplant process.

Psychiatric assessment and support of the entire family unit are highly beneficial, if not critical. Travel and extended-stay accommodation arrangements should be made in advance to minimize confusion and anxiety at the time of transplantation. Because extended preoperative hospitalization is often required in addition to the transplant procedure, financial counseling and support assistance are necessary for most patients.

Operative Procedure
Adequate preoperative preparation for liver transplantation includes provisions for significant perioperative life support. Blood bank resources, including packed red blood cells, platelets, fresh-frozen plasma, and cryoprecipitate to replace two patient blood volumes, should be available. Upper extremity, large-bore intravenous lines, central venous access lines, and an arterial catheter for blood gas and blood pressure measurements are necessary. An underpatient warming blanket and blood and intravenous fluid warmers assist in the difficult temperature management of small recipients. Provisions should be made for inotropic support using dopamine, dobutamine, and epinephrine. As in all complex operative procedures, extensive preoperative and intraoperative communication among the surgical, nursing, and anesthesia team members is invaluable.

Critical junctures in the operative procedure occur at several intervals. Blood loss must be carefully avoided; all losses should be replaced, especially when the native diseased liver is being removed. Previous operative procedures and concurrent portal hypertension complicate this goal. When the native diseased liver is removed, hemodynamic stability often decreases because venous blood return from the lower extremities of the portal system is diminished as a result of the division of the intrahepatic inferior vena cava and portal vein. This problem persists throughout the anhepatic phase (phase without the liver). Careful and extensive flushing of the transplant liver to remove hyperkalemic preservation solutions is necessary to avoid cardiac arrhythmias when circulation to the allograft is restored. After implantation, the body temperature must be returned to normal by vigorous warming, and coagulation function must be reestablished by judicious administration of coagulation factors. The overall operative procedure may require 6 to 18 hours of diligent monitoring and care by the operative team. However, careful operative and anesthetic coordination allows the surgical procedure to proceed without difficulty in most circumstances.

Surgical Techniques
Successful transplantation requires not only meticulous surgical technique but also appropriate donor selection and postoperative care. The surgical options include (1) whole organ transplantation, (2) reduced-size liver transplantation, (3) living related donor transplantation, and (4) auxiliary transplantation.

Whole Organ Transplantation
Replacement of the diseased liver with a size-matched allograft is the standard procedure for older children and adults. In infant recipients, however, an insufficient number of size-matched organs is available for anatomic replacement. Reliance on size-matched livers for transplantation led to a pretransplant waiting list mortality rate of 25% to 50% in many pediatric transplant centers. Even when organs are available from infant donors, the long-term quality and survival of these allografts are still poor. When suitable size-matched donors are available, however, successful transplantation is technically possible.

Whole organ transplantation involves anatomic replacement of the liver with direct vascular reconstruction. Biliary continuity is re-established using a Roux-en-Y hepaticojejunostomy, and an internal biliary Silastic stent is placed because of the small size or absence of the extrahepatic biliary tree in small children (Figure 38-1). Reliance on whole organ replacement techniques does not appear to be feasible for all potential pediatric recipients because the supply of adequate infant donor organs is insufficient. When the outcomes of whole organ and reduced-size liver transplants have been compared, the relative difference in morbidity and mortality has not been significant (Asensio et al, 2001). In many cases a reduced-size liver transplant is done so that the waiting time to transplant is shortened.

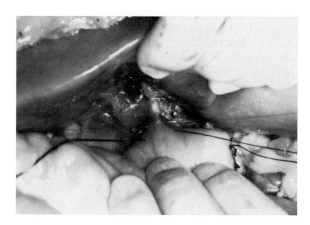

FIGURE **38-1**
Placement of an internal biliary Silastic stent.

Reduced-Size Liver Transplantation. Segmentation of the liver into fully functional but reduced-size allografts has allowed liver transplantation into the smallest recipients. Division along the known anatomic planes in the hepatic parenchyma allows the preparation of various-size liver allografts from larger donor livers (Figures 38-2 and 38-3). Donor to recipient weight ratios of 4:1 are possible with left lobe (segments 1 to 4) reduced-size grafts, and 10:1 ratios are possible using the left lateral segment (segments 2 and 3). Right lobe allografts (segments 5 to 8) are less commonly used in children because of the increased thickness of the right hepatic lobe.

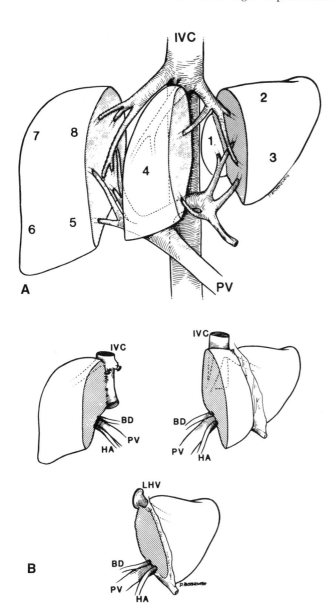

FIGURE **38-2**
Segmental anatomy of the human liver. **A,** Functional allografts can be constructed from segments that have discrete vascular supply and bile drainage. **B,** In practice, the right lobe graft (*upper left*) consists of segments 5 to 8, the left lobe graft (*upper right*) of segments 1 to 4, and the left-lateral segment graft (*lower*) of segments 1 to 3. *IVC,* inferior vena cava; *PV,* portal vein; *HA,* hepatic artery; *LHV,* left hepatic vein, BD, bile duct. From Emond JC, et al. [1989]. Reduced size orthotopic liver transplantation: Use in the management of children with chronic liver disease. *Hepatology,* 10[5], 867–872. Reprinted with permission.

Survival in infants who receive reduced-size allografts is significantly improved over those who receive whole organ transplants (Ryckman et al, 1991a). Survival is improved in these cases because there are fewer life-threatening complications in the postoperative period, including a lower incidence of vascular thrombosis, and the risk of primary nonfunction or biliary complications is not increased.

Split Liver Transplantation. Division of a single donor liver into two usable reduced-size allografts has also been undertaken The results of this procedure, known as split liver grafting, are not as successful as reduced-size allografts, but they are nearly equivalent to whole organ transplantation with respect to survival and complication rates. Some researchers have reported an increase in graft loss after split liver transplantation, but no difference in the ultimate survival rate is seen between whole grafts and split grafts (Langham et al, 2001).

Living Donor Liver Transplantation (LDLT). The use of living related donors for small children has also become a primary mode of transplantation for children. It is especially useful in children experiencing multiple organ system failure and liver failure (Mack et al, 2001). Organ and patient survival results are equivalent to those for reduced-size transplantation. The immunologic advantages of living related donor liver transplants reduce the overall incidence of rejection, although this is not apparent in the initial patient series. Morbidity in the donor is minimal but not absent; death of the donor is rare but possible after the donor hepatectomy.

These options are designed to increase the donor pool to meet the needs of an increasing transplant population. These innovative techniques need continued re-evaluation in light of the donor to recipient mismatch seen in pediatrics and the progressively increasing need for donor organs.

Auxiliary Liver Transplantation. Placement of a second liver in an auxiliary position in the abdomen has been used as a treatment option for metabolic diseases or acute hepatic failure. In infants and small children, the lack of available intraabdominal space to accommodate the transplanted liver mass limits this option. In older children, replacement of the left lobe of the liver using a left lateral segment allograft has successfully corrected metabolic disease without requiring total removal of the recipient's native liver. In acute hepatic failure, recovery of the native liver has been reported while function was supported by the auxiliary graft. Further uses of this technique need to be evaluated. The use of isolated hepatocytes as cellular transplants is also currently under laboratory investigation (Balladur et al, 1995; Hoofnagle et al, 1995).

Postoperative Care

The postoperative care of the liver transplant patient does not differ from that of patients having other extensive operative procedures. Particular attention to temperature management often requires the use of overhead radiant warmers and heating blankets. Intravenous fluid support to maintain central venous pressures of 8 to 10 cm H_2O should ensure adequate perfusion. The hematocrit should be maintained at 35%, and a urine output of 1 to 2 ml/kg/hour is expected. Prophylactic antibiotics directed against *S. epidermidis,* enterococci, and enteric organisms are administered preoperatively, intraoperatively, and for several postoperative doses. Antifungal and antiherpesvirus prophylaxis is also administered. Ventilatory assistance should

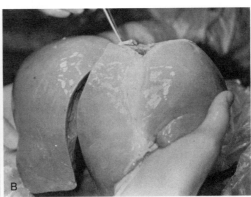

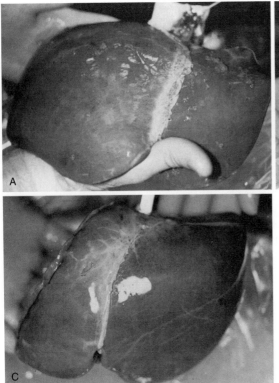

Reduced-sized liver transplant, left lobe allograft surgical preparation. **A,** Whole liver from 25-kg donor before reduction. **B,** Division of liver along interlobar anatomic plane into right and left lobe sections. **C,** Prepared left lobe allograft.

FIGURE **38-3**

be discontinued when adequate blood gases are maintained, organ function is documented, and fluid balance is adequate.

Monitoring of coagulation parameters best assesses the function of the transplanted organ. An increasing Factor VII level establishes hepatocellular recovery. Rapid and accurate daily assessment of allograft blood flow can be done using real-time ultrasonography at the bedside. Episodes of hypotension, acidosis, fever, or deterioration of hepatocellular enzyme or coagulation profiles require immediate and vigorous investigation. Vascular complications also can arise with liver transplantation; these can be detected by use of Doppler ultrasonography (Ganschow et al, 2001).

Immunosuppressive Management

In addition to prednisone, primary immunosuppressive management in infants and children includes cyclosporine or tacrolimus. Azathioprine is used in some centers as part of a cyclosporine-based initial immunotherapy program. It is usually discontinued early in the post-transplant period. Rejection is treated with steroid pulses, steroid recycling, or the monoclonal anti-T-cell antibody muromonab-CD3 (Orthoclone OKT3). Daily monitoring of immunosuppressive medications is necessary for proper dose adjustment in infants and children in whom intestinal absorption is variable. One of the major side effects of immunosuppressive therapy is arterial hypertension; this complication must always be anticipated as an essential feature of postoperative care (Ganschow et al, 2001).

Postoperative Complications

Many complications after liver transplantation are heralded by an increase in hepatocellular enzymes, often associated with malaise, fever, leukocytosis, and jaundice. This clinical picture defines hepatic allograft dysfunction, but it does not separate allograft rejection from other allograft complications such as primary nonfunction, bile duct abnormalities, hepatic artery thrombosis, or allograft infection. The use of real-time and Doppler ultrasonography to assess hepatic vasculature and the use of computed tomography (CT) to assess allograft structure are often necessary. Allograft biopsy is definitive when the cause of the graft abnormality is rejection; it can strongly support the diagnosis of viral infection or cholangitis when the characteristic histologic markers and microscopic appearance are seen. Definitive diagnosis of the cause of the allograft dysfunction should precede immunologic manipulation. Selected complications unique to liver transplantation are outlined in the following sections.

Primary Nonfunction.   Primary nonfunction is defined as a failure of the transplant allograft to recover function despite successful operative implantation. Careful evaluation of the donor allograft, using frozen section biopsy, can assist in identifying failures associated with primary nonfunction, such as allograft stenosis (Markin et al, 1993; Strasberg et al, 1994). Since the introduction of University of Wisconsin preservation solution, initial nonfunction of the transplanted allograft is uncommon. In our experience, initial nonfunction occurs in 2% of cases, regardless of allograft type. Hepatic allograft preservation for up to 24 hours can be accomplished; however, preservation times of less than 12 hours are associated with excellent organ function after reperfusion. When primary nonfunction occurs, rapidly increasing levels of hepatocellular enzymes and bilirubin are accompanied by failure of functional recovery, manifested by an uncorrectable coagulopathy. Treatment with prostaglandin E_2 has been helpful in restoring hepatocellular function in nonrandomized trials in primary nonfunction, although controlled trials to support its use have not been undertaken. Retransplantation is required if no functional improvement is recognized within 48 hours.

Rejection.   Acute cellular rejection occurs in up to 95% of patients treated by conventional immunosuppressive protocols using prednisone, cyclosporine, and azathioprine (Ryckman et al, 1991b). In our experience, when sequential induction immunotherapy using Orthoclone OKT3, prednisone, and azathioprine is combined with delayed introduction of cyclosporine, the incidence of rejection is reduced to 46% (Ryckman et al, 1991b). Rejection episodes are treated aggressively with methylprednisolone or Orthoclone OKT3 and are reversible in 95% of cases. When medical therapy for rejection fails, retransplantation is required.

Bile Duct Complications.   Biliary leak or stricture formation at the site of the surgical anastomosis or within the liver parenchyma can result from prolonged or incomplete ischemia preservation or from viral infection; however, these complications most often occur after hepatic artery thrombosis. Treatment is individualized and includes anastomotic revision, percutaneous dilation and internal stent placement, or retransplantation. Bile duct disruption with intrahepatic biloma formation can also occur. Adequate drainage using percutaneous techniques is necessary at the time of diagnosis to prevent the formation of an intrahepatic abscess. Resolution may occur with prolonged drainage, although allograft replacement is often required because of the extensive bile duct injury. Associated infection complications are common with all bile duct abnormalities, most often with a combination of enteral bacteria and fungal organisms. Vigorous antimicrobial treatment must accompany restoration of unobstructed bile flow (Peclet et al, 1994).

Hepatic Artery Thrombosis.   Clotting within the arterial circulation of the transplanted liver occurs in approximately 15% of all patients, with the incidence inversely proportional to the recipient's size at the time of transplantation and the age of the liver donor. Early thrombosis manifests with signs of fulminant hepatic failure, biliary leak or stricture, or systemic sepsis. Immediate thrombectomy is occasionally successful. When ischemia allograft damage has occurred, retransplantation is nearly always required. Late thrombosis can manifest similarly or may be silent. The incidence of arterial thrombosis is lower with reduced-size allografts, possibly because of the improved stability of the donor, the larger size of the arterial vasculature in these older donors, or the direct implantation of the hepatic artery into the infrarenal aorta (Ryckman et al, 1991b).

Retransplantation.   In all cases of irreversible liver failure after transplantation, retransplantation is the only option that allows survival. The use of reduced-size liver allografts has greatly improved the likelihood of a replacement allograft being located within the abbreviated time frame imposed by allograft failure. Retransplantation rates of 15% are common in pediatric series involving small infant recipients (Ryckman et al, 1991b). Survival after retransplantation is similar to survival after primary transplantation and is directly related to the severity of the recipient's illness before the operation.

Long-Term Survival of Transplantation
Survival after liver transplantation is directly related to the severity of the patient's illness before surgical therapy. Despite

the serious complications regularly encountered in these individuals, the overall survival rate is rewarding. The current overall survival rate for pediatric transplantation is about 80% (Ryckman et al, 1991a). Improvements in immunosuppressive therapy, anesthetic and perioperative management, and innovative surgical procedures such as reduced-size or living related liver transplantation have all improved patient survival (Ryckman et al, 1991a, 1991b). Survival has historically been diminished by the following factors: (1) small patient size and weight, (2) previous extensive operative procedures, and (3) severe disease at the time of transplantation. Improved preoperative care, careful donor selection, use of innovative technical procedures, and evolving immunosuppressive management promise further increases in recipient survival.

Improved survival of infants and children after transplantation has allowed health care professionals to focus on the overall goals of complete rehabilitation with appropriate growth and development, social reintegration, enhanced self-esteem, and improved quality of life. Recent advances in post-transplant management have been directed at minimizing complications related to immunosuppression, enhancing growth velocity, and promoting normalcy and lifestyle improvement (Sokal, 1995). Increased energy and motor dexterity, a decrease in the number of medications and hospitalizations, success in school, and attainment of satisfying peer relationships have been seen in our pediatric liver transplant population, as well as in other centers, and these attributes have contributed to the perception of an improved quality of life.

After transplantation, establishment of a satisfactory lifestyle should remain as important a goal as patient survival. Currently, all of our surviving recipients have returned to a normal lifestyle for their age and have shown satisfactory developmental progress consistent with their age and developmental status before transplantation. This experience has been seen in other centers as well.

RENAL TRANSPLANTATION IN INFANTS AND CHILDREN

Through the vast strides made with extensive experience in older children and adults, renal transplantation in infants and children has become an increasing reality. Recent advances in the techniques of dialysis and the management of end-stage renal disease (ESRD) in infants have allowed many patients with complex urologic or hereditary abnormalities to reach the age and size at which transplantation is possible. These advances have allowed the implementation of renal transplantation, along with dialysis, as a complementary treatment in the care of infants with irreversible renal dysfunction.

Etiology
Acute renal failure in infants is most often the consequence of hemodynamic instability, hypoxia, or malperfusion, resulting in acute tubular necrosis. Most of these infants either recover sufficient function for normal long-term survival or die of multisystem failure. Chronic renal failure is uncommon in infants. Congenital nephrosis, dysplasia-hypoplasia, and other anatomic abnormalities associated with complex urogenital malformations are the common causes of ESRD in infants. In children younger than 5 years of age who have glomerulonephritis, 46% have a congenital cause for ESRD. Lupus nephritis and recurrent pyelonephritis, which are more common in older patients, are uncommon causes of ESRD in the infant. Hereditary causes of renal failure are important to identify in planning the appro-

priate overall treatment strategy; evaluation of other family members and provision of genetic counseling, when needed, must also be considered. Appropriate identification of the cause of the ESRD also allows assessment of the potential for recurrence within a transplant allograft and consideration of living related donor transplantation.

Pretransplant Management

A better understanding of fluid and electrolyte management and the introduction of dialysis techniques suitable for small infants have significantly improved the management of infants with renal failure. These advances, coupled with improvements in infant nutritional support and medical management, allow extended survival for the infant with ESRD.

Dialysis

Dialysis is indicated in infants, as in older children, if complications of medical management of ESRD occur, namely, hyperkalemia, volume overload, acidosis, intractable hypertension, and uremic symptoms, such as vomiting. In addition, dialysis may be necessary to allow administration of adequate protein as part of an extensive nutritional resuscitation plan. However, there is no requirement that dialysis be undertaken before transplantation in infants or children. In the North American Pediatric Renal Transplant Cooperative Study (NAPRTCS), 22% of children underwent transplantation without previous dialysis (McEnery et al, 1992). If dialysis is undertaken, peritoneal dialysis is preferred for the following reasons: (1) it avoids the multiple transfusions associated with hemodialysis, (2) it allows smoother gradual correction of electrolyte abnormalities, preventing cerebral disequilibrium syndrome in small infants; and (3) it is easier to perform. Hemodialysis can be used in infants with an unsuitable peritoneal cavity or a peritoneal infection; however, the construction and maintenance of adequate vascular access in small infants and children are difficult. Use of centralized venous catheters rather than arteriovenous fistulas is our preferred mode for hemodialysis access in small children, although infection and vascular clotting difficulties complicate this therapy. One of the major complications of long-term dialysis is cardiovascular disease. This complication accounts for about 25% of the mortality in children on dialysis versus receiving a renal transplant (Chavers & Schnaper, 2001). More research is needed to obtain an accurate account of cardiovascular disease and of death from this cause in children with ESRD.

Nutritional Support

The need for vigorous nutritional support of the infant with uremia has been verified by the well-documented growth retardation seen in infants and children with ESRD. The cause of growth disturbance is multifactorial and includes both protein and calorie insufficiency, renal osteodystrophy, aluminum toxicity, acidosis, impaired somatomedin activity, and insulin resistance. Because the most intense period of growth occurs during the first 2 years of life, careful nutritional support during that time is essential. According to the recent NAPRTCS findings, despite extensive nutritional efforts, the mean height for all patients at the time of transplantation was 2.2 standard deviations (SD) below the appropriate age- and sex-adjusted mean for normal children. This growth deficit was greater (-2.8 SD) in children younger than 5 years of age. Transplantation afforded a $+0.8$ SD increase in growth over the first post-transplant year; however, this accelerated growth then

reached a stable plateau. After 2 to 3 years, the mean weight values were comparable to those in normal children (McEnery et al, 1992). If epiphyseal closure has occurred, additional bone growth (bone age older than 12 years) is often not achieved. Normalization of growth rarely occurs with the introduction of either hemodialysis or peritoneal dialysis.

The importance of efforts to normalize nutritional parameters is emphasized by the adverse impact of uremia on the developing nervous system in the infant. Monitoring of the head circumference has been suggested as a means to identify the infant at risk, with subsequent initiation of dialysis, nutritional support, or transplantation if this parameter deviates from the normal curve.

Transplant Management

Preoperative Evaluation. In addition to assessment of nutritional parameters, extensive evaluation of the patient's urinary tract and immunologic status is necessary before transplantation. The increased incidence of urinary tract abnormalities as the primary cause of ESRD in infants and children necessitates investigation of the urinary tract for sites of obstruction and the presence of ureteral reflux; the functional state and capacity of the urinary bladder must also be determined. This investigation is best accomplished by obtaining an intravenous pyelogram or sonogram to evaluate the upper urinary tract and a voiding cystourethrogram to assess bladder and reflux parameters. Any questions related to bladder function or structure require cystometry and cystoscopy. In infants with long-standing oliguric ESRD, the bladder capacity may appear very small. In the absence of an abnormal obstructive or a neuromuscular pathologic condition of the bladder, adequate enlargement of the bladder with normal urinary production is to be expected. Any surgical correction of urethral obstruction or augmentation of bladder size should be undertaken far in advance of transplantation. Preoperative sterilization of the urinary tract and the development of unobstructed urinary outflow should be the ultimate goals of evaluation and reconstruction. Although complex anomalies of the urogenital tract often require many extensive operative procedures to augment, reconstruct, or create an acceptable lower urinary tract, virtually all children with such anomalies can undergo successful reconstruction with continent urinary reservoirs without the use of intestinal conduits (Sheldon et al, 1994).

Immunologic assessment includes tissue typing and panel reactive antibody analysis. Patients should be monitored periodically for the development of a positive crossmatch to their potential donor or the development of positive cytotoxic antibody to a panel of random donors to assess immunologic reactivity. In addition, reactivity to cytomegalovirus, Epstein-Barr virus, herpes simplex virus, and hepatitis should be investigated. Childhood immunizations should be current, and immunization against the hepatitis B virus should be instituted when indicated. Any immunizations with live virus vaccines should be given well in advance of transplantation because their use is contraindicated in the early post-transplant period.

Selection of the appropriate donor source for transplantation is a decision for the transplant team and family to consider together. A living related donor kidney from an immediate family member has the advantage of a low incidence of postoperative acute tubular necrosis; improved histologic matching, leading to fewer rejection episodes and the need for less immunosuppression; and the possibility of extended organ function. In addition, the operative procedures required for preparation and the transplant procedure can be scheduled around the needs of the patient, simplifying preoperative care and potentially avoiding the complications of dialysis. Parents account for most donors; siblings younger than 18 years of age are not considered. Currently about half of children receive a living related donor kidney. Cadaveric kidneys are successfully transplanted in infants and children, with improved results when sequential immunotherapy and cyclosporine or tacrolimus is used. The unpredictability of donor organ availability and the need to establish a negative antibody cross-match for cadaver transplantation make surgical planning more difficult.

The size of the allograft, cadaveric or living related, is important. Adult kidneys from small-size donors can be transplanted into infants weighing as little as 5 kg with good technical success. Cadaveric organs from pediatric donors older than 4 years of age are most appropriate and should be used preferentially in pediatric recipients when possible. However, a progressive decrease in 1-year graft survival has been observed when kidneys from donors younger than 3 years of age have been used. This decrease in graft and patient survival is related to the donor organ source, because infants and children younger than 5 years old who receive organs from older children and adults enjoy similar survival to the overall pediatric population using living related donors. Caution should be exercised when using donors younger than 3 years of age until the factors responsible for this decreased graft survival are defined. The decision to use a cadaveric donor is often strengthened by the likelihood of disease recurrence in the transplanted kidney. In small infants, a cadaveric kidney may be recommended for short-term improvement, with the use of a living related donor kidney reserved for the later expected growth needs of the developing child, when the larger kidney can be more easily implanted.

Because of the relatively small number of suitable cadaveric allografts for the pediatric population, ABO-incompatible living donors have been successfully used. Shishido and colleagues (2001) have reported use of such donors from 1989 to the present. When the immunoglobulin and isoagglutinin titers are followed, patient survival was 100% with no antibody-related rejection. More research at other centers is needed to support these findings.

Operative Procedure.   Preparation for transplantation should include the placement of adequate large-bore intravenous lines and the largest Foley catheter possible. Central venous lines are used in all infants and children to ensure vascular access and a route for postoperative immunosuppressive delivery. Perioperative prophylactic antibiotics are administered.

Transplantation in infants and small children can be undertaken through a generous retroperitoneal approach or transabdominal placing of the allograft in the peritoneal cavity posterior to the right or left colon. Retroperitoneal placement allows maintenance of postoperative peritoneal dialysis and should be strongly considered with cadaveric allografts when size permits. The arterial anastomosis should be to the distal aorta using a Carrel patch, and venous outflow of the allograft should be to the inferior vena cava or common iliac vein. Ureteral implantation using the Lich external ureteroneocystostomy avoids a cystotomy and minimizes postoperative blood clots in the bladder, which may obstruct the Foley catheter.

Anesthetic management of the infant and small child during both liver and kidney transplantation is complex. The intravascular blood volume must be augmented during allograft implantation to allow restoration of flow to the kidney without sudden sequestration of blood in the allograft, precipitating hypotension. In addition, blood sequestered in the lower extremities during caval and aortic occlusion is acidotic and hyperkalemic. Efforts to remove the hyperkalemic graft preservation solution before implantation are necessary to avoid massive potassium infusion with reconstitution of allograft perfusion. Blood volume loading to a central venous pressure of 13 to 15 cm H_2O and administration of bicarbonate, calcium, and insulin-glucose mixtures may be necessary. Vasopressors (dopamine, dobutamine, epinephrine) should be immediately available in the operating room.

Postoperative Management.   Fluid and electrolyte monitoring every 15 to 30 minutes is necessary immediately after transplantation, because adult kidneys can excrete the equivalent of the infant's blood volume within a single hour. Careful attention to serum concentrations of calcium, phosphorus, and magnesium, in addition to electrolytes, is necessary. Glucose-free urine replacement fluids minimize hyperglycemia and attendant osmotic diuresis in the recipient. Maintenance of catheter patency is essential, and any episode of decreased urinary output should be rapidly investigated to exclude Foley catheter occlusion and bladder distention.

Immunosuppression.   Many immunosuppressive regimens are available, and they all share a similar strategy. Our current preference is sequential immunotherapy using antilymphocyte globulin, azathioprine, and steroids at the time of transplantation, with the introduction of cyclosporine after demonstration of stable renal function. Maintenance immunotherapy uses cyclosporine, azathioprine, and steroids. It is hoped that by using multiple agents, steroid dosing can be minimized and growth parameters maximized in infants and children.

Overall, half of all transplant recipients have a bout of rejection within 2 months of transplantation. Factors that increase the likelihood of rejection or long-term graft loss include the use of cadaveric donors rather than living related donors, use of a kidney from a donor younger than 5 years of age, allowing the kidney to remain in cold storage longer than 24 hours, African American race, and delayed graft function caused by acute tubular necrosis. Rejection episodes are treated with steroids or monoclonal anti-T-cell agents, such as Orthoclone OKT3. As with liver transplantation, tacrolimus can be used in place of cyclosporine, and in conjunction with steroids.

Basiliximab is another medication being added to tacrolimus and prednisone to reduce the chance of acute rejection. In a randomized controlled trial, the group of children that received basiliximab in addition to other immunosuppressive agents showed a rejection rate of 26%; the rate was 43% in the group that did not receive basiliximab (Swiatecka-Urban et al, 2001). More research is needed in this area.

Post-Transplant Management.   Post-transplant management requires careful screening for rejection and for recurrence of the primary renal disease, as well as prevention of immunosuppression-related complications. Any pre-existing hypertension is augmented by the immunosuppressive drugs cyclosporine, tacrolimus, and prednisone. Careful attention to pretransplant control of hypertension and dietary management improves post-transplant management. Antihypertensive control is especially important to preserve all possible renal function when using small allografts in infants. Development of hypertension more than 3 months after transplantation suggests the possibility of renal artery stenosis and warrants ultrasonographic Doppler flow studies and arteriography in questionable cases. Transluminal angioplasty has been successful in managing most of these cases; surgical correction is reserved for angioplasty failures. High-resolution ultrasonography is assisting in the early detection of arterial compromise in the allografts. Research is under way to examine the use of this technology to reduce vascular complications (Herz et al, 2001). However, the procedure requires anesthesia and is not without risk.

Most long-term complications are related to infection and occur within the first 6 post-transplant months. During this time immunosuppression is greater, as is susceptibility to life-threatening infection. The use of organs from donors who had prior exposure to cytomegalovirus and Epstein-Barr virus in infants and children who are seronegative enhances the risk of these specific infections. Expanded use of antiviral prophylaxis with ganciclovir and acyclovir has diminished the intensity of these infections and their associated morbidity or mortality. Trimethoprim-sulfamethoxazole is used for *Pneumocystis carinii* pneumonia prophylaxis. Chronic steroid toxicity that manifests as posterior subcapsular cataracts, excessive weight gain, hyperlipidemia, or aseptic necrosis of the bone must be carefully sought and treated.

Results of Renal Transplantation. The overall results of renal transplantation in children are similar to those in adults. Overall, the 1-year transplant graft survival rate is 75% to 100%, regardless of whether living related or cadaveric allografts are used. These optimistic results further support the need for rapid transplantation in children with ESRD to avoid the secondary growth and developmental consequences.

OTHER TRANSPLANTS

Hepatic and renal transplants are the common types of transplantation in the pediatric population. However, other types of transplantation are growing in number.

Cardiac Transplants

Newborn and infant cardiac diseases are often related to genetic factors (Towbin & Lipshultz, 1999). These problems carry a high mortality rate. Loma Linda has reported that 75% of its pediatric patients who have undergone transplantation since 1999 required the procedure because of congenital heart disease (del Rio, 2000). Of these the most common cause was hypoplastic left heart. Of the children who underwent this procedure, a 77% survival rate was reported in the neonatal population. This rate was higher than that for older children with cardiomyopathy (63% survival rate) (del Rio, 2000). Pediatric or adolescent heart donors are ideal for newborn and infant recipients, because older hearts tend to have the beginnings of atherosclerotic changes (UNOS, 2001). The survival rate for adolescents undergoing transplantation is 58% from older donors and 85% from younger ones (UNOS, 2001). It is extrapolated that the same differences would hold true for the newborn and infant recipients and donors.

With the advent of effective immunosuppressive agents that can be safely used in newborns and infants, cardiac transplants in those age groups are becoming more common. The most common complication, graft coronary artery disease, also carries the highest morbidity and mortality rates (Luiart, 2001).

Another therapy used either before or after transplantation is extracorporeal membrane oxygenation (ECMO). The Extracorporeal Life Support Organization (ELSO) Registry reports that of 95 centers that responded to a questionnaire (81% response rate), 36 did neonatal and pediatric cardiac transplants, and of these, 29 centers use ECMO to support cardiac transplant patients (Hopper et al, 1999). The survey found that there is no consistency among the centers in the way ECMO is used in this population. This area is in need of further research.

Intestinal Transplants

Intestinal transplants also are increasingly being used in newborns and infants. Children requiring intestinal grafts are those who have experienced intestinal failure secondary to other life-threatening illnesses. Because of their need for total parenteral nutrition (TPN), some of the children may also have liver failure, resulting in a need for liver and small bowel allografts (Bueno et al, 2000). The number of children requiring such transplants is growing, therefore it is important to increase the donor pool through preservation of the head of the pancreas and the sparing of the duodenal area. Composite liver and small bowel allografts have shown promise in reducing morbidity and mortality (Bueno et al, 2000), but further research is needed to determine pretransplantation and post-transplantation treatment protocols.

Children with short bowel syndrome constitute another group that requires intestinal transplants. The syndrome may arise from complications of necrotizing enterocolitis (NEC). Bowel resection is performed in most of these infants, but some go on to develop short bowel syndrome in which only a small portion of the bowel, if any, is functional. The only choices basically are a life of TPN or a transplant. In a retrospective study, University of Miami researchers reported good outcomes for prematurely born infants who developed NEC and then went on to have short bowel syndrome and, ultimately, intestinal transplants (Vennarecci et al, 2000). These researchers found that survival without TPN was possible and that the reported quality of life was improved. However, this was one center reporting on 10 patients with NEC who had had, on average, five intestinal surgeries before the transplant, among whom transplantation resulted in a 60% survival rate (Vennarecci et al., 2000). Although these results are encouraging, more research is needed.

Other centers throughout the world have reported small bowel transplantation in small children. Most of these procedures are for short bowel syndrome, intractable neonatal diarrhea, Hirschsprung's disease, or combined liver and bowel disease (Jan et al, 1999). Whatever the reason, immunosuppressive therapy with tacrolimus, azathioprine, and corticosteroids is a cornerstone of therapy. This treatment improves the survival rate and reduces the overall rejection rate in children with intestinal failure (Jan et al, 1999).

Stem Cell and Bone Marrow Transplantation

Stem cells are cells that can rapidly divide but that are not yet committed to a specific function. They are referred to as pluripotent because they are not specialized. Rather, they can be induced to divide and supply missing types of cells. As they become specialized, stem cells are considered to be multipotent. They can serve multiple specialized purposes. When certain immune factors are missing, the stem cells can reproduce and make up for this gap. Genes turn on and off the cellular division. Some of the findings from the Human Genome

Project will help us to better understand the role genes play in this process.

Stem cells are present in the umbilical cord. These undifferentiated cells can boost the immune system in ways other cells cannot. They can be extracted from the cord blood to form blood cells such as platelets, white blood cells, and red blood cells, as well as other hematologic and immunologic cells. When stem cells were injected into a newborn suffering from, for example, beta-thalassemia, B-lymphocytes and natural killer cells increased to levels above the normal amounts found in neonatal blood. However, in this same condition, when neonatal blood from a related donor was used as therapy, the granulocyte/macrophage colony-forming units, the erythroid colony-forming units, the erythroid burst-forming units, and the long-term culture initiating cells all increased to levels higher than those found in cord blood (Liu et al, 1999). This may mean that neonatal blood transfusions, in some instances, are as good if not better than cord blood. Further research is needed to support these findings. Beta-thalassemia is but one condition for which stem cell transplants are used. More of the transplants are done for severe immunosuppression.

Umbilical cord blood transplants (UCBT) and stem cell transplants (SCT) are growing in number, and allogeneic bone marrow transplants (BMT) are no longer the only treatment available. Reports from 121 transplant centers in 29 countries indicate that the overall survival rate for unrelated UCBT is comparable to that for BMT (Gluckman, et al, 2001). These patients are not all children, but no specific data are re-ported separately for the pediatric population. It is an area of further study for pediatrics, and specifically for newborns and infants.

Other research has compared early postnatal bone marrow transplants to in utero transplantation of the same tissue for the treatment of severe combined immunodeficiency (SCID). The researchers found that the early postnatal bone marrow transplants were more successful with regard to graft-versus-host reactions and survival without problems than the in utero procedures (Kane et al, 2001). In addition, SCT shows promise as a successful treatment for SCID, one of the more serious immunologic problems (see Chapters 29 and 30 for more information on stem cells).

Anytime transplantation is performed, immunosuppressive therapy is required to reduce the possibility of rejection. Because this therapy suppresses vital factors that act as the body's defense against infection, there is always concern that the infant may contract a nosocomial infection or other disease. Safeguards must be in place to ensure protection against infection. The use of steroids also can have adverse effects on the metabolic and endocrine systems.

Families must be aided in their efforts to understand the condition, the treatment, and the long-term consequences of the selected therapies. For the most part, the family needs help in coping with life-threatening illness. Once the infant is home, the parents may feel overwhelmed by their responsibility to manage technologic devices and medications. The nurse must make sure that appropriate referrals are made for such services as genetic counseling, if appropriate, psychologic and financial counseling, home care services, and community support services.

ORGAN PROCUREMENT

A problem common to all types of transplantation is donor organ availability. This problem is intensified in small pediatric recipients by a relative maldistribution of donors and recipients, because the most common pediatric organ donor is in the midchildhood to teenage years. This problem is most significant for liver, heart, and lung transplant recipients, because the donor organ must be a special size; that is, matched to the size of the diseased organ to be removed. The increasing discrepancy between the supply and demand for organs has forced the creation of more criteria for the selection of recipients and donors, and more policies and procedures have had to be developed for the organ procurement process.

Organ procurement and distribution are monitored and managed through the United Network for Organ Sharing (UNOS), a congressionally mandated organization. Computer-generated scoring systems take into account tissue or blood type matching, organ size, disease severity, and donor location to direct distribution of allografts. The ultimate donor organ selection and acceptance are the responsibilities of the transplant team. However, UNOS has made the pediatric population a priority for liver, kidney, and heart transplants (UNOS, 2001).

A surgical team composed of specialists in multiple organ harvest and preservation undertakes operative removal of the donor organ. Multiple organs, including the heart, lung, liver, pancreas, kidneys, and intestine, can all be sequentially harvested from a single donor using hypothermic preservation techniques. Other tissue grafts, such as cornea, skin, bone, heart valves, and tendons, can be removed after the solid perfused organs have been removed successfully. Simple hypothermic sterile packaging is used to preserve the organs for transport to the recipient's transplant center.

Preservation times have been significantly prolonged by the University of Wisconsin preservation solution; cold ischemic preservation times exceed 48 hours for kidney allografts, 18 hours for liver allografts, and 24 hours for pancreas allografts. Heart and heart-lung preservation times are limited to 4 to 6 hours.

The current success of transplantation has led to a vast discrepancy between donor organ availability and the rapidly increasing recipient waiting lists. Only through increased donor organ acquisition, achieved by creative surgical options and improved professional and community education, can the goals and success of pediatric transplantation be offered to all potential recipients.

Three databases have been established to track transplants for the pediatric age group. They are NAPRTCS (pediatric kidney transplants), SPLIT (liver transplants), and the Pediatric Heart Transplantation Study Group. UNOS (2001) reports that survival and success rates are higher in centers that do transplants on a routine basis. They house the data that can help health professionals inform families about available transplant centers. These databases also provide useful information to health professionals and the families they serve.

SUMMARY

Transplantation offers the possibility of relief from the complications of end-stage liver and renal failure in infants and small children. However, these procedures treat the primary disease only at the cost of the potential complications of long-term immunosuppressive treatment. Only through the development of new and innovative transplant techniques and through further research into the mechanisms of transplant tolerance can the hope for safe and successful transplantation become reality for all patients with end-stage organ failure. Increasing emphasis is being placed on other types of transplants in the pediatric population. These include cardiac, intestinal, bone marrow, and stem cell transplants. Only time will tell what new horizons will be reached in the newborn and infant populations and in the ability to "grow our own organs" for transplant.

REFERENCES

Asensio M et al (2001). Comparative study of reduced-size and whole liver transplantation in children. *Circulation pediatrics*, 14(3), 116-120.

Balladur P et al (1995). Transplantation of allogenic hepatocytes without immunosuppression: long-term survival. *Surgery*, 117(2), 189-194.

Bueno J et al (2000). Composite liver-small bowel allografts with preservation of donor duodenum and hepatic biliary system in children. *Journal of pediatric surgery*, 35(2), 291-295.

Chavers B, Schnaper HW (2001). Risk factors for cardiovascular disease in children on maintenance dialysis. *Advances in renal replacement therapies*, 8(3), 180-190.

Colombani PM, McDonald RA (2001). *Report of the OPTN/UNOS pediatric transplant committee to the board of directors*. OPTN/UNOS Pediatric Transplant Committee: San Diego.

del Rio MJ (2000). Transplantation in complex congenital heart disease. *Progressive pediatric cardiology*, 11(2), 107-113.

Emond JC et al (1989). Reduced-size orthotopic liver transplantation: use in the management of children with chronic liver disease. *Hepatology*, 10(5), 867-872.

Emond JC et al (1990). Transplantation of two patients with one liver: analysis of a preliminary experience with "split-liver" grafting. *Annals of surgery*, 212(1), 14-22.

Ganschow R et al (2001). Intensive care management after pediatric liver transplantation: a single-center experience. *Pediatric transplantation*, 4(4), 273-279.

Gluckman E et al (2001). Results of unrelated umbilical cord blood hematopoietic stem cell transplant. *Transfusion clinical biology*, 8(3), 146-154.

Herz DB et al (2001). High-resolution ultrasound characterization of early allograft hemodynamics in pediatric living-related renal transplantation. *Journal of urology*, 166(5), 1853-1858.

Hoofnagle JH et al (1995). Fulminant hepatic failure: summary of a workshop. *Hepatology*, 21(1), 240-252 (review).

Hopper AO et al (1999). Extracorporeal membrane oxygenation for perioperative support in neonatal and pediatric cardiac transplant. *Artificial organs*, 23(11), 1006-1009.

Jan D et al (1999). Up-to-date evolution of small bowel transplantation in children with intestinal failure. *Journal of pediatric surgery*, 34(5), 841-843.

Kane L et al (2001). Neonatal bone marrow transplantation for severe combined immunodeficiency. *Archives of disease in childhood (fetal & neonatal)*, 85, F110-F113.

Langham MR Jr et al (2001). Graft survival in pediatric liver transplantation. *Journal of pediatric surgery*, 36(8), 1205-1209.

Li Liu J et al (1999). Human neonatal blood: stem cell content, kinetics of cd34+ cell decline and ex vivo expansion capacity. *British journal of haematology*, 104(1), 178-185.

Luiart H (2001). Pediatric cardiac transplantation: management issues. *Journal of pediatric nursing*, 16(5), 320-331.

Mack CL et al (2001). Living donor liver transplantation for children with liver failure and concurrent multiple organ system failure. *Liver transplant*, 7(10), 890-895.

Malatack JJ et al (1987). Choosing a pediatric recipient for orthotopic liver transplantation. *Journal of pediatrics*, 111(4), 479-489.

Markin RS et al (1993). Frozen section evaluation of donor livers before transplantation. *Transplantation*, 56(6), 1403-1409.

McEnery PT et al (1992). Renal transplantation in children: a report of the North American Pediatric Renal Transplant Cooperative Study. *New England journal of medicine*, 326(26), 1727-1732.

Peclet MH et al (1994). The spectrum of bile duct complications in pediatric liver transplantation. *Journal of pediatric surgery*, 29(2), 214-220.

Ryckman FC et al (1991a). Segmental orthotopic hepatic transplantation as a means to improve patient survival and diminish waiting list mortality. *Journal of pediatric surgery*, 26(4), 422-428.

Ryckman FC et al (1991b). The use of monoclonal immunosuppressive therapy in pediatric renal and liver transplantation. *Clinical transplantation*, 5, 189.

Sheldon CA et al (1994). Renal transplantation into the dysfunctional bladder: the role of adjunctive bladder reconstruction. *Journal of urology*, 152(3), 972-975.

Shishido S et al (2001). ABO-incompatible living donor kidney transplantation in children. *Transplantation*, 72(6), 1037-1042.

Sokal EM (1995). Quality of life after orthotopic liver transplantation in children: an overview of physical, psychological, and social outcome. *European journal of pediatrics*, 154(3), 171-175 (review).

Strasberg SM et al (1994). Selecting the donor liver: risk factors for poor function after orthotopic liver transplantation. *Hepatology*, 20(4 part 1), 829-838 (review).

Swiatecka-Urban A et al (2001). Basiliximab induction improves the outcome of renal transplants in children and adolescents. *Pediatric nephrology*, 16(9), 693-696.

Towbin JA, Lipshultz SE (1999). Genetics of neonatal cardiomyopathy. *Current opinions in cardiology*, 14(3), 250-262.

United Network for Organ Sharing (UNOS) (2001). United Network for Organ Sharing rules and organ availability for children: current policies and future directions. *Pediatric transplantation*, 5(5), 311-316.

Vennarecci G et al (2000). Intestinal transplantation for short gut syndrome attributable to necrotizing enterocolitis. *Pediatrics*, 105(2), E25.

CHAPTER 39

ASSESSMENT AND MANAGEMENT OF THE SUBSTANCE-EXPOSED NEWBORN AND INFANT

DEBORAH L. FIKE

Drug abuse by women of childbearing age is on the rise at all levels of society, and as a result, more and more pregnancies are complicated by substance abuse. This chapter discusses the effects of prenatal exposure to tobacco, cocaine, heroin, alcohol, methamphetamine, and 3,4 methylenedioxymethamphetamine (MDMA, or "Ecstasy"). The effects of each substance are considered separately. However, nurses should realize that often several substances are abused simultaneously, making it difficult to ascertain which substance causes which effect. This determination may be further complicated by an interactive effect of two or more drugs, by adulterants used to dilute illicit drugs, or by both of these factors.

The physical, psychosocial, and financial concerns related to substance abuse do not end with birth but continue throughout childhood. Through long-term prospective studies, health care professionals have become knowledgeable about the deleterious perinatal effects of substance abuse. It is now the responsibility of those professionals to educate the public about these grave and far-reaching consequences.

DEFINITIONS

The following definitions are used in this chapter:
- *Low birth weight (LBW):* 2500 g or less regardless of gestational age (Fletcher, 1999)
- *Preterm:* Born before 37 completed weeks of gestation (Fletcher, 1999)
- *Small for gestational age (SGA):* Infants whose birth weight is more than two standard deviations below the mean or less than the 10th percentile of a population-specific birth weight versus gestational age plot (Anderson & Hay, 1999)

NURSING CONSIDERATIONS

Nurses are in a pivotal position to effect change through dissemination of health-related information to the diverse individuals with whom they work. Nursing education includes a liberal base of interviewing techniques, active listening and, of course, the nursing process. Nurses are able to polish these skills daily by working with their patients.

Because of the rapid and widespread growth of substance abuse, all nurses must be taught interviewing strategies that enhance self-reporting of tobacco, alcohol, and drug use. When such interviews are conducted with all patients, nurses become adept at detecting subtle cues or inferences that may be explored with further questioning. However, even with the best interviewing strategies, substance abuse is underreported, particularly the use of negatively sanctioned substances such as alcohol and street drugs. Women often underreport such use because they do not want to receive health teaching on the merits of stopping and because they know that substance use during pregnancy is socially unacceptable. They also may fear loss of their infants through child protection laws. Although underreporting is a problem, if women are not asked about substance use, they do not spontaneously divulge the information. Until a better screening method for substance use is developed, a thorough history is the best available tool to elicit the information.

Prenatal education about substance abuse is essential. Programs that provide information before conception, such as during health classes in high school or during routine gynecologic examinations, would be beneficial. The overall emphasis should be on promoting a healthier lifestyle for young women of childbearing age. This strategy could ameliorate the problem of fetal damage caused by drug exposure during the first 8 weeks of pregnancy, the period during which birth defects can occur even before a woman realizes that she is pregnant. Educational programs, therefore, should focus on young, nonpregnant women who are sexually active. These programs should emphasize that all substances of abuse, including tobacco and alcohol, should be avoided during the sexually active years when conception can take place.

When a woman becomes pregnant and begins receiving prenatal care, the importance of abstinence from substance use can be reinforced. Pregnant women should be informed that use might harm the fetus during all trimesters of pregnancy. For example, alcohol consumption or cocaine use may cause disruption of organogenesis during the first trimester, may increase the risk of spontaneous abortion during the second trimester, and may create the potential for intrauterine growth restriction (IUGR), as well as interfere with brain maturation, during the third trimester. For these reasons, there is no safe time to ingest alcohol or use cocaine during pregnancy. Nurses can and should launch their own personal anti–substance abuse campaign.

Prevention is truly the key to reducing the number of drug-affected infants. Programs to achieve this goal vary. Admittedly, the "just say no" slogan was a simplistic view of the drug problem. However, a drug prevention program targeted at young children can be influential in forming attitudes that may dissuade future substance use. If such use is negatively sanctioned by society (e.g., smoke-free buildings, mandatory prison time for driving under the influence, and the "three strikes and you're out" policy for repeat offenders), individuals may be less likely to use such substances. Unlike other disease processes, drug-induced anomalies are irreversible. For example, once a child is born impaired with fetal alcohol syndrome or fetal alcohol effects, there is no cure; the damage is lifelong. Other substances, such as cocaine, heroin, and tobacco, have not been correlated with as predictable a pattern of aberrant behavior and appearance as that associated with alcohol. However, tobacco, cocaine, and heroin have been associated with significant fetal harm (e.g., learning delays, irritability, and IUGR) that persists into later life.

TOBACCO

History

Tobacco dependence is the number one public health problem in the world today (Cody, 2001). According to the World Health Organization, there are 1.1 billion smokers worldwide and 10,000 tobacco-related deaths per day. Each day in the United States, 6000 young people start smoking, a 50% increase since 1988. Approximately 43% of children 2 to 11 years of age are exposed to environmental tobacco smoke (American Academy of Pediatrics [AAP], 1998, 2001).

In the past, the prevalence of smoking among those 18 to 24 years of age was lower than among adults 25 to 44 years of age. By 1998, however, the prevalence of smoking in the younger age group had increased to equal that for the older adults (Centers for Disease Control and Prevention [CDC], 2001). Smoking is three times more prevalent among women with nine to 11 years of education than among women with 16 or more years, and it is highest among those living below the poverty level. The smoking prevalence is highest among American Indians/Alaska Natives, followed by African Americans (CDC, 2001).

Despite increased knowledge about the dangers of smoking, many women who smoke have difficulty abstaining from tobacco use during pregnancy. Approximately 25% of women continue to smoke during pregnancy (Eyler & Behnke, 1999; Howard & Lawrence, 1999).

A common consequence of tobacco use is addiction to nicotine. One puff on a cigarette produces peak nicotine levels in the brain within 10 seconds, resulting in activation of the brain circuitry that regulates pleasure. Most smokers report a true enjoyment, associated with a sense of relaxation during stress, especially with the first cigarette of the day (CDC, 2001).

Nicotine dependence is a primary, chronic disease. Psychosocial, environmental, and genetic factors influence its development and manifestations, and emergence of the disease is common after as few as 100 cigarettes (AAP, 2001).

To overcome the strong addictive properties of nicotine, the pregnant woman must be motivated and supported during her attempts to quit. She must be educated about the risks smoking poses to her pregnancy, such as the association between tobacco use and low birth weight, prematurity, and placental abruption. The practical implications also must be explained, such as the myriad complications of prematurity, which range from mild learning disabilities to death.

The effect of cigarette exposure on the pregnant woman and her developing fetus may be the most underrated, at least in public opinion (Eyler & Behnke, 1999). One reason is that few individuals recognize the vast array of dangers. Tobacco-induced hazards are discussed in the following section as they relate to various stages in the developing child's life (fetus, infancy, and childhood).

Risk Factors

Cigarette smoking has been associated with a variety of untoward effects during pregnancy, including placenta previa, abruptio placentae, and loss of the pregnancy. Periconceptual cigarette smoking has been found to interfere with attempts to conceive. This effect appears to be dose dependent in that the reduction in fertility is reversible if the woman stops smoking (Lee, 1998).

A relationship between smoking and spontaneous abortion has been documented in both animal and human studies. The risk of pregnancy loss before 20 weeks' gestation is 33% higher in women who smoke than in those who do not (Lee, 1998; Wagner et al, 1998; Ostrea et al, 1999). The mechanism of this association is not completely understood, although studies support the theory that it may be related to the vasoactive effects of nicotine on the umbilical arteries. Nicotine reduces prostacyclin production in the umbilical artery and diminishes that artery's capacity for vasodilation. Another possible effect is binding of carbon monoxide, resulting in inhibition of oxygen release into the fetal tissues by carboxyhemoglobin. These conditions affect fetal nutrition and oxygen transport, especially in conditions that cause asphyxia (Wagner et al, 1998; Ostrea et al, 1999). Other studies attribute the higher rate of abortion to abnormalities in placental development and dysfunction of the hormones that sustain pregnancy (Ostrea et al, 1999).

A correlation has been found between abruptio placentae and placenta previa and abnormalities of the placenta. Women who smoked for longer than 6 years had an increased incidence of placenta previa of 14.3% and of placental abruption of 72%. The ratio of placental weight to birth weight is higher for smokers than nonsmokers; this suggests that placental hypertrophy is a compensatory response to fetal hypoxia. The placentas of smokers show histologic damage consistent with hypoxia, including necrosis and inflammation of the decidua, diminished intervillous space, retroplacental hematomas, and calcification and fibrin deposition. Early placental morphologic studies revealed increased thickness of the villous membrane, which can adversely affect gas and metabolite exchange to the developing fetus (Lee, 1998; Jauniaux et al, 1999; Ostrea et al, 1999).

Classification of tobacco as a teratogen remains controversial. Various studies examining an association between cigarette smoking during pregnancy and congenital malformations have produced conflicting results (Ostrea et al, 1999). The British Perinatal Mortality Survey suggested an association between maternal smoking and congenital heart defects, but the U.S. Collaborative Perinatal Project was unable to confirm these findings (Ostrea et al, 1999). An increased risk of cleft lip and palate has been suggested, but the difference between infants of smokers and those of nonsmokers has not been shown to be clinically significant (Lee, 1998). Except for IUGR, no consistent evidence has confirmed teratogenicity (Bauer, 1999). The inconsistency of the reports suggests that cigarette smoking per se may not be a cause of congenital malformations in infants (Ostrea et al, 1999).

A more recent study by Jauniaux and colleagues (1999) evaluated the distribution of cotinine, a metabolite of nicotine, in fetal fluids. These researchers reported that cotinine was found throughout the fetal fluids. This study demonstrated fetal susceptibility early in gestation that could lead to chronic toxic exposure. The three different sources of exposure that make the fetus susceptible are the maternal circulation, skin absorption, and gastrointestinal reabsorption of urine. Tobacco carcinogens are transformed into metabolites that might react with deoxyribonucleic acid (DNA) and induce subsequent cellular damage in human tissues. It is hypothesized that this damage at the genetic level may contribute to the impairment of fetoplacental development, and that it explains the possible teratogenic effect of cigarette smoking (Jauniaux et al, 1999). Further study is needed in this area.

Causes of Intrauterine Hazards

The tobacco in cigarettes is composed primarily of leaves from the plant *Nicotiana tabacum*. The smoke from tobacco contains more than 4000 compounds, which can be categorized into two groups, those of the gas phase and those of the particulate phase. Chemicals in the gas phase are particles smaller than 0.1 μm, which pass through a filter pad. The smoke particles of the particulate phase can be collected on the filter pad (Lee, 1998).

More than 30 of the compounds found in cigarette smoke have been associated with adverse health effects. Of those, carbon monoxide from the gas phase and nicotine from the particulate phase have received the most attention (Lee, 1998).

Carbon monoxide is a colorless, odorless gas found in 1% to 5% of cigarette smoke. Compared with oxygen, it has a 200-fold affinity for hemoglobin. Carbon monoxide binds hemoglobin to form carboxyhemoglobin, which reduces the oxygen-carrying capacity of the blood. Carbon monoxide also increases the binding of hemoglobin to oxygen, impairing the release of oxygen into the tissues. As a result, the fetus experiences intrauterine hypoxia (Lee, 1998).

Nicotine is a pale yellow alkaloid that is both water and lipid soluble. Because it has a low boiling point, it is vaporized as tobacco is smoked. Nicotine is absorbed through the lungs from cigarette smoke, and it moves rapidly out of the bloodstream into the intracellular space. It is metabolized primarily in the liver into cotinine, which is pharmacologically inactive. The kidneys eliminate nicotine and its metabolites (Lee, 1998; Jauniaux et al, 1999).

The plasma half-life of nicotine is approximately 40 minutes. However, cotinine may persist in the bloodstream for several days after smoking, despite a half-life of 15 to 30 hours. Serum concentrations of cotinine are tenfold higher than those of nicotine and therefore are a better index of nicotine exposure. Because cotinine is a biologic metabolite, samples cannot be contaminated by environmental nicotine, therefore its presence in biologic fluids indicates exposure (Lee, 1998; Milerad et al, 1998; Jauniaux et al, 1999).

Cotinine can be found in a number of body fluids, including plasma, urine, and saliva (Milerad et al, 1998). The study by Jauniaux and colleagues (1999) that examined the distribution of cotinine in fetal fluids provided evidence that cotinine accumulates in the early fetal circulation and fluids in measurable concentrations as early as 7 weeks' gestation. Results also demonstrated a positive linear correlation between the number of cigarettes a mother smoked per day and the concentration of cotinine in the maternal urine. The maternal or fetal serum cotinine concentration was not dependent on the number of cig-

arettes smoked per day and could be influenced by other factors, such as the nicotine content of the cigarette brand and the time elapsed between the last cigarette smoked and the sampling. The results of this study indicate that cotinine levels may be used as markers in the epidemiology of maternal-fetal tobacco exposure during pregnancy (Jauniaux et al, 1999).

Fetal Hazards

Low Birth Weight.   Maternal smoking has been documented as the responsible factor in reduced birth weight among term infants (Lee, 1998; Wagner et al, 1998; Bauer, 1999; Becker et al, 1999; Windham et al, 2000). Women who smoke during pregnancy are estimated to face twice the risk of LBW infants than those who do not smoke (Windham et al, 2000). At birth, a consistent average decrement in weight of 150 to 200 g is seen (Lee, 1998; Windham et al, 2000). Growth inhibition also affects length and head circumference, with most infants born symmetrically small (Bauer, 1999). In addition, a dose-response relationship has been demonstrated between the number of cigarettes smoked and the decline in birth weight and the percentage of LBW infants (Ostrea et al, 1999).

Low birth weight accounts for half of all infant deaths and for long-term morbidity for many of the survivors. Maternal smoking contributes to approximately 5% of perinatal deaths and 46,000 LBW births per year. Aligne and Stoddard (1997) calculated the estimated medical costs of LBW births related to maternal smoking; they determined the direct medical costs to be approximately $1.2 billion and the loss of life costs to be $3.7 billion.

Strong evidence supports the importance of cessation of smoking before and during pregnancy. Studies have shown that the reduction in birth weight can be diminished or prevented if the mother stops smoking during pregnancy (Lee, 1998). Compared with the infants of persistent smokers, the difference in birth weight was significant when smoking was stopped by as late as 16 weeks' gestation. Even past 16 weeks' gestation, cessation of smoking was found to be associated with higher birth weights than those for infants of persistent smokers (Ostrea et al, 1999).

Examination of the subcutaneous fat deposition and lean body mass in infants of smokers and nonsmokers assessed the growth deficit in infants. The two groups showed no difference in skin fold measurements or the calculated cross-sectional fat area of the upper arm. These results suggest that the decline in birth weight of infants of mothers who smoke is primarily a decrease in lean body mass, whereas deposition of subcutaneous fat is fairly unaffected (Ostrea et al, 1999).

Most of the longitudinal studies have shown that the growth restrictions seen at birth resolve by 18 to 24 months of age, with catch-up growth in both weight and head growth generally occurring within the first year. Length frequently lags behind and may not reach normal percentiles until the second year of life (Bauer, 1999).

Neurobehavioral Effects.   Newborns exposed to nicotine in utero frequently display soft neurologic signs. Variations in tone have been seen, including both hypotonia and hypertonia. Fine tremors are common and may persist into the first month of life (Bauer, 1999).

Early behavioral dysfunction has been described, including impaired attention, poor orientation, and hyperactivity (Bauer, 1999). One of the early studies on the relationship of prenatal tobacco use to infant behavior and development used the

Brazelton Neonatal Assessment Scale (BNAS). This study compared infants born to women who smoked consistently throughout pregnancy with those born to nonsmokers. The women were matched on maternal age, socioeconomic status, and parity. The infants exposed to cigarettes scored higher on auditory habituation; they acclimated themselves to repeated auditory stimulation to remain asleep, thus conserving energy. However, these infants scored lower on the orientation items with auditory components; they had difficulty focusing and becoming alert. They also scored lower on consolability (Brazelton, 1999; Eyler & Behnke, 1999; Ostrea et al, 1999).

Picone and colleagues found that in utero exposure impaired neonatal habituation, orientation, consolability, autonomic regulation, and orientation to sound and is associated with a heightened Moro reflex and tremors (Wagner et al, 1998; Eyler & Behnke, 1999).

Cognitive effects and receptive language delays that persisted to school age have been described. These effects often occurred with polydrug exposure (Bauer, 1999). Environmental influences that affect infant development must also be considered. These influences may include the social-emotional interactions of caregivers and extended family and friends with the child and the teaching and learning experiences available that affect the child's development (Eyler & Behnke, 1999). The life of a polysubstance user is disorganized and chaotic. Low self-esteem and altered parenting abilities are likely, and physical abuse is common. Studies are beginning to show that changes in cognitive and neurobehavioral development are as much a result of the environment as of the substance used.

Premature Birth.
Maternal smoking has been suggested as a risk factor for preterm labor, but earlier studies failed to show a significant relationship (Ostrea et al, 1999). Windham and colleagues (2000) found sufficient evidence to indicate that maternal smoking is moderately associated with preterm delivery. In addition to their findings, which demonstrated a doubled rate of preterm births (which they defined as less than 35 weeks' gestation) among heavy smokers, other studies are reporting a closer association with delivery before 33 weeks' gestation (Windham et al, 2000).

Premature rupture of membranes (PROM) occurs more frequently in mothers who smoke but appears to be dose related. Studies showed that women who smoked 20 or more cigarettes per day had a 1.4% incidence of PROM; the incidence was 0.6% in women who smoked one to five cigarettes per day and 0.3% in women who did not smoke (Lee, 1998).

Fetal Death and Neonatal Mortality.
Epidemiologic studies have noted a significant effect of maternal smoking on late fetal death and neonatal mortality. Compared with infants of nonsmokers, among first-born infants of mothers who smoked, the risk of fetal death and neonatal mortality was 25% higher if the mother smoked less than one pack per day and 56% higher if the mother smoked more than one pack per day. For second and subsequent births, the risk of late fetal death and neonatal mortality was 30% higher for infants of mothers who smoked (Ostrea et al, 1999).

Risk Factors in Infancy and Childhood
Second-Hand Smoke.
Second-hand smoke, or environmental tobacco smoke (ETS), is a major cause of morbidity and mortality among American children. People exposed to ETS are subjected to most of the components found in main-

stream smoke, but the pattern and amount of exposure are different (Windham et al, 2000). Nonsmokers with ETS exposure have been shown to have cotinine concentrations, although, on an average, one or two levels of magnitude lower than those of active smokers. Infants born to mothers exposed to ETS were also found to have a decrement in mean birth weight, although of a smaller magnitude than that of infants born to mothers who smoked during pregnancy (Windham et al, 2000).

Ownby and colleagues (2000) examined infants and children exposed to ETS by individuals other than parents to determine if this exposure was significant. The researchers followed a cohort of infants from birth to 2 years of age, using questionnaires concerning the amount of ETS exposure and bimonthly urinary cotinine-creatinine ratios. The results showed that smoking by adults other than parents was significantly related to ETS exposure, a finding that demonstrated the need for all those who have regular contact with infants to reduce smoking.

Several studies have shown that infants and children exposed to ETS are adversely affected, especially their respiratory health. However, because women who smoke during pregnancy are likely to continue smoking after delivery, it is difficult to study the independent effects of in utero exposure to maternal smoking and postnatal ETS exposure (Gilliland et al, 2001).

Little is known about the effect of ETS exposure on the child's subsequent smoking behavior. Recent studies have demonstrated that maternal smoking during pregnancy may increase the probability of smoking in adolescents. The results also suggested that the risk was related to the cotinine content of their saliva 6 years earlier. These data suggest that the systemic effects of ETS exposure during pregnancy and early in life may lead to an increased risk of addiction to tobacco (Becker et al, 1999; AAP, 2001).

Respiratory Effects.
In utero smoke exposure represents a different insult to lung development than postnatal smoke exposure. In utero smoke exposure is not associated with direct contact between inhaled smoke and the airway. Postnatal smoke is a true inhalational insult in that the infant directly inhales sidestream cigarette smoke. However, it cannot be determined which exposure is responsible for the alterations in lung and airway morphology (Elliot et al, 1998).

Substantial evidence indicates that exposure to tobacco smoke adversely affects children's respiratory health by diminishing lung growth and function and by increasing the risk of respiratory infection and respiratory symptoms, including wheezing and exacerbation of asthma (Elliot et al, 1998; Gilliland et al, 2001).

Nicotine exposure has been shown to interfere with the growth and morphology of fetal alveolar pneumocytes. A significant decrease in the number of type I pneumocytes was found, as well as an increase in the number of type II pneumocytes. However, the type II cells lacked microvilli on the alveolar surface. Nicotine was also found to interfere with the formation of elastic tissue, which led to the development of emphysema-like damage to the neonatal lungs (Lee, 1998).

In utero exposure to maternal smoking adversely affects postnatal lung function and increases the occurrence of asthma. A growing number of reports suggests that this exposure is associated with deficits in lung function at birth that may persist into young adulthood. Reports also suggest that the changes in airway dimensions and the deficits in small airway function may predispose children to wheezing during respiratory infections or other illnesses that produce inflammation, subsequent bronchial hyperactivity, and airflow obstruction. Chronic increased bronchial hyperactivity may then contribute to persistent wheezing and a greater predisposition to asthma. In addition, in utero exposure may affect the development and maturation of the pulmonary immune system (Gilliland et al, 2001).

Sudden Infant Death Syndrome.   Numerous epidemiologic studies have identified maternal smoking during pregnancy and nursing as a risk factor for sudden infant death syndrome (SIDS). The consistency of these findings and the strength of the statistical association suggest a causal relationship in some cases (Elliot et al, 1998; Milerad et al, 1998). In other cases, mounting evidence indicates that a certain gene plays a role in the development of SIDS by controlling the development of the brainstem (Hunt, 2001).

The exact mechanism by which maternal smoking increases the risk of SIDS has not yet been determined. Elliot and colleagues (1998) documented changes in airway wall dimensions in infants who had died and who had been exposed to consistently high levels of maternal smoking; these changes were not seen in infants who had died of the same cause but who had had no exposure to maternal cigarette smoking. These researchers hypothesized that the increased airway wall thickness may contribute to exaggerated airway narrowing and abnormalities in neonatal lung function, thereby increasing the risk of SIDS.

A study by Franco and colleagues (1999) demonstrated that infants born to mothers who smoked had higher arousal thresholds for auditory challenges, as well as more frequent obstructive sleep apnea, than infants born to nonsmoking mothers. Maternal cigarette smoke influences fetal brain development. It primarily acts in brainstem tissues that are rich in cholinergic nicotinic binding receptors. These areas are associated with the regulation of arousal and cardiopulmonary integration, and changes in these tissues could account for the diminished arousability (Franco et al, 1999). Although the relationship between these results and SIDS has yet to be determined, the findings must be considered a possible contributor to the disorder.

Wisborg and colleagues (2000) studied the association between smoking during pregnancy and SIDS using prospectively collected data. Despite the small number of cases, and controlling for possible confounders, they were able to document a statistically significant association, which showed that the risk increased with the number of cigarettes smoked per day.

Milerad and colleagues (1998) examined the cotinine levels in infants diagnosed with SIDS. All infants examined had cotinine concentrations indicative of exposure to nicotine before death. Although cotinine concentrations were also found in infants who had died of known infections, the median levels were significantly lower than in the SIDS victims. These researchers were unable to determine if the levels of cotinine found in SIDS victims were high enough to adversely affect physiologic functions; however, growing evidence indicates that fetal exposure to maternal smoking makes infants more vulnerable to hypoxic stress (Milerad et al, 1998).

Breastfeeding.   In addition to crossing the placenta, nicotine is excreted in the milk of lactating women. Becker and colleagues (1999) examined infants of mothers who smoked, comparing the urinary cotinine levels of the breastfed infants with those of the infants who were not breastfed. The researchers found that the cotinine levels were much higher in the breastfed infants, on average, five times higher. Although this is likely to be due to a combination of inhaled and ingested nicotine and cotinine, breast milk is the major contributor to an infant's urinary cotinine level (Becker et al, 1999). It is not clear whether ingested tobacco products play a role in any adverse effects on respiratory health. However, the risk of respiratory illness was seven times higher in infants who were not breastfed compared with those breastfed by mothers who smoked; this suggests that ingested components did not place infants at greater risk for respiratory problems (Becker et al, 1999).

Recommendations
When the results of abundant studies focusing on the effects of maternal smoking on pregnancy and the effects of ETS on the health of infants and children are considered, promotion of a tobacco-free environment appears to be essential to the well-being of infants and children. The American Academy of Pediatrics (AAP) Committee on Substance Abuse has recommended many ways to fight ETS, including not smoking, promoting a smoke-free environment in public places, rejecting products that advertise tobacco, and supporting antismoking programs. Pediatricians should inform parents about the dangers of ETS and the availability of various smoking cessation methods. The AAP considers nicotine to be contraindicated during lactation, but this finding currently is the subject of controversy among experts in the field (Becker et al, 1999; Howard & Lawrence, 1999; AAP, 2001).

COCAINE

History
Cocaine, the primary alkaloid extract from the leaves of the shrub *Erythroxylon coca,* has been recognized since the mid-1850s for its stimulant effects. The drug was first used by the aboriginal peoples of South America as a euphoric stimulant and to forestall hunger in times of famine. Cocaine was extracted and identified by German chemist Albert Nieman. A period of time followed in which cocaine was proclaimed as a cure-all, and its use became widespread. Before its adverse effects were recognized, it was a major ingredient in the original Coca-Cola (Malanga & Kosofsky, 1999; Ostrea et al, 1999; Askin & Diehl-Jones, 2001).

During the past decade, as cocaine's availability rose and its cost fell, use of the drug increased dramatically in the United States. In 1998 the National Household Survey on Drug Abuse found that approximately 1.7 million Americans were current (at least once per month) cocaine users. The rate was highest (2%) among those 18 to 25 years old, significantly higher than in 1997. A parallel rise in cocaine use was seen among pregnant women, and cocaine now is among the illicit drugs most often used by women of reproductive age (Beckman & Brent, 1999; Askin & Diehl-Jones, 2001; National Institute on Drug Abuse [NIDA], 2001).

Common Attributes of Women Who Use Cocaine
It is important to recognize that the picture of a "typical" drug addict is no longer valid. Cocaine use transcends social class, and users are found in all economic brackets. However, several common social and lifestyle factors have been identified in a large number of cocaine users. The lives of women who use cocaine have been described as "chaos in action." These women

are disorganized, less likely to have adequate prenatal care, and more likely to be polydrug users; they consume alcohol or smoke, have a lower socioeconomic standard, are more likely to be malnourished, and are more likely than nonusers to have a sexually transmitted infection. Additional studies have linked violence, physical abuse, and sexual abuse with the use of cocaine (Kaltenbach & Finnegan, 1998; Miller & Boudreaux, 1999; Ostrea et al, 1999; Askin & Diehl-Jones, 2001).

Mechanism of Action

Cocaine is a central nervous system (CNS) stimulant that blocks the reuptake of neurotransmitters, especially dopamine and norepinephrine, which accumulate at the synaptic cleft. This leads to prolonged stimulation of the corresponding receptors, which produces the effects of norepinephrine and dopamine stimulation. These effects include tachycardia, hypertension, arrhythmia, diaphoresis, and tremors (norepinephrine), as well as increased alertness, euphoria or an enhanced feeling of well-being, sexual excitement, and heightened energy (dopamine). Cocaine also interferes with the uptake of tryptophan, which affects serotonin biosynthesis. Because serotonin regulates the sleep-wake cycle, a reduced level is associated with a diminished need for sleep (Mirochnick et al, 1997; Wagner et al, 1998; Ostrea et al, 1999; Askin & Diehl-Jones, 2001).

Cocaine also is the only known local anesthetic that is found naturally. Its anesthetic properties arise from the inhibition of peripheral nerve conduction and the prevention of norepinephrine uptake (Ostrea et al, 1999). Long-term use of cocaine can lead to depletion of central dopamine stores, which explains the dysphoria and drug craving experienced during withdrawal (Mirochnick et al, 1997).

Route of Administration

The primary routes of cocaine administration are oral, intranasal, intravenous, and inhalation. The oral route, also called "chewing," produces a peak effect in 45 to 90 minutes. Cocaine can also be rubbed directly onto mucous membranes. Intranasal use, or "snorting," involves inhalation of cocaine powder into the nostrils, where it is absorbed into the bloodstream through the nasal tissues. Peak effect is reached in 15 to 30 minutes, and the high lasts 60 to 90 minutes. Intravenous use, also called "mainlining" or "injecting," releases the drug directly into the bloodstream and heightens the intensity of its effects. Smoking involves inhalation of cocaine vapor or smoke into the lungs, where absorption into the bloodstream occurs as quickly as with injection; peak effect is attained in 60 to 90 seconds, but the high lasts only for about 5 to 10 minutes. The intense high is followed by a down period as the drug's effects wear off. This down period may be so unpleasant that more cocaine is used to re-experience the high, or other drugs are used. Consequently, the use of cocaine promotes the abuse of other drugs (Ostrea et al, 1999; NIDA, 2001).

Cocaine hydrochloride is the most common available form of cocaine. In its acid state, it is a water-soluble white powder that can be snorted or injected. Cocaine hydrochloride usually is mixed with starch, glucose, phencyclidine (PCP), heroin, or amphetamines, and its purity ranges from 20% to 80% (Ostrea et al, 1999; Askin & Diehl-Jones, 2001; NIDA, 2001).

Since the mid-1980s a freebase form of cocaine, known as crack, has been available. Crack cocaine is processed with ammonia or baking soda and heated to remove the hydrochloride; the result is a paste that, when dried, forms a rocklike substance that can be smoked. The term "crack" is derived from the crackling sound generated when the substance is prepared or smoked. Crack is less expensive than cocaine and quickly produces a powerful high, factors that have contributed to its popularity among young people (Ostrea et al, 1999; Askin & Diehl-Jones, 2001; NIDA, 2001).

Metabolism

Enzymes in the liver and plasma, called cholinesterases, metabolize cocaine. These enzymes transform cocaine into two main derivatives, benzoylecgonine and ethyl methylecgonine. Both of these derivatives are water soluble and are excreted in urine and sweat. Crack cocaine is metabolized into anhydroecgonine methyl ester, which is also detectable in urine (Ostrea et al, 1999; Askin & Diehl-Jones, 2001).

The systems involved in cocaine metabolism generally are less mature in the neonate, meaning that cocaine and its metabolites can remain in the infant for a longer period. The metabolites themselves are known to be toxic, which may put the fetus or neonate particularly at risk. Metabolites can be found in an adult's urine 72 hours after drug use. However, they may remain for up to 2 weeks in an infant, especially if the infant is premature (Ostrea et al, 1999; Askin & Diehl-Jones, 2001).

Effects on Pregnancy

Maternal cardiovascular adaptation to pregnancy appears to influence the physiologic responses to cocaine, and pregnancy appears to increase the toxicity of cocaine. Animal studies have demonstrated that when identical doses of cocaine were given to pregnant and nonpregnant sheep, a twofold greater hypertensive response occurred. This response was thought to be dependent on the hormonal environment of pregnancy (Plessinger & Woods, 1998). In addition, plasma cholinesterase, which inactivates cocaine, is comparatively deficient in pregnant women (Mirochnick et al, 1997).

Maternal use of cocaine has been associated with several complications, including spontaneous abortion, which has been found to occur in 25% to 38% of pregnancies complicated by cocaine use. Cocaine may alter the hormonal environment in a manner that threatens early pregnancy and implantation. In early pregnancy, human chorionic gonadotropin (hCG) maintains the endometrium by maintaining corpus luteal production of progesterone. Investigators have demonstrated a decrease in hCG production after cocaine ingestion, which suggests that cocaine could alter the milieu of early pregnancy, resulting in spontaneous abortion (Plessinger & Woods, 1998; Ostrea et al, 1999).

The incidence of stillbirth is five to 10 times higher among women who continue to use cocaine late into the third trimester. This rate has been credited to abruptio placentae, placental infarcts, or hemorrhage. It has been suggested that placental vasoconstriction associated with an abrupt hypertensive episode can precipitate placental separation from the uterine lining. The incidence of associated fetal death is significant once this occurs (Plessinger & Woods, 1998; Ostrea et al, 1999).

Effects on the Fetus

Although numerous clinical studies have linked prenatal cocaine use with a variety of adverse fetal effects, methodologic limitations have made establishing a causal relationship between these effects and maternal cocaine use problematic. It is difficult not only to determine the timing, frequency, and dose of cocaine, but also to dissociate the harmful effects of other factors (e.g., low socioeconomic status, poor nutrition, polydrug use, infections, and lack of prenatal care) from the effects of cocaine use alone. Consequently, the issue of how much risk to the fetus is associated with cocaine use during pregnancy remains unresolved. However, a growing body of literature supports the theory that cocaine is a developmental toxicant (Plessinger & Woods, 1998; Wagner et al, 1998; Bauer, 1999; Beckman & Brent, 1999).

The adverse effects of cocaine in the pregnant woman and fetus are thought to arise primarily from vascular disruptive events, which are caused by the vasoconstrictive effects of cocaine on both the maternal and fetal vasculature (Plessinger & Woods, 1998; Beckman & Brent, 1999). The uterine arteries normally are fully dilated during pregnancy, and the vasoconstriction caused by cocaine may compromise fetal growth and development. Animal studies have shown that maternal blood pressure rises within 5 minutes after cocaine infusion, accompanied by an increase in uterine vascular resistance and a decrease in uterine blood flow. The result is a reduced supply of oxygen and nutrients to the fetus. Cardiovascular effects seen in the fetus include hypertension, tachycardia, hypoxia, and increased cerebral blood flow (Beckman & Brent, 1999; Ostrea et al, 1999).

Cocaine easily and rapidly crosses the placenta by simple diffusion because it is lipophilic and of low molecular weight. Cocaine is not significantly metabolized during maternal-fetal transfer; consequently, once in the fetal circulation, cocaine and its metabolites are widely distributed and are detectable in a variety of human fetal tissues. Although the fetal concentration is only one fourth to one ninth of the maternal concentration, elimination of cocaine and its metabolites is much slower in the fetus, which increases the risk of cocaine toxicity (Beckman & Brent, 1999; Malanga & Kosofsky, 1999; Ostrea et al, 1999; Askin & Diehl-Jones, 2001).

Premature Birth. Premature birth reportedly has occurred in approximately 25% of the pregnancies of cocaine users, a rate three to four times higher than that for nonusers (Ostrea et al, 1999). One theory is that cocaine increases myometrial contractile activity, which may lead to an increase in PROM (Plessinger & Woods, 1998). However, not all studies have been able to demonstrate a clear-cut link between cocaine use and premature delivery; some studies suggested instead that a more precise explanation would be a combination of polydrug use and environmental factors (Wagner et al, 1998; Askin & Diehl-Jones, 2001).

Intrauterine Growth Restriction and Low Birth Weight. Studies have reported lower birth weights and smaller body length and head circumference in infants prenatally exposed to cocaine. It has been suggested that placental vasoconstriction, leading to diminished fetal nutrition, is the cause. However, newer studies again implicate polydrug use and environmental factors as a more accurate explanation (Wagner et al, 1998; Askin & Diehl-Jones, 2001). A study by Eyler and colleagues (1998) found significant growth restriction in infants exposed to cocaine. However, once the findings were adjusted for polydrug use, no significant differences were seen.

Cerebral Effects. Studies have suggested a higher incidence of intracerebral hemorrhage or infarction in infants exposed prenatally to cocaine. These defects may be related to the vascular disruptive effects of cocaine. Cerebral blood velocity is higher in cocaine-exposed infants, and when this ef-

fect is combined with cocaine-associated fetal hypertension, a higher incidence of defects is seen (Plessinger & Woods, 1998; Beckman & Brent, 1999; Malanga & Kosofsky, 1999).

A study by Frank and colleagues (1999) demonstrated that ultrasonographic findings suggestive of vascular injury to the CNS are related to the extent of prenatal cocaine exposure. They found more evidence of hemorrhages than cysts, which suggests that these effects occurred closer to delivery, perhaps within hours or days. The researchers speculated that exposed infants show less adaptive vasoregulation in response to the hypoxic-ischemic stress of labor, especially when stress is increased by an increase in maternal blood pressure. Given that previous studies have been inconsistent in finding a clear-cut association, perhaps because of failure to consider dose effects or environmental factors (or both), further research in this area is necessary.

Cocaine as a Teratogen

Cocaine has been implicated as a potential teratogen when ingested during pregnancy. Although it is difficult to document this definitively because of confounding variables, such as polydrug use, correlations between the use of cocaine and congenital anomalies must be considered. The mechanisms most likely involved are vascular disruption and oxygen free radical formation. If the blood supply is compromised by vasoconstriction during a critical period of organogenesis, oxygenation and nutrition of fetal tissue may be impaired. This impairment during a critical time in organ formation may restrict the growth and development of cells, resulting in disruption or absence of growth (Wagner et al, 1998; Ostrea et al, 1999; Askin & Diehl-Jones, 2001).

Several structural cardiac defects in the neonate are thought to be associated with prenatal cocaine exposure, including ventricular septal defect, auricular septal defect, cardiomegaly, hypoplastic right or left side of the heart, and absent ventricle. Cocaine has also been known to cause neonatal arrhythmias, altered electrocardiographic results, diminished cardiac output, coarctation of the aorta, peripheral pulmonic stenosis, patent ductus arteriosus, and aortic valve prolapse (Plessinger & Woods, 1998). Although some of these defects are found frequently in premature infants, the significant documentation of their occurrence in full-term infants exposed prenatally to cocaine suggests a teratogenic effect.

Other anomalies thought to be related to prenatal cocaine exposure are genitourinary tract defects, renal defects, neural tube defects, and skeletal defects (Plessinger & Woods, 1998; Ostrea et al, 1999).

Effects on the Neonate

Gastrointestinal Effects. Prenatal cocaine exposure has been associated with several gastrointestinal problems, including necrotizing enterocolitis and intestinal perforation. The vasoconstrictive effects of cocaine alter fetal intestinal blood flow, resulting in ischemic-hypoxic events. These events have the potential to initiate the "diving" reflex, which results in shunting of blood away from the mesenteric arteries. The shunting of blood can lead to bowel wall ischemia and inflammation and focal areas of necrosis (Plessinger & Woods, 1998; Wagner et al, 1998).

Ophthalmic Effects. Alterations in the visual system have been observed after prenatal exposure to cocaine. Most commonly seen are hypoplasia of the optic nerve, delayed visual maturation, profound eyelid edema, nystagmus, and/or strabismus. Blindness and retinopathy of prematurity have also been noted but less often. Follow-up studies discovered visual motor disturbances, indicated by difficulty copying straight lines, circles, and more complex forms, as well as evidence of impaired visual-tracking and abnormal visual evoked potentials. All defects are thought to be consequences of the hypertensive, vasoconstrictive, ischemic, and hemorrhagic effects of cocaine (Church et al, 1998; Plessinger & Woods, 1998).

Hearing Effects. Clinical studies have suggested that varying degrees of hearing impairment can be a consequence of prenatal cocaine exposure. Developmental delays in auditory brainstem response maturation have been observed, probably reflecting impaired neural growth. The sensorineural hearing loss seen in animal studies, as well as the peripheral hearing loss and deafness noted in human studies, are probably the result of damage to the auditory sensory receptor cells or the auditory nerve, or both (Church et al, 1998).

Long-Term Outcomes

As mentioned earlier, methodologic limitations have made it difficult to establish a causal relationship between adverse fetal effects and maternal cocaine use. Researchers are now studying children who were exposed prenatally to cocaine, looking for neurobehavioral and developmental changes.

Singer and colleagues (2001) studied children at 1 year of age who were exposed to cocaine prenatally, looking for an association between the level of fetal cocaine exposure and developmental precursors of speech-language skills. They documented significant behavioral teratogenic effects on the attentional abilities underlying the auditory comprehension skills that are considered precursors of receptive language. Children who were more heavily exposed were more likely to be classified as mildly delayed in language skills. Parents or health care workers can easily evaluate most of the items that were delayed. Most often seen were localizing to sounds, visually following an object, attending to toys or books, and playing social games.

Karmel and colleagues (1998) compared the neurobehavioral performance of different groups of infants with CNS injury, one group consisting entirely of cocaine-exposed infants. Belcher and colleagues (1999) also looked at neurobehavioral performance, but in infants with prenatal cocaine or polydrug exposure or both. Both studies obtained similar results. At birth, several abnormalities were noted among all groups, including hypertonicity, increased jitteriness, poorer state control, and increased deficits in visual attention. Most of the problems were transient and resolved by 1 month of age, except for jitteriness in the cocaine-exposed group, although it was significantly diminished. By 1 year of age, any lingering effects were absent. Based on these results, an assumption was made that prenatal exposure to cocaine had affected the developing nervous system in some way, despite the fact that cognitive skills were within normal range.

Arendt and colleagues (1999) investigated the effects of prenatal cocaine exposure on the motor development of young children at 2 years of age. The results of this study showed that these children performed less well on a standardized test of motor development, especially hand use and eye-hand coordination, indicating a lag in motor development beyond the neonatal period. However, the findings also reinforced the results of previous studies and current theory that motor development is a product of the interaction of genetic attributes, biologic maturation, and environmental stimulation (Arendt et al, 1999).

Richardson (1998) followed infants prenatally exposed to cocaine, examining their physical, cognitive, and behavioral development at birth and at 1 and 3 years of age, controlling for other factors that affect child development. The consistent finding was that CNS deficits result from prenatal cocaine exposure. First trimester cocaine use was found to be associated at 3 years of age with reduced head circumference, lower IQ, and increased fussiness and difficultness and behavior problems. At birth, cocaine exposure was related to poorer autonomic stability and a greater number of abnormal reflexes. During the 1-year follow-up, the children were found to be more fussy and difficult, and at 3 years, there were indications of cognitive and short-term memory deficits. An increase in behavior problems also was seen (Richardson, 1998). Richardson concluded that definite signs of subtle CNS effects existed. These effects were more difficult to detect at younger ages, but as the children grew older, they became more detectable. Further study of these children is planned at 7 years of age (Richardson, 1998).

Eyler and colleagues (1998) also found deficits in state regulation, attention, and responsiveness among cocaine-exposed neonates, but they were unable to attribute the changes to cocaine use alone, because polydrug use was common in their subjects. Their study emphasized the importance of considering the amount and duration of drug exposure, as well as the interactive effects of the drugs used. These researchers also noted their concern about infants who demonstrated alterations in attention and responsiveness and the impact of these alterations on the caregiver, whose parenting abilities may already be compromised by drug use (Eyler et al, 1998).

A study by Chasnoff and colleagues (1998) examined the outcome at 4 to 6 years of age of children prenatally exposed to cocaine. The results confirmed findings of smaller head circumferences, although less statistically significant results were found, suggesting a trend toward catch-up growth. This study also documented significant neurobehavioral deficiencies in the neonatal period. However, long-term follow-up consistently showed normal global cognitive development. Minimal direct influence on cognitive development by prenatal cocaine exposure was seen, as measured with the Stanford-Binet test; however, the home environment, as measured on the Home Screening Questionnaire, was found to be the single most important predictor of cognitive development (Chasnoff et al, 1998).

Chasnoff and colleagues also found that in this study population, 60% of the women who had used cocaine during pregnancy continued their use 6 years after delivery, adding another risk factor with the potential to impair the child's development. In the home environment, a correlation was found between the mother's continuing drug use and the child's IQ and behavioral problems at 6 years of age, resulting in the conclusion that prenatal cocaine or polydrug exposure did not have a direct effect on global cognitive functioning, but rather a strong indirect effect as mediated through the home environment (Chasnoff et al, 1998).

Prenatal/polydrug exposure was found to have a significant direct effect on the children's behavior at 4, 5, and 6 years of age. Clinically significant levels of behavior were found on one or more scales of the Child Behavior Checklist. Also, a neurobehavioral difficulty that consistently has been documented with cocaine-exposed infants is a deficiency in state regulation capabilities. Chasnoff and colleagues (1998) found that 6 years later, these children continued to demonstrate behaviors associated with regulatory difficulties, including difficulty managing impulses and frustration and difficulty with tension regulation and arousal.

Teachers have long reported problems with the behavior of children exposed prenatally to cocaine. Delaney-Black and colleagues (1998) reported that teachers blinded to prenatal cocaine-exposure status identified more problem behaviors among exposed children. Although these researchers were unable to document a definitive causal relationship between prenatal cocaine exposure and behavior problems, it was clear that significant changes occurred in these children. The study's findings also suggested, as other studies have, that other maternal and environmental factors played a significant role in the behavior. The results of this study are important because they lend credence to what educators have reported: the cocaine-exposed child, for whatever reason, is at risk for problem behaviors (Delaney-Black et al, 1998).

To summarize the most recent studies, significant, long-term neurobehavioral changes clearly are found in children who were exposed to cocaine in utero, although at this time no definitive consensus exists as to the exact problems. However, most studies indicate that these changes cannot be isolated to cocaine exposure, but rather are related more to polydrug use and the influence of the environment.

Leventhal and colleagues (1997) found an association between maternal cocaine use and the occurrence of maltreatment, primarily neglect, and placement outside the home. These results clearly indicate that women who use cocaine during pregnancy are at increased risk for parenting failure, thus increasing the risk of child neglect and abuse. The authors concur with recommendations from previous studies that continued efforts are needed to provide services not only to the children but also to their parents to improve the child's nurturing environment and reduce the rate of parenting failure.

Recommendations

The AAP recommends that pediatricians provide developmental monitoring, through the process of surveillance, in which the performance of skilled, longitudinal observations is emphasized. More developmental surveillance of cocaine-exposed infants is needed, because even the relatively small effects on attention and auditory comprehension that have been documented can have large population effects on the number of children needing long-term intervention services.

Current studies emphasize how important it is for practitioners, as well as researchers, to consider postnatal factors, particularly the adequacy of the home environment, including maternal IQ and psychological status, in their evaluation and treatment of children with a history of prenatal drug exposure. Also, it is essential that as a risk factor for atypical motor development, prenatal drug exposure be considered as a marker for other potential problems that can have a negative impact on a child's development. Continued, diligent observation of the child's behavioral and cognitive, as well as physical, development is needed (Arendt et al, 1999). Therefore, it is vital for practitioners, caregivers, educators, and researchers to monitor the progress of these children, examining all areas of risk, so that appropriate interventions can be put into place that will enhance optimal performance.

Breastfeeding

Significant amounts of cocaine have been found in human milk, which puts the infant at serious risk of toxicity. In a 2-week-old infant who was breastfed five times over a 4-hour period, during which the mother ingested cocaine, distinct irritability, vomiting, and diarrhea began 3 hours after the first breastfeeding. Tremors and changes in behavioral state and reflexes also were noted. Twelve hours after the mother's last dose, urine testing showed large amounts of cocaine and metabolites, which persisted for 60 hours. Another case involved a mother who applied cocaine to her nipples, using it as a local anesthetic. Three hours after breastfeeding, the infant was found gasping, choking, and cyanotic, and seizure activity also was documented. Although the mother's milk tested negative for cocaine, the infant's urine tested positive for the drug (Howard & Lawrence, 1998; Ostrea et al, 1999).

The AAP considers cocaine to be contraindicated during breastfeeding. Based on the toxicity exhibited by infants after breastfeeding, maternal cocaine use during breastfeeding must be strongly discouraged (Howard & Lawrence, 1998).

Sudden Infant Death Syndrome (SIDS)

Studies have not shown prenatal exposure to cocaine to be an independent risk factor for SIDS, although concurrent opiate exposure appears to increase the risk. However, abnormal breathing patterns have been observed in cocaine-exposed infants, including a higher respiratory rate, a diminished end-tidal partial pressure of carbon dioxide (PCO_2) and a shift to the left of the breathing response curve to carbon dioxide (CO_2). Increased apneic density and periodic breathing have also been documented (Ostrea et al, 1999; Frank et al, 2001).

Lustbader and colleagues (1998) found that postnatal use of cocaine by mothers or other adults in the infants' environment exposes infants and young children to crack/cocaine smoke during critical periods of growth and development. Passive exposure likely occurs in much the same way as with second-hand cigarette smoke. Children exposed passively to cocaine were found to have a significant increase in the incidence of upper and lower respiratory symptoms. This increase may be related to irritation of the airway mucosa by exposure to cocaine smoke. Although information about exposure to nicotine cigarette smoke in the home was lacking, the incidence of cigarette smoking among crack/cocaine abusers generally is higher. The researchers therefore were unable to attribute respiratory changes solely to cocaine. One assumption made was that an increased risk of SIDS must be considered, although a causal relationship between SIDS and cocaine has not been supported (Lustbader et al, 1998; Ostrea et al, 1999; Frank et al, 2001).

Mortality and Morbidity of Cocaine-Exposed Infants

Greene and colleagues (1998) found that in utero, cocaine exposure or polydrug exposure (or both) is associated with significant increases in morbidity and length of hospital stay. Morbidity includes poor prenatal care, low birth weight, prematurity, microcephaly, and meconium-stained amniotic fluid.

Behnke and associates (1997) found that cocaine-exposed infants had an across the board increase in the use of hospital resources, as well as higher hospital charges and longer stays. Total hospital charges for a group of cocaine-exposed infants were more than double those for a nonexposed group. More frequent admissions to the neonatal intensive care unit (NICU) were noted, usually related to decreased birth weight, prematurity, and sepsis workups, and these admissions required longer stays. Also, discharge often was delayed because of family and social problems identified at birth. Interventions to reduce hospital stays, thus reducing costs, should be directed toward improved prenatal care for addicted mothers, leading to improved outcomes for their infants (Behnke et al, 1997).

Clinical Management

In contrast to infants exposed to opioids in utero, an abstinence syndrome for infants exposed prenatally to cocaine has not been identified. Rather, it is believed that the manifestations seen at birth reflect the continuing toxic effects of the drug itself (Askin & Diehl-Jones, 2001).

Pharmacologic therapy is recommended for narcotic withdrawal, but infants exposed solely to cocaine do not usually require such treatment. Reducing environmental stimulation and using techniques such as swaddling and flexed positioning are effective strategies for managing signs of CNS irritation (Ostrea et al, 1999; Askin & Diehl-Jones, 2001).

Infants exposed to cocaine may need small, frequent feedings and may require additional calories to gain weight. These infants also may have poor coordination of suck and swallow, as well as tongue thrusting and oral hypersensitivity, requiring a patient, calm approach to feeding (Howard & Lawrence, 1998; Ostrea et al, 1999; Askin & Diehl-Jones, 2001).

The safety of the cocaine-exposed infant must be of major concern to members of the health care team. The infant's home environment and the mother's well-being must be assessed, and appropriate referrals (e.g., social services) must be made as needed (Askin & Diehl-Jones, 2001).

HEROIN

History

The use of opium probably dates back about 6000 years. Hippocrates made one of the earliest references to complications of opium use in the perinatal period, mentioning "uterine suffocation" as a possible consequence. By the late nineteenth and early twentieth century, reference to the passively addicted infant is evident in reports describing the diffusion of morphine through the placenta and its transmission through breast milk (Ostrea et al, 1999).

Morphine and codeine, the naturally occurring opiates, are derived from the seed of the unripe poppy plant, *Papaver somniferum*. They were used as analgesics and soporifics (Malanga & Kosofsky, 1999; Ostrea et al, 1999).

Heroin (diacetylmorphine), a semisynthetic opioid, was first introduced in 1874. It became popular because of the rapid onset of its CNS effects. By the 1950s heroin had replaced morphine as the drug of choice among abusers, and opioid use during pregnancy began to emerge as a significant problem. By the mid-1970s numerous articles had begun to appear in the literature identifying the perinatal complications of heroin use. However, heroin has received little attention during the past 12 to 15 years, because researchers, health care providers, politicians, and policy makers have focused their attention on the impact of the cocaine epidemic (Kaltenbach et al, 1998; Ostrea et al, 1999).

Heroin is making a comeback as a drug of choice for addicts. The National Household Survey on Drug Abuse showed a fourfold increase in heroin use between 1990 and 1995 (Kaltenbach et al, 1998). According to the 1998 survey, which may actually underestimate illicit heroin use, nearly 130,000 people reportedly used heroin within the month preceding the survey. The report also estimated that there were 81,000 new heroin users in 1997, most under age 26. The 1998 Drug Abuse Warning Network estimated that 14% of all drug-related emergency room episodes involved heroin, and episodes among youths 12 to 17 years of age nearly quadrupled (NIDA, 2001f). This increase in use has been attributed both to the lower cost of heroin and to its improved purity. Furthermore, it includes a new generation of middle-class suburbanites. Because most drug-abusing women are of reproductive age, this represents a significant pool of potentially pregnant women (Kaltenbach et al, 1998).

Mechanism of Action

Heating morphine with acetyl anhydride produces heroin. The result is an off-white or pale brown powder that can be sniffed, smoked, or injected parenterally with a hypodermic needle (Kenner & D'Apolito, 1997; D'Apolito, 1998; Jorgensen, 1999; NIDA, 2001f). Heroin is approximately 25 times stronger than morphine. It is lipophilic and of low molecular weight, which allows the drug to cross the placenta easily. It is present in fetal tissue within 1 hour of administration (Kenner & D'Apolito, 1997; D'Apolito, 1998; Wagner et al, 1998). It is metabolized in the liver into morphine and is excreted in the urine. Some of the metabolized drug is excreted into bile, therefore small amounts of morphine are excreted in the feces (D'Apolito, 1998).

The most common route of administration is intravenous injection, known as "mainlining." This route provides the greatest intensity and the most rapid onset of euphoria (7 to 8 seconds). This brief but intense high is followed by a drowsy, detached, peaceful period of several hours, which is followed by an intense craving for more of the drug. Intramuscular injection produces a slower onset of euphoria (5 to 8 minutes). Sniffing or smoking heroin does not produce a "rush" as quickly or as intensely as intravenous injection; peak effects are felt within 10 to 15 minutes. Nonetheless, researchers for the National Institute on Drug Abuse (NIDA) have confirmed that all three forms of administration are addictive (NIDA, 2001f).

Although injection continues to be the predominant method of heroin use among addicts, researchers have seen a shift in administration routes from injection to sniffing and smoking. One of the larger groups of heroin users comprises those over 30 years of age. However, with the availability of inexpensive, high-purity heroin that can be sniffed or smoked instead of being injected, new, young users are being lured to the drug. It has also been appearing in more affluent communities (NIDA, 2001f).

Common Attributes of Women Who Use Heroin

Women addicted to heroin generally have myriad personal and family problems that affect their health and that of their fetuses. They frequently must cope with many financial, social, and psychologic difficulties. Many of these women are homeless or live in inadequate housing. Food may be scarce or perhaps not a priority. The result is a poorly nourished woman with inadequate prenatal care and poor personal hygiene who is at risk of contracting an infectious disease (Kaltenbach et al, 1998; Bauer, 1999).

A high percentage of heroin-dependent women are single heads of households, have less than a high school education, and are progeny of substance-abusing parents. The incidence of physical abuse and sexual molestation is high. Many have poor self-esteem and have difficulty with interpersonal relationships (Kaltenbach et al, 1998; Bauer, 1999).

Risk Factors

The heroin-dependent woman is at high risk for infection with the human immunodeficiency virus (HIV) and for viral hepatitis as the result of both needle sharing and unsafe sexual practices. Infections account for a high percentage of complications. Those most frequently seen are hepatitis A, B, and C, tuberculosis, bacterial endocarditis, septicemia, cellulitis, and sexually transmitted infections (Kaltenbach et al, 1998; Bauer, 1999; Coghlan et al, 1999).

The form of heroin available to the addict, "street" heroin, may be mixed with other drugs or with substances such as sugar, starch, powdered milk, mannitol, quinine, amphetamines, strychnine, or procaine-lidocaine. These substances themselves can have deleterious effects on the fetus (Wagner et al, 1998; NIDA, 2001f).

Because heroin abusers do not know the actual strength of the drug or its true content, they are at risk of overdose or death (NIDA, 2001f). Also, the sterility of heroin is unclear, and the drug frequently is tainted with bacteria, fungi, or viruses. A separate risk factor that can jeopardize the health of the fetus is whether the mother has contracted HIV or viral hepatitis, increasing the risk of transmission of these viruses to the fetus and neonate (Wagner et al, 1998; NIDA, 2001f).

Effects on the Fetus

Asphyxia and Fetal Distress.   Intrauterine asphyxia is possibly the single greatest risk to the fetus, as evidenced by a high incidence of meconium-stained amniotic fluid, fetal distress, low Apgar scores, neonatal aspiration pneumonia, and intrauterine death (Kaltenbach et al, 1998; Ostrea et al, 1999). The predisposition to asphyxia underscores the need for repeated evaluation of fetal well-being during pregnancy. Fetal asphyxia in the pregnant addict may occur secondary to a number of factors. Several studies have suggested that opiates affect both quiet sleep and rapid eye movement (REM) sleep, which is associated with a hyperactive state that causes an increase in fetal oxygen consumption (Kaltenbach et al, 1998; Ostrea et al, 1999). Another possible cause of asphyxia is fetal withdrawal, which usually coincides with the mother's withdrawal. Fetal withdrawal results in hyperactivity and an increase in catecholamines, resulting in increased oxygen consumption by the fetus that can lead to asphyxia (Kaltenbach et al, 1998; Ostrea et al, 1999).

The fetus mirrors the mother's withdrawal response, therefore maternal detoxification is not recommended before 14 weeks' gestation because of the risk of inducing abortion; it also should not be done after 32 weeks because of possible withdrawal-induced stress. Generally, the pregnant addict is placed on methadone maintenance and given prenatal care, nutritional assistance, and counseling. After the infant is delivered, detoxification may be attempted (Kaltenbach et al, 1998; Ostrea et al, 1999).

Meconium-stained amniotic fluid, which frequently is found in the pregnant addict, is a manifestation of fetal distress. Aspiration of meconium may account for the increased incidence of meconium aspiration syndrome and persistent pulmonary hypertension (PPHN) of the newborn (Weiner & Finnegan, 1998; Ostrea et al, 1999).

Effects on the Neonate

Low Apgar Scores.   The infants of opioid-dependent mothers show a high incidence of low Apgar scores. This may be related to intrauterine asphyxia or to the effects of narcotics the

mother received before delivery. Often the pregnant addict uses heroin before entering the hospital, which can result in neonatal depression. However, caution must be exercised with the use of narcotic antagonists to reverse the respiratory depression in these infants because narcotic antagonists can precipitate an acute withdrawal in the infant (Kaltenbach et al, 1998; Ostrea et al, 1999).

Low Birth Weight.   Human and animal studies have shown that heroin can affect fetal growth. A significant decrease in weight, length, and head circumference can be seen during the first months of life. However, by the age of 2 years, only length remained less than that of children of the same age in the general population. The exact mechanism by which heroin inhibits growth is unknown; although growth inhibition may be a direct effect of the drug, it may actually be an indirect effect of the mother's nutritional status.*

Infants of pregnant women in methadone programs reportedly had higher birth weights than those exposed to heroin. However, this may reflect the better prenatal care and nutrition these women receive (Ostrea et al, 1999).

Heroin as a Teratogen

In general, heroin is not believed to be teratogenic to the fetus. Although a few studies have shown an increase in the incidence of congenital anomalies, no consistent pattern has been seen. A study of 830 heroin-addicted mothers showed a significant increase in the number of infants with congenital anomalies, but the researchers were unable to determine if these findings were a true effect of heroin or were related to polydrug use, because most of the subjects did not abuse heroin only (Wagner et al, 1998; Weiner & Finnegan, 1998; Ostrea et al, 1999).

Because it is generally accepted that heroin and methadone are not teratogenic, the pregnant woman is maintained on methadone until delivery. A cross-dependence exists between heroin and methadone, which helps prevent fetal withdrawal. The benefit of methadone over heroin is that methadone can be prescribed by exact dose, can be given orally, and does not exert the mood-altering effects of heroin. The methadone level can be maintained at a more constant value, thus in utero fetal withdrawal is avoided. Women in methadone programs are provided with support services such as counseling, prenatal care, and assistance for food and shelter (Wagner et al, 1998; Weiner & Finnegan, 1998; Ostrea et al, 1999).

Sudden Infant Death Syndrome

The risk of SIDS is more than twice as high for heroin-exposed infants. These infants show an altered sleep pattern characterized by more REM sleep than quiet sleep. Auditory brainstem evoked responses have shown decreased conductance time, and abnormal heart rate and breathing patterns have been observed. Respiratory rates are increased, with low end-tidal volume PCO_2 and a shift to the left of the breathing response to CO_2. It has been suggested that these abnormalities increase the predisposition to SIDS (Wagner et al, 1998; Ostrea et al, 1999).

Another question undergoing investigation is whether the increased risk of SIDS is the result of a direct effect by the narcotic on the development of the respiratory center in the brainstem, or whether it is caused by a comprised home environ-

---

*Kenner & D'Apolito, 1997; Ostrea et al, 1997, 1999; Bauer, 1999; D'Apolito, 1998; Kaltenbach et al, 1998; Wagner et al, 1998; and Weiner & Finnegan, 1998.

ment with a mother who is under the influence of a narcotic, or whether it arises from a combination of these two factors (Wagner et al, 1998).

Respiratory Problems

Retained fetal lung fluid (RFLF) is among the leading pulmonary problems seen in heroin-addicted infants. The condition may occur secondary to the narcotic's inhibitory effects on the reflex clearance of fluid by the lungs (Ostrea et al, 1999).

The incidence of respiratory distress syndrome (RDS) among heroin-exposed infants generally is lower than would be expected, possibly because of enhanced fetal maturation from chronic stress. Chronic stress hastens lung maturity by stimulating the fetal adrenal gland to produce glucocorticoids, which in turn facilitate the production of surfactant in the lungs (Wagner et al, 1998; Ostrea et al, 1999).

Heroin-exposed infants have a higher incidence of meconium aspiration. As the fetus passes meconium during periods of fetal distress, aspiration may occur, leading to pneumonia or PPHN or both. Approximately 30% of cases of aspiration pneumonia result from meconium aspiration in these infants.

These respiratory problems (meconium aspiration, PPHN, and RDS) together account for more than 50% of the deaths among heroin-exposed infants (Wagner et al, 1998; Ostrea et al, 1999).

Sepsis

Pregnant addicts have a high incidence of infection, and a correspondingly high incidence of infection is seen in their infants. Many of the neonatal infections, such as sepsis, necrotizing enterocolitis, and gastroenteritis, are nonspecific in nature. Some infections, including hepatitis and sexually transmitted infections such as syphilis, gonorrhea, herpes, and group B streptococcal and HIV infection, are related to the mother's antenatal lifestyle and problems (Ostrea et al, 1999).

Neurobehavioral Effects

Some evidence suggests that long-term neurologic and developmental abnormalities are associated with intrauterine opiate exposure. Testing of these infants at 1 month and 2 years of age showed increased muscle tone, excessive movements, and problems with coordination and balance. By 7 to 12 years of age, no significant neurologic differences were found between children living with biologic parents and those living with foster families (Kenner & D'Apolito, 1997; D'Apolito, 1998). Difficulty with consolability and cuddling and other signs of poor state control and lability have also been seen. These problems can result in difficulties with infant-caregiver interactions or infant-mother bonding, or both. These infants are more likely to elicit consolation because they cry more often, but they are less easy to cuddle because of increased tone. They are also less readily maintained in an alert state and become increasingly less responsive to stimuli, especially visual and auditory stimuli. Because these are the primary means by which an infant initiates and maintains social interaction, these impairments may affect infant-mother interaction (Wagner et al, 1998; Eyler & Behnke, 1999; Ostrea et al, 1999).

Opiate-exposed infants have been shown to have lower scores on intelligence and language tests compared with a nonexposed control group. The differences widened with advancing age but were less apparent in children who were adopted or were placed in foster homes. It is difficult to say if these findings are completely explained by a direct effect of heroin, by

maternal health status during pregnancy, by polydrug use, or by later environmental conditions (Wagner et al, 1998; Coghlan et al, 1999; Eyler & Behnke, 1999).

Neonatal Abstinence Syndrome (NAS)

Abuse of heroin results in addiction, which is characterized by psychologic and physical dependence (D'Apolito, 1998; Ostrea et al, 1999). The fetus experiences withdrawal from heroin when intake is reduced and also in the neonatal period, because the newborn is no longer exposed after delivery (D'Apolito, 1998). Drug withdrawal in the mother heralds concomitant withdrawal in the fetus, which may lead to an increased risk of fetal distress and demise (D'Apolito, 1998; Wagner et al, 1998).

Neonatal abstinence syndrome (NAS) is described as a generalized disorder characterized by CNS hyperirritability, gastrointestinal dysfunction, respiratory distress, and autonomic dysfunction manifested by vague symptoms such as yawning, hiccups, sneezing, mottled color, and fever (Weiner & Finnegan, 1998). The origin of NAS is the abnormal uterine environment. The continuing or episodic transfer of addictive substances from the maternal to the fetal circulation, during which time the fetus goes through a biochemical adaptation to the drugs, threatens the growth and survival of the fetus. At delivery the abrupt removal of the drug precipitates the onset of symptoms. The infant continues to metabolize and excrete the drug, so that withdrawal signs occur when critically low tissue levels have been reached (Weiner & Finnegan, 1998).

The onset of withdrawal symptoms usually occurs within the first 72 hours after birth, often within the first 24 to 48 hours. However, the onset varies widely and depends on several factors, such as the type of substance and amount used by the mother, the time and duration of drug exposure, the drug elimination half-life, and the routes of drug metabolism and excretion in both the mother and fetus. Other factors that may also affect the rate and extent of drug transfer to the fetus include lipid solubility, molecular mass, protein binding, placental blood flow and permeability, degree of ionization, and the type of transfer (AAP, 1998a; Weiner & Finnegan, 1998; Tran, 1999; Ostrea et al, 1999; D'Apolito & Hepworth, 2001).

Infants exposed to opiates typically show more withdrawal symptoms than do infants exposed to other drugs, with methadone and heroin having the highest incidence (60% to 90% and 50% to 80%, respectively). Heroin is not stored in appreciable amounts by the fetus, therefore signs of heroin withdrawal appear quickly, usually within 24 to 48 hours after birth. However, methadone is stored in the fetal lungs, liver, and spleen, which facilitates the slower decline of methadone levels and results in a later onset of symptoms, possibly as late as 4 weeks (AAP, 1998a; Weiner & Finnegan, 1998; Ostrea et al, 1999; Tran, 1999).

Withdrawal symptoms may last up to 4 to 6 months. The prolonged symptoms usually are milder than the initial ones and consist of irritability, tremors, hypertonicity, sneezing, hiccups, and regurgitation. This persistence is related directly to the initial severity and is more prolonged in infants with severe withdrawal. No correlation has been seen between the severity of withdrawal and the infant's gender, race, or Apgar score or the mother's age or parity (Weiner & Finnegan, 1998; Ostrea et al, 1999; Tran, 1999).

Neurologic Signs. Neurologic signs are the most common symptoms of NAS, and they appear early. They include signs of CNS excitability, such as hyperactivity, irritability, tremors, and hypertonicity (Weiner & Finnegan, 1998; Ostrea et al, 1999; D'Apolito & Hepworth, 2001). Initially the infant may appear only to be restless. Tremors develop, which at first are mild and occur only when the infant is disturbed, but which eventually occur spontaneously without any external stimulation. High-pitched cry, increased muscle tone, and irritability progress to the point of inconsolability (Weiner & Finnegan, 1998; Ostrea et al, 1999).

Abstinence-associated seizures have been reported in about 1% of heroin-exposed infants and in about 5% to 7% of infants exposed to methadone. The onset occurs most often at 1 to 2 weeks. These seizures are most likely to be generalized motor seizures or myoclonic jerks, and they may occur even during NAS treatment. Abnormal electroencephalographic results tend to occur only during the active seizure, and the short-term prognosis is favorable (Weiner & Finnegan, 1998; Kandall, 1999).

Gastrointestinal Signs.   These infants have a suck that is disorganized, reduced in rate and sucking pressure, and poorly coordinated with swallowing. They appear incessantly hungry and suck frantically on their fists or fingers. However, they often have difficulty feeding because of coordination problems, resulting in poor nutrient intake, excessive weight loss, and suboptimum weight gain. Also common are vomiting and diarrhea, which can be severe enough to cause not only profound weight loss but also alterations in electrolytes and pH, as well as dehydration (Kaltenbach et al, 1998; Weiner & Finnegan, 1998; Kandall, 1999; Ostrea et al, 1999).

Respiratory Signs.   Respiratory signs most common in NAS include tachypnea, irregular respirations, rhinorrhea, a stuffy nose, nasal flaring, chest retractions, intermittent cyanosis, and apnea. These symptoms may become more severe if the infant regurgitates, aspirates, or develops aspiration pneumonia. Some evidence of transient abnormalities of lung compliance and tidal volume has been seen in opiate-exposed infants, which suggests that opioids may alter fetal development of the respiratory system. Alkalosis may be seen as a result of hyperventilation, and it may cause a decline in ionized calcium levels, which could lead to tetany (Weiner & Finnegan, 1998; Ostrea et al, 1999).

Signs of Autonomic Dysfunction.   Infants undergoing withdrawal exhibit signs such as frequent sneezing, yawning, mottling of the skin, tearing, and excessive generalized sweating. Sweating may be caused by the predominantly central-neurogenic stimulation of sweat glands induced by heroin withdrawal. Occasionally fever may be seen with the increased neuromuscular activities of tremors (Weiner & Finnegan, 1998; Kandall, 1999; Ostrea et al, 1999).

Diagnosis.   The diagnosis of NAS depends on a thorough maternal history, including medication and drug use and social habits; maternal and infant toxicology screens; and the infant's clinical presentation. Differentiating signs of drug withdrawal from those of infectious or metabolic disorders may be difficult. No clinical signs should be attributed only to withdrawal without appropriate assessment and diagnostic tests to rule out other causes, such as hypoglycemia, hypocalcemia, hypomagnesemia, and hypothermia (AAP, 1998a; Weiner & Finnegan, 1998: Tran, 1999).

Several scoring tools are available to assist the caregiver in evaluating and treating neonatal abstinence. One tool, the

NICU Network Neurobehavioral Scale (NNNS), was developed for the National Institutes of Health (NIH) as part of a neurobehavioral assessment battery for drug-exposed and high-risk infants. The NNNS was developed for use in the NIH Maternal Lifestyle Study, and it is the "offspring" of the Neonatal Behavioral Assessment Scale (NBAS). Although this tool provides a comprehensive evaluation of drug-exposed infants, the examiner must be certified in its use. It is extremely useful as a basis for consultation between clinician and parent, enabling them to mutually evaluate the infant and arrive at an appropriate plan of care that includes parental needs and anticipatory guidance, but it may be too time-consuming to be used as a bedside tool (Boukydis & Lester, 1999).

The Neonatal Abstinence Scoring System (NASS) is a widely used withdrawal severity scale for newborns that is objective and comprehensive. This tool measures 32 items, each assigned a weight of one to five points. Point summation yields a total score that represents the severity of withdrawal. However, this tool is cumbersome; its all-inclusiveness undermines its usefulness; and standard administration stipulates that scoring be done by the nurse caring for the infant, which precludes the possibility of blinded assessment (Zahorodny et al, 1998).

Zahorodny and colleagues (1998) have tested a newer method for rapid assessment of neonatal withdrawal, the Neonatal Withdrawal Inventory (NWI). The NWI consists of a standardized sequence of clinical care and assessment procedures, followed by evaluation of withdrawal severity with an eight-point checklist. Using the NASS as the standard, testing found the NWI to be reliable and valid. It can be administered and scored in 10 minutes or less by any clinician trained in its use, making it a highly efficient and flexible diagnostic method. It can be used under case-blinded conditions and is based entirely on structured observation, thus reducing potential sources of error. Also, withdrawal severity can be easily analyzed into its CNS, autonomic, gastrointestinal, and behavioral parameters, which allows investigators to track these aspects of withdrawal across time and in response to various treatments.

Loretta Finnegan's system, also called the Neonatal Abstinence Scoring System, monitors the infant in a comprehensive and objective way. It can be used to assess the onset, progression, and resolution of symptoms and can also be used to monitor the infant's clinical response to the pharmacotherapy used to control the symptoms of NAS. This system uses 21 symptoms most commonly observed in withdrawal, rated on a one to five point scale based on the symptom's clinical significance. Infants are initially assessed 2 hours after birth and every 4 hours afterward. If scores increase to eight or higher, scoring every 2 hours is instituted. The need for medication is indicated when the total score is eight or higher for three consecutive scorings or when the average of any three consecutive scores is eight or higher (Weiner & Finnegan, 1998; Tran, 1999). Although this system has been one of the most familiar and most frequently used, some institutions are adopting newer tools.

Treatment

Supportive Therapy.   The initial treatment of an infant with withdrawal symptoms should be mainly supportive, because drug therapy may prolong hospitalization and may not be necessary for infants with mild symptoms. Supportive therapy includes swaddling, reducing external stimulation such as light and noise, and maintaining a calm, quiet environment (D'Apolito, 1999; Tran, 1999).

A study by Maichuk and associates (1999) examined the use of positioning to reduce the severity of NAS in infants. These researchers confirmed that even the most highly agitated infants can enjoy a significant reduction in distress by being laid in the prone position for sleeping. The newborns who were undergoing narcotic withdrawal experienced significantly lower levels of distress and lower abstinence scores when placed in the prone position for sleeping, compared with infants who were kept in the supine position, a 30% difference, overall.

Rocking beds, combined with auditory stimulation, have been used to quiet irritable full-term infants, with the soothing effects of rocking being attributed to movements felt by the infant while in utero. Waterbeds, although nonoscillating, have been used to improve neurobehavioral functioning in opiate-exposed infants. It has been hypothesized that the rocking bed, combined with maternal intrauterine sounds, may reduce symptoms of withdrawal and promote neurobehavioral functioning in infants who have been exposed to drugs. D'Apolito (1999) studied 14 full-term methadone-exposed infants (placing seven in regular beds and seven in rocking beds), expecting to see improved sleep, less motor disturbance, and improved neurobehavioral organization among infants placed in the rocking beds. However, these outcomes were not observed. The results of the study suggested that the type of rocking bed therapy used might be too stimulating for infants experiencing withdrawal. The total average withdrawal symptoms had increased by the seventh day of life among the infants in the rocking beds, who also showed an increase in sleep disturbance. It is possible that the combination of motion and intrauterine sounds was too stimulating, and that one or the other alone actually may have improved the outcomes.

Pharmacologic Therapy. The decision to use drug therapy must be individualized, based on both the severity of withdrawal symptoms and an assessment of the risks versus benefits. Although drug therapy is known to reduce symptoms of withdrawal, the effects on long-term morbidity are unknown at present. Infants with confirmed drug exposure who do not have signs of withdrawal do not require drug therapy (AAP, 1998a; Tran, 1999).

Approximately 50% to 70% of infants that have been exposed to opiates require the use of pharmacologic agents to control withdrawal symptoms. Indications for the initiation of drug therapy include the following symptoms: seizure activity, poor feeding, severe diarrhea and vomiting that results in excessive weight loss and dehydration, inability to sleep, and fever that is unrelated to infection. If the Neonatal Abstinence Scoring System by Finnegan and associates is used, drug therapy should be started when the total score is eight or higher for three consecutive scorings or when the average of any three consecutive scores is eight or higher (AAP, 1998a; Weiner & Finnegan, 1998; Tran, 1999).

If pharmacologic management is needed, a drug should be selected from the same class as the drug causing the withdrawal symptoms. Guidelines to adequate therapy include a normal temperature curve; the ability to sleep between feedings and administration of medications; a decrease in activity, crying, and motor instability; and weight gain. Several pharmacologic agents have been used for therapy with favorable results, including paregoric, tincture of opium, morphine, methadone, phenobarbital, chlorpromazine, clonidine, and finally, diazepam (Table 39-1) (AAP, 1998a; Tran, 1999; Lipshitz et al, 2001).

Paregoric. Paregoric, which contains anhydrous morphine (0.4 mg/ml), was one of the first drugs used to treat NAS. Infants treated with paregoric had improved sucking patterns, resulting in increased nutrient consumption and better weight gain, as well as better seizure control than was obtained with phenobarbital or diazepam. Despite these beneficial effects, the use of paregoric has declined during recent years because of the known and potential toxic effects of its ingredients. Paregoric contains the isoquinoline derivatives noscapine and papaverine, which are antispasmodics. It also contains other potentially toxic compounds that include camphor, a CNS stimulant that is eliminated from the body slowly. It has a high concentration of ethanol (44% to 46%), a CNS depressant, and anise oil, which may cause habituation. Benzoic acid, an oxidative product of benzyl alcohol, is present and may compete for bilirubin binding sites or cause "gasping baby syndrome," which is characterized by severe acidosis, CNS depression, respiratory distress, hypotension, kidney failure, and death in small premature infants. Glycerin, another component, may cause severe diarrhea. In addition, large doses of paregoric and a long duration of use may be needed to control symptoms (AAP, 1998a; Kandall, 1999; Tran, 1999; Lifshitz et al, 2001).

Tincture of Opium. Tincture of opium (10 mg/ml) is the preferred drug for the treatment of opiate withdrawal because of its limited toxic effects. Tincture of opium should be used as a 25-fold dilution with water. Once diluted, it contains the same concentration of morphine equivalent as paregoric and is stable for 2 weeks. Tincture of opium can be administered according to the same morphine-equivalent dosage as paregoric (0.4 mg/ml) without the toxic additives or high alcohol content (AAP, 1998a; Tran, 1999).

Morphine. The parenteral form of morphine contains sodium bisulfite and phenol, both of which have been associated with adverse effects in infants. However, the amount of additives in standard doses of morphine may not be large enough to affect the newborn significantly (AAP, 1998a).

An oral preparation of morphine is available in concentrations of 2 and 4 mg/ml; this preparation has less alcohol and fewer additives than paregoric. As of this time, there have been no reported studies about the use of morphine in NAS, nor have any comparison studies been done with paregoric. If oral morphine is used, it is important to provide the same amount of morphine-equivalent as that in paregoric (AAP, 1998a; Tran, 1999).

Methadone. Methadone has been used extensively in adults to reduce withdrawal symptoms and to help addicts abstain from heroin use. It has also been used effectively in the treatment of NAS, but the use of methadone may be limited by several factors. For example, infants usually are not discharged from the hospital while they are taking methadone because of the potential for maternal abuse, therefore therapy generally is tapered and discontinued before the addicted infant is discharged from the hospital. Also, because of the long half-life of methadone in infants (about 26 hours), dose titration is difficult, and prolonged hospitalization is required (AAP, 1998a; Tran, 1999).

Phenobarbital. Phenobarbital has been used extensively for the treatment of opiate or barbiturate withdrawal in infants, and it is the drug of choice for nonnarcotic-related withdrawal symptoms. It is especially effective in controlling irritability and insomnia. It may also be used as an additional drug when tincture of opium is not effective (AAP, 1998a; Tran,

TABLE 39-1	Pharmacologic Management of Neonatal Abstinence Syndrome	
Drug	**Advantages**	**Disadvantages**
Paregoric (0.4 mg/ml anhydrous morphine)	Improved sucking patterns, better seizure control, diminished bowel motility and loose stools	Large doses and long duration of therapy are required to control symptoms. Drug contains toxic ingredients that can cause serious side effects in the neonate.
Tincture of opium (10 mg/ml)	Limited toxic effects; when used as a 25-fold dilution with water, contains the same concentration of morphine equivalent as paregoric and is stable for 2 weeks	Drug does not control loose stools.
Morphine sulfate	Lower alcohol content and fewer additives than paregoric	Drug contains additives that have been associated with adverse effects in infants, although the amounts may not be large enough to cause significant side effects. No reported studies are available about use for neonatal abstinence syndrome (NAS). No current comparison studies with paregoric are available.
Methadone	Has been used effectively to treat NAS	Infants are not discharged from the hospital while undergoing methadone therapy because of the potential for maternal abuse; therapy must be tapered and discontinued before discharge. Long half-life makes dose titration difficult. Use of drug results in prolonged hospitalization.
Phenobarbital	Has been used extensively for treatment of opiate or barbiturate withdrawal; effective in controlling irritability and insomnia; serum levels easily obtained	At high doses drug impairs sucking reflex. Tolerance to sedation develops. Induction of enhanced drug metabolism occurs. Drug is effective only for control of CNS symptoms. No effect is seen on gastrointestinal symptoms.
Chlorpromazine	Effective in controlling gastrointestinal and CNS symptoms	Adverse effects can include cerebellar dysfunction, lower seizure threshold, and hematologic abnormalities. Elimination is slow; half-life is 3 days. Titration is difficult.
Clonidine	Used effectively in treatment of withdrawal symptoms in opiate-addicted adults; small trials show effective reduction in most symptoms, except poor sleep, with no adverse effects; duration of treatment is significantly shorter	Drug has limited use in neonates; additional studies are needed in infants before routine use can be recommended.
Diazepam	Effective when used in conjunction with paregoric or phenobarbital; helps control symptoms of tremulousness, abnormal sucking, and irritability	Drug is not effective as a single agent. Elimination of drug and metabolites is lengthy (takes longer than 1 month). Late-onset seizures are common. Drug contains additives that may result in cerebral and hepatic dysfunction and hyperosmolarity.

1999; Lifshitz et al, 2001). The disadvantages of phenobarbital include impairment of the sucking reflex with high doses, development of tolerance to sedation, and induction of enhanced drug metabolism. Also, phenobarbital is effective only for control of CNS symptoms and has no effect on gastrointestinal symptoms. If phenobarbital is used, plasma concentrations must be measured 24 to 48 hours later; the desired level is 20 to 30 mg/L. The maintenance dosage should be adjusted according to the plasma concentrations and the infant's symptomatology as determined by abstinence scores (AAP, 1998a; Weiner & Finnegan, 1998; Tran, 1999).

Chlorpromazine. Chlorpromazine has proved to be effective in controlling gastrointestinal and CNS symptoms of NAS. However, its use has been limited by adverse effects, such as cerebellar dysfunction, reduced seizure threshold, and hematologic abnormalities. Also, the drug is eliminated very slowly in the neonate, having a reported half-life of 3 days, which makes dose titration very difficult (AAP, 1998a; Tran, 1999).

Clonidine. Clonidine, a nonnarcotic medication, has been used effectively in the treatment of withdrawal symptoms in adults addicted to opiates. However, its use in neonates is limited. In an open trial with seven neonates, clonidine was shown to be effective in reducing most NAS symptoms except poor sleep (AAP, 1998a; Tran, 1999). Neither hypotension nor other adverse effects were noted, and the duration of therapy was significantly shorter than with phenobarbital. Although clonidine appears to be effective for treatment of NAS, additional studies in infants are needed before routine use can be recommended.

Diazepam. Diazepam has proved effective for the treatment of NAS in opiate-exposed infants when used in conjunction with paregoric or phenobarbital, but it has never been used successfully as a single agent. Although diazepam helps control symptoms such as tremulousness, abnormal sucking behavior, and irritability, it is no longer used to treat NAS for several reasons. First, because newborns have a limited capacity to metabolize and excrete diazepam, elimination of the drug and its metabolites is prolonged, requiring longer than 1 month. Second, adverse effects, such as late-onset seizures, are common. Third, the parenteral formulation contains benzyl alcohol, sodium benzoate, ethyl alcohol, and propylene glycol, which may cause cerebral and hepatic dysfunction and hyperosmolarity in infants (AAP, 1998; Tran, 1999).

ALCOHOL

History

Alcohol is perhaps the first exogenous substance discovered by human beings that leads to altered states of consciousness. The earliest fermented beverage, wine, and, later, with the advent of distillation techniques, distilled spirits, were thought to be an "elixir of life" and were widely credited with medicinal properties in early European cultures, a practice that has persisted well into current times (Malanga & Kosofsky, 1999).

Although the consumption of alcohol can easily be traced to biblical times, the adverse effects on offspring of excessive alcohol consumption during pregnancy began to be suspected only about 200 years ago (Beckman & Brent, 1999). In the early 1970s, the features and problems of fetal alcohol syndrome were described by Jones and colleagues in the United States and by Lemoine and associates in France (Eyler & Behnke, 1999).

With the exception of caffeine, alcohol is used by more people and in larger amounts than any other psychoactive substance. Beer and wine are standard beverages with meals in many parts of the world (Howard & Lawrence, 1998). In late 1989, federal law began requiring warnings on all alcohol-containing beverages stating that women should not consume such beverages during pregnancy because of the risk of birth defects (Bauer, 1999). Despite these warning labels and other educational programs, the consumption of alcohol has increased. Although drinking during pregnancy declined in the late 1980s, the rates of alcohol use have again increased, especially that for frequent drinking (CDC, 1998; Jorgensen, 1999; Ostrea et al, 1999). Studies by the Centers for Disease Control and Prevention (CDC) have shown that alcohol use by pregnant women in the United States increased significantly from 1991 to 1995, with more than a 400% increase in the rate of heavier drinking. Heavier drinking was considered to be seven or more drinks per week or five drinks on any one occasion (CDC, 1998; Ostrea et al, 1999).

The use of alcohol among students in eighth through twelfth grades has also increased steadily. Nearly 80% of high school seniors report having used alcohol at some time in their life, and binge drinking (five or more drinks at one time) is common (AAP, 1998). Many young people do not consider wine, wine coolers, or beer to be alcohol, a fact that should influence the way a nurse questions a teenager about drinking.

The increase in the use of alcohol by young adults and pregnant women emphasizes the need for education and programs aimed at eliminating alcohol use during pregnancy, thereby preventing its devastating effects on the fetus.

Common Attributes of Women Who Use Alcohol

Based on CDC studies (1998), the characteristics of women most likely to indulge in moderate to heavy drinking during pregnancy are (1) unmarried, (2) employed or a student, and (3) annual income of $10,000 or less. Conversely, the moderate to heavy drinking group also includes women earning $50,000 or more who are college educated, who smoke, who are of minority race or ethnicity, and who have no prenatal care. Children with fetal alcohol syndrome or fetal alcohol effects are more likely to be born to an older woman who is multiparous. This is thought to be the case because the longer the woman drinks, the more alcohol it takes to achieve the effects she wants from alcohol consumption and the more damage is done to her organs, resulting in reduced liver and renal clearance of alcohol. The woman may be malnourished, because alcohol gradually replaces food. Possible associated diseases such as hepatitis, HIV infection, and sexually transmitted disease also affect the health of the mother and her child (Kenner & D'Apolito, 1997; Eyler & Behnke, 1999).

Polysubstance use, especially use of cocaine, may be common among individuals who drink heavily. These other substances reduce the uncomfortable side effects of an alcohol hangover, and the alcohol diminishes the loss of the effects of the other substances as the drug levels decrease. Pregnant women who abuse alcohol, especially if other drugs are also involved, often delay or eliminate prenatal care (Kenner & D'Apolito, 1997). Frequently, the woman has turned to drugs to dispel anxiety or depression. Drugs may also be an escape from poverty, personal problems, or feelings of hopelessness. If these issues are unresolved, they may contribute to long-term problems for mother and child (Kenner & D'Apolito, 1997).

Mechanism of Action

Ethyl alcohol (ethanol) is an analgesic with a depressant effect on the CNS. It is absorbed rapidly by diffusion across the mucosa of the stomach and intestines and usually is cleared by the bloodstream in about 1 hour in adults and 2 hours in newborns. The liver metabolizes approximately 95% of ethanol, and the kidneys and lungs filter the remaining 5%. Acetaldehyde, the metabolite of ethanol, is thought to be more toxic than ethanol itself (Howard & Lawrence, 1998; Ostrea et al, 1999).

An unimpeded bidirectional placental transfer of ethanol takes place during pregnancy. Alcohol is distributed quickly and nearly equally in maternal and fetal tissues. Fetal ethanol is metabolized and eliminated by the maternal liver. The amniotic fluid is considered a reservoir for ethanol, which increases the availability of the drug for the fetus. Fetal ethanol metabolism is half that of the adult. As a result, a major pathway for fetal ethanol clearance is back diffusion to the maternal system. Once the infant is born, this pathway is gone, and infants with high ethanol levels may appear intoxicated until the immature fetal liver can complete metabolism (D'Apolito, 1998; Ostrea et al, 1999).

Effects on Pregnancy

Ethanol has been found to cause impairment of normal placental function. It interferes with the transport of amino acids across the placenta to the fetus. It also has been shown to inhibit DNA synthesis and protein synthesis, in addition to impairing cellular growth, differentiation, and migration. Consequently, embryonic organization is altered, resulting in intrauterine growth restriction and chronic fetal hypoxia (Weiner & Finnegan, 1998; Ostrea et al, 1999).

Alcohol has been associated with a higher incidence of spontaneous abortion; the increase in spontaneous abortion among alcoholic pregnant women is as high as 52% of pregnancies. A large prospective study of pregnant women found alcoholic women to have a 2.3 times higher incidence of three or more spontaneous abortions than nonalcoholics. One single variable that correlated highly with spontaneous abortion was an extremely heavy episode of drinking during the early first trimester (D'Apolito, 1998; Ostrea et al, 1999). Other studies have not always shown an association between spontaneous abortion and alcohol use in light to moderate drinkers (Ostrea et al, 1999).

An increased risk of stillbirth has not been shown, even among women classified as heavy drinkers. However, the risk of abruptio placentae reportedly is greater (D'Apolito, 1998; Ostrea et al, 1999).

An increase in the occurrence of aneuploidy was found in the abortuses of women who consumed two or more drinks per week. Studies of mice showed that preovulatory alcohol exposure did not increase the incidence of abortion or aneuploidy, but alcohol administration shortly after ovulation did result in an increase in aneuploidy. Another study demonstrated that a single "binge" (three drinks at one time, or 2 drinks less than when a woman is not pregnant) resulted in the production of aneuploid embryos, which have a high risk of being spontaneously aborted during the first trimester. These studies lend credence to the theory that the high rate of spontaneous abortion among alcoholic women may be related to a single episode of heavy drinking around the time of conception (Ostrea et al, 1999). Another area of research concerns the possibility of a genetic connection with maternal metabolism and alcohol. The theory is that a woman's metabolism or the way in which she metabolizes alcohol may have as much to do with the effect on the developing fetus as does the actual amount of alcohol.

Fetal Effects

It is well known that infant development is directly impaired by fetal exposure to alcohol and that absolute alcohol is equally detrimental, be it derived from beer, wine, or liquor. Alcohol consumption during pregnancy results in growth restriction, physical anomalies, and CNS dysfunction (D'Apolito, 1998; Ostrea et al, 1999). The period in gestation during which the fetus is most vulnerable to the effects of alcohol, the areas of the brain that are most affected, and the threshold exposure for these events remain vague (Wagner et al, 1998). Animal models suggest that microcephaly secondary to diminished brain growth appears to be dose dependent late in gestation. A critical period for teratogenicity appears to be around the time of conception, when developing tissue is highly vulnerable, because anomalies characteristic of teratogenic effects on the anterior neural tube and surrounding structures frequently are seen (Malanga & Kosofsky, 1999). Both in vitro and animal studies support the premise that alcohol predominately interferes with the development of cells that are exiting mitosis at the time of exposure, leaving the remaining cell populations unharmed. This could explain some of the variability in the structural and behavioral anomalies (Wagner et al, 1998).

Animal studies have suggested that in utero alcohol exposure may cause fetal malnutrition and chronic fetal hypoxia by inducing hypoglycemia at high blood alcohol levels. Alcohol reduces the number of adrenergic receptors on the hepatic plasma membrane, interfering with carbohydrate metabolism and prenatal and postnatal growth. A dose-dependent contraction of the umbilical cord in vitro and diminished fetal placental flow in vivo have been seen with alcohol exposure, and these further contribute to fetal hypoxia (Ostrea et al, 1999).

Also described with alcohol use during pregnancy are abnormal fetal heart rate patterns, a decrease in fetal breathing movements, and a decrease in fetal movements. A reduction of the neurotransmitters in the human brain has also been seen, as have a decrease in the myelination process and decreases in fetal hippocampal nitric oxide synthase activity (Ostrea et al, 1999).

A number of factors appear to determine the outcome of a pregnancy in which the mother consumes alcohol. One in question is the amount of alcohol considered safe to consume during pregnancy. A large prospective study of 31,000 pregnancies was undertaken in an attempt to answer this question. A drink was defined as $1\frac{1}{2}$ ounces of distilled spirits, 5 ounces of wine, or 12 ounces of beer. Consumption of one or more drinks per day was associated with an increased risk of giving birth to an infant with growth restriction. The mother's age, parity, and health, as well as specific fetal susceptibility, contribute to the infant's outcome, but the potential for harm to the fetus is much greater with large amounts of maternal alcohol consumption. Nonetheless, current data do not support the concept of a "safe level" of alcohol consumption, below which no fetal damage occurs, during pregnancy (Committee on Substance Abuse & Committee on Children with Disabilities, 2000).

Use of both alcohol and cocaine by a pregnant woman poses an additional risk to the developing fetus. When the two are used together, a unique metabolite, cocaethylene, is formed. Cocaethylene is reported to be 10 times more potent than cocaine alone, and it readily crosses the placenta. The plasma concentrations of cocaethylene are higher, and it has a longer half-life. Cocaethylene intensifies the euphoric effects of cocaine and possibly increases the risk of sudden death. Animal studies have shown that cocaethylene affects brain growth in rat pups exposed during the third trimester. These findings suggest that cocaethylene may be more toxic in its effects on the fetus (Plessinger & Woods, 1998; Weiner & Finnegan, 1998; Jorgensen, 1999; NIDA, 2001).

Neurodevelopmental Disorders

In the early 1970s Jones and colleagues in the United States and Lemoine and colleagues in France first described the dysmorphic features, growth restriction, and CNS problems of infants with fetal alcohol syndrome. More recently, alcohol exposure in utero has been linked to a variety of other neurodevelopmental problems with new terminology. The term "fetal alcohol effects" is used to describe children with a variety of problems but not the full complement of fetal alcohol syndrome (Eyler & Behnke, 1999; Committee on Substance Abuse & Committee on Children with Disabilities, 2000).

Fetal Alcohol Syndrome. Fetal alcohol syndrome (FAS) may be the most commonly recognized cause of environmentally induced mental deficiency. Each year several hundred children are born with full FAS, and many more are born with more subtle fetal alcohol effects. FAS is considered to be one of the three most common known causes of mental restric-

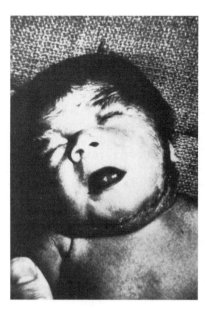 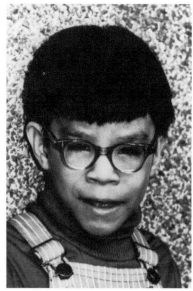 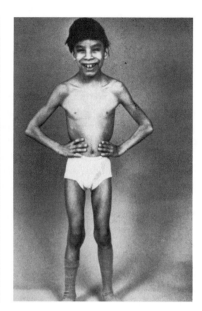

FIGURE **39-1**
Fetal alcohol syndrome (FAS). From Streissguth AP et al (1985). Natural history of the fetal alcohol syndrome: a 10-year follow-up of eleven patients. *Lancet*, 2(8445), 85-91.

tion and the only one that is completely preventable (Bauer, 1999; Beckman & Brent, 1999). Of all the drugs of recreational abuse, alcohol is the only one that is obviously teratogenic (Bauer, 1999).

The term fetal alcohol syndrome refers to a constellation of physical, behavioral, and cognitive abnormalities (Kenner & D'Apolito, 1997; Ostrea et al, 1999; Autti-Ramo, 2000; Committee on Substance Abuse & Committee on Children with Disabilities, 2000). The incidence of FAS is estimated to be 5.2 per 10,000 live births in the United States. The prevalence varies, depending on geographic location and specific population. The highest reported incidence of FAS occurs in the Native American and African American populations and among those with low socioeconomic status. For alcohol-abusing women, the risk of FAS increases with increasing maternal age and parity. If an older sibling has been diagnosed with FAS, the risk of a younger sibling having it is 406 times greater (Ostrea et al, 1999; Committee on Substance Abuse & Committee on Children with Disabilities, 2000).

Three specific criteria have been defined for the diagnosis of FAS, and an infant must have an abnormality in each category.
- Prenatal and postnatal growth restriction in relation to weight, length, or head circumference below the 10th percentile when corrected for gestational age
- CNS involvement, which includes signs of neurologic abnormalities (e.g., irritability in infancy, hyperactivity during childhood), developmental delay, hypotonia, or intellectual impairment (e.g., mental restriction)
- Characteristic facial dysmorphology (at least two of the three must be present): microcephaly (i.e., head circumference below the 3rd percentile), microphthalmia or short palpebral fissures, poorly developed philtrum, thin upper lip (i.e., vermilion border), and flattening of the maxilla (Kenner & D'Apolito, 1997; Ostrea et al, 1999; Autti-Ramo, 2000)

In addition to the short palpebral fissures, smooth philtrum, thin vermilion border, and hypoplastic maxilla, other dysmorphic features seen are epicanthal folds, broad nasal bridge, flat-

tened midfacies, short upturned or beaklike nose, micrognathia, and abnormal palmar creases (Figure 39-1) (Kenner & D'Apolito, 1997; Ostrea et al, 1999; Autti-Ramo, 2000).

Fetal Alcohol Effects. The term fetal alcohol effects (FAE) originally was developed to describe abnormalities observed in animal studies, but it was adopted by clinicians to describe children with a variety of problems, including growth deficiency, behavioral mannerisms, and delays in motor and speech performance, who lacked the full complement of FAS diagnostic criteria (Committee on Substance Abuse & Committee on Children with Disabilities, 2000). Although the term is widely used, no generally accepted definition exists for the diagnosis of FAE; however, it generally is associated with a wide range of developmental disorders of varying severity and complexity. An early definition, suggested by the Research Society on Alcohol, was "any condition thought to be secondary to alcohol exposure in utero." However, this definition was cumbersome and allowed for a wide divergence in interpretation. In 1996 the Institute of Medicine issued a report proposing that the terms "alcohol-related neurodevelopmental disorder" (ARND) and "alcohol-related birth defects" (ARBD) be used to describe conditions involving a history of maternal alcohol exposure (defined as substantial regular intake or heavy episodic drinking). This terminology uses a pathophysiologic basis for the diagnostic categories to describe conditions resulting from prenatal alcohol exposure (Figure 39-2) (Autti-Ramo, 2000; Committee on Substance Abuse & Committee on Children with Disabilities, 2000).

Long-Term Effects

Effects on Growth. Fetal alcohol exposure has both physical and psychologic long-term effects. One outcome that has been overlooked is that for approximately 69% of these children, their mothers will have died of complications related to alcohol abuse by the child's fourth birthday (Kenner & D'Apolito, 1997).

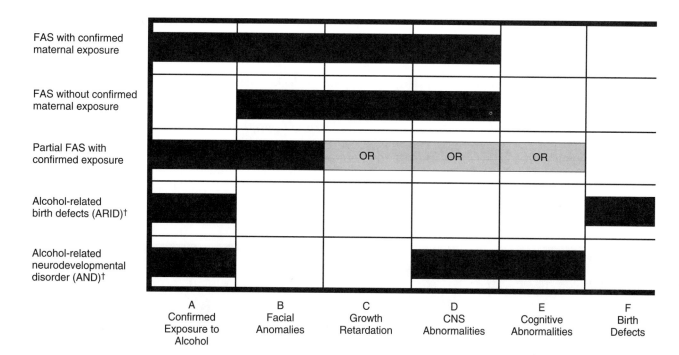

	A Confirmed Exposure to Alcohol	B Facial Anomalies	C Growth Retardation	D CNS Abnormalities	E Cognitive Abnormalities	F Birth Defects
FAS with confirmed maternal exposure	■	■	■	■		
FAS without confirmed maternal exposure		■	■	■		
Partial FAS with confirmed exposure	■	■	OR	OR	OR	
Alcohol-related birth defects (ARID)†	■					■
Alcohol-related neurodevelopmental disorder (AND)†	■			■		

*Adapted from Fetal alcohol syndrome: diagnosis, epidemiology, prevention, and treatment, 1996: 4-5. Letter designations in the figure indicate the following:

A. Confirmed maternal alcohol exposure indicates a pattern of excessive intake characterized by substantial, regular intake or heavy episodic drinking. Evidence of this pattern may include frequent episodes of intoxication, development of tolerance or withdrawal, social problems related to drinking, legal problems related to drinking, engaging in physically hazardous behavior while drinking, or alcohol-related medical problems such as hepatic disease.

B. Evidence of a characteristic pattern of facial anomalies that includes features such as short palpebral fissures and abnormalities in the premaxillary zone (eg, flat upper lip, flattened philtrum, and flat midface).

C. Evidence of growth retardation, including at least one of the following:
   • low birth weight for gestational age
   • decelerating weight over time not caused by nutrition
   • disproportional low weight to height

D. Evidence of CNS neurodevelopmental abnormalities, including at least one of the following:
   • decreased cranial size at birth
   • structural brain abnormalities (eg, microcephaly, partial or complete agenesis of the corpus callosum, cerebellar hypoplasia)
   • neurological hard or soft signs (as age appropriate), such as impaired fine motor skills, neurosensory hearing loss, poor tandem gait, poor eye-hand coordination

E. Evidence of a complex pattern of behavior or cognitive abnormalities that are inconsistent with developmental level and cannot be explained by familial background or environment alone, such as learning difficulties; deficits in school performance; poor impulse control; problems in social perception; deficits in higher level receptive and expressive language; poor capacity for abstraction or metacognition; specific deficits in mathematical skills; or problems in memory, attention, or judgment.

F. Birth defects associated with alcohol exposure include:

Cardiac	Atrial septal defects	Aberrant great vessels
	Ventricular septal defects	Tetralogy of Fallot
Skeletal	Hypoplastic nails	Clinodactyly
	Shortened fifth digits	Pectus excavatum and carinatum
	Radioulnar synostosis	Klippel-Feil syndrome
	Flexion contractures	Hemivertebrae
	Camptodactyly	Scoliosis
Renal	Aplastic, dysplastic, hypoplastic kidneys	Ureteral duplications
	Horseshoe kidneys	Hydronephrosis
Ocular	Strabismus	Refractive problems
	Retinal vascular anomalies	secondary to small globe
Auditory	Conductive hearing loss	Neurosensory hearing loss
Other	Virtually every malformation has been described in some patient with FAS. The etiologic specificity of most of these anomalies to alcohol teratogensis remains uncertain.	

†Alcohol-related effects indicate clinical conditions in which there is a history of maternal alcohol exposure, and where clinical or animal research has linked maternal alcohol ingestion to an observed outcome. There are two categories, alcohol-related neurodevelopmental disorder and alcohol-related birth defects, which may co-occur. If both diagnosis are present, then both diagnoses should be rendered.

FIGURE 39-2
Diagnostic classification of fetal alcohol syndrome (FAS) and alcohol-related effects. Redrawn from Committee on Substance Abuse and Committee on Children with Disabilities (2000). Fetal alcohol system and alcohol-related neurodevelopmental disorders. *Pediatrics*, 106(2), 358-361. Reprinted with permission.

Postnatal growth restriction and delayed motor performance are hallmarks of prenatal alcohol exposure; these children are growth restricted with respect to weight, height, and head circumference. Weight to height ratios were especially decreased. Because of the small mouth, CNS problems, and hypotonia, many of the infants may have difficulty feeding, resulting in failure to thrive (Figures 39-3 and 39-4) (Kenner & D'Apolito, 1997; Ostrea et al, 1999).

Cerebral Effects.   Slow growth of head circumference may indicate slow brain growth. Neurologic findings on magnetic resonance imaging (MRI) have shown a significant decrease in the cerebellar vermis, cerebral vault, basal ganglia, and dien-

cephalons. Other anomalies have been found, including complete callosal agenesis, hypoplastic corpus callosum, and hydrocephalus (Kenner & D'Apolito, 1997; Ostrea et al, 1999).

Ophthalmologic Effects.   Ophthalmologic abnormalities are common in children with FAS. These consist primarily of fundal anomalies and optic nerve hypoplasia, which have been attributed to competition of ethanol with retinal at the same ADH-binding sites. Other problems include strabismus, severe myopia, cataracts, glaucoma, persistent hyperplastic primary vision, and increased tortuosity of retinal vessels with reduced vascular branching hydrocephalus (Kenner & D'Apolito, 1997; Ostrea et al, 1999).

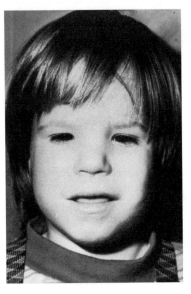 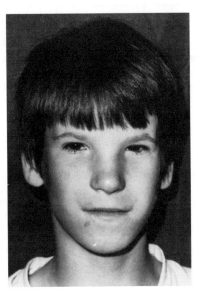 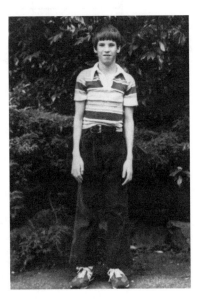

FIGURE **39-3**
Fetal alcohol syndrome (FAS) in the older child. From Streissguth AP et al (1985). Natural history of the fetal alcohol syndrome: a 10-year follow-up of eleven patients. *Lancet*, 2(8445), 85-91.

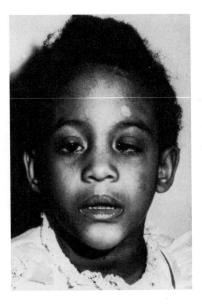 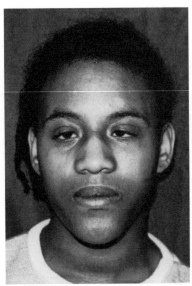 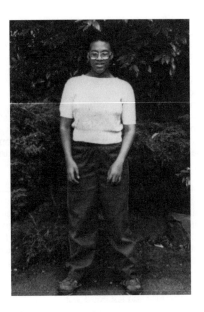

FIGURE **39-4**
Adult fetal alcohol syndrome (FAS). From Streissguth AP et al (1985). Natural history of the fetal alcohol syndrome: a 10-year follow-up of eleven patients. *Lancet*, 2(8445), 85-91.

Skeletal Effects.   Skeletal structural problems may be associated with FAS and usually are seen as scoliosis or flexion contractures. If the genitourinary system is affected because of these abnormalities, urinary tract infections or hydronephrosis, or both, are a possibility (Kenner & D'Apolito, 1997).

Hearing Effects.   FAS may be one of the more common causes of childhood hearing, speech, and language disorders. Four types of hearing disorder have been associated with FAS:
- Developmental delay in auditory maturation
- Sensorineural hearing loss
- Intermittent conductive hearing loss from recurrent serous otitis media
- Central hearing loss (70% of these children have conductive hearing loss secondary to recurrent serous otitis media, which may be related to craniofacial anomalies and eustachian tube dysfunction seen in FAS)

Most children with FAS have central hearing function injuries that are a serious concern. Such children have difficulty attending to and comprehending conversation in the presence of competing sounds such as conversations or noises in the classroom and social environment. This impairment may make language seem chaotic and incomprehensible and can lead to speech and language pathology, inattention, learning problems, and disruptive behaviors (Church & Abel, 1998; Ostrea et al, 1999).

Effects on Equilibrium.   Abnormal balance, coordination, and ataxia problems have been seen in children with FAS, and these problems appear to be related to cerebellar dysfunction. Studies have looked for evidence of alcohol damage to the vestibular system, but no compelling evidence has been found that the condition is a vestibular problem (Church & Abel, 1998).

Effects on Speech and Language.   Children with FAS typically are developmentally delayed in language acquisition and expressive and receptive language. Specific problems include poor syntactic or grammatical abilities, poor semantic abilities, and poor memory abilities. Other studies have reported depressed performance on sentence combining, word ordering, and grammatical comprehension and difficulty interpreting the pragmatic intent of statements (Church & Abel, 1998; Ostrea et al, 1999). Church and Abel (1998) observed expressive and receptive language delays in 86% of children with FAS.

Speech disorders associated with FAS include deficits in fluency, lack of intonation, and voice dysfunctions, such as hypernasality or a harsh voice, slurred speech, and poor articulation. These pathologic conditions are probably the result of a combination of CNS, hearing, and oral-motor defects. The study by Church and Abel (1998) found that 95% of children with FAS had significant speech pathology. Therefore children with FAS should be thoroughly evaluated and should undergo early intervention for hearing, speech, and language disorders.

Behavioral and Cognitive Effects.   Children exposed prenatally to alcohol may manifest cognitive, behavioral, and psychologic problems that cause lifelong disabilities. These manifestations may vary with age and circumstances. A study by Streissguth and colleagues that traced the natural history of alcohol-affected children into adulthood demonstrated the profound, pervasive, and persistent nature of the disorder. Abnormal cognitive functioning manifested itself many ways, including specific mathematical deficiency, difficulty with abstraction (e.g., time and space, cause and effect), and problems with generalizing from one situation to another. Poor attention and concentration skills, memory deficits, and impaired judgment, comprehension, and abstract reasoning also were seen. Behavioral issues, such as impulsivity and hyperactivity, and conduct problems, such as lying, stealing, stubbornness, and oppositional behavior, were common and were different from those found in other forms of mental restriction (Eyler & Behnke, 1999; Committee on Substance Abuse & Committee on Children with Disabilities, 2000).

Autti-Ramo (2000) followed children exposed to alcohol in utero for 12 years, with many of the same results, including deficits in attention, naming, receptive language, and visuomotor function. She also discovered that none of the existing special education classes was appropriate for all the children; rather, each child needed individual support. A surprising discovery was that the children with ARND often required more special education than the children with FAS. This was most likely a result of later identification and treatment, which emphasizes the need to consider fetal alcohol exposure as a learning difficulty factor, even if a child does not merit a diagnosis of FAS.

Autti-Ramo's study also found that many of the behavioral problems shown by alcohol-exposed children might be diminished or prevented if alcohol-exposed infants are identified and if their well-being is attended to on a continuing basis.

Breastfeeding.   Alcohol passes freely into breast milk, appearing quickly in fore and hind milk at levels equivalent to or higher than maternal serum levels. A significant and uniform intensity of odor to the milk has been noted between 30 and 60 minutes after alcohol ingestion. Infants' suckling rate increases, but less milk is obtained in the presence of alcohol. High amounts of maternal alcohol consumption have been found to suppress lactation. Acetylaldehyde, the toxic metabolite of alcohol, does not pass into milk. Currently the AAP considers maternal ethanol use to be compatible with breastfeeding, although it recognizes that adverse effects may occur (Howard & Lawrence, 1998, 1999).

Recommendations

Based on the medical, surgical, behavioral, custodial, and judicial services required, fetal alcohol exposure takes an economic toll on the individual, family, and society. Annual cost estimates for the United States range from $75 million to $9.7 billion, and the total lifetime cost of caring for a typical child with FAS may be as high as $1.4 million (Committee on Substance Abuse & Committee on Children with Disabilities, 2000).

The diagnosis of FAS is based on observation of physical findings, neurologic and cognitive effects, and a history of alcohol exposure. Nonetheless, many times a diagnosis may not be made because of lack of knowledge about how to make the diagnosis or because of physician reluctance to label the mother an alcohol user. Affected children may not be diagnosed until they come to the attention of a teacher who begins to see some of the cognitive and behavioral problems in school. If an infant is diagnosed early, monitoring and intervention can begin immediately, providing the opportunity for better outcomes and eligibility for special services (Kenner & D'Apolito, 1997; Stoler & Holmes, 1999; Autti-Ramo, 2000).

Pediatricians must be educated about the wide range of potential fetal effects of alcohol and about the importance of early recognition is. As Auti-Ramo (2000) demonstrated, infants and children with FAE often have more secondary disabilities than do children with FAS. The most likely reason is that the children with FAE were diagnosed late and therefore were not eligible for special services. Without accurate prevalence figures, the magnitude of the problem will be underestimated, and fewer resources may be allocated to the identification and treatment of women at risk and to services for affected children (Stoler & Holmes, 1999).

METHAMPHETAMINE

Drugs of choice vary over time and by geographic region. In recent years, methamphetamine, also known as "ice," "crank," "crystal," or "speed," has become a highly prevalent drug of abuse. In 1996 the National Household Survey on Drug Abuse reported that 4.9 million people have tried the drug at some time. Methamphetamine is a derivative of amphetamine and is prepared through the reduction of ephedrine or pseudoephedrine. Ease of synthesis, availability, and affordability, as well as a prolonged high, have made it an increasingly popular drug of choice (Ostrea et al, 1999; Smeriglio & Wilcox, 1999; Marwick, 2000).

Methamphetamine is a powerfully addictive substance that stimulates the CNS, producing increased alertness, sleeplessness, euphoria, and exhilaration. The drug metabolizes slowly, and the high lasts 8 to 24 hours (the high with cocaine lasts only 20 to 30 minutes) (Ostrea et al, 1999; Smeriglio & Wilcox, 1999; Marwick, 2000).

Currently little is known about the drug's effects on and mechanism of action in the fetus and neonate, but research is under way. It is not known how dangerous the drug is, but there is no basis for thinking methamphetamine is safe. Early studies have suggested that infants born to mothers who used the drug had significantly lower birth weight, length, and head circumference, but no significant increase was seen in the occurrence of congenital anomalies. Abnormalities such as altered sleep patterns, tremors, poor feeding, hypertonia, tachypnea, a high-pitched cry, and hyperreflexia, in addition to neurobehavioral changes, were also suggested. However, polydrug use is as common with methamphetamine users as with those who use other drugs, so it cannot be determined if these abnormalities are a result of methamphetamine use alone (Ostrea et al, 1999; Marwick, 2000).

ECSTASY (3,4 METHYLENEDIOXYMETHAMPHETAMINE)

The drug 3,4 methylenedioxymethamphetamine (MDMA), popularly known as "Ecstasy," is a "designer" drug that has become increasingly popular over the past two decades. The drug appeals to young people, who believe it enhances empathy and closeness to others. MDMA, which combines methamphetamines with hallucinogenic properties, is also known as "X-TC," "Adam," "Clarity," and "Lover's Speed." It was first used in the United States in the late 1970s as an adjunct to psychotherapy (Schwartz & Miller, 1997; Mueller & Korey, 1998; National Clearinghouse for Alcohol and Drug Information, 2001).

Common effects of MDMA include sweating, tachycardia, muscle spasms (including jaw clenching), and fatigue. Serious adverse effects include serious or fatal heat injury; fluid and electrolyte imbalance, especially hyponatremia; and dysfunction of the CNS, cardiac, muscular, renal, and hepatic systems (Schwartz & Miller, 1997; Henry et al, 1998; Baggott et al, 2000). MDMA has been shown to affect the serotonergic and dopaminergic neurons of the brain, causing a calcium-independent flood of serotonergic neuron release into the synaptic cleft while inhibiting serotonin reuptake. This results in the euphoria and stimulus effects of MDMA (Rochester & Kirchner, 1999).

Few studies have been done on the effects of MDMA on the fetus and neonate. The results of a study by Broening and colleagues (2001) using neonatal rats suggested that MDMA may pose a risk to the developing brain by inducing long-term deleterious effects on learning and memory. This raises concerns about the safety of MDMA when exposure occurs during stages of brain development comparable to the human late fetal period.

It previously was thought that MDMA toxicity required multiple exposures, but subsequent studies have shown that a single exposure to a high dose can induce the same adverse effects. In animal studies, signs of toxicity have been seen, such as behavioral changes and altered cerebral function. A particularly worrying feature emerging with MDMA toxicity is chronic psychosis, which reportedly responds poorly to therapy (Kelly, 2000).

McElhatton and colleagues (1999) conducted a prospective follow-up study of infants exposed to MDMA in utero. Their results indicated an association with a significantly increased risk of congenital defects, with cardiovascular and musculoskeletal anomalies predominant. Although this small case series had insufficient statistical power to confirm a causal relationship, the results are sufficient to justify further study.

POLYDRUG USE

As discussed throughout this chapter, polydrug use is common among pregnant women. The impact of drugs on the outcome of pregnancy depends on the type of drug used, the frequency and gestational period of use, and associated medical, nutritional, psychologic, and economic factors (Stichler et al, 1998). Studies on the effects of prenatal drug exposure have been difficult to evaluate, because few women addicts use only one drug. Furthermore, only a small number of studies have been done that report on the effects of polydrug exposure on newborns. Early studies suggested that tremors and startles, increased muscle tone, and greater irritability were among the most frequent symptoms of polydrug exposure (D'Apolito & Hepworth, 2001; Lester et al, 2001). A study by D'Apolito and Hepworth (2001) provided data about the most prominent symptoms of withdrawal found in a group of infants exposed to a variety of both legal and illegal drugs during pregnancy. Their results indicated that infants exposed to combinations of opiates, depressants, sedatives, and stimulants prenatally may experience more prominent symptoms of increased tone, increased respiratory rate, disturbed sleep, fever, excessive sucking, and watery or loose stools during withdrawal.

Sweeny and colleagues (2000) examined whether engaging pregnant substance abusers in an integrated program of prenatal care and substance abuse treatment would improve neonatal outcomes. Babies from the treatment group were reported to be 2 weeks farther along in gestation and to weigh 400 g more than the control group. These babies also had higher Apgar scores, fewer NICU admissions, and shorter hospitalizations. The researchers concluded that the neonatal outcome is significantly improved for infants born to substance abusers who receive substance abuse treatment and prenatal care concurrently.

CARE OF INFANTS WITH CENTRAL NERVOUS SYSTEM MANIFESTATIONS

Neonatal intervention is largely supportive and depends on the type of substance the mother has abused (Table 39-2). Infants born to women who abuse various substances are irritable and easily excited by sensory stimuli. The caregiver, therefore, should regulate the environment of these infants so as to reduce the amount and variety of sensory input. This can be done by dimming the nursery lights and reducing noise. If the nursery lights cannot be altered, a blanket can be placed over the infant's incubator to shield the baby from the bright lights. Many types of noise can be eliminated, for example, by speaking softly at the bedside, keeping radio and intercom volumes low, silencing alarms after responding, and closing incubator doors quietly. Infants exposed to drugs in utero benefit from a private or isolation room or a quieter area of the nursery.

The frequency of nursing intervention should be minimized by grouping care to the level of infant tolerance and by using electronic monitoring capabilities for routine vital signs. Unnecessary handling should be avoided. Routine laboratory work should be assessed individually and discontinued if unnecessary. Nurses can use infant behavioral cues as a basis for directing the amount of stimulation to be given. Infants have their own unique personalities; thus, the caregiver learns each infant's signals.

The amount of visual, auditory, and kinesthetic stimulation should be individually tailored to meet the infant's needs. The infant must be able to set the pace and tone of the interaction. An understanding of the infant's behavioral cues must be shared with the parents so that they can understand the basis for their child's behavior, which will help them to be more responsive to their infant's needs (Kenner & D'Apolito, 1997; Weiner & Finnegan, 1998).

CARE RELATED TO GASTROINTESTINAL MANIFESTATIONS

Infants who have been exposed to substances in utero often have a low birth weight and a poorly coordinated suck-swallow reflex. They also may experience abdominal cramping with diarrhea. Intense crying frequently is misinterpreted as hunger, and overfeeding creates abdominal distention, vomiting, and diarrhea. In these situations, infants should be fed smaller amounts more frequently. Often feedings every 3 hours are well tolerated, although this can be assessed on an individual basis. Because adequate nutrition is essential, accurate intake and output records must be kept. An indwelling nasogastric (NG) feeding tube often is helpful. Although bolus feedings are desirable because of their physiologic nature, the infant may be unable to finish the bottle; the remaining milk can be instilled via NG tube. Nipple feeding assisted by gavage reduces expenditure of calories and allows calories to be used for growth. An indwelling NG tube may also be used for the infant's benefit if a feeding is needed during nighttime sleep. Rest can then be maintained while nutrition is provided. Care must be taken to do what is best for the infant, not what is most convenient for the caretaker; feeding tubes should not be used indiscriminately. Sucking needs can be met with a pacifier or hand sucking during gavage feedings. Daily measurements of weight and head circumference should be obtained to track growth. Weight measurements are most accurate if the infant is weighed at the same time each day and with the same scale

(Kenner & D'Apolito, 1997; Weiner & Finnegan, 1998; D'Apolito & Hepworth, 2001).

CARE RELATED TO RISK OF INFECTION

Infants born to substance-abusing women are at risk of developing an infection as a result of exposure to maternal pathogens. These infants often are poorly nourished in utero and are more susceptible to infectious processes because of diminished immunocompetence. Care should be taken to maintain universal isolation precautions, because the incidence of hepatitis and HIV infection is higher among these women and their infants. Common signs and symptoms suggestive of sepsis are temperature instability, hypotonicity, color changes (pale or mottled), feeding intolerance, episodes of apnea, and bradycardia. Skin excoriations from episodes of crying and flailing may result from rubbing the nose, knees, and elbows against bed linens. The infant should be positioned so that these areas are protected, and the infant should be comforted consistently. Excoriations should be kept clean and dry and should be assessed periodically for infection. Tegaderm or its equivalent can be used to protect excoriated areas on knees and elbows from further breakdown (Kenner & D'Apolito, 1997; Weiner & Finnegan, 1998).

IDENTIFICATION OF THE SUBSTANCE-EXPOSED INFANT

Substance exposure in the neonate and infant often is difficult to identify. Mothers frequently do not admit that they take drugs because they fear the consequences of admitting to the use of an illegal substance. Recall usually is inaccurate, especially for details such as when, how often, and how much (Kwong & Shearer, 1998; Ostrea et al, 1999; Lester et al, 2001).

The AAP recommends that a comprehensive medical and psychosocial history that includes specific information about maternal drug use should be included in every newborn evaluation. Although maternal self-reporting frequently underestimates drug exposure, and maternal urine screening during pregnancy fails to identify many cases of drug use, laboratory screening should be seen as only a potential adjunct to a thorough history. The AAP also suggests that screening is needed when certain maternal characteristics are present. These include no or limited prenatal care, previous unexplained fetal demise, precipitous labor, abruptio placentae, hypertensive episodes, severe mood swings, cerebrovascular accidents, myocardial infarction, and repeated spontaneous abortions. Infant characteristics that may suggest maternal drug use include prematurity, unexplained intrauterine growth restriction, neurobehavioral abnormalities, urogenital anomalies, and atypical vascular incidents, such as cerebrovascular accidents, myocardial infarction, and necrotizing enterocolitis in an otherwise healthy full-term infant (AAP, 1998b; Buchi, 1998; Reinarz & Ecord, 1999).

Laboratory Tests
Urine Analysis. Urine has been the most commonly used specimen for neonatal drug testing because the collection is noninvasive; drugs and their metabolites usually are present in higher concentrations than in serum because of the concentrating ability of the kidneys; and urine usually is devoid of protein and other cellular constituents. However, this method has several limitations. The interval for drug detection depends on many variables, such as the individual drug metabolism, the infant's hydration status, and the route and frequency of ingestion.

TABLE 39-2   Summary of Potential Effects of Maternal Substance Abuse on Pregnancy and the Neonate

Effects	Tobacco	Cocaine	Heroin	Alcohol	Methamphetamines	3,4 Methylenedioxymethamphetamine (MDMA/Ecstasy)
Pregnancy-associated risks	Placental vasoconstriction Placenta previa Placental abruption Large placental to fetal ratio Spontaneous abortion	Placental vasoconstriction Spontaneous abortion Placental infarct Placental abruption Possible developmental toxicant	Placental vasoconstriction Intrauterine asphyxia Unsterile injections Unknown substances mixed with heroin Increased risk for hepatitis Increased risk for human immunodeficiency virus	Impaired placental function Inhibition of DNA and protein synthesis Impaired cellular growth, differentiation, and migration Placental abruption Spontaneous abortion	Research is ongoing.	Research is ongoing.
Direct fetal hazards	Prematurity Premature rupture of membranes Exposure to carcinogens Decreased birth weight Decreased head circumference Intrauterine hypoxia Reduced oxygen-carrying capacity of the blood Impaired ability to release oxygen into tissues	Prematurity Increased incidence of stillbirth Increased heart rate Increased blood pressure Increased cerebral blood flow Intrauterine hypoxia Meconium staining Teratogenic effects	Intermittent hypoxia from periodic withdrawal Increased incidence of stillbirth Increased breech position Increased meconium staining Increased asphyxia/fetal distress	Intrauterine growth restriction Chronic fetal hypoxia Microcephaly secondary to decreased brain growth Abnormal fetal heart rate patterns Decreased fetal breathing movements Decreased fetal movement Teratogenic effects	Research is ongoing.	Increased risk to developing brain
Infant hazards	Increased sudden infant death syndrome Increased respiratory distress syndrome Hypotonia/hypertonia Fine tremors Heightened Moro reflex Poor orientation Impaired attention Impaired consolability	Hypertonic effects Decreased head circumference Increased jitteriness Easy to overstimulate Altered state control Altered attention and responsiveness Difficulty with consolability Hyperextension Agitation Increased intracerebral hemorrhage/infarction	Neonatal abstinence syndrome Decreased respiratory distress syndrome Lower Apgar scores Neonatal depression Decreased birth weight Decreased length Decreased head circumference Increased incidence of aspiration pneumonia	Low birth weight Fetal alcohol syndrome/fetal alcohol effects Cerebral anomalies Cataracts Glaucoma Optic nerve hypoplasia Fundus anomalies Strabismus Myopia Scoliosis Flexion contractures Increased risk of nonspecific infections	Decreased birth weight Decreased length Decreased head circumference Altered sleep patterns Tremors Poor feeding Hypertonic Tachypnea High-pitched cry Hyperreflexia	Altered cerebral function

Hazards persisting into childhood	Impaired autonomic regulation Impaired orientation to sound Impaired lung growth and function Emphysema-like damage to lungs Impaired development and maturation of pulmonary immune system Decreased school performance Receptive language delays Exposure to second-hand smoke Possible increased risk of addiction to tobacco Impaired lung function Increased risk of upper respiratory infections with wheezing Increased occurrence of asthma	Cardiac defects Cardiac arrhythmias Necrotizing enterocolitis Intestinal perforation Optic nerve hypoplasia Delayed visual maturation Profound eyelid edema Nystagmus/strabismus Hearing impairment Attention deficit difficulties Abnormal play patterns Difficulty with concentration Delayed language skills Delayed motor development Cognitive and short-term memory deficits Decreased intelligence quotient (IQ) Increased behavior problems Difficulty managing impulses and frustration Visual motor disturbances Continued decreased head circumference	Increased incidence of meconium aspiration Retained fetal lung fluid Difficulty with consolability and cuddling Poor state control Difficulty with infant-caregiver bonding Persistent decreased weight, length, and head circumference Increased muscle tone Difficulty with coordination and balance	Central nervous system dysfunction Irritability Tremors Poor feeding Easy to overstimulate Attention deficit difficulties Learning disorders Cognitive impairment Impaired judgment Postnatal growth restriction Decreased weight Decreased height Decreased head circumference Decreased scores on IQ and language tests Hearing deficits Difficulty with balance and coordination Delayed language acquisition Delayed expressive and receptive language Poor memory abilities Impaired comprehension Impaired abstract reasoning Impulsivity Hyperactivity Conduct problems (e.g., lying, stealing)	Research is ongoing. Deficits in learning and memory

Most illegal drugs can be detected in urine only within 48 to 72 hours after use. Therefore the longer after birth that urine is collected and tested, the greater the likelihood of a false-negative result. Also, if the mother has abstained for a few days before delivery, the infant's urine may test negative. If a positive result is obtained, confirmatory testing must be done, because other substances, such as over-the-counter medications and herbal preparations, can produce a positive result (Buchi, 1998; Kwong & Shearer, 1998; Ostrea et al, 1999; Reinarz & Ecord, 1999).

Meconium Analysis.　In the fetus, drugs of abuse are metabolized into water-soluble products in the liver and then excreted in the urine or bile. These metabolites accumulate in the meconium during gestation, either by direct deposition from the biliary tree or through fetal ingestion of amniotic fluid. Meconium is not normally excreted in utero, which allows for concentration of the metabolite in the sample. Consequently, meconium analysis has several advantages over urine testing in newborns. It has a large interval for detection of intrauterine drug exposure, as early as the sixteenth week of gestation. It also has high sensitivity and specificity, and the sample can be obtained with ease in a noninvasive manner. The disadvantages are that the test is more expensive to perform, and some hospitals are not set up to run it, which means the samples must be sent out, possibly delaying diagnostic results (Buchi, 1998; Kwong & Shearer, 1998; Ostrea et al, 1999; Reinarz & Ecord, 1999).

Hair Analysis.　Hair analysis, one of the most recent additions to drug testing, is based on the principle that illegal substances and their metabolites in blood become incorporated into the hair follicle and grow into the cuticle and hair shaft. Once the drug is deposited in the hair shaft, it remains for an indefinite period. Because hair grows at the rate of 1 to 2 cm per month, the deposited drugs follow the growth of the hair shaft, with the hair closest to the scalp being the most recently exposed. Thus sectional analysis can be done by month to provide information on the duration and time of drug use. However, several drawbacks limit the usefulness of this technique. First, a sufficient sample requires an amount of hair of as much as 10 mg. Even if a newborn has enough hair to collect an adequate specimen, the mother may be reluctant to allow the infant's hair to be cut. Second, the possibility exists that external contamination of the hair may occur, and third, hair analysis is more difficult to perform, and only a few laboratories currently are available to do the analysis (Buchi, 1998; Kwong & Shearer, 1998; Ostrea et al, 1999; Reinarz & Ecord, 1999).

Other Methods of Analysis.　Several methods currently are under investigation as possible drug testing techniques, including analysis of gastric contents, nail clippings, perspiration, and saliva. However, these types of specimens have not been commonly used for drug detection, and further testing and refinement are needed to improve reliability (Ostrea et al, 1999; Reinarz & Ecord, 1999).

Legal Implications

Studies have shown that many drug-using mothers are unable to care for their infants properly or that their environments are unsafe for their infants. As a result, many institutions have taken measures to identify these infants, and child protective agencies have acted to separate them from their mothers at birth (MacMahon, 1997). In some locales, public attitudes have encouraged criminal prosecution of the mother. Several states have mandatory reporting policies regarding drug-exposed infants, and in some stated these cases must be reported to criminal justice agencies as child abuse or neglect (MacMahon, 1997; Buchi, 1998).

The AAP considers the practice of performing drug screening for the primary purpose of detecting illegal use as unethical. The AAP recommends that drug screening be done only as part of a medical evaluation to assist in the diagnosis of drug exposure, thus ensuring prompt and proper treatment. When the test is ordered, the mother should be informed that it is being done and that all infants who meet certain guidelines are screened routinely to ensure appropriate treatment (MacMahon, 1997; AAP, 1998b; Reinarz & Ecord, 1999).

A study by MacMahon (1997) followed the judicial placement of newborns with positive toxicologic screens, the mothers' compliance with court orders, and the eventual placement of the infants. The study's findings support the idea that identifying and reporting maternal substance abuse during pregnancy can be associated with beneficial changes in the infants' environment and with successful rehabilitation of the mother when the reporting process is accompanied by judicial investigation, provision of rehabilitative and supportive services, and long-term involvement of the courts or social services without criminal prosecution.

The dilemma of defining high-risk behavior is strengthened by physicians' general lack of knowledge about addiction and about referral options, a lack of confidence in treatment programs, and an assumption that substance use is not prevalent among their patients. These factors result in a low rate of interaction between families and physicians on substance abuse problems. Consequently, the problem is approached from a purely legal avenue, resulting in the child being lost in a quagmire of bureaucracy. Instead, access to treatment for these families should be improved, allowing the family the opportunity to receive support. However, should the family fail to take advantage of these opportunities, consequences should be tightened to protect the child (Chasnoff, 1998). Still, if there are no beneficial outcomes of reporting these situations, the practice cannot be condoned.

Some institutions have made it a practice to obtain toxicology screens for the purpose of gathering evidence against the drug-using mother. However, this practice currently is being challenged in court. In Charleston, South Carolina, as a result of a joint effort by the hospital and the police, several women were arrested after testing positive for cocaine. In March, 2001, in *Ferguson v City of Charleston*, the U.S. Supreme Court ruled that a state hospital's order to give a patient a drug test without the patient's consent for the sole purpose of obtaining evidence of a patient's criminal conduct is a violation of the patient's Fourth Amendment rights. The Court reasoned that administering such diagnostic tests without obtaining informed consent constituted an unreasonable search. Although they ruled that drug testing without consent is a violation, the justices eventually sent this case back to the lower court to decide if any of the women involved had actually given consent to the drug tests (Greenhouse, 2001; Supreme Court of the United States, 2001). Health care professionals must closely follow this case, because the final outcome may require changes in practice.

NURSING ASSESSMENT OF THE SUBSTANCE-USING MOTHER

With today's abbreviated hospital stays, the admission protocol for all women should include a systematic routine assessment for substance abuse. The foundation for this form of intervention should be a staff of well-educated nurses. In-services and continuing education programs could be a vehicle to augment the staff's expertise in detecting signs of abuse.

Nurses gather data through all available means. They need to systematically observe and interview all women entering the health care system for signs of substance abuse, such as track marks on the arms from injections, an inflamed nasal septum from cocaine use, alcohol on the breath, and tobacco stains on the fingers. Beyond observational data comes interview data. Drug history taking obtained by a more structured interview and in a nonthreatening environment significantly improves the rate of maternal admission to illegal drug use (Ostrea et al, 1997).

Women, especially pregnant women, frequently underreport smoking, drinking, and drug use. However, self-reporting is the best method available to date, and if no questions are asked about use of these substances, no information will be elicited. To increase self-reporting, the nurse must create a comfortable atmosphere that encourages the woman to disclose sensitive information (Box 39-1). This atmosphere can be created by applying the following principles. Interviews should be conducted in a private office and should start with generic questions covering factual information (e.g., name, address); they should progress to the most sensitive information at the end of the interview (e.g., substance use). Questions should be open ended and phrased in a manner to permit discussion. The interviewer should expect the patient to be open and honest. This attitude is subtly conveyed to the woman and becomes a self-fulfilling prophecy.

A woman's tobacco, alcohol, and drug use patterns resemble those of her partner, and past use parallels current practices. As the interview begins, the nurse should tell the woman that the questions she will be asked are asked of everyone. The ordering of the questions is important; they should begin with questions about the partner's use, proceed to the woman's past use, and, finally, center on the woman's current use. Box 39-2 presents a list of questions that can be used effectively to obtain accurate information from a substance-using mother.

The nurse's questions should be nonjudgmental and should give the woman permission to report drinking. If the woman is

having two drinks per day, but she is asked if she has three or four drinks per day, then she will feel more comfortable self-reporting drinking. Questions are also phrased so that the answer is more than "yes" or "no" and so that some discussion ensues. If the woman responds to any of the questions with ambiguous answers, such as, "I'm a social drinker" or "I use crack for recreation," the responses must be clarified with respect to amount and frequency of use (Weiner et al, 1985).

If a woman becomes angry about the questions or refuses to answer, it may be because the questions have come uncomfortably close to her personal use and she is not willing to discuss

---

BOX 39-1

Effective Interview Techniques

1. Create a comfortable atmosphere.
2. Conduct the interview in a private office or area.
3. Ask open-ended questions.
4. Phrase questions in a way that allows discussion.
5. Begin with generic questions about factual information (e.g., name, address).
6. Progress to the most sensitive questions (e.g., substance abuse) at the end of the interview.
7. Use nonjudgmental questions.
8. When discussing substance use, begin with questions about the partner's use, follow with questions about the woman's past use, and end with questions about the woman's current use.
9. The interviewer should expect the woman to be open and honest; the interviewer's attitude is subtly conveyed to the woman and becomes a self-fulfilling prophecy.

BOX 39-2

Effective Interview Questions to Ask the Substance-Using Mother

The following questions are more likely to elicit accurate information than vague questions such as, "Do you drink?" or "You don't smoke, do you?"

1. "I would like to begin by asking a few questions about your partner's habits."
2. "How many packs of cigarettes per day does your partner smoke?"
3. "How often does your partner drink beer, wine coolers, malt liquor, or hard liquor?" (*Note:* Several alcoholic beverages are itemized because many individuals do not realize that wine coolers and beer contain enough alcohol to harm the fetus.)
4. "How many drinks does your partner have at one time?"
5. "Does he party?" If the answer is yes, ask:
   - "Does he ever do pot, crack/cocaine, or other drugs when he's out with his friends?"
   - "What do you do when he is partying?"
   If the answer to the party question is no, ask:
   - "When was the last time he used pot, crack/cocaine, or other drugs?" (*Note:* Women whose partners use drugs are more likely to use drugs themselves. Questions about the partner's behaviors should be explored to identify women at risk for substance use. Pregnant women sometimes find it hard to admit their use for fear of harm to the fetus or recriminations from the health professional, but exposure to substances by the partner is acceptable.)
6. "Think back over the 6 months just before you knew you were pregnant, then please answer the following questions." (*Note:* If the woman admits to use before the pregnancy, it may have continued before she realized she was pregnant. Use may be continuing, but the woman may be afraid to admit it.)
   - "How many packs of cigarettes per day do you smoke?"
   - "How often do you drink beer, wine coolers, whiskey, or other drinks containing alcohol?"
   - Do you have three or four drinks at a time?" (*Note:* Asking about drinking large amounts may help the woman feel comfortable about disclosing that she has one or two drinks per night. This question also may reveal a binge drinking pattern of three or more drinks at a time for a pregnant woman.)
   - "When was the last time you used pot, crack/cocaine, or other drugs?

this. She may also react out of shock at being questioned. Her response should be noted and evaluated by the nurse. If the nurse feels that she is perhaps using substances and not disclosing it, the subject can be brought up again later in the course of her prenatal care.

Once substance abuse has been identified, the nurse can begin counseling by exploring with the patient the risks of continuing the addiction.

NURSING INTERVENTION FOR THE SUBSTANCE-USING MOTHER

Interventions for Families

It is imperative that members of the health care team approach drug-using families in a nonjudgmental manner. It is appropriate to acknowledge the mother's actions and the resultant effects on the infant, but it must be done factually. Scare tactics and threats are counterproductive in that they heighten maternal anxiety and may exacerbate the abuse. The clinician, therefore, should avoid dwelling on what damage may have already been sustained and instead focus on the potential good that could occur from detoxification or, in the case of heroin, transference to methadone (Robinson, 1999).

Other family members may have a wide range of needs, possibly related to their feelings about the mother's actions. However, it is important for the health team member to support the mother and not to allow family members to play one against another (Robinson, 1999).

Interventions to Enhance Mother-Baby Bonding

Influencing the parenting effectiveness of substance-dependent women requires a comprehensive approach. First and foremost is the need to successfully assess substance abuse problems and to make appropriate treatment referrals. Before these women can be taught effective parenting techniques, they must commit to recovery efforts. Lasting improvements in the mother-child relationship are not feasible until the mother's pre-existing problems have been addressed (Davis, 1997).

French and colleagues (1998) determined that nurses can help mothers recognize and respond to the behavioral cues of their newborns by demonstration, thus enhancing mother-infant interactions. Appropriate nursing intervention includes educating parents, pointing out infant cues and explaining their significance. The mother should also be shown when the infant appears receptive to interaction. These mothers may misinterpret infant irritability as dislike, but it is important to emphasize that the infant lacks the cognitive abilities to "dislike" her and that the infant, when irritable, simply needs extra patience and understanding rather than avoidance or resentment. It is important to involve other family members in the infant's care to lend assistance to both mother and baby. These women have frail coping reserves and need help to care adequately for their infants. A trusting nurse-patient relationship can help immensely. Discharge should be interdisciplinary and should include follow-up care.

The ultimate goal is to reduce or eliminate substance abuse among women, especially during pregnancy. Improved outcomes have been reported for infants and children who live in a supportive and nurturing environment. In addition, early intervention has helped improve outcomes for children with deficits caused by prenatal drug exposure (D'Apolito, 1998).

VALUE CONFLICTS FOR HEALTH PROFESSIONALS

It is common for the health team member to experience a wide range of emotional responses when working with substance-exposed infants. These feelings may vary from sincere empathy to anger and frustration. However, care must focus on serving the best interests of the child while supporting the family as much as possible (Robinson, 1999). Recognition and discussion of the difficulties faced by professionals who treat infants exposed to drugs in utero are critical to the delivery of quality care.

Because of the negative label frequently attached to drug addiction, many health care providers are uncomfortable with openly discussing relevant issues with their patients. However, if substance issues are not discussed, many women will fail to receive needed services and referrals.

Discussing substance abuse as a disease helps to take the value judgment away from the conversation and allows the woman to be less defensive. Defensive behaviors are part of the addictive disorder and must be dealt with professionally and objectively (Davis, 1997).

SUMMARY

Infants who have been exposed to substances in utero present a challenge for the neonatal nurse; accurate assessment is vital in order to anticipate and plan for the problems that may occur. More is being learned about these neonates every day, but many of the long-term risks are still unknown. The care of these infants is much more complex because of the pattern of maternal polydrug use, and each neonate may have slightly different clinical manifestations. The management principles outlined in this chapter provide a sound basis for care, regardless of the combination of maternal drugs to which the neonate has been exposed.

REFERENCES

Aligne CA, Stoddard JJ (1997). Tobacco and children: an economic evaluation of the medical effects of parental smoking. *Archives of pediatrics and adolescent medicine,* 151, 648-653.

American Academy of Pediatrics (AAP) Policy Statement (1998a). Neonatal drug withdrawal (RE9746). *Pediatrics,* 101(6), 1079-1088.

American Academy of Pediatrics (AAP) Policy Statement (1998b). Tobacco, alcohol, and other drugs: the role of the pediatrician in prevention and management of substance abuse (RE9801). *Pediatrics,* 101(1), 125-128.

American Academy of Pediatrics (AAP) Policy Statement (2001). Tobacco's toll: implications for the pediatrician (RE0041). *Pediatrics,* 107(4), 794-798.

Anderson MS, Hay WW (1999). Intrauterine growth restriction and the small-for-gestational-age infant. In Avery GB, Fletcher MA, MacDonald MG, editors. *Neonatology: pathophysiology and management of the newborn,* ed 5. Lippincott Williams & Wilkins: Philadelphia.

Arendt R et al (1999). Motor development of cocaine-exposed children at age two years. *Pediatrics,* 103(1), 86-92.

Askin DF, Diehl-Jones B (2001). Cocaine: effects of in utero exposure on the fetus and neonate. *Journal of perinatal and neonatal nursing,* 14(4), 83-102.

Autti-Ramo I (2000). Twelve-year follow-up of children exposed to alcohol in utero. *Developmental medicine and child neurology,* 42, 406-411.

Baggott M et al (2000). Chemical analysis of ecstasy pills (research letter). *Lancet,* 284(17), 2190.

Bauer CR (1999). Perinatal effects of prenatal drug exposure: neonatal aspects. *Clinics in perinatology*, 26(1), 87-106.

Becker AB et al (1999). Breastfeeding and environmental tobacco smoke exposure. *Archives of pediatrics and adolescent medicine*, 153, 689-691.

Beckman DA, Brent RL (1999). The effects of maternal drugs in the developing fetus. In Avery GB, Fletcher MA, MacDonald MG, editors. *Neonatology: pathophysiology and management of the newborn*, ed 5. Lippincott Williams & Wilkins: Philadelphia.

Behnke M et al (1997). How fetal cocaine exposure increases neonatal hospital costs. *Pediatrics*, 99(2), 204-208.

Belcher HME et al (1999). Sequential neuromotor examination in children with intrauterine cocaine/polydrug exposure. *Developmental medicine and child neurology*, 41, 240-246.

Boukydis CFZ, Lester BM (1999). The NICU network neurobehavioral scale: clinical use with drug-exposed infants and their mothers. *Clinics in perinatology*, 26(1), 213-230.

Brazelton TB (1999). Behavioral competence. In Avery GB, Fletcher MA, MacDonald MG, editors. *Neonatology: pathophysiology and management of the newborn*, ed 5. Lippincott Williams & Wilkins: Philadelphia.

Broening HW et al (2001). 3,4-Methylenedioxymethamphetamine (Ecstasy)-induced learning and memory impairments depend on the age of exposure during early development. *The journal of neuroscience*, 21(9), 3228-3235.

Buchi KF (1998). The drug-exposed infant in the well-baby nursery. *Clinics in perinatology*, 25(2), 335-350.

Centers for Disease Control and Prevention (CDC), National Center on Birth Defects and Developmental Disabilities (1998a). Fetal alcohol syndrome: prevention activities. Retrieved online June 4, 2001, at http://www.cdc.gov/ncbddd/fas/fasprev.htm

Centers for Disease Control and Prevention (CDC), National Center on Birth Defects and Developmental Disabilities (1998b). Fetal alcohol syndrome fact sheet. Retrieved online June 4, 2001, at http://www.cdc.gov/ncbddd/fas/default.htm

Centers for Disease Control and Prevention (CDC) (2001c). Women and smoking: a report of the surgeon general, 2001: pattern of tobacco use among women and girls—fact sheet. Retrieved online June 1, 2001, at http://www.gov/tobacco/sgr_forwomen/factsheet_tobaccouse.htm

Centers for Disease Control and Prevention (CDC), National Center for Chronic Disease Prevention and Health Promotion (2001d). Cigarette smoking among adults: United States, 1998. Retrieved online June 4, 2001, at http://www.cdc.gov/tobacco/research_data/adults_prev/ccmm4939_fact_sheet.html

Centers for Disease Control and Prevention (CDC), National Center for Chronic Disease Prevention and Health Promotion (2001e). Pattern of tobacco use among women and girls: fact sheet. Retrieved online June 4, 2001, at http://www.cdc.gov/tobacco/sgr_forwomen/factsheet_tobaccouse.htm

Chasnoff IJ (1998). Silent violence: is prevention a moral obligation? (commentary). *Pediatrics*, 102(1), 145-147.

Chasnoff IJ et al (1998). Prenatal exposure to cocaine and other drugs: outcome at four to six years. *Annals of the New York Academy of Sciences*, 846, 314-328.

Church MW, Abel EL (1998). Fetal alcohol syndrome: hearing, speech, language, and vestibular disorders. *Obstetrics and gynecology clinics of North America*, 25(1), 85-97.

Church MW et al (1998). Effects of prenatal cocaine on hearing, vision, growth, and behavior. *Annals of the New York Academy of Sciences*, 846, 12-28.

Cody MM (2001). Is there help for a smoker? understanding nicotine replacement therapy. *The American journal for nurse practitioners*, April, 32-41.

Coghlan D et al (1999). Neonatal abstinence syndrome. *Irish medical journal*, 92(1), 232-233, 236.

Committee on Substance Abuse and Committee on Children with Disabilities (2000). Fetal alcohol syndrome and alcohol-related neurodevelopmental disorders. *Pediatrics*, 106(2), 358-361.

D'Apolito K (1998). Substance abuse: infant and childhood outcomes. *Journal of pediatric nursing*, 13(5), 307-316.

D'Apolito K (1999). Comparison of a rocking bed and standard bed for decreasing withdrawal symptoms in drug-exposed infants. MCN, *The American journal of maternal child nursing*, 24(3), 138-144.

D'Apolito K, Hepworth JT (2001). Prominence of withdrawal symptoms in polydrug-exposed infants. *Journal of perinatal and neonatal nursing*, 14(4), 46-60.

Davis SK (1997). Comprehensive interventions for affecting the parenting effectiveness of chemically dependent women. *Journal of obstetric, gynecologic, and neonatal nursing*, 26(5), 604-610.

Delaney-Black V et al (1998a). Prenatal cocaine exposure and child behavior. *Pediatrics*, 102(4), 945-950.

Delaney-Black V et al (1998b). Prenatal coke: what's behind the smoke? *Annals of the New York Academy of Sciences* 846, 277-288.

Elliot J et al (1998). Maternal cigarette smoking is associated with increased inner airway wall thickness in children who die from sudden infant death syndrome. *American journal of respiratory and critical care medicine*, 158, 802-806.

Eyler FD, Behnke M (1999). Early development of infants exposed to drugs prenatally. *Clinics in perinatology*, 26(1), 107-150.

Eyler FD et al (1998). Birth outcome from a prospective matched study of prenatal crack/cocaine use. I and II, Interactive and dose effects on health and growth. *Pediatrics*, 101(2), 229-241.

Fletcher MA (1999). Physical assessment and classification. In Avery GB, Fletcher MA, MacDonald MG, editors. *Neonatology: pathophysiology and management of the newborn*, ed 5. Lippincott Williams & Wilkins: Philadelphia.

Franco P et al (1999). Prenatal exposure to cigarette smoking is associated with a decrease in arousal in infants. *Journal of pediatrics*, 135(1), 34-38.

Frank DA et al (1999). Level of in utero cocaine exposure and neonatal ultrasound findings. *Pediatrics*, 104(5), 1101-1105.

Frank DA et al (2001). Growth, development, and behavior in early childhood following prenatal cocaine exposure. *Journal of the American Medical Association*, 285(12), 1613-1626.

French ED et al (1998). Improving interactions between substance-abusing mothers and their substance-exposed newborns. *Journal of obstetric, gynecologic, and neonatal nursing*, 27(3), 262-269.

Gilliland FD et al (2001). Effects of maternal smoking during pregnancy and environmental tobacco smoke on asthma and wheezing in children. *American journal of respiratory and critical care medicine*, 163, 429-436.

Greene O et al (1998). Perinatal outcome after cocaine and polydrug exposure. *Annals of the New York Academy of Sciences*, 846, 396-398.

Greenhouse L (2001). Justices, 6-3, bar some drug tests. *New York Times*, March 22.

Henry JA et al (1998). Low-dose MDMA ("Ecstasy") induces vasopressin secretion (research letter). *Lancet*, 351, 1784.

Howard CR, Lawrence RA (1998). Breastfeeding and drug exposure. *Obstetrics and gynecology clinics of North America*, 25(1), 195-217.

Howard CR, Lawrence RA (1999). Drugs and breastfeeding. *Clinics in perinatology*, 26(2), 447-478.

Hunt CE (2001). Increased risk of SIDS in younger siblings of SIDS patients tied to genetics. *American journal of critical care medicine*, 164, 246-357.

Jauniaux E et al (1999). Maternal tobacco exposure and cotinine levels in fetal fluids in the first half of pregnancy. *Obstetrics and gynecology*, 93(1), 25-29.

Jorgensen KM (1999). The drug-exposed infant: physiology, signs, and symptoms. *NANN central lines*, 15(2), 1-2, 8-9, 11.

Kaltenbach K, Finnegan L (1998). Prevention and treatment issues for pregnant cocaine-dependent women and their infants. *Annals of the New York Academy of Sciences*, 846, 329-334.

Kaltenbach K et al (1998). Opioid dependence during pregnancy: effects and management. *Obstetrics and gynecology clinics of North America*, 25(1), 139-151.

Kandall SR (1999). Treatment strategies for drug-exposed neonates. *Clinics in perinatology*, 26(1), 231-243.

Karmel BZ et al (1998). Neonatal neurobehavioral assessment and Bayley I and II scores of CNS-injured and cocaine-exposed infants. *Annals of the New York Academy of Sciences*, 846, 391-395.

Kelly P (2000). Does recreational Ecstasy use cause long-term cognitive problems? *Western journal of medicine*, 173, 129-130.

Kenner C, D'Apolito K (1997). Outcomes for children exposed to drugs in utero. *Journal of obstetric, gynecologic, and neonatal nursing*, 26(5), 595-603.

Kwong TC, Shearer D (1998). Detection of drug use during pregnancy. *Obstetrics and gynecology clinics of North America*, 25(1), 43-57.

Lee M (1998). Marijuana and tobacco use in pregnancy. *Obstetrics and gynecology clinics of North America*, 25(1), 65-83.

Lester BM et al (2001). The maternal lifestyle study: drug use by meconium toxicology and maternal self report. *Pediatrics*, 107(2), 309-317.

Leventhal JM et al (1997). Maltreatment of children born to women who used cocaine during pregnancy: a population-based study. *Pediatrics*, 100(2). Retrieved online May 31, 2001, at http://www.pediatrics.org/cgi/content/full/100/2/e7

Lifshitz M et al (2001). A four-year survey of neonatal narcotic withdrawal: evaluation and treatment. *Israel Medical Association Journal*, 3(1), 17-20.

Lustbader AS et al (1998). Incidence of passive exposure to crack/cocaine and clinical findings in infants seen in an outpatient service. *Pediatrics*, 102(1). Retrieved online May 31, 2001, at http://www.pediatrics.org/cgi/content/full/102/1/e5

MacMahon JR (1997). Perinatal substance abuse: the impact of reporting infants to child protective services. *Pediatrics*, 100(5). Retrieved online May 31, 2001, at http://www.pediatrics.org/cgi/content/full/100/5/e1

Maichuk GT et al (1999). Use of positioning to reduce the severity of neonatal narcotic withdrawal syndrome. *Journal of perinatology*, 19(7), 510-513.

Malanga CJ, Kosofsky BE (1999). Mechanisms of action of drugs of abuse on the developing fetal brain. *Clinics in perinatology*, 26(1), 17-33.

Marwick C (2000). NIDA [National Institute on Drug Abuse] seeking data on effect of fetal exposure to methamphetamine (Medical News & Perspectives). *Journal of the American Medical Association*, 283(17), 2225-2226.

McElhatton PR et al (1999). Congenital anomalies after prenatal Ecstasy exposure (research letter). *Lancet*, 354, 1441.

Milerad J et al (1998). Objective measurements of nicotine exposure in victims of sudden infant death syndrome and in other unexpected child deaths. *Journal of pediatrics*, 133(2), 232-236.

Miller JM, Boudreaux MC (1999). A study of antenatal cocaine use: chaos in action. *American journal of obstetrics and gynecology*, 180(6), 1427-1431.

Mirochnick M et al (1997). Elevated plasma norepinephrine after in utero exposure to cocaine and marijuana. *Pediatrics*, 99(4), 555-559.

Mueller PD, Korey WS (1998). Death by "Ecstasy": the serotonin syndrome? *Annals of emergency medicine*, 32(3), 377-380.

National Clearinghouse for Alcohol and Drug Information (2001). Prevention works: Ecstasy. Retrieved online June 4, 2001, at http://www.health.org/govpubs/prevalert/v3i25.htm

National Institute on Drug Abuse (NIDA), National Institutes of Health (2001a). Cocaine abuse and addiction. Retrieved online June 4, 2001, at http://www.drugabuse.gov/ResearchReports/Cocaine/cocaine.html

National Institute on Drug Abuse (NIDA), National Institutes of Health (2001b). Cocaine abuse and addiction. Retrieved online June 4, 2001, at http://www.drugabuse.gov/ResearchReports/Cocaine/cocaine3.html

National Institute on Drug Abuse (NIDA), National Institutes of Health (2001c). Cocaine abuse and addiction. Retrieved online June 4, 2001, at http://www.drugabuse.gov/ResearchReports/Cocaine/cocaine4.html

National Institute on Drug Abuse (NIDA), National Institutes of Health (2001d). Cocaine abuse and addiction. Retrieved online June 4, 2001, at http://www.drugabuse.gov/ResearchReports/Cocaine/cocaine5.html

National Institute on Drug Abuse (NIDA), National Institutes of Health (2001e). Crack and cocaine. Retrieved online June 4, 2001, at http://www.drugabuse.gov/infofax/cocaine.html

National Institute on Drug Abuse (NIDA), National Institutes of Health (2001f). Heroin: abuse and addiction. Retrieved online June 4, 2001, at http://www.drugabuse.gov/drugpages/heroin.html

Ostrea EM et al (1997). Mortality within the first 2 years in infants exposed to cocaine, opiate, or cannabinoid during gestation. *Pediatrics*, 100(1), 79-83.

Ostrea EM et al (1999). The infant of the drug-dependant mother. In Avery GB, Fletcher MA, MacDonald MG, editors. *Neonatology: pathophysiology and management of the newborn*, ed 5. Lippincott Williams & Wilkins: Philadelphia.

Ownby DR et al (2000). Passive cigarette smoke exposure of infants. *Archives of pediatrics and adolescent medicine*, 154, 1237-1241.

Plessinger MA, Woods JR (1998). Cocaine in pregnancy: recent data on maternal and fetal risks. *Obstetrics and gynecology clinics of North America*, 25(1), 99-118.

Reinarz SE, Ecord JS (1999). Drug-of-abuse testing in the neonate. *Neonatal network*, 18(8), 55-61.

Richardson GA (1998). Prenatal cocaine exposure: a longitudinal study of development. *Annals of the New York Academy of Sciences*, 846, 144-152.

Robinson TMS (1999). Perinatal substance abuse: working with neonates and families. *Neonatal network*, 18(2), 68-70.

Rochester JA, Kirchner JT (1999). Ecstasy (3,4 methylenedioxymethamphetamine): history, neurochemistry, and toxicology. *Journal of the American Board of Family Practice*, 12, 137-142.

Schwartz RH, Miller NS (1997). MDMA (Ecstasy) and the rave: a review. *Pediatrics*, 100(4), 705-708.

Singer LT et al (2001). Developing language skills of cocaine-exposed infants. *Pediatrics*, 107(5), 1057-1064.

Smeriglio VL, Wilcox HC (1999). Prenatal drug exposure and child outcome: past, present, future. *Clinics in perinatology*, 26(1), 1-16.

Stichler JF et al (1998). Examining the "cost" of substance abuse in pregnancy: patient outcomes and resource utilization. *Journal of perinatology*, 18(5), 384-388.

Stoler JM, Holmes LB (1999). Under-recognition of prenatal alcohol effects in infants of known alcohol abusing women. *Journal of pediatrics*, 135(4), 430-436.

Supreme Court of the United States (March 21, 2001). *Ferguson et al v City of Charleston et al* Available online at http://supct.law.cornell.edu/supct/html/99-936.ZS.html

Sweeny PJ et al (2000). The effect of integrating substance abuse treatment with prenatal care on birth outcome. *Journal of perinatology*, 4, 219-224.

Tran JH (1999). Treatment of neonatal abstinence syndrome. *Journal of pediatric health care*, 13(6 part 1), 295-300; quiz, 301-302.

Wagner CL et al (1998). The impact of prenatal drug exposure on the neonate. *Obstetrics and gynecology clinics of North America*, 25(1), 169-194.

Weiner SM, Finnegan LP (1998). Drug withdrawal in the neonate. In Merenstein GB, Gardner SL, editors. *Handbook of neonatal intensive care*, ed 4. Mosby: St Louis.

Weiner L et al (1985). Training professionals to identify and treat pregnant women who drink heavily. *Alcohol health and research world*, 10, 32-35.

Windham G et al (2000). Prenatal active or passive tobacco smoke exposure and the risk of preterm delivery or low birth weight. *Epidemiology*, 11(4), 427-433.

Wisborg K et al (2000). A prospective study of smoking during pregnancy and SIDS. *Archives of disease in childhood* 83(3), 203-206.

Zahorodny W et al (1998). The neonatal withdrawal inventory: a simplified score of newborn withdrawal. *Journal of developmental and behavioral pediatrics*, 19(2), 89-93.

CHAPTER 40

CARE OF THE EXTREMELY-LOW-BIRTH-WEIGHT INFANT

CAROLE KENNER

The extremely-low-birth-weight (ELBW) infant is a frequent resident of most neonatal intensive care units (NICUs) these days. Technology has grown exponentially, to the extent that the age of viability, although still hovering at 23 weeks, could conceivably drop lower. Genetic knowledge is providing the tools to "fix" errors of metabolism and repair defects in utero. Cloning of human tissues is possible. What the NICU will look like in another decade and which infants will be cared for there cannot be accurately predicted. One certainty is that very-low-birth-weight (VLBW) infants and ELBW neonates will be part of this new population.

The care of these infants has been detailed in each of the system chapters. The ethical and legal dilemmas were addressed in Chapter 3. This chapter is an overview, a quick reference for risk factors, typical problems, and some of the long-term outcomes for these infants. The chapter also addresses the areas where nurses need to contribute to the scientific basis for nursing care.

VLBW AND ELBW INFANTS

The term very-low-birth-weight infant refers to one who is born weighing less than 1500 g (Table 40-1). The extremely-low-birth-weight infant is one who is born weighing less than 1000 g. These infants have unique problems because of their very vulnerable state of development.

Many years ago, all children were viewed as "little adults," and their care usually reflected a variation on adult care. However, over the past 30 years, it has become clear that children are not small adults; they are a special population of patients who require very specialized treatment.

The same change occurred with respect to the neonatal population. In the late 1960s health care professionals realized that neonates, especially those who were sick and premature, required more specialized care than simply general pediatrics. It now is well recognized that the growing subset of neonates born at 23 to 28 weeks is an exception to the general neonatal "rules." These infants are premature according to their gestational age, and generally they are VLBW or ELBW neonates. The two designations are not always interchangeable. For example, in underdeveloped countries, a few infants may be of low birth weight (weighing less than 2500 g) because of intrauterine growth restriction and maternal malnutrition. Some VLBW and ELBW infants, therefore, are not premature, although the majority are. Whatever the reason for the low-birth-weight (LBW) status, these neonates require highly specialized care if they are to survive and thrive.

RISK FACTORS

Many risk factors appear to contribute to low birth weight. Some of these factors require further investigation to determine their precise effects. However, many factors are known.

- *Culture:* American-born white infants, for example, are less likely to be LBW neonates than American-born black infants (Southgate & Pittard, 2001). The exact reason is unclear.
- *Maternal nutritional status:* If the mother's nutritional status is poor, the infant is more likely to be born underweight. Researchers are just beginning to follow the birth weights of women with a history of eating disorders to determine if the mother's birth weight might somehow be related to the birth weights of her children. Women who are underweight when they become pregnant may give birth to LBW infants.
- *Maternal history of problem pregnancies or known risk factors (e.g., age disparity):* These risk factors include maternal age under 15 or over 35 years; a history of spontaneous abortions or premature births, or a history in the family of other infants who were classified as LBW neonates; and perinatal infections that easily cross the placenta, such as rubella, syphilis, cytomegalovirus (CMV), human immunodeficiency virus (HIV), and herpes simplex virus (Southgate & Pittard, 2001).
- *Altitude:* Infants born high in the Andes of South America or in Denver, Colorado, in the United States are known to be under the established norms for their gestational age, and the difference may push the infant into the 10th percentile on typical growth charts. New growth charts, redrawn by Lubchenco, reflect a downward trend for infants born in regions higher than 2000 m above sea level (Southgate & Pittard, 2001).
- *Substance abuse:* Mothers who smoke or drink alcohol or who abuse cocaine or other illegal substances are known to give birth to infants affected by intrauterine growth restriction (IUGR). These infants may or may not be premature.
- *Pregnancy-induced hypertension:* This condition, especially when it occurs early in gestation, can result in low birth weight.

TABLE **40-1**	Percentage of All Infants Born at Very-Low-Birth-Weight*: Selected Years, 1970-1994							
	YEAR							
Category	1970	1975	1980	1985	1990	1992	1993	1994
Total	1.2	1.2	1.2	1.2	1.3	1.3	1.3	1.3
Race/Ethnicity[†]								
White	1	0.9	0.9	0.9	1	1	1	1
Black	2.4	2.4	2.5	2.7	2.9	3	3	3
Hispanic	—	—	1	1	1	1	1.1	1.1
Age of Mother (years)								
Under 15	—	3.1	3.4	3.1	3.2	3.1	3.6	3.4
15 to 19	—	1.8	1.7	1.8	1.8	1.8	1.8	1.7
20 to 24	—	1.1	1.1	1.2	1.3	1.3	1.3	1.3
25 to 29	—	0.9	1	1	1.1	1.1	1.1	1.2
30 to 34	—	1	1	1.1	1.2	1.2	1.2	1.2
35 to 49	—	1.2	1.2	1.3	1.4	1.5	1.5	1.6

*Before 1979, very-low-birth-weight was defined as less than 1500 g; since 1979, very-low-birth-weight has been defined as infants weighing less than 1500 g.
[†]Percentages are based on the race and ethnicity of the mother. Percentages of very-low-birth-weight by ethnicity are not available before 1980. Birth figures for Hispanic infants in 1980 are based on data from 22 states that reported Hispanic origin of the mother on the birth certificate. Other figures for Hispanic infants are based on reporting from 23 states and the District of Columbia in 1985; 48 states and the District of Columbia in 1990; 49 states and the District of Columbia in 1992; and 50 states and the District of Columbia in 1993 and 1994.
Sources: National Center for Health Statistics (1996). Health, United States, 1995. Table 11 for totals and race/ethnicity breakdowns for 1970-1993. Public Health Service: Hyattsville, MD; **1975** data from Table 1-37, Vital Statistics of the United States, 1975, **1980** data from Table 13 (1982). Monthly Vital Statistics Report, vol. 31, no. 8, supplement. National Center for Health Statistics: Hyattsville, MD; **1985** data from Table 17 (198). Monthly Vital Statistics Report, vol. 36, no.4, supplement. National Center for Health Statistics: Hyattsville, MD; **1990** data from Table 13 (1993). Monthly Vital Statistics Report, vol. 41, no. 9, supplement. National Center for Health Statistics: Hyattsville, MD; **1992** data from Ventura SJ et al (1994). Advance report of final natality statistics, 1992. Tables 24 and 44. Monthly Vital Statistics Report, vol. 43, no. 5, supplement. National Center for Health Statistics: Hyattsville, MD; **1993** data from Ventura SJ et al (1995). Advance report of final natality statistics, 1993. Tables 24 and 44. Monthly Vital Statistics Report, vol. 44, no. 3, supplement. National Center for Health Statistics: Hyattsville, MD; **1994** data from Ventura SJ et al (1996). Advance report of final natality statistics, 1994. Tables 24 and 44. Monthly Vital Statistics Report, vol. 44, no. 11, supplement. National Center for Health Statistics: Hyattsville, MD.

- *Higher order multiple pregnancies:* Twins or a higher number of fetuses are more likely than the singleton pregnancy to produce an LBW infant.
- *Genetic factors:* Short maternal stature is related to low birth weight and the occurrence of congenital malformations or syndromes, including errors of metabolism.
- *Placental changes:* Placental risk factors for low birth weight include an aged placenta; cord anomalies that reduce vascular blood flow to the fetus; torsion of the placental vessels; chronic maternal conditions that affect the placental blood flow; and abnormalities of implantation, such as placenta accreta (Box 40-1).

In summary, any condition, maternal or fetal, that adversely affects the vascularity of the placenta or cord or the delivery of nutrients to the developing fetus has the potential to restrict growth and may lead to the delivery of an LBW, a VLBW, or an ELBW infant. Premature birth often accompanies a low birth weight. The risk factors for prematurity generally are the same as those listed above. However, the anticipated problems are slightly different for the too-low-birth-weight, or premature, infant.

LBW VERSUS PREMATURITY

The LBW, VLBW, or ELBW infant is one who has not grown in utero according to the established norms. This infant has been competing for nutrients, including oxygen, during gesta-

tional development. Whether the cause is maternal illness or infection or multiple gestations, the result is a stressed fetus. A stressed fetus generally develops more quickly than a premature or LBW infant. Many neonatal nurses remember the first time they saw the wizened, "old" baby that was small for gestational age (SGA); these babies just look old and worried. For a long time it has been thought that these infants would have fewer respiratory complications, even if born prematurely, because their lungs were forced to mature quickly. However, current research is not clearly supporting this notion. Some SGA infants do have respiratory problems, including bronchopulmonary dysplasia (BPD). This is an area ripe for research.

Growth-restricted infants have few nutrient stores, and if they are born prematurely, the scenario worsens. These neonates have no areas of brown fat for thermoregulation, and their labile metabolic state adds to their thermal problems. Low oxygen levels, which are tolerated better in utero than in extrauterine life, lead to problems such as some degree of asphyxia; respiratory depression, if the infant is close to term; possible passage of meconium in utero, leading to meconium aspiration; polycythemia and elevated erythropoietin levels, the body's attempt to produce more oxygen-carrying cells and to protect the fetus; and hypoglycemia and hypocalcemia. All these factors lead to a decrease in blood flow to tissues and developing organ systems; one of the seriously vulnerable systems is the developing brain.

BOX 40-1

Placental Findings with Idiopathic Growth Restriction

Uteroplacental Blood Flow
Diminished blood flow
Increased vascular resistance
Absent spiral artery remodeling
Atherosis of vessels of parietal deciduas

Fetoplacental Blood Flow
Diminshed branching of umbilical arteries and veins
Increased irregularity of luminal size
Abnormal umbilical Doppler flow studies
Decreased number of placental arterial vessels
Decreased size of placental vessels
Decreased artery to villus ratio

Interface of Maternal and Fetal Circulations
Cytotrophoblastic hyperplasia
Thickened basement membrane
Chronic villitis

From Southgate WM, Pittard WB II (2001). Classification and physical examination of the newborn infant. In Klaus MH, Fanaroff AA, editors. Care of the high-risk neonate, ed 5. WB Saunders: Philadelphia.

If an infant is LBW and premature, the brain is very vulnerable to the effects of diminished oxygen levels. Pain research has shown that the "wiring" of the brain is affected by both intrauterine and extrauterine events and that the capabilities of sensation are present early in gestation (see Chapter 42 for more information on pain in the neonate). These infants are vulnerable to intracranial bleeding (Chapter 37) because of the friability of the neurologic tissue, especially in the growing germinal matrix. The neurodevelopmental and neurobehavioral outcomes of these infants are also areas of growing concern. These outcomes likewise are affected not only by insults that occur in utero, but also by those that occur during the first few weeks of extrauterine life.

More attention is focusing on the physical environment of the NICU and the impact of that environment on the developing neonate. Issues underlying this reassessment include the development of retinopathy of prematurity (ROP) secondary to diminished oxygen levels and exposure to direct bright lights; the development of hearing loss and auditory damage secondary to increased noise levels in the NICU; and the development of an increased neurologic network when painful procedures are performed repeatedly without the benefit of analgesia or anesthesia, a condition that leaves these children supersensitive to painful stimuli for life.

More research is under way to design individualized care that will promote the growth and development of sick, premature, or growth-restricted infants. Health professionals must be more aware of their daily procedures and of the impact of these procedures on the developing neonate. For example, a study by Lott and colleagues (2001) conducted with VLBW infants showed that a simple, routine procedure, such as flushing an umbilical artery catheter (with the line in either the high or low position), changed the cerebral blood flow patterns seen on Doppler sonograms.

Another area of concern is the skin. The skin of a very premature VLBW or ELBW infant is very thin and gelatinous. The barrier function for heat (thermoregulation) and for invading organisms is absent. These infants are at risk for fluid losses (i.e., insensible losses caused by thermal factors, exposure to radiant warmers, and sometimes care procedures). They also require the most use of equipment and technologic devices, which puts them at risk of skin abrasions caused by tape or invasive procedures (Chapter 34). The risk of infection is high, because these infants have an immature immune system; because they often lack the protection of passive immunity; or because a perinatal infection has been passed on in utero. Skin breakdown, another pathway for infection, occurs more frequently in these neonates if nutritional status is allowed to continue to decline after birth.

Premature VLBW or ELBW infants also are very vulnerable to iatrogenic complications, including side effects of medications such as diuretics and antibiotics. Steroids, which are used to promote lung development, are also known to suppress the immune system and to alter fluid and electrolyte balance.

CARE OF VLBW AND ELBW INFANTS

Specific methods of care have been provided in each of the systems chapters. This section is meant only to outline the key areas of care. The nurse must keep in mind that the infant is part of a family unit and will grow up within a cultural context. The family must be included as partners in the care of their infant, and they must help the nurse understand the cultural influences that should be a part of that care.

The following are the key areas of care:

- *Airway:* What is the infant's respiratory status? Are supports needed? Is meconium aspiration a consideration? Is the infant at risk for the development of BPD?

- *Thermoregulation:* This is always a priority consideration, along with the airway. Keep the infant warm and protected from cold stress, particularly evaporative and convective heat losses. If necessary, rewarm the infant gradually and open the isolette only for a specific reason, not just to check on the infant. The use of kangaroo care in the delivery room, if feasible, is a valuable aid to this process. The use of kangaroo care as an intervention to reduce morbidity with VLBW infants requires further research (Conde-Agudelo et al, 2001).

- *Fluid and electrolytes:* Considerable fluid loss can occur, especially through insensible losses. The metabolism may be either exceedingly high or exceedingly low, depending on other factors such as gestational age, severity of illness, and intrapartal complications. Adjust fluid management according to the infant's gestational age, weight, and general condition (see Chapter 24). Some NICUs use swamping (piping highly humidified air into the isolette) when the infant is under a radiant warmer an effort to reduce insensible water losses and promote thermoregulation.

- *Metabolic considerations:* Closely monitor blood glucose levels; if the level falls below 40 mg/dl, intervention is needed. Rapid or high-concentration boluses are not advisable, because rebound hypoglycemia can occur (Southgate & Pittard, 2001). Calcium levels are often labile; monitor these levels and supplement when needed. The most vulnerable period for metabolic complications is the first 72 hours after birth.

- *Polycythemia:* It may be necessary to reduce the cellular mass, because the presence of too many cells further impedes vascular blood flow. A partial exchange with saline may be needed.

- *Cardiac considerations:* Many VLBW and ELBW infants have a patent ductus arteriosus (PDA). Observe the infant for the de-

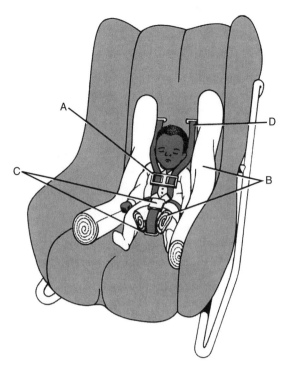

FIGURE **40-1**
Positioning of premature infant in car seat. **A,** Positioning of the retainer clip on the child's chest. **B,** Blanket rolls on both sides of trunk and between crotch strap and infant. **C,** Distance of 5 ½ inches or less from crotch strap to seat back. **D,** Distance of 10 inches or less from lower harness strap to seat bottom. From Hirata T et al (2000). Prematurity. In Jackson PL, Vessey JA, editors. *Primary care of the child with a chronic condition,* ed 3. Mosby: St Louis.

BOX 40-2

Safe Transportation of Premature Infants

1. The infant should be placed in the rear seat of the car with observation by an adult.
2. Infants who are younger than 1 year of age or who weigh less than 20 pounds must ride facing the rear.
3. Infants who are older than 1 year of age and who weigh more than 20 pounds should ride in rear seats approved for higher weights.
4. A car seat for young children should never be placed in the front passenger seat of any vehicle with a passenger-side air bag.
5. The car seat's retainer clip should be positioned on the infant's chest.
6. Blanket rolls should be used inside the car seat for head and lateral trunk control.
7. Rolls should be placed between the crotch strap and the infant to reduce slouching.
8. The safety seat should be reclined at a 45-degree angle to prevent the head from dropping forward.
9. If the infant's head drops forward, the seat should be titled back and/or a clot roll should be wedged under the base of the safety seat.
10. Use of convertible car seats with a shield, abdominal pads, or arm rests that would contact the infant's face or neck during impact should be avoided.
11. An infant should never be left unattended in a car seat.

From Hirata T et al (2000). Prematurity. In Jackson PL, Vessey JA, editors. *Primary care of the child with a chronic condition, ed 3. Mosby: St Louis. Adapted from the Committee on Injury and Poison Prevention and the Committee on the Fetus and Newborn (1996). Safe transportation of premature and low birth weight infants.* Pediatrics, 97, 758-760.

---

gree of severity. Listen for murmurs and consider if the PDA appears to opening and closing. Some of these infants respond favorably to indomethacin therapy, but others require surgical ligation. Fowlie (2001) conducted a systematic review of intravenous indomethacin therapy and the outcomes for VLBW infants. No significant adverse effects (e.g., increased incidence of intracranial hemorrhage) were found after its use for PDA correction. More research is needed to support these conclusions.

- *Immunocompromised status:* Determine if any infections are present and begin appropriate therapy. Remember that other treatments, procedures, and conditions may aggravate the problem (e.g., steroid therapy; use of blood products, leading to thrombocytopenia or lymphocytopenia; antibiotic therapy; invasive procedures; loss of the skin barrier or the presence of a minimal skin barrier; changes in the pH of the skin as a result of bathing practices).
- *Nutrition:* Although enteral feeding, especially with breast milk, provides nutritional and immune protection, it may not be feasible. Closely monitor electrolytes, trace minerals, and other nutrients to facilitate growth. If enteral feeding is impossible, total parenteral nutrition (TPN) can be used. Calculate fluids and nutrients according to the infant's weight, gestational age, and condition (Chapters 24 and 25). If nutritional health is not promoted, the infant will be even more vulnerable to insults from the environment and infectious agents.
- *Skin:* Use as little tape as possible. Apply emollients (e.g., Aquaphor) to prevent drying and minimize fluid losses. Change the infant's position frequently to prevent abrasions and pres-

sure areas and assess the skin frequently for improvement or deterioration.
- *Neurodevelopment:* Neurodevelopment can be promoted if the potential impact of the environment is recognized. Protect the infant from overstimulation in the form of noise, light, or disruption of the sleep-wake pattern (Chapter 17). Observe the infant's reactions to procedures, whether positive or negative, and use that information to adapt the baby's care so as to reduce adverse reactions and increase positive ones.
- *Family care:* Teach the family the unique features of their infant and of the infant's care. Show them how they can participate. Find out what cultural rituals might be important. For example, some African American families like to "oil" their babies. If this is the case and emollients are being used, let the family members apply these to the skin. Also recognize that the family may be in a state of shock that their infant weighs, for example, only 750 g. Talk to them about their feelings if they are grieving the loss of the anticipated child. If the infant is not expected to live but may go home, determine what home care, hospice, or end of life care needs the family might have. Also determine what social and financial support is available (Chapters 8, 9, and 47). If the infant is to go home whether sick or well, talk to the family about the transition to home and what it means to family members. What do they view as needed to ease this transition? (See Chapter

BOX 40-3

Summary of the Primary Care Needs of Premature or Low-Birth-Weight Infants

Health Care Maintenance

Growth and Development

1. Use corrected age to plot height, weight, and head circumference.
2. Preterm infants who are appropriate or average for gestational age (AGA) follow growth patterns similar to those of full-term infants.
3. Infants who are small for gestational age (SGA) tend to be smaller children.
4. Catch-up growth occurs within the first year to after 3 years of age and may be prolonged to adolescence in ELBW infants.
5. Head circumference should be monitored for abnormal growth.
6. VLBW and ELBW infants are at high risk for neurologic, cognitive, or learning abnormalities.
7. The incidence of abnormal development increases with decreasing birth weight.
8. Corrected age should be used to assess development.
9. Transient neuromuscular abnormalities may be present in the first year.

Diet

1. Breastfeeding is recommended.
   - Special concerns about the transmission of the human immunodeficiency virus, cytomegalovirus, and hepatitis B virus in breast milk must be addressed.
   - Feeding problems such as real hypersensitivity and gastroesophageal reflux are common.
2. Fortification of breast milk or a higher-caloric formula may be needed for ELBW and SGA infants for several weeks after hospital discharge.
3. Multivitamins should be given to infants who weigh less than 2.5 kg and to those with chronic illness or poor growth.
4. All preterm infants should receive 2 to 4 mg/kg/day of iron for the first year of life.

Safety

1. Anticipatory guidance is based on developmental age.
   - Recommendations for car seat use include using blanket rolls for support, observing the infant while driving, and avoiding care seat models with lap pads or shields.
   - Air travel should be delayed until an infant tolerates lower environmental oxygen concentrations.
   - Parents should be trained in cardiopulmonary resuscitation (CPR) for infants at high risk for apnea.

Immunizations

1. All immunizations should be administered at the chronologic ages recommended by the American Academy of Pediatrics.
   - Infants should be given inactive polio virus (IPV) while still in the hospital.
   - The effectiveness of the hepatitis B vaccine is unknown in infants weighing less than 2 kg.
2. Preterm infants with long-term pulmonary or cardiac problems and their caretakers should receive the influenza vaccine each fall.
3. Varicella-zoster immune globulin should be given to infants born at less than 28 weeks' gestation who are exposed to varicella while hospitalized.
4. Breastfeeding infants of mothers who test positive for hepatitis B surface-antigen should receive hepatitis B immune globulin.

Screening

1. *Vision:* Assessment of fixation, following, and alignment and funduscopic examination are recommended. Ophthalmologic follow-up is necessary for infants with ROP or other adverse visual findings.
2. *Hearing:* Screening is recommended for all infants, particularly those with risk factors that are identified before hospital discharge. Screening should be repeated within 3 months of age if initial results are abnormal or equivocal.

Continued

46.) Teach the family about car seat safety (Figure 40-1 and Box 40-2) and special considerations for their premature infant.
- *Long-term complications:* Consider the following questions: What long-term outcomes are anticipated for these infants? Are they likely to have a physical or cognitive disability? Examine the current research for pertinent evidence in this important area of care.

LONG-TERM OUTCOMES

Despite 20 years of experience, much is still unknown about the long-term outcomes of VLBW and ELBW infants. The picture is not clear, nor are the authorities in agreement. Some researchers suggest that almost half of all VLBW infants will have a major physical or neurologic disability.

A long-term complication that may develop while the infant is still in the NICU is necrotizing enterocolitis (NEC). This complication arises when enteral feedings, especially calorically dense formulas, are introduced. The more immature the infant and the lower the birth weight, the more likely NEC is to develop. The VLBW or ELBW infant is at risk for intestinal perforations and may require surgical intervention. In

some cases the surgery leaves the infant with short bowel syndrome, with all its accompanying digestion and nutritional problems (see Chapter 26).

High-density formulas should be introduced slowly, and the infant should be observed for intolerance or abdominal distention. More NICUs are now using trophic feedings to wean the infant gradually from TPN to enteral feedings without increasing the occurrence of NEC. Once NEC develops, depending on its severity, the long-term consequences may include poor growth patterns, short bowel syndrome, and many nutritional deficits that require supplementation.

Foster and Cole (2001) conducted a systematic review of studies in which oral immunoglobulin was used in an attempt to prevent NEC in premature and LBW infants. They found no significant difference in the incidence of NEC between infants who received oral immunoglobulin and those who did not.

Another complication related to digestion is gastroesophageal reflux (GER). The lack of muscle tone in premature infants is greatest in the area of the lower esophagus. This hypotonia allows food to reverse flow (reflux) from the gastric area up to the esophagus. Continuation of the pattern can lead

BOX 40-3

Summary of the Primary Care Needs of Premature or Low-Birth-Weight Infants—cont'd

3. *Dental:* Prolonged intubation affects palate and dentition.
   - Routine fluoride supplementation is recommended after 6 months corrected age.
4. *Blood pressure:* Hypertension screenings should be done at 1, 2, 6, 12, and 24 months of age and then routinely in childhood.
   - Children whose blood pressure is above 95% for three screenings should be considered hypertensive, and the reason should be identified.
5. *Hematocrit:* Hematocrit values should be checked based on the infant's history, nutritional status, and symptoms.
6. *Urinalysis:* Routine screening is recommended.
7. *Tuberculosis:* Routine screening is recommended.

Condition-Specific Screening
1. *Hernia and testicular screening:* Infants should be screened for inguinal hernia and undescended testicles.

Common Illness Management
Differential Diagnosis
1. Risk of infection, particularly respiratory infection, is increased.
   - Respiratory syncytial virus (RSV), herpes simplex virus (HSV), chlamydia, group B streptococci, *Staphylococcus aureus,* and *Escherichia coli* must all be considered possible pathogens.
   - Risk for *Streptococcus pneumoniae* and *Haemophilus influenzae* type b infections must be evaluated.
   - Possible sepsis must be identified early.

Developmental Issues
Sleep Patterns
1. Children may have disorganized sleep patterns.

Toileting
1. Toileting readiness is based on developmental age.
   - Increased muscle tone may impede toilet training.

Discipline
1. Children should be assessed for vulnerable child syndrome.
   - Limits should be set as for any other child.
   - The incidence of child abuse is higher than with other children; shaken baby syndrome should also be considered.

Child Care
1. Home care or small day care programs are recommended.

Schooling
1. These children have a higher incidence of educational problems. School readiness should be ascertained before a child enters kindergarten.
   - Psychometric testing is indicated for poor school performance.

Sexuality
1. Preterm children have normal offspring.
   - Standard developmental counseling is advised. The incidence of SGA and prematurity is higher in the children of women who were SGA at birth.

Transition to Adulthood
1. Pre-existing developmental or behavior problems may become exaggerated. Concerns of parental overprotection, adolescent low self-esteem, correction of cosmetic deformities, and parental communication should be addressed.
   - These children's self-perception of quality of life is good.

Special Family Concerns
1. Special family concerns include grief, attachment issues as a result of prolonged hospitalization, financial considerations, and concerns about developmental outcomes.

From Hirata T et al (2000). Prematurity. In Jackson PL, Vessey JA, editors. Primary care of the child with a chronic condition, *ed 3. Mosby: St Louis.*

to the formation of scar tissue in the esophagus, intolerance of feedings, and poor growth. For some families, GER is familial and not simply related to low birth weight or prematurity.

ROP is another long-term complication in VLBW and ELBW infants. The longer oxygen therapy is needed, the more likely the infant is to develop some degree of ROP. Close follow-up examinations are necessary if problems are to be detected and corrected early (Chapter 36). Vitamin A supplementation is a potential protective therapy. Darlow and Graham (2001) did a meta-analysis of studies that examined vitamin A supplementation in VLBW infants in relation to outcomes. They found that less oxygen was used and there was a tendency toward less ROP in infants who received such supplementation. Askie and Henderson-Smart (2001) performed a systematic review of studies of unrestricted oxygen use and outcomes in LBW infants. They found that if oxygen levels were not monitored closely, morbidity in this population rose. Oxygen levels, therefore, must be watched and controlled carefully.

A systematic review done by Subamanian and Henderson-Smart (2001) examined oxygen levels as they related to nasal continuous positive airway pressure (CPAP) and the impact on the use of intermittent positive pressure ventilation. They

found that although nasal CPAP may be useful for supporting ventilation in VLBW infants, no evidence indicates that it reduces morbidity in this group. More research is needed in this area.

Anemia is another problem. The infant at first may be polycythemic, but even in healthy term infants, the hematocrit level falls as the transition to extrauterine life continues. Unfortunately for sick, underweight, and premature infants, most of the long-term anemia is iatrogenic, occurring secondary to invasive procedures, drawing of blood, and stress. Nurses must be aware of these factors and act as advocates to eliminate unnecessary procedures. The hematocrit level must be monitored closely, especially during the first few months of life. The nurse should observe for signs of anemia, such as poor growth, tachycardia, or tachypnea, and intervene as needed (Chapter 28).

Renal function is compromised in VLBW and ELBW infants. This may or may not be a long-term complication, depending on the severity of the compromise. During the infant's stay in the NICU, it is imperative that nurses give medications with careful consideration of renal function. For example, gentamicin is a nephrotoxic drug. If renal function is compromised, a toxic level of this drug can be reached quite quickly, leading to permanent renal and auditory damage. The nurse should consider where the drug is metabolized and cleared through the body. If the site is the renal system and if output is severely diminished, use of the medication may need to be suspended temporarily.

Other genitourinary problems are related to prematurity, including undescended testes and inguinal hernia. Both conditions are amendable to corrective surgery, if needed, when the child's condition is stable (Hirata et al, 2000) (Chapter 33).

Growth patterns remain altered throughout life for VLBW and ELBW infants. Small stature is common. Ford and colleagues (2000) found that even at adolescence, the rate of catch-up growth is slow. Often walking is delayed as well. Lacey (2001) found that for some of these children, walking may be delayed by several months but that most walk by 18 months of age.

Neurodevelopment is a major consideration. Some researchers report that by 2 years of age, these infants have 64% normalcy (Piecuch et al., 1997). Others suggest that 75% will be relatively free of cognitive problems (Vohr & Msall, 1997). Doyle and Casalaz (2001) studied the neurodevelopmental outcomes of 351 infants at age 14 years. They found that 25% of the infants survived. Of these, 10% had cerebral palsy; 6% had bilateral blindness; 5% were deaf, and 46% had an intelligence quotient (IQ) of less than one standard deviation below the norms compared with a control group. These researchers concluded that overall, the outcomes at 14 years of age were not generally positive. More research needs to be done in this area.

School performance problems have been documented, and delayed speech and language development may be a contributing factor. Visuomotor and perceptual problems, as well as hyperactive behavior, also are seen. Reading and comprehension levels are lower in some instances. School readiness may be compromised by immaturity or the family's overprotectiveness (vulnerable infant/child syndrome), which reduces the opportunities to socialize with other children (Hirata et al, 2000). These children need to be referred for early intervention services, and an individualized family service plan must be devised. Families must be taught the ways to assess their child for developmental difficulties and behavioral cues that might signal problems (Chapters 17, 31, and 45). The primary care needs of these children must be reinforced (Box 40-3), and their families must be included in this care plan.

SUMMARY

This chapter presented a brief overview of the problems and long-term consequences of very low birth weight and extremely low birth weight. It also discussed the care required for these infants. Only time will tell if our predictions for outcomes are true, but one thing is certain: nurses and parents can make a difference if they are aware of the potential problems and know how to detect or recognize them early.

REFERENCES

Askie LM, Henderson-Smart DJ (2001). Restricted versus liberal oxygen exposure for preventing morbidity and mortality in preterm or low birth weight infants (Cochrane Review). The Cochrane Library, 4, 2001. Update Software: Oxford.

Conde-Agudelo A et al (2001). Kangaroo mother care to reduce morbidity and mortality in low birth weight infants (Cochrane Review). The Cochrane Library, 4, 2001. Update Software: Oxford.

Darlow BA, Graham PJ (2001). Vitamin A supplementation for preventing morbidity and mortality in very low birth weight infants (Cochrane Review). The Cochrane Library, 4, 2001. Update Software: Oxford.

Doyle LW, Casalaz D (2001). Outcome at 14 years of extremely low birth weight infants: a regional study. Archives of disease in child and fetal and neonatal education, 85(3), F159-F164.

Ford GW (2000). Very low birth weight and growth into adolescence. Archives of pediatric adolescent medicine, 154, 778-784.

Foster J, Cole M (2001). Oral immunoglobulin for preventing necrotizing enterocolitis in preterm and low birth weight neonates (Cochrane Review). The Cochrane Library, 4, 2001. Update Software: Oxford.

Fowlie PW (2001). Intravenous indomethacin for preventing mortality and morbidity in very low birth weight infants (Cochrane Review). The Cochrane Library, 4, 2001. Update Software: Oxford.

Hirata T et al (2000). Prematurity. In Jackson PL, Vessey JA, editors. Primary care of the child with a chronic condition, ed 3. Mosby: St Louis.

Lacey J (2001). Very low birth weight preterm infants walk later than term infants, but most are walking by 18 months. Australian journal of physiotherapy, 47(1), 65.

Lott JW (2001). Personal communication.

Piecuch R et al (1997). Outcome of extremely low birth weight infants (500-999 grams) over a 12 year period. Pediatrics, 100, 633-639.

Southgate WM, Pittard WB II (2001). Classification and physical examination of the newborn infant. In Klaus MH, Fanaroff AA, editors. Care of the high-risk neonate, ed 5. WB Saunders: Philadelphia.

Subramaniam P et al (2001). Prophylactic nasal continuous positive airway pressure for preventing morbidity and mortality in very preterm infants (Cochrane Review). The Cochrane Library, 4, 2001. Update Software: Oxford.

Vohr BR, Msall ME (1997). Neuropsychological and functional outcomes of very low birth weight infants. Seminars in perinatology, 31(3), 377-386.

CHAPTER

41

DIAGNOSTIC PROCESSES

CATHERINE THEORELL, SHERYL MONTROWL

Care of the neonate typically involves numerous diagnostic procedures and tests to identify dysfunction related to birth, prematurity, illness, or congenital malformations. This chapter highlights the commonly used methods for developing a medical or surgical diagnosis in the newborn and infant. The nursing implications for appropriate assessment of preprocedural and postprocedural care also are discussed.

Diagnostic imaging has assumed an increasingly important role in neonatal diagnosis and the assessment, evaluation, and follow-up of neonatal care. Technologic advances since the 1970s have resulted in a variety of imaging modalities that demonstrate not only the internal structure but also the function of organ systems in the fetus and neonate. The spectrum of diagnostic imaging methods includes radionuclide imaging, ultrasonography, and magnetic resonance imaging, as well as conventional roentgenologic techniques. With such an array of imaging modalities available, complex, problem-oriented decision making is required to determine which techniques should be used and which omitted in a particular clinical situation. In addition, diagnostic imaging examinations are expensive, with ultrasonography being the least expensive and magnetic resonance imaging the most expensive. As the public, the government, private insurers, and the health care system have become increasingly cost conscious, health care providers have faced growing pressure to make efficacious and cost-effective decisions about the use of imaging examinations.

The selection of a particular imaging examination should be based on the inherent patient risks, the likelihood that the examination will establish or refute a working diagnosis, the potential benefit to the patient, and the risk of liability if the examination is requested or if the examination is not requested (Swischuk, 1997a, 1997b; Juhl et al, 1998). In selecting an imaging examination, the clinician must carefully consider how much the examination will affect the certainty of the differential diagnosis and whether the information derived from the examination will alter the diagnostic approach or choice of treatment. Diagnostic certainty never reaches 100%. Because of the cost, imaging examinations with a low diagnostic yield or those that only duplicate information that can be obtained from other, less expensive methods must be omitted. The acceptable level of compromise depends on the specific clinical problem, the type of imaging abnormality, and the experience of the radiologist (Swischuk, 1997b). To minimize the risks and maximize the diagnostic benefit from

any imaging examination, the diagnostic procedure must be tailored to the specific clinical problem under consideration. For these reasons, diagnostic approaches vary among radiologists and institutions (Hilton & Edwards, 1994; Swischuk, 1997a, 1997b).

The roles of the nurse, neonatologist, nurse practitioner, and radiologist are critically interrelated in diagnostic imaging. It is essential that the history, clinical presentation, physical examination, and laboratory data be understood so that the imaging modalities selected are the ones properly indicated for the diagnostic evaluation and subsequent therapy of the individual newborn.

After the neonatologist or nurse practitioner orders a diagnostic imaging examination, the radiologist evaluates whether the examination is indicated, what views should be obtained, what sequence of examinations is necessary, and whether contrast or supplementary examinations are (Swischuk, 1997a, 1997b; Juhl et al, 1998).

Nurses should be aware of the rationale for the selection and sequencing of these diagnostic evaluations, the indications for various imaging modalities, the need for patient preparation, and the biophysical principles involved in producing the image. The nurse ensures that the correct newborn undergoes the procedure, monitors the newborn during and after the procedure, and minimizes changes in the thermal environment. The nurse may also be responsible for preparing information about the infant that is essential to the interpretation of imaging examinations. For example, the gestational, postnatal, and corrected gestational ages are important considerations when interpreting bone density, and the perinatal history is an important consideration when interpreting intracranial calcifications or hemorrhages (Swischuk, 1997a). In addition, the nurse must often act as a liaison between the medical staff and the parents. The relationship the nurse establishes with the family often provides an opportunity to inform the parents of the benefits and risks of the procedure and allows the parents to express their questions and concerns. Armed with a thorough understanding of these concepts, the nurse is able to coordinate the acquisition of diagnostic information with minimal disruption to patient care. A knowledge of patient preparation, proper positioning, and the potential risks of each procedure forms the basis of the care plans and parent teaching. These plans of care and acknowledgment of risks facilitate the development of unit policies and procedures.

DIAGNOSTIC IMAGING IN INFANTS

Diagnostic imaging in newborns and infants is unique, differing in several ways from the procedures used for older children and adults. Infants and newborns are not just small adults for whom smaller films and less exposure are all that is required. Significant differences exist, not just in size, but also in the origin and imaging appearance of disease entities, anatomic proportions, exposure factors, radiation protection, and methods of immobilization (Hilton & Edwards, 1994; Swischuk, 1997a, 1997b; Huda et al, 2001).

Conditions Requiring Diagnostic Imaging

Pathologic conditions commonly encountered in adults often are not found in infants, and many abnormal conditions are exclusive to the newborn period. Examples of these pathologic conditions are the congenital abnormalities of the newborn, such as atresias of the gastrointestinal (GI) tract, severe congenital heart defects, surgical causes of respiratory distress, spina bifida, and bilateral choanal atresia. These lesions, which are lethal if left untreated, often are symptomatic in the first days after birth. Medical problems related to premature and postmature birth, intrauterine growth disturbances, nonlethal developmental defects, genetic abnormalities, and perinatal asphyxia are of greatest concern in the newborn period. In addition, malignant tumors, such as neuroblastoma and Wilms' tumor, may appear in the newborn period and up to approximately 4 years of age. Certain infections, such as cytomegalovirus (CMV), toxoplasmosis, and syphilis, have a distinct radiographic and ultrasonographic presentation if exposure occurred in utero rather than in the neonatal period (Hilton & Edwards, 1994; Swischuk, 1997a, 1997b; Fanaroff & Martin, 2002).

Anatomic Proportions

The anatomic proportions of infants are very different from those of adults, and the younger the infant, the more marked the differences. A thorough knowledge of these proportions is essential for correct patient positioning to limit field exposure and for accurate interpretation of diagnostic imaging (Hilton & Edwards, 1994; Dowd, 1999). It is important that only the area in question, but the whole of the area in question, appear in the imaging field.

As shown in Figure 41-1, the newborn's head is large in proportion to the body, and the cranial vault is large in proportion to the area of the face. The neck is short, and the diaphragm is high. The kidneys are low, about midway between the diaphragm and symphysis pubis. The abdomen is large because of the relative size of the liver and stomach. The pelvic cavity is very small, and the bladder extends above the symphysis pubis. The chest, pelvis, and limbs are small in proportion to the abdomen (Hilton & Edwards, 1994; Swischuk, 1997a, 1997b).

In an anteroposterior (AP) projection, the neonate's lungs appear wider than they are long and much higher up in the thoracic cavity than is normally expected (Hilton & Edwards, 1994; Swischuk, 1997a, 1997b). The diaphragm is located just below the level of the nipples. On a lateral projection, the posterior aspect of the lungs may extend to twice the depth of the anterior part (Swischuk, 1997a, 1997b).

The newborn's abdomen bulges laterally wider than the pelvis, and the bulge contains abdominal organs displaced by the large liver and stomach. Care must be taken to include this area of the abdomen in the imaging field (Hilton & Edwards, 1994; Swischuk, 1997a, 1997b). Irradiation should encompass

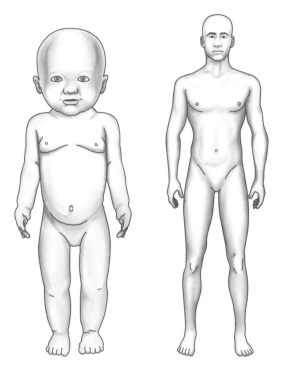

FIGURE 41-1
Proportional anatomic differences between a neonate and an adult.

the smallest possible body area consistent with production of the necessary information (Dowd, 1999). Often the field is too large, particularly in premature infants and newborns. Arms and legs should not appear on the abdominal film, nor should half the skull and abdomen appear on a chest film (Figure 41-2) (Hilton & Edwards, 1994; Swischuk, 1997a, 1997b; Fanaroff & Martin, 2002).

TYPES OF DIAGNOSTIC IMAGING

Diagnostic imaging methods are limited to the demonstration of pathologic features no smaller than a few millimeters in diameter, whereas biochemical and histologic methods document disease at a molecular or cellular level. It is commonly thought that diagnostic imaging provides only anatomic information; however, a significant amount of physiologic data may be derived from studies such as barium examinations or urography, as well as from dynamic radionuclide, ultrasonographic, and molecular imaging (Abramoff et al, 2000; Weissmann & Seidel, 2000; Bushong, 2001; Weissleder & Mahmood, 2001).

The four major diagnostic imaging methods are x-ray (roentgenologic) imaging, radionuclide imaging, ultrasonographic imaging, and magnetic resonance imaging (Treves, 1995; Bushong, 1996, 1999, 2000, 2001; Juhl, 1998). This chapter discusses each of these imaging modalities in relation to the biophysical principles responsible for producing the image, the potential risks of the procedure, and the nursing care of the newborn or infant undergoing such an examination. Table 41-1 summarizes the types of diagnostic imaging commonly used for neonates.

X-Ray Imaging (Roentgenology)

The principles of conventional radiography have not changed since the discovery of x-rays in the late 1800s. However, the equipment and techniques have become far more sophisti-

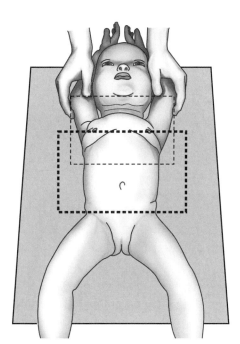

FIGURE **41-2**
Neonatal radiographs should be limited to only the area of interest. Total body radiographs should be avoided. The top box (*light dashed lines*) defines the area of interest for an anteroposterior chest radiograph. The bottom box (*heavy dashed lines*) defines the area of interest for an anteroposterior abdominal film. The gonad shield has been omitted for illustrative purposes.

cated; current radiographic methods include tomography, fluoroscopy, computed tomography, and digital radiography.

Roentgenologic Biophysical Principles

X-rays are a form of electromagnetic energy that travel at the speed of light (about 300,000 km [186,000 miles] per second). Other forms of electromagnetic energy include gamma rays, radio waves, microwaves, and visible light (Figure 41-3). Only x-rays and gamma rays have enough energy to produce an ion pair by separating an orbital electron from its parent atom (Bushong, 1996, 1999, 2000, 2001; Alpen, 1998; Juhl, 1998). The amount of radiation present is measured by detection of such ionization. Radiation exposure is measured either in units of coulombs per kilogram (C/kg) or in roentgens (1 R/258/ C/kg). Although the roentgen is no longer an official scientific unit, it is still widely used in radiology. The rad is the unit of measure for the amount of radiation absorbed by the body (Alpen, 1998; Juhl, 1998; Dowd, 1999; Bushong, 2001).

When an x-ray beam is directed toward a part of the body, differential absorption of the x-ray photons by different types of body tissue occurs. A beam of x-ray photons is variously attenuated as it passes through the body tissues, producing a shadow image that is recorded on photographic film; the absorbed x-ray photons interact with the tissue, causing ionization in the body (Alpen, 1998; Juhl, 1998; Dowd, 1999; Bushong, 2001). Bone and metal fragments absorb x-ray photons and therefore appear white on the radiographic film, whereas air-containing structures, such as lungs and gas-filled bowel, absorb few x-ray photons and appear black. Soft tissues and blood vessels appear as intermediate shades of gray.

A radiograph gives a two-dimensional projection of three-dimensional structures. An x-ray tube is positioned to direct the x-ray beam through the part of the neonate to be examined so as to record different views or projections on the film. This simple imaging technique can distinguish only among air, fat, and tissues with densities approximately equal to those of water or metals, but it continues to be enormously valuable and is still the diagnostic imaging method most often used in neonatal care.

X-ray photons are generated in the tungsten anode of the tube when it is bombarded by a stream of high-energy electrons emitted from the cathode (Figure 41-4) (Alpen, 1998; Juhl, 1998; Dowd, 1999; Bushong, 2001). The energy, or penetrating power, of the resulting x-ray photons is a function of the electron energy, which is controlled by the voltage gradient across the cathode-anode gap. In diagnostic radiology, this gradient usually is 60 to 120 kilovolts (kV) (Hilton & Edwards, 1994; Juhl, 1998; Dowd, 1999; Bushong, 2001). Low kilovoltage x-rays have poor penetrating ability, whereas higher kilovoltage x-rays have deeper penetrating ability. The kilovoltage across the cathode-anode gap, therefore, controls the penetration of the x-ray beam.

The milliamperage (mA) indicates the amount of current applied to the cathode filament (Alpen, 1998; Bushong, 2001). The greater the current, the more electrons are produced for transmission across the cathode-anode gap, and the greater the number of x-ray photons generated by the anode in a finite time. The product of the exposure time and the milliamperage given to the cathode filament controls the amount, or dose, of x-rays and is expressed in milliampere-seconds (mAs) (Alpen, 1998; Juhl, 1998; Dowd, 1999; Bushong, 2001).

Early radiographs required an exposure time of as long as 30 minutes to produce a satisfactory image (Juhl, 1998; Bushong, 2001). It is not surprising, then, to find reports of radiation injury in the early days of radiology. Reports of superficial skin and tissue damage, hair loss, and anemia were common among patients and their physicians because of the prolonged exposure times and the low-energy radiation that was available. The development of an interrupterless transformer by H.C. Snook in 1907 and progressive improvements in the cathode ray tube resulted in a marked decline in reports of radiation injury. Since that time, improvements in film sensitivity and fluorescent screens have further reduced exposure times, to the point where the average exposure time for a chest radiograph is approximately one twentieth of a second (Alpen, 1998; Juhl, 1998; Dowd, 1999; Bushong, 2001). The short exposure time diminishes image blurring caused by involuntary and cardiovascular motion and reduces the neonate's exposure to radiation. However, it also is important to limit the cross-sectional area of the x-ray beam to the region of interest to reduce unnecessary irradiation of adjacent organs (Alpen, 1998; Bushong, 2001; Dowd, 1999; Juhl, 1998).

Conventional radiographic images commonly have been recorded with large-size photographic film enclosed in an aluminum or plastic lightproof cassette. The film is compressed between fluorescent screens that emit visible light when exposed to x-rays. The fluorescence from the phosphor screens, rather than the direct effect of x-rays on the photographic emulsion, produces most of the image on the film (Alpen, 1998; Juhl, 1998; Bushong, 2001). Other diagnostic imaging methods also use ionizing radiation.

Xeroradiography. Xeroradiography is a radiographic imaging technique used to evaluate soft tissue. With this technique, the electrical charge of a photoconductive plate is altered in

TABLE 41-1   Diagnostic Imaging Methods Commonly Used for Neonates

Technique	Indications and Advantages	Limitations	Potential Risks	Comments	Cost
Roentgenologic Techniques					
Radiographic imaging	Most frequently used initial diagnostic screening mode	Detects only four different levels of photon absorption (air, fat, water, and mineral); two-dimensional (2D) projection of three-dimensional (3D) structures	Ionizing radiation; thermal stress of cool film plate	Proper positioning of infant is essential; child must be monitored during procedure	$
Xeroradiographic imaging	Used to evaluate soft tissue structures	Tissue structures defined by relative amounts of air, fat, water and minerals; seldom used since advent of newer diagnostic imaging methods	Higher level of ionizing radiation than with routine radiographs	Proper positioning of infant is essential; child must be monitored during procedure	$$
Fluoroscopic imaging	Used to evaluate motion or function of cardiovascular, gastrointestinal, and genitourinary systems; may be used to guide therapeutic or diagnostic procedures	Images rely on greater radiation and/or movement of contrast material; improper diagnostic sequencing may delay informational yield; contrast material may have physiologic consequences	Much higher level of ionizing radiation than with routine radiographs; thermal stress of cool radiology environment	Proper positioning of infant is essential; child must be monitored during procedure	$$-$$$$
Computed tomography (CT)	Used to provide detailed, superior characterization of various soft tissue densities that cannot be detected by conventional radiographs	Motion artifact may cause blurring of scans; radiation dose depends on scan time; contrast material may have physiologic consequences	Ionizing radiation; thermal stress of cool environment	Proper positioning of infant is essential; child must be monitored during procedure	$$$
Ultrasound Imaging	Does not use ionizing radiation, but rather uses sound waves to depict anatomic and functional motion of tissue; sound waves can be directed in a beam in a variety of planes; portable; different graphic displays are available	Ultrasound technique is operator dependent; does not provide as much information on organ function such as urography; reveals less anatomic detail than CT; scan is adversely affected by the presence of bone and air	Thermal stress may occur with application of cool scanning gel to infant's skin; there are no known deleterious effects from clinical use of ultrasound imaging	Proper positioning of infant is essential; child must be monitored during procedure	$
Radionucleotide Imaging	Used to trace anatomic proportions and a wide range of physiologic functions in virtually every organ in the body Amount of ionizing radiation emitted by injected agent is significantly less than the amount required for corresponding radiograph	Diagnostic yield depends on uptake of radionucleotide by different organs; radionucleotides are rarely organ specific; limited anatomic resolution	Thermal stress during nucleotide scanning	Proper positioning of the infant is essential; maximum radiation exposure is not always the organ of interest; child must be monitored during procedure	$$

Continued

TABLE 41-1 Diagnostic Imaging Methods Commonly Used for Neonates—Cont'd

Technique	Indications and Advantages	Limitations	Potential Risks	Comments	Cost
Positron Emission Tomography (PET) and Single Photon Emission Computed Tomography (SPECT)	Both techniques have greater sensitivity and qualifications of the distribution and density of radioactivity to depict the "metabolic" function of tissue; 3D imaging is possible with computer reconstruction; dose of nucleotide is the same; artifactual lesions can be eliminated Amount of ionizing radiation emitted by injected agents (carbon 11, oxygen 15, nitrogen 13) is significantly less than the amount required for corresponding radiograph	PET scanning requires access to a cyclotron to produce the positrons used in scans	Thermal stress during nucleotide scanning	Proper positioning of infant is essential; child must be monitored during procedure	$$$$$ $
Magnetic Resonance Imaging (MRI)	Uses magnetic fields and radio waves to produce images; the region of the body scanned can be controlled electronically, and hardware does not limit scanning sites; scans are free of high-intensity artifacts; newer scanning techniques can quantify many pathologic conditions	Availability and cost; limited use in unstable infants on life support; monitoring equipment must be free from interference with magnetic field	Does not use ionizing radiation to produce images; limited access to infant during procedure	Proper positioning is essential; must be monitored during procedure	$$$$$ $

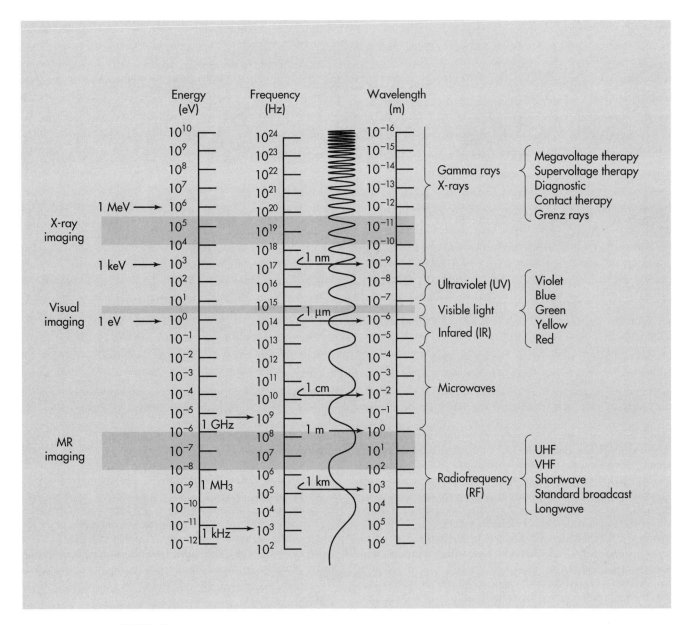

FIGURE **41-3**
The electromagnetic spectrum extends over 25 orders of magnitude. The chart illustrates the values of frequency, energy, and wavelength and identifies some common regions of the spectrum. From Bushong SC (2001). *Radiologic science for technologists,* ed 7. Mosby: St Louis.

proportion to the intensity of the transmitted radiation image (Alpen, 1998; Juhl, 1998; Dowd, 1999; Bushong, 2001). The image is recorded on the plate rather than on x-ray film. With soft tissue structures that differ only slightly in density, this method provides much better contrast than conventional radiography. It also provides an "edge effect" at the margins of discontinuous structures and therefore is indicated for the detection of nonmetallic foreign bodies and for evaluation of complex upper airway abnormalities in the neonate (Hilton & Edwards, 1994; Swischuk, 1997a; Juhl, 1998). Despite these benefits, the risks associated with this imaging technique must be considered. The radiation exposure involved is six to 12 times greater than that with conventional radiographs (Hilton & Edwards, 1994; Swischuk, 1997a; Alpen, 1998; Juhl, 1998).

Fluoroscopic Imaging.   Thomas Edison developed the fluoroscope in 1898 (Bushong, 2001). He focused on the use of flu-

orescent materials in this new imaging modality. During the period of his investigation, Edison analyzed the fluorescent properties of more than 1800 materials, including zinc cadmium sulfide and calcium tungstate, both of which are still used. Edison halted his research in this area when his assistant and long-time friend, Clarence Dally, suffered severe x-ray burns that required bilateral upper extremity amputation. Dally's subsequent death in 1904 is considered the first x-ray fatality (Juhl, 1998; Dowd, 1999; Bushong, 2001).

Fluoroscopic imaging is a radiologic technique used to evaluate the motion of an organ system. After passing through the patient, the fluoroscopic x-rays interact with the input phosphor of the image intensifier tube. The input phosphor converts the incident x-rays into visible light, which causes the photocathode to emit electrons (Alpen, 1998; Juhl, 1998; Dowd, 1999; Bushong, 2001). These electrons are accelerated and focused by electrodes in the image intensifier onto the

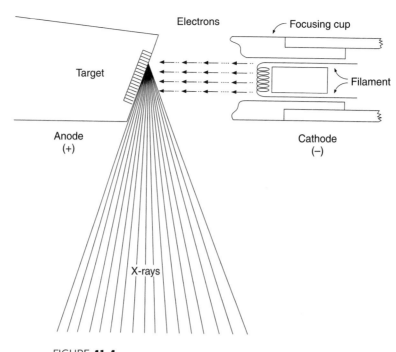

FIGURE **41-4**
Generation of x-ray photons in a tungsten anode-cathode tube.

output phosphor to produce visible light that can be viewed directly through an optical system or by a television system (Alpen, 1998; Dowd, 1999; Bushong, 2001). Fluoroscopic images can be recorded on film or videotape. Videotape recording of fluoroscopy has become essential. It is easier and safer to rerun videotape several times to evaluate dysfunction than to prolong the radiation exposure from fluoroscopy.

During a fluoroscopic examination, the anatomic structure may be evaluated by obtaining a spot film, which is produced by photographing the output phosphor on 100-mm or 105-mm film. This type of intensifier optical-coupled spot film camera reduces the radiation dose to the infant by at least 75% compared with a conventional spot film device (National Council on Radiation Protection [NCRP], 1993a, 1993b, 1993c; Juhl, 1998; Dowd, 1999; Bushong, 2001). Videotapes are used to record motions, and spot films are used to document anatomy. Although fluoroscopy has many advantages, the radiation dose delivered in 1 minute of fluoroscopy is equivalent to that of more than 30 105-mm spot films or more than eight conventional radiographs (NCRP, 1993a, 1993b, 1993c; Alpen, 1998; Dowd, 1999).

Electronic intensification of the faint fluoroscopic image allows fluoroscopy to be performed in subdued lighting. Improved intensifier systems have made invasive catheter studies, such as cardiac angiography, much easier to perform (Dowd, 1999; Bushong, 2001).

Fluoroscopically guided cytologic biopsy of the lung, bone, pancreas, and lymph nodes has become possible with percutaneous needle insertion. With the aid of fluoroscopy, arteriovenous malformations can be embolized; arterial stenoses can be dilated with balloon catheters; and plastic stents can be inserted to provide drainage through biliary strictures (Hilton & Edwards, 1994; Swischuk, 1997a). These surgical-radiologic procedures are needed for only a relatively small proportion of neonates; however, all fluoroscopic procedures depend on high-quality image intensification, and all require cooperation among the neonatal, surgical, and radiologic teams to achieve the best results.

Conventional X-Ray Tomography. Tomography is a radiologic method of imaging a "slice" of tissue at a specific level. Coordinated movement of the x-ray tube and film cassette gives a defined image in the two-dimensional plane of interest, whereas the structures in front of or behind this plane are blurred out (Alpen, 1998; Juhl, 1998; Bushong, 2000). Tomography is useful in many circumstances, but its usefulness has been overshadowed by the development of computed tomography (CT).

Computed Tomography. CT was first developed in 1961 by Oldendorf, and by 1973 it had become a recognized diagnostic imaging tool (Bushong, 2000). CT scanning obtains cross-sectional images rather than the shadow images of conventional radiography. Conventional radiography is based on variable attenuation of the x-ray beam as it passes through tissue. Because only the sum total of this attenuation is available for recording on the film, conventional radiography can detect only differences of 10% attenuation (Juhl, 1998; Bushong, 2000, 2001). Conventional radiographs, therefore, cannot produce a detailed characterization of various soft tissue densities. The densities that can be visualized on conventional radiographs are air, fat, soft tissue, and bone. CT passes multiple, highly collimated beams through the same cross-sectional slice of tissue at different angles during different intervals of time. In CT scanning, a fan x-ray beam from a source rotating about the infant passes through the body, and the exit transmission of x-ray beam intensity is monitored by a series of detectors (Alpen, 1998; Bushong, 2000). The x-ray beam "cuts a slice" from 3 to 13 mm thick through the infant. The exit transmission at any angle can be used to calculate the average attenuation coefficient along the length of the x-ray beam. By measuring the exit transmission at a large number of angles around the infant, a complex series of mathematic equations can be solved by computer to calculate and determine the mass attenuation coefficient of small (approximately $0.5 \times 0.5 \times 10$ mm) volume elements, or voxels. The final cross-sectional image is made up of a display of the gray scale value of every voxel, which can be projected on a cathode ray tube and recorded photographically (Alpen, 1998; Juhl, 1998; Bushong, 2000, 2001). Bone is the densest, absorbs the largest amount of x-rays, and appears white; air is the least dense and appears black; soft tissues are displayed as intermediate shades of gray. CT scanning has the ability to separate spatial and contrast resolution and is much more sensitive to tissue densities than conventional radiographs. CT can distinguish differences in attenuation coefficients as small as 0.1%; it also detects changes in density in very small areas of tissue and allows identification of various components of soft tissue, such as subarachnoid space, white matter, gray matter, and ventricles (Alpen, 1998; Juhl, 1998; Bushong, 2000, 2001). CT of the body is technically more difficult than cranial examination because of cardiac and respiratory motion; however, a modern body scanner can complete a scan in 2 to 4 seconds, which reduces movement artifact. In the neonate, the rapid heart and respiratory rates limit the usefulness of this technique for thoracic examination.

With CT the density, or contrast resolution, depends on the radiation dose and scan time (Alpen, 1998; Juhl, 1998; Bushong, 2000, 2001). As the radiation dose (i.e., scan time) increases, the number of photons collected in each area increases and the statistical noise decreases, resulting in better contrast resolution. CT demonstrates tissue structure with precise clarity, showing superior anatomic detail compared with conventional radiographic imaging (Alpen, 1998; Juhl, 1998; Bushong, 2001). CT permits two-dimensional visualization of entire anatomic sections of tissue, which aids the determination of the extent of the disease or malformation. Anatomic and physiologic information can be visualized despite overlying gas and bone. Contrast enhancement can measure blood flow and help define pathologic abnormalities (Swischuk, 1997a, 1997b; Bushong, 2000). Bolus injection of contrast material allows excellent visualization of vascular structures.

As good as CT is as an imaging modality, it is still not a radiologic microscope; CT does have its drawbacks. It also uses ionizing radiation, and because the computers require a cool room for proper equipment performance, the neonate's environment is altered significantly, a circumstance that must be considered.

Digital Radiography and Digital Vascular Imaging.   Digital radiography is the term used to describe techniques that use computers to produce projectional images similar to those of conventional radiography (Bushong, 2001). Although standard CT instruments have been designed to produce two-dimensional images of two-dimensional body slices, they can also be used to project three-dimensional structures into two-dimensional images that are similar to conventional radiographs. These projections do not have the fine detail of conventional radiographs, but because the pictorial data are stored in the computer, the image can be manipulated and subtle features can be enhanced (Bushong, 2001).

Another method of digital radiography converts the image intensifier picture to digital signals that can be stored and manipulated. The most important use of this method is to obtain

---

BOX 41-1

Radiopharmaceuticals Used in Neonatal Diagnostic Imaging

- Technetium 99m
  Sulfur or tin colloid: Used for imaging liver, spleen, bone marrow, ventilation, and gastrointestinal bleeding
  Albumin microspheres: Used for imaging lung perfusion
  Pyrophosphate, diphosphate: Used for imaging skeletal and myocardial infarcts
  Pertechnetate: Used for imaging thyroid, brain, and gastrointestinal tract
  Diethylenetriaminepentaacetic acid (DTPA) glucoheptonate: Used for imaging kidney and brain
  Hepatoiminodiacetic acid (HIDA): Used for imaging biliary system
- Iodine 131: Used for imaging thyroid and fibrinogen and for clot localization
- Xenon 131, krypton 81m: Used for imaging lung ventilation
- Thallium 201: Used for imaging myocardial perfusion and for testicular localization

---

digital subtraction images of the heart and major arteries from data recorded before and after the injection of angiographic contrast material (Bushong, 2001). This method is much less invasive than catheterization, although the technique is new and the equipment is expensive. It has been used on a very limited basis in the neonate.

Radiographic Contrast Agents

Plain radiography can differentiate only four kinds of body tissue: tissue containing gas (lung and bowel), fatty tissue and tissue containing calcium (bone or pathologic calcifications), and tissues of water density (solid organs, muscle, and blood). To demonstrate blood vessels that are in solid organs or surrounded by muscle or to demonstrate other hollow structures, artificial radiographic contrast agents must be introduced. The contrast medium may be negative or positive and may be injected, swallowed, or administered as an enema (Hilton & Edwards, 1994; Swischuk, 1997a, 1997b).

Negative contrast media absorb less radiation than adjacent soft tissues and therefore cast a darker radiographic image. Gases such as air, oxygen, and carbon dioxide can be used as negative contrast media. Because negative media provide a limited amount of contrast for conventional radiography, they are seldom used (Swischuk, 1997a, 1997b; Fanaroff & Martin, 2002).

Positive contrast media use elements with a high atomic number, which absorb much more radiation than surrounding soft tissues and therefore cast a lighter image. Barium and iodine are the two elements currently used. Barium sulfate, a relatively stable, nontoxic compound, is the major contrast agent used for outlining the walls of the GI tract. Iodine-containing salts that are excreted by the kidneys are used for a wide variety of urographic and angiographic studies. The kidneys also excrete the newer nonionic, iodine-containing media. Because of their lower osmolality, these agents are less painful than iodine-containing salts when injected into arteries, and they are rapidly replacing the older contrast agents (Box 41-1) (Hilton & Edwards, 1994; Swischuk, 1997a, 1997b; Fanaroff & Martin, 2002).

Ionizing Radiation Interactions with Tissue

When an infant undergoes a radiologic procedure, most of the radiation passes through the infant's body and strikes the fluorescent screens encompassing the film. The roentgen (or C/kg) is a measure of how many x-rays were present. For the infant, the more important quantity is the number of x-rays that stop in the body and how much energy they deposit. The radiation dose (rad) is a measure of the energy deposited. X-rays that pass through the infant are attenuated by photoelectric absorption and Compton scattering (Alpen, 1998; Juhl, 1998; Dowd, 1999; Bushong, 2001).

Photoelectric absorption involves the complete interaction and absorption of the incoming x-ray photon by the atom. The photon energy is transferred to one of the orbital electrons, which is then ejected as a photoelectron (Alpen, 1998; Bushong, 2001). The ejected electron leaves a vacancy in one of the inner orbits, and an outer orbit electron immediately fills this vacancy. The difference in binding energies between the outer orbit and the inner orbit is released as a characteristic x-ray (Alpen, 1998; Juhl, 1998; Dowd, 1999; Bushong, 2001). The attenuation of the photoelectric effect depends on the atomic number of the material and the amount of incoming energy. The photoelectric interaction declines rapidly with increasing energy and increases rapidly with increasing atomic number (Alpen, 1998; Bushong, 2001). This is why lead is such an effective shield and bone is so much more absorptive than soft tissue.

Compton scattering is the phenomenon in which only part of the energy of the incoming x-ray photon is transferred to the atom; this reduces the energy of the original photon and produces a scattered electron (Bushong, 2001). The scattered electron has a range of less than 1 mm in tissue. The reduced-energy x-ray photon can do exactly what the original x-ray photon could do; it can interact with another atom, causing a photoelectric effect and transferring all its energy to set an electron in motion, or it can itself undergo the Compton effect, scattering an electron and creating a new x-ray photon that has still further reduced energy (Alpen, 1998; Juhl, 1998; Bushong, 2001). Through these two processes, all the energy eventually is transferred to electrons to set them into high-velocity motion. At low photon energies (less than 60 kV), photoelectric interactions predominate. At approximately 140 kV, the photoelectric and Compton interactions transfer equal energy to tissue; at more than approximately 200 kV, most of the energy transfer to tissue is through the Compton interaction (Alpen, 1998; Dowd, 1999; Bushong, 2001). Most neonatal diagnostic radiographs use photon energies between 60 and 100 kV (Hilton & Edwards, 1994; Swischuk, 1997a, 1997b; Fanaroff & Martin, 2002).

X-ray photons with energies greater than 1.02 million electron volts (meV) cause both a photoelectric and a Compton effect and have an additional capability as well. In the vicinity of the atom, the incoming x-ray photons disappear and, in the process, create new matter in the form of one electron and one positron (Alpen, 1998; Dowd, 1999; Bushong, 2001). A positron is a particle of the same size and mass as an electron, but the positron has one unit of positive charge. To create this pair, exactly 1.02 meV of energy is consumed in the conversion of energy into matter. If the incoming x-ray photon has more energy than 1.02 meV, the residual energy is distributed equally to the electron and the positron in the form of kinetic energy (Alpen, 1998; Dowd, 1999; Bushong, 2001).

The effects of the electron when placed in high-velocity orbit are the same as those previously described for the photoelectric and Compton effects. The positron effects are different. The positron expends some of its energy interacting with atoms of the material in which it has been set in motion. Eventually it meets an electron, and the two annihilate each other. When this occurs, both the electron and the positron disappear and two gamma rays appear, each with 0.51 meV of energy (NCRP, 1993a, 1993b, 1993c; Alpen, 1998; Dowd, 1999; Bushong, 2001).

With ionizing radiation, electrons are removed from their atoms and endowed with energies 14 to 20,000 times greater than those in ordinary biochemical reactions (Alpen, 1998; Juhl, 1998; Dowd, 1999; Bushong, 2001). These electrons can maraud through tissue for some distance and can break any kind of chemical bond in the body (NCRP, 1993a, 1993b, 1993c; Dowd, 1999; Bushong, 2001). In biochemical systems the reactions are carefully controlled, often by a special geometric juxtaposition of the reactants. A high-speed electron is akin to a bull in a china shop; it can break anything, anywhere. Once it has ripped an electron out of an atom in a molecule, the molecule itself is placed at such a high energy level that it can produce all kinds of chemical reactions that would never have been possible without ionizing radiation (NCRP, 1993a, 1993b, 1993c; Alpen, 1998; Dowd, 1999; Bushong, 2001).

X-rays and gamma rays are identical in nature except that, in general, x-rays are made in high-voltage machines, whereas gamma rays originate from the nuclei of atoms. Radiations emitted from such naturally unstable atoms as uranium commonly are more energetic per unit than x-ray photons. For example, gamma rays commonly are measured in millions of electron volts (meV) per photon, whereas x-rays commonly are measured in 50 to 100 kiloelectron volts (keV) (50,000 to 100,000 electron volts). Gamma rays from unstable nuclei do all the things that x-rays do; that is, they can undergo photoelectric and Compton effects, and they can produce high-energy electrons and positrons (Dowd, 1999; Bushong, 2001).

Other radiation decay products also create particulate radiation called alpha and beta rays. Beta rays are not truly rays but high-speed electrons emitted from the nuclei of decay products of uranium (Alpen, 1998; Dowd, 1999; Bushong, 2001). Once emitted from the nuclei, beta particles act the same as any high-speed electron. Alpha rays are also not rays and are unlike beta particles. Alpha particles are emitted from the nuclei of uranium. Alpha particles are the "stripped" nuclei of helium and consist of any two protons. Ultimately, the two protons find two electrons in the environment and become helium gas. Most beta particles have energies of about 1 meV, although they are always accompanied by beta particles of lesser energies ranging down to nearly zero. Alpha particles, however, have energies of about 5 meV (Alpen, 1998; Dowd, 1999; Bushong, 2001). X-rays and gamma rays, which pass through the body and do not produce effects on tissue, have no biologic effect. However, alpha and beta particles interact at every millimeter along their path through tissue, so that if they gain access to tissue, biologic harm is guaranteed (NCRP, 1993a, 1993b, 1993c; Dowd, 1999; Bushong, 2001).

Biologic damage from ionizing radiation depends on the amount of energy deposited in a particular tissue. X-rays and gamma rays produce harmful effects only to the extent that they put high-speed electrons in motion. If the same number of electrons are put in motion by gamma rays from plutonium or from deposited radionuclide or by agents from external x-rays, the biologic effects are the same (NCRP, 1993a, 1993b, 1993c; Dowd, 1999; Bushong, 2001).

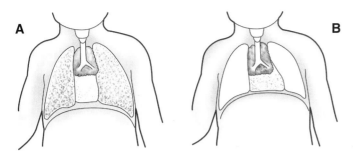

FIGURE **41-5**
Differences in appearance between inspiration (**A**) and expiration (**B**) in a neonatal chest radiograph. On full inspiration, the diaphragm is located at the eighth rib, and the lungs appear larger and darker. During expiration, the diaphragm is at or above the seventh rib, and the lung fields appear smaller and lighter. The heart size may also appear larger on expiratory films.

Factors Affecting Radiographic Quality

Interpretation of a neonatal radiograph requires a rapid evaluation to determine whether the radiograph is technically satisfactory. Several factors determine the technical quality of a radiograph, including film exposure, phase of respiration, motion, tube angulation, and infant positioning. If one of these factors is unsatisfactory, the film may be misinterpreted. When nurses have an understanding of these factors, the technical quality of radiographs is improved.

Film Exposure.   A reasonable criterion for judging film exposure is satisfactory visualization of the dorsal intervertebral disk spaces through the entire cardiothymic silhouette (Hilton & Edwards, 1994; Swischuk, 1997a, 1997b; Fanaroff & Martin, 2002). If the film is underexposed, the dorsal disk spaces are lost, and the lungs and other structures have a homogeneous, "whitewashed" appearance. If the film is overexposed, the pulmonary vascular markings are progressively lost until the lungs have a black, "burned out" appearance (Hilton & Edwards, 1994; Swischuk, 1997a, 1997b).

Phase of Respiration.   The phase of respiration at the time the film is obtained affects the appearance of the radiograph considerably (Figure 41-5). On an expiratory film, the heart may appear grossly enlarged, the lung fields may appear opaque (which may simulate diffuse atelectasis), and the diaphragm is located above the seventh rib (Hilton & Edwards, 1994; Swischuk, 1997a, 1997b). On an inspiratory film, the diaphragm is at the eighth rib, the cardiothymic diameter is normal, and the pulmonary vascularity is prominent. The right hemidiaphragm is slightly higher than the left. If the right hemidiaphragm is at or above the level of the seventh rib, the film was obtained in the expiratory phase or the infant has hypoaerated (Hilton & Edwards, 1994; Swischuk, 1997a, 1997b).

Motion.   If the infant moves just as the radiograph is made, the resulting film is blurred. Motion causes blurring of the hemidiaphragms, the cardiovascular silhouette, and all fine pulmonary detail (Hilton & Edwards, 1994; Swischuk, 1997a, 1997b). Movement blur on diagnostic images can be prevented by fast imaging and adequate immobilization.

Speed.   A short exposure time is essential for obtaining clear images. This can be achieved by limiting the duration of exposure to the energy source and by increasing the use of computed imaging.

Immobilization.   The nursing staff is primarily responsible for ensuring adequate immobilization during diagnostic imaging. Inadequate immobilization is an important cause of poor quality on neonatal images. Proper immobilization techniques improve image quality, shorten the examination time, and eliminate the need for repeat studies (Hilton & Edwards, 1994; Swischuk, 1997a, 1997b). Proper immobilization may be less traumatic than manual restraint alone. An immobilization board may be required, or tape, foam rubber blocks and wedges, towels, diapers, or clear plastic acetate sheets may be used.

Physical risks to neonates are associated with immobilization. The type of restraint or an ill-designed immobilization device may cause trauma. Tape or plastic sheets may cause skin and soft tissue damage if not applied and removed carefully. Also, thermal stress may be a factor when a neonate is placed on a noninsulated board or film cassette. The nurse should position and immobilize the infant properly so that the technician can center the tube, position the beam, and make the exposure. If the nurse and the technician work together, superior results are achieved with greater speed and less disruption than if they worked separately.

Infants lie still only when they are very ill. Otherwise, they greatly resent being forcibly restrained, especially in an unusual position. A number of immobilization devices are available, but the best means is a pair of adequately protected adult hands (Hilton & Edwards, 1994; Swischuk, 1997a, 1997b).

Tube Angulation.   Another factor that affects radiographic quality is angulation of the x-ray tube, along with improper field limitation. Often on neonatal films, the infant's chest appears mildly lordotic, with the medial clavicular ends projected on or above the dorsal vertebrae. This results in a rather peculiar chest configuration. The preossified anterior arcs of the upper ribs are positioned superior to the posterior arcs (Figure 41-6). The lordotic projection tends to increase the apparent transverse cardiac diameter, making it difficult to determine the size of the heart. Lordotic projections result when the x-ray tube is angled cephalad, when the x-ray beam is centered over the abdomen, or when an irritable infant has arched the back at the time of the film exposure (Hilton & Edwards, 1994; Swischuk, 1997a, 1997b). If the x-ray tube is angled caudad or the x-ray beam is centered over the head, the anterior rib arcs are angulated sharply downward in relation to the posterior arcs (Hilton & Edwards, 1994; Swischuk, 1997a, 1997b).

Infant Positioning.   Proper infant positioning is important to radiographic quality and interpretation. If the infant is rotated, a false impression of a mediastinal shift may be created (Figure 41-7) (Hilton & Edwards, 1994; Swischuk, 1997a, 1997b). The direction and degree of rotation can be estimated by comparing the lengths of the posterior arcs of the ribs from the costovertebral junction to the lateral pleural line at a given level. The infant is rotated toward the side with the greatest posterior arc length (Hilton & Edwards, 1994; Swischuk, 1997a, 1997b).

Another measurement for determining the degree of rotation is the distance from the medial aspect of the clavicles to the center of the vertebral body at the same level. If the infant is properly positioned, the medial aspects of the clavicles should be equidistant from the center of the vertebral body (Hilton & Edwards, 1994; Swischuk, 1997a). The distance is

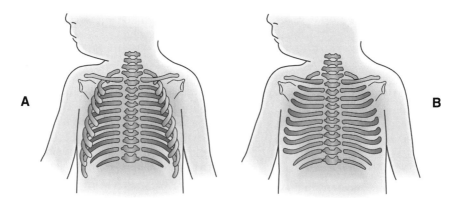

FIGURE **41-6**
Skeletal position in a normally positioned radiograph (**A**) and in a film obtained with cephalad positioning of the x-ray tube (**B**).

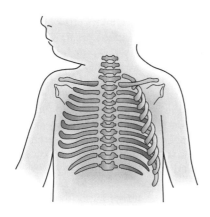

FIGURE **41-7**
Skeletal configuration in a film obtained with the infant rotated to the right.

greater on the side toward which the infant is rotated. On a lateral view, rotation can be readily determined by observing the amount of offset between the anterior tips of the right and left sets of ribs.

Before any chest film is interpreted, these factors must be systematically evaluated. Through experience this evaluation becomes automatic, and the film can be scanned rapidly.

Radiologic Projections

Radiologic projections are the geometric views of the radiograph, and they vary among institutions and radiologists. They can be customized to the specific infant or clinical condition. For example, the skull may require a simple AP film to make the diagnosis of a fracture, whereas a complete skull series may be necessary for evaluation of congenital malformations. In the neck and upper airway, a lateral film in inspiration with the infant's head extended may be sufficient for the evaluation of stridor, or a xeroradiograph of the soft tissue structures of the neck may be required. Because the radiation dose is much greater with a xeroradiograph than with a plain lateral neck film, the indications for this examination should be clear (Swischuk, 1997b).

For evaluation of the spine, the AP projection is most commonly used. Oblique views of the spine usually are difficult to obtain in infants because it is difficult to position and immobilize babies. Also, the diagnostic information gained does not outweigh the risk of the greater radiation exposure required to obtain such views. For evaluation of congenital hip dysplasia,

an AP view of the entire pelvis and both hips is required. Gonadal exposure should be minimized with proper shielding during radiographic examination of the hips. Assessment of skeletal maturation in the infant requires an AP film of the left hemiskeleton, and a long bone series requires a film of the upper and lower extremities (Hilton & Edwards, 1994; Swischuk, 1997a, 1997b).

Chest radiographs are the most frequently performed diagnostic imaging procedure in the neonatal intensive care unit (NICU). In most cases an AP projection from a supine position is satisfactory for evaluating the infant's chest, heart, and lung fields. Lateral projections of the chest often are poorly positioned, have diminished technical quality, and require greater radiation exposure of the infant. For the experienced radiographer, an AP film in the supine position is sufficient in most cases. In rare cases a lateral chest film with esophageal barium contrast may be requested for evaluation of the left atrium of the heart (Hilton & Edwards, 1994; Swischuk, 1997a, 1997b).

Abdominal x-ray films also are frequently obtained in the NICU. The most commonly used radiographic projections are the AP and cross-table lateral views (Hilton & Edward, 1994; Swischuk, 1997a). Because the infant's abdomen is relatively cylindric, a lateral view provides more information than it does in an older child or adult. AP views define the gas pattern, intestinal displacement, some masses, and ascites, whereas the cross-table lateral view is recommended in the diagnosis of intestinal perforation, pneumoperitoneum, and portal venous air (Hilton & Edwards, 1994; Swischuk, 1997a).

Exposure Factors in Infancy

Numerous radiographic variables are involved in x-ray exposure. The x-ray machine, films, screens, types of cassette, and processing methods, as well as the radiologist's preference, may vary greatly from one department and institution to another. However, a few general principles can be stated:

1. Exposure time should be kept short to prevent movement blur and to limit the radiation dose.
2. Radiographic technicians should be knowledgeable about factors and variables that affect exposure so that repeat films occasioned by poor technique on the initial radiograph can be avoided.
3. A repeated infant x-ray is the major cause of the largest dose of unnecessary radiation (Hilton & Edwards, 1994; Swischuk, 1997a, 1997b); every possible precaution should be taken to ensure that the first attempt produces a film of diagnostic quality.

4. Before a repeat is done, the film should be shown to the radiologist or neonatologist who requested it; although the technical quality may not be ideal, the film may provide sufficient information.

Radiation exposure can also be reduced by using other diagnostic imaging modalities, when possible, that do not use ionizing radiation to create an image (e.g., ultrasonography, magnetic resonance imaging) (Swischuk, 1997a, 1997b). If radiologic imaging is the best diagnostic approach for the infant's condition, it may be important to "customize" the examinations, to limit the area examined, and to reduce the number of follow-up films. The radiologist and technician should be knowledgeable about the rapid technologic advances in film-screen combinations, filtration, projections, and film processing, which can help produce a film of fine diagnostic quality while minimizing radiation exposure (Swischuk, 1997a, 1997b; Alpen, 1998).

Ideally there would be no "routine" radiologic examinations, just problem-oriented procedures. However, there is a logical approach to radiographic examinations. Plain films should be obtained first. Then, if indicated, a dye contrast study (e.g., excretory urograph) should be performed, because the contrast material is rapidly eliminated from the body. Last, barium contrast studies should be obtained (Hilton & Edwards, 1994; Swischuk, 1997a, 1997b). Barium contrast studies are performed after the others because (1) barium interferes with any nuclear scintigraphic scans, body computed tomograms, and ultrasonographic scans, and (2) barium is slowly eliminated from the GI tract, which delays further diagnostic evaluation. Additional radiation exposure is possible if the barium must be completely eliminated before the next imaging procedure (Hilton & Edwards, 1994; Swischuk, 1997a, 1997b).

Adequate patient preparation is another means of reducing radiation exposure (Hilton & Edwards, 1994; Swischuk, 1997a, 1997b). If GI and genitourinary (GU) imaging are both to be performed, the GU examination should be scheduled first. Although each institution has its own policies, in preparation for a GU examination such as excretory urography, the infant should be kept on nothing by mouth (NPO) status for no longer than 3 hours; this can be accomplished by withholding the early morning feeding and scheduling the examination for 8 A.M. No preparation is necessary for excretory urography in infants with abdominal masses, trauma, or GU emergencies. If the infant has impaired renal function, the radiologist and the neonatologist should discuss the condition thoroughly so that the risks of this procedure are minimized. For an infant who has been feeding, the baby is prepared for a GI contrast study by keeping the child on NPO status for no longer than 3 hours before the examination. Generally, if a contrast study of the entire GI tract has been requested, the lower GI series is performed before the upper GI series (Hilton & Edwards, 1994; Swischuk, 1997a, 1997b). This allows time for elimination of the barium in the colon and prevents the barium from interfering with the diagnostic quality of the upper GI study. Colon preparation usually is unnecessary in the neonate and should be avoided in infants with an acute abdominal condition and in those suspected of having Hirschsprung disease (Swischuk, 1997a, 1997b).

Collaborative Care
Radiation Protection. Any radiation is considered harmful to the infant, and all efforts must be made to reduce radiation exposure without forgoing diagnostic information. Radiation exposure can have both genetic and somatic effects (NCRP, 1993a, 1993b, 1993c; Dowd, 1999; Bushong, 2001). Reduction

of radiation exposure should be the goal for sites that are sensitive genetically (gonads) and somatically (eyes, bone marrow). Although there is no evidence that somatic damage (e.g., carcinogenesis or cataracts) occurs as a result of low-dose diagnostic radiologic procedures, dose reduction should be accomplished for the site examined and for the rest of the body (Dowd, 1999). Methods of reducing radiation exposure include performing examinations only when they are clinically indicated, selecting the appropriate imaging modality, using the lowest radiation dose that achieves an image of diagnostic quality, avoiding repeat examinations, reducing the number of films obtained, using appropriate projections with tight field limitation, ensuring proper positioning and immobilization, and shielding the gonads (NCRP, 1993a, 1993b, 1993c; Hilton & Edwards, 1994; Alpen, 1998; Dowd, 1999).

If the gonads are not within the area of interest, gonadal exposure depends on the adequacy of field limitation. The maximum gonadal dose occurs when the gonads are unshielded and exposed to the primary x-ray beam. This dose declines rapidly as the distance from the gonads to the primary beam increases. Gonadal exposure in an AP film that includes the gonads can be reduced by 95% with proper contact shielding (Dowd, 1999). The gonads should be shielded whenever they are within 5 cm of the primary x-ray beam.

Contact gonadal shields are easy to make from 0.5-mm thick lead rubber sheets, and they should be sized for gender and age (Figure 41-8) (Swischuk, 1997a, 1997b). In males, proper positioning of the shield avoids obscuration of any bony detail of the pelvis if the upper edge of the shield is placed just below the pubis and if the testicles have descended into the scrotum. In females, the position of the ovaries varies with bladder distention. Because of their anatomic location, the ovaries cannot be shielded without obscuring lower abdominal and pelvic structures. The lower margin of the gonad shield should be placed at the level of the pubis, and the upper margin should cover at least the lower margin of the sacroiliac joints (Hilton & Edwards, 1994; Swischuk, 1997a, 1997b).

Radiation Safety. The three ways to reduce radiation exposure of personnel are (1) shorten the duration of radiation exposure; (2) increase the distance from the radiation source; and (3) provide radiation shielding between the nurse and the radiation source (NCRP, 1993a, 1993b, 1993c; Alpen, 1998; Dowd, 1999; Bushong, 2001). Portable radiologic examinations are the most common form of diagnostic imaging routinely performed in the NICU. During these procedures, there is a tendency for all the nurses to leave the room when an exposure is being produced; consequently, other infants may be left unattended for that short period. Because of this practice, parents have expressed fear about their infants facing environmental radiation hazards.

Using the example of an infant who receives two radiologic examinations per shift, the total dose outside a 30-cm (1 foot) radius of the primary beam is 70 microroentgens (μR). If the staff nurse worked a 250-day work year and held an infant who received two x-ray examinations per shift, the cumulative dose would be 18,000 μR (18 mrad) per year (1000 μR = 1 mrad). This value is considerably lower than the background radiation in a building, which amounts to 100 to 150 mrad per year (Dowd, 1999; Bushong, 2001).

Other radiologic studies done in the NICU have found that within 1.82 m (6 feet) of the target, an unshielded person receives 100 mrad *per hour of exposure*. Because the duration of exposure is approximately 0.1 second, the radiation dose is

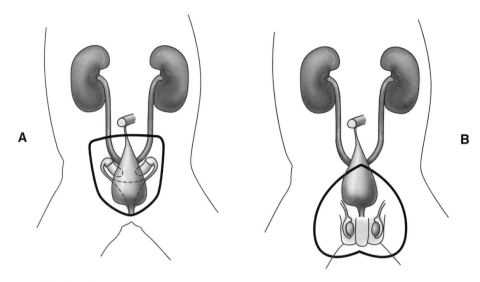

FIGURE **41-8**
Anatomic placement of gonad shield for female infants (**A**) and for male infants (**B**).

0.003 mrad per exposure. This amount of radiation is far below the safety limit of 500 mrad per year. At this rate of radiation exposure, a full-time staff nurse would have to be exposed to more than 6000 x-rays each day to reach the radiation safety limit per year (NCRP, 1993a, 1993b, 1993c).

It appears that if certain basic radiation precautions are observed, nurses and other NICU personnel need not leave the room during x-ray exposures. However, staff members should stay 30 cm (1 foot) or farther from the infant being radiographed. Care must be taken to ensure that if a horizontal beam film is obtained (e.g., in a cross-table lateral projection), no one is in the direct x-ray beam, because the radiation dose in the primary beam is considerably higher than in the scattered portion. When a horizontal beam is used, it should not be directed at any other patient or person. Any employee within 30 cm (1 foot) of the incubator or one who is holding the infant for the exposure should wear a lead apron and gloves.

The x-ray beam must be confined to the area within the cassette's edges. An infant causes little scatter, but an adult's hands can easily come within the field of primary radiation and cause scatter. It is important to position and secure the infant properly while keeping the hands out of the x-ray beam. If correct radiographic technique is used, the dose to the nurse's lead-protected hands is approximately 0.01 mSv. (millisieverts). The annual dose limit to the hands of nondesignated personnel is 500 mSv.

Table 41-2 summarizes the process of systematic interpretation of radiographic images in the neonate.

Radionuclide Imaging

The use of radioisotopes has brought a new dimension to diagnostic imaging, because they can be used to trace a wide range of physiologic functions in virtually every organ in the body, thereby complementing conventional radiography and ultrasonographic imaging. The difference between conventional radiography and radionuclide imaging is that with the former, images are produced by the transmission of radiation, whereas with the latter, images are produced by the emission of radiation (gamma rays) previously introduced into the body and recorded on film or in a computer (Figure 41-9) (Treves, 1995; Alpen, 1998; Juhl, 1998; Dowd, 1999; Bushong, 2001).

Radionuclide studies yield both physiologic information and anatomic representations of the distribution of radioactivity, depending on the selective uptake of radionuclide by different organs of the body (Treves, 1995; Dowd, 1999; Bushong, 2001). The primary disadvantage of radionuclide imaging is the limited anatomic resolution to diameters greater than 2 cm.

Biophysical Principles. Relatively small amounts of radioactivity are used in radionuclide imaging, and the radiation hazard is significantly smaller than for corresponding conventional radiographic investigations (Treves, 1995; Dowd, 1999; Bushong, 2001). The radioactive substance injected usually is distributed throughout the body, and the site of maximum radiation is not always the organ under investigation (Treves, 1995; Dowd, 1999; Bushong, 2001). For example, the thyroid gland selectively concentrates radioactive iodine, even if this compound is being used to study another organ. In this case, thyroid iodine uptake can be blocked pharmaceutically. The kidneys excrete the radioactive phosphonate agents used for skeletal scanning, and the maximum radiation dose is to the bladder mucosa (Treves, 1995; Dowd, 1999). Promoting diuresis can reduce this dose effect. The radiation hazards in radionuclide imaging, therefore, are affected by the physiologic distribution of the agent and its physical half-life, the dose of radionuclide administered, and the pharmacologic half-life in the body (Treves, 1995; Dowd, 1999).

Choice of Nucleotide. With nuclear diagnostic imaging, several factors help determine the amount of energy actually deposited in the tissue and may influence the choice of radionuclide. These factors include the following (Treves 1995; Dowd, 1999):

- Route of entry
- Fraction of the administered dose that actually reaches the tissue
- Rate of biologic removal of the radionuclide
- Amount of radiation the tissue of interest receives from the portion of the radionuclide deposited in tissues other than the one of interest
- Number of microcuries of radionuclide taken in

TABLE 41-2 Radiographic Interpretation

Technical Evaluation	Characteristics
Film density and contrast	The intravertebral disk spaces should be visible through the cardiothymic silhouette. Underexposed films appear whitish with progressive loss of spaces; overexposed films have a "burned out" appearance with loss of pulmonary vascular markings.
Phase of respiration	The respiratory phase affects the appearance of the lung fields. During expiration, the cardiothymic silhouette appears larger, and the lung fields appear more opaque; the hemidiaphragms usually are at the level of the seventh rib. During inspiration, the cardiothymic silhouette is normal, pulmonary vascularity is seen, and the lung fields are clear. Adequate inspiration puts the right hemidiaphragm at the level of the posterior eighth rib; the right hemidiaphragm usually is slightly higher than the left during basal breathing.
Motion	Radiology personnel must check for motion at the time the film is taken. Motion is detected by blurring of the hemidiaphragms and cardiothymic silhouette. Motion obscures all fine pulmonary vascular detail, which makes the films unsatisfactory for evaluation of the lung fields.
Tube angulation and patient positioning	Anteroposterior (AP) films of the newborn appear lordotic, with the medial ends of the clavicles projecting on or above the second dorsal vertebra. If the tube has been angled cephalad, the lordosis is exaggerated, with the anterior arcs of the ribs positioned superior to the posterior arcs. The cardiothymic silhouette appears larger because the view is through the transverse diameter of the heart. This occurs if the infant arches during the procedure or if the beam has been centered over the abdomen. Caudad angulation of the beam over the head results in distortion of the chest, with the anterior ribs arcs angled sharply downward in relation to the posterior arcs.
Rotation of the patient	Assessment of rotation is critical in determining whether mediastinal shift is present. Lateral rotation may lead to the false impression of a mediastinal shift. The trachea shifts toward the side of the rotation, and the contours of the heart are altered. The direction and degree of rotation are estimated by comparing the lengths of the posterior arcs of the ribs on both sides. The side with the longest posterior arc is the side to which the patient is rotated. Rotation also results in unequal lengths of the clavicles when they are measured from the medial aspects to the center of the vertebral body at the same level. The patient is rotated to the side with the longer clavicle.
Heart size and pulmonary vascularity	These features are difficult to determine in the newborn in the first 24 hours of life because of the dynamic cardiovascular alterations that occur during this period. Changes in the transitional circulation are associated with an increase in pulmonary blood flow and in blood return to the left atrium, a decrease in blood return and lower pressure in the right atrium, and changes in systemic and pulmonary arterial pressures. The newborn's heart size is relatively larger in the first 48 to 72 hours because of those rapid changes. Heart size can be accurately assessed only during basal breathing. After the first 24 hours, a cardiothoracic ratio above 0.6 is the upper limit of normal. Fetal lung fluid is reabsorbed, and the air spaces are filled with air on inspiration. The resorption of lung fluid enhances the appearance of the pulmonary lymphatics, resulting in an apparent increase in vascularity at birth. Transient tachypnea of the newborn is characterized by perihilar streaky infiltrates with increased pulmonary vascularity and good lung inflation.
Cardiothymic silhouette	The cardiac configuration is difficult to determine in the newborn largely because of the variation in size and shape of the thymus. The aortic knob and main pulmonary artery are obscured by the thymus, which frequently has a wavy border. A tuck may be seen in the left lobe of the thymus at the lateral margin of the right ventricle, a feature called a sail sign. The apex of the heart has a more cephalad position and assumes a more caudal position over time. The elevation of the apex is due to the relative right ventricular hypertrophy of the fetus. After birth, as the left ventricle becomes more prominent, the cardiac apex descends. The thymus involutes rapidly under the stress of delivery and over the next 2 weeks of life may enlarge slightly.
Aeration of the lungs	Satisfactory inspiration positions the hemidiaphragms at the posterior arcs of the eighth rib. Expansion and radiolucency of the right and left sides are equal. If the sides are not comparable, a right and left lateral decubitus film should be obtained to evaluate for fluid levels or air. The lungs may bulge slightly through the ribs. On lateral projection, the hemidiaphragms should be smoothly domed. The AP and transverse diameters of the chest vary with age and disease. In a normal newborn, the AP and transverse diameters are equal. Over time, the transverse diameter increases, giving the chest cavity an oblong appearance. Air-trapping diseases produce a more rounded configuration, whereas hypoaeration results in a more flattened AP diameter. With hypoaeration, the right hemidiaphragm is located at the seventh rib, the posterior arcs have a more downward slope, and the transverse diameter of the chest is reduced. Laterally, hypoaeration results in increased doming of the diaphragm. With hyperaeration, the hemidiaphragm is located below the level of the ninth rib, the diaphragm is flattened, and the posterior rib arcs are horizontal. Hyperaeration also results in greater bulging of the lungs through the intercostal spaces and an increased diameter of the upper thorax.

Continued

TABLE 41-2 Radiographic Interpretation—cont'd

Technical Evaluation	Characteristics
Pulmonary infiltrates	Films should be evaluated for areas of increased pulmonary lucency or density. The characteristics and distribution of densities may lead to a diagnosis. Infiltrates should be described with regard to their distribution (unilateral, bilateral) and nature (alveolar, reticulated, diffuse, nondiffuse, patchy, streaky).
Mediastinal shift	The examiner evaluates for mediastinal shift by determining if the trachea, heart, and mediastinum are in normal position. In general, the shift occurs toward the side with the diminished lung volume or away from the hemithorax with the increased lung volume. Rotation of the patient must first be excluded.
Liver size	The edges of the liver should be clearly defined, and the size of the organ should correlate well with the size determined by palpation. The position of the liver may be altered by congenital malformations such as situs inversus. If insufficient gas is present in the abdomen, the size of the liver cannot be determined. Atelectasis obscures the upper margin of the liver. Radiographically, the size of the liver is not altered by the phase of respiration, as it is during palpation. Liver size may vary with progression of right-sided heart failure.
Abdominal gas pattern	Swallowing air produces gas in the stomach. The gas pattern must be interpreted in light of the infant's history. In the newborn, stomach air is present, with progression of air through the small bowel at 3 hours of life and rectal air by 6 hours. With bowel obstruction, gaseous distention progresses until at some point the bowel is blocked; beyond that point there is a paucity of air or a gasless bowel. Lack of haustra in the colon makes it distinguish the small and large bowels on the radiograph. A gasless abdomen may be seen with prolonged gastrointestinal decompression, severe dehydration, acidosis, oversedation, brain injury, diaphragmatic hernia, midgut volvulus, and esophageal atresia. Marked aerophagia may be due to mechanical ventilation, tracheoesophageal fistula, necrotizing enterocolitis, and mesenteric vascular occlusion. Free peritoneal air rises to the highest level and outlines superior structures, therefore it is best demonstrated on a left lateral decubitus film.
Catheter and tube positions	All catheter and tube positions should be evaluated and reported each time a radiograph is made. The position of these devices may provide clues to the underlying disease, and malpositioning of tubes and catheters may be life threatening. The trachea is positioned to the right in the midmediastinum, anterior and slightly to the right of the esophagus. The carina is located at T4. In the right aortic arch, the trachea is found slightly to the left of the vertebral column. Endotracheal tubes optimally are placed in the midtrachea. If the tip is too low (below T4) or too high (above the thoracic inlet), ventilation is suboptimal. Inadvertent esophageal intubation has occurred when the tip of the tube is below T4 but is still in the midline or when the trachea can be visualized apart from the tube. Nasogastric (NG) tube placement should be reported. NG tubes may be too short (seen in the distal esophagus) or too long (seen in the duodenum or jejunum), or they may be coiled in the esophagus (tracheoesophageal atresia). The location of vascular catheters must be evaluated. Central catheters should be placed with the tip in the superior part of the inferior cava. Umbilical artery catheters ideally should be located in the high (T6-T9) or low (L3-L5) position, away from major arterial branches. Umbilical venous catheters should be positioned with the tip in the inferior vena cava and not in a hepatic branch.
Bony structures	The skeleton should be evaluated, especially the general configuration of the thoracic cage. Normally, over time, the cephalic portion of the thoracic cage becomes rounded and the transverse diameter increases. Hyperaeration exaggerates cephalic rounding, and the horizontal position of the rib arcs. Hypoaeration reduces the diameter of the upper thorax and increases the inferior slope of the rib arcs (bell-shaped thorax). The radiograph must be evaluated for fractures, dislocations, hypodensities, or other lucencies. Persistent elevation of the scapula and an ipsilateral elevated diaphragm (which occur secondary to phrenic nerve injury) may accompany Erb's palsy. Scans should be done for vertebral, rib, and other bony anomalies. Rib aplasia is associated with hemivertebrae, and complete or partial aplasia of the clavicles may be a manifestation of chromosomal abnormality. The proximal humeri can yield information related to congenital infections such as in rubella, syphilis, and cytomegalovirus infection. The bone density should be evaluated in relation to film penetration.

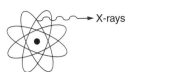 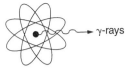

FIGURE **41-9**
X-rays are produced outside the nucleus of artificially excited atoms; gamma rays are produced inside the nucleus of radioactive atoms.

- Careful calculation of the average energy of the beta particles emitted, of any ancillary gamma rays emitted, and of any loss of radiation out of the specific tissue
- Metabolic or other factors that might alter the distribution of the radionuclide in various tissues of the human population studied

Estimation of the true dose of energy delivered to a specific tissue by radionuclide exposure, plutonium contamination, or external x-ray exposure, therefore, involves serious technical considerations and requires the efforts of physicists skilled in such measurements.

Nearly all radionuclides used in medicine are artificially produced in nuclear reactors. The most versatile of these compounds is technetium 99m (^{99m}Tc), which has many ideal physical properties, including the following (Treves, 1995; Dowd, 1999):

1. It is nontoxic and nonallergenic.
2. It is easily bound to other physiologic compounds.
3. It is relatively inexpensive.
4. It circulates in the blood, and small amounts accumulate in the gastric mucosa, salivary glands, and thyroid tissue.
5. It is excreted primarily in the feces and urine but can also be found in sweat and tears.
6. It does not accumulate in the brain (except in the choroid plexus) unless the blood-brain barrier has been disrupted.
7. It has a short physical half-life (6 hours), long enough for tests to be completed while allowing high initial radioactivities to be administered within an acceptable radiation hazard.
8. It emits only gamma photons, which can be detected by the sodium iodide crystals of gamma cameras.

Despite the wide use of technetium, it is not suitable for all investigations, and a number of alternative isotopes are available (Box 41-1).

The ideal instrument for detecting the radiation emission of the radionuclide is the gamma camera. With this camera, images are rapidly acquired and dynamic studies are easily performed and quantified. Multiple views from various projections can be obtained. The camera consists of a large crystal of sodium iodide protected by a heavy lead collimator. The shielded crystal is placed over the target organ, and the gamma photons emitted from the body strike it and are converted into light scintillations. The pinhole and converging collimators allow the image to be magnified without loss of resolution. These light scintillations are manipulated electronically to define the distribution and intensity of the radioactivity. The final copy of the image is produced on film or stored on videotapes or magnetic disk (Treves, 1995; Alpen, 1998; Dowd, 1999; Bushong, 2001).

Because radiopharmaceuticals are rarely organ specific, interference from radioactivity outside the organ of interest is always a factor. Advances in computer processing similar to CT have been developed to eliminate this interfering background data, thereby increasing the accuracy of derived data. Two types of computer-enhanced radionuclide imaging are available: single photon emission computed tomography (SPECT) and positron emission tomography (PET). Both modalities have significant advantages over conventional planar radionuclide imaging in that (1) the sensitivity and qualification of the distribution and density of radioactivity are much greater; (2) three-dimensional imaging is possible with computer reconstruction; (3) the dose of radionuclide is the same; and (4) artifactual lesions can be eliminated.*

Single Photon Emission Computed Tomography (SPECT). With SPECT, a gamma camera is rotated 360 degrees around the infant, and a series of equally spaced, cross-sectional images is obtained and stored in the computer. These images are used to reconstruct a series of cross-sectional slices at right angles to the axis of rotation of the camera. Each cross-sectional slice comprises a series of squares arranged in a matrix. Using a mathematic model, the computer can readily reconstruct these cross-sectional slices in other planes, such as the lateral or coronal plane. The image is then viewed directly from the computer screen or formatted on film. This type of computer-enhanced emission tomography scan uses the standard gamma-emitting radionuclides such as technetium, thallium, gallium, and iodine (Treves, 1995; Lewis et al, 2000).

Positron Emission Tomography (PET). With PET, a different type of radiopharmaceutical, called a positron, is used. Positrons are the same size and shape as electrons but have a positive charge. Typical positrons used in this type of imaging are carbon 11, oxygen 15, and nitrogen 13. Using the metabolic nucleotide from oxygen, carbon, or nitrogen, PET scans create images that depict the "metabolic" function of tissue such as the brain (Treves, 1995; Dowd, 1999; Bushong, 2001; Lin et al, 2001; Weissleder, 2001). SPECT is widely available for general use, but PET scanning is available only at large university medical centers with access to a cyclotron, which can produce the short-lived positrons required for this imaging modality. Continued advances in particle physics enhance the development of the technique as a research tool in the study of cerebral blood flow and physiology. The recent substitution of fluorine in the glucose molecule has been very useful in the study of cerebral metabolism in neonates after intracranial hemorrhage (Swischuk, 1997a; Peterson et al., 2000; Rushe et al, 2001). Although this modality is not used frequently in clinical medicine, nurses should understand its potential as a research tool.

Collaborative Care. The care of a neonate undergoing a radionuclide scan requires knowledge about the patient's history and clinical manifestations, the type of nuclear scan requested, and the radiopharmaceutical used. In general, the doses of radiopharmaceuticals are based on the infant's body weight, and the total whole body irradiation is considerably less than that with a conventional radiograph. The infant poses no radioactivity hazard for the nursing staff or other neonates. Linen, diapers, and body excreta can be disposed of in the usual manner. Nurses should be aware that the radionuclide can concentrate in areas other than the organ of interest so that the proper agents for blocking thyroid iodine uptake can be administered or diuresis can be promoted.

*Treves, 1995; Swischuk, 1997a, 1997b; Bellenger et al., 2000; Lewis et al, 2000; Bushong, 2001; Tierney et al, 2001; and Weisslleder, 2001.

Ultrasonographic Imaging

With neonates, ultrasonography frequently is used in the evaluation and treatment of internal anatomic structures. Unlike conventional radiography, ultrasonography does not involve the emission of ionizing radiation. Instead, sound waves are used to evaluate tissue densities, the movement of tissues, and blood flow (Swischuk, 1997a, 1997b; Bushong, 1999, 2001; Fanaroff & Martin, 2002). The images can be recorded on videotape, photographic film, light-sensitive paper, or magnetic disks.

Biophysical Principles. By definition, ultrasound is any sound that has a frequency greater than 20,000 cycles per second (Hz), which exceeds the audible range of human hearing (20 to 20,000 Hz) (Bushong, 2001). Ultrasonography uses high-frequency sound waves (3.5 to 10 MHz). For echocardiography and Doppler studies, the ultrasound frequencies range in the millions of cycles per second (Bushong, 1999). Ultrasonography has the following advantages as a diagnostic tool (Swischuk, 1997a, 1997b; Bushong, 1999, 2001; Fanaroff & Martin, 2002):

1. It emits no ionizing radiation and has no known deleterious somatic or genetic effects, therefore follow-up examinations may be repeated at will.
2. Ultrasound waves can be directed as a beam.
3. Sound waves obey laws of reflection and refraction.
4. Ultrasound waves are reflected by objects of small size.
5. Ultrasonography can be used in a variety of transverse, longitudinal, sagittal, or oblique planes.
6. Ultrasonography is considerably less costly than either CT or magnetic resonance imaging.
7. Ultrasound equipment is easily portable.
8. The examination is relatively painless and well tolerated.
9. Sedation is rarely required.
10. Ultrasonography relies on acoustic impedance of tissue to demonstrate anatomy.
11. Ultrasonography is diagnostically accurate.

The following are the principal disadvantages of ultrasonography (Bushong, 1999, 2001):

1. It is operator dependent.
2. It does not provide as much information on organ function as urography.
3. It has limited value as a screening procedure for "acute abdominal distress"; rather, the examination should focus on a particular area of interest.
4. CT is superior in demonstrating the extent of disease, because ultrasonography demonstrates a smaller area of interest and less anatomic detail.
5. Bone, excessive fat, and gas artifacts adversely affect ultrasonography.

Because of these drawbacks, certain parts of the body, such as the brain, must be imaged through an ultrasound "window," such as the anterior fontanel. In addition, because sound waves are poorly propagated through a gaseous medium, the transducer must have airless contact with the surface being examined, and parts of the body that contain large amounts of air are difficult to examine.

High-frequency sound passes through the body tissues at a fairly constant speed of approximately 1500 m/second, or 1.5 mm/microsecond (Bushong, 1999, 2001). Using electronic mechanisms, it is possible to time the passage of an ultrasound impulse to within a fraction of a microsecond so that the distance between an ultrasound transducer and a reflecting interface of tissue can be determined to a fraction of a millimeter. The transducer converts electrical energy into ultrasonographic energy and acts as both the emitter of the initial impulse and the receiver of the reflected impulse.

The velocity of sound wave transmission is the product of the sound frequency and the wavelength. The speed at which sound is transmitted varies, depending on the density and compressibility of the medium (Bushong, 1999, 2001). The velocity of sound transmission is low in a gaseous medium because of the large compressibility and low density of the substance. Sound does not exist in the vacuum of outer space but is readily transmitted through objects of greater density, such as water or metal. This principle can be readily illustrated with the use of a tuning fork. When struck, the tuning fork vibrates and emits sound that can be easily heard. However, when the vibrating tuning fork is placed against the mastoid bone of the cranium, the sound is transmitted to the ear much more readily and is perceived as being louder.

Frequency and wavelength are inversely proportional in ultrasonography (Bushong, 1999, 2001). That is, as the ultrasound frequency increases, the wavelength decreases. The ability to distinguish objects of small size with ultrasonography is directly related to the sound wavelength. High-frequency ultrasonography uses short wavelengths and results in better image resolution than is seen with low frequency, long-wavelength ultrasonography. This is the case because as the ultrasound frequency increases, the degree of interaction with the conducting medium increases, and absorption of the ultrasound beam is increased. Therefore at higher ultrasound frequencies, less tissue penetration occurs. For example, ultrasound examinations of the eye typically use frequencies of about 10 MHz, whereas an examination of deep structures of the abdomen uses frequencies of about 2.5 MHz (Bushong, 1999).

The frequency-dependent characteristic of ultrasonography results in its highly directional and collimated nature, which enhances its imaging ability (Bushong, 1999). As the frequency of sound increases, its dispersion from the source is reduces and its transmission becomes more like that of a collimated beam. This becomes apparent when experimenting with a household stereo. The woofers, which produce low-frequency bass sound, fill the entire room with sound. A person's perception of these low-frequency sounds does not change, no matter where the person stands in the room. However, the higher frequency sound produced by the tweeters does not disperse as well in the room and can best be heard when the person is positioned directly in front of the speakers. In addition, low-frequency sounds seem at times to penetrate and reverberate in the body, which is not true with higher frequency sounds.

These same principles govern ultrasound transmission through tissue. At higher ultrasound frequencies, the beam becomes more collimated in a forward direction. As the ultrasound frequency is increased, the ability to distinguish small objects increases, but the penetrability of the beam decreases. For these reasons, the highest frequency transducer is chosen to provide the greatest depth for the tissue or organ imaged.

Ultrasonography also is useful as a diagnostic imaging method because it is reflected at tissue interfaces. A principle called "sonic momentum" describes the velocity of sound transmitted through tissue. Sound transmission through different tissues varies with sound velocity, the freedom of motion of the molecules (density), and the sound waves' compressibility. The way sound travels through a tissue often is referred to as the acoustic impedance of that tissue. As a sound wave travels through a homogeneous tissue, it continues in a straight line. When the sound wave reaches an interface between two tissues with different acoustic impedances, it undergoes reflection

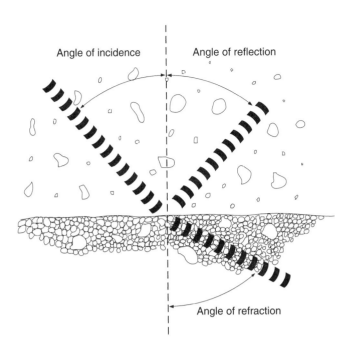

Angle of incidence   Angle of reflection

Angle of refraction

FIGURE **41-10**
The reflection and refraction of ultrasound.

and refraction (Figure 41-10) (Bushong, 1999, 2001). The amount of sound reflected depends on the degree of difference between the two tissues; the greater the disparity, the greater the reflection. Diagnostic ultrasound has little interest in the refracted wave but is primarily interested in the intensity of the reflected beam relative to the original sound wave (Bushong, 1999, 2001).

The major patterns of ultrasound reflection are anechoic, echoic, and mixed. An anechoic structure, which is described as sonar lucent, is a structure in which the acoustic medium is homogeneous and the sound waves are unimpeded. An anechoic structure may be fluid filled (bladder), cystic (hydronephrosis), or solid (lymphoma), as long as the tissue is homogeneous. Cystic structures usually have sharp echogenic margins anteriorly and posteriorly. Echoic structures are inhomogeneous and reflect sound waves. These tissues generally are solid and have a variety of densities (typical Wilms' tumor) or may be cystic (hemorrhagic Wilms' tumor). A mixed pattern of reflections has the combined qualities of anechoic and echoic tissues. In addition, ribs and calculi may cause imaging artifacts on an ultrasonographic image. These dense structures prevent further penetration of the ultrasound beam and cause a band-like region of decreased sound transmission beyond that point, called acoustic shadowing (Bushong, 1999).

Applying these principles to clinical practice, it is known that ultrasound is propagated differently in various human tissues and is reflected from each acoustic interface (Bushong, 1999, 2001). A stationary interface results in a reflected ultrasound wave that has the same frequency as the transmitted wave. When the tissue interface is moving (e.g., the movement of red blood cells in a vessel), the reflected ultrasound wave has a shifted frequency directly proportional to the velocity of the reflecting blood cells, in accordance with a principle called the Doppler effect. If the movement of the blood cells is toward the transducer, the frequency of the reflected wave is higher than the transmitted frequency. Conversely, movement of blood away from the transducer results in a lower frequency of the reflected wave (Bushong, 1999, 2001). The difference

between the transmitted frequency and the reflected frequency is called the Doppler shift. It is the principle of sound frequency shifts that allows the application of the mathematic relationship between the velocity of the target and the Doppler frequency to calculate flow. This is used most commonly in the echocardiographic evaluation of the heart and in cerebral blood flow determinations (Bushong, 1999, 2001).

Modes of Ultrasonography.   Currently there are five modes of ultrasonic imaging: two static modes (A-mode and B-mode), two dynamic modes (M-mode and real-time), and one Doppler mode. The two static and two dynamic modes use a pulse-echo transducer, which sends ultrasound waves for 0.0001 second and then waits for the reflected sound for 0.999 second. The first and most intense reflection of a sound wave occurs at the transducer-patient interface. At each succeeding tissue interface, reflection of the sound wave diminishes in intensity as the tissue is penetrated. The time required for the pulse to be reflected to the transducer and its returned intensity indicate the position of the interface; the reflection is indicated as a blip on the video display screen (Bushong, 1999, 2001).

In A-mode, ultrasonic images are displayed on the video screen as a series of vertical blips that represent the returning echoes. The distance between these blips is proportional to distances between the tissue interfaces, and the height of each blip is proportional to the intensity of the reflected beam. Thus distal reflections produce lower blips (Bushong, 1999). The main purpose of A-mode imaging is to measure depths of interfaces and to detect their separation accurately. A-mode ultrasonography is primarily used in echoencephalography to determine the cranial midline; it also is used for ultrasonically guided aspiration techniques such as amniocentesis. The advantages of A-mode are that it relies on axial resolution; it is relatively inexpensive; and it is easy to use. The primary disadvantage of this mode is that is requires frequent calibration (Bushong, 1999).

B-mode, or brightness mode, ultrasonic imaging displays information as dots, with the brightness of the dot corresponding to the distance of the reflecting interface from the transducer (Figure 41-11, A and B). Advances in microcomputers and electromechanical coupling have resulted in a compound B-mode image (Bushong, 1999). This is achieved when the spatial position and direction of the ultrasound beam are coupled to the video display screen and the B-mode pulses are individually stored while the transducer is moved about the body. The image that appears on the video display screen, therefore, is the summation of many individual B-mode lines. The spatial resolution of this type of imaging varies considerably and depends on the transducer's characteristics and the electromechanical linkages available commercially. This mode of imaging has become widely used, especially for intracranial and abdominal examinations. The B-mode transducer can be moved linearly to provide a rectangular scan view or it can be angled to provide a sector scan (Bushong, 1999).

M-mode, or motion mode, is an imaging process that incorporates pulse-echo ultrasonography to define tissue movement. If an ultrasound transducer is operated in A-mode over the heart, it detects a number of vertical blips from stationary objects, which indicate the motionless interfaces of the tissue. The amplitude of these blips is proportional to the intensity of the echo. The magnitude of the moving objects represents the degree of movement of tissue interface. If this A-mode scan is converted into a B-mode scan, the image is transformed into a number of dots, some of which are fixed and some of which are moving. If this image is driven on the X-axis according to time,

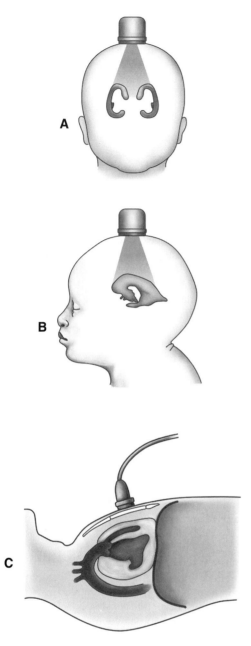

FIGURE **41-11**

A, Ultrasound display pattern defining the sagittal sections of ventricular shape and size using brightness (B mode) imaging. **B,** Ultrasound display pattern defining the shape and size of lateral ventricles in the neonate using B-mode imaging. **C,** M-mode ultrasound display pattern produces a strip chart for tracing moving tissue interfaces such as appear in the heart.

as in a chart recording, a tracing of the dots results (Figure 41-11, *C*). The stationary dots trace a regular pattern according to the motion of the tissue interface. The Y-axis is the depth of the tissue plane. This type of imaging is used primarily to monitor heart function and can be synchronized with the electrocardiograph (Bushong, 1999).

Real-time ultrasonic imaging is another dynamic form of examining tissues. Real-time is considered the ultrasonic fluoroscope and has several advantages over B-mode imaging, including the following:

1. Real-time ultrasonography units cost considerably less than B-mode units.

2. Acquisition of real-time images is much less dependent on operator skill.
3. Real-time examinations take less time because the imaging technique is relatively easy.
4. Portable versions of real-time units are readily available.

The transducer used for real-time ultrasonography is longer than the one used for B-mode imaging, therefore more gel is needed. The real-time transducer is moved over the surface until the anatomic region of interest is found. The dynamic image is recorded on videotape, and the examiner obtains stop-action frames by taking sequential photographs of the display. The disadvantages of real-time ultrasonography are that (1) the ultrasound beam interacts with tissue interfaces from only one direction, whereas B-mode transducers can move while storing the image from many directions, and (2) lateral resolution is superior in B-mode imaging compared with real-time imaging (Bushong, 1999).

The popularity of real-time ultrasonography as an imaging modality has generated three types of real-time transducer devices—mechanical, linear array, and phased array—with displays that have distinct characteristics. The mechanical transducer was the first real-time device developed. This transducer is motorized so that the ultrasound beam is mechanically swept across the field in an oscillating fashion. Each sweep results in one image frame, and as many as 15 frames per second can be obtained. The transducer can be moved linearly for a rectangular view or in an angulated fashion for a sector view (Bushong, 1999). The mechanical transducer was not popular in the early days of real-time ultrasonography because of the limitation of frame rate per second, restricted field of view, and distortion. In recent years, manufacturers have improved this transducer by increasing the frame rate, expanding the viewing field, and reducing the distortion.

The linear array transducer device has a line of 32 transducers aligned in a single case. Because each transducer is only 2 mm wide, the overall length of the transducer case is 64 mm. In linear array, each transducer is energized in sequence from 1 to 32. This provides 32 image lines over the pulse of ultrasound, called sequential linear array. If four or five contiguous transducers are energized simultaneously, each pulse of the ultrasound results in four or five scan image lines, called segmental linear array. In a typical system, the transducers are fired in an overlapping pattern so that numbers 1 through 5, then 2 through 6, 3 through 7, and so on are segmentally, then sequentially energized (Bushong, 1999). This type of transducer device provides for greater image line density and improved image quality over sequential linear array devices. As with the mechanical devices, sequential and segmental linear array devices have poor lateral resolution.

Phased-array real-time ultrasonic imaging is similar to linear array in that it incorporates segmental excitation of the transducer elements. The transducers are segmentally sequenced and have programmable electronic circuitry to incorporate delay lines, so that the excitation and reception of the ultrasound waves by each element can be timed precisely. This delay allows a plane of sound waves from the transducer to be directed, or "phased." The result is a sector scan with a maximum sector angle of 90 degrees (Bushong, 1999). The scan line rate, frame rate, and depth of scan can be selected. The electronic delay lines on the receiver circuitry allow some depth of focusing through synchronization of the returning reflected pulses. The transducer size is smaller than with linear array, and axial resolution is good. As with real-time imaging, lateral resolution is poor but can be improved with acoustic focusing.

Biologic Effects of Ultrasonography. Ultrasonic imaging was introduced into obstetric practice in 1966. Since that time, despite the widespread use of this imaging modality and the use of multiple scans during an individual pregnancy, there have been no reports of manifested injury or late effects in human beings (or fetuses) exposed to diagnostic levels of medical ultrasound (Bushong, 1999). In the laboratory, however, it has been shown that much higher levels of ultrasound can produce measurable tissue effects. The levels of ultrasound energy required to produce these effects are approximately 1000 times greater than those used in diagnostic medical ultrasonography. In vitro, the mechanism of action of the ultrasonic effects on tissue is presumed to be increased tissue temperature, cavitation, and various viscous stresses on the tissue (Bushong, 1999, 2001).

The thermal effects of ultrasonography occur because of the molecular agitation and relaxation processes caused by the passing sound waves (Bushong, 1999, 2001). Extremely high levels of ultrasound are required to produce even a measurable increase in tissue temperature. The effects of the elevation in tissue temperature occur not only with ultrasonography but also with fever or hyperthermia. At the local tissue level, significant changes in tissue temperature, regardless of the cause, result in structural changes in macromolecules and membranes and alter the rates of biochemical reactions. The thermal effects of diagnostic medical ultrasonography do not result in any increase in tissue temperature.

High levels of experimental ultrasound can also result in alteration in the structure and function of macromolecules and cells without an increase in tissue temperature. These changes can result from cavitation, which occurs when tiny bubbles of gas are formed during the molecular relaxation after sound wave agitation (Bushong, 1999, 2001). As the cavitation increases, more energy is absorbed from the incident ultrasound beam. This is thought to cause disruption of molecular bonds and the production of free hydrogen and hydroxide radicals resulting from the dissociation of water vapor. Cavitation effects have not been observed with the levels of sound used in diagnostic medical ultrasonography (Bushong, 2001).

Every tissue has a specific density, and the density of tissues on either side of an interface may not be equal. As ultrasound waves interact along this tissue interface, the differences in density result in stress exerted on the tissue boundary. This tissue boundary stress results in small-scale fluid motions called microstreaming (Bushong, 1999). It is theoretically possible that microstreaming can disrupt membranes and cells in the region of the interface. Microstreaming has been observed in vitro only after exposure to extremely high levels of ultrasound.

Experimental evidence has shown that ultrasound in sufficiently high doses can degrade macromolecules and may produce chromosomal aberrations and cause cellular death. To induce these effects in living tissue, however, ultrasound intensities of 10 W/cm^2 exposure over considerable periods of time are necessary. The absolute minimum dose level that has been reported to have an observable effect in experimental specimens is 100 mW/cm^2, and then only after many hours of continuous ultrasonographic application (Bushong, 1999, 2001). The intensity range of diagnostic ultrasound is 1 to 10 mW/cm^2, and examinations using this modality frequently require only a few minutes of ultrasound exposure. There are no reports of human chromosomal effects or of changes in prenatal or neonatal death rates after exposure to ultrasound, nor is there evidence that ultrasound induces latent malignant disease. For these reasons, the use of ultrasonic imaging has grown in all areas of medicine, and its uses in neonatal care are increasing rapidly.

Indications for ultrasonography in neonatal intensive care commonly include evaluation of brain parenchyma and ventricular size, myocardial function and structure, cholelithiasis, choledochal cysts, intestinal duplication, renal neoplasms, urinary tract dilation and duplication, pelvic masses, and skeletal anomalies of the spine and hips (Fanaroff & Martin, 2002).

Collaborative Care. The care of a neonate undergoing a diagnostic ultrasound examination ensures that any disruption of the infant's microenvironment is minimal. The infant's temperature can be maintained more easily if the ultrasound examination can be performed by using the transducer in the incubator. Although this method is technically more cumbersome for the ultrasonographer, cooperation between the ultrasonographer and the nurse facilitates the procedure. The transducer gel should be warmed to the same temperature as the infant's incubator to minimize heat loss. Placing a diaper or other pad under the imaged area, as well as removing the gel quickly and drying the skin after the scan, also helps to reduce heat loss caused by wet blankets or skin.

Having an understanding of the imaging examination to be performed allows the nurse to more accurately position the infant and move electrodes, tape, or other artifacts that limit the surface area to be scanned. The nurse's assistance in performing an ultrasound examination is important for monitoring the infant's tolerance of the procedure and for providing information that may be of diagnostic importance to the ultrasonographer. In addition, the nurse's presence at the bedside allows for immediate visual feedback and interpretation of the extent of the pathologic condition that may be present. This knowledge enables the nurse to better support the infant's parents as they make decisions on further diagnostic testing and treatment after their discussions with the medical staff. Interaction with the ultrasonographer at the bedside may also help the nurse to anticipate the infant's immediate and long-term future health care needs.

Magnetic Resonance Imaging

The theoretic basis for magnetic resonance imaging (MRI) is a development of research conducted since the 1940s for studying atomic nuclear structure, which resulted in the awarding of the Nobel Prize for physics in 1952 to Edward Purcell and Felix Block. In addition to the advances in atomic nuclear research, other developments were necessary, such as superconductivity and advances in computer programming, before this concept could be applied to diagnostic imaging.

As an imaging modality, MRI has several advantages over CT and ultrasound (Bushong, 1996, 2001; Huda et al, 2001; Lansberg et al, 2001; Peled & Yeashurun, 2001; Schierlitz et al, 2001):

1. Like ultrasonography, MRI does not use ionizing radiation to produce the image, but rather uses magnetic fields and radio waves.
2. The magnetic resonance image depends on three separate molecular parameters that are sensitive to changes in structure and bioactivity rather than on x-ray photon interaction with tissue electrons as in CT.
3. The region of the body imaged with MRI is not limited by the gantry geometry, as it is with CT, but can be controlled electronically, allowing imaging in transverse planes and in true sagittal, coronal, and oblique planes.
4. Magnetic resonance images are free of the high-intensity artifacts produced in CT scans by sharp, dense bone or metallic surgical clips.

The principal disadvantages of MRI are its high cost and limited availability. Its use for clinically unstable infants on life support also is restricted, because the strong magnetic field can interfere with monitoring devices, and access to the infant is limited during the procedure (Swischuk, 1997a, 1997b; Lansberg et al, 2001; Peled & Yeashurun, 2001; Schierlitz et al, 2001).

Despite the disadvantages of MRI, its clinical applications are rapidly expanding. The image quality is excellent, with the advances in the use of surface coils, and more sensitive head and body coils allow structures such as cranial nerves and small joints to be evaluated more precisely. The increased use of gating, fast scanning, and diffusion-weighted and magnetization transfer imaging have improved MRI evaluation of many tissues and structures and have identified many pathologic conditions that previously could not be quantified.*

Biophysical Principles. All particles in an atom have either a positive or a negative charge, or a "spin," like a tiny spinning top. The total spin of the protons and neutrons on the nucleus is the sum of the individual spins. Moving charges create magnetic fields, thus the nucleus of an atom develops north and south magnetic dipoles (Bushong, 1996, 2001; Juhl, 1998; Dowd, 1999). In most materials such as soft tissue, these little spinning magnetic dipoles are randomly oriented (Figure 41-12, A). This random orientation causes all the spins and magnetic forces to cancel in the material so that the net magnetic force is zero. However, if the material is placed in a strong magnetic field, the magnetic dipoles align themselves, much like a compass needle aligns itself with the Earth's magnetic field. The alignment of these magnetic dipoles produces a net magnetic force or vector that is oriented parallel to the direction of the imposed magnetic field (Figure 41-12, B). Not all magnetic dipoles become aligned; some are in constant thermal motion so that nuclei are continually knocked out of alignment (Bushong, 1996, 2001; Juhl, 1998).

In MRI, the strong magnetic field is imposed to align the molecular magnetic dipoles, and radio frequency pulses then are applied. The known specific frequency of these radio waves displaces the net magnetic moment by an amount determined by the strength and duration of the pulse. The frequency is directly proportional to the strength of the magnetic field and is known as the resonant frequency. After the pulse, the protons emit radio frequencies as they return to their original orientation. Therefore the frequency of signals emitted by the protons after the application with radio frequency waves reflects their position in the tissue. Although in theory any stable nuclei can be used, hydrogen is the most abundant and has the strongest resonance (Bushong, 1996, 2001; Juhl, 1998).

When protons are placed in a magnetic field, proton alignment does not occur instantaneously but rather increases exponentially with a time constant characterized by T_1, or spin-lattice relaxation time, which reflects the interaction of the hydrogen nucleus with its molecular environment (Bushong, 1996, 2001; Juhl, 1998). T_1 characterizes the return of the net magnetization from its displaced position to its normal vertical position resulting from spin-lattice interactions. To form an image, the radio frequency pulses must be applied repetitively. After each radio frequency pulse, the net magnetic force of the

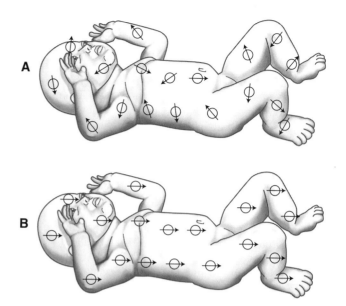

FIGURE **41-12**

A, All the magnetic moments are randomly oriented in the body so that the net magnetic charge is zero. **B,** Applied radio frequency pulses align the magnetic moments along a predetermined axis. The rate at which the atoms return to their "normal" magnetic moment after the radio frequency is stopped is characteristic for physiologic and pathologic tissues and is responsible for creating the magnetic resonance image.

sample is reduced; therefore too rapid a radio frequency repetition depletes the magnetization of the tissue, and an image cannot be produced. Thus radio frequency pulses are sequenced with a certain time interval to allow the magnetic force to be reestablished. The longer the time interval, the greater the magnetic force and the longer the imaging time (Bushong, 1996, 2001; Juhl, 1998).

After exposure to the radio frequency pulse has occurred, the signal emitted from the sample of protons decays exponentially with a time constant referred to as T_2, or spin-spin relaxation time. T_2 reflects the magnetic interactions between protons. It characterizes the exponential loss of signal caused by dephasing or desynchronization of magnetic force, which results from spin-spin interactions (Bushong, 1996, 2001; Juhl, 1998; Dort et al, 2001). The interval between the application of a radio frequency pulse and the emitted signal depends on the alignment and synchronization of magnetic dipoles. A strong magnetic force results in a long interval for the emitted signal after the pulse; this explains the contrast between tissues with different values of T_2 changes. T_1 is not equal to T_2, because each nucleus is not located within identical magnetic fields. Each hydrogen nucleus is subject to different local magnetic fields because of the presence or absence of other hydrogen nuclei (Bushong, 1996, 2001; Dort et al, 2001).

The third variable that affects image resolution with MRI is spin density. Spin density refers to the strength of the signal received from the nuclei before any of the decay processes have taken place (Bushong, 1996, 2001; Juhl, 1998; Dort et al, 2001). This strength is proportional to the number of nuclei within the detection volume of the scanner. Spin density is an indication of hydrogen concentration in the tissue.

A magnetic resonance image results from the mixture of these three properties (T_1, T_2, and spin density) unique to each

*Bushong, 1996, 2001; Nolte et al, 2000; Fogel et al, 2001; Huppi et al, 2001; Sinson et al, 2001; and Swischuk, 1995.

tissue. The values of T_1 and T_2 for various tissues have been defined. A wide range of values exists among various types of tissue, and considerable differences have been documented between pathologic and normal tissue (Juhl, 1998; Dort et al, 2001). Each number defined for the relaxation times (T_1 and T_2) for various tissues depends on the primary external magnetic field and thus may vary from scanner to scanner. The visual projection of the magnetic resonance image is similar to that obtained in CT. By controlling the gradient field of radio frequency pulses, a series of projections at uniform angles through the tissue can be collected. The computer can then reconstruct the image and can emphasize the individual T_1, T_2, or spin density parameters to further define detail (Bushong, 1996, 2001; Juhl, 1998; Dort et al, 2001).

The spatial resolution of an MRI scan compares favorably to that with CT. If the object scanned is of high tissue contrast, a lesion as small as 1 mm can be defined. As more data are collected on this imaging modality, even greater spatial resolution and enhanced three-dimensional images are being obtained. As stronger magnetic fields are used, the emitted signals become stronger, and greater resolution may be possible using even higher radio frequency pulses (Bushong, 1996, 2001; Dort et al, 2001).

MRI is better able than CT to detect differences between low-contrast structures. The difference in T_1 and T_2 MRI between biologic tissues frequently is 10% or more. For example, on CT scans, the x-ray photon attenuation coefficient between gray and white matter is approximately 0.5%, whereas the differences in T_1, T_2, and spin density between gray and white matter are great, allowing for more accurate definition of these two tissues (Bushong, 1996, 2001; Dort et al, 2001). Thus MRI has become the diagnostic imaging mode of choice for certain neurologic conditions such as multiple sclerosis, cerebral infarctions, and periventricular leukomalacia. MRI may be useful in the early diagnosis of periventricular leukomalacia, before the characteristic cystic lesions have developed (Krishnamoorthy et al, 2000; Peterson et al, 2000; Sie et al, 2000; Huppi et al, 2001; Tierney et al, 2001).

Safety of Magnetic Resonance Imaging.   MRI scanning uses three kinds of fields associated with the imaging process: (1) a static, moderately strong magnetic field; (2) a switched, weaker magnetic field gradient; and (3) radio frequency waves. The energies associated with the imaging process are approximately 10^{-8} eV/quantum, which are too weak to cause ionization or breakage of chemical bonds (Bushong, 1996, 2001; Dowd, 1999). Energies associated with body temperature elevations are 100,000 to 1 million times greater, therefore these temperature effects are far more disruptive to chemical bonds than the energy associated with MRI (Bushong, 1996, 2001).

In the laboratory, biologic responses in animals, chromosomes, plant seeds, and molecular specimens have shown effects only after extremely high intensities of MRI energy. A dose-response relationship apparently exists, although the biologic threshold is exceedingly high. In human beings, tests for genetic damage have proved negative, and studies of workers in particle accelerators exposed to static magnetic fields six to seven times greater than those used with MRI have shown no detrimental effect (Bushong, 1996, 2001; Dowd, 1999). Long-term studies of human beings exposed to radio frequency waves have not demonstrated any deleterious effect (Bushong, 1996, 2001; Dowd, 1999).

TABLE **41-3**	Common Electrolyte and Chemistry Values
Parameter	**Normal Value**
Serum Electrolytes	
Sodium (Na)	135 to 145 mEq/L
Potassium (K)	4.5 to 6.8 mEq/L
Chloride (Cl)	95 to 110 mEq/L
Carbon dioxide (CO_2)	20 to 25 mmol/L
Serum Chemistries	
Blood urea nitrogen (BUN)	6 to 30 mg/dl
Calcium (Ca)	7 to 10 mg/dl
Creatinine (Cr)	0.2 to 0.9 mg/dl
Glucose (G)	40 to 97 mg/dl
Magnesium (Mg)	1.5 to 2.5 mg/dl
Phosphorus (P)	5.4 to 10.9 mg/dl

Data from Fanaroff A, Martin R (1987). Neonatal-perinatal medicine: diseases of the fetus and infant, ed 4. Mosby: St Louis; Cohen S et al (1991). Maternal, neonatal and women's health nursing. Springhouse: Springhouse, PA; Kenner C et al (1988). Neonatal surgery: a nursing perspective. Grune & Stratton: Orlando, FL; and Streeter NS (1986). High risk neonatal care. Aspen: Rockville, MD.

The hazards of MRI relate primarily to any ferromagnetic objects (e.g., tools, oxygen cylinders, watches, bank cards, pens, and paper clips) that are accelerated toward the center of the magnetic field. The magnetic propulsion of these objects can result in projectile damage, therefore any patient with a pacemaker or an extensive metal prosthesis should be excluded from this imaging technique. In addition, MRI has not been fully tested with pregnant women.

Collaborative Care.   The care of a neonate who requires an MRI scan includes careful preparation and elimination of any ferromagnetic objects brought near the magnetic field. The infant's condition must be clinically stable, because the strong magnetic field affects some monitoring devices, and visualization of the neonate is impossible during the scan. Surface respiratory monitors and possibly an esophageal stethoscope may be used. An MRI scan is degraded by motion, therefore the infant must be positioned comfortably and safely in the magnetic cylinders. Because the infant must remain motionless for several minutes, an MRI scan is best done after the infant has been fed and is sleeping. If the infant is unable to remain motionless for the duration of the scan, oral chloral hydrate sedation may be recommended.

LABORATORY VALUES

A wide variety of laboratory tests can be used in both the diagnosis and care of the newborn. The values given in this chapter represent the broader normal ranges, but values in a specific chapter may vary slightly, depending on the range the author considers to be within normal limits. Every attempt has been made to provide consistent diagnostic and laboratory values. However, many hospitals have compiled their own list of acceptable laboratory test values, therefore specific laboratories should be contacted when evaluating results (Tables 41-3 to 41-20).

CARDIAC PROCEDURES

Electrocardiography

Electrocardiography is a noninvasive diagnostic tool used with neonates. It is most useful in the diagnosis and management of cardiac arrhythmias or in conjunction with other diagnostic measures to evaluate cardiac function, specifically the circulatory demands placed on individual heart chambers. In the neonatal period, however, electrocardiography is less helpful in evaluating cardiac anomalies associated with significant ventricular enlargement (Flanagan et al, 1999).

Echocardiography

Echocardiography, another noninvasive diagnostic procedure, commonly is used in the evaluation of the structure and function of the heart. This information can be important not only in the preoperative assessment of cardiac defects but also in the postoperative evaluation of procedures. High-frequency sound waves send vibrations to the structures in the heart, which reflect energy, which is transmitted into a visual image. Echocardiography may be used prenatally as early as 11 weeks' gestation when used transvaginally or 18 weeks' gestation when used transabdominally (Patel et al, 2002).

Single dimension echocardiography allows the evaluation of anatomic structures, including valves, chambers, and vessels. Two-dimensional echocardiography provides more in-depth information about relationships between the heart and the great vessels (Flanagan et al, 1999).

Doppler echocardiography is used in various forms in the evaluation of characteristics of blood flow through the heart, valves, and great vessels. It can measure not only cardiac output but also flow velocity changes, as demonstrated in stenotic lesions. Regurgitation through insufficiently functioning valves can also be identified. Doppler studies can be used to show regurgitation through insufficiently functioning valves or to identify shunting, as through a patent ductus arteriosus (Zahka & Lane, 2002).

Cardiac Catheterization

Historically, cardiac catheterization in the neonate was used for the diagnosis of congenital heart disease. With the advent of more sophisticated echocardiography, especially Doppler echocardiography, cardiac catheterization is used increasingly as a therapeutic modality. The use of radiopaque dye allows for clarification of congenital heart disease and helps to provide data that cannot be obtained from echocardiography.

TABLE **41-4**	Normal Hematologic Values						
	GESTATIONAL AGE (WEEKS)						
	28	**34**	**Full-Term Cord Blood**	**Day 1**	**Day 3**	**Day 7**	**Day 14**
Hemoglobin (g/dl)	14.5	15	16.8	18.4	17.8	17	16.8
Hematocrit (%)	45	47	53	58	55	54	52
Red cells (mm^3)	4	4.4	5.25	5.8	5.6	5.2	5.1
MCV (μm^3)	120	118	107	108	99	98	96
MCH (pg)	40	38	34	35	33	32.5	31.5
MCHC (%)	31	32	31.7	32.5	33	33	33
Reticulocytes (%)	5-10	3-10	3-7	3-7	1-3	0-1	0-1
Platelets (×10^3/mm^3)			290	192	213	248	252

From Klaus MH, Fanaroff AA (2001). Care of the high-risk neonate, ed 5. WB Saunders: Philadelphia.
MCV, Mean corpuscular volume; MCH, mean corpuscular hemoglobin; MCHC, mean corpuscular hemoglobin concentration.

TABLE **41-5**	White Cell and Differential Counts in Premature Infants					
	BIRTH WEIGHT					
	UNDER 1500 g			**1500 TO 2500 g**		
	1 Week Old	**2 Weeks Old**	**4 Weeks Old**	**1 Week Old**	**2 Weeks Old**	**4 Weeks Old**
Total Count (×10^3/mm^3)						
Mean	16.8	15.4	12.1	13	10	8.4
Range	6.1-32.8	10.4-21.3	8.7-17.2	6.7-14.7	7.0-14.1	5.8-12.4
Percentage of Total						
Polymorphs						
Segmented	54	45	40	55	43	41
Unsegmented	7	6	5	8	8	6
Eosinophils	2	3	3	2	3	3
Basophils	1	1	1	1	1	1
Monocytes	6	10	10	5	9	11
Lymphocytes	30	35	41	9	36	38

From Klaus MH, Fanaroff AA (2001). Care of the high-risk neonate, ed 5. WB Saunders: Philadelphia.

Immobilization and constant monitoring of the neonate are required during cardiac catheterization. The infant must be restrained to maintain supine positioning. Electrocardiographic electrodes must also be placed to provide constant monitoring of vital signs. Sedation may be considered to maintain proper positioning during the procedure.

A local anesthetic is administered at the insertion site. A radiopaque catheter is inserted into an arm or leg vessel by percutaneous puncture or cut-down. Under fluoroscopy, the catheter is visualized and passed into the heart. Contrast medium is injected through the catheter to allow visualization of the various cardiac structures. Selected chambers and vessels of the heart can be evaluated for size and function. Intracardiac pressures and oxygen saturations can also be measured during this procedure. The use of balloons during catheterization can facilitate procedures such as septostomy, angioplasty, and valvuloplasty (Flanagan et al, 1999; Patel et al, 2002).

After the necessary information has been obtained, the catheter is carefully removed. If a cut-down was performed, the vessel is ligated and the skin is sutured. Pressure should be applied over a percutaneous puncture site to enhance clot formation. For continued bleeding problems, pressure dressings may be applied to the insertion site; these must be checked frequently for active bleeding. After cardiac catheterization the vital signs should be measured frequently and compared with precatheterization baseline values. Evaluation of localized bleeding or of signs of hypotension resulting in changes in heart rate and blood pressure is essential. Assessment of the insertion site and affected extremity for bleeding, color, peripheral pulses, temperature, and capillary refill should continue for at least 24 hours after the procedure. In addition, the nurse must monitor for complications of catheterization, including hypovolemia (as a result of bleeding or fluid loss during the procedure), infection, thrombosis, or tissue necrosis.

GENETIC TESTING

Chromosome Analysis

Karyotyping and Banding.   Analysis of chromosome composition can assist in identification of various genetic disorders. A blood specimen is obtained from the infant and used to harvest an actual set of chromosomes. During active cell division, usually during metaphase, the chromosomes are photographed and then arranged in pairs by number. The chromosomes are also separated into regions, bands, and subbands. The end result, a karyotype with banding, is evaluated for the appropriate number of pairs, chromosome size, and structure. Specific genetic disorders can be associated with abnormal numbers of chromosomes (e.g., trisomy 21) or an abnormal chromosome structure, as in cri du chat syndrome, which reflects loss of part of the short arm of chromosome 5 (Kuller et al, 1996). Abnormal genes on the chromosomes can also cause genetic disorders, such as Duchenne muscular dystrophy, an X-linked recessive disorder.

TABLE 41-6   Summary of Normal Urinary Laboratory Values

	Age of Infant	Normal Value
Ammonia	2 to 12 months	4 to 20 µEq/min/m²
Calcium	1 week	Under 2 mg/dl
Chloride	Infant	1.7 to 8.5 mEq/24 hours
Creatinine	Newborn	7 to 10 mg/kg/day
Glucose*	Preterm	60 to 130 mg/dl
	Full-term	12 to 32 mg/dl
Glucose (renal threshold)	Preterm	2.21 to 2.84 mg/ml
	Full-term	2.20 to 3.68 mg/ml
Magnesium		180 ± 10 mg/1.73 m²/dl
Osmolality	Infant	50 to 600 mOsm/kg
Potassium		26 to 123 mEq/L
Protein		Under 100 mg/m²/dl
Sodium		0.3 to 3.5 mEq/dl (6 to 10 mEq/m²)
Specific gravity	Newborn	1.006 to 1.008

From Ichikawa I (1990). Pediatric textbook of fluids and electrolytes. Williams & Wilkins: Baltimore.

TABLE 41-7   Electrocardiographic Data Pertinent to the Neonate*

Parameter	AGE			
	Birth to 24 Hours	1 to 7 Days	8 to 30 Days	1 to 3 Months
Heart rate (beats/min)	119 (94 to 145)	133 (100 to 175)	163 (115 to 190)	154 (124 to 190)
PR interval (sec)	0.1 (0.07 to 0.12)	0.09 (0.07 to 0.12)	0.09 (0.07 to 0.11)	0.1 (0.07 to 0.13)
P wave amplitude II	1.5 (0.8 to 2.3)	1.6 (0.8 to 2.5)	1.6 (0.08 to 2.4)	1.6 (0.8 to 2.4)
QRS duration (sec)	0.065 (0.05 to 0.08)	0.06 (0.04 to 0.08)	0.06 (0.04 to 0.07)	0.06 (0.05 to 0.08)
QRS axis (degrees)	135 (60 to 180)	125 (80 to 160)	110 (60 to 160)	80 (40 to 120)
R amplitude V_{4R} (mm)	8.6 (4 to 14.2)	—	6.3 (3.3 to 8.5)	5.1 (1.1 to 10.1)
R amplitude V_1 (mm)	11.9 (4.3 to 21)	—	11.1 (3.3 to 18.7)	11.2 (4.5 to 18)
R amplitude V_5 (mm)	10.2 (4 to 18)	10.7 (3.4 to 19)	11.9 (3.5 to 27)	13.6 (7.3 to 20.7)
R amplitude V_6 (mm)	3.3 (2.3 to 7)	5.1 (2.2 to 13.1)	6.7 (1.7 to 20.5)	8.4 (3.6 to 12.9)
S amplitude V_{4R} (mm)	3.8 (0.2 to 13)	—	1.8 (0.8 to 4.6)	3.4 (0- to 9.3)
S amplitude V_1 (mm)	9.7 (1.1 to 19.1)	—	6.1 (0 to 15)	7.5 (0.5 to 17.1)
S amplitude V_5 (mm)	11.9 (0.24)	6.8 (3.6 to 16.2)	4.8 (2.7 to 12.3)	4.7 (2 to 12.7)
S amplitude V_6 (mm)	4.5 (1.6 to 10.3)	3.3 (0.8 to 9.9)	2 (0.6 to 9)	2.4 (0.8 to 5.8)

From Fanaroff A, Martin R (1987). Neonatal-perinatal medicine: diseases of the fetus and infant, ed 4. Mosby: St Louis; and Liebman J, Plonsey R (1977). Electrocardiography. In Moss AJ et al, editors. Heart disease in infants, children and adolescents, ed 2. Williams & Wilkins: Baltimore.
*Mean (5th to 95th percentile).

TABLE 41-8	Time of First Void in 500 Infants					
	395 FULL-TERM INFANTS		**80 PRETERM INFANTS**		**25 POSTTERM INFANTS**	
Hours Since Delivery	**Number of Infants**	**Cumulative (%)**	**Number of Infants**	**Cumulative (%)**	**Number of Infants**	**Cumulative (%)**
Under 1	51	12.9	17	21.2	3	12
1 to 8	151	51.1	50	83.7	4	38
9 to 16	158	91.1	12	98.7	14	84
17 to 24	35	100	1	100	4	100
Over 24	0	—	0	—	0	—

From Clark DA (1977). Times of first void and first stool in 500 newborns. Pediatrics, 60, 457-459.

TABLE 41-9	Time of First Stool in 500 Infants					
	395 FULL-TERM INFANTS		**80 PRETERM INFANTS**		**25 POSTTERM INFANTS**	
Hours Since Delivery	**Number of Infants**	**Cumulative (%)**	**Number of Infants**	**Cumulative (%)**	**Number of Infants**	**Cumulative (%)**
Under 1	66	16.7	4	5	8	32
1 to 8	169	59.5	22	32.5	9	68
9 to 16	125	91.1	25	63.8	5	88
17 to 24	29	98.5	10	76.3	3	100
24 to 48	6*	100	18†	98.8	0	‡
Over 48	0	—	1†	100	0	—

From Clark DA (1977). Times of first void and first stool in 500 newborns. Pediatrics, 60, 457-459.
At 25 to 28, 33, and 37 hours.
† Five infants stooled more than 36 hours after birth, at 38, 39, 40, 42, and 47 hours.
‡ At 59 hours.

TABLE 41-10	Acid-Base Status						
Determination	**Sample Source**	**Birth**	**1 Hour**	**3 Hours**	**24 Hours**	**2 Days**	**3 Days**
Vigorous Term Infants (Vaginal Delivery)							
pH	Umbilical artery	7.26					
	Umbilical vein	7.29					
PCO$_2$ (mm Hg)	Arterial	54.4	38.8	38.3	33.6	34	35
	Venous	42.8					
O$_2$ saturation	Arterial	19.8	93.8	94.7	93		
	Venous	47.6					
pH	Left atrial		7.30	7.34	7.41	7.39	7.38
CO$_2$ content (mEq/L)	—	—	20.6	21.9	21.4	Temporal artery	Temporal artery
Premature Infants							
	Capillary (skin puncture)						
pH	<1250 g				7.36	7.35	7.35
Pco$_2$ (mm Hg)					38	44	37
pH	>1250 g				7.39	7.39	7.38
Pco$_2$ (mm Hg)					38	39	38

From Schaffer AJ (1971). Diseases of the newborn, ed 3. WB Saunders: Philadelphia.
pH, Hydrogen ion concentration; PCO$_2$, partial pressure of carbon dioxide; O$_2$, oxygen; CO$_2$, carbon dioxide.

Fluorescence In Situ Hybridization. Chromosomes can be further analyzed using fluorescence in situ hybridization (FISH) to detect syndromes that are not visible to the naked eye. The FISH process allows fluorescent-coated DNA probes to detect submicroscopic chromosomal deletions. It can be used with interphase and metaphase cells. FISH testing is limited in that the particular chromosome to be assessed must be identified (McLean, 1999; Schwartz & Dickerman, 2002).

Bone marrow cells may be analyzed for chromosomes if a more rapid evaluation is required. Skin fibroblast analysis is required when an infant has been transfused, making lymphocyte analysis inaccurate. In cases such as stillbirth, tissue biopsy

TABLE 41-11	Selected Chemistry Values in Preterm and Full-Term Infants	
Constituent	**Preterm Infant**	**Full-Term Infant**
Alkaline phosphatase (U/L) (mean ± SD)[8]	207 ± 60 to 320 ± 142	164 ± 68
Ammonia (μg/dl)[1]		90 to 150
Base, excess (mmol/L)[1]		−10 to −2
Bicarbonate, standard (mmol/L)[2]	18 to 26	20 to 26
Bilirubin, total (mg/dl)		
Cord[2]	Under 2.8	Under 2.8
24 Hours old	1 to 6	2 to 6
48 Hours old	6 to 8	6 to 7
3 to 5 Days old	10 to 12	4 to 6
1 Month or older	Under 1.5	Under 1.5
Bilirubin, direct (mg/dl)[2]	Under 0.5	Under 0.5
Calcium, total (mg/dl), week 1[3,4]	6 to 10	8.4 to 11.6
Ceruloplasmin (mg/dl)[1]		1 to 3 months: 5 to 18
Cholesterol (mg/dl)		
Cord[2]		45 to 98
3 Days to 1 year old		65 to 175
Creatine phosphokinase (U/L)		
Day 1[5]		44 to 1150
Day 4		14 to 97
Creatine (mg/dl)	10 days : 1.3 ± 0.07	1 to 4 days: 0.3 to 1
	1 month: 0.6 ± 0.05	Over 4 days: 0.2 to 0.4
Ferritin (μg/dl)		
Neonate[1]		25 to 200
1 Month old		200 to 600
2 to 5 Months old		50 to 200
Over 6 months old		7 to 142
Gamma-glutamyl transferase (GGT) (U/L)[6]		14 to 131
Glucose (mg/dl)		
Under 72 hours old[7,9]	20 to 125	30 to 125
Over 72 hours old	40 to 125	40 to 125
Lactate dehydrogenase (U/L)[6]		357 to 953
Magnesium (mg/dl)[4]		1.7 to 2.4
Osmolality (mOsm/L)[1]		275 to 295 (may be as low as 266)
Phosphorus (mg/dl)		
Birth[4]		4.5 to 8.7
Day 5		4.2 to 7.2
1 Month old		4.5 to 6.5
Aspartate aminotransferase (SGOT/AST) (U/L)[7]		24 to 81
Alanine aminotransferase (SGPT/ALT) (U/L)[7]		10 to 33
Triglycerides (mg/dl)[2]		10 to 140
Urea nitrogen (mg/dl)[1]	3 to 25	4 to 12
Uric acid (mg/dl)[2]		3 to 7.5
Vitamin A (μg/dl) (mean ± SD) (under 10 μg/dl indicates very low hepatic vitamin A stores)[10]	16 ± 1	23.9 ± 1.8
Vitamin D		
25-hydroxycholecalciferol (ng/ml)*[11,12]		20 to 60
1,25-dihydroxycholecalciferol (pg/ml)*[11,12]		40 to 90

From Fanaroff AA, Martin RJ (2002). Neonatal-perinatal medicine, ed 7. WB Saunders: Philadelphia.

*Serum levels are affected by race, age, season, and diet

[1]Tietz NW, editor (1988). Textbook of clinical chemistry. WB Saunders: Philadelphia.

[2]Wallach JB (1983). Interpretation of pediatric tests. Little, Brown: Boston.

[3]Meites S (1975). Critical reviews of clinical laboratory science, 6, 1.

[4]Nelson N et al (1987). Scandinavian journal of clinical laboratory investigations, 47, 111.

[5]Drummond LM (1979). Archives of disease in childhood, 54, 362.

[6]Statlan BE et al (1978). Clinical chemistry, 24, 1010 (abstract).

[7]Cornblath M, Schwartz R, editors (1976). Disorders of carbohydrate metabolism, ed 2. WB Saunders: Philadelphia.

[8]Glass L et al (1982). Archives of disease in childhood, 57, 373.

[9]Heck LJ et al (1987). Pediatric research, 110, 119.

[10]Shenai JP et al (1981). Journal of pediatrics, 99, 302.

[11]Cooke R et al (1990). Journal of pediatrics, 116, 423.

[12]Lichtenstein P et al (1986). Pediatrics, 77, 883.

TABLE 41-12 Plasma Albumin and Total Protein in Preterm Infants from Birth to 8 Weeks

Gestation (weeks)	26	27	28	29	30	31	32	33	34	35	36	37	38	39	40	41	42
Albumin gm/dl																	
Reference Range (95% confidence limits)	—	1.18 to 3.06	1.09 to 2.87	1.20 to 2.74	1.63 to 2.75	1.08 to 3.20	1.38 to 3.14	1.44 to 3.34	0.53 to 3.87	1.15 to 3.87	1.96 to 3.44	1.50 to 4.10	1.89 to 4.15	2.07 to 4.15	2.07 to 4.05	2.04 to 3.90	2.08 to 3.90
Corrected Age																	
26 to 28 weeks' gestation		2.13	2.10	2.58	2.29	2.39				2.73			2.82				
29 to 31 weeks' gestation					2.02	2.14	2.44	2.44	2.54							3.35	
32 to 34 weeks' gestation								2.35	2.42	2.46	2.38	2.44					
Total Protein gm/dl																	
Reference range (95% confidence limits)	—	1.28 to 7.94	3.03 to 5.03	2.18 to 5.84	2.64 to 5.80	3.26 to 5.66	3.63 to 5.81	3.57 to 5.87	3.57 to 6.59	1.52 to 8.62	3.85 to 6.91	4.69 to 6.95	3.32 to 9.16	4.17 to 8.25	4.26 to 8.08	3.73 to 8.47	3.24 to 8.76
Corrected age																	
26 to 28 weeks' gestation		4.07	4.45	4.84	4.49	4.45				4.41							
29 to 31 weeks' gestation					3.93	4.42	4.70	4.82	4.51				4.55				
32 to 34 weeks' gestation								4.54	4.93	4.78	4.86	4.81				4.96	

From Fanaroff A, Martin R (2002). Neonatal-perinatal medicine: diseases of the fetus and infant, ed 7. Mosby: St Louis; and Reading RF et al (1990). Early human development, 22, 81.

TABLE 41-13	Plasma Immunoglobulin (Ig) Concentrations* in Premature Infants (25-28 Weeks' Gestation)			
Age (months)	N	IgG (mg/dl)	IgM (mg/dl)	IgA (mg/dl)
0.25	18	251 (114-552)	7.6 (1.3-43.3)	1.2 (0.07-20.8)
0.5	14	202 (91-446)	14.1 (3.5-56.1)	3.1 (0.09-10.7)
1	10	158 (57-437)	12.7 (3-53.3)	4.5 (0.65-30.9)
1.5	14	134 (59-307)	16.2 (4.4-59.2)	4.3 (0.9-20.9)
2	12	89 (58-136)	16 (5.3-48.9)	4.1 (1.5-11.1)
3	13	60 (23-156)	13.8 (5.3-36.1)	3.4 (0.6-15.6)
4	10	82 (32-210)	22.2 (11.2-43.9)	6.8 (1-47.8)
6	11	159 (56-455)	41.3 (8.3-205)	9.7 (3-31.2)
8-10	6	273 (94-794)	41.8 (31.1-56.1)	9.5 (0.9-98.6)

From Ballow M et al (1986). Development of the immune system in very low birth weight (less than 1500 g) premature infants: concentrations of plasma immunoglobulins and patterns of infections. Pediatric research, 20, 899-904.
*The figure given is the geometric mean; the normal ranges, which are in parentheses, were determined by taking the antilog of (mean logarithm ± 2 SD of the logarithms).

TABLE 41-14	Plasma Immunoglobulin (Ig) Concentrations* in Premature Infants (29-32 Weeks' Gestation)			
Age (months)	N	IgG (mg/dl)	IgM (mg/dl)	IgA (mg/dl)
0.25	42	368 (186-728)	9.1 (2.1-39.4)	0.6 (0.04-1)
0.5	35	275 (119-637)	13.9 (4.7-41)	0.9 (0.01-7.5)
1	26	209 (97-452)	14.4 (6.3-33)	1.9 (0.3-12)
1.5	22	156 (69-352)	15.4 (5.5-43.2)	2.2 (0.7-6.5)
2	11	123 (64-237)	15.2 (4.9-46.7)	3.4 (1.1-8.3)
3	14	104 (41-268)	16.3 (7.1-37.2)	3.6 (0.8-15.4)
4	21	128 (39-425)	26.5 (7.7-91.2)	9.8 (2.5-39.3)
6	21	179 (51-634)	29.3 (10.5-81.5)	12.3 (2.7-57.1)
8-10	16	280 (140-561)	34.7 (17-70.8)	20.9 (8.3-53)

From Ballow M et al (1986). Development of the immune system in very low birth weight (less than 1500 g) premature infants: concentrations of plasma immunoglobulins and patterns of infections. Pediatric research, 20, 899-904.
*The figure given is the geometric mean; the normal ranges, which are in parentheses, were determined by taking the antilog of (mean logarithm ± 2 SD of the logarithms).

specimens can be used for chromosome testing because viable lymphocytes are absent (Jones & Cahill, 1994).

Sweat Chloride Test

The sweat chloride test is used to evaluate for and confirm the diagnosis of cystic fibrosis. During the procedure the skin is stimulated with pilocarpine and a small electrical current for 5 minutes. The sweat is collected on a 2 × 2-inch gauze pad or filter paper for 30 minutes. Over this 30-minute period, 75 mg of sweat must be produced to ensure an appropriate sweat rate (National Committee for Clinical Laboratory Standards, 1994). A sweat chloride level below 40 mEq/L is normal. Levels between 60 and 165 mEq/L are considered diagnostic for cystic fibrosis (Wilford & Taussig, 1998). Sweat tests can be inaccurate if an inadequate amount of sweat is produced; if the sweat evaporates; or if the patient has edema.

GASTROINTESTINAL PROCEDURES

Barium Enema

A barium enema is used in the evaluation of the structure and function of the large intestine. The diagnosis of disorders such as Hirschsprung disease and meconium plug syndrome can easily be supported by the use of this procedure.

For the enema procedure, either air or a contrast solution (e.g., barium sulfate) is instilled and a series of films are taken under fluoroscopy. The infant must be well restrained, starting in the supine position. As the contrast solution is instilled, its flow through the bowel is observed as the infant's position is changed. A series of abdominal x-ray films should be taken once the bowel has been filled with contrast solution. Follow-up films may also be necessary to document evacuation of the contrast solution from the bowel. Evaluation of the bowel is essential after this procedure to prevent constipation or obstruction. Assessment of bowel elimination is an important nursing concern after barium enema.

Upper Gastrointestinal Series with Small Bowel Follow-Through

As with the barium enema, barium sulfate or some other water-soluble contrast solution is used for the upper GI series with small bowel follow-through. However, the contrast solution is swallowed so that the upper gastrointestinal tract can be examined. The three main areas examined are (1) the esophagus

TABLE **41-15**	Plasma-Serum Amino Acid Levels in Premature and Term Newborns (μmol/L)		
Amino Acid	**Premature (First Day)**	**Newborn 16 (Before First Feeding)**	**16 d-4 mo**
Taurine	105-255	101-181	
OH-proline	0-80	0	
Aspartic acid	0-20	4-12	17-21
Threonine	155-275	196-238	141-213
Serine	195-345	129-197	104-158
Asp + Glut	655-1155	623-895	
Proline	155-305	155-305	141-245
Glutamic acid	30-100	27-77	
Glycine	185-735	274-412	178-248
Alanine	325-425	274-384	239-345
Valine	80-180	97-175	123-199
Cystine	55-75	49-75	33-51
Methionine	30-40	21-37	31-47
Isoleucine	20-60	31-47	31-47
Leucine	45-95	55-89	56-98
Tyrosine	20-220	53-85	33-75
Phenylalanine	70-110	64-92	45-65
Ornithine	70-110	66-116	37-61
Lysine	130-250	154-246	117-163
Histidine	30-70	61-93	64-92
Arginine	30-70	37-71	53-71
Tryptophan	15-45	15-45	
Citrulline	8.5-23.7	10.8-21.1	
Ethanolamine	13.4-10.5	32.7-72	
Alpha-amino-*n*-butyric acid	0-29	8.7-20.4	
Methylhistidine			

From Klaus MH, Fanaroff AA (2001). Care of the high-risk neonate, ed 5. WB Saunders: Philadelphia; Dickinson JC et al (1965). Ion exchange chromatography of the free amino acids in the plasma of the newborn infant. Pediatrics, 36, 2; Dickinson JC et al (1970). Ion exchange chromatography of the free amino acids in the plasma of infants under 2,500 gm at birth. Pediatrics, 45, 606; and Behrman RE (1977). Neonatal-perinatal diseases of the fetus and infant, ed 2. Mosby: St Louis.

(for size, patency, reflux, and presence of a fistula or swallowing abnormality), (2) the stomach (for anatomic abnormalities, patency, and motility), and (3) the small intestine (for strictures, patency, and function).

Follow-up x-ray films may be desirable to evaluate both the emptying ability of the stomach and intestinal motility as the contrast material moves through the small bowel. Again, care of the infant includes assessment of temperature and cardiac and respiratory status throughout the procedure. The nurse should be alert for reflux or vomiting, which can be accompanied by aspiration. Evacuation of contrast material from the bowel remains a concern after upper GI series with small bowel follow-through and should be monitored by the nurse. It is also possible for fluid to be pulled out of the vascular compartment and into the bowel, resulting in hypotension. It is imperative that the health care team assess the infant for signs of these complications.

Rectal Suction Biopsy

Rectal biopsy is a procedure commonly used to help determine the presence or absence of ganglion cells in the bowel (the latter condition is seen in Hirschsprung disease). Before a rectal biopsy, it is essential to obtain bleeding times, prothrombin time, partial thromboplastin time, and platelet counts, as well as a spun hematocrit, to ensure that the infant is in no danger of excessive bleeding.

The infant is positioned supine with the legs held toward the abdomen. Small specimens of rectal tissue from the mucosal and submucosal levels are excised with a suction blade apparatus inserted through the anus into the bowel. The section of the pathology department that deals with the composition of ganglion cells evaluates the specimens.

Care of the infant after rectal suction biopsy should focus on assessments for bleeding or intestinal perforation. These assessments should include evaluation of vital signs for increased heart rate or decreased blood pressure, fever, persistent guaiac-positive stools, or frank rectal bleeding.

Liver Biopsy

Open or closed liver biopsy may be required for neonates. Open liver biopsy is a surgical procedure that requires general anesthesia, whereas a closed liver biopsy may be done using local anesthesia. As with the rectal biopsy, coagulation studies are essential, including bleeding time, platelet count, and spun hematocrit. Preoperative care may include sedation of the infant, requiring frequent monitoring of vital signs. Throughout the procedure, assessment of vital signs is essential for identifying changes in hemodynamics or respiratory status. After the procedure, assessment of vital signs for signs and symptoms of hemorrhage is essential. Indications of hemorrhage include decreases in the hemoglobin and hematocrit, which makes laboratory monitoring an important element of postbiopsy care.

TABLE 41-16 Urine Amino Acid Levels in Normal Newborns (µmol/L)	
Amino Acid	**µmol/d**
Cysteic acid	Tr-3.32
Phosphoethanolamine	Tr-8.86
Taurine	7.59-7.72
OH-proline	0-9.81
Aspartic acid	Tr
Threonine	0.176-7.99
Serine	Tr-20.7
Glutamic acid	0-1.78
Proline	0-5.17
Glycine	0.176-65.3
Alanine	Tr-8.03
Alpha-aminoadipic acid	
Alpha-amino-n-butyric acid	0-0.47
Valine	0-7.76
Cystine	0-7.96
Methionine	Tr-0.892
Isoleucine	0-6.11
Tyrosine	0-1.11
Phenylalanine	0-1.66
Beta-aminoisobutyric acid	0.264-7.34
Ethanolamine	Tr-79.9
Ornithine	Tr-0.554
Lysine	0.33-9.79
1-Methylhistidine	Tr-8.64
3-Methylhistidine	0.11-3.32
Carnosine	0.044-4.01
Beta-aminobutyric acid	
Cystathionine	
Homocitrulline	
Arginine	0.088-0.918
Histidine	Tr-7.04
Sarcosine	
Leucine	Tr-0.918

From Klaus MH, Fanaroff AA (2001). Care of the high-risk neonate, ed 5. WB Saunders: Philadelphia; Meites S, editor (1997). Pediatric clinical chemistry: a survey of normals, methods, and instruments. American Association for Clinical Chemistry: Washington, DC; and Fanaroff AA, Martin RJ, editors (1997). Neonatal-perinatal medicine: diseases of the fetus and infant, ed 6. Mosby: St Louis.

The biopsy site must be evaluated for signs of active bleeding, ecchymosis, swelling, or infection.

GENITOURINARY PROCEDURES

Cystoscopy

Cystoscopy permits direct visualization of the urinary structures, including the bladder, urethra, and urethral orifices, allowing diagnosis of abnormalities in the structure of the bladder and urinary tract.

Cystoscopy is performed using general anesthesia. Preparation of the urethral opening with an antiseptic solution is followed by sterile draping. The lubricated cystoscope is inserted through the urethra, and the urinary structures are examined.

As with any patient who has had anesthesia, postprocedural care includes vital sign assessment. However, particular atten-

tion should be paid to assessing for adequate urinary output, the presence of hematuria, and signs of infection (Pagana & Pagana, 2001).

Excretory Urography and Intravenous Pyelography

Excretory urography and intravenous pyelography complement cystoscopic evaluation because they allow the examiner not only to evaluate structures but also to focus on the function of those structures. Small amounts of contrast media are injected by the intravenous route, and as the contrast material is excreted through the urinary system, a sequence of x-ray films is taken. These films reflect the configuration of organs and the rate of excretion of the contrast media.

Excretory urography and intravenous pyelography are relatively safe for use in neonates and should cause no postprocedural complications.

Voiding Cystourethrogram

The purpose of a voiding cystourethrogram is to visualize the lower urinary tract after instillation of contrast media through urethral catheterization. The infant's bladder is emptied after catheterization and then filled with the contrast media. Serial films under fluoroscopy in a variety of positions are taken during voiding. After voiding, additional films are obtained. Pathologic results of a voiding cystourethrogram demonstrate residual urine in the bladder, such as with a neurogenic bladder, posterior valve obstructions, or vesicourethral reflux.

As with cystoscopy, the infant should be evaluated for hematuria; the baby also should be checked for signs of infection (fever, cloudy or sedimented urine, foul-smelling urine) in the event of contaminated catheterization.

Electroencephalography

An electroencephalographic examination records the electrical activity of the brain. Numerous electrodes are placed at precise locations on the infant's head to record electrical impulses from various parts of the brain. This procedure can be important for diagnosing lesions or tumors, for identifying nonfunctional areas of the brain, or for pinpointing the focus of seizure activity.

The infant may require sedation during this procedure to prevent crying or movement. As much equipment as is safely possible should be removed to reduce electrical interference. Also, calming procedures, such as reducing light stimulation or warming the environment, may help quiet the infant during electroencephalography. The infant should be closely observed throughout the procedure for any signs of seizure activity.

RESPIRATORY PROCEDURES

Pulse Oximetry

Pulse oximetry is a widely used, noninvasive method of monitoring arterial blood oxygenation saturations (SaO_2). The SaO_2 is the ratio of oxygenated hemoglobin to total hemoglobin. A single probe, attached to an infant's extremity or digit, uses light emitted at different wavelengths, which is absorbed differently by saturated and unsaturated hemoglobin. The change in the light during arterial pulses is used to calculate the oxygen saturation. Pulse oximetry saturations reflect a more accurate measure of actual hemoglobin saturation. Saturations obtained by blood gas sample are calculated using a hemoglobin of 15 g% (Goetzman & Wennberg, 1999).

TABLE 41-17 Cerebrospinal Fluid Values of Healthy Term Newborns

Component	AGE			
	Birth to 24 Hours	1 Day	7 Days	Over 7 Days
Color	Clear or xanthochromic	Clear or xanthochromic	Clear or xanthochromic	
Red blood cells (cells/mm^3)	9 (0 to 1070)	23 (6 to 630)	3 (0 to 48)	
Polymorphonuclear leukocytes (cells/mm^3)	3 (0 to 70)	7 (0 to 26)	2 (0 to 5)	
Lymphocytes (cells/mm^3)	2 (0 to 20)	5 (0 to 16)	1 (0 to 4)	
Protein (mg/dl)	63 (32 to 240)	73 (40 to 148)	47 (27 to 65)	
Glucose (mg/dl)	51 (32 to 78)	48 (38 to 64)	55 (48 to 62)	
Lactate dehydrogenase (IU/L)	22 to 73	22 to 73	22 to 73	0 to 40

From Klaus MH, Fanaroff AA (2002). Neonatal-perinatal medicine: diseases of the fetus and infant, ed 6. Mosby; St Louis; Naidoo BT (1968). South African medical journal, 42, 932; and Neches W et al (1968). Pediatrics, 41, 1097.

TABLE 41-18 Cerebrospinal Fluid Values in Very Low-Birth-Weight Infants on Basis of Birth Weight

	≤1000 G		1001-1500 G	
	Mean ± SD	Range	Mean ± SD	Range
Birth weight (g)	763 ± 115	550 to 980	1278 ± 152	1020 to 1500
Gestational age (wk)	26 ± 1.3	24 to 28	29 ± 1.4	27 to 33
Leukocytes/mm^3	4 ± 3	0 to 14	6 ± 9	0 to 44
Erythrocytos/mm^3	1027 ± 3270	0 to 19,050	786 ± 1879	0 to 9750
PMN leukocytes (%)	6 ± 15	0 to 66	9 ± 17	0 to 60
MN leukocytes (%)	86 ± 30	34 to 100	85 ± 28	13 to 100
Glucose (mg/dl)	61 ± 34	29 to 217	59 ± 21	31 to 109
Protein (mg/dl)	150 ± 56	95 to 370	132 ± 43	45 to 227

PMN, polymorphonuclear; MN mononuclear.
Modified from Rodriquez AF, Kapian SL, Mason EO: Cerebrospinal fluid values in the very low birth weight infant. Journal of pediatrics 116:871, 1990.

TABLE 41-19 Cerebrospinal Fluid Values in Very-Low-Birth-Weight Infants (1001-1500 g) by Chronologic Age

Component	POSTNATAL AGE (days)					
	0-7		8-28		29-84	
	Mean ± SD	Range	Mean ± SD	Range	Mean ± SD	Range
Birth weight (gm)	1428 ± 107	1180 to 1500	1245 ± 162	1020 to 1480	1211 ± 86	1080 to 1300
Gestational age at birth (wk)	31 ± 1.5	28 to 33	29 ± 1.2	27 to 31	29 ± 0.7	27 to 29
Leukocytes/mm^3	4 ± 4	1 to 10	7 ± 11	0 to 44	8 ± 8	0 to 23
Erythrocytes/mm^3	407 ± 853	0 to 2450	1101 ± 2643	0 to 9750	661 ± 1198	0 to 3800
PMN (%)	4 ± 10	0 to 28	10 ± 19	0 to 60	11 ± 19	0 to 48
Glucose (mg/dL)	74 ± 19	50 to 96	59 ± 23	39 to 109	47 ± 13	31 to 76
Protein (mg/dL)	136 ± 35	85 to 176	137 ± 46	54 to 227	122 ± 47	45 to 187

Modified from Rodriquez AF, et al. Journal of pediatrics 116: 971, 1990.

Proper placement of the probe should be assessed regularly, because movement, environmental light, edema, and diminished perfusion can reduce the accuracy of readings. The probe should be rotated every few hours to prevent skin breakdown at the site.

End-Tidal Carbon Dioxide Monitoring

End-tidal carbon dioxide (CO_2) monitoring is used routinely in pediatrics and in adult intensive care units. Its use in neonates, especially the smaller baby, is not yet practical as a continuing therapy because the adapters are heavy and create excess

| TABLE 41-20 | Thyroid Function in Full-Term and Preterm Infants |

	SERUM T$_4$ CONCENTRATION IN PREMATURE AND TERM INFANTS					SERUM FREE T$_4$ INDEX IN PREMATURE AND TERM INFANTS				
	ESTIMATED GESTATIONAL AGE (WEEKS)									
	30 to 31	32 to 33	34 to 35	36 to 37	Term	30 to 31	32 to 33	34 to 35	36 to 37	Term
Cord										
Mean	6.5*	7.5‡	6.7‡	7.5	8.2			5.6	5.6	5.9
SD	1	2.1	1.2	2.8	1.8			1.3	2	1.1
N	3	8	18	17	17			12	10	14
12 to 72 Hours Old										
Mean	11.5‡	12.3‡	12.4‡	15.5†	19	13.1§	12.9§	15.5§	17.1	19.7
SD	2.1	3.2	3.1	2.6	2.1	2.4	2.7	3	3.5	3.5
N	12	18	17	15	6	12	14	14	14	6
3 to 10 Days Old										
Mean	7.7‡	8.5‡	10‡	12.7†	15.9	8.3§	9§	12¶	15.1	16.2
SD	1.8	1.9	2.4	2.5	3	1.9	1.8	2.3	0.7	3.2
n	7	8	9	9	29	6	9	5	4	11
11 to 20 Days Old										
Mean	7.5†	8.3‡	10.5	11.2	12.2	8*	9.1¶	11.8	11.3	12.1
SD	1.8	1.6	1.8	2.9	2	1.6	1.9	2.7	1.9	2
n	5	11	9	9	8	5	8	8	5	8
21 to 45 Days Old										
Mean	7.8‡	8‡	9.3‡	11.4	12.1	8.4*	9¶	10.9		11.1
SD	1.5	1.7	1.3	4.2	1.5	1.4	1.6	2.8		1.4
n	11	17	13	5	5	11	17	5		5
46 to 90 Days Old		30 to 73 weeks					34 to 35 weeks			
Mean		9.6			10.2	9.4				9.7
SD		1.7			1.9	1.4				1.5
n		16			17	13				10

From Cuestas RA (1982). Journal of pediatrics, 92, 963.
*$p < 0.05$
†$p < 0.005$
‡$p < 0.001$
§$p = 0.001$
‖$p = 0.025$
¶$p = 0.01$
#$p = 0.005$
For comparison of premature and term infants (t test).

dead space in the ventilator system. End tidal CO_2 monitoring is most useful during intubation procedures for determining if endotracheal intubation rather than esophageal intubation has occurred (Yorgin & Rhee, 1998; Goetzman & Wennberg, 1999).

Bronchoscopy

Bronchoscopy of the newborn is performed to visualize the upper and lower airways and to collect diagnostic specimens. The procedure can be done in the NICU using a flexible bronchoscope, or it can be performed under general anesthesia in the operating room using either a flexible or rigid bronchoscope. The flexible bronchoscope is preferable for examining the lower airways of an intubated patient or for examination of a patient with mandibular hypoplasia. A rigid bronchoscope is more advantageous in situations requiring removal of foreign bodies and for evaluation of patients with H-type tracheoesophageal fistula (TEF), laryngotracheoesophageal clefts, and bilateral abductor paralysis of the vocal cords (Wood, 1998). Examination of structures by direct visualization provides the opportunity to identify congenital anomalies, obstructions, masses, or mucous plugs and to evaluate stridor or respiratory dysfunction.

Bronchoscopy done at the bedside requires the nurse to assist with positioning, sedation, and monitoring of vital signs. Whether the infant undergoes flexible or rigid bronchoscopy, respiratory and cardiovascular monitoring should be continued in the immediate postprocedural period. Possible complications related to these procedures include bronchospasm, laryngeal spasms, laryngeal edema, or pneumothorax or bradycardia resulting in hypoxia.

SUMMARY

Marked technical advances over the past two decades have produced a variety of imaging methods for the diagnosis, treatment, and evaluation of neonates. Sizable expenditures have been directed toward improving image presentation and quality on the assumption that a trained clinical eye can make diagnostic use of the data provided. Investigations are useful only insofar as they reduce the diagnostic uncertainty. The final product of any radiologic imaging procedure is not a set of photographic pictures, but a diagnostic opinion that should be beneficial to the infant's management. Before initiating any imaging method, physicians should consider whether further information is really needed, and they should select the imaging technique that will give the required information with sufficient reliability and with minimal risk to the patient. The value of any diagnostic imaging examination must be balanced against the potential hazards. In addition to care of the newborn during and after a procedure, nursing care of newborns and infants undergoing diagnostic procedures requires a knowledge of the expected outcomes and methods so that the best result possible is obtained. Nurses also must be knowledgeable about normal values for the laboratory tests commonly used in the care of newborns and infants.

REFERENCES

Abramoff MD et al (2000). MRI dynamic color mapping: a new quantitative technique for imaging soft tissue motion in the chest. *Investigative ophthalmology and visual science*, 41(11), 3256-3260.

Alpen EL (1998). *Radiation biophysics*, ed 2. Prentice Hall: Englewood Cliffs, NJ.

Bellenger NG et al (2000). Comparison of left ventricular ejection fraction and volumes in heart failure by echocardiography, radionucleotide ventriculography and cardiovascular magnetic resonance: are they interchangeable? *European heart journal*, 21(16), 1387-1396.

Bushong SC (1996). *Magnetic resonance imaging: physical and biologic principles*, ed 2. Mosby: St Louis.

Bushong SC (1999). *Essentials of imaging series: diagnostic ultrasound*. McGraw Hill: New York.

Bushong SC (2000). *Essentials of imaging series: computed tomography*. McGraw Hill: New York.

Bushong SC (2001). *Radiologic science for technologists: physics, biology and protection*, ed 7. Mosby: St Louis.

Dort JC et al (2001). Screening for cerebellopontine angle tumours: conventional MRI versus T2 fast spin echo MRI. *Canadian journal of neurological sciences* 28(1), 47-50.

Dowd SB (1999). *Practical radiation protection and applied radiobiology*, ed 2. WB Saunders: Philadelphia.

Fanaroff AA, Martin RJ, editors (2002). *Neonatal-perinatal medicine*, ed 7. Mosby: St Louis.

Flanagan MF et al (1999). Cardiac disease. In Avery GB et al, editors. *Neonatology: pathophysiology and management of the neonate*, ed 5. JB Lippincott: Philadelphia.

Fogel MA et al (2001). Evaluation and follow-up of patients with left ventricular apical to aortic conduits with 2D and 3D magnetic resonance imaging and Doppler echocardiography: a new look at an old operation. *American heart journal*, 141(4), 630-636.

Goetzman BW, Wennberg RP (1999). *Neonatal intensive care handbook*. Mosby: St Louis.

Hilton S, Edwards DK III (1994). *Practical pediatric radiology*, ed 2. WB Saunders: Philadelphia.

Huda W et al (2001). Radiation doses to infants and adults undergoing head CT examinations. *Medical physics*, 28(3), 393-399.

Huppi PS et al (2001). Microstructural brain development after perinatal cerebral white matter injury assessed by diffusion tensor magnetic resonance imaging. *Pediatrics*, 1107(3), 455-460.

Jones OW, Cahill TC (1994). Basic genetics and patterns of inheritance. In Creasy RK, Resnik R, editors. *Maternal-fetal medicine*, ed 3. WB Saunders: Philadelphia.

Juhl JH et al, editors (1998). *Paul and Juhl's essentials of radiologic imaging*, ed 7. Lippincott-Raven: Philadelphia.

Krishnamoorthy KS et al (2000). Diffusion-weighted imaging in neonatal cerebral infarction: clinical utility and follow-up. *Journal of child neurology*, 15(9), 592-602.

Kuller JA et al (1996). *Prenatal diagnosis and reproductive genetics*. Mosby: St Louis.

Lansberg MG et al (2001). Evolution of cerebral infarct volume assessed by diffusion-weighted magnetic resonance imaging. *Archives of neurology*, 58(4), 613-617.

Lewis PJ et al (2000). Does performing image registration and subtraction in ictal brain SPECT help localize neocortical seizures? *Journal of nuclear medicine*, 41(10), 1619-1629.

Lin JW et al (2001). Improving PET-based physiological quantification through methods of wavelet denoising. *IEEE transactions on biomedical engineering*, 48(2), 202-212.

McLean SD (1999). Congenital anomalies. In Avery GB et al, editors. *Neonatology: pathophysiology and management of the neonate*, ed 5. JB Lippincott: Philadelphia.

National Committee for Clinical Laboratory Standards (1994). *Sweat testing: sample collection and quantitative analysis: approved guideline*. The Committee: Wayne, PA.

National Council on Radiation Protection and Measurements (1993a). Risk estimates for radiation protection. NCRP Report No. 15. National Council on Radiation Protection: Bethesda, MD.

National Council on Radiation Protection and Measurements (1993b). Research needs for radiation protection. NCRP Report No. 117. National Council on Radiation Protection: Bethesda, MD.

National Council on Radiation Protection and Measurements (1993c). A practical guide to the determination of human exposure to radiofrequency fields. NCRP Report No. 119. National Council on Radiation Protection: Bethesda, MD.

Nolte UG et al (2000). Rapid isotropic diffusion mapping without susceptibility artifacts: whole brain studies using diffusion-weighted single-shot STEAM MR imaging. *Magnetic resonance in medicine*, 44(5), 731-736.

Pagana KD, Pagana TJ (2001). *Mosby's diagnostic and laboratory test reference*. Mosby: St Louis.

Patel CR et al (2002). Fetal cardiac physiology and fetal cardiovascular assessment. In Fanaroff AA, Martin RJ, editors. *Neonatal-perinatal medicine*, ed 7. Mosby: St Louis.

Peled S, Yeashurun Y (2001). Superresolution in MRI: application to human white matter fiber tract visualization by diffusion tensor imaging. *Magnetic resonance in medicine*, 45(1), 29-35.

Peterson BS et al (2000). Regional brain volume abnormalities and long-term cognitive outcome in preterm infants. *Journal of the American Medical Association* 284(15), 1939-1947.

Rushe TM et al (2001). Neuropsychological outcome at adolescence of very preterm birth and its relation to brain structure. *Developmental medicine and child neurology*, 43(4), 226-233.

Schierlitz L et al (2001). Three-dimensional magnetic resonance imaging of fetal brains. *Lancet*, 357(9263), 1177-1178.

Schwartz S, Dickerman LH (2002). Genetic aspects of perinatal disease and prenatal diagnosis. In Fanaroff AA, Martin RJ, editors. *Neonatal-perinatal medicine*, ed 7. Mosby: St Louis.

Sie LT et al (2000). Value of fluid-attenuated inversion recovery sequences in early MRI of the brain in neonates with a perinatal hypoxic-ischemic encephalopathy. *European radiology*, 10(10), 1594-1601.

Sinson G et al (2001). Magnetization transfer imaging and proton MR spectroscopy in the evaluation of axonal injury: correlation with clinical outcome after traumatic brain injury. *American journal of neuroradiology*, 22(1), 143-151.

Swischuk LE (1997a). *Imaging of the newborn, infant, and young child*, ed 4. Williams & Wilkins: Baltimore.

Swischuk LE (1997b). *Differential diagnosis in pediatric radiology*, ed 3. Williams & Wilkins: Baltimore.

Tierney MC et al (2001). PET evaluation of bilingual language compensation following early childhood brain damage. *Neuropsychologia*, 39(2), 114-121.

Treves ST, editor (1995). *Pediatric nuclear medicine*, ed 2. Springer-Verlag: New York.

Weissleder R, Mahmood U (2001). Molecular imaging. *Radiology*, 219(2), 316-333.

Wiessmann M, Seidel G (2000). Ultrasound perfusion imaging of the human brain. *Stroke*, 13(10), 2421-2425.

Wilford BS, Taussig LM (1998). Cystic fibrosis: general overview. In Taussig LM, Landau LI, editors. *Pediatric respiratory medicine*. Mosby: St Louis.

Wood RE (1998). Diagnostic and therapeutic procedures in pediatric pulmonary patients. In Taussig LM, Landau LI, editors. *Pediatric respiratory medicine*. Mosby: St Louis.

Yorgin PD, Rhee KH (1998). Gas exchange and acid-base physiology. In Taussig LM, Landau LI, editors. *Pediatric respiratory medicine*. Mosby: St Louis.

Zahka KG, Lane JR (2002). Approach to the neonate with cardiovascular disease. In Fanaroff AA, Martin RJ, editors. *Neonatal-perinatal medicine: diseases of the fetus and infant*, ed 7. Mosby: St Louis.

CHAPTER 42

IDENTIFICATION, MANAGEMENT, AND PREVENTION OF NEWBORN/INFANT PAIN

MARLENE WALDEN, LINDA STURLA FRANCK

INTRODUCTION

Acute pain is a highly complex, dynamic, subjective experience that is generally useful to the growing infant by warning the infant of danger and limiting exposure to further injury. It is important that children learn effective methods of preventing and coping with the everyday pains of growing up. Furthermore, untreated acute, recurrent, or chronic pain related to disease or medical care may have significant and lifelong physiological and psychological consequences. As with all other medical conditions, the first step in the treatment process is the accurate diagnosis of the problem. Thus pain assessment provides the foundation for all pain treatment. This chapter reviews the developmental neurophysiology of pain, discusses methods to assess pain in infants, highlights factors that influence the pain experience and discusses evidence-based strategies for managing infant pain.

DEFINING PAIN AND DISTRESS IN INFANTS AND CHILDREN

Pain is defined by the International Association for the Study of Pain (IASP) as "an unpleasant sensory and emotional experience associated with actual or potential tissue damage or described in terms of such damage" (Merskey, 1979). The IASP definition also states that pain is always subjective and is learned through experiences related to injury in early life. This definition is problematic when considering infants who are incapable of self-report and who may not have had previous experience with injury. Anand and Craig (1996) propose that pain perception is an inherent quality of life that appears early in development to serve as a signaling system for tissue damage. This signaling includes behavioral and physiologic responses, which are valid indicators of pain that can be inferred by others. Broadening the definition of pain to include behavioral and physiologic indicators in addition to self-report can benefit preverbal, non-verbal, or cognitively impaired individuals who are experiencing pain by providing objective pain assessment.

The phrase "pain and distress" is used to describe pain and pain-related fear, anxiety, and agitated behavior that often are exhibited by children in pain. This phrase acknowledges that the pain experience comprises affective and emotional as well as sensory aspects. However, although degree of pain-related distress is highly correlated with pain intensity, measurement of distress may reflect other emotional reactions; thus caution must be used to infer pain from global measures of distress in the absence of other indicators of pain.

DEVELOPMENTAL NEUROPHYSIOLOGY OF PAIN

The basic mechanisms of pain perception in infants and children are similar to those of adults and include: a) transduction and transmission; and b) perception and modulation. However, because of neurophysiologic and cognitive immaturity, some differences exist. A brief review is presented here and emphasizes the developmental and maturational changes that occur during infancy and childhood. For a more in-depth discussion of the pathophysiology of pain, the reader is referred to the numerous reviews in the literature (Fitzgerald & Anand 1993; Wall & Melzack, 1994).

Peripheral Transduction and Transmission

Noxious mechanical, thermal, or chemical stimuli excite primary afferent fibers that transmit information about the potentially injurious stimuli from the periphery to the dorsal horn of the spinal cord. A-delta (large, myelinated, and fast-conducting) and C (small, unmyelinated and slow-conducting) fibers are primarily responsible for pain impulse transmission (nociception). However, these signals can be amplified or attenuated by activation of surrounding neurons in the periphery and spinal cord. For example, tissue injury causes the release of inflammatory mediators (e.g., potassium, bradykinin, prostaglandins, cytokines, nerve growth factors, catecholamines, and substance P) that sensitize A-delta and C fibers and recruit other neurons (silent nociceptors) and results in hyperalgesia. Stimulation of A-beta fibers that signal nonpainful touch and pressure can compete with the transmission of nociception in the dorsal horn of the spinal cord, thus reducing the intensity of the perceived pain.

Central Mechanisms and Modulation

Neurotransmitters in the spinal cord either amplify (e.g., substance P, calcitonin gene-related peptide, neurokinin A) or attenuate (e.g., endogenous opioids, norepinephrine, serotonin, GABA, glycine) pain information from the periphery. Central sensitization occurs when excitatory amino acids act on NMDA receptors to induce prolonged depolarization and windup.

Nociceptive sensory input reaches the thalamus through second order neurons in the spinothalamic, spinoreticular, and spinomeosencephalic tracts and is then widely distributed throughout the brain. The perception, emotional interpretation, and cognitive meaning of nociceptive stimuli occurs within a distributive neuromatrix; the no one 'pain center' exists. The sensory-discriminative, affective-motivational, and evaluative dimensions of pain perception are mediated by past experience and the context of the painful event. For example, nociceptive stimuli activate areas of the limbic system thought to control emotion, particularly anxiety. Thus differences in physiological, biochemical, and psychological factors influence the perception of pain, thus making it an individual phenomenon.

Descending modulation occurs when efferent projections from supraspinal areas such as the periaqueductal grey, raphe nucleus, and locus coeruleus release inhibitory neurotransmitters. The major neurotransmitters that mediate descending inhibition are norepinephrine, serotonin, endogenous opioids, GABA, and acetylcholine.

Neurodevelopment of Pain Perception

Infants, even prematurely born infants, have the neurological capacity to perceive pain at birth (Fitzgerald & Anand 1993). The peripheral and central structures necessary for nociception are present and functional early in gestation (between the first and second trimesters). Functional maturation of the fetal cerebral cortex has been demonstrated by: (1) electroencephalogram (EEG) patterns and cortical evoked potentials; (2) measurement of cerebral glucose use that shows maximal metabolic rates in sensory areas of the brain; and (3) well-defined periods of sleep and wakefulness that are regulated by cortical functioning from 28 weeks of gestation. The newborn infant possesses a well-developed hypothalamic-pituitary-adrenal axis and can mount a fight-or-flight response with the release of catecholamines and cortisol. Cortisol and endorphin levels have been shown to increase during intrahepatic transfusion in 23- to 34-week old fetuses (Giannakoulopoulos et al, 1994), thus demonstrating an appropriate hormonal response to needling of the fetal abdomen.

Research suggests that some differences in nociceptive processes between infants and adults exist. For example, pain impulse transmission in neonates occurs primarily along nonmyelinated C fibers rather than myelinated A-delta fibers. Less precision also occurs in pain signal transmission in the spinal cord, and descending inhibitory neurotransmitters are lacking (Fitzgerald & Anand 1993). Thus young infants may perceive pain more intensely than older children or adults because their descending control mechanisms are immature and thus limit their ability to modulate the experience.

Pathophysiology of Acute Pain

Although pain can serve as a warning of injury, the effects of pain are generally deleterious. Pain evokes negative physiological, metabolic, and behavioral responses in infants (Anand 1998). These responses include increased heart rate, respiratory rate, and blood pressure and increased secretion of catecholamines, glucagon, and corticosteroids. The catabolic state induced by acute pain may be more damaging to infants who have higher metabolic rates and fewer nutritional reserves than adults. Pain leads to anorexia and causes poor nutritional

intake, delayed wound healing, impaired mobility, sleep disturbances, withdrawal, irritability, and developmental regression. Premature infants who underwent cardiac surgery and who received less anesthesia had more postoperative complications (Anand & Hickey, 1992) and prolonged pain may increase neonatal morbidity and mortality (Anand 1998; Anand et al, 1999).

Learning about pain occurs with the first pain experience and has profound effects on subsequent pain perception and responses. Memory of pain in infants is evident from differences in responses to painful vaccination in infants who had undergone unanesthetized circumcision in comparison to infants who were uncircumcised or who received analgesia during circumcision (Gunnar et al, 1995; Taddio et al, 1995a; Taddio & Ohlsson, 1997). Findings from two studies suggest that the pain experience in the Neonatal Intensive Care Unit (NICU) may alter the normal course of development of pain expression in toddlers and preschoolers (Grunau et al, 1994a; 1994b). Animal research suggests that pain and stress in the neonatal period result in altered pain sensitivity, decreased weight gain, decreased ability to learn, and increased preference for alcohol (Anand & Plotsky, 1995; Anand et al, 1999). Humans and animals do not become tolerant to pain and are likely sensitized to the effects of pain over time. Thus recognition and treatment of pain is important for the immediate well being of the infant for their optimal long-term development.

CLINICAL ASSESSMENT OF PAIN

Presently, no easily administered, widely accepted, uniform technique exists for assessing pain in infants, although it is an area of active research. Assessment techniques can be classified as behavioral observation or physiological measures. A multidimensional assessment of pain in infants is more accurate than dependence on a single parameter (Stevens & Koren, 1998). Composite pain measures use more than one parameter to assess the pain experience, usually physiologic and behavioral indicators. The following discussion highlights some of the important features of each type of pain assessment.

Behavioral Observation of Pain

Pain assessment tools that measure pain-related behavior are used for preverbal infants alone or to supplement physiological measures. One caution in using behavioral observation tools is that health care providers consistently underestimate pain in infants who because of illness or immaturity display less pain behavior than healthy fullterm infants, even when the painful stimulus is the same (Page & Halvorson, 1991). The use of standardized, multidimensional assessment tools and the provision of staff education produce pain assessments that more closely reflect actual pain intensity.

Another issue with the use of behavioral observation to assess pain is discriminating between distress and agitation due to causes other than pain (e.g., hunger, wet diaper). Assessment methods such as the COMFORT scale (Ambuel et al, 1992) measure the infant's global behavioral distress, which may be pain-related. In situations in which the source of pain is clearly identifiable (e.g., procedural pain), global distress scales may be a better indicator of the overall impact of the experience than would a specific measure of pain intensity. In other situations, in which the source of pain is unclear, measures of distress may confound the assessment of pain. However, even when it is unclear whether the infant's distress is due to pain or other factors, the distress must be assessed and treated because such distress decreases the infant's coping ability.

Physiological Measures of Pain

Pain is a stressor that activates the compensatory mechanisms of the autonomic nervous system. Sympathetic nervous system (SNS) stimulation produces the fight-or-flight response, which includes tachycardia, peripheral vasoconstriction, diaphoresis, pupil dilation, and increased secretion of catecholamines and adrenocorticoid hormones (Fitzgerald & Anand 1993). Although these parameters are sensitive to changes in pain intensity, they reflect a global response to pain-related stress and are not unique to pain. For example, alterations in these parameters can occur in infants because of crying or handling. The precise measurement of physiological and hormonal responses to pain is generally invasive, expensive, and slow; therefore it is not appropriate for clinical assessment of pain. Thus although clinicians generally associate pain with changes of 10% to 20% in noninvasively measured physiological parameters (i.e., heart rate, blood pressure, and respiratory rate), no standard pain assessment tools that rely exclusively on these parameters exist.

Selection of a Pain Assessment Tool

Selection of an appropriate clinical pain assessment method should be based first on the developmental age of the infant, and second, on the type of pain or medical condition where specific pain assessment tools exist (e.g., for procedural pain or postoperative pain). The validity and reliability of the measures, the specific dimensions of pain that are measured (e.g., intensity, location, quality), and the feasibility of use in the clinical setting are equally important considerations in choosing a pain assessment tool. Published infant-specific pain assessment tools that may be useful in a variety of clinical settings are listed in Table 42-1. The reader is also referred to reviews that compare the psychometric properties of some of these pain assessment tools (Franck & Miaskowski, 1997; Stevens & Franck, 2001; Stevens et al, 2000).

Behavioral Pain Tools. Infants are preverbal and thus cannot communicate their pain in words. In the absence of self-report, behavioral and physiological parameters are used to infer pain in infants. Behavioral indicators of pain include facial expression, cry, gross motor movement, changes in behavioral state, or changes in behavior patterns such as sleep. Because the preterm infant's response to pain is less robust than that of a fullterm infant, the health care provider needs to be cognizant of the more subtle pain cues in premature infants. These cues include less crying; weaker facial grimacing; and limp, flaccid, listless posturing.

Facial expression has been the most comprehensively studied behavioral pain assessment measure. It is the most reliable and consistent indicator of pain across populations and types and as such should be considered the gold standard of behavioral responses for pain in infants. The facial expression of the infant who experiences acute pain consists of the following characteristics: eyes forcefully closed; brows lowered and furrowed; nasal roots broadened and bulged; deepened nasolabial furrow; a square mouth; and a taut, cupped tongue (Grunau & Craig, 1987).

An evaluation of procedural pain in infants through assessment of facial expression can be performed with the Neonatal Facial Coding System (NCFS), which is a valid and reliable coding system for quantifying facial actions associated with acute pain in infancy. Grunau and colleagues (1998) recently established the feasibility of using the complete NCFS in real time at the bedside. The Infant Body Coding System (IBCS; Craig et al, 1984) is a behavioral measure for assessing gross motor activity in infants. However, body activity appears less specific to pain than facial expression in the preterm and fullterm infant (Craig et al, 1993).

Other behavioral assessment tools with preliminary validity in preterm and/or fullterm infants include the Postoperative Pain Score (Barrier et al, 1989), the Liverpool Infant Distress Scale (LIDS; Horgan & Choonara, 1996) for postoperative pain, and the Neonatal Infant Pain Scale (NIPS; Lawrence et al, 1993) for procedural pain. Behavioral assessment tools developed from studies of older infants include the Modified Behavioral Pain Scale (MBPS; Taddio et al, 1995b) for use in infants aged 4 to 6 months who are undergoing immunizations and the Neonatal Assessment of Pain Inventory (NAPI; Schade et al, 1996) for use with children ages 1 to 36 months.

Multidimensional Pain Tools. Multidimensional tools that include behavioral observation and quantification of physiological parameters include the CRIES (Krechel & Bildner, 1995; Schiller, 1998) and the Pain Assessment Tool (PAT; Hodgkinson et al, 1994) developed for postoperative pain and the Scale for Use in Newborns (SUN; Blauer & Gertsmann, 1998) developed for procedural pain. The Behavioral Pain Score (BPS; Pokela, 1994) and the Distress Scale for Ventilated Newborn Infants (DSVNI; Sparshott, 1995) were specifically developed to assess the responses of ventilated newborn infants to procedural pain.

The infant pain assessment tool that has been most widely validated in premature and fullterm infants during procedural pain is the Premature Infant Pain Profile (PIPP; Stevens et al, 1996). The PIPP is a seven-indicator measure that includes behavioral, physiologic, and contextual indicators. Gestational age and behavioural state of the infant are taken into consideration in the scoring. This measure had initial validity and reliability determined by four retrospective data sets. Clinical validation that included the establishment of interrater and intrarater reliability was determined prospectively (Ballantyne et al, 1999). Clinical utility has been established by comparing the PIPP and the CRIES. The PIPP primarily has been used to evaluate procedural pain in preterm neonates greater than 28 weeks' gestational age. Recently, the PIPP has been validated for evaluating postoperative pain in neonates and for determining the efficacy of pain-relieving interventions in premature infants (Eriksson et al, 1999; Stevens et al, 1999).

Factors that Influence Pain

Pain is unique among neurological functions because of the degree of plasticity in pain neurophysiology. Although structural and functional maturity is reached at an early age, anatomic and functional changes occur throughout life and are related to the effects of each pain experience. This plasticity means that the perception and meaning of pain are unique to each individual and are determined not by maturation alone but are influenced by many individual and contextual factors. Currently available methods to assess pain in infants do not adequately or quantitatively incorporate all aspects of the context of pain that influence the pain experience. Thus the clinician must remain cognizant of the ways in which perception of pain may be positively or negatively influenced by these factors and subjec-

TABLE 42-1	Clinical Assessment of Infant Pain		
Measure	**Age Level**	**Indicators**	**Pain Stimulus**
Behavioral pain score	Preterm and fullterm neonates	Facial expression, body movements, response to handling/consolability	Procedural pain in ventilated neonates
Clinical Scoring System	Infants aged 1 to 7 months	Sleep facial expression, cry motor activity-excitability, digit flexion, sucking, tone, consolability sociability	Postoperative pain
CRIES	Fullterm neonates	Crying, oxygen saturation, heart rate, blood pressure, expression, Sleeplessness	Postoperative pain
Distress Scale for Ventilated Newborn Infants	Preterm and fullterm neonates	Facial expression, body movement, color, heart rate, blood pressure, oxygen saturation	Procedural pain in ventilated neonates
Neonatal Facial Coding System (NFCS)	Preterm and fullterm neonates, infants 4 months	Facial muscle group movement: brow bulge, eye squeeze, nasolabial furrow, open lips, stretch mouth, lip purse, taut tongue, chin quiver	Procedural pain
Infant Body Coding System	Preterm and fullterm neonates	Hand foot, arm, leg, head, torso, motor activity	Procedural pain
Liverpool Infant Distress Scale (LIDS)	Fullterm infants	Spontaneous movements, spontaneous excitability flexion of fingers and toes, facial expression, quantity of crying, quality of crying, sleep	Postoperative pain
Modified Behavioral Pain Scale	Infants aged 2 to 4 months	Facial expression, cry, gross motor movement	Immunization pain
Neonatal Assessment of Pain Inventory (NAPI)	Infants aged 1 to 36 months	Smiling, sleeping, response to touch, crying, respirations	Postoperative pain
Neonatal Infant Pain Scale (NIPS)	Preterm and fullterm neonates	Facial expression, cry breathing pattern, arms, legs, state of arousal	Procedural pain
Pain Assessment Tool (PAT)	Fullterm neonates	Posture, tone, sleep pattern, expression, color, cry, respirations, heart rate, oxygen saturation, blood pressure, nurses' perception of infant pain	Postoperative pain
Premature Infant Pain Profile (PIPP)	Preterm and fullterm neonates	Gestational age, behavioral state, heart rate, oxygen saturation, brow bulge, eye squeeze, nasolabial furrow	Procedural pain
Scale for Use in Newborns (SUN)	Preterm and fullterm infants	Movement, tone, facial expression, behavioral state, breathing,	Procedural pain

From Franck LS et al. Pain assessment in infants and children. *Pediatric clinics of North America 2000;47(3):487-512.*

tively incorporate them into the assessment of pain. These factors do not influence pain in isolation but are listed separately for clarity.

Biological Factors.   Genetic variation leads to differences in the amount and type of neurotransmitters and receptors that are available to mediate pain. Recent advancements in molecular biology have allowed for investigation of the genes responsible for pain perception and modulation. Gender may also influence pain perception. Reports of sex differences in pain response in the newborn period are inconsistent (Stevens et al, 1999).

Previous pain experience leads to alterations in pain signal processing that may be reversible or permanent. Studies of premature infants (Johnston & Stevens, 1996; Stevens et al, 1999)

suggest that previous pain experience is the most important factor accounting for differences in response to the acute pain of heelstick. Infants who were subjected to more frequent painful procedures in the NICU had decreased behavioral and increased cardiovascular responses than infants who experienced less pain, even after controlling for gestational age-related differences in pain expression.

Behavioral State.   The behavioral state of the infant, ranging from deep sleep to awake and crying, acts as a moderator of behavioral pain responses. The behavioral state of the infant immediately before the painful stimulus affects the robustness of the response. Infants in awake states demonstrate more robust reactions to pain than infants in sleep states. Infants in a deep sleep state will show less vigorous facial expression in response to heelstick than infants who are alert or aroused before the heelstick (Stevens et al, 1994). Term and healthy preterm newborns who were handled or immobilized before heelstick exhibited greater physiologic and behavioral reactivity, thus indicating that previous stress may result in greater instability in response to pain (Porter et al, 1998).

Gestational Age. Gestational age affects infant pain responses, with younger infants displaying fewer and less vigorous behavioral responses to pain (Stevens et al, 1994; Stevens et al, 1996; Stevens et al, 1999). However, the interaction between gestational age and pain experience has not been well studied. Because younger infants are often subjected to more painful procedures, the pain responses of younger infants may represent an effect of pain experience more so than of age (Stevens et al, 1999).

Pain Characteristics. Pain characteristics such as the source or cause of the pain (acute injury, disease), location, and timing of pain influence the perception and response to pain. Most research has focused on the responses to acute pain caused by single noxious stimuli. However, pain commonly occurs over a prolonged period or is recurrent in nature. Because of the tremendous plasticity within pain processing systems, these factors will significantly impact the infant's experience of pain.

Parents. Nurses who care for the infant in pain must care for the infant's family as well. Parents have many concerns and fears about their infants' pain and about the drugs used in the treatment of pain. Parents may fear the effects of pain on their children's development. They may also fear that their infant may become "addicted" to the analgesics (Franck et al, 2000). Nurses must be prepared to respond to questions from parents and encourage parent participation in providing nonpharmacologic comfort measures to their infants. Parents must be reassured that they are expected to ask questions about their infants' pain management.

Practitioner Factors. The knowledge, attitudes, and beliefs of health care professionals have played a major factor in the undertreatment of pain in both adults and children, despite emerging scientific evidence. Fear of addiction and disproportionate concern for side effects have resulted in severe underuse of opioid analgesics for acute postoperative pain for infants and children.

Lack of education about pain in nursing and medical education is a major cause of myths and biases that impede appropriate assessment and management of pain in infants. Research has shown that infant pain management is strongly influenced by a nurse's biases, personal experiences with pain, and area of specialization. Nurses must examine closely their own beliefs and attitudes about pain, explore the impact that their attitudes might have on their patient care, and challenge their beliefs to determine whether they are science-based or tradition-based. Hester (1998) describes an "illusion of certainty" in which providers assume they know the level of a patient's pain without having to measure it based on the illness or procedure, without regard to the individual patient's experience. Use of validated pain assessment tools results in greater consistency in provider ratings of pain and may more accurately reflect pain experienced by preverbal infants.

Implementing Clinical Assessment of Pain in Infants

Despite the substantial evidence that the pain experience of infants can be assessed in the clinical setting, pain assessment is not routinely performed in most NICU settings. Implementing an effective pain assessment program is more complex than simply selecting an appropriate assessment tool. Pain assessment must be viewed by the health care team as an integral component of quality patient care and numerous organizational, provider, and patient barriers must be overcome (AHCPR, 1992). Successful implementation is determined by the degree of collaboration among the health care team and family to achieve a shared goal of decreased pain for the infant. It requires resources for education, team building, development of processes, documentation of outcomes, and change management. For these reasons, continuous quality improvement strategies are useful for successful implementation of pain assessment for infants in the clinical setting (AHCPR, 1992; Friedrichs et al, 1995; Furdon et al, 1998).

Common themes are noted in reports of successful implementation of all clinical pain assessment programs related to the content of the program, the organizational structure to support improved pain assessment, and the process by which the change process is initiated and sustained. These factors are relevant to implementation of pain assessment programs in inpatient and outpatient settings. The fundamental elements include: 1) multidisciplinary collaboration; 2) staff education about pain pathophysiology, assessment, and management; 3) staff participation in the development of a setting-specific protocol; 4) simple-to-use, standardized, routine pain assessment for all patients; 5) formal documentation of pain assessment in the medical record; 6) mutual goal setting for pain control between health care provider and family; and 7) monitoring of adherence and effect of pain assessment on pain management. No data on the cost or economic impact of implementing standardized pain assessment in the NICU setting exist. Research is needed to evaluate the cost and effectiveness of pain assessment on an organizational as well as on an individual level.

MANAGEMENT OF NEONATAL PAIN

The goals of pain management in infants are (1) to minimize intensity, duration, and physiologic cost of the pain experience; and (2) to maximize the infant's ability to cope with and recover from the painful experience. Depending on duration and severity, pain may be successfully managed with nonpharmacologic and/or pharmacologic therapies.

Nonpharmacologic Management

Painful procedures in the NICU are unavoidable; therefore it is vital that caregivers assist infants to cope with and recover from necessary but painful clinical procedures. Nonpharmacologic strategies to prevent pain should be employed whenever possible including such strategies as grouping blood draws to minimize the number of venipunctures per day, establishing central vessel access to minimize vein and artery punctures, and limiting adhesive tape and gentle removal of tape to minimize epidermal stripping. Nonpharmacologic strategies such as hand or blanket swaddling, nonnutritive sucking, and oral sucrose may help minimize neonatal pain and stress while maximizing the infant's own regulatory and coping abilities.

Swaddling. Minimizing the physiologic cost of pain can be achieved by providing proper support to the infant during the procedure. This support includes providing containment for preterm infants to limit excessive, immature motor responses.

Swaddling is thought to reduce pain by providing gentle stimulation across the proprioceptive, thermal, and tactile sensory systems. Two studies have been conducted in the preterm population using different methods of swaddling. A hand swaddling technique known as "facilitated tucking" (holding the infant's extremities flexed and contained close to the trunk), implemented before the heelstick procedure, was shown to reduce pain responses in preterm neonates as young as 25 weeks' gestational age (Corff et al, 1995). In that study, preterm infants in the post-heelstick recovery phase demonstrated significantly reduced heart rates and crying, and more stability in sleep-wake cycles in the hand-swaddled position.

A similar containment study conducted by Fearon et al (1997) used blanket swaddling for nesting. The researchers examined the effectiveness of blanket swaddling after a heel lance in younger (less than 31 weeks' postconceptual age) and older (at or older than 31 weeks' postconceptual age) preterm infants. Trends showed that blanket swaddling was effective for reducing heart rate and negative facial displays in the post-heelstick phase for the older infants and increased oxygen saturation levels in younger infants.

Nonnutritive Sucking (NNS).   NNS is the provision of a pacifier into the mouth to promote sucking without the provision of breastmilk or formula for nutrition. Franck (1987) found that pacifiers were ranked by NICU as the first choice of pain intervention. NNS is thought to produce analgesia through stimulation of orotactile and mechanoreceptors when a pacifier is introduced into the infant's mouth. NNS is hypothesized to modulate transmission or processing of nociception through mediation by the endogenous nonopioid system (Blass et al, 1987; Gunnar et al, 1988).

NNS has been shown to reduce behavioral pain responses in term infants during immunizations (Blass, 1997) and heel lances in term and preterm infants (Blass & Shide, 1994; Field & Goldson, 1984; Miller & Anderson, 1993). One study found that NNS reduced composite pain responses in preterm infants during heel lances (Stevens et al, 1999). However, pain relief was greater in infants who received both NNS and sucrose. Compared to blanket swaddling (Campos, 1989) or rocking (Campos, 1994) during painful procedures, NNS reduced duration of cry and soothed infants more rapidly. Unlike with blanket swaddling, however, a rebound in distress occurred when the NNS pacifier was removed from the infants' mouths. Therefore the efficacy of NNS is immediate but appears to terminate almost immediately upon cessation of sucking.

Sucrose.   Sucrose with and without NNS has been the most widely studied nonpharmacological intervention for infant pain management. Sucrose is a disaccharide the comprises fructose and glucose. A systematic review and metaanalysis of four studies of term infants and one study of preterm infants ($N = 271$) on the efficacy of sucrose for relieving pain revealed that sucrose is associated with statistically and clinically significant reductions in crying after a painful stimulus. The pain reduction response is particularly evident when 2 milliliters of sucrose are administered approximately 2 minutes before the painful stimulus (Stevens et al, 1997). This 2-minute time interval appears to coincide with endogenous opioid release triggered by the sweet taste of sucrose (Stevens et al, 1999). In a second systematic review, smaller doses of sucrose (as little as

0.05 milliliters) are shown to be effective in decreasing the percent of occurrence of facial expressions of pain when administered in either single or triple oral applications to preterm neonates between 25 and 34 weeks' gestation (Johnston et al, 1997; Stevens & Ohlsson, 1998).

Although relatively few contraindications to the provision of swaddling and nonnutritive sucking for management of pain in neonates exist, the absolute safety of sucrose has not been determined. Sucrose should be used with caution in extremely preterm neonates, critically ill newborns, neonates with unstable blood glucoses, and infants at risk for necrotizing enterocolitis. Furthermore, sufficient evidence of the safety of repeated doses of sucrose in neonates to recommend its widespread use for repeated painful procedures is lacking (Walden, 2001).

In general, nurses should begin with nonpharmacologic interventions before progressing to pharmacologic agents. However, nonpharmacologic interventions may not be appropriate for situations in which severe or prolonged pain is assessed.

Pharmacologic Management

Pharmacologic agents are often required to alleviate moderate to severe procedural, postoperative, or disease-related pain in neonates. Systemic analgesia, epidural anesthesia and analgesia, topical anesthetics, nonopioid analgesia, and adjunctive medications will be reviewed.

Opioids.   Opioid analgesics are considered the gold standard for pain relief. The most commonly used drugs for analgesia and sedation in neonates are provided in Table 42-2.

Opioids are often the preferred choice to manage moderate to severe pain in neonates. Advantages of opioid therapy include: (1) prolonged clinical experience with their use in preterm and fullterm neonates; (2) analgesic potency without a ceiling effect; (3) ability to produce sedation in ventilated patients; (4) few hemodynamic side effects; and (5) availability of antagonist drugs such as naloxone to reverse adverse side effects (Anand et al, 2000).

Morphine.   Morphine is the most widely studied opioid analgesic in critically ill and postoperative neonates. Mean elimination half-life following single-dose administration of morphine ranges between 2.6 and 14 hours (Bhat et al, 1990, 1994). Differences exist in the pharmacokinetics of morphine administered to premature neonates in the first week of life (Bhat et al, 1990). After bolus administration, neonates of less than 40 weeks' gestation have longer elimination half-lives and delayed clearance of morphine than older neonates. In addition, plasma proteins in premature neonates unbind approximately 80% of morphine. This unbound morphine may account for its increased central nervous system concentrations. When morphine was administered as a continuous infusion, plasma concentrations were three times greater, and the elimination half-life was seven times longer in neonates than in older infants and children.

Concurrent illness such as renal failure may significantly impact morphine clearance and lead to the rapid accumulation of morphine metabolites (Faura et al, 1998). Other studies have demonstrated that continuous infusion of morphine is effective and postoperatively well tolerated in neonates (Farrington et al, 1993).

Effective concentrations of morphine for analgesia and sedation are inconclusive and dependent on the age of the pa-

TABLE 42-2	Commonly Used Drugs for Analgesia and Sedation in Neonates	
Drug	**Intermittent Doses**	**Infusion Dose**
Opioid Analgesics		
Morphine	0.05 to 0.1 mg/kg/dose IV repeated every 4 hours as needed	Loading Dose: 0.1 mg/kg/dose IV infused over 1½ hours Maintenance Dose: 0.015 to 0.020 mg/kg/hour IV
Fentanyl	1 to 4 mcg/kg/dose IV repeated every 2 to 4 hours as needed	Loading Dose: 1 mcg/kg IV Maintenance Dose: 0.5 mcg/kg/hour up to 4 mcg/kg/hour IV
Methadone	0.05 to 0.2 mg/kg/dose IV repeated every 6 to 12 hours as needed	
Nonsteroidal Antiinflammatory Drugs		
Acetaminophen	10 to 15 mg/kg/dose PO repeated every 6 to 8 hours as needed 20 to 25 mg/kg/dose PR repeated every 6 to 8 hours as needed	
Benzodiazepines		
Midazolam	0.05 to 0.1 mg/kg/dose IV every 2 to 4 hours prn	Loading Dose: 0.05 to 0.2 mg/kg IV Maintenance Dose: 0.2 mcg/kg/minute up to 0.6 mcg/kg/minute
Miscellaneous Agents		
Chloral Hydrate	Intermittent Dose: 20 to 40 mg/kg/dose every 4 to 6 hours as needed PO/PR Single Dose: 30 to 75 mg/kg/dose PO/PR	

Adapted from Zenk K et al (2000). Neonatal medications & nutrition: a comprehensive guide. Santa Rosa, CA: NICU Ink.

tient. Research in this areas started in the early 1980s and continues today.

Morphine has few effects on the neonatal cardiovascular system in the well hydrated neonate. Hypotension, bradycardia, and flushing are part of the histamine response to morphine and can be decreased by slow intravenous bolus administration (over 10 to 20 minutes) and optimizing intravascular fluid volume (Anand et al, 2000; Stoelting, 1995). Although relatively uncommon, the effects of histamine release may also cause bronchospasm in infants with chronic lung disease (Anand et al, 2000). Enterohepatic recirculation of morphine may contribute to rebound increases in plasma levels and late respiratory depression (Bhat et al, 1990, 1992). Decreased intestinal motility and abdominal distention may also occur causing a delay in the establishment of enteral feeding in preterm neonates (Saarenmaa et al, 1999). The effect of morphine on gastrointestinal motility is hypothesized to be dose-dependent, and tolerance of enteral feeds may be improved by priming the gut with small volumes of milk and lower does of morphine (Anand et al, 2000).

Despite relatively few side effects, fullterm and especially preterm neonates remain susceptible to morphine toxicity that results from gradually increasing plasma concentrations. Close monitoring and individual titration of the amount and frequency of doses for all neonates receiving morphine therapy is therefore important (Anand et al, 2000).

Fentanyl. Randomized clinical trials in neonates have found fentanyl is approximately 13 to 33 times more potent than morphine (Ionides et al, 1994; Saarenmaa et al, 1999).

Fentanyl is probably the most widely used analgesic in neonates and offers two distinct advantages over morphine (Anand et al, 2000). First, fentanyl causes less histamine release than morphine and may be more appropriate for infants with hypovolemia or hemodynamic instability, congenital heart disease, or ex-preterm infants with chronic lung disease (Anand et al, 2000). Secondly, fentanyl blunts increases in pulmonary vascular resistance. This finding makes it potentially useful in managing pain in neonates with persistent pulmonary hypertension, in neonates during extracorporeal membrane oxygenation (ECMO), and in neonates following cardiac surgery (Anand et al, 2000).

Fentanyl has a more rapid onset and shorter duration of action compared with morphine and must be administered as a continuous infusion or as an intravenous bolus every 1 to 2 hours. Fentanyl is a highly lipophilic compound that crosses the blood-brain barrier more rapidly and has a longer elimination half-life than morphine (6 to 32 hours after a single-dose administration of fentanyl) (Anand et al, 2000). Accumulation of fentanyl in fatty tissues with extended use may prolong its sedative and respiratory depressant effects and may be responsible for the rebound increase in plasma levels observed following discontinuation of therapy in neonates (Anand et al, 2000). The liver metabolizes more than 90% of fetanyl.

Little is known about the relationship of fentanyl plasma concentrations to analgesia in neonates. Roth et al (1991) reported that mean effective plasma concentrations for fentanyl in neonates whose gestational age was less than 34 weeks was 1.7 ng/ml, whereas that of neonates whose gestational age was over 34 weeks required 2.1 ng/ml. In adults, mean effective concentration for postoperative analgesia is reduced, at 0.6 ng/ml.

Rarely, fentanyl can significantly reduce chest wall compliance (stiff chest syndrome). This naloxone-reversible side effect can be prevented by slow infusion (as opposed to rapid bolus administration), administration of doses less than 3 mcg/kg, or concomitant use of muscle relaxants.

The administration of fentanyl is associated with a modest increase in intracranial pressure (Anand et al, 2000). Caution is therefore recommended for administration of fentanyl to patients with intracranial pathology.

Increased intraabdominal pressure can triple the elimination half-life of fentanyl, probably because of reduced hepatic artery blood flow. Although it has only been demonstrated for fentanyl, increased intraabdominal pressure probably occurs with other opioids that are metabolized by the liver. Because many neonates experience increased intraabdominal pressure, elimination is an important consideration in administering opioids to neonates.

Prevention of Opioid Withdrawal Symptoms.

Neonates who require opioid therapy for an extended period of time may develop physical dependence. Opioid dependence and withdrawal may occur after as little as 48 hours of a continuous morphine infusion but generally does not develop until after 4 to 5 days of therapy (Anand et al, 2000). In general, infants who receive opioid therapy for more than 5 days should be weaned slowly, usually by a dose reduction of 10% to 20% per day, depending on duration of therapy and presence of clinical symptoms of withdrawal (Franck & Vilardi, 1995; Suresh & Anand, 1998). Rapid weaning of opioids may lead to withdrawal symptoms such as irritability, crying, increased respiratory rate, jitteriness, hypertonicity, vomiting, diarrhea, sweating, skin abrasions, seizures, yawning, stuffy nose, sneezing, and hiccups. Abstinence scoring methods commonly used in the care of the infant with prenatal drug exposure must be used in assessing the infant during the opioid weaning (Franck & Vilardi, 1995).

Methadone.

Methadone is a synthetic opioid that produces prolonged analgesia and has good oral bioavailability, thus making it an attractive option to treat postoperative pain in neonates (Berde et al, 1991) and prevent neonatal abstinence syndrome (Maas et al, 1990). When an infant is being weaned from opioid therapy to a longer-acting oral medication such as Methadone, the starting dose of Methadone should be calculated to provide a dose equivalent to the dose of opioid the neonate is receiving (AAP et al, 2000). Further weaning should then be accomplished based on frequent reassessment to ensure that the patient is free of pain and withdrawal symptoms. Studies are needed to further establish the pharmacokinetics and dosing requirements of methadone in neonates.

Epidural Anesthesia and Analgesia.

Epidural anesthesia and analgesia is a relatively new option available to manage surgical and postoperative pain in many NICUs. Morphine or fentanyl administered alone or in combination with local anesthetics into the epidural space can provide good intraoperative anesthesia and postoperative analgesia after abdominal or lower extremity surgery (Ochsenreither, 1997). Epidural analgesia should not be used in patients with sepsis or local infection at insertion site, thrombocytopenia or other known coagulopathy, increased intracranial pressure, suspected neurologic disease or malformations of the vertebral column, and infants

who cannot tolerate a decrease in systemic vascular resistance such as tetralogy of fallot (Ochsenreither, 1997).

Use of epidural analgesia may potentially expedite extubation (Murrell et al, 1993; Sethna & Koh, 2000; Valley & Bailey, 1991). Because opioids added to local anesthetic infusions act directly on the neurons in the spinal cord, lower doses of local anesthetic are required for epidural administration, and fewer opioid-related side effects are generally seen. Opioid-related side effects can still occur and require careful monitoring of the patient for side effects such as respiratory depression or urinary retention. Catheter-related side effects include catheter migration, infection, occlusion, neural injury/paresthesia, catheter breakage upon removal, or hematoma formation at site of insertion (Ochsenreither, 1997). Anesthetic-related side effects include injection into the cerebrospinal fluid that results in a high block with muscle paralysis or injection into a blood vessel resulting in seizures, hypotension, dysrhythmia, or cardiac arrest (Ochsenreither, 1997).

Epidural anesthesia and analgesia requires specially trained health care personnel and involves appropriate and close observation (AAP et al, 2000). In addition to monitoring for opioid-related, catheter-related, and anesthetic-related side effects, nursing care of neonates who are receiving epidural analgesia includes regular inspection of the catheter site for leakage, drainage, hematoma, and erythema. The infusate, dose, and rate of the infusion should be carefully checked and the area should be kept clean and dry (Ochsenreither, 1997).

Topical Application of Local Anesthetics

EMLA Cream.   EMLA cream (eutectic mixture of local anesthetics, lidocaine, and prilocaine; Astra Pharmaceuticals, London) is approved for use in infants at birth with a gestational age of 37 weeks or greater for a variety of clinical procedures. EMLA produces topical anesthesia when applied as a cream to the surface of intact skin and then covered with an occlusive dressing (Stoelting, 1995). The primary concern with the use of EMLA is methemoglobinemia caused by prilocaine toxicity (Sethna & Koh, 2000). Neonates, particularly preterm neonates, are at increased risk due to a thinner stratum corneum and less active NADH-dependent methemoglobin reductase enzymes that result in higher plasma levels (Sethna & Koh, 2000). Neonates with anemia, sepsis, hypoxemia, or metabolic acidosis and who are receiving other methemoglobin-inducing drugs such as acetaminophen, phenytoin, phenobarbital, or nitroprusside may also be at increased risk for development of systemic toxicity (Sethna & Koh, 2000). Although it is not routinely recommended for use in preterm neonates, one study found that a single dose of 0.5 grams EMLA cream applied for 60 minutes to the intact skin of preterm infants older than 30 weeks' gestation did not result in significant increases in blood methemoglobin concentrations (Taddio et al, 1995c). In addition to the risk of methemoglobinemia, local skin reactions have been noted with EMLA cream and have included blanching, redness, and transient purpuric lesions (Sethna & Koh, 2000). Policies and procedures regarding application of EMLA cream should be established to maximize pain relief while minimizing the potential side effects.

Three primary factors determine the effectiveness of EMLA cream: dose, size of application area, and duration of exposure (Sethna & Koh, 2000). The recommended dose in neonates is 0.5 to 2 grams applied to the procedure site one hour before the procedure and covered with an occlusive dressing (Anand et al, 2001). Studies suggest that EMLA cream reduces pain associated with circumcision in male newborns as evidenced by shorter crying times and reduced facial activity and increases in heart rate (Taddio & Ohlsson, 1997). Taddio et al (1998) also suggests that EMLA cream reduces pain in neonates during venipuncture, arterial puncture, and percutaneous venous catheter placement. EMLA has not been shown, however, to be effective in managing pain associated with the heelstick procedure (Taddio et al, 1998).

Nonopioid Analgesics

Acetaminophen. Acetaminophen is a nonopioid analgesic for short-term management of mild to moderate pain in neonates. Acetaminophen has been commonly administered in neonates as an oral or rectal preparation. A new intravenous injectable preparation has been developedbut is currently not available in the United States (Anand et al, 2000). When acetaminophen is administered concurrently with opioid analgesia, the effect is additive and allows a reduction in dosages of both drugs and resulting in fewer adverse side effects (Menon et al, 1998).

Little information is available on the pharmacokinetics of acetaminophen administration in neonates, especially administration by the rectal route. However, studies in adults have demonstrated greater than 80% bioavailability for orally administered acetaminophen (Depre et al, 1992). In children, peak concentrations of analgesic effect are reached in 30 to 60 minutes. The elimination half-life in newborns is estimated to be less than or equal to 4.9 hours. Acetaminophen is metabolized almost entirely by hepatic conjugation that is then renally eliminated.

Although acetaminophen has been demonstrated to significantly reduce pain responses during skin excision and comfort scores at six hours following the circumcision procedure (Howard et al, 1994), other studies have failed to demonstrate efficacy resulting from acute tissue injury of heelstick and postoperative pain relief after cardiac surgery (Shah et al, 1998; Van Lingen et al, 1999). The results from these studies suggest that acetaminophen may be more appropriate for mild to moderate dull, continuous pain resulting from inflammatory conditions than acute, tissue-damaging or severe noxious stimuli (Anand et al, 2000).

At therapeutic doses, acetaminophen is well tolerated and has a low toxicity (Olkkola & Hamunen, 2000). Because acetaminophen does not inhibit prostaglandin synthesis in tissues other than the brain, common side effects of nonsteroidal anti-inflammatory drugs—such as inhibition of platelet function, renal insufficiency, and gastrointestinal irritation—do not occur (Anand et al, 2000). The primary concern of acetaminophen is liver damage, but this should not be a concern in neonates if standard doses are used (Berde et al, 1991).

Use of Adjunctive Drugs. In the NICU, the use of sedatives, alone or in combination with analgesics, is controversial. Although sedatives suppress the behavioral expression of pain, they have no analgesic effects and can even increase pain. Sedatives should only be used when pain has been ruled out. When administered with opioids, sedatives may allow more optimal weaning of opioids in critically ill, ventilator-dependent neonates who have developed tolerance from prolonged opioid therapy. No research has been done to determine the safety or efficacy of combining sedatives and analgesics for the treatment of pain in infants.

The most commonly administered sedatives in the NICU are benzodiazepines and chloral hydrate.

Benzodiazepines

Midazolam. Midazolam is a short-acting benzodiazepine that has increasingly been used in the NICU to provide sedation for mechanically ventilated neonates. Midazolam is preferred over other benzodiazepines because of its water solubility, rapid clearance, and shorter elimination half-life (6.5 hours) (Jacqz-Aigrain et al, 1992). Recent concern about the safety of midazolam in neonates has been reported because of the large number of adverse neurologic effects associated with midazolam in term and preterm neonates (Adams et al, 1997; Magny et al, 1994; Ng et al, 2000). Transient neurologic effects after boluses and/or infusions of midazolam include impaired level of consciousness, lack of visual following, hypertonia, hypotonia, choreic movements, dyskinetic movements, myoclonus, epileptiform activity, abnormalities in electroencephalograms, and cerebral hypoperfusion (Ng et al, 2000). A study by Anand et al (1999) also found a higher incidence of poor neurological outcome as defined by death, severe intraventricular hemorrhage, and periventricular leukomalacia in ventilated preterm neonates treated with midazolam.

Diazepam. Diazepam is not recommended for administration in neonates because of its very prolonged half-life (20 to 50 hours), its long-acting metabolites, and concern about the benzyl alcohol content. The dose of benzyl alcohol preservative in diazepam is, however, below the dose known to cause fatal toxicity in premature neonates (100 to 400 mg/kg/day). Diazepam displaces bilirubin from albumin-binding sites, thereby increasing the neonate's risk of kernicterus (Anand et al, 2000).

Chloral Hydrate. Chloral hydrate has been used in single doses to sedate neonates during pulmonary function, radiographic, and other diagnostic testing for which the patient must lie still. The onset of action is approximately 30 minutes and the lasts about 2 to 4 hours, depending on the dose (Anand et al, 2000). Although clinically effective, concern has been raised about the potential carcinogenic and genotoxic effects of chloral hydrate administered to animals. Chloral hydrate has also been used in repeated doses to sedate neonates on mechanical ventilation. Alternative sedatives (i.e., benzodiazepines) should be used when possible because chloral hydrate has other gastrointestinal side effects and may be associated with direct hyperbilirubinemia. The extremely long half-life (greater than 72 hours) of chloral hydrate increases the risk of toxicity with repeated administration, which may be manifest as increased agitation.

Management of Specific Pain Types

Pain management techniques may vary based on pain type and clinical situation. This section will review special issues related to procedural pain, postoperative pain, preemptive analgesia for mechanical ventilation, and pain management at end of life.

Procedural Pain. It has been estimated that newborn infants, particularly those born preterm, are routinely subjected to an average of 61 invasive procedures performed from admission to discharge, with some the youngest or sickest infants experiencing over 450 painful procedures during their hospital stays (Barker & Rutter, 1995). These frequent, invasive, and noxious procedures occur randomly in the NICU and many times are not routinely managed with either pharmacologic or nonpharmacologic interventions (Anand et al, 1996). Anand

TABLE 42-3   Suggested Management of Painful Procedures Commonly Performed in the NICU

Procedures	Pacifier with Sucrose	Swaddling, Containment, or Facilitated Tucking	EMLA Cream	Subcutaneous Infiltration of Lidocaine	Opioids	Other
Diagnostic Procedures						
Arterial puncture	✓	✓	✓	✓		Consider venipuncture; skin-to-skin contact with mother; mechanical spring-loaded lance
Heel lancing	✓	✓				
Lumbar puncture	✓	✓	✓	✓		Use careful physical handling
Venipuncture	✓		✓		✓	
Therapeutic Procedures						
Central venous line placement	✓	✓	✓	✓	✓	Consider general anesthesia
Chest tube insertion	✓			✓	✓	Anticipate need for intubation and ventilation in neonates spontaneously breathing; consider short acting anesthetic agents; avoid midazolam
Gavage tube insertion	✓	✓				Gentle technique and appropriate lubrication
Intramuscular injection	✓	✓	✓			Give drugs intravenously, whenever it is possible
Peripherally inserted central catheter placement	✓	✓	✓		✓	
Endotracheal intubation					✓	Various combinations of atropine, ketamine, thiopental sodium, succinylcholine chloride, morphine, fentanyl, nondepolarizing muscle relaxant; consider topical lidocaine spray
Endotracheal suction	Sucrose optional	✓			✓	
Surgical Procedures						
Circumcision	✓		✓			Mogen clamp preferred over Gomco clamp; dorsal penile nerve block, ring block, or caudal block using plain or buffered lidocaine; consider acetaminophen for postoperative pain

From Anand et al, 2001.

and the International Evidenced-Based Group for Neonatal Pain (2001) provide guidelines for preventing and treating neonatal procedural pain. Strategies for the management of diagnostic, therapeutic, and surgical procedures commonly performed in the NICU are summarized in Table 42-3.

Local anesthesia may not be sufficient for procedures that affect deeper tissue, such as chest tube insertion or surgical cut down of vessels. Central analgesia is then required to prevent pain. For the nonventilated patient, in whom concern for the respiratory depressant effects of opioids exists, one half the standard dose may be administered. The infant's respiratory status and responsiveness to pain stimuli can then be assessed before further drug administration. For the infant who is receiving opioid analgesics on a regular basis, a controlled infusion of a bolus dose may be required to provide adequate analgesia during an invasive procedure.

Postoperative Pain. Adequate analgesia is important during the immediate postoperative period for the optimal recovery of the patient. Unrelieved pain can interfere with ventilation and delay weaning. Use of low-dose continuous infusion of opioid analgesics can provide more constant, effective pain relief with less medication than intermittent scheduled doses of opioids (Truog & Anand 1989).

Preemptive Analgesia for Mechanical Ventilation. Opioids are frequently used to sedate, promote respiratory synchrony, produce physiologic stability, and relieve pain or discomfort in ventilated neonates (Anand et al, 1999). In a multicenter trial of 67 ventilated preterm infants between 24 and 33 weeks' gestation, Anand et al (1999) found that preemptive analgesia using morphine and midazolam reduced pain responses and stabilized vital signs. This study also found that morphine—but not midazolam—reduced the risk of death or adverse neurological morbidity as evidenced by a grade 3/4 intraventricular hemorrhage or periventricular leukomalacia.

Pain Management at End-of-Life (EOL). Pain management at end-of-life (EOL) primarily centers on the provision of opioids to minimize pain and nonpharmacologic therapies to enhance the infant's comfort level (Walden et al, 2001). Pain assessment is extremely difficult in neonates at end of life. Therefore caregivers must often consider risk factors for pain and rely on physiologic measures such as increases in heart rate and decreases in oxygen saturation to make pain management decisions.

Continuous infusions of opioid therapy such as morphine and fentanyl are often required to manage pain at EOL and should be titrated to desired clinical response (analgesia) (Anand et al, 2000). Opioid doses well beyond those described for standard analgesia are often required for infants who are in severe pain or who have developed tolerance (decreasing pain relief with the same dosage over time) after the prolonged use of opioids (Partridge & Wall, 1997).

Physiologic comfort measures may palliate pain and distressing symptoms in infants at EOL and include reduction of noxious stimuli, organization of care giving, and positioning and containment strategies (Walden et al, 2001). See Chapter 9 for more information on EOL.

NEONATAL NURSE'S ROLE AND RESPONSIBILITIES

Providing comfort and relieving pain are two primary goals of nursing care. To accomplish these goals, neonatal nurses must: (1) prevent pain when possible; (2) assess pain in their neonatal patients who cannot verbalize their subjective experience of pain; (3) provide relief or reduction of pain through implementation of nonpharmacologic and/or pharmacologic measures; and (4) assist the infant in coping when pain cannot be prevented.

The effective management of infant pain requires nurses to collaborate with each other, with physicians, and with the infant's parents. Nurses must effectively communicate assessments and recommendations in an objective, concise manner and advocate for pain relief strategies with responsible health care team members.

Neonatal nurses must remain informed about professional standards and clinical guidelines related to pain assessment and management in neonates. The nurse should also participate in ongoing pain education and review of new research and scientific developments.

SUMMARY

Pain in neonates is often assessed and managed inadequately in large proportion of neonates in the NICU. It is clear, however, that caring for infants in pain requires attention not only to the immediate effects but also to the long-term developmental consequences of pain and pain treatment. Through ongoing research, objective assessment, effective collaboration, and systematic application of treatment plans, nurses will achieve greater comfort for individual patients and add to the body of knowledge in this rapidly evolving field.

REFERENCES

Adams MM et al (1997). A series of neonatal patients with paradoxical seizure-like reactions to bolus intravenous injections of midazolam. *Pediatric research*, 41, 134A.

Agency for Health Care Policy and Research (AHCPR). (1992). *Acute pain management guidelines*. Rockville, MD: Author.

Ambuel B et al (1992). Assessing distress in pediatric intensive care environments: the COMFORT scale. *Journal of pediatric psychology*, 17(1), 95-109.

American Academy of Pediatrics et al (2000). Prevention and management of pain and stress in the neonate. *Pediatrics*, 105(2), 454-461.

Anand KJ (1998). Neonatal analgesia and anesthesia: introduction. *Semin perinatol*, 22(5), 347-349.

Anand K et al (1996). Routine analgesic practices in 109 neonatal intensive care units (NICUs). *Pediatric research*, 39, 192A.

Anand KJ et al (1999). Analgesia and sedation in preterm neonates who require ventilatory support: results from the NOPAIN trial: Neonatal Outcome and Prolonged Analgesia in Neonates. *Arch pediatr adolesc med*, 153(4), 331-338.

Anand KJS et al (2000). Systemic analgesic therapy. In Anand K et al, *Pain in neonates*, ed 2, Amsterdam: Elsevier Science.

Anand KJ, Craig KD (1996). New perspectives on the definition of pain. *Pain*, 67(1), 3-6; discussion 209-211.

Anand KJ, Hickey PR (1992). Halothane-morphine compared with high dose sufentanil for anesthesia and post-operative analgesia in neonatal cardiac surgery. *New England journal of medicine*, 326 (1), 1-9.

Anand KJS & the International Evidence-Based Group for Neonatal Pain. (2001). Consensus statement for the prevention and management of pain in the newborn. *Archives of pediatric adolescent medicine*, (155), 173-180.

Anand KJS, Plotsky PM (1995). Repetitive neonatal pain alters weight gain and pain threshold during development in infant rats. *Critical care medicine*, 23(Suppl.), A22.

Ballantyne M et al (1999). Validation of the premature infant pain profile in the clinical setting. *Clinical journal of pain*, 15(4), 297-303.

Barker DP, Rutter N (1995). Exposure to invasive procedures in neonatal intensive care unit admissions. *Archives of disease in childhood*, 72(1), F47-F48.

Barrier G et al (1989). Measurement of post-operative pain and narcotic administration in infants using a new clinical scoring system. *Intensive care medicine*, 15(Suppl. 1), 537-539.

Berde CB et al (1991). Comparison of methadone and morphine for prevention of postoperative pain in 3-7 year old children. *Journal of pediatrics*, 119(1, Part 1), 136-141.

Bhat R et al (1990). Pharmacokinetics of a single dose of morphine in preterm infants during the first week of life. *Journal of pediatrics*, 117(3), 477-481.

Bhat R et al (1992). Morphine metabolism in acutely ill preterm newborn infants. *Journal of pediatrics*, 120, 795-799.

Bhat R et al (1994). Postconceptual age influences pharmacokinetics and metabolism of morphine in sick neonates. *Pediatric research*, 35(4, Part 2), 81A.

Blass E (1997). Milk-induced hypoalgesia in human newborns. *Pediatrics*, 99, 825-829.

Blass E et al (1987). Interactions between sucrose, pain and isolation distress. *Pharmacology, biochemistr,y & behavior*, 26(3), 483-489.

Blass E, Shide D (1994). Some comparisons among the calming and pain relieving effects of sucrose, glucose, fructose and lactose in infant rats. *Chemical senses*, 19, 239-249.

Blauer T, Gerstmann D (1998). A simultaneous comparison of three neonatal pain scales during common NICU procedures. *Clinical journal of pain*, 14(1), 39-47.

Campos RG (1989). Soothing pain-elicited distress in infants with swaddling and pacifiers. *Child development*, 60(4), 781-792.

Campos RG (1994). Rocking and pacifiers: two comforting interventions for heelstick pain. *Research in nursing & health*, 17, 321-331.

Corff K et al (1995). Facilitated tucking: a nonpharmacologic comfort measure for pain in preterm neonates. *Journal of obstetric, gynecologic, and neonatal nursing*, 24, 143-147.

Craig KD et al (1984). Developmental changes in infant pain expression during immunization injections. *Soc Sci Med*, 19(12), 1331-1337.

Craig KD et al (1993). Pain in the preterm neonate: behavioural and physiological indices. *Pain*, 52(3), 287-299.

Depre M et al (1992). Tolerance and pharmacokinetics of propacetamol, a paracetamol formulation for intravenous use. *Fundamentals in clinical pharmacology*, 6, 259-262.

Eriksson M et al (1999). Oral glucose and venepuncture reduce blood sampling pain in newborns. *Early human development*, 55(3), 211-218.

Farrington EA et al (1993). Continuous intravenous morphine infusion in postoperative newborn infants. *American journal of perinatology*, 10(1), 84-87.

Faura CC et al (1998). Systematic review of factors affecting the ratios of morphine and its major metabolites, *Pain*, 74, 43-53.

Fearon I et al (1997). Swaddling after heel lance: age-specific effects on behavioral recovery in preterm infants. *Journal of developmental and behavioral pediatrics*, 18, 222-232.

Field T, Goldson E (1984). Pacifying effects of nonnutritive sucking on term and preterm neonates during heelstick procedures. *Pediatrics*, 74(6), 1012-1015.

Fitzgerald M, Anand KJS (1993). Developmental neuroanatomy and neurophysiology of pain. In Schechter NL et al (Eds.), *Pain in infants, children, and adolescents*, Baltimore: Williams & Wilkins.

Franck LS (1987). A national survey of the assessment of pain and agitation in the national intensive care unit. *Journal of obstetric, gynecologic, and neonatal nursing*, 16(6), 387-393.

Franck LS et al (2000). Plasma norepinephrine levels, vagal tone index, and flexor reflex threshold in premature neonates receiving intravenous morphine during the postoperative period: a pilot study. *Clinical journal of pain*, 16(2), 95-104.

Franck LS, Miaskowsi C (1997). The use of intravenous opioids to provide analgesia in critically ill, premature neonates: a research critique. *Journal of pain and symptom management*, 15(1), 41-69.

Franck L, Vilardi J (1995). Assessment and management of opioid withdrawal in ill neonates. *Neonatal network*, 14(2), 39-48.

Friedrichs JB et al (1995). Where does it hurt? An interdisciplinary approach to improving the quality of pain assessment and management in the neonatal intensive care unit. *Nursing clinics of North America*, 30(1), 143-159.

Furdon SA et al (1998). Outcome measures after standardized pain management strategies in postoperative patients in the neonatal intensive care unit. *Journal of perinatal and neonatal nursing*, 12(1), 58-69.

Giannakoulopoulos X et al (1994). Fetal plasma cortisol and □-endorphin response to intrauterine needling. *Lancet*, 344(8915), 77-81.

Grunau RV et al (1994a). Pain sensitivity and temperament in extremely low-birth-weight premature toddlers and preterm and full-term controls. *Pain*, 58(3), 341-346.

Grunau RVE et al (1994b). Early pain experience, child and family factors, as precursors of somatization: a prospective study of extremely premature and fulltern children. *Pain*, 56(3), 353-359.

Grunau RV et al (1998). Bedside application of the Neonatal Facial Coding System in pain assessment of premature neonates. *Pain*, 76(3), 277-286.

Grunau RV, Craig KD (1987). Pain expression in neonates: facial action and cry. *Pain*, 28(3), 395-410.

Gunnar MR et al (1988). Adrenocortical activity and behavioral distress in human newborns. *Developmental psychobiology*, 21(4), 297-310.

Gunnar MR et al (1995). Neonatal stress reactivity: predictions to later emotional temperment. *Child development*, 66(1), 1-13.

Hester NO (1998). Assessment: the cornerstone for successful management of intractable pain. *Colorado nurse*, 98(1), 11.

Hodgkinson K et al (1994). Measuring pain in neonates: evaluating an instrument and developing a common language. *Australian journal of advance nursing*, 12(1), 17-22.

Horgan M, Choonara I (1996). Measuring pain in neonates: an objective score. *Paediatric nursing*, 8(10), 24-27.

Howard CR et al (1994). Acetaminophen analgesia in neonatal circumcision: the effect on pain. *Pediatrics*, 93, 641-646.

Ionides SP et al (1994). Plasma beta-endorphin concentrations and analgesia-muscle relaxation in the newborn infant supported by mechanical ventilation. *Journal of pediatrics*, 125, 113-116.

Jacqz-Aigrain E et al (1992). Pharmacokinetics of midazolam during continuous infusion in critically ill neonates. *Eur j clin pharmacol*, 42, 329-332.

Johnston C et al (1997). Effectiveness of oral sucrose and simulated rocking on pain response in preterm neonates. *Pain*, 72, 193-199.

Johnston CC, Stevens BJ (1996). Experience in a neonatal intensive care unit affects pain response. *Pediatrics*, 98(2), 925-930.

Krechel SW, Bildner J (1995). Cries: A new neonatal postoperative pain measurement score. Initial testing of validity and reliability. *Pediatric anaesthesia*, 5, 53-61.

Lawrence J et al (1993). The development of a tool to assess neonatal pain. *Neonatal network*, 12(6), 59-66.

Maas U et al (1990). Infrequent neonatal opiate withdrawal following maternal detoxification during pregnancy. *Journal of pediatric medicine*, 18(2), 111-118.

Magny JF et al (1994). Midazolam and myoclonus in neonate. *Eur j pediatr*, 153, 389-392.

Menon G et al (1998). Practical approach to analgesia and sedation in the neonatal intensive care unit. *Seminars in perinatology*, 22, 417-424.

Merskey H (1979). Pain terms: a list with definitions and notes on usage recommended by the IASP Subcommittee on Taxonomy. *Pain*, 6(3), 249-252.

Miller H, Anderson G (1993). Nonnutritive sucking: effects on crying and heart rate in intubated infants requiring assisted mechanical ventilation. *Nursing research*, 42, 305-307.

Murrell D et al (1993). Continuous epidural analgesia in newborn infants undergoing major surgery. *Journal of pediatric surgery*, 28(4), 548-553.

Ng E et al (2000). Intravenous midazolam infusion for sedation of infants in the neonatal intensive care unit. *Neonatal modules of the Cochrane database of systematic reviews*, electronic 1-20.

Ochsenreither J (1997). Epidural analgesia in infants. *Neonatal network*, 16, 79-84.

Olkkola K, Hamunen K (2000). Pharmacokinetics and pharmacodynamics of analgesic drugs. In Anand K et al, *Pain in neonates*, ed 2, Amsterdam: Elsevier Science.

Page GG, Halvorson M (1991). Pediatric nurses: the assessment and control of pain in preverbal infants. *Journal of pediatric nursing*, 6(2), 99-106.

Partridge JC, Wall SN (1997). Analgesia for dying infants whose life support is withdrawn or withheld. *Pediatrics*, 99(1), 76-79.

Pokela M (1994). Pain relief can reduce hypoxemia in distressed neonates during routine treatment procedures. *Pediatrics*, 93(3), 379-383.

Porter FL et al (1998). The effect of handling and immobilization on the response to acute pain in newborn infants. *Pediatrics*, 102(6), 1383-1389.

Roth B et al (1991). Analgesia and sedation in neonatal intensive care using fentanyl by continuous infusion. *Developmental pharmacology and therapeutics*, 17, 121-127.

Saarenmaa E et al (1999). Advantages of fentanyl over morphine in analgesia for ventilated newborn infants after birth: a randomized trial. *Journal of pediatrics*, 134, 144-150.

Schade JG et al (1996). Comparison of three preverbal scales for postoperative pain assessment in a diverse pediatric sample. *Journal of pain and symptom management*, 12(6), 348-359.

Schiller C (1998). Clinical utility of two neonatal pain assessment measures. Master of Science in Nursing Thesis, University of Toronto, unpublished.

Sethna N, Koh J (2000). Regional anesthesia and analgesia. In Anand K et al, *Pain in neonates*, ed 2, Amsterdam: Elsevier Science.

Shah V et al (1998). Randomized controlled trial of paracetamol for heel prick pain in neonates. *Archives of diseases in childhood, fetal, neonatal edition*, 79, F209-211.

Sparshott M (1995). Assessing the behaviour of the newborn infant. *Paediatric nursing*, 7(7), 14-16, 36.

Stevens BJ et al (1994). Factors that influence the behavioral pain responses of premature infants. *Pain*, 59(1), 101-109.

Stevens B et al (1996). Premature infant pain profile: development and initial validation. *Clinical journal of pain*, 12, 13-22.

Stevens B et al (1997). The efficacy of sucrose for relieving procedural pain in neonates: a systematic review and meta-analysis. *Acta paediatrica*, 86, 837-842.

Stevens B et al (1999). The efficacy of developmentally sensitive interventions and sucrose for relieving procedural pain in very low birth weight neonates. *Nursing research*, 48, 35-43.

Stevens B et al (2000). Pain assessment in neonates. In Anand K et al, *Pain in neonates*, ed 2, Amsterdam: Elsevier Science.

Stevens BJ, Franck LS (2001). Assessment and management of pain in neonates. *Paediatric drugs*, 3(7), 539-558.

Stevens B, Koren G (1998). Evidence-based pain management for infants. *Current opinion in pediatrics*, 10(2), 203-207.

Stevens B, Ohlsson A (1998). Sucrose in neonates undergoing painful procedures. *Neonatal modules of the Cochrane database of systematic reviews*, electronic 1-13.

Stoelting R (1995). *Handbook of pharmacology & physiology in anesthetic practice*. Philadelphia: Lippincott, Williams, & Wilkins.

Suresh S, Anand K (1998). Opioid tolerance in neonates: mechanisms, diagnosis, assessment, and management. *Seminars in perinatology*, 22 (5), 425-433.

Taddio A et al (1995a). Effect of circumcision on pain responses during vaccination in male infants. *Lancet*, 345, 291-292.

Taddio A et al (1995b). A revised measure of acute pain in infants. *Journal of pain and symptom management*, 10, 456-463.

Taddio A et al (1995c). Safety of lidocaine-prilocaine cream in the treatment of preterm neonates. *Journal of pediatrics*, 127, 1002-1005.

Taddio A et al (1998). A systematic review of lidocaine-prilocaine cream (EMLA) in the treatment of acute pain in neonates. *Pediatrics*, 101(2), [Electronic database, 299].

Taddio A, Ohlsson A (1997). Lidocaine-prilocaine cream (EMLA) to reduce pain in male neonates undergoing circumcision: *Neonatal modules of the Cochrane database of systematic reviews*. [Electronic database].

Truog R, Anand KJS (1989). Management of pain in the postoperative neonate [Review]. *Clinics in perinatology*, 16(1), 61-78.

Valley RD, Bailey AG (1991). Caudal morphine for postoperative analgesia in infants and children: A report of 138 cases. *Anesthesia and analgesia*, 72(1), 120-124.

Van Lingen RA et al (1999). Pharmacokinetics and metabolism of rectally administered paracetamol in preterm neonates *Archives of diseases in childhood, fetal neonatal edition*, 80, F59-63.

Walden M (2001). Pain assessment and management: guideline for practice. Glenview, Illinois: National Association of Neonatal Nurses.

Walden M et al (2001). Comfort care for infants in the neonatal intensive care unit at end of life. *Newborn and infant nursing reviews*, 1, 97-105.

Wall PD, Melzack R (1994). *Textbook of pain*, ed 3, New York: Churchill Livingstone.

Zenk K et al (1999). *Neonatal medications & nutrition: a comprehensive guide*. Santa Rosa, CA: NICU Ink.

PRINCIPLES OF NEWBORN AND INFANT DRUG THERAPY

BETH SHIELDS

INTRODUCTION

Newborn and infant pharmacology requires an understanding of the impact of immature organ system on drug clearance. This chapter will review the basic principles of newborn and infant drug therapy. Discussion of the nursing implications is included.

GENERAL PRINCIPLES OF DRUG THERAPY

The individualization of drug therapy in infants and children is essential because of rapid and variable maturation of all physiologic and pharmacologic processes. This is particularly true for both preterm and fullterm infants. The phrase therapeutic orphans, coined over 25 years ago, stresses the relative lack of drug safety and efficacy information in the pediatric population (Shirkey, 1968). Twenty-five years later, published literature on the use of medications in the pediatric population remains sparse. Thirty-eight percent of medications listed in the 1991 *Physician's Desk Reference* contain FDA-approved labeling for use in pediatric patients, with even fewer (19%) medications providing information for use in the neonatal population (Gilman & Gal, 1992). Therapeutic regimens are often supported by case reports, small studies, or past experiences of a particular clinician. Conducting well-controlled trials is difficult because of ethical constraints, and the market for use in neonates and children is quite small in many cases. Advances in medical care have provided for the survival of younger infants, thus resulting in an even more pharmacologically challenging population.

PEDIATRIC LABELING

Over the past several years, legislation has been passed to encourage labeling for medications commonly used in the pediatric population. This legislation includes the Food and Drug Modernization Act, the Food and Drug Administration (FDA) Pediatric Studies Rule, and draft guidelines by the FDA for the clinical investigation of medicinal products in the pediatric population. The goal of new legislation is to encourage the systematic collection of efficacy, safety, and pharmacokinetic and pharmacodynamic data among the pediatric population. The Food and Drug Modernization Act contains incentives to encourage pharmaceutical companies to perform pediatric studies. One of the strongest incentives of this act is a six-month patent extension awarded to a product if pediatric labeling is obtained (Brummel, 2001; Hubbard, 2000; Spielberg, 2001).

PEDIATRIC DOSING METHODS

Infants are not small adults and as such cannot simply be given a portion of an adult dose. Drug dosages must be prescribed for each infant on an individual basis. Their unique pharmacotherapeutic requirements predispose this population to errors in individual dosage calculations. Guidelines have been developed in an attempt to prevent dosing errors in this diverse patient population (American Academy of Pediatrics, 1998; Institute for Safe Medication Practices, 1998).

Several dosing methods have been used to calculate the optimal drug dose for both preterm and fullterm infants. Pediatric dosage handbooks employ dosing methods based on age, body weight, and body surface area (BSA) as well as pharmacokinetic dosing (Taketomo et al, 2000; Young & Mangum, 2000). Each method provides only an estimate, and dosages must constantly be reevaluated and adjusted according to clinical efficacy and toxicity.

To calculate a drug dosage based on age or body weight, it is important to understand the meaning of terms commonly used in the pediatric population (Table 43-1). Because of ease of calculation, dosing based on weight (mg/kg/dose or mg/kg/day) is the most common method. Weight-based dosing is expressed as a dosage range versus an absolute dose. Dosing based on BSA (mg/m^2/dose) requires both a weight and height to accurately assess an infant's BSA. Lack of appropriate pediatric dosing information makes this method impractical except with steroids and chemotherapeutic agents. Pharmacokinetic dosing will be discussed in detail in the following sections.

ADVERSE DRUG EFFECTS

Like the elderly, infants are prone to adverse drug events (ADEs). An ADE is an injury (both preventable and not preventable) that results from the use of a drug (Kaushal et al, 2001). The sick premature infant is exposed to multiple drugs while in the neonatal intensive care unit. Unique drug delivery factors—including individual dosage calculations, preparation

TABLE 43-1	Pediatric Drug Dosing: Age/Weight Terminology
Term	**Definition**
Gestational age (GA)	By dates: number of weeks from the onset of mother's last menstrual period until birth
	By exam: assessment of gestation (time from conception until birth) by a physical and neuromuscular examination
Low-birth-weight (LBW)	Birth weight of <2500 grams
Very-low-birth-weight (VLBW)	Birth weight of <1500 grams
Small-for-gestational-age (SGA)	Birth weight <10th percentile for GA
Appropriate for gestational age (AGA)	Birth weight between 10th and 90th percentile for GA
Large for gestational age (LGA)	Birth weight >90th percentile for GA
Postnatal age (PNA)	Chronological age (in days) after birth
Postconceptional age (PCA)	GA at birth plus PNA
Preterm infant	<37 completed weeks GA at birth
Fullterm infant	38 to 42 weeks GA at birth
Neonate	0 to 28 days PNA
Infant	1 month to 1 year of age
Child	1 to 12 years of age

Data from Behram & Shiono, 1997.

of small doses from concentrated commercial solutions, and slow IV rates-also make neonates more prone to ADEs.

Neonates are particularly predisposed to ADEs because of immature metabolic and excretion pathways as well as potential drug exposures during pregnancy, delivery, and lactation. A study that included eight hundred infants exposed to medications through breast milk revealed that 11% of infants experienced ADEs. The rate of adverse events rose to approximately 16% when multiple medications were used during breastfeeding (Howard & Lawrence, 2001).

Several classic neonatal ADEs have occurred because of lack of knowledge or forethought regarding developmental differences between neonates and older infants and children. Examples of such ADEs include chloramphenicol-associated gray baby syndrome, neonatal gasping syndrome that was after the administration of large volumes of flush solution, and numerous case reports of ADEs caused by absorption of drugs through the skin of newborn infants (Besunder et al, 1988; Gupta & Waldhauser, 1997; Kaushal et al, 2001; Stewart & Hampton, 1987; Zenk, 1994).

DEVELOPMENTAL PHARMACOKINETICS

Pharmacokinetics is the study of a drug concentration versus time and encompasses the absorption, distribution, metabolism, and elimination (ADME) of a drug and its metabolites in the body. Developmental pharmacokinetics—or the change in

the ADME of drugs with organ maturation—is a well-known phenomenon (Table 43-2). To fully comprehend the ADME of drugs, pharmacokinetic terminology must be applied. Standard pharmacokinetic terminology is used when describing the ADME of medications (Table 43-3).

In addition to the pharmacokinetics of a drug, the pharmacodynamics of a particular medication is also important. Pharmacodynamics is the relationship between the pharmacokinetics of a drug and its therapeutic or toxic effects in a specific patient. Pediatric drug dosing regimens are influenced by both the effect of the body on a drug (pharmacokinetics) as well as the effect of a drug on the body (pharmacodynamics) (Figure 43-1) (Besunder et al,1988; McLeod & Evans,1992; Stewart & Hampton, 1987).

Absorption

Absorption refers to the translocation of a drug from the site of administration into the systemic circulation (Besunder et al, 1988). With the exception of the intravenous route, all other routes of administration require a drug to cross membranes in order to reach the systemic circulation and exert its pharmacological effects. Bioavailability is the pharmacokinetic term that has been used to describe the extent to which a drug enters the systemic circulation (McLeod & Evans, 1992). Drugs administered via the intravenous route are 100% bioavailable. In most instances, drugs administered via other routes are less than 100% bioavailable, which should be considered when making dosing conversions between various routes of administration.

Drug absorption depends on the physiochemical properties of the drug—including molecular weight, degree of ionization, lipid solubility, and drug formulation characteristics. In addition, patient-dependent factors, many of which are age-related, affect drug absorption. (Massanari et al, 1997; Stewart & Hampton, 1987).

Medications are administered to infants via many routes including oral (PO), intravenous (IV), intramuscular (IM), percutaneous, and rectal administration. Each route of administration presents its own unique challenge with regard to drug absorption. Parenteral administration (IV, IM) of drugs is important when a rapid response is desired or clinical status precludes oral absorption. Muscle tone, muscle mass, and regional blood flow to the area influence absorption of medications from an IM injection. Neonates, particularly premature neonates, may have significantly decreased muscle mass, as muscle mass is directly proportional to an infant's gestational age (Besunder et al, 1988; Massanari et al, 1997). Hypoxemia, sepsis, shock, or congestive heart failure may compromise blood flow to the muscle tissue. The IM injection of a medication may result in a delay in peak serum concentrations due to poor or erratic absorption. Medications commonly administered to neonates via the IM route include vitamin K, ampicillin, and gentamicin.

Absorption from the gastrointestinal tract depends on factors including gastric acidity, gastric emptying time, bacterial colonization of the gastrointestinal tract, intestinal transit time and permeability, and biliary and pancreatic function (Besunder et al, 1988; McLeod & Evans, 1992; Stewart & Hampton, 1987). The gastric pH in neonates differs significantly from that in adults. The maturation of gastric pH differs in preterm versus term infants and seems to correlate with postnatal age rather than postconceptional age. The gastric pH at birth approaches 6 to 8 because of the presence of residual amniotic fluid, falls to approximately 1.5 to 3 several hours after birth, and then slowly increases over the next 10 days in

TABLE 43-2	Developmental Pharmacokinetics in the Neonate		
Route of Administration	**ADME**	**Alteration in Kinetics**	**Therapeutic Implication**
Oral	Absorption	Prolonged gastric emptying time	Delayed oral absorption; decrease serum peak concentrations
Oral	Absorption	Relative achlorhydria	Increased absorption of basic drugs; decreased absorption of acidic drugs
Intramuscular	Absorption	Decreased muscle mass, decreased muscle blood flow, decreased muscle activity	Decreased/erratic drug absorption
Percutaneous	Absorption	Decreased thickness of stratum corneum; increased skin hydration, increased BSA/weight ratio	Increased percutaneous absorption, increased systemic toxicity
All*	Distribution	Increased ECF and TBW	Increased doses (mg/kg) for water-soluble drugs
All*	Distribution	Decreased plasma protein binding (PPB)	Increased volume of distribution, increased free fraction
All*	Metabolism	Immature hepatic enzyme activity	Decreased drug clearance
All*	Excretion	Immature glomerular and tubular function	Decreased drug clearance

*All routes of administration include oral, parenteral, percutaneous, and rectal.
Data from Besunder et al 1988; Massanari et al, 1997, McLeod & Evans, 1992; Stewart & Hampton, 1987.

TABLE 43-3	Pharmacokinetic Terminology	
Pharmacokinetic Term	**Abbreviation**	**Definition**
Bioavailability	F	The extent to which a drug enters the systemic circulation
Volume of distribution	Vd	The relation between the amount of drug in the body and the measured plasma concentration
Clearance	Cl	The ability of eliminating organs to remove a drug from the blood or plasma
Elimination half-life	$t^{1/2}$	The time required for half the amount of drug present in the blood to disappear
Steady state concentration	Cp_{ss}	A concentration at which the rate of drug administration is equal to the rate of drug elimination

Data from Winter, 1994.

term infants. The lack of gastric acid output early in postnatal life is called *relative achlorhydria*. Gastric pH will reach adult values by two years of age (Besunder et al, 1988; Stewart & Hampton, 1987). Gastric pH affects drug ionization and drug absorption. Unionized particles, are those which pass through membranes. In general, a more basic environment (higher gastric pH) will decrease the absorption of acidic drugs (i.e.,

phenytoin, phenobarbital) and favor the oral absorption of more basic or acid-labile drugs (i.e.,, ampicillin, penicillin, and erythromycin).

Most drugs are absorbed in the small intestine. Therefore gastric emptying time will play an important role in both the rate and extent of oral drug absorption. Gastric emptying time is delayed in the neonatal patient, especially in the premature infant. Gastric emptying may be prolonged up to six to eight hours, and may not attain adult values until six to eight months of age. Oral absorption may also be delayed in the neonate because of decreased intestinal transit time and activity of pancreatic enzymes as well as low concentrations of intraluminal bile acids. In addition, medications such as metoclopramide, which increase gastric emptying time, must also be taken into account (Besunder et al, 1988; Stewart & Hampton, 1987).

Percutaneous absorption or absorption through the skin depends on skin integrity, blood flow to the skin, thickness of the epidermal layer (i.e., stratum corneum), skin hydration, and the ratio of surface area per kg of body weight (BSA to weight ratio) (Stewart & Hampton, 1987). Percutaneous absorption may be increased substantially in newborn infants because of an underdeveloped stratum corneum, smaller amounts of subcutaneous fat, and increased skin hydration. Maturation of premature skin is related to postnatal age, and the attainment of an epidermal layer similar to a fullterm neonate occurs within three weeks of postnatal life (Massanari et al, 1997). The greater the BSA to weight ratio, the greater the absorption of a drug is on a per-kilogram basis with topical medications. The ratio of a newborn's skin to body surface area is approximately three times that of an adult. Therefore after the topical application of the same dose of a drug to a newborn and an adult, the newborn infant will absorb three times as much drug on a mg/kg basis (Besunder et al, 1988; Massanari et al, 1997). Systemic toxicity has been described in neonates after the administration of topical iodine, hexachlorophene, salicylic acid, epinephrine, and corticosteroids (Massanari et al, 1997; Rutter, 1987; Zenk, 1994). The rectal mucosa may serve as a site of

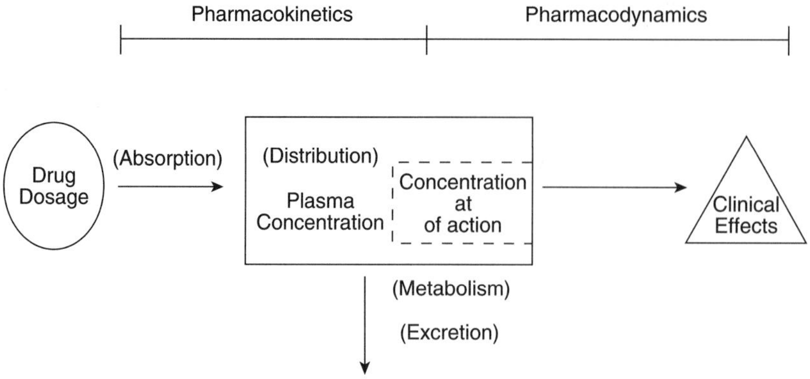

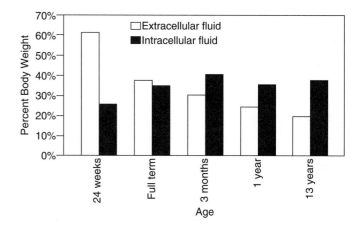

FIGURE **43-1**
Relationship between pharmacokinetics and pharmacodynamics. From *Pediatrics in Review*, 13(11), 420.

drug absorption in neonates who are unable to take medications by mouth, and in whom rapid IV access cannot be achieved. Rectal absorption is dependent on regional blood flow, retention of the drug in the rectum, and chemical properties of the drug. The rectal route of administration results in less efficient absorption when compared to the oral route, and in many instances higher mg/kg doses will be required (Besunder et al, 1988; Van Lingen et al, 1999). Medications commonly administered via the rectal route in infants include acetaminophen, diazepam, chloral hydrate, and sodium polystyrene sulfonate.

Distribution

Once a medication has reached the blood stream, it will distribute among various organs, fluids, and tissues. The distribution of drugs within the body is influenced by many factors—including total body water, total body fat, plasma and tissue binding, membrane permeability, and the infant's hemodynamic status (Massanari et al, 1997). The pharmacokinetic term used to describe the relation between the amount of drug in the body and the measured plasma concentration is the apparent volume of distribution (Vd) (Besunder et al, 1988).

Total body water can be divided into intracellular and extracellular spaces. As a neonate matures, both the total body water and the extracellular space decrease. Conversely, the intracellular space will increase as the neonate ages. At birth, a fullterm neonate is approximately 80% water, with 45% as extracellular and 35% as intracellular fluid. By one year of age a child is approximately 60% water, with 20% extracellular and 40% intracellular fluid (Massanari et al, 1997) (Figure 43-2). Body fat is approximately 1% of the total body composition of a premature infant at 29 weeks' gestational age, increases to approximately 15% at term, and is 25% of total body composition between one to two years of age (Massanari et al, 1997). These changes in the total body composition of the newborn will influence the distribution of water and lipid soluble drugs. Water-soluble medications have a much higher volume of distribution in neonates than in adults; therefore neonatal dosing is higher on a per-kilogram basis (i.e., gentamicin, vancomycin). Fat-soluble medications have a much smaller distribution volume in a neonate than in an adult. Neonatal dosing of medications that are fat-soluble is lower on a per-kilogram basis.

Several physiologic variables can produce both quantitative and qualitative differences in plasma and tissue binding of

FIGURE **43-2**
Changes in total body water distribution with age. From *The Journal of Pediatric Pharmacy Practice*, 2(3),143.

drugs. In general, neonatal plasma protein binding of drugs is decreased in comparison to adults. The decrease in plasma protein binding in neonates is a result several factors, including the decreased formation of plasma proteins by the immature neonatal liver. Serum albumin and serum total proteins are decreased during infancy and rise slowly over the first year of life to adult values. Albumin is the major drug-binding protein in plasma and binds primarily to acidic drugs (i.e., phenobarbital, phenytoin). In addition, drugs bind to globulins, alpha-1 acid glycoprotein, lipoproteins, and other plasma proteins. Fetal albumin has a decreased binding affinity for drugs. A lower plasma pH may decrease protein binding of acidic drugs, and the presence of endogenous substances may compete for protein binding sites. Endogenous substances in the neonate include free fatty acids and bilirubin, as well as transplacentally acquired interfering substances such as hormones and pharmacologic agents (Massanari et al, 1997; McLeod & Evans, 1992).

The decreased plasma protein binding seen in neonates has several therapeutic consequences. Reduction in the protein binding of drugs leads to an increase in the unbound or active component of a drug. Pharmacologic and toxic effects are directly related to the concentration of free drug in the body. Patients with hepatic dysfunction or renal failure have alterations in protein binding and will also have increased amounts of free or unbound drug (Besunder et al, 1988).

Metabolism

Most drugs are fat-soluble and require biotransformation into more water-soluble substances before they can be eliminated from the body. This process of biotransformation occurs mainly in the liver, but other tissues may also be involved. Drug metabolism by the liver depends on factors such as hepatic blood flow, rate of extraction, and hepatic enzyme activity. Drug metabolism may produce inactive as well as active drug metabolites. Many enzymatic pathways are available for drug metabolism, and enzymatic pathways mature in the neonate at different rates.

The two main types of drug metabolism are Phase I (nonsynthetic) and Phase II (synthetic) reactions. Phase I reactions include oxidation, reduction, methylation, hydrolysis, and hydroxylation. The cytochrome P450 mixed-function oxidase system is responsible for most Phase I reactions. Phase II reactions include conjugation with glycine, glucuronic acid, and sulfate. Phase I reactions appear to mature more rapidly, meeting or exceeding adult capacity by six months of age. Phase II reactions reach adult levels in children by 3 to 4 years of age. Maturation of these enzymatic pathways will affect neonatal metabolism of medications and thereby affect the clinical response to medications. Examples of drug toxicity in neonates with immature metabolic pathways include the gray baby syndrome, caused by decreased capacity to glucuronidate chloramphenicol, and neonatal gasping syndrome in neonates decreased capacity for glycination of the benzyl alcohol found in flush solutions (Massanari et al, 1997; McLeod & Evans, 1992; Stewart & Hampton, 1987).

Neonates may use different pathways to metabolize drugs than older infants and children use. These alternate metabolic pathways may result in a modified pharmacologic response to medications. For example, neonates are not able to metabolize morphine adequately to its 6-glucuronide (20 times more active than morphine as an analgesic). Because glucuronidation is limited in neonates, they may require more of the parent drug per weight to produce adequate analgesia (Chay et al, 1992). Theophylline, a drug commonly used for the treatment of apnea of prematurity, presents another example of altered metabolic pathways. Theophylline is oxidized to inactive components in adults but is N-methylated to caffeine, a pharmacologically active agent in the neonate.

Maturation of hepatic enzymes may also be influenced by prenatal or postnatal exposure to enzyme-inducing (i.e., phenobarbital, phenytoin, rifampin) or enzyme-inhibiting (i.e., cimetidine, erythromycin) agents. One drug may alter the metabolism of another medication, thereby increasing or decreasing effectiveness, creating toxicity, or producing subtherapeutic levels. Drug activity may also be interfered with by concurrent disease states. Congestive heart failure results in alterations in blood flow to the liver, thereby decreasing the metabolism of medications that require hepatic biotransformation. Interferences such as these are referred to as drug-disease state interactions (McLeod & Evans, 1992; Stewart & Hampton, 1987).

Elimination

Systemic clearance (Cl) is the ability of the eliminating organs, (kidney, liver, lung, skin) to remove a drug from the blood or plasma (McLeod & Evans, 1992). Drugs and their metabolites are primarily eliminated by the kidneys. The principle renal

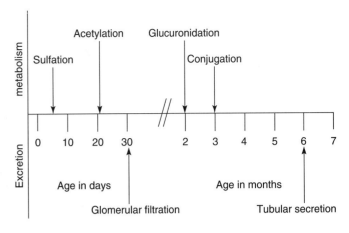

FIGURE **43-3**
The time line of expected maturation of metabolic pathways in the neonate to six-month-old infant. From *The Journal of Pediatric Pharmacy Practice*, 2(3), 145.

mechanisms responsible for drug excretion include glomerular filtration, tubular secretion, and tubular reabsorption, all of which are immature at birth (Massanari et al, 1997). Overall renal function increases with age, although as with hepatic metabolism, the maturation rate of individual physiologic functions varies (Figure 43-3). Glomerular filtration matures several months before tubular secretion; tubular reabsorption is the last to mature. The glomerular filtration rate is lower in infants than in adults and is significantly lower in premature infants than in those born at term. The glomerular filtration is directly proportional to gestational age after 34 weeks' gestation. The increase in glomerular filtration after birth depends on postconceptional age and is influenced by increased cardiac output, decreased peripheral vascular resistance, increased mean arterial pressure, and increased surface area for filtration. The clinical importance of increases in glomerular filtration become apparent when one examines drugs excreted primarily by filtration such as gentamicin and vancomycin. Tubular reabsorption and secretion are also decreased in the neonate.

Ampicillin, a drug commonly used in the neonatal population, undergoes tubular secretion. Therefore drugs excreted primarily via the renal route must have extended dosing intervals in comparison to adult dosing (Besunder et al, 1988; Massanari et al, 1997).

It is clear that most drugs undergo renal excretion; however, it is often important to describe how plasma drug concentrations will change (increase or decrease) with time. With few exceptions (i.e., phenytoin), the serum concentration of drugs change in proportion to the change in dosage. This concept is called first-order or linear kinetics. The majority of medications used in neonates (i.e., aminoglycosides, vancomycin, phenobarbital, caffeine, and theophylline) follow this type of kinetics (McLeod & Evans, 1992). In contrast, a drug that follows zero-order or nonlinear pharmacokinetics may exhibit a rapid rise in serum concentration in response to a small increase in dose. A proportional increase in clearance is not seen with a dosage increase; rather, serum concentrations become excessively elevated with small dosage increases.

The elimination half-life (t ½) of a drug refers to the time it takes for half the amount of drug in the blood to be eliminated (Besunder et al, 1988). The volume of distribution and clearance of a medication are determinants of a drug's half-life.

Half-life is an important factor in determining the appropriate interval between drug doses. Drugs with a long half-life are given at less frequent dosing intervals, whereas those with shorter half-lives may need to be given via a continuous infusion (McLeod & Evans, 1992).

With constant drug dosing, the elimination half-life will determine the time to reach the so-called steady-state serum concentration (McLeod & Evans, 1992). Steady state refers to the time at which the rate of drug administration equals the rate of drug elimination. When drug concentrations are monitored in clinical practice, steady-state concentrations should be obtained. Steady-state concentrations are reached in approximately five half-lives. This factor explains the rationale for administering a loading dose for medications with long half-lives. A loading dose is a single dose of a medication that is used to rapidly attain a serum concentration and therefore the desired clinical effect (McLeod & Evans, 1992). A loading dose produces a higher circulating concentration earlier in the therapeutic course as opposed to waiting five half-lives. In neonates, loading doses are commonly administered for theophylline, caffeine, phenobarbital, dilantin, and digoxin.

THERAPEUTIC DRUG MONITORING

Therapeutic drug monitoring (TDM) is the use of serum drug concentrations and pharmacokinetic and pharmacodynamic principles to regulate drug dosages. TDM in the neonatal population presents several unique challenges. These challenges include the precise delivery of very small doses, the availability of blood for measurement of drug concentrations, interference of endogenous substances with drug assays, frequent changes in neonatal pharmacokinetic parameters, and the extrapolation of therapeutic serum concentrations from adult data to the neonatal population (Gal, 1988).

TDM is used for drugs in which a correlation between the measured plasma concentration and drug efficacy or toxicity exists. Drugs with narrow therapeutic indexes are ideal candidates for TDM. A drug exhibits a narrow therapeutic index if the plasma concentration required for therapeutic effects is relatively close to the concentration known to produce toxicity. Drugs that use TDM in the neonatal population include theophylline, caffeine, phenobarbital, phenytoin, gentamicin, vancomycin, and digoxin (McLeod & Evans, 1992; Gal, 1988). TDM allows the clinician to aim for a therapeutic range, which is usually safe and effective, with minimal drug toxicity. The therapeutic range can be applied to the majority of patients; however, some patients respond to serum concentrations outside this range, and others experience toxic effects within or below the defined therapeutic range.

With the exception of drugs administered via a continuous infusion, drug concentrations in the plasma are not static. The time of blood sampling relative to the time of drug administration is of utmost importance. For some medications both trough and peak concentrations are monitored, whereas other medications routinely monitor trough concentrations (Table 43-4). Obtaining levels once a patient achieves steady-state concentrations provides the most accurate information with regard to drug efficacy or toxicity. Obtaining serum concentrations may require significant volumes of blood in a neonate; therefore assessing the patient's clinical status is also of great importance. Patients with altered organ function or rapidly changing clinical status may require closer monitoring of serum concentrations than do other patients.

TABLE **43-4**	Neonatal Therapeutic Drug Monitoring	
Drug	**Trough Serum Concentration**	**Peak Serum Concentration**
Theophylline (AOP)	6 to 12 mcg/ml	
Caffeine	5 to 20 mcg/ml	
Phenobarbital	20 to 40 mcg/ml	
Phenytoin	8 to 15 mcg/ml	
Gentamicin	<2 mcg/ml	4 to 12 mcg/ml
Vancomycin	5 to 10 mcg/ml	25 to 40 mcg/ml
Digoxin	0.9 to 2 mcg/ml	

In general, elevation of a trough concentration reflects an inability of the body to eliminate a medication, and the dosing interval should be extended. Conversely, if the trough concentration is below a desired level, the dosage interval should be shortened. Subtherapeutic or elevated peak levels necessitate actual dosage adjustment instead of a dosing interval change.

Certain medications such as phenytoin are highly plasma protein-bound. For these medications, two types of assays are available, including total and free serum concentrations. Free levels indicate the amount of free, unbound drug that is available to exert its effects on target tissues. When free phenytoin serum assays are not available, caution must be used in the interpretation of total serum concentrations. Levels may be falsely interpreted as low when the actual amount of active drug is adequate or toxic.

FETAL AND INFANT EXPOSURE TO MATERNAL MEDICATIONS

Fetal Exposure

Virtually any medication or substance given to the mother, either intentionally or inadvertently, can cross the placental membrane. The amount of drug that passes into the fetal circulation depends on several factors—including the molecular weight, protein binding, lipid solubility, and ionization of the drug; maternal drug serum concentrations; and integrity of the placental barrier. Physiologic changes during pregnancy can affect absorption, distribution, metabolism, and excretion of medications in the mother. Specific alterations during pregnancy include decreased gastrointestinal motility, a decreased plasma albumin concentration, increased extracellular fluid volumes, increased renal elimination, and an inhibition of the metabolic inactivation in the liver late in pregnancy.

The consequence of fetal exposure to a medication may be deleterious effects on the exposed fetus or may result in minimal or no adverse outcomes. Labeling a drug as a teratogen indicates the potential of a medication to produce congenital malformations in an infant. A medication may not be a teratogen but may produce other untoward effects on the infant, such as respiratory depression or sedation seen with maternal narcotic administration just prior to delivery. The FDA (1980) published definitions that indicate pregnancy risk categories for certain medications. Drug companies have been required since 1983 to assign each medication a risk category (Box 43-1) (Brent, 2001; Yaffe, 1998).

Lactation Exposure

An often-overlooked source of exposure to medications is transfer from the maternal circulation into breast milk. The safety and potential risks to the nursing infant must be consid-

Pregnancy Risk Categories

Definition*

Category A:

Controlled studies in women fail to demonstrate a risk to the fetus when exposed in the first trimester; possibility of fetal harm appears remote.

Category B:

Either animal-reproduction studies have not demonstrated a fetal risk but no controlled studies in pregnant women exist or animal-reproduction studies have shown an adverse effect that was not confirmed in controlled studies in women in the first trimester.

Category C:

No controlled studies in women or animals available or studies in animals have revealed adverse effects on the fetus. Drugs should be given only if the potential benefit outweighs the potential risk.

Category D:

Positive evidence of human fetal risk; benefits of use in pregnant women may outweigh risk because of-life threatening or serious disease state.

Category X:

Studies in animals or human beings have demonstrated fetal abnormalities or evidence of fetal risk based on human experience exists; risk outweighs any potential benefit. Drugs are contraindicated in women who are or may become pregnant.

*Definitions used by the United States Food and Drug Administration, adapted from Federal Register (1980), 44, 37434-37467.

TABLE 43-5	Drugs Contraindicated During Breastfeeding
Drug	**Reported or Possible Effect**
Amphetamines	Irritability, poor sleeping
Anticancer drugs	Possible immunosuppression, questionable effects on growth
Cocaine	Cocaine intoxication
Heroin	Tremors, restlessness, vomiting, poor feeding
Lithium	Cyanosis, poor muscle tone, ECG changes
Marijuana	Structural changes in nursing brain in laboratory animals
Phencylidine (PCP)	Potent hallucinogen
Radioactive compounds	Radioactivity in breast milk

Data from Committee on Drugs, 1994; Howard & Lawrence, 2001; Ito, 2000.

The list does not contain information on every available drug, because some drugs may not have any information available in the literature. Specific medications are considered contraindicated in the breastfeeding infant (American Academy of Pediatrics, 1994; Ito, 2000) (Table 43-5).

MEDICATION ADMINISTRATION

Once an appropriate drug dosage is established, the optimal route and method of drug administration is also of utmost importance. Many commercially available dosage forms are not suitable for use in the pediatric patient population. Developmental considerations with regard to medication administration must also be considered.

Oral Administration

Many drugs prescribed for infants and children are not available in suitable oral dosage forms. Oral medications are administered to an infant via a nipple, dropper, syringe, or feeding tube. The preferred dosage form for infants is an alcohol-free, sugar-free, and dye-free liquid preparation. However, orally administered medications may only be commercially available as tablets or capsules or as concentrated oral solutions or suspensions. Osmolality must be considered in providing neonatal oral medications. High-osmolality substances administered to the neonate have been associated with many adverse effects, including the development of necrotizing enterocolitis and decreased intestinal transit time. It is important to stagger neonatal oral medication administration to avoid simultaneous administration of highly osmolar medications.

Preparation of small therapeutic doses from concentrated commercial oral solutions may be difficult. An oral product may be concentrated in such a way that accurate measuring of a neonatal dose is difficult. Alteration (dilution) of an adult dosage form raises issues regarding compatibility and stability. In many instances, oral suspensions must be extemporaneously prepared with commercially available tablets or capsules. Commonly prescribed oral medications that are not commercially available in a liquid formulation include rifampin, captopril, spironolactone, and lorazepam. Oral preparations are formulated from available literature on in vitro drug stability.

ered during maternal drug use. Maternal drug use includes over-the-counter drugs, prescription drugs, illicit drugs, and, more recently, herbal products. A recent survey of 14,000 breastfeeding women revealed that 79% took at least one medication, and each woman averaged of 3.3 different medications during the course of breastfeeding their infants (Howard & Lawrence, 2001). Once transferred into breast milk, the infant must than excrete maternal drug. An infant's ability to metabolize and excrete a particular drug changes with the age of the infant. The reduced ability to metabolize drugs is magnified in the preterm, ill, and low-birth-weight infant.

The pH and size of a drug molecule, protein-binding properties, lipid and water solubility, and diffusion rate will all influence the quantity of drug that passes from maternal serum into breast milk. Additional considerations include the time the medication is taken in relation to the period of nursing, the amount or dose of medication, the pharmacokinetics of the drug, the length of nursing, and the amount of milk ingested. For example, for medications with short elimination half-lives, administering a dose after breastfeeding may decrease drug exposure to the infant.

The American Academy of Pediatrics Committee on Drugs periodically publishes guidelines regarding the transfer of drugs and chemicals into human milk. These guidelines include a list of medications and chemicals for which data concerning the transfer of a substance into the mother's milk and the subsequent effects to expect in the nursing infant are available.

Some ingredients necessary for the preparation of these medications may not be readily available and therefore make acquisition of the drugs difficult after discharge from the hospital. For infants, the dose of an oral medication is often a small fraction of the smallest commercial tablet size. Patient-specific dose unit dose powder can be prepared by crushing the tablet, adding a diluent (i.e., lactose), and weighing the patient. In addition, liquid-containing capsules may require the administration of a small portion of the capsule contents.

Oral medications may also contain silent or inactive ingredients that supply the "delivery system" of the drug or serve to flavor, sweeten, and preserve the drug. Such inert ingredients may be harmless in adults but may, when administered frequently to neonates, result in toxicity (American Academy of Pediatrics Committee on Drugs, 1985).

Intravenous Administration

The most effective means of rapid drug delivery in a critically ill neonate is IV administration. Lack of appropriate concentrations from drug manufacturers as well as small doses and delivery volumes all complicate the delivery of IV medications. Furthermore, IV medication delivery is often delayed, prolonged, or incomplete in the neonatal patient. Factors known to affect the rate and completeness of drug delivery include the site of injection, intravenous flow rate, type of infusion system, fluid volume, and properties of the drug solution such as specific gravity, pH and osmolality. A slow flow rate, distal drug delivery site, and large infusion volume delay intravenous drug delivery. A major impact of delayed drug delivery is the potential for subtherapeutic plasma concentrations or even clinical failure with some medications. This is particularly important for medications that may require TDM. Incomplete medication administration may occur, thus delaying peak serum concentrations by several hours. If a peak serum concentration is much lower than expected, infusion system error should be ruled out as a cause before dosage adjustments are made (Gal, 1988; Massanari et al, 1997).

Several techniques are currently used to administer IV medications in the neonatal population and include IV push, IV buretrol, IV retrograde, and IV syringe pump. The infusion device, IV tubing, container holding the medication (i.e., syringe, IV bag), dead space at injection ports, and IV in-line filters will affect drug delivery. Patient-specific factors such as body position and vascular occlusion may also affect IV drug delivery (Carl et al, 1995; Chen & Martinez, 1998; Jew et al, 1997).

Administration of medications using the IV push method allows rapid drug delivery but is not appropriate for many medications. Ampicillin, furosemide, and maintenance-dose theophylline are examples of medications that may be given IV push in the neonate. The IV buretrol method is simple and allows easy dilution of a drug in the primary IV fluids. Potential disadvantages of the IV buretrol method include the fact that medications may not reach the patient for a prolonged period of time, particularly if the primary IV flow rate is not high. In addition, part of the dose may be inadvertently discarded with IV tubing changes, and the drug must be compatible with the primary IV fluid to which it is added.

Another technique—one that was started in the early 1970s—is the IV retrograde system. The IV retrograde infusion system consists of extension tubing with two three-way stopcocks. When a drug is introduced into the system, the stopcock closest to the patient is turned off to the patient end of the system. The medication is given through the stopcock and forced to move in the direction opposite the usual direction of flow (i.e., retrograde). Simultaneously, the distal stopcock is turned off to the pump end of the system, and a syringe is attached to accept the displaced maintenance fluid. This displaced fluid is discarded. After the drug is in the tubing, the stopcocks are positioned to allow normal flow of maintenance fluid, and the medication is infused at the rate set for the maintenance fluid. This method can yield inconsistent delivery but allows delivery of medications with minimal extra volume (Figure 43-4).

Drug delivery with a syringe pump and microbore tubing is the preferred method of IV drug administration in the neonatal population. A syringe pump allows absolute control over the rate of drug delivery with minimal IV fluid volume, at a rate that is independent of the primary IV rate (Figure 43-5). Precise tim-

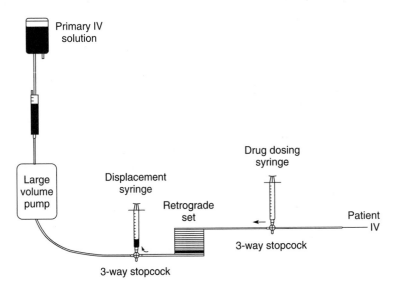

FIGURE **43-4**
Set for retrograde administration of medication. From *Critical Care Nurse*, 17(4), 69.

ing of drug delivery allows for accurate measurement of drug levels for medications that employ TDM. The use of microbore tubing allows the use of minimal volumes of flush solution. In addition to intermittent medications, continuous infusion medications such as pressors and inotropes may be administered via a syringe pump. Continuous infusion rates of less than 1 ml/hr are frequently employed for continuous infusion medications with IV syringe pumps. A potential disadvantage of a syringe pump is the capital expense required to purchase the pump. In addition, if minimal mixing with the primary IV fluid will occur, medications must be diluted to a safe concentration before administration (Carl et al, 1995; Gura, 1999; Jew et al, 1997).

Many of the problems that plague commercially available oral medications can also be found in commercial IV medications. IV medications may be available in concentrations that prohibit accurate measurement and administration of small neonatal doses. In selection of parenteral medications, not only drug concentration but also preservatives and other ingredients in the parenteral preparation are factors. Benzyl alcohol is a common preservative added to parenteral drug products. Severe toxicity has been reported in neonates after the use of flush solutions that contain benzyl alcohol. Whenever possible, preservative-free parenteral products should be used in the neonatal population for the first two months of life.

The osmolality of a drug solution is an important delivery factor. Tissue irritation or pain at the injection site can occur when a drug solution with an osmolality significantly different from that of the serum (275-295 mOsm/kg) is administered intravenously. Infiltration of a hypotonic or hypertonic solution can cause trauma and necrosis of the injection site (Jew et al, 1997).

Premature infants typically have fluid restrictions as well as limited intravenous access, and the question of IV drug compatibilities often comes into play. Drug compatibility involves the question of both physical (visual) and chemical (nonvisual) compatibilities. Two drugs are physically incompatible when turbidity, cloudiness, or a precipitate is formed when two or more drugs are mixed together. An example of a physical incompatibility results when calcium gluconate and sodium bicarbonate-containing or phosphorous-containing solutions are mixed in the same IV solution or IV tubing. Chemical incompatibility implies a loss of potency or formation of a toxic byproduct when two or more substances are mixed. Epinephrine and sodium bicarbonate are chemically incompatible when coinfused (Trissel, 2001).

IV drug compatibility is not clearcut. This is true because of the influence of alterations in drug concentration, order of drug infusion, pH, and temperature. For these reasons, reference books and articles may provide conflicting information with regard to drug compatibilities (Taketomo et al, 2000; Trissel, 2001; Young & Mangum, 2000; Zenk, 1992). Drug incompatibilities can be minimized by infusing medications at the port closest to the patient rather than adding drugs to IV or hyperalimentation solutions. Limited contact between drugs and IV fluids will decrease the likelihood of physical and chemical instability and allow the simultaneous administration of multiple medications.

Extravasation and infiltration are used interchangeably in the literature; both terms reflect a leakage of IV fluid or medication out of a vein and into surrounding tissues (Flemmer & Chan, 1993). Extravasation in neonates with circulatory compromise can lead to significant morbidity, functional impairment, or cosmetic defects. The extent of damage that follows such an event depends on the extravasated substance and the volume of the fluid that has leaked into the interstitium. Many medications (i.e., potassium, calcium, parenteral nutrition, dopamine) that are incorporated into the drug regimens of patients in the neonatal intensive care unit are capable of causing tissue damage if extravasation occurs. The use of small or superficial venous access sites should be avoided for administration of these agents unless absolutely necessary. The best prevention is close attention to the IV site where the medication is infusing. Rapid and appropriate therapy becomes critical with the extravasation of IV fluids and medications. The mechanism by which IV fluids and medications cause tissue necrosis varies, and this will effect treatment options. The degree of cellular injury is often directly related to the physiochemical characteristics of the infusant—including osmolarity, pH, and molecular weight.

The treatment of extravasation injuries that result from infiltration of medications and IV solutions involves the use of specific antidotes. Three possible antidotes—hyaluronidase, phentolamine, and topical nitroglycerin—have been studied most extensively in the neonatal population (Table 43-6). Hyaluronidase, an enzyme that destroys tissue cement, is no longer a treatment option because its production was recently discontinued. Phentolamine competitively blocks alphaadrenergic receptors, thus relaxing smooth vascular muscle. Phentolamine has been proven effective in treating infiltrates of vasoconstrictive medications. For optimal efficacy, phentolamine should be administered within twelve hours of the infiltration episodes (Flemmer & Chan, 1993; Siwy and Sadove, 1987, Taketomo et al, 2000; Young & Mangum, 2000). With the recent removal of hyaluronidase from the marketplace, the use of topical nitroglycerin may become more widespread. Several case reports of use of topical nitroglycerin in the neonatal population have been published (Flemmer & Chan, 1993; Wong et al, 1992).

Aerosol Administration

The importance of aerosolized medications has increased in infants with reactive airway disease and neonatal chronic lung disease. The rationale for aerosol medication delivery includes

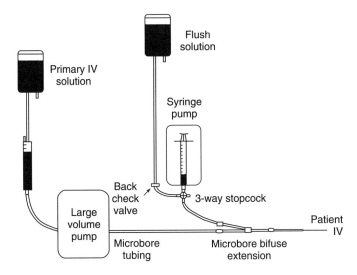

FIGURE **43-5**
Syringe pump delivery of medication for patients with medication volumes <60 ml. From *Critical Care Nurse*, 17(4), 69.

TABLE **43-6**	Extravasation Treatment
Extravasated Drug/Fluid	**Treatment**
Parenteral nutrition	Topical nitroglycerin
Calcium	Topical nitroglycerin
Dopamine	Phentolamine, topical nitroglycerin
Dobutamine	Phentolamine
Epinephrine	Phentolamine

Data from Flemmer & Chan, 1993; Taketomo et al, 2000; Young & Mangum, 2000.

direct delivery to the target organ (lungs) with decreased systemic adverse drug effects. The therapeutic efficacy of aerosolized medications depends on delivery of an adequate dose to the target sites within the lung. The primary factors that influence lung deposition include particle size, the infant's breathing pattern, and the efficiency of the aerosol delivery system. The available methods to aerosolize medications in the neonate include nebulization (jet or ultrasonic) or a metered-dose inhaler (MDI) with a spacing device. Studies have revealed conflicting results with regard to the optimal method of aerosol drug delivery in the neonate (Cole 2000; Sivakumar et al, 1999).

Aerosol delivery varies in young infants. Age-related variables include anatomical and physiological differences as well as the unpredictability of patient cooperation. With respect to anatomical considerations, nasal breathing results in an unpredictable loss of drug particles. In addition, the smaller oropharynx reduces the amount of aerosol that reaches the lower airway. The smaller airway may be further compromised by inflammation, edema, mucus, bronchoconstriction, and distorted airway growth and remodeling (Cole, 2000).

Medication Administration in ECMO

Extracorporeal membrane oxygenation (ECMO) is a highly technical and invasive technique used to treat respiratory failure when conventional means and technologies fail. ECMO has become a more frequently used mode of medical management for neonatal patients—including those with persistent pulmonary hypertension, meconium aspiration, sepsis, respiratory distress syndrome, pneumonia, and congenital diaphragmatic hernia. Patients who undergo ECMO are often treated with numerous medications—including antibiotics, sedatives, analgesics, inotropes, diuretics, and antiepileptics.

Medications may be administered to ECMO patients either into the ECMO circuit before or after the filter or directly into the patient. Varying pharmacokinetics may be observed, depending on the actual site of injection. Distribution and delivery of medication are more consistent when drugs are injected after the filter. Administration into this site places the patient at risk for development of air emboli, and administration of medications here should be done with great caution. Medications injected directly into the reservoir or before the filter usually result in a prolonged time of actual drug delivery to the patient and incomplete drug administration. A large part of the ECMO circuit consists of disposable polyvinyl chloride tubing. The amounts of tubing and other components of the circuit contribute to a large surface area with the potential for drug binding. Binding of drugs to the ECMO circuit results in an increase in the neonate's volume of distribution. In addition to the pharmacokinetic influences of ECMO, drugs such as heparin, fentanyl, and phenobarbital bind to the ECMO circuit, thus resulting in a reduced amount of bioavailable drug for the patient. Once the circuit becomes saturated with these medications, the medications reach the infant's circulation. Therefore increased doses may be required initially when these medications are used or when the circuit is changed during ECMO therapy (Noerr, 1996).

Interpretation of pharmacokinetic parameters in this type of patient is often difficult because of the influences of the site of injection, flow rate of the ECMO circuit, and clinical status and organ function of the patient. Gentamicin and vancomycin are two antibiotics that are commonly administered to infants on ECMO. Pharmacokinetics for these agents vary, not only with the ECMO circuit but also with the clinical status of the infant—including altered renal function in a sick infant. In addition, pharmacokinetics was found to vary with the infant's gestational age, postnatal age, and weight. Peak effect for these patients is often delayed, thus resulting in false interpretation of serum peak levels for aminoglycoside antibiotics (Buck, 1995, 1998; Noerr, 1996).

Patients placed on ECMO often have underlying hepatic and renal dysfunction secondary to hypoxic insults. The physiologic effects of ECMO further compound this dysfunction. Renal function often continues to deteriorate during ECMO. Dosing adjustments need to be made for any medications cleared renally.

SUMMARY

The individualization of drug therapy is critical in the neonatal population. The neonatal population presents a unique challenge with regard to both medication dosing and administration. Drug dosing on a mg/kg basis is the most common method because of the ease of calculation. A lack of large, well controlled trials in this unique patient population results in drug dosing based on extrapolation from the adult literature or anecdotal experience. Furthermore, developmental pharmacokinetics—or the change in absorption, distribution, metabolism, and elimination of drugs—creates a population whose drug dosing is constantly changing. Once an appropriate dosing regimen is determined, the optimal drug administration technique is equally important.

REFERENCES

American Academy of Pediatrics Committee on Drugs (1985). "Inactive" ingredients in pharmaceutical products. *Pediatrics*, 76(4), 635-643.

American Academy of Pediatrics Committee on Drugs (1994). The transfer of drugs and other chemicals into human milk. *Pediatrics*, 93(1), 137-150.

American Academy of Pediatrics Committee on Drugs and Committee on Hospital Care (1998). Prevention of medication errors in the pediatric inpatient setting. *Pediatrics*, 102(2), 428-429.

Behram RE, Shiono PH (1997). Neonatal risk factors. In Fanaroff AA, Martin RJ, *Neonatal-Perinatal Medicine*, ed 6, St Louis: Mosby.

Besunder JB et al (1988a). Principles of drug biodisposition in the neonate: part I (review). *Clinical pharmacokinetics*, 14(4), 189-216.

Besunder JB et al (1988b). Principles of drug biodisposition in the neonate: part II (review). *Clinical pharmacokinetics*, 14(4), 261-286.

Brent RL (2001). Addressing environmentally caused human birth defects. *Pediatrics in review*, 22(5), 153-165.

Brummel GL (2001). The FDA drug approval process: focus on pediatric labeling. *Neonatal network*, 20(3), 49-51.

Buck ML (1995). Assessment of gentamicin dosing intervals in neonates receiving extracorpeal membrane oxygenation. *Pharmacotherapy*, 15, 384-388.

Buck ML (1998). Vancomycin pharmacokinetics in neonates receiving extracorpeal membrane oxygenation. *Pharmacotherapy*, 18, 1082-1086.

Carl J et al (1995). Fluid delivery from infusion-pump syringes. *American journal of health-system pharmacy*, 52, 1428-1432.

Chay PC et al (1992). Pharmacokinetic-pharmacodynamic relationships of morphine in neonates. *Clinical pharmacology and therapeutics*, 51(3), 334-342.

Chen JL, Martinez CM (1998). Filtration recommendations for IV medications. *American journal of health system pharmacists*, 55, 1313-1314.

Cole CH (2000). Special problems in aerosol delivery: neonatal and pediatric considerations. *Respiratory care*, 45(6), 646-651.

Flemmer L, Chan J (1993). A pediatric protocol for management of extravasation injuries. *Pediatric nursing*, 19(4), 355-358.

Gal P (1988). Therapeutic drug monitoring in neonates: problems and issues. *Drug intelligence and clinical pharmacy*, 22, 317-323.

Gilman JT, Gal P (1992). Pharmacokinetic and pharmacodynamic data collection in children and neonates: a quiet frontier. *Clinical pharmacokinetics*, 23, 1.

Gupta A, Waldhauser LK (1997). Adverse drug reactions from birth to early childhood. *Pediatric clinics of North America*, 44(1), 79-93.

Gura KM (1999). Intravenous drug administration guidelines for pediatric patients 1999. *The journal of pediatric pharmacy practice*, 4(2), 80-106.

Howard CR, Lawrence RA (2001). Xenobiotics and breastfeeding. *Pediatric clinics of North America*, 48(2), 485-505.

Hubbard WK (2000). International conference on harmonization: clinical investigation of medicinal products in the pediatric population. *The journal of pediatric pharmacy practice*, 5(3), 114-121.

Institute for Safe Medication Practices. (1998). Draft guidelines for preventing medication errors in pediatrics. *The journal of pediatric pharmacy practice*, 3(4), 189-202.

Ito S (2000). Drug therapy for breast-feeding women. *The New England journal of medicine*, 343(2), 118-126.

Jew R et al (1997). Clinical implications of IV drug administration in infants and children. *Critical care nurse*, 17(4), 62-70.

Kaushal R et al (2001). Medication errors and adverse drug events in pediatric inpatients. *Journal of the American Medical Association*, 285(16), 2114-2120.

Massanari MA et al (1997). Age-based competency assessment of pharmacists in pediatrics, part II: application of developmental pharmacokinetics to pediatric pharmacy practice. *The journal of pediatric pharmacy practice*, 2(3), 139-158.

McLeod HL, Evans WE (1992). Pediatric pharmacokinetics and therapeutic drug monitoring. *Pediatrics in review* 13(11), 413-421.

Noerr B (1996). ECMO and pharmacotherapy. *Neonatal network*, 15(6), 23-31.

Rutter N (1987). Percutaneous drug absorption in the newborn: Hazards and uses. *Clinics in perinatology*, 14(4), 911-930.

Shirkey H (1968). Therapeutic orphans. *Journal of pediatrics*, 72, 119.

Sivakumar D et al (1999). Bronchodilator delivered by metered dose inhaler and spacer improves respiratory system compliance more than nebulizer-delivered bronchodilator in ventilated premature infants. *Pediatric pulmonology*, 27, 208-212.

Siwy BK, Sadove AM (1987). Acute management of dopamine infiltration injury with Regitine. *Plastic and reconstructive surgery*, 80(4), 610-612.

Spielberg SP (2001). Pediatric therapy for the new millenium. *Journal of pediatric pharmacology and therapeutics*, 6, 6-9.

Stewart CF, Hampton EM (1987). Effect of maturation on drug disposition in pediatric patients [Review]. *Clinical pharmacy*, 6(7), 548-564.

Taketomo CK et al (2000). *Pediatric Dosage Handbook*, ed 7, Hudson, Ohio: Lexi-Comp.

Trissel LA (2001). Drug stability and compatibility issues in drug delivery. In Trissel LA (Ed.), *Handbook of injectable drugs*, ed. 11, pp. 17-22. Bethesda: American Society of Health-System Pharmacists.

United States Food and Drug Administration. (1980). Drug use in pregnancy risk categories. *Federal Register*, 44, 3734-3767.

Van Lingen RA et al (1999). Pharmacokinetics and metabolism of rectally administered paracetamol in preterm neonates. *Archives of diseases of childhood fetal and neonatal edition*, 80, F59-F63.

Winter ME (1994). In Koda-Kimble MA, *Basic clinical pharmacokinetics*, ed 3, Vancouver, WA: Applied Therapeutics.

Wong A et al (1992). Treatment of peripheral tissue ischemia with topical nitroglycerin ointment in neonates. *The journal of pediatrics*, 121(6), 980-983.

Yaffe S (1998). Introduction. In Briggs GE et al (Eds.), *Drugs in pregnancy and lactation*, ed 5, Baltimore: Williams & Wilkins.

Young TE, Mangum B (2000). *Neofax*, ed 13, Raleigh, NC: Acorn.

Zenk K (1992). Y-site compatibility of drugs commonly used in the NICU. *Neonatal pharmacology quarterly*, 1(2), 13-22, NICU Ink.

Zenk K (1994). Challenges in providing pharmaceutical care to pediatric patients. *American journal of hospital pharmacy*, 51, 688-694.

COMPLEMENTARY THERAPIES

Nadine Annette Kassity, Jamieson E. Jones, Carole Kenner, Armenda Turner, Michael J. Hayes

INTRODUCTION

Complementary and alternative medicine (CAM) is a growing trend in this country and abroad (Eisenberg et al, 1998). Such a topic is included in a neonatal text because although little research has been done in the area of CAM as it applies to the newborn, many of the families we serve use these therapies, and some health professionals are beginning to apply the concepts of holistic care and alternative modalities to this population. In fact, this emerging area of medicine has become so important that the National Institutes of Health (NIH) created the National Center for Complementary and Alternative Medicine (NCCAM). Monies are now set aside for in-depth research of CAM therapies. We, as health professionals, need to recognize these therapies as well as the gaps in our scientific knowledge regarding CAM. CAM is a part of the integrative health care movement. In the neonatal unit, CAM therapies may add critical support to neonatal care by adding more nurturing elements one would expect around newborns, thus softening the high-tech environment. This chapter will briefly describe some of the most popular and promising CAM therapies and explore how these options are used in the neonatal intensive care unit (NICU) and other infant populations and will point towards fruitful areas for further study.

COMPLEMENTARY AND ALTERNATIVE MEDICINE (CAM)

The merging of complementary and alternative therapies with mainstream Western medicine is often called integrative medicine. In this new approach, health professionals are expanding to look at health from a holistic perspective. Thus in the West two streams of view are now being integrated—one that views disease as having specific causative agents and another that views the mind-body connection as all-powerful. According to the mind-body perspective, disease results from disharmony of the mind and body. In treating disease, practitioners of mind-body medicine look at many factors, including the nature of relationships—such as the relationship between the parents and the infants and the dynamic between the healer and patient. This new integrative, holistic model has thus increasingly challenged our profession to broaden our definitions of healing to include all aspects of relationship as part of health and wholeness.

In neonatal care, complementary therapies may be especially useful in helping to minimize some of the iatrogenic complications of development that are associated with prematurity. The high-tech environment may at times cause infants to be overwhelmed and touch-deprived or excessively stimulated. CAM therapies may provide balance to support the amazing technological advances we have made.

Alternative medicine, like conventional medicine, has pros and cons, promotes good ideas and bad ones, and promises to hold both benefits and risks. To keep an open skeptical mind will allow examination of our current medical model with its focus on the "cure" and allow us to broaden our perspective on healing and health. Nursing and nursing care is naturally compatible with CAM as we tend to use a holistic approach to care. The operative word "care" connotes a friendlier, humanistic value than the word *cure* does. Caring (communication, sensitivity, holistic approach) are some of the hallmarks of our profession. Much of CAM is based on expanding these areas as well as broadening our awareness of many different subtleties in healing.

In our exploration of complementary therapies, we use the complementary categories that were established by the National Center for Complementary and Alternative Medicine (NCCAM):

Lifestyle Therapies (Developmental Care)
Aromatherapy, Music, Light, Kangaroo Care, Cobedding
Biomechanical Therapies
Massage, Reflexology, Osteopathy/Cranial Sacral Therapy
Bioenergetic Therapies
Acupuncture, Energy Healing, Healing Touch, Reiki
Biochemical Therapies
Herbs and Supplements; Homeopathy

Although some practices could fit in more than one, the categories are useful. For instance, some view homeopathy as a vibrational medicine because its effect is energetic rather than biochemical. Likewise, many practitioners reflexology and cranial sacral therapy are believed by to affect the energy balance of the patient. Also, some consider other techniques alternative therapies that focus more on environmental manipulation. These fall into the realm of either Developmental Care (Chapter 18) or the NICU environment, discussed in Chapter 16.

LIFESTYLE THERAPIES (DEVELOPMENTAL CARE)

Aromatherapy

Aromatherapy uses aromatic and essential oils from herbs and flowers as treatments to alter a person's mood or behavior and to facilitate physical, mental, or emotional well-being. People respond immediately and involuntarily to scents, which release neurotransmitters in the brain and cause calming, sedating, pain-reducing, stimulating, or euphoric effects. Truck drivers are known to use peppermint aromatherapy to keep them awake during long night drives. A month-long Japanese study of aromatherapy found that when the air in an office for keypunch operators was scented with Jasmine, error rates dropped 33%; the scent was also found to increase efficiency and relieve stress among employees.

Lavender, of all the essential oils, has been the most studied by health care providers. Various studies mention the use of lavender on pillows in order to alleviate insomnia, as well as to help ICU patients cope with stress. Another oil, Brazilian guava, has been found to have analgesic effects and is being further investigated. A variety of oils are used for diaper rashes, such as lavender sitz baths, almond oils, and beeswax. Aromatherapies are often recommended for colic. They are believed to reduce infant anxiety as well as parental stress, which many feel plays a role in colic. Could NICU staff use this anxiety-relief and stress reduction technique as well?

Researchers have found that newborns have an acute sense of smell. Indeed, the natural odor that emanates from the mother forms part of the complex bonding process. Dr. Hisanobu Sugano, director of the Life Science Institute at Moa Health Science Foundation in Fukuoka, Japan demonstrated through his numerous studies in subtle energies and aromatherapy that newborns could correctly identify their mothers' milk from nine other specimens. Several other experiments have shown that when used and unused breast pads are placed on either side of the newborn's head, the newborn will turn more often to the side of the used pad. Within a week after birth, the newborn can discern its mother's milk on a breast pad from the milk of other mothers.

The different calming or stimulating effects of CAM therapies could be a fruitful area for further research. With the fragrance perception of newborns, is it possible to manipulate the scents to achieve effects from olfactory stimulants, anxiolytics, or enhanced attachment? In some cultures this process is already done. For instance, Filipino families often leave mother's clothing in the newborn's crib to calm the child in her absence. Could we use peppermint in isolettes as an "olfactory caffeine"—a stimulant to minimize or eliminate apnea and bradycardia events in preemies? Could we use lavender rather than sedatives for sleep? Could chamomile help regulate sleep-wake cycles? If a newborn is having sleepless nights, might this be mitigated using olfaction?

Music Therapy

For several years now of media attention has turned toward what is called the Mozart effect, which in our field has focused on music used to soothe and stimulate developing infants in addition to its use in the in utero state. (Campbell, 1997). For the past 10 years, music therapy has been used in the NICU to mediate stress and promote positive development. We know that by the eighteenth week of gestation the auditory capabilities of the fetus are present (Cheour-Luhtanen et al, 1996). Some studies have measured heart rate changes in the fetus, even at this early age, when exposed to certain music through the womb. Lullabies have been linked with infants for as long as history. Music therapy carries this tradition over into the NICU. When music is used as a therapy after birth, it is defined as the use of controlled music given at certain intervals and doses.

Music therapy aims to produce quiet, regular rhythms. Music has been shown to promote neurological development and to promote language development if words accompany the music (Standley, 2001; Wagner, 1994). Music with or without vocalization has been shown to sooth a crying infant or to decrease a heart rate and increase oxygen saturation levels (Caine, 1991; Cassidy & Standley, 1995; Standley, 1998). In the first meta-analysis of music therapy studies of premature infants, Standley (2001) reported that the observed state, heart and respiratory rates, oxygen saturation levels, weight gain, length of stay, feeding rate, and nonnutritive sucking rates were all positively influenced by music therapy. Music may even alleviate some of the distress that ambient noise in the NICU may cause (see Chapter 16). Attempts have been made to cover the noise in the NICU by using sound to negate other sounds. These masks are aimed at sound reduction as well as minimizing vestibular stimulation. Hospital noise is markedly differently from in utero acoustics or from the sound of soothing music (Ernst, 1996).

Based on experience rather than evidence from controlled studies, Standley (2001), a certified music therapist, suggests the following guidelines for music in the NICU:

Music Selection: sounds in the NICU should be soothing, constant, stable, and relatively unchanging to reduce alerting responses

Volume level: in the 65 to 70 dB (Scale C) range is recommended. *Note: male hearing acuity is less developed than female acuity.*

Maximum time/day for continuously playing music: 1.5 hours (alternating ½ hour on and ½ hour off).

Approval for auditory stimuli: daily approval of the nurse providing care to the infant should be obtained for provision of music stimulation*

Light Therapy

This area of research is just beginning to flourish. Certainly, neonatologists have done much to show the scientific significance of phototherapy. Aside from the classically recognized effects of diminishing bilirubin and activation of vitamin D, numerous studies have shown this therapy's effect on thyroid stimulation alterations in renal and vascular parameters, increased gut transit times, and a host of other metabolic alterations. Could it be such an intellectual challenge to think that other wavelengths of light might have other physiological effects? This is the basis for the field of color and light therapy.

For the last few years regulation of ambient lighting in the NICU has been a major concern. Research in this area falls under the category of NICU design and is discussed in the NICU environment chapter in this text. Constant exposure to light can result in disorganization of the infant's state (Jones et al, 2001; Rivkees, 1997). For this reason, procedural lighting and blanket covers are used to shield infants in isolettes from direct light. More research is needed to determine whether light therapy—exposing the infant to varying light cycles—alters Circadian rhythms or physiologic stability. The rationale for studies of the effects of light on the neonate is to determine its effects on endocrine functions. Assessing and stretching our current understanding could expand light, color, and/or other wavelengths for newborns and staff.

Kangaroo Care

Kangaroo Care (KC) started in the mountains of Bogata, Columbia, about 20 years ago. It builds on a practice that may

---

*Used with permission from Standley J (2001). Music Therapy for the Neonate. *Newborn and Infant Nursing Reviews*, 1(4), 211-216.

be older than recorded history. The intervention was to place the newborn skin-to-maternal skin, usually on the chest between the mother's breasts. Mothers used it as a means to keep a newborn warm. For the last decade skin-to-skin care has undergone numerous studies to determine its effect on physiologic stability and bonding. The two best-known researchers in this area are Drs. Gene Cranston Anderson (1989, 1991) and Susan Luddington-Hoe (1993, 1996). Engler and Ludington-Hoe (1999) conducted a survey of 1133 NICUs known to exist in the United States to determine what percentage of those NICUs used KC. They found 82% of the units practiced some form of skin-to-skin care.

To date, studies indicate that KC can positively affect both the mother and the infant. When a parent holds the infant against his or her skin, the infant's breathing, oxygen saturation, and heart rate become more regular; the flexion and tone improve; and the sleep state becomes less disorganized (Gale et al, 1993). KC seems to promote not only a sensory dialogue for the infant and caregiver but also a method of central nervous system regulation of the autonomic motor and state systems. Mounting evidence in favor of KC to promote physiologic stability encouraged more studies of this therapy with very immature, unstable infants (Eichel, 2001). Future studies most likely will focus on specific subsets of neonates and the effects it has on physiologic stability and length of stay.

Co-bedding

Co-bedding of twins and higher order multiples (HOM) is a growing practice. The rationale is that during their gestational development, multiple-gestation fetuses lived side-by-side. Once born, they are normally separated and put in a single beds, partly because of concerns over infection and because of the size of standard infant beds. Studies that are underway examine the practice of co-bedding on physiologic stability, soothing, motoric organization, proprioceptive stimulation, and enhanced growth (Altimier & Lutes, 2001). One completed study (Altimier & Lutes, 2001) focused on premature twins and higher-order multiples admitted to a large Midwestern tertiary center. Twenty-three sets of twins, 4 sets of triplets, and 1 set of quadruplets were included. The control group consisted of 15 sets of twins, 7 sets of triplets, and 2 sets of quadruplets. A randomized control design was used. All infants were infection-free, weighed less than 1500 grams, and were admitted to a NICU. The following co-bedding protocol was followed:

Twins and HOM being cared for in the same NICU were put together when stability was achieved.

Oxygen requirement was limited to nasal cannula only.

IVs, gavage feeding, cardiopulmonary monitoring, pulse oximetry, and phototherapy were permitted.

All equipment, clothing, and chart forms were color-coded to match each twin/multiple. The twins and HOM wore hospital identification bands at all times.

Positioning of twins or HOM in the womb was replicated, if this was known. Otherwise, siblings were placed them side-by-side, facing each other, facing the other one's back, or in a head-to-toes position. Repositioning of one or more infants was considered if infant(s) appeared restless.

One blanket was lightly swaddled around the twins and HOM; hands were free to reach their own face or a sibling to facilitate each other's motor organization.

Care giving was clustered to address all infants' needs during the same interaction. (Infant in most awake state received care first).

If one infant demonstrated temperature instability, the temperature probe was placed on that infant, otherwise on the smallest infant. All infants were dressed/undressed depending on their individualized thermoregulatory needs.*

The results demonstrated that the co-bedded group had a more positive growth rate in grams and in head circumference than the control group. No differences in nosocomial rates or in thermal needs were noted between the two groups (Altimier, Lutes, 2001). More research is needed in this area to substantiate these findings. Cobedding is considered a developmentally supportive care strategy (Nyqvist & Lutes, 1998). Before this therapy is completely embraced, further research needs to determine the benefits and safety in this population of neonates.

Infant Massage

Massage develops the expression of our first language—touch. There are many types of massage from the gentle, superficial, friction, pressure, kneading, containment, vibration and percussion to the more intense manipulations of Rolfing.

Infant massage has been the focus of many research studies. However, most have been done on fullterm, healthy newborns. Recently infant massage has been used in the neonatal units on infants who are in the recovery phase of their treatment. Researchers have focused on massage as a way to reduce stress and to increase bonding/attachment when a parent performs massage.

Fields (1995) has promoted extensive research in infant massage since the 1970s. She has focused much of her research on the premature infant. Nevertheless, she found that massaged infants have a 47% greater weight gain and better-organized sleep states; moreover, they are more responsive to social stimulation, have more organized motor development, and are commonly discharged 6 to 10 days earlier from the hospital. This allows the newborn to go home earlier and also alleviates significant cost for the parents. Kirpatrick (2001, personal communication) has found in her NICU experience that massage helps postoperative edema through stimulation of cardiac and lymphatic activity and decreases the need for postoperative narcotics. This action leads to a more organized physiological state.

Field's study (1995) of cocaine-exposed newborns suggests that touch therapy increases vagal activity, which in turn releases the food absorption hormones gastrin and insulin, which may explain the weight gain in the premature infant. Massage stimulates the parasympathetic nervous system. If an infant is more attentive, it may follow that more stimulation from the parent is elicited, thus improving the dyad interactions and performance on the infant developmental assessment tools (Fields, 1995). Infant massage also depends on respect for the infant's readiness. Consideration of timing and readiness for infant massage is very important. Massage should be state-dependent; for example, the deep sleep state is not the best time for a massage. A time when the infant is fussy, however, may be the perfect time. Being aware of the baby and his or her receptivity and alertness is important in determining the best time for a massage rather than relying on a predetermined time. The type and amount of massage depends on the infant's gestational age, degree of illness or stability, and ability to engage.

---

*Used with permission from Altimier L, Lutes L (2001). Cobedding Multiples. *Newborn and Infant Nursing Reviews*, 1(4), 205-206.

Field has also suggested many benefits to the "massager"—such as lower stress hormone levels and decreased depression.

Uses of massage are expanding and undergoing research. Concerns as to whether infant massage can produce overstimulation and therefore adverse effects have been raised. Further research is needed through controlled trials to determine the benefits as well as the risks of this alternative therapy.

Reflexology

Reflexology is an ancient form of healing, somewhat similar to traditional acupuncture. It is a healing method based on the principle that there are reflexes in the hands and feet specific to each organ, gland, function, and part of the human body. The goal of reflexology is to stop or reverse the negative chain reactions that occur within the mind-body and to restore the energy balance. Applying pressure to these points can also bring about stress relief by improving circulation and minimizing pain. This modality can be considered the opposite of the heelstick blood draw; it involves the same area but a reverse technique.

The presumed mechanisms in reflexology, from a Western medical perspective, are: 1) that the treatment of reflex zones stimulates the body's blood flow; 2) that pressure to these points increases the body's production of endorphins; and 3) that it assists in the elimination of waste materials (Launso, 1995). However, research strongly suggests the presence of a mind-body link in which psychological and physical aspects are indivisible (Pert, 1986). Reflexologists believe that health problems occur when the flow of life energy (chi) is blocked or disturbed and that it is alleviated when the flow of chi is restored by manipulation of the reflex points.

Reflexology may be useful in a neonatal unit to help balance and soothe the patient's bioenergy, which might decrease periods of fussiness or disorganization. Reflexology may also benefit the infant by increasing blood flow to specific organ sites, increasing perfusion to the kidneys, and increasing cardiac output.

Osteopathy/Cranio-Sacral Therapy

Osteopathy is a system of medicine based on the premise that the body has within it an inherent therapeutic potency. The body is its own medicine chest. Most of the biomechanical manipulations in the pediatric osteopathic community come under the healing category of cranio-sacral therapy. A practitioner of cranial-sacral therapy works with the subtle pressure fluctuations of the cerebral-spinal fluid to optimize a patient's health. Moreover, a practitioner may gently realign cranial bones to bring them into the proper relationship.

Osteopaths believe that many problems begin at birth. They feel that birth (labor and delivery) is one of the most traumatic experiences and that skeletal strains on the newborn can cause problems throughout life. Recognition and treatment of these dysfunctions in the immediate postpartum period is considered an essential preventative measure. In the cranio-sacral system, misalignment of structure that is not corrected can lead to potential alterations in function. The occipital area is believed to sustain most of the trauma during delivery. A complex study by Frymann (1998) explores the relationship between symptomotology in the newborn and the anatomic physiologic disturbances of the CS system. The study suggests that strains within the unfused fragments of the occipital bones produce problems in the nervous system (i.e., vomiting), hyperactive parastalsis, tremor, hypertonicity, and irritability. Frymann (1998) reports that compression of the

hypoglossal nerve can cause newborn's failure to grasp the nipple and suck effectively. If symptoms are left untreated, these newborns may exhibit tongue thrust and may have deviant swallowing patterns, speech problems, and even malocclusion. Problems such as sucking-swallowing difficulties and recurrent reflux after birth are so common that many mothers and doctors consider them to be normal. According to cranial sacral theory, these can be easily rectified. When the vagus nerve is compressed, for example, recurrent vomiting or reflux can occur. Decompress the condylar parts of the occiput, and the vomiting stops. If descending motor tracks are compromised, the newborn may cry incessantly and grow up to have attention deficit syndrome. In temporal bone development, misalignment may cause recurrent otitis media. If the sphenoids are involved, the child may have headaches. Until the structural cause of the problem is recognized and addressed, the underlying pathophysiology will not change. Osteopaths often feel that every child should be structurally evaluated after any type of trauma, especially birth.

This field presents some interesting opportunities for research. What portals of understanding could this field open in this search for intraventricular hemorrhage (IVH)? Little progress has been made in understanding the etiology or evolvement of IVH. Could daily CS therapy assist in developing a more womblike analogue for brain and spinal development? Could they palpate and help guide the developmental energies in the CS system by tuning in with their "knowing fingers," tracking the system to retrace its normal developmental pattern, and bringing the memory of health to play? As osteopathy's founder, Dr. Andrew Still, once said, "To find health should be the objective of the doctor. Anyone can find a disease."

BIOENERGETIC THERAPIES

Acupuncture

Acupuncture is part of a complex system known as traditional Chinese medicine (TCM) that has been practiced in China for some two thousands years. This is an energy-based approach to a patient rather than a disease-oriented diagnostic and treatment model. The main concept behind this system is that of energy in the body called chi (immeasurable by current instrumentation in Western science) (Chien et al, 1991; Freeman, 2001a), which underlies and supports all aspects of the physical body. This energy circulates throughout the body along specific pathways called meridians. Obstructions in the flow of chi may cause disease. Acupuncturists rebalance the flow of energy by gently placing thin, solid, disposable, metallic needles into the skin along the meridians where chi is blocked. These needles are either briefly left in place or are stimulated with electricity heat, laser, or moxibustion (burning of the moxa herb over the acupuncture point).

Acupuncture has shown promising results in use for anesthesia, postoperative pain, and addiction recovery. In the West, acupuncture has been used since the early 1970s for various forms of addiction and withdrawal in expectant mothers (Bullock et al, 1989) as well as for infants to help reduce the residual effects of drug exposure in cases of prenatal substance abuse (Brumbaugh, 1993). Researchers are currently considering whether acupuncture can help treat colic, constipation, diminished postoperative urine output, apnea, and bradycardia as well as whether it can improve cardiac output and control postoperative pain. Currently in China, acupuncture is used to treat infants with jaundice (augmenting hepatic chi), skin problems, teething, ear infections, constipation, conjunctivitis, and peripheral nerve injury (Jun et al, 1995).

Acupressure, which is similar to acupuncture, appears more popular in pediatric patients because it does not involve the use of needles. Acupressure involves applying pressure at acupuncture points along the 14 major energy meridians to promote the flow of chi. Numerous studies show that acupressure, like acupuncture, stimulates physical reactions in the body, such as changes in brain activity and blood chemistries, in addition to enhancing immune and endocrine functions.

Healing Touch

Healing touch (HT) is an energy-based therapy developed by Mentgen and the American Holistic Nurses Association in the late 1980s; its practitioners are certified. It is another therapy that reaches out to the essence of being human—that is, our desire to be touched. Touch conveys and connotes caring and is the way parents and children have bonded throughout history. It is a way for nurses to convey to their patients and families that they care for them as people. Using touch as a therapy requires a belief that the human being is an energy system that can be balanced through touch. Along with traditional medicine, healing touch promotes a calm, restful state and relieves discomfort, which helps support the body, mind, and spirit's natural healing process. Healing occurs as the energy system returns to a state of balance (Wardell & Mentgen, 1999).

This therapy is considered experimental and requires parental consent. During a HT session infants are not to be disturbed. They usually are scheduled for at least two sessions per week that last from 15 to 40 minutes. HT consists first of a hand scan to assess the infant's condition. This assessment is done by gently and slowly moving a hand from head to toes to detect changes in the infant's energy field. Once the assessment is completed, a variety of techniques can be used: energy field centering, comfort infusion, energy infusion or modulation, modified magnetic unruffling, spiral healing light, and halo. All of these use the hands-on or moving of the hands over the body to balance the energy field of the infant. Comfort infusion is a technique that parents can be taught. It is believed to relieve pain by draining the pain away. Parents place the left palm over the infant, encouraging the pain to move through their palm up through their body and out their right hand. When parents no longer sense pain, the right hand is placed palm on or over the infant and the left one turned upward to infuse healing energy. This technique empowers parents to actively participate in care of their infants.

In any of these modes, the infant may be observed to calm down (if unsettled before HT), relax, and even fall into a sleep state. The spiral healing light uses a visualized light beam for those infants who are very compromised. A beam of healing light is visualized flowing through the crown chakra "energy center" down the arm and out the first two fingers and thumb as they are held together. Starting at the center of the infant's body, the beam is slowly directed in a clockwise spiral that expands to cover the whole body. The healing light touches every cell of the body and infuses healing energy. When the edges of the body are reached, the spiral is brought back to the center of the body while the practitioner visualizes the healing beam of light, thus giving the infant strength and energy to help the cells release excess fluid, carbon dioxide, bilirubin, or infection. When the center of the body is reached, a clear blue healing light is visualized as flowing through the practitioner's hand and is held over the infant's crown, thus washing away what has been released.

Energy-based healing is growing in popularity in hospitals and medical and nursing school curricula around the country. Results of completed healing touch studies support its use in depression, cancer, pain, and other conditions. It adds a spiritual dimension to our increasingly high-tech health care system.

Reiki

Reiki is another form of energy healing. Energy is transferred from the hands of a practitioner to a patient using a sequence of hand positions above the body. The objectives of Reiki are to restore the body's energy balance and flow, assisting with the natural ability of the body to heal itself, provide relaxation, reduce stress levels, and enhance the feeling of overall well-being, similar to HT. Stein (1995) explains that Reiki relaxes and heals by clearing energy meridians and chakras (vortices of energy along the spine), thus restoring balance, relieving pain, and accelerating the healing process. Respiration slows; blood pressure decreases; emotional clearing and calming occurs. Blockages are dissolved and the vibrational frequency of the body increases.

Few studies of Reiki have been done in the United States. In one 1998 study of Reiki in New Hampshire, more than 872 patients underwent a 15-minute Reiki treatment both before and after surgery (Alandydy & Alandydy, 1999). The patients reported an increased sense of relaxation, reduction in stress, and a possible enhancement of the natural healing ability of their bodies.

Reiki treatments are applicable for pregnancy and infancy in many situations. Simply increasing relaxation and improve the body's healing ability could be valuable in many circumstances. Additionally, Reiki could be used to assist in babies who are recovering from acute infections to enhance respiratory efforts and possibly decrease bronchial spasms. Reiki treatments can enhance circulation and perfusion and provide a calming atmosphere for the infant.

BIOCHEMICAL INTERVENTIONS

Homeopathy

Respecting the innate wisdom of the body is the basic idea behind homeopathy. The premise is to honor the symptoms of illness that one's body experiences as it responds to defend, heal, and/or protect itself against stress or infection. The way a homeopath views this process is that the body's internal wisdom will defend and heal itself by choosing a beneficial response. Homeopathy is based on the "like cures, like principle:" a symptom in a patient is treated with a remedy that causes this same symptom, thus further stimulating the body's current responses. Homeopaths explain that when a truly effective therapy is underway, a temporary exacerbation of certain symptoms may appear. This idea contrasts with the suppression theory of conventional medicine, which homeopaths feel works on disease suppression rather than elimination. A homeopath's use of the principle of similars tries to minimize the wisdom of the body rather than suppress its symptoms (Ullman, 1999). Homeopathic remedies are an enigma to those unaware of the concepts of the energetic memory of water, the potentizing successions or "vigorous stimulation," that enhances the memory of the water, which appears to physical science as a mere series of dilutions.

A review of 89 clinical studies showed that patients who were given a homeopathic medicine were 2.45 times more likely to improve than those who received placebos. (Linde et al, 1997). These findings were based on the efficacy of homeopathic remedies in healing and treating a variety of conditions such as asthma, ear infections, childbirth, postsurgical complications, sprains, and rheumatoid arthritis.

Homeopathy can be considered a catalyst to "jump start" the body and its healing process. Professional homeopaths prescribe medicine that is very patient-specific and is based on that patient's past health history, past medical treatments, genetic inheritance, and the totality of the physical, emotional, and mental/spiritual symptoms. Unfortunately, titrating individualized medicine(s) for everyone, especially newborns, is not always easy. It sometimes takes more than a single visit to a homeopath to find the correct remedy to start the healing process (Linde et al, 1997). Chubby babies require different constitutional remedies from small or low birth-rate babies, as do babies who sleep through the night compared to those who do not. Some research on homeopathic remedies for pregnant women has been done. One must keep in mind that a mother who receives homeopathic remedies during pregnancy and childbirth will pass its benefits onto the fetus. Postnatal treatment of the mother will also benefit the child if he or she is breastfed (Linde et al, 1997).

Infants that endure traumatic labors with bruising or other injury (i.e., postnatal IV infiltrates) are considered to benefit from a remedy called arnica, which aims to optimize the body's attempts to heal its wounds, both physical and psychological. In addition to arnica, hypericum perforadtum can be used for IV burns for the mother or newborn during hospitalization.

Homeopathic remedies such as arnica, staphysagria, and calendula can help circumcised newborns heal from the physical and psychological trauma of circumcision. Chamomilla is the most effective of many remedies suggested for colic and is also the most common remedy for teething pain in older infants. Other remedies for teething pain may include calcarea carbonica, calcarea phosphorica, and silicea. Magnesium phosphorica relieves the symptoms of gas, bloating, and burping. Nux vomica may be used when the woman has ingested alcohol or therapeutic or recreational drugs and the newborn exhibits colicky behavior. Aethusa is used for newborns who are intolerant of milk or who reflux shortly after milk has been ingested. Calendula given externally for diaper rash will soothe the newborn's bottom and help fight infection. In Europe, carbovege is a homeopathic remedy used for apnea and bradycardia in the infant. Homeopathy offers much to learn and much that health care professionals could assimilate into our practices to broaden current medical understandings.

HERBAL MEDICINE

The use of botanical medicine is ancient. Hippocrates (466-377 B.C.) integrated herbal medicine into his teaching and his practice. The World Health Organization estimates that about 75% of the world population relies on botanical medicines; indeed, 30% of Americans also use botanical remedies, and the practice is growing in popularity (Aketele, 1985, Barrett et al, 1999; Duke, 1991). Substances first isolated from plants account for approximately 25% of the Western pharmacopoeia and another 25% is derived from modification of chemicals first found in natural products (Barrett et al, 1999; Freeman, 2001b). Digitalis, the ever-popular echinacea, and caffeine are all are herbal and have effects and side effects (Boullata & Nace, 2000).

It behooves health care professionals to be familiar with the expanding field of herbal medicine. "Historically, economically, theoretically, and methodologically, herbal medicine (Phytomedicine) occupies a unique position in the growing debate surrounding the use of complementary and alternative medicine (CAM)."

The bulk of phytomedicineal research has been conducted in Germany, where the medical and social culture accepts herbal medicine. In Germany, tens of millions of prescriptions are written for herbal medicines each year, and tens of millions more over-the-counter treatment courses are self-directed. In the United States herbal medicines are classified as food supplements and are often available without a prescription. They receive minimal regulatory governing from the Food and Drug Administration. Herbal remedies sold in the United States require no proof of efficacy, safety, potency, or standardization and may vary considerably from brand to brand (Gurley et al, 2000; ISMP, 1998; Klepser & Klepser, 1999). For instance, a sampling of 24% of over 2600 traditional Chinese medicines (herbs) at the Institute for Safe Medicine contained a therapeutic drug adulterant, and over 50% contained two or more adulterants—including antiinflammatory, analgesic, and diuretic agents (Huang et al, 1997). moreover, some Americans mistakenly believe that a natural herb is necessarily a safe herb. On the contrary, some are potent drugs (Barrett et al, 2001). In taking family history, nurses should ask whether any herbal substances are regularly used or were used during pregnancy. Knowing what, if any, herbal remedies nursing mothers use is essential, because the substances can be passed through breast milk to children.

With some imagination, the scope for herbal medicine could be integrated into current practice. Parents of neonates have been known to ask about aloe vera as a skin protectant or for its use with burns and skin irritations, as it has long been used as a folk remedy. Other creams made from comfrey, platain, or marigold can be used for rashes and cradle cap. Calendula is used in Russia for conjunctivitis. Tree tea oil is an antifungal. Dandelion has diuretic properties, and chamomile is an antispasmatic, as are herbs like valerian, fennel, antiseed, and cardamon. Peppermint stimulates bile flow and lowers lower-esophageal spinetic pressure. Milk thistle increases enterohepetic circulation. Tripola increases intestinal peristalsis. Kava can be used to induce oral numbness, which would be helpful with endotracheal tube discomfort. St. John's wort is used for nervous unrest and for its more common use, depression. Immune stimulants such as echinacea and astragalus and all of the herbs in this discussion will surely be studied more extensively in adults before their use is standardized for children and infants. For gastrointestinal problems, for example, the aim in herbal medicine is to relax the abdominal musculature through the use of carminative and antispasmodic herbs such as fennel, aniseed, or cardamon. Caffeine is the leading herb therapy in the United States and is used for apnea and bradycardia in infants. Marked expansion can come out of photomedicines if we remain open-minded to the worldwide wisdom accrued through its extensive use.

RESEARCH

CAM is growing in its use in neonatal care. Unfortunately, for a variety of reasons, little systematic research has supported its use. We need to encourage our researchers to conduct the studies necessary to move these modalities safely into the mainstream. Currently, many in the medical community condemn these therapies without even making a genuine scientific inquiry into their efficacy. As health professionals we can either help gain the evidence to support these practices or watch them be incorporated in possibly unsystematic, unhealthy ways.

Because of the lack of broad research in these areas, many aspects of how CAM therapies work are not yet fully understood from a Western perspective. Nevertheless, some exciting developments have occurred. Thus far, much of the research on CAM has focused on psychoneuroimmunology (PNI) effects and have examined how various complementary therapies affect the stress response. For many years bench researchers have studied stress responses in animals and in humans. We know that two pathways mediate the body's response to a stress. These are the sympathetic-adrendal-medullary (SAM) pathway and the hypothalamic-pituitary-adrenal (HPA) pathway. Each feeds information into the body to put it in "flight or fright" or "calm" mode. In the newborn a stressor such as a cool environment within the delivery room activates the stress response pathway. The body responds by releasing cortisol. This in turn activates the hypothalamus, which either sends signals down directly to the body via SAM or indirectly through the HPA axis. If SAM is followed, the sympathetic pathway is activated and stimulates the adrenal medulla and then the sympathetic postganglionic neurons. Finally, norepinehrine is released. If the HPA axis is stimulated, the anterior pituitary is stimulated; adrenal cortex follows; and finally cortisol is released. Often these events are used as outcome measures in CAM research. (Figure 44-1).

As research continues, CAM therapies may give us many new insights into the nature of the mind-body and the overall complexities of health and healing. For instance, if no biochemical mechanisms exist in some CAM therapies, what are the mechanisms of action? If it is subtle energy, what can we do to measure it? Some scientists for example, have begun to look at the heart rhythms and brain waves of energy healers to detect subtle changes in the overall patterning. In other cases, researchers are turning to double-blind studies to determine whether a CAM therapy is effective, even if the mechanism through which it works is not yet understood. CAM therapies have been traditionally viewed with suspicion by mainstream medicine. However, researchers and practitioners increasingly are looking at these therapies as new areas for scientific inquiry and discovery.

SUMMARY

We must ask questions but remain open to the way we find answers. Modern culture is predisposed to expect answers upon demand. CAM therapies show us that how we think—not just what we think—affects medical progress. We believe that CAM has important potential for the health care field; CAM therapies are relevant to current medical practice because of their global applicability and our need to understand their impact. It is exciting to observe the complexion of our profession changing so dramatically. The process can be infectiously inspiring as the search for a new sense in health care is struggling to be born. The information of this article is merely the tip of an iceberg.

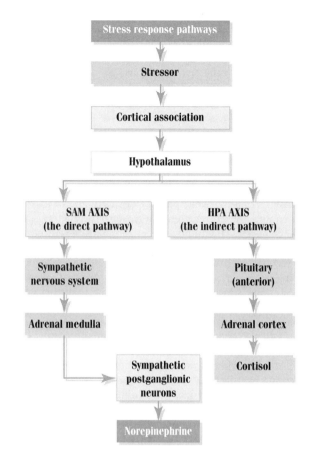

FIGURE **44-1**

Stress response pathways. From Freeman LW, Lawlis GF (2001). *Mosby's complementary and alternative medicine: a research-based approach*, St Louis: Mosby.

REFERENCES

Aketele O (1985). The WHO Traditional Medicine Program: Policy and Implementation. International Traditional Health Newsletter, 1(1), Geneve, Switzerland: World Health Organization.

Alandydy P, Alandydy K (1999). Performance brief: using reiki to support surgical patients. *Journal of nursing care & quality*, 13(4):89-91.

Altimier L, Lutes L (2001). Cobedding multiples. *Newborn and infant nursing reviews*, 1(4), 205-206.

Anderson GC (1989) Skin-to-skin: kangaroo care in Western Europe. *American journal of nursing*, 89, 662-666.

Anderson GC (1991). Current knowledge about skin-to-skin (Kangaroo) care for preterm infants. *Journal of perinatology*, 11 (3), 216-226.

Barrett B et al (1999). Assessing the risks and benefits of herbal medicine: an overview of scientific evidence. *Alternative therapies*, 5(4), 40-49.

Barrett S et al (2001). The herbal minefield. http://www.quackwatch.com/01QuackertyRelatedTopics/herbs.html.

Boullata JL, Nace AM (2000). Safety issues with herbal medicine. *Pharmacolotherapy*, 20, 257-269.

Brumbaugh AG (1993). Acupuncture: new perspectives in chemical dependency treatment. *Journal of substance abuse treatment*, 10(1), 35-43.

Bullock ML et al (1989). Controlled trial of acupuncture for severe recidivistic alcoholism. *Lancet* 1, 1435-1439.

Caine J (1991). The effects of music on the selected stress behaviors, weight, caloric and formula intake, and length of hospital stay of premature and low birth weight neonates in a newborn intensive care unit. *Journal of music therapy*, 28, 180-192.

Campbell D (1997). *The Mozart effect*. New York: Avon Press.

Cassidy JW, Standley JM (1995). The effect of music listening on physiological responses of premature infants in the NICU. *Journal of music therapy*, 32, 208-227.

Cheour-Luhtanen M et al (1996). The ontogenetically earliest discriminative response of the human brain. *Psyhcophysiology*, 33, 478-481.

Chien CH et al (1991). Effect of emitted bioenergy on biochemical functions of cells. *American journal of Chinese medicine*, 19(3-4), 285-292.

Duke JA (1991). Promising phytomedicinals. *Journal of naturopathic medicine*, 2, 48-52.

Eichel P (2001). Kangaroo care. *Newborn and infant nursing reviews*, 1(4), 224-228.

Eisenberg DM et al (1998). Trends in CAM use in the United States, 1990-1997: results of a follow-up national survey, *Journal of the American Medical Association*, 280, 1569-1575.

Engler A, Ludington SM (1999). Kangaroo care in the United States: a national survey. *Journal of investigative medicine*, 47(2), 168A.

Ernst E (1996). *Complementary medicine: an objective appraisal*. Oxford, England: Butterworth-Heinemann.

Fields TM (Ed.) (1995). *Touch in early development*. Mahwah, NJ: Lawrence Erlbaum Associates.

Freeman LW (2001a). Acupuncture. In Freeman LW, Lawlis GF (Eds.) *Mosby's complementary and alternative medicine: a research-based approach*. St Louis, Mosby.

Freeman LW (2001b). Herbs as medical intervention. In Freeman LW, Lawlis GF (Eds.) *Mosby's complementary and alternative medicine: a research-based approach*. St Louis, Mosby.

Frymann VM (1998). *The collected papers of Viola M. Frymann, DO: legacy of osteopathy to children*. Ann Arbor, MI: Edward Brothers, Inc.

Gale G et al (1993). Skin-to-skin (kangaroo) holding of the intubated premature infant. *Neonatal network*, 12(6), 49-57.

Gurley BJ et al (2000). Content versus label claims in ephedra-containing dietary supplements. *American journal of health-systems pharmacy*, 57, 963-969.

Huang WF et al (1997). Adulteration by synthetic therapeutic substances of traditional Chinese medicines in Taiwan. *Journal of clinical pharmacology*, 37, 344-350.

Institution for Safe Medication Practices (ISMP). (1998). An overview of herbal medicines and adverse events. ISMP Medication Safety Alert! August 26, 1998. http://www.ismp.org

Jones J et al (2001). Complementary care alternatives for the NICU. *Newborn and infant nursing reviews*, 1(4), 207-210.

Jun H et al (1995). Electric acupuncture treatment of peripheral nerve injury. *Journal of traditional Chinese medicine*, 15(2), 114-117.

Kirpatrick G (2001). Personal Communication.

Klepser BT, Klepser ME (1999). Unsafe and potentially safe herbal therapies. *American journal of health-systems pharmacy*, 56, 125-138.

Launso L (1995). A description of reflexology practice and clientele in Denmark. *Complementary therapy medicine*, 3(4), 206-211.

Linde K et al (1997). Are the clinical effects of homeopathy placebo effects? Metaanaylsis of placebo-controlled trials. *Lancet*, 350 (9081), 834-843.

Ludington-Hoe SM, Golant SK (1993). *Kangaroo care: the best you can do for your preterm infant*. New York: Bantam Books.

Ludington-Hoe SM, Swinth J (1996). Developmental aspects of Kangaroo Care. *Journal of obstetric, gynecologic, and neonatal nursing*, 25(8), 691-703.

Nyqvist KH, Lutes LM (1998). Cobedding twins: a developmentally supportive care strategy. *Journal of obstetric, gynecologic, and neonatal nursing*, 27(4), 450-456.

Pert CB (1986). The wisdom of the receptors: neuropeptides, the emotions and bodymind. *Advances*, 3(3): 8-16.

Rivkees SA (1997). Developing circadian rhythmicity. *Pediatric endocrinology*, 44(2), 467-487.

Standley JM (1998). The effect of music and multimodal stimulation on physiologic and developmental responses of premature infants in neonatal intensive care. *Pediatric nursing*, 24, 532-538.

Standley JM (2001). Music therapy for the neonate. *Newborn and infant nursing reviews*, 1(4), 211-216.

Stein D (1995). *Essential reiki*. Freedom, CA: The Crossing Press, Inc.

Ullman D (1999). Homeopathy A-Z. Carlsbad, CA: Hay House, Inc.

Wagner M (1994) *Introductory Musical Acoustics*. Raleigh, NC: Contemporary Publishing.

Wardell DW, Mentgen J (1999). Healing touch: an energy-based approach to healing. *Imprint*, 45(2), 34-35, 51.

CHAPTER

45

SYSTEMATIC ASSESSMENT AND HOME FOLLOW-UP: A BASIS FOR MONITORING THE NEWBORN AND INFANT'S INTEGRATION INTO THE FAMILY

NIA R. JOHNSON-CROWLEY, LANA CONRAD

INTRODUCTION

Going home. For parents invested in the day-to-day struggles of their preterm infant within the neonatal intensive care unit (NICU), those two words are guaranteed to make them sit up and take notice. Comments such as "finally," "You mean we really can take her home—with us?," "I can't believe this!," "You're sure it's OK—you're really sure?," or "I don't believe I'm ready for this." All reflect the joy, disbelief, anxiety, and ambivalence that many of these parents feel. After days, weeks, and possibly months in the NICU, an important goal is finally reached: the child is coming home with them.

During their infants' stays in the hospital, parents come to depend on the supportive environment of the NICU to understand and cope with the behavior and care of their infants. Doctors, nurses, nutritionists, and other hospital personnel have been on hand to ensure that their preterm infant not only survived but survived in the best possible condition, thus setting the stage for as normal a developmental outcome as possible. Knowledge that they must now assume the responsibility that heretofore the hospital personnel assumed for the care of their babies can undermine even the most stalwart person's confidence in his or her parenting ability (Wasserman, 2000). Parents need continued availability of support during the transition between hospital and home and in the ongoing weeks and months as they begin to integrate the new infant into the family unit (Gray et al, 2000). Parents need this support not just for their own confidence but because research has shown that no matter how easy or traumatic the infant's stay in the NICU, the home environment has the greatest influence on how well a given preterm infant develops and thrives from hospital discharge to adolescence (Berlin et al, 1995; Holditch-Davis et al, 2000).

This chapter explores the importance of home follow-up for preterm infants after hospital discharge. Areas discussed include the preterm infant's vulnerability for developing problems that affect later positive outcomes, how parents want and need further monitoring and support when their infant comes home, and the value of nurses in providing this follow-up. The importance of systematic assessment and the use of intervention programs that include the needs of the parents are discussed. Finally, examples of assessments and an intervention program found to be successful with this population are presented.

NEED FOR HOME FOLLOW-UP OF PRETERM INFANTS

It has long been known that disabling neurodevelopmental conditions are prevalent among infants of low birth weight (Blackburn, 1995; Hack et al, 2000; Halsey et al, 1996; Saigal et al, 1999; Thompson et al, 1997). However, research has shown that perinatal and neonatal complications do not account alone for these neurodevelopmental conditions (Holditch-Davis et al, 2000; Magill-Evans & Harrison, 1999). Sameroff (1981), in one of the first reviews of longitudinal studies for this population, found that 20% to 50% of low-birth-weight infants demonstrate developmental problems in later years. In addition, he found that the variables that most strongly predicted these outcomes were measures of the infant's home environment (Sameroff, 1981). Some 30 years later these findings continue to be salient in more recent research (Holditch-Davis et al, 2000; Magill-Evans & Harrison, 1999).

Research studies have provided strong correlations between cognitive development and the quality of a child's care giving relationships and overall environment, for both fullterm and preterm infants (Berlin et al, 1995; Thompson et al, 1997; Zeanah et al, 1997). Although the majority of studies are interested in cognitive development (e.g., language development and school performance), factors which affect these outcomes such as attention problems (impulsiveness, distractibility and hyperactivity)—behaviors which parents and care givers often find problematic—have been less studied. However, Spiker and colleagues (1992) found that preterm infants who grow up in more positive environments—specifically positive social environments—had fewer behavioral problems overall, including attention disorders.

Preterm infants are especially vulnerable because of both their biologic status (i.e., being preterm) and environmental factors that interact to put them at high risk for later problems (Holditch-Davis et al, 2000; Thompson et al, 1994). In fact, Greenberg and Crnic (1988) noted that the preterm infants in their study were more strongly influenced by their environments in terms of positive outcomes than were the fullterm infants. These studies suggest that ensuring positive environmental conditions after discharge is especially important for the promotion of normal development for preterm infants.

Within the home environment, the parent-infant interaction was found to be the best predictive factor for later positive development in preterm infants. Barnard and associates (1989), in their investigation of several research programs that study these interactive qualities for both fullterm and preterm infants, stated that "In general, high-quality interactions during the first years of life tend to be positively linked to the infant's subsequent cognitive and linguistic competence and to more secure attachments to major caregivers." Later research confirms that these findings continue to hold true (Holditch-Davis, 2000; Magill-Evans & Harrison, 1999). Many of these studies identified certain behavioral characteristics that may account for parent-infant interaction difficulties seen in preterm infants and in their parents, thus resulting in less desirable development outcomes. The next section explores these characteristics and their effects on parenting.

PRETERM INFANT CHARACTERISTICS AND THEIR EFFECT ON CAREGIVER INTERACTION

Studies that compare fullterm and preterm infants found preterm infants to be different from their fullterm counterparts in several ways—ways that have a tremendous influence on the parent-infant interaction. First, preterm infants as a group were found to be less neurologically mature than fullterm infants. As a result of this lack of maturity, preterm infants are less regulatory (organized) in their behavior, which makes it harder to understand and predict how they will behave. This lack of neurologic maturity is directly related to how premature they are; the younger the preterm infant gestationally, the less mature and the more disorganized the infant's behavior. Second, preterm infants as a group exhibited a lower level of behavioral social responsiveness, were less persistent and adaptable, and tended to respond to stimuli in more negative ways than did fullterm infants (Magnusson, 1995).

As a result of these characteristics, such infants give hard-to-read cues, thus making it difficult for their parents to know when to feed them, when to soothe them, when to leave them alone, and when to play with them. Preterm infants, sensitive to stimuli and limited in energy reserves, respond to their parents' attempts to interact by turning away, dropping off to sleep, or crying inconsolably; parents see such behavior as negative and difficult to handle and understand. If parent-infant interaction is seen as a sort of dance in which each participant (parent and infant) must give clear and readable cues that can be read by the partner, must be motorically and neurologically alert to respond quickly and positively to the partner's cues, and must retain enough energy to keep the dance going in a smooth and rhythmic way, it is easy to see why interacting (dancing) with a preterm infant may not be the positive experience that most parents expect it to be. Because parents often expect their preterm infants to behave like full-term infants, they become confused when this does not occur. In essence, parents are dancing with a partner who does not hold up his or her side of the dance duo, which results in dyssynchrony and discord. Even the most positive mothers and fathers can lose confidence in their ability to parent. In addition, more recent research suggests that the child as an active participant in the social environment (e.g., this dance), is continuously influencing or self-correcting the flow of this dance or interaction, and in turn is influencing the caregiver and their relationship. Thus "a poor-

quality social environment interferes with self-correction [by the child], and a more positive environment enhances it" (Holditch-Davis et al, 2000).

These characteristics of giving unclear cues and being more negative and less socially responsive may also account for the report by parents of preterm infants that it is more difficult to care for their children and that they have more difficult temperaments than fullterm infants. Several researchers have studied the temperament of preterm infants. In general, their findings suggest that the older (born at 34 to 37 weeks' gestation), heavier (weight, >1200 g), and healthier preterm infants show no differences in temperament from fullterm infants by parent report, whereas the younger (born at less than 34 weeks' gestation), lighter (weight, <1200 g), and sicker preterm infants are described by parents as being more difficult in temperament than those in reports by parents of fullterm infants. Patteson and Barnard (1990), after reviewing several of these studies, concluded that some basis for the report of preterm infants' having a more difficult temperament existed, especially as it related to the lower birth weight infants and those with health problems—specifically, respiratory problems.

Riese (1988), Schraeder and Tobey (1989), and Washington and associates (1986) also studied how stable the preterm infant temperament characteristics were over time. Infants in all three studies averaged 1200 grams and were essentially healthy, growing preterm infants. Findings from Riese (1988) and Washington and associates (1986) suggested that temperament characteristics are less stable for preterm infants than for fullterm infants over the first year of life. Riese reported that by 18 to 24 months, preterm infants were as stable in temperament as the fullterm infants (Riese, 1988; Washington et al, 1986). Schraeder and Tobey's findings (1989) differed; they found preterm infants to be rated as more difficult in temperament characteristics up to 4 years of age. However, this was related to conditions of the home environment. The more optimal and positive the home environment, the less difficult the preterm infant was rated by the parent (Schraeder & Tobey, 1989).

Washington and associates (1986) found temperament ratings to be related to the sensitivity of the parent. Ratings of preterm infants as a group varied throughout the year (i.e., they were less stable); however, the more sensitive the caretaker toward the infant, the less difficult the preterm infant was rated by 12 months of age. Washington and associates (1986) questioned whether altering the environment (i.e., the behavior of the caretaker) changed the caretaker's perception of the infant or whether the infant changed (i.e., became less irritable, more responsive) because the caretaker became more sensitive. Their conclusion was that "temperament, at least early on in life, is not a fixed construct but a reflection both of the changing transactions between caretakers and infants accompanying growth and development, and the discontinuities of the infant's biobehavioral organization" (Washington et al, 1986).

In a later study, Zahr (1991) supported earlier work that found a link between temperament and characteristics of the parent-infant interaction. Studying a set of preterm infant-mother dyads (n = 49) from low socioeconomic backgrounds, Zahr reported that the more positive the mother-infant interaction, the less likely that the child's temperament would be perceived as difficult at 4 and 8 months of age and the more social support the mother had. Although birth weight and length of hospitalization also correlated with the positiveness of mother-infant interaction at 4 months of age, only temperament and social support correlated with how well the infant and mother interacted at 8 months of age (Zahr, 1991).

Thomas and Chess (1977) earlier described this mix of infant characteristics and environmental conditions, such as a sensitive caregiver, a "goodness of fit" between the child and the parent. Schraeder and Tobey suggested enhancing this goodness of fit by having nurses help parents assess and understand their preterm infant's style" of behavior so that parents could better adapt their own behavior and environmental conditions to help the infant adapt and respond better, thus creating a more optimal parent-infant interaction (Schraeder & Tobey, 1989).

More recent studies specifically aimed at determining whether preterm children as a group differ greatly in temperament and behavior from fullterm infants have resulted in conflicting findings. For instance, Gennaro and associates (1992) used secondary analysis of common variables among three cohort study groups to analyze the effects of perinatal factors and NICU influences on infant temperament. Although, as a group, preterm infants in each cohort sample were "significantly more difficult [in temperament] that the comparison groups of fullterm infants," by parent report at 6 months, perinatal variables (mechanical ventilation, length of hospital stay, infant birth weight, and gestational age) did not predict well which infants would be perceived as having a difficult temperament. They found that "infants who were the smallest, sickest, and exposed longest to the multiple, often noxious stimuli in neonatal intensive care nurseries in each cohort were not necessarily the infants who had the most difficult temperaments." They concluded that parents could now be assured that "no particular perinatal or neonatal event contributes to this behavioral style" (Gennaro et al, 1992).

Oberklaid and associates (1991), however, in their longitudinal study of a group of infants found little difference in temperament between preterm and fullterm infants up to age 6 years. Over all the five time periods in which temperament data were gathered (4 and 8 months in infancy and as young toddlers, older toddlers, preschoolers, and early school age children), "the only difference in any temperament rating was in the young toddler age group, when preterm subjects had a tendency to be less intense than control [fullterm] subjects . . . [and] significantly more likely to be rated as having an easy temperament" (Oberklaid et al, 1991).

Researchers of these most recent studies acknowledge that although preterm infants may be described as more difficult in temperament initially, this perception moderates over time. When problems attributed to a more difficult temperament persist, other factors such as maternal depression, stress, infant illness, medical complications, inadequate support systems, and/ or dysfunctional parent-child relationships have been identified as possible correlates. However, how the infant's temperament is influenced by or influences these factors has not been conclusively determined and is a matter for further research (Gennaro et al, 1992; Oberklaid et al, 1991; Zahr, 1991). However, such inconsistency of findings may be due more to difficulties of defining and measuring the trait of temperament, and lack of agreement between caregiver and observer reports of infant temperament.

In conclusion, studies from the past two decades to have compared preterm and fullterm infants and continue to provide evidence that preterm infants have some characteristics, such as harder-to-read behavioral cues, low responsiveness, and less predictability, that may make them seem more difficult in temperament and make it harder for their parents to care for them, especially during the early weeks and months at home. In addition, these characteristics seem to strongly affect the adaptation between these infants and their caregivers. However, parents who are aware, understand, and adapt to the behavioral and temperament characteristics of their preterm infant report that their preterm infants are easier to parent and more enjoyable at later ages. Unfortunately, not all parents are able to adapt. The next section describes four conditions in which parents do not adapt and that may occur more often in families with preterm infants than in families with fullterm infants.

PARENTAL RESPONSE TO THEIR PRETERM INFANT'S BEHAVIOR

Parental burnout, super parent syndrome, vulnerable child syndrome, and higher potential for child abuse are four phenomena described in the literature as maladaptive responses by parents possibly related to the behaviors of preterm infants. Beckwith and Cohen (1980) first described parental burnout in their follow-up study of preterm infants. They found that the level of maternal responsiveness changes over time and is related to the infant's behavior. The more responsive the mother, the more likely the fullterm infant is to be responsive. However, they found that the mothers of preterm infants who had more health problems and who were more premature tended to become less socially responsive over the first year of life. The authors concluded that some reinforcement from the infant was needed to keep the mother responding to her infant's behavior in a positive way. If this reinforcement did not occur, the mother responded less and less over time. Furthermore, they found that the length of time parents will respond is limited without any reinforcement. If no reinforcement is forthcoming, parents become exhausted trying and eventually "burn out" (Beckwith & Cohen, 1980).

Other studies have supported these findings (Zeanah et al, 1997). Holditch-Davis and Thoman (1988) reported similar findings in their study, but they concluded that the early lack of responsiveness and low stimulation by the parent was not maladaptive but appropriate, in view of the preterm infant's low tolerance for stimulation. They cautioned, however, that if this parental behavior continued and did not change as the infant grew older, the infant would suffer developmentally (Holditch-Davis & Thoman, 1988). In their later research, these predictions held, especially when the infant exhibited early developmental problems, such as language delays and low IQ (Holditch-Davis et al, 2000). Beckwith and Cohen's phenomenon of burnout may be the result of the parents' not adapting their behavior to the infant as he or she grew older, as suggested by Holditch-Davis and Thoman. Whatever the reason, these studies suggest the need for monitoring the interaction between the parent and preterm infant.

Maygary (1987), in discussing Beckwith and Cohen's "burnout," described how some parents, when confronted with this low social responsiveness in their infant, become "hyperactive" in their interactions—that is, in compensating for the lower level of social responsiveness of the preterm infant, the parent tries harder and harder to get the infant to respond. As the parent heightens his or her response, the infant withdraws further, becoming less and less responsive in an attempt to deal with the increased stimulation. This "super parent syndrome," as Maygary described it, leads to the parental burnout described by Beckwith and Cohen, in which the parent eventually gives up when the responsiveness needed by the infant does not occur. When maladaptation between the infant and the caregiver occurs, as in the case of parental burnout and the super parent syndrome, the positive integration of the infant into the family unit suffers.

Importantly, studies show that parents can be taught to be more sensitive to their infants, thus preventing many later problems. For instance, when parents are taught about their infant's sleep-wake organization and appropriate ways of responding to their easily overstimulated infant, they provide more sensitive care giving to their infant, and disturbances in the parent-infant interaction such as burnout and super parent syndrome do not occur (Kang et al, 1995; Zelle, 1995).

Vulnerable child syndrome (VCS), a term first coined by Green and Solnit in 1964, has been associated with preterm infants. In this phenomenon, parents continue to see their infants as vulnerable (susceptibility to a negative outcome) despite evidence to the contrary—that the infant is physically and developmentally normal. This results in maladaptive behavior on the part of both the parent (usually the mother) and the infant. Reported parental behaviors include overprotectiveness (i.e., less willingness to leave infant alone, discouragement of infant exploration), skewed perception of the infant's capabilities, and frequent visits to the hospital or clinic. Behaviors reported in infants and children include less exploration, infantilization, separation anxiety, and psychosocial problems such as somatic complaints and problems in school.

However, Scheiner and associates (1985) found no greater degree of overprotectiveness in mothers of preterm infants than they did in mothers of fullterm infants, which led them to suggest that VCS is most likely related to certain personality characteristics of the parent or family and other situational events rather than an infant's prematurity *per se*. A later study by Culley and colleagues (1989) supported the work of Scheiner and associates (1985) and concluded that "illness or prematurity in itself does not lead to the [vulnerable child] syndrome" but that "graduates of the NICU had more concerns about their children's health status than did parents of children born at term." In addition, mothers who had a positive supportive relationship reported less of a sense of vulnerability of their preterm infants (Culley et al, 1989).

Work by Schraeder and associates (1992) that investigated caregivers' perception of vulnerability, parental subjective stress, and child temperament in 39 very-low-birth-weight [VLBW] and 30 normal-birth-weight [NBW] children at 7 years of age found "caregivers of healthy normal school-aged VLBW children did not view their children as more vulnerable than parents of NBW children" (Schraeder et al, 1992). However, caregivers who viewed their children as vulnerable, whether they were VLBW or NBW, perceived their children as more negative in temperament and reported themselves as having higher levels of subjective stress. In addition, no significant correlation between those caregivers who reported more vulnerability in their children and the number of reports of visits and telephone calls to the doctor existed (Schraeder et al, 1992).

Schraeder and associates concluded that "temperament dimensions made significant contributions to parental perceptions of child vulnerability over and above birth weight status, supporting the hypothesis that child temperament is a factor in parental perceptions of child vulnerability" but that further research was needed to determine whether child temperament or parental perception was the antecedent construct. They also surmised from their findings that "it is possible that both parental perceptions of child vulnerability and medical care-seeking behaviors by parents who express fears for the child's health and well-being are responses to stress" and that more research into parental (maternal) depression and anxiety related to stress was needed (Schraeder et al, 1992). Other studies have also reported a link between high levels of stress in families and cognitive and behavioral outcomes of preterm infants (Future of Children, 1998; Thompson et al, 1994).

Another phenomenon reported to be associated with preterm infants is child abuse. As with the other three phenomena discussed, reasons for the increase risk of abuse seem to be the combination of infant behavioral characteristics (irritability, lack of clear cues, and low social responsiveness) and certain parental experiences and characteristics (e.g., lack of social support, history of violence as a child or with a spouse, insensitivity to the child, annoyance or anger when the infant cries). However, rather than reacting with a lack of responsiveness to the infant (parental burnout), an increase in infant stimulation (super parent syndrome), or over protectiveness (vulnerable child syndrome), the parent instead abuses the child (Future of Children, 1998).

THE NEED FOR HOME FOLLOW-UP PROGRAMS

Much evidence supports providing prevention and intervention programs for families with preterm infants. Patteson and Barnard (1990), in a comprehensive review of intervention programs, found 16 of the 19 studies identified had positive outcomes. Elements believed to be effective in producing these positive results included the use of both hospital and home contacts or home contacts alone and the enlistment and involvement of the parent in the intervention and in interaction with the child. Urging further research in the area of infant intervention, Patteson and Barnard (1990) stated that continued focus should be on "testing ways to help parents cope with the emotional crises of having a low-birth-weight infant, enhancing positive interactions with their infant, and increasing their knowledge of infant developmental and care needs."

Many researchers who study preterm infants and their families have supported the findings of Patteson and Barnard for continued monitoring and follow-up for these families after discharge. Several of these researchers themselves have been involved in home intervention studies and demonstrated significant results in the cognitive and behavioral outcomes for preterm infants when the needs of the family and infant are met (Bakewell-Sachs & Porth, 1995; Kang et al, 1995; Zahr, 1994; Zelle, 1995). In addition, continued research with some of these targeted groups, show positive differences as these children mature into adolescents. For instance, Olds and colleagues, in a 15-year follow-up of their nurse home visitation program, reported that adolescents who had been born to women who were unmarried and from families of low socioeconomic status (SES) had fewer episodes of troubling behavior—such as running away, arrests, and convictions than did those in the comparison group. In addition, they engaged in fewer destructive health activities, such as cigarette smoking and alcohol consumption, as well as having fewer sexual partners, than those in the comparison group. The parents of these adolescents also reported fewer behavior problems related to the use of drugs and alcohol (Olds et al, 1998a).

These findings suggest the need for follow-up and assessment of the home environment to identify any characteristics or situations that might lead to the maladaptive behaviors previously described. In addition, research from the last 30 years has given us a pretty good idea of what kinds of follow-up is needed and how best to deliver it. For this to occur, agencies and health care providers must be persuaded to the need for follow-up and assessment in the home. Once assessment has been completed, intervention strategies can be identified to assist families in recognizing and understanding the behavior of their infants and in meeting the needs of both the infants and the families. The question becomes "are parents interested in follow-up, and if so, what kind do they want and need?" This next section explores that question.

NEEDS OF PARENTS WITH A PRETERM INFANT: WHAT DO THEY WANT AND NEED? WHAT ARE THEY GETTING?

The birth of an infant is a major event in the life of a family. Researchers have documented that the parenting role begins in pregnancy and evolves throughout the first weeks and months at home (Bryan, 2000; Schumacher & Meleis, 1994). The first year of life has been shown to be a critical time for the adaptation of a new infant into the family milieu. This adaptation requires enormous amounts of energy and adjustment on the part of the parents and does not always occur smoothly. As discussed previously, preterm infants seem especially vulnerable to this adaptation process because of the conditions of birth and certain characteristics that affect the care giving they receive. Parental care giving characteristics have a significant impact on the positive development of their children, either fullterm or preterm (Zeanah et al, 1997). Parental perception and support play a critical role in determining the effectiveness of the care giving provided infants. Therefore, examining what parents of preterm infants encounter during the first few weeks and months at home, what they need to provide growth-fostering care to their infant, and what they feel they actually are receiving is important.

Parents of preterm infants convey that their parenting is different than with a fullterm infant. Rather than a time of joy, the birth of a preterm baby is one of fear and anxiety. Rather than a process of parental role development, it is a process of grief, dominated by feelings of loss, anger, and resentment. Although hope emerges as the infant survives, these fragile threads can be broken and destroyed should a setback occur. Although parents anxiously await the first feelings of attachment to their infant, other feelings such as shame and guilt may emerge from their lack of affective responses to the "little stranger" in the NICU. Rather than a responsive, alert infant, parents are faced with an infant whose response to parental touch and voice is one of withdrawal and bodily system overload. As lights flash, bells ring, buzzers go off, and hospital personnel rush to intervene with the infant's decreased heart rate and lack of breathing, parents learn firsthand what they subconsciously believe—that they do not belong there and that their infant does not want them.

Faced with a dramatically different birth process and infant than expected, parents form a wall of detachment to deal with the dichotomy of reality versus fantasy. Above all else, although parents of preterm infants worry about their own adaptability to parenthood in much the same way as parents of full-term infants, the intensity of the situation clearly delineates the parents of preterm infants from their counterpart parents of fullterm infants. Their feelings regarding whether their infants will survive, whether they will have confidence and competence to deal with the normal everyday responsibilities of parenting, and whether they have the ability to cope with even

the slightest changes and challenges (stresses) that occur are extremely intense.

As already stated, parents of preterm infants can learn to adapt and deal with all these issues if they have the support and help consistent with their needs and those of the infant. Although most of this adaptation occurs over the weeks and months at home, the positive relationship between parent and child can get a significant boost from measures instituted in the hospital setting (Zelle, 1995). The NICU environment can aid in the development of the parent and the child when it is flexible enough to adjust its procedures and interventions to the biologic development and rhythms of the infant and to the needs and schedules of the parents and other supportive family members. For instance, spacing intrusive (and exhausting) procedures to allow for the infant's recovery, varying levels of light and dark to promote normal levels of infant sleep and awake times, and timing awake times so that they coincide with parent visits all combine to promote normal infant development and positive parent-infant interactions.

Chapter 46 describes the importance of support for parents to help them cope and manage the stress of the NICU environment, preventing "learned helplessness" that so often occurs. Giving time and attention to really listen to parents, communicating clearly, and teaching effectively all are factors that parents see as important. When support is given and stress is reduced, parents become confident in their ability to care for the infant and are more likely to become actively involved in his or her care—one step toward a positive parent-infant interaction and optimal infant development. Promotion of normal infant development and positive parent-infant interaction are the two key elements that form a basis for the infant's appropriate development and set the stage for coping with the transition from hospital to home and later integration into the family unit.

All parents faced with taking their new infants home have questions and concerns about the care that they should provide. Parents of preterm infants are no different in this regard. Where they differ is in what kinds of concerns and questions they have and the need for an earlier and longer period of continued monitoring and support to ensure the healthy development of the preterm infant (Kavanaugh et al, 1995). Several studies have documented these differences and are discussed in the following sections.

Koral (1987), in a study of gestational age and parents' perception, found that parents with preterm infants differed significantly from those with fullterm infants in their ability to respond to or recognize cues involving four behaviors—crying, feeding, spitting, and sleeping. No correlation with parents' age, educational level, and income existed. Koral concluded that members of the health care team needed to work together to provide guidance and special teaching to parents of preterm infants, especially in the area of feeding, with which parents had the most difficulties. The nurse has a pivotal role in this process.

Kenner (1990), in qualitative research involving interviews after hospital discharge with parents of preterm and fullterm infants, identified five major issues that surround the parents' transition from hospital to home: (1) parent-child development, which involved parental and child role expectations, separation of parent and child, and the transition into parenthood; (2) anticipatory grief, related to concern for the infant's health and fear of infant death; (3) stress and coping, related to the parents' ability to deal with the stresses of having a preterm infant; (4) social support, involving parents' perception of whether sources of support were positive or negative; and (5) informational needs, regarding the care and development of the infant to cope with the transition from hospital to home. This information was viewed as important by the parents in their ability to cope with the stresses of a preterm birth.

Kenner (1990) concluded that professionals must view parents as individuals that their concerns during and after hospital discharge need to be determined and that care related to those concerns should be provided. Follow-up visits after hospital discharge was recommended as one way to address parental concerns and provide the information they needed (Kenner et al, 1996).

McKim (1993) also examined mothers' perception, related to information needed and information received, as well as support available and support received. She found that parents of preterm infants perceived the need for—but did not receive—information related to crying and spitting up—a finding similar to Koral's (1987) finding. In addition, reports from both primiparous and multiparous mothers in the sample identified the areas of noisy breathing, infant behavior, infant illness, and prematurity in general for which they needed information and did not receive it, which is similar to Kenner's (1990) findings. McKim found that the mothers who needed support but did not receive it were more anxious and less confident about their care giving. Multiparous mothers stated they needed less information than primiparous mothers early on but later requested a need for more information. This may relate to multiparous mothers' receiving less support at home because they are seen as experienced and not needing information. Finally, in regard to support from health professionals, many mothers reported an increase in confidence and a decrease in anxiety when they received a visit from the public health nurse during the first week after discharge (McKim, 1993).

Using qualitative research similar to Kenner's, Baker (1989), addressed six specific research questions involving parent interviews before and after hospital discharge. The questions involved parental expectations, concerns, feeding, and the general characteristics of the transition period. As in Kenner's study, Baker found several underlying themes that characterized the parents' concerns in one degree or another. They included ambivalence before discharge, impact of the infant on the family, issues of parental competence, infant vulnerability, feeding issues, continued pervasiveness of problems related to the infant's prematurity, and recognition of the possible positive outcomes of the birth of a preterm infant (e.g., stronger marital ties, increased belief in self, and ability to cope).

In addition, several issues discussed previously in this chapter were also mentioned by the parents in Baker's study, such as their preterm infant's being difficult to care for and their own failure to anticipate the emotional and physical toll that results from having the infant at home. Parents said that their needs for information and support to cope after discharge were significant, yet they judged the teaching and professional support received before discharge to be inconsistent. Those who did establish a supportive relationship with the staff reported being less anxious. Once again, the nurses were noted to be key factors in this regard. In addition, parents reported that when they had a chance to participate more fully in their infant's care, they felt more competent in caring for their infants and less anxious about the infants' forthcoming discharges (Baker, 1989).

The studies of both Brooten and associates (1989) and Kavanaugh and associates (1995) found that greater concerns for parents of preterm infants around the area of feedings ex-

isted. Specifically, questions of "getting enough" (milk), increasing "weight gain," and reading "infant cues" were among some of the most frequent areas of concerns addressed in this population. Although mothers of fullterm infants have addressed similar concerns as well, these two studies found that the frequency and intensity of concern were greater for the mothers of preterm infants.

Finally, parents are not the only ones to experience difficulty coping and adjusting to the birth of a premature infant. Whereas the birth of a fullterm infant in most cases is a positive event during which network members rally to support the family, the birth of a preterm infant causes confusion and ambivalence in network members, thus leaving them unsure of their roles and how to respond. This may result in an increase in maternal distress rather than the buffering effects usually seen. Grandparents report reactions similar to those of parents with regard to the birth of a preterm infant. Although parents received most of their information about the preterm infants directly from nurses, doctors, and support groups, grandparents relied on the parents to keep them informed. This puts an added stress on the already overstressed parents to provide information. Grandparents who are given access to information experience reduced anxiety. They are then more available emotionally to aid their own children (the infant's parents). Although this true, the issue of legality and hospital policies sometimes preclude the provision of this information to persons other than the parents or legal guardians. Research needs to be done to study the feasibility of giving grandparents access to information as one way to reduce parental stress. What is clear from all these studies is that parents of preterm infants desire follow-up from the NICU environment, that they have questions and concerns that currently are not being met, and that they look to health professionals to provide these services, especially nursing staff, who have 24-hour contact with the infant (Wereszczak et al, 1997). This becomes especially relevant today with earlier discharges and increased survival of VLBW and ELBW infants (Gray et al, 2000; Hack et al, 1999; Thompson et al, 1997; Zelle, 1995).

IMPORTANCE OF NURSE FOLLOW-UP

Nurses are in key positions to make a difference for parents of preterm infants. In many of the previous studies cited, nurses in the NICU were identified as important sources of information and support in the early weeks after the preterm birth. These studies emphasized the need for nurses to help parents cope with the stress in the hospital environment and make the transition home easier (Gray et al, 2000; Zelle, 1995).

Nursing has been synonymous with skill and caring. In the NICU environment, this caring is delivered in a stressful, technical, yet hopeful world. Parents of preterm infants have many concerns, problems, and needs. They have identified the nurse as a key person to help them deal with these issues. They want and need the caring provided by nursing. This is not surprising in view of the fact that the nurse is usually the first person with whom parents come in contact in the NICU environment and is there when they see their child for the first time. Throughout their infant's hospital stay, parents develop a close and often intense relationship with the nurse who provides the primary care for their children. When they leave the hospital, they want and need this relationship to continue (Kenner et al, 1996).

Other reasons why nurses may be best suited to provide the follow-up to the family after the preterm infant is discharged exist. First, studies have documented that nursing intervention makes a difference. Olds and colleagues (1998b) found that prenatal and postpartum home visitation by nurses promoted the health and development in a group of socially disadvantaged mothers and their infants. The best outcome measures were obtained on mothers and infants who had nursing visits both prenatally and postnatally through the first 2 years of the infant's life. The investigators concluded that community health nurses could play a key role in reducing unfavorable outcomes of childbearing by socially disadvantaged women, provided they had reasonable caseloads, focused efforts, and augmented training.

Another major study tested nursing intervention protocols with socially and medically high-risk families. This model of newborn nursing intervention demonstrated that nursing intervention during the first 3 months of life improved parent-infant interaction (Barnard et al, 1983a, 1983b). A reanalysis of this study, comparing fullterm and preterm infants, demonstrated that preterm infants and their mothers involved in the nursing intervention study did better than the fullterm infants and mothers, although both benefited. They also did better in a previously reported comparison of fullterm and preterm infants without nursing follow-up (Barnard et al, 1984). What was interesting in this study was that the preterm infants did not seem healthier than their fullterm counterparts during the 3 months of nursing intervention. However, at the 10-month evaluation, no parent-infant interaction differences were noted, and the preterm infants scored higher on the Bayley Psychomotor Index. These results led the investigators to conclude that the nursing intervention helped to sustain the preterm infants and their mothers as well as improve the parents' interaction and stimulation over the first year (Barnard et al, 1984). This positive "delay effect" of improved parent-infant interaction was also reported in another intervention home follow-up program (Rauh et al, 1988).

Further support for nursing follow-up came from a study by Ross (1984), in which public health nurses made home visits to low-income families with premature infants. Nursing interventions involved emotional support, instruction on the care and development of preterm infants, and a physical examination. In addition, a pediatric therapist visited monthly to advise the family on feeding and stimulation of the infant. The results showed that infants who received the home intervention had significantly higher scores on the Bayley Mental Scales and on the Home Observation for Measurement of the Environment (HOME) inventory (a measurement of the animate and inanimate home environment) than did a matched set of control infants (Ross, 1984).

A second reason why nurses may be best suited for follow-up was given in a study by Brooten and associates (1986) that demonstrated that nursing intervention could be excellent and cost-effective. They also implemented an intensive hospital teaching program delivered by nurses with master's degrees who were specially trained to work with preterm infants and their families. Their study included stable, healthy preterm infants and involved teaching parents about health concerns, care giving activities, and behavioral characteristics of infants born preterm. Follow-up after early hospital discharge included close telephone contact and some home visiting. Brooten and associates demonstrated that stable, healthy preterm infants who were discharged early and monitored by nurses knowledgeable in the special needs of preterm infants fared as well as a set of matched infants not discharged early, with a documented savings of $18,560 per infant for the early-discharge group (Brooten et al, 1986).

More recently, support for earlier discharges of preterm infants is growing as studies demonstrate the benefits to the preterm infants and their families as well as the savings in cost to the community (Shapiro, 1995). This movement toward earlier discharge will only continue to grow as new studies are demonstrating that transitional procedures for preterm infants, such as moving from an isolette to an open crib, can be done safely at lower weights, thereby setting the stage for preterm babies to go home sooner (Medoff-Cooper, 1994; Zelle, 1995).

Olds and his colleagues reported another comprehensive home intervention study that demonstrated cost-effectiveness but was not tied to early discharge. They also used trained registered nurses who followed up a group of poor, unmarried, teenaged primiparous women ($n = 400$) from pregnancy until the infants were 2 years of age. Some of the infants were preterm. The nurses in the study "systematically addressed the health, behavioral and psycho-social conditions that lead to poor maternal and child outcomes" (Olds et al, 1993). This study demonstrated a savings of $801 per family for government costs, determined by such factors as reduction in later pregnancies and treatment of child abuse. They also demonstrated that their intervention program "saved the most money when it was delivered to women in the lowest social classes" (Olds et al, 1993). Continued follow-up of these children and replication of this program in other sites show that comprehensive, systematic, and structured intervention by trained, skilled nurses can make a difference in the outcome of children at risk, (Olds et al, 1998a; 1998b).

A word of caution—all the studies demonstrating improved family outcomes and cost savings had in place a structured and organized home intervention program that followed preterm infants and their families beyond the infants' first year of life (Future of Children, 1998; Shapiro, 1995). Although cost-effectiveness should never be the primary reason for providing service delivery, in this age of rising health care costs, the fact that an intervention service can give quality care, improve family outcomes, and be cost-effective can only add to its attractiveness and feasibility. The fact that in a review of successful home intervention studies that involved pregnant women and young children "programs which employ professionals (especially nurses) and are based on more comprehensive service models stand a greater chance of influencing qualities of parental care giving and the child's intellectual functioning than do narrowly focused programs staffed by paraprofessionals" (Olds and Kitzman, 1993) should make us as nurses stand up, take notice, and demand further support for a service we apparently do so well.

Nurse home follow-up is not a new phenomenon. Most states have in place some form of community health nursing services. Most of these nursing services give priority to high-risk groups. However, in a survey of infants discharged from the NICU in one metropolitan city, fewer than half the preterm infants have any record of public health nurse follow-up. Of those who received visits, the average number of visits was two (Johnson-Crowley & Sumner, 1987a). From the reports of parents and researchers studying preterm infant outcome, two visits would not be enough in a majority of the cases. Additionally, in a recent analysis of the effectiveness of home visiting programs, evaluators noted that "many links in a fairly long chain must be in place before positive results can be observed, including a well-implemented program and accurate assessment in a well-designed study," (Future of Children, 1999). Even when these elements were present, evaluators further reported that "somewhere between 20% and 30% of those families that accepted the offers of service failed to successfully engage in their programs," thus suggesting the need for simultaneous support from other community institutions to be successful (Future of Children, 1999).

Thus nurses involved in home intervention need to do a better job of reporting and evaluating systematically the population they serve and the services they perform and include their programs as part of a more of a more global, community supportive network. In a research review of intervention programs that involve preterm infants from disadvantaged backgrounds, "programs that provide home intervention by nurses through public or private agencies [were excluded because they] do not have an evaluation component and are difficult to quantify" (Zahr, 1994). Clearly, we must, as nurses, start documenting, evaluating, and publicizing our activities along standardized research lines and must collaborate effectively and consistently and with the needs of the family in mind rather than imposing our own agenda (Future of Children, 1999). When these elements are in place, we will be able to influence public, private, and governmental opinion to gain support for nursing home intervention for preterm infants or, for that matter, for all populations.

Conversations with community health nurses across the nation provide general agreement that they may have little knowledge of the NICU environment from which preterm infants come and are unaware of new research findings that would tailor their services to those needed by preterm infants and their families (Johnson-Crowley & Sumner, 1987a). Many of the researchers cited here would agree that nursing intervention and follow-up of high-risk groups, either socially disadvantaged or preterm, require nurses specially trained to follow those groups (Barnard et al, 1987; Brooten et al, 1986; Future of Children, 1993; Olds et al, 1993; 1998b; Shapiro, 1995; Zahr, 1994). In addition to receiving special training, nurses also need to be sensitive to the diverse culture contexts within in which they work (Gross, 1996) and the challenges of working with socially and physically high-risk populations while instigating a program of intervention successfully (Kitzman et al, 1997).

Nurses in the NICU environment may seem to be the logical choice to fulfill this role. As mentioned, parents eagerly want and expect these nurses to provide services to help them understand and cope with their preterm infants. Most NICU nurses, however, would agree that they have little knowledge of community-based follow-up and would feel ill prepared to perform home visitation without additional training. Because both NICU nurses and community health nurses possess knowledge and skill to help families with preterm infants, a collaborative model that blends the knowledge of both these nurses would be ideal, thereby ensuring that consistent information and support are given as the parents move from the hospital environment to the home environment. Such a collaborative model has been implemented successfully between hospital and community nurses (Zelle, 1995).

Research continues to demonstrate the need for home follow-up of preterm infants and their families that is feasible and cost-effective. Nurses supported by a large body of research findings now have a great opportunity to see that this service is provided. Throughout this text, collaboration among nurses within the hospital setting is advocated. This collaboration must extend into the community. Hospital nurses and community nurses must work together to promote an early, smooth, and continued transition from hospital to home for preterm infants and their families. Because of limitations of time and resources, alternate and innovative ways to provide resources and follow-up must also be considered, such as using the Internet and telecommunications to deliver interventions (Gray et al, 2000). Most importantly, hospital and community nurses need to collaborate with nurse researchers in their fields to ensure that populations served and services given are documented systematically and effectively. This documentation will allow for comparisons within and among home intervention programs so that services may be individualized for infants and their families and we provide the appropriate "nurse dose" (Brooten and Naylor, 1995)—what they need, when they need, and how they need services. This then will allow us to further refine what important components are necessary for any given home follow-up program. The following section describes what we currently know are important components for any successful home intervention program.

SYSTEMATIC ASSESSMENTS

An important component of any follow-up with families is the use of systematic assessment. Systematic assessment is the use of validated measures to organize the collection of information that can be used to promote strengths, identify concerns, and suggest areas for further evaluation or referral (Barnard et al, 1983a). Bailey and Simeonsson (1988) identified the home environment and parent-infant interaction as important areas to include in any family assessment related to early intervention. Hardy-Brown and colleagues (1987) also advocated assessing the home environment because "assessment of the infant's actual living situation (in contrast to hospital evaluation alone) can permit the most pertinent interventions to be recognized and administered quickly." Barnard and Douglas (1974) identified child rearing and nurturing as two areas in which nursing could make the biggest contributions to families—areas that heretofore were largely neglected but in which parents and professionals identified a need for information and help.

Tekolste and Bennett (1987) supported the findings of Barnard and Douglas (1974) by identifying areas in which nurses can make a difference in home follow-up care with preterm infants and their families. Areas included (1) monitoring and providing support, instructions, and problem solving in the areas of feeding, weight gain and growth, sleeping, and developmental and behavioral concerns; and (2) the concept of the nurse as a complementary liaison with the primary care physician (Tekolste and Bennett, 1987; Gray et al, 2000). On the basis of these findings, it seems logical to use measures that assess those areas needed and not being universally monitored, such as sleep-wake organization, parent-infant interaction, and conditions of the home environment.

Nursing Child Assessment Satellite Training Scales
An important aspect of any assessment measure is that it be married to the realities of the health care system—that is, the measure should be easy to use, complement current practice, provide information (for both professional and client), and assess factors found through research to be predictive of a child's later development. In addition, measures should address areas of parent concern to ensure the interest and motivation of the parent in incorporating whatever recommendations are warranted from the assessment (Delerian, 1988). The Nursing Child Assessment Satellite Training (NCAST) Scales are examples of assessment measures that fit these criteria. Developed under the direction of Dr. Kathryn Barnard, a nurse, they result from her examinations of characteristics present in families early on that predicted later child outcomes. In addition to assessing the areas of sleep-wake organization, feeding, parent-

infant interaction, and the home environment, these scales are useful as a clinical tool to (1) provide information and support to the parent; (2) document the infant's and parent's current behavior; and (3) provide information about predictability of behavior over time, support for positive behavior, and improvement in problem areas when repeated measurements of the same assessment are used (Johnson-Crowley & Sumner, 1987a; Ruff, 1987).

Another advantage is that assessments completed over time generate a picture of the child's changing behavior in a realistic way. This cuts down on exaggeration or understatement of the infant's problems and helps produce a more realistic perception of the infant for the parents.

Professionals find these assessments clinically useful because they help organize the home visit and give them a baseline from which to identify the following (Johnson-Crowley & Sumner, 1987a, 1987b):

1. The developing sleep-wake patterns.
2. The appropriateness of the amount and type of infant feedings.
3. Areas of strength to build the parents' confidence in the care of their infant.
4. Problem areas and relay areas of concern to the parent.
5. When and where further assessments need to be performed.
6. Documented evidence of the behavior of the parent and the child, especially parent-child interaction.

Studies using these scales have found correlations with later cognitive performance and behavioral outcomes (Holditch-Davis et al, 2000; Zahr, 1991). Thus the NCAST scales are valuable tools for identifying and preventing problems before they occur. Although these assessments were originally designed from observations of a population of fullterm infants, they have been validated and found extremely useful with preterm infants and their families, (Barnard, 1985; Barnard et al, 1987; Farel et al, 1991; Johnson-Crowley, 1988; Johnson-Crowley & Sumner, 1987a; Slater et al, 1987; Sumner & Spietz, 1994a, 1994b). The four NCAST assessments are described in the following sections.

NCAST Sleep-Activity Record.

The Sleep-Activity Record (SAR) is a 24-hour record that requires the parent (or care giver) to keep an hour-by-hour record of the infant's sleep and activity for up to 1 week (Barnard, 1980, 1999). Originally developed for use with fullterm newborns, the SAR has now been adapted and found useful for "recording accurate data in a systematic way to improve self-regulation in pregnant women and infants during the first three years," (Barnard, 1999). The record comprises four major sections: 1) a place to record demographic information; 2) a section for both day and night recordings of daily sleep and activities; 3) three columns on the right for recording type, frequency, and total amounts of these sleep and activities; and 4) suggested symbols to use to record behaviors, along with a summary area to record averages (Figure 45-1). The use of symbols is an advantage by making it useful for parents and caregivers who have low education, difficulty reading, or are non-English speaking (Johnson-Crowley, 1988).

Because the SAR is completed over 24 hours and can be filled out week after week, it generates a picture of the child's "increasing temporal integration of activities" (Barnard, 1999). This means that over time, the neuromaturational behavior of the infant—a relative decrease in the amount of feedings and night awakenings in infants as they grow and mature—is recorded. With this decrease comes an increase in the amount of time spent awake and more time for play and parent-infant interaction. Parents have found the SAR useful in organizing their activities and providing an ongoing view of their infants' changing behaviors, which is an important process for parents of preterm infants, in whom developmental strides may be slow and seemingly nonexistent at times (Johnson-Crowley, 1986).

Nursing Child Assessment Feeding Scale.

Whereas the SAR scale gives a picture of the amount and frequency of feedings the infant is getting, the Nursing Child Assessment Feeding Scale (NCAFS) assesses certain tasks that the parent and the child have for ensuring a positive interactional relationship during feeding, so that the feeding is set in as positive an atmosphere as possible for both parent and child (Barnard & Kelly, 1990; Sumner & Spietz, 1994a). For preterm infants and their families—who may experience feeding as a long, arduous, and often negative process—this scale can provide a very important way to change conditions so that the feeding is a more positive experience. If parents realize that during the early months of life the feeding episode may provide the only times the preterm infant is awake and one of the only times the parent and infant are together and interacting for any length of time, it becomes additionally important that this be as pleasant a time as possible (especially for the parent), because it may set the stage for later interactions (Johnson-Crowley & Sumner, 1987a).

Areas of assessment include the infant's ability to provide clear cues to the parent and respond appropriately and positively to the parent's attempt to interact. For the parents, their ability during the feeding to be sensitive to the infant's cues, respond sympathetically to any distress the infant might experience, provide social and emotional activities that are affectionate and social in nature, and present activities that enhance the infant's cognitive development is assessed as well.

The NCAFS works well as a follow-up to the use of the SAR should any feeding difficulties be identified. For instance, a review of the SAR reveals that a breastfeeding preterm infant is getting fewer than the recommended number of feedings per day, and discussions with the parent reveal difficulties in getting the infant to eat. The NCAFS may reveal areas in the parent-infant interaction that may be affecting this, such as the parent's inability to read the infant cues (Johnson-Crowley & Sumner, 1987a, 1987b). The use of the NCAFS after discussion of the SAR is an example of how assessment measures can complement and build on one another, thus providing information related to a similar topic (in this case, feeding) but in different areas. In this way a more comprehensive view of the parent, infant, and the situation is obtained by using multiple assessment measures, which makes assessment, intervention, and evaluation easier and more complete.

Nursing Child Assessment Teaching Scale.

The Nursing Child Assessment Teaching Scale (NCATS) assesses the interaction between parent and child while the parent is teaching the child a simple task (Barnard & Kelly, 1990; Sumner & Spietz, 1994b). The parent chooses the task and how he or she wishes to present and teach the task to the child. The areas assessed are similar to those in the NCAFS scale just described but center around a different topic—teaching instead of feeding. Both the NCAFS and NCATS have been shown to be reliable and valid measurements of the parent-infant interaction. Although both assessments measure parent-infant interaction, analysis of the assessments has shown that they offer

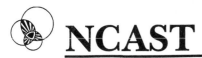

NCAST SLEEP/ACTIVITY RECORD

Date of Recording _____

Pregnant Woman /Parent /Caregiver	Infant / Child	Sleep Concerns of Parent/Child

Name STACIE

Age 17

Expected date of delivery _____

Usual Bedtime 12 midnight

Usual Awakening 9 am

Child's Name MASON

Gestational Age at Birth 31 weeks

Child's Age (wks./mo.) 5 weeks (36 CGA)

Child's Sex ☒ Male ☐ Female

Location of Child
During Day ☒ Home ☐ Child Care Other _____
During Night ☒ Home ☐ Child Care Other _____

Number of people sleeping in same room as baby ___1___

Do you have any concerns about your sleep or your baby's sleep? ☒ Yes ☐ No
If yes specify:
☐ Getting to Sleep   ☐ Waking Up at Night
☐ Sleeping Too Much   ☒ Sleeping Too Little
☐ Sleeping Wrong Time
☒ Other, specify: POOR FEEDING

DAY TIME (6AM to 6PM)

SUMMARY

Day of Week	Hrs of Sleep	# of sleep segs	# of feeds
Wed	5.25	6	3
Thurs	6.75	6	3
Fri	7	5	3
Sat	7.5	3	2
Sun	6.25	5	3
Mon	5.5	4	3
Tues	6.25	4	3
DAY TIME TOTALS	44.5	33	20
Average Day Time (divide by 7)	6.4	4.7	2.8

NIGHT TIME (6PM to 6AM)

Day of Week	Hrs of Sleep	# of sleep segs	# of feeds
Wed	7	3	2
Thurs	7.5	3	2
Fri	8	3	2
Sat	7.5	3	2
Sun	5	2	3
Mon	6.25	2	2
Tues	7	3	2
NIGHT TIME TOTALS	48.25	19	15
Average Night Time (divide by 7)	6.9	2.7	2.1
Average Day Time (from above)	6.4	4.7	2.8
24 HOUR TOTALS	13.3	7.4	4.9

Symbols
— Sleep
■ Feeding
X Crying
O Awake
• Visitors

Summary
Avg total sleep/d = 13.4
Avg # feedings/d = 4.9
Avg # sleep seq/d = 7.4

FIGURE **45-1**
Sleep-Activity Record (SAR) completed by mother of preterm infant. From Barnard KE (1999). *Beginning rhythms: the emerging process of sleep wake behaviors and self-regulation.* Seattle: NCAST Publications, University of Washington.

different and important glimpses of the parent-infant interaction (Barnard et al, 1989; Farel et al, 1991; Gross et al, 1993; Sumner & Spietz, 1994a, 1994b).

Other differences also exist. First, the NCAFS (feeding) assessment takes as long as a feeding lasts, possibly 15 minutes to more than an hour; the NCATS (teaching) assessment is brief, usually lasting between 1 and 5 minutes. The NCAFS is validated for use up to 12 months of an infant's life, whereas the NCATS can be performed up to 36 months (Barnard et al, 1989). The investigators point out that the feeding situation, because it occurs six times a day, 7 days a week, may be a more familiar, well-rehearsed situation that places few demands on the parent-child pair. The teaching situation, in contrast, set up by the observer, is more novel in approach and places some stress on the parent-child interaction, possibly resulting in more restrictive behavior on the part of the parent (Barnard & Kelly, 1990; Barnard et al, 1989). Barnard and colleagues (1989) note that "added together, the two scales give us a richer look at the interactive patterns than either taken separately, but each can be used independently when the situation calls for or allows only one." In addition, the NCAFS (feeding) is useful for measuring parent-infant interaction only as long as the infant and parent are involved in the feeding situation. When the infant is older (older than 1 year), most parents allow infants to feed themselves while parents are engaged in other activities. At this time, the NCATS may be useful to get a more accurate picture of the parent-infant interaction, especially related to cognitive development (Gross et al, 1993).

Home Observation for Measurement of the Environment (HOME). The HOME is no longer a part of the NCAST assessment package. However, it is a reliable and valid adjunct to the NCAST assessments. This instrument—designed by Caldwell, Bradley, and their colleagues—measures "the quality and quantity of support for cognitive, social and emotional development available to the child in the home environment" (Bradley & Caldwell, 1988). This assessment is administered using a combination of interview and observation. Both the animate (i.e., people) and the inanimate (e.g., toys) aspects of the home environment are assessed (Caldwell & Snyder, 1978). A review of several studies using the HOME assessment measure has demonstrated that the HOME is a powerful predictor of later cognitive skills both in fullterm and preterm infants (Bradley & Caldwell, 1988; Gottfried, 1984; Holditch-Davis et al, 2000). Its ease of use, broad perspective, and extensive use in research make it a popular assessment measure in clinical practice.

Used together in any home follow-up program, the SAR, NCAFS, NCATS, and HOME assessments offer a way for the health care professional to monitor the ongoing integration of the preterm infant into the family unit by identifying strengths that increase a parent's confidence and competence, assessing systematically those areas found problematic for this population, providing organization to clinical practice, planning individual intervention, measuring outcomes, and most importantly, providing a way to give support and direction to the parents in relation to care giving for their children.

HOME-BASED PROTOCOLS OF CARE FOR PRETERM INFANTS AND THEIR FAMILIES

In home follow-up of preterm infants and their families, the assessment component must be attached to a plan of prevention and intervention. This plan should entail a predesigned set of protocols outlining strategies of care. Protocols set up plans of care that are based on the population being served but allow flexibility for individual, cultural, and familial differences. For instance, in the case of the preterm infant, these protocols of care would involve instructions for monitoring weight and growth parameters. Feeding issues and sleep-wake organization would also be included. It is critical that any set of protocols be based on the needs and wants of preterm infants and their families, but they should also include components important to the growth and development of any infant. Protocols have been found to be extremely useful in organizing nursing practice and creating satisfaction in providing care and increasing optimal parenting (Barnard, 1985; Olds et al, 1993). In a report on five nurse entrepreneurs, four of the five described the use of nursing protocols as an aid to their practices (Hartman, 1988).

Nursing Systems toward Effective Parenting—Preterm

Nursing Systems toward Effective Parenting—Preterm (NSTEP-P) is an example of parent-focused home follow-up intervention program designed specifically to address the problems of parenting a preterm infant. A component of this program is specific protocols of care that help the nurse get organized, thus allowing him or her to meet the needs of the family in a way that is comfortable, thorough, supportive, and efficient, thereby increasing nurse satisfaction. The original NSTEP-P program was developed in 1984 through a Continuing Education Grant from Maternal-Child Health Service (Grant #MCJ-009035-01-0), the University of Washington, Department of Parent and Child Nursing, under the direction of Dr. Kathryn Barnard, to test the efficacy of providing nursing services to preterm infants and their families. The nursing protocol that was an integral part of the program was based on research of preterm infants, parenting, and "ecology" of infants and families previously discussed in this chapter (Barnard, 1985).

This home follow-up program was tested in six sites across the nation, involving 23 public health nurses, making eight home visits at specific times. Evaluation data for 76 mothers and their preterm infants were collected and analyzed. The results from this research indicated that the program was successful. Nurses reported that it was helpful to their practices. In addition, measures used to assess parent-infant interaction (NCAFS and NCATS) demonstrated that the techniques used to modulate the infant's sleep-wake state had significantly improved the parent-child interaction. Additional measures of family function, perceived support, and child growth and development were all positive. Follow-up of a subset of these children revealed higher scores on the NCATS, NCAFS, and HOME measurements at 24 months of chronologic age than at 5 months of corrected age. Denver Developmental Screening Test (DDST) scores revealed that 95% of the children tested normal at 24 months of chronologic age in the area of fine motor, gross motor, and personal-social development. In the area of language, 100% of the children were normal (Johnson-Crowley, 1987).

A later multisite field experiment that involved NSTEP-P with a group of low-education mothers and their preterm infants was also found to be a "potent intervention to improve the interactive competence of less well-educated mothers to complement the improved social responsiveness of preterm infants and to establish synchronized growth fostering interaction" (Kang et al, 1995).

The following section describes the organization and content of the current NSTEP-P program as an example of what a successful intervention program for preterm infants and their families might include.

Overview.   The need to assist parents in learning how to manage their preterm infants after hospital discharge spurred nurse researchers and nurse clinicians to develop the NSTEP-P protocols of care. The overall framework for the NSTEP-P program is the therapeutic relationship in which the nurse structures the interaction to be sensitive to the parents' need while providing information that will help them learn parenting techniques for the preterm infant who has difficulty feeding, whose state regulation is not well organized, and who tends not to be responsive to the caregiver (Johnson-Crowley & Sumner, 1987b).

The protocols designed as part of the NSTEP-P program are intended to complement a health agency's current strategy of care, allowing use of the agency's routines as well as to incorporate any existing preterm follow-up programs in the community. Although comprehensive in scope, the NSTEP-P program is not designed to take the place of visits to the physician. In fact, an important part of this program is to monitor families to ensure that they continue to see their physicians for well child checkups or for specific health concerns (Johnson-Crowley, 1988).

Content.   The content of the program is built on the established characteristics and problems of the preterm infant reported in research and focuses on two main areas: Content for the Family and Content for the Health Professional.

Content for the Family.   Health-related concerns: These issues relate to feeding and nutrition, safety and temperature, illness and infection control, and growth and development. Special health problems more common to the preterm infant—such as anemia, hernias, and vision and hearing problems—are also included.

State modulation: This involves infant state organization, alertness, maintaining state arousal, and stimulation related to the state of the infant.

Parent-infant interaction: This covers behavioral cues, behavioral differences, importance in developing social competence in children, and the preterm infant's effect on his or her caregiver.

Infant's environment: This includes stimulation as provided by the animate and inanimate environment, elements of parent involvement, the important roles of fathers and siblings, stimulation of the preterm infant, and the importance of playing with and enjoying the infant.

Parental coping and support: This involves parental support (family and professional networks), problem solving, stress appraisal, parental coping, and the challenges of parenting a preterm infant.

As might be expected, issues involving health and state modulation (especially in relation to feeding) take priority early in the program; less time is spent discussing the other content areas. Later, as the problems and concerns in health and state modulation resolve, the content areas of parent-infant interaction and the infant's environment become more paramount. Parental coping and support continues to be a focus throughout the entire home visit program.

Content for the Health Professional.   Therapeutic process: This involves contract setting, therapeutic relationships, and closure (termination) with families.

Intervention strategies: These involve the use of systematic assessments, prescriptions of care, and integrated handouts.

Structured protocols: These involve the organization of practice, step-by-step home visiting instructions, and detailed record keeping.

Systematic assessments are given special emphasis because they are critical to the delivery and evaluation of the NSTEP-P program. During delivery of the program, assessments (infant health, parent-infant interaction, parental support, and the home environment) identify potential problems before they develop and delineate when intervention would be most effective. During evaluation, systematic assessments document accomplishment of program goals and promote professional accountability. Assessments found to be important to the success of the NSTEP-P program are anthropometric measures—including height, weight, and head circumference—as well as measures of developmental assessment; the NCAST assessment measures, including the SAR, NCAFS, NCATS, and HOME; and the Network Survey, a measurement of the family's support network, including a section assessing support from family, friends, and coworkers; and a section assessing support from health agencies and health professionals.

Structure.   The NSTEP-P program involves a series of home visits starting from hospital discharge to 5 months of corrected age. One visit is designed to be made before the infant's discharge from the hospital to aid in the transition to home, and check-in visits can be scheduled between 9 and 12 months of corrected age to monitor the progress of the family. More visits are made in the beginning, when the parents are most anxious and desirous of contact. As the infant matures and parental confidence increases, the visits are spaced further apart. More visits may occur during the home visit program and after the program has concluded, depending on the needs and wants of the family. This allows for flexibility and takes into account the individual differences and needs of each family.

Format.   Presentation of the content information is formulated around a structured format that is consistent from visit to visit. This format—which includes a brief introduction, review of previous content, presentation of new content, summary of the visit, anticipatory guidance, nursing prescriptions, and termination—provides structure for the NSTEP-P families during a period of family disorganization and disequilibrium. This structure and consistency allow nurses and parents to know what to expect with each visit, which reduces the possibility of ambiguity, confusion, and miscommunication. Having clearly defined role expectations helps lessen the parent's need to mobilize additional energy for the nurse's visits. However, built-in flexibility allows for the content of the program to be arranged visit-to-visit according to the needs and wants of each family.

Parent Handouts.   Handouts are an important source of information for parents. When designed well (a key point), handouts present much of the information—some of it complex—in a format that is easy to read and geared to the interest and education level of the parent. Whenever possible, pictures rather than words are used to convey the information. This is critical, because parents who might be exhausted and overburdened do not need pages of materials to read, when important information can be presented simply, visually, and attractively. Figure 45-2 presents an example of one handout—Cues Baby Uses During Interaction—which conveys informa-

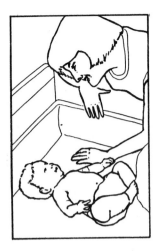

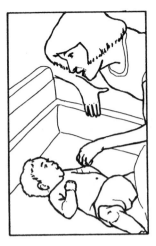

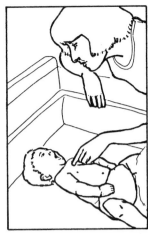

Your baby uses eye contact and his winning smile to reach out to you.

Baby's excitement builds quickly. He smiles and waves his arms and legs.

He shows more excitement by making noises, bringing his hands to his mouth, sucking, or clasping his hands.

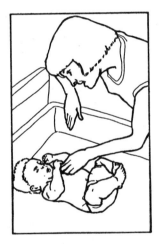

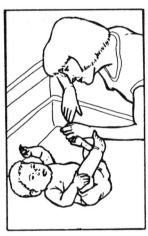

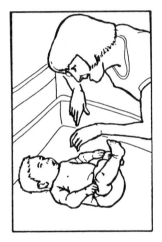

As he gets overwhelmed and needs a break from the interaction.

He turns away. You notice his need for a break and stop talking and touching. You look and wait.

He makes contact again with you to begin the whole cycle again.

FIGURE **45-2**

Cues baby uses during interaction. From Johnson-Crowley N, Sumner G (1987). *Protocol manual: nursing systems toward effective parenting—Preterm.* Seattle: NCAST Publications, University of Washington. Adapted from *Infant Development Program*, Johnson & Johnson, 1976.

tion about the give and take (synchrony) that occurs during the interaction between the parent and infant.

Designed for parents with an eighth grade education, these handouts would be a problem for parents who cannot read at an eighth grade level or for those who do not read English. However, because the protocol requires that the content of the handouts be explained fully, most professionals have found them applicable for those with less than an eighth grade education. Parents who do not read English often have found another family member to translate the information if they see the value in that information.

Most handouts present information related to the content, but handouts can be used in additional ways, such as (1) an av-

enue for assessment of the infant by the nurse or parent; (2) a means for the nurse to model appropriate behavior for the parent; (3) a way to transmit information to other members of the family or support network; and (4) a record for the parent and nurse of the home visit. In the NSTEP-P program all five of these functions—providing information, assessing the infant, modeling behavior, relaying information to other family members, and recording the visit—are promoted in a positive and supportive way through handouts. They are an important part of the NSTEP-P protocols of care (Johnson-Crowley, 1988b).

The NSTEP-P program is an example of what should be included in any quality parent-focused follow-up program for preterm infants and their families. Important components to keep in mind for any follow-up program of this population include the following:

Home visiting to monitor and provide support.

Identification of problem areas, providing interventions, and evaluating outcomes; are based on measures for systematically assessing the infant and family.

Protocols of care are structured, flexible, and consistent from visit to visit.

Parent involvement is essential in all aspects of care, including assessment, intervention, and evaluation.

Content encompassing important areas for normal growth and development yet specific to the needs and problems of preterm infants.

Research-based and research-supported.

Those programs that include these important components help ensure not only that their NICU graduates survive but also that they develop optimally and as normally as possible—one of the most important considerations for all health professionals, parents, and families. Finally, any program of care is only as good as the person providing the intervention. Thus anyone desiring to provide services and interventions described here need to make sure they have the knowledge, experience, skills and training necessary—including documented training and skill in all assessment measures, knowledge and understanding of preterm infants and their families experiences during and after hospitalization, and training and understanding of the techniques to deliver the intervention services. Most importantly, competent assessment and intervention includes the ability to understand the cultural context of the families with whom they are working, so they can "understand and support families from diverse backgrounds and work to promote good parenting in ways that are meaningful to the families they are trying to help," (Gross, 1996).

ADVANCED PRACTICE NURSES INTO LONG-TERM CARE: NURSES NEED TO KNOW THIS

Neonatal Nurse Practitioners and Clinical Nurse Specialists have been well established the role of caring for neonates as skilled, cost-effective health care professionals in the literature. Adequate evidence to support their knowledge base and clinical expertise allows them to be accepted by peers and professionals as practitioners in an advanced practice role in the traditional NICU setting. (Hunsberger et al, 1992; Mitchell-DeCenso et al, 1996; Schultz et al, 1994). It has been suggested that advance practice nurses expand their role into complimentary areas such as primary care and case management. Strodtbeck et al (1998) note that many changes with hospital reorganization, amalgamation, downsizing, cross training, and shifts to a primary care focus for medical care in the past few years have created new opportunities for nontraditional NICU roles for nurses and NNPs in neonatal follow-up, case management, quality improvement, and community hospital care.

Earlier interest in the follow-up of neonates dates back to Brooten et al (1986), who reported a randomized control trial in which very-low-birth-weight NICU graduates were followed via home visits by Perinatal Clinical Nurse Specialists. CNSs made routine visits at 1 week and at 1, 9, 12, and 18 months. Extensive telephone follow-up and availability to the families was also provided. The infants in the CNS group were smaller at discharge and were discharged sooner than the routine NICU infants, with significant cost savings for early discharge, as noted earlier in this chapter. Beal et al (1999), also note that

follow-up support for parents (education, emotional support, and coordination of care) can facilitate transitions from the NICU to home.

NNPs have also been reported in the literature as participating in various primary care roles following neonates after discharge from the NICU (Beal et al, 1999). Noting that consistency of care and consistent follow-up are key concerns for the NICU graduate, Beal et al surveyed a sample of 505 American Neonatal Nurse Practitioners to collect practitioners thoughts on the evolution of the NNP role to follow-up care of neonates. The vast majority agreed that the NICU follow-up role was important, and approximately half of the sample felt they were qualified to participate in the role, although the authors found many NNPs felt their programs did not incorporate enough didactic learning or clinical opportunities focused on infant follow-up needs. Based on this study, the authors suggest that NNPs who feel their programs do not provide adequate preparation for post-NICU care could complete a pediatric nurse practitioner program or work with primary care providers to mentor NNPs into a new aspect of their roles (Beal et al, 1999).

Most often, nurses who work in a follow-up clinic or long term care practice in a collaborative agreement with a physician (usually a neonatologist or pediatrician). In addition to acquired knowledge and expertise with perinatal assessment, general physical assessment, disease process (inclusive of long term neonatal sequelae), and general management of the neonate, nurses may need to incorporate additional learning in selected areas or "program/clinic specific" assessment for follow-up issues. However, common areas of needed expertise focus on the following topics adapted from the NCC study guidelines (2000) and Beal et al (1999):

Neonatal assessment (inclusive physical, behavioral, developmental assessments)

Nutritional assessment

Assessment of parent child interaction, family integration, and communication

Assessment of home management for special needs infants (home oxygen, g-tube feeding, etc.)

Parent education

Emergency measures health management or pediatric screening assessment

Management and referral service for long-term development problems or issues beyond the scope of primary care

It is apparent from the literature that a role exits for advanced practice nurses to practice primary care for neonatal follow-up. Although documentation of the role is scant and the definition of the role varies with the age of infants to be followed as well as with the scope of practice, support from professional organizations is growing for nurses to practice in primary care. The National Association of Neonatal Nurses (NANN) practice of neonatal follow-up care by qualified health care professionals, including neonatal nurses knowledgeable in special needs of the infant (NANN, 1997). The National Association of Pediatric Nurse Associates and Practitioners (NAPNAP) position is that the discharge and follow-up of newborns by a primary care provider is essential and includes pediatric nurse practitioners as primary care providers (NAPNAP, 1997).

Needless to say, each nurse who is considering a expansion of his or her practice needs to consider on an individual basis. What does the scope of practice involve? What specifically will be my role? Am I qualified for the role? If not, what do I need to do to acquire the skills and expertise, and where do I get it?

SUMMARY

The birth of a preterm infant is a dramatic and frightening event. Before parents really begin to cope with the trauma of their infant's birth and survival, they must bring their infant home. Because of their vulnerability, preterm infants need further monitoring and support to ensure positive developmental outcomes. Nurses have been shown to make a difference when providing home intervention with families who have a high-risk infant. Any intervention program should include parent involvement, systematic assessment, and protocols of care as part of the intervention. Both systematic assessment measures and intervention programs designed with the needs and problems of preterm infants and their families have proven to be valuable resources in the provision of home follow-up with this population to ensure optimal developmental outcomes. Parents and their preterm infants deserve help and support as they make the transition from hospital to home and integrate their new infant into the family unit. Nurses can play a key role in this process.

For information about the NCAST Assessments and the NSTEP-P parent handouts, contact Anita Spietz, NCAST, WJ-10, University of Washington, Seattle, WA 98195; 206-543-8528, FAX: 206-685-3284.

REFERENCES

Bailey DB, Simeonsson RJ (1988). *Family assessment in early intervention.* Columbus, OH: Merrill.

Baker AL (1989). *The transition home for preterm infants: parents' perceptions.* Unpublished master's thesis, Yale University School of Nursing, New Haven, CT.

Bakewell-Sachs S, Porth S (1995). Discharge planning and home care of the technology-dependent infant. *Journal of obstetric, gynecologic, and neonatal nursing,* 24(1), 77-83.

Barnard KE (1980). Sleep organization and motor development in prematures. In Sell EJ (Ed.), *Follow-up of the high-risk newborn: a practical approach.* Springfield, IL: Charles C Thomas.

Barnard KE (1985). *Nursing systems toward effective parenting—Preterm.* Final report supported by Maternal and Child Health Training, Grant #MCH-009035, Bureau of HCDA, HRSA, PHS, and DHHS, Washington, DC.

Barnard KE (1999). *Beginning rhythms: the emerging process of sleep-wake behaviors and self-regulation.* Seattle: NCAST, University of Washington.

Barnard KE et al (1984). Developmental changes in maternal interactions with term and preterm infants. *Infant behavior and development,* 7, 101-113.

Barnard KE et al (1983a). *Final report: newborn nursing models* (Grant #RO1 NU-00719-03). Seattle: NCAST Publications.

Barnard KE, Douglas HB (1974). *Child health assessment, part 1: a literature review.* Seattle: NCAST Publications.

Barnard KE et al (1983b). An ecological paradigm for assessment and intervention. In Brazelton TB, Lester BM (Eds.), *New approach to developmental screening of infants.* New York: Academic Press.

Barnard KE et al (1989). Measurement and meaning of parent-child interaction. In Morrison F et al (Eds.), *Applied Developmental Psychology* (Vol. III, pp. 39-80). New York: Academic Press.

Barnard KE et al (1987). Helping parents with preterm infants: field test of a protocol. *Early child development and care,* 27, 255-290.

Barnard KE, Kelly JF (1990). Assessment of parent-infant interaction. In Meisels SJ, Shonkoff JP (Eds.), *Handbook of early childhood intervention.* Cambridge, UK: Cambridge University Press.

Beal JA et al (1999). The role of the neonatal Nurse Practitioner in post NICU follow-up. *Journal of perinatal and neonatal nursing,* 13, 78-89.

Beckwith L, Cohen SE (1980). Interactions of preterm infants with their caregivers and test performance at age 2. In Field TM et al (Eds.), *High-risk infants and children: adult and peer interactions.* New York: Academic Press.

Berlin LJ et al (1995). Examining observational measures of emotional support and cognitive stimulation in black and white mothers of preschoolers. *Journal of family issues,* 16(5), 664-686.

Blackburn S (1995). Problems of preterm infants after discharge. *Journal of obstetric, gynecologic, and neonatal nursing,* 24(1), 43-49.

Bradley RH, Caldwell BM (1988). Using the HOME inventory to assess the family environment. *Pediatric nursing,* 14(2), 97-102.

Brooten D et al (July-August, 1989). Clinical specialist pre- and post-discharge teaching of parents of very low birth weight infants. *Journal of obstetric, gynecologic, and neonatal nursing,* 316-322.

Brooten D et al (1986). A randomized clinical trial of early hospital discharge and home follow-up of very-low-birth-weight infants. *New England journal of medicine,* 315, 934-939.

Brooten D, Naylor MD (1995). Nurses' effect on changing patient outcomes. *Image,* 27(2), 95-99.

Bryan AA, (2000). Enhancing parent-child interaction with a prenatal couple intervention. *Maternal child nursing,* 25(3), 139-144.

Caldwell BM, Snyder C (1978). *HOME-Home observation for measurement of the environment.* Seattle: NCAST Publications.

Culley BS et al (1989). Parental perception of vulnerability of formerly premature infants. *Journal of pediatric health care,* 3, 237-245.

Delerian D (1988). *Focus on patient education.* Seminar presented by The Continuing Education Project, Seattle, WA.

Farel AN et al (1991). Interaction between high-risk infants and their mothers: the NCAST as an assessment tool. *Research in nursing and health,* 14, 109-118.

The Future of Children: Home Visiting, 3(3) (Winter, 1993). Los Altos, CA: Center for the Future of Children, The David and Lucile Packard Foundation.

The Future of Children: Protecting Children from Abuse and Neglect, 8(1) (Spring, 1998). Los Altos, CA: Center for the Future of Children, The David and Lucile Packard Foundation.

The Future of Children: Home Visiting: Recent Program Evaluations, 9(1) (Spring/Summer, 1999). Los Altos, CA: Center for the Future of Children, The David and Lucile Packard Foundation.

Gennaro S et al (1992). Perinatal factors and infant temperament: a collaborative approach. *Nursing Research,* 41(6), 375-377.

Gottfried A (1984). *Home environment and early cognitive development.* New York: Academic Press.

Gray JE et al (2000). *Pediatrics,* 106(6), 1308-1324.

Green M, Solnit AJ (1964). Reactions to the threatened loss of a child: a vulnerable child syndrome. *Pediatrics,* 34, 58-66.

Greenberg MT, Crnic KA (1988). Longitudinal predictors of developmental status and social interaction in premature and fullterm infants at age two. *Child development,* 59, 554-570.

Gross D (1996). What is a "good parent?" *Maternal child nursing,* 21(July/August), 178-182.

Gross D et al (1993). What does the NCATS measure? *Nursing research,* 42(5), 260-265.

Hack M et al (1999). Functional limitations and special health care needs of 10- to14-year-old children weighing less than 750 grams at birth. *Pediatrics,* 106, 554-560.

Halsey CL (1996). Extremely low-birth-weight children and their peers: a comparison of school-age outcomes. *Archives of pediatric and adolescent medicine,* 150, 790-794.

Hardy-Brown K et al (1987). Home based intervention: catalyst and challenge to the therapeutic relationship. *Zero to three,* 8, 8-12.

Hartman K (Ed.). (1988). Nurses offer home health-care alternatives—part II. *NAACOG Newsletter,* 15(5), 4-8.

Holditch-Davis D et al (2000). Developmental problems and interactions between mothers and prematurely born children. *Journal of pediatric nursing,* 15(3), 157-167.

Holditch-Davis D, Thoman EB (1988). The early social environment of premature and fullterm infants. *Early human development,* 17(2-3), 221-232.

Hunsberger M et al (1992). Definition of an advanced nursing practice role in the NICU: the clinical nurse specialist/neonatal practitioner. *Clinical nurse specialist*, 6, 91-96.

Johnson-Crowley N (1986). Guidelines for nursing intervention NCASA record with prematures. *NCAST National News*, II(2), 2-4.

Johnson-Crowley N (1987). *NSTEP-P: A home visit program for preterm infants and their families*. Poster session presented at the Fifth Biennial National Training Institute for National Center for Clinical Infant Programs, Washington, DC.

Johnson-Crowley N (1988). *NSTEP-P: A Home visit program for preterm infants and their families*. Presentation at the Annual Pediatric Nursing Conference, Chicago.

Johnson-Crowley N, Sumner GA (1987a). *Concept manual: nursing systems toward effective parenting—Preterm*. Seattle: NCAST Publications.

Johnson-Crowley N, Sumner GA (1987b). *Protocol manual: nursing systems toward effective parenting—Preterm*. Seattle: NCAST Publications.

Kang R et al (June, 1995). Preterm infant follow-up project: a multi-site field experiment of hospital and home intervention programs for mothers and preterm infants. *Public health nursing*, 12, 171-180.

Kavanaugh K et al (1995). Getting enough: mothers' concerns about breastfeeding a preterm infant after discharge. *Journal of obstetric, gynecologic, and neonatal nursing*, 24(1), 23-32.

Kenner C (1990). Caring for the NICU parent. *Journal of perinatal and neonatal nursing*, 4(3), 78-87.

Kenner C et al (1996). Parenting in the NICU. In Zaichkin J (Ed.), *Newborn intensive care: what every parent needs to know*. Petaluma, CA: NICU Ink.

Kitzman H et al (1997). Challenges experienced by home visitors: a qualitative study of program implementation. *Journal of community psychology*, 25(1), 95-109.

Koral PA (1987). *Parents' perceptions of the premature infant*. Unpublished master's thesis, University of Cincinnati College of Nursing and Health, Cincinnati, OH.

Magill-Evans J, Harrison MJ (1999). Parent-child interactions and development of toddlers born preterm. *Western journal of nursing research*, 21(3), 292-312.

Magnusson D (1995). Individual development: a holistic, integrated model. In Moen P et al (Eds.) *Examining lives in context: perspectives on the ecology of human development*. Washington, DC: American Psychological Association.

Maygary D (1987). Parent-infant interaction. In Johnson-Crowley N, Sumner GA (Eds.), *Nursing systems toward effective parenting—Preterm*. Seattle: NCAST Publications.

McKim E (1993). The information and support needs of mothers of premature infants. *Journal of pediatric nursing*, 8(4), 233-244.

Medoff-Cooper B (1994). Transition of the preterm infant to an open crib. *Journal of obstetric, gynecologic, and neonatal nursing*, 23(4), 329-335.

Mitchell-DiCenso A et al (1996). A controlled trial of nurse practitioners in neonatal intensive care units. *Pediatrics*, 98, 1143-1148.

NANN- National Association of Neonatal Nurses. (1997). Position paper on early discharge and follow-up. *Neonatal network*, 16, 67-70.

NAPNAP- National Association of Pediatric Nurse Associates and Practitioners. (1997). Position statement on newborn discharge and follow-up care. *Journal of pediatric health care*, 11, 147-148.

NCC, National Certification Corporation. (2000). Guide to NCC certification: neonatal nurse practitioner. Chicago: The National Certification Corporation for the Obstetric, Gynecologic, and Neonatal Nursing Specialties.

Oberklaid F et al (1991). Temperament and behavior of preterm infants: a six-year follow-up. *Pediatrics*, 87(6), 854-861.

Olds DL et al (1993). Effect of prenatal and infancy nurse home visitation on government spending. *Medical care*, 31(2), 155-174.

Olds DL et al (1998a). Long-term effects of nurse home visitation on children's criminal and antisocial behavior: 15-year follow-up of a randomized controlled trial. *JAMA: Journal of the American Medical Association*, 280(14), 1238-1244.

Olds DL et al (1998b). The promise of home visitation: results of two randomized trials. *Journal of community psychology*, 26(1), 5-21.

Olds DL, Kitzman HK (1993). Review of research on home visiting for pregnant women and parents of young children. In *The future of children: home visiting*, 3(3) (Winter, 1993). Los Altos, CA: Center for the Future of Children, The David and Lucile Packard Foundation.

Patteson DM, Barnard KE (1990, Spring). Parenting of low-birthweight infants: a review of issues and interventions. *Infant mental health journal*, 37-56.

Rauh VA et al (1988). Minimizing adverse effects of low birthweight: four-year results of an early intervention program. *Child development*, 59(3), 544-553.

Riese M (1988). Temperament in fullterm and preterm infants: stability over ages 6 to 24 months. *Journal of developmental and behavioral pediatrics*, 9(1), 6-11.

Ross G (1984). Home intervention of premature infants of low-income families. *American journal of orthopsychiatry*, 54(2), 263-270.

Ruff CC (1987). How well do adolescents mother? MCN; *Journal of maternal child nursing*, 12, 249-253.

Saigal S et al (1999). School difficulties at adolescence in a regional cohort of children who were extremely low birth weigh. *Pediatrics*, 105, 325-331.

Sameroff AJ (1981). Longitudinal studies of preterm infants. In Friedman S, Sigman M (Eds.), *Preterm birth and psychological development*. New York: Academic Press.

Scheiner A et al (1985). The vulnerable child syndrome: fact and theory. *Developmental and behavioral pediatrics*, 6(5), 298-301.

Schraeder BD et al (1992). Vulnerability and temperament in very low birth weight school-aged children. *Nursing research*, 41(3), 161-165.

Schraeder BD, Tobey GY (1989). Preschool temperament of very-low-birth-weight infants. *Journal of pediatric nursing*, 4(2), 119-126.

Schultz JM et al (1994). Nurse practitioners effectiveness in the NICU. *Nurse Manager*, 25, 50-53.

Schumacher KL, Meleis AI (1994). Transitions: a central concept in nursing. *Image: journal of nursing scholarship*, 26(2), 119-127.

Shapiro C (1995). Shortened hospital stay for low-birth-weight infants: nuts and bolts of a nursing intervention project. *Journal of obstetric, gynecologic, and neonatal nursing*, 24(1), 56-62.

Slater MA et al (1987). Neurodevelopment of monitored versus non-monitored very low birth weight infants: the importance of family influences. *Developmental and behavioral pediatrics*, 8(5), 278-285.

Spiker D et al (1992). Reliability and validity of behavior problem checklists as measures of stable traits in low birthweight, premature preschoolers. *Child development*, 63, 1481-1496.

Strodtbeck F et al (1998). Coping with transition: neonatal nurse practitioner education for the 21st century. *Journal of pediatric nursing*, 13, 272-278.

Sumner G, Spietz A (1994a). *NCAST caregiver/parent-child interaction feeding manual*. Seattle: NCAST Publications, University of Washington, School of Nursing.

Sumner G, Spietz A (1994b). *NCAST caregiver/parent-child interaction teaching manual*. Seattle: NCAST Publications, University of Washington, School of Nursing.

Tekolste KA, Bennett FC (1987). State of the art, the high risk infant: transitions in health, development, and family during the first years of life. *Journal of perinatology*, 7(4), 368-377.

Thomas A, Chess S (1977). *Temperament and development*. New York: Brunner/Mazel.

Thompson RJ, Jr et al (1994). Developmental outcome of very low birthweight infants as a function of biological risk and psychosocial risk. *Journal of developmental and behavioral pediatrics*, 15, 232-238.

Thompson RJ, Jr. et al (1997). Developmental outcome of very low birthweight infants at four years of age as a function of biological risk and psychosocial risk. *Journal of developmental and behavioral pediatrics*, 18, 91-96.

Washington J et al (1986). Temperament in preterm infants: style and stability. *Journal of the American academy of child psychiatry, 25*(4), 493-502.

Wasserman W (2000). Complications. *New Yorker,* 87-109.

Wereszczak J et al (1997). Maternal recall of neonatal intensive care unit. *Neonatal network, 16*(4), 33-40.

Zahr L (1991). Correlates of mother-infant interaction in premature infants from low socioeconomic backgrounds. *Pediatric nursing, 17*(3), 259-264.

Zahr L (1994). An integrative research review of intervention studies with premature infants from disadvantaged backgrounds. *Maternal-child nursing journal, 22*(3), 90-101.

Zelle RS (1995). Follow-up of at-risk infants in the home setting: consultation model. *Journal of obstetric, gynecologic, and neonatal nursing, 24*(1), 51-55.

Zeanah CH et al (1997). Infant development and developmental risk: a review of the past 10 years. *Journal of the American academy of child and adolescent psychiatry, 36*(2), 165-178.

CHAPTER 46

TRANSITION TO HOME

CAROLE KENNER, GAIL A. BAGWELL, LISA SPANGLER TOROK

INTRODUCTION

In the United States, in 1999, 467,211 infants were born with some degree of prematurity. Of these infants, approximately 12.7% were very-low-birth-weight infants—that is, those that weighed less than 1500 grams at birth. Of those 12.7%, approximately 22,815 were extremely-low-birth-weight infants—weighing less than 1000 grams. (Ventura et al, 2001). Modern health care and technology have improved the survival rates of the micropremie. Survival rates for micropremies with birth weights between 500 and 750 grams improved from 32% in 1988 to 54% in 1996, and the survival rates for micropremies with birth weights of 751 to 1000 grams improved from 65% in 1988 to 86% in 1996. (Lemons et al, 2001; Stevenson et al, 1998).

The technology necessary to support these infants requires complex equipment and professional skill. The result is survival and finally discharge after a prolonged hospitalization. The neonatal intensive care unit (NICU) contains not only premature infants. The multiple neonatal problems that bring an infant to a NICU have been described, in depth, throughout the preceding chapters. The one common factor when caring for these infants is the parent. Parents also require complex care during and following the infant's discharge.

This chapter focuses on the infant and parents and the transition to home for the family unit. Although the NICU label is used throughout the chapter, it actually refers to either a level II or a level III unit, because these authors have found that, for parents, the transition to home from a NICU or special care unit is similar. We believe that parents are not visitors and that they are an integral part of their infant's care during the hospital stay. We also believe that many neonatal nurses are now caring for past NICU graduates through the first year of life; thus the transition to home has extended well beyond the immediate NICU stay. We also recognize that we transition to home may be even more difficult if the infant requires technology in the home. We have included evidence to support what the transition is like for these mothers.

THE NEONATAL INTENSIVE CARE UNIT EXPERIENCE

Try to remember the first time you walked into the NICU. What were your thoughts and feelings? We know what ours were—an overwhelming urge to flee. Time seemed to be running. People were rushing and talking loudly; alarms were buzzing, intercoms were blaring, and doors were slamming. We suddenly felt tense, on edge, and fearful of our ability to survive in such an environment. We were almost immobilized—yet we recognized some of the ventilators, intravenous pumps, and monitors. Surely, with this passing acquaintance, we could learn to work in this environment and actually care for the critically ill infant. Then we walked over to an incubator and peered in at a premature infant—born at 28 weeks' gestation and weighing less than 1000 grams—who looked as though she had been through a war. Scratches and cuts were visible. Tape cut into the infant's face to hold an endotracheal tube in place. The right arm was pinned to the bed to hold an intravenous line in place, and her legs were restrained to prevent dislodgment of an umbilical arterial line that was being used for blood gas sampling. Our hearts sank. We could never be responsible for providing care to this type of infant. We tried to summon the courage to walk—if not run—out of there.

If we, as beginning professionals, could not at first face the unit or the responsibility of care, what must parents feel? They have the additional fear of the death of a family member. For the most part, they lack the knowledge about the medical diagnosis, equipment, treatments, and routines necessary to support neonates. The mothers must, in addition, make a physiologic and psychological postpartum adjustment. They are also in need of care, yet most express the need to put aside their own time for healing to focus on their infants. For the fathers, the need to run between two units (the postpartum and the NICU) is an added stress even if these units are in the same institution. The parents' concern for their partners and their children often forces them between the two. For the family with other children at home, the stress becomes even greater. Who can take charge of the children? How long will it be necessary for another person to help out with family responsibilities? Is someone who can or will step in to help even available? These are very real family concerns. Along with these concerns comes the assumption of the new parental role. This role adjustment occurs for both first-time and experienced parents. It requires a change from a previous functional pattern to a new one. This change marks a developmental passage or transition.

PARENTAL TRANSITION

Transition involves change—leaving behind the familiar and trying something new. Throughout life, events necessitate change. These life changes are often viewed as turning points. Taking on a new role requires energy, commitment, and most of all a change in the pattern of functioning—thus a transition. A new role requires an adjustment, a setting of new priorities, and an examination of new expectations. This transition can be negative or positive, depending on the perceptions of the person involved in the transition. The role of parent is a good example of the transition process. Once a pregnancy is confirmed, the mother and father begin the task of examining their individual roles. For first-time parents, this means considering what it will be like to be a mother or father to a dependent infant. For parents with other children, the new infant will bring a unique personality and another dimension to the already formed family unit. This infant, too, will require role adjustment on the part of the parents.

Maternal Role

Rubin (1973) examined the development of the maternal role. She referred to pregnancy as having a cognitive style, because it is during pregnancy that women question their personal identity. She suggested that women develop their maternal identity in relationship to the developing fetus and newborn (Mercer, 1995, 1998; Rubin, 1984). It is the infant's identity that really brings this maternal identity to fruition (Rubin, 1984). If an infant is premature or sick and does not fit the image of the robust fullterm infant, women lose their normal frames of reference for the development of their own role expectations and the expectations of their infants as well.

Bonding is a natural outgrowth of this process. During the postpartum period, mothers continue to embellish their maternal identity in relationship to their growing infants. Rubin (1984) called this the claiming process. Claiming happens as the mother looks for familial characteristics in her infant. She examines the infant's behavior and appearance to tie the image of this infant with the family unit. When the infant lacks common familial characteristics—because of prematurity or illness—the task of claiming is made difficult. If the infant has been transferred to a distant NICU, the lack of spatial proximity to and repeated contacts with the infant add further to the potential for a difficult adjustment. It is through learning about the infant's routine and unique characteristics that the image moves away from the fantasy child created during the gestation and into the realm of reality of the actual infant (Rubin, 1984).

Bialoskurski et al (1999) showed that attachment in a NICU was not automatic but an individualized process, the timing of which is difficult to assess. They stated that attachment is not a simple process and can be affected by many factors such as the infant's health status, the mother, the environment, and the nursing care that the infant and family receives. They describe the attachment process as being both overt and covert. Overt attachment is easily observed, whereas covert attachment is not visible to the observer. Both overt and covert attachment have three types: immediate, delayed, and problematic.

The immediate process of attachment occurs with wanting of the pregnancy, positive maternal feelings, seeing the infant soon after birth, immediate contact with the infant after birth, and being unable to have other children. Delayed attachment occurs with a premature infant, uncertain outcomes, a handi-capped child, poor maternal health, prolonged ventilation of the infant, the attitude of their partners, a lack of social support, drug dependency, and taking-one-day-at-a-time attitude. This study found that delayed attachment is a way for families to cope with the possibility that the infant might not survive. Problematic attachment occurs when a mother is unable to keep the infant, has drug dependency, experiences a break in the relationship with their partner, gives birth to a handicapped infant, or has ambiguous maternal feelings (Bialoskurski et al, 1999).

Attachment, which is usually considered dyadic, because a triadic relationship in the NICU, in which NICU personnel—especially nurses—can alter the process. Nurses can hinder or facilitate a mother's attachment to her infant by encouraging mother-infant touch or by forbidding it. Physical contact strengthens the attachment process (Bialoskurski et al 1999).

Bruns et al (1999) studied the maternal role in the NICU and at home for medically fragile infants and found that mothers required expertise not only in care giving but also in communication with health care professionals to take their children home. Worrier, novice learner, and expert were roles that mothers assumed in the NICU. In the communication realm mothers were decision makers, information collector, advocate and negotiator.

The mother of a premature infant is also a premature mother. Not only are the binding-in and claiming processes affected; the mother herself is a "premie" as well. Her pregnancy has ended before her own needs are fulfilled. Some or all of the social rituals that socialize mothers into their impending role and prepare them for their new responsibilites—such as baby showers, parenting classes, and birth announcements—may have been forgotten with the birth of a premature or ill infant. Friends and family who would normally be happy to help celebrate the joyous occasion of birth with the exuberant parents may feel uncomfortable and helpless around them. Their support may not be offered, thus leaving the parents more alone and isolated. Thus the transition to a new role becomes more difficult.

Role Theory

Mercer (1981) used Rubin's concepts of social and cognitive learning coupled with role theory to examine facts that affected the maternal role. She developed a theoretical framework for studying role acquisition. On the basis of her research, Mercer described role acquisition as a staged process that occurs gradually over the infant's first year of life (Mercer, 1995, 1998). The variables that affect this process are: (1) maternal age; (2) maternal perceptions of the birth experience; (3) early maternal-infant separation; (4) support system; (5) maternal self-concept; (6) maternal personality traits; (7) maternal illness; (8) childrearing attitudes; (9) infant temperament; (10) infant illness; (11) cultural influences; and (12) socioeconomic level. Many researchers have found that the characteristics of a premature or sick neonate are different enough from the expected term newborn that parental—especially maternal attachment—is affected (Miles et al, 1998; Singer et al, 1999).

In part, this discrepancy between the infant's actual behavior and the infant's expected behavior may arise from the lack of experience on the part of the mothers. If one does not know what to expect, it is difficult to plan or respond in less than an anticipatory or contrived manner. Role models may be missing; thus the normal process of change that transpires with a new role is not perceived as normal at all.

Whenever change occurs—leaving the familiar and moving toward an uncharted path—feelings of lower self-esteem, decreased confidence, and decreased ability to cope are expected—even for events that are not tied to an illness or a problem, such as marriage or a new career. When there is an illness or a problem, it is reasonable to assume that these negative feelings may be even more intensely felt. For parents of a NICU infant, the transition may have two phases—one associated with becoming parents at the time of birth and the other occurring at the time of discharge.

Although the time of NICU discharge is the overriding goal for the health care professional and the family, the actual transition to home can be a time of crisis for the family. The actual assumption of the new parental role can be quite overwhelming. Some researchers and clinicians view this transition as a crisis rather than just a developmental passage to a new functional level.

Transition as a Crisis

The idea that a crisis is a state of disequilibrium is based on the postulate that humans strive for homeostasis by constantly using coping mechanisms to maintain equilibrium. When a situation that upsets the equilibrium arises, a person employs the usual coping mechanisms to solve the problem. When the usual coping methods do not return the person to a state of equilibrium, a crisis evolves. The outcome of a crisis depends on whether resources are available to support the individuals undergoing the crisis. Even when a healthy newborn is brought into a family, a crisis can ensue. For premature or sick infants, however, the meaning to the family usually is viewed as a crisis. A crisis usually lasts 4 to 6 weeks, and crisis intervention is most effective when used during this period. When intervention is applied as close to the time of the crisis as possible, it becomes even more effective. The aim of crisis intervention is not to restructure a person's personality but to help the person deal with the present problem and to rely on history only as it pertains to the present situation. Many things can initiate a crisis in a family. Families see bringing a premature or ill infant who has been in the NICU as a crisis. Contemplating taking home a medically fragile infant or one that is technology-dependent may create a crisis situation for a parent (Scholtes et al, 1994).

For neonatal nurses, knowing when a family is in crisis and its causes is very important. When an impending or a true crisis is recognized, neonatal nurses can implement interventions that will help prevent or alleviate it. Anticipatory planning for future crises involves reviewing with the family their coping strategies and how they handled the crisis. Coping, then, is the process by which an individual regulates stress. An outcome of coping is usually either control over the stress or being taken over by the stress, as in learned helplessness.

For many parents, the NICU reinforces learned helplessness. Parents express the need to understand their role and what is expected of them in relationship to their infants' care needs; yet they feel "in the way" and unable or incapable of caring for their infants. Thus they learn to be helpless. However, at the time of discharge, the picture changes. The parents are told, "Now it is your turn" (Figure 46-1). It is no wonder that this discharge can be cognitively appraised as being a stress. Nor is it unusual that parents feel helpless and hopeless when it comes to accepting total responsibility for their infants.

Parents are very vocal about their feelings regarding their NICU care and preparation for discharge when given the op-

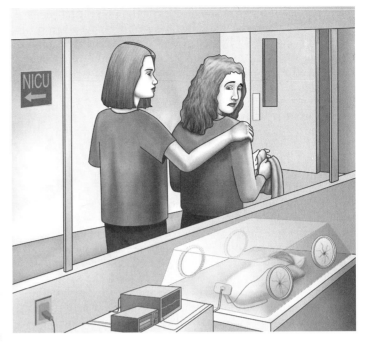

FIGURE **46-1**
Leaving the neonatal intensive care unit (NICU).

portunity to discuss their concerns. Another way to meet the needs of those who are problem-focused copers is to present them with transition programs such as one case management–home care program in Utah called Welcome Home (Scholtes et al, 1994). This program was specifically designed to enable parents of medically fragile infants in the NICU to learn how to take care of their children before discharge. After discharge, community resources that were known to the parents before the discharge was completed were made available to the parents. Parents who went through this program felt less of a crisis upon discharge than did parents who had no support. Costello and Chapman (1998) showed that mothers who participated in a care-by-parent program in which they roomed for 12 to 48 hours outside the NICU felt that their readiness to care for their infants was confirmed, as was the infant's readiness for discharge. This helps to decrease the mother's uncertainty in caring for her infant at home. A transitional care unit at Rainbow Babies and Children's Hospital was developed as a quality improvement project to look at innovative models of care and environments in order to transition infants home. The results of this project showed that a transitional care unit decreased the length of stay, decreased the number of readmissions (30% in 1992 to 6% in 1997), increased the discharges to home from 69% to 87%, improved parental satisfaction, and had a positive impact on the staff (Forsythe, 1998).

Parental Concerns

Kenner (1988) and Bagwell and associates (1990) found that parents from level II and III units had similar concerns. Their concerns fell into five categories: (1) informational needs; (2) grief; (3) parent-child development; (4) stress and coping; and (5) social support.

Informational Needs.   The informational needs of parents include how to provide routine newborn care; how to recognize normal newborn characteristics, both physical and behavioral; how to keep the infant healthy after discharge; their own responsibilities about how to provide care; the equipment used on their infant while in the NICU; and a complete explanation of the medical diagnosis and the expected prognosis (McKim, 1993a).

Parents want to feel that they are important enough to know what is really wrong with their infant (Kenner, 1988; Kenner et al, 1996). One family stated, "The only time that the physicians really asked us our opinion or told us about the baby's condition was when they were obligated to get informed consent for an experimental treatment." Another family said, "We would ask the nurses about the baby's apnea, but they said they had to check with the physicians and they would have to talk to us." Other comments included, "I never understood why nurses just came over and turned off our baby's sounding alarms without seemingly looking at the baby;" "No one told me how difficult it would be to breastfeed a premie;" "I did not realize how different from my other children the sleep cycle would be for my premie." These are just a few examples of information that the parents wanted. Parents felt better about their role and the information about their infant's care if they were considered part of the care team. Barker (1995) referred to this as viewing parents as partners in their children's care.

Grief. The category of grief was first called anticipatory grief (Kenner, 1988)—the rationale being that parents expressed the loss of their expected child once the reality of the neonatal problem shattered their hopes and fantasies. However, as time went on, parents continued to grieve but in the form of anticipating that the infant would eventually die if he or she were sick enough to require special or NICU care. They continued to anticipate this death or at least that the infant would get sick again and require hospitalization after discharge. Their perceptions suggest that the concept seems more appropriately considered grief than anticipatory grief. The process of grief and the period of mourning begin once the infant does not meet the parents' expectations of the fantasy or ideal child. If the parents have other children, they speak of how different this child is from their others or how different the infant is from their expectations. Although the parents anticipate further problems, it is probably not anticipatory grief but rather a continuation of the grief process. Another component of grief seems to be for the loss of the expected parenting role—that is, their normal, familiar role. This feeling may not be different from that of parents of normal, healthy infants, because the homecoming of those infants also requires a role adjustment. This assumption is an area still in need of further research.

Parent-Child Development. This category refers to the parents' and children's role expectations. Earlier in the chapter, role theory was examined. For anyone making a transition or entering a new level of functioning or a new stage of life, certain expectations about what is to come exist. New parents of healthy infants make adjustments in how they carry out the tasks of daily living once their newborn is at home. Each time a new member is introduced into the family, adjustments are made. When a problem with the infant that requires special care arises, parents may have to set aside their ideal expectations of their roles. The hospitalization may reinforce their roles or may hinder them.

Parents learn a lot about parenting by observing health care professionals. They learn what is valued. When a mother calls the unit for a progress report, she is usually told the infant's weight, amount of feedings, stooling patterns, percentage of oxygen, and how many times apnea occurred. It is not surprising that during home follow-up, parents, particularly mothers, want more information about feeding, formula, breastfeeding, elimination patterns (especially constipation), fear of the infant's losing weight (many say they have been told that if the infant loses weight, rehospitalization may be necessary), and whether the infant's breathing pattern seems normal. Nurses also may communicate to parents that the parents are not capable of caring for their infants. One family said, "I read all the literature about bonding and knew it was important to hold the baby, but we were not allowed;" "One nurse would say 'maybe in a couple of hours, maybe 4,' but that time would never come;" and "We were in the unit for 3 days before we held the baby, and he was the least sick of any of the infants in the nursery." This family was from a level II unit, and the infant was experiencing some periods of apnea. Thermoregulation was not a concern in this case. The parents felt that they were not needed, not important, and certainly not capable of parenting their infant. These feelings only add to the stress of having a sick infant (Kenner, 1995).

Stress and Coping. For many families, no warning that a problem is pending with the infant's birth or that the infant will be sick is available. Therefore they are unprepared, and reality of a sick neonate comes suddenly. The expected feelings of joy and the months of anticipation are replaced by sharply contrasting feelings of fear, shock, and overwhelming sadness. The family experiences disbelief that there could be a problem. Even when a premature or complicated birth is expected or a neonatal problem is diagnosed *in utero*, many parents still do not believe that a problem will occur. They are usually angry that their infant is sick. Demystification is the understanding of the medical condition—that is, having the informational needs about the prognosis and plan of treatment met. The conditional acceptance is integration of the infant's problem into the family. Even if this is a time-limited condition, the illness must be incorporated into the family's attitude about the unit and the demands that are facing them.

Adaptation coping is necessary for reaching a stage of conditional acceptance. This form of coping comes about through the identification of the family's stresses from their own perspective. It also requires a determination of the resources that are available to the family. These resources might be parent support groups, parent hotlines, extended family members, friends, financial resources, or home care. Adaptation also requires a change of attitude. Information and acknowledgment of feelings before and after discharge both help to ease the transition process to home and into the role of parent. Acknowledging that other parents have been scared about assuming responsibility for their infants' care and introducing them to successful parents decreases stress and increases coping.

Peeples-Kleiger (2000) studied the hospitalization in the neonatal intensive care as a traumatic stressor on parents and their adaptation. She used the American Psychiatric Association's *Diagnostic and Statistics Manual of Mental Disorders* (1994) definition for traumatic stressor of "actual or threatened death or serious injury, or a threat to the physical integrity of self or others" in looking at the NICU hospitalization as a traumatic stressor. She drew the following conclusions:

- Families that acknowledge the severity of the problem and talk about it cope better than those who do not.

- Parents must learn to manage one's feelings in order to adapt.
- Parents must learn that traumatic events will lead to involuntary memories for weeks, months, and years to come.
- Parents must learn that trauma-related symptoms such as lack of sleep and edginess can occur at any point, even after the crisis.
- Parents will feel helpless and may have unchanneled aggression related to the helplessness.
- Parents will need to learn to rebuild their lives and resolve their grief.

Continued stress, feelings of failure, and grieving for the loss of the fantasy child all has the potential for leading to maternal and paternal depression. Singer et al (1999) showed that psychological stress experienced by mothers of VLBW infants continued well past discharge. Parenting stress for mothers of infants with bronchopulmonary dysplasia or chronic lung disease extended to the infants' third year. Therefore for the health of the family, implementation of interventions is imperative. Ehrhard (1982) conducted a case study to "investigate the physical and neurodevelopmental sequelae of an extremely premature very-low-birth-weight infant" (p. i). When she finished her case study, she shared the information with the parents. The mother cried and stated, "Why didn't they tell me all this? I never really understood what he went through. This information helps me to understand my child and his needs." Thus as the researcher answered her research question, the parents received a lot of information as well. They got reassurance from a neonatal clinical nurse specialist that they had not caused the infant's problem and that they were not bad parents for feeling frustrated. These parents benefited by the follow-up. These serendipitous findings illustrate the need for parent care both in and out of the hospital setting. These findings now almost 20 years later still hold true.

Social Support.   Parents expressed the feeling that social support had both positive and negative facets. They meant that they saw the NICU nurses as having a lot of power and the potential to explain their infants' progress. They also believed that nurses had the potential to explain why medical treatment plans changed when house staff changes took place in teaching institutions. Nonetheless, parents did not feel that, for the most part, nurses fulfilled their role as advocates. The NICU nurses did not anticipate that the parents might be confused, and the parents readily admitted that they were too confused or intimidated by the health professionals to ask questions. They assumed that the nurses knew how they felt. They also thought that the nurses were working too many shifts in a row or too many long hours to be bothered with their seemingly trivial concerns. Some parents went so far as to describe the nurse's role as providing expert infant care but not parent care. Other parents expressed frustration over having to reorient nurses to their infant's condition. They often did not see the same nurse twice, even during a prolonged stay. Although the parents saw the potential for support, they did not feel that the support was always given. Primary nurses for continuity and mother-baby nurses for the level II parents were viewed as helpful for support.

The physician's role was viewed as being for infant care and not for the support of the family. For most families, the physician was the gatekeeper regarding what they were allowed to know about their infant. Physicians even regulated communication to parents via the nursing staff. Even after discharge, parents believed that the physician's permission was necessary

to make even the smallest change in the infants' routines that had been established in the hospital. These feelings might be tied to the parents' need for structure and their attempt to continue the safety of the NICU at home. Parents also viewed nurses as gatekeepers of information. The nurses would let parents know when it was not appropriate, for instance, to hold the infant, but only occasionally did they say when parents could hold the infant. Once again, support for their parenting role was not always seen as readily given. Unfortunately, a side effect of this perception is the parents' sense of a lack of trust that they can provide care or a feeling that the truth about their infants' conditions is being withheld from them.

The positive side of support was also expressed: the caring attitude by some professionals, the friendly hug, and the taking time to talk with the parents, even if it was about something other than their infants' problems. Acknowledgments of the mother's own physical discomfort conveyed a caring and supportive attitude. The availability of a phone number and the potential for a home visit were viewed as positive. Positive social support affects parents' views of their children's care. Van Riper (2001) studied parental well-being in relationship to the family provider relationship. She found that parents that had positive relationships with the child's care giver in the NICU and viewed the care as family-centered had more satisfaction with the care. For many parents, the home visit provides a way to vent feelings that otherwise must often be suppressed around family and friends (McKim, 1989, 1993b).

Parents also believed that many times family and friends withdrew their support. As previously mentioned, family and friends often believe that at discharge the crisis is past. For other parents, family and friends were afraid to approach the parents for fear of doing the wrong thing. Still other times, parents felt that their family and friends wanted to tell them what they were doing wrong and how they should parent their infants. For instance, the advice several mothers got included statements such as "Don't breastfeed your premie; he will get sick. Don't allow visitors; they will only make the baby sick." Positive reaction from family and friends included comments about how well the parents were doing with their infants, how well they were coping, and how normal their feelings of inadequacy are. Social support differs, however, by whether it is professional or personal.

Social support is an important aspect of coping and managing stress. If support is not provided, family functioning and health may suffer. Once social support needs are identified, a plan of action must be implemented. Because there are both positive and negative aspects of social support, it is probably more correct to term this category as social interaction. There is an interaction between at least two people; and whether it is positive or negative; support is determined by the recipient (McKim et al, 1995).

The five categories of parental concerns just discussed may represent a taxonomy for transitional care follow-up. These categories form the basis for transition to home.

INTERVENTION STRATEGIES

Many interventions can alleviate a crisis situation for a family of a premature infant at discharge. The NICU nurse—in the role of primary nurse, clinical nurse specialist, or neonatal nurse practitioner—can advocate for positive parental discharge. Recognizing parents' for information about their infants and the required at-home care facilitates development of a collaborative, interdisciplinary plan of care, including discharge and follow-up. This type of collaborative plan should include the parents' demonstrating competence and comfort with routine newborn care. Mothers, in particular, need support and reassurance, even after discharge (Bagwell et al, 1990; Kenner, 1988; Scholtes et al, 1994). The nurse needs to ensure that the parents are completely comfortable bathing, feeding, and diapering their infant and with administering any special care procedures, such as medication or oxygen therapy. The parents also need to be taught how the NICU infant's temperament differs from that of a normal newborn. Good discharge teaching includes all this as well as developmental information.

Parents also need continuity of care. Many parents express the frustration of trying to build a rapport with medical staff, who change monthly, and with nurses, who change daily. This situation will not necessarily improve, as more nurses work part-time flexible hours or work from agencies that float them between several intensive care units.

Parents also need to be informed and reminded that even though their infant is 6 months old by chronological age, she or he may be only 3 months old by conceptional age. Thus the infant may act more like a 3-month-old than like a 6-month-old. Tips on helping the infant adapt to home should also be included in the discharge information. Parents of former premature infants have offered such advice as leaving radios and lights on to help the infant adapt to the new environment. This need for increased stimuli may change as NICU infants begin to recognize a developmentally supportive environment (Cicco et al, 1996). Nursing research is needed in this area to determine whether NICU infants require more lights or noise at home.

Parents often report that they feel supported and reassured if a professional in addition to family or friends advise them. Neonatal Nurse Practitioners (NNPs) are often responsible for follow-up care. Follow-up nurses recognize that failure to use available community resources or follow professional advice may be related to coping difficulties. If this is true, avoidance of these failures may stop the cycle of stress and coping difficulties. Scheduling home visits at frequent intervals is a good strategy for assessing the family's progress (Chapter 47).

Care-by-parent units have been another way to alleviate parental anxiety and to decrease the chance for a crisis. Programs such as the previously discussed Utah program for parents of medically fragile infants, care-by-parent units, and transitional care units seem to help ease the transition home and increase parental confidence (Costello & Chapman, 1998; Forsythe, 1998; Scholtes et al, 1994). Some NICUs have a modified version of this type of care-by-parent or a transition unit. The ones cited in the articles by Costello & Chapman, (1998), Forsythe (1998), and Scholtes et al (1994) were well staffed with experienced nurses. In the modified units these areas usually has less staff, and parents are expected to provide more of the care. The irony is that parents feel very afraid of doing this. It may be their first attempt at being on their own with their infant. They need reassurance, discharge teaching, and role modeling; however, when NICUs are busy, the least experienced nurses are assigned to the transition unit. Also, changing health care environment and hospital budget cuts have resulted in many transitional units being supplemented with nonlicensed patient care assistants (PCAs) to help decrease the number of registered nurses needed and thus to decrease costs. The rationale is that these infants are "growers" who require minimal care. Nevertheless, some of these infants get sick again, many times because of inept assessments that

have allowed a minor problem to get out of hand. It would not be considered a good idea to assign a beginning-level nursing student to the most inexperienced clinician to learn nursing care—yet this is precisely what is done with parents. Parents need confident, well seasoned clinicians who value the need for parental education. Parenting is not a natural function, especially with a fragile neonate. Parents need reassurance; they need to gain self-confidence; they need someone who will recognize their needs without their having to verbalize them; and they need to know what to expect of their infants. If the infant is premature, what is the normal pattern of sleep? How long will it take for the infant's head to look like that of a fullterm neonate? These are only a couple of examples of behavioral characteristics that parents need to know to understand their infants' developmental pattern of growth. State modulation and developmentally supportive environments are other areas that should be explored with parents.

Family Care

The concept of the family as a unit is another point addressed in care-by-parents or transition units. The father and siblings are often forgotten during discharge preparation. More research is needed to determine fathers' concerns and the supports they need to prepare for their infants' discharge. Also, is information given differently to fathers than to mothers? Some fathers have expressed the feeling that they were given factual, detailed information on the infant's condition, whereas the mother received very little direct information from either the nursing or the physician staff (Bagwell et al, 1990; Kenner, 1988; McKim, 1993a). Most fathers want to participate in care and decision making.

Siblings must also adjust to the infant, who may not seem real to them until they are able to visit the infant in the NICU. Many units now encourage sibling visits to help ease the infant into the family well before the actual discharge.

Communication

Communication is a key element to successful relationships. It is a new focus for medical care. Classes and seminars in bedside manner are being conducted in medical schools across the United States. One reason for this is consumer pressure to have physicians display a caring attitude. Another factor is that malpractice cases are brought against physicians more often when communication has broken down between the physician and the patient. Suing "friendly, trustworthy" physician is more difficult than suing one who may be viewed as efficient but not concerned or personable.

Nurses are expert communicators. The art of nursing has revolved around the ability to convey care and personal attention to the client. Unfortunately, because of today's health care crisis, nursing shortages have resulted in staff mixes and use of unskilled personnel, coupled with economic constraints resulting in shortened hospital stays; nurses are also falling into the trap of assembly line health care delivery. However, nurses have the advantage of being able to identify and assess a family's needs and to convey these needs to other health care team members. Being an advocate for the family is an essential part of preparing a family for discharge. Follow-up, in essence, is allowing an open line of communication among health care professionals, the health care delivery system, and the family. It allows a partnership to develop between the health care team and the family. It gives the family back some control. Follow-up moves the family away from the learned helplessness acquired in the hospital to a more participative role. Nurses are often sought out by families who want to vent feelings and concerns-as long as the family feels that the nurses care enough to be concerned. Parents need to be able to openly express their concerns about their infants' appearance and about their feelings of helplessness without fear of being judged as bad parents. Nonverbal cues can get in the way of communication. The nurse's expertise, knowledge, and use of medical terminology without explanations all convey the nurse's need to be in control. Someone has to be in control, but relinquishing some control to the family does not lessen one's credibility as a professional. It conveys to the family that they have a role in their infants' care and that they are important too.

Another facet to this communication system is the other health care team members. Nurses cannot afford to withhold information that might help the physicians, social workers, and financial counselors who work with the family. Nurses need to convey information and coordinate the assessment data. Application of the nursing process may sound trite, but it is important in terms of not only collecting data but also using the data to identify problems, make nursing diagnoses, and develop a plan of care before and after discharge.

Long-Term Implications for the Family Unit

The breakdown of communication or of family functioning can lead to a less than optimal environment for the infant and child to grow. Studies have documented that the infant of very low birth weight, in particular, is at risk for child abuse, neglect, nonorganic failure to thrive, and developmental and behavioral problems found that the caregivers of these infants experienced more daily stress than did the average caregiver.

Collaboration between pediatric medical follow-up, parent support or psychosocial assessments at home, and obstetrical follow-up for the mother is essential. Each health care professional has something to contribute to the family's overall well-being. It is essential not to compete but to work with other professionals for the good of the family. This means that turf issues must be settled behind the scenes. It also means that each profession must share information that it receives from the family. It is not unusual during a home visit for the family to say; "I did not tell the OB [or pediatrician] about my concern over changing from cloth diapers to disposables because I did not want to bother him about that. Yet I am afraid to make even the smallest change in my baby's routine set up by the hospital." These statements demonstrate the need for a discharge protocol for the family.

Miles and Holditch-Davis (1995) and Wereszczak and associates (1997) found in retrospective research studies that the NICU stay has long-lasting effects on mothers of premature infants. When the children are 3 years old, these mothers experience what these researchers term compensatory parenting. This parenting style is overcompensation for feeling sorry for or guilty about having an infant in the NICU. They reported trying to provide special experiences and more stimulation to foster development with these children. At the same time they have shielded their children from other life situations to protect them from further hurt (Miles & Holditch-Davis, 1995). These researchers suggest that prospective research is needed to determine when or how this parenting style evolves. The other research that is needed is testing of interventions during and after the infants' NICU stay and continuing until preschool to determine what helps mothers coping with their special infants.

Technology-Dependent infants

In recent years the number of technology-dependent infants discharged home has increased, because of the many early discharge programs available or the survival of the extremely-low-birth-weight infants with chronic conditions. Alhough a fair amount is written about setting up early discharge programs and the positive financial rewards associated with early discharge, little research is available to look at the effects of having a technology-dependent infant at home.

Spangler-Torok applied the concepts of transition to this unique population. Spangler-Torok (2001) studied mothers receiving and caring for their technology-dependent infants in the home. The experiential descriptions were from eight mothers, aged 17 to 42, who were the primary caretakers of their technology-dependent infants. All of the mothers were interviewed within the first four weeks of receiving their infant into the home. Although this was a phenomenological study, it provides support for the concepts of the Kenner Transition Model.

Information Needs.   Mothers in this study understood the need to learn information regarding care and equipment so that the infant could be discharged. Mothers described moving from learning care to making judgments regarding the infant's health. Gathering information is a way of seeking control of the situation. The mothers in this study sought information to make an overwhelming experience more manageable. The mothers described initial fear of caring for the infant at home and their ability to move beyond the fear and do what needed to be done. As more information was gathered, mothers described using their judgment with infant health decisions. When receiving and caring for a technology-dependent infant in the home, more information seems to give mothers more control, confidence, and peace of mind.

Grief.   The mothers in this study feared the infant becoming ill and requiring rehospitalization. Several of the mothers voiced concern that the infant may die. Mothers grieved over the loss of the "ideal" pregnancy and infant. Mothers would report that they were managing the home care experience, "but this is not what I planned for." Mothers grieved about the life their infants would have and vowed to give them "as normal a life as possible." Mothers worried about what others would think. Would they think it was something I did while I was pregnant that caused this to happen to the baby? Mothers felt the need to "warn" others that the baby was different before they approached the infant.

Parent-Child Role Development.   Once they were at home, mothers in this study believed that they were getting to know their infants and that their infants were getting to know them as their mothers. Mothers reported learning things about their infants that they didn't know until they were home, like when their fussy times were. Mothers believed as they learned more about infant preferences and health-related behaviors they were able to make appropriate adjustments to infant care.

Regardless of whether they had other children, the mothers saw a need to adjust the parenting role and expectation to accommodate the premature infant. They realized this infant was different and require special care—in some instances, more vigilant care. They discussed how the increased needs of this infant took time away from other children and spouses but acknowledged that being home was easier than extended hospital visits. Most of the mothers in this study quit their jobs or school to care for the infant, which was not planned if the infant had been healthy. The mothers discussed lifestyle changes since infant came home from the hospital such as decreased number of outings, staying indoors more, and limiting visitors to the home.

Stress and Coping.   Mothers in this study acknowledged that receiving and caring for a technology-dependent infant in the home is a lot of work. One mother stated it is "a ton of work . . . ten times more work than a normal infant." Mothers report more time is needed with infant care as well as with supplemental tasks such as dealing with insurance companies, managing supplies, and checking equipment. A lot of time is required to prepare infant for outings, and time is needed for infant to readjust to home after outings. Mothers reported problems with infant digestion and temperament when away from home. "She may require two or three days to recover from an outing to the doctor's office." All of the mothers described the extra work and time the infant required but most felt it was worth it to have infant home with them.

Two mothers described being overwhelmed with infant care in the home and felt they faced too many demands. One mother felt torn between caring for the infant and spending time with her other children. She is "only one person" and can "only be in one place at a time." She appreciates the break the home nurses provide but feels guilty that infant receives care from others. Another mother describes frustration in dealing with the equipment. She has a "hard time looking" at the feeding tube but is less bothered by the tracheotomy. She gets angry when husband gravitates towards Holly, the "normal" twin, and leaves all the work for Grace to her. This mother is afraid that infant will pick up on her frustration with the equipment and feel that she doesn't love her.

Social Interaction.   Several mothers in this study attributed their ability to care for this infant at home to the support of family and friends. Mothers stated they could focus on infant care because others were handling household chores and running errands for them. One mother described how strangers who heard of their situation were delivering food to them. The same mother felt that their experience was probably easier than others because "so many people have pitched in to do things." In describing her experience, on mother stated "we just needed a lot of family." Having people come and help seems to make the experience more manageable for some of the mothers.

One mother described being supported by the home care nurses. "It's wonderful to have the nursing staff here, because when you want to break down and cry, they're there to tell you, rub your hand, or your shoulder and say 'you're doing a good job, don't think that you're not; you are.'" She is thankful for them and uses the nurses for other things so that she can spend time with the infant.

Although some mothers spoke of the assistance they received, others described the lack of support from family and friends. A mother spoke of being "annoyed" with her husband. She discussed how supportive they were of each other during infant's hospitalization and that she had assumed that would continue once they were home. Unfortunately, she described his lack of support and assistance with infant care and home management. "Hey, we have special circumstances here, this isn't just your average baby and you need to help me," she said. Another mother describes a lack of support from husband, children, and friends. She says her husband helps with the cooking, but it takes her three times as long to clean up. Although her 12-year old daughter is old enough to help, she doesn't. She also wonders why friends have not come to see her. She believes they are afraid to see the baby and therefore do not visit. She sometimes feels alone in her responsibility for the baby.

The experiences of mothers receiving and caring for their technology-dependent infants in the home support the Kenner Transition Model (1998). Mothers saw the need for information before the infant was discharged and after the infant was home. Mothers grieved for the child they had envisioned during pregnancy and worried what others would think about infant's special needs. Once they were home, mothers felt they learned more about their infant's likes and dislikes. They also saw the need for an adjustment in roles and responsibilities. Mothers reported increased work and worries when caring for the infant in the home. Two mothers expressed feelings of being overwhelmed. Many mothers reported that the support and assistance of others made the experience more manageable. Two mothers reported lack of support and problems coping with the increased demands.

It appears that the transition to home for this ever-growing population is even more fraught with stress and information needs. Nurses who advocate for their parents and infants and who are responsible for either providing or arranging care after discharge can make all the difference in the families' long-term outcomes. What will the transition be? It is up to you as the neonatal nurse to decide.

SUMMARY

The interventions discussed have been shown to have some effect in decreasing parental anxiety and thus lessening the crisis situation of the transition from the NICU to home. More research is needed to help determine whether specific way to alleviate the crisis situation for a family taking home a premature infant exists. Existing studies also must be replicated to demonstrate that the interventions are as effective as the original research suggests. A specific research question to be considered is whether all parents of premature infants need as extensive interventions as described or whether only parents of extremely ill or premature infants need such interventions. None of the existing studies address which group of parents are more at risk for crisis problems. The results of such a study might show that all parents, not only the parents of extremely ill or premature infants, need these types of interventions.

REFERENCES

American Psychiatric Association. (1994). *Diagnostic and statistical manual of mental disorders,* ed 4, Washington, DC: Author.

Bagwell GA et al (1990). *Parent transition from a special care nursery to home: a replicative study.* Unpublished master's thesis, University of Cincinnati College of Nursing and Health; Cincinnati, OH.

Barker JG (1995). Parents as partners in the NICU. *Neonatal network,* 14(1), 9-10.

Bialoskurski M et al (1999). The nature of attachment in a Neonatal Intensive Care Unit. *Journal of perinatal and neonatal nursing,* 13(1), 66-77.

Bruns DA et al (1999). What is and what should be: maternal perceptions of their roles in the NICU. *Infant toddler intervention: the transdisciplinary journal,* 9(3), 281-298.

Cicco R et al (1996). *Making NICUs more developmentally appropriate for infants: parents and families.* Paper presented at the Physical and Developmental Environment of the High Risk Neonate, University of South Florida College of Medicine, Clearwater Beach, FL.

Costello A, Chapman J (1998). Mothers' perceptions of the care-by-parent program prior to hospital discharge of their preterm infants. *Neonatal network*, 17(7), 37-42.

Ehrhard EM (1982). *The sequelae of an infant born at 24-25 weeks' gestation.* Unpublished master's thesis, University of Cincinnati College of Nursing and Health; Cincinnati, OH.

Forsythe P (1998). New practices in the transitional care center improve outcomes for babies and their families. *Journal of perinatology,* 18(6), S13-17.

Kenner C (1995). The transition to parenthood. In Gunderson LP, Kenner C (Eds.), *Care of the 24-25 week gestational age infant: small baby protocol,* ed. 2, Petaluma, CA: NICU Ink.

Kenner CA (1988). *Parent transition from the newborn intensive care unit (NICU) to home.* Unpublished doctoral dissertation, Indiana University; Indianapolis, IN.

Kenner C et al (1996). Parenting in the NICU. In Zaichkin J (Ed.), *Newborn intensive care: what every parent needs to know.* Petaluma, CA: *NICU Ink.*

Lemons JA et al (2001). Very Low birthweight outcomes of the National Institute of Child Health and Human Development Neonatal Research Network, January 1995 through December 1996. *Pediatrics,* 107(1), E1-8.

McKim E (1989). *The support needs of mothers of premature infants.* Presented at the Third International Nursing Research Symposium, McGill University School of Nursing, Montreal, Quebec, Canada.

McKim E (1993a). The information and support needs of mothers of premature infants. *Journal of pediatric nursing,* 8(4), 233-244.

McKim EM (1993b). The difficult first week at home with a premature infant. *Public health nursing,* 10(2), 89-96.

McKim EM et al (1995). The transition to home for mothers of healthy and initially healthy newborns. *Midwifery,* 11, 184-194.

Mercer RT (1981). A theoretical framework for studying factors that impact on the maternal role. *Nursing research,* 30(2), 73-77.

Mercer RT (1995). *Becoming a mother: research from Rubin to the present.* New York: Springer Publishers.

Mercer RT (1998). Maternal role attainment. In Tomey AM, Alligood MR (1998). *Nursing theorists and their work,* ed 4. St Louis: Mosby.

Mercer RT, Ferketich SL (1990). Predictors of family functioning eight months following birth. *Nursing research,* 39(2), 39-82.

Miles MS, Holditch-Davis D (1995). Compensatory parenting: how mothers describe parenting their 3-year-old, prematurely born children. *Journal of pediatric nursing,* 10(4), 243-253.

Miles MS et al (1998). Maternal concerns about parenting prematurely born children. *MCN American journal of maternal child nursing,* 23(2), 70-75.

Peeples-Kleiger MJ (2000). Pediatric and neonatal intensive car hospitalization as traumatic stressor: Implications for intervention. *Bulletin of the Menninger Clinic,* 64(2), 257-280.

Rubin R (1984). *Maternal identity and the maternal experience.* New York: Springer.

Scholtes PF et al (1994). Management of medically fragile infants and children. *Physician executive,* 20(9), 41-43.

Singer LT et al (1999). Maternal psychological distress and parenting stress after the birth of a very-low-birth-weight infant. *Journal of American Medical Association,* 281(9), 799-805.

Spangler-Torok L (2001). *Maternal perceptions of the technology-dependent infant.* Unpublished dissertation, Cincinnati: University of Cincinnati College of Nursing; Cincinnati, OH.

Stevenson DK et al (1998). Very-low-birth-weight outcomes of the National Institute of Child Health and Human Development Neonatal Research Network, January 1993-December 1994. *American journal of obstetrics and gynecology,* 179(6), 1632-1639.

Van Riper M (2001). Family-provider relationships and well-being in families with preterm infants in the NICU. *Heart & Lung,* 30(1), 74-84.

Ventura SJ et al (2001). Births: final data for 1999. *National vital statistics report,* 49(1), 1-99.

Wereszczak J et al (1997). Maternal recall of neonatal intensive care unit. *Neonatal network,* 16(4), 33-40.

HOME- AND COMMUNITY-BASED CARE

STEPHANIE L. DURFOR, MICHELE MURPHY-RATCLIFF

INTRODUCTION

For the family of a sick newborn, the time that the infant spends in a neonatal intensive care unit (NICU) is stressful. Although parents often have feelings of inadequacy and helplessness about their ability to care for their children, they anxiously await the time when they can take their children home. For many of these families, home care represents a desirable alternative to prolonged costly hospitalization and family separation.

Dramatic advances in medical technology have contributed to increased survival of infants with chronic medical conditions needing long-term care. Of the estimated 4 million infants born in the United States annually, more than 250,000 require some form of special care. Approximately 230,000 low-birth-weight infants (less than 2500 g) are born each year (Pellegrino, 1998). Low birth weight is a principle predictor of infant survival and potential morbidity.

Although the majority of infants who require ongoing care—preterm and fullterm infants with birth asphyxia, sepsis, respiratory distress, major congenital anomalies, metabolic problems, and hyperbilirubinemia—are also hospitalized for special care, home health care has become one alternative method of health care delivery for infants and children.

DEVELOPMENT OF HOME CARE

Home health care options for neonates and infants have grown in response to rising hospital costs, emotional need of families, and technologic advances. The trend toward home-based care has been influenced most by developmental philosophy, technologic advances, family emotional health, and cost efficiency. The factor that has created the greatest pressure to expand the home care industry is cost efficiency.

United States health care expenditures are about $1 billion per day (Pellegrino, 1998). The gross national production portion dedicated to health care is greater in the United States than most other countries (Pellegrino, 1998). Two billion dollars are spent each year on NICU care (Pellegrino, 1998). Third-party payers are unable to sustain the high costs of maintaining medically fragile infants in acute care facilities. These infants quickly exhaust insurance benefits and hospital resources. Institutions faced with unsustainable expenses are eagerly seeking more cost-effective systems to provide quality care. Home care is a less expensive alternative.

Financial savings related to neonatal home care have been well documented. In 1976, Pinney and Cotton described a home management program for infants with bronchopulmonary dysplasia (BPD); this program had resulted in a savings of $18,000 per patient. Donn (1982) documented the cost effectiveness of home management of patients with BPD. This study reported an average per-patient savings of $60,690. Brooten and associates (1986) demonstrated that early hospital discharge of infants of very low birth weight to follow-up home care provided by a hospital-based nurse specialist could realize a net savings of $18,560 for each infant. Thilo and colleagues (1987) found substantial cost savings for families and health insurance carriers when infants were discharged from NICUs with home oxygen therapy. This group reported a savings of $33,370 per patient.

In a home phototherapy study, Eggert and associates (1985) found home phototherapy to be feasible, safe, effective, and cost-effective. They compared costs between home and in-hospital phototherapy. The results indicated home phototherapy provided a potential savings of $73,152 over a year after treating 254 infants (Eggert et al, 1985). A study in 1986 also concluded that home phototherapy is effective, safe, and cost-effective, showing a savings of $430 per patient treated by home phototherapy in comparison with hospital phototherapy (Grabert et al, 1986).

In 1991, Fields and colleagues (1991b) evaluated home care costs and the cost effectiveness of home care for respiratory technology–dependent children. The study, conducted in a Medicaid Model Waiver Program in Maryland, compared the difference between the established Medicaid reimbursements for a long-term care institution and actual Medicaid reimbursements for home care. The mean annual home care costs were $109,836 (with a standard deviation of $20,781) for ventilator-dependent children and a mean cost of $63,650 (standard deviation, $12,350) for oxygen-dependent children with tracheostomies. The home care costs, in comparison with standard Medicaid long-term institutional care, represented an annual savings of approximately $79,000 per ventilator-dependent patient and $83,000 per oxygen-dependent patient with a tracheostomy (Fields et al, 1991b).

Several studies of home care for technology-dependent children have shown home care to be more cost-effective than institutional care. Home care may save as much as a half million dollars per year, or about 50% of the inpatient costs.

Many investigators have addressed the emotional aspect of home care for infants. The process of parent-infant bonding is dramatically altered when a child is hospitalized in a NICU. The authoritarian setting and the confusion of an acute care unit create barriers to the normal bonding activities of parents and neonate. Parents often feel as if the hospitalized infant belongs to the hospital staff. Parents feel ownership of their infant only after they are able to take the child home.

Prolonged infant hospitalization has been shown to be associated with failure to thrive, with child abuse, and with parental feelings of inadequacy. When early discharge can be facilitated, parents begin to resolve negative feelings surrounding the birth of their children. Home care can restore to some parents a positive self-image and allows them to regain feelings of control over their lives and the life of their child. Uniting parents and their children in the home enhances the process of bonding and attachment. Families often take pride in their accomplishments as the infant grows and develops. If medical and nursing treatments are required, parents may develop an increased sense of satisfaction from their involved loving care in the home. Family members can become accomplished in oxygen administration, gavage feedings, respiratory treatments, dressing changes, and various other tasks that are rewarding to them.

Since the 1980s, concern has been expressed regarding the adverse developmental consequences for children of prolonged institutional care. In the past, it was believed that acute care facilities offered major advantages in terms of available services for a child with special care requirements. As more investigations were conducted, a greater appreciation of the deleterious effects of prolonged hospitalization on development has been noted. Improvements in developmental performance and in social interactions have been documented after discharge to home care with consistent caregivers.

Technologic advances have made neonatal and infant care in the home not only possible but also safe and efficient. Procedures that were previously limited to in-hospital settings can now be performed in the home. Oxygen administration, respiratory care, mechanical ventilation, phototherapy, intravenous therapy, and alternative modes of nutritional support are just a few of the modalities available to children in the home environment. Manufacturers of health care products are making available supplies and equipment that make home care feasible. Monitor manufacturers, oxygen supply companies, and intravenous product suppliers have developed designs specific to home care. Portable equipment has become a major market focus for the health care product industry. Although the technology is available to support the home care, it nonetheless requires a family that is able—physically and emotionally—to turn their home into a mini-NICU.

Nurses who are doing home care must feel comfortable in troubleshooting the equipment. They must teach the families to do the same. For example, if oxygen is being used at home that the nurse must know how to swap a tank and to teach the family this skill as well. Ventilators are now sometimes brought into the home; therefore the nurse must know the manufacturer's instructions for its use in this environment. Troubleshooting of this equipment may require consultation with the technical support from the ventilator company. The family must also have this information.

As technology for home therapy expands, the need for additional home care agencies and support personnel becomes essential. Home care systems have been established in response to the demand for increasingly complex and highly technical care in the home. Entrepreneurial endeavors, proprietary home health care agencies, and hospital-based programs have been introduced into the field of home care to provide the resources and the services necessary to meet the increasing need.

In attempts to shift costs from the expensive in-patient setting to the home, hospitals are creating home care services. Neonatal home care programs are being developed to address comprehensive discharge planning, parental and family education and skills development, cardiopulmonary resuscitation instruction, and appropriate follow-up. Home follow-up and program evaluation are essential elements of neonatal home care programs. Brooten and associates (1986) described one model of home follow-up of very-low-birth-weight infants. Early discharge of these infants with home follow-up by perinatal nurse specialists was concluded to be safe and cost-effective and to provide potential benefits to society in regard to potential reduction in child abuse and foster placement.

In 1991, Fields and colleagues (1991a) described an independent community-based care management model. Children in this report received home care coordinated by a community-based consortium of public and private organizations that was developed to provide case management for respiratory-disabled children in the home or alternative living facilities. This model offered maximized regional experience and expertise, case management with no financial self-interest in coordinating services, improved regional quality assurance of home care, and decreased reliance on tertiary care centers, thus allowing easier access to community-based resources.

All Aboard the 2010 Express: A 10-Year Action Plan to Achieve Community-Based Service Systems for Children and Youth with Special Health Care Needs and their Families, published by the Department of Health and Human Services (DHHS, 2001) addresses the objectives of Healthy People 2010. The main thrust of the infant and family objectives is to build community programs to support the health care needs of this vulnerable population. The Omnibus Budget and Reconciliation Act of 1989 mandated funds to support maternal child health care needs (DHHS, 2001). From that time building strategic partnerships with communities and with parents to provide care in the community and home settings has been emphasized. A new definition now exists for children with special health care need— "children with special health care needs are those who have or are at increased risk for a chronic physical, developmental, behavioral, or emotional condition and who also require health and related services of a type or amount beyond that required by children generally." (DHHS, 2001). This definition broadens the services that are covered or expected—such as transportation, respite care, and early intervention.

For the first time the concept of family-centered care is now applied to home care. The family becomes integral to the decision-making for their infant's care. Family Voices is a grass-roots volunteer group that lends support to families (DHHS, 2001). The term medical home is used to define the community care that is given to infants and their families. It provides support to families and coordination of multidisciplinary services. One of families' complaints is that care is very fragmented. Nurses who provide case management or care coordination can readily help families to provide comprehensive care—both primary and acute. Often we forget that former NICU patients still require ongoing primary care, just as any other child does. The Neonatal Nurse Practitioner (NNP) often now cares for infants through the first year of life. More nurses are becoming dually certified as Pediatric Nurse Practitioners (PNPs) and NNPs to meet the combination of well child and chronic care. Another important aspect of this care is the cultural component. Because the care is delivered in the home and done within the context of the family, the family values and cultural believes are even more important considerations than when the infant is hospitalized. Nurses need to provide culturally sensitive and competent care. About one-quarter of all uninsured children who have special care needs have no designated physician (DHHS, 2001). State Children's Health Insurance Program, or S-CHIP, and Health Insurance Portability Act (HIPAA) have helped to extend some coverage for a portion of the child with special care needs; however a lot of children and families nonetheless go without health care coverage. The implications for home care are that if these children are discharged from the hospital while they are still in need of medical care they sometimes fall through the cracks once they reach the home. They find that the coverage they thought they had—either insurance or physician—does not exist. Thus home care may or may not be feasible. Use of Early and Periodic Screening, Diagnostic and Treatment (EPSDT) can sometimes gain support for the need for home care services.

As the home care industry rapidly expands, issues concerning quality of care are being addressed. In 1988, the Joint Commission on Accreditation of Healthcare Organizations (JCAHO) developed accreditation standards for home care providers, These standards are comprehensive and focus on patient care, safety, infection control, quality assurance, management, administration, and governance. Specific standards apply to equipment management services, equipment selection, setup and maintenance, and client education. Standards pertaining to related medical supplies that are delivered to and used in the home environment have also been established. The JCAHO accreditation is awarded to home care companies that demonstrate compliance with recommended standards of practice.

TYPES OF HOME CARE

Home care, for most practical purposes, is classified as short-term, long-term, or hospice care. Other programs involve respite care, day care, and foster care.

Short-Term Care

Short-term care is considered by many health care services to be less than 6 months in duration. Short-term care of an infant at home may include phototherapy for hyperbilirubinemia (Madlon-Kay, 2001), administration of supplemental oxygen to treat respiratory distress, home monitoring for apnea of the premature infant, medication administration for various neonatal conditions, and alternative feeding methods such as gavage for nutritional support. The primary caregivers in the home usually attend to these treatment modalities. Parents and families are carefully instructed in the use of any equipment placed in the home to administer health care. Extensive teaching before hospital discharge must convey the precise reasons for the therapy, the necessity for close observation of the infant by the caregivers, and the importance of communication and supervision by the primary care physician. In situations of short-term home care, the condition is usually self-limiting, and the home therapy can be discontinued at a predetermined end point.

Long-Term Care

The point at which care becomes long-term is determined by the nature of the health care needs of the individual. The providers of extended care and the insurers paying for the care also arbitrarily set the time frame for long-term care. In general, long-term care indicates that the duration of the condition and the need for care will exceed 6 months. Long-term home care addresses situations for children with disease processes such as BPD, short bowel or short gut syndrome, congenital heart disease, physical and cosmetic defects, neurologic and metabolic disorders, and numerous other prolonged pathologic conditions.

Upon discharge, these children may require home care services performed by professional home care agencies or programs. Families gradually become integrated into the health care routine. The family's responsibility changes as the condition of an infant changes. The primary care physician must be closely involved and should be able to rely comfortably on the caregiver's judgment for making assessments and alterations in the home care plan. Long-term home care requires open communication among the family, community physicians, tertiary resources, community health care providers, home medical equipment providers, and financial providers. Many hospital records are now incorporating discharge notes, especially nursing case management notes or orders for the actual discharge and home care follow-up plan. These notes are a good vehicle for communication among the community health care providers and the discharging hospital.

Hospice Care

Despite dramatic developments in medical expertise and technology, a significant number of neonates who are admitted to special care units do not survive. Infant mortality in the United States has declined dramatically since 1960, but this trend leveled off in the 1990s (Stricklin, 1993). Congenital anomalies are the leading cause of infant mortality in the United States and are also a major contributor to childhood morbidity, long-term disability, and loss of years of potential life. The proportion of infant deaths attributed to birth defects has remained significantly high. Our Human Immunodeficiency Virus (HIV) epidemic is improving but still takes it toll on the neonatal population. Those infants require specialized home care and in some instances palliative care. In addition, with technological advances the ability to prolong lives has increased. Infants who are born dying due go home where they need end-of-life (EOL) care. When it becomes clear that an infant will no longer benefit from acute intervention, plans for health care should focus on physical and emotional comfort. The transition from acute care to palliative care involves concepts of hospice.

Hospice care is a philosophy of caring when cure is no longer a reasonable expectation. This care is not strictly a kind of terminal care but rather an effort to maximize current quality of life without giving up all interest in a cure. Hospice provides comfort measures and focuses on alleviation of symptoms. Whether the infant is terminally or chronically ill, the ultimate goal is to provide an environment that comforts the child and supports the family.

Hospice home care can be provided by a variety of models. Programs have been developed to use parents as primary caregivers and hospital-based personnel as facilitators and resource support. Terminal care can be shifted from hospital-based medical management to community-supported home nursing. Essential to the success of these types of programs, however, is the family's desire and their confidence in their ability to care for the child at home. In addition, they must be assured of regularly scheduled home visits and the availability of program personnel to respond when needed (Lauer & Camitta, 1980). Community caregivers with hospital coordination constitute a successful support system for families who elect to care for their dying child or a child with a disabling disease or condition for which no curative therapy is known (Martin, 1985).

Institutions dedicated to the care of the terminally ill have become an important alternative care approach and an accepted part of the health care field in the United States. Hospice facilities caring for children are currently increasing in number, but access to hospice care still has several barriers. Most facilities require a physician's certification that the child will die within 6 months. It is very often difficult to predict the remaining time that a child has left. Another serious barrier is the lack of financial reimbursement for care or the inadequacy of the reimbursement to cover the cost of hospice care (Rhymes, 1990). This area of neonatal and infant care is relatively new but a much needed one. For a comprehensive review of EOL and palliative care, see Chapter 9.

Respite Care

At the time of the infant's discharge from the hospital, many parents do not perceive a need for relief or respite care. If comprehensive discharge teaching has been accomplished, parents often feel anxious and ready to assume responsibility for their child. Over the course of time, however, parents find that many of their expected support systems are unavailable to assist with a sick infant. Relatives, friends, and babysitters often feel inadequate and are unable to assume the responsibility of caring for an infant with special needs.

The daily routine for parents may be time-consuming and exhausting. Practical problems that were not issues during hospitalization arise. Family and friends outside of the household cannot appreciate the constant strain that is experienced by the immediate family. Social activities become restricted and ungratifying. Even routine outings such as grocery shopping become cumbersome. The child is often too fragile to take to the store, and appropriate childcare is often scarce. The resulting fatigue and frustration can threaten the quality of care provided for the child and other family members.

Social and emotional support can be provided to families in a variety of ways. Respite or relief care can be sought from willing family members, friends, the community, and health care facilities.

Use of homemaker home health aides has been successful in providing assistance for families caring for high-risk infants in the home. Parents need to maintain time for them. Privacy and recreation for parents are essential if the parents are to meet the challenge of caring for a sick infant at home successfully. Various community services are making available relief care for overburdened families. Families should be encouraged to seek out and take advantage of any available family or community source of respite care.

Day Care

Models of special day care centers are emerging across the country. These facilities offer a protected environment, medical technology, and professional nursing care in a day care setting. One such facility is Kangaroo Kids Center in Santa Ana, California. This center, established in 1989, offers a comprehensive program for medically fragile children in a day care center. Open 16 hours each day, Kangaroo Kids Center addresses the child's nursing care needs as well as the developmental and psychosocial needs of the entire family.

A similar model of day care is offered by the Community Health Programs at The Children's Hospital in Denver, Colorado. Kidstreet—a day care facility for medically fragile children—opened in August, 1992. This center offers day care for children 6 weeks to 6 years of age who need the services of medicine, nursing, occupational therapy, speech/language therapy, and psychosocial support for families. As a result of the successful provision of cost-effective, safe, high technology day care, a second center was opened in February, 1995 (The Children's Hospital Practice Update, 1995).

Day care for medically fragile, technology-dependent infants is a concept with great potential for future growth. This new alternative offers a much needed care delivery system to special-needs infants and their families. This avenue of care also presents nurses with a challenge and an opportunity to expand professional knowledge and nursing expertise.

Foster Care

Parents and families of infants with complex medical conditions and complex health care needs may find themselves unable to assume the responsibility of caring for their children. The child's health status requires monitoring, compliance with medical and developmental protocols, and timely interventions. These demands are often beyond the capabilities of birth families.

The number of low-birth-weight infants and infants with developmental delays born to teenagers, substance-using mothers, and homeless women continue to grow rapidly. Because of the circumstances surrounding the birth and the dysfunctional dynamics of these families, many infants are assumed to be at high risk for abuse, neglect, and abandonment. For these infants and children, medical foster care is an option.

Medical foster care for medically fragile infants can be provided through a variety of programs. Buenvenidos Children's Center, Inc., in eastern Los Angles County developed Bienvenidos Children's Center to provide medical foster care. This program, in coordination with the Los Angeles County Department of Children's Services and community-based agencies, helps parents become more competent and self-assured in appropriately caring for their medically fragile child in their home.

The Medical Foster Parent Program of the Children's Home and Aid Society of Illinois and La Rabida Children's Hospital and Research Center in Chicago offers another type of medical foster care. This program is designed to locate families and facilitate foster care for medically dependent children under the custody or guardianship of the Illinois Department of Children and Family Services. These children are medically ready for discharge, but their families are either unable or unwilling to care for them.

Medical foster care poses a unique challenge for health care providers, child welfare professionals, and foster families. The successful development and management of medical foster services depend on the ability of all related community systems to be committed, flexible, creative, and aggressive in arriving at solutions that will facilitate the transition of these children from hospital to home care.

CRITERIA FOR HOME CARE

Some hospitals throughout the country are developing specialized outreach/home care services as an extension of their inpatient services. Regardless of how services are to be provided, the decision to facilitate early discharge from hospital care to home care must be based on standards that are safe and that provide effective ongoing therapy. The infant, the family, the home equipment, and the follow-up health care system must meet criteria for discharge to home care.

Infant Criteria

The infant's home health care needs must be assessed as to technical feasibility and medical requirement. Nutritional support must be evaluated. How does the infant feed and how frequently? How often does the infant require gavage feedings, and which feeding techniques are required? Pharmacologic support assessment must be evaluated. What medication does the infant need and how often? What are the desired and adverse effects of these drugs? Does the infant require supplemental oxygen, respiratory therapy treatments, or chest physical therapy? The assessment of the level of care required must be matched to the ability and skills of the home care providers. It must be determined before discharge that care in the home will be safe and meet the needs of the infant and family.

The specific criteria for discharge of special groups of children—such as those with BPD, short bowel or gut syndrome, neurologic disease, cardiac disease, and other pathologic conditions—are addressed in the preceding chapters.

Family Criteria

The assessment of the family's commitment to home care is perhaps the most critical factor determining the success or failure of home health care. After extensive discharge teaching, skills development, and repetitive occasions of care giving, the family must want the child at home and under their care. They must be willing and able to devote the time and energy required to meet the physical and emotional needs of the child. These factors are essential for the well-being of the family unit.

To prepare families for the discharge of their sick or high-risk infant, NICU personnel must begin teaching them as soon as the neonate is admitted to the unit. Once the family is confident and capable of meeting the needs of the infant, a home assessment should be completed. Basic facilities such as heat, water, telephone, electricity, and transportation must be available. Appropriate support systems must be set up in the home, including the technology necessary for the delivery of care. The operation of phototherapy lights or blankets, oxygen delivery systems, portable suction equipment, respiratory and cardiac monitoring systems, ventilators, and numerous other devices must be thoroughly understood by the caregivers. Clear instructions need to be given to the family members by the providers of the home care technology. Ideally, the parents should bring the equipment to the hospital, or the equipment company can help transport it to the hospital before discharge. The rationale is that the parents can be taught on their own equipment. If a problem arises, it can usually be identified before the infant's discharge. The parents should spend at least 24 hours providing total care before discharge. This time under health professional's supervision helps the family gain confidence in their care giving abilities. They can also be reassured that they have the proper equipment.

Home Equipment Criteria

The most common equipment needs for neonates are cardiopulmonary monitoring, oxygen, suction, and feeding implements. The family's first decision making question is how to select a home care equipment company. Most hospital discharge planners or the nurse responsible for the discharge can make recommendations. Burstein (1995) outlined the criteria for selecting a home care pulmonary equipment company. These criteria (Box 47-1) can be used for other types of equipment suppliers as well.

Once the supplier has been selected and the necessary equipment identified, parent education can begin. This education should include neonatal cardiopulmonary resuscitation (CPR). The parents should be given written instructions to take home and a checklist for the CPR procedure that can be clearly posted. If parents cannot read, visual charts outlining the steps should be made available.

A cardiopulmonary monitor is the most common equipment needed in the home. Infants who should be placed on this type of monitoring are those whose sibling died of sudden infant death syndrome (SIDS) or who are at risk for SIDS. These infants are usually monitored until age 6 to 12 months (Burstein, 1995). An infant on home oxygen or one who has neurologic impairment is at risk for apneic or bradycardic episodes. Most of these monitors have built-in impedance pneumography capabilities that allow strips to be watched or viewed by home care nurses. In some instances, these can be sent via computer modems. The parents should be told that when an episode of apnea or bradycardia occurs, they must mark on the strip the infant's color, activity, and what they had to do, if anything, to stop the episode (Burstein, 1995). Burstein (1995) made two important points about this type of monitor. For infants on mechanical ventilation, chest excursion that is detected by the monitor because breathing does not allow the alarm to sound until the heart rate is affected, as in the NICU. Also, for infants who have tracheostomies, the monitoring is to identify episodes in which breathing may stop as a result of mucus plugs or thickened secretions. The survival instinct of the infant to struggle to breathe will not allow the respiratory monitor alarm to sound as movement is detected. It is the cardiac portion of the monitor that at a much later stage detects bradycardia. Parents need to understand these delays and how to respond.

Suctioning equipment is needed for patients with tracheostomies. This equipment requires electricity and running

---

BOX 47-1

Criteria for Selecting A Home Care Pulmonary Equipment Accreditation by the Joint Commission on Accreditation of Healthcare Organizations (JCAHO)

Location: within an hour's driving radius of home
Availability of equipment and supplies required for care
Experience with equipment required for care
24-hour on-call service for emergencies
Professional home care clinicians or staff*
Record system available to communicate with physician
Availability of back-up equipment on site
Experience with similar clinical situations
Acceptance of assignment on insurance benefits

Some areas may require professional services to be contracted. Contracted professionals must be available on 24-hour on-call basis.
From Czervinske MP, Barnhart SL (Eds.) (2002). Perinatal and pediatric respiratory care, ed 2, Philadelphia: WB Saunders.

water. One type of suctioning equipment must be portable and battery-powered for trips to and from the clinic and other excursions out of the home. It should have a regulator valve to adjust the amount of suction. If the valve is not present, negative pressure can be very great and cause mucosal trauma to the nasopharyngeal and tracheal tissues. The battery-powered suction machines can be recharged much like portable phones with a direct A/C adapter into a wall outlet or via a cigarette lighter adapter (Burstein, 1995). Most run about 2 hours without recharging. The recharging process takes about 12 hours. The other type of suctioning equipment can be a stationary set-up. Parents should be taught clean suctioning technique, which is used as long as no danger of cross-contamination with other infectious agents in the home exists, as may be the case when siblings are ill. Nosocomial infections and cross-contamination are very real possibilities when the infant is hospitalized. The parents should also be taught sterile technique, which should be used only when illness that may put the infant at risk for cross-contamination is present in the home.

Suctioning should be taught according to the physician/practitioner's orders. Usually this is done on an as-needed basis. Signs that indicate the need for suctioning are the same as those used by health professionals in the NICU: restlessness, decreased color, coughing, increased respiratory effort, or sounds of congestion. In general, suctioning is necessary every 2 to 4 hours. Parents should keep a log of the timing of the suctioning and the type of secretions obtained. In addition to the suctioning equipment, parents will need a 50-pound per square inch (PSI) portable air compressor and possibly compressed oxygen with portable reservoir. Portable or stationary oxygen devices vary in size and the amount of time that they will last. They are classified as sizes AA through K. G, H, and K are large and stationary, whereas the others are portable. The oxygen tanks for these devices differ from those of liquid oxygen in that they can be stored and will not leak if the shut-off valve is left on. They are larger and are filled under high pressure so they are more difficult to move. A slight danger from pressure occurs if they are accidentally dropped or damaged. The liquid oxygen is more portable and smaller in size. It does not require external electricity or battery-powered sources. The cylinder is small and filled under very little pressure. The liquid oxygen must be moved from the base of the chamber to a portable reservoir. It is more costly than gas pressure oxygen cylinders.

These infants often also need an oxygen concentrator. The concentrator is like the old-fashioned mix-box used in the NICU to mix air and oxygen to achieve the desired oxygen concentration. It separates oxygen from nitrogen in room air and collects oxygen (Burstein, 1995). The concentrations that are possible with these home devices are between 45% and 95% (Burstein, 1995). They cannot deliver very low flow rates such as 0.5 L/minute. They are electrically powered. Portable units are needed outside the home. A back-up gas oxygen cylinder is necessary for electrical failures and for excursions outside the home. It is beyond the scope of this chapter to detail the exact procedure for the suctioning and care of the tracheostomy tube. The equipment needed for an infant with a tracheostomy is listed in Box 47-2.

Humidification of the airway is necessary for infants with artificial airways, regardless of whether they are on oxygen. If the airway is not humidified, mucus membranes may dry and crack, creating areas that may become infected. Volume jet nebulizers can provide humidification with a 50-PSI portable air com-

pressor. Humidification levels of 35% to 100% can generally be achieved (Burstein, 1995). This compressor should be capable of providing high- or low-pressure aerosol. This capability is important if the infant requires a mist tent at night but during the day is connected to a tracheostomy collar or other airway devices. Some companies suggest use of a heat and moisture exchanger (HME), which can be used for travel and is used by itself and not in conjunction with other humidifying devices. It can be attached to the airway without intermediate equipment (Burstein, 1995).

Mechanical ventilation is another area of home care. Information on home use of ventilators can be obtained from the National Center for Home Mechanical Ventilation. The physician or practitioner on the basis of infant's need orders the specific type of ventilator. The decision also takes into consideration the family's lifestyle. If the family anticipates movement from home to other areas or other relatives' homes, a portable unit may be best. All portable units must have an internal and external battery. An emergency back-up unit must be available—whether it be housed in the home or at immediate dispatch from the equipment company does not matter as long as it is available for times when equipment failures occur with the portable device. Battery backup is also necessary. Usually a 12-volt battery with 74-amp/hour potential is sug-

---

BOX 47-2

Equipment Supply List for Tracheostomy Patient

Heat and moisture exchangers (1 to 2 boxes per month) apnea-bradycardia monitor
Electrodes (2 pairs)
Lead wire (2 pairs)
Belts (2 each)
Tracheostomy tubes (same size) (4 per month)
Tracheostomy tubes (one size smaller) 1 each
Velcro tracheostomy ties (2 boxes per month)
Twill tape (1 roll)
Free-standing suction machine (1 each)
Portable suction machine
Suction connecting tubing (4 per month)
Suction catheters (4 cases per month)
DeLee traps (6 each)
50-PSI portable air compressor
Jet nebulizers (4 per month)
Corrugated aerosol tubing (100-ft roll)
Tracheostomy collars (4 per month)
Liquid oxygen with portable reservoir (as needed)
Oxygen connecting tubing (4 each)
Sterile water (2 to 3 cases per month)
Normal saline, 3-ml vials (2 boxes month)
Heat and moisture exchangers (1 to 2 boxes per month)
Scissors (2 pairs)
Nonsterile gloves (2 boxes per month)
Manual resuscitation bags (2 each)
Sterile cotton-tipped applicators (2 boxes per month)
Hydrogen peroxide (2 bottles per month)
Stethoscope

From Czervinske MP, Barnhart SL (Eds.) (2002). Perinatal and pediatric respiratory care, ed 2, Philadelphia: WB Saunders.

gested; such a battery can go about 18 to 20 hours without recharge.

These areas of home care monitoring are the most common. Specific instructions on which equipment is necessary and how to use it in each situation should be obtained from a home health care agency who is to provide care, the hospital equipment vendors, and the home health care equipment vendors. Nurses who are responsible for discharge should be very familiar with the advantages and disadvantages of the equipment that the family will need. The family's lifestyle and capabilities also have to be considered when an infant is sent home on equipment.

Home care equipment and supplies must fit the patient just as it did in the hospital. The nurse responsible for the discharge must make sure that the child's size is considered when ordering equipment. For example, if the infant is now 12 pounds, do you still use a premie stethoscope? If the child has a tracheostomy, is there a back-up of proper size?

Ideally the nurse should make a home visit before the discharge to assess the home environment for safety hazards. For example, is the house/apartment too hot or cold? Either condition can lead to apneic spells. Are there exposed wires in the house? Peeling paint? Open flames used for cooking when oxygen is going to be used in the house? Are there any strong or chemical odors that may be harmful to a child with respiratory compromise? Is there an emergency phone? All aspects of the home and the community setting should be considered when discharging the infant and family.

Follow-Up System Criteria

Criteria for home care cannot be complete without accurate assessment of the availability of follow-up after discharge. Environmental conditions and social supports are two of the strongest influences on the ability of the parents to nurture their child in the home.

Hospital-based programs that provide home health services may establish home health visits. Community-funded home health care agencies are often available to provide some home follow-up. The departments of public health and other publicly funded agencies can be of assistance with home care follow-up.

The visiting resource person must be appropriately knowledgeable about the physical and emotional needs of the family. To be effective, the home visitor should be sensitive to cultural and ethnic differences and incorporate knowledge about them into the follow-up plan.

Public Law 99-457 regarding education of the handicapped mandates that services be available for NICU graduates. These children must be referred to early intervention programs to promote the most positive development possible. Any infant who has a developmental delay, is at risk for a developmental problem, or has a condition with a high probability for developmental problems, such as Down syndrome, is eligible (Stepanek, 1996). Resources for information in early intervention services include National Early Childhood Technical Assistance System (NEC*TAS), 137 East Franklin Street, Suite 500, Chapel Hill, NC 27514, 919-962-2001 and Technical Assistance for Parents Program (TAPP), 95 Berkley Street, Suite 104, Boston, MA 02116, 617-482-2915 (Stepanek, 1996).

Families are taught the value of developmental care in most NICUs today. They expect nurses to teach them how to continue these strategies in the home. Teach them how to watch the behavioral cues and assess their home environment for excessive noise or light levels, for disruptions to the sleep-wake cycles, and potential for excess handling from overzealous friends and relatives. Teaching the family how to protect the infant and to assist in promoting positive growth gives them back some control over the situation that they may have felt somewhat powerless to this point. Help them to advocate for the child's well-being. This includes how to support behaviorally appropriate feedings and other aspects that promote positive development (see Chapter 25). Developmental care in the home is a growing trend.

FUTURE TRENDS

One of the new trends that started in the adult population but is beginning to reach into infant care is the movement of telehealth. Telehealth care refers to a variety of venues—videoconferencing, Personal Digital Assistants (PDAs), computer connection through the telephone lines to transmit data. Telehealth has been used with infants with special care needs (Farmer & Muhlenbruck, 2001). Unfortunately our reimbursement system for such services is low (Farmer & Muhlenbruck, 2001). This technology gives infants and family in very rural settings or isolated communities to receive health care and follow-up services that might not otherwise be possible. We need studies to demonstrate the effectives of this form of health in the neonatal/infant population. Only time will tell if this trend will continue.

SUMMARY

Home care needs are increasing. The expertise required of those nurses involved in home care is also increasing. The family is central to the adequate provision of home care. They must be knowledgeable about the care and safety issues surrounding the interventions they are to provide. Equipment must be demonstrated as how to work it, troubleshoot, or when to get help. This is all part of the family's education. Close follow-up by qualified health professionals is necessary if this care is to be successful. We need more evidence to support the value—fiscally and physically—to determine best practices.

REFERENCES

Brooten D et al (1986). A randomized clinical trial of early hospital discharge and home follow-up of very-low-birth-weight infants. *New England journal of medicine*, 315(15), 934-939.

Burstein L (1995). Home care. In Barnhart SL, Czervinske MP (Eds.), *Perinatal and pediatric respiratory care*. Philadelphia: WB Saunders.

Department of Health and Human Services (DHHS) (2001). *All Aboard the 2010 Express: A 10-Year Action Plan to Achieve Community-based Service Systems for Children and Youth with Special Health Care Needs and their Families*. Rockville, MD: DHHS.

Donn S (1982). Cost effectiveness of home management of bronchopulmonary dysplasia [Letter]. *Pediatrics*, 70(2), 330-331.

Eggert LD et al (1985). Home phototherapy treatment of neonatal jaundice. *Pediatrics*, 76(4), 579-584.

Farmer JE, Muhlenbruck L (2001). Telehealth for children with special health care needs: promoting comprehensive systems of care. *Clinical pediatrics* (Phila), 40(2), 92-93.

Fields AI et al (1991a). Outcome of home care for technology-dependent children: success of an independent, community-based case management model. *Pediatric pulmonology*, 11(4), 310-317.

Fields AI et al (1991b). Home care cost-effectiveness for respiratory technology-dependent children. *American journal of diseases of children*, 145(7), 729-733.

Grabert BE et al (1986). Home phototherapy. *Clinical pediatrics*, 25(6), 291-294.

Lauer ME, Camitta BM (1980). Home care for dying children: a nursing model. *Journal of pediatrics*, 97(6), 1032-1035.

Madlon-Kay DJ (2001). Home health nurse clinical assessment of neonatal jaundice: Comparison of 3 methods. *Archives of pediatric and adolescent medicine*, 155(5), 583-586.

Martin BB (1985). Home care for terminally ill children and their families. In Corr CA, Corr DM (Eds.), *Hospice approaches to pediatric care*. New York: Springer.

Pellegrino ED (1998). Rationing health care: the ethics of medical gatekeeping. In Monagle JF, Thomasma DC. *Health care ethics: critical issues for the 21st century*. Gaithersburg, MD: Aspen Publishers, Inc.

Pinney MA, Cotton EK (1976). Home management of bronchopulmonary dysplasia. *Pediatrics*, 58(6), 856-859.

Rhymes J (1990). Hospice care in America. *Journal of the American Medical Association*, 264(3), 369-372.

Stepanek JA (1996). Early intervention services for the high-risk infant. In Ahman E (Ed.) *Home care for the high-risk infant*, ed. 2, Gaithersburg, MD: Aspen Publishers, Inc.

Stricklin ML (1993). *The cost effectiveness of maternal-child home health care*. Paper presented to Clinton Health Care Reform Task Force, 1993, Visiting Nurse Associations of America.

Thilo EH et al (1987). Home oxygen therapy in the newborn: cost and parental acceptance. *American journal of diseases of children*, 141(7), 766-768.

APPENDIX

A PREEMIE'S BILL OF RIGHTS

I deserve . . .

I deserve . . . your recognition that I may be completing many months of my physical and neurological development outside the protection of my mother's womb. Even as you give me the life sustaining care I so badly need, as much as possible I deserve to have the boundaries, quiet, warmth, gentle stimulation, dim lighting and fetal positioning I would have in my mother's womb.

I deserve . . . to be understood and treated as the individual I am. I deserve to have my language of cues and signals understood by you, my caregiver. My grimaces, hand stretches, frowns, and hiccups are as meaningful as any words, but delivered in the only language I know.

I deserve . . . periods of uninterrupted quiet so I can use my energy to grow and not hopelessly trying to overcome excess light, noise, and overstimulation.

I deserve . . . the positive energy of love . . . your kind thoughts and words as you care for me . . . my father's soft touch . . . my mother's gentle words . . . a volunteer's quiet rocking. I deserve these things because in your heart you know their worth, even through their absolute clinical value will never be proven.

I deserve . . . your understanding that what is normal and routine for you, as my caregiver, is abnormal and frightening for my mom and dad. So please answer kindly, no matter how many times they ask the same question. They deserve your support and the support of other families as they go through the roller coaster experience of the NICU.

I deserve . . . your recognition that my parents are an integral part of my caregiving team and should be allowed and encouraged to the best of their ability to help care for me during my stay in your hospital.

I deserve . . . your understanding that part of your job is to help me bond with my family as we learn to trust each other and as they prepare to bring me home.

I deserve . . . continuity of care from the NICU to my home . . . from my neonatologist to my primary care giver . . . so together my family and I can reach our full potential.

You deserve my thanks and recognition. I am here because of YOU!

Courtesy of Read McCarty, founder of The Wee Make a Difference Foundation, and founder and retired CEO of Children's Medical Ventures, Inc. The Foundation is dedicated to making the practice of developmentally supportive, family-centered care the standard of care in the NICU.

HISTORY:
Age:_____ G_____ P_____ AB _____
NSVD_____ C/S_____
GA:_____ APGARS_____/_____
B/W_____
Special Family Needs/Requests:

CONSULTS

SKIN / WOUND CARE / SPECIAL NEEDS

RESPIRATORY
Vent:_____ FIO2:_____ PIP/PEEP_____
CPAP:_____ FIO2:_____ PEEP_____
NC:_____ FIO2:_____ LPM_____
Hood_____ FIO2:_____ Weaning Orders:_

Surfactant Doses:_____
Aerosol:_____ CPT: _____
ABG:_____ CBG:_____

VS / BLD GLUCOSE
TPR:_____ BP: _____
Bld Gluc._____

FLUIDS   TOTAL FLUIDS:
CVC_____ @_____
PICC_____ @_____
PAL_____ @_____
UAC_____ @_____
PIV_____ @_____
Additional Fluids
_____ @_____
_____ @_____
_____ @_____
_____ @_____
_____ @_____
UAC Level_____ UVC Level____
CVL Drsg. Change:_____
NUTRITION   NPO_____
TPR_____ Nutrition:____
COG_____ _____
OG/NG_____ _____
PO_____ Amt/Freq: ____
LABS PENDING | RADIOLOGY

CULTURES

MISC
Neomap Review Date:_____ / SHIFT_____
Isolette Change Date: _____
Phototherapy:
Spot _____   K-PAD _____
Bank_____
Wallaby_____

Tour SCN with family_____
MD/ARNP _____
1st Feed _____

DIAGNOSTIC STUDIES

FIGURE **A-1**
Neocare map. Courtesy of Florida Hospital, Orlando, FL.

NEOMAP

Aspect of Care	DAY 1 Date:	Init.	DAY 2 Date:	Init.	DAY 3 Date:	Init.
RESPIRATORY - Optimal gas exchange and perfusion at minimal settings.	Respiratory support as needed. CXR. Surfactant per protocol. Suction PRN. Continuous pulse oximeter, monitor blood gases.		Respiratory support as needed. Suction PRN. Continuous pulse oximeter, monitor blood gases.		⟶	
CARDIAC - Optimal perfusion without pressor agents. Heart rate within normal limits.	Assess perfusion (capillary refill, pulses, BP x4 extremities.) Vital signs per protocol.		Assess perfusion (capillary refill, pulses). Vital signs per protocol.		Assess perfusion (capillary refill, pulses) Vital signs per protocol. Assess for PDA. ECHO?	
NUTRITION / FLUIDS - Adequate fluid/electrolyte and hydration status. Progress toward all nipple feeds.	NPO. Establish IV access, provide fluid needs. Blood glucose per protocol. Initial weight/head circumference.		Maintain IV access. Consider PICC. Consider feeds. Blood glucose per protocol. Daily weights and head circumference.		Maintain IV access. Consider feeds. Blood glucose per protocol. Daily weights and head circumference. Assess feeding tolerance. Offer pacifier.	
ELIMINATION - cc/kg output within acceptable range while on continuous fluids. No less than 6 wet diapers in 24 hours when off IVF.	I&O, calculate urine output every day and PRN. Utilize appropriate diapers per developmental / clinical needs.		⟶		⟶	
THERMAL REGULATION - Temperature maintained within normal limits.	Radiant warmer on ISC and K-pad, if necessary. Shield with plastic and use humidity as indicated.		Consider double-wall isolette on ISC. K-pad as necessary.		⟶	
NEURODEVELOPMENT - Progress toward oral-motor readiness with subsystem stability.	Cluster care/minimal handling. Narcotics prior to painful procedures. Offer pacifier for consoling and during procedures. Maintain flexion using developmental supports. Minimize sensory stimulation by decreasing exposure to light and noise.		⟶		⟶	
SKIN INTEGRITY - Minimal skin irritation. Integrity of epidermal barrier maintained.	Assess skin integrity. Bathe when stable. Minimal tape usage. Tegaderm under adhesives as needed. Cord care per protocol.		Minimal tape usage. Tegaderm under adhesive as needed. Cord care per protocol. Bathe with warm sterile water prn. Eucerin/Aquaphor prn.		⟶	
INFECTION - No signs nor symptoms of infection.	Admission labs as ordered. Antibiotics as ordered. Hand washing per protocol, always before and after patient contact.		Check Gentamycin level. Hand washing per protocol. Monitor results of cultures.		Monitor results of cultures. Hand washing per protocol.	
FAMILY SUPPORT - Optimal family involvement and knowledge.	Admission packet given. Discuss breast feeding. Explain equipment / unit routines including hand washing protocol. Provide support for initial contact.		Encourage and facilitate communication with MD/ ARNP. Introduce concept of Kangaroo Care. Reinforce unit routine information. If breast feeding, arrange to introduce parents to a Lactation Consultant. Discuss collection and storage of breask milk.		Discuss signs of stress and soothing techniques. Encourage involvement in care as appropriate. Reinforce information regarding collection and storage of breast milk.	
DISCHARGE PLANNING - Family will demonstrate ability to perform basic skills needed post discharge.	Initial assessment of family needs/referrals as needed. Family supports identified.		Assessment of family needs. Family supports identified. Interdisciplinary Assessment tool completed by Clinical Care Coordinator.		Assessment of family needs. Family supports identified. Teach as appropriate: Take a temperature_____ Diaper change_____ Cord care_____ Skin care_____ Use of bulb syringe_____	

Before performing these routines, a physician's order must be received for those activities requiring an order.

SIGNATURE	INITIALS	SIGNATURE	INITIALS

CODE - VARIANCE SOURCE:

	A. Patient/Family	B. Caregiver / Clinician	C. Hospital	D. Community
1. Event not applicable	3. Patient condition	10. Physician's order	20. Information/Data availability	30. Placement delay
2. Unpredicted event	4. Patient/family decision	11. Caregivers decision	21. Supplies/Equipment availability	31. Transportation delay
	5. Patient/family availability	12. Caregiver action	22. Department overbooked/closed	32. Community-other
	6. Patient/family cognition		23. Delayed/incorrect medication/fluids	33. Home Healthcare delay
	7. Mother's condition		24. Bed Availability	

FIGURE **A-2-01**
Courtesy of Florida Hospital, Orlando, FL.

DAY 4 Date:	Init.	DAY 5 Date:	Init.	DAY 6 Date:	Init.	DAY 7 Date:	Init.
⟶		⟶		⟶		⟶	
Assess perfusion (capillary refill, pulses). Vital signs per protocol.		⟶		⟶		⟶	
Maintain IV access. Blood glucose per protocol. Daily weights & head circumference. Assess feeding tolerance. Offer pacifier.		⟶		⟶		Florida Infant Screen Weekly length assessment	
⟶		⟶		⟶		⟶	
⟶		Double-wall isolette with ISC & K-pad if necessary.		⟶		Double-wall isolette as necessary. D/C K-pad if temperature stable.	
⟶		⟶		⟶		⟶	
⟶		⟶		⟶		⟶	
⟶		⟶		⟶		⟶	
Discuss signs of stress and soothing techniques. Encourage involvement in care as appropriate.		⟶		⟶		⟶	
Teach as appropriate: Take a temperature_____ Diaper change_____ Cord care_____ Skin care_____ Use of bulb syringe_____		⟶		⟶		⟶	

DATE	CODE	VARIANCE	CAUSE	ACTION	DATE RESOLVED

FIGURE **A-2-02**
Courtesy of Florida Hospital, Orlando, FL.

Aspect of Care	DAY 14 Date:	Init.	Date:	Init.	Date:	Init.
	Gestational Age:		Gestational Age: 30 weeks		Gestational Age: 32 weeks	
RESPIRATORY - Optimal perfusion and gas exchange at minimal settings.	Respiratory support as needed. Monitor blood gases as needed. Continuous pulse oximeter.		⟶		⟶	
CARDIAC - Optimal perfusion without pressor agents. Heart rate within normal limits.	Assess perfusion (capillary refill, pulses). Vital signs per protocol.		⟶		⟶	
NUTRITION / FLUIDS - Adequate fluid/electrolyte and hydration status. Progress toward all nipple feeds.	Maintain IV access. Advance feeds as tolerated. Offer pacifier with gavage feeds. Blood glucose per protocol. Daily weights and head circumference. Weekly length assessment.		⟶		⟶ Assess po readiness.	
ELIMINATION - cc/kg output within acceptable range while on continuous fluids. No less than 6 wet diapers in 24 hours when off IVF.	I&O. Calculate urine output daily and PRN. Utilize appropriate diapers per developmental / clinical needs.		⟶		⟶	
THERMAL REGULATION - Temperature maintained within normal limits.	Double-walled isolette with ISC as needed. Change isolette weekly.		⟶		DWI. D/c ISC if > 15000 gms. Change isolette weekly.	
NEURODEVELOPMENT - Progress toward oral-motor readiness with subsystem stability.	Cluster care/minimal handling. Narcotics prior to painful procedures. Offer pacifier for consoling and during procedures. Maintain flexion using developmental supports. Minimize sensory stimulation by decreasing exposure to light and noise.		⟶		⟶	
SKIN INTEGRITY - Minimal skin irritation. Integrity of epidermal barrier maintained.	Minimal tape usage. Tegaderm under adhesives as needed. Bathe with mild soap prn. Eucerin prn.		⟶		⟶	
INFECTION - No signs nor symptoms of infection.	Hand washing per protocol, always before and after patient contact.		⟶		⟶	
FAMILY SUPPORT - Optimal family involvement and knowledge.	Reinforce signs of stress and soothing techniques. Encourage involvement in care as appropriate. Consider Kangaroo Care.		Encourage involvement in care as appropriate. Kangaroo Care.		⟶	
DISCHARGE PLANNING - Family will demonstrate ability to perform basic skills needed post discharge.	Teach as appropriate: Taking a temperature _____ Diaper change_____ Skin care_____ Use of bulb syringe_____		Return demonstration of: Taking a temperature _____ Diaper change _____ Skin care _____ Use of bulb syringe _____		Discuss clothing needs.	

Before performing these routines, a physician's order must be received for those activities requiring an order.

SIGNATURE	INITIALS	SIGNATURE	INITIALS

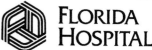

FLORIDA HOSPITAL

NEONATAL CARE MAP

665-NNCM (12/01)

FIGURE **A-2-03**
Courtesy of Florida Hospital, Orlando, FL.

Date:	Init.	Date:	Init.	Date:	Init.	Date:	Init.
Gestational Age: 33 weeks		Gestational Age: 34 weeks		Gestational Age: 36 weeks		Gestational Age: 37-40 weeks	
⟶		⟶		Consider d/c pulse oximeter.		⟶	
⟶		⟶		⟶		⟶	
Maintain IV access. Assess po readiness. Full feeds. Offer pacifier with gavage feeds. Daily weights and head circumference. Weekly length assessment.		Assess readiness for increased frequency of po feeds. Maintain IV access. Full feeds. Offer pacifier with gavage feeds. Daily weights and head circumference. Weekly length.		Assess fluid needs. Full feeds. Consider gavage prn/po with cues. Daily weights and head circumference. Weekly length.		PO all feeds. Daily weights and head circumference. Weekly length.	
Diaper checks if no IV.		⟶		⟶		⟶	
DWI. Change isolette weekly. Dress in light clothing.		⟶		Assess readiness for open crib. Provide containment by swaddling.		Open crib. Dress in appropriate clothing.	
Cluster care. Offer pacifier for consoling. Maintain flexion using developmental supports. Minimize sensory stimulation by decreasing exposure to light and noise.		⟶		Cluster care. Place in supine position. Provide containment by swaddling.		Cluster care. Place in supine position.	
Bathe prn. Eucerin prn. Minimal tape usage. Protective barriers for diaper area.		⟶		⟶		⟶	
⟶		⟶		⟶		⟶	
Encourage involvement in care as appropriate. Kangaroo care.		⟶		⟶		⟶	
Bath demonstration. Discuss feeding techniques with family. Encourage family to schedule CPR training.		Family doing baby care / feeding. Demonstration of medication administration and return demonstration by family.		Family doing baby care / feeding. Teach as appropriate: Formula preparation_____ Adequate I&O_____ Circumcision care_____ Signs&symptoms of illness_____ Car seat instruction_____ Prescriptions to family.		Teach as appropriate: Formula preparation_____ Adequate I&O_____ Circumcision care_____ Signs&symptoms of illness_____ Car seat instruction_____	

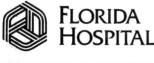

FLORIDA HOSPITAL

NEONATAL CARE MAP

665-NNCM (12/01)

FIGURE **A-2-04**
Courtesy of Florida Hospital, Orlando, FL.

CRITICAL PATHWAYS

Critical pathways are not a new concept. They have become the buzzword with health care reform. They are a method for multidisciplinary identification and measurement of patient outcomes. Critical pathways allow for anticipating the normal course of events or progress that a patient with a specific problem should follow. They are management plans that have a time frame for achievement of "milestones" according to a sequence of multidisciplinary interventions. All multidisciplinary teams may use the same plan because it is reflective of holistic care and not nursing versus medical care. This tool may be referred to as clinical pathways, care maps, or multidisciplinary action plans, to name a few (Ignatavicius & Hausman, 1995). The salient features of any of these tools are patient outcomes, timelines, collaboration, and comprehensive care aspects. Because these are generally developed by different disciplines, there is a built-in "ownership" by health professionals responsible for managing the care versus turf issues over certain aspects of the care. These pathways help meet the Joint Commission on Accreditation of Healthcare Organizations (JCAHO) requirements for documentation or tracking of a patient's continuum of care. Ignatavicius & Hausman (1995)* outlined highlights of JCAHO Requirements.

Highlights of JCAHO Continuum of Care Requirements for 1995

- Have a process to facilitate patients' access to the appropriate clinical service and caregiver(s), based on assessed need.
- Perform an assessment before accepting patients into a given service or setting.
- Ensure as part of the admissions process that patients and families are appropriately informed about the care that will be provided.
- Assure continuity of care: a logical progression of service from assessment and diagnosis through planning and treatment.
- Assure that all care is coordinated by the health professionals in the various settings.
- Refer, transfer, or discharge the patient to the appropriate provider if assessment data indicate that a patient needs another level of care.
- Consider all the patient's care needs in the discharge plan to assure continuity of care.
- Make sure there is an exchange of appropriate patient and clinical information when patients are admitted, referred, transferred, or discharged.
- Assure that decisions to provide or deny care or service are based on the needs of the patient.

If an institution or unit is trying to develop a critical pathway, educational and motivational steps must precede this process. Ignatavicius & Hausman (1995) outlined a method for starting the development and facilitating the implementation processes of this tool.

Clinical Pathway Program

1. Educate and obtain support from staff and physicians.
2. Form the interdisciplinary teams:
   A. Steering committee and pathway-specific group
   B. A group to identify potential obstacles to implementation

---

* Ignatavicius DD, Hausman KA (1995). *Clinical pathways for collaborative practice*. Philadelphia: WB Saunders.

3. Data collection: Determine patient population, Diagnostic Related Groups, International Code of Diseases—9 code to focus on those who are:
   A. High volume
   B. High cost
   C. High risk
   D. Difficult to manage
4. Use continuous quality improvement methods and tools to select.
   A. Pareto charts
   B. Statistical process control chart
5. Determine which ICD-9 code is most predictable.
6. Determine staff interest.
7. Select pathways to develop.
8. Develope format for pathway.
9. Select interdisciplinary clinical experts for pathways team.
10. Collect clinical pathway data:
    A. Medical record review for practice patterns
    B. Literature review
    C. Comparison with other intitutions
    D. Practice guidelines
11. Write the pathway:
    A. Review by staff
    B. Review as necessary
12. Develop variance analysis system:
    A. Information needed to measure compliance with the pathway
    B. Outcomes measurement
    C. Clinical and financial measurements
13. Present pathway to hospital committees for approval; incorporate revisions.
14. Develop implementation plan.
15. Provide in-service staff.
16. Use pilot pathway for 3 to 6 months; revise as needed.
17. Monitor variances:
    A. Develop automated data collection if possible
    B. Present variance data to staff and physicians

REGIONAL NURSERY DIRECTORS' RECOMMENDATIONS FOR INFANTS DISCHARGED LESS THAN 48 HOURS AFTER UNCOMPLICATED VAGINAL DELIVERY AND INFANTS DISCHARGED LESS THAN 72 HOURS AFTER UNCOMPLICATED C-SECTION

It is the goal of this committee that all health care professionals have the means necessary to provide optimal care for mother–infant dyad without financial constraints and without compromising the quality of care.

It is our recommendation that all infants as described above should have an assessment after discharge, at 2 to 5 days of age, as directed by their primary care physician. A pathway flow chart has been developed for follow-up of these infants and is enclosed. This pathway is recommended as a guideline for care in this region.

Home care content should be consistent in the region and include, at a minimum, the following:

1. Physical assessment, including rectal/axillary temperature.
2. Parental interaction evaluation.
3. Home environment assessment with assessment of equipment available to the mother for care of her infant.
4. All infants should be weighed (visiting nurse must have a scale).
5. Documentation of the future follow-up appointment with primary care physician/visiting nurse.

6. Evaluation and documentation of pulse, respirations, and capillary refill.

7. Check for femoral pulses and respiratory effort (e.g., retractions, grunting).

8. Careful history of output since discharge from hospital, including urine and stool. Specific and complete feeding history, including type, times, and volume of feeding.

9. Visiting nurse must have inpatient information from hospital stay of mother and infant during home visit.

10. Forms should be the same, or similar in format, for all visiting nurses, and the forms sent to the primary care physician should be consistent.

11. The forms for metabolic screens have number, date, and time.

12. General education of the family.

Credentialing* of home care nurses should include the following:

1. The Consortium for Advancement of Perinatal Practice (CAPP). Mother and Baby I and II programs or equivalent.

2. Not less than 2000 hours of newborn care experience over 3 years' time.

---

*Didactic content and clinical skills verification for the professional nurse providing perinatal home care is based on standards published by the Association of Women's Health, Obstetric, and Neonatal Nurses (AWHONN).

3. Basic Cardiac Life Support (BCLS) certified. Neonatal Resuscitation Certification recommended, not required.

4. Skill in drawing blood, specifically for metabolic screens and bilirubin.

5. Cross-training in mother and infant care.

6. One third of continuing educational time related to mother and infant.

7. Five supervised home visits.

The third-party payors must provide the home care nurses with the means to obtain prenatal, intrapartum, postpartum, and nursery in-patient information that is available at the time of the home visit.

Postdischarge assessment as described above should be a reimbursable professional service. This assessment should be provided by physicians, nurses, or a hospital perinatal service. Home assessment visits should be a part of all hospital perinatal services.

All home care forms in the region should be consolidated into one user-friendly form for nurse, physicians, and third-party payors.

A regional data base is needed to evaluate the impact of early discharge. This should include information on emergency room visits and readmissions before the infant is 28 days of age and all visits to the primary care physician's office before the infant is 2 weeks of age.

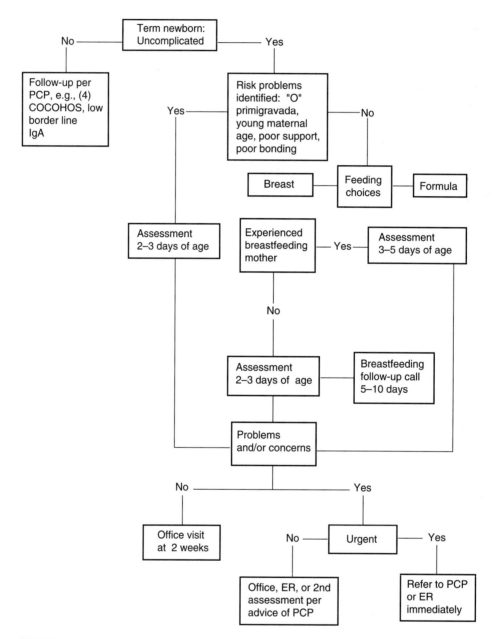

FIGURE **A-3**
Clinical pathway for follow-up of infants of uncomplicated vaginal full-term delivery. From Ignatavicius DD & Hausman KA (1995). *Clinical pathways for collaborative practice*. Philadelphia: WB Saunders.

Birth to 36 months: Girls
Length-for-age and Weight-for-age percentiles

NAME _____

RECORD # _____

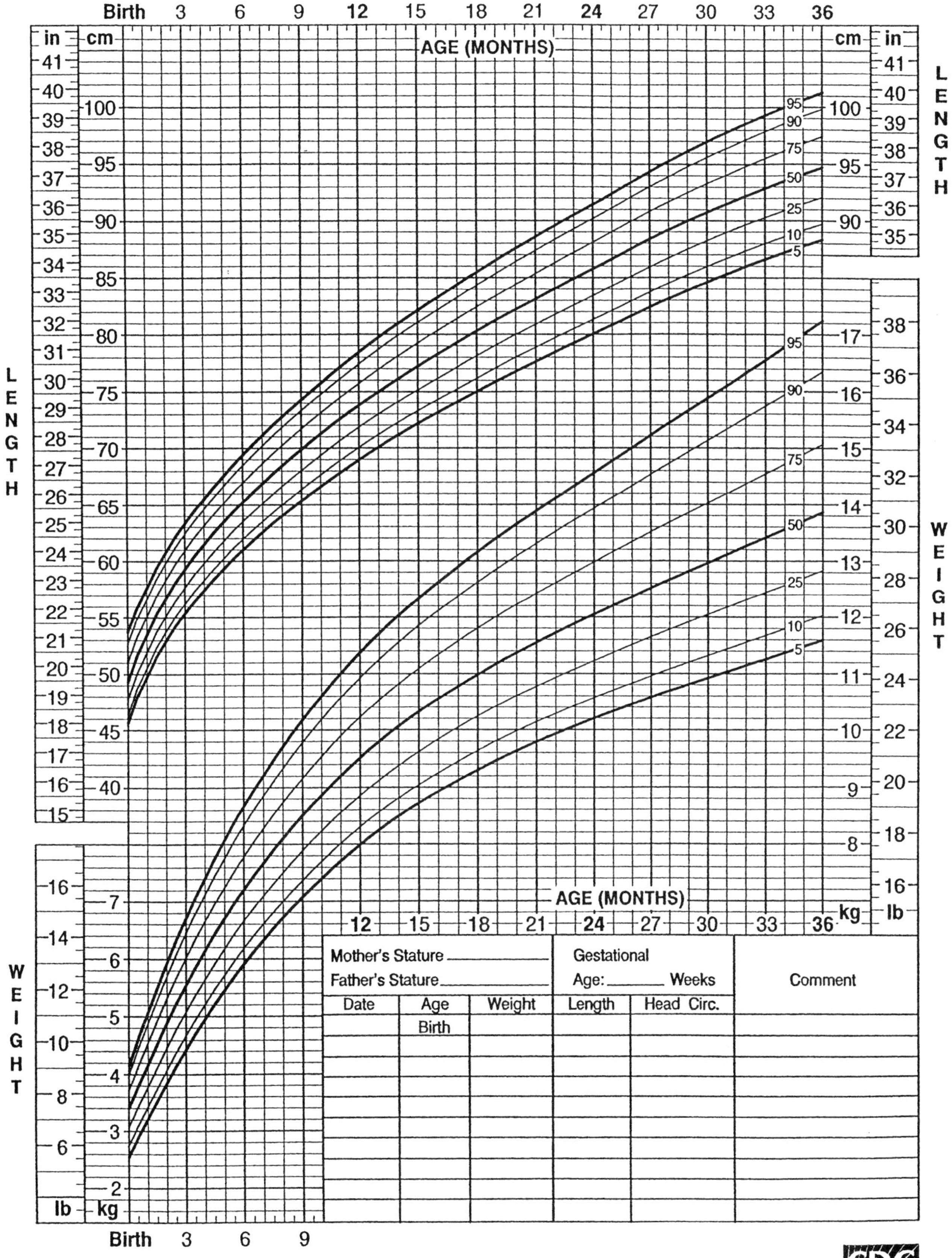

FIGURE **A-4**

Birth to 36 months: girls' length-for-age and weight-for-age percentiles. Developed by the National Center for Health Statistics in collaboration with the National Center for Chronic Disease Prevention and Health Promotion (2002). www.cdc.gov/growthcharts.

Birth to 36 months: Girls
Head circumference-for-age and
Weight-for-length percentiles

NAME _____

RECORD # _____

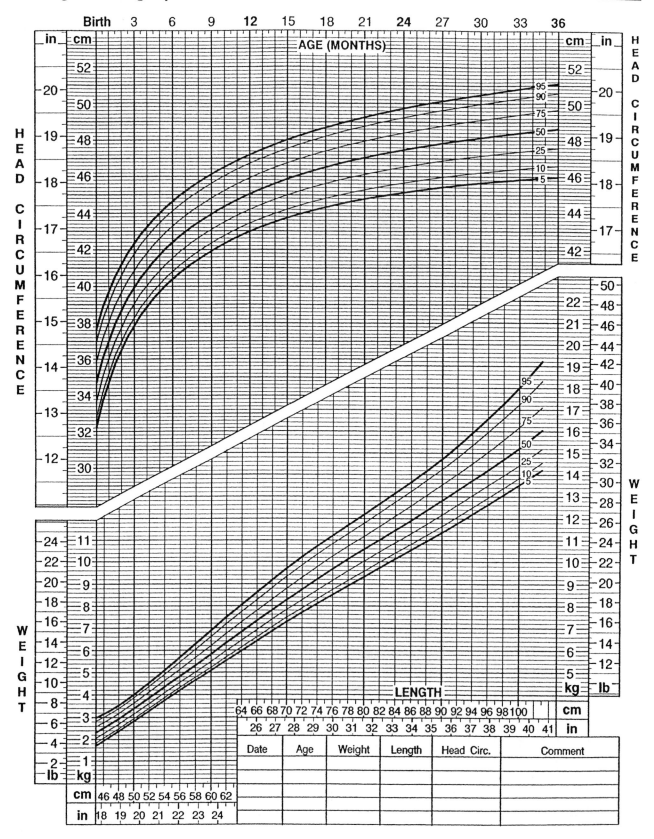

FIGURE **A-5**

Birth to 36 months: girls' head circumference-for-age and weight-for-length percentiles. Developed by the National Center for Health Statistics in collaboration with the National Center for Chronic Disease Prevention and Health Promotion (2002). www.cdc.gov/growthcharts.

Birth to 36 months: Boys
Length-for-age and Weight-for-age percentiles

NAME ____________________

RECORD # ____________

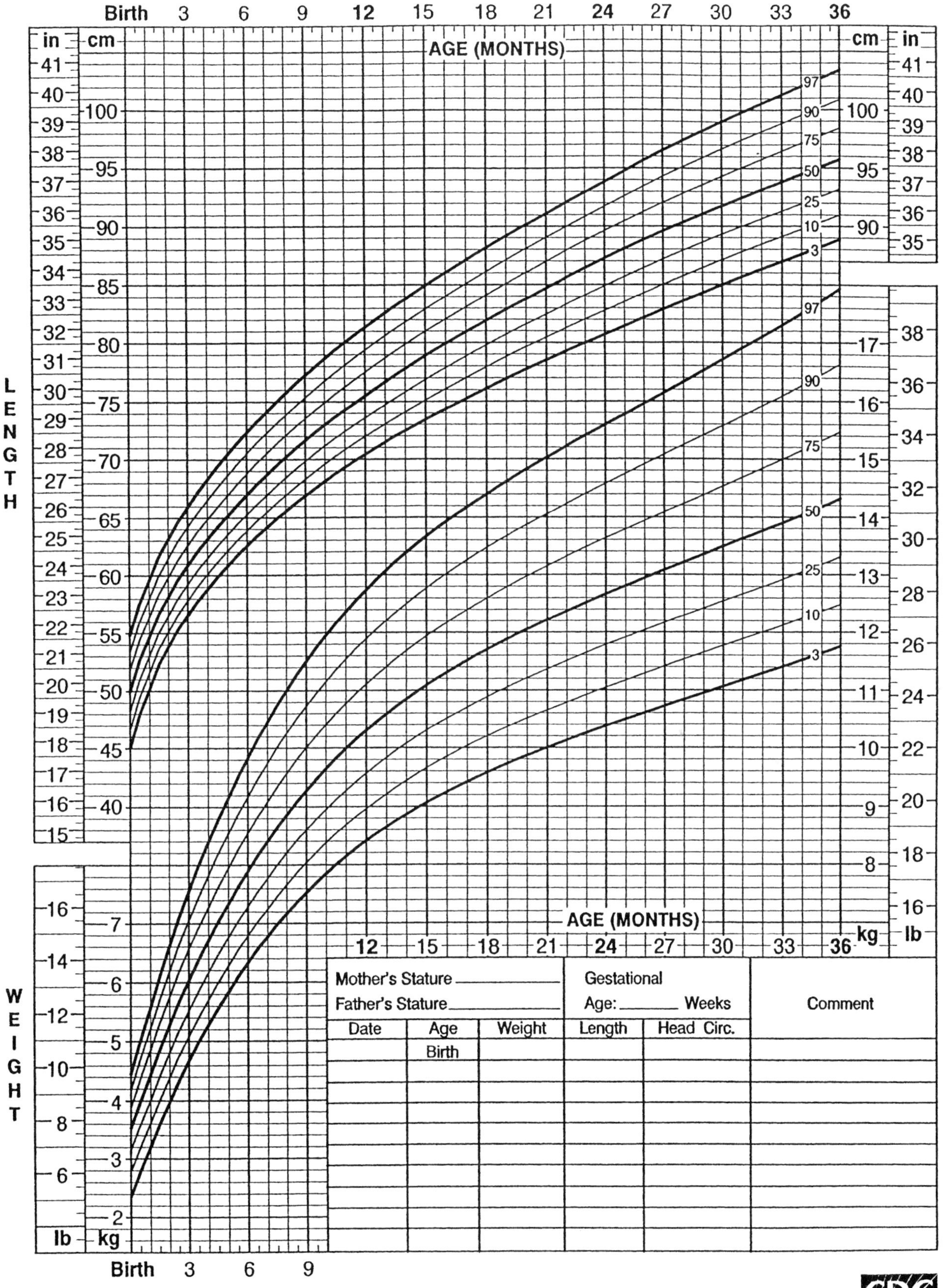
Birth 3 6 9 12 15 18 21 24 27 30 33 36
AGE (MONTHS)
LENGTH
WEIGHT
in
cm
kg
lb
97
90
75
50
25
10
3
Mother's Stature ____
Father's Stature ____
Gestational Age: ____ Weeks
Comment
Date
Age
Weight
Length
Head Circ.
Birth

CDC

FIGURE **A-6**

Birth to 36 months: boys' length-for-age and weight-for-age percentiles. Developed by the National Center for Health Statistics in collaboration with the National Center for Chronic Disease Prevention and Health Promotion (2002). www.cdc.gov/growthcharts.

Birth to 36 months: Boys
Head circumference-for-age and
Weight-for-length percentiles

NAME _____

RECORD # _____

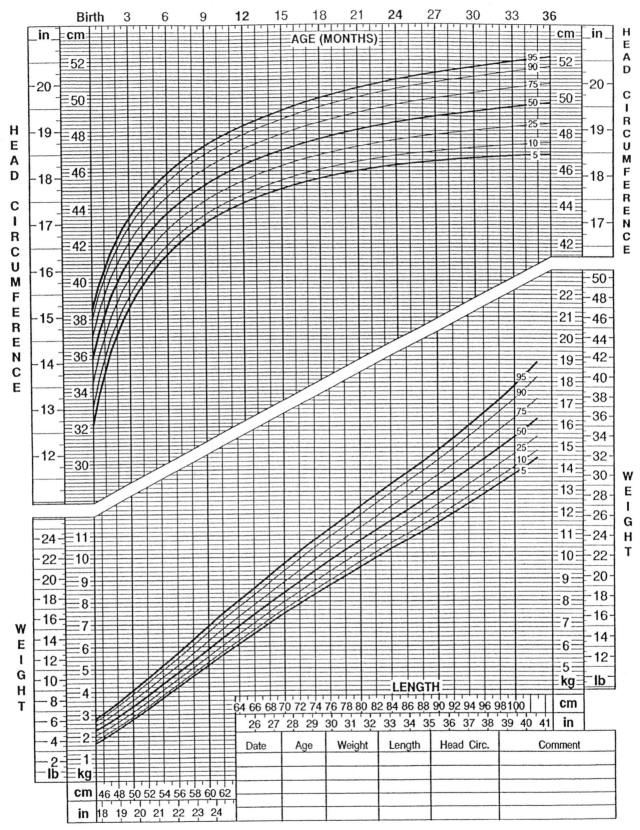

FIGURE **A-7**

Birth to 36 months: boys' head circumference-for-age and weight-for-length percentiles. Developed by the National Center for Health Statistics in collaboration with the National Center for Chronic Disease Prevention and Health Promotion (2002). www.cdc.gov/growthcharts.

Index

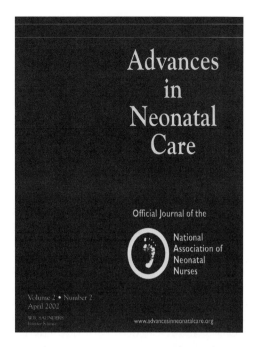

NEWBORN AND INFANT NURSING REVIEWS

RECEIVE 15% OFF YOUR SUBSCRIPTION TO THE JOURNAL WHEN YOU PURCHASE THE BOOK!

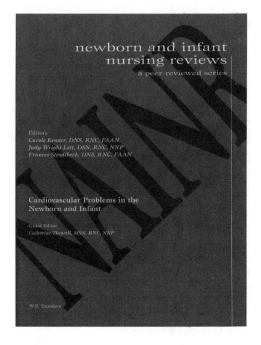

Editors
CAROLE KENNER, DNS, RNC, FAAN
JUDY WRIGHT LOTT, DSN, RNC, NNP
FRANCES STRODTBECK, DNS, RNC, FAAN

Full-text Internet access included when you subscribe!

Newborn and Infant Nursing Reviews provides critical reviews of neonatal nursing subjects of interest to clinicians, educators, and researchers. Each quarterly issue of the journal follows a specific content outline, which includes presentation of a case study related to the issue topic and articles on background (literature review), physiology/pathophysiology, diagnosis/treatment, nursing implications/applications, research/advances/new developments, clinical/evidence-based research, and point-counterpoint related to the main issue topic.

Subscriber Information
Volume 2, 2002
ISSN 1527-3369
Published quarterly

Subscription Rates
Individual: $73.00   Individual: $62.05
Institution: $102.00   Institution: $86.70
Student: $37.00*   Student: $31.45*

Prices subject to change without notice. All prices are in US dollars and payable in US funds.

*Please supply, on school letterhead, your name, dates of study, and signature of academic advisor. Orders will be billed at the individual rate until proof of status is received.